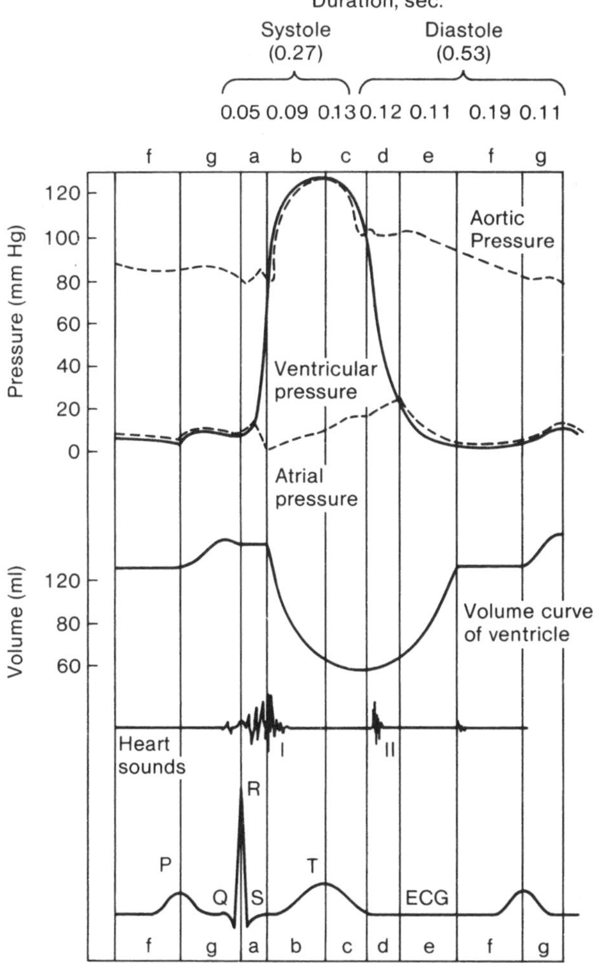

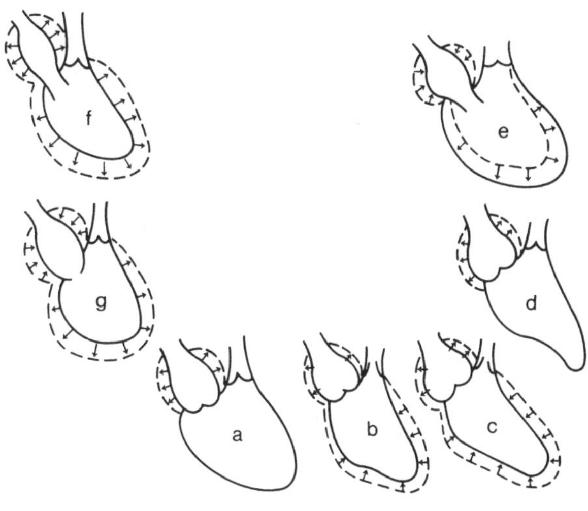

The cardiac cycle, illustrating the changes in aortic, left ventricular, and left atrial pressures, and in left ventricular volume, in relation to the phonocardiogram and the electrocardiogram. The duration of each phase at a heart rate of approximately 75 beats/min is indicated at the top of the figure. a, isovolumetric ventricular contraction; b, rapid ventricular ejection; c, slow ventricular ejection; d, isovolumetric relaxation; e, rapid ventricular filling; f, diastasis; g, atrial contraction; I, first heart sound; II, second heart sound. Insets: Changes in the configuration of the left atrium, mitral valve, left ventricle, and aortic valve during various phases of the cycle. (Adapted from Wiggens. [1952]. *Circulatory dynamics.* New York: Grune & Stratton.)

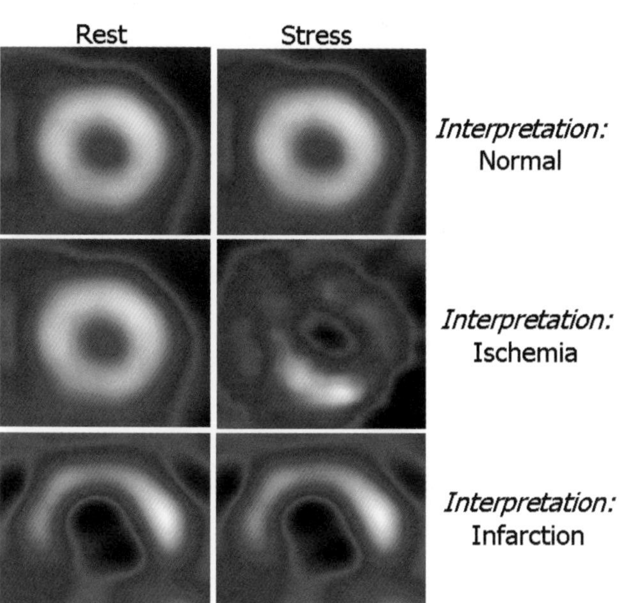

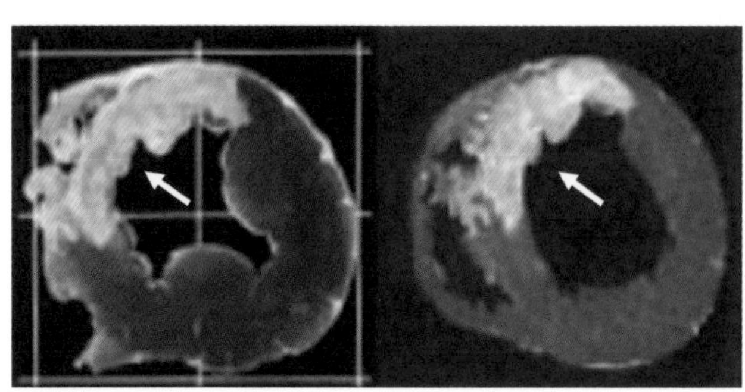

EDITION 6

Car

Susan L. W
Professor and
School of Nurs
University of W
Seattle, Washi

Erika S. Si
Professor
Department of
Department of
University of C
San Francisco

Sandra A
Associate Prof
Department o
School of Nur
University of W
Seattle, Wash

Elizabeth
Associate Pro
Biobehaviora
University of W
School of Nu
Clinical Nurs
University of Washington Medical Center
Colonel USAFR NC IMA, Director
Clinical Investigations Facility David Grant Medical Center
Travis AFB, California

Wolters Kluwer Health | Lippincott Williams & Wilkins
Philadelphia • Baltimore • New York • London
Buenos Aires • Hong Kong • Sydney • Tokyo

Acquisitions Editor: Hilarie Surrena
Product Director: Renee Gagliardi
Design Coordination: Holly McLaughlin
Compositor: Aptara, Inc.

351 West Camden Street
Baltimore, MD 21201

530 Walnut Street
Philadelphia, PA 19106

Printed in China.

9 8 7 6 5 4 3 2 1

Library of Congress Cataloging-in-Publication Data

Cardiac nursing / [edited by] Susan L. Woods . . . [et al.].
p. ; cm.
Includes bibliographical references and index.
ISBN 978-0-7817-9280-6 (alk. paper)
1. Heart—Diseases—Nursing. I. Woods, Susan L.
[DNLM: 1. Heart Diseases—nursing. 2. Heart Diseases—prevention & control—Nurses' Instruction. WY 152.5 C2672 2009]
RC674.C3 2009
616.1'20231—dc22

2009021310

DISCLAIMER

Care has been taken to confirm the accuracy of the information present and to describe generally accepted practices. However, the authors, editors, and publisher are not responsible for errors or omissions or for any consequences from application of the information in this book and make no warranty, expressed or implied, with respect to the currency, completeness, or accuracy of the contents of the publication. Application of this information in a particular situation remains the professional responsibility of the practitioner; the clinical treatments described and recommended may not be considered absolute and universal recommendations.

The authors, editors, and publisher have exerted every effort to ensure that drug selection and dosage set forth in this text are in accordance with the current recommendations and practice at the time of publication. However, in view of ongoing research, changes in government regulations, and the constant flow of information relating to drug therapy and drug reactions, the reader is urged to check the package insert for each drug for any change in indications and dosage and for added warnings and precautions. This is particularly important when the recommended agent is a new or infrequently employed drug.

Some drugs and medical devices presented in this publication have Food and Drug Administration (FDA) clearance for limited use in restricted research settings. It is the responsibility of the health care provider to ascertain the FDA status of each drug or device planned for use in their clinical practice.

To purchase additional copies of this book, call our customer service department at (800) 638-3030 or fax orders to (301) 223-2320. International customers should call (301) 223-2300. Visit Lippincott Williams & Wilkins on the Internet: http://www.lww.com. Lippincott Williams & Wilkins customer service representatives are available from 8:30 am to 6:00 pm, EST.

LWW.COM

Contributors

Sushama D. Acharya, MS
Doctoral Student, Epidemiology, Interventionist SMART Trial
University of Pittsburgh
Pittsburgh, Pennsylvania

Gaylene Altman, PhD, RN
Associate Professor
Department of Biobehavioral Nursing and Health Systems
School of Nursing
University of Washington
Seattle, Washington

Bradley E. Aouizerat, PhD, MAS
Associate Professor
School of Nursing and Institute for Human Genetics
University of California San Francisco
San Francisco, California

Kathleen A. Berra
Stanford Prevention Research Center
Stanford University School of Medicine
Stanford, California

Susan Blancher, MN, ARNP
Cardiology Nurse Practitioner
Virginia Mason Medical Center
Seattle, Washington

Jean Marie Blue Verrier, MN, ARNP
Cardiology Nurse Practitioner/Acute Care Nurse Practitioner
Swedish Physician Division/Summit Cardiology
Seattle, WA
Clinical Instructor
Department of Biobehavioral Nursing
School of Nursing
University of Washington

Eleanor F. Bond, PhD, RN, FAAN
Professor
Susan and Michael Cummings Term Professor in Nursing
Department of Biobehavioral Nursing and Health Systems
School of Nursing
University of Washington
Seattle, Washington

Lora E. Burke, PhD, MPH, FAHA, FAAN
Professor of Nursing and Epidemiology
University of Pittsburgh School of Nursing and Graduate School of Public Health
Pittsburgh, Pennsylvania

Robert L. Burr, MSEE, PhD
Research Professor
Department of Biobehavioral Nursing and Health Systems
School of Nursing
University of Washington
Seattle, Washington

Mary M. Canobbio, MN, RN, FAAN
Lecturer, UCLA School of Nursing
Administrative Coordinator, Programs, Research, Development
Ahmanson/UCLA Adult Congenital Heart Disease Center
Los Angeles, California

Peter J. Cawley, MD
Acting Assistant Professor of Medicine
Division of Cardiology
Department of Medicine
University of Washington School of Medicine
Seattle, Washington

Michael A. Chen, MD, PhD
Assistant Professor of Medicine
Division of Cardiology
Harborview Medical Center
University of Washington School of Medicine
Seattle, Washington

Susanna G. Cunningham, BScN, MA, PhD
Professor
Department of Biobehavioral Nursing and Health Systems
School of Nursing
University of Washington
Seattle, Washington

Michaelene Hargrove Deelstra, MSN, ARNP
Cardiology/Acute Care Nurse Practitioner
Swedish Physician Division/Summit Cardiology
Seattle, Washington
Clinical Instructor
Department of Biobehavioral Nursing and Health Systems
School of Nursing
University of Washington
Seattle, Washington

Cheryl R. Dennison, PhD, ANP
Associate Professor
Department of Health Systems and Outcomes, Johns Hopkins University School of Nursing
Division of Health Sciences Informatics, Johns Hopkins University School of Medicine
Baltimore, Maryland

Sandra B. Dunbar, DSN, RN, FAAN, FAHA
Charles Howard Candler Professor
Nell Hodgson Woodruff School of Nursing
Emory University
Atlanta, Georgia

Joan M. Fair, PhD, ANP
Consulting Assistant Professor
Stanford Research Prevention Center
School of Medicine
Stanford University
Stanford, California

Linda Felver, PhD, RN
Associate Professor
School of Nursing
Oregon Health and Science University
Portland, Oregon

Polly E. Gardner, MN, ACNP, ARNP, FAHA
Cardiology Nurse Practitioner
Seattle Cardiology
Clinical Instructor, Department of Biobehavioral Nursing and Health Systems
School of Nursing
University of Washington
Seattle, Washington

Rebecca A. Gary, PhD, RN
Assistant Professor
Nell Hodgson Woodruff School of Nursing
Emory University
Atlanta, Georgia

Donna Gerity, MN, RN
Clinical Nurse Specialist
Seattle Cardiology
Seattle, Washington

Mark Hawk, MSN, ACNP
Health Sciences Assistant Clinical Professor, School of Nursing
University of California San Francisco
San Francisco, California

Nancy Houston Miller, BSN, RN
Associate Director, Stanford Cardiac Rehabilitation Program
School of Medicine
Stanford University
Stanford, California

Jon S. Huseby, MD
Internal Medicine, Pulmonary and Critical Care Medicine
Polyclinic
Swedish Hospital Cherry Hill Campus
Clinical Professor of Pulmonary and Critical Care Medicine
School of Medicine
University of Washington
Seattle, Washington

Carol Jacobson, MN, RN
Director
Quality Education Services
Clinical Faculty, School of Nursing
University of Washington
Seattle, Washington

M. Kaye Kramer, DrPH, MPH, BSN, CCRC
Director, Diabetes Prevention Support Center
University of Pittsburgh Diabetes Institute
3512 Fifth Avenue, 3rd floor
Pittsburgh, Pennsylvania

Shannon M. Latta, MN, RN
Clinical Instructor
Department of Biobehavioral Nursing and Health Systems
School of Nursing
University of Washington
Seattle, Washington

Denise LeDoux, MN, ARNP
Cardiology Nurse Practitioner
Overlake Internal Medicine Associates
Bellevue, Washington

Barbara S. Levine, PhD, CRNP, CS
Nurse Practitioner
Cardiovascular Healthcare Consultants
Paoli, Pennsylvania

Helen Luikart, MS, RN
Clinical Research Coordinator
Division of Cardiovascular Medicine
Stanford University
Clinical Heart Transplant Coordinator
Stanford Hospital and Clinics
Stanford, California

Simone K. Madan, PhD
Clinical Professor and Clinical Psychologist
University of California San Francisco
San Francisco, California

Kirsten Martin, BSN, MS, RN
Nursing Faculty
Los Medanos College
Pittsburg, California

Diana E. McMillan, PhD, RN
Associate Professor, Faculty of Nursing
Helen Glass Centre for Nursing
University of Manitoba
Winnipeg, Manitoba

Margaret M. McNeill, PhD, RN, CCRN, CCNS, NE-BC
Colonel, United States Air Force, Nurse Corps
Master Clinician, Critical Care Nursing
79th Medical Wing
Andrews Air Force Base, Maryland

Philip Moons, PhD, RN
Center for Health Services and Nursing Research
Catholic University of Leuven
Leuven, The Netherlands

Nancy Munro, MN, CCRN, ACNP
Acute Care Nurse Practitioner
Critical Care Medicine Department
National Institutes of Health
Bethesda, Maryland

Jonathan Myers, PhD
Clinical Professor
VA Palo Alto Health Care System
Stanford University School of Medicine
Palo Alto, California

Katherine M. Newton, PhD, RN
Assistant Professor
Department of Biobehavioral Nursing and Health Systems
School of Nursing
University of Washington
Seattle, Washington

Kathy P. Parker, PhD, RN, FAAN
Dean and Professor, School of Nursing
University of Rochester
Rochester, New York

Susan L. Reed, MN, CCRN, ARNP
Cardiology Nurse Practitioner
Swedish Heart and Vascular Institute
Swedish Heart and Vascular Clinic
Seattle, Washington

Joseph O. Schmelz, PhD, RN, CIP, FAAN
Director, Institutional Review Board & Associate Professor/Research, School of Nursing
University of Texas Health Science Center at San Antonio
San Antonio, Texas

Kawkab Shishani, PhD
Associate Professor
Community Health Department
The Hashemite University
Jordan

Min Sohn, PhD, ACNP
Assistant Professor
Department of Nursing and Health Sciences
California State University, East Bay Hayward
California

Laurie A. Soine, PhD, ARNP, ACNP
Nurse Practitioner, Nuclear Cardiology
Teaching Associate
Department of Radiology
University of Washington Medical Center
Seattle, Washington

Beverly Dyck Thomassian, MPH, RN, BC-ADM, CDE
Diabetes Nurse Specialist and President
Diabetes Educational Services
Chico, California

Patricia K. Tuite, MSN, RN, CCRN
Instructor
Acute and Tertiary Care Department
University of Pittsburgh
Pittsburgh, Pennsylvania

Melanie Warziski Turk, PhD, RN
Assistant Professor
Duquesne University
Pittsburgh, Pennsylvania

Kyeongra Yang, PhD, MPH, RN
Assistant Professor
Department of Health and Community Systems
School of Nursing
University of Pittsburgh
Pittsburgh, Pennsylvania

About the Editors

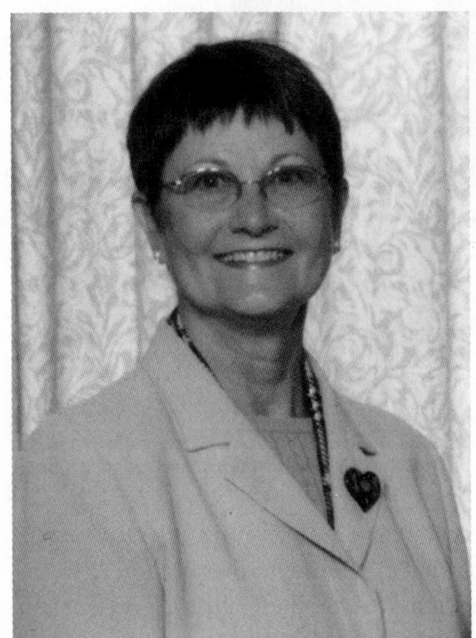

Susan L. Woods, PhD, RN, FAHA, FAAN

Susan has been on the faculty at the University of Washington, School of Nursing since 1975, where she has taught both undergraduate and graduate courses. She is currently Professor of Biobehavioral Nursing and Health Systems and the Associate Dean for Academic Services in the School of Nursing. Her clinical and research focus has been in all aspects of cardiac nursing, particularly in measurement of cardiovascular variables and chronobiology. Susan was a founding board member of the Commission on Collegiate Nursing Education (CCNE) and was a member of the 2008–2009 CCNE Accreditation Standards Committee. She has been the recipient of the Distinguished Research Award from the American Association of Critical Care Nursing and the Katherine Lembright Award from the American Heart Association Council on Cardiovascular Nursing. Susan has also received the Alumni All-Around Award from Oregon Health Science University, where she obtained a PhD in Nursing. She is a fellow in the American Academy of Nursing and the American Heart Association. Susan has two children, Jaime Rose Navetta and Jennifer Mary Ferrer, and is married to Jim Woods. She enjoys traveling, gardening, swimming, and collecting shells.

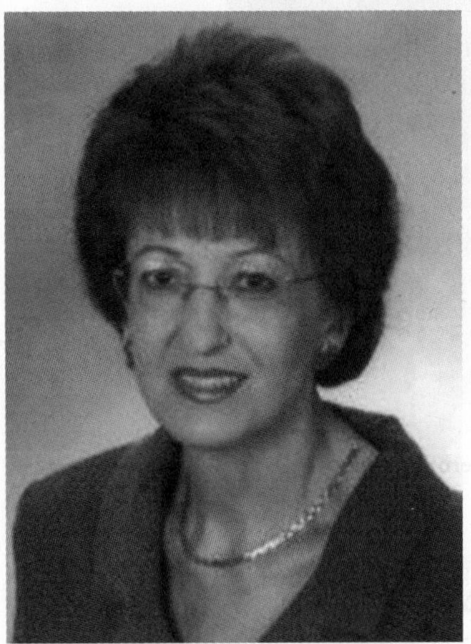

Erika S. Sivarajan Froelicher, MA, MPH, PhD, RN, FAAN

Erika has advanced degrees in nursing, public health, and epidemiology. During more than 30 years of nursing and public health experience, she has been an emergency room nurse, a psychiatric nurse, a center director, a researcher, an epidemiologist, and a university professor. As a consultant, she has advised hospitals, businesses, and foundations in the areas of nursing and cardiac care. Currently, she serves on the editorial board of *Heart and Lung, Human Kinetics, Cardiovascular Nursing,* and *European Journal for Cardiovascular Nursing* and is both a Founding and Associate Editor for *Journal of Cardiovascular and Pulmonary Rehabilitation* as well as having acted as a reviewer for many other medical and nursing journals.

Erika has presented papers and given invited lectures on coronary disease prevention and rehabilitation to more than 100 national and international groups. Her articles and abstracts have appeared in such publications as *New England Journal of Medicine, Circulation, Heart and Lung, American Journal of Nursing, Advanced Journal for Nursing Scholarship, Patient Education and Counseling,* and *Circulation.* As coauthor, she has published books on critical care nursing and cardiac care.

She has dedicated herself to research and teaching in nursing and medicine internationally in Asia, Europe, South America, Canada, Australia the middle East (Jordan, Lebanon and Saudi Arabia), and Africa through consultation, collaborative research, and guest faculty as visiting professor in Hong Kong, University of Basel Switzerland, University of Natal South Africa, and the University of Vienna a Fulbright Scholar 2005–2006 at the University of Jordan and continues her teaching and research as a Visiting Professor, among others.

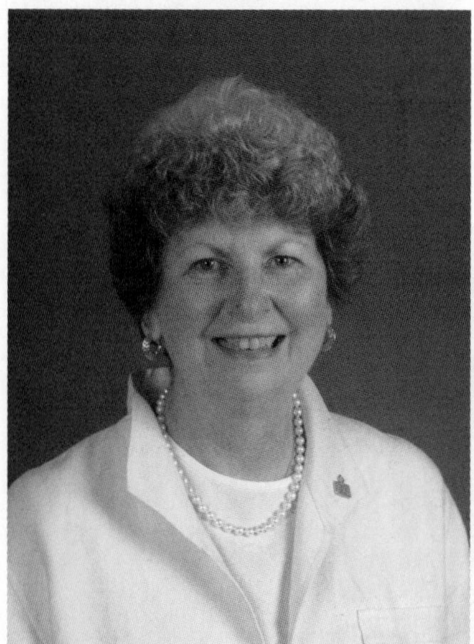

Sandra Adams (Underhill) Motzer, PhD, RN, FAHA, FAAN

Sandra is a diploma graduate from Washington Hospital Center School of Nursing, Washington, DC. She earned her BSN and MN at the University of Washington and her PhD at Oregon Health Sciences University, Portland. She completed a postdoctoral fellowship at the University of Washington. She was a founding coeditor of the journal *Progress in Cardiovascular Nursing,* is a charter Fellow of the American Heart Association's Council on Cardiovascular Nursing as well as the American Heart Association (FAHA), and a fellow of the American Academy of Nursing (FAAN). She is a past president of the Puget Sound Chapter of the American Association of Critical Care Nurses and is active in Sigma Theta Tau at the international and local levels. She has taught cardiovascular nursing for many years at all academic levels and in the community. Before retiring in 2008, she directed the master's-level medical—surgical nurse educator and clinical nurse specialist tracks at the University of Washington School of Nursing. She taught graduate-level courses in advanced pathophysiology, practice teaching, and, for the clinical nurse specialist and nurse educator students, clinical specialization and role development. Her funded research involved the effects of chronic health disturbances on immune function across the menstrual cycle and the effects of exercise on sleep in persons with heart failure. Sandy and her husband Tim enjoy hiking, beach walking, and traveling.

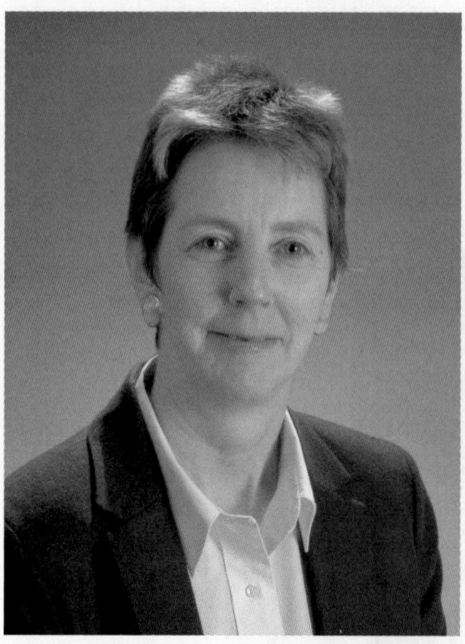

Elizabeth J. Bridges, PhD, RN, CCNS, FCCM, FAAN

Elizabeth has been a critical care nurse for the past 25 years, including 25 years active and reserve duty in the US Air Force. Her clinical research focuses on the integration of hemodynamic monitoring into the care of critically ill patients and the care of critically ill patients in military, unique, and austere environments. Specifically, she is studying functional hemodynamic monitoring, hemodynamic monitoring at altitude, aspects of thermal stress, and the maintenance of body temperature in critically ill patients under field conditions and long-distance aeromedical transport, factors that affect the efficacy of CPR under field conditions, and interventions to prevent decubitus ulcer formation during long-distance aeromedical transport. Elizabeth also served as the Director, Deployed Combat Casualty Care Research Team and was responsible for all Department of Defense human research in Afghanistan.

Preface to the 6th Edition

Cardiac Nursing continues to be *the* reference book for nurses caring for patients who have or are at risk for developing cardiac disease. *Cardiac Nursing*, Sixth Edition, provides the basic and advanced nurse with the most comprehensive evidence-based practice information. We believe that bedside nurses, clinical nurse specialists, nurse practitioners, nurse educators, and nurse researchers all will benefit from the content in this edition. We also support the Scope and Standards for Cardiovascular Nursing from the Task Force of Cardiovascular Nursing Organization Representatives, the summary of which appears on p. xi.

About This Edition

Global perspectives of cardiovascular disease have been enhanced in all chapters where appropriate and by the addition of a new chapter on global cardiovascular health (Chapter 43), which enhances the usefulness and generalizability of the content. A majority of the national clinical protocols were replaced with evidence-based protocols. Numerical citations were reintroduced to allow for more rapid identification of content related to specific areas. One new chapter on mechanical assist devices (Chapter 26) has been added. Other chapters, for example, Chapter 5 on pathophysiology of atherosclerosis and acute coronary syndrome and Chapter 24 on heart failure and cardiogenic shock, have been combined and reorganized to allow for more comprehensive coverage of the materials. There have been many changes in the care of cardiac patients since the fifth edition. Thus, all chapters have been updated to reflect the most current evidence-based practice guidelines.

Content and Organization

The emphasis on health promotion, health maintenance, and disease management has been maintained throughout the text. By adding, reorganizing, and revising chapters and content, the sixth edition will help all cardiac nurses provide care more confidently and effectively within the changing health care and economic environment across all practice settings. There are five parts in this edition:

PART ONE: ANATOMY AND PHYSIOLOGY. Includes chapters on anatomy and physiology, cardiopulmonary circulation, and the regulation of cardiac output and blood pressure.

PART TWO: PHYSIOLOGIC AND PATHOPHYSIOLOGIC RESPONSES. Includes chapters on genetics; atherosclerosis and acute coronary syndrome; hematopoiesis, coagulation, and bleeding; fluid and electrolyte and acid—base balances and imbalances; sleep; and aging.

PART THREE: ASSESSMENT OF HEART DISEASE. Includes chapters on history taking and physical examination; laboratory tests; radiologic examination of the chest; echocardiography; nuclear imaging, magnetic resonance imaging, and computed tomography imaging; electrocardiography; arrhythmias and conduction disturbances; heart rate variability; cardiac electrophysiologic procedures; exercise testing; cardiac catheterization; and hemodynamic monitoring.

PART FOUR: PATHOPHYSIOLOGY AND MANAGEMENT OF HEART DISEASE. Includes chapters on acute coronary syndrome; interventional cardiology techniques; heart failure and cardiogenic shock; cardiac surgery; mechanical assist devices; sudden cardiac death and cardiac arrest; pacemakers and implantable defibrillators; acquired valvular heart disease; pericardial, myocardial, and endocardial disease; and congenital heart disease.

PART FIVE: HEALTH PROMOTION AND DISEASE PREVENTION. Includes chapters on the assessment and management of coronary heart disease risk factors and disease prevention; psychosocial interventions; smoking cessation and relapse prevention; hypertension; hyperlipidemia; activity and exercise; obesity; diabetes and metabolic syndrome; adherence; complementary and alternative medicine; disease management models; and global cardiovascular health.

The Tradition of Excellence

The sixth edition continues our tradition of excellence in nursing care found in the previous five editions by having more than 90% of the chapters written by cardiac nursing experts. The "red book" maintains our nursing philosophy by organizing the content within the framework of the nursing process and includes numerous nursing care plans. Where possible, the rationale and evidence for treatments and interventions are included.

We sincerely appreciate all the comments we received about the previous editions. We hope you find that the sixth edition lives up to our standard of excellence of the past five editions and that it becomes your primary reference source for cardiac nursing.

Susan L. Woods, PhD, RN, FAHA, FAAN
Erika S. Sivarajan Froelicher, MA, MPH, PhD, RN, FAAN
Sandra Adams (Underhill) Motzer, PhD, RN, FAHA, FAAN
Elizabeth J. Bridges, PhD, RN, CCNS, FCCM, FAAN

Standards of Cardiovascular Nursing Practice

Standards of Practice

STANDARD 1. ASSESSMENT
The cardiovascular registered nurse collects comprehensive data pertinent to the patient's health or the situation.

STANDARD 2. DIAGNOSIS
The cardiovascular registered nurse analyzes the assessment data to determine the nursing diagnoses or health-related issues.

STANDARD 3. OUTCOMES IDENTIFICATION
The cardiovascular registered nurse identifies expected outcomes for a plan individualized to the patient or the situation.

STANDARD 4. PLANNING
The cardiovascular registered nurse develops a plan that prescribes strategies and alternatives to attain expected outcomes.

STANDARD 5. IMPLEMENTATION
The cardiovascular registered nurse implements the identified plan.

STANDARD 5A: COORDINATION OF CARE
The cardiovascular registered nurse coordinates care delivery.

STANDARD 5B: HEALTH TEACHING AND HEALTH PROMOTION
The cardiovascular registered nurse employs strategies to promote health and a safe environment.

STANDARD 5C: CONSULTATION
The advanced practice registered nurse and the cardiovascular registered nurse provide consultation to influence the identified plan, enhance the abilities of others, and effect change.

STANDARD 5D: PRESCRIPTIVE AUTHORITY AND TREATMENT
The advanced practice registered nurse uses prescriptive authority, procedures, referrals, treatments, and therapies in accordance with state and federal laws and regulations.

STANDARD 6. EVALUATION
The cardiovascular registered nurse evaluates progress towards attainment of outcomes.

STANDARD 7. QUALITY OF PRACTICE
The cardiovascular registered nurse systematically enhances the quality and effectiveness of nursing practice.

STANDARD 8. EDUCATION
The cardiovascular registered nurse attains knowledge and competency that reflects current nursing practice.

STANDARD 9. PROFESSIONAL PRACTICE EVALUATION
The cardiovascular registered nurse evaluates one's own nursing practice in relation to professional practice standards and guidelines, relevant statutes, rules, and regulations.

STANDARD 10. COLLEGIALITY
The cardiovascular registered nurse interacts with and contributes to the professional development of peers and colleagues.

STANDARD 11. COLLABORATION
The cardiovascular registered nurse collaborates with patient, family, and others in the conduct of nursing practice.

STANDARD 12. ETHICS
The cardiovascular registered nurse integrates ethical provisions in all areas of practice.

STANDARD 13. RESEARCH
The cardiovascular registered nurse integrates research findings into practice.

STANDARD 14. RESOURCE UTILIZATION
The cardiovascular registered nurse considers factors related to safety, effectiveness, cost, and impact on practice in the planning and delivery of nursing services.

STANDARD 15. LEADERSHIP
The cardiovascular registered nurse provides leadership in the professional practice setting and the profession.

Contents

PART I

Anatomy and Physiology 1

CHAPTER 1

Cardiac Anatomy and Physiology 1

Eleanor F. Bond

CHAPTER 2

Systemic and Pulmonary Circulation and Oxygen Delivery 42

Elizabeth J. Bridges • Joseph O. Schmelz

CHAPTER 3

Regulation of Cardiac Output and Blood Pressure 69

Elizabeth J. Bridges

PART II

Physiologic and Pathologic Responses 97

CHAPTER 4

Genetics 97

Bradley E. Aouizerat

PART I

Anatomy and Physiology

CHAPTER 1

Cardiac Anatomy and Physiology

Eleanor F. Bond*

An understanding of cardiac anatomy is helpful for understanding cardiac physiology and the functional consequences of disease. This chapter describes normal human adult cardiac anatomy, cellular structure, and ultrastructure. The chapter also discusses electrical, mechanical, and metabolic activities that underlie cardiac pump performance. The coronary circulation is described and discussed in the context of its linkage to changing demands of cardiac tissue for nutrient delivery and waste removal. Finally, integrated cardiac performance is discussed.

GENERAL ANATOMIC DESCRIPTION

The heart is a hollow muscular organ encased and cushioned in its own serous membrane, the pericardium. It lies in the middle mediastinal compartment of the thorax between the two pleural cavities. Two thirds of the heart extends to the left of the body's midline (Fig. 1-1).

The heart consists of four muscular chambers, two atria and two ventricles, and associated structures. The right heart (right atrium and ventricle) receives blood from the body and pumps it into the low-pressure pulmonary arterial system. The left heart (left atrium and ventricle) receives oxygenated blood from the lungs and pumps it into the high-pressure systemic arterial system. Interatrial and interventricular septa separate the right from the left atrium and the right from the left ventricle.

The long axis of the heart is directed obliquely, leftward, downward, and forward. Any factor changing the shape of the thorax changes the position of the heart and modifies its directional axis. Respiratory alterations in the diaphragm and the rib cage constantly cause small changes in the cardiac axis. With a deep inspiration, the heart descends and becomes more vertical. Factors that may cause long-term axis variations in healthy people include age, weight, pregnancy, body shape, and thorax shape. A tall, thin person usually has a more vertical heart, whereas a short, obese person usually has a more horizontal heart. Pathologic conditions of the heart, lungs, abdominal organs, and other structures influence the cardiac axis.

The surfaces of the heart are used to reference its position in relation to other structures and to describe the location of damage, as in a myocardial infarction. The right ventricle and parts of the right atrium and the left ventricle form the anterior (or sternocostal) cardiac surface (Figs. 1-1 and 1-2). The right atrium and ventricle lie anteriorly and to the right of the left atrium and ventricle in the frontal plane. Thus, when viewed from the front of the body, the heart appears to be lying sideways, directed forward and leftward, with the right heart foremost.

The small portion of the lower left ventricle that extends anteriorly forms a blunt tip composed of the apical part of the interventricular septum and the left ventricular free wall. Because of the forward tilt of the heart, movement of this apex portion of the left ventricle during cardiac contraction usually forms the *point of maximal impulse*, which can be observed in healthy people in the fifth intercostal space at the left midclavicular line, 7 to 9 cm from midline. The sternum, costal cartilages of the third to sixth ribs, part of the lungs, and, in children, the thymus, overlie the anterior cardiac surface.

The left atrium and a small section of the right atrium and ventricle comprise the base of the heart, which is directed backward and forms the posterior surface of the heart (Fig. 1-3). The thoracic aorta, esophagus, and vertebrae are posterior to the heart. The inferior or diaphragmatic surface of the heart, composed chiefly of the left ventricle, lies almost horizontally on the upper surface of the diaphragm (Fig. 1-4). The right ventricle forms a portion of the inferior cardiac surface.

The right atrium forms the lateral right heart border; therefore, the right atrium and right lung lie close together. The entire right margin of the heart extends laterally from the superior vena cava along the right atrium and then toward the diaphragm to the cardiac apex. The lateral wall of the left ventricle and a small part of the left atrium form most of the left heart border. This portion of the left ventricle is next to the left lung and sometimes is referred to as the *pulmonary surface.*

The coronary [or atrioventricular (AV)] sulcus (groove) is the external landmark denoting the separation of the atria from the ventricles. The AV sulcus encircles the heart obliquely and contains coronary blood vessels, cardiac nerves, and epicardial fat. The aorta and pulmonary artery interrupt the AV sulcus anteriorly. The anterior and posterior interventricular sulci separate the right and left ventricles on the external heart surface. The *crux* of the heart is the point on the external posterior heart surface where

*The material in this chapter was originally co-authored with Carol Jean Halpenny.

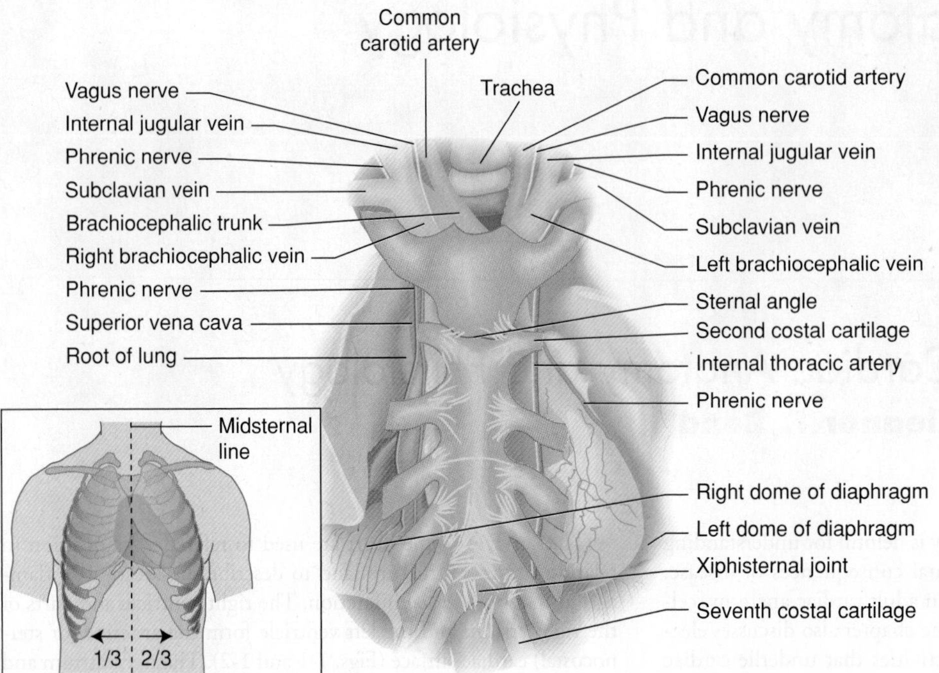

■ **Figure 1-1** Location of the heart and pericardium. This dissection exposes the pericardialsac posterior to the body of the sternum from just superior to the sterna angel to the level of the xiphisternal joint. The pericardial sac is approximately one third to the right of the midsternal line and two thirds to the left. (From Moore, K. L., & Dalley, A. F. [2005]. *Clinically oriented anatomy* [5th ed., p. 145]. Philadelphia: Lippincott Williams & Wilkins.)

the posterior interventricular sulcus intersects the coronary (AV) sulcus externally and where the interatrial septum joins the interventricular septum internally.

The average adult heart is approximately 12 cm long from its base at the beginning of the root of the aorta to the left ventricular apex. It is 8 to 9 cm transversely at its greatest width, and 6 cm thick anteroposteriorly. Tables have been derived to indicate normal ranges of heart size for various body weights and heights.[1]

The adult male heart comprises approximately 0.43% of body weight, typically 280 to 350 g, with an average weight of 300 g. The adult female heart comprises approximately 0.40% of body weight, 230 to 300 g, with an average weight of 250 g.[2,3] Age, body build, frequency of physical exercise, and heart disease influence heart size and weight.

CARDIAC STRUCTURES

Fibrous Skeleton

Four adjacent, dense, fibrous connective tissue rings, the annuli fibrosi, surround the cardiac valves and provide an internal supporting structure for the heart. The annuli are attached together and connected by a central fibrous core (Fig. 1-5). Each annulus and valve has a slightly different orientation, but the entire

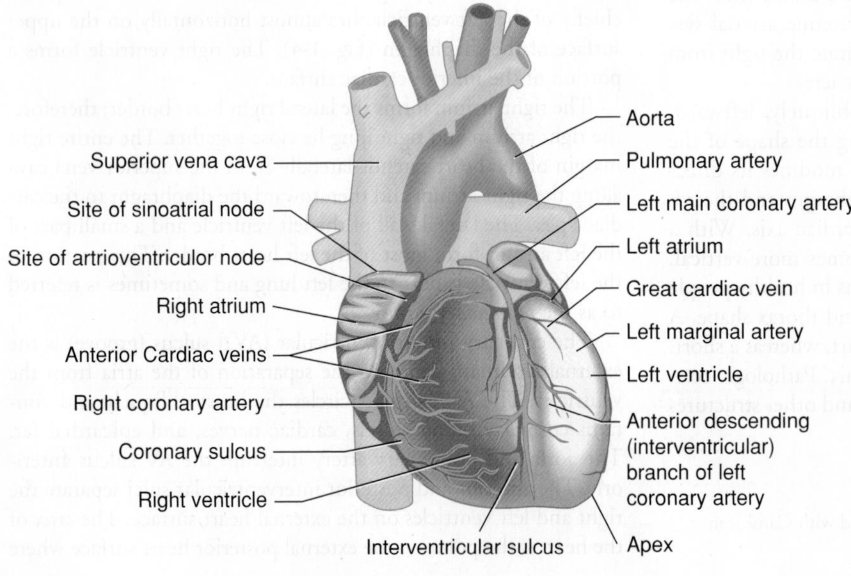

■ **Figure 1-2** Anterior view of the heart, illustrating the cardiac structures. The pericardial sac has been cut open. (From Anatomical Chart Company, General Anatomy, 2008-05-14 0614, 2008-07-13 1449.)

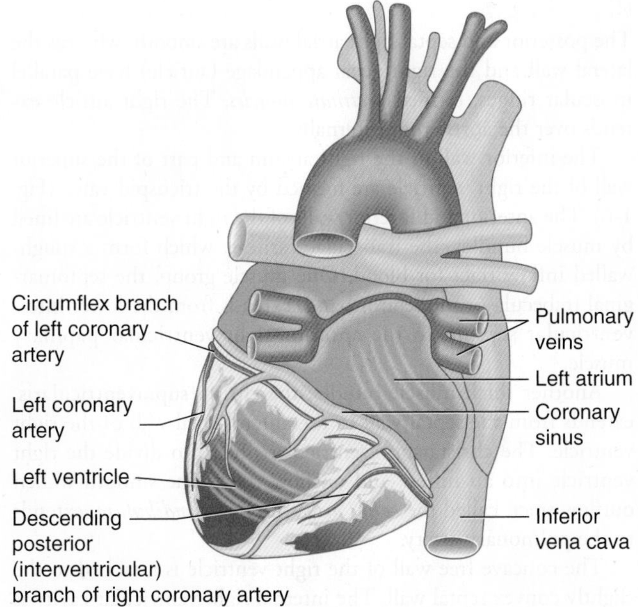

■ **Figure 1-3** Posterior view of the heart. (From Anatomical Chart Company, General Anatomy, 2008-05-14 0614, 2008-07-13 1449.)

connective tissue structure, termed the *fibrous skeleton*, is oriented obliquely within the mediastinum.

The fibrous skeleton divides the atria from the ventricles. It provides the attachment site for some of the atrial and ventricular cardiac muscle fibers. A portion of the fibrous skeleton extends downward between the right atrium and left ventricle, forming the upper or membranous part of the interventricular septum.

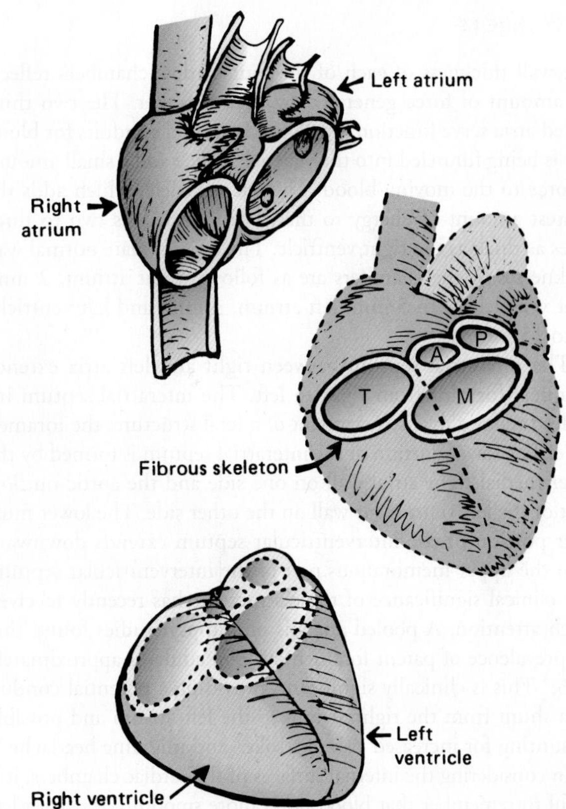

■ **Figure 1-5** Schematic view of the fibrous skeleton, illustrating the attachment of the cardiac valves and chambers. The four annuli and their extensions lie in different planes, so it is impossible to depict them accurately on a plane surface. T, tricuspid valve; M, mitral valve; A, aortic valve; P, pulmonic valve. (Adapted from Rushmer, R. F. [1976]. *Cardiovascular Dynamics* [p. 77]. Philadelphia: WB Saunders.)

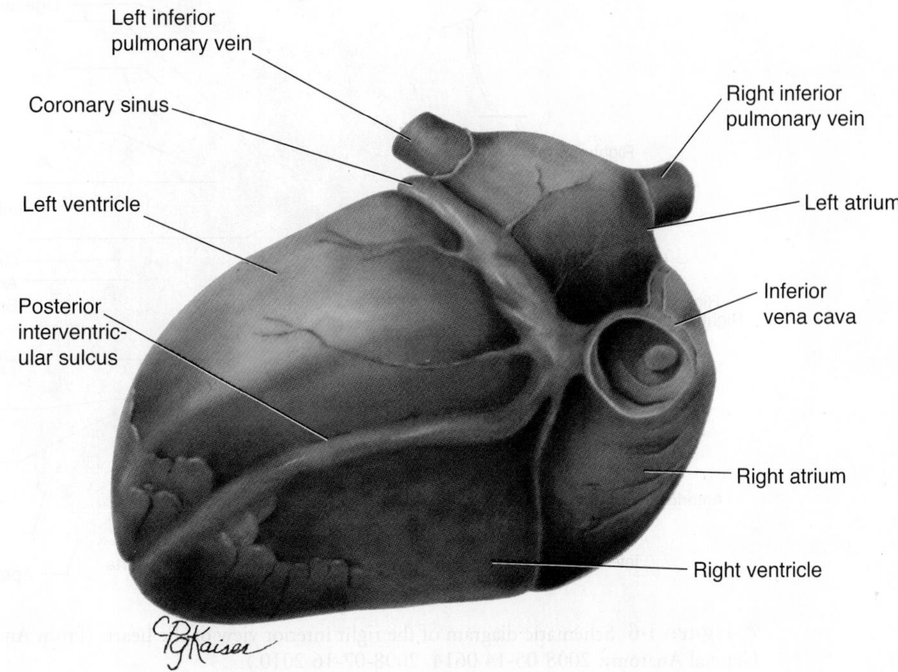

■ **Figure 1-4** Inferior or diaphragmatic heart surface.

Chambers

The wall thickness of each of the four cardiac chambers reflects the amount of force generated by that chamber. The two thin-walled atria serve functionally as reservoirs and conduits for blood that is being funneled into the ventricles; they add a small amount of force to the moving blood. The left ventricle, which adds the greatest amount of energy to the flowing blood, is two to three times as thick as the right ventricle. The approximate normal wall thicknesses of the chambers are as follows: right atrium, 2 mm; right ventricle, 3 to 5 mm; left atrium, 3 mm; and left ventricle, 13 to 15 mm.

The interatrial septum between right and left atria extends obliquely forward from right to left. The interatrial septum includes the fossa ovalis, a remnant of a fetal structure, the foramen ovale. The lower portion of the interatrial septum is formed by the lower medial right atrial wall on one side and the aortic outflow tract of the left ventricular wall on the other side. The lower muscular portion of the interventricular septum extends downward from the upper membranous part of the interventricular septum. The clinical significance of these structures has recently received much attention. A pooled analysis of autopsy studies found that the prevalence of patent foramen ovale in adults is approximately 26%.[4] This is clinically significant, providing a potential conduit for a shunt from the right atrium to the left atrium and possibly accounting for increased risk of stroke[5] and migraine headache.[6]

In considering the internal surfaces of the cardiac chambers, it is useful to remember that blood flows more smoothly and with less turbulence across walls that are smooth rather than ridged. Blood pools in appendages or other areas out of the direct blood flow path.

Right Heart

The posterior and septal right atrial walls are smooth, whereas the lateral wall and the right atrial appendage (auricle) have parallel muscular ridges, termed *pectinate muscles*. The right auricle extends over the aortic root externally.

The inferior wall of the right atrium and part of the superior wall of the right ventricle are formed by the tricuspid valve (Fig. 1-6). The anterior and inferior walls of the right ventricle are lined by muscle bundles, the trabeculae carneae, which form a rough-walled inflow tract for blood. One muscle group, the septomarginal trabecula or moderator band, extends from the lower interventricular septum to the anterior right ventricular papillary muscle.

Another thick muscle bundle, the christa supraventricularis, extends from the septal wall to the anterolateral wall of the right ventricle. The christa supraventricularis helps to divide the right ventricle into an inflow and outflow tract. The smooth-walled outflow tract, called the *conus arteriosus* or *infundibulum*, extends to the pulmonary artery.

The concave free wall of the right ventricle is attached to the slightly convex septal wall. The internal right ventricular cavity is crescent or triangle shaped. The right ventricle also forms a crescent laterally around the left ventricle. Right ventricular contraction causes the right ventricular free wall to move toward the interventricular septum. This bellows-like action is effective in ejecting large and variable volumes into a low-pressure system (Fig. 1-7).

Venous blood enters the right atrium from the upper and the lower posterior parts of the atrium through the superior and

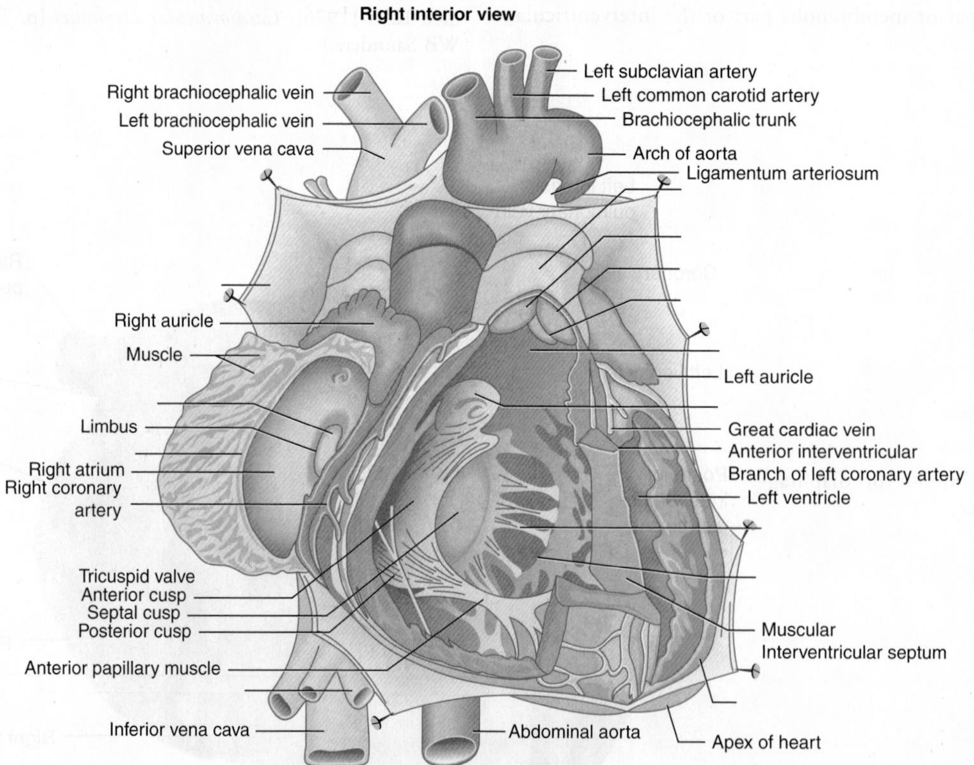

■ **Figure 1-6** Schematic diagram of the right interior view of the heart. (From Anatomical Chart Company, General Anatomy, 2008-05-14 0614, 2008-07-16 2010.)

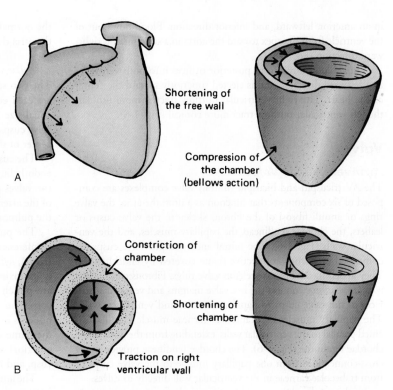

■ Figure 1-7 Right and left ventricular contraction. (A) Right ventricular contraction. Right ventricular ejection of blood is accomplished primarily by shortening and movement of the free wall toward the interventricular septum. Note the crescent shape of the right ventricle. (B) Blood is ejected from the left ventricle primarily by a reduction in the diameter of the chamber. There is some ventricular shortening. (Adapted from Rushmer, R. [1976]. *Cardiovascular dynamics* [p. 92]. Philadelphia: WB Saunders.)

Shortening of the free wall
Compression of the chamber (bellows action)
A
Constriction of chamber
Shortening of chamber
Traction on right ventricular wall
B

inferior venae cavae. Most of the venous drainage from the heart enters the right atrium through the coronary sinus, which is located between the entrance of the inferior vena cava into the right atrium and the orifice of the tricuspid valve. Blood flows medially and anteriorly from the right atrium through the tricuspid orifice into the right ventricle.

Blood enters the right ventricle in an almost horizontal but slightly leftward, anterior, and inferior direction. It is ejected superiorly and posteriorly through the pulmonary valve (Fig. 1-8).

Left Heart

The left atrium is a cuboid structure that lies between the aortic root and the esophagus. The left atrial appendage, or auricle, extends along the border of the pulmonary artery. The walls of the left atrium are smooth except for pectinate muscle bundles in the atrial appendage.

The left ventricle has a cone-like or oval shape, bordered by the generally concave left ventricular free wall and interventricular septum. The mitral valve and its attachments form the left ventricular inflow tract. The outflow tract is formed by the anterior surface of the anterior mitral valve cusp, the septum, and the aortic vestibule. The lower muscular interventricular septum and free walls of the left ventricle are deeply ridged with trabeculae carneae muscle bundles, so most of the interior surface of the ventricle is rough. The upper membranous septum and aortic vestibule region have smooth walls. The interventricular septum is functionally and anatomically a more integral part of the left ventricle than the right ventricle. The septum is triangular, with its base at the aortic area. The upper septum separates the right atrium from the left ventricle and is often called the *AV septum.*

Blood is ejected from the left ventricle mainly by circumferential contraction of the muscular wall, that is, by decreasing the diameter of the cylinder (see Fig. 1-7). There is some longitudinal shortening. The ventricular cavity has a small surface area in relation to the volume contained, but high pressure can be developed because of the amount of ventricular muscle, the shape of the cavity, and the way the muscles contract.

Four pulmonary veins return blood from the lungs to openings in the posterolateral wall of the left atrium. Blood is directed obliquely forward out of the left atrium and enters the left ventricle

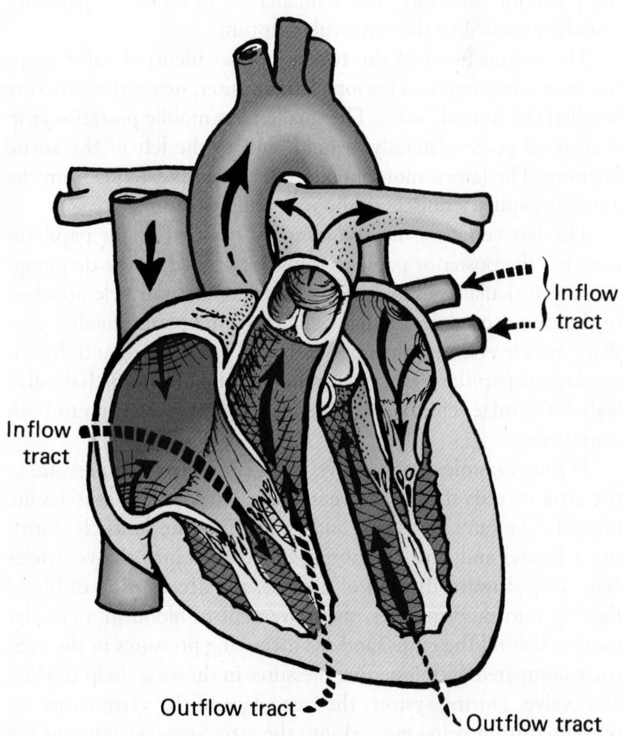

■ Figure 1-8 Blood flow through cardiac chambers and valves.

in an anterior, leftward, and inferior direction. Blood flows out of the ventricle from the apex toward the aorta in a superior and rightward direction (Fig. 1-8).

Thus, blood flows from posterior orifices into both ventricles in a leftward direction and is ejected superiorly toward the center of the heart. The right ventricular outflow tract is more tubular; the left ventricular outflow tract more conical (Fig. 1-8).

Valves

Atrioventricular Valves

The AV tricuspid and bicuspid (mitral) valve complexes are composed of six components that function as a unit: the atria, the valve rings or annuli fibrosi of the fibrous skeleton, the valve cusps or leaflets, the chordae tendineae, the papillary muscles, and the ventricular walls (Fig. 1-6). The mitral and tricuspid valve cusps are composed of fibrous connective tissue covered by endothelium. They attach to the fibrous skeleton valve rings. Fibrous cords called *chordae tendineae* connect the free valve margins and ventricular surfaces of the valve cusps to papillary muscles and ventricular walls. The papillary muscles are trabeculae carneae muscle bundles oriented parallel to the ventricular walls, extending from the walls to the chordae tendineae (Fig. 1-6). The chordae tendineae provide many cross-connections from one papillary muscle to the valve cusps or from trabeculae carneae in the ventricular wall directly to valves.

In the adult, the tricuspid orifice is larger (approximately 11 cm in circumference, or capable of admitting three fingers) than the mitral orifice (approximately 9 cm in circumference, or capable of admitting two fingers). The combined surface area of the AV valve cusps is larger than the surface area of the valvular orifice because the cusps resemble curtain-like, billowing flaps.

Most commonly, there are three tricuspid valve cusps: the large anterior, the septal, and the posterior (inferior). There are usually two principal right ventricular papillary muscles, the anterior and the posterior (inferior), and a smaller set of accessory papillary muscles attached to the ventricular septum.

The arrangement of the two triangular bicuspid valve cusps has been compared to a bishop's hat, or miter; hence the structure is called the "mitral" valve. The smaller, less mobile posterior cusp is situated posterolaterally, behind, and to the left of the aortic opening. The larger, more mobile anterior cusp extends from the anterior papillary muscle to the ventricular septum.

The left ventricle most commonly has two major papillary muscles: the posterior papillary muscle attached to the diaphragmatic ventricular wall and the anterior papillary muscle attached to the sternocostal ventricular wall. Thus, the posteromedial papillary muscle extends to the posterolateral valve leaflet, and the anterolateral papillary muscle extends to the anteromedial valve leaflet. Chordae tendineae from each papillary muscle go to both mitral cusps.

During diastole, the AV valves open passively when pressure in the atria exceeds that in the ventricles. The papillary muscles are relaxed. The valve cusps part and project into the ventricle, forming a funnel and thus promoting blood flow into the ventricles (Fig. 1-8). Toward the end of diastole, the deceleration of blood flowing into the ventricles, the movement of blood in a circular motion behind the cusps, and the increasing pressures in the ventricle compared with lessening pressures in the atria, help to close each valve. During systole, the free edges of the valve cusps are prevented from being everted into the atria by contraction of the papillary muscles and tension in the chordae tendineae. Thus, in the normal heart, blood is prevented from flowing backward into the atria despite the high systolic ventricular pressures.

Semilunar Valves

The two semilunar (pulmonary [or pulmonic] and aortic) valves are each composed of three cup-shaped cusps of approximately equal size that attach at their base to the fibrous skeleton. The valve cusps are convex from below, with thickened nodules at the center of the free margins.

The cusps are composed of fibrous connective tissue lined with endothelium. The endothelial lining on the nonventricular side of the valves closely resembles and merges with that of the intima of the arteries beyond the valves. The aortic cusps are thicker than the pulmonic; both are thicker than the AV cusps.

The pulmonary valve orifice is approximately 8.5 cm in circumference. The pulmonic valve cusps are termed *right anterior* (right), *left anterior* (anterior), and *posterior* (left). The aortic valve is approximately 7.5 cm in circumference. The sinuses of Valsalva are pouch-like structures immediately behind each semilunar cusp. The coronary arteries branch from the aorta from two of the pouches or sinuses of Valsalva. The aortic cusps are designated by the name of the nearby coronary artery: *right coronary* (right or anterior) aortic cusp, *left coronary* (left or left posterior) aortic cusp, and *noncoronary* (posterior or right posterior) aortic cusp.

The aortic and pulmonic semilunar valves are approximately at right angles to each other in the closed position. The pulmonic valve is anterior and superior to the other three cardiac valves. When closed, the semilunar valve cusps contact each other at the nodules and along crescent arcs, called *lunulae,* below the free margins. During systole, the cusps are thrust upward as blood flows from an area of greater pressure in the ventricle to an area of lesser pressure in the aorta or the pulmonary artery. The effect of the deceleration of blood in the aorta during late systole on small circular currents of blood in the sinuses of Valsalva helps passively to close the semilunar valve cusps. Backflow into the ventricles during diastole is prevented because of the cusps' fibrous strength, their close approximation, and their shape.

CARDIAC TISSUE

The heart wall is composed mainly of a muscular layer, the myocardium. The epicardium and the pericardium cover the external surface. Internally, the endocardium covers the surface.

Epicardium and Pericardium

The epicardium is a layer of mesothelial cells that forms the visceral or heart layer of the serous pericardium. Branches of the coronary blood and lymph vessels, nerves, and fat are enclosed in the epicardium and the superficial layers of the myocardium.

The epicardium completely encloses the external surface of the heart and extends several centimeters along each great vessel, encircling the aorta and pulmonary artery together. It merges with the tunica adventitia of the great vessels, at which point it doubles back on itself as the parietal pericardium. This continuous membrane thus forms the pericardial sac and encloses a potential space, the pericardial cavity (Fig. 1-1). The serous parietal pericardium lines the inner surface of the thicker, tougher fibrous pericardial membrane. The pericardial membrane extends beyond the serous pericardium and is attached by ligaments and loose connections to

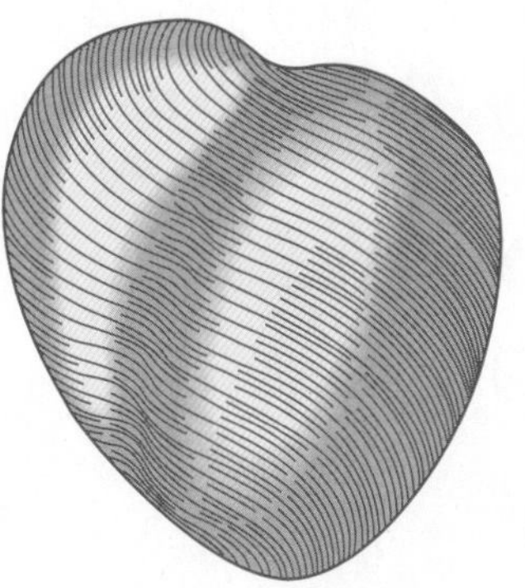
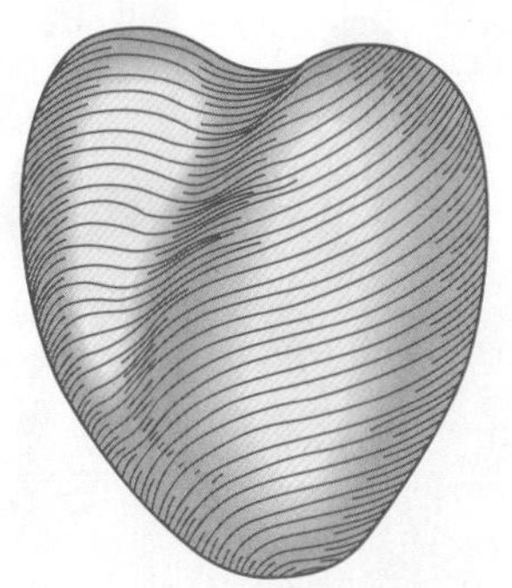
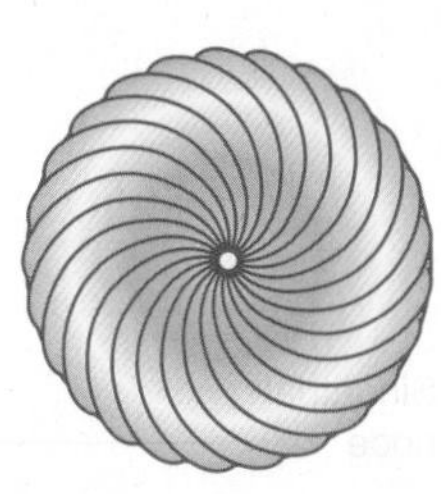

■ **Figure 1-9** Schematic view of spiral arrangement of ventricular muscle fibers. (From Katz, A. [2006]. *Physiology of the heart* [4th ed., p. 8]. Philadelphia: Lippincott Williams & Wilkins.)

the sternum, diaphragm, and structures in the posterior mediastinum.

The pericardial cavity usually contains 10 to 30 mL of thin, clear serous fluid. The main function of the pericardium and its fluid is to lubricate the moving surfaces of the heart. The pericardium also helps to retard ventricular dilation, helps to hold the heart in position, and forms a barrier to the spread of infections and neoplasia.

Pathophysiological conditions such as cardiac bleeding or an exudate-producing pericarditis may lead to a sudden or large accumulation of fluid within the pericardial sac. This may impede ventricular filling. From 50 to 300 mL of pericardial fluid may accumulate without serious ventricular impairment. When greater volumes accumulate, ventricular filling is impaired; this condition is known as cardiac tamponade. If the fluid accumulation builds slowly, the ventricles may be able to maintain an adequate cardiac output by contracting more vigorously. The pericardium is histologically similar to pleural and peritoneal serous membranes, so inflammation of all three membranes may occur with certain systemic conditions such as rheumatoid arthritis.

Myocardium

The myocardial layer is composed of cardiac muscle cells interspersed with connective tissue and small blood vessels. Some atrial and ventricular myocardial fibers are anchored to the fibrous skeleton (see Fig. 1-5). The thin-walled atria are composed of two major muscle systems: one that surrounds both of the atria and another that is arranged at right angles to the first and that is separate for each atrium.

Each ventricle is a single muscle mass of nested figure eights of individual muscle fiber path spirals anchored to the fibrous skeleton.[7,8] Ventricular muscle fibers spiral downward on the epicardial ventricular wall, pass through the wall, spiral up on the endocardial surface, cross the upper part of the ventricle, and go back down through the wall (Fig. 1-9). This vortex arrangement allows for the circumferential generation of tension throughout the ventricular wall; it is functionally efficient for ventricular contraction. Some fiber paths spiral around both ventricles. The fibers form a fan-like arrangement of interconnecting muscle fibers when dissected horizontally through the ventricular wall.[8] The orientation of these fibers gradually rotates through the thickness of the wall (Fig. 1-10).

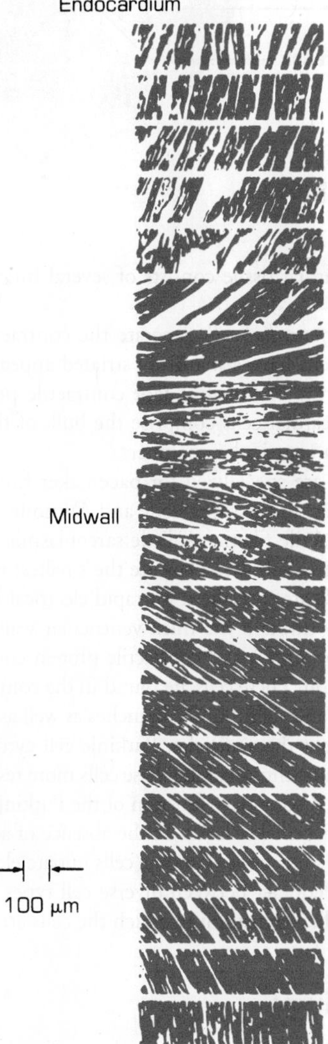

■ **Figure 1-10** Changing ventricular muscle fiber angles at different depths. Reconstructed from a series of microphotographs. (From Streeter, D. D., Jr, Spotnitz, H. M., & Patel, D. P., et al. [1969]. Fiber orientation in the canine left ventricle during diastole and systole. *Circulation Research*, *24*, 342–347, with permission of the American Heart Association, Inc.)

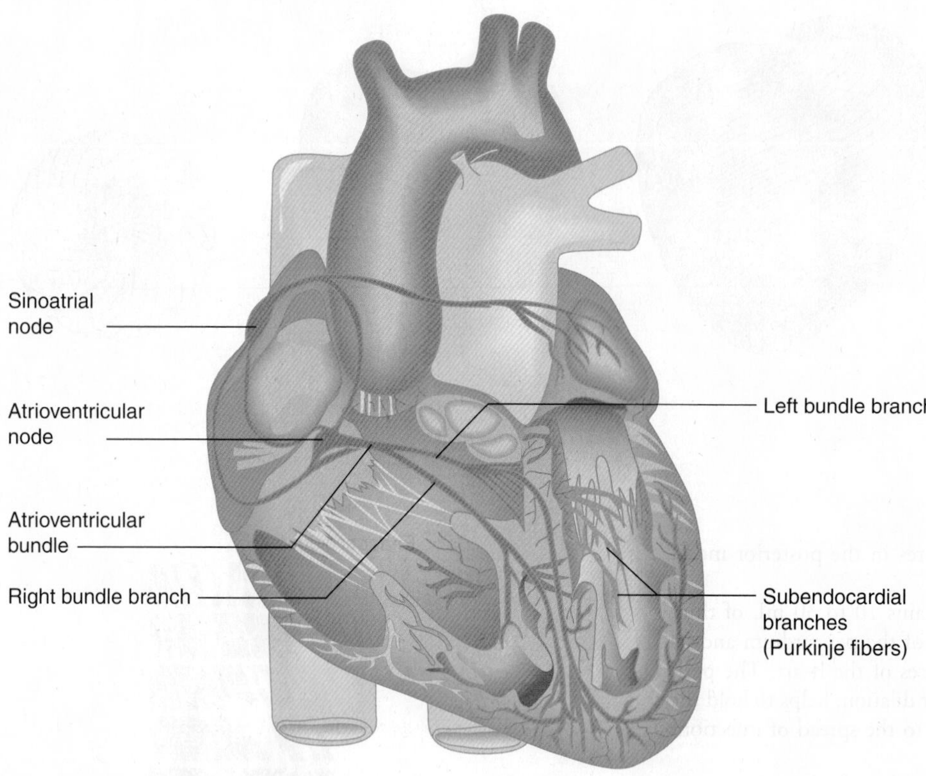

■ **Figure 1-11** Schematic illustration of the human cardiac conducting system. (From LifeART image © 2007 Lippincott Williams & Wilkins.)

The myocardial tissue consists of several functionally specialized cell types.

Working myocardial cells generate the contractile force of the heart. These cells have a markedly striated appearance caused by the orderly arrays of the abundant contractile protein filaments. Working myocardial cells comprise the bulk of the walls of both atrial and both ventricular chambers.

Nodal cells are specialized for pacemaker function. They are found in clusters in the sinus node and AV node. These cells contain few contractile filaments, little sarcoplasmic reticulum (SR), and no transverse tubules. They are the smallest myocardial cells.

Purkinje cells are specialized for rapid electrical impulse conduction, especially through the thick ventricular wall. The large size, elongated shape, and sparse contractile protein composition reflect this specialization. These cells are found in the common His bundle and in the left and right bundle branches as well as in a diffuse network throughout the ventricles. Purkinje cell cytoplasm is rich in glycogen granules; thus, making these cells more resistant to damage during anoxia. A secondary function of the Purkinje cells is to serve as a potential pacemaker locus. In the absence of an overriding impulse from the sinus node, Purkinje cells initiate electrical impulses.

In areas of contact between diverse cell types, there is usually an area of gradual transition in which the cells are intermediate in appearance.

Endocardium

The endocardium is composed of a layer of endothelial cells and a few layers of collagen and elastic fibers. The endocardium is continuous with the tunica intima of the blood vessels.

Conduction Tissues

In the normal sequence of events, the specialized nodal myocardial cells depolarize spontaneously, generating electrical impulses that are conducted to the larger mass of working myocardial cells (Fig. 1-11). The sequential contraction of the atria and ventricles as coordinated units depends on the anatomic arrangement of the specialized cardiac conducting tissue. Small cardiac nerves, arteries, and veins lie close to the specialized conducting cells, providing neurohumoral modulation of cardiac impulse generation and conduction.

Keith and Flack[9] first described the sinus node in 1907.[9,10] The sinus node lies close to the epicardial surface of the heart, above the tricuspid valve, near the anterior entrance of the superior vena cava into the right atrium. The sinus node is also referred to as the *sinoatrial node.* It is approximately 10 to 15 mm long, 3 to 5 mm wide, and 1 mm thick. Small nodal cells are surrounded by and interspersed with connective tissue. They merge with the larger working atrial muscle cells.

Bachmann[11] originally described an interatrial myocardial bundle conducting impulses from the right atrium to the left atrium. James[12] presented evidence for three *internodal conduction pathways* from the sinus node to the AV node. It is unclear whether the pathways have functional significance.[13,14] It is generally believed that the cardiac impulse spreads from the sinus node to the AV node via cell-to-cell conduction through the atrial working myocardial cells.[15]

Tarawa[16] initially described the AV node in 1906. It is located subendocardially on the right atrial side of the central fibrous body, in the lower interatrial septal wall. The AV node is close to the septal leaflet of the tricuspid valve and anterior to the coronary sinus. A group of fibers connects the AV node to working myocardial cells in the left atrium.[17] The AV node is approximately 7 mm long, 3 mm wide, and 1 mm thick.[18] Nodal fibers are interspersed with normal working myocardial fibers; it is difficult to precisely identify the AV node boundaries. There are several zones of specialized conducting tissue in the AV junction area: the compact AV node, a transition zone containing small nodal and larger working atrial myocardial cells, the penetrating AV bundle, and the branching AV bundle.[19,20]

Fibers from the AV node converge into a shaft termed the *bundle of His* (also called the *penetrating AV bundle* or *common bundle*). It is approximately 10 mm long and 2 mm in diameter.[18] The bundle of His passes from the lower right atrial wall anteriorly and laterally through the central fibrous body, which is part of the fibrous skeleton.

As first noted by His in 1893,[21] the His bundle provides the only cellular connection between the atria and ventricles and is of pivotal functional importance. Cardiac impulse transmission is slowed at this site, providing time for atrial contraction to dispel blood from the atria into the ventricles. This slowing boosts ventricular volume and increases the cardiac output during subsequent ventricular contraction. At the membranous septal region of the heart, the right atrium and left ventricle are opposite each other across the septum, with the right ventricle in close proximity. Three of the four cardiac valves are nearby.[22] Thus, pathology of the fibrous skeleton, tricuspid, mitral, or aortic valves can affect functioning of one or more of the other valves or may affect cardiac impulse conduction. Dysfunction of the AV conducting tissue may affect the coordinated functioning of the atria and ventricles.

Abnormal accessory pathways, termed *Kent bundles*, occasionally join the atria and ventricles through connections outside the main AV node and His bundle.[23,24] Tracts from the His bundle to upper interventricular septum (termed *paraspecific fibers of Mahaim*) sometimes occur and are also abnormal.[25,26] AV conduction is accelerated when impulses bypass the delay-producing AV junction and travel instead through these abnormal connections. When accelerated AV conduction occurs, cardiac output often decreases because there is inadequate time for atrial contraction to boost ventricular filling.[27]

The His bundle begins branching in the region of the crest of the muscular septum (Fig. 1-11). The right bundle branch typically continues as a direct extension of the His bundle. The right bundle branch is a well-defined, single, slender group of fibers approximately 45 to 50 mm long and 1 mm thick. It initially courses downward along the right side of the interventricular septum, continues through the moderator band of muscular tissue near the right ventricular apex, and then continues to the base of the anterior papillary muscle. If a small segment of the bundle is damaged, the entire distal distribution is affected because of the right bundle's thinness, length, and relative lack of arborization.

The left bundle branch arises almost perpendicularly from the His bundle as the common left bundle branch. This common left bundle, approximately 10 mm long and 4 to 10 mm wide, then divides into two discrete divisions, the left anterior bundle branch and the left posterior bundle branch. The left anterior bundle branch, or left anterior fascicle, is approximately 25 mm long and 3 mm thick. It usually arises directly from the common left bundle after the origin of the posterior fascicle and close to the origin of the right bundle. It branches to the anterior septum and courses over the left ventricular anterior (superior) wall to the anterior papillary muscle, crossing the aortic outflow tract. Anterior and septal myocardial infarctions and aortic valve dysfunction often affect the left anterior bundle branch.

The large, thick, left posterior bundle branch, or left posterior fascicle, arises either from the first portion of the common left bundle or from the His bundle directly. The left posterior fascicle goes inferiorly and posteriorly across the left ventricular inflow tract to the base of the posterior papillary muscle; it then spreads diffusely through the posterior inferior left ventricular free wall. It is approximately 20 mm long and 6 mm thick. This fascicle is often the least vulnerable segment of the ventricular conducting system because of its diffuseness, its location in a relatively protected nonturbulent portion of the ventricle, and its dual blood supply (Table 1-1).

Three, rather than two, major divisions of the left bundle branch are sometimes found, with a group of fibers ramifying from the left posterior fascicle and terminating in the lower septum and apical ventricular wall.[20] This trifascicular configuration of the bundles explains some conduction defects involving partial bundle-branch block. Sometimes instead of three discrete bundles the common left bundle fans out diffusely along the septum and the free ventricular wall.[28]

Purkinje fibers, first described in 1845, form a complex network of conducting tissue ramifications that provide a continuation of the bundle branches in each ventricle.[29] The Purkinje fibers course down toward the ventricular apex and then up toward the fibrous rings at the ventricular bases. They spread over the subendocardial ventricular surfaces and then spread from the endocardium through the myocardium; thus, spreading from inside outward, providing extensive contacts with working myocardial cells, and coupling myocardial excitation with muscular contraction.

CORONARY CIRCULATION

The heart is continuously active. Like all tissues, it must receive oxygen and metabolic substrates; carbon dioxide and other wastes must be removed to maintain aerobic metabolism and contractile activity. However, unlike other tissues, it must generate the force to power its own perfusion. The heart requires continuous perfusion.

Coronary Arteries

The major coronary arteries in humans are the right coronary artery and the left coronary artery, sometimes called the *left main coronary artery.* These arteries branch from the aorta in the region of the sinus of Valsalva (Figs. 1-12 and 1-13). They extend over the epicardial surface of the heart and branch several times. The branches usually emerge at right angles from the parent artery.[30] The arteries plunge inward through the myocardial wall and undergo further branching. The epicardial branches exit first. The more distal branches supply the endocardial (internal) myocardium. The arteries continue branching and eventually become arterioles, then capillaries. Partially because the blood supply originates more distally, the endocardium is more vulnerable to compromised blood supply than is the epicardial surface.

There is much individual variation in the pattern of coronary artery branching. In general, the right coronary artery supplies the right atrium and ventricle. The left coronary artery supplies much of the left atrium and ventricle. The following discussion describes the most common arterial pattern. Table 1-1 lists the major cardiac structures, their usual arterial supply, and some common variations (e.g., either the right or the left coronary artery may supply the AV node).

Table 1-1 ■ AREA SUPPLIED BY COMMON ARTERIES*

Structure	Usual Arterial Supply	Common Variants
Right atrium	Sinus node artery, branch of RCA (55%)	Sinus node artery, branch of L circumflex (45%)
Left atrium	Major L circumflex†	Sinus node artery, branch of L circumflex (45%)
Right ventricle		
Anterior	Major RCA Minor LAD	
Posterior	Major RCA; posterior descending branch of RCA Minor LAD (ascending portion)	Posterior descending may branch from L circumflex (10%) LAD terminates at apex (40%)
Left Ventricle		
Posterior (diaphragmatic)	Major L circumflex, posterior descending branch of RCA Minor LAD (ascending portion)	Posterior descending may branch from L circumflex (10%) LAD terminates at apex (40%)
Anterior	L coronary artery; L circumflex and LAD	
Apex	Major LAD	
Intraventricular septum	Major septal branches of LAD Minor posterior descending branch of RCA and AV nodal branch of RCA	Minor posterior descending may branch from L circumflex, AV nodal may branch from L circumflex
Left ventricular papillary muscles		
Anterior	Diagonal branch of LAD; other branches of LAD, other branches of L circumflex	Diagonal may branch from circumflex
Posterior	RCA and L circumflex	RCA and LAD
Sinus node	Nodal artery from RCA (55%)	Nodal artery from L circumflex (45%)
AV node	RCA (90%)	L circumflex (10%)
Bundle of His	RCA (90%)	L circumflex (10%)
Right bundle	Major LAD septal branches Minor AV nodal artery	
Left anterior bundle	Major LAD septal branches Minor AV nodal artery	
Left posterior bundle	LAD septal branches and AV nodal artery	

*Percentages in parentheses denote frequency of occurrence in autopsy studies.
†Major and minor refer to degree of predominance of an artery in perfusing a structure.
RCA, right coronary artery; LAD, left anterior descending artery; L, left; LV, left ventricle; AV, atrioventricular.
Data from James, T. N. (1961). *Anatomy of the coronary arteries.* New York: Paul B. Hoeber; James, T. N. (1978). Anatomy of the coronary arteries and veins. In J. W. Hurst (Ed.), *The heart* (4th ed., pp. 32–47). New York: McGraw-Hill.

Individual anatomic variation should be considered in analyzing patient data. For example, angiographic visualization of the left circumflex artery might show severe stenosis. Although it is not likely that AV node and His bundle perfusion would be affected (because the right coronary artery typically perfuses these structures), in approximately 10% of cases the structures would be at risk. Thus, angiographic information is validated with clinical data. Also, apparently attenuated or narrowed vessels may be normal anatomic variants.

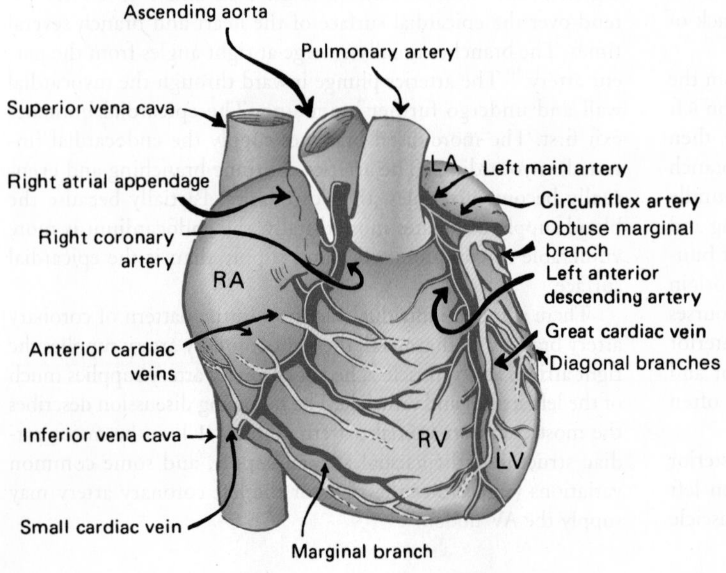

■ **Figure 1-12** Principal arteries and veins on the anterior surface of the heart. Part of the right atrial appendage has been resected. The left coronary artery arises from the left coronary aortic sinus behind the pulmonary trunk. RA, right atrium; RV, right ventricle; LA, left atrium; LV, left ventricle. (Adapted from Walmsley, R., & Watson, H. [1978]. *Clinical anatomy of the heart* [p. 203]. New York: Churchill Livingston.)

Vessel Dominance

Dominance (or *preponderance*), a term commonly used in describing coronary vasculature, refers to the distribution of the terminal portion of the arteries. The artery that reaches and crosses the *crux*

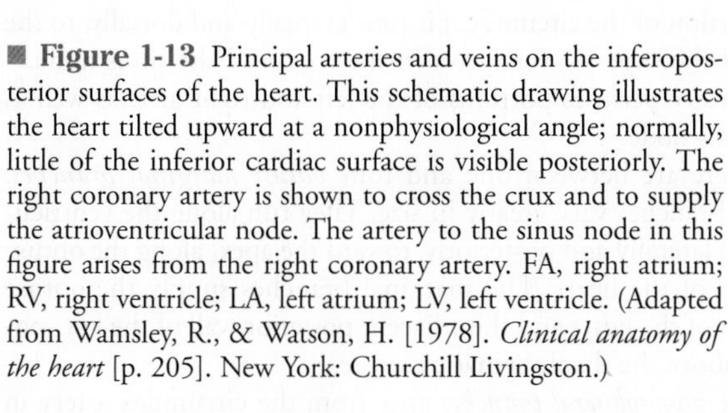

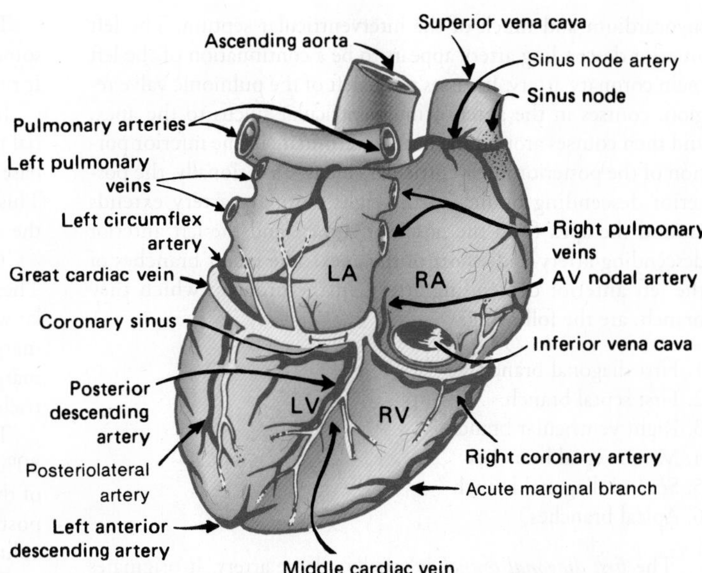

■ **Figure 1-13** Principal arteries and veins on the inferoposterior surfaces of the heart. This schematic drawing illustrates the heart tilted upward at a nonphysiological angle; normally, little of the inferior cardiac surface is visible posteriorly. The right coronary artery is shown to cross the crux and to supply the atrioventricular node. The artery to the sinus node in this figure arises from the right coronary artery. FA, right atrium; RV, right ventricle; LA, left atrium; LV, left ventricle. (Adapted from Wamsley, R., & Watson, H. [1978]. *Clinical anatomy of the heart* [p. 205]. New York: Churchill Livingston.)

(where the right and left AV grooves cross the posterior interatrial and interventricular grooves) is said to be *dominant.* In approximately 85% of cases, the right coronary artery crosses the crux and this is "dominant." The term can be confusing because in most human hearts, the left coronary artery is of wider caliber and perfuses the largest proportion of myocardium. Thus, the dominant artery usually does not perfuse the largest percentage of myocardial mass. The dominant artery supplies the posterior diaphragmatic interventricular septum and diaphragmatic surface of the left ventricle.

Right Coronary Artery

The right coronary artery supplies the right atrium, right ventricle, and a portion of the posterior and inferior surfaces of the left ventricle. It supplies the AV node and bundle of His in 90% of hearts, and the sinus node in 55% of hearts.[30] It originates behind the right aortic cusp and passes behind the pulmonary artery, coursing in the right AV groove laterally to the right margin of the heart and then posteriorly. The major branches of the right coronary artery, in order of origin, are as follows:

1. Conus branch
2. Sinus node artery
3. Right ventricular branches
4. Right atrial branch
5. Acute marginal branch
6. AV nodal branch
7. Posterior descending branch
8. Left ventricular branch
9. Left atrial branch

The *conus branch* is small; in 60% of cases it exits within the first 2 cm of the right coronary artery. It sometimes originates as a separate vessel with an ostium within a millimeter of the right coronary artery.[31] The branch proceeds centrally to the left of the pulmonic valve. It supplies the upper part of the right ventricle, near the outflow tract at the level of the pulmonic valve. When the conus branch anastomoses with a right ventricular branch of the left anterior descending artery, the resulting structure is called the *circle of Vieussens,* an important collateral link between left and right coronary arteries.

The sinus node artery arises from the right coronary artery in 55% of cases.[31] It proceeds in the opposite direction from the conus branch, coursing cranially and to the right, encircling the superior vena cava. It usually has two branches: one supplies the sinus node and parts of the right atrium and the other branches to the left atrium.

The right coronary artery courses along the AV groove, giving rise next to one or more *right ventricular branches* that vary in length and distribute to the right ventricular wall. The *right atrial branch* proceeds cranially toward the right heart border and it perfuses the right atrium.

The *acute marginal branch* is a fairly large branch of the right coronary artery. It originates at the acute margin of the heart near the right atrial artery and courses in the opposite direction, toward the apex. It perfuses the inferior and diaphragmatic surfaces of the right ventricle and occasionally the posterior apical portion of the interventricular septum.

The *AV nodal branch* is slender and straight. It originates at the crux and is directed inward toward the center of the heart. It perfuses the AV node and the lower portion of the interatrial septum.

The *posterior descending branch* is an important branch of the right coronary artery. It supplies the posterosuperior portion of the interventricular septum. It exits at the crux and courses in the posterior interventricular sulcus.

The *left ventricular branch* originates just beyond the crux. It runs centrally in the angle formed by the left posterior AV groove and the posterior interventricular sulcus. It perfuses the diaphragmatic aspect of the left ventricle.

A *left atrial branch* may course in the posterior left AV groove, perfusing the left atrium.

Left Coronary Artery

The left main coronary artery arises from the aorta in the ostium behind the left cusp of the aortic valve. This artery passes between the left atrial appendage and the pulmonary artery. Typically, it then divides into two major branches: the *left anterior descending artery* and *left circumflex artery.*

Left Anterior Descending Artery. The left anterior descending artery supplies portions of the left and right ventricular myocardium and much of the interventricular septum. The left anterior descending artery appears to be a continuation of the left main coronary artery. It passes to the left of the pulmonic valve region, courses in the anterior interventricular sulcus to the apex, and then courses around the apex to terminate in the inferior portion of the posterior interventricular sulcus. Occasionally, the posterior descending branch of the right coronary artery extends around the apex from the posterior surface and the left anterior descending artery ends short of the apex. The major branches of the left anterior descending artery, in the order in which they branch, are the following:

1. First diagonal branch
2. First septal branch
3. Right ventricular branch
4. Minor septal branches
5. Second diagonal branch
6. Apical branches

The *first diagonal branch* is usually a large artery. It originates close to the bifurcation of the left main coronary artery and passes diagonally over the free wall of the left ventricle. It perfuses the high lateral portion of the left ventricular free wall. Several smaller diagonal branches may exit from the left side of the left anterior descending artery and run parallel to the first diagonal branch. The one referred to as the *second diagonal branch* takes its origin approximately two thirds of the way from the origin to the termination of the left anterior descending artery. This second diagonal branch perfuses the lower lateral portion of the free wall to the apex.

The number of septal branches varies. The *first septal branch* is the first to exit the left anterior descending artery. The others are referred to as *minor septal branches.* The septal branches exit at a 90-degree angle. They then course into the septum from front to the back and caudally. Together, the septal branches perfuse two thirds of the upper portion of the septum and most of the inferior portion of the septum. The remaining superoposterior section of the septum is supplied by branches from the posterior descending artery, which usually derives from the right coronary artery.

There can be one or more *right ventricular branches.* One branch runs toward the conus branch of the right coronary artery; it can anastomose into the circle of Vieussens.

The final branches are the *apical branches.* These branches perfuse the anterior and diaphragmatic aspects of the left ventricular free wall and apex.

Circumflex Artery. The *circumflex artery* supplies blood to parts of the left atrium and left ventricle. In 45% of cases, the circumflex artery supplies the major perfusion of the sinus node; in 10% of cases, it supplies the AV node.[31] The circumflex artery exits from the left main coronary artery at a near-right angle and courses posteriorly in the AV groove toward, but usually not reaching, the crux. If the circumflex reaches the crux, it gives rise to the posterior descending artery. In the 15% of cases in which this occurs, the left coronary artery supplies the entire septum and possibly the AV node.[31] The branches of the circumflex artery, in order of origin, are as follows:

1. Atrial circumflex branch
2. Sinus node artery
3. Obtuse marginal branches
4. Posterolateral branches

The *atrial circumflex branch* is usually small in caliber but sometimes is as wide as the remaining portion of the circumflex. It runs along the left AV groove, perfusing the left atrial wall.

In 45% of cases, the *sinus node artery* originates from the initial portion of the circumflex; it runs cranially and dorsally, to the base of the superior vena cava in the region of the sinus node.[31] This artery perfuses portions of the left and right atria as well as the sinus node.

There are between one and four *obtuse marginal branches.* These branches vary greatly in size. They run along the ventricular wall laterally and posteriorly, toward the apex, along the obtuse margin of the heart. The marginal branches supply the obtuse margin of the heart and the adjacent posterior wall of the left ventricle above the diaphragmatic surface.

The *posterolateral branches* arise from the circumflex artery in 80% of cases.[31] These branches originate in the terminal portion of the circumflex artery and course caudally and to the left on the posterior left ventricular wall, supplying the posterior and diaphragmatic wall of the left ventricle.

The *posterior descending* and AV nodal arteries occasionally arise from the circumflex. When they do, the entire septum is supplied by branches of the left coronary artery.

Coronary Capillaries

Blood passes from arteries into arterioles, then into capillaries, where exchange of oxygen, carbon dioxide, metabolic compounds, and waste materials takes place. The heart has a dense capillary network with approximately 3,300 capillaries per mm^2 or approximately 1 capillary per muscle fiber.[32] Blood flow through coronary capillaries is regulated according to myocardial metabolic needs.

When myocardial cells hypertrophy, the cell radius increases. The capillary network; however, does not appear to proliferate.[33] The same capillaries must perfuse a larger tissue mass. The diffusion distance is increased. Thus, with hypertrophy, the mass of tissue to be perfused is increased but the efficiency of exchange is diminished.

Coronary Veins

Most of the venous drainage of the heart is through epicardial veins. The large veins course close to the coronary arteries. Two veins sometimes accompany an artery.[30] The major veins feed into the great cardiac vein, which runs alongside the circumflex artery, becomes the coronary sinus, and then empties into the right atrium (Fig. 1-13). An incompetent (incompletely shut) semilunar valve, called the valve of Vieussens, marks the junction between the great cardiac vein and the coronary sinus. A similar structure, the Thebesian valve, is also incompetent and is found at the entry of the coronary sinus into the right atrium. Venous blood from the right ventricular muscle is drained primarily by two to four anterior cardiac veins that empty directly into the right atrium, bypassing the coronary sinus (Fig. 1-12).

The *Thebesian veins* empty directly into the ventricles (Fig. 1-14). These are more common on the right side of the heart, where the pressure gradient is favorable for such flow. Only a small amount of venous blood is returned directly to the left ventricle. When blood is returned to the left ventricle, this flow is a component of physiologic shunt, or unoxygenated blood entering the systemic circulation. Many collateral channels are found in the venous drainage system.

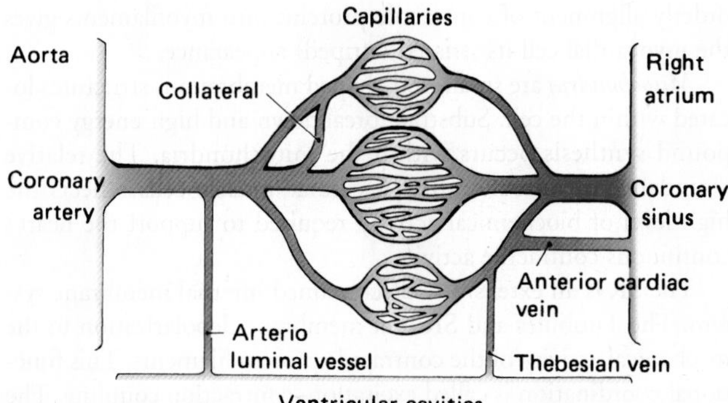

■ **Figure 1-14** Schematic model of coronary circulation. As in other circulatory beds, the coronary circulation includes arteries, capillaries, and veins. Some veins drain directly into the ventricles. Collateral channels may link arterial vessels. Art, arterial. (Adapted from Ruch, T. C., & Patton, H. D. [1974]. *Physiology and biophysics* [20th ed., Vol 2, p. 249]. Philadelphia: WB Saunders.)

Lymph Drainage

Cardiac contraction promotes lymphatic drainage in the myocardium through an abundant system of lymphatic vessels, most of which eventually converge into the principal left anterior lymphatic vessel. Lymph from this vessel empties into the pretracheal lymph node and then proceeds by way of two channels to the cardiac lymph node, the right lymphatic duct, and then into the superior vena cava.[34]

The importance of a normally functioning lymphatic system in maintaining an appropriate environment for cardiac cell function is frequently overlooked. Although complete cardiac lymph obstruction is rarely observed, experimental acute and chronic lymphatic impairment causes myocardial and endocardial cellular changes, particularly when occurring in conjunction with venous congestion.[34] Experimentally induced myocardial infarction in animals with chronically impaired lymphatic drainage causes more extensive cellular necrosis, an increased and prolonged inflammatory response, and a greater amount of fibrosis than infarction in animals without lymphatic obstruction.[34]

CARDIAC INNERVATION

Sensory nerve fibers from ventricular walls, the pericardium, coronary blood vessels, and other tissues transmit impulses by way of the cardiac nerves to the central nervous system. Motor nerve fibers to the heart are autonomic. Sympathetic stimulation accelerates firing of the sinus node, enhances conduction through the AV node, and increases the force of cardiac contraction. Parasympathetic stimulation slows the heart rate, slows conduction through the AV node, and may decrease ventricular contractile force.

Sympathetic preganglionic cardiac nerves arise from the first four or five thoracic spinal cord segments. The nerves synapse with long postganglionic fibers in the superior, middle, and cervicothoracic or stellate ganglia adjacent to the spinal cord. Most postganglionic sympathetic nerves to the heart travel through the superior, middle, and inferior cardiac nerves. However, several cardiac nerves with variable origins have been identified.[33,35]

Parasympathetic preganglionic cardiac nerves arise from the right and left vagus nerves and synapse with postganglionic nerves close to their target cardiac cells.

Both vagal and sympathetic cardiac nerves converge in the cardiac plexus. The cardiac plexus is situated superior to the bifurcation of the pulmonary artery, behind the aortic arch, and anterior to the trachea at the level of tracheal bifurcation. From the cardiac plexus, the cardiac nerves course in two coronary plexuses along with the right and left coronary blood vessels.

Sympathetic fibers are richly distributed throughout the heart. Right sympathetic ganglia fibers most commonly innervate the sinus node, the right atrium, the anterior ventricular walls, and to some extent the AV node. Most commonly, left sympathetic ganglia fibers extensively innervate the AV junctional area and the posterior and inferior left ventricle.[35]

A dense supply of vagal fibers innervates the sinus node, AV node, and ventricular conducting system. Consequently, many parasympathetic ganglia are found in the region of the sinus and AV nodes. Vagal fibers also innervate both atria and, to a lesser extent, both ventricles.[35] Right vagal fibers have more effect on the sinus node; left vagal fibers have more effect on the AV node and ventricular conduction system. However, there is overlap. The clinical importance of vagal stimulation for ventricular function continues to be debated. Although neurotransmitters from cardiac nerves are important modulators of cardiac activity, the success of cardiac transplantation illustrates the capacity of the heart to function without nervous innervation.

MYOCARDIAL CELL STRUCTURE

Myocardial cells are long, narrow, and often branched. A limiting membrane, the sarcolemma, surrounds each cell. Specialized surface membrane structures include the intercalated disc, nexus, and transverse tubules (T-tubules). Major intracellular components are contractile protein filaments (called myofibrils), mitochondria, sarcoplasmic recticulum (SR), and nucleus. There is a small amount of cytoplasm, called *sarcoplasm* (Fig. 1-15).

The cell membrane or *sarcolemma* separates the intracellular and extracellular spaces. The sarcolemma is a thin phospholipid bilayer studded with proteins. Across the barrier of the sarcolemma are marked differences in ionic composition and electrical charge. The embedded proteins serve multiple functions. Embedded receptors bind extracellular substances; this binding in turn activates or inhibits cell electrical, contractile, metabolic, or other functions. Embedded ion channels regulate membrane ion permeability and electrical function. Various carrier proteins facilitate uptake of metabolic substrates such as glucose. Some sarcolemma proteins add structural stability, anchoring the cell's internal and external structural elements.

Structurally, each myocardial cell is distinct. An *intercalated disc* forms a junction between adjacent cells. A specialized type of cell-to-cell connection, the *nexus* (sometimes called the *gap junction*), is present in the intercalated disc. The nexus is the site of direct exchange of small molecules. The nexus also provides a low-resistance electrical path between cells, thus facilitating rapid impulse conduction. Physiologic conditions alter the permeability of the nexus. For example, two substances that vary with physiological state are adenosine triphosphate (ATP)-dependent and cyclic adenosine monophosphate (cAMP)-dependent protein kinases. Both alter nexus permeability.[36,37] Because of these

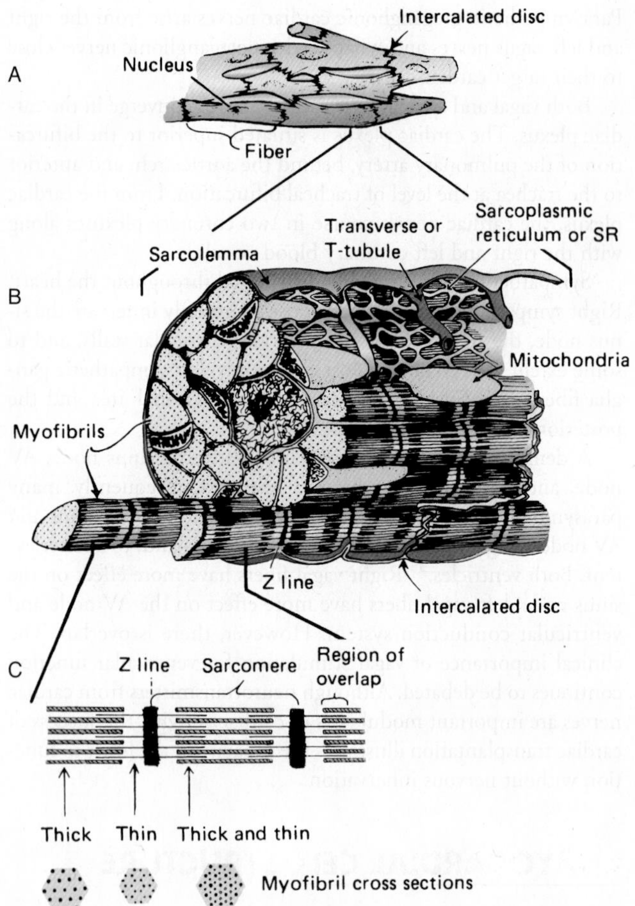

■ **Figure 1-15** The microscopic structure of working myocardial cells. (A) Working myocardial cells as seen under the light microscope. Note the branching network of fibers and intercalated discs. (B) Schematic illustration of the internal structure of the working myocardial cell. Note the striated appearance of the myofibrils, the intimate association of the sarcoplasmic reticulum (SR) with the myofibrils, the presence of T-tubules, and the large number of mitochondria. (C) Structure of the sarcomere, illustrating alignment of thick and thin filaments. Cross sections taken at three different positions along the sarcomere illustrate a region with only thick filaments, a region with only thin filaments, and a region of overlap where the thick and the thin filaments interdigitate. (Adapted from Braunwald, E., Ross, J., & Sonneblick, E. [1976]. *Mechanisms of contraction of the normal and failing heart* [2nd ed., p. 3]. Boston: Little, Brown.)

junctions, the heart functions as a syncytium of electrically coordinated cells, although anatomically the cells are discrete.

Another specialized membrane structure, the *T-tubule system,* is an extensive network of membrane-lined tubes systematically tunneling inward through each cell. T-tubules are formed by sarcolemma invaginations and are continuous with the surface membrane. The T-tubule lumen contains extracellular fluid. The T-tubular network carries electrical excitation to the central portions of myocardial cells, allowing near-simultaneous activation of deep and superficial parts of cells.

Myofibrils are long, rod-like structures that extend the length of the cell. They contain the contractile proteins, which convert the chemical energy of ATP into mechanical energy and heat. Muscle contraction involves generation of force, shortening, or both. The orderly alignment of contractile proteins into myofilaments gives the myocardial cell its striated (striped) appearance.

Mitochondria are small, rod-shaped membranous structures located within the cell. Substrate breakdown and high-energy compound synthesis occurs within the mitochondria. The relative abundance of mitochondria in cardiac muscle cells reflects the high level of biochemical activity required to support the heart's continuous contractile activity.

The SR is an extensive, self-contained internal membrane system. The T-tubules and SR link membrane depolarization to the mechanical activity of the contractile protein filaments. This functional coordination is called excitation–contraction coupling. The SR is the major storage depot for calcium ion, which releases then takes up calcium ions with each contraction of the heart.

The *nucleus* contains the genetic material of the cell. The nucleus is the site where new proteins are synthesized.

MYOCARDIAL CELL ELECTRICAL CHARACTERISTICS

There is an electrical potential difference across the sarcolemma; it is measured in millivolts (mV). During the interim between excitations, the intracellular space is negative compared with the extracellular space. This potential difference is called the *membrane resting potential.* During excitation, the potential difference changes: the inside of the cell becomes less negative or slightly positive compared with the extracellular space. This type of potential difference change is called *depolarization.* After depolarization, the cell membrane *repolarizes,* or returns to the resting potential value. The normal depolarization–repolarization cycle is known as the *action potential.* The action potential is the signal evoking contraction. Until the cell repolarizes sufficiently, there can be no action potential. If the potential difference becomes more negative than the usual resting potential, the membrane is said to be *hyperpolarized.* The more hyperpolarized the membrane, the more current is required to evoke an action potential.

Some myocardial cells have *automaticity,* that is, an intrinsic ability to depolarize spontaneously and initiate an action potential. The action potential generated in such a cell is then propagated throughout cardiac tissue. Depolarization of one cardiac cell initiates depolarization of adjacent cells and evokes contraction.

There are approximately 19 billion cells in the adult heart; these cells must depolarize in an orderly sequence if the heart is to undergo a coordinated contraction that is able to add force to moving blood. Impulses generated in ectopic sites in the heart are less likely to depolarize in an orderly sequence and less likely to contract in an orderly fashion that effectively pumps blood.

Basis for Myocardial Excitation: Characteristics of Biologic Membranes

Intracellular and extracellular spaces are separated by a thin insulating membrane, the sarcolemma. These spaces have very different ionic compositions. The intracellular space contains high concentrations of potassium ion (positively charged) and protein (negatively charged) and has low concentration of sodium ion (positively charged). The extracellular space consists of high concentrations of sodium ion and chloride ion (negatively charged); extracellular potassium ion concentration is low.

Table 1-2 ■ APPROXIMATE INTRACELLULAR AND EXTRACELLULAR ION CONCENTRATIONS AND ACTIVITIES IN CARDIAC MUSCLE*

Ion†	Extracellular Concentration‡	Intracellular Concentration§11	Ratio of Extracellular to Intracellular Concentration	E_1	Intracellular Activity#
Na^+	145 mM	15 mM	9.7	+60 mV	7.0 mM
K^+	4 mM	150 mM	0.027	−94 mV	125 mM
Cl^-	120 mM	5 mM	24	−83 mV	15 mM
Ca^{2+}	2 mM	10^{-4} M	2×10^4	+129 mV	8×10^{-6} mM

*Values given are approximations and vary according to the cardiac tissue, species, and method used for measurement.
†Na^+, sodium; K^+, potassium; Cl^-, chloride; Ca^{2+}, calcium.
‡mM, millimolar.
§11Most of the intracellular calcium is bound to proteins or sequestered in intracellular organelles; thus, total intracellular calcium content approximates 1 to 2 mm. During contraction, measurable intracellular calcium concentration approximates 10^{-5} mm.
¶E_1, equilibrium potential; mV, millivolt.
#Median values from summarized data; these values should be considered as subject to revision. Concentrations and equilibrium potentials from Sperelakis, N. (1979). Origin of the cardiac resting potential. In R. M. Berne (Ed.), *Handbook of physiology, section 2: The cardiovascular system, vol 1, the heart* (p. 193). Bethesda: American Physiological Society. Activities are approximations from Lee, C. O. (1981). Ionic activities in cardiac muscle cells and application of ion-sensitive microelectrodes, *American Journal of Physiology, 10,* H461, H464 and Fozzard, H. A., & Wasserstrom, J. A. (1985). Voltage dependence of intracellular sodium and control of contraction. In P. P. Zipes, & J. Jalife. *Cardiac electrophysiology and arrhythmias* (p. 52.). Orlando: Grune & Tratton.

For each ion, concentration differences across the sarcolemma are determined by the sarcolemma's permeability to that ion and the balance of forces moving the ion from one to the other side of the membrane. Electrical and concentration differences are maintained by a number of active and passive processes. Typical concentration differences are outlined in Table 1-2.

The sarcolemma is composed of phospholipid molecules. Each molecule consists of a charged hydrophilic (water-attracting) globular head and a noncharged hydrophobic (water-repelling) tail. The molecules organize into thin sheets, with the heads oriented in a consistent direction. Two sheets are aligned tail-to-tail to form a double layer (bilayer). The tails form the core of the sheet, and the heads are directed outward in both directions. The result is a 7- to 9-nm, high-resistance, insulated barrier to ionic movement.

Proteins embedded within the phospholipid bilayer may compose more than half the mass of the membrane. Proteins function as receptors, channels, pumps, or structural stabilizers. The proteins may be inserted into the intracellular or extracellular side of the bilayer or span its full thickness. Some of the proteins contain a water-filled pore that spans the membrane, connecting the intracellular and extracellular spaces and forming a channel through which ions can pass. Membrane channels open and close in response to a stimulus (electrical, mechanical, or chemical), allowing passage of specific ions when open. The opening and closing properties of a channel are called its *gating* characteristics. The ability of a channel to selectively allow passage of certain ions while restricting other ions is called its *selectivity* property. Many ion channels are named after the ion for which they have selectivity. Some common types are sodium channels, potassium channels, and calcium channels (Fig. 1-16).

Mechanisms of Ion Distribution across the Myocardial Membrane

Ions are distributed across the sarcolemma according to the membrane permeability to the ion and the electrical and diffusion forces on the ion. For each ion that can penetrate the membrane,

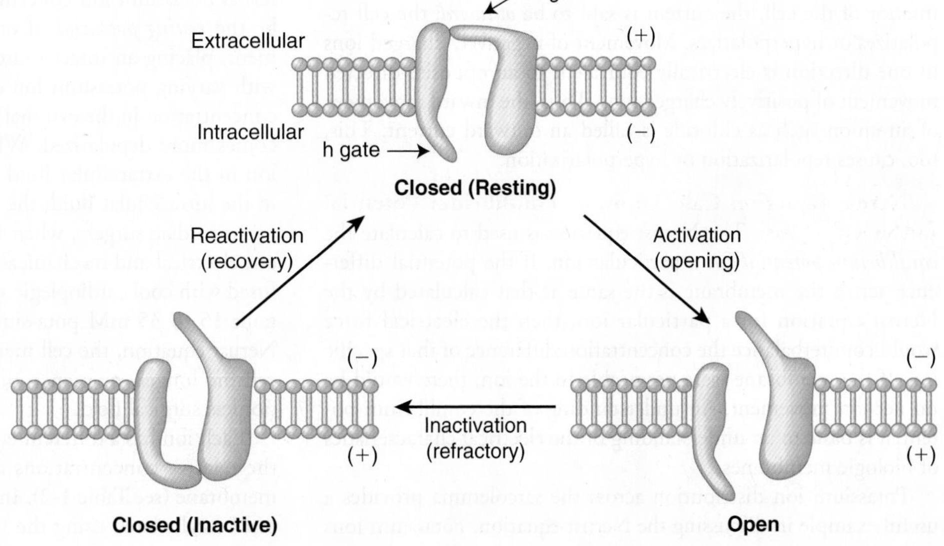

■ **Figure 1-16** Three states of a voltage-gated ion channel. Depicted are the two closed and one open state. Transition between these states (*arrows*) open the channel (*activation*), close the channel in a refractory state where it cannot be reopened (*inactivation*), and reactivate the channel by ending this refractory state (*recovery*). (From Katz, A. [2006]. *Physiology of the heart* [4th ed., p. 376]. Philadelphia: Lippincott Williams & Wilkins.)

there is a continual movement toward equilibrium. When equilibrium is reached, forces driving ion movement are balanced, and there is no additional net change in the ion distribution. The Nernst equation, discussed later, is useful in understanding the relationship between electrical and diffusional forces driving ion movement. It is useful to remember that the permeability properties of the living membrane change continually.

Diffusional Force

Particles in solution move, or diffuse, from an area of higher concentration to an area of lower concentration. In the case of uncharged, soluble molecules, diffusion proceeds until there is a uniform distribution of the molecules within the solution. The solution is then said to be in equilibrium. At equilibrium, there is still particle movement within the solution, but no net change in overall particle distribution. Charged particles also diffuse. The diffusion of charged particles is influenced not only by the concentration gradient but also by the electrical field.

Electrical Force and Current

Like charges repel, and opposite charges attract. Positively charged particles flow toward negatively charged particles and regions; similarly, negatively charged particles are attracted to positive ions and regions. The electrical (or electromotive) force difference between regions is called the *potential difference* and is expressed in volts (1 mV = 0.001 V). The net flow of charges is called *current* (measured in amperes). *Resistance* is the opposition to the flow of current, measured in ohms. Ohm's law (electromotive force = current × resistance) describes the relation among current, voltage, and resistance.

When charged particles have different concentrations in the solutions separated by a cell membrane, and some of the particles are able to permeate the membrane and others are not, an electrical force is established. This force influences the distribution of all other charged particles. The potential difference across biologic membranes is described by comparing the interior of the cell with the external solution. In the typical quiescent or resting myocardial cell, the potential difference is –70 to –90 mV; that is, the cell interior is negative with respect to the exterior. When positively charged ions move from the extracellular fluid to the intracellular fluid, the current is said to be *inward.* With inward current, the cell interior becomes less negative, that is, it depolarizes. When positively charged ions flow into the extracellular space from the interior of the cell, the current is said to be *outward*; the cell repolarizes or hyperpolarizes. Movement of negatively charged ions in one direction is electrically equivalent to an opposite-directed movement of positively charged ions. Thus, the inward movement of an anion such as chloride is called an outward current. This, too, causes repolarization or hyperpolarization.

Nernst Equation Calculation of Equilibrium Potential for Specific Ions. The Nernst equation is used to calculate the *equilibrium potential* for a particular ion. If the potential difference across the membrane is the same as that calculated by the Nernst equation for a particular ion, then the electrical force would counterbalance the concentration difference of that specific ion. If the membrane were permeable to the ion, there would be no net ion movement. An understanding of the equilibrium potential is basic to an understanding of the electrical characteristics of biologic membranes.

Potassium ion distribution across the sarcolemma provides a useful example in discussing the Nernst equation. Potassium ions (positively charged) are more concentrated in the sarcoplasm than in the extracellular space. To balance the force of the concentration difference, the inside of the myocardial cell would need to be approximately −94 mV compared with outside of the membrane. That charge, −94 mV, is known as the potassium ion equilibrium potential or the Nernst potential for potassium ion. The resting myocardial membrane is permeable to potassium ions. The large concentration gradient is maintained because the actual voltage across the membrane between activation cycles, approximately –90 mV (inside negative), is close to the Nernst potential for potassium ions in the myocardial cell, and thus nearly sufficient to retain potassium ions within the cell. The slow outward trickle of potassium ions is corrected by a membrane pump that moves potassium ions back into the cell (and moves sodium ions out of the cell). If the resting potential were –94 mV, there would be no net potassium ion movement.

The following illustrates the Nernst equation calculation of the equilibrium potential for potassium ion:

$$E_K = \frac{RT}{FZ_K} \mathrm{Ln} \frac{[K^+]_o}{[K^+]_i}$$

where E_K = equilibrium potential for K^+
R = gas constant
T = absolute temperature
F = the Faraday (number of coulombs per mole of charge)
Z_K = the valence of K^+ (+1)
$[K^+]_o$ = K^+ concentration outside the cell (e.g., 4 mM)
$[K^+]_i$ = K^+ concentration inside the cell (e.g., 155 mM)

Converting from the natural log to the base 10 log and replacing the constants measured at 37°C with numeric values, the equation becomes approximately as follows:

$$E_K = 61 \log_{10} \frac{[K^+]_o}{[K^+]_i}$$

$$E_K = 61 \log_{10} \frac{4}{155} = -97 \text{ mV}$$

According to the Nernst equation, the higher the potassium ion concentration in the external solution, the more depolarized is the *potassium equilibrium potential.* If the resting membrane were highly permeable to potassium ion, then the higher the external potassium ion concentration, the more depolarized would be the *resting potential.* If one were to perform such an experiment, placing an intact muscle cell in a dish bathed in solutions with varying potassium ion concentrations as the potassium ion concentration in the external solution is raised, the membrane becomes more depolarized. When the concentration of potassium ion in the extracellular fluid becomes equal to the concentration in the intracellular fluid, the membrane potential is 0 mV.

In cardiac surgery, when it is important to have a heart without electrical and mechanical activity, the organ is sometimes perfused with cool cardioplegic solution. The perfusate typically contains 15 to 35 mM potassium. As would be predicted from the Nernst equation, the cell membranes depolarize. The depolarized cells no longer experience an action potential, resulting in a motionless surgical field.

Each ion has a different equilibrium potential that depends on the relative concentrations of that ion on the two sides of the membrane (see Table 1-2). In each case, the equilibrium potential can be calculated using the Nernst equation. For example, given typical sodium ion concentrations as in Table 1-2, the equilibrium potential for sodium ion is approximately +60 mV. This means that if the membrane were permeable to sodium ion, then the membrane potential would have to be +60 mV to halt net inward sodium current. At typical resting potentials of −90 mV, a large electromotive force favors inward sodium current. The sodium concentration is markedly higher in the extracellular space than it is in the intracellular space. Thus, diffusion forces also favor inward sodium current. At rest, however, there is minimal net movement of sodium ion because the sodium channels are closed. When the channels open during activation, the diffusional and electrical forces combine to produce a large, but transient, inward current carried by sodium ion. The result is rapid depolarization.

The chloride ion concentration is higher in the extracellular space than in the intracellular space. Thus, diffusional force favors inward movement of chloride ion. However, the resting membrane potential is at approximately the chloride ion equilibrium potential. Thus, the negative potential opposes the net inward movement of chloride ion. The resting muscle membrane is permeant to chloride ion, but there is scant net chloride ion movement.

The sarcoplasmic calcium ion concentration is extremely low. Calcium ions are actively removed from the sarcoplasm. Calcium ions are taken up into the SR and pumped outward to the extracellular space. The extracellular calcium ion concentration is in the millimolar range, approximately 10,000 times higher than the intracellular concentration. Thus, a powerful concentration gradient would move calcium ions inward if a path were available. A powerful electrical force also favors inward movement. The calcium ion equilibrium potential calculated from the Nernst equation is more positive than +100 mV. However, the resting membrane is not permeant to calcium ion. As with the sodium ion, the opening of a calcium ion channel evokes a large inward current. This inward current happens during activation. An increase in intracellular calcium ion signals metabolic and contractile changes.

Calculating Membrane Resting Potential. At high extracellular potassium ion concentrations, the Nernst equation for potassium ion predicts resting membrane potential with good accuracy. In and below the physiological range of external potassium ion concentrations, the membrane potential is slightly less negative than would be predicted based on potassium ion concentrations. This state occurs because at very low external potassium ion concentrations, the membrane is slightly permeable to sodium ion. Because concentration and electrical gradients for sodium ion both favor inward sodium ion movement, an increase in sodium ion permeability allows an inward trickling of sodium ions (an inward current). The membrane depolarizes, becoming several millivolts more positive than the potassium ion equilibrium potential. The ratio of potassium and sodium permeabilities determines the extent to which the resting membrane potential deviates from the potassium ion equilibrium potential. Equations have been developed to predict resting membrane potential based on the relative permeabilities and concentrations of various ions. These computations assume that the membrane is in a steady state and that there are no active ion pumps producing current.

Typically, cardiac muscle cell resting membrane potential is approximately −90 mV. Excitation and propagation of excitation depend on the resting membrane potential. The more negative the resting membrane potential, the more current is required to initiate excitation, but the speed and amplitude of the subsequent depolarizing excitation are greater. The less negative is the resting membrane potential, the less is the current required to initiate excitation but the speed and amplitude of depolarization are reduced. If the resting potential is substantially depolarized, the cell can be impossible to activate.

The resting membrane potential is altered by changes in the ionic milieu on either side of the membrane and by hormones or drugs that alter the relative permeabilities of potassium or sodium ion. Factors that alter the action of the sodium–potassium pump alter the resting membrane potential. These include insulin and epinephrine (hyperpolarizing influences) and digoxin-like drugs (depolarizing influence).

Ionic Activity. Although electrochemical gradients are most frequently explained in terms of chemical concentration gradients, it is actually each ion's chemical activity that affects most cellular functions. Ionic activity reflects interactions between ions as well as the ion concentration. An ion's activity is equal to its concentration times its activity coefficient. It is possible to make reasonably accurate measurements of ionic activities within cells. However, most descriptions of ion movements are based on ion concentration.

Ion Movement Across the Myocardial Cell Membrane

Passive Ion Movement. Ions traverse the sarcolemma passively through membrane-bound, water-filled pores called *channels*. When a channel is open, any ions that are able to pass through the channel move according to the concentration and electrical gradient, as constrained by the channel dimensions. When the channel is closed, ions do not penetrate. The opening and closing properties of an ion channel are referred to as its *gating* characteristics. The signal to open may be a change in the electrical field (voltage-gated channel) or a change in the chemical milieu (receptor-gated channel). Changes in the internal or external milieu may modify channel gating. Also, there can be time-dependent effects. For example, a small depolarization opens the sodium channel; it closes after a few milliseconds.

An important channel characteristic is its ability to allow passage of some ions while excluding others. This is called *selective permeability*. A theoretical model of an ionic channel is given in Figure 1-16.

The sodium channel is common in excitable cells and has been well characterized. In Nobel prize–winning work, Hodgkin and Huxley[38] described the sodium current of the squid giant axon. According to them, at rest, the membrane potential is negative, perhaps −90 mV, extracellular sodium ion concentration is high, and intracellular concentration low. Electrical and diffusion gradients favor inward sodium ion movement. Because the sodium channel is closed, there is no path for the ions to travel. With a small depolarization the sodium channel opens. This opening of the sodium channel in response to a small depolarizing current is sometimes described as opening the *activation (or m) gate*. When the activation gate opens, the sodium channel is then open; an inward depolarizing of sodium ion flows. Because both the electrical and concentration gradients are significant and favor inward movement, this inward current is intense. After a few milliseconds, however, another gate (sometimes called the *inactivation* or *h gate*) closes, halting the current. The h gate remains closed until the membrane is restored to a sufficiently negative voltage. At that time, the inactivation gate opens but no current flows because the activation gate has closed. With the closing of either gate, current is halted. To summarize, the sodium channel is conceptualized as having two gates. At resting membrane potential, the channel is closed because the activation gate is closed. Depolarization opens that gate but, after a brief lag, the inactivation gate closes, again closing the channel. Repolarization opens the inactivation gate but closes the activation gate.

Scores of channels have been described, each with characteristic gating and selectivity profiles. The mixing of channel types in various membranes can produce a rich repertoire of biologic operating characteristics. The membrane of vertebrate cardiac muscle is especially complex, with a diverse mix of channels. The result is a dynamic, responsive membrane that can be finely tuned to varying operating conditions. Some of the other major channels of the vertebrate heart are described later in this chapter.

Active Ion Transport. Any movement of ion against its electrochemical gradient is said to be *active movement* or *active transport.* To move any ion against its electrochemical gradient requires energy. The energy may be stored in ATP. In some cases, the energy stored in one ion's electrochemical gradient can be expended to power the movement of another ion against its electrochemical gradient. The former ion is said to be moving "downhill" or in the direction of a lower energy state. The ion that is moved against the gradient is said to be transported "uphill."

Sodium–Potassium–Adenosine Triphosphatase Pump. At resting potential, there is a slight inward trickle of sodium ions. During activation, there is transient inward sodium current. Sodium–potassium pumps on the cardiac muscle membrane (as well as on many other types of membranes) moves sodium ion back out of the cell in exchange for an inward movement of potassium ions. Both ions are moving against a concentration gradient. The pump is powered by the energy stored in ATP; hence, the pump is known as the *sodium–potassium pump* or *sodium—potassium–ATPase.* This pump helps to re-establish the resting concentrations of intracellular sodium and potassium after cardiac depolarization. The ratio of sodium ions pumped out to potassium ions pumped in is usually 3:2. This ratio of 3:2 results in a net outward charge movement, hyperpolarizing the membrane. A primary regulator of this pump is the intracellular sodium ion concentration. Other factors influencing pump activity include extracellular sodium concentration and intracellular and extracellular potassium concentration. Digoxin-like drugs block the sodium–potassium pump.[39] Epinephrine and insulin both stimulate the sodium–potassium pump, causing uptake of potassium into cells. Clinicians capitalize on this feature when they administer insulin and glucose to the hyperkalemic patient. Epinephrine and insulin can be associated with hypokalemia.

Sodium–Calcium Exchange. Another important cardiac membrane pump is the sodium–calcium pump. Calcium ion moves across the sarcolemma into the cell to activate contraction. It must be removed. Although there is some harvesting of calcium ion into the intracellular sequestering sites such as SR, the inward movement and storage cannot go on unopposed. Calcium ion is moved back into the extracellular space by means of an exchange pump. The energy stored in the sodium gradient powers the movement of calcium ion. In other words, sodium ion is moved downhill to pump calcium ion uphill.[40] Usually, this exchange mechanism transports three sodium ions into the cell for one calcium ion transported out of the cell. In this situation, the pump is electrogenic, but the direction or ratios of transmembrane ion exchanges may be reversed or changed. When the concentration of intracellular sodium ion is increased (e.g., when the use of digoxin-like drugs has partially blocked the sodium–potassium–ATPase pump), there is less energy stored in the sodium gradient. This exchange mechanism does not promote as great a sodium influx and calcium efflux. There is then more calcium ion stored in the SR and more calcium ion released during activation, with net positive inotropic effects.

Calcium ATPase Pumps. The cardiac SR actively pumps calcium ion uphill into its core in a process that hydrolyzes ATP as an energy source. An active calcium pump in the cardiac sarcolemma also extrudes calcium ion from the cell. The latter may be more important in vascular tissue than in cardiac muscle.

CARDIAC ACTION POTENTIAL

Each structural cardiac cell type (e.g., working myocardial, nodal, Purkinje cells) has characteristic action potential features. Electrically, there are two general types of cardiac cells: *fast-* and *slow-response* cells. Fast-response cells (e.g., Purkinje and working myocardial cells) have a fairly constant resting membrane potential, a rapid depolarization, and then a period of sustained depolarization (called *plateau phase*) before repolarizing to resting potential. Impulse conduction to adjacent cells is rapid. Slow-response cells (e.g., sinus and AV nodal cells) slowly and spontaneously depolarize during the interim prior to the action potential, and have a shorter, nonprominent plateau phase that merges into a slow repolarization period. These cells conduct more slowly (Fig. 1-17). Ionic current differences account for varying action potential shape.

In the following sections, the cardiac action potential is described. Table 1-3 summarizes the electrophysiological properties of the various tissue types.

Fast-Type Myocardial Action Potentials

The fast response type cell has a five-phase action potential (Fig. 1-18). Phase 0 is the initial period of rapid depolarization, the action potential upstroke. Membrane potential changes from resting potential (approximately −90 mV) to a value positive to 0 mV (e.g., +30 mV). After this brief (<1 to 2 milliseconds) phase, the cell repolarizes slightly (phase 1) and then there is a period of sustained depolarization called the *plateau phase* (phase 2). In phase 3, repolarization becomes rapid, returning the membrane to resting potential. Phase 4 is the interval between action potentials; the resting potential is fairly constant. The cardiac action potential may take hundreds of milliseconds. Duration and amplitude of each phase depends on the opening and closing of various ion channels, which in turn depends on the ionic and neurohormonal milieu. Conduction to adjacent cells is rapid.

Phase 0: Action Potential Upstroke

The working myocardial cell action potential is initiated by an inward current flowing primarily by way of the low-resistance nexus. This small current depolarizes the cell to threshold (approximately −70 mV; Fig. 1-19). Once threshold voltage is reached, the

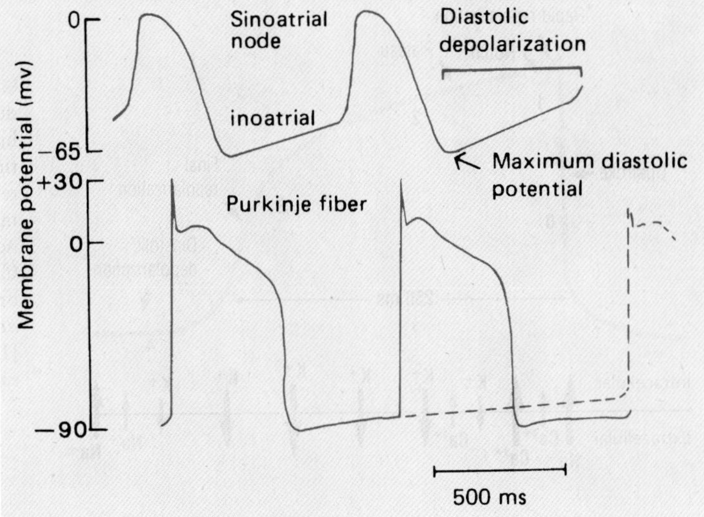

■ **Figure 1-17** Action potentials of sinus node cells and Purkinje cells. Purkinje cells are not discharged by impulses from the sinus node or elsewhere, the Purkinje diastolic depolarization progresses enough to attain threshold. (Adapted from Vassale, M. [1976]. *Cardiac physiology for the clinician* [p. 35]. New York: Academic Press.)

sodium channel activation gate opens; thus, opening the sodium channel followed by a large inward current carried by sodium ions. The depolarizing current opens more sodium channels, producing the propagating, regenerating, swift depolarization of the action potential upstroke. Peak voltages attained are +30 to +40 mV, approaching but not attaining the sodium equilibrium potential (approximately +65 mV). Depolarization closes the inactivation gate. The channel closes, halting the current and stopping depolarization.

The maximal velocity of phase 0 depolarization is sometimes called V_{max} (to be distinguished from the contractile variable, maximal shortening velocity, also called V_{max}). The speed of impulse conduction through the myocardium depends on V_{max} for the individual cells. V_{max} reflects sodium channel activity. Factors that alter the resting potential or the sodium gradient alter V_{max}. Such factors include ionic milieu and certain drugs, including many antiarrhythmic drugs. Class I antiarrhythmic agents (lidocaine, quinidine, procainamide, etc.) block the fast sodium channel, slowing the rate of phase 0 depolarization.

Generally, the more negative is the resting membrane potential, the faster is V_{max}, and the greater is the amplitude of depolarization. Hyperpolarization opens the inactivation gate. When depolarization opens the activation gate, the sodium channel is open, and the current is intense. Conversely, if the membrane potential preceding threshold depolarization is less negative, inactivation may be incompletely removed; V_{max} is slower. Hyperkalemia causes such depolarization; this condition is associated with arrhythmias.

Table 1-3 ■ CARDIAC ACTION POTENTIAL PROPERTIES*

	Fast-Conducting Tissue			Slow-Conducting Tissue	
	Purkinje	Atrial Muscle	Ventricular Muscle	Sinus Node	Atrioventricular Node
Resting potential	−90 to −95 mV	−80 to −90 mV	−80 to −90 mV	−50 to −60 mV	−60 to −70 mV
Activation threshold	−70 to −60 mV			−40 to −30 mV	
Action potential					
Rate of phase 0 (V_{max})	500 to 800 V/s	100 to 200 V/s	100 to 200 V/s	1 to 10 V/s	5 to 15 V/s
Amplitude	120 mV	110 to 120 mV	110 to 120 mV	60 to 70 mV	70 to 80 mV
Overshoot	30 mV	30 mV	30 mV	0 to 10 mV	5 to 15 mV
Duration	300 to 500 ms	100 to 300 ms	200 to 300 ms	100 to 300 ms	100 to 300 ms
Diastolic depolarization		Not prominent		Prominent	
(major ion) Depolarizing current		Na^+		Ca^{2+}	
Channel blocked by	Tetrodotoxin, type I antiarrhythmics, or sustained depolarization at −40 mV			Mn^{2+}, La^{3+}, verapamil, nifedipine, other inorganic substances, type IV antiarrhythmics	
Effect of adrenergic stimulation	Not pronounced			Pronounced	

*Values are approximations and vary with methods and specific tissue used.

Adapted from Bigger, J. T. (1984). Electrophysiology for the clinician. *European Heart Journal, 5*(Suppl. B), 1–9; Opie, L. (1984). *The heart* (p. 44). Orlando: Grune & Stratton; Sperelakis, N. (1979). Origin of the cardiac resting potential. In R. E. Berne (Ed.), *Handbook of physiology, section 2: The cardiovascular system, vol 1, the heart* (p. 190). Bethesda, MD: American Physiological Society; Zipes, D. P. (1984). Genesis of cardiac arrhythmias. In E. Braunwald (Ed.), *Heart disease* (2nd ed., p. 615). Philadelphia: WB Saunders.

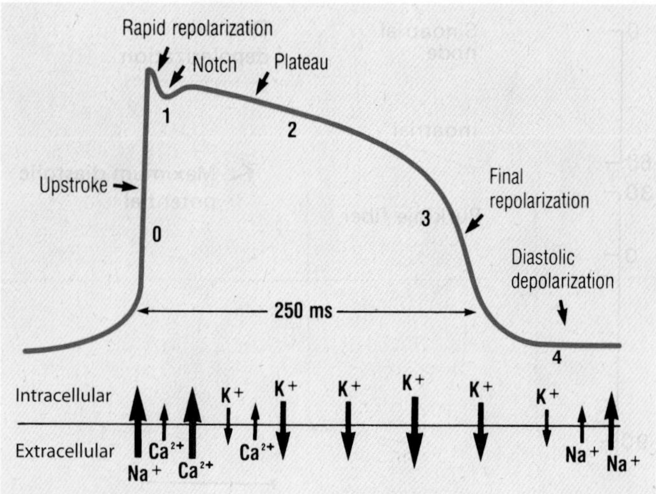

■ **Figure 1-18** Schematic illustration of major ionic movements during a Purkinje cell action potential, with the cell depicted as exhibiting spontaneous depolarization. Arrows indicate approximate times when the indicated ion movement influences membrane potential. Pumps, exchanges, and leaks are not illustrated. Under normal physiologic conditions, Purkinje cells do not exhibit spontaneous depolarization. (Adapted from Ten Eick, R. E., Baumgarten, C. M., & Sunger, D. H. [1981]. Ventricular dysrhythmia: Membrane basis of currents, channels, gates and cables. *Progress in Cardiovascular Disease, 24*, 159; Fozzard, H. A. & Gibbons, W. R. [1973]. Action potential and contraction of heart muscle. *American Journal of Cardiology, 31*, 183.)

Phase 1: Early Repolarization

The rapid upstroke ceases when sodium channels close spontaneously after a few milliseconds (caused by inactivation). Another transient current is activated, the transient outward current. This outward current is carried primarily by potassium ion (moving outward) but also by chloride ion (moving inward) and results in the slight repolarization of the cell to approximately +10 mV. When the voltage is positive, both the concentration gradient and the electrical force (inside positive) favor outflow of the positively charged potassium ion from the cell, an outward current. Similarly, with chloride ion, when the membrane potential is positive, the electrical gradient amplifies the concentration gradient, both favoring inward movement of the negatively charged chloride ion. Inward movement of negative ions is electrically indistinguishable from an outward movement of positive ions; both are called *outward currents.*

Phase 1 ends with the closure of the current-bearing channels. A "notch" appears on the action potential profile. The voltage of the notch region has important effects on subsequent gating of other channels and can affect the shape of the remainder of the action potential.

Phase 2: Action Potential Plateau

During the plateau, little net current flows. Inward (depolarizing) and outward (repolarizing) currents are nearly balanced; there is little change in membrane voltage. Inward currents are carried by sodium and calcium ions. Calcium ion in turn evokes additional calcium ion release from internal stores; contraction ensues. Outward currents are carried by potassium ion. Over time, calcium channels inactivate, repolarizing outward potassium currents predominate and the membrane repolarizes. This phase ends when the calcium channels close.

During the plateau, sodium currents travel through fast sodium channels that failed to inactivate and through at least two types of calcium channels. Both types of calcium channels open with depolarization, and then close spontaneously after a period of time. β-Adrenergic agonists potentiate calcium currents, increasing plateau amplitude and duration. Ultimately, the result is increased sarcoplasmic calcium ion concentration, which in turn has a positive inotropic effect on contraction. Calcium channel blockers, acidosis, and ATP depletion are negative inotropes, diminishing calcium currents, reducing plateau amplitude and duration, and diminishing the force generated during contraction.

The counterbalancing outward current is carried by potassium ion through multiple channel types. One type of potassium channel that is important in disease is the ATP-sensitive potassium current. This potassium channel is activated or opened when the ATP concentration falls, such as during ischemia, which in turn greatly shortens the duration of the plateau and hastens the onset of the rapid repolarization phase. Shortened depolarization decreases the calcium current and thus the contractile force (a negative inotropic influence).

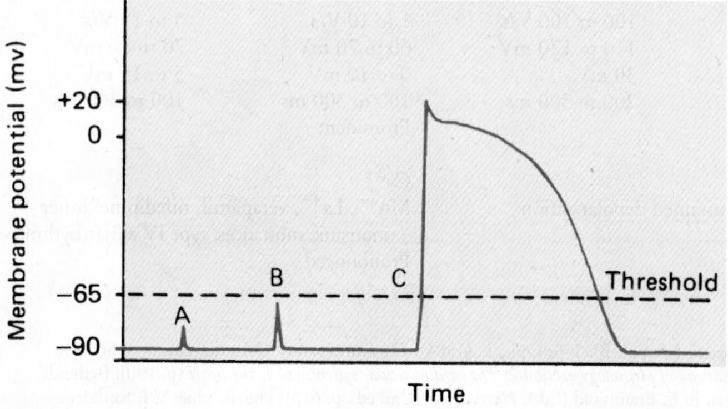

■ **Figure 1-19** Schematic illustration of the initiation of an action potential when the membrane potential is depolarized to threshold. Small depolarizing stimuli (*A* and *B*) that fail to reach threshold (dashed line) are unable to initiate an action potential. When depolarization reaches threshold *(C)*, a regenerative action potential is produced. Once the latter begins, further depolarization becomes independent of the initial stimulus. (From Katz, A. [2006]. *Physiology of the heart* [4th ed., p. 395]. Philadelphia: Lippincott Williams & Wilkins.)

The plateau phase distinguishes working myocardial cells from skeletal muscle cells and neuronal tissue. The plateau provides for greater inward calcium currents in cardiac muscle. Because the cell is refractory to stimulation for the duration of phase 2 and much of phase 3, cardiac muscle cannot experience tetany.

Phase 3: Late Rapid Repolarization

The calcium currents that sustained the plateau eventually stop when the calcium channels close and repolarization proceeds unopposed, caused by outward potassium ion movement. As membrane voltage becomes increasingly negative, sodium channel inactivation is removed. The sodium channel can once again be activated (as soon as a small depolarization opens the activation gate).

Phase 4: Interim Between Action Potentials

During rapid repolarization (phase 3), the membrane potential is restored to the resting potential. Phase 4 is the period between the end of rapid repolarization and the start of the next action potential. During phase 4, the membrane is permeable to potassium ion. The membrane voltage is close to the potassium equilibrium potential. The type of potassium channel open during this phase is called the *inward rectifier* (so called because it allows inward current more readily than outward current). Because the membrane potential is slightly more positive than the potassium equilibrium potential, potassium trickles outward.

Slow-Type Myocardial Action Potentials

Slow-response cells, such as cells of the sinus and AV nodes, spontaneously depolarize between action potentials. The action potential upstroke of depolarization is slower; the plateau phase is shorter and nonprominent; repolarization is slower; the maximum repolarization potential achieved is less negative than that in fast-response cells.

Phase 0 depolarization is slower in the slow-response cells; it is primarily carried by calcium ion rather than sodium ion. The transition between the depolarization rate before and after reaching threshold is less abrupt in the in slow-response cells. Phase 1 is absent: there is no large transient outward potassium current and no notch in the action potential. Phase 2 is present, but abbreviated. Slow repolarization begins after the maximal positive voltage. As in other cells, potassium efflux evokes repolarization in slow myocytes. Phase 3 repolarization is similar to that in fast myocytes, although the rate of repolarization is slower and the maximal diastolic potential attained is less negative than in fast-response cells. During phase 4, the slow-response cells continually depolarize toward threshold. Maximal negative voltage at the start of phase 4 is approximately –60 mV, termed the *maximal diastolic potential* (see Fig. 1-17). Phase 4 spontaneous depolarization is caused by the following sequence of currents: a nonselective channel opens, allowing inward sodium current; outward potassium current declines after some depolarization; transient (T)-type calcium channels open, allowing inward calcium current; long-lasting (L)-type calcium channels open, again allowing inward calcium current and evoking the action potential upstroke, phase 0.

Ionic currents flowing in slow-type myocytes are modulated by autonomic innervation. Adrenergic stimulation increases the repolarizing potassium current, causing the cell to repolarize to a more negative potential, and the action potential to proceed more swiftly. Acetylcholine, the parasympathetic mediator, slows the phase 4 depolarizing currents.

Action Potential of the Sinus Node Cells

Cells in the sinus node spontaneously depolarize to threshold more rapidly than do other automatic cardiac cells. Thus, the slope of phase 4 is steeper in sinus node cells and these cells normally set the pace for cardiac contraction.

Action Potential of Purkinje-Type Cells

The Purkinje cell action potential is similar to that of the working myocardial cell, although the plateau duration is somewhat prolonged. Hypoxia and acidosis in ischemic Purkinje cells may produce conditions in which the fast sodium channel is not opened. Phase 0 depolarization is then due to slow channel activation, carried primarily by calcium ion.

Action Potential of Atrial Cells

Atrial working myocardial cells undergo rapid depolarization. These cells have essentially no plateau period, but repolarization is slower than in Purkinje cells (Fig. 1-20). The total action potential duration of atrial cells is shorter than that of Purkinje cells. Atrial muscle cells do not spontaneously depolarize under physiologic conditions. Spontaneous depolarization can occur under nonphysiological conditions.

Cells in the Atrioventricular Node

In general, spontaneously depolarizing cells of the AV node are similar to sinus node cells in the rate of phase 0 depolarization and of maximal repolarization voltage (see Fig. 1-20). The AV node has several types of cells with different electrophysiological characteristics; these are termed *atrionodal*, *nodal*, and *nodal-His*. These are located in the upper, middle, and lower junctional areas, respectively.[41]

Cells in the Bundle of His

The electrophysiological characteristics of His bundle cells closely resemble those of Purkinje cells in the distal conducting system. The duration of the His bundle action potential, however, is slightly less than that of cells in the Purkinje network. The most rapid period of depolarization and the longest period of repolarization occur in Purkinje cells at the distal end of the conducting system (Fig. 1-20).

Refractory Periods

The period after depolarization, during which it is difficult or impossible to re-excite the cell, is termed the *refractory period* (Fig. 1-21). Refractoriness reflects the effects on depolarization of time and voltage requirements for the activation, inactivation, and recovery of ion channels.

During the *effective refractory period*, no action potential can be initiated by an external electrical stimulus. The duration of this

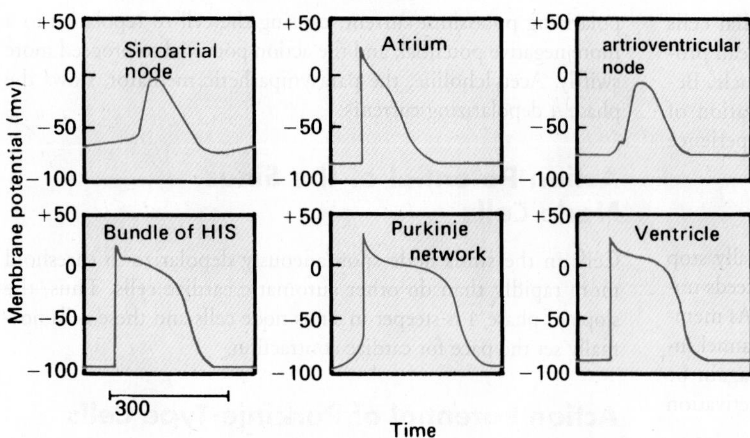

■ **Figure 1-20** Characteristic action potentials in different regions of the heart. See text for description. (From Katz, A. [2006]. *Physiology of the heart* [4th ed., p. 414]. Philadelphia: Lippincott Williams & Wilkins.)

period depends on the time it takes to remove inactivation from the sodium and calcium channels. The effective refractory period extends from phase 0 through the middle of phase 3.

During the *relative refractory period*, only a stimulus greater than normal can initiate an action potential. The relative refractory period occurs during the latter part of repolarization (late phase 3). Under certain conditions, a stimulus can initiate an action potential during the last part of phase 3 and the beginning of phase 4. Cardiac arrhythmias may occur during when this happens, especially when pathophysiological situations, such as ischemia, promote abnormal refractory periods.

The entire period between depolarization and complete repolarization is termed the *full recovery time*. Under normal conditions, cardiac cells are not depolarized until they have had time to recover fully from the previous depolarization. Usually, cells with long refractory periods have long action potential durations. The upper limits of normal heart rate responses and the time allowed for ventricular filling depend on normal cardiac electrical refractoriness.

SARCOLEMMAL IONIC CURRENTS

The currents that combine to orchestrate the action potential can be studied independently. Neurohormonal and ionic milieu, pharmacologic agents, and pathologic processes variably influence each current. Techniques such as the patch clamp and molecular biology have extended our understanding of channels types and hold the promise of increasing our understanding of important issues such as the generation of arrhythmias in disease states. New treatments are being developed. Some of the major channels are discussed individually (Table 1-4).

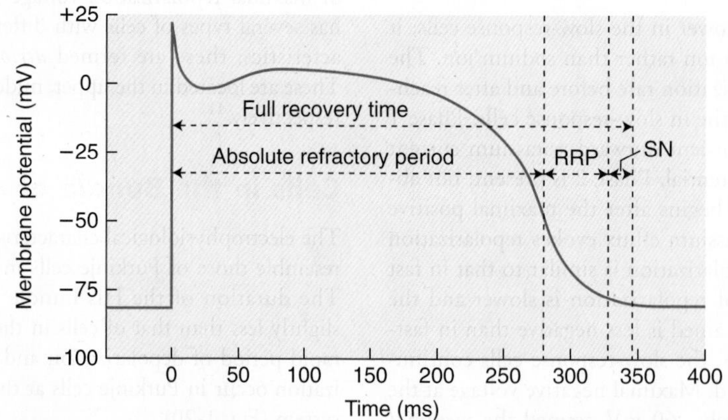

■ **Figure 1-21** Refractory periods. Closing of the h gates immediately after membrane depolarization causes the absolute refractory period, during which no stimulus regardless of its strength is able to initiate a propagated action potential. This is followed by a relative refractory period (RRP) during which only stimuli that exceed the normal threshold can cause a propagated action potential. The functional refractory period, which includes the absolute and relative refractory periods, is followed by a supernormal (SN) period, during which subthreshold stimuli slightly less than those that reach the normal threshold can generate a propagated action potential. Action potentials generated during the relative refractory and supernormal periods are small and slowly rising because of incomplete recovery of the sodium channels. The full recovery time begins with depolarization and ends after the supernormal period, when normal stimuli produce normally propagated action potentials. (From Katz, A. [2006]. *Physiology of the heart* [4th ed., p. 397]. Philadelphia: Lippincott Williams & Wilkins.)

Table 1-4 ■ CARDIAC IONIC CURRENTS

Current*	Charge Carrier	Activation Mechanism	Function
Inward Currents			
I_{Na}	Na^+	Voltage	AP upstroke
I_{Ca} (I_{Si}, I_{Caf}, I_{Cas})	Ca^{2+}	Voltage	AP plateau E–C coupling AP upstroke Sinus pacemaker
$I_f(I_h)$	Na^+ and K^+	Voltage	Spontaneous depolarization
I_{ti} ($I_{t'}$, $I_{Na,K}$)	Na^+ and K^+	?$[(Ca^{2+}]_i$	After-depolarization
Outward Currents			
I_K (I_x, I_{x1}, I_{x2})	K^+ (Na^+)	Voltage	Repolarization
I_{to}	K^+	Voltage, ?$[Ca^{2+}]$	Early repolarization
I_{K1}	K^+	Voltage	Resting potential Repolarization ?Plateau potential
$I_{K_{Ca}}$	K^+	$[Ca^{2+}]_i$	Repolarization
$I_{K_{Ach}}$	K^+	ACh, ? voltage	Inhibition
Pump/Exchange Currents			
I_p	Na^+, K^+	$[K^+]$, $[Na^+]$	Na^+–K^+–ATPase pump
$I_{Na,\,Ca}$	Na^+, Ca^{2+}	$[Ca^{2+}]$, $[Na^+]$	Na^+–Ca^{2+} exchange
Background Currents			
$I_{b_{Na}}$	Na^+	?	Inward leakage
$I_{b_{Ca}}$	Ca^{2+}	?	? Inward leakage
? $I_{b_{Cl}}$	Cl^-	?	?

*Currents identified in multicellular preparations are labeled I and currents identified in single-cell preparations are labeled i. Some of these currents are speculative (see text).
Ach, acetylcholine; AP, action potential; E–C, excitation–contraction; [ ], concentration of ion indicated.
Adapted from Brown, H. F. (1982). Electrophysiology of the sinoatrial node. *Physiology Review, 62*(2), 505–530; Nobel, D. (1981). The surprising heart. *Journal of Physiology, 353,* 43; Opie, L. (1984). *The heart* (p. 47). Orlando: Grune & Stratton; and Reuter, H. (1984). Ion channels in cardiac cell membranes. *Annual Review of Physiology, 46,* 474.

Inward Currents

The inward currents are carried by sodium or calcium ions moving into the cell. For each ion, there are several different types of channels, each with its own gating characteristics.

Fast Inward Current I_{NA}

The fast sodium current is activated to cause rapid depolarization in phase 0 of fast-response cells. It was discussed in some detail previously. Briefly, the sodium channel opens with depolarization to threshold (−70 to −60 mV), but quickly closes because of inactivation. Repolarization is necessary to remove the inactivation.[38] The fast sodium current is blocked by the puffer fish poison tetrodotoxin. Many antiarrhythmic agents, particularly class I agents, alter this current.

Calcium Currents

The two major types of calcium channels are termed L (long-lasting) and T (transient). The L current activates with depolarizations beyond –40 mV and then slowly inactivates. The T current activates at –70 mV and rapidly diminishes. Both channels probably contribute to maintaining the plateau phase of the cardiac action potential. The T channels contribute to spontaneous depolarization in pacemaker cells and the L channels contribute to the action potential upstroke in these cells. These currents may be potentiated by β-adrenergic (catecholamine) stimulation and diminished by acetylcholine and acidosis.[36] The current is blocked by inorganic compounds such as lanthanum, cobalt, nickel, and manganese. Organic charged tertiary amines, such as verapamil, block the slow channel. The block depends on membrane potential and rate of stimulation. Organic dihydropyridines, such as nifedipine, also block this channel.

Pacemaker Current

Pacemaking results from the combination of at least four currents. There is a time-dependent inactivation of the potassium current, and thus a loss of outward current (which would tend to hyperpolarize). This inactivation alone does not produce depolarization; channels that carry ions with an equilibrium potential positive to the membrane potential also must open. The currents involved are I_h, I_{Ca}, and background sodium current. I_h channels open at negative (hyperpolarized) potentials (hence the designation "h"), close at positive potentials, and allow passage of both sodium (hence a depolarizing influence) and potassium. Gating is slow. Similarly, a sodium leak current occurs and is a depolarizing influence. Calcium channels are activated with depolarization. With increasing depolarization, the calcium T channels open, carrying inward depolarizing calcium current (I_{Ca}).[42]

Transient Diastolic Inward Current I_{ti}

The transient diastolic inward current is a nonselective current that carries both sodium and potassium and may be activated by intracellular calcium. It is not normally active but may be involved in initiating delayed depolarizations and triggering arrhythmias in Purkinje and ventricular muscle cells, particularly when extracellular potassium concentration is low. Other inward currents have been identified. Sodium and calcium "leak" currents and the sodium–calcium exchange mechanisms can generate small inward currents.

Outward Currents

A cell can experience outward current in two primary ways: (1) potassium can flow out of the cell or (2) chloride can flow inward. Both ways tend to repolarize the membrane that had been depolarized and to stabilize the resting membrane potential. There are many types of potassium currents in cardiac muscle.

Outward Rectifying Current I_K

The outward rectifying current causes repolarization after an action potential. It opens slowly after depolarization, so it is also called the *delayed rectifying current.* It carries potassium, and it closes with repolarization. It also may be labeled I_x, and has been subdivided into I_{x1} early rapid component and I_{x2} late slower component.

Background Outward Current I_{K1}

This potassium current flows through channels that close with depolarization and open with repolarization. Thus, when the cell is depolarized during the plateau phase, the channel is closed. Were the channel open, potassium would flow outward, resulting in a repolarization. This repolarization would abort the plateau and halt the calcium current, which activates contraction. Hence, it is efficient that this channel is closed during depolarization. It is open with repolarization and serves to stabilize the membrane potential close to the potassium equilibrium potential. It is sometimes called the *inward rectifier* because it is highly permeant to inward potassium currents but less permeant to outward currents. When the membrane is depolarized and potassium can flow outward, the channel closes. It is sensitive to the extracellular potassium concentration.

Transient Outward Current I_{to}

This potassium current is linked with early (phase 1) rapid repolarization. It opens when a cell is depolarized after a period of hyperpolarization, and it closes quickly.

Other Potassium Currents

A nonvoltage-dependent potassium current, which is activated by an increase in the intracellular calcium concentration (I_{Kca}), may participate in the maintenance of the plateau and in repolarization. This current may be the same as or similar to the transient outward current (I_{to}).

Of potential importance in the diseased heart is the ATP-dependent potassium channel. This channel opens when the ATP concentration falls to 10% to 20% of normal.[41] The action potential becomes abbreviated during ischemia. This channel may account for such a phenomenon. It opens when the ATP level drops, shortens the action potential duration, and results in less contraction when the substrate needed for contraction is unavailable.[43]

Acetylcholine activates potassium channels whose outward currents decrease during depolarization. Although this phenomenon may be related to potentiation of the background outward potassium current (I_{K1}), there is evidence for a separate voltage-responsive potassium current (I_{KACh}), whose channels are regulated by muscarinic cholinergic receptors.

Other outward currents have been identified. The sodium–potassium–ATPase pump usually generates a small outward current (I_p).

FACTORS MODIFYING ELECTROPHYSIOLOGIC FUNCTION

Factors that alter cardiac cell depolarization and repolarization do so by affecting the rates of voltage changes, the magnitudes of voltage changes, or the timing of the phases of the cardiac action potential. Such changes affect cardiac impulse generation, impulse conduction, or both, and reflect the effects of environmental alterations on transcellular ionic fluxes.

Impulse generation, or *automaticity*, is influenced by a cardiac cell's maximal diastolic repolarization, threshold level, and rate of spontaneous depolarization to threshold (slope of phase 4). If maximal diastolic repolarization becomes more negative, if threshold becomes less negative, or if the slope of phase 4 becomes less steep, the rate at which the entire cell is spontaneously depolarized can become slower; opposite effects can lead to a more rapid rate of spontaneous depolarization.

Cardiac impulse conduction velocity is influenced by the rate of depolarization (slope of phase 0), the magnitude of depolarization (amplitude of phase 0), the distance from resting potential to threshold level, the action potential and refractory period durations, and the resistance to current flow. If the rate or amplitude of phase 0 is decreased, the difference between resting potential and threshold is increased, the action potential or refractory periods are lengthened, or the resistance to current flow is increased, the rate of conduction can slow. For example, Purkinje cells have faster conduction velocities than nodal cells because the Purkinje cells have rapid sodium channels that create fast and large depolarization.

The responsiveness of cardiac cells is described by the relation between the membrane potential before rapid depolarization and the maximal velocity of conduction during rapid depolarization. Cardiac cell excitability is described by the current required to alter the membrane potential from resting to threshold.[44] Although once threshold is reached, the cell rapidly depolarizes, the amplitude of the action potential can be decreased if the distance between the resting potential and the threshold potential is less than usual. Stimuli that are insufficient to depolarize a cell to threshold are not effective in initiating action potentials, but such stimuli can have an effect on ionic movements; in pathophysiological situations, these stimuli may influence cardiac arrhythmia generation and conduction.

Cardiac impulse generation, conduction, or both can be altered by the effects on cardiac cells of changes in the ratio of extracellular to intracellular ionic concentrations, acid–base changes, sympathetic and parasympathetic stimulation, myocardial stretch, cooling, ischemia, and heart rate changes. These factors often affect different cardiac cells in different ways; the following section discusses general selected examples of some of these alterations. (The effects of alterations in extracellular ionic concentrations on cardiac electrical and mechanical functions are discussed in Chapter 7.)

Adrenergic and Cholinergic Effects

Catecholamines

This broad class of biologically active compounds includes many endogenous hormones and neurotransmitters (epinephrine, norepinephrine, and dopamine) as well as pharmacological agents.

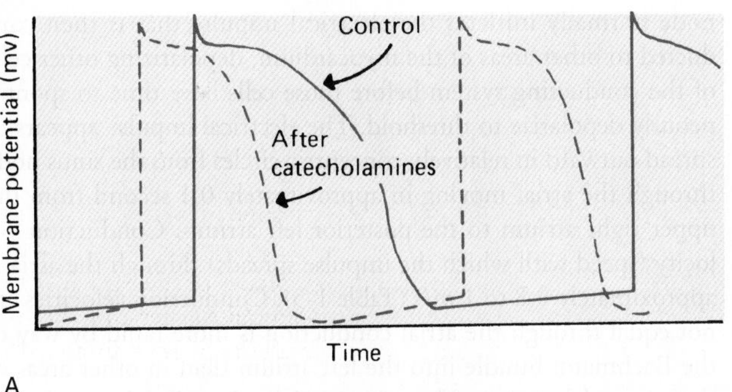

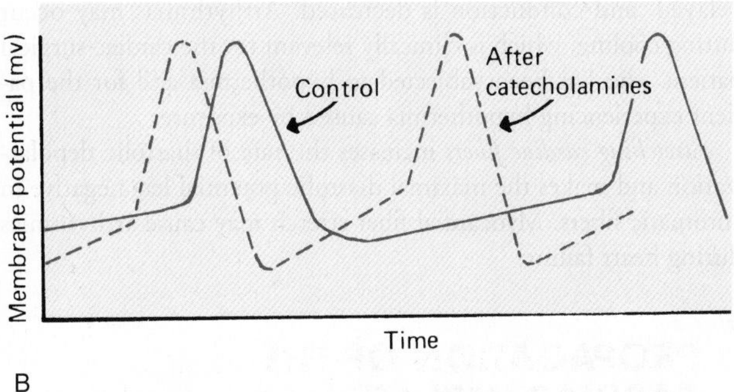

■ **Figure 1-22** Schematic illustration of the general electrophysiological effects of catecholamines on (A) Purkinje cells and (B) sinus node cells. (From Katz, A. [2006]. *Physiology of the heart* [4th ed., p. 449]. Philadelphia: Lippincott Williams & Wilkins.)

These compounds have metabolic, endocrine, central nervous system, and other actions. In the heart they are generally excitatory, increasing the strength and/or the frequency of contraction. In the blood vessels, these substances can evoke constriction or dilation. There are several receptor subtypes producing complex and sometimes conflicting effects on cardiac cell action potentials. Generally, catecholamines increase the magnitude and rate of diastolic depolarization in both Purkinje and sinus nodal cells. Repolarization becomes faster, and the action potential duration is shortened. The increased rate of sinus node spontaneous depolarization (slope of phase 4) appears to be the most important mechanism by which adrenergic stimulation increases heart rate (Fig. 1-22). Catecholamines increase the amplitude and rate of rise of phase 0 in junctional cells, which increases conduction velocity through the AV node. Catecholamines also increase myocardial contractility. Most of catecholamine effects on the cardiac action potential are caused by stimulation of β-adrenergic receptors.

Acetylcholine

The cholinergic effects of parasympathetic (vagal) nerve stimulation are more pronounced on the sinus node, AV node, and atrial muscle than on ventricular muscle. Acetylcholine slows the rate of diastolic depolarization (slope of phase 4) in sinus node cells. The heart rate is slowed (Fig. 1-23). The sinus node action potential duration and refractory period are both shortened. There is a decreased rate of rise and amplitude of phase 0 in AV nodal cells in response to acetylcholine, leading to slowed AV conduction. The AV refractory period may also be prolonged. Atrial contractile strength is decreased. Cholinergic cardiac receptor stimulation inhibits cardiac catecholamine effects by inhibiting the β-adrenergic effects of cAMP and inhibiting prejunctional norepinephrine release.

Effects of Acidosis and Alkalosis

Acidosis slows repolarization and prolongs the action potential duration in Purkinje fibers. Cardiac calcium channels are blocked by acidosis, resulting in a cardiac action potential with a slower rate of rise, amplitude, and duration.[5] Acidosis decreases contractility by decreasing calcium ion influx and decreasing the sensitivity of the myofibrils to calcium ion.[45] Alkalosis can shorten the action potential duration. Purkinje automaticity is increased owing to an increased rate of diastolic depolarization.[44]

Other Effects

The action potential duration is related to the length of the preceding diastolic interval. When heart rate increases (thus the interval between successive cardiac impulses decreases), then repolarization is usually also faster. The action potential is shorter in duration. At slower heart rates, the action potential duration lengthens.

In experimental situations, the effects of *warming the heart* are somewhat similar to adrenergic effects (e.g., diastolic depolarization is increased in automatic fibers). *Cooling the heart* depresses spontaneous depolarization in automatic cells. Repolarization is

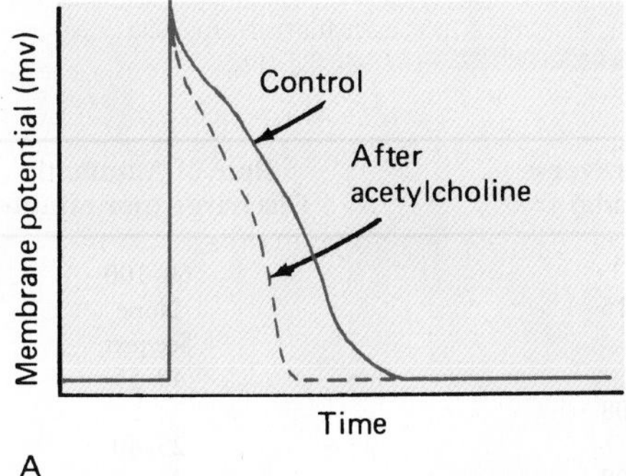

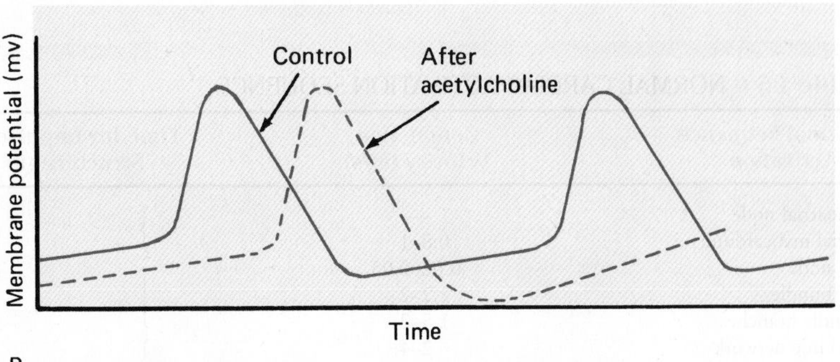

■ **Figure 1-23** Schematic illustration of the general electrophysiological effects of acetylcholine (vagal stimulation) on (A) atrial muscle cells and (B) sinus node cells. (From Katz, A. M. [1977]. *Physiology of the heart* [pp. 362, 363]. New York: Raven Press.)

delayed, and conduction is decreased. Arrhythmias may occur during cooling, which is clinically relevant for the cardiac surgical patient who has been subjected to hypothermia and for the patient experiencing hypothermia caused by exposure.

Stretching cardiac fibers increases the rate of diastolic depolarization and makes the maximal diastolic potential less negative in automatic fibers. Myocardial fiber stretch may cause arrhythmias during heart failure.

PROPAGATION OF THE CARDIAC IMPULSE

The spread of the cardiac impulse through the heart depends upon several factors, including (1) anatomic characteristics of the conducting system, (2) structural characteristics of cells (e.g., cardiac cell type and diameter, arrangement of low-resistance intercalated discs, and contiguity to other cells capable of conducting current), and (3) electrophysiological state of the cell membrane (i.e., resting and threshold potentials, ionic concentrations and conductances, rate and magnitude of depolarization and repolarization, duration of the action potential and the refractory period). As in a battery, there is energy stored across the cell membrane. When one segment of the membrane depolarizes, positive charge enters the cell, and an electrical circuit is established along the cell.[5]

In general, current flows more easily inside the cell and to adjacent cells across the intercalated discs at tight junctions than laterally across adjacent, highly resistant areas of cell membranes. If the current is sufficient to depolarize adjacent cells, a wave of depolarization is propagated and spreads rapidly from cell to cell. Thus, the cardiac tissue behaves essentially as a syncytium, although propagation may be somewhat discontinuous.[46]

As the impulse spreads through the heart, it depolarizes tissue that has recovered and is excitable, but it cannot depolarize tissue that is still refractory. Because the cardiac impulse spreads rapidly through the atria, slowly through the AV junction, and then rapidly through the ventricles, both atria contract almost synchronously, the ventricles have time to receive blood from the contracting atria, and then both ventricles contract almost synchronously.

Atrial Conduction

Sinus node cells normally have the fastest rate of spontaneous depolarization and thus set the pace of cardiac excitation. The sinus node normally initiates the electrical impulse that is then conducted to other areas of the myocardium, depolarizing other cells of the conducting system before those cells have time to spontaneously depolarize to threshold. The electrical impulse appears to spread outward in relatively concentric circles from the sinus node through the atria, moving in approximately 0.1 second from the upper right atrium to the posterior left atrium. Conduction velocity (speed with which the impulse spreads) through the atria is approximately 0.8 to 1 m/s (Table 1-5). Conduction velocities are not equal through the atria; conduction is more rapid by way of the Bachmann bundle into the left atrium than in other areas of the interatrial septum. There are specialized conduction pathways in the atrium as in the ventricle, but the functional significance of the atrial fibers is less clear. Generally, the impulse travels radially within the atria. Atrial repolarization spreads in the same direction as depolarization.

Junctional Conduction

The cardiac impulse is not conducted through the connective tissue of the cardiac skeleton, so cardiac muscle tissue in the AV junction provides the only pathway for electrical conduction from the atria to the ventricles. Conduction velocity through the AV node is approximately 0.05 m/s, although in some areas it has been found to be as slow as 0.02 m/s.

The rate of impulse conduction through the AV junction is influenced by the atrial site at which the impulse enters the junctional area.[47] An initial normal slowing of conduction through the AV junction with a later increase in the speed of conduction is correlated with electrophysiological differences in atrionodal, nodal, and nodal-His cells.[48] Other mechanisms have been postulated for the slowing of conduction through the junction, including the small size of the junctional conducting cells and the amounts of connective tissue interspersed among conducting cells.

The term *decremental conduction* describes the condition when a propagating impulse becoming successively weaker. The extent that decremental conduction normally occurs in the AV junction is debatable. Decremental conduction can lead to AV blocks. Slowing of the cardiac impulse at the AV junction prevents the atria and ventricles from contracting simultaneously and protects the ventricles from the abnormally fast heart rates that can be generated in the atria under abnormal situations. Preexcitation syndromes are evoked when there are accessory junctional pathways.[27]

Table 1-5 NORMAL CARDIAC ACTIVATION SEQUENCE

Normal Sequence of Activation	Conduction Velocity (m/s)	Time for Impulse to Traverse Structure (in seconds)	Rate of Automatic Discharge (per minute)
Sinoatrial node	—	} ~0.15	60–100
Atrial myocardium	0.8–1		None
AV node	0.02–0.05		See text
AV bundle	1.2–2	} ~0.08	40–55
Bundle branches	1.5–2		
Purkinje network	2–4	} ~0.08	25–40
Ventricular myocardium	0.3–1		None

AV, atrioventricular; m, meters; s, second; ~, approximately.
Adapted from Katz, A. M. (1977). *Physiology of the heart* (p. 259). New York: Raven Press.

Ventricular Conduction

The excitation impulse travels quickly through the His-Purkinje system. The His-Purkinje cells have the most rapid conduction velocities in the heart, approximately 1.5 to 2 m/s in the His bundle and 2 to 4 m/s in the Purkinje system.[44] The cardiac impulse next spreads rapidly (approximately 0.08 seconds), in a sequential manner from the common His bundle through the bundle branches, then through the extensive ramifications of the Purkinje fiber system, and finally through ventricular muscle. Ventricular activation occurs in three general phases: septal depolarization, apex depolarization, and basal depolarization (Fig. 1-24). The depolarization wave moves through the interventricular septum from left to right. The middle left septal area and the anterior and posterior left paraseptal areas are depolarized within the first 0 to 10 milliseconds.[49]

Most of the left and right ventricular muscle is depolarized within 20 to 40 milliseconds.[49] Activation spreads from the endocardium toward the epicardium. Although the impulse travels more rapidly through left ventricular tissue, the right ventricular wall is thinner. Thus, the full thickness of the right ventricle generally depolarizes prior to the left. The first epicardial depolarization usually occurs in the lower right ventricular wall.

A

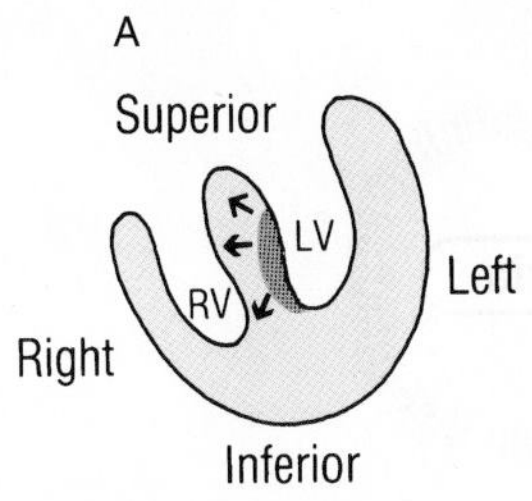

B

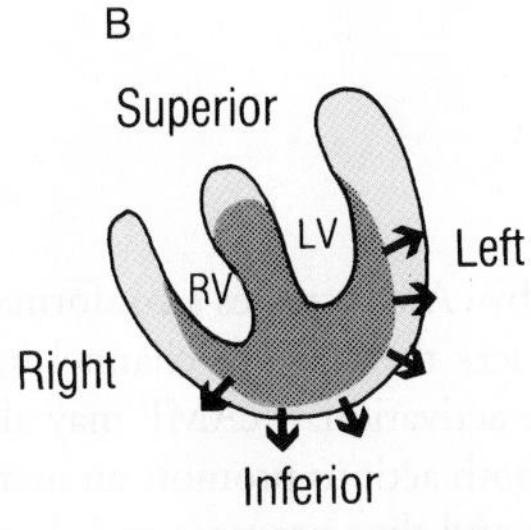

C

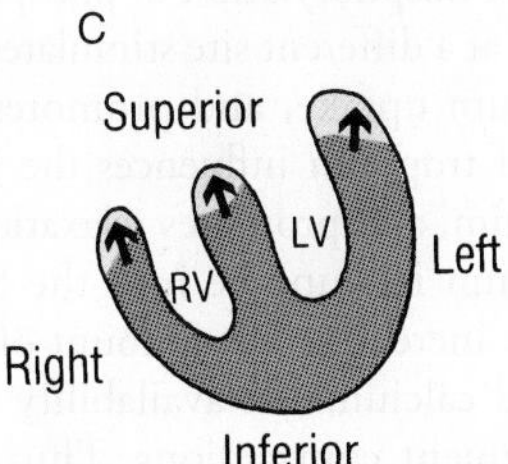

■ **Figure 1-24** Schematic illustration of the sequence of ventricular depolarization. See text for description. RV, right ventricle; LV, left ventricle. (From Katz, A. [2006]. *Physiology of the heart* [4th ed., pp. 447–448]. Philadelphia: Lippincott Williams & Wilkins.)

Purkinje fibers are sparsely distributed in the basal (upper) sections of the ventricles and septum, particularly in the right ventricle and the septum. The basal and posterior portions of both ventricles and the basal interventricular septum are the last areas to be activated, at approximately 80 milliseconds.[49]

Although Purkinje fibers conduct the cardiac impulse more rapidly than other cardiac cells, Purkinje cells in the distal terminations of the conducting system have longer action potential durations and refractory periods than do ventricular muscle fibers (see previous). Because conduction is slower in cells with longer action potential durations and refractory periods, the conduction velocity of the cardiac impulse is slowed at the point where Purkinje fibers connect with ventricular muscle cells. In theory, the distal Purkinje fibers then function like a gate, the length of the refractory period in distal Purkinje fibers normally controlling the rate at which ventricular muscle fibers depolarize.[50] Excitation–contraction coupling and the rate of cardiac contraction may be controlled by this gating mechanism. The clinical importance of this gating mechanism is not clear.

Ventricular repolarization proceeds in general from the epicardium to the endocardium and spreads from the ventricular bases to the apices.[51] Thus, ventricular repolarization proceeds in a direction that is opposite to the direction of depolarization; thus, the QRS and T waves are generally oriented in the same direction under normal circumstances. All portions of the ventricle recover at approximately the same time. However, ventricular repolarization is not homogeneous; under pathophysiological conditions, this may help create situations that promote ventricular arrhythmias.

Excitation–Contraction Coupling

Electrical excitation (i.e., depolarization of the myocardial cell membrane during the action potential) causes cardiac muscle contraction. Linking of electrical and mechanical activity is called *excitation–contraction coupling.* As identified by Ringer more than 100 years ago, an increase in cytosolic calcium concentration is necessary to trigger this process.[52] An increase in intracellular calcium ion concentration occurs with electrical excitation. Intracellular calcium ion in turn is the key that initiates contractile protein interaction during contraction. Calcium ion removal turns off the process and results in relaxation of the contractile apparatus. Thus, calcium ion is the link between electrical excitation and mechanical contraction. Calcium ion flows inward across the cell membrane during the action potential. Intracellular calcium ion stimulates release of calcium ion from internal stores such as the SR. Removal of calcium ion from the myoplasm evokes relaxation. The mechanisms by which ionic fluxes across the sarcolemma evoke contraction and relaxation are illustrated in Figure 1-25.

Calcium influx across the sarcolemma in response to cardiac membrane depolarization triggers calcium release by the SR.[17] The terminal cisternae of the SR press closely on the T-tubule. Bridges or "feet" spanning the distance between the two membrane systems are visible with electron microscopy.[53] These structures, called *ryanodine receptors* (because of binding properties), communicate the signal for SR calcium ion release.

The primary cardiac contractile proteins are actin, myosin, troponin, and tropomyosin. In cardiac cells, tropomyosin inhibits actin–myosin interaction. When calcium ion binds with troponin following electrical excitation, this alters tropomyosin in such a way that the resting inhibition by tropomyosin ceases. Myosin interacts with actin, binding and forming crossbridges.

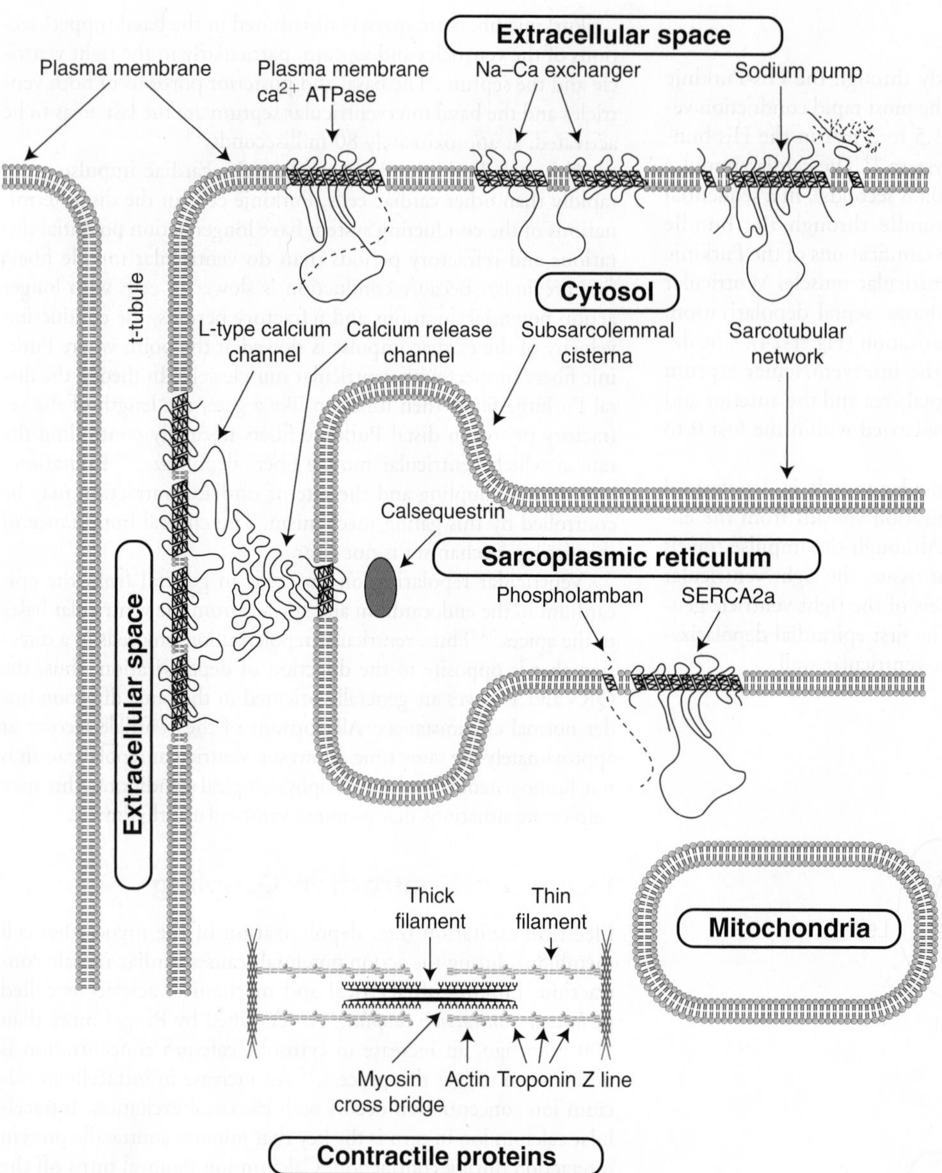

■ **Figure 1-25** Schematic diagram showing extracellular and intracellular calcium cycles that control cardiac excitation–contraction coupling and relaxation. Major structures and calcium "pools" (bold capital letters). (From Katz, A. [2006]. *Physiology of the heart* [4th ed., p. 194]. Philadelphia: Lippincott Williams & Wilkins.)

Calcium exerts some effects by combining with the intracellular protein *calmodulin.* In cardiac myocardial cells, the calcium–calmodulin complex promotes calcium ion binding to troponin and thus promotes contraction. Calcium–calmodulin also may stimulate calcium ion pumps on the SR and sarcolemma and may stimulate sodium–calcium exchange; these actions help remove calcium ion from the cytosol. Calcium–calmodulin influences the synthesis and breakdown of cAMP and may promote sarcolemmal calcium influx. Calcium may exert several other effects, either directly or by combining with other intracellular proteins, and thus may modulate myocardial cell contraction and relaxation through several different mechanisms.

Stimulation of β-adrenergic receptors on the cardiac cell membrane influences transmembrane calcium fluxes and cardiac contraction through the intracellular production of cAMP from ATP. cAMP in turn initiates several reactions involving intracellular protein phosphorylation (transfer of high-energy phosphates) by protein kinases. Phosphorylation of a sarcolemmal calcium channel membrane protein by cAMP creates a conformation or pore diameter change that places the calcium channel in a functional state available for voltage activation.[54] cAMP may also facilitate the SR release of calcium. Both actions promote an increased cytosolic calcium concentration and thus promote muscle contraction.

Phospholamban is an SR membrane protein that activates the SR calcium pump. Phosphorylation of phospholamban by cAMP and by calmodulin at a different site stimulates the calcium pump, increases SR calcium uptake, and promotes relaxation. cAMP phosphorylation of troponin influences the interaction between troponin and calcium, and promotes relaxation.

Although calcium ion uptake into the SR promotes relaxation, mechanisms increasing the amount of calcium ion in the SR cause increased calcium ion availability for tension generation during subsequent contractions. Thus, the increased rate and strength of contraction produced by β-adrenergic stimulation and other combined chronotropic–inotropic mechanisms appear to be matched by mechanisms that enhance the rate of cardiac relaxation.[54]

Calcium ion, the initiator and regulator of contraction, is the major link between excitation and contraction. The intracellular calcium concentration is directly and indirectly influenced by the amount of calcium transported in and out of the cell across the sarcolemma.[54] Calcium sarcolemmal fluxes are affected by the membrane potential and by sodium and potassium ion concentrations and transcellular fluxes. Conversely, potassium flux through the calcium-regulated potassium channel and sodium flux during sodium–calcium exchange are affected by the intracellular concentration of calcium ion.

MECHANICAL CHARACTERISTICS OF CARDIAC CELLS

Overview of Contraction

As seen in Figure 1-15, the myofibril is composed of a series of repeating units, called *sarcomeres*. Sarcomeres are the basic functional and structural units of the myofibril. Dark-staining Z lines mark the ends of the sarcomere. Attached to the Z line are the thin filaments. The center of the sarcomere is composed of the dark-appearing thick filaments. Interdigitating thin and thick filaments overlap to a variable extent. Shortening alters the amount of thick and thin filament overlap: filament proteins interact causing the filaments slide past one another.

The individual thick and thin filaments do not themselves change in length; the sarcomere (and the muscle as a whole) shortens. If shortening of the sarcomere (or the muscle cell) is prevented, the interaction of thick and thin filaments is manifested as tension or force generation. Such a contraction is termed *isometric*. When a stimulated muscle is allowed to shorten, tension is not increased, and the contraction is said to be *isotonic* (Fig. 1-26). In the heart, early systolic contraction is primarily isometric, that is, tension increases and muscle length remains fairly constant. Later in systole, the contraction is primarily isotonic, that is, the heart muscle shortens and the blood is expelled into the aorta, whereas little additional tension is developed.

Molecular Basis for Contraction

The *thick filaments* are composed primarily of the protein myosin. Myosin is large, consisting of six subunits: two heavy chains and four light chains per molecule. The two heavy chain subunits are coiled to form a long, rod-like tail at one end. At the opposite end of the long myosin heavy chain, a head protrudes from each subunit. Groups of myosin tails are arranged to form the rigid backbone of the thick filament. The heads are the site of ATP breakdown and interaction with the thin filaments. Heads project outward in a spiral along the length of the thick filament. At the center of the filament, the molecules reverse direction, leaving a bare region from which no heads protrude. The small light chains are nestled in the angle between head and tail, two per heavy chain. Both heavy and light chains are members of multigene families and exist in several forms, called *isoforms*. Variation in isoform composition may modify the rate or intensity of myosin chemical activity, which may modify the contractile properties of the tissue. Age, mechanical loading, or metabolic or hormonal state may modify isoform composition.

The *thin filaments* are composed of bead-shaped molecules of the protein actin arranged in an intercoiled, double-stranded chain. Two other proteins, troponin and tropomyosin, are located on the thin filaments at periodic intervals (Fig. 1-27). Actin interacts with the thick-filament protein, myosin, resulting in the transduction of the chemical energy of ATP into mechanical energy. Troponin and tropomyosin are called *regulatory proteins* because they modify the interaction of actin and myosin (Figs. 1-28, 1-29).

Myosin is an enzyme that breaks down the high-energy ATP molecule. During the resting state, the products of ATP breakdown remain bound to the myosin head. When myosin interacts with actin, the rate of ATP turnover is greatly increased. The chemical energy released from ATP is converted to the mechanical energy of contraction and heat.

According to the *cross-bridge theory*, a bond or crossbridge forms during muscle contraction, linking thick and thin filaments. The protuberant myosin head contains an actin-binding site and forms the crossbridge. This crossbridge is capable of binding,

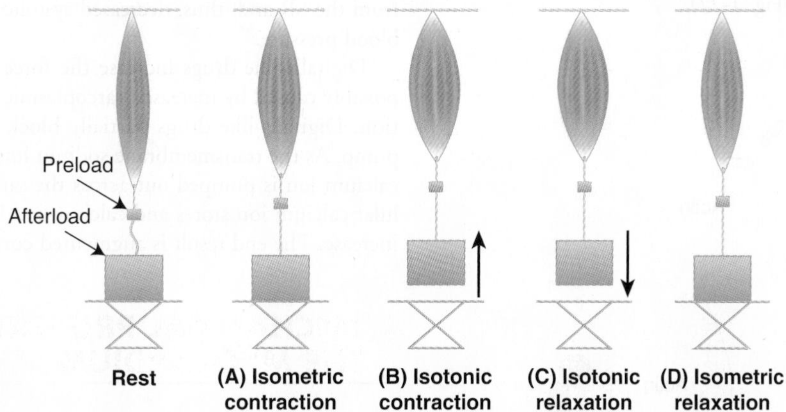

Figure 1-26 Cycle of contraction and relaxation in an afterloaded skeletal muscle. A small preload stretches the resting muscle, while the heavier afterload rests on a support until after the muscle has started to contract. The first phase in the cycle is isometric contraction (A), during which tension developed by the muscle increases until it equals the afterload. In the second phase, isotonic contraction (B), the muscle shortens while lifting the afterload. Relaxation is initially isotonic when the afterload is lowered to the support (C). Isometric relaxation (D) begins when the afterload reaches the support and continues until muscle tension returns to zero. (From Katz, A. [2006]. *Physiology of the heart* [4th ed., p. 322]. Philadelphia: Lippincott Williams & Wilkins.)

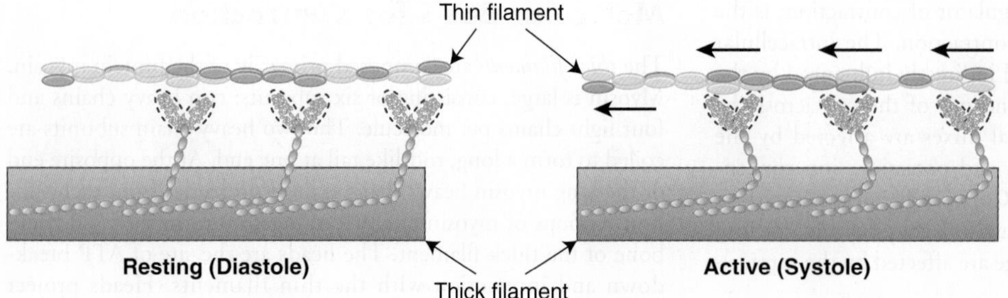

■ **Figure 1-27** In resting muscle (right), the crossbridges project almost at right angles to the longitudinal axis of the thick filament. In active muscle (left), the crossbridges interact with the thin filaments, which are drawn toward the center of the sarcomere. (From Katz, A. [2006]. *Physiology of the heart* [4th ed., p. 106]. Philadelphia: Lippincott Williams & Wilkins.)

flexing, releasing, and binding again, thus pulling the thin filament toward the center of the sarcomere in an isotonic contraction. If the muscle is held at a fixed length and is unable to shorten (an isometric contraction), tension is generated by the pulling of the crossbridge.

When the muscle is relaxed during diastole, actin–myosin interaction is inhibited by tropomyosin and troponin. Depolarization initates inward calcium ion currents across the sarcolemma and T-tubule membranes; calcium ion is then released from within the SR. The increased sarcoplasmic calcium ion concentration is in turn a trigger for contraction. Calcium ion binds troponin; tropomyosin rotates in a manner such that resting inhibition to cross-bridge formation is removed, and crossbridges form (see Fig. 1-27).

At relaxation, sarcoplasmic calcium ion concentration is very low. When calcium ion concentration rises, contraction occurs. The sarcoplasmic calcium ion concentration determines the forcefulness of contraction. Figure 1-30 illustrates the relationship; the higher the sarcoplasmic calcium ion concentration the greater the tension the heart muscle can generate until a saturating concentration is attained.

Molecular Basis for Relaxation

Contraction ceases when calcium ion is removed from the sarcoplasm. Troponin releases its bound calcium ion; tropomyosin returns to the position in which actin and myosin interaction was blocked. The cell relaxes (see Fig. 1-27).

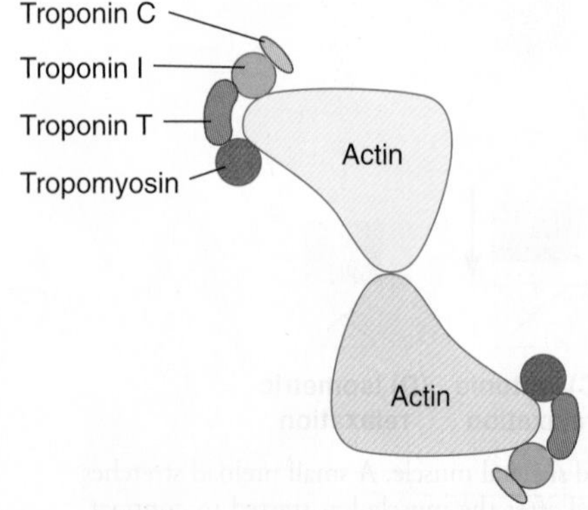

■ **Figure 1-28** Cross section of the thin filament in resting muscle at the level of a troponin complex showing relationship between actin, tropomyosin, and the three components of the troponin complex. (From Katz, A. [2006]. *Physiology of the heart* [4th ed., p. 110]. Philadelphia: Lippincott Williams & Wilkins.)

Removal of calcium ion is essential in relaxation. Two mechanisms are important in this process. The SR pumps calcium ion into its core. This is an active process and requires chemical energy from ATP breakdown. Also, calcium ion is pumped outward across the sarcolemma. This removal process is also an active process because calcium ions must be moved against electrical and concentration gradients. Rather than using ATP directly, this process uses the energy stored in the sodium ion gradient. In conjunction with sodium ion moving inward down its concentration gradient, calcium ion is forced outward. The sodium ion gradient, in turn, is maintained by the sodium–potassium pump, which is powered by ATP.

The ATP required for the calcium ion removal from the sarcoplasm and for the cycling of crossbridges may be depleted, for example, in myocardial ischemia. When this happens, crossbridges form and are not broken and the muscle becomes stiff.

Modulation of Sarcoplasmic Calcium Ion Concentration

Interventions that alter sarcoplasmic calcium ion concentration alter the force generated during contraction. For example, β-adrenergic drugs, such as epinephrine, may increase inward calcium current through calcium channels opened during the action potential, increasing sarcoplasmic calcium ion concentration and thus the force of contraction. Certain antiarrhythmic drugs such as procainamide are associated with decreased calcium ion release from the SR and, thus, decreased systolic tension generation and blood pressure.[55]

Digitalis-like drugs increase the force of contraction. This is possibly caused by increased sarcoplasmic calcium ion concentration. Digitalis-like drugs partially block the sodium–potassium pump. As the transmembrane sodium ion gradient decreases, less calcium ion is pumped out across the sarcolemma. The intracellular calcium ion stores and calcium ion level during contraction increase. The end result is augmented contractile strength.

MECHANICAL PROPERTIES OF THE MYOCARDIUM

The heart is a pump. It functions to add energy to the flowing blood, thus propelling the blood through the systemic and pulmonary circulations. The performance of the heart as a pump can be described in terms of the cardiac output (*CO*). CO is the volume of blood pumped by one ventricle in 1 minute. CO is equal to the stroke volume (*SV*), or volume of blood pumped with each beat times the number of cardiac contractions (heart rate, *HR*) in

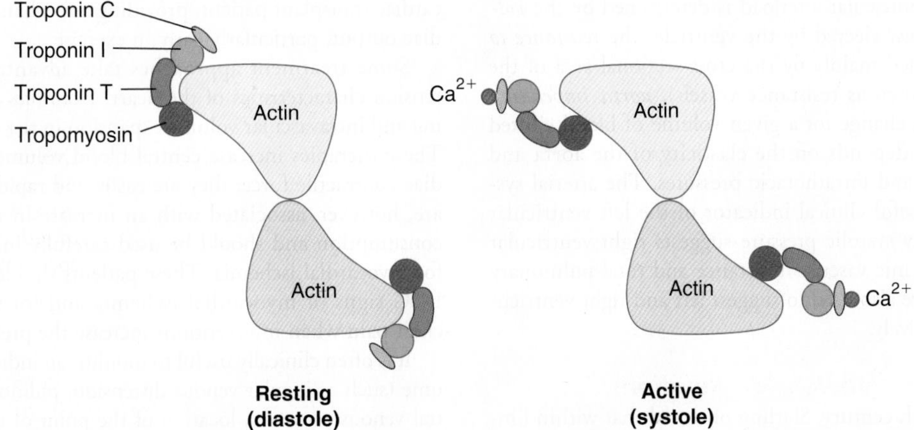

■ **Figure 1-29** Cross section of a thin filament at a region containing the troponin complex in resting (left) and active (right) muscle. At rest, the troponin complex holds the tropomyosin molecules toward the periphery of the groove between adjacent actin strands, which prevents actin from interacting with the myosin crossbridges. In active muscle, calcium binding to troponin C weakens the bond linking troponin I to actin. Loosening of this bond rearranges the regulatory proteins so as to shift tropomyosin deeper into the groove between the strands of actin, thereby exposing active sites on actin for interaction with the myosin crossbridges. (From Katz, A. [2006]. *Physiology of the heart* [4th ed., p. 117]. Philadelphia: Lippincott Williams & Wilkins.)

1 minute (CO = SV × HR). Typical normal values in a 70-kg man at rest (HR: 68 beats/min; SV: 80 mL) produce a cardiac output of 5,440 mL/min or 5.4 L/min.

Stroke volume is determined by the degree of ventricular filling during diastole (preload), the force against which the ventricle must pump (afterload), the contractile state of the myocardium, and heart rate. In the remainder of this section, these factors are discussed in more detail, and the manner in which they interact to influence the mechanical function of the heart is described.

Preload and Afterload

Preload is the distending force that stretches the ventricular muscle immediately before electrical excitation and contraction. Figure 1-31 further defines preload and illustrates the role of preload in the contraction of a simple muscle preparation. Left ventricular end-diastolic pressure is the left ventricular preload. In the absence of pathologic mitral valve changes, left atrial pressure is an indicator of left ventricular preload. In order to make clinical judgments about left ventricular preload, clinicians measure the pulmonary artery pressures and the pulmonary artery occlusion pressure. If there is no pulmonary hypertension as well as no mitral valve pathology, then these pressures are useful indices of left ventricular preload. Central venous pressure, in the absence of tricuspid valve disease, is an index of right ventricular preload (see Chapter 21).

A related term describing cardiac mechanical function is *afterload.* Afterload is the force that opposes ventricular ejection (i.e., the forces that the muscle must overcome to move the blood during

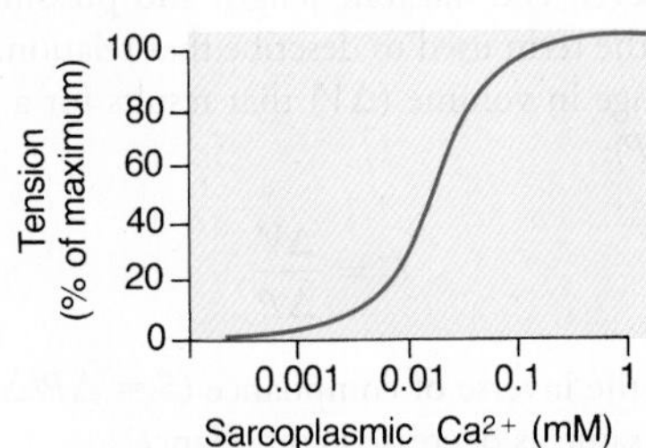

■ **Figure 1-30** The calcium ion (Ca^{2+}) concentration versus tension relation. The higher the sarcoplasmic Ca^{2+} concentration, the more tension the heart muscle is able to generate until a maximum level is attained. Note the range of intracellular Ca^{2+} is significantly lower than the 1- to 2-mM concentration in the extracellular space.

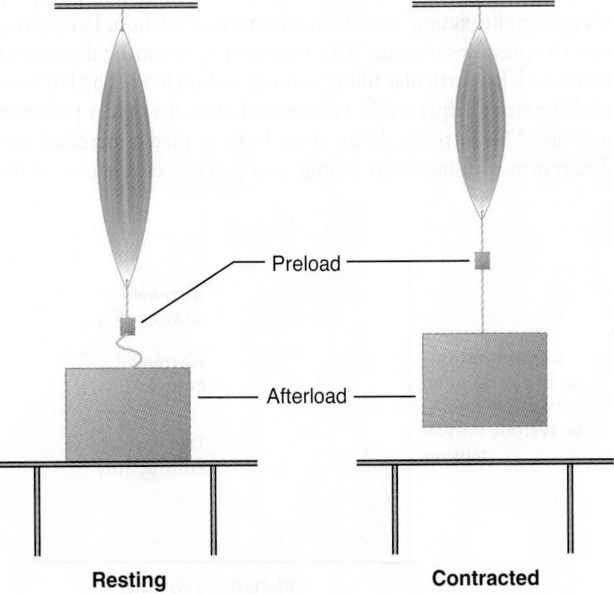

■ **Figure 1-31** Preload and afterload. A preload is supported by a resting muscle before it begins to contract (left). An afterload, such as a weight resting on a support, is not encountered by the muscle until developed tension exceeds its weight (right). (From Katz, A. [2006]. *Physiology of the heart* [4th ed., p. 83]. Philadelphia: Lippincott Williams & Wilkins.)

contraction). Left ventricular afterload is determined by the *volume and mass of blood* ejected by the ventricle, the *resistance to blood flow* (determined mainly by the cross-sectional area of the small arterioles, known as resistance vessels), *aortic impedance* (amount of pressure change for a given volume of blood ejected into the aorta; this depends on the elasticity of the aorta and branching arteries), and intrathoracic pressures. The arterial systolic pressure is a useful clinical indicator of the left ventricular afterload; pulmonary systolic pressure suggests right ventricular afterload. Total systemic vascular resistance and total pulmonary vascular resistance are also used to suggest left and right ventricular afterload, respectively.

Preload Role: Length–Tension Relationship

Early in the twentieth century, Starling observed that within limits, an increase in left ventricular volume at the end of diastole resulted in the generation of increased active pressure and increased volume pumped during the ensuing contraction. Beyond a certain volume, this mechanism is no longer operational; increased end-diastolic volume results instead in decreased pressure developing and a decreased volume of blood being ejected.[56] This property is known as *Starling's law of the heart* or the *length–tension relation of cardiac muscle* (or sometimes, the *Frank-Starling law of the heart*). This property is commonly illustrated in a graph (Fig. 1-32). Although the left ventricular *volume* at the end of diastole is a factor that determines the subsequent force of contraction, clinicians measure pressure increments, not volume. However, the volume and the pressure are related, as discussed later (see "Compliance" section).

The length–tension mechanism is useful; it likely contributes to overall matching of the left and right ventricular outputs. For instance, if a person reclines after being in a standing position (or elevates the legs when in a reclining position), the volume of blood returning to the heart transiently increases. The right ventricle is stretched and increases its force of contraction, pumping a larger stroke volume into the pulmonary circulation. Pulmonary vascular pressures increase. This increased right ventricular output increases left ventricular filling volume and preload. The left ventricle pumps a larger stroke volume and arterial vascular pressures increase. This intrinsic ability of the heart to match increased cardiac return with increased volume pumped is useful in case of the cardiac transplant patient, providing a mechanism to increase cardiac output, particularly early in exercise.

Some treatment approaches take advantage of the length–tension characteristics of the heart. Examples of this are leg raising and intravascular volume expansion in the patient with shock. These therapies increase central blood volume and improve cardiac contractile force; they are easily and rapidly accessible. They are, however, associated with an increase in myocardial oxygen consumption and should be used carefully in the patient at risk for myocardial ischemia. These patients should be monitored for ECG signs of myocardial ischemia and for symptoms such as chest pain when interventions increase the preload.

It is often clinically useful to monitor an indicator of cardiac volume (such as jugular venous distension, pulmonary artery or central venous pressures, location of the point of maximum impulse) and a concurrently measured indicator of the tension generated (such as cardiac output). The length–tension relationship characterizes the mechanical functioning of the heart and can be helpful in judging the efficacy of therapies (see Fig. 1-32). Positive inotropic factors, that is, factors that increase the contractility of the heart, such as sympathetic stimulation, alter the length–tension relation, so that a higher tension is generated at the same left ventricular end-diastolic volume. In the failing heart, the same stretch generates much less tension and cardiac output does not substantially increase with volume. The heart is said to be refractory to inotropic stimulation; it could be said that the Starling curve is reduced.

The cross-bridge theory of muscle contraction partly accounts for the cardiac muscle length–tension relationship. Tension generated by muscle is proportional to the number of crossbridges formed. At short lengths, thin filaments overlap one another and interfere with cross-bridge formation. Maximal tension development occurs in the range of muscle lengths at which the myosin crossbridge regions maximally overlap the thin filaments without the thin filaments overlapping one another. If the muscle is stretched still further, then the region of cross-bridge overlap is diminished and less tension is developed.[57]

Other factors also contribute to the shape of the Starling curve. For example, when the heart is stretched, more cells may be brought into parallel with the axis of shortening and may be able to contribute more effectively to the total development of force within the ventricle. Calcium ion, which grades the force of contraction, may enter the sarcoplasm in larger quantities for longer periods of time. Contractile filaments may be more sensitive to calcium ion at longer sarcomere lengths.

Compliance. Starling's law of the heart relates end-diastolic length, rather than end-diastolic pressure, to the strength of contraction. However, end-diastolic length and pressure are related. *Compliance* is the term used to describe that relation. Compliance (C) is the change in volume (ΔV) that results for a given change in pressure (ΔP):

$$C = \frac{\Delta V}{\Delta P}$$

Stiffness (S) is the inverse of compliance ($S = \Delta P/\Delta V$). Increased stiffness is the same as decreased compliance.

Cardiac compliance is determined by inherent properties of the cardiac muscle tissue, cardiac chamber geometry, and the state of the pericardium. Myocardial tissue is stiffer with hypoxia, ischemia, and scarring, such as after a myocardial infarction.[58] (curve 2 in Fig. 1-33). Infiltrative myocardial diseases such as

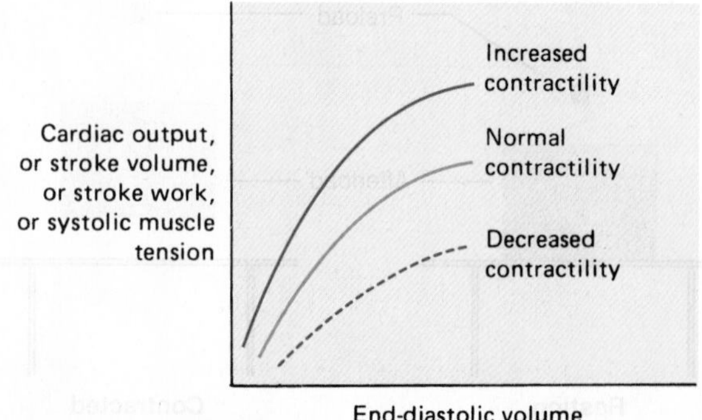

Figure 1-32 The length–tension relation of the heart. End-diastolic volume determines the end-diastolic length of the ventricular muscle fibers and is proportional to the tension generated during systole as well as to cardiac output, stroke volume, and stroke work. A change in cardiac contractility causes the heart to perform on a different length–tension curve.

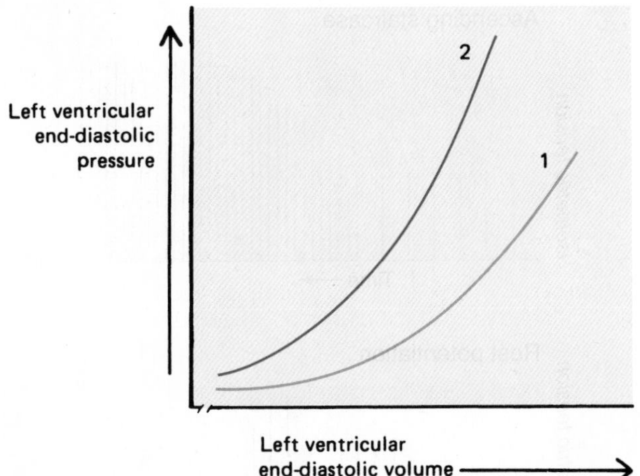

■ **Figure 1-33** The stiffness of the left ventricle. Stiffness is the slope of the pressure–volume relation. Curve 1 represents normal stiffness; curve 2 represents an increase in stiffness such as that which might occur after a myocardial infarction. In both cases, increases in volume result in increased pressure and an increased increment in pressure for a given increment in volume. Compliance is the inverse of stiffness. (Adapted from Forrester, J. S., & Diamone, G. A. [1973]. Clinical application of left ventricular pressures. In E. Corday, & H. J. C. Swan [Eds]. *Myocardial infarction: New perspectives in diagnosis and management* [pp. 143–148]. Baltimore: Williams & Wilkins.)

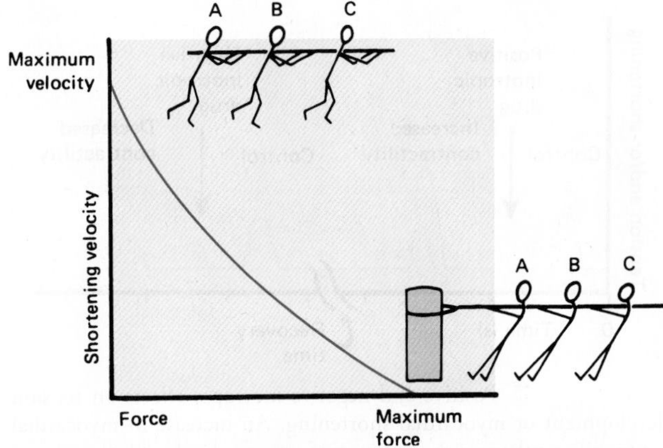

■ **Figure 1-34** Approximation of the force–velocity of shortening relation of cardiac muscle. Velocity of shortening is maximal with extremely light afterload. Shortening is impossible with large afterload. (Adapted from Katz, A. M. [1977]. *Physiology of the heart* [pp. 87, 126]. New York: Raven Press.)

amyloidosis increase muscle stiffness. Geometry changes that result in increased stiffness include hypertrophy. When operating at a more distended volume, the heart is invariably stiffer: it requires larger increments in filling pressure to achieve a given increment in volume (Fig. 1-33). Pericardial conditions that increase cardiac stiffness include pericarditis and tamponade. The ability of the cardiac muscle to relax, expand, and stretch in response to increased volume is called "lusitropy."

Implications for Patient Care. It is important to consider left ventricular compliance in patient care. In monitoring preload, the nurse commonly measures indices of ventricular filling *pressures*. Yet, therapeutic goals are related to achieving *volume* changes that will take advantage of the length–tension relation of the heart to maintain or increase cardiac output. The pressure change is important, too, because elevated ventricular filling pressures may result in pulmonary congestion and edema. For example, immediately following a myocardial infarction, myocardial stiffness may be increased[59] (Fig. 1-33). The same end-diastolic volume may be accompanied by such a markedly increased end-diastolic pressure that signs of left ventricular failure, such as crackles, appear. In this case, inotropic agents, which increase the force of contraction, would be of little or no benefit. Unloading therapies, which may decrease the end-diastolic volume, can eliminate the damaging increase in end-diastolic pressures. Furthermore, decreased ventricular pressures throughout diastole may improve coronary artery filling. Better coronary perfusion can improve tissue oxygenation and further diminish stiffness.

Afterload Role: Force–Velocity Relationship

The heart's ability to shorten is influenced by the amount of pressure above preload it must actively generate. With a smaller afterload, the heart is able to contract more rapidly. Contraction is much slower against very large afterload. This interaction is referred to as the *force–velocity of shortening relation*, or simply the *force–velocity relation* (Fig. 1-34). Changes in the initial muscle length or changes in contractility can alter the force–velocity relation.

At the molecular level, the rate of cycling of crossbridges may be equated to the speed of shortening. Generation of tension may be equated to attachment and pulling by the crossbridges. The amount of tension the muscle can generate is determined by the number of crossbridges the muscle is able to form. The crossbridge formation is determined in part by the preload, or the amount of diastolic stretch placed on the muscle. Once a critical amount of force equivalent to the afterload, or force opposing ejection, is generated, the muscle shortens. The speed of that shortening may be equated with the speed of cycling of crossbridges and is determined in part by the afterload.

Effect of Afterload on the Volume Ejected by the Ventricle. In addition to influencing the speed of shortening, afterload is related to extent of shortening. Increases in systemic vascular resistance, at a constant end-diastolic pressure, result in decreased volume pumped by the left ventricle. When pumping against decreased aortic pressure, the left ventricle pumps a larger stroke volume. Note that this effect primarily occurs in individuals with impaired cardiac contractile function.

Implications for Patient Care. It is important to consider the force–velocity relation in myocardial performance. Vasopressors that increase vascular resistance increase the afterload. Because of the inverse nature of the force–velocity relation, development of greater force is accompanied by a slower velocity of shortening. There may be a concomitant decrease in stroke volume and cardiac output. Further, there is an increase in the oxygen requirements of the cardiac tissue when afterload is increased.

Conversely, therapies that decrease afterload are associated with faster, more extensive shortening and a larger stroke volume. The cardiac output increases. Increases in cardiac output achieved in this manner have the unique advantage of decreasing myocardial oxygen consumption. Reduced afterload, however, may be associated with decreased coronary perfusion pressure.

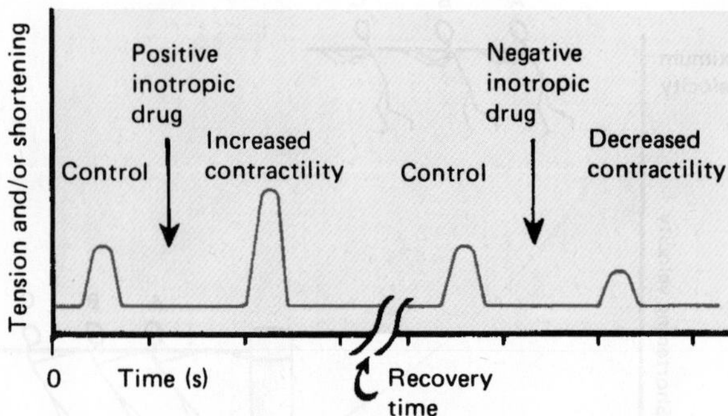

■ **Figure 1-35** Positive and negative inotropic effects on tension development or myocardial shortening. An increase in myocardial contractility enhances the amount of tension developed, the rate of shortening, or both, without an increase in initial cardiac muscle length. A decrease in myocardial contractility reduces the amount of tension developed, the rate of shortening, or both, without a decrease in initial cardiac muscle length. (From Katz, A. [2006]. *Physiology of the heart* [4th ed., pp. 285–286]. Philadelphia: Lippincott Williams & Wilkins.)

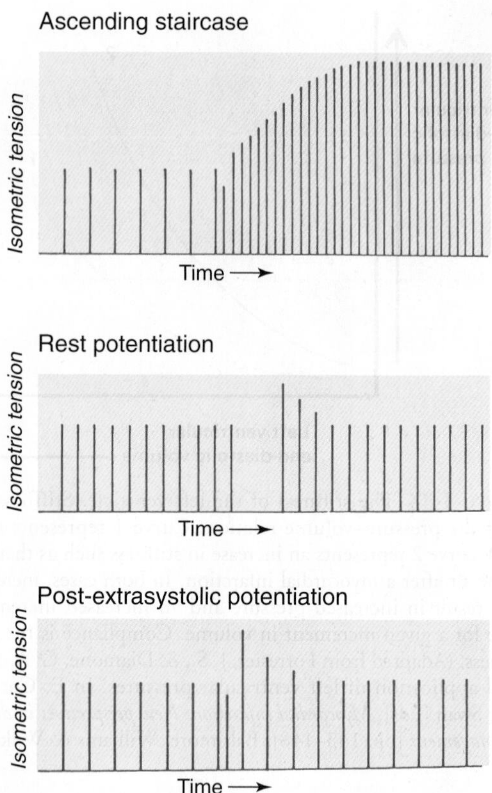

■ **Figure 1-36** Changes in isometric force generated in cardiac muscle when the stimulation frequency is altered. (From Feigl, E. O. [1974]. *Physiology and biophysics* [20th ed., Vol 2, p. 37]. Philadelphia: WB Saunders.)

Contractility of Cardiac Muscle

Contractility describes the heart's ability to contract; it describes the ability of the heart muscle to shorten, develop tension, or both. Altered contractility is a change in the ability of the heart to contract independent of variations induced by altering either preload or afterload (see Fig. 1-32; Fig. 1-35). In Figure 1-32, the curves other than "normal" represent alterations in contractility.

Contractility is a property intrinsic to the muscle. Its physiological basis is not well understood. Although contractility is difficult to define or measure, it is a property of critical importance because abnormalities in contractility are a major problem in the failing heart. Many therapies are designed to enhance contractility.

Contractility is not equivalent to cardiac performance, which can be influenced by valvular function and circulating blood volume as well as by myocardial contractility. *Inotropic agents* affect the contractility of the heart. Positive inotropic agents, which increase contractility, include sympathetic stimulation, excess thyroid hormone, exogenous epinephrine, norepinephrine, dopamine, dobutamine or isoproterenol infusions, and calcium salt infusion. Digitalis-like drugs have positive inotropic action. Increased contractility increases myocardial oxygen consumption. Agents such as catecholamines increase both contractility and afterload and result in substantial increase in myocardial oxygen consumption. Negative inotropic agents decrease contractility; these include myocardial hypoxia, ischemia, acidosis, barbiturates, alcohol, propranolol, and possibly lidocaine.

Treppe

Heart rate is the fourth major determinant of the force of contraction. Alteration in the force of contraction with heart rate is called the *Treppe* or the *staircase phenomenon.* In an experimental preparation with the preload held constant, the faster the rate of stimulation, the stronger is the force of contraction. Conversely, in the same preparation, slower rates of stimulation result in less forceful contraction. In the intact organism, as heart rate increases, there is decreased time for filling. The Treppe phenomenon provides some compensation for the decrement (Fig. 1-36). Treppe is an intrinsic property of the heart muscle, independent of hormones or innervation. It is present in the transplanted heart. The physiological basis for Treppe may be rate-driven variations in sarcoplasmic calcium ion concentration.

Two other types of rate-related alterations occur in force of contraction. A pause augments the force of the ensuing beat. This is called *rest potentiation.* After an extra beat, the force of the ensuing contraction is increased. This effect is called *postextrasystolic potentiation.* The manner in which variations in cardiac rate or rhythm induce changes in cardiac output in the intact heart is complex. Rate-related variations in force of contraction and filling interact; the stroke volume depends on that complex interaction.

Cardiac Reserve

The interaction of the mechanical properties of the heart can be illustrated by considering the reserve capacity of the heart. *Cardiac reserve* refers to the ability of the heart to increase its output. In the healthy person, the reserve capacity is used to meet demands for increased blood flow, such as during exercise. Normal cardiac output is 5.5 L/min in a healthy, 70-kg man. This can be increased with activity to about 18 L/min. Heart disease often limits the total possible output and the patient may have to rely on reserve capacity simply to maintain a normal cardiac output at rest. The two components of cardiac reserve are increase in heart rate and stroke volume.

Heart rate increases often increase the cardiac output. However, as the heart beats more rapidly, there is less time for filling. The rate-related increase in force of contraction partially compensates for the lower end-diastolic filling. At rates exceeding about 180 beats/min, diastole is shortened and the diastolic filling is decreased. Stroke volume is then decreased, as predicted by the Starling relation. Furthermore, the coronary arteries are perfused during diastole, and a fast heart rate decreases coronary blood flow, which may result in ischemia, and in turn decrease myocardial compliance and contractility. The stiff ventricle requires greater filling pressures to expand it to the same diastolic volume and may operate at a smaller volume, further decreasing stroke volume, as defined by the Starling relation.

During diastole, the heart can fill to a larger volume than usual, thereby increasing its stroke volume. This is sometimes called the *diastolic cardiac reserve*. Increases in diastolic volume are accompanied by increases in end-diastolic pressure. Left ventricular end-diastolic pressures beyond approximately 20 to 25 mm Hg typically result in pulmonary congestion. The more dilated the ventricle, the more oxygen it requires; this may be a limiting problem in the patient with coronary artery disease.

The heart also has *systolic reserve*, an ability to eject a larger percentage of the end-diastolic volume. Increased contractility and decreased afterload increase stroke volume and cardiac output. Increases in velocity of contraction or contractility make extra demands on the heart in terms of oxygen requirements and pose risk for the patient with coronary artery disease.

Factors involved in mechanical performance interact continuously. For example, an increase in afterload decreases the stroke volume. This in turn results in a larger volume of blood in the heart at the end of systole. The addition of an unchanged amount of blood during the subsequent diastole increases the end-diastolic volume. The ensuing contraction is more forceful, and stroke volume is increased owing to the Starling effect.

In hemorrhage, the filling pressure may diminish; the stroke volume decreases as predicted by the Starling relationship. However, the afterload (ventricular wall tension) may also decrease. This tends to raise the stroke volume. Adrenergic outflow also contributes to increased stroke volume. The cardiac output may increase despite decreased filling pressures.

Assessment of the Pump Performance

Assessment of the patient includes the evaluation of numerous indices of overall pump performance as follows:

- urine output, mental status, skin color, and temperature are indices of the adequacy of cardiac output to various organs and tissues;
- cardiac output may be measured directly;
- left ventricular preload is estimated from the pulmonary artery occlusion pressure;
- systemic vascular resistance (index of left ventricular afterload) is calculated; and
- mean arterial blood pressure is the product of cardiac output and vascular resistance.

These observations measure end products of many interacting variables that together compose the reserve capacity of the cardiovascular system. In making these assessments, the nurse not only should ask whether blood flow and pressure are adequate but also should probe more deeply.

- How much of the patient's reserve capacity must be used to maintain the current level of functioning?
- Is the patient already tachycardic, with a dilated left ventricle?
- Is the patient's heart already receiving a high level of endogenous catecholaminergic stimuli?
- How much of the patient's reserve capacity is left? Of the reserve capacity left, how much can be used in planning the patient's care?
- What is the cost of the patient's current functional state in terms of myocardial oxygen consumption?

MYOCARDIAL METABOLISM

The chemical energy of ATP powers myocardial contraction, ion pumping, and many other activities. ATP is broken down (hydrolyzed) into adenosine diphosphate and inorganic phosphate. With hydrolysis, chemical energy is transformed into mechanical energy and heat. Because the heart is continuously active, ATP must be continuously available. The usual intramyocardial cellular concentrations of ATP (estimated at 5 mM) are sufficient to power contraction mechanical activity for only a few beats.

Creatine phosphate is a backup source of high-energy phosphate to replenish the ATP supply. However, energy stores in ATP and creatine phosphate together supply enough energy only for several minutes of activity. Thus, the heart depends on ongoing ATP synthesis. This occurs in a series of efficient, but complex, enzyme-dependent reactions. The bulk of myocardial ATP is synthesized in an aerobic environment. Myocardial cells have large amounts of mitochondria, the sites of aerobic synthesis of ATP.

Free fatty acids are the preferred myocardial fuel, particularly when the patient is in the fasting state. *Glucose* or its storage form, glycogen, can serve as an additional substrate for energy metabolism. Whereas glucose contributes only 15% to myocardial ATP synthesis in the fasting patient, its role increases to nearly 50% in the postprandial state. *Amino acids* play a minor role in energy metabolism of the heart. In starvation, however, amino acid intermediates are metabolized to maintain energy stores.

PHYSIOLOGY OF THE CORONARY CIRCULATION

Under normal conditions at rest, the heart extracts a large amount of oxygen from the blood perfusing the heart: the difference in oxygen content between coronary arterial and coronary sinus blood is approximately 11.4 mL O_2/100 mL blood.[60] The total oxygen content of arterial blood is normally approximately 20 mL O_2/100 mL blood, so this represents extraction of more than 50% of the arterial oxygen content. It is difficult to extract much more oxygen than this, yet the oxygen requirement of the heart may increase many fold. This additional oxygen can be supplied only by increasing coronary blood flow. Coronary blood flow is proportionate to myocardial metabolism and oxygen consumption.

Determinants of Myocardial Oxygen Consumption

Several factors contribute to the oxygen needs of the heart. A small and relatively constant volume is used in the "housekeeping" activities of heart cells. "Housekeeping" activities are independent of contraction and include repair or replacement of intracellular proteins and maintenance of the ionic environment.

Each cardiac contraction involves ionic movement across cell membranes. The oxygen required for electrical depolarization and repolarization is small,[61] accounted for by the cycling of pumps that maintain sodium, potassium, and other ionic distributions.

In addition to these two fairly constant and low requirements for oxygen, factors related to activity and the state of the heart that determine how much oxygen the heart needs. These factors, which include intramyocardial tension, heart rate, shortening, and contractile state, constitute the major determinants of myocardial oxygen consumption ($M\dot{V}O_2$).

Intramyocardial Tension

The *law of Laplace* is used to calculate intramyocardial tension. This law states that intramyocardial tension is proportional to the internal pressure within the ventricular cavity times the ventricular cavity radius; it is inversely proportional to the ventricular wall thickness. An increase in left ventricular afterload causes the left ventricle to develop more pressure during the systolic period, thereby increasing intramyocardial tension and oxygen consumption. An increase in the preload or filling pressures of the left ventricle increases tension because both internal pressure and the radius of the ventricular cavity are increased and the thickness is decreased. Again, $M\dot{V}O_2$ is increased.

Heart Rate

Increased heart rate (at the same preload and afterload) increases $M\dot{V}O_2$. Each beat represents the generation of tension by the myocardium.

Shortening

In an *isotonic twitch*, there is a component of the oxygen consumption that is proportional to the amount of shortening by a muscle. That is, there is a metabolic cost that is related to shortening. This is sometimes called the *Fenn effect* and is a characteristic of cardiac as well as of skeletal muscle. In cardiac muscle, a contraction with a large amount of shortening is one that expels a large stroke volume. Increased myocardial shortening increases $M\dot{V}O_2$.

Contractile State

Contractility correlates with the amount of oxygen consumed by the heart. Positive inotropic factors increase $M\dot{V}O_2$ and negative inotropic agents decrease $M\dot{V}O_2$.

Pressure Versus Volume Work

Work done by the heart is proportional to the pressure generated times the volume pumped (stroke work = [mean arterial pressure – left atrial pressure] × stroke volume). Pressure generated is a component of intramyocardial tension as described by the Laplace relationship, and contributes to overall $M\dot{V}O_2$. The size of the stroke volume is related to the amount of myocardial shortening, and thus it too contributes to $M\dot{V}O_2$. Although equal amounts of work can be obtained by altering pressure or volume, the cost in terms of $M\dot{V}O_2$ is much greater for high-pressure work than for high-volume work. Thus, cardiac work is not well correlated with $M\dot{V}O_2$.

Indices of Myocardial Oxygen Consumption

There is no single accurate indicator of myocardial oxygen requirements. Ideally, such an indicator would take into account all major $M\dot{V}O_2$ determinants. The pressure–rate product and tension–time index are often used to estimate $M\dot{V}O_2$. The pressure–rate product is calculated by multiplying the heart rate by the systolic or mean arterial pressure and dividing by 100. The tension–time index (more appropriately should be called the pressure–time index) is calculated by multiplying the area under the left ventricular pressure curve by heart rate. Both pressure–rate product and tension–time index take heart rate (a major $M\dot{V}O_2$ determinant) into account. Because pressure, not tension, is included in these indicators, the other factors in the Laplace equation (i.e., ventricular cavity radius, ventricular wall thickness) must be constant if these indices are to accurately predict $M\dot{V}O_2$.

Myocardial Oxygen Supply

Control of Coronary Blood Flow

Flow of blood in the coronary circulation is, as in all vascular beds, proportional to the perfusion pressure and inversely proportional to the resistance of the bed. Resistance in the coronary bed is altered by compression on it during systole and by metabolic, neural, and hormonal factors. Coronary artery disease can impose significant resistance.

The pressure difference that drives cardiac perfusion is the gradient between aortic pressure and right atrial pressure because most of the coronary perfusion returns to the right atrium. Because the heart develops its own perfusion pressure, a fall in aortic pressure can reduce coronary perfusion, which in turn may further decrease cardiac function and pressure development. A cycle of deterioration may result. The coronary circulation, however, is autoregulated. This means that changes in the perfusion pressure over a range of pressures (approximately 60 to 180 mm Hg) make little difference in the amount of blood flowing to the heart if the other factors influencing perfusion are held constant.

During systole, myocardial wall tension is high. This compresses the coronary arteries, preventing perfusion. Thus, the heart has the unique property of receiving most of its blood flow during diastole (Fig. 1-37). Rapid heart rates decrease the time spent in diastole and may impinge on coronary perfusion.

Intramyocardial tension tends to be highest in the subendocardial regions of the left ventricle. Thus, $M\dot{V}O_2$ is probably

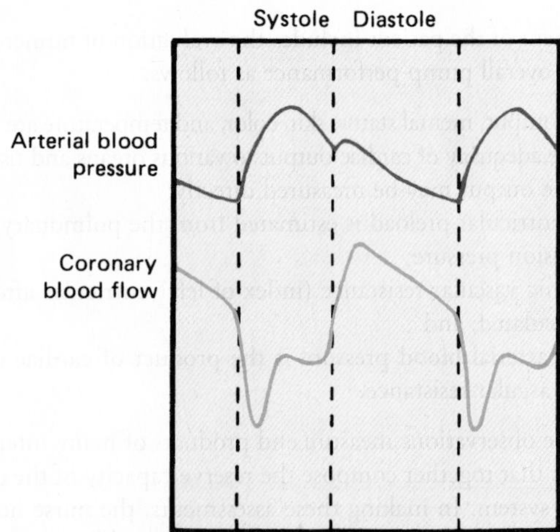

■ **Figure 1-37** Effect of systolic compression on coronary blood flow. Note the decrease in flow during systole and the increase during diastole. (From Folkow, B., & Neil, E. [1971]. *Circulation* [p. 421]. Oxford: Oxford University Press.)

highest in this region; yet systolic compression is also greatest here, which in part explains why this area has an increased incidence of infarction. In transmural infarctions (i.e., ones that involve the full thickness of the left ventricular wall), the area of involvement is typically greater on the subendocardial surface than on the subepicardial surface. Another factor contributing to this infarction pattern is the coronary artery distribution. Because arteries enter the myocardium on the epicardial surface and plunge inward through the wall, the most easily compromised distal segments of the coronary arteries perfuse the endocardium.

The coronary arteries are innervated by α-sympathetic and parasympathetic fibers. The direct effects of neural outflow are the same in the coronary bed as in other systemic beds; α-adrenergic stimulation (or norepinephrine) constricts arteries and parasympathetic (vagal) stimulation dilates them. Pharmacologic doses of the β-adrenergic drug isoproterenol dilate the coronary artery bed. Often, however, the direct effect of neural outflow on the coronary bed is masked because the autonomic nervous system also affects myocardial metabolism and contractility, and the effect of these latter factors predominates.

Local metabolic conditions are the predominant determinants of coronary perfusion. Increased metabolism or hypoxia leads to vasodilation and increased myocardial blood flow. The mechanism that mediates this effect is unknown.

With atherosclerosis, significant resistance can develop in the coronary arteries. Lesions that occupy more than two thirds of the vessel's cross-sectional area may impinge on flow at rest. Such lesions can prevent the increases in flow necessary when myocardial oxygen demand increases.

Collateral Circulation

Collateral arteries are interarterial vessels that can connect two branches of a single coronary artery or connect branches of the right coronary artery with branches of the left. In the human heart, collaterals are found through the full thickness of the myocardium, with the highest density near the endocardial surface. Although they are present at birth, collaterals do not become functionally significant unless the myocardium experiences hypoxic or ischemic insult. Before transformation, the collateral arteries are very narrow. They are devoid of smooth muscle and therefore are unable to respond to pharmacologic or metabolic vasoactive substances. After being stimulated to develop, the collateral tracts increase in diameter and develop a smooth muscle layer until, ultimately, the vessels are histologically similar to arterioles. When fully developed, these vessels are able to vasodilate when nitrates are administered and may autoregulate.[51] The time course from ischemic insult until significant enlargement is seen may be as short as 9 days.[62]

Three conditions are correlated with collateral development: coronary artery disease, chronic myocardial hypoxia, and myocardial hypertrophy. In coronary artery disease, the collateral diameter increases in proportion to the severity of coronary artery narrowing. Functionally significant increases in collateral structure are seen with a 75% or greater reduction in the luminal diameter of a major vessel. Chronic hypoxic myocardium is seen in patients with anemia, cyanotic heart disease, and chronic obstructive pulmonary disease.[63] There is also an increase in collateral diameter in hypertrophied hearts.[64] Attempts to stimulate development of collaterals with exercise programs have not been successful.[51] Collaterals frequently disappear after successful aortocoronary bypass grafting.[65]

Blood flow through collateral vessels may contribute significantly to myocardial perfusion. Patients with similar coronary occlusions have smaller areas of infarction when collateral development has occurred. Patients with abundant and well-developed collaterals sometime have a totally occluded coronary artery but no evidence of infarction. Blood flow through collateral vessels may be insufficient to meet increased demand, such as during exercise, and is insufficient to prevent necrosis in most cases.

Clinical Implications

It is important to analyze the effect of altered clinical states on the myocardial oxygen need. It is useful to consider the Laplace relation when evaluating oxygen demand in clinical states. For example, *hypertrophy of ventricular muscle* results in an increase in the thickness of the ventricular wall. This is advantageous in that wall tension is lower for the same left ventricular cavity size (same end-diastolic volume); hence, oxygen consumption is decreased. However, development of hypertrophy is a double-edged sword. At the same time that wall tension is decreased, the mass of tissue requiring oxygen is increased; the net result may well be a greater oxygen demand by the heart. Furthermore, because hypertrophy tends to increase the size of the muscle cells without increasing the tissue capillarity, diffusional distances are increased. The supply of oxygen to the interior of the fiber may be significantly impaired.

With *cardiac dilation*, left ventricular radius is increased. A larger end-diastolic volume is associated with higher end-diastolic pressure and increased pressure generation during systole. The Laplace relationship predicts that both factors lead to increased intramyocardial wall tension. Stretching of the heart wall is associated with decreased wall thickness, further increasing intramyocardial wall tension.

THE CARDIAC CYCLE

Every ventricular contraction that propels blood to the body or the lungs is the result of the sequential activation of the cardiac chambers through the coordinated functioning of electrical and mechanical factors. This section describes the changing cardiac pressures and volumes that coincide with the time sequence of cardiac events. An understanding of normal or abnormal cardiac functioning depends on familiarity with the cardiac cycle, which is represented graphically in Figure 1-38.

For the sake of simplicity, this description of events occurring during the cardiac cycle begins with events in the left heart. Figure 1-38 should be referred to frequently to obtain an understanding of what is occurring concurrently with respect to electrical activity; atrial, ventricular, and aortic pressures; atrial and ventricular volumes; valvular activity; and heart sounds.

Some general points about pressure and timing are useful to remember. Blood flows from the chamber with greater pressure to the chamber with lower pressure. When valves are open between two chambers, pressures in both chambers change until they are approximately equal. When valves between two chambers are closed, the pressures in the chambers change relatively independently of each other.

Ventricular systole and diastole divide the cardiac cycle into two major phases. The cardiac cycle can be further subdivided into several separate periods during systole and diastole. Because the cardiac cycle is continuous, the description of these periods can begin at any point.

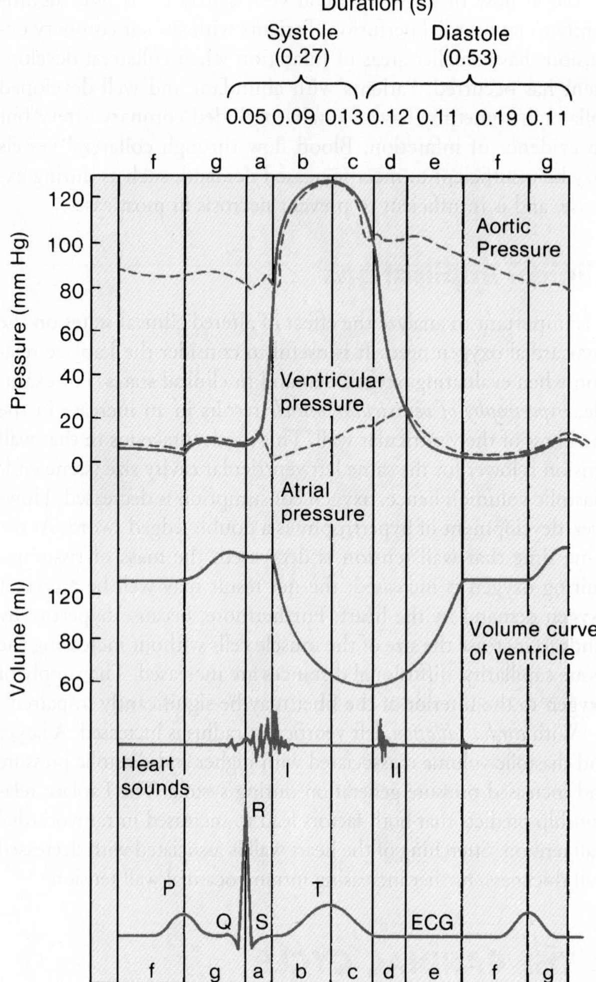

■ **Figure 1-38** The cardiac cycle, illustrating the changes in aortic, left ventricular, and left atrial pressures, and in left ventricular volume in relation to phonocardiogram and the ECG. The duration of each phase at a heart rate of approximately 75 beats/min is indicated at the top of the figure. A, isovolumetric ventricular contraction; b, rapid ventricular ejection; c, slow ventricular ejection; d, protodiastole and isovolumetric relaxation; e, rapid ventricular filling; f, diastasis; g, atrial contraction; I, first heart sound; II, second heart sound. (Adapted from Wiggers C. J. [1952]. *Circulatory dynamics* [p. 57]. New York: Grune and Stratton.)

Left Ventricular Cardiac Events

Ventricular Systole

Isovolumic Ventricular Contraction (Period a, Fig. 1-38). Ventricular contraction follows ventricular depolarization (reflected by the ECG QRS wave). Ventricular pressure increases rapidly. At the onset of this phase, pressures in the atrium and ventricle are approximately equal, but atrial pressure decreases with atrial muscle relaxation. Closure of the mitral valve buffers the atria from the high ventricular pressures.

The mitral valve closes when the ventricle contracts. Pressure in the ventricle becomes higher than in the atrium. The aortic valve remains closed until left ventricular pressure exceeds aortic pressure. Bulging of the cardiac valves due to abrupt ventricular pressure increases may cause slight increases in atrial and aortic pressures recorded during this period.

During the brief time when both mitral and aortic valves are closed, there are no actual changes in ventricular volume because no blood is flowing into or out of the ventricle. The ventricle changes shape during this period. The apparent increase in ventricular volume recorded on the ventricular volume curve in Figure 1-38 occurs when ventricular volume is calculated based on ventricular circumference.

The *isovolumic* or *isovolumetric period* is also termed the *isometric phase* of ventricular contraction because tension is increasing rapidly, but the muscle fibers do not shorten much until they overcome the afterload of aortic pressure. Muscle contraction is not completely isometric, however, because the ventricles change dimensions.

Rapid Ventricular Ejection (Period b, Fig. 1-38). Ventricular muscle contraction continues, and the aortic valve remains open as long as left ventricular pressure exceeds aortic pressure. The aorta and left ventricle are essentially a common cavity at this time. Ventricular pressure continues to increase rapidly during the initial part of this period, and then rises less rapidly to approximately the systolic pressure (120 mm Hg in the figure) later during this period.

Ventricular volume decreases rapidly during ventricular ejection; two thirds or more of the stroke volume is ejected during this approximately 0.09-second period (Table 1-6). Aortic flow reaches peak velocity early in the rapid ejection period before the point of maximal ventricular pressure. Aortic pressure may actually slightly exceed ventricular pressure during the latter period of rapid ventricular ejection, but blood continues to flow into the aorta because of the forward momentum of the blood. Much of the stroke volume is accommodated in the elastic proximal aorta.

The left atrium is relaxed at this time. Atrial pressure slowly begins to increase as blood from the lungs accumulates in the atrium. Ventricular repolarization begins.

Reduced Ventricular Ejection (Period c, Fig. 1-38). Ventricular and aortic pressures begin to decrease approximately 0.13 seconds before the end of ventricular contraction. During this time, ventricular muscle fibers are no longer contracting as forcefully as during the previous period. The fibers have reached a shorter length. Ventricular volume continues to fall, although at a

Table 1-6 ■ DURATION OF CARDIAC CYCLE PERIODS*

Cycle Phase	Duration (in seconds)
Isometric contraction	0.05
Maximal ejection	0.09
Reduced ejection	0.13
Total systole	0.27
Protodiastole	0.04
Isometric relaxation	0.08
Rapid inflow	0.11
Diastasis	0.19
Atrial systole	0.11
Total diastole	0.53

*Numbers shown are for heart rate of approximately 75 beats/min.
From Scher, A. M. (1974). Mechanical events of the cardiac cycle. In T. C. Ruch, & H. D. Patton (Eds.), *Physiology and biophysics* (20th ed., Vol. II, pp. 102–116). Philadelphia: WB Saunders.

slower rate than during rapid ejection. Blood continues to flow into the aorta. This period of reduced ventricular ejection comprises approximately the latter two thirds of the total ejection period (see Table 1-6). Atrial pressure and volume continue to increase. Ventricular repolarization is usually complete by this time, as indicated by the end of the T wave.

Ventricular Diastole

Protodiastole (Initial Part of Period d, Fig. 1-38). As ventricular muscle relaxation begins, there is a brief period before ventricular pressure becomes lower than aortic pressure when no blood is being ejected from the ventricle. Blood flow momentarily reverses. This backflow at a time when ventricular pressure is becoming less than aortic pressure facilitates the closure of the aortic valve. The second heart sound occurs. During this time, a slight transient decrease in atrial pressure may occur, reflecting the effect of ventricular relaxation.

Isovolumic Ventricular Relaxation (Latter Part of Period d, Fig. 1-38). Ventricular pressure decreases rapidly as the ventricle relaxes. There is no change in ventricular volume during this period when all the cardiac valves are closed. After closure of the aortic valve, aortic pressure increases by a few millimeters of mercury, and the incisura or dicrotic notch is noted on the aortic pressure tracing. Atrial pressure continues to increase as the atrium continues to receive pulmonary venous blood.

Rapid Ventricular Filling (Period e, Fig. 1-38). The AV (mitral) valve opens when atrial pressure exceeds ventricular pressure. The ventricle fills rapidly with blood that has been accumulating in the atrium, but ventricular pressure continues to decrease during this period because ventricular relaxation continues. Most of the blood that was sequestered in the atrium during systole is emptied into the ventricle by the time the ventricle reaches maximal diastolic size. Atrial pressure decreases as the atria empty but remains slightly greater than ventricular pressure throughout this period.

Late Diastole (Diastasis; Period f, Fig. 1-38). The mitral valve remains open, and pressures in the atrium and ventricle equilibrate in the time after rapid ventricular filling and before the beginning of atrial contraction. Blood from the lungs continues to enter the left ventricle passively, so ventricular volume and pressure slowly increase. Coronary artery blood flow usually is maximal during late diastole. The beginning of atrial depolarization is indicated by the upstroke of the ECG P wave.

Atrial Contraction (Period g, Fig. 1-38). Atrial muscle contraction follows atrial depolarization and results in an increase in left atrial pressure. Ventricular volume and pressure are increased slightly as the atrium forces much of its remaining blood into the ventricles. Between 15% and 25% of the end-diastolic ventricular volume consists of blood that has been ejected from the atrium during atrial contraction. The contribution of atrial contraction to total ventricular volume depends on venous return and heart rate; it is greater at faster heart rates. This atrial contribution to ventricular volume may be lost when the atria and ventricles are electrically and mechanically dissociated, such as during atrial fibrillation or complete heart block. Aortic pressure continues to decrease as blood in the aorta flows into the periphery. Toward the end of this period, the ventricles begin to depolarize. Diastole ends with the onset of ventricular contraction. The cardiac cycle is repeated.

Right Ventricular Cardiac Cycle

The sequence of events in the right ventricle during the cardiac cycle is exactly the same as in the left ventricle, but the timing of events in the two ventricles is slightly different. Right ventricular and pulmonary artery pressures are much lower than left ventricular and aortic pressures and right atrial pressures are usually slightly less than left atrial pressures.

Several factors lead to differences in the timing of events between the right and left heart. Contraction of the left ventricle begins before contraction of the right ventricle. Left ventricular isovolumetric contraction and relaxation last longer than right ventricular isovolumetric contraction and relaxation, presumably because the left ventricle must develop more contractile force to overcome higher systemic pressures. Right ventricular ejection begins before, lasts longer than, and ends after left ventricular ejection. Thus, right ventricular filling and ejection periods are longer than left ventricular periods, but the durations of left and right ventricular electromechanical systole are almost equal.

Cardiac Valvular Events and Normal Heart Sounds

Valvular Events

The differences in timing of right and left ventricular events lead to differences in timing of right and left valvular events. The AV valves close at the onset of ventricular systole. The mitral valve normally closes before the tricuspid valve because left ventricular contraction begins before right ventricular contraction.

The aortic and pulmonic valves open when ventricular pressures exceed arterial pressures. The pulmonic valve opens before the aortic valve. Right ventricular isovolumetric contraction is shorter than left ventricular isovolumetric contraction.

The aortic and pulmonic valves close when ventricular pressures fall below arterial pressures. The aortic valve closes before the pulmonic valve. The right ventricular ejection period is longer than the left.

The AV valves open during diastole when ventricular pressures are lower than atrial pressures. The tricuspid valve opens before the mitral valve because of the more rapid isovolumetric right ventricular relaxation.

Normal Heart Sounds

The specific mechanisms responsible for heart sounds are disputed. Sudden accelerations and decelerations of blood, turbulent blood flow, and the movements of valves, heart walls, and blood vessels may all produce vibrations and sounds audible at the body surface.

First Heart Sound. Mitral valve closure and oscillations in the movement of blood in the ventricles are associated with vibrations of the entire valvular apparatus and of atrial and ventricular walls. This creates the early components of the first heart sound. Later components of the first heart sound may be due to the acceleration of blood ejected into the aorta.

Second Heart Sound. The second heart sound actually begins before semilunar valve closure. The mechanisms responsible for the second heart sound include arterial blood flow decelerations caused by ventricular relaxation, blood vessel wall vibrations, and semilunar valvular vibrations.

Pulmonic valve closure follows aortic valve closure and leads to a two-component sound, which is accentuated during inspiration.

During inspiration, the time between closure of the aortic and pulmonic valves is increased, probably because a decrease in pulmonary vascular impedance leads to a longer right ventricular ejection time.

Clinical Applications of Cardiac Events

Systolic Events

The stroke volume is the volume ejected by the ventricle in a single contraction. Stroke volume multiplied by the number of cardiac cycles per minute (heart rate) equals the cardiac output. A typical volume ejected by the ventricle is 60 to 130 mL/m^2 body surface area/s, illustrated by the ventricular volume downstroke of Figure 1-38. The stroke volume, which is the difference between the ventricular end-diastolic and end-systolic volume, is approximately 24 to 36 mL/beat/m^2 of body surface area.

The *ejection fraction* is the percentage of total ventricular volume ejected during each contraction (i.e., stroke volume divided by end-diastolic volume). The ejection fraction is a frequently used index of ventricular function; normally, it is greater than 55% and usually is approximately 65%.

The maximal rate of left ventricular force development and rise of left ventricular pressure over time (peak d*P*/d*t*) occurs during isovolumic ventricular contraction. Peak d*P*/d*t* is sometimes used as a clinical measure of ventricular contractility.

Diastolic Events

Diastole comprises a greater portion of the cardiac cycle (approximately 65%) than does systole (approximately 35%) at normal heart rates (see Table 1-6). At faster heart rates, both systole and diastole are shortened, diastole proportionally more so than systole. For example, at a heart rate of 180 beats/min, diastole comprises approximately 40% and systole approximately 60% of the cardiac cycle. At fast heart rates, diastolic filling is increasingly important in terms of the decreased amount of time available for ventricular and coronary artery filling, which may lead to impaired myocardial functioning.

The jugular venous and the carotid arterial pulses normally reflect right and left heart events, respectively. All cardiovascular assessment and treatment plans intimately depend on an appreciation of the cardiac cycle.

REFERENCES

1. Ungerleider, H., & Clark, C. (1939). Study of the transverse diameter of the heart silhouette with prediction table based on the teleroentgenogram. *American Heart Journal, 17*, 92–102.
2. Reiner, L., Mazzoleni, A., Rodriguez, F. L., et al. (1959). The weight of the human heart. I. Normal cases. *AMA Archives of Pathology, 68*, 58–73.
3. Smith, H. (1928). The relation of the weight of the heart to the weight of the body and of the weight of the heart to age. *American Heart Journal, 4*, 79–93.
4. Windecker, S., & Meier, B. (2002). Patent foramen ovale and atrial septal aneurysm: When and how should they be treated? *ACC Current Journal Review, 11*, 97–101.
5. Overell, J. R., Bone, I., & Lees, K. R. (2000). Interatrial septal abnormalities and stroke: A meta-analysis of case-control studies. *Neurology, 55*, 1172–1179.
6. Milhaud, D., Bogousslavsky, J., van Melle, G., et al. (2001). Ischemic stroke and active migraine. *Neurology, 57*, 1805–1811.
7. Robb, J., & Robb, R. (1942). The normal heart: Anatomy and physiology of the structural limits. *American Heart Journal, 23*, 455–467.
8. Streeter, D. D., Jr., Spotnitz, H. M., Patel, D. P., et al. (1969). Fiber orientation in the canine left ventricle during diastole and systole. *Circulation Research, 24*, 339–347.
9. Keith, A., & Flack, M. (1907). The form and nature of the muscular connections between the primary divisions of the vertebrate heart. *Journal of Anatomy and Physiology, 41*, 172–189.
10. Silverman, M. E., & Hollman, A. (2007). Discovery of the sinus node by Keith and Flack: On the centennial of their 1907 publication. *Heart, 93*, 1184–1187.
11. Bachmann, G. (1916). The inter-auricular time interval. *American Journal of Physiology, 41*, 309–320.
12. James, T. N. (1963). The connecting pathways between the sinus node and A-V node and between the right and the left atrium in the human heart. *American Heart Journal, 66*, 498–508.
13. Scher, A., & Spach, M. (1979). Cardiac depolarization and repolarization and the electrocardiogram. In R. Berne (Ed.), *Handbook of physiology. Section 2. The cardiovascular system, vol 1, the heart* (pp. 357–392). Bethesda, MD: American Physiological Society.
14. Spach, M., & Barr, R. (1976). Cardiac anatomy from an electrophysiological viewpoint. In C. Nelson & D. Geselivitz (Eds.), *The theoretical basis of electrocardiography* (pp. 3–20). Oxford: Clarendon Press.
15. Fawcett, D. (1986). *A textbook of histology*. Philadelphia: WB Saunders.
16. Tarawa, S. (1906). *Das Reisleitungs system des Saugetierherzens [The conduction system of the mammalian heart]*. Jena, Germany: Gustav Fischer.
17. Fabiato, A. (1983). Calcium-induced release of calcium from the cardiac sarcoplasmic reticulum. *American Journal of Physiology, 245*, C1–14.
18. Titus, J. L., Daugherty, G. W., & Edwards, J. E. (1963). Anatomy of the normal human atrioventricular conduction system. *American Journal of Anatomy, 113*, 407–415.
19. Anderson, R. H., Becker, A. E., Brechenmacher, C., et al. (1975). The human atrioventricular junctional area. A morphological study of the A-V node and bundle. *European Journal of Cardiology, 3*, 11–25.
20. Hecht, H. H., Kossmann, C. E., Childers, R. W., et al. (1973). Atrioventricular and intraventricular conduction. Revised nomenclature and concepts. *American Journal of Cardiology, 31*, 232–244.
21. His, W. (1893). Die Thätigkeit des embryonalen Herzens und deren Bedeutung für die Lehre von der Herzbewegung beim Erwachsenen. [The function of the embryonic heart and its significance in the interpretation of the heart action in the adult]. Arbeit aus der Medizin Klinik zu Leipzig, 14–50.
22. Hudson, R. E. (1967). Surgical pathology of the conducting system of the heart. *British Heart Journal, 29*, 646–670.
23. Kent, A. (1914). The right lateral auriculo-ventricular junction of the heart. *Journal of Physiology, 48*, 22–24.
24. Kent, A. F. (1893). Researches on the structure and function of the mammalian heart. *Journal of Physiology, 14*, i2–254.
25. Mahaim, I. (1947). Kent's fibers and the A-V paraspecific conduction through the upper connections of the bundle of His-Tawara. *American Heart Journal, 33*, 651–653.
26. Mahaim, I., & Winston, M. (1941). Recherches d'lanatomic comparee et du pathologic experimentale sur les connexions hautes du faisceau de His-Tawara. *Cardiologia, 5*, 189–260.
27. Anderson, R. H., Becker, A. E., Brechenmacher, C., et al. (1975). Ventricular preexcitation. A proposed nomenclature for its substrates. *European Journal of Cardiology, 3*, 27–36.
28. Massing, G. K., & James T. N. Anatomical configuration of the His bundle and bundle branches in the human heart. *Circulation, 53*, 609–621.
29. Purkinje, J. (1845). Mikroskopisch-neurologische beobachtungen. *Arch Anat Physiol Wiss Med, 12*, 281–295.
30. James, T. (1961). *Anatomy of the coronary arteries*. New York: Paul B Hoeber.
31. Kelly, A. E., & Gensini, G. G. (1975). Coronary arteriography and left-heart studies. *Heart Lung, 4*, 85–98.
32. Wearn, J. (1940). Morphological and functional alterations of the coronary circulation. *Bulletin of the New York Academic Medicine, 17*, 754–777.
33. Armour, J., & Hopkins, D. (1984). Anatomy of the efferent autonomic nerves and ganglia innervating the heart. In W. Randall (Ed.), *Nervous control of cardiovascular function* (pp. 20–45). New York: Oxford University Press.
34. Miller, A. (1982). *Lymphatics of the heart*. New York: Raven Press.
35. Randall, W. (1984). Selective autonomic innervation of the heart. In W. Randall (Ed.), *Nervous control of cardiovascular function* (pp. 46–67). New York: Oxford University Press.
36. Sperelakis, N. (1984). Hormonal and neurotransmitter regulation of Ca^{++} influx through voltage-dependent slow channels in cardiac muscle membrane. *Membrane Biochemistry, 5*, 131–166.
37. De Mello, W. (1989). Effect of isoproterenol and 3-isobutyl-1-methylxanthine on junctional conductance in heart cell pairs. *Biochimica et Biophysica Acta, 1012*, 291–298.

38. Hodgkin, A. L., & Huxley, A. F. (1952). Currents carried by sodium and potassium ions through the membrane of the giant axon of Loligo. *Journal of Physiology, 116*, 449–472.
39. Glynn, I. M. (1993). Annual review prize lecture. 'All hands to the sodium pump'. *Journal of Physiology, 462*, 1–30.
40. Langer, G. A. (1982). Sodium-calcium exchange in the heart. *Annual Review of Physiology, 44*, 435–449.
41. Noma, A., & Shibasaki, T. (1985). Membrane current through adenosine-triphosphate-regulated potassium channels in guinea-pig ventricular cells. *Journal of Physiology, 363*, 463–480.
42. DiFrancesco, D. (1981). A new interpretation of the pace-maker current in calf Purkinje fibres. *Journal of Physiology, 314*, 359–376.
43. Nichols, C. G., Ripoll, C., & Lederer, W. J. (1991). ATP-sensitive potassium channel modulation of the guinea pig ventricular action potential and contraction. *Circulation Research, 68*, 280–287.
44. Singer, D. H., Baumgarten, C. M., & Ten Eick, R. E. (1981). Cellular electrophysiology of ventricular and other dysrhythmias: Studies on diseased and ischemic heart. *Progress in Cardiovascular Diseases, 24*, 97–156.
45. Donaldson, S. K., Goldberg, N. D., Walseth, T. F., et al. (1987). Inositol trisphosphate stimulates calcium release from peeled skeletal muscle fibers. *Biochimica et Biophysica Acta, 927*, 92–99.
46. Spach, M. S., & Kootsey, J. M. (1983). The nature of electrical propagation in cardiac muscle. *American Journal of Physiology, 244*, H3–H22.
47. Maylie, J., & Morad, M. (1984). Ionic currents responsible for the generation of pace-maker current in the rabbit sino-atrial node. *Journal of Physiology, 355*, 215–235.
48. de Carvalho, A., & de Almeida, D. (1960). Spread of activity through the atrioventricular node. *Circulation Research, 8*, 801–809.
49. Durrer, D., van Dam, R. T., Freud, G. E., et al. (1970). Total excitation of the isolated human heart. *Circulation, 41*, 899–912.
50. Weidmann, S. (1982). Cardiac cellular physiology and its contribution to electrocardiography. *Japanese Heart Journal, 23* (Suppl.), 12–16.
51. Cohen, M. (1985). *Coronary collaterals: Clinical and experimental observations.* Mt Kisco, New York: Futura.
52. Ringer, S. (1883). A further contribution regarding the influence of the different constituents of the blood on the contraction of the heart. *Journal of Physiology, 4*, 29–42.
53. Franzini-Armstrong, C. (1973). Studies of the triad. IV. Structure of the junction in frog slow fibers. *Journal of Cell Biol, 56*, 120–128.
54. Sperelakis, N. (1979). Propagation mechanisms in heart. *Annual Review of Physiology, 41*, 441–457.
55. Hunter, D. R., Haworth, R. A., & Berkoff, H. A. (1982). Cellular calcium turnover in the perfused rat heart: Modulation by caffeine and procaine. *Circulation Research, 51*, 363–370.
56. Patterson, S. W., & Starling, E. H. (1914). On the mechanical factors which determine the output of the ventricles. *Journal of Physiology, 48*, 357–379.
57. Gordon, A. M., Huxley, A. F., & Julian, F. J. (1966). The variation in isometric tension with sarcomere length in vertebrate muscle fibres. *Journal of Physiology, 184*, 170–192.
58. Lewis, B. S., & Gotsman, M. S. (1980). Current concepts of left ventricular relaxation and compliance. *American Heart Journal, 99*, 101–112.
59. Hood, W. B., Jr., Bianco, J. A., Kumar, R., et al. (1970). Experimental myocardial infarction. IV. Reduction of left ventricular compliance in the healing phase. *Journal of Clinical Investigation, 49*, 1316–1323.
60. Regan, T. J., Frank, M. J., Lehan, P. H., et al. (1963). Myocardial blood flow and oxygen uptake during acute red cell volume increments. *Circulation Research, 13*, 172–181.
61. Klocke, F. J., Braunwald, E., & Ross, J., Jr. (1966). Oxygen cost of electrical activation of the heart. *Circulation Research, 18*, 357–365.
62. Siepser, S. L., Kaltman, A. J., Mills, N., et al. (1972). Coronary collateral flow after traumatic fistula between right coronary artery and right atrium. *New England Journal of Medicine, 287*, 754–756.
63. Zimmerman, H. A. (1952). The coronary circulation in patients with severe emphysema, cor pulmonale, cyanotic congenital heart disease, and severe anemia. *Diseases of the Chest, 22*, 269–273.
64. Barmeyer, J. (1971). Postmortem measurement of intercoronary anastomotic flow in normal and diseased hearts: A quantitative study. *Vascular Surgery, 5*, 239–248.
65. Levin, D. C., Beckmann, C. F., Sos, T. A., et al. (1981). The effect of coronary artery bypass on collateral circulation. *Radiology, 141*, 317–322.

CHAPTER 2

Systemic and Pulmonary Circulation and Oxygen Delivery

Elizabeth J. Bridges / Joseph O. Schmelz

The structural and functional characteristics of the systemic circulation determine the continuous adjustments in flow, pressure, and resistance that occur in each vascular bed and that are vital determinants of tissue function. Blood flow and nutrient exchange in various vascular beds are affected by the structural and metabolic characteristics of the vascular bed, the physical factors that affect flow and the exchange of materials across the blood vessel wall, the local factors originating from the metabolically active cells and vascular endothelium that regulate flow to individual vascular beds, and local and systemic neuroendocrine regulation. The combined regulation of cardiac output, blood pressure, and systemic vascular resistance determines tissue blood flow and, ultimately, the survival of each organ system and the body as a whole. This chapter describes the basic anatomy and physiology of the systemic and pulmonary circulation; Chapter 3 describes the overall regulation of cardiac output and blood pressure.

STRUCTURAL CHARACTERISTICS OF THE VASCULATURE AND LYMPHATICS

Blood vessels are usually classified in the following manner: aorta, large arteries; main arterial branch, small arteries, arterioles; terminal arterioles, capillaries, postcapillary venules; venules, small veins, main venule branch, large veins, and the vena cava.[1–3] These classifications are based on structural characteristics such as diameter, wall thickness, and the presence of muscle. Although blood vessel diameter is often used to characterize different vessels, it is not an appropriate criterion to use for classification, because differences in vessel size reflect the state of vessel contraction as well as differences between organ systems and species.[3,4]

With the exception of the capillaries, the systemic vasculature is composed of three layers: the tunica intima or internal layer, which consists of the endothelium and the basal membrane; the tunica media, which consists of smooth muscle and a matrix of collagen, elastin, and glycoproteins; and the tunica adventitia, which consists of connective tissue (Fig. 2-1). The muscularis in the artery is a concentric ring, which allows for vasoconstriction. In contrast, the venous musculature is organized into small bundles at right angles.[5] In the larger arteries and veins, the tunica adventitia also contains blood vessels that supply the vessel wall (vasa vasorum).[3] The vascular endothelium, which is a metabolically active barrier, is a primary mediator of vascular function and is discussed in detail.

Arteries

Arteries in which the media contains smooth muscle and elastin are called *elastic arteries*.[3] Because of the considerable amount of elastin, these large conducting arteries are able to distend to twice their unloaded length. The ability of the capacitive arteries to distend is important in cushioning pulsatile flow, such that the blood flow to the organs/tissue is almost a constant flow. During systole, the aorta and proximal large vessels store approximately 50% to 60% of the stroke volume. During diastole, the distended vessels recoil and move the remaining blood to the periphery. This phenomenon is referred to as a "Windkessel function," which is the transformation of pulsatile flow in the central arteries to constant flow in the periphery.[6] As the arteries approach the periphery, they become smaller in diameter, and there is a relative decrease in elastin and a relative increase in smooth muscle in the tunica media.[7,8] These peripheral arteries are referred to as *muscular arteries*.

The small arteries (prearteriolar vessels with a diameter less than 500 mm) receive nervous stimulation primarily from noradrenergic stimuli, with the nerve terminals located in the adventitia. Unlike the larger arteries, in which sympathetic neural constriction is activated by α_1 and postsynaptic α_2 receptors, the small arteries are noradrenergically constricted mainly by the postsynaptic α_2 receptors.[8,9] The small arteries are also sensitive to endothelium-derived relaxing and contracting factors. Of clinical importance, abnormal small artery wall structure is an independent predictor of cardiovascular events (e.g., stroke, myocardial infarction, death).[10,11] However, it may be possible to reverse these changes with vasodilator therapy.[12]

Microvascular Bed

The term *microcirculation* denotes the vascular and lymphatic microcirculation. The vascular microcirculation consists of (1) large and small arterioles (*precapillary resistance vessels*); (2) terminal arterioles, which in many tissues serve as so-called precapillary sphincters; and (3) other precapillary structures such as capillaries; and (4) nonmuscular venules, known collectively as the exchange vessels, and muscular venules (postcapillary resistance vessels). The term *lymphatic microvasculature* refers specifically to the terminal lymphatic vessels.

Arterioles

As the vessel diameter decreases from the small arteries to the arterioles, the number of smooth muscle layers decreases from approximately six layers in the 300-μm vessels to a single layer of irregularly dispersed smooth muscle in the 30- to 50-μm vessels.[7] At this point, the vessels are referred to as *arterioles*. The smallest arteriolar branches (8 to 20 μm in diameter) are called the *terminal arterioles*.[13] In some cases, smooth muscle extends beyond the intersection of the terminal arterioles with the nonmuscular capillaries into structures known as *precapillary sphincters*.[14] The terminal arterioles and precapillary sphincters control the distribution of blood supply to the exchange vessels.[15]

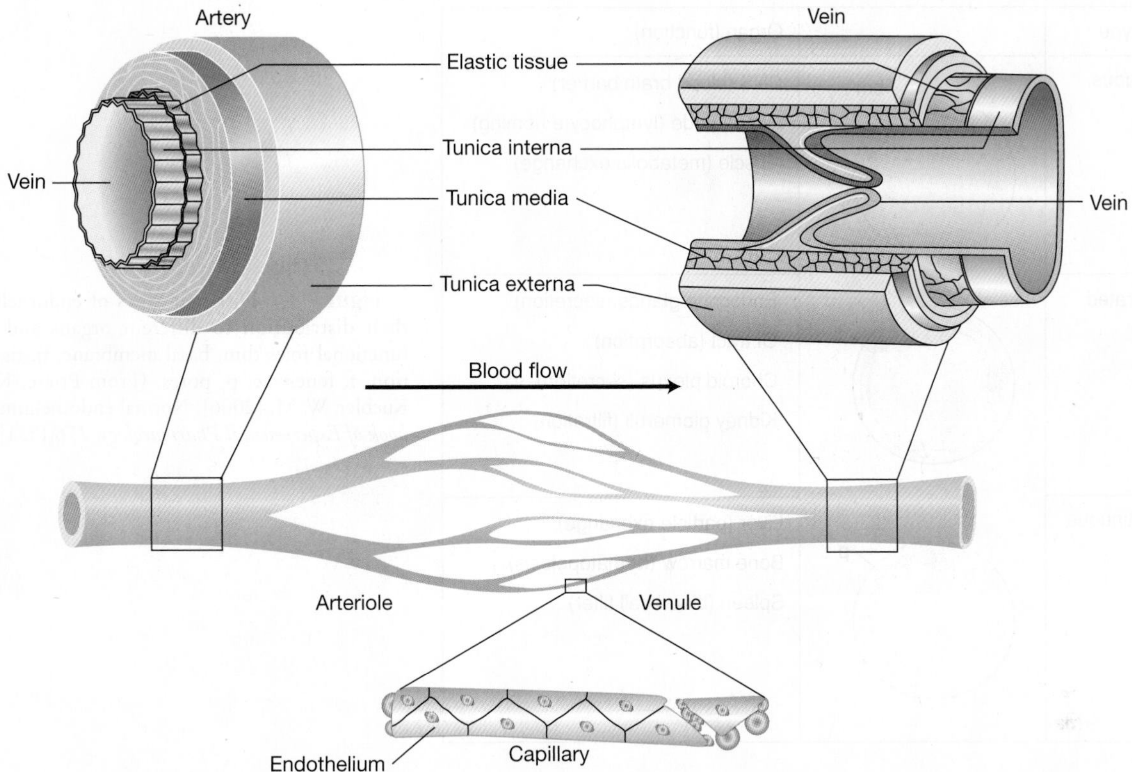

■ **Figure 2-1** Schematic drawing of the major structural characteristics of the principal segments of blood vessels. The relative amounts of elastic tissue and fibrous tissues are largest in the aorta and least in small branches of the arterial tree. Small vessels have more prominent smooth muscle in the media. Capillaries consist only of endothelial cells. The walls of the veins are much like the arterial walls, but are thinner in relation to their caliber. (From iDAMS 3746-08-17.)

Capillaries

Capillaries branch from terminal arteriolar segments. The capillary wall consists of endothelial cells and basal lamina; there is no tunica media or adventitia. Capillary diameter is 4 to 8 mm, which is just large enough to allow the deformable red blood cells to pass through.[14,16] Not all exchange vessels in an area are simultaneously open. During periods of increased metabolism, capillary recruitment increases the number of open and perfused exchange vessels, thereby decreasing the distances for diffusion between exchange blood vessels and cells, as well as increasing the total surface area for exchange between the capillaries and cells.[13]

In microvascular beds located in the ears, fingers, and toes in humans and many other mammals, there are arteriovenous vascular channels that bypass the exchange vessels and allow blood to flow directly from arterioles to venules.[13] These arteriovenous anastomoses, which are richly innervated by the sympathetic nervous system, are important in local temperature control in these areas and even of the whole body in some conditions.[17]

Exchange Vessel Endothelium

The endothelium of exchange vessels in various organs contains at least four different structures that determine the rate of filtration and bulk transport of water and solutes and the exchange of larger molecules (Fig. 2-2). The structure of the membrane (continuous, fenestrated, discontinuous and tight junction) varies depending on the location of the vascular bed.[18] All four types of endothelium have a continuous basement membrane, with the exception of the discontinuous endothelium.

Continuous endothelium is found in skin; skeletal, smooth, and cardiac muscle; and the lungs. There are several mechanisms by which substances pass through continuous endothelium. Water and solutes pass through intercellular junctions (40 to 1 Å) driven predominantly by a pressure gradient (ΔP) driving fluid out of the vessels. This outward flow is partly counterbalanced by forces drawing water back into the vessels. Lipid-soluble substances (CO_2, O_2) pass directly through the cell by diffusion; cytoplasmic vesicles transport solutes and water back and forth through the endothelium; and vesicles intermittently fuse to create channels in the cell. The junctions between the cells are responsible for the high permeability of the membrane to "ultrafiltrate," or protein-free fluid, and for the rapid diffusion of small ions. The continuous endothelium is relatively impermeable to plasma proteins and large molecules.

Fenestrated vascular endothelium is located in the gastrointestinal mucosa, glands, renal glomerular capillaries, and peritubular capillaries. The endothelium has openings (fenestrae) that expose the basement membrane (renal glomerular capillaries) or are covered by a thin diaphragm (gastrointestinal mucosa, renal peritubular capillaries). The fenestrated endothelium has a higher permeability to water and small solute molecules than continuous endothelium, whereas its permeability to plasma proteins is low, similar to continuous endothelium.[13]

Discontinuous endothelium is located in the hepatic cells, bone marrow, and splenic sinusoids. Discontinuous endothelium contains gaps in the endothelium and basement membrane and is permeable to proteins and other large molecules.

Phenotype		Organ (function)
Continuous	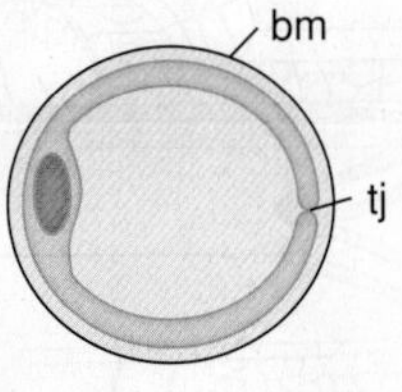 bm tj	CNS (blood brain barrier) Lymph node (lymphocyte homing) Muscle (metabolic exchange)
Fenestrated	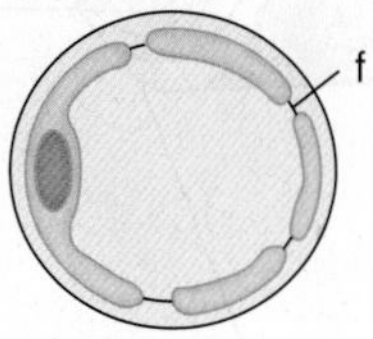 f	Endocrine glands (secretion) GI tract (absorption) Choroid plexus (secretion) Kidney glomeruli (filtration)
Discontinuous	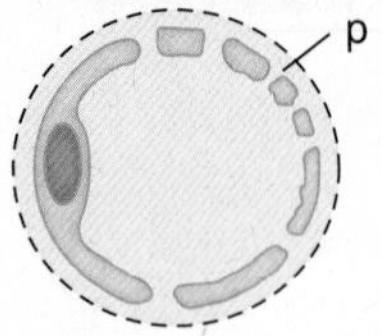 p	Liver (particle exchange) Bone marrow (hematopoiesis) Spleen (blood cell filter)

■ **Figure 2-2** Different types of endothelial cells, their distribution to different organs and specific functional roles (bm, basal membrane, tj, tight junction, f, fenestrae, p, pores. (From Priese, K. R., & Kuebler, W. M. [2006]. Normal endothelium. *Handbook of Experimental Pharmacology, 176*[Pt. 1], 1–40.)

Tight-junction endothelium is located in the central nervous system and retina. It is the least permeable. The endothelial cells are connected by tight junctions that effectively restrict passage of all substances. Water- and lipid-soluble molecules pass directly through the endothelium, whereas ions and lipid-insoluble substances, such as glucose and amino acids, are transported by membrane carriers.[19]

Venules

Venous capillaries extend to the postcapillary venules (nonmuscular, 7 to 50 μm) and collecting venules. Along with the capillaries, the nonmuscular venules act as exchange vessels. Smooth muscle reappears in venules that are approximately 30 to 50 μm in diameter. These venules, which receive adrenergic innervation, are referred to as the muscular venules, postcapillary resistance vessels, or capacitance vessels.[2,13,16] As discussed later in the section on microcirculation, postcapillary resistance tends to be far less than precapillary resistance and has almost no effect on overall systemic vascular resistance. The veins contain approximately 70% of total blood volume, with approximately 25% of this volume in the venules.[2]

Veins

In general, veins have a larger diameter and thinner, more compliant walls than arteries at equivalent branches of the vascular tree.[2] However, the thickness of the venous walls is variable. For example, the veins in the legs and feet, which withstand the high hydrostatic pressure associated with standing, are thick-walled, whereas the veins near or above the level of the heart are thin-walled. The veins contain all three vascular layers found in the arteries; however, these layers are often indistinct.[3] Superficial veins form a rich anastomosis with deeper veins via vessels that perforate the muscles. These perforating veins allow venous return from cold skin to be diverted to warm muscle, providing a thermal short circuit, and they are particularly important for function of the muscle pump, which is described in Chapter 3.

Venous Valves

With the exception of the intrathoracic and intracerebral veins, the medium-sized veins contain valves that are oriented in the direction of blood flow, thus preventing retrograde blood flow into the muscle.[2] The presence of competent valves, in conjunction with the muscle pump in the lower extremities, is crucial to the ability to stand erect and in maintaining a reasonably low capillary pressure, because the valves interrupt the hydrostatic column that extends from the right atrium to the feet after each leg muscle contraction.[20] After humans with normal valvular function stand up, the valves in dependent veins initially interrupt the hydrostatic column. However, over a period of approximately 2 to 3 minutes, as the veins fill with blood, the valves can no longer interrupt the hydrostatic column as volume continues to accumulate. At this time, there is a displacement of approximately 600 mL of blood from the central circulation into the legs and pelvic organs.[21] In conditions in which blood flow is high, the hydrostatic effects associated with the loss of valvular function occur within 2 to 3 seconds. If the hydrostatic effects are not overcome by the muscle pump in the lower extremities, arterial hypotension, and syncope result. This phenomenon is readily seen in the soldier who faints while standing motionless at attention. There is also some evidence that there are microscopic venous valves located in the small veins and also in the post-capillary venules.[22] These microscopic valves may play a protective role against venous hypertension when there is valvular insufficiency in larger veins.

Venoconstriction

In contrast to the arteries, not all veins constrict when exposed to norepinephrine. For example, the postcapillary venules ranging from 0.007 to 2 mm in diameter do not have smooth muscle and therefore cannot constrict.[23] Most of the larger venules and small veins (including veins in the skeletal muscle) contain some smooth muscle,[2] but they are sparsely innervated and are not considered sites of vasoconstriction. The lack of venoconstriction in the skeletal muscle is important because the leg veins do not constrict in orthostasis. The splanchnic organs (liver, gastrointestinal tract, pancreas, and spleen) are the exception because they are richly innervated by sympathetic noradrenergic fibers and are capable of venoconstriction. In addition, the veins in the skin respond to thermoregulatory reflexes. In humans, significant venoconstriction occurs only in the splanchnic circulation; in response to thermoregulatory reflexes, the veins in the skin constrict and dilate.[17,24,25]

Lymphatics

The lymphatics are a system of thin-walled vessels that collect and conduct lymph through active contraction of the lymphatic microvasculature to the central circulation.[26–28] Lymph consists primarily of ultrafiltrate and proteins that have been filtered from exchange vessels. The initial lymphatic vessels (also known as terminal lymphatics or lymph capillaries), which consist of endothelialized tubes, originate in large, blind-terminal bulbs located in the connective tissue of most organ systems.[29] The lymphatic capillaries empty into collecting lymphatics, which in turn empty into transporting lymphatic vessels (Fig. 2-3). The central lymphatic vessels empty into the left and right lymphatic ducts, which empty into the subclavian veins.

A very small and transient pressure gradient between the interstitium and the terminal lymphatics promotes fluid movement into the lymphatics. Beginning at the level of the collecting capillaries, there are bicuspid valves, and the larger lymphatics contain smooth muscle that spontaneously contracts in a rhythmic manner.[30] The primary mechanism underlying the peristaltic like lymphatic flow is the intrinsic contraction of the lymphangions, which are the functional unit of lymphatic vessels, consisting of the valve and portion of the vessel surrounding the valve. The intrinsic contraction remains active during rest, anesthesia, and immobilization.[31] Lymphatic flow is also facilitated by lymph formation, skeletal muscle contractions (e.g., walking, foot flexing), respiration, fluctuations of central venous pressure, gastrointestinal peristalsis, and arterial pulsations.[32]

Vascular Smooth Muscle

Vascular smooth muscle contains the contractile filaments, actin and myosin; however, unlike striated smooth muscle (cardiac), the filaments are not organized in any fashion.[33] Although the sarcoplasmic reticulum is not as prominent in vascular smooth muscle as in cardiac muscle, it serves as the primary intracellular source of calcium.[34] Additionally, the amount of myosin in smooth muscle is approximately one-fifth that found in striated muscle. Despite this lower amount of myosin, smooth muscle develops higher force per cross-sectional area than striated muscle. Vascular smooth muscle also usually contracts more slowly than striated muscle, and it maintains tonic contractions with lower energy [adenosine triphosphate (ATP)] expenditure.

Smooth muscle is characterized as "phasic" and "tonic." Phasic vascular smooth muscle, which is capable of high shortening velocities, is located in the portal veins. Tonic vascular smooth muscle is located in most of the small arteries and arterioles and has a slower shortening velocity, but it is capable of maintaining sustained vascular tone.[35] As in cardiac and skeletal muscle, contraction of vascular smooth muscle is related to the formation and release of crossbridges by the cyclic attachment and detachment of the heads of the contractile protein myosin with actin (see Chapter 1). Tonic contractions allow for the maintenance of a basal vascular tone, which is crucial for the maintenance of arterial blood pressure. These tonic contractions are the result of a "latch bridge," which is a slowing in the cross-bridge cycling rate. Other possible mechanisms for the tonic contraction include increased calcium sensitivity and inhibition by agonists of proteins (e.g., caldesmon) that bind actin and interfere with the inhibitory effects of calcium–calmodulin.[36]

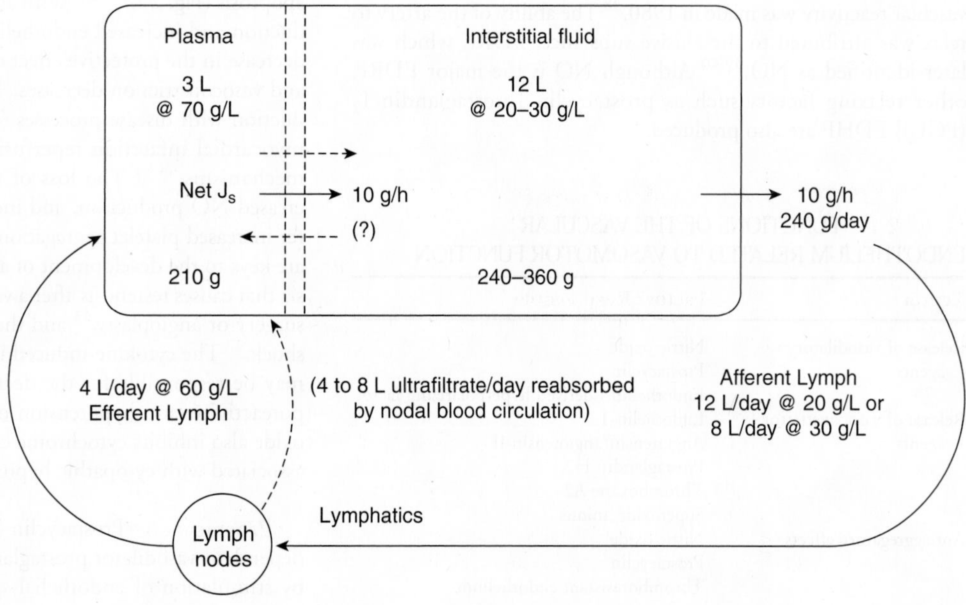

Figure 2-3 Steady-state distribution and circulation of fluid (ultrafiltrate) and plasma proteins in a normal human (weight, 65 kg). The double-dashed line between plasma and interstitial fluid represents exchange vessel endothelium. The weights at the bottoms of the boxes represent the total content of each. (From Renkin, E. M. [1986]. Some consequences of capillary permeability to macromolecules: Starling's hypothesis reconsidered. *American Journal of Physiology, 250*, H706–H710.)

LOCAL REGULATION

In addition to the systemic factors that affect vascular resistance, there are local factors that control resistance. These factors include autacoids, endothelium-derived vasoactive substances, local metabolic factors that match blood flow (oxygen transport) to metabolism, autoregulation (see Chapter 3), and local heating and cooling.

Autacoids

The autacoids (vasoactive substances) include histamine, serotonin, prostaglandin, and bradykinin. These factors most often compete with adrenergic (vasoconstrictive) effects and exert a local vasodilatory effect, which can improve tissue perfusion. The autacoids are not involved in systemic regulation of blood pressure or total peripheral resistance; however, they initiate or modify the vascular response to other stimuli.

Endothelium-Derived Vasoactive Substances

The vascular endothelium, which is a single layer of squamous cells in the tunica intima that lines the entire vascular tree, modulates vascular tone by secreting dilator and constrictor substances. In addition, the endothelium affects platelet adhesion and aggregation and under basal conditions substances secreted by the endothelium affect the clotting cascade.[37] The endothelium is also involved in the regulation of vascular smooth muscle proliferation.[37] The proposed functions of the vascular endothelium (Table 2-1) require an intact endothelium.[38] The control of vascular tone involves cross talk between the vasodilators nitric oxide (NO), prostaglandins, and endothelial-derived hyperpolarizing factor (EDHF) and the vasoconstrictors endothelin-1 and prostacyclin (Fig. 2-4). A discussion of each of these factors related to vascular control follows. A summary of the stimuli that cause the release of each of the factors is presented in Table 2-2.

Endothelium-Derived Relaxing Factors

The seminal observation that endothelium is a key mediator of vascular reactivity was made in 1980.[38] The ability of the artery to relax was attributed to the elusive substance, EDRF, which was later identified as NO.[39,40] Although NO is the major EDRF, other relaxing factors such as prostacyclin [prostaglandin I_2 (PGI_2)] EDHF are also produced.

Table 2-1 ■ FUNCTIONS OF THE VASCULAR ENDOTHELIUM RELATED TO VASOMOTOR FUNCTION

Action	Factors Responsible
Release of vasodilatory agents	Nitric oxide Prostacyclin Endothelium-derived hyperpolarizing factor
Release of vasoconstrictor agents	Endothelin-1 Angiotensin/angiotensin II Prostaglandin H2 Thromboxane A2 Superoxide anions
Antiaggregatory effects	Nitric oxide Prostacyclin Thromboresistant endothelium

Nitric Oxide. NO is a gas with an extremely short half-life (seconds) that diffuses into vascular smooth muscle cells and causes vasodilation.[40–42] NO production is stimulated by the enzyme nitric oxide synthase (NOS). There are two constitutive forms of NOS: endothelial NOS (eNOS) and neurological NOS (nNOS). Inducible NOS (iNOS), which is present only under pathological conditions, generates 100- to 1000-fold more NO than the constitutive forms.

Shear stress and vasoactive substances are the primary factors involved in the release of NO for control of vasomotor tone (Fig. 2-5). The activation of eNOS is different for these two mechanisms. Shear stress through G proteins (Gs) leads to eNOS activation, which via the inositol triphosphate (IP_3) pathway causes hyperpolarization of the endothelial cells, which allows calcium to flow into the cell.[43,44] The increased intracellular calcium binds to calmodulin, which releases eNOS from the inhibitory protein calveolin. The eNOS catalyzes the conversion of L-arginine to NO. After NO is formed in the endothelial cells, it diffuses out of the endothelial cell to the vascular smooth muscle and as described below causes vasodilation. Nitric oxide also has secondary vasodilatory effects through the inhibition of the release of the vasoconstrictor endothelin-1 (ET_1), although this beneficial effect decreases with age.[45,46]

Autocoids and hormones cause the release of NO from the endothelium (Fig. 2-6).[47] These substances (Table 2-2) cause the release of IP_3, which leads to an increase in intracellular calcium and subsequently stimulates the release of NO. Additionally, NO decreases sympathetic vasoconstriction by inhibiting the release of norepinephrine at the supraspinal, spinal, and synaptic levels.[48] Clinically, nitrovasodilators (e.g., nitroglycerin and sodium nitroprusside) cause vasodilation by the donation of NO or NO-like compound.[49,50] Of note, nitroglycerin-induced coronary artery vasodilation does not require the presence of an intact endothelium. In addition, ACE inhibitors, calcium channel blockers, statins, and phosphodiesterase inhibitors indirectly stimulate NO release or enhance its bioavailability.[51]

Nitric oxide also inhibits platelet activation, aggregation, and adhesion (i.e., anticoagulant/profibrinolytic phenotype), leukocyte adhesion,[52] vascular smooth muscle proliferation, and it inhibits endothelial cell apoptosis but stimulates vascular smooth muscle apoptosis (Fig. 2-6).[37,53] With aging there is a decrease in NO production and increased endothelial cell apoptosis, which leads to a decrease in the protective effect of NO against platelet aggregation and vasoconstriction decreases. There is also diminished NO production with disease processes (e.g., hypertension, diabetes, postmyocardial infarction reperfusion injuries) and altered defense mechanisms.[44,54] The loss of the protective endothelium, decreased NO production, and increased NO degradation may foster increased platelet aggregation and vascular proliferation, which are keys to the development of atherosclerosis,[55] intimal hyperplasia that causes restenosis after a vascular intervention such as bypass surgery or angioplasty,[53] and the procoagulant state seen in septic shock.[37] The cytokine-induced increase in NO synthesis by iNOS may be responsible for the decreased vascular tone, vascular hyporeactivity, and hypotension observed in septic shock.[56] Nitric oxide also inhibits cytochrome c oxidase, which may be one factor associated with cytopathic hypoxia in sepsis.[57,58]

Prostacyclin. Prostacyclin (PGI_2) is a cyclooxygenase (COX) dependent vasodilator prostaglandin, which is released transiently by stimulation of endothelial-specific receptors. Prostacyclin receptor stimulation causes an increase in intracellular calcium,

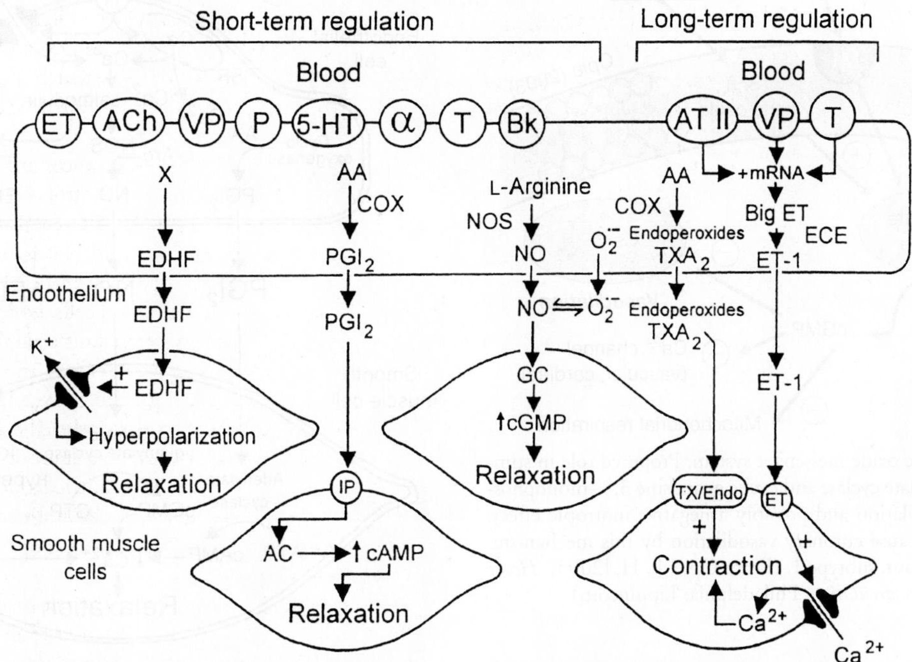

■ **Figure 2-4** Activation of endothelial receptors can stimulate NO synthase (NOS, with the production of nitric oxide [NO]) and cyclooxygenase (COX), which produces prostacyclin (PGI_2) from arachidonic acid (AA) and can lead to the release of EDHF. NO causes relaxation by activating the formation of cyclic GMP (cGMP) from guanosine triphosphate (GTP) by soluble guanylate cyclase (GC). PGI_2 causes relaxation by activating adenylate cyclase (AC) leading to the formation of cyclic AMP (cAMP). EDHF causes hyperpolarization and relaxation by opening K^+ channels. Any increase in cytosolic calcium (including that induced by calcium ionophore A23187) causes the release of relaxing factors. In certain blood vessels, contracting substances can be released from the endothelial cells, which include superoxide anions (O_2^-), thromboxane A_2 (TXA_2), endoperoxides, and possibly ET_1. Thromboxane A_2 and endoperoxides activate specific receptors (TX/Endo) on the vascular smooth muscle, as does ET_1. Such activation causes an increase in intracellular Ca^{2+} leading to contraction. The production of ET_1 (catalyzed by endothelin converting enzyme [ECE]) can be augmented by angiotensin II (ATII), vasopressin (VP), or thrombin (T). The neurohumoral mediators that cause the release of endothelium-derived relaxing factors (and sometimes contracting factors) through activation of specific endothelial receptors (circles) include acetylcholine (ACh), adenosine diphosphate (P), bradykinin (BK), endothelin (ET), adrenaline (α), serotonin (5HT), T, and VP. (From Vanhoutte, P. M. [1999]. How to assess endothelial function in human blood vessels. *Journal of Hypertension, 17,* 1047–1058.)

Table 2-2 ■ ENDOTHELIUM-DERIVED VASODILATING AND VASOCONSTRICTING FACTORS

Factors	Stimuli
Vasodilating Factors	
Nitric oxide Endothelium-derived relaxing factor Prostacyclin Endothelium-derived hyperpolarizing factor	Acetylcholine, histamine, arginine vasopressin, epinephrine, norepinephrine, bradykinin, adenosine diphosphate, serotonin (from aggregating platelets), thrombin (from coagulation cascade)
Vasoconstricting Factors	
Endothelium-derived contracting factor	Physical stimuli (mechanical stretch), arachidonic acid (endothelial injury and platelet aggregation), serotonin, adenosine platelet diphosphate
Endothelin-1	Thrombin, interleukin-1, epinephrine, angiotensin II, arginine vasopressin
Prostanoids	Endothelin-1, endothelial membrane damage
Superoxide anions	Physical stress (e.g., shear stress, postischemic reperfusion), chemical endothelial stimulants (bradykinin, cytokines)

which activates phospholipase A_2 and subsequently releases arachidonic acid. Under basal conditions the arachidonic acid is then metabolized by COX-1, which results in the production of prostaglandin H2 (PGH_2) and subsequently PGI_2.[59] Prostacylin binds to receptors on vascular smooth muscle and platelets and through G-protein mediated activation of adenylate cyclase increases cyclic adenosine monophosphate (cAMP) (Fig. 2-7). Increased cAMP stimulates potassium-induced cellular hyperpolarization and the phosphorylation of protein kinase A (PKA), which increases calcium extrusion from the cell and causes vasodilation and also inhibits platelet activation.[59] Prostacylin also act through peroxisome proliferator-activated receptor (PPAR)β/δ, which causes a decrease in intracellular calcium and subsequent vasodilation and platelet inhibition through mechanisms that are still being studied. There is cross talk between PGI_2 and NO and they have synergistic vasodilatory and antithrombotic actions. Prostacyclin increases NO release and, concomitantly, NO prolongs the effect of prostacyclin by inhibiting its breakdown.[59,60]

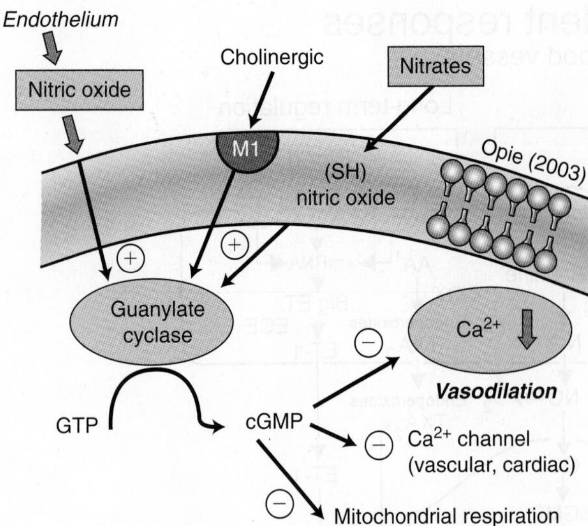

■ **Figure 2-5** Nitric oxide messenger system. Proposed role in stimulating soluble guanylate cyclase and cyclic guanosine 3,5′-monophosphate to cause vasodilation and possibly a negative inotropic effect. Antianginal nitrates cause coronary vasodilation by this mechanism. M1, muscarinic receptor, subtype 1. (From Opie, L. H. [2004]. *Heart physiology: From cell to circulation*. Philadelphia: Lippincott.)

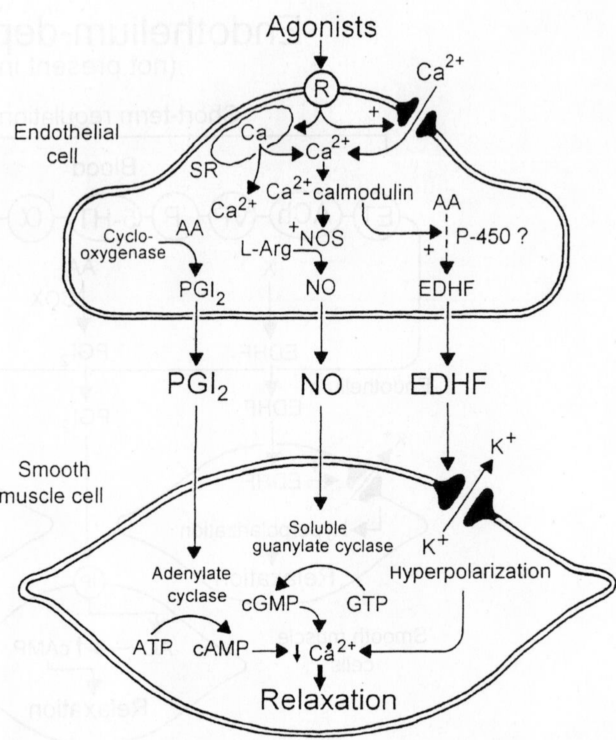

■ **Figure 2-7** Schematic summarizing the release of relaxing factors from endothelial cells and their effect on vascular smooth muscle cells. Ach, acetylcholine; A23187, calcium ionophore A21837; BK, bradykinin; B2, bradykinin B2 receptor; cAMP, cyclic adenosine monophosphate; cGMP, cyclic guanosine monophosphate; EDHF, endothelium-derived hyperpolarizing factor; EET, epoxyeicosatrienoic acid; K^+; potassium channel; M1, M3, muscarinic M1 or M3 receptor subtypes; NOS, nitric oxide synthase; PGI_2, prostacyclin; P450, cytochrome P450 monooxygenase; TBA, tetrabutylammonium; TEA, tetraethylammonium. The *broken line* indicates the action of an inhibitor or an antagonist. (From Mombouli, J. V., & Vanhoutte, P. M. [1999]. Endothelial dysfunction: From physiology to therapy. *Journal of Molecular Cell Cardiology, 31*, 61–74.)

Endothelium-Derived Hyperpolarizing Factors. Vasodilation of arterioles is also mediated by non-NO/non-prostanoid EDHFs.[61,62] EDHF may be the predominant mechanism for vasodilation in smaller diameter vessels (i.e., resistance arteries <300 μm) in contrast to larger vessels where NO is the dominant vasodilator.[63] There are four putative EDHFs: the enzyme cytochrome p450 monooxygenase (cytochrome P-450), potassium, hydrogen peroxide, and C-type natriuretic peptide.[62] EDHFs, which may be considered a mechanism as much as a factor,[63] are synthesized in response to wall shear stress or the binding of bradykinin and acetylcholine or substance P to endothelial cell receptors. EDHF diffuses from the endothelium to the vascular smooth muscle where it

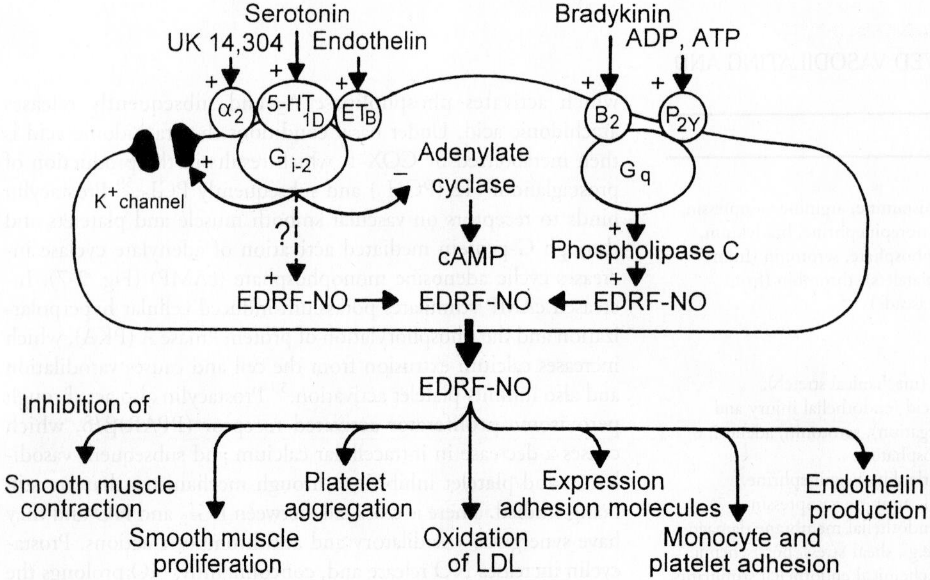

■ **Figure 2-6** Postulated signal transduction processes in a normal endothelial cell. Activation of the cell causes the release of NO, which has important protective effects in the vascular wall. α, alpha-adrenergic; 5-HT, serotonin receptor; EDHF, endothelium-derived hyperpolarizing factor; ET, endothelin receptors; B, bradykinin receptor; P, purinoreceptor; G, coupling proteins; cAMP, cyclic adenosine monophosphate; NO, nitric oxide; LDL, low-density lipoproteins; +, activation; –, inhibition. (Modified from Vanhoutte, P. M. [1999]. Endothelial dysfunction and vascular disease. In J. A. Panza, & R. O. Cannon (Eds.), *Endothelium, nitric oxide and atherosclerosis*. New York: Futura Publishing.)

causes endothelium-dependent hyperpolarization, which in turn decreases cytosolic calcium and causes vasorelaxation through the various mediator-specific pathways (Fig. 2-8).[61]

In hypertension or hypercholesterolemia, when NO-mediated vasodilation is decreased, there may be a compensatory upregulation of EDHF-mediated vasorelaxation.[64] Of note, there may be gender-specific EDHF compensatory response, with increased EDHF activity in females but not in males.[62] However, oxidative stress associated with atherosclerosis, hyperhomocysteinemia, and possibly poorly controlled diabetes can decrease this compensatory response.[64–66]

Endothelium-Derived Contracting Factors

The endothelium-derived contracting factors include ET_1, the vasoconstrictor prostanoids, PGH_2, the precursor of thromboxane A2 (TXA_2); superoxide anions (O_2^-); and components of the renin–angiotensin–aldosterone system. These substances are released in response to vasoconstrictive stimuli (see Fig. 2-4). Vasoconstriction also occurs as a result of a decrease in endothelial production of NO.

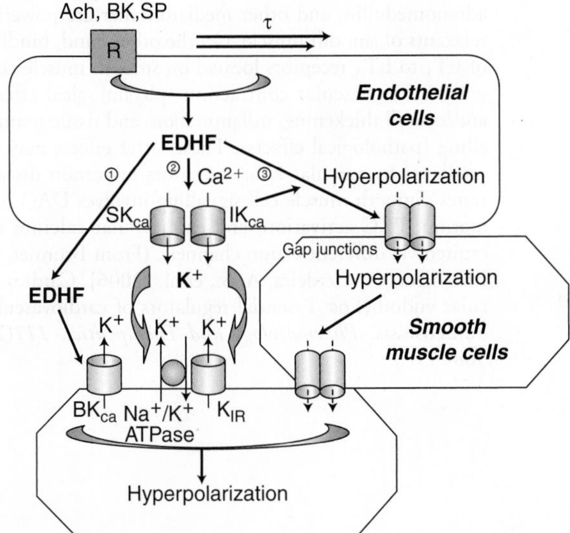

■ **Figure 2-8** Schematic description of the main hyperpolarizing mechanisms mediated by endothelium-derived hyperpolarizing factor (EDHF). The binding of acetylcholine (Ach), bradykinin (BK), and substance P (SP) to their endothelial receptors and the increase in wall shear stress (τ) promote the synthesis of EDHF. EDHF can then hyperpolarize the smooth muscle cells by three principal pathways. EDHF can passively diffuse from the endothelium to activate calcium-activated potassium (K_{Ca}) channels of large conductance (BK_{Ca}) located on the smooth muscle cells thereby promoting the release of K^+ and membrane hyperpolarization. EDHF can act in an autocrine manner to facilitate the activation of the endothelial K_{Ca} channels of small (SK_{Ca}) and intermediate (IK_{Ca}) conductance directly mediated by Ca^{2+} inducing the release of K^+ and the hyperpolarization of the endothelial cells. Then, the hyperpolarization is transmitted electronically through the myoendothelial gap junctions into the smooth muscle cell layer and/or the K^+ released from the endothelial SK_{Ca} and IK_{Ca} channels into the myoendothelial space activates the Na^+/K^+ ATPase and the inward rectifying potassium channels (K_{IR}) located on the smooth muscle cells promoting the release of K^+ and subsequent hyperpolarization of these cells. EDHF can enhance gap junctional communication. Finally, the smooth muscle cells hyperpolarization decreases the open-state of voltage-gate Ca^{2+} channels lowering cytosolic Ca^{2+} and thereby provoking vasorelaxation. (From Bellien, J., Thuillez, C., & Joannides, R. [2008]. Contribution of endothelium-derived hyperpolarizing factors to the regulation of vascular tone in humans. *Fundamental of Clinical Pharmacology, 22*(4), 363–377.)

Endothelin-1. In humans there are three isoforms of endothelin.[67] ET_1, which is the primary isoform in the cardiovascular system, is thought to be the most potent vasoconstrictor known. ET_1 is an amino acid peptide that binds to vascular smooth muscle membrane receptors ET_A (located on vascular smooth muscle) and ET_B (located on vascular smooth muscle and endothelial surfaces). Binding of ET_1 to the ET_A and ET_B receptors on the vascular smooth muscle activates the phospholipase C (PLC)-IP_3 pathway, which increases intracellular calcium and the phosphorylation of myosin kinase and causes prolonged muscle contraction. In contrast, under normal resting conditions, the circulating plasma level of ET_1 is very low and it acts locally, in a paracrine fashion, to cause vasodilation through the endothelial synthesis of NO and PGI_2.[68,69] The production of ET_1 can be augmented by shear stress, angiotensin II (AII), vasopressin, oxygen free radicals, thrombin, and platelet-derived transforming growth factor and inhibited by NO, atrial natriuretic polypeptide, B-type natriuretic peptide, and prostacylin[70] (Fig. 2-9).

The effects of ET_1 are important clinically. In pathological conditions such as heart failure, increased ET_1 levels are associated with increased morbidity and mortality[71] and may play an important role in the disease pathogenesis.[64] For example, ET_1 stimulates the renin–angiotensin–aldosterone system, which enhances the conversion of angiotensin I to AII, causing a synergistic augmentation of vasoconstriction and sodium retention.[70] In addition, in heart failure, ET_1 has an negative inotropic effect.[68] ET_1 may play a role in salt-sensitive hypertension although the mechanism remains unclear.[68,72] Unfortunately antagonism of ET_1 receptors has not been found to improve outcomes for patients with heart failure or hypertension.[73–75] ET_1 levels are increased with hypercholesterolemia and increased ET_1 levels may be a marker for endothelial dysfunction. Possible pathological mechanisms for ET_1 in atherosclerosis and restenosis after angioplasty include increased fibrous tissue formation, inhibition of eNOS formation, stimulation of platelet aggregation, vascular smooth muscle proliferation, and inflammation of the vessel wall.[69,76,77] There is also a link between ET_1 and idiopathic pulmonary arterial hypertension and inhibition of ET_1 has been shown to improve outcomes for these patients.[78,79]

Prostanoids. Two prostanoids that have vasoconstrictive actions are PGH_2 and TXA_2. Similar to prostacyclin, arachidonic acid is converted by COX-1 to PGH_2. PGH_2 is then converted to TXA_2 by thromboxane synthase or as discussed above, to prostacyclin.[80] TXA_2, which acts in a paracrine fashion, causes platelet activation, vasoconstriction, and smooth muscle proliferation, and it is thought to play an important role in the pathogenesis of myocardial infarction. The rationale for the administration of COX-1 antagonists [e.g., nonsteroidal anti-inflammatory drugs (NSAIDs), aspirin] in cardiovascular disease is to inhibit platelet production of TXA_2, which reduces cardiovascular morbidity and mortality;[81,82] however, in patients where there is incomplete TXA_2 inhibition, there is still a risk for cardiovascular events.[83] A negative side effect of the COX-1 antagonists is that they are toxic to the gastric mucosa.

Because of the negative side effects of COX-1 antagonists, the use of selective PGH2 or COX-2 inhibitors (coxibs), which are not toxic to the gastrointestinal tract, were evaluated. However, several studies of coxibs found an increased incidence of adverse

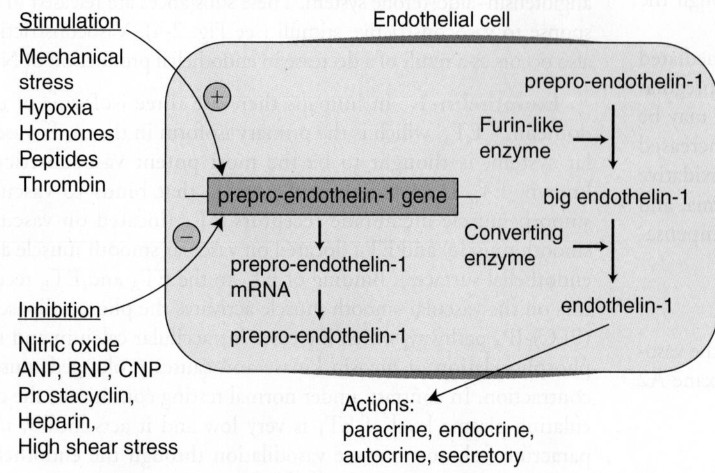

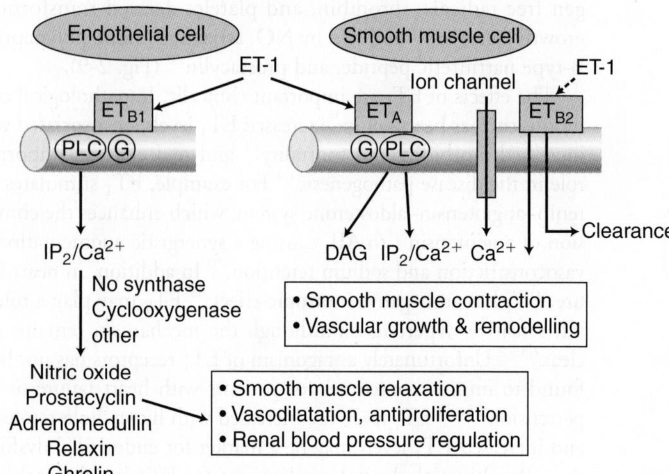

Figure 2-9 A. Synthesis of endothelin receptors (ET) and its regulation. The release of active ET_1 is controlled via regulation of gene transcription and/or endothelin converting enzyme activity. ET_1 synthesis is stimulated by several factors, of which hypoxia seems to be the most important. ET_1 formation is down regulated by activators of the NO/cGMP pathway and other factors. **B.** Vascular actions of ET. In healthy blood vessels, the main action of ET_1 is indirect vasodilation mediated by ET_B receptors located on endothelial cells. Their activation generates a Ca^{2+} signal via PLC that turns on the generation of nitric oxide (NO), prostacyclin, adrenomedullin, and other mediators that are powerful relaxants of smooth muscle. On the other hand, binding of ET_1 to ET_A receptors located on smooth muscle cells will lead to vascular contraction (physiological effect) and/or wall thickening, inflammation, and tissue remodelling (pathological effects). These latter effects may be mediated by vascular ET_{B2} receptors in certain disease states. Smooth muscle cell signalling involves DAG formation, PKC activation, and extracellular calcium recruited via different cation channels. (From Brunner, F., Bras-Silva, C., Cerdeira, A. S., et al. [2006]. Cardiovascular endothelins: Essential regulators of cardiovascular homeostasis. *Pharmacology and Therapeutics, 111*(2), 508–531.)

serious cardiovascular events, including myocardial infarction and stroke.[84,85] This increased risk resulted in the Food and Drug Administration requiring labeling of all selective and nonselective NSAIDs to reflect the possibility of an increased risk for myocardial infarction and stroke with their use.[86] It is important to note that the increased risk varies depending on the medication[87–89] and a prospective clinical trial is ongoing to determine the cardiovascular risk of selective and nonselective NSAIDS. The probable mechanism of these adverse effects is that while COX-2 inhibitors do not inhibit thromboxane they do inhibit vascular prostacyclin causing increased systolic blood pressure and platelet activation, which increases the likelihood of thrombus formation.[90–92]

Reactive Oxygen Species. In response to physical stresses, such as oscillatory shear stress, postischemic reperfusion, and chemical endothelial stimulants (bradykinin, cytokines, AII), the endothelium and vascular smooth muscle produce reactive oxygen species (ROS), which are metabolites of oxygen. Example of ROS include superoxide (O_2^-), hydrogen peroxide, and peroxynitrite ($ONOO^-$), which is the product of NO and O_2^-.[93] These ROS inhibit NO, EDHF, and prostacyclin pathways and guanalyl cyclase (Fig. 2-10), increase calcium mobilization and the production of the vasoconstrictors PGH_2 and TXA_2, decrease NO-mediated vasorelaxation, and play a role in endothelial dysfunction.[64,93] Pathological effects of ROS that contribute to the development of atherosclerosis include stimulation of vascular smooth muscle proliferation and migration, endothelial apoptosis, altered vasomotor reactivity, oxidation of low-density lipoprotein, which causes cholesterol accumulation in macrophages, the upregulation of adhesion molecules and the creation of a proinflammatory state.[94,95] In contrast antioxidant systems, such superoxide dismutase (SOD) and glutathione peroxidase, scavenge, and inactivate ROS. SOD are enzymes that breaks down the free radicals into nontoxic substances and inhibits the breakdown of NO by superoxide anions, inhibits pathologic ET_1 production and augments endothelial relaxation.[95] Clinically, ACE inhibitors, which prevent angiotensin II from inducing oxidative stress, may improve NO availability,[96,97] and statins, which inhibit ROS formation have been found to improve cardiovascular outcomes.[98] However, studies and meta-analyses failed to find any beneficial effects from supplemental antioxidants (Vitamin C and Vitamin E) in the reduction of cardiovascular mortality or death.[99–101]

Local Metabolic Control of Blood Flow

Local metabolic factors that control arteriolar resistance play a role in matching blood flow (oxygen transport) to metabolism. These

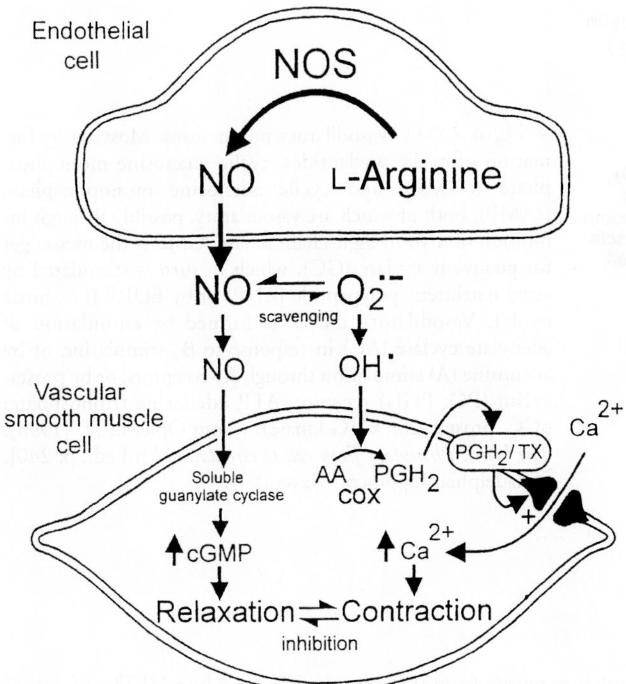

■ **Figure 2-10** Interactions between nitric oxide (NO) and superoxide anions (O_2^-). Superoxide anions cause contraction of vascular smooth muscle by scavenging endothelium-derived NO and by activating the production of vasoconstrictor prostaglandins in the vascular smooth muscle cells, presumably after transformation of hydroxyl radicals (OH^-). AA, arachidonic acid; COX, cyclooxygenase; cGMP, cyclic guanosine monophosphate; NOS, nitric oxide synthase; PGH_2, endoperoxides; TX, thromboxane. (From Vanhoutte, P. M. [1999]. Endothelial dysfunction and vascular disease. In J. A. Panza & R. O. Cannon (Eds.), *Endothelium, nitric oxide and atherosclerosis*. New York: Futura Publishing.)

factors may accumulate in low-flow conditions and cause vasodilation by inhibition of basal tone. The increased flow that occurs as a result of the vasodilation is referred to as *reactive hyperemia*. Metabolic factors that have been shown to interact and contribute to reactive hyperemia include adenosine and ATP, NO, prostaglandins, and potassium.[102–104] An increase in flow-dependent shear stress on the endothelium has also been shown to cause vasodilation in skeletal muscle and venules. This vasodilation is mediated in part by the release of NO and prostaglandin.[105]

NEUROHUMORAL STIMULATION

In addition to stimulation by endothelium-derived vasodilating and vasoconstricting factors, neurohumoral factors bind with receptors on vascular smooth muscle. The effects of this stimulation vary throughout the vascular system.

Adrenergic Stimulation

α-Adrenergic Stimulation

The α-adrenergic receptors, which are a series of G_q protein-coupled receptors that bind epinephrine and norepinephrine, are generally categorized as α_1 and α_2 receptors.[106] Molecular cloning techniques have lead to a further division of the α-receptor subtypes. The α_1-adrenergic receptors, which are now characterized as subtypes α_{1A}, α_{1B}, and α_{1D}, are located in arteries, arterioles, and cutaneous and visceral veins. The α_{1A} receptors are responsible for vessel contraction. The α_{1B} receptors are thought to contribute to the maintenance of basal vascular tone and arterial blood pressure in conscious animals and are sensitive to exogenous agonists. Finally, the α_{1D} receptors also play a role in vascular contraction, although they have a lesser effect than the α_{1B} receptors.[107]

The α_2 receptors, which have presynaptic and postsynaptic functions, are characterized as $\alpha_{2A/D}$, α_{2B}, and α_{2C}. The $\alpha_{2A/D}$ and α_{2B} receptors are present in large arteries but are located with greater density on the terminal arterioles, which act as precapillary sphincters to control the number of open capillaries and total capillary blood flow. The $\alpha_{2A/D}$ receptors play the primary role in vasoconstriction.[108,109] The α_{2B} receptors also play a role in vasoconstriction and may contribute to the onset of hypertension. The α_{2C} receptors are responsible for venoconstriction.[107,110]

Whereas stimulation of the presynaptic α_2 receptors inhibits norepinephrine, stimulation of the postsynaptic α_2 receptors located on the vascular smooth muscle causes norepinephrine release and subsequent vasoconstriction. However, the α_2-mediated vasoconstriction is attenuated by the α_2 presynaptic inhibition of norepinephrine release. In addition, in contrast to α_1 receptor stimulation, the effect of norepinephrine on α_2 in terminal arterioles is inhibited by metabolites, thus fostering metabolic vasodilation even when vasoconstrictor tone to blood vessels in the skeletal muscle is high.

β-Adrenergic Stimulation

In the heart, β_1 receptors predominate (80%), although there are also a smaller number of β_2 receptors (20%), with the β_2 receptors playing a role in coronary vasodilation.[111] Of note, the β_2 vasodilation is impaired in severely atherosclerotic coronary vessels.[112] There is also a small number (<1%) of β_3 adrenergic receptors in cardiomyocytes.[113] The β_3 receptors, which mediate negative inotropy via a NO-dependent pathway,[114] become important during heart failure when they are up-regulated and while protective may contribute to functional degradation of the failing heart.[113,115]

In vascular smooth muscle, the β-adrenergic receptors are predominantly of the β_2-subtype. Stimulation of these receptors causes vasorelaxation[116] via activation of Gs protein, which binds to adenylate cyclase and catalyzes the conversion of ATP to cAMP. cAMP in turn activates PKA, which then phosphorylates myosin light-chain kinase (MLCK) (Fig. 2-11). Phosphorylation decreases MLCK's affinity for calmodulin, which decreases the promotion of the myosin kinase–calmodulin–calcium complex. Failure to form the calmodulin–calcium complex inhibits cross-bridge formation with subsequent vascular relaxation.[117] β_2-Adrenergic stimulation also decreases intracellular calcium by hyperpolarization of the vascular smooth muscle, which decreases the influx of calcium into the cell, increases cAMP-mediated extrusion of calcium from the cell, and promotes calcium uptake by the sarcoplasmic reticulum.[118] There is also a β_2-mediated release of NO, which is thought to involve the cAMP/PKA pathway.[117] The β_3 receptors in the vascular smooth muscle may mediate vasodilation, with the effects vary depending on the vascular bed.[114,119]

Vasopressin

Vasopressin, which is synthesized in the hypothalamus, is released in response to increased plasma osmolality and decreased blood

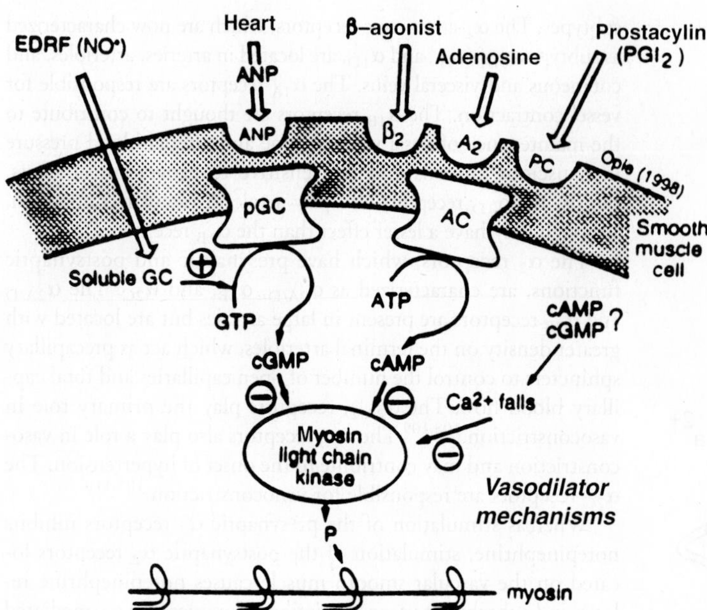

■ **Figure 2-11** Vasodilatory mechanisms. Most act by formation of cyclic nucleotides, cyclic guanosine monophosphate (cGMP), and cyclic adenosine monophosphate (cAMP), both of which are vasodilatory, possibly through inhibition of myosin light-chain kinase. GMP is the messenger for guanylate cyclase (GC), which in turn is stimulated by atrial natriuretic polypeptide (ANP) or by EDRF (i.e., nitric oxide). Vasodilatory cAMP is formed by stimulation of adenylate cyclase (AC) in response to β_2-stimulation or by adenosine (A) stimulation through A_2-receptors, or by prostacyclin (PO; PGI_2) receptor. ATP, adenosine triphosphate; pGC, prostacyclin C (G kinase). (From Opie, L. H. [1998]. *The heart: Physiology from cell to circulation* [3rd ed., p. 240]. Philadelphia: Lippincott-Raven.)

pressure and cardiac output and exogenous vasopressin is used to treat refractory hypotension.[120] There are three types of vasopressin receptors, with V1 receptors located on vascular smooth muscle. V1 receptor stimulation causes the activation of PLC, which catalyzes the conversion of IP_3, and subsequently causes calcium release from the sarcoplasmic reticulum.[121] The increased intracellular calcium causes vasoconstriction (Fig. 2-12). If the sympathetic and renin–angiotensin systems are in intact, vasopressin has minimal effect on vascular control. However, if these systems are impaired, vasopressin plays a larger role in acute blood

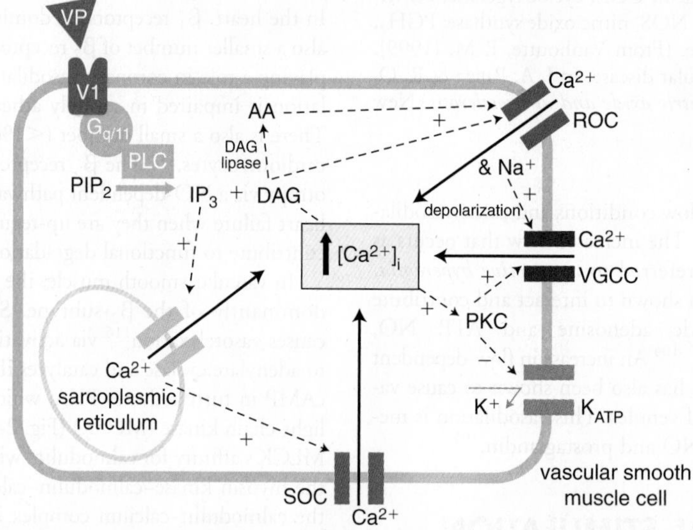

■ **Figure 2-12** A schematic showing the pathways of intracellular calcium (Ca^{2+}) elevation following the binding of vasopressin (VP) to the V1 receptor (*V1R*) on a vascular smooth muscle cell. The weighting of the black solid arrows demonstrates the relative importance of the different pathways. V1Rs are coupled through Gq/11 to phospholipase C (PLC), which hydrolyzes phosphatidyl inositol bisphosphonate (PIP2) to produce inositol triphosphate (IP_3) and diacylglycerol (DAG). The latter, in turn, stimulates the activity of protein kinase C (PKC). A transient increase in intracellular Ca^{2+} is produced by the action of IP_3 on the sarcoplasmic reticulum, whereas a sustained increase is triggered by influx of extracellular Ca^{2+}. Store-operated channels (*SOCs*), activated by intracellular store depletion, appear to play a minor role in comparison to voltage-gated calcium channels (VGCCs) and receptor operated channels (ROCs). VGCCs are opened by cell membrane depolarization, secondary to cation influx via ROCs and the PKC-mediated closure of adenosine triphosphate-sensitive potassium (KATP) channels. PKC can also open VGCCs directly. The opening of ROCs is G protein-dependent via PLC, with a downstream mechanism involving DAG and arachidonic acid (AA). They have significant permeability to Ca^{2+}, which is likely to contribute directly to contraction. (From Barrett, L. K., Singer, M., & Clapp, L. H. [2007]. Vasopressin: Mechanisms of action on the vasculature in health and in septic shock. *Critical Care Medicine, 35*(1), 33–40.)

pressure control. Exogenous vasopressin may be beneficial in refractory vasodilatory shock when there is a relative vasopressin deficiency (e.g., septic shock, intraoperative hypotension).[122] During cardiopulmonary resuscitation, vasopressin increases coronary and cerebral blood flow, and is part of the protocol for resuscitation of ventricular fibrillation.[123,124]

Intracellular Signals for Vasodilation and Vasoconstriction

The two major messengers for vasodilation are the intracellular nucleotides cAMP and cyclic guanosine monophosphate (cGMP). The primary messenger for vasoconstriction is IP_3.

Cyclic Guanosine Monophosphate. Nitric oxide, atrial natriuretic peptides, and nitrovasodilators (e.g., nitroglycerin and nitroprusside) activate membrane bound or soluble guanylate cyclase, which generates cGMP from guanosine triphosphate. The cGMP then activates phosphokinase G, which is thought to decrease intracellular calcium and subsequently cause vasorelaxation by (1) increasing the uptake or extrusion of calcium by the cytoplasm, (2) inhibiting calcium release from the sarcoplasmic reticulum, (3) regulating the levels of IP_3, (4) inhibiting calcium-activated potassium channels, and (5) decreasing contractile protein sensitivity to calcium.[125–127] Phosphokinase G also directly inhibits MLCK, thus inhibiting contraction. Additionally, cGMP hyperpolarizes the cell, which further decreases intracellular calcium.[43] Nitric oxide also, independent of cGMP, increases the uptake of cytosolic calcium into the sarcoplasmic reticulum.[127]

Inositol Triphosphate. In response to vasoconstrictor stimuli (e.g., norepinephrine, AII, and endothelin), the enzyme PLC located in the cell wall splits phosphatidyl inositol into IP_3 and diacylglycerol (Fig. 2-13). IP_3 is the primary messenger for vasoconstriction and acts on a special calcium-receptor channel on the sarcoplasmic reticulum to release calcium, which as described below leads to contraction. Conversely, cGMP inhibits the accumulation of IP_3, which leads to a decrease in cytosolic calcium levels and vasorelaxation.[128]

CALCIUM

The major endpoint of extrinsic neurohormonal factors and local regulation of vascular tone involves a cascade of messengers that influence calcium movement in and out of the cell or sarcoplasmic reticulum, thus influencing the contractile process.[129] Knowledge of the role of calcium is important because the modulation of calcium flux is the focus of pharmacologic control of vascular resistance.

As with cardiac and skeletal muscle, the changes in intracellular calcium are responsible for vascular smooth muscle contraction and relaxation. However, unlike skeletal and cardiac muscle in which calcium reverses the inhibitory effect of troponin on the actin–myosin interaction, vascular smooth muscle cross-bridge formation and muscle contraction result from the indirect activation of myosin by calcium.[35,130]

Sources of Calcium

The increased intracellular calcium comes from an influx of calcium across the sarcolemma and from the sarcoplasmic reticulum.[130] The calcium influx across the sarcolemma is through voltage-gated ion channels, which are altered by the activation of the IP_3-regulated channels or ryanodine receptors. These receptors display calcium-induced calcium release.[129,131]

Calcium Signaling

The increased intracellular calcium binds with calmodulin, a small protein found in the cytosol of vascular smooth muscle. The calcium–calmodulin complex activates the enzyme MLCK, which in turn phosphorylates the light protein chains of the myosin head. The phosphorylation activates the myosin (increases the ATPase activity) such that the myosin can interact with actin. The process of phosphorylation is considered the primary mechanism of smooth muscle contraction. Conversely, a decrease in the cytoplasmic calcium concentration inactivates the MLCK and permits

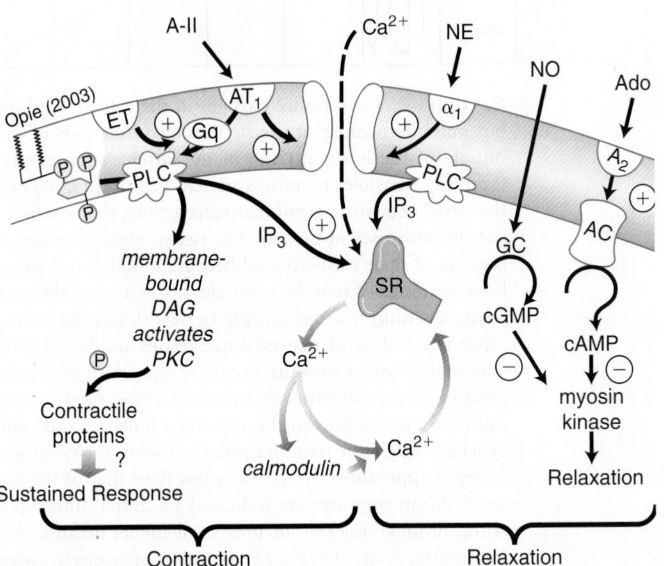

■ **Figure 2-13** Protein kinase C (PKC)-linked receptors in vascular smooth muscle. For example, the α1-agonist signalling system is coupled via a G protein to phospholipase C (PLC), which breaks down phosphatidylinositol 4,5-biphosphate (PIP2) to 1,2-diacylglycerol (DAG) and inositol 1,4,5-triphosphate (IP_3). DAG is thought to translocate protein kinase C from cytosol to the sarcolemma, thereby activating protein kinase C. signals beyond protein kinase C are not clear. IP_3 releases calcium from the sarcoplasmic reticulum to initiate contraction in vascular smooth muscle. Other vasoconstrictors such as angiotensin II and endothelin act by the same signal system. (From Opie, L. H. [2004]. *The heart: Physiology from cell to circulation* [4th ed., p. 206]. Philadelphia: Lippincott Williams & Wilkins.)

dephosphorylation of myosin by the enzyme myosin light-chain phosphatase. The dephosphorylation facilitates the detachment of myosin from actin, resulting in relaxation.[130]

The cytoplasmic calcium concentration is decreased through uptake of calcium into the sarcoplasmic reticulum and transport out of the cell across the plasma membrane by Ca^{2+}-ATPase exchanger or a probable Na^{+}/Ca^{2+} exchanger.[34] Additionally, calcium is decreased by closure of the membrane calcium channels through hyperpolarization[132] or pharmacologically with calcium channel blockers.

VOLUME AND FLOW DISTRIBUTION

Resistance

The pressure decrease from the aorta to the small arteries is relatively small, approximately 25 mm Hg (Fig. 2-14).[133] As much as 50% of the peripheral resistance appears to occur proximal to vessels with diameters of 100 mm. This finding indicates the primary sites for peripheral vascular resistance are the small arteries and the arterioles, although the exact location of the resistance vessels remains equivocal.[134]

Alterations in the diameter of the terminal arterioles or precapillary blood vessels control capillary and venous pressures, microvascular blood flow and exchange, and postcapillary venous volume.[135,136] Although the radius of the capillaries is considerably smaller than the radius of the arterioles, the resistance is lower because of the increase in cross-sectional area.

Volume Distribution

At rest, the systemic veins contain as much as 60% to 80% of the total blood volume, with 25% to 50% of this volume in the small veins (<1 mm in diameter). One-fourth of the total blood volume is in the capacious splanchnic circulation. Although the cross-sectional area is largest at the end of the capillaries, the largest volume of blood, as demonstrated in Figure 2-15, is in the venules because of the combination of cross-sectional area and the length of the venules.[137] The remainder of the blood is distributed in the aorta and systemic arteries (10%), the capillaries (5%), and the pulmonary bed and heart (15% to 25%).[2]

Blood Flow

Definition of Flow

Blood flow ($\dot{Q}$) is expressed in terms of volume of blood per unit of time (volume/time). For example, the cardiac output, which is defined as the liters of blood pumped out of the left ventricle into the systemic circulation each minute, is usually expressed as liters per minute.

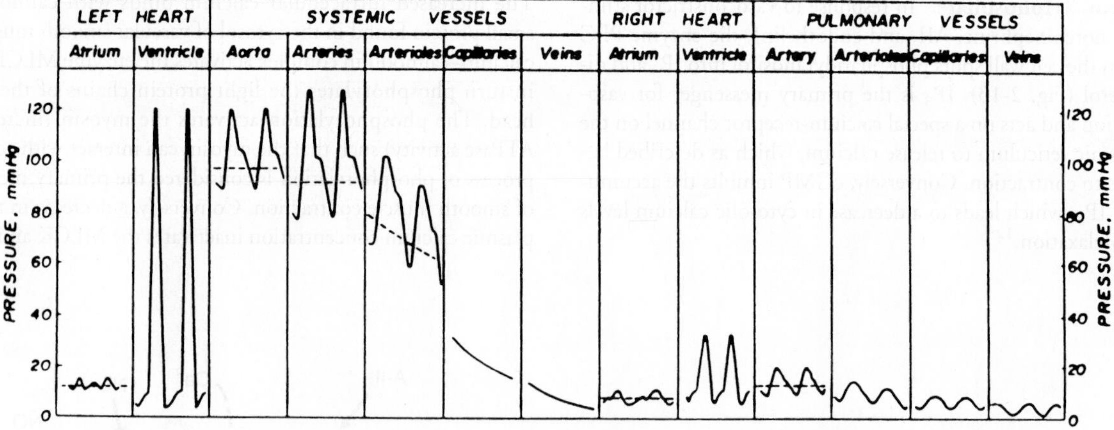

■ Figure 2-14 Pressure changes in the human cardiovascular system. In the left atrium, the pressure is low but pulsatile because of the rhythmic contractions of the atrial muscle. The main generator of pressure is the muscle of the left ventricle; in the latter cavity, the pressure alternates with each cardiac cycle from near 0 mmHg (diastole) to approximately 120 mm Hg (systole). When the pressure in the ventricle exceeds that in the aorta, the aortic semilunar valve opens, the ventricle and aorta become a common chamber, and the pressure in both rises in unison. The rise in aortic pressure causes an expansion of the aorta and the large arteries because of their elasticity and because blood enters the arterial trees faster than it leaves it through the small-bore arterioles. When the ventricle starts to relax, the aortic valve closes. As the ventricle continues to relax, the pressure within it drops quickly to near 0, but the pressure in the aorta falls slowly throughout ventricular diastole as the distended arterial tree recoils and blood continues to flow to the capillaries through the arterioles. The major loss of pressure occurs at the arterioles because of the high resistance to flow that they offer. The pressure in the capillaries and veins decreases further to approximately 0 mmHg in the great veins entering the right atrium; the flow in the systemic capillaries and veins is relatively nonpulsatile. The right side of the heart generates a pressure pattern similar to that in the systemic circulation, but the systolic pressure in the pulmonary artery is approximately six times less than that of the aorta, and the flow in the pulmonary capillaries is pulsatile. Mean pressures are indicated by dotted lines. In large arteries, the mean pressure is lower than in the aorta, although the systolic pressure is higher because of reflection of the pulse waves. (From Shepherd, J. T., & Vanhoutte, P. M. [1979]. *The human cardiovascular system: Facts and concepts* [p. 78]. New York: Raven Press.)

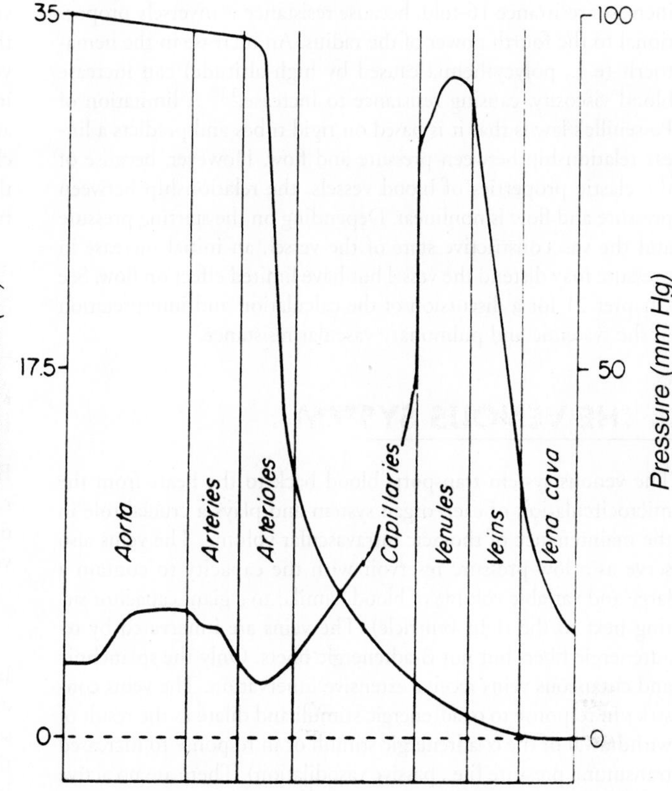

■ **Figure 2-15** Changes in estimated blood volume (%) and blood pressure (mm Hg) in consecutive segments of the systemic blood vessels. Note that the volume is predominantly in the venules. The pressure is high in the aorta and arteries, falls rapidly in the arterioles, and then falls more slowly from the capillaries to the vena cava. (From Scher, A. M. [1989]. The veins and venous return. In H. D. Patton, A. Fuchs, B. Hille, et al. [Eds.], *Textbook of physiology, Vol. 2* [21st ed., p. 880]. Philadelphia: WB Saunders.)

Determinants of Flow

Nonturbulent flow ($\dot{Q}$) in a segment of an isogravitational blood vessel (i.e., a blood vessel on the same horizontal level) is determined by the pressure difference (ΔP) between the inflow and outflow ends of that segment divided by the resistance (R) to flow provided by that segment. The relationship that demonstrates that flow will change as the result of a change in pressure or the change in resistance across a vascular bed is expressed in the following equation:

$$\dot{Q} = \frac{\Delta P}{R}$$

Substituting physiological values into this equation gives:

$$\text{CO} = \frac{\text{MAP} - \text{RAP}}{\text{SVR}}$$

where MAP − RAP is the difference between the mean arterial pressure (MAP; as an indicator of aortic or upstream pressure) and right atrial pressure (RAP; downstream pressure) divided by the systemic vascular resistance (SVR).

Pressure. Blood pressure is the force exerted by the blood in a blood vessel. Clinically, pressure is expressed as millimeters of mercury, torr, or centimeters of H_2O. The relationship between these various measures is:

$$1 \text{ mm Hg} = 1 \text{ torr} = 1.36 \text{ cm } H_2O$$

Pressure in blood vessels has three components: (1) static pressure, which is related to the fullness of the vascular system at zero flow; (2) hydrostatic pressure, which is equal to the height of the column of liquid (h) multiplied by the density of the liquid (p) multiplied by the gravitational force (g), hydrostatic pressure = pgh; and (3) dynamic pressure, which is the pressure generated by the heart and is equal to flow multiplied by resistance (pressure = flow × resistance). The static pressure and the hydrostatic pressure are added to the dynamic pressure to give blood pressure. The hydrostatic pressure, and particularly the effect of the height of the fluid column, is especially important in the upright position, because the fluid column between the heart and the feet may add an additional 100 mm Hg of hydrostatic pressure to the dynamic pressure (100 mm Hg). In the systemic circulation, blood flows from the aorta, where the MAP is 100 mm Hg, to the right atrium (mean pressure = 0 to 6 mm Hg). Blood pressure control is discussed in Chapter 3.

Resistance. Based on an analogy to Ohm's law, resistance (R) is equal to a pressure gradient (ΔP) divided by blood flow ($\dot{Q}$):

$$R = \frac{\Delta P}{\dot{Q}}$$

According to Poiseuille's law for laminar nonpulsatile flow of a substance with uniform viscosity, vascular resistance is proportional to a constant ($8/\pi$), the viscosity of the blood (η), and the length of the vessel (L). It is inversely proportional to the fourth power of the radius (r^4):

$$R = \frac{8L\eta}{\pi r^4}$$

Thus, the resistance to flow depends on only the dimension length (L) and radius (r) of the vessel and the viscosity (η) of the fluid. The radius of the blood vessel is the primary factor determining resistance in the vascular system. For example, if all other factors are held constant, decreasing the vessel radius by 50%

increases resistance 16-fold, because resistance is inversely proportional to the fourth power of the radius. An increase in the hematocrit (e.g., polycythemia caused by high altitude) can increase blood viscosity, causing resistance to increase.[138] A limitation of Poiseuille's law is that it is based on rigid tubes and predicts a linear relationship between pressure and flow. However, because of the elastic properties of blood vessels, the relationship between pressure and flow is nonlinear. Depending on the starting pressure and the vasoconstrictive state of the vessel, an initial increase in pressure may distend the vessel but have limited effect on flow. See Chapter 21 for a discussion of the calculation and interpretation of the systemic and pulmonary vascular resistance.

THE VENOUS SYSTEM

The venous system transports blood back to the heart from the microcirculation of each organ system and plays a crucial role in the maintenance of thoracic intravascular volume. The veins also serve as a low-pressure reservoir with the capacity to contain a large and variable volume of blood (similar to a giant capacitor sitting next to the right ventricle). The veins are innervated by α-adrenergic fibers but not β-adrenergic fibers. Only the splanchnic and cutaneous veins receive extensive innervation. The veins constrict in response to α-adrenergic stimuli and dilate as the result of withdrawal of the α-adrenergic stimuli or in response to increased transmural pressure (i.e., passive vasodilation). There are no active vasodilatory mechanisms in the veins.[23]

Venous Pressure and Resistance

In the supine position, the pressure generated by the heart in the large arteries is approximately 100 mm Hg. However, as demonstrated in Figure 2-14, the pressure decreases across the arterioles and capillaries, with a resultant pressure in the small veins of only 15 to 20 mm Hg. The right atrial pressure is approximately 0 to 5 mm Hg (depending on position, the state of hydration, and cardiac output). Thus, the pressure driving blood flow from the left side of the heart to the capillaries is approximately 80 mm Hg, whereas the driving pressure from the postcapillary vessels to the right atrium is only 15 to 20 mm Hg (difference between the postcapillary vessels and the right atrium). Interestingly, in the upright position this gradient is unchanged, despite the addition of hydrostatic pressure (determined by the height of a continuous column of blood between any given point and the heart).

Skeletal muscle contractions in the extremities (the muscle pump) and respiration (respiratory pump) play an essential role in propelling venous blood from the veins to the right atrium (see Chapter 3). In addition, the venous valves prevent backward flow into the muscle. Valvular function is particularly important during standing and exercise and the pathogenesis of venous insufficiency. The valves also promote the one-way flow of blood through perforating veins that lie between the superficial and deep veins.

Venous Compliance

When empty, the thin walls of the veins are flattened and the vessels are elliptical. As the veins fill with blood, they passively change to a circular shape. Because of this passive accommodation to an increase in volume, the veins are capable of receiving large volumes of fluid with only small increases in transmural pressure; that is, they are compliant. Because of their ability to serve as a volume reservoir, the veins are referred to as capacitance vessels. At increased pressures, the veins become distended and less compliant; thus, any given pressure change is associated with a smaller change in volume. Because of the compliant nature of the veins, the venous system plays an important role in altering thoracic intravascular volume.[24]

MICROCIRCULATORY EXCHANGE

Flow Through the Microvascular Circulation

Blood flow ($\dot{Q}$) through the microcirculation (or any organ) is directly related to the difference in pressure between the arterial end of the vascular segment (P_A) and venous pressure (P_v) and is inversely related to vascular resistance (R_T).[13,14]

$$\text{Flow} = \frac{P_A - P_V}{R_T}$$

In the absence of changes in arterial pressure (P_A), changes in local vascular resistance and intravascular pressure are caused by vasodilation and vasoconstriction of the arterioles. Any alteration in the tone of the muscular venules contributes little to the change in resistance.

Microvascular Transport Mechanisms

Solutes and water passively move across the endothelium as the result of two processes, diffusion and ultrafiltration. Diffusion is the result of the random kinetic motion of ions and molecules. Diffusion results in the net transport of substances along a concentration gradient from high to low concentration. Ultrafiltration is the combined movement of fluid and solutes in a unilateral direction through a membrane, except that the movement of the solutes is restricted by the membrane. The driving force for ultrafiltration is the difference between hydrostatic pressure and oncotic pressure across the membrane. Ultrafiltration is the primary mechanism for controlling plasma and interstitial fluid volume.[13]

Diffusion

Concentration gradients, created by the production or consumption of specific substances, are the primary driving forces for diffusion (with the exception of the tight-junction capillaries, which are affected by electrical gradients). Because diffusion in or out of a blood vessel creates a concentration gradient along the vessel, diffusion exchange is strongly influenced by blood flow, particularly for those substances that rapidly diffuse through the membrane wall.[14,139] The rate of diffusion of a solute across the capillary wall (J_s) is proportional to the concentration gradient, that is, the difference between the concentration in the plasma (C_p) and interstitial concentration (C_i), the permeability (P_s) of the endothelium to the solute, and the surface area (A) available for exchange.

$$J_s = P_s A (C_p - C_i)$$

For substances that diffuse rapidly through the capillary endothelium (e.g., O_2, CO_2), the transport of the solute depends on the concentration gradient and blood flow (through the delivery or removal of the substance). The rate of diffusion (J_s) is described as *flow-limited.*

$$J_s = (C_a - C_i)\dot{Q}$$

where C_a is the concentration of the substance in the arterial blood, C_i is the concentration of the substance in the interstitium, and $\dot{Q}$ is the rate of blood flow. Flow-limited diffusion has potentially important implications for oxygen delivery in the setting of decreased oxygen delivery (e.g., cardiogenic shock or during severe exercise when flow rates are so high that diffusion is limited). However, most substances have intermediate endothelial permeability, and the rate of diffusion depends on endothelial permeability and flow.[13]

Most solutes, including small lipophilic and hydrophilic molecules and macromolecules, move through membranes of exchange vessels by diffusion. The route of diffusion depends on the type of membrane (continuous, fenestrated, discontinuous, and tight-junction) and the characteristics of the substance (e.g., lipid soluble, ionic, large macromolecule). Water diffuses through the endothelium primarily through intercellular clefts.[140,141] Lipid-soluble substances, such as O_2, CO_2, and anesthetic gases, which pass easily through the lipid bilayer of the microvascular wall, diffuse relatively rapidly through the endothelium. Small hydrophilic solutes, such as ions and simple sugars, pass primarily through fenestrae, junctions between cells, or intracellular clefts. The primary mode of macromolecular transport is through vesicles or possibly large pores.[141] The transport or movement of the macromolecules into the interstitium contributes to interstitial oncotic pressure.

Ultrafiltration

Starling's hypothesis of microvascular fluid exchange is described by the following equation[142–145]:

$$\frac{J_v}{A} = L_p([P_c - P_i] - \sigma[\pi_c - \pi_i])$$

J_v/A = fluid filtration across the capillary wall per unit area
L_p = hydraulic permeability of the capillary wall
P_c = global value for capillary pressure
P_i = global value for interstitial pressure
σ = osmotic reflection coefficient
π_c = global value for capillary oncotic pressure
π_i = global value for interstitial oncotic pressure

In Starling's initial conceptualization of ultrafiltration, it was thought that at the arterial end of the capillary, the net forces favored the movement of fluid out of the vessel (filtration). Somewhere in the middle of the vessel, an equilibrium point was reached at which there was neither a gain nor a loss of fluid. Finally, on the venous end of the exchange vessel, the net forces favored reabsorption. Although the validity of Starling's equation has been repeatedly confirmed, the conceptualization of upstream filtration and downstream reabsorption has been questioned.[145] In general, the forces opposing filtration do not exceed capillary pressure, and filtration occurs along the entire length of the exchange vessel.[146] The net filtration is necessary to wash out the proteins that are continuously diffusing out of the vessels into the interstitium.[146,147] The ultrafiltrate and proteins that cross the vessel wall into the interstitial fluid are subsequently removed by the lymphatic system.

The primary direction of ultrafiltration is out of the vessel (filtration versus reabsorption), with the rate of fluid movement across a short segment of exchange vessel (J_v/A) having a curvilinear relationship to the net pressure difference (i.e., limited fluid movement at low P_c) across the vessel wall.[145] In Starling's initial conceptualization, the net pressure difference reflected the algebraic sum of four pressures: intravascular (capillary) pressure (P_c), interstitial fluid pressure (P_i), plasma oncotic pressure (π_c), and interstitial oncotic pressure (π_i). The true pressure opposing filtration (P_o) is not simply plasma oncotic pressure, but rather oncotic plasma pressure minus interstitial oncotic pressure plus interstitial hydrostatic pressure and the reflection coefficient:

$$P_o = \sigma(\pi_p - \pi_i) + P_i$$

However, the effective oncotic force that opposes fluid filtration across the microvessel wall is the local oncotic pressure difference across the endothelial surface glycocalyx (the structure that covers the entire capillary endothelium and is the primary filter for proteins) and not the global difference between the oncotic pressure in the plasma and tissue.[148] Models of this new conceptualization suggest that the oncotic pressure opposing filtration is greater than estimated from blood–tissue protein concentration differences, and transcapillary fluid flux is smaller than predicted from the original Starling equation. Therefore, in the Starling equation, the pressures P_i and π_i are the local hydrostatic pressure behind the glycocalyx and oncotic pressure on the tissue side of the matrix layer, respectively, and not the values from the tissue space.[148,149]

Capillary pressure (P_c) is the primary force behind filtration. Mean capillary pressure (P_c) is determined by the arterial and venous pressures and the ratio of postcapillary resistance (R_v) to precapillary resistance (R_a), as described by the following equation:[150]

$$P_c = (P_v + P_a) \times \frac{R_v}{R_a}$$

where P_v is venous pressure, P_a is arterial pressure, R_v is postcapillary midpoint resistance, and R_a is precapillary midpoint resistance (where $R_v + R_a = R_{Total}$). An increase in either P_a or P_v results in an increase in P_c, unless counteracted by a decrease in the R_v/R_a ratio. The lower the R_v/R_a ratio (i.e., increased precapillary resistance or decreased postcapillary resistance) the lower the capillary pressure. It is the adjustment in R_v/R_a ratio, primarily through regulation of precapillary resistance (R_a) in the skeletal muscle and skin, that constitutes the primary effector mechanism for the central nervous system-mediated control of plasma volume.[151,152] However, the centrally mediated decrease in mean capillary pressure occurs only to the extent allowed by local autoregulatory adjustments.

In response to hypovolemic hypotension, compensatory precapillary vasoconstriction (increased R_a) decreases the mean P_c, and the net pressure in the downstream (venous) segment of the exchange vessel favors transient reabsorption. This autotransfusion is the result of a change in the ratio of the postcapillary to precapillary resistance on mean capillary pressure.[153] Of note, this response is decreased in older individuals, which may impair their response to orthostasis or hemorrhage.[154]

In addition to the hydrostatic and oncotic forces, two other factors affect fluid movement across the exchange vessel: the hydraulic conductivity of the wall (L_p) and the reflection coefficient (σ). Hydraulic conductivity is a measure of the permeability of the exchange vessel to fluid, with the highest L_p values for fenestrated endothelia and lowest for tight-junction endothelia.[13] Hydraulic conductivity is difficult to measure and is estimated by the capillary filtration coefficient. The capillary filtration coefficient, which is equal to the product of hydraulic conductivity and the available area (L_pA), is expressed as milliliters of net filtrate formed in 100 g of tissue per minute for each milliliter increase in mean capillary filtration pressure (ml × min^{-1} mm Hg^{-1} × 100 g^{-1}). The capillary filtration coefficient is a useful indicator of capillary permeability.[147] A decrease in the capillary filtration coefficient, for example by a decrease in the area available for exchange, reduces the rate of net capillary filtration for any given net filtration pressure. The second factor, the reflection coefficient (σ), represents the osmotic pressure exerted by a difference in the concentration gradient of a substance across a membrane (oncotic effect of the concentration gradient) and the greater the ratio of the solute size to pore size, the greater the ratio.[155]

The reflection coefficient is close to 1 for tight-junction endothelium, which is completely impermeable to protein. In normal systemic exchange vessels in the skin and skeletal muscle, with continuous or fenestrated endothelium, the reflection coefficient ranges from 0.8 to 0.95 for albumin and total protein,[146,147] which indicates that these vessels are not completely impermeable to proteins. In the lungs, the reflection coefficients are, in general, lower for albumin (0.5 to 0.6) and protein (0.5 to 0.7).[147] In cases of injury to the endothelium, the reflection coefficient is markedly reduced, allowing increased movement of large molecules (e.g., protein) out of the exchange vessels.

THE LYMPHATIC SYSTEM

Removal of fluid and plasma proteins from the interstitium by the terminal lymphatics is essential in the maintenance of equilibrium in microvascular-interstitial exchange.[155] Depending on the protein concentration in the lymph, 8 to 12 L/day of lymph, which reflects net filtration caused by movement of fluid out of the vascular bed, is removed from the interstitium by the lymphatic system[144,155] (see Fig. 2-3). Approximately 4 to 8 L of the ultrafiltrate is directly reabsorbed from the lymphatic vessels back into the blood vessels, and the remaining 4 L of efferent lymph, which includes all of the filtered protein, is delivered back to the central circulation.[144,147] This high level of lymphatic flow supports the idea that filtration (return of lymph to the systemic vasculature) occurs along the entire length of lymphatic bed and not just in the central circulation.

PULMONARY CIRCULATION

Gross Anatomy

The primary function of the pulmonary circulation is to expose the blood to alveolar air so that oxygen can be taken up by the blood and carbon dioxide can be excreted. The pulmonary circulation is in series with the systemic circulation and receives the same cardiac output, approximately 5 to 6 L/min at rest for an adult weighing 70 kg. The pulmonary circulation has only 10% the capacity of the systemic circulation, yet it must accommodate the same ejected volume.

Although pulmonary blood flow is equal to that of the systemic system, its vascular resistance is seven to eight times lower than systemic resistance. The pulmonary vascular bed is regulated by passive factors, such as lung volume, and active factors, such as alveolar gas. These mechanisms alter pulmonary vascular resistance.

Pulmonary blood volume decreases or is diverted to the systemic circulation in conditions such as generalized systemic vasodilation, the standing position, positive end-expiratory pressure, or circulatory shock. Conditions that increase pulmonary blood volume include generalized systemic vasoconstriction, the supine position, mitral stenosis, and left heart failure.[156]

The pulmonary circulation originates from the base of the right ventricle, extends 5 cm, and divides into the right and left pulmonary arteries. As the pulmonary artery rises, the right pulmonary artery is positioned posterior to the aorta and superior vena cava and anterior to the right mainstem bronchus. The left pulmonary artery extends over the left main bronchus and divides into lobar branches. The pulmonary arteries and segmental and lobar branches are composed of elastic arteries to maintain low vascular resistance. These arteries contain smooth muscle with the capability of vasoconstriction and vasodilatation. The muscular arteries have internal and external elastic laminae with a layer of smooth muscle cells. The acinour and supernumerary arteries (precapillary arteries) are muscular. Increases in pulmonary vascular resistance come from the precapillary arteries. Arterioles are vessels with a thin intima and a single elastic lamina. These vessels make up the accessory branches of the respiratory tree and end at the alveolar capillary network (see Table 2-3 for abbreviations used in this section).

Cellular and Hormonal Effects

The pulmonary vascular bed is lined with endothelium. In the pulmonary vasculature, the primary endothelium relaxing factors released by the endothelial cells are NO and prostacyclin

Table 2-3 ■ ABBREVIATIONS

V_T	Tidal volume
V_E	Expired volume
V_D	Dead space volume
V_A	Alveolar volume
P_A	Alveolar pressure
P_a	Arterial pressure
P_v	Venous pressure
PA_{O2}	Alveolar partial pressure of oxygen
PA_{CO2}	Alveolar partial pressure of carbon dioxide
PA_{O2}	Arterial partial pressure of oxygen
Pa_{CO2}	Arterial partial pressure of carbon dioxide
$P\bar{v}O_2$	Mixed venous partial pressure of oxygen
PCO_2	Partial pressure of carbon dioxide
PO_2	Partial pressure of oxygen
FI_{O2}	Fraction of inspired oxygen
PI_{O2}	Pressure of inspired oxygen
P_{50}	Partial pressure of oxygen at which Hgb is 50% saturated
Sa_{O2}	Arterial blood saturation
Ca_{O2}	Oxygen content of arterial blood
Cv_{O2}	Oxygen content of mixed venous blood
$C(a-v)_{O2}$	Difference between arterial and venous oxygen content
$S\bar{v}O_2$	Mixed venous oxygen saturation
O_2ER	Oxygen extraction ratio
Sp_{O2}	Pulse oximetry oxygen saturation
$\dot{V}/\dot{Q}$	Ventilation–perfusion ratio
$\dot{V}O_2$	Oxygen consumption
$\dot{D}O_2$	Oxygen delivery
$\dot{Q}O_2$	Oxygen transport
WOB	Work of breathing
Hgb	Hemoglobin

(PGI_2). Nitric oxide plays an important role in baseline pulmonary vasodilation where it is most likely the common pathway for producing pulmonary vasodilation.[156] Nitric oxide-mediated vasodilation maintains low basal pulmonary vascular resistance, and it can cause further vasodilation in response to receptor-mediated stimulation.[157] Additionally, NO counteracts hypoxic pulmonary vasoconstriction (HPV), but its release is decreased with chronic hypoxia and primary pulmonary hypertension.[158] There is no evidence that EDHF exists in the pulmonary circulation.

Circulating factors that cause pulmonary vasoconstriction include endothelin, superoxide anion (O_2^-), TXA_2, serotonin, PGH_2, and angiotensin. Factors that cause vasodilation include histamine, bradykinin, and substance P. In addition, circulating catecholamines induce vasoconstriction via $\alpha 1$ receptors (mediated by norepinephrine and epinephrine), whereas α_2 and β_2 receptors stimulation causes vasodilation (mediated by epinephrine). Vasoconstriction predominates in response to sympathetic stimulation.

The pulmonary vascular endothelium also plays a role in activation of vasoactive substances. For example, 80% of angiotensin I is converted to AII during one pass through the pulmonary circulation. This conversion is caused by the presence of angiotensin-converting enzyme, which is located on the endothelial surface.[159] ACE inhibitors cover this enzyme and thus interfere with it action. Pulmonary vascular ACE also deactivates the peptide bradykinin. Other factors that may be altered as they pass through the pulmonary circulation include atrial natriuretic peptide and the endothelins.[156]

Physiology

Respiration is a process consisting of four major events: (1) pulmonary ventilation, which is the bulk movement of air between the atmosphere and the alveoli in the lungs; (2) diffusion of gases (O_2 and carbon dioxide) across the respiratory membrane between the alveoli and blood; (3) transport of gases to and from the cells of the body; and (4) other non-gas exchange functions (e.g., hormonal activity).

Maintenance of adequate tissue oxygenation depends on complex mechanisms, including transport of oxygen, microvascular control (systemic and local), and intact metabolic cellular function. Figure 2-16, which illustrates the processes by which oxygen is transported from the atmosphere to the mitochondria, demonstrates the pressure gradient from 150 mm Hg in the atmosphere to 1 mm Hg at the mitochondria.

Ventilation is the process of the exchange of air between the atmosphere (external environment) and alveoli. It involves the distribution of air into the pulmonary structures of the tracheobronchial tree to the alveoli of the lung. Air flow in the conducting airways (first 17 airway generations) is along a pressure gradient. Air moves from higher outside pressure (atmospheric) to lower airway pressure (sub-atmospheric). As air enters the alveolar region of the lung, the movement of gases becomes less dependent on the pressure gradient and diffusion becomes increasingly important.[156]

Diffusion is the process of movement of gases from an area of high partial pressure to an area of low partial pressure. Toward the end of the airways, at the alveoli, diffusion is the driving force

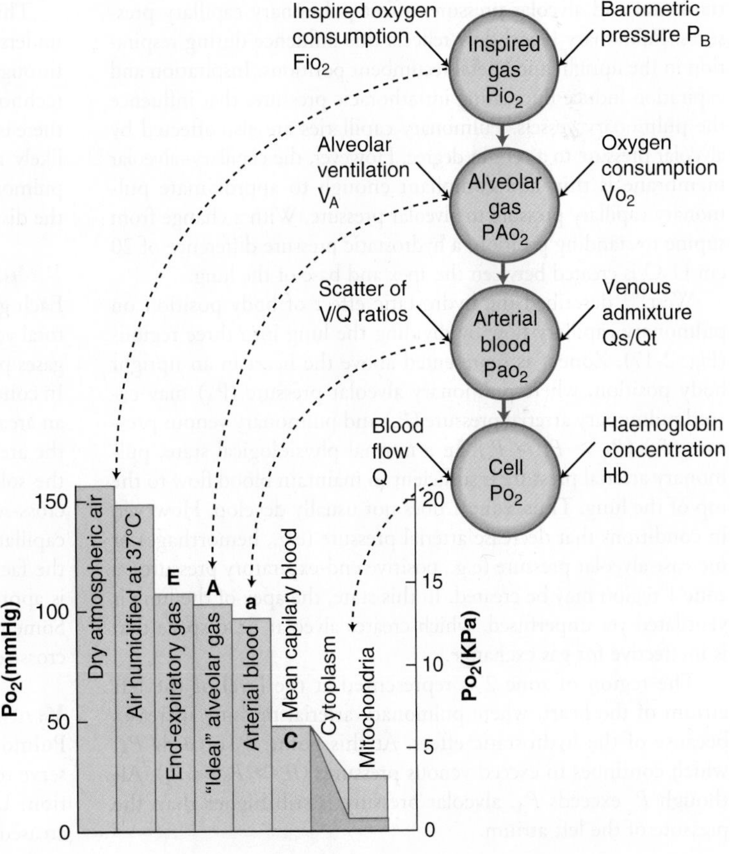

■ **Figure 2-16** The oxygen cascade. On the left is shown the oxygen cascade with PO_2 falling from the level in the ambient air down to the level in the mitochondria. On the right is a summary of the factors influencing oxygenation at different levels in the cascade. (From Lumb, A. B. [Ed.] [2005]. *Nunn's applied respiratory physiology* [6th ed.]. Philadelphia: Elsevier.)

behind the movement of oxygen and carbon dioxide across the alveolar membrane into the pulmonary capillaries.

Perfusion is the process of transporting gases to and from the cells of the body. This event includes mixed venous blood flow to the pulmonary capillaries where gases are exchanged between the alveoli and blood, and blood flow to the systemic capillaries where gases are exchanged between the blood and the surrounding body fluids.

Other lung functions that affect respiration but do not involve gas exchange include hormonal activity and the work of breathing. Work of breathing is the metabolic demand of breathing. It includes the energy needed to move the lung and chest wall and results in a demand for oxygen.

Dead Space

Ventilation must keep pace with the constant demand to replenish oxygen and eliminate carbon dioxide exchanged in the alveoli. Dead space is the volume of inspired air that does not participate in gas exchange. The volume of gas in a normal breath is measured as the tidal volume (V_T). This volume is multiplied by the number of breaths per minute to calculate minute volume (V_E). Minute volume represents the total volume of air moved through the airways to and from the alveoli. A portion of this volume will reach the alveoli where gas exchange can occur (alveolar volume), while the remainder will stay in the conducting airways and will not contribute to gas exchange (anatomic dead space) ($V_T = V_A + V_A$). In disease states, some lung regions may continue to receive ventilation but will not get normal blood flow. The result is wasted ventilation, adding to dead space volume (physiologic dead space).[160]

Lung Zones

Because the alveolar air spaces surround collapsible capillaries, intrapleural and alveolar pressures affect pulmonary capillary pressures. Pulmonary blood flow reflects this influence during respiration in the upright and lateral recumbent positions. Inspiration and expiration induce fluctuating intrathoracic pressures that influence the pulmonary vessels. Pulmonary capillaries are also affected by alveolar pressure to a certain degree. However, the capillary–alveolar membrane is thin and compliant enough to approximate pulmonary capillary pressure to alveolar pressure. With a change from supine to standing position, a hydrostatic pressure difference of 20 cm H_2O is created between the apex and base of the lung.

West[161] described the hydrostatic effect of body position on pulmonary capillary flow by dividing the lung into three regions (Fig. 2-17). Zone 1 is represented above the heart in an upright body position, where pulmonary alveolar pressure (P_A) may exceed pulmonary arterial pressure (P_a) and pulmonary venous pressure (P_v) ($P_A > P_a > P_v$). In a normal physiological state, pulmonary arterial pressure is sufficient to maintain blood flow to the top of the lung. Thus, zone 1 does not usually develop. However, in conditions that decrease arterial pressure (e.g., hemorrhage) or increase alveolar pressure (e.g., positive end-expiratory pressure), a zone 1 region may be created. In this state, the apex of the lung is ventilated yet unperfused, which creates alveolar dead space that is ineffective for gas exchange.

The region of zone 2 is represented at the level of the left atrium of the heart, where pulmonary arterial pressure increases because of the hydrostatic effect. At this point, P_a exceeds P_A, which continues to exceed venous pressures ($P_a > P_A > P_v$). Although P_a exceeds P_A, alveolar pressure is still higher than the pressure of the left atrium.

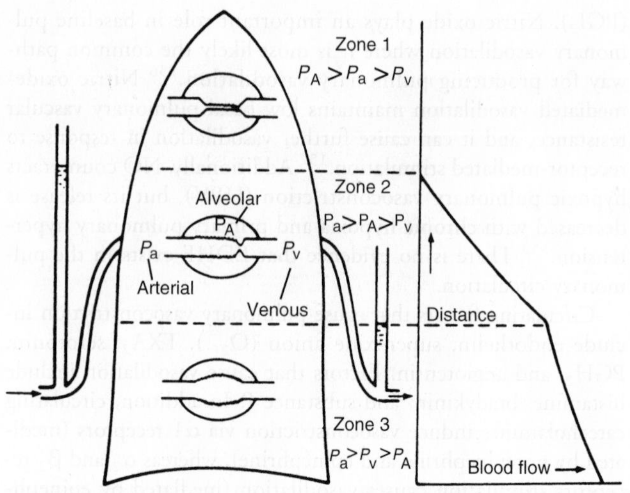

■ **Figure 2-17** Model to explain the zones of the lungs. P_A, alveolar pressure; P_a, pulmonary arterial pressure; P_v, pulmonary venous pressure. (From West, J. B. [1979]. *Respiratory physiology: The essentials* [2nd ed., p. 43]. Baltimore: Williams & Wilkins.)

The region of zone 3, below the left atrium, is where both P_a and left atrial pressures exceed P_A ($P_a > P_v > P_A$). Blood flow, which is determined by the difference between arterial and venous pressures, is increased markedly in this region of the lung because of capillary distention. The zone 3 region creates a continuous column of fluid between the pulmonary artery and the left atrium. Reliable pulmonary artery pressure measurements can be obtained when the tip of the pulmonary artery catheter is located in zone 3.

This general model of blood flow distribution is adequate for understanding the range of ventilation and perfusion relationships throughout the lung as a whole. However, high-resolution imaging technology has found that within a given isogravitational plane, there is greater heterogeneity than explained by the West zones most likely related to the asymmetrical branching of the bronchial and pulmonary vascular anatomy, and that gravity plays less of a role in the distribution of blood flow than previously thought.[162–166]

Diffusion

Each gas in a mixture of gases behaves as if it alone occupies the total volume and exerts a partial pressure independent of the other gases present. Diffusion is the process of movement of molecules. In conditions in which a gas has an area of high concentration and an area of low concentration, the net diffusion of gas will be from the area of high to low. In addition to the difference in pressure, the solubility of the gas in the body fluid (primarily water), the cross-sectional area of the exchange surface (alveolar–pulmonary capillary interface), and the distance the gas must travel are among the factors that affect the net diffusion in fluids. Carbon dioxide is approximately 20 times more soluble in water than in oxygen. Some pathological conditions (e.g., pulmonary edema) can affect cross-sectional area and distance.

Ventilation–Perfusion Matching

Pulmonary precapillary vasomotor and bronchiolar responses serve to match pulmonary capillary perfusion to alveolar ventilation. Unlike in the systemic circulation where hypoxemia, decreased pH, or increased amounts of carbon dioxide cause local vasodilation, any of these conditions in the pulmonary circulation may cause arteriolar vasoconstriction. In well-ventilated regions, there is little vasoconstriction in response to deoxygenated blood. In poorly ventilated areas where the amount of alveolar oxygen is less than normal, such as when a bronchus is obstructed, vasoconstriction occurs and blood is shunted to other lung areas.

Distribution of pulmonary blood flow in normal adults is normally controlled to a greater extent by the hydrostatic pressure gradient discussed earlier. Active control of pulmonary circulation, for example hypoxic vasoconstriction, serves a useful role in diverting blood flow to areas of the lung with more abundant oxygen, thus improving gas exchange. In contrast to peripheral vasculature, which vasodilates in response to hypoxia, pulmonary vessels constrict (e.g., HPV) to shunt blood away from poorly ventilated areas to match perfusion and ventilation.[167] HPV occurs within seconds in response to alveolar hypoxia and decreased mixed venous (pulmonary arterial) PO_2, with alveolar PO_2 exerting a greater effect.[156] The exact mechanism of HPV is unknown; however, the most likely cause is hypoxia-induced vascular smooth muscle hyperpolarization, which leads to increased intracellular calcium and subsequent vasoconstriction.[168–170] Other factors that are endothelium dependent, and may modulate hypoxic vasoconstriction and cause vascular remodeling, include inhibition of NO production, decreased effect of prostacyclin and increased endothelin.[156,171] Of clinical importance, while inhaled NO has been used to acutely treat pulmonary hypertension, its effectiveness is equivocal,[172] and a recent meta-analysis recommended that NO not be used for the treatment of acute respiratory distress syndrome.[173] In contrast, phosphodiesterase inhibitors, which enhance NO-mediated vasodilation have been found to improve outcomes.[174,175] In addition, endothelin receptor antagonists have become first-line therapy for pulmonary arterial hypertension[176] and intravenous prostacylin is reserved for severely ill patients.[175,177]

When blood flow to a region of the lung is decreased, there is also a decrease in alveolar CO_2. The bronchial smooth muscle responds to the decreased alveolar CO_2 levels by constricting; thus, shifting ventilation away from a poorly perfused area. This response occurs in conditions such as prolonged high altitude or in patients with chronic obstructive pulmonary disease or prolonged pulmonary hypertension.[178]

Ventilation and perfusion must occur in equal proportion in the various regions of the lung to achieve adequate gas exchange. Gas exchange determines the levels of alveolar oxygen partial pressure (PA_{O_2}) and carbon dioxide partial pressure (PA_{CO_2}). An adequate alveolar PO_2 depends on a balance of two factors: the rate of removal of oxygen by the pulmonary arterial blood and the rate of replenishment of oxygen by alveolar ventilation. An adequate PA_{CO_2} depends on the rate of removal of carbon dioxide by alveolar ventilation. A key concept used to understand pulmonary gas exchange is the ventilation–perfusion ratio ($\dot{V}/\dot{Q}$). The concentration of gases (i.e., oxygen, carbon dioxide, nitrogen) in the various regions of the lung is determined by the ratio of the rate of ventilation to the rate of perfusion (blood flow). Obstruction to ventilation or perfusion leads to alteration in this ratio and, consequently, the composition of gases. Inequality in ventilation–perfusion hinders the lungs' ability to replenish oxygen and remove carbon dioxide. Impairment of gas exchange can result in a decrease in Pa_{O_2} and an increase in tissue PCO_2. Clinically, these conditions can result in hypoxemia.

Causes of Arterial Hypoxemia

There are six sources of arterial hypoxemia:

- Decreased partial pressure of inspired oxygen
- Decreased percentage of inspired oxygen (decreased fraction of inspired oxygen, FI_{O_2})
- Diffusion limitation
- Hypoventilation
- $\dot{V}/\dot{Q}$ mismatch
- Shunt

Decreases in the atmospheric pressure related to higher altitude result in a proportional decrease in the partial pressure of inspired oxygen (PI_{O_2}). These conditions are common to high-altitude locations and air travel; however, they are rarely encountered in the clinical setting. Decreased percentage of inspired oxygen (FI_{O_2}) occurs in situations in which other gases may displace oxygen and lower the overall percentage of oxygen below 21% (e.g., diagnostic testing, fire). Diffusion limitation can potentially cause abnormal diffusion of oxygen across the alveolar–capillary membrane. Diffusion limitation can be caused by increases in the thickness of the diffusion pathway and/or decreased transit time through the pulmonary circulation. Hypoventilation can result in a decrease in alveolar PO_2 caused by insufficient gas exchange between the external environment and the alveoli. Hypoventilation can result from trauma to the chest wall, paralysis of the respiratory muscles, and medications such as morphine sulfate and barbiturates, which depress the respiratory center.[179]

Matching ventilation of the alveoli with perfusion of the pulmonary capillary bed is a delicate balance. $\dot{V}/\dot{Q}$ matching is a dynamic process with different distributions occurring simultaneously within the regions of the lungs. In disease, there are a myriad of $\dot{V}/\dot{Q}$ relationships exemplified by regions receiving excessive ventilation (dead space), normal ventilation and perfusion (ideal), and excessive perfusion (shunt).

Shunt refers to the condition when blood passes into the systemic circulation without passing through a ventilated region of the lung. Under normal conditions, there exists a small physiological shunt because of the difference in PO_2 between alveolar gas and end-capillary blood. Physiologically, mixed venous blood from the pulmonary arterial bed mixes with capillary blood from pulmonary venous beds, thereby lowering the end-capillary PO_2. This difference can become larger in conditions such as ventricular septal defect, in which greater amounts of venous blood are added to arterial blood across the defect, resulting in a lower Pa_{O_2}.

An important clinical characteristic of a shunt is that the hypoxemia cannot be completely resolved by placing the patient on an inspired oxygen fraction (FI_{O_2}) of 100%. Because the shunt blood bypasses the ventilated regions of the lung, it is not exposed to the higher alveolar PO_2. In patients with shunt, the arterial PCO_2 may be low, normal, or high, depending on the capacity to increase respiratory drive in response to hypoxemia.

Gas Transport

Gas Exchange

In the lungs, oxygen and carbon dioxide equilibrate across the alveolar–capillary membranes by simple passive diffusion, moving from an area of greater partial pressure to a region of lesser partial pressure. The partial pressure of oxygen in pulmonary arterial blood (venous blood from the body) is approximately 40 mm Hg, whereas pulmonary alveolar partial pressure of oxygen is approximately 100 mm Hg; thus, oxygen diffuses into the blood. The partial pressure of systemic arterial oxygen is slightly less than 100 mm Hg because of the admixture of oxygenated and deoxygenated blood. Blood from pulmonary veins is mixed with some deoxygenated blood from bronchial veins, and in the left heart it is mixed with deoxygenated blood from thebesian veins draining cardiac muscle tissue (physiological shunt).

Carbon dioxide is removed in the pulmonary capillaries. The partial pressure of carbon dioxide in pulmonary arterial blood (systemic venous blood) is 46 mm Hg and that of blood leaving the lung (which becomes systemic arterial blood) is 40 mm Hg. The release of carbon dioxide is aided by the conversion of hemoglobin (Hgb) to oxyhemoglobin.

Oxygen reaching the tissues must dissociate from Hgb and pass out of the red blood cells and move to the mitochondria. Just as in the lungs, once the oxygen molecule leaves the cell, passive diffusion becomes the driving force in the movement of oxygen. Unlike the relatively short distances encountered in the lung, the oxygen diffusion from the blood to the mitochondria in the target cell is much greater. The partial pressure of oxygen at the arterial end of the capillary, approximately 90 mm Hg, quickly drops to approximately 30 mm Hg in the tissues and to approximately 1 to 3 mm Hg in the mitochondria.[156] Factors other than diffusion that influence oxygen delivery include the rate of oxygen delivery, the position of the P_{50} (right or left shift), and the rate of cellular oxygen consumption.[180]

Transport of carbon dioxide in the blood begins with the diffusion of carbon dioxide out of the tissue cells. The P_{CO_2} of the tissues (50 mm Hg) is greater than the Pa_{CO_2} in systemic capillaries (46 mm Hg). Thus, carbon dioxide diffuses from the tissues into the blood. The P_{CO_2} in the tissues is proportional to the amount of energy expended. Once carbon dioxide has diffused into the capillaries, a series of chemical reactions can occur. Carbon dioxide is carried in the blood by three mechanisms. Approximately 6% of carbon dioxide is carried in the dissolved state, 20% to 25% combines with Hgb, and the remainder (approximately 70%) of it combines with hydrogen to form bicarbonate. In the normal physiological state, an average of 4 mL of carbon dioxide is transported from the tissues to the lungs in each 100 mL of blood. The amount of carbon dioxide carried in the blood can greatly alter the acid–base balance and must be carefully monitored in the critically ill patient. The diffusion of carbon dioxide into the blood is determined by two factors, the Pco_2 of the tissues and the oxygen content of the blood; both factors are in turn determined by the environment of the tissues. Thus, the physiochemical state that results from this exchange of gases is controlled by the metabolic demands of the tissues.

Oxygen Cascade

The oxygen cascade describes the partial pressure gradient for oxygen as it moves from air (P_{IO_2}= 149 mm Hg at 37°C at sea level) through the respiratory tract where it is humidified to the alveolus (P_{AO_2}= 100 mm Hg), across the alveolar–capillary membrane to arterial blood (P_{AO_2} = 90 to 100 mm Hg) and the capillaries (P_{O_2}= 30 to 40 mm Hg) and then into the tissues and finally to the cytoplasm and the mitochondria. The oxygen concentration at the tissue level varies based on the organ, by regional variations in perfusion, oxygen consumption, and the distance from the capillary. Mitochondrial function is generally not impaired until cellular oxygen drops below 1 to 2 mm Hg.[181]

Oxygen diffuses from the capillary to the mitochondria along a concentration gradient. In 1919, Krogh[182] defined a model of oxygen delivery that is characterized by a tissue cylinder surrounding each capillary. The Krogh model was based on the idea that oxygen consumption takes place along the capillary, with a progressive decrease in oxygen from the artery to the vein. This longitudinal oxygen gradient suggests that cells receiving oxygen from the venous end of the capillary would be at increased risk for decreased oxygen delivery under conditions of decreased flow or arterial oxygen. Current research indicates that while there is a longitudinal delivery gradient there is less heterogeneity than originally conceived.[183] In addition, oxygen delivery occurs not only along the capillaries, but also from the arterioles. The current models also suggest that oxygen consumption occurs not only within the tissue, but also in the arteriolar endothelium.[184,185] The implication of these findings is the need to redefine the radial gradient for oxygen delivery to include endothelial oxygen consumption and account for the relatively homogeneous delivery gradients.[184,185]

Mitochondrial Respiration

Ninety percent of the body's oxygen consumption occurs in the mitochondria. Inside the mitochondria the hydrogen ions produced during glycolysis are passed to the electron transport chain and through the step-wise process of oxidative phosphorylation they combine with molecular oxygen (dioxygen) to form water. The final step in the process is the reduction of oxygen by cytochrome a_3. Under aerobic conditions, the electron transport chain produces three ATP molecules during this process. Of clinical importance, mitochondrial respiration may be disrupted in sepsis by NO, which inhibits cytochrome a,a_3 and pyruvate dehydrogenase, which is responsible for the conversion of pyruvate.[57,186,187]

Oxygen Delivery, Consumption, Extraction

Oxygen Delivery

The delivery of adequate oxygen for normal cellular function depends not only on the total amount of oxygen in the arterial blood (arterial oxygen content) but also on the ability of the heart to provide adequate blood flow (cardiac output). Oxygen delivery ($\dot{D}O$) is defined as the transport of oxygen to the tissues per minute. Oxygen delivery is determined by the combined processes of ventilation and diffusion (pulmonary function), Hgb-binding capacity, convective movement of blood (cardiac function), microvascular distribution, and delivery of oxygen to the mitochondria (passive diffusion).

Cardiac Output. Cardiac output is a main determinant of oxygen delivery. Decrease in blood flow decreases the supply of oxygen to the cells, thereby initiating a series of compensatory mechanisms to increase oxygen transport and extraction. Careful monitoring of the determinants of cardiac output (preload, afterload, and contractility) and heart rate are necessary to optimize oxygen delivery. Arterial oxygen content and cardiac output are combined in the oxygen delivery ($\dot{D}O2$) equation to measure the amount of oxygen delivered to the tissues in a given unit of time. Further discussion of the clinical implications of the oxygen consumption–delivery relationship is presented in Chapter 21.

Hemoglobin. In the red blood cell, the Hgb molecule acts as an oxygen-binding site responsible for carrying 97% of the oxygen in the blood. Hgb is a protein of four subunits of porphyrin and iron. The molecule is composed of two α and two β polypeptide chains, each with an iron-containing heme molecule capable of binding oxygen. Theoretically, 1 g of Hgb is capable of transporting 1.39 mL of oxygen. However, some of the heme sites are in an alternate form (methemoglobin) that is not capable of combining with oxygen. The maximum amount of oxygen that can be transported is approximately 1.34 to 1.36 mL/g of Hgb (some authors suggest this number may be lower, approximately 1.31 mL/g).[156] Hgb has a unique chemical structure that accounts for the differences in the speed at which oxygen binds with Hgb (affinity). Oxygen affinity increases as more Hgb is saturated with oxygen, so that the affinity of the last heme unit is greater than the first unit. This relationship explains the nonlinear curve represented in the oxyhemoglobin dissociation (or equilibrium) curve.[138]

Partial Pressure of Oxygen. Alveolar oxygen diffuses into the pulmonary capillaries. The amount of oxygen transferred depends on the mechanics of the ventilation–perfusion relationship of the lungs and the amount of inspired oxygen. The majority (97%) of the oxygen transported by the blood is bound to Hgb. The remaining 3% of the oxygen transported by the blood (0.3 mL/dL) comprises oxygen dissolved in plasma. The Pa_{O2}, a measurement of oxygen tension, is simply a reflection of the patient's plasma oxygenation. The Pa_{O2} is an indication of the patient's capacity for bonding oxygen to Hgb and the ability of oxygen to be released into the interstitial tissues. The body's plasma may carry a small percentage of the arterial oxygen, but measurement of its oxygen tension is an indirect method for determining the patient's oxygen–Hgb affinity.

Arterial Oxygen Saturation. As the partial pressure of oxygen in the pulmonary capillaries increases, oxygen binds with Hgb to form oxyhemoglobin. After leaving the pulmonary circulation, arterial blood can be sampled to measure the partial pressure of oxygen Pa_{O2}. Because oxygen binds with Hgb in a predictable manner, the saturation of Hgb in the arterial blood (Sa_{O2}) can be calculated (or measured directly by co-oximetry). The quantity of oxyhemoglobin, reflecting the amount of Hgb bound to oxygen, is measured as oxygen saturation. Saturation can be expressed as a percentage when multiplied by 100.

Oxyhemoglobin Dissociation Curve. The essential relationship between Pa_{O2} and Sa_{O2} is graphically illustrated by the oxyhemoglobin dissociation curve (Fig. 2-18). The sigmoid, or S, shape of this curve reflects the optimal conditions that facilitate oxygen loading in the lungs and oxygen release to the tissues. To describe these processes in relation to the curve, the curve is often divided into two segments: the association segment and the dissociation segment.

The upper portion of the curve, or the association segment, represents oxygen uptake, where large decreases in Pa_{O2} elicit only small decreases in Sa_{O2}. For example, in the association segment of the curve, a 40% decrease in the Pa_{O2} (mm Hg) from 100 to 60 results only in a 7% decrease in oxygen saturation. The association segment also represents the body's protective mechanism to ensure that, even with a substantial decrease in Pa_{O_2}, adequate arterial oxygen content is available for transport to the cells. The lower portion of the curve, or the dissociation segment, reflects the release of oxygen to the tissues. Here, small changes in Pa_{O2} result in large changes in Sa_{O2}, protecting the tissues by releasing large amounts of oxygen with minimal changes in oxygen tension.

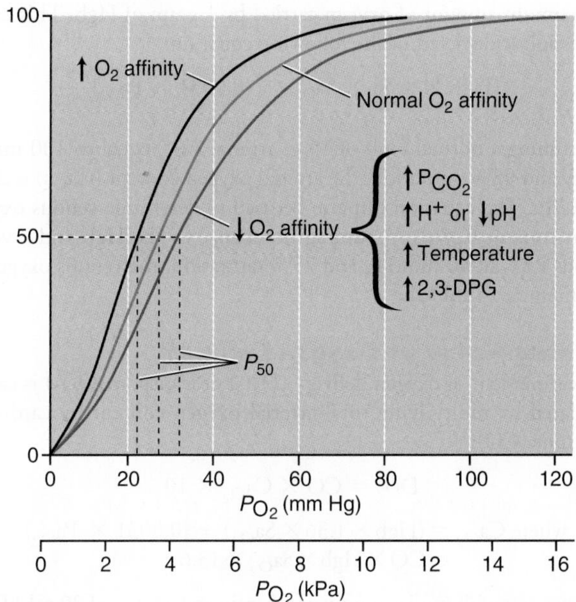

■ **Figure 2-18** Changes in O_2 affinity of the O_2 saturation curve. Three curves are shown with progressively decreasing O_2 affinity indicated by increasing P_{50}. (From Hlastala, M. P., & Berger, A. J. [2001]. *Physiology of respiration* [2nd ed., p. 99]. New York: Oxford University Press.)

Unlike in the association segment, a 40% decrease in the Pa_{O2} causes a 20% decrease in oxygen saturation.

Changes in oxyhemoglobin affinity affect the oxyhemoglobin dissociation curve and need to be considered in tissue oxygen assessment. Increased affinity, caused by hypothermia, alkalosis, or decreased levels of 2,3-diphosphoglycerate (also referred to as biphosphoglycerate), decreases oxyhemoglobin affinity, shifting the curve to the right and thus allowing more oxygen to be released. In this way, tissue oxygenation is enhanced in the presence of decreased saturation and increased demand.

Change in the Pa_{CO2} and pH also cause shifts in the Hgb dissociation curve; this is termed the *Bohr effect*.[156,188] As blood perfuses through the lungs, carbon dioxide diffuses from the blood to the alveoli. As a result of this movement of carbon dioxide, the Pa_{CO2} is reduced, and there is a subsequent increase in pH. The Hgb dissociation curve shifts to the left, thus increasing the binding of Hgb to oxygen and allowing greater oxygen transport to the tissues. At the tissue level, however, carbon dioxide displaces oxygen from the hemoglobin. The Hgb dissociation curve shifts to the right at the tissue level, facilitating higher oxygen delivery to the tissues (opposite to what occurs in the lungs). Shifts in the oxygen–Hgb dissociation curve have greater affects on events in the tissues than in the lungs because the relationships in the lungs are described in the flat upper position of the curve.

The P_{50}, which is an index of right and left shifts of the dissociation curve, describes the Pa_{O2} at which Hgb is 50% saturated. A higher than normal P_{50} value indicates a lower than normal affinity for oxygen. Under normal conditions (37°C, pH 7.40, Pco_2 40 mm Hg, and normal Hgb), the P_{50} is 27 mm Hg.

Blood Oxygen Content. Blood oxygen content reflects the amount of oxygen dissolved in plasma ($0.0031 \times Po_2$) and the amount bound to Hgb ($1.36 \times Hgb \times Sa_{O2}$), where 1.36 is the maximum amount of oxygen carried by 1 gram of Hgb. This expression is depicted in the following equation:

$$(\text{Hgb} \times \underset{97\%}{1.36 \times \text{Sa}_{O_2}}) + (\underset{3\%}{0.0031 \times \text{Pa}_{O_2}})$$

Assuming a normal Hgb of 15 g, arterial Pa_{O_2} equal to 100 mm Hg, and 98% saturation, the arterial oxygen content (Ca_{O_2}) is 20 mL/dL. The equation can also be used to determine venous oxygen content (Cv_{O_2}). Assuming no change in the Hgb and a venous Pa_{O_2} of 40 mm Hg and 75% saturation, the venous oxygen content is 15 mL/dL.

Measurement of Oxygen Delivery

Measurement of oxygen delivery ($\dot{D}O_2$) or transport ($\dot{Q}O_2$) is calculated by multiplying total arterial oxygen content by cardiac output (CO):

$$\dot{D}O_2 = CO \times Ca_{O_2} \times 10$$

$$\text{where } Ca_{O_2} = (\text{Hgb} \times 1.36 \times Sa_{O_2}) + (0.0031 \times Pa_{O_2})$$
$$= CO \times \text{Hgb} \times Sa_{O_2} \times 13.6$$

In patients with cardiac output of 5 L/min and a Ca_{O_2} of 20 mL/dL, arterial oxygen delivery ($\dot{D}O_2$) is 1,000 mL of oxygen/min or on average 500 to 650 ml/min/m^2. Critical oxygen delivery, which reflects the point where oxygen delivery fails to satisfy metabolic needs for oxygen has not been definitively identified. Critical $\dot{D}O_2$ has been estimated to be less than 7 ml/kg/min in awake, healthy young adults and 330 ml/min/m^2 in anesthetized older adults.[189–191]

Delivery of oxygen to support aerobic metabolism can be limited anywhere along the route from the environment through the alveolar–pulmonary interface, the systemic circulation, and the capillary–tissue junction to the mitochondria. Hypoxia is the shortage of oxygen at the tissue level. Hypoxia can be classified as (1) *hypoxic hypoxia*, caused by a decreased PO_2; (2) *anemic hypoxia*, caused by decreased Hgb; (3) *ischemic (stagnant) hypoxia*, caused by a lack of blood flow to the tissue; and (4) *histotoxic (cytopathic) hypoxia*, normal oxygen delivery; however, the cell is unable to process the oxygen and produce ATP.

Oxygen Consumption

Oxygen consumption ($\dot{V}O_2$) is the body's demand for oxygen and is defined as the amount of oxygen consumed at the tissue level per minute. Oxygen consumption can be calculated by determining the difference between the quantity of oxygen carried by the arterial system to the tissues (Ca_{O_2}) and the quantity remaining in the blood returning in the venous system to the lungs (Cv_{O_2})[180]:

$$\dot{V}O_2 = (CO \times Ca_{O_2} \times 10) - (CO \times Cv_{O_2} \times 10)$$
$$\dot{V}O_2 = Ca_{O_2} \times Cv_{O_2}$$

By combining the factors, the preceding can be simplified to the following equation:

$$\dot{V}O_2 = CO \times \text{Hgb} \times 13.6 \times (Sa_{O_2} \times S\bar{v}_{O_2})$$

This equation is a restatement of the Fick equation, placing $\dot{V}O_2$ on the left instead of cardiac output. This formula identifies all components of oxygen supply and demand. In a patient with normal values in a relatively steady state, normal $\dot{V}O_2$ is on average between 200 and 250 mL/min (or estimates of 3.5 mL/kg), as shown in the following equation:

$$\dot{V}O_2 = 5 \text{ L/min} \times 15 \text{ g/dL} \times 13.6\ (0.98 - 0.75)$$
$$\dot{V}O_2 = 234 \text{ mL/min}$$

Oxygen consumption is affected by several factors. Blood flow depends on the cardiac output and on the degree of constriction of the vascular bed in the tissue (vasoregulatory mechanisms). Low Hgb decreases the amount of available oxygen to be delivered to the tissues. Reduced Pa_{O_2} can affect the driving force needed to load the oxygen molecule on the Hgb. Decreased Sa_{O_2} affects the affinity between oxygen and Hgb, enhancing the release of oxygen to the tissues. The metabolic rate of the tissues also affects the affinity of oxygen to be released.

Oxygen Extraction Ratio

The percentage of oxygen extracted by the tissues is a useful indicator of the balance between oxygen delivery and consumption. Oxygen extraction represents the difference between arterial and venous oxygen contents (normal 5 mL/dL or 25%) and is known as the $C(a\text{–}v)_{O_2}$ difference or oxygen extraction ratio (O_2ER). This ratio increases in pathological conditions characterized by an imbalance between oxygen delivery and VO_2. O_2ER is increased by factors such as decreased cardiac output, increased oxygen consumption (e.g., shivering), anemia, and decreased arterial oxygenation. O_2ER is decreased in conditions where VO_2 is relatively low in proportion to oxygen delivery, such as in sepsis, hypothermia, high-flow states, peripheral shunting, or cytopathic hypoxia.[180,187]

REFERENCES

1. Wiedeman, M. (1963). Dimensions of blood vessels from distributing artery to collecting vein. *Circulation Research, 12*, 375–378.
2. Rothe, C. (1983). Venous system: Physiology of the capacitance vessels. In J. Shepherd & F. Abboud (Eds.), *Handbook of physiology. The cardiovascular system. Peripheral circulation and organ blood flow* (pp. 397–452). Bethesda, MD: American Physiological Society.
3. Rhodin, J. (1980). Architecture of the vessel wall. In D. Bohr, A. Somlyo, & H. Sparks (Eds.), *Handbook of physiology* (pp. 1–31). Bethesda, MD: American Physiological Society.
4. Rhodin, J. (1981). Anatomy of the microcirculation. In R. Effros, H. Schmid-Schonbein & J. Ditzel (Eds.), *Microcirculation* (pp. 11–17). New York: Academic Press.
5. Dalton, S. R., Fillman, E. P., Ferringer, T., et al. (2006). Smooth muscle pattern is more reliable than the presence or absence of an internal elastic lamina in distinguishing an artery from a vein. *Journal of Cutaneous Pathology, 33*, 216–219.
6. O'Rourke, M. F. (2007). Arterial aging: Pathophysiological principles. *Vascular Medicine, 12*, 329–341.
7. Mulvany, M., & Aalkjeær, C. (1990). Structure and function of small arteries. *Physiology in Review, 70*, 922–961.
8. Mulvany, M. (1996). The Seventh Heymans Memorial Lecture Ghent, February 18, 1995. Physiological aspects of small arteries. *Archives of International Pharmacodynamic Therapeutics, 331*, 1–31.
9. Faber, J. (1988). In situ analysis of alpha-adrenoreceptors on arteriolar and venular smooth muscle in rat skeletal muscle microcirculation. *Circulation Research, 62*, 37–50.
10. Rizzoni, D., Porteri, E., Boari, G. E., et al. (2003). Prognostic significance of small-artery structure in hypertension. *Circulation, 108*, 2230–2235.
11. De Ciuceis, C., Porteri, E., Rizzoni, D., et al. (2007). Structural alterations of subcutaneous small-resistance arteries may predict major cardiovascular events in patients with hypertension. *American Journal of Hypertension, 20*, 846–852.
12. Mulvany, M. J. (2007). Small artery structure: Time to take note? *American Journal of Hypertension, 20*, 853–854.
13. Renkin, E. (1989). Microcirculation and exchange. In H. Patton, A. Fuches, B. Hille, et al. (Eds.), *Textbook of physiology* (pp. 860–878). Philadelphia: WB Saunders.
14. Renkin, E. (1984). Control of microcirculation and blood-tissue exchange. In E. Renkin & C. Michel (Eds.), *Handbook of physiology* (pp. 627–687). Bethesda, MD: American Physiological Society.
15. Sarelius, I. H., Cohen, K. D., & Murrant, C. L. (2000). Role for capillaries in coupling blood flow with metabolism. *Clinical Experiments in Pharmacology and Physiology, 27*, 826–829.

16. Simionescu, M., & Simionescu, N. (1984). Ultrastructure of the microvascular wall: Functional correlations. In E. Renkin & C. Michel (Eds.), *Handbook of physiology: Microcirculation* (pp. 41–101). Bethesda, MD: American Physiological Society.
17. Charkoudian, N. (2003). Skin blood flow in adult human thermoregulation: How it works, when it does not, and why. *Mayo Clinics Proceeding, 78*, 603–612.
18. Pries, A. R., & Kuebler, W. M. (2006). Normal endothelium. *Handbook of Experimental Pharmacology, 1,* (176, Pt. 1):1–40.
19. Schneeberger, E. E., & Lynch, R. D. (2004). The tight junction: A multifunctional complex. *American Journal of Physiology and Cellular Physiology, 286*, C1213–C1228.
20. Raju, S., Fredericks, R., Lishman, P., et al. (1993). Observations on the calf venous pump mechanism: Determinants of postexercise pressure. *Journal of Vascular Surgery, 17*, 459–469.
21. Rowell, L. (1993). *Human cardiovascular control.* New York: Oxford University Press.
22. Caggiati, A., Phillips, M., Lametschwandtner, A., et al. (2006). Valves in small veins and venules. *European Journal of Vascular and Endovascular Surgery, 32*, 447–452.
23. Rowell, L. (1986). *Human circulation: Regulation during physical stress.* New York: Oxford University Press.
24. Hainsworth, R. (1986). Vascular capacitance: Its control and importance. *Review of Physiology and Biochemistry, 105*, 101–173.
25. Rowell, L., O'Leary, D., & Kellogg, D. (1996). Integration of cardiovascular control systems in dynamic exercise. In L. Rowell & J. Sheperd (Eds.), *Handbook of physiology. Exercise: Regulation and integration of multiple systems* (pp. 770–838). Bethesda, MD: Oxford University Press.
26. Aukland, K. (2005). Arnold Heller and the lymph pump. *Acta Physiologica Scandinavia, 185*, 171–180.
27. Zawieja, D. (2005). Lymphatic biology and the microcirculation: Past, present and future. *Microcirculation, 12*, 141–150.
28. Muthuchamy, M., & Zawieja, D. (2008). Molecular regulation of lymphatic contractility. *Annals of the New York Academy of Sciences, 1131*, 89–99.
29. Schmid-Schonbein, G. (1990). Microlymphatics and lymph flow. *Physiology in Review, 70*, 987–1028.
30. Gashev, A. A. (2008). Lymphatic vessels: Pressure- and flow-dependent regulatory reactions. *Annals of the New York Academy of Sciences, 1131*, 100–109.
31. Olszewski, W. L. (2002). Contractility patterns of normal and pathologically changed human lymphatics. *Annals of the New York Academy of Sciences, 979*, 52–63.
32. Gashev, A. A. (2002). Physiologic aspects of lymphatic contractile function: Current perspectives. *Annals of the New York Academy of Sciences, 979*, 178–187.
33. Small, J., & Gimona, M. (1998). The cytoskeleton of the vertebrate smooth muscle cell. *Acta Physiologica Scandinavia, 164*, 341–348.
34. Somlyo, A., & Somlyo, A. (2002). The sarcoplasmic reticulum: Then and now. *Novartis Foundation Symposia, 246*, 258–268; discussion 268–271, 272–276.
35. Horowitz, A., Menice, C., Laporte, R., et al. (1996). Mechanisms of smooth muscle contraction. *Physiology in Review, 76*, 967–1003.
36. Griendling, K. K., Harrison, D., & Alexander, R. (2008). Biology of the vessel wall. In V. Fuster, R. Walsh, & M. F. O'Rourke (Eds.), *Hurst's the heart.* New York: McGraw-Hill.
37. Wiel, E., Vallet, B., ten Cate, H. (2005). The endothelium in intensive care. *Critical Care Clinics, 21*, 403–416.
38. Furchott, R., & Zawadzki, J. (1980). The obligatory role of endothelial cells in the relaxation of arterial smooth muscle by acetylcholine. *Nature, 288*, 373–376.
39. Ignarro, L. J., Buga, G. M., Wood, K. S., et al. (1987). Endothelium-derived relaxing factor produced and released from artery and vein is nitric oxide. *Proceedings of the National Academy of Sciences USA, 84*, 9265–9269.
40. Palmer, R., Ferrige, A., & Moncada, S. (1987). Nitric oxide release accounts for the biological activity of endothelium-derived relaxing factor. *Nature, 327*, 524–526.
41. Luscher, T. F. (1991). Endothelium-derived nitric oxide: The endogenous nitrovasodilator in the human cardiovascular system. *European Heart Journal, 12*(Suppl. E), 2–11.
42. Moncada, S., Palmer, R., & Higgs, E. (1991). Nitric oxide: Physiology, pathophysiology, and pharmacology. *Pharmacology in Review, 43*, 109–142.
43. Cohen, R. (2000). Role of nitric oxide in vasomotor regulation. In J. Loscalzo & J. Vita (Eds.), *Contemporary cardiology: Nitric oxide and the cardiovascular system* (pp. 105–122). Totowa, NJ: Humana Press.
44. Moncada, S., & Higgs, E. A. (2006). Nitric oxide and the vascular endothelium. *Handbook of Experimental Pharmacology*, 213–254.
45. Vanhoutte, P. M. (2000). Say NO to ET. *Journal of the Autonomic Nervous System, 81*, 271–277.
46. Alonso, D., & Radomski, M. W. (2003). The nitric oxide-endothelin-1 connection. *Heart Failure Review, 8*, 107–115.
47. Busse, R., & Fleming, I. (2006). Vascular endothelium and blood flow. *Handbook of Experimental Pharmacology*, 43–78.
48. Iida, N. (1999). Nitric oxide mediates sympathetic vasoconstriction at supraspinal, spinal, and synaptic levels. *American Journal of Physiology, 276*, H918–H925.
49. McHugh, J., & Cheek, D. J. (1998). Nitric oxide and regulation of vascular tone: Pharmacological and physiological considerations. *American Journal of Critical Care, 7*, 131–140.
50. Ignarro, L. J. (2002). After 130 years, the molecular mechanism of action of nitroglycerin is revealed. *Proceedings of the National Academy of Science USA, 99*, 7816–7817.
51. Ignarro, L. J. (2002). Nitric oxide as a unique signaling molecule in the vascular system: A historical overview. *Journal of Physiology and Pharmacology, 53*, 503–514.
52. Loscalzo, J. (2001). Nitric oxide insufficiency, platelet activation, and arterial thrombosis. *Circulation Research, 88*, 756–762.
53. Ahanchi, S. S., Tsihlis, N. D., & Kibbe, M. R. (2007). The role of nitric oxide in the pathophysiology of intimal hyperplasia. *Journal of Vascular Surgery, 45*(Suppl. A), A64–A73.
54. Friedewald, V. E., Giles, T. D., Pool, J. L., et al. (2008). The Editor's Roundtable: Endothelial dysfunction in cardiovascular disease. *American Journal of Cardiology, 102*, 418–423.
55. Behrendt, D., & Ganz, P. (2002). Endothelial function. From vascular biology to clinical applications. *American Journal of Cardiology, 90*, 40L–48L.
56. Fernandes, D., & Assreuy, J. (2008). Nitric oxide and vascular reactivity in sepsis. *Shock, 30*(Suppl. 1), 10–13.
57. Galkin, A., Higgs, A., & Moncada, S. (2007). Nitric oxide and hypoxia. *Essays in Biochemistry, 43*, 29–42.
58. Trzeciak, S., Cinel, I., Phillip Dellinger, R., et al. (2008). Resuscitating the microcirculation in sepsis: The central role of nitric oxide, emerging concepts for novel therapies, and challenges for clinical trials. *Academy of Emergency Medicine, 15*, 399–413.
59. Mitchell, J. A., Ali, F., Bailey, L., et al. (2008). Role of nitric oxide and prostacyclin as vasoactive hormones released by the endothelium. *Experimental Physiology, 93*, 141–147.
60. Mollace, V., Muscoli, C., Masini, E., et al. (2005). Modulation of prostaglandin biosynthesis by nitric oxide and nitric oxide donors. *Pharmacology in Review, 57*, 217–252.
61. Bellien, J., Thuillez, C., & Joannides, R. (2008). Contribution of endothelium-derived hyperpolarizing factors to the regulation of vascular tone in humans. *Fundamentals of Clinical Pharmacology, 22*, 363–377.
62. Lushka, L., Agewall, S., & Kublickiene, K. (2008). Endothelium-derived hyperpolarizing factor in vascular physiology and cardiovascular disease. *Atherosclerosis*; doi:10.1016/j.atherosclerosis.2008.06.008.
63. Feletou, M., & Vanhoutte, P. M. (2006). Endothelium-derived hyperpolarizing factor: Where are we now? *Arteriosclerosis and Thrombosis Vascular Biology, 26*, 1215–1225.
64. Feletou, M., & Vanhoutte, P. M. Endothelial dysfunction: A multifaceted disorder (The Wiggers Award Lecture). *American Journal of Physiology Heart Circulation Physiology, 291*, H985–H1002.
65. Feletou, M., & Vanhoutte, P. M. (2007). Endothelium-dependent hyperpolarizations: Past beliefs and present facts. *Annals of Medicine, 39*, 495–516.
66. Yang, Q., Yim, A. P., & He, G. W. (2007). The significance of endothelium-derived hyperpolarizing factor in the human circulation. *Current Vascular Pharmacology, 5*, 85–92.
67. Yanigisawa, M., Kurihara, H., & Kimura, S. (1988). A novel potent vasoconstrictor peptide produced by vascular endothelial cells. *Nature, 332*, 411–415.
68. Shah, R. (2007). Endothelins in health and disease. *European Journal of Internal Medicine, 18*, 272–282.
69. Stauffer, B. L., Westby, C. M., & DeSouza, C. A. (2008). Endothelin-1, aging and hypertension. *Current Opinion in Cardiology, 23*, 350–355.

70. Brunner, F., Bras-Silva, C., Cerdeira, A. S., et al. (2006). Cardiovascular endothelins: Essential regulators of cardiovascular homeostasis. *Pharmacology Therapeutics, 111*, 508–531.
71. Masson, S., Latini, R., Anand, I. S., et al. (2006). The prognostic value of big endothelin-1 in more than 2,300 patients with heart failure enrolled in the Valsartan Heart Failure Trial (Val-HeFT). *Journal of Cardiac Failure, 12*, 375–380.
72. Feldstein, C., & Romero, C. (2007). Role of endothelins in hypertension. *American Journal of Therapeutics, 14*, 147–153.
73. O'Connor, C. M., Gattis, W. A., Adams, K. F., Jr., et al. (2003). Tezosentan in patients with acute heart failure and acute coronary syndromes: Results of the Randomized Intravenous TeZosentan Study (RITZ-4). *Journal of the American College of Cardiology, 41*, 1452–1457.
74. Anand, I., McMurray, J., Cohn, J. N., et al. (2004). Long-term effects of darusentan on left-ventricular remodelling and clinical outcomes in the EndothelinA Receptor Antagonist Trial in Heart Failure (EARTH): Randomised, double-blind, placebo-controlled trial. *Lancet, 364*, 347–354.
75. Sica, D. A. (2008). Endothelin receptor antagonism: What does the future hold? *Hypertension, 52*, 460–461.
76. Van Guilder, G. P., Westby, C. M., Greiner, J. J., et al. (2007). Endothelin-1 vasoconstrictor tone increases with age in healthy men but can be reduced by regular aerobic exercise. *Hypertension, 50*, 403–409.
77. Ivey, M. E., Osman, N., & Little, P. J. (2008). Endothelin-1 signalling in vascular smooth muscle: Pathways controlling cellular functions associated with atherosclerosis. *Atherosclerosis, 199*, 237–247.
78. Rubin, L. J., Badesch, D. B., Barst, R. J., et al. (2002). Bosentan therapy for pulmonary arterial hypertension. *New England Journal of Medicine, 346*, 896–903.
79. Denton, C. P., Pope, J. E., Peter, H. H., et al. (2008). Long-term effects of bosentan on quality of life, survival, safety and tolerability in pulmonary arterial hypertension related to connective tissue diseases. *Annals of Rheumatic Diseases, 67*, 1222–1228.
80. Le Brocq, M., Leslie, S. J., Milliken, P., et al. (2008). Endothelial dysfunction: From molecular mechanisms to measurement, clinical implications, and therapeutic opportunities. *Antioxidants and Redox Signals, 10*, 1631–1674.
81. Antithrombotic Trialists' Collaboration (2002). Collaborative meta-analysis of randomised trials of antiplatelet therapy for prevention of death, myocardial infarction, and stroke in high risk patients. *BMJ, 324*, 71–86.
82. Ridker, P. M., Cook, N. R., Lee, I. M., et al. (2005). A randomized trial of low-dose aspirin in the primary prevention of cardiovascular disease in women. *New England Journal of Medicine, 352*, 1293–1304.
83. Eikelboom, J. W., Hankey, G. J., Thom, J., et al. (2008). Incomplete inhibition of thromboxane biosynthesis by acetylsalicylic acid: Determinants and effect on cardiovascular risk. *Circulation, 118*, 1705–1712.
84. Bombardier, C., Laine, L., Reicin, A., et al. (2000). Comparison of upper gastrointestinal toxicity of rofecoxib and naproxen in patients with rheumatoid arthritis. VIGOR Study Group. *New England Journal of Medicine, 343*, 1520–1528.
85. Bresalier, R. S., Sandler, R. S., Quan, H., et al. (2005). Cardiovascular events associated with rofecoxib in a colorectal adenoma chemoprevention trial. *New England Journal of Medicine, 352*, 1092–1102.
86. U.S. Food and Drug Administration. (2005). *Alert for healthcare professionals: Non-selective non-steroidal antiinflammatory drugs (NASIDs).* Silver Spring, MD: U.S. Department of Health and Human Services.
87. McGettigan, P., & Henry, D. (2006). Cardiovascular risk and inhibition of cyclooxygenase: A systematic review of the observational studies of selective and nonselective inhibitors of cyclooxygenase 2. *Journal of the American Medical Association, 296*, 1633–1644.
88. Warner, J. J., Weideman, R. A., Kelly, K. C., et al. (2008). The risk of acute myocardial infarction with etodolac is not increased compared to naproxen: A historical cohort analysis of a generic COX-2 selective inhibitor. *Journal of Cardiovascular Pharmacology and Therapies, 13*(4), 252–260.
89. Roumie, C. L., Mitchel, E. F., Jr., Kaltenbach, L., et al. (2008). Nonaspirin NSAIDs, cyclooxygenase 2 inhibitors, and the risk for stroke. *Stroke, 39*, 2037–2045.
90. Grosser, T., Fries, S., & FitzGerald, G. A. (2006). Biological basis for the cardiovascular consequences of COX-2 inhibition: Therapeutic challenges and opportunities. *Journal of Clinical Investigations, 116*, 4–15.
91. Funk, C. D., & FitzGerald, G. A. (2007). COX-2 inhibitors and cardiovascular risk. *Journal of Cardiovascular Pharmacology, 50*, 470–479.
92. Friedewald, V. E., Jr., Bennett, J. S., Packer, M., et al. (2008). The editor's roundtable: Nonsteroidal antiinflammatory drugs and cardiovascular risk. *American Journal of Cardiology, 102*, 1046–1055.
93. Harrison, D., Griendling, K. K., Landmesser, U., et al. (2003). Role of oxidative stress in atherosclerosis. *American Journal of Cardiology, 91*, 7A–11A.
94. Forstermann, U. (2008). Oxidative stress in vascular disease: Causes, defense mechanisms and potential therapies. *Nature Clinical Practice, 5*, 338–349.
95. Bonomini, F., Tengattini, S., Fabiano, A., et al. (2008). Atherosclerosis and oxidative stress. *Histology and Histopathology, 23*, 381–390.
96. Hornig, B., Landmesser, U., Kohler, C., et al. (2001). Comparative effect of ace inhibition and angiotensin II type 1 receptor antagonism on bioavailability of nitric oxide in patients with coronary artery disease: Role of superoxide dismutase. *Circulation, 103*, 799–805.
97. McQueen, M. J., Lonn, E., Gerstein, H. C., et al. (2005). The HOPE (Heart Outcomes Prevention Evaluation) Study and its consequences. *Scandinavian Journal of Clinical Laboratory Investigations Supplement, 240*, 143–156.
98. Landmesser, U., Bahlmann, F., Mueller, M., et al. (2005). Simvastatin versus ezetimibe: Pleiotropic and lipid-lowering effects on endothelial function in humans. *Circulation, 111*, 2356–2363.
99. Lonn, E., Bosch, J., Yusuf, S., et al. (2005). Effects of long-term vitamin E supplementation on cardiovascular events and cancer: A randomized controlled trial. *Journal of the American Medical Association, 293*, 1338–1347.
100. Vivekananthan, D., Penn, M., Sapp, S., et al. (2003). Use of antioxidant vitamins for the prevention of cardiovascular disease: Meta-analysis of randomised trials. *Lancet, 361*, 2017–2023.
101. Bjelakovic, G., Nikolova, D., Simonetti, R. G., et al. (2008). Systematic review and meta-analysis: Primary and secondary prevention of gastrointestinal cancers with antioxidant supplements. *Alimentary Pharmacology and Therapies, 28*(6), 689–703.
102. Marshall, J. M. (2002). Roles of adenosine in skeletal muscle during systemic hypoxia. *Clinical and Experimental Pharmacology and Physiology, 29*, 843–849.
103. Ralevic, V. (2002). Hypoxic vasodilatation: Is an adenosine-prostaglandins-NO signalling cascade involved? *Journal of Physiology (London), 544*, 2.
104. Ray, C. J., Abbas, M. R., Coney, A. M., et al. (2002). Interactions of adenosine, prostaglandins and nitric oxide in hypoxia-induced vasodilatation: In vivo and in vitro studies. *Journal of Physiology (London), 544*, 195–209.
105. Koller, A., & Bagi, Z. (2002). On the role of mechanosensitive mechanisms eliciting reactive hyperemia. *American Journal of Physiology, 283*, H2250–H2259.
106. Flavahan, N., Cooke, J., Shepherd, J., et al. (1987). Human postjunctional alpha-1 and alpha-2 adrenoreceptors: Differential distribution in arteries and limbs. *Journal of Pharmacology and Experimental Therapeutics, 241*, 361–365.
107. Civantos Calzada, B., & Aleixandre de Artinano, A. (2001). Alpha-adrenoceptor subtypes. *Pharmacology Research, 44*, 195–208.
108. Kable, J., Murrin, L., & Bylund, D. B. (2000). In vivo gene modification elucidates subtype-specific functions of alpha (2)-adrenergic receptors. *Journal of Pharmacology and Experimental Therapeutics, 293*, 1–7.
109. Kanagy, N. L. (2005). Alpha(2)-adrenergic receptor signalling in hypertension. *Clinical Science (London), 109*, 431–437.
110. Leech, C. J., & Faber, J. E. (1996) Different alpha-adrenoceptor subtypes mediate constriction of arterioles and venules. *American Journal of Physiology, 270*, H710–H722.
111. Feigl, E. O. (1998). Neural control of coronary blood flow. *Journal of Vascular Research, 35*, 85–92.
112. Barbato, E., Piscione, F., Bartunek, J., et al. (2005). Role of beta2 adrenergic receptors in human atherosclerotic coronary arteries. *Circulation, 111*, 288–294.
113. Gauthier, C., Seze-Goismier, C., & Rozec, B. (2007). Beta 3-adrenoceptors in the cardiovascular system. *Clinical Hemorheology and Microcirculation, 37*, 193–204.
114. Gauthier, C., Leblais, V., Kobzik, L., et al. (1998). The negative inotropic effect of B3-Adrenoreceptor stimulation is mediated by activation of nitric oxide synthase pathway in human ventricle. *Journal of Clinical Investigations, 102*, 1377–1384.
115. Moniotte, S., Kobzik, L., Feron, O., et al. (2001). Upregulation of beta(3)-adrenoreceptors and altered contractile response to inotropic amines in human failing myocardium. *Circulation, 103*, 1649–1655.

116. Lands, A. M., Arnold, A., McAuliff, J. P., et al. (1967). Differentiation of receptor systems activated by sympathomimetic amines. *Nature, 214*, 597–598.
117. Queen, L. R., & Ferro, A. (2006). Beta-adrenergic receptors and nitric oxide generation in the cardiovascular system. *Cellular and Molecular Life Sciences, 63*, 1070–1083.
118. Sperelakis, N., Tohse, N., Ohya, Y., et al. (1994). Cyclic GMP regulation of calcium slow channels in cardiac muscle and vascular smooth muscle cells. *Advances in Pharmacology, 26*, 217–252.
119. Rozec, B., & Gauthier, C. (2006). Beta3-adrenoceptors in the cardiovascular system: Putative roles in human pathologies. *Pharmacologic Therapeutics, 111*, 652–673.
120. Treschan, T., & Peters, J. (2006). The vasopressin system: Physiology and clinical strategies. *Anesthesiology, 105*, 599–612.
121. Barrett, L., Singer, M., & Clapp, L. (2007). Vasopressin: Mechanisms of action on the vasculature in health and septic shock. *Critical Care Medicine, 35*, 33–40.
122. Dellinger, R. P., Levy, M. M., Carlet, J. M., et al. (2008). Surviving Sepsis campaign: International guidelines for management of severe sepsis and septic shock: 2008. *Critical Care Medicine, 36*, 296–327.
123. Wenzel, V., & Lindner, K. H. (2002). Arginine vasopressin during cardiopulmonary resuscitation: Laboratory evidence, clinical experience and recommendations, and a view to the future. *Critical Care Medicine, 30*, S157–S161.
124. American Heart Association. (2005). American Heart Association guidelines for cardiopulmonary resuscitation and emergency cardiovascular care. *Circulation, 112*, IV1–IV203.
125. Loscalzo, J., & Vita, J. (2000). *Contemporary cardiology: Nitric oxide and the cardiovascular system.* Totowa, NJ: Humana Press.
126. Yao, X., & Huang, Y. (2003). From nitric oxide to endothelial cytosolic Ca^{2+}: A negative feedback control. *Trends in Pharmacological Science, 24*, 263–266.
127. Cohen, R. A., & Adachi, T. (2006). Nitric-oxide-induced vasodilatation: Regulation by physiologic s-glutathiolation and pathologic oxidation of the sarcoplasmic endoplasmic reticulum calcium ATPase. *Trends in Cardiovascular Medicine, 16*, 109–114.
128. Komalavilas, P., & Lincoln, T. (2000). Regulation of intracellular Ca+2 by cyclic GMP-dependent protein kinase in vascular smooth muscle. In P. J. Kadowitz & D. McNamara (Eds.), *Nitric oxide and the regulation of peripheral circulation* (pp. 15–32). Boston: Birkhauser.
129. Berridge, M. J. (2008). Smooth muscle cell calcium activation mechanisms. *Journal of Physiology, 95*(11), 5165–5177.
130. Somlyo, A. P., & Somlyo, A. V. (1994). Signal transduction and regulation in smooth muscle. *Nature, 372*, 231–236.
131. Berridge, M. (2002). The endoplasmic reticulum: A multifunctional signalling organelle. *Cell Calcium, 32*, 235–249.
132. Patterson, A., Henrie-Olsen, J., & Brenner, R. (2002). Vasoregulation at the molecular level: A role for the beta1 subunit of the calcium-activated potassium (BK) channel. *Trends in Cardiovascular Medicine, 12*, 78–82.
133. Sheperd, J., & Vanhoutte, P. (1979). *The human cardiovascular system. Facts and concepts.* New York: Raven Press.
134. Christensen K. L., & Mulvany, M. J. (2001). Location of resistance arteries. *Journal of Vascular Research, 38*, 1–12.
135. Duling, B. (1981). Coordination of microcirculatory function with oxygen demand in skeletal muscle. In A. Kovach, J. Hamar, & L. Szabo (Eds.), *Advances in physiology: Cardiovascular physiology: Microcirculation and capillary exchange* (pp. 1–16). Budapest: Akademiai Kaido.
136. Duling, B. R., & Klitzman, B. (1980). Local control of microvascular function: Role in tissue oxygen supply. *Annual Review of Physiology, 42*, 373–382.
137. Scher, A. (1989). The veins and venous return. In H. Patton, A. Fuchs, & B. Hille (Eds.), *Textbook of physiology* (pp. 879–886). Philadelphia: WB Saunders.
138. Hlastala, M., & Berger, A. (2001). *Physiology of respiration.* New York: Oxford University Press.
139. Crone, E., & Levitt, D. (1984). Capillary permeability to small solutes. In E. Renkin & C. Michel (Eds.), *Handbook of physiology* (pp. 411–466). Bethesda, MD: American Physiological Society.
140. Curry, R. (1984). Mechanics and thermodynamics of transcapillary exchange. In E. Renkin & C. Michel (Eds.), *Handbook of physiology* (pp. 309–374). Bethesda, MD: American Physiological Society.
141. Michel, C. (1996). Transport of macromolecules through microvascular walls. *Cardiovascular Research, 32*, 644–653.
142. Starling, E. (1896). On the absorption of fluids from the connective tissue spaces. *Journal of Physiology (London), 19*, 312–316.
143. Landis, E. (1927). Micro-injection studies of capillary permeability II. *American Journal of Physiology, 82*, 217–238.
144. Renkin, E. (1986). Some consequences of capillary permeability to macromolecules: Starling's hypothesis reconsidered. *American Journal of Physiology, 250*, H706–H710.
145. Michel, C. (1997). Starling: The formulation of his hypothesis of microvascular fluid exchange and its significance after 100 years. *Experimental Physiology, 82*, 1–30.
146. Levick, J. (1997). Fluid exchange across the endothelium. *International Journal of Microcirculation and Clinical Experiences, 17*, 241–247.
147. Aukland, K., & Reed R. (1993). Interstitial-lymphatic mechanisms in the control of extracellular fluid volume. *Physiology in Review, 73*, 1–78.
148. Weinbaum, S., Tarbell, J. M., & Damiano, E. R. (2007). The structure and function of the endothelial glycocalyx layer. *Annual Review of Biomedical Engineering, 9*, 121–167.
149. Hu, X., & Weinbaum, S. (1999). A new view of Starling's Hypothesis at the microstructural level. *Microvascular Research, 58*, 281–304.
150. Pappenheimer, J. (1984). Contributions to microvascular research of Jean Leonard Marie Poiseuille. In E. Renkin, & C. Michel (Eds.), *Handbook of physiology* (pp. 1–10). Bethesda, MD: American Physiological Society.
151. Mellander, S. (1978). On the control of capillary fluid transfer by precapillary and postcapillary vascular adjustment. *Microvascular Research, 15*, 319–330.
152. Aukland, K., & Nicolaysen, G. (1981). Interstitial fluid volume: Local regulatory mechanisms. *Physiological Reviews, 61*, 556–643.
153. Lanne, T., & Lundvall, J. (1992). Mechanisms in man for rapid refill of the circulatory system in hypovolaemia. *Acta Physiologica Scandinavia, 146*, 299–306.
154. Olsen, H., Vernersson, E., & Lanne, T. (2000). Cardiovascular response to acute hypovolemia in relation to age. Implications for orthostasis and hemorrhage. *American Journal of Physiology, 278*, H222–H232.
155. Levick, J. (1991). Capillary filtration-absorption balance reconsidered in light of dynamic extravascular factors. *Experimental Physiology, 76*, 825–857.
156. Lumb, A. (2005). *Nunn's applied respiratory physiology.* Philadelphia: Elsevier.
157. Cooper, C. J., Landzberg, M. J., Anderson, T. J., et al. (1996). Role of nitric oxide in the local regulation of pulmonary vascular resistance in humans. *Circulation, 93*, 266–271.
158. Ricciardolo, F. L., Sterk P. J., Gaston, B., et al. (2004). Nitric oxide in health and disease of the respiratory system. *Physiology in Review, 84*, 731–765.
159. Brew, K. (2003). Structure of human ACE gives new insights into inhibitor binding and design. *Trends in Pharmacological Science, 24*, 391–394.
160. Weinberger, S., Cockrill, B., & Mandel, J. (2008). *Principles of pulmonary medicine.* Philadelphia: Saunders/Elsevier.
161. West, J. (1963). Distribution of gas and blood in the normal lung. *British Medical Bulletin, 19*, 53–58.
162. Glenny, R. W. (1998). Blood flow distribution in the lung. *Chest, 114*, 8S–16S.
163. Hlastala, M. P., & Glenny, R. W. (1999). Vascular structure determines pulmonary blood flow distribution. *News in Physiological Science, 14*, 182–186.
164. Galvin, I., Drummond, G. B., & Nirmalan, M. (2007). Distribution of blood flow and ventilation in the lung: gravity is not the only factor. *British Journal of Anaesthesia, 98*, 420–428.
165. Glenny, R. (2008). Last word on Point:Counterpoint: Gravity is/is not the major factor determining the distribution of blood flow in the human lung. *Journal of Applied Physiology, 104*, 1540.
166. Hughes, M., & West, J. B. (2008). Last word on Point:Counterpoint: Gravity is/is not the major factor determining the distribution of blood flow in the human lung. *Journal of Applied Physiology, 104*, 1539.
167. Michiels, C. (2004). Physiological and pathological responses to hypoxia. *American Journal of Pathology, 164*, 1875–1882.
168. Mauban, J. R., Remillard, C. V., & Yuan J. X. (2005). Hypoxic pulmonary vasoconstriction: Role of ion channels. *Journal of Applied Physiology, 98*, 415–420.
169. Moudgil, R., Michelakis, E. D., & Archer, S. L. (2005). Hypoxic pulmonary vasoconstriction. *Journal of Applied Physiology, 98*, 390–403.
170. Aaronson, P. I., Robertson, T. P., Knock, G. A., et al. (2006). Hypoxic pulmonary vasoconstriction: Mechanisms and controversies. *Journal of Physiology, 570*, 53–58.

171. Gurney, A. M. (2002). Multiple sites of oxygen sensing and their contributions to hypoxic pulmonary vasoconstriction. *Respiratory Physiology & Neurobiology, 132,* 43–53.
172. Griffiths, M. J., & Evans, T. W. (2005). Inhaled nitric oxide therapy in adults. *New England Journal of Medicine, 353,* 2683–2695.
173. Adhikari, N. K., Burns, K. E., Friedrich, J. O., et al. (2007). Effect of nitric oxide on oxygenation and mortality in acute lung injury: Systematic review and meta-analysis. *BMJ, 334,* 779.
174. Kanthapillai, P., Lasserson, T., & Walters, E. (2004). Sildenafil for pulmonary hypertension. *Cochrane Database Systematic Reviews,* CD003562.
175. Liu, C., Liu, K., Ji, Z., et al. (2006). Treatments for pulmonary arterial hypertension. *Respiratory Medicine, 100,* 765–774.
176. Price, L. C., & Howard, L. S. (2008). Endothelin receptor antagonists for pulmonary arterial hypertension: rationale and place in therapy. *American Journal of Cardiovascular Drugs, 8,* 171–185.
177. Paramothayan, N. S., Lasserson, T. J., Wells, A. U., et al. (2005). Prostacyclin for pulmonary hypertension in adults. *Cochrane Database Systematic Reviews,* CD002994.
178. Levitzky, M. (2007). *Pulmonary physiology.* New York: McGraw-Hill.
179. Pinsky, M. (2002). Role of cardiorespiratory system in delivering oxygen. In W. Sibbald, K. Messmer, & M. Fink (Eds.), *Tissue oxygenation in acute medicine* (pp. 3–13). Berlin: Springer-Verlag.
180. Leach, R. M., & Treacher, D. F. (2002). The pulmonary physician in critical care: Oxygen delivery and consumption in the critically ill. *Thorax, 57,* 170–177.
181. Wilson, D. F. (2008). Quantifying the role of oxygen pressure in tissue function. *American Journal of Physiology of Heart Circulation Physiology, 294,* H11–H13.
182. Krogh, A. (1999). The number and distribution of capillaries in muscles with calculations of the oxygen pressure head necessary for supplying the tissue. *Journal of Physiology, 52,* 409–415.
183. Tsai, A. G., Johnson, P. C., & Intaglietta, M. (2007). Is the distribution of tissue pO(2) homogeneous? *Antioxidants and Redox Signals, 9,* 979–984.
184. Tsai A. G., Johnson P. C., & Intaglietta, M. (2003). Oxygen gradients in the microcirculation. *Physiology in Review, 83,* 933–963.
185. Tsai, A. G., Friesenecker, B., Cabrales, P., et al. (2006). The vascular wall as a regulator of tissue oxygenation. *Current Opinion in Nephrology and Hypertension, 15,* 67–71.
186. Erusalimsky, J. D., & Moncada, S. (2007). Nitric oxide and mitochondrial signaling: From physiology to pathophysiology. *Arteriosclerosis, Thrombosis, and Vascular Biology, 27,* 2524–2531.
187. Fink, M. P. (2002). Bench-to-bedside review: Cytopathic hypoxia. *Critical Care, 6,* 491–499.
188. Jensen, F. B. (2004). Red blood cell pH, the Bohr effect, and other oxygenation-linked phenomena in blood O2 and CO2 transport. *Acta Physiologica Scandinavia, 182,* 215–227.
189. Shibutani, K., Komatsu, T., Kubal, K., et al. (1983). Critical level of oxygen delivery in anesthetized man. *Critical Care Medicine, 11,* 640–643.
190. Ronco J. J., Fenwick J. C., Tweeddale M. G., et al. (1993). Identification of the critical oxygen delivery for anaerobic metabolism in critically ill septic and nonseptic humans. *Journal of the American Medical Association, 270,* 1724–1730.
191. Lieberman, J. A., Weiskopf, R. B., Kelley S. D., et al. (2000). Critical oxygen delivery in conscious humans is less than 7.3 ml O2 × kg(−1) × min(−1). *Anesthesiology, 92,* 407–413.

CHAPTER 3

Regulation of Cardiac Output and Blood Pressure

Elizabeth J. Bridges

This chapter reviews the neurohumoral control of the cardiovascular system as it relates to the rapid and more long-term control of cardiac output and blood pressure and the local control of blood flow (autoregulatory, metabolic, autacoid). Several models of cardiac function are presented, including the relationship between cardiac output and central venous pressure, the Krogh model of the effect of distribution of blood volume on cardiac output, and the arterial baroreflex responses to decreased and increased blood pressure.

AFFERENT INPUT AND RECEPTOR

Arterial Baroreceptors

The arterial baroreceptors are responsible for the reflex control of blood pressure. These baroreceptors are undifferentiated nerve fibers located in the adventitia of the carotid sinus (at the bifurcation of the carotid artery) and the aortic arch (between the arch of the aorta and the bifurcation of the subclavian artery; Fig. 3-1). The receptors are mechanoreceptors that respond to distortion or a change in transmural pressure or stretch of the vascular bed in which they are located. For example, the carotid baroreceptors are sensitive to external compression or massage, both of which unload them (decrease transmural pressure). Although baroreceptors are often referred to as "pressoreceptors," they in fact do not sense pressure directly, but instead only indirectly through change in stretch.

The baroreceptors respond to two types of input: static input (i.e., mean arterial pressure) and phasic input (i.e., pulsatile changes). Therefore, the baroreceptors are responsive to mean arterial pressure, pulse pressure, and the number of pulses per minute (e.g., heart rate).[1] The static response has a threshold effect, that is, below a certain threshold of mean arterial pressure (20 to 50 mm Hg), the receptor stops firing. Above this threshold there is an increase in rate of receptor firing in proportion to the increase in mean pressure, until a plateau of the output is reached at saturation. The phasic response increases when the rate of change of pressure rises (increasing pressure) and decreases when the rate of change in pressure decreases.

Cardiopulmonary Receptors

Cardiopulmonary or low-pressure baroreceptors are located in the atria, ventricles, and pulmonary arteries and veins, with the cardiac baroreceptors providing the primary afferent input for the vagal cardioreflex.[2,3] The properties of the cardiopulmonary baroreceptors are similar to those of the arterial baroreceptors, that is, a decrease in transmural pressure in the chamber or vessel results in a decrease in the firing rate of receptors, and vice versa.

Input to the central nervous system from the ventricular receptors, which are sensitive to mechanical and chemical stimuli, is through nonmyelinated vagal afferents (C fibers).[4] In response to an increase in ventricular pressure, the mechanoreceptors were previously thought to stimulate a depressor response (decreased heart rate/vasodilation). The depressor reflex causes a decrease in heart rate, and may play a role in the alteration in vascular tone;[5] although this response is less than the vascular response induced by increases in carotid or coronary arterial pressure. The ventricular mechanoreceptors appear to play a role only in protection from gross overdistention, possibly during myocardial ischemia.[6,7] Chronic activation of cardiac receptors in heart failure cause increased activation of hypothalamic paraventricular neurons, which may contribute to resetting of the baroreceptor reflex and a sustained increase in sympathetic activation.[8]

Bezold-Jarisch Reflex

The Bezold-Jarisch reflex, which is the most commonly used model to explain the triggering of vasovagal (neurocardiogenic) syncope, is manifested as a triad of symptoms (bradycardia, apnea, and hypotension).[9] Neurocardiogenic syncope is thought to occur as a result of excessive venous pooling and a decrease in peripheral venous return. The decreased venous return leads to a hypercontractile state that stimulates the cardiac mechanoreceptors (particularly those in the inferoposterior wall of the left ventricle).[10] This hypercontractile state mimics hypertension and causes a paradoxical inhibitory or depressor reflex causing a vagally mediated decrease in heart rate and withdrawal of sympathetic stimulation to the peripheral vasculature with subsequent vasodilation.[11] Stimulation of this reflex may occur with pathological conditions, such as myocardial infarction, administration of thrombolytic therapy, hemorrhage, aortic stenosis, or syncope. It is important to note that vasovagal syncope may also occur in patients with transplanted (denervated) hearts; thus, factors other than those traditionally attributed to the Bezold-Jarish reflex must be considered.[9] Figure 3-2 characterizes the numerous putative causes of vasovagal syncope. During an acute inferoposterior myocardial infarction (particularly because of right coronary artery occlusion) and at the time of reperfusion of these infarctions, the transient bradycardia observed is thought to be a manifestation of the depressor effect of vagal receptors located in the inferoposterior wall of the left ventricle.[12] Recent research also suggests that this response occurs with more proximal lesions involving the right ventricle.[13] During ischemia, these receptors, which are mechanosensitive or chemosensitive, may be distorted by bulging of the ventricular wall during systole[14] or by the presence of reactive oxygen species, serotonin, bradykinin, thromboxane A_2, or adenosine.[15–17] During thrombolytic therapy, the occurrence of vagally mediated bradycardia may be an indicator of reperfusion and sustained vessel patency, particularly with an inferior myocardial infarction.[18] These receptors are also thought to mediate the

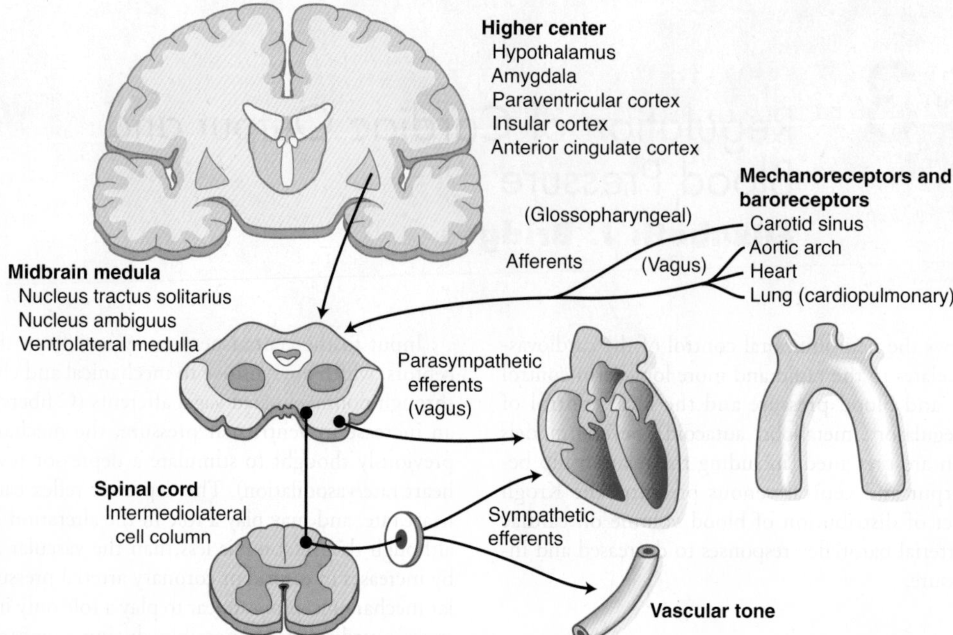

■ **Figure 3-1** Autonomic nervous system regulation of cardiovascular hemodynamic responses. The baroreceptors (mechanoreceptors), which are located in the carotid sinus, in the aortic arch, and in the heart and lungs, send afferent impulses to the nucleus tractus solitarius. The vagal fibers to the heart arise from the vagal nucleus in the brainstem. This nucleus is governed by the nucleus tractus solitarius, which is the main receiving station for afferent information from the peripheral mechanoreceptors and chemoreceptors. The medullary centers also receive input from higher brain centers. The vagal nerve alters heart rate through its effect on the sinoatrial and atrioventricular nodes. Sympathetic fibers innervate the sinoatrial and atrioventricular nodes and the ventricular myocardium, and affect heart rate and contractility. In addition, the sympathetic fibers innervate the vasculature, and thus alter vascular tone. (From Fenton, A. M., et al. [2000]. Vasovagal syncope. *Annals of Internal Medicine, 133*, 714–725.)

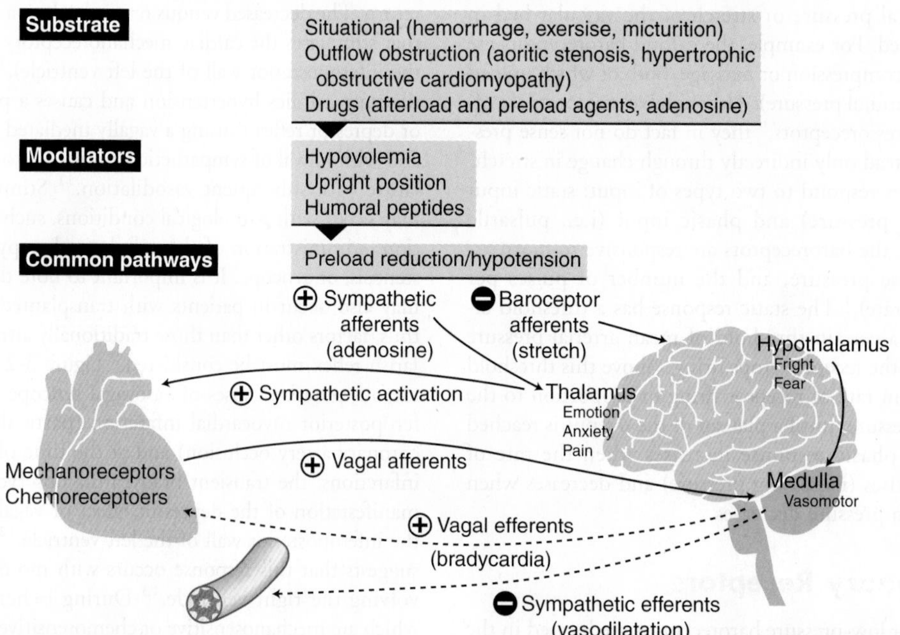

■ **Figure 3-2** The Bezold-Jarisch reflex indicates that the neurocardiogenic reflex is initiated by cardiac mechanoreceptor activation. This information is transmitted by the vagal afferents to the cardiovascular respiratory center in the medulla. The negative feedback response is transmitted by an activation of the vagal efferents and an inhibition of the sympathetic efferents. Inputs to the medulla may originate from extracardiac locations as well as directly from the higher central nervous system. (From Fenton, A. M., et al. [2000]. Vasovagal syncope. *Annals of Internal Medicine, 133*, 714–725.)

reflex bradycardia and hypotension that occur during coronary angiography, particularly during injection of contrast material into the arteries that supply the inferoposterior surface of the left ventricle (e.g., circumflex, right coronary artery).[19]

In severe aortic stenosis, some patients experience exertional syncope and even sudden death. The probable mechanism of the syncope is an exercise-induced increase in left ventricular pressure, which is extreme because of high aortic valve resistance, despite a decrease in aortic blood pressure. This high left ventricular pressure stimulates the ventricular baroreceptors and is manifested by a Bezold-Jarisch response.[20–23] Once these patients undergo surgical correction of the stenosis, however, the normal sympathetic vasoconstrictor response to exercise is restored. Similarly, in patients with hypertrophic cardiomyopathy, this abnormal response may be the cause of syncope, exercise-induced paradoxical peripheral vasodilation, or sudden cardiac arrest.[24–26] Finally, in cases of severe hemorrhage or during head-up tilt (particularly in patients receiving a concurrent infusion of isoproterenol), the ventricular depressor reflex is thought to be initiated by the acute distortion of the ventricular mechanoreceptors by a forceful ventricular contraction on a relatively empty ventricle or simply forceful contraction alone.[27] In a trauma model, inhibition of Bezold-Jarisch mediated bradycardia with β-adrenergic blockade may aid in resuscitation.[28]

Chemoreceptors

Peripheral chemoreceptors located in the carotid and aortic bodies are sensitive to decreased arterial Pa_{O_2} or an increase in Pa_{CO_2} or $[H^+]$, whereas central chemoreceptors, which are located in the medulla are sensitive to increased Pa_{CO_2}.[29] Stimulation of these receptors leads to hyperventilation and sympathetic activation, which causes vasoconstriction in most vascular beds, except the brain and heart. While an increase in blood pressure is an outcome of the chemoreflex, an increase in baroreceptor stimulation (i.e., increased arterial blood pressure) inhibits the chemoreflex response. Conversely, the chemoreflexes potentiate the baroreflex-mediated vasoconstriction in response to decreased arterial blood pressure.[30] In hypertension and sleep apnea, the peripheral chemoreflex response to hypoxemia is enhanced, with a resultant increase in sympathetic activation. Of clinical importance, there is a strong relationship between hypertension and sleep apnea (i.e., individuals with sleep apnea have a high prevalence of hypertension).[31] In heart failure, both the peripheral and central chemoreflex responses may be enhanced, as manifested by increased sympathetic activation.[32] This enhanced response may contribute to genesis of sleep apnea in these patients, which is associated with a poorer prognosis.[33–35] (See Chapter 8 for discussion of the relationship between sleep apnea and cardiovascular disease.)

CENTRAL NERVOUS SYSTEM REGULATION

The *nucleus tractus solitarius* is an ovoid area located in the medulla that receives efferent input from cardiovascular, respiratory, and gastrointestinal sites (see Fig. 3-1). The *nucleus tractus solitarius* serves as the first relay station for reflexes (e.g., baroreceptor reflex, central and peripheral arterial chemoreceptors, and skeletal muscle receptors [ergoreceptors]) that control circulation and respiration.[36] From the *nucleus tractus solitarius*, there are multiple projections to areas such as: (1) the ventrolateral medulla, which is responsible for sympathetic efferent activity; (2) the *nucleus ambiguus* or "cardioinhibitory center" of the medulla, which is the location of the cell bodies of the vagal parasympathetic nerves; and (3) the median preoptic nuclei, which affect the release of vasopressin. The output from the medulla depends on the perturbation of the system (i.e., an increase or decrease in blood pressure). From the central nervous system, the efferent arm of the rapid control of blood pressure operates through the autonomic nervous system. From the carotid sinus, afferent input to the nucleus tractus solitarius in the medulla is through the carotid sinus nerve (nerve of Hering), which joins the ninth cranial nerve (glossopharyngeal). The sensory input from the aortic arch is through the 10th cranial nerve (vagus). Through synaptic connections to areas located in caudal and rostral ventrolateral medulla and *nucleus ambiguus*, sympathetic and parasympathetic output, respectively, is modified by afferent feedback from the baroreceptors. Output from the lateral ventrolateral medulla, which is directly projected to spinal sympathetic outflow via the bulbospinal (or medullospinal) tract, is responsible for maintaining tonic sympathetic activity, and thus resting arterial blood pressure.[37,38] In addition, baroreceptor signals are transmitted to the forebrain. Paraventricular nuclei in the forebrain play a role in the release of vasopressin in response to a sustained decrease in blood pressure and increased osmolarity (or hypernatremia) and influences the sympathoexcitatory vasomotor neurons in the medulla.[39,40] The excitation or inhibition of the sympathetic and parasympathetic systems depends on the direction of the change in arterial blood pressure. An example of the reflex response (increased parasympathetic activity in the heart and sympathetic activity in the heart and vasculature) to increased blood pressure is summarized in Figure 3-3.[41] Of clinical importance, the baroreceptor reflex is reset at a higher point in hypertension, which is associated with adrenergic overdrive, decreased ability of cardiopulmonary receptors to control renin release and altered control of blood pressure and blood volume.[42]

AUTONOMIC NERVOUS SYSTEM REGULATION

The autonomic nervous system, which is one branch of the peripheral nervous system, is responsible for coordination of body functions that ensure homeostasis. The autonomic nervous system is further divided into two major components: the sympathetic nervous system and the parasympathetic nervous system (Fig. 3-4).

Sympathetic Nervous System

Efferent projections from the hypothalamus and medulla terminate in the intermediolateral cells located in the gray matter of the thoracic and lumbar (thoracolumbar) sections of the spinal column (specifically, T-1 to L-2). Hence, the sympathetic nervous system is often referred to as the thoracolumbar division of the autonomic nervous system. The neuronal cell bodies, which are located in the spinal column, are generally the origin of short preganglionic efferent fibers that innervate postsynaptic sympathetic neurons located in three general groupings of ganglia (a group of nerve cell bodies). The paravertebral ganglia are located in a bilateral chain-like structure adjacent to the spinal column. This chain extends from the superior cervical ganglia, located at the level of the bifurcation of the carotid artery, to ganglia located in the

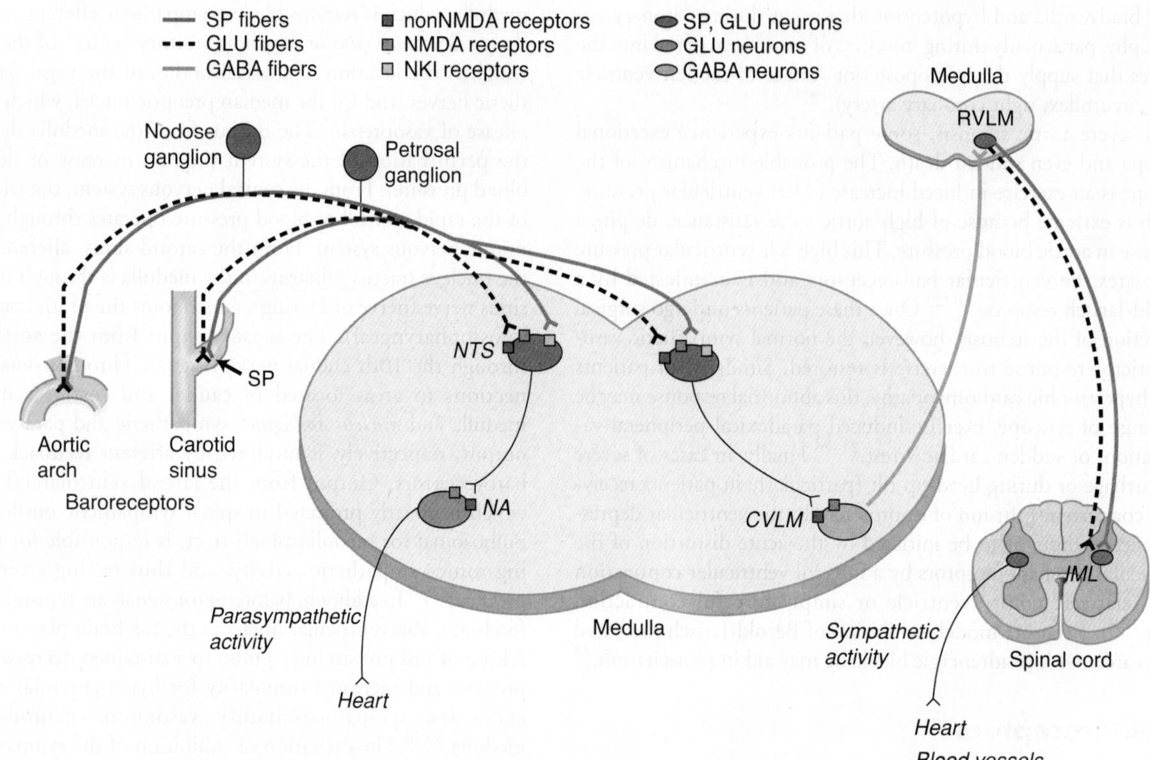

■ **Figure 3-3** Schematic diagram indicating the baroreflex arc. Baroreceptor afferents, with cell bodies in the petrosal and nodose ganglia, are activated by high blood pressure (stretch) and excite neurons in the nucleus tractus solitarius (NTS). These neurons then activate neurons within the nucleus ambiguus (N. AMB) to increase parasympathetic activity to the heart or activate neurons in the caudal ventrolateral medulla (CVLM), which in turn inhibit presympathetic neurons in the rostral ventrolateral medulla (RVLM). This inhibition of RVLM neurons reduces activation of sympathetic preganglionic neurons in the intermediolateral cell column (IML) of the spinal cord, reducing sympathetic activity to the heart and vessels. Glutamate (GLU) has been identified as an excitatory neurotransmitter at many synapses in the reflex arc, while gamma-aminobutyric acid (GABA) has been identified as an inhibitory neurotransmitter at the RVLM. SP has been identified in presumptive baroreceptor fibers: in the carotid sinus and aortic arch, in fibers and neurons within the petrosal and nodose ganglia, in fibers and neurons in the NTS, within neurons in the RVLM, and in fibers in the IML. Release of SP within the NTS, RVLM, and IML has been found to excite neurons within the regions through activation of NK1 receptors. (From Helke, C. J, & Seagard, J. L. (2004). Subtance P in the baroreflex: 25 years. *Peptides, 25*(3), 413–423.)

sacral region. The prevertebral ganglia, which lie midline and anterior to the aorta and vertebral column, include the celiac, aorticorenal, and superior and inferior mesenteric ganglia. The third group of ganglia comprises the previsceral or terminal ganglia, which are located close to the target organs of the sympathetic nervous system. The previsceral ganglia have long preganglionic fibers and short postganglionic fibers. In contrast, the paravertebral and prevertebral ganglia give rise to long postganglionic fibers, which extend to the target organs of the sympathetic nervous system (e.g., heart, lungs, vascular smooth muscle, liver, kidneys, bladder, and reproductive organs; see Fig. 3-4). Of particular importance to the control of blood pressure are the sympathetic receptors located in the heart, vasculature, kidneys, and renal medulla.

Adrenoreceptors

At the target organs, the postganglionic fibers terminate at the neuroeffector junction and are separated from the adrenergic receptors (adrenoreceptors) by only a small junctional gap or cleft. The adrenoreceptors have been classified into two general groups: α-adrenergic receptors and β-adrenergic receptors. The receptor groups are further divided into general subtypes, β_1, β_2, and β_3 and α_1 and α_2 (Table 3-1).[43,44] Based on molecular cloning techniques, the α-receptors are further subdivided, with the α_1 subclassified as (α_{1A}, α_{1B}, α_{1D}).[45] The α_1-adrenergic receptors, which are now characterized as subtypes α_{1A}, α_{1B}, and α_{1D}, are located in arteries, arterioles, and cutaneous and visceral veins. The α_{1A} receptors are responsible for vessel contraction. The α_{1B} receptors are thought to contribute to the maintenance of basal vascular tone and arterial blood pressure in conscious animals and are sensitive to exogenous agonists. Finally, the α_{1D} receptors also play a role in vascular contraction, although they have a lesser effect than the α_{1B} receptors.[46] The α_2 receptor has also been subclassified (α_{2A}, α_{2B}, and α_{2C}). The α_2 receptors, which have presynaptic and postsynaptic functions, are characterized as $\alpha_{2A/D}$, α_{2B}, and α_{2C}. The $\alpha_{2A/D}$ and α_{2B} receptors are present in large arteries but are located with greater density on the terminal arterioles, which act as precapillary sphincters to control the number of open capillaries and total capillary blood flow. The $\alpha_{2A/D}$ receptors play the primary role in vasoconstriction.[47,48] The α_{2B} receptors also play a role in vasoconstriction and may contribute

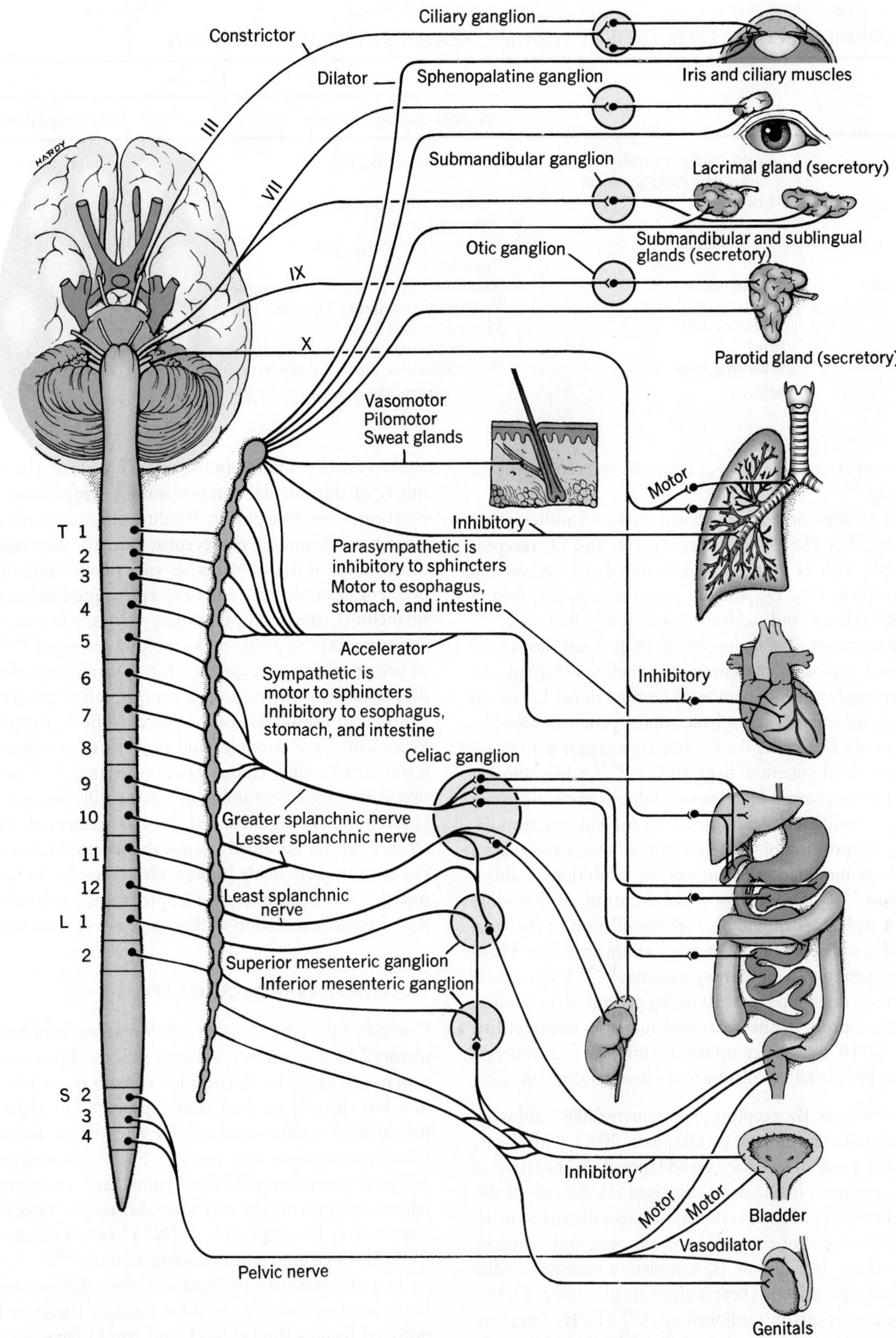

■ **Figure 3-4** The autonomic nervous system. Parasymphathetic (craniosacral) divisions send long preganglionic fibers that synapse with a second nerve in ganglia located close to or within the organs that are then innervated by short postganglionic fibers. The sympathetic (thoracolumbar) division sends relatively short preganglionic fibers to the chains of paravertebral ganglia and to certain outlying ganglia. The second cell then sends relatively long postganglionic fibers to the organs they innervate. (From Rodman, M. J. & Smith, D. W. [1985]. *Pharmacology and drug therapy in nursing* [3rd ed., p. 302]. Philadelphia: JB Lippincott.)

Table 3-1 ■ CARDIOVASCULAR EFFECTS OF AUTONOMIC NERVOUS SYSTEM INNERVATION

Organ	Site	Effects: Sympathetic Stimulation	Effects: Parasympathetic Stimulation
Heart	Sinoatrial/atrioventricular nodes, His-Purkinje system	+ Chronotrope (β_1, β_2)	– Chronotrope
	Myocardium	+ Inotrope (β_1, β_2, presynaptic α_1, presynaptic α_{2c})	– Inotrope (minor)
	Coronary arteries	Vasoconstriction (α_{1D}, α_2) Vasodilation (β_2)	Dilation
Systemic vasculature	Skeletal muscle	Vasodilation ($\beta_1 < \beta_2$, β_3, presynaptic α_2) Vasoconstriction (postsynaptic α_2)	—
	Splanchnic bed	Vasoconstriction (α, α_2)	—
	Renal	Vasoconstriction (α_1)	—
	Cutaneous veins	Vasoconstriction (postjunctional α_1, α_2)	Vasodilation

to the onset of hypertension. The α_{2C} receptors are responsible for venoconstriction.[46,49]

The effects of dopamine are mediated by two families of receptors (D_1 and D_2). The D_1-like receptors (D_1 and D_5 receptor subtypes) couple with G proteins to activate adenyl cyclase and the D_2-like receptors (D_2, D_3, and D_4 receptor subtypes) inhibit adenyl cyclase release and activate potassium channels.[50,51] Dopamine is a precursor of norepinephrine. In the heart, dopamine exerts its indirect inotropic and chronotropic effects through the release of norepinephrine. Stimulation of postjunctional D_1 receptors in the renal, mesenteric, and splenic arteries produces vasodilation and natriuresis. Defects in the D_1 and D_5 receptor may be associated with the development of hypertension.[50,52] Stimulation of prejunctional D_2 receptors in blood vessels inhibits norepinephrine release causing vasodilation. Additionally, in the kidneys stimulation of the D_2 receptor inhibits norepinephrine release and plays a synergistic role in modulating natriuresis via inhibition of aldosterone secretion.[52–55] Exogenous administration of low-dose dopamine (<4 μg/kg per minute) causes vasodilation of the renal and splanchnic vascular beds and increases sodium excretion. However, low-dose dopamine is not reno-protective.[56–58] Intermediate doses of exogenous dopamine (2 to 10 μg/kg per minute) stimulate β_1-adrenergic receptors in the heart and increases contractility. Higher doses (>10 μg/kg per minute) stimulate α-adrenergic receptors in the peripheral vasculature and cause vasoconstriction.

Heart. In the heart, β_1 receptors predominate (80%), although there are also a smaller number of β_2 receptors (20%), with the β_2 receptors playing a role in coronary vasodilation.[59] Stimulation of the β_1 and β_2 receptors in the heart increases: (1) the rate of discharge of the sinoatrial node, (2) conduction across the atrioventricular node, and (3) speed of contraction in the atria and ventricles (chronotropic effect). In addition, β_1 stimulation increases cardiac contractility (inotropic effect). There is also a small number (<1%) of β_3 adrenergic receptors in cardiomyocytes.[60] The β_3 receptors, which mediate negative inotropy via a nitric oxide-dependent pathway,[61] become important during heart failure when they are upregulated and while protective may contribute to functional degradation of the failing heart.[60,62] There are small number (approximately 14%) of α_1 receptors located in the atria and ventricles.[63] Stimulation of the α_1 receptors creates a modest inotropic response.[64]

Vasculature. Sympathetic stimulation of the arterial tree extends to the level of the terminal arterioles and is also present on capacitance vessels, primarily in the splanchnic bed. The primary transmitter of the vascular smooth muscle sympathetic neuroeffector junction is norepinephrine. Binding of norepinephrine to the vascular smooth muscle α_1 receptor initiates vasoconstriction. The distribution of the α_1 subtypes varies depending on the vascular bed. For example, α_{1A} adrenoreceptors predominate in coronary, splanchnic, renal, and pulmonary vessels, whereas central arteries and veins express all three α_1 receptor subtypes.[46,65] Stimulation of presynaptic α_2 receptors inhibits norepinephrine release and decreases vasoconstriction, a process called *passive vasodilation.* Conversely, stimulation of the postsynaptic α_2 receptors, which are located on large arterioles and perhaps most importantly on the terminal arterioles, causes vasoconstriction.[49] This vasoconstriction determines the number of open capillaries, and thus capillary blood flow. The α_2-mediated vasoconstriction of the terminal arterioles can be inhibited by metabolic vasodilators (e.g., oxygen, potassium), particularly in the skeletal muscles. In vascular smooth muscle, the β-adrenergic receptors are predominantly of the β_2-subtype. Stimulation of these receptors causes vasorelaxation.[44]

Cutaneous Vasculature

Control of the cutaneous circulation arises from both thermoregulatory and nonthermoregulatory reflexes. The cutaneous circulation has an extensive distribution of both α_1 and α_2 adrenoreceptors, but virtually no β adrenoreceptors.[66] The glabrous skin (e.g., palms/soles) is innervated only by vasoconstrictive nerves. In contrast, nonglabrous skin receives both vasoconstrictive and vasodilator innervations.[67] The sympathetic vasoconstrictor nerves release norepinephrine and may also release vasoconstrictive cotransmitters (neuropeptide Y [NPY] or adenosine triphosphate [ATP]), which augments vasoconstriction.[68,69]

In a thermoneutral environment, the cutaneous resistance vessels in the acral regions (e.g., ears) are tonically constricted, whereas the nonacral regions (limbs, head, and trunk) have minimal constriction.[70,71] Vasodilation in the acral regions is primarily caused by withdrawal of vasoconstrictive tone (passive vasodilation), whereas vasodilation in nonacral regions is the result of an active process, which is sympathetically (but not adrenergically) mediated. Within a "neutral zone," thermoregulation is controlled entirely by changes in cutaneous vasomotor tone.[72] An active increase in adrenergic tone causes vasoconstriction in response to hypothermia. Conversely, a decrease in adrenergic stimulation causes passive vasodilation and is responsible for 10% to 20% of vasodilation in response to hyperthermia.[67,68,73] Cholinergic nerves, which innervate the sweat glands, release a yet to be described co-transmitter that may be functionally linked to the large and important active cutaneous vasodilation seen in heat stress.[69,73,74] Additionally, under conditions of hyperthermia, nitric oxide is necessary for the vasodilatory response.[69] Endothelial nitric oxide (eNOS) is responsible for vasodilation in response to local cutaneous heating,[75] whereas neuronal nitric oxide (nNOS) is responsible for vasodilation in response to whole-body heating.[76] The cutaneous veins constrict in response to local cold and are reflexly constricted in response a decrease in skin or core body temperature.[77]

Nonthermoregulatory control of the cutaneous circulation via the arterial and cardiopulmonary baroreflexes plays a role in blood pressure control. For example, under normothermic conditions, "unloading" of the baroreflex causes cutaneous vasoconstriction. Because of the normally low cutaneous blood flow during normothermia, this vasoconstriction contributes little to blood pressure maintenance. However, under conditions of hyperthermia and during exercise, when there is significant blood flow to the cutaneous vasculature, baroreflex-mediated vasoconstrictive may offset thermoregulatory vasodilation and play an important role in maintenance of blood pressure.[67,73] Of note, the baroreflex sensitivity is not impaired by whole-body heating as previously thought; however, heat stress may decrease peripheral vasoconstrictor responsiveness, which contributes to an increased susceptibility to orthostatic intolerance.[78]

Neurotransmitters

The sympathetic postganglionic fibers that innervate the arterial tree are in general noradrenergic (i.e., release norepinephrine). The only exceptions are the postganglionic fibers that innervate the sweat glands (sudomotor neurons), which have acetylcholine as their neurotransmitter and the extrapyramidal system, which has dopamine as the primary neurotransmitter. Norepinephrine is synthesized from tyrosine and is stored in sympathetic nerve terminals. In response to neuronal stimulation, the "packets" or quanta of norepinephrine are extruded from the axon vesicles by exocytosis. The vesicular release of norepinephrine is enhanced by angiotensin II and cold, whereas the prejunctional effects of potassium, decreased PO_2, heat, autacoids (adenosine, bradykinin, serotonin, and prostaglandins), nitric oxide, and acetylcholine inhibit its release[79] (Fig. 3-5). The neurotransmitters diffuse over varying small distances, depending on the width of the junctional cleft, to receptors located on effector organs. Norepinephrine is also considered a systemic hormone because of its spillover into the interstitial space.

Parasympathetic Nervous System

The second branch of the autonomic nervous system is the parasympathetic nervous system. The primary parasympathetic outflow is through four cranial nerves (III, VII, IX, and X). Of importance to blood pressure and cardiac output control, cardiac vagal (cranial nerve X) *motorneurons* are located in the nucleus ambiguus and dorsal vagal nucleus of the medulla. In addition, there are cell bodies located in the spinal cord gray matter at S-2 through S-4. Hence, the parasympathetic nervous system is referred to as the *craniosacral* branch of the autonomic nervous system. In contrast to the sympathetic nervous system, the preganglionic fibers of the parasympathetic nervous system are long fibers, synapsing on ganglia that are close to or directly attached to the effector organ. The postsynaptic fibers are relatively short, in contrast to the fibers of the sympathetic nervous system.

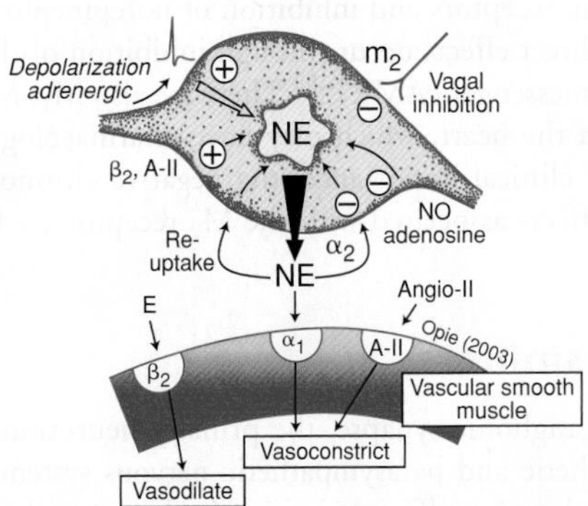

■ **Figure 3-5** Role of neuromodulation in arteriolar constriction and dilation. Norepinephrine is released from the storage granules of the terminal neurons into the synaptic cleft that separates the terminals from the arterial wall. Norepinephrine has predominantly vasoconstrictive effects acting through postsynaptic α_1 receptors. In addition, norepinephrine stimulates presynaptic α_2 receptors to invoke feedback inhibition of its own release, to modulate excess release of NE. Parasympathetic cholinergic stimulation inhibits the release of norepinephrine and thereby indirectly causes vasodilation. Circulating epinephrine stimulates vascular vasodilatory β_2 receptors, but also presynaptic receptors on the nerve terminal that promotes release of norepinephrine. Angiotensin II, formed ultimately in response to renin released from the kidneys, is also powerfully vasoconstrictive, acting both by inhibition of norepinephrine release (presynaptic receptors, schematically shown to the left of the terminal neuron) and also directly on arteriolar receptors. E, epinephrine; NE, norepinephrine; A-II, angiotensin II; M2, muscarinic receptor, subtype 2. (From Opie, L. H. [2003]. *The heart: Physiology from cell to circulation* [4th ed., p. 25]. Philadelphia: Lippincott Williams & Wilkins.)

Receptors

In the parasympathetic nervous system, the nerve fibers are cholinergic, which means they liberate acetylcholine. Despite a common neurotransmitter (acetylcholine), stimulation of various receptors in the parasympathetic nervous system causes different effects. The reason for the variable response is that there are two general types of cholinergic receptors: nicotinic and muscarinic.

Preganglionic cholinergic receptors, which are found in the sympathetic and parasympathetic nervous systems, are nicotinic. The nicotinic receptors are located on autonomic ganglia and skeletal muscle endplates. Stimulation of the nicotinic receptors is excitatory and short-term (milliseconds). These receptors are blocked by curare. In clinical practice, blockade of the nicotinic receptors with various neuromuscular-blocking agents (e.g., succinylcholine, pancuronium) causes musculoskeletal paralysis (blockade at the skeletal muscle endplate) and may potentially cause hypotension because of blockade at the autonomic ganglia.[80]

The primary postganglionic receptor in the heart, smooth muscle, and glandular tissue is muscarinic. These receptors are stimulated by muscarine and can be antagonized by atropine and scopolamine. There are subtypes of the muscarinic receptors that result in varied responses. The primary muscarinic receptors in the heart are the muscarinic subtype 2 (M_2), which are specifically associated with vagal nerve endings in the heart. The M_2 receptors have direct and indirect negative inotropic and chronotropic effects.[81] The direct effects are secondary to occupation of the β-adrenergic receptors and inhibition of norepinephrine release, and the indirect effects occur through inhibition of the adrenergic second messenger cAMP.[82,83] There are also M_1, M_3, and M_5 receptors in the heart, which may have pharmacologic implications.[84] Of clinical importance, the negative chronotropic and inotropic effects associated with the M_2 receptor are blocked by atropine.

Co-transmitters

At the preganglionic synapse, the primary neurotransmitter for the sympathetic and parasympathetic nervous systems is acetylcholine. At the neuroeffector junction in the sympathetic nervous system, the primary neurotransmitters are norepinephrine and its precursor, dopamine, whereas the primary neurotransmitter of the postganglionic fibers of the parasympathetic nervous system is acetylcholine. However, other neurotransmitters that augment or modify the effects of the primary neurotransmitter are co-released, and are referred to as *co-transmitters* (Fig. 3-6).[85–87] The most prominent co-transmitters in the sympathetic nervous system ganglia are NPY and ATP.[86,88] Vasoactive intestinal peptide (VIP) is the prominent co-transmitter in the parasympathetic nervous system ganglia and nonadrenergic, noncholinergic nerves.[89]

Neuropeptide Y

NPY is an amino acid peptide released with norepinephrine from sympathetic nerve terminals. NPY has direct pressor effects and also exerts a prejunctional modulation of the release of other neurotransmitters. For example, NPY inhibits the release of acetylcholine from vagal nerve endings, thus attenuating the effects of the parasympathetic system on heart rate, atrioventricular conduction, and atrial contractility.[90,91] In addition, NPY potentiates the postjunctional contractile effects of norepinephrine. In the mesentery, 30% of the sympathetic nervous system induced vasoconstriction depends on NPY,[92,93] although the role of NPY varies depending on the vascular bed. NPY is also associated with vascular remodeling (Y1 receptor) and angiogenesis (Y2). Pharmacologic strategies that promote angiogenesis but inhibit the pro-atherosclerotic effects of NPY may be useful in preventing or treating pathological vascular remodeling.[94,95]

Vasoactive Intestinal Peptide

VIP is present in the peripheral and central circulation, where it acts as a nonadrenergic, noncholinergic neurotransmitter, or neuromodulator. Endogenous VIP is a potent vasodilator, although its effects vary in different vascular beds. It is released in response to vagal stimulation in the heart, where it produces coronary vasodi-

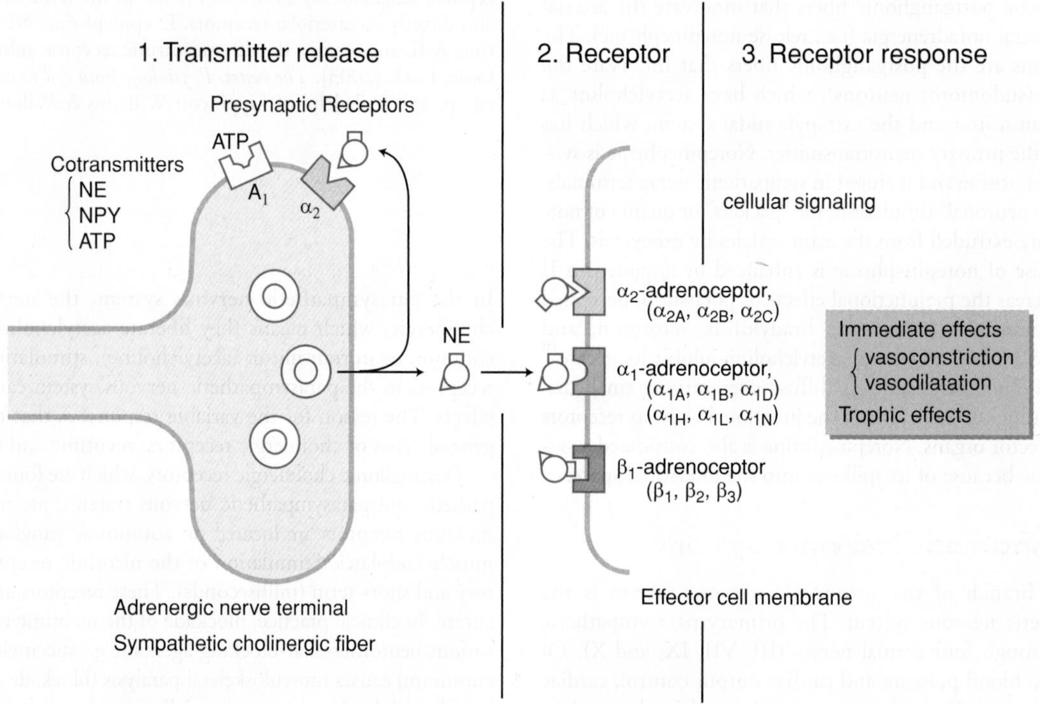

Figure 3-6 Diagram of the sympathetic nerve and adrenergic neuroeffector mechanism. (1) Transmitter release from the sympathetic terminal. Sympathetic nerve may contain three cotransmitters, that is, norepinephrine (NE), neuropeptide Y (NPY), and adenosine triphosphate (ATP). Release of main transmitter NE may be presynaptically modulated by α_2-adrenoreceptor, A_1 adenosine receptor, and so on. (2) Adrenoreceptors on the effector cell membrane. There are α- and β-adrenoreceptors and subtypes α_1 (α_{1A}, α_{1B}, and α_{1D}; α_{1H}, α_{1L}, and α_{1N}), α_2 (α_{2A}, α_{2B}, and α_{2C}), and β_1, β_2, and β_3. There may be regional differences in the population of adrenoreceptors. (3) Effector responses. Sympathetic nerves have both immediate effects—contraction and dilation, differing from vessel to vessel—as well as long-term trophic effect on blood vessels. (From Tsuru, H. et al. [2002]. Role of perivascular sympathetic nerves and regional differences in the features in sympathetic innervation of the vascular system. *Japanese Journal of Pharmacology, 88*[1], 9–13.)

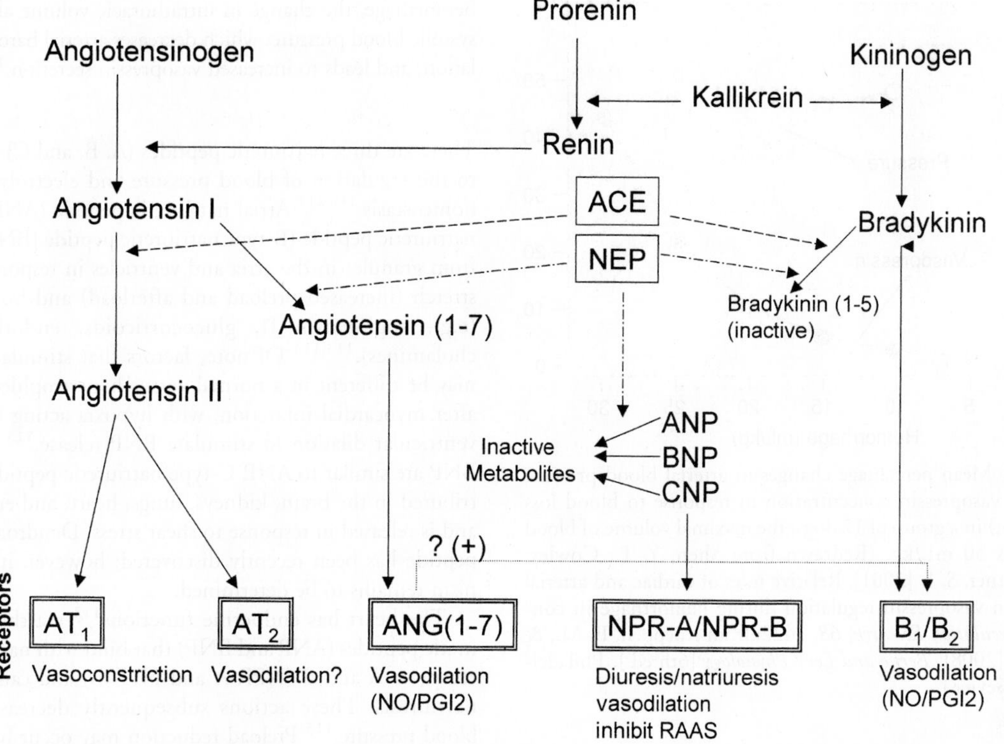

■ **Figure 3-7** Interaction of the renin–angiotensin–aldosterone system (RAAS), kallikrein–kinin system (KKS), and natriuretic peptides.

lation (effect greater on the arteries than the veins) as well as positive inotropic (particularly in the right atria and ventricle) and chronotropic effects.[96,97] VIP-induced peripheral vasodilation is caused by increased calcium-extrusion or sequestration induced by VIP or natriuretic protein-C receptor stimulation. This peripheral vasodilation enhances the VIP-mediated inotropic effects.[98]

SYSTEMIC HORMONES

In addition to the rapid control of arterial pressure by the autonomic nervous system, hormones such as epinephrine and arginine vasopressin (AVP) directly and indirectly affect the baroreceptor reflex and play an important role in the rapid control of blood pressure. Three interrelated systems (natriuretic peptide system, renin–angiotensin–aldosterone system [RAAS], and the kallikrein–kinin system [KKS]) also contribute to the regulation of the arterial blood pressure and fluid volume (Fig. 3-7). Finally, a spillover of norepinephrine into the systemic circulation also affects blood pressure and cardiac output.

Epinephrine

In response to physical or emotional stressors (mental stress, exercise, hyperthermia, hypoglycemia), epinephrine is secreted into the plasma by the adrenal medulla, causing the plasma level of epinephrine to increase. Epinephrine stimulates β_1 receptors in the heart and has positive chronotropic and inotropic effects. The net effect of this cardiac stimulation is an increase in cardiac output. Epinephrine also acts on the vasculature and stimulates the β_2 receptors in the skeletal muscles and splanchnic arterioles, which cause vasodilation in these two large regions and potentially large decrements in the systemic vascular resistance. In the skin and kidneys, epinephrine stimulates the α-adrenergic receptors and causes vasoconstriction.[99]

Exogenously administered epinephrine has dose-specific effects. Low-dose epinephrine (0.1 mcg/kg per minute) stimulates the β_1 and β_2 adrenoreceptors and causes vasodilation and increased heart rate and contractility. Increased doses (>0.2 mcg/kg per minute) stimulate the α-adrenoreceptors and increases vascular resistance and blood pressure.[100] Knowledge of these dose-specific effects is important, and although epinephrine is often administered for its vasoconstrictive effects, it may cause vasodilation with a smaller dose.

Arginine Vasopressin

AVP, or antidiuretic hormone (ADH), is a neurotransmitter synthesized in the hypothalamus and released from the neurohypophysis of the pituitary gland (posterior pituitary gland). Vasopressin is primarily released in response to changes in plasma osmolality; however, AVP may also be released in response to a decrease in blood volume or blood pressure. As the osmolality increases, AVP secretion increases. In humans, the primary effect of AVP is its antidiuretic effect, which is caused by stimulation of water absorption at the distal and collecting tubules of the kidney.[101,102] The change in water absorption affects plasma osmolality. Vasopressin is exquisitely sensitive to changes in osmolality; for example, a 5- to 10 mOsm increase in osmolality causes an increase in plasma AVP.[103,104] The close relation between osmolality and AVP maintains plasma osmolality within 1% of normal under most conditions.[105,106]

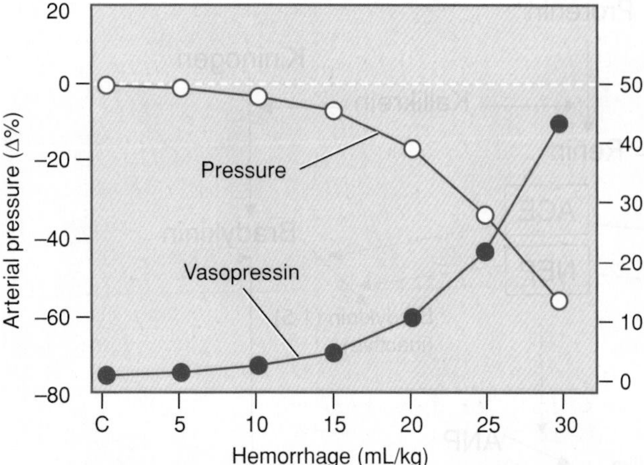

■ **Figure 3-8** Mean percentage changes in arterial blood pressure and in plasma vasopressin concentration in response to blood loss (0.5 mL/kg/min) in a group of 12 dogs; the maximal volume of blood withdrawn was 30 mL/kg. (Redrawn from Shen, Y.-T., Cowley, A. W., J., & Vatner, S. F. [2001]. Relative roles of cardiac and arterial baroreceptors in vasopressin regulation during hemorrhage in conscious dogs. *Circulation Research, 68*, 1422; from Koeppen, B. M., & Stanton, B. A. [2008]. *Berne and Levy Physiology* [6th ed.]. Philadelphia: Mosby Elsevier.)

The sensitivity of the baroreceptor system is less than that of the osmoreceptors, as demonstrated by the large (5% to 10%) isoosmotic change in plasma volume required before vasopressin secretion is altered. However, during hemorrhage (plasma volume decreased by >5% to 10%), plasma levels of vasopressin are increased, in some cases 100-fold[107] (Fig. 3-8). In this case, vasopressin acts in a manner similar to renin and norepinephrine, causing vasoconstriction and playing a supporting role to the sympathetic nervous system in the maintenance of blood pressure. The primary reflex controllers of the plasma volume-mediated release of vasopressin are the arterial baroreceptors and not the cardiac receptors.[70,108] In hemorrhage, the change in intrathoracic volume alters the arterial systolic blood pressure, which decreases arterial baroreceptor stimulation, and leads to increased vasopressin secretion.[109]

Natriuretic Peptides

There are three natriuretic peptides (A, B, and C) that contribute to the regulation of blood pressure and electrolyte and volume homeostasis.[110,111] Atrial natriuretic peptide (ANP)[112] and brain natriuretic peptide (B-type natriuretic peptide [BNP]) are released from granules in the atria and ventricles in response to increased stretch (increased preload and afterload) and hormonal stimuli (e.g., angiotensin II, glucocorticoids, endothelin I, catecholamines).[113,114] Of note, factors that stimulate BNP release may be different in a normal versus hypertrophied ventricle and after myocardial infarction, with hypoxia acting independent of ventricular dilation to stimulate BNP release.[113] The actions of BNP are similar to ANP. C-type natriuretic peptide is widely distributed in the brain, kidneys, lungs, heart, and endothelial cells, and is released in response to shear stress. Dendroaspis natriuretic peptide has been recently discovered; however, its exact mechanism remains to be determined.

The heart has endocrine functions[113] via the cardiac natriuretic peptides (ANP and BNP) that bind with natriuretic peptide receptors A and B (NPR-A and NPR-B) and cause diuresis and natriuresis. These actions subsequently decrease preload and blood pressure.[115] Preload reduction may occur because of shifting of fluid from the intravascular to the extravascular space (increased vascular endothelial permeability) and possibly increased capillary hydrostatic pressure along with natriuresis.[110,116] Additionally, ANP and BNP decrease sympathetic tone to the peripheral vasculature both centrally and peripherally, inhibit the RAAS by inhibiting angiotensin II-stimulated sodium and water transport in the proximal tubules, inhibit endothelin-1 production, improve ventricular relaxation, and lower the activation threshold for the vagal afferents, which suppresses the reflex tachycardia and vasoconstriction associated with the decrease in preload and cardiac output[117,118] (Fig. 3-9). In severe heart failure, increased

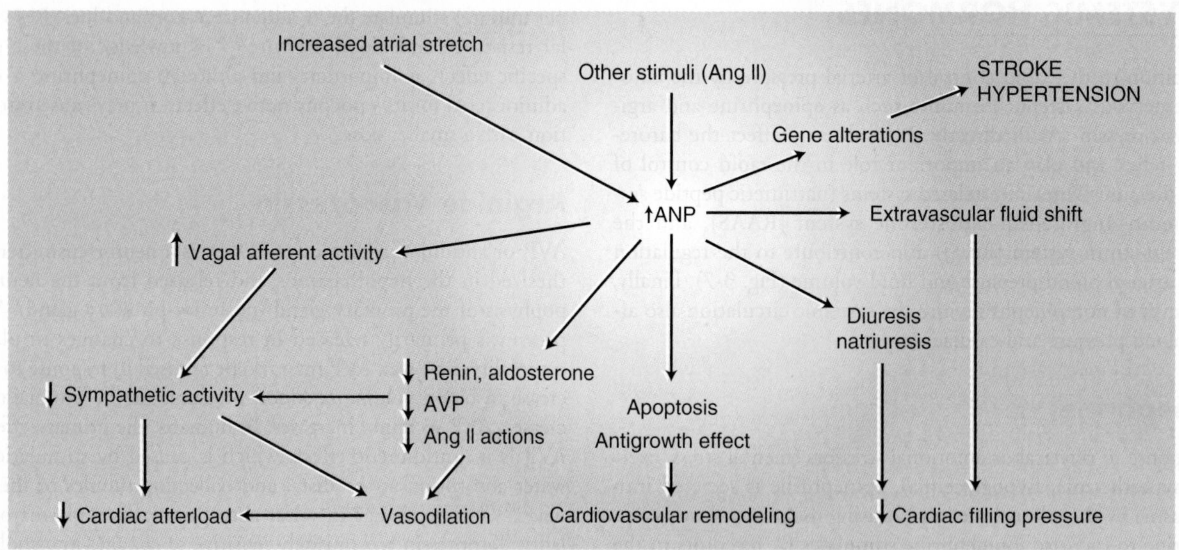

■ **Figure 3-9** Schematic representation of the regulation and function of atrial natriuretic peptide (ANP). Along with the classical circulatory effects, the new emerging functional properties of the atrial natriuretic peptides are shown. AVP, vasopressin; ANG II, angiotensin II. (From Rubattu, S., & Volpe, M. [2001]. The atrial natriuretic peptide: A changing view. *Journal of Hypertension, 19*, 1925.)

levels of ANP may offset the detrimental effects of increased angiotensin–aldosterone and the sympathetic nervous system.[111,119]

Clinically, the short-term administration of intravenous BNP nesitiride (Natrecor) has been shown to improve hemodynamic function and decrease symptoms of acute decompensated heart failure compared with standard therapy[120–122]. However, meta-analyses indicate that there may be increased risk of worsening renal failure and increased 30-day mortality;[123–125] thus caution must be taken when administering this medication.[126]

C-type natriuretic peptide, which is stored in endothelial cells, acts in a paracrine fashion and binds to natriuretic peptide receptor C (NPR-C), which is located in vascular smooth muscle. Note that other texts refer to binding to NPR-A.[91] CNP couples to inhibitory G proteins (G_i) and causes inhibition of adenylate cyclase and activation of phospholipase-C leading to vasodilation. ANP also binds to NPR-C with similar inhibitory effects.[117] Recent research suggests that CNP may be an endothelium-dependent hyperpolarizing factor, with actions in the peripheral and coronary vasculature[117,127–129] (see Chapter 2). The peripheral vascular effect of CNP decreases venous return and subsequently decreases cardiac filling pressures, cardiac output, and arterial blood pressure. Unlike ANP and BNP, CNP has minimal renal actions.[130] CNP is a potent coronary vasodilator and also has an antimitogenic effect on vascular smooth muscle, which may be protective against atheroma development and restenosis.[131] Additionally, in an experimental model of myocardial infarction, CNP administration decreased the size of the infarct and myocardial dysfunction and protected against ischemic reperfusion injury, with possible mechanisms including CNP/NPR-C related coronary vasodilation and decreased heart rate.[127]

Renin–Angiotensin–Aldosterone System

The RAAS plays an important role in the long-term control of arterial blood pressure, regional blood flow, and sodium balance. The RAAS acts in a cascade fashion, initiated by the stimulation of renin release from the kidney. Renin is stored in and released from the juxtaglomerular cells near the renal afferent arterioles. Renin release is stimulated by three mechanisms. First, renin release occurs in response to increased sympathetic nervous system stimulation of the afferent and efferent arterioles in the renal glomeruli. The β-adrenergic receptors in the cells of the juxtaglomerular apparatus are sensitive to neurally released and systemic catecholamines. This neurally mediated response can be blocked by β-adrenergic blockers (e.g., propranolol). Second, renin release is stimulated by decreased renal perfusion pressure, distending the afferent arterioles (intrarenal baroreceptor pathway). Below a mean arterial pressure of 80 to 90 mm Hg, renin secretion is a steep and linear function of renal perfusion pressure. Finally, decreased sodium chloride concentration in the macula densa, which is located in the early distal tubule, stimulates the juxtaglomerular apparatus to secrete renin. Increased blood pressure decreases renin release by activating the baroreceptors causing a decrease in sympathetic tone, increasing pressure in the renal arterioles, and decreasing sodium chloride reabsorption in the proximal tubule, causing increased sodium chloride to reach the macula densa.

Angiotensin II is released through the proteolytic effects of renin on the plasma protein, angiotensinogen, which is synthesized and released into the plasma from the liver. Renin converts angiotensinogen to angiotensin I. Angiotensin I, which is inactive, is converted to angiotensin II by an angiotensin-converting enzyme (ACE) located in the plasma and vascular endothelium (primarily pulmonary).[132] Pharmacologically, ACE inhibitors exert their effect at this level of the RAAS.[133]

Angiotensin II has two receptors (AT1 and AT2). The classic actions of angiotensin II, which are primarily mediated through AT1, include vasoconstriction and stimulation of aldosterone release. Angiotensin II causes vasoconstriction of the arterioles through a direct effect on the vascular smooth muscle and indirectly affects vascular tone by stimulating the formation of superoxide anions, which inhibit nitric oxide-mediated vasodilation, and by inducing endothelin-1 formation to cause further vasoconstriction.[134–136] Angiotensin receptor blockers work primarily on the AT1 receptors.

The renal and splanchnic circulations are particularly sensitive to angiotensin II. Angiotensin II increases vascular resistance and stimulates the heart indirectly through its potentiating actions on the sympathetic nervous system. These effects include: (1) accelerating the synthesis and release of norepinephrine; (2) delaying neuronal reuptake of norepinephrine; (3) directly stimulating the sympathetic ganglia; and (4) facilitating the response to sympathetic activity and vasoconstrictor drugs.[70]

Angiotensin II also has a long-term effect on blood pressure through stimulation of aldosterone synthesis and secretion, which increases blood volume. Aldosterone, a mineralocorticoid synthesized and secreted by the adrenal cortex, increases sodium reabsorption in the loop of Henle and decreases sodium excretion, which together lead to retention of water and expansion of blood volume. The change in blood volume is a slow process, which is important in the long-term control of blood pressure. Angiotensin II may also play a role in a sustained increase in sympathetic vasomotor or cardiac sympathetic activity by modification of sympathetic nervous system activity perhaps by action at the level of the paraventricular nucleus.[8,37] This latter mechanism may contribute to long-term control of sympathetic activity.

In 2000 ACE2 was discovered.[137,138] This enzyme hydrolyzes angiotensin (Ang) I to produce Ang-(1-9), which is subsequently catalyzed by neutral endopeptidase 24.11 (NEP) to produce Ang-(1-7). Angiotensin II can also be converted to Ang-(1-7). The receptor for Ang-(1-7) is Mas, which is located in the vascular wall and in myocardial cells. Ang-(1-7) has antiproliferative and vasodilator effects, which counterbalance the effects of the RAAS.[139] The role of Ang-(1-7) and the potential therapeutic benefit of Ang-(1-7) remains under investigation.

Kallikrein–Kinin System

The tissue KKS plays a role in blood pressure control and has protective cardiovascular effects. Kinins (e.g., bradykinin and kallidin or lys-BK), which are produced by the action of the enzyme hK1 (a kallikrein) on kininogens, bind with B_1 and B_2 receptors. Bradykinin is inactivated rapidly (<15 seconds) by ACE. Binding of kinins with the inducible B_1-receptor, which is up-regulated during inflammation and tissue injury, causes the release of nitric oxide and prostacyclin (PGI_2) from endothelial cells and subsequent vasodilation. The constitutive B_2 receptors play a role in pathological conditions such as pain, inflammation and hypertension. Stimulation of the B_2 receptor causes the release of nitric oxide and PGI_2 and may be cardioprotective via vasodilation and anti-ischemic and antiproliferative effects.[140,141] Bradykinin plays a role in blood pressure regulation via antagonism of angiotensin-induced vasoconstriction and vasodilation (decreased vascular resistance), diuresis and natriuresis.[140,142]

A deficient KKS (decreased levels of hK1 and kininogen deficiency and altered B_1 and B_2 genotypes) plays a role in the pathogenesis of hypertension through altered sodium excretion.[140,143] Bradykinin, which is released during ischemia, may also play a cardioprotective role in myocardial infarction and heart failure. After a myocardial infarction, ACE inhibition decreases cardiac dilation and failure by decreasing angiotensin II, but also by preventing the breakdown of kinins. Possible mechanisms for the KKS effect include increasing coronary blood flow and the promotion of angiogenesis and cardiac regeneration, which decrease the infarct size and inhibit ventricular remodeling.[140,143,144] The beneficial effects of the KKS suggest the possible role for pharmacological treatment of hypertension, postmyocardial infarction, and heart failure.[140,145] However, kinins may contribute the adverse side effects (e.g., increased microvascular permeability, cough, and angioedema) associated with ACE inhibitors.[146]

Interaction Between the KKS, RAAS, and Natriuretic Hormones

The KKS, RAAS, and the natriuretic hormones interact via the actions of ACE and neuropeptidase (NEP) (see Fig. 3-7). ACE stimulates the conversion of angiotensin I to angiotensin II and degrades kinins. NEP is involved in the metabolism of ANP, BNP, CNP, bradykinin, endothelin-1, and angiotensin II and also stimulates the formation of angiotensin (1–7) from angiotensin I. Angiotensin (1–7) has vasodilatory and antiproliferative effects that inhibit ACE and also counteract the actions of angiotensin II.[147] Angiotensin (1–7) also enhances the effects of bradykinin. Kallikrein, which is the enzyme involved in the formation of bradykinin, may also stimulate the conversion of prorenin to renin.[148,149] Renin subsequently causes the conversion of angiotensinogen to angiotensin I. Exploitation of the physiological interactions between these three systems may be useful in the treatment of heart failure and hypertension. For example, ACE inhibition exerts its antihypertensive effects by decreasing angiotensin II, increasing angiotensin (1–7) levels and potentiating the effects of bradykinin by increasing its level and through direct effect on the B_2-receptor.[146,147] Triple vasopeptidase inhibitors, which inhibit NEP as well as ACE and endothelin-1-converting enzyme may offer a multimodal approach to the management of cardiovascular disease.[146] However, side effects may limit the utility of some of these medications. For example, omapatrilat (an ACE/NEP inhibitor), which decreased the risk of death and hospitalization in chronic heart failure compared to ACE inhibition alone,[150] was removed from development because of an increased incidence of angioedema,[151] possibly due to increased bradykinin or increased endothelin-1-induced nitric oxide production.[146]

Norepinephrine Spillover

Approximately 80% of the norepinephrine secreted at the neuroeffector junction is either taken-up by sympathetic neurons (neuronal reuptake) or broken-down by the enzymes monoamine oxidase or catechol-*O*-methyl transferase. The remaining 20% may spill into the systemic circulation. The spillover is usually proportional to the increase in sympathetic nervous system activation; thus, the plasma norepinephrine level can be used as an approximate indicator of SNS activity.[152] Factors such as the nerve-firing rate, blood flow, neuronal uptake of norepinephrine, capillary permeability, and width of the junctional cleft can also affect the level of plasma norepinephrine. The width of the junctional cleft is particularly important in the pulmonary vasculature, where spillover is predominantly the result of the wide junctional clefts and not of a high rate of sympathetic nervous system activation or norepinephrine release.[153–155]

ARTERIAL BLOOD PRESSURE

Systolic and diastolic blood pressures describe the high and low values of pressure fluctuations around the mean of the arterial pressure wave. The mean arterial pressure (MAP) in the ascending aorta depends on the cardiac output and SVR:

$$MAP = CO \times SVR$$

whereas arterial distensibility and left ventricular stroke volume determine the amplitude and contour of the pressure wave.[156] The peak systolic pressure is determined by the volume and velocity of left ventricular ejection (i.e., the larger the SV, the larger the pulse pressure at any given distensibility), peripheral arterial resistance, the distensibility of the arterial wall, the viscosity of blood, and the end-diastolic volume in the arterial blood.[157] During diastole, arterial pressure decreases until the next ventricular contraction, so the minimal diastolic pressure is determined by factors that affect the magnitude and rate of the diastolic pressure drop including blood viscosity, arterial distensibility, peripheral resistance, and the length of the cardiac cycle. Central blood pressure measurements (aorta and carotid), which reflect both the antegrade pressure and the reflected pressure, may be different from peripheral blood pressure measurements (see Chapter 21).[158]

During systole, the elastic walls of the aorta and large arteries stretch as more blood enters than runs off into the periphery. Thus, a portion of the stroke volume is stored in the relatively distensible aorta during systole. During diastole, there is passive elastic recoil of the arterial walls, causing continued, but decreasing, ejection of blood out of the aorta and into the peripheral arteries. The elastic recoil transforms pulsatile flow into more continuous flow in the smaller vessels and explains why the blood pressure does not drop to zero during periods of no flow (e.g., diastole).

Pulse pressure is the difference between the systolic and diastolic pressures. The aortic pulse pressure is directly proportional to left ventricular stroke volume and inversely related to arterial compliance, with changes in stroke volume responsible for most acute changes.

$$\text{Pulse pressure} \cong \text{Stroke volume/arterial compliance}$$

A normal pulse pressure at the brachial artery is approximately 40 mm Hg. A higher pulse pressure may reflect where the pressure is measured in the body (increased pulse pressure in the periphery). Ejection velocity also affects the pulse pressure, whereas the SVR does not affect the pulse pressure as it affects both systolic and diastolic pressures.

HEART RATE

Control of Heart Rate

The intrinsic heart rate at rest, without any neurohumoral influence, is approximately 100 to 120 beats per minute. The heart rate in the intact, resting person reflects a balance between the

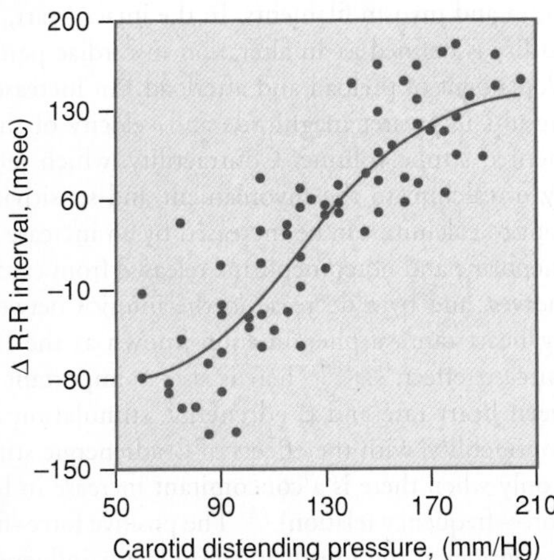

Figure 3-10 Stimulus–response curve for the cardiac arm of the baroreflex determined during application of positive and negative pressures over the anterior aspect of the neck in humans. Relations between carotid distending pressure and changes in *R-R* interval are presented. Data are the mean responses of 10 trials for each subject at each level of neck pressure and suction. The stimulus variable varies depending on the method used to assess baroreflex sensitivity. In this case, the stimulus is carotid sinus pressure (systolic pressure minus neck pressure). (From Rea, R. F., & Eckberg, D. L. (1987). Carotid baroreceptor-muscle sympathetic response in humans. *American Journal of Physiology, 253*(6, Pt. 2), R929–R934.)

tonically active sympathetic and parasympathetic nervous systems, with the parasympathetic nervous system predominating.[159–161] The predominance of the parasympathetic nervous system is manifested by a resting heart rate that is lower than the intrinsic rate. Parasympathetic predominance may also be demonstrated by abolishing the vagal influence with the administration of atropine. See Chapter 17 for a discussion of the effects of neural control on heart rate variability.

Vagal stimulation of the sinoatrial and atrioventricular nodes leads to a rapid (within one to two beats) decrease in heart rate. When vagal stimulation is discontinued, the heart rate increases rapidly. The rapid response to vagal stimulation and the presence of a large amount of cholinesterase (the enzyme that degrades the acetylcholine that is released from the parasympathetic fibers) allows the vagus nerve to exert beat-to-beat control of heart rate. Conversely, the heart rate response to sympathetic stimulation is gradual in onset, and once the sympathetic stimulation is terminated, the heart rate slowly decreases.[160]

There is an inverse relation between heart rate and arterial blood pressure (Fig. 3-10).[162,163] The inverse changes in heart rate are in response to baroreceptor stimulation, with the response most pronounced over a mean arterial pressure of 70 to 160 mm Hg. The alterations in heart rate are achieved by a reciprocal relationship between sympathetic and parasympathetic cardiac stimulations.

Changes in heart rate also occur as a result of chemosensor reflexes (Pa_{O_2} and Pa_{CO_2}) mediated by the carotid chemoreceptors. For example, a relatively slight excitation of the chemoreceptors leads to stimulation of the vagal center in the medulla and a decrease in heart rate. This response, which is seldom seen clinically, is considered the primary reflex effect of chemosensor stimulation. With increased levels of stimulation (e.g., a marked decrease in Pa_{O_2}), a secondary reflex is initiated that leads to depression of the primary chemoreceptor reflex and an increase in heart rate. This reflex is caused by pulmonary hyperventilation, which leads to hypocapnia and activation of pulmonary stretch receptors. The chemosensor reflex plays only a minimal role in the control of heart rate because the primary and secondary reflexes tend to offset one another.[36] In heart failure, abnormal central and peripheral chemosensor responses may contribute to sympathetic overactivity and suppression of baroreceptor function.[164,165]

Respiratory Sinus Arrhythmia

There is a direct relation between heart rate and respiration. During inspiration the heart rate increases, then it decreases during expiration. This respiratory-induced cyclical variation in heart rate is referred to as a *respiratory sinus arrhythmia.* There is an ongoing debate whether this arrhythmia is due to a central mechanism, a baroreflex, or a combination of both.[166] The effector arm of this response is via vagal cardiac nerve activity. Respiratory activity phasically alters vagal motorneuron responsiveness, with decreased vagal output during inspiration compared to expiration.[167]

Heart Rate and Cardiac Output

The relationship between heart rate and cardiac output is defined by the equation: cardiac output = stroke volume × heart rate. The effect of heart rate on cardiac output can vary over a wide range because of changes in stroke volume. A small increase in heart rate causes an increase in cardiac output and a decrease in stroke volume. The decrease in stroke volume is due to the effect of increased cardiac output on the peripheral volume, and a subsequent decrease in central venous pressure.[168,169] In this case, the increase in heart rate is not the direct cause of the decrease in stroke volume. Only when the heart rate exceeds 150 beats per minute does the cardiac output decrease, due to inadequate diastolic filling time and decreased stroke volume. Conversely, below a heart rate of 50 beats per minute, the stroke volume is relatively fixed, and a further decrease in heart rate causes a decrease in cardiac output.[159,170–172]

INTRINSIC CARDIAC CONTROL

In addition to cardiac control through the autonomic nervous system and systemic hormones, cardiac output is modified by the intrinsic factors: preload, afterload, and contractility. The following discussion focuses on how these factors affect cardiac output.

Preload

At the level of the muscle fiber, preload is defined as the force acting to stretch the ventricular fibers at end-diastole. Preload is related to cardiac output by the Frank–Starling law of the heart (length–tension relationship), which states that an increase in myocardial muscle fiber length is associated with an increase in the force of contraction,[173,174] and the subsequent increase in stroke volume and cardiac output.[175,176] Preload induced changes in cardiac output allow for beat-to-beat equalization of right and left ventricular stroke volume. In the case of preload-/afterload-dependent changes in contractile function, the mechanism of increased contractile force is known as length-dependent activation, whereby the myofilaments increase their sensitivity to cytosolic calcium as the sarcomere length increases to maximum.[177,178] This mechanism is contrary to traditional descriptions of Starling's law of the heart, which had maximal cardiac function occurring at an sarcomere length where there was optimal overlap of actin and myosin.[179]

Afterload

In muscle fiber experiments, preload is the tension in the muscle before contraction and afterload is the additional tension that must develop in the muscle during contraction before shortening occurs.[173,180] At the level of the ventricle, afterload is defined as ventricular wall tension during the shortening phase of contraction and reflects the sum of the forces against which the ventricle must act to eject blood. However, given the heterogeneous direction of myocardial fibers and the torsion or twisting of the ventricle during systole, a single measure of ventricular wall tension is inadequate to define afterload. In the intact system in vivo, afterload is defined as the pressure in the aorta during systole.[181] The aortic blood pressure is essentially equal to left ventricular pressure during the ejection phase of systole; thus, these values are interchangeable. The key factors that affect aortic blood pressure during ejection are arterial compliance, arterial resistance, and the reflection of pulse waves from the periphery.

As described by the force–velocity relation, for any given preload there is an inverse relation between afterload and muscle shortening, and thus stroke volume.[182] Although this relationship is observed in the isolated muscle fiber, it is not clinically apparent in people with normal cardiac function.[168] However, in individuals with a chronically depressed inotropic state (e.g., heart failure, cardiomyopathy), a steady state with altered ventricular dimensions (hypertrophy, dilatation) and maximal use of the length–tension relation occurs. Therefore, in these people in the face of an increase in afterload, the reserve provided by the length–tension relationship is exhausted and stroke volume decreases acutely.[183,184] These findings help to explain the use of afterload-reducing agents in patients with heart failure.

In clinical practice, systemic vascular resistance, which is often considered *the* indicator of afterload, is used interchangeably with afterload. This conceptualization is incorrect because afterload can change independently of vascular resistance. For example, in a patient who has experienced a severe hemorrhage, despite the fact that the systemic vascular resistance is increased (often to extreme), afterload is actually decreased. Recalling the original definition of afterload as the additional tension that develops in the muscle during contraction before shortening occurs helps to clarify this area of confusion. The tension or stress that develops in the ventricular wall according to the Laplace relation is:

$$T = \frac{PR}{2h}$$

where T is average circumferential wall stress (force/cross-sectional area), P is intraventricular pressure, R is the radius of curvature of the wall, and h is wall thickness. In hemorrhage, the radius of the ventricle is decreased, and if the compensatory actions of increased heart rate and systemic vasoconstriction are inadequate to maintain pressure, the intraventricular pressure also decreases. Thus, despite an increase in systemic vascular resistance, ventricular afterload decreases.

Contractility

Contractility refers to the intrinsic properties of cardiac myocytes that reflect the activation, formation, and cycling of crossbridges between actin and myosin filaments. In the intact heart, a change in contractility is defined as an alteration in cardiac performance that is independent of preload and afterload. An increase in contractility results in greater magnitude and velocity of shortening and augmented stroke volume. Contractility, which reflects the availability of calcium to the myofilament and sensitivity of the myofilament to calcium, can be increased by an increase in circulating epinephrine and norepinephrine released from cardiac sympathetic nerves, and by a decrease in the interval between beats (increasing heart rate), a phenomenon known as the Bowditch treppe (staircase) effect.[185,186] There is also an important relationship between heart rate and β-adrenergic stimulation and myocardial contractility, with the effects of β-adrenergic stimulation expressed only when there is a concomitant increase in heart rate (positive force–frequency relation).[187] The positive force–frequency relation is considered the fourth intrinsic factor influencing myocardial contractility, along with length-dependent activation, basal force frequency effect, and direct positive inotropic effect of myocardial β-adrenergic receptor stimulation.[182] Clinically, loss of the force–frequency relationship during heart block and downregulation of β-adrenergic stimulation during heart failure contributes to impaired cardiac function.[185,186] In patients with diastolic dysfunction, the positive force–frequency relation is maintained, whereas the positive force–relaxation relation is impaired, resulting in decreased stroke volume with increasing heart rate.[188]

EXTRINSIC CONTROL: PERICARDIAL LIMITATION

Under normal resting conditions, the pericardium has little or no effect on cardiac filling; however, during acute increases in cardiac volume, the pericardium affects ventricular interaction and plays a role in the compensatory increase or decrease in stroke volume between the two ventricles.[189] Additionally, in the face of increased filling pressures, the pericardium restricts cardiac filling, which is important in preventing excessive dilation during acute increases in cardiac volume.[190] Under conditions of acute failure, the pericardium augments ventricular interaction with decreased stroke volume.[191,192] In chronic cardiac dilation, however, there is growth of new pericardial tissue or slippage of the collagen fibers, and the pericardium actually enlarges in size and mass. As a result of this pericardial distortion or remodeling, there is limited increase in pericardial constraint in chronic cardiac dilation.[193,194]

After pericardiectomy there is an increase in the maximal cardiac output, O_2 consumption, and left ventricular end-diastolic segment length.[195] The increase in cardiac output is caused by an increase in stroke volume, which is caused by an increase in end-diastolic volume and myocardial fiber length, as described by the Frank–Starling law of the heart.[196] However, the effects of pericardiectomy on stroke volume and cardiac output are apparent only during exercise.[195,197]

Cases in which the pericardium has been opened and reapproximated, pericardial constraint increases because of development of adhesions between the pericardium and the heart.[198] The increased constraint is manifested as an increase in intraventricular pressure for any given volume, which reflects an increase in juxtacardiac pressure.[199] Consideration of the increased juxtacardiac pressure is important in the interpretation of hemodynamic data (increased pressure for any given volume) in postcardiac surgery patients who have had pericardial reapproximation.

LONG-TERM CONTROL OF BLOOD PRESSURE

The mechanism for the long-term control of blood pressure has traditionally been considered to involve fluid volume regulation, with the mechanism being renal pressure diuresis–natriuresis.[200,201] There are alternative models which suggest that volume diuresis–natriuresis and central baroreceptors play a role in long-term blood pressure control. This section presents the pressure diuresis–natriuresis model, introduces the alternative models of long-term arterial blood pressure control, and discusses the importance of basal tone on the maintenance of blood pressure.

Pressure Diuresis–Natriuresis Model

The classic model of long-term blood pressure control is based on the principle that arterial pressure is maintained at a level required by the kidneys to excrete a volume of urine approximately equivalent to the daily fluid intake (minus extrarenal fluid losses).[200,202] The kidneys sense a change in blood volume through the arterial pressure.[200,203] According to this model, that arterial pressure and not fluid volume is sensed is demonstrated in disease processes associated with a combination of increased extracellular volume and decreased arterial pressure (e.g., heart failure or cirrhosis with ascites). In these cases, the kidneys retain fluid despite expanded fluid volume. Based on this hypothesis, an increase in renal perfusion pressure causes a decrease in sodium reabsorption and an increase in sodium and water excretion. This model may involve autoregulation of renal medullary blood flow, although the exact mechanism remains unknown.[201,204] According to this model, as long as sodium and water intake remained stable, the enhanced sodium excretion will decrease extracellular volume and blood volume, and arterial pressure will decrease. Additionally, an increase in systemic vascular resistance and subsequent increase in renal perfusion pressure would not cause a long-term increase in arterial pressure, unless renal function was impaired.[200]

Alternative Models of Long-Term Blood Pressure Control

An alternative model for long-term blood pressure control suggests that the pressure diuresis–natriuresis mechanism may play less of a role under normal circumstances than previously conceptualized; rather that volume diuresis–natriuresis may be the primary mechanism for long-term blood pressure role.[205] According to this model sodium excretion is based on extracellular volume, with the renin system playing a key role.

Another model suggests that while the sympathetic nervous system, through the sinoaortic baroreceptor reflex, plays the primary role in the rapid regulation of blood pressure it may also play a role in long-term blood pressure control.[206–208] The clinical importance of the involvement of the sympathetic nervous system in long-term blood pressure control may be in the development to hypertension. Resetting of the baroreflex at a higher pressure threshold may limit their ability to buffer changes in blood pressure and increased sympathetic nervous system activity at any given pressure.[209,210] Further research is needed to support this model.[206,211]

Baroreflex independent control of the blood pressure via a central baroreceptor (rather than a pressor–sensor in the kidney) has been proposed, with the primary goal of maintaining cerebral blood flow.[212,213] The paraventricular nuclei in the hypothalamus may also play a role in modulating renal sympathetic nerve activity.[8]

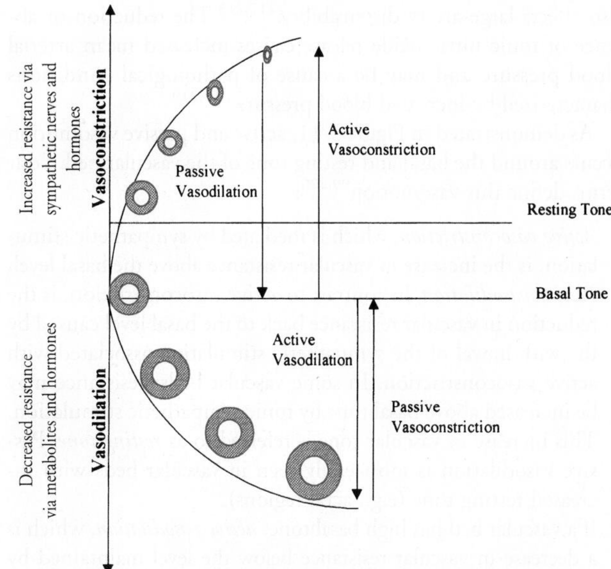

Figure 3-11 Schematic of active and passive changes in vascular resistance. The vascular bed is tonically constricted (basal tone) as a result of neurohumoral and local factors (autoregulation). In addition, some vascular beds have a higher level of tone (resting tone) indicating sympathetic nervous system stimulation. Passive vasodilation is the passive release of sympathetic nervous system stimulation, dilating the vessel toward basal tone. Passive vasoconstriction is the release of active vasodilatory stimuli. Active vasodilation is vascular dilation below basal tone and active vasoconstriction is constriction above basal tone. (Courtesy of Loring B. Rowell, University of Washington, Seattle, WA.)

Basal Tone

All arterioles exhibit a basal level of vasoconstriction or tone. Basal tone, which is the intrinsic level of vascular tone, is independent of neural or humoral influences and serves as the baseline around which neural or humorally mediated vasoconstriction or vasodilation occurs (Fig. 3-11). Basal tone varies among organs; it is lowest in the kidneys and highest in the skeletal muscles, heart, and brain.[214] The maintenance of arteriolar tone through tonic rhythmic vasoconstriction is essential for the maintenance of blood pressure. For example, it is estimated that if this basal myogenic tone were eliminated, a minimal cardiac output of 60 to 75 L/min would be required to maintain a normal blood pressure.[99,214] In contrast, if the sympathetic input associated with resting tone were withdrawn, the blood pressure would decrease only from 100 to 86 mm Hg. This small decrease in blood pressure occurs because the vascular bed with the highest resting tone (skeletal muscle) normally receives only 15% of the cardiac output.

Nitric oxide (eNOS and nNOS) affects basal arteriolar and microvascular tone, with a greater effect in larger resistance vessels (>200 μm) than in smaller resistance vessels (<200 μm).[215,216] Recent research suggests that nNOS generated nitric oxide is important for the regulation of basal vasomotor tone, which influences blood pressure, and eNOS generated nitric oxide affects the dynamic alterations in blood flow distribution.[215] Nitric oxide also affects large-artery distensibility.[217,218] The reduction or absence of tonic nitric oxide release causes increased mean arterial blood pressure and may be a cause of pathological conditions characterized by increased blood pressure.[218,219]

As demonstrated in Figure 3-11, active and passive vasomotion occurs around the basal and resting tone of the vascular bed. Four terms define this vasomotion[99,220]:

1. *Active vasoconstriction*, which is mediated by sympathetic stimulation, is the increase in vascular resistance above the basal level.
2. *Passive vasodilation*, in contrast to active vasoconstriction, is the reduction in vascular resistance back to the basal level caused by the withdrawal of the sympathetic stimulation associated with active vasoconstriction. In some vascular beds, resistance may be increased above basal tone by tonic sympathetic stimulation. This increase in vascular tone is referred to as *resting tone.* Passive vasodilation is most easily seen in vascular beds with increased resting tone (e.g., acral regions).
3. If a vascular bed has high basal tone, *active vasodilation*, which is a decrease in vascular resistance below the level maintained by basal tone, may occur (i.e., vasodilation beyond that which exists after all neural and hormonal influences are removed). In this case, the vasodilation is not merely the result of withdrawal of sympathetic tone, because this action causes passive vasodilation.
4. *Passive vasoconstriction* is caused by withdrawal of the stimulation causing active vasodilation.

The skeletal muscle arterioles have a high basal tone and therefore are capable of a wide range of vasoconstriction and vasodilation, because there is an increased level of basal tone to be modulated. In contrast, the renal vasculature has a low basal and resting tone that can be markedly increased through sympathetic stimulation, but has little capability to undergo active vasodilation because there is so little basal tone to inhibit.

LOCAL REGULATION OF SYSTEMIC MICROVASCULAR BEDS

Arteriolar resistance vessels are partially constricted under normal circumstances by a tonic rhythmic myogenic tone, and this level of tone is modulated by neurogenic or other factors that cause active vasoconstriction or vasodilation. In the intact organism, blood flow and vascular hydrostatic pressure in the microvasculature of each organ system are controlled by complex interrelations among the effects of physical factors, locally released substances, circulating hormones, and above all by neurotransmitters secreted in response to central activation of the sympathetic nervous system. The relative predominance of local versus centrally mediated control of the microvascular bed varies among vascular beds, and it also varies among resistance, precapillary, and postcapillary blood vessels within a given vascular bed.

The large- and medium-sized arterioles, which are the predominant sites of vascular resistance, are primarily under the control of the sympathetic nervous system and centrally mediated neurohumoral factors (e.g., angiotensin II). These vascular segments are influential in the control of arterial blood pressure and, by virtue of their position; they control the total amount of blood entering a specific vascular area; and therefore, the distribution of blood flow between the different vascular beds. The terminal arterioles or precapillary vascular segments control the number of open capillaries and are under sympathetic nervous system and local control.[221] Local control mechanisms (autoregulation) that affect the terminal arterioles may have a substantial influence on exchange vessel pressures and flows and on the vascular tissue exchange of fluid and solutes.

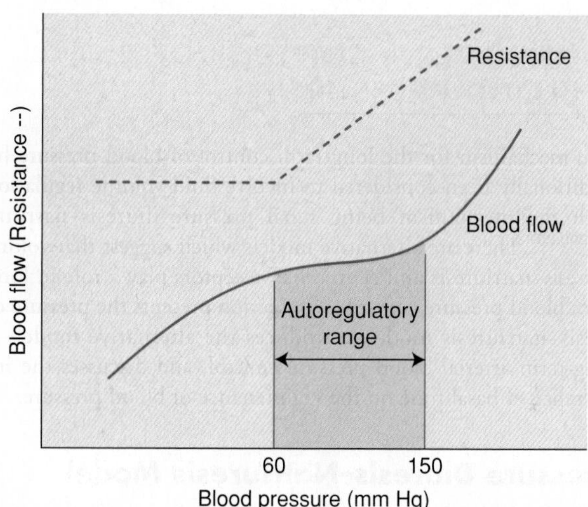

Figure 3-12 A schematic representation of autoregulation. The blood flow is relatively constant between an arterial pressure of 60 and 150 mm Hg because of an active increase in resistance. Below a mean pressure of 60 mm Hg and above 150 mm Hg, the flow is directly related to pressure.

Autoregulation

Autoregulation, which appears to occur in all organs except the lung, is the intrinsic tendency of an organ or vascular bed to maintain constant blood flow through alteration in its arteriolar tone, despite changes in arterial pressure. Autoregulation can occur in some organs over a range of perfusion pressure of 60 to 80 mm Hg to an upper limit of 150 mm Hg (Fig. 3-12), and is independent of neural and hormonal control. There are three hypotheses to explain autoregulation: the myogenic, metabolic, and tissue pressure hypotheses.[222,223] It appears that none of these mechanisms works in isolation and, as described later, the tissue pressure hypothesis may apply only in pathological conditions. A recent model suggests that myogenic and metabolic regulations overcome myogenic (shear-induced) effects.[224]

Myogenic Hypothesis

The myogenic hypothesis refers to the acute reaction of a blood vessel to a change in intraluminal pressure. For example, increasing intraluminal pressure between 20 and 120 mm Hg causes a pressure-induced stretch in vascular smooth muscle, which results in vasoconstriction and a decrease in the flow.[222,225] However, above an intraluminal pressure of 140 mm Hg the blood vessels dilate.[224] Shear stress, which is also associated with increased pressure, causes an increase in the release of endothelial niric oxide and subsequent vasodilation (see Chapter 2). Conversely, when the intraluminal pressure is decreased, the stimulus for the myogenic response is decreased, the vessel dilates, and blood flow is returned toward control levels. Recent research suggests that, in isolation the myogenic response exerts only a small autoregulatory response.[224]

Metabolic Hypothesis

The metabolic hypothesis is based on the idea that the concentration of metabolites and metabolic substrates (e.g., ATP, potassium, hydrogen, O_2, CO_2, adenosine) in the interstitial space controls vascular tone. In this case, the vascular smooth muscle acts as a chemosensor. According to this hypothesis, a decrease in blood flow leads to an increase in the local concentration of a metabolite and causes vasodilation and increased blood flow.[223,226] For example, red blood cells release ATP in response to increased oxygen demand. Increased venular ATP may trigger an upstream response that causes arteriolar vasodilation.[224,227,228] The metabolic hypothesis has been suggested as a mechanism for autoregulation in organs or tissues where the primary function of blood supply is to support local metabolism. In this case, there is a close relation between blood flow and metabolic needs. However, in organ systems with high blood flow (e.g., kidney, skin), where blood flow occurs in excess of metabolic needs, there is a limited relationship between blood flow and metabolism,[99] and the metabolic hypothesis as a factor in the autoregulatory control of blood flow has not been supported. A combination of metabolic and myogenic responses generate autoregulatory flow changes despite the opposing effects of shear.[224]

An important point is that metabolic autoregulation is not the same as metabolically induced active and reactive hyperemia (increased blood flow), which occur in response to increased metabolic demand (e.g., intestinal vasculature during digestion or cardiac and skeletal muscle during activity) or interruption of blood flow to a vascular bed, respectively.[223] Active hyperemia is the adaptive increase in blood flow in response to changes in the local metabolic rate caused by variation in the functional activity of the surrounding cells. In response to this change in functional status, the vascular resistance decreases almost immediately. In addition, there is an increase in the number of perfused capillaries (capillary recruitment) in response to metabolic stimulation. The magnitude of the reactive hyperemia response depends on the duration of the vascular obstruction and the metabolic rate of the given vascular bed. Unlike "pure" metabolic autoregulation, this response is a combination of three components: (1) passive changes in vessel diameter caused by a change in transmural pressure; (2) a myogenic response to the change in transmural pressure; and (3) a metabolic component.[223,229,230]

Tissue Pressure Hypothesis

The tissue pressure hypothesis states that an increase in external pressure (e.g., interstitial pressure) decreases transmural pressure (pressure inside minus pressure outside the vessel), which passively decreases the vessel diameter and decreases flow.[223] The effect of external compression on blood flow normally occurs during ventricular systole, when the coronary arteries are compressed. Clinically, the effect of transmural compression is more likely to be observed in organs constrained in a rigid container (e.g., brain, where increased cerebrospinal fluid pressure may compress cerebral vessels) or a stiff capsule (e.g., kidney).[99,223] In the lung, vascular compression caused by increased external (alveolar) pressure, such as with the application of high levels of positive end-expiratory pressure, may also affect blood flow.

Under physiological conditions, tissue pressure probably does not play a major role in the control of blood flow, but it may be particularly important under pathological conditions such as edema, hemorrhage into the interstitial space, or cellular swelling caused by injury or hypoxemia (compartment syndrome).[223] In the latter cases, external compression may decrease blood flow below a physiologically safe level.

VENOUS SYSTEM

The primary functions of the venous system are to return blood from the capillaries to the heart and to serve as a reservoir that counterbalances the transient imbalance between cardiac output and venous return. However, because of its capacious nature, the venous system serves not only as a reservoir, storing approximately 70% of the total blood volume (approximately 33% of total blood volume is stored in the splanchnic bed—liver, stomach, spleen, and intestines), but also as a buffer against changes in cardiac output and blood pressure. The venous system plays both an active (venoconstriction) and, more importantly, a passive role in the maintenance of thoracic blood volume.

Neurohumoral Stimulation

The only neural control of veins is through the α-adrenergic fibers of the sympathetic nervous system.[231] Release of norepinephrine from α-adrenergic fibers causes constriction in the splanchnic and cutaneous veins, whereas withdrawal of sympathetic stimulation results in passive vasodilation. The cutaneous veins are densely innervated with α-adrenergic receptors, predominantly postsynaptic α_2-receptors.[68,232] There is limited β-adrenergic stimulation in the cutaneous veins and the veins of the skeletal muscle and the small venules have virtually no innervation. Epinephrine is the primary humoral factor that affects the veins, with actions on cutaneous vessels and, more importantly, splanchnic vessels. Given the preponderance of α-adrenergic receptors on the veins, epinephrine stimulation causes venoconstriction.

Passive Versus Active Effects

Neurohumoral stimulation primarily affects the most capacious volume reservoirs (splanchnic and cutaneous venous bed). The question is whether translocation of blood from the venous system is primarily the consequence of active venoconstriction or of the passive effects that stem from the substantial changes in venous transmural pressure caused by arteriolar vasoconstriction or vasodilation.

Changes in upstream arteriolar tone alter downstream venous transmural pressure and the volume of blood that flows through the venous system. For example, arteriolar vasodilation increases blood flow into the highly capacious postcapillary venous beds, and the increase in their transmural venular pressure passively expands their volume. Given that total blood volume is constant, an increase in blood volume in the peripheral venous system means a decrease in the volume of the central veins that fill the heart. Conversely, vasoconstriction decreases flow into the postcapillary venous system, venous transmural pressure decreases, and the elastic recoil of the veins passively expels their volume toward the central thoracic veins.[231]

The magnitude of passive change in venous transmural pressure depends on where the changes occur along the venous volume–pressure curve. For example, as demonstrated in Figure 3-13, at a low venous transmural pressure, the pressure–volume curve is steep. A small change in distending pressure causes a large change in volume, that is, arteriolar vasodilation, which increases venous blood flow and venous transmural pressure, which causes a larger increase in venous volume expansion when the veins are

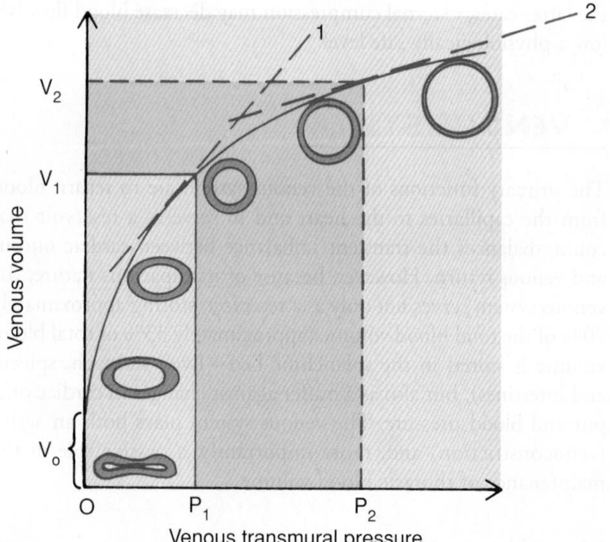

■ **Figure 3-13** Typical volume–pressure curve of an isolated vein. Dashed lines (1 and 2) show the compliance ($\Delta V/\Delta P$) at two venous transmural pressures, P_1 and P_2. Note that compliance varies with pressure, being greatest at the lower pressures (line 1) and decreasing as the pressure increases (line 2). V_0 is the unstressed volume, which is the volume contained at 0 transmural pressure. The change in volume from V_2 to V_1 is the passive effect of changing pressures from P_2 to P_1. Note how changing cross-sectional geometry contributes to passive emptying. (From Rowell, L. B. [1986]. *Human circulation: Regulation during physical stress* [p. 46]. New York: Oxford University Press.)

not initially distended compared with the volume expansion that would occur if the veins were fully distended with decreased compliance. Conversely, passive vasoconstriction translocates a larger volume of blood to the central circulation when venular volume is normal or increased, in contrast to a situation such as hemorrhage, in which the volume is already diminished (e.g., no further volume to move into the central circulation).

The passive effects of an alteration in blood flow on venous volume are exemplified in a study that evaluated the effect of a pacing-induced increase or decrease in cardiac output on central venous pressure.[169] A decrease in cardiac output, which resulted in a 17-mm Hg decrease in arterial pressure, was associated with a 3.9-mm Hg increase in central venous pressure. The increase in central venous pressure reflects the decrease in venous flow and transmural pressure associated with the decrease in cardiac output and the resultant passive recoil of the veins and the translocation of their blood centrally. The relation between venous volume and cardiac output is addressed further in the sections on the relation between cardiac output and central venous pressure, and the Krogh model.

The dominance of passive venous volume mobility can be altered in conditions such as hemorrhage, in which active venoconstriction of the richly innervated splanchnic veins can also play a role in the translocation of blood back to the central circulation.[99,233,234] In a study that examined the effects of a 27% decrease in cardiac output, with and without the presence of reflexes, active constriction of the splanchnic veins accounted for 21% of the translocated blood volume, whereas passive vasodilation accounted for the remaining 79%.[235] Thus, when active and passive effects are combined, the passive effects of decreased blood flow on venous volume mobility exceed the effect of simultaneous active venoconstriction.[70,235]

RELATION BETWEEN CARDIAC OUTPUT AND CENTRAL VENOUS PRESSURE—RETROGRADE VERSUS ANTEGRADE MODELS

In the 1950s, Guyton et al.[236–238] developed a model in which central venous pressure was presumed to affect cardiac output in a retrograde fashion. However, an opposing conceptualization is a model of the anterograde relationship between cardiac output and central venous pressure, that is, cardiac output affects central venous pressure.[70,239,240] A recent point–counterpoint discussion has failed to resolve these opposing models, with issues around the concept of mean circulatory pressure, the clarification of the components of the pressure gradient (mean circulatory pressure vs. right atrial pressure) and its effect on cardiac output, and the application of the models in static versus dynamic states.[241–245]

There are several implications of this discussion for clinical practice. For example, does increasing heart rate increase cardiac output? In experiments, an increase in cardiac output secondary to an increase in heart rate was limited by a decrease in central venous pressure.[172] Consideration of the resistive and capacitive properties of the arteries and veins within the context of an antegrade model may help to explain this effect.[99,168] In response to increased blood flow (increased cardiac output), transmural pressure in the veins rises, and thus their volume rises as well. The consequent shift in blood volume from the central to the peripheral veins lowers the central venous pressure.[73,168,169] If cardiac output continues to increase, the central venous pressure approaches 0 mm Hg, and eventually the central venous vasculature collapses, making it impossible to increase cardiac output further. This inverse relationship constitutes an autolimitation on our ability to increase cardiac output when there is no extra cardiac force available to match increased venous return with cardiac output. Factors that offset this autolimitation and allow us to stand and exercise are the muscle pump and the respiratory pump.

Muscle Pump

Initially when standing, there is an immediate translocation of 500 to 700 mL of blood to the periphery, which causes a decrease in central venous pressure and cardiac output and if allowed to continue could cause a person to faint. To offset this effect, contraction of the skeletal muscles in the legs causes compression of the veins and generates a gradient for flow between the venous beds and the right atrium, which can expel blood against the 100 mm Hg venous hydrostatic pressure that develops during quiet standing. The muscle pump, with a pumping capability *equal to that of the left ventricle*, is so important (particularly with exercise) that it is often referred to as the "second heart."[73,246,247] Clinically, encouraging the patient to actively contract their calf muscles when arising from bed will augment the muscle pump and potentially decrease the risk for orthostasis.

Respiratory Pump

The respiratory pump augments the effect of the muscle pump on venous blood flow.[248,249] The pressure difference promoting flow from the venules to the right atrium is affected by changes in intrathoracic and intra-abdominal pressures. During inspiration,

■ **Figure 3-14** (*Right*) The Krogh model divides the circulation between two circuits, one compliant (C_1) and the other noncompliant (C_2). (*Left*) The relation between the change in organ venous volume and blood flow through a compliant organ (C_1) and a noncompliant organ (C_2). The volume of blood available to the heart is determined by the distribution of blood flow between such circuits. For example, in hyperthermia there is increased blood volume in the compliant vascular beds of the skin, and the amount of blood available to the heart is decreased. (From Rowell, L. B. [1986]. *Human circulation: Regulation during physical stress* [p. 60]. New York: Oxford University Press.)

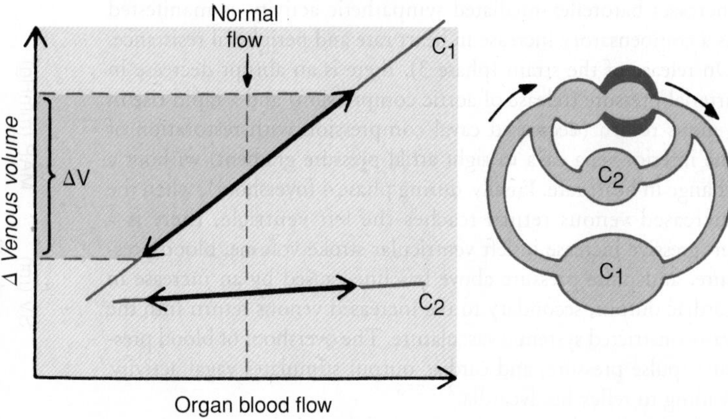

the diaphragm descends and intrathoracic pressure decreases and intra-abdominal pressure increases. These pressure changes create a gradient for blood flow from the point where the vena cava enters the thoracic cavity to the right atrium and thereby increases venous return to the heart. During expiration, the diaphragm relaxes and intrathoracic pressure increases, whereas intra-abdominal pressure decreases. The increased intrathoracic pressure impedes thoracic venous flow; however, there is an increase in blood flow from the lower extremities. During mechanical ventilation, the relation between the respiratory cycle and venous return is reversed.[250] These ventilatory-induced changes in preload have been exploited to aid in determining if a patient will respond to a fluid bolus with a clinically significant increase in stroke volume (see Chapter 21).

As described by the Krogh model (Fig. 3-14), the relative distribution of the cardiac output to compliant vascular beds (splanchnic—liver, gastrointestinal tract, pancreas, and the skin) and the remaining noncompliant vascular beds affects cardiac filling pressures.[70,231,251] For example, the administration of an α-adrenergic agent to a patient who is vasodilated will cause vasoconstriction of vessels leading into compliant vascular beds (e.g., splanchnic), which results in a passive collapse of the vascular bed with translocation of blood into the central circulation and a subsequent increase in blood return to the heart. However, a decrease in blood flow to the splanchnic region is not risk-free; as decreased gastrointestinal tract perfusion and ischemic bowel can occur if the vasoconstrictor-induced decrease in flow is too great. Conversely, the Krogh model is also useful for understanding the potentially negative consequences of recreational hyperthermia (i.e., hot tub or sauna) on coronary blood flow and cardiac output in a person with coronary artery disease. With hyperthermia, the highly compliant cutaneous vascular bed dilates, with up to 60% of the cardiac output directed to the skin to facilitate heat dissipation.[67,73] Generally, the redistribution of blood volume does not compromise oxygen delivery to vital organs. However, in individuals with compromised coronary circulation, there is a potential for a decrease in blood volume available to the heart and a subsequent decrease in cardiac output and coronary artery perfusion. The effects of environmental thermal stress plus exercise can also precipitate problems. In this case, the ability to increase cardiac output is limited by the decrease in central venous pressure and stroke volume, which is caused by vasodilation of the cutaneous vascular bed and the subsequent large increase in venous volume. This finding has important implications for exercise programs that are a part of cardiac rehabilitation and highlights the need for control of ambient temperature to maximize the benefits of exercise.[70,99]

VALSALVA MANEUVER

Extreme changes in intrathoracic pressure (Valsalva maneuver) also have potentially serious consequences for patients with cardiovascular disease. The Valsalva maneuver, which is a deep breath followed by straining to expire against a closed glottis, causes an abnormal increase in intrathoracic pressure. The hemodynamic response to the sudden increase in intrathoracic pressure associated with the Valsalva maneuver can be subdivided into four phases[252–254] (Fig. 3-15). During the initial phase (phase 1: strain phase), which is produced by forcefully exhaling against a closed glottis, there is a transient increase in arterial systolic and diastolic pressures due to aortic compression caused by increased intrathoracic pressure, and a marked decrease in venous return subsequent to compression of the vena cava and a decrease in pulse pressure and heart rate. During the remainder of the strain phase (phase 2), there is a progressive decrease in blood pressure and cardiac output due to a decrease in venous return and left ventricular filling and stroke volume subsequent to compression of the vena cava. The decrease in cardiac output and arterial pulse pressure, which

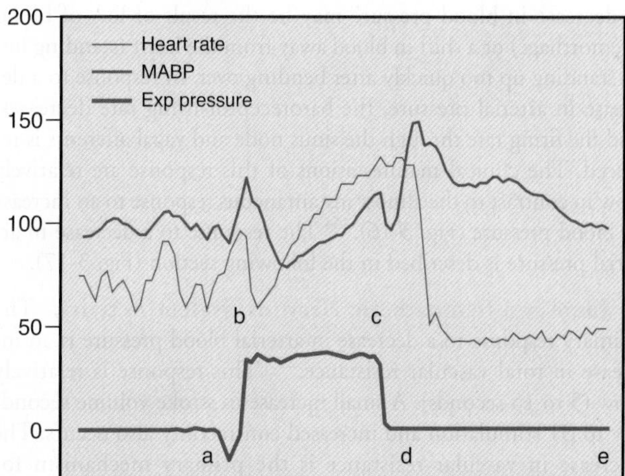

■ **Figure 3-15** The normal hemodynamic response to a Valsalva maneuver. Phase 1: a–b, phase 2: b–c, phase 3: c–d, and phase 4: d–e. MABP, mean arterial blood pressure; Exp pressure, expiratory pressure. (From Freeman, R. [1997]. Noninvasive evaluation of heart rate variability. In P. A. Low [Ed.], *Clinical autonomic disorders* [2nd ed., p. 302]. Philadelphia: Lippincott-Raven.)

increases baroreflex-mediated sympathetic activity, is manifested as a compensatory increase in heart rate and peripheral resistance. On release of the strain (phase 3), there is an abrupt decrease in arterial pressure (release of aortic compression) and a rapid rise in venous return (decreased caval compression with restoration of the inferior vena cava to right atrial pressure gradient) without a change in heart rate. Finally, during phase 4 (overshoot), when the increased venous return reaches the left ventricle, there is a progressive increase in left ventricular stroke volume, blood pressure, and pulse pressure above baseline caused by an increase in cardiac output, secondary to the increased venous return into the vasoconstricted systemic vasculature. The overshoot of blood pressure, pulse pressure, and cardiac output stimulates vagal activity, leading to reflex bradycardia.[255,256]

In the clinical setting, the effects of the Valsalva maneuver may be observed when a patient strains during defecation or vomiting.[257] It is the reflex bradycardia and the sequelae of the Valsalva maneuver (cardiac arrhythmias, sudden cardiac arrest, cerebral and subarachnoid hemorrhage, rupture of a dissecting aortic aneurysm) that are observed clinically.[258] Patients who may be at increased risk for an adverse response to the Valsalva maneuver include those with cardiac disease (e.g., heart failure) and older individuals.[254,259] Interventions to protect this high-risk group from the sequelae of the Valsalva maneuver (e.g., positioning, and avoiding straining during a bowel movement or vomiting) should be performed.

OVERALL CONTROL

Baroreflex Control of Blood Pressure

The arterial baroreflex is the primary mechanism of control for the short-term or rapid control of arterial blood pressure.[260–263] Neurohumoral factors (predominantly the control of sodium excretion) are primarily responsible for long-term or slower blood pressure control, although the sympathetic nervous system may also play a role in long-term control of blood pressure.

Arterial Baroreceptor Response to Decreased Arterial Pressure

A decrease in blood pressure may be the result of loss of blood (hemorrhage) or a shift in blood away from the heart (standing up) or standing up too quickly after bending over. In response to a decrease in arterial pressure, the baroreceptor-firing rate decreases, and the firing rate through the sinus node and vagal afferents is reduced. The clinical manifestations of this response are relatively slow in contrast to the almost instantaneous response to an increase in blood pressure (Fig. 3-16).[264] The response to a decrease in arterial pressure is described in the following section (Fig. 3-17).

Increased Sympathetic Nervous System Activity. The primary response to a decrease in arterial blood pressure is an increase in total vascular resistance.[265] This response is relatively slow (5 to 15 seconds). A small increase in stroke volume secondary to β1 stimulation and increased contractility also occurs. The increase in vascular resistance is the primary mechanism for restoring blood pressure, because an increase in heart rate is relatively ineffective in raising cardiac output. As described previously, if the cardiac output increases without an increase in peripheral vascular tone, then the central venous pressure decreases. The sympathetic nervous system-mediated vasoconstriction decreases blood flow to the splanchnic region, thereby causing a passive release of 300 to 500 mL of blood from its capacious veins into the central circulation.[70,266,267] An individual who experiences dizziness or faints after bending over and then standing up to quickly is first exposed to increased blood pressure in the head followed by a rapid decrease. In this case, the dizziness is caused by an exaggerated rate of blood flow to the legs compared to an individual who moves from supine to upright.[268,269] The mechanism for this unique response to a "push–pull" maneuver has not been identified, but it may include myogenic vasodilation during the head down phase or rapid refilling of the emptied veins. In this case, the relatively slow sympathetic response cannot offset these effects.

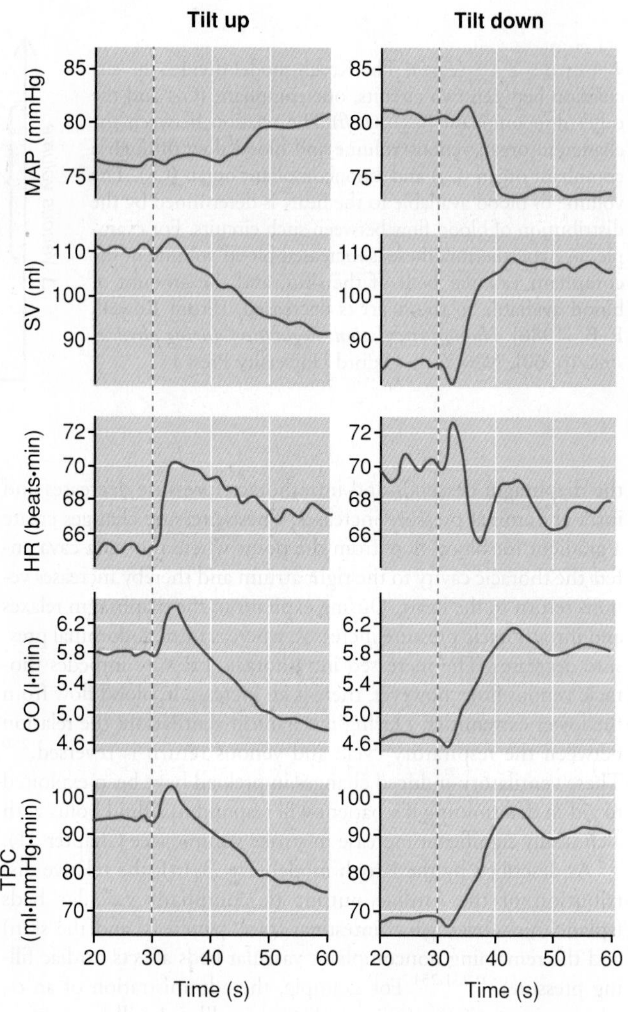

■ **Figure 3-16** Average response to 30° head-up tilt and tilt back to supine position in seven subjects (41 experiments). (From Toska, K., & Walløe, L. [2002]. Dynamic time course of hemodynamic responses after passive head up tilt and tilt back to supine position. *Journal of Applied Physiology, 92*, 1674.)

Decreased Vagal Activity Causing an Increase in Heart Rate. The cardiovagal arm of the baroreflex involves modulation of the heart rate. An increase in heart rate is not a primary compensatory response to a decrease in blood pressure,[265] although altered vagal function is associated with lower blood pressure.[270] As described by the cardiac output–central venous pressure relation, an increase in heart rate-induced central venous pressure is of limited efficacy in increasing the cardiac output and offsetting the decrease in blood pressure.

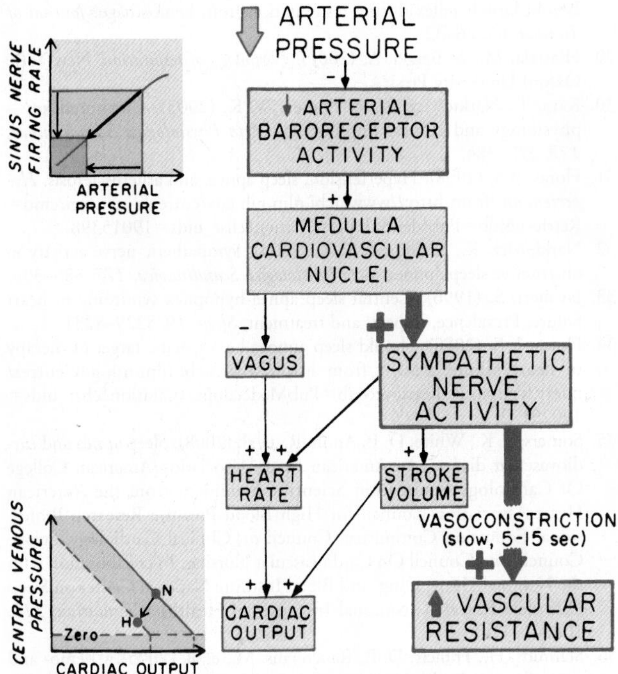

Figure 3-17 Summary of how the arterial baroreflex restores blood pressure back toward normal during arterial hypotension. Correction is by relatively slow (5 to 15 seconds) vasoconstriction. Increased heart rate has little or no effect if cardiac filling pressure is low and cardiac output cannot be increased, for reasons illustrated in the small graph next to "cardiac output" (central venous pressure vs. cardiac output). When normal (N) cardiac output increases, central venous pressure falls. When both cardiac output and central venous pressure are low during hemorrhage (H), cardiac output cannot rise much without collapsing central veins as central venous pressure goes to 0. (From Rowell, L. B. [1993]. *Human cardiovascular control* [p. 57]. New York: Oxford University Press.)

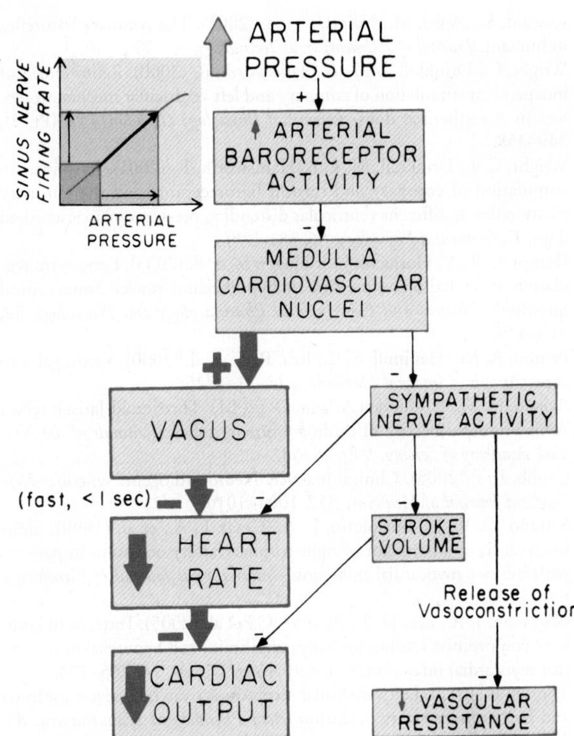

Figure 3-18 Summary of how the arterial baroreflex restores blood pressure back toward normal after sudden hypertension. Correction is rapid and achieved by immediate vagal activation and reduced heart rate and cardiac output. Release of tonic vasoconstriction is slow and has a minimal effect because only skeletal muscle has significant tonic vasoconstriction to be withdrawn in resting humans. (From Rowell, L. B. [1993]. *Human cardiovascular control* [p. 58.]. New York: Oxford University Press.)

Arterial Baroreceptor Response to Increased Arterial Pressure

An acute increase in blood pressure results in increased stimulation of the sinoaortic baroreceptors. The increased baroreceptor-firing rate increases sinus and vagal afferent input into the nucleus tractus solitarius of the medulla (see Figs. 3-1 and 3-3). In response to the increased baroreceptor input, the following occur (Fig. 3-18):

1. A rapid (within one beat) decrease in heart rate, secondary to a sudden increase in vagal tone.
2. A secondary decrease in stroke volume due to the negative inotropic effects of the increased vagal tone (minor effect).
3. A sympathetic nervous system-mediated decrease in vascular tone (minor effect).

The net result or this response is a decrease in heart rate, with a subsequent decrease in cardiac output and blood pressure. The most important point is that the response, which occurs within one beat, is mediated by a vagally induced decrease in heart rate and cardiac output.[271] Passive vasodilation due to a decrease in sympathetic tone occurs only in the skeletal muscles, and thus does not contribute greatly to the sudden lowering of arterial blood pressure.[70]

The rapid baroreflex response is extremely important in the protection of the cerebral vessels[272]. An impaired baroreflex response can be observed in patients after a stroke, where over 70% of these individuals exhibit increased blood pressure.[273] There is also a decrease in baroreflex-mediated buffering with aging,[162,274] which may place older individuals at increased risk for the negative effects of blood pressure perturbations. Of clinical importance, older individuals may have an altered response to vasoactive medications, such as greater blood pressure response to any given does of nitroprusside.[162,275–277]

REFERENCES

1. Scher, A. (1989). Cardiovascular control. In H. Patton, A. Fuchs, B. Hille, et al. (Eds.), *Textbook of physiology. Circulation, respiration, body fluids, metabolism, and endocrinology* (pp. 972–990). Philadelphia: WB Saunders.
2. McMahon, N. C., Drinkhill, M. J., Myers, D. S., et al. (2000). Reflex responses from the main pulmonary artery and bifurcation in anaesthetised dogs. *Experimental Physiology, 85*, 411–420.
3. Minisi, A. J. (1998). Vagal cardiopulmonary reflexes after total cardiac deafferentation. *Circulation, 98*, 2615–2620.
4. Hainsworth, R. (1995). Cardiovascular reflexes from ventricular and coronary receptors. *Advances in Experimental Medicine and Biology, 381*, 157–174.

5. Kincaid, K., Ward, M., Nair, U., et al. (2005). The coronary baroreflex in humans. *Journal of Extracorporeal Technology, 37*, 306–310.
6. Wright, C., Drinkhill, M. J., & Hainsworth, R. (2000). Reflex effects of independent stimulation of coronary and left ventricular mechanoreceptors in anaesthetised dogs. *Journal of Physiology (London), 528*(Pt. 2), 349–358.
7. Wright, C. I., Drinkhill, M. J., & Hainsworth, R. (2001). Responses to stimulation of coronary and carotid baroreceptors and the coronary chemoreflex at different ventricular distending pressures in anaesthetised dogs. *Experimental Physiology, 86*, 381–390.
8. Dampney, R. A., Horiuchi, J., Killinger, S., et al. (2005). Long-term regulation of arterial blood pressure by hypothalamic nuclei: Some critical questions. *Clinical and Experimental Pharmacology and Physiology, 32*, 419–425.
9. Fenton, A. M., Hammill, S. C., Rea, R. F., et al. (2000). Vasovagal syncope. *Annals of Internal Medicine, 133*, 714–725.
10. Aviado, D. M., & Guevara Aviado, D. (2001). The Bezold-Jarisch reflex. A historical perspective of cardiopulmonary reflexes. *Annals of the New York Academy of Science, 940*, 48–58.
11. Grubb, B. P. (2005). Clinical practice. Neurocardiogenic syncope. *New England Journal of Medicine, 352*, 1004–1010.
12. Serrano, C. V., Jr., Bortolotto, L. A., Cesar, L. A., et al. (1999). Sinus bradycardia as a predictor of right coronary artery occlusion in patients with inferior myocardial infarction. *International Journal of Cardiology, 68*, 75–82.
13. Goldstein, J. A., Lee, D. T., Pica, M. C., et al. (2005). Patterns of coronary compromise leading to bradyarrhythmias and hypotension in inferior myocardial infarction. *Coronary Artery Disease, 16*, 265–274.
14. Thoren, P. (1972). Left ventricular receptors activated by severe asphyxia and by coronary artery occlusion. *Acta Physiologica Scandinavica, 85*, 455–463.
15. Fu, L. W., Guo, Z. L., & Longhurst, J. C. (2008). Undiscovered role of endogenous thromboxane A2 in activation of cardiac sympathetic afferents during ischaemia. *Journal of Physiology, 586*, 3287–3300.
16. Fu, L. W., Phan, A., & Longhurst, J. C. (2008). Myocardial ischemia-mediated excitatory reflexes: A new function for thromboxane A2? *American Journal of Physiology Heart and Circulatory Physiology, 295*(6), H2530–H2540.
17. Longhurst, J. C., Tjen, A. L. S. C., & Fu, L. W. (2001). Cardiac sympathetic afferent activation provoked by myocardial ischemia and reperfusion. Mechanisms and reflexes. *Annals of the New York Academy of Science, 940*, 74–95.
18. Chiladakis, J. A., Patsouras, N., & Manolis, A. S. (2003). The Bezold-Jarisch reflex in acute inferior myocardial infarction: Clinical and sympathovagal spectral correlates. *Clinical Cardiology, 26*, 323–328.
19. Perez-Gomez, F., & Garcia-Aguada, A. (1977). Origin of ventricular reflexes caused by coronary arteriography. *British Heart Journal, 39*, 967–973.
20. Mark, A. L., Kioschos, J. M., Abboud, F. M., et al. (1973). Abnormal vascular responses to exercise in patients with aortic stenosis. *Journal of Clinical Invest, 52*, 1138–1146.
21. Mark, A., Abboud, F., Schmid, P., et al. (1973). Reflex vascular response to left ventricular outflow obstruction and activation of ventricular baroreceptors in dogs. *Journal of Clinical Investigations, 52*, 1147–1153.
22. Mark, A., & Mancia, G. (1983). Cardiopulmonary baroreflexes in humans. In J. Sheperd & F. Abboud (Eds.), *Handbook of physiology. Section 2. The cardiovascular system* (pp. 795–813). Bethesda, MD: American Physiological Society.
23. Omran, H., Fehske, W., Rabahieh, R., et al. (1996). Valvular aortic stenosis: risk of syncope. *Journal of Heart Valve Disease, 5*, 31–34.
24. Prasad, K., Williams, L., Campbell, R., et al. (2008). Episodic syncope in hypertrophic cardiomyopathy: Evidence for inappropriate vasodilation. *Heart, 94*, 1312–1317.
25. Thaman, R., Elliott, P. M., Shah, J. S., et al. (2005). Reversal of inappropriate peripheral vascular responses in hypertrophic cardiomyopathy. *Journal of the American College of Cardiology, 46*, 883–892.
26. Lim, P. O., Morris-Thurgood, J. A., & Frenneaux, M. P. (2002). Vascular mechanisms of sudden death in hypertrophic cardiomyopathy, including blood pressure responses to exercise. *Cardiology in Review, 10*, 15–23.
27. Lee, T. M., Chen, M. F., Su, S. F., et al. (1996). Excessive myocardial contraction in vasovagal syncope demonstrated by echocardiography during head-up tilt test. *Clinical Cardiology, 19*, 137–140.
28. Wisbach, G., Tobias, S., Woodman, R., et al. (2007). Preserving cardiac output with beta-adrenergic receptor blockade and inhibiting the Bezold-Jarisch reflex during resuscitation from hemorrhage. *Journal of Trauma, 63*, 26–32.
29. Hlastala, M., & Berger, A. (2001). *Physiology of respiration*. New York: Oxford University Press.
30. Kara, T., Narkiewicz, K., & Somers, V. K. (2003). Chemoreflexes—physiology and clinical implications. *Acta Physiologica Scandinavica, 177*, 377–384.
31. Floras, J. S. (2008). Hypertension, sleep apnea, and atherosclerosis. *Hypertension*, from http://www.ncbi.nlm.nih.gov/entrez/query.fcgi?cmd=Retrieve&db=PubMed&dopt=Citation&list_uids=19015398.
32. Narkiewicz, K., & Somers, V. K. (2003). Sympathetic nerve activity in obstructive sleep apnoea. *Acta Physiologica Scandinavica, 177*, 385–390.
33. Javaheri, S. (1996). Central sleep apnea-hypopnea syndrome in heart failure: Prevalence, impact, and treatment. *Sleep, 19*, S229–S231.
34. Floras, J. S. (2008). Should sleep apnoea be a specific target of therapy in heart failure? *Heart*, from http://www.ncbi.nlm.nih.gov/entrez/query.fcgi?cmd=Retrieve&db=PubMed&dopt=Citation&list_uids=19029172.
35. Somers, V. K., White, D. P., Amin, R., et al. (2008). Sleep apnea and cardiovascular disease: An American Heart Association/American College Of Cardiology Foundation Scientific Statement from the American Heart Association Council for High Blood Pressure Research Professional Education Committee, Council on Clinical Cardiology, Stroke Council, and Council On Cardiovascular Nursing. In collaboration with the National Heart, Lung, and Blood Institute National Center on Sleep Disorders Research (National Institutes of Health). *Circulation, 118*, 1080–1111.
36. Schmidt, H., Francis, D. P., Rauchhaus, M., et al. (2005). Chemo- and ergoreflexes in health, disease and ageing. *International Journal of Cardiology, 98*, 369–378.
37. Dampney, R. A., Coleman, M. J., Fontes, M. A., et al. (2002). Central mechanisms underlying short- and long-term regulation of the cardiovascular system. *Clinical and Experimental Pharmacology and Physiology, 29*, 261–268.
38. Pilowsky, P. M., & Goodchild, A. K. (2002). Baroreceptor reflex pathways and neurotransmitters: 10 years on. *Journal of Hypertension, 20*, 1675–1688.
39. Stocker, S. D., Osborn, J. L., & Carmichael, S. P. (2008). Forebrain osmotic regulation of the sympathetic nervous system. *Clinical and Experimental Pharmacology and Physiology, 35*, 695–700.
40. Coote, J. H. (2007). Landmarks in understanding the central nervous control of the cardiovascular system. *Experimental Physiology, 92*, 3–18.
41. Helke, C. J., & Seagard, J. L. (2004). Substance P in the baroreceptor reflex: 25 years. *Peptides, 25*, 413–423.
42. Grassi, G., Trevano, F. Q., Seravalle, G., et al. (2006). Baroreflex function in hypertension: Consequences for antihypertensive therapy. *Progress in Cardiovascular Disease, 48*, 407–415.
43. Bylund, D. B., Eikenberg, D. C., Hieble, J. P., et al. (1994). International Union of Pharmacology nomenclature of adrenoceptors. *Pharmacology in Review, 46*, 121–136.
44. Lands, A. M., Arnold, A., McAuliff, J. P., et al. (1967). Differentiation of receptor systems activated by sympathomimetic amines. *Nature, 214*, 597–598.
45. Guimaraes, S., & Moura, D. (2001). Vascular adrenoceptors: An update. *Pharmacology in Review, 53*, 319–356.
46. Civantos Calzada, B., & Aleixandre de Artinano, A. (20010. Alpha-adrenoceptor subtypes. *Pharmacology Research, 44*, 195–208.
47. Kable, J., Murrin, L., & Bylund, D. B. (2000). In vivo gene modification elucidates subtype-specific functions of alpha (2)-adrenergic receptors. *Journal of Pharmacology and Experimental Therapeutics, 293*, 1–7.
48. Kanagy, N. L. (2005). Alpha(2)-adrenergic receptor signalling in hypertension. *Clinical Science (London), 109*, 431–437.
49. Leech, C. J., & Faber, J. E. (1996). Different alpha-adrenoceptor subtypes mediate constriction of arterioles and venules. *American Journal of Physiology, 270*, H710–H722.
50. Banday, A. A., & Lokhandwala, M. F. (2008). Dopamine receptors and hypertension. *Current Hypertension Report, 10*, 268–275.
51. Missale, C., Nash, S. R., Robinson, S. W., et al. (1998). Dopamine receptors: from structure to function. *Physiology in Review, 78*, 189–225.
52. Zeng, C., Armando, I., Luo, Y., et al. (2008). Dysregulation of dopamine-dependent mechanisms as a determinant of hypertension: studies in dopamine receptor knockout mice. *American Journal of Physiology Heart and Circulatory Physiology, 294*, H551–H569.
53. Jose, P. A., Eisner, G. M., & Felder, R. A. (2003). Regulation of blood pressure by dopamine receptors. *Nephron Physiology, 95*, 19–27.

54. Jose, P. A., Eisner, G. M., & Felder, R. A. (2003). Dopamine and the kidney: A role in hypertension? *Current Opinion on Nephrology Hypertension, 12*, 189–194.
55. Zeng, C., Eisner, G. M., Felder, R. A., et al. (2005). Dopamine receptor and hypertension. *Current Medical and Chemical Cardiovascular Hematology Agents, 3*, 69–77.
56. Kellum, J., & Decker, J. (2001). Use of dopamine in acute renal failure: A meta-analysis. *Critical Care Medicine, 29*, 1526–1531.
57. Marik, P. E. (2002). Low-dose dopamine: A systematic review. *Intensive Care Medicine, 28*, 877–883.
58. Friedrich, J. O., Adhikari, N., Herridge, M. S., et al. (2005). Meta-analysis: Low-dose dopamine increases urine output but does not prevent renal dysfunction or death. *Annals of Internal Medicine, 142*, 510–524.
59. Feigl, E. O. (1998). Neural control of coronary blood flow. *Journal of Vascular Research, 35*, 85–92.
60. Gauthier, C., Seze-Goismier, C., & Rozec, B. (2007). Beta 3-adrenoceptors in the cardiovascular system. *Clinical Hemorheology and Microcirculation, 37*, 193–204.
61. Gauthier, C., Leblais, V., Kobzik, L., et al. (1998). The negative inotropic effect of B3-Adrenoreceptor stimulation is mediated by activation of nitric oxide synthase pathway in human ventricle. *Journal of Clinical Investigations, 102*, 1377–1384.
62. Moniotte, S., Kobzik, L., Feron, O., et al. (2001). Upregulation of beta(3)-adrenoreceptors and altered contractile response to inotropic amines in human failing myocardium. *Circulation, 103*, 1649–1655.
63. Bristow, M., Monobe, W., Pasmussen, R., et al. (1988). Alpha-1 adrenergic receptors in the nonfailing and failing human heart. *Journal of Pharmacology and Experimental Therapeutics, 247*, 1039–1045.
64. Franchini, K., & Cowley, A. J. (1996). Autonomic control of cardiac function. In D. Robertson, P. Low, & R. Polinsky (Eds.), *Primer on the autonomic nervous system* (pp. 42–48). San Diego: Academic Press.
65. Rudner, X. L., Berkowitz, D. E., Booth, J. V., et al. (1999). Subtype specific regulation of human vascular alpha(1)-adrenergic receptors by vessel bed and age. *Circulation, 100*, 2336–2343.
66. Borbujo, J., Garcia-Villalon, A., Valle, J., et al. (1989). Postjunctional alpha-1 and alpha-2 adrenoreceptors in human skin arteries. An in vitro study. *Journal of Pharmacology and Experimental Therapeutics, 249*, 284–287.
67. Johnson, J., & Proppe, D. (1996). Cardiovascular adjustments to heat stress. In M. Fregly & C. Blatteis (Eds.), *Handbook of physiology: Section 4. Environmental physiology* (pp. 215–243). New York: Oxford University Press.
68. Charkoudian, N. (2003). Skin blood flow in adult human thermoregulation: How it works, when it does not, and why. *Mayo Clinics Proceeding, 78*, 603–612.
69. Kellogg, D. L., Jr. (2006). In vivo mechanisms of cutaneous vasodilation and vasoconstriction in humans during thermoregulatory challenges. *Journal of Applied Physiology, 100*, 1709–1718.
70. Rowell, L. (1993). *Human cardiovascular control*. New York: Oxford University Press.
71. Pergola, P. E., Kellogg, D. L., Jr., Johnson, J. M., et al. (1994). Reflex control of active cutaneous vasodilation by skin temperature in humans. *American Journal of Physiology, 266*, H1979–H1984.
72. Savage, M. V., & Brengelmann, G. L. (1996). Control of skin blood flow in the neutral zone of human body temperature regulation. *Journal of Applied Physiology, 80*, 1249–1257.
73. Rowell, L., O'Leary, D., & Kellogg, D. (1996). Integration of cardiovascular control systems in dynamic exercise. In L. Rowell & J. Sheperd (Eds.), *Handbook of physiology, exercise: Regulation and integration of multiple systems* (pp. 770–838). Bethesda, MD: Oxford University Press.
74. Kellogg, D. L., Jr., Pergola, P. E., Piest, K. L., et al. (1995). Cutaneous active vasodilation in humans is mediated by cholinergic nerve cotransmission. *Circulation Research, 77*, 1222–1228.
75. Kellogg, D. L., Jr., Zhao, J. L., & Wu, Y. (2008). Endothelial nitric oxide synthase control mechanisms in the cutaneous vasculature of humans in vivo. *American Journal of Physiology Heart and Circulatory Physiology, 295*, H123–H129.
76. Kellogg, D. L., Jr., Zhao, J. L., & Wu, Y. (2008). Neuronal nitric oxide synthase control mechanisms in the cutaneous vasculature of humans in vivo. *Journal of Physiology, 586*, 847–857.
77. Joyner, M. J., & Dietz, N. M. (2003). Sympathetic vasodilation in human muscle. *Acta Physiologica Scandinavica, 177*, 329–336.
78. Crandall, C. G., Cui, J., & Wilson, T. E. (2003). Effects of heat stress on baroreflex function in humans. *Acta Physiologica Scandinavica, 177*, 321–328.
79. Vanhoutte, P., & Leusen, I. (1981). *Vasodilatation*. New York: Raven Press.
80. Palmer, T. (2008). Agents acting at the neuromuscular junction and autonomic ganglia. In L. L. Brunton & J. S. Lazo (Eds.), *Goodman & Gilman's the pharmacological basis of therapeutics*. New York: McGraw Hill.
81. Myslivecek, J., & Trojan, S. (2003). Regulation of adrenoceptors and muscarinic receptors in the heart. *General Physiology and Biophysics, 22*, 3–14.
82. Brodde, O. E., & Michel, M. C. (1999). Adrenergic and muscarinic receptors in the human heart. *Pharmacology in Review, 51*, 651–690.
83. Brodde, O. E., Bruck, H., Leineweber, K., et al. (2001). Presence, distribution and physiological function of adrenergic and muscarinic receptor subtypes in the human heart. *Basic Research in Cardiology, 96*, 528–538.
84. Myslivecek, J., Novakova, M., & Klein, M. (2008). Receptor subtype abundance as a tool for effective intracellular signalling. *Cardiovascular & Hematological Disorders Drug Targets, 8*, 66–79.
85. Burnstock, G. (2004). Cotransmission. *Current Opinion in Pharmacology, 4*, 47–52.
86. Burnstock, G. (2007). Physiology and pathophysiology of purinergic neurotransmission. *Physiology in Review, 87*, 659–797.
87. Burnstock, G. (2008). Non-synaptic transmission at autonomic neuroeffector junctions. *Neurochemistry International, 52*, 14–25.
88. Tsuru, H., Tanimitsu, N., & Hirai, T. (2002). Role of perivascular sympathetic nerves and regional differences in the features of sympathetic innervation of the vascular system. *Japanese Journal of Pharmacology, 88*, 9–13.
89. Burnstock, G. (1996). Purines and cotransmitters in adrenergic and cholinergic neurones. *Progress in Brain Research, 68*, 193–203.
90. Herring, N., Lokale, M. N., Danson, E. J., et al. (2008). Neuropeptide Y reduces acetylcholine release and vagal bradycardia via a Y2 receptor-mediated, protein kinase C-dependent pathway. *Journal of Molecular and Cellular Cardiology, 44*, 477–485.
91. Herring, N., & Paterson, D. J. (2009). Neuromodulators of peripheral cardiac sympatho-vagal balance. *Experimental Physiology, 94(1)*, 46–53. Epub 2008 Oct 22.
92. Han, S., Yang, C. L., Chen, X., et al. (1998). Direct evidence for the role of neuropeptide Y in sympathetic nerve stimulation-induced vasoconstriction. *American Journal of Physiology, 274*, H290–H294.
93. Westfall, T. C., McCullough, L. A., Vickery, L., et al. (1998). Effects of neuropeptide Y at sympathetic neuroeffector junctions. *Advances in Pharmacology, 42*, 106–110.
94. Abe, K., Tilan, J. U., & Zukowska, Z. (2007). NPY and NPY receptors in vascular remodeling. *Current Topics in Medicinal Chemistry, 7*, 1704–1709.
95. McDermott, B. J., & Bell, D. (2007). NPY and cardiac diseases. *Current Topics in Medicinal Chemistry, 7*, 1692–1703.
96. Henning, R. J., & Sawmiller, D. R. (2001). Vasoactive intestinal peptide: Cardiovascular effects. *Cardiovascular Research, 49*, 27–37.
97. Dvorakova, M. C. (2005). Cardioprotective role of the VIP signaling system. *Timely Topics in Medicine, 9*, E33.
98. Lundberg, J. M. (1996). Pharmacology of cotransmission in the autonomic nervous system: Integrative aspects on amines, neuropeptides, adenosine triphosphate, amino acids and nitric oxide. *Pharmacology in Review, 48*, 113–178.
99. Rowell, L. (1996). *Human circulation: Regulation during physical stress*. New York: Oxford University Press.
100. Westfall, T. C., & Westfall, D. P. (2008). Adrenergic agonists and antagonists. In L. Brunton, K. Parker, N. Murri, et al. (Eds.), *Goodman & Gilman's pharmacology*. New York: McGraw-Hill.
101. Barrett, L., Singer, M., & Clapp, L. (2007). Vasopressin: Mechanisms of action on the vasculature in health and septic shock. *Critical Care Medicine, 35*, 33–40.
102. Treschan, T., & Peters, J. (2006). The vasopressin system: Physiology and clinical strategies. *Anesthesiology, 105*, 599–612.
103. Bie, P. (1980). Osmoreceptors, vasopressin, and control of renal water excretion. *Physiology in Review, 60*, 961–1048.
104. Ramsay, D. J., Thrasher, T. N., & Bie, P. (1988). Endocrine components of body fluid homeostasis. *Comparative Biochemistry and Physiology, 90*, 777–780.
105. Voisin, D. L., & Bourque, C. W. (2002). Integration of sodium and osmosensory signals in vasopressin neurons. *Trends in Neuroscience, 25*, 199–205.

106. Bourque, C. W. (2008). Central mechanisms of osmosensation and systemic osmoregulation. *Nature Reviews, 9*, 519–531.
107. Shen, Y. T., Cowley, A. W., Jr., & Vatner, S. F. (1991). Relative roles of cardiac and arterial baroreceptors in vasopressin regulation during hemorrhage in conscious dogs. *Circulation Research, 68*, 1422–1436.
108. Thrasher, T. N., Chen, H. G., & Keil, L. C. (2000). Arterial baroreceptors control plasma vasopressin responses to graded hypotension in conscious dogs. *American Journal of Physiology, 278*, R469–R475.
109. Thrasher, T. N., Keil, L. C. (2000). Systolic pressure predicts plasma vasopressin responses to hemorrhage and vena caval constriction in dogs. *American Journal of Physiology, 279*, R1035–R1042.
110. Levin, E. R., Gardner, D. G., & Samson, W. K. (1998). Natriuretic peptides. *New England Journal of Medicine, 339*, 321–328.
111. Rubattu, S., Sciarretta, S., Valenti, V., et al. (2008). Natriuretic peptides: An update on bioactivity, potential therapeutic use, and implication in cardiovascular diseases. *American Journal of Hypertension, 21*, 733–741.
112. de Bold, A. J., Borenstein, H. B., Veress, A. T., et al. (1981). A rapid and potent natriuretic response to intravenous injection of atrial myocardial extract in rats. *Life Sciences, 28*, 89–94.
113. Clerico, A., Recchia, F. A., Passino, C., et al. (2006). Cardiac endocrine function is an essential component of the homeostatic regulation network: Physiological and clinical implications. *American Journal of Physiology Heart and Circulatory Physiology, 290*, H17–H29.
114. Ruskoaho, H. (1992). Atrial natriuretic peptide: Synthesis, release, and metabolism. *Pharmacology in Review, 44*, 479–602.
115. Dhingra, H., Roongsritong, C., & Kurtzman, N. A. (2002). Brain natriuretic peptide: Role in cardiovascular and volume homeostasis. *Seminars in Nephrology, 22*, 423–437.
116. Sabrane, K., Kruse, M. N., Fabritz, L., et al. (2005). Vascular endothelium is critically involved in the hypotensive and hypovolemic actions of atrial natriuretic peptide. *Journal of Clinical Investigations, 115*, 1666–1674.
117. Rose, R. A., & Giles, W. R. (2008). Natriuretic peptide C receptor signalling in the heart and vasculature. *Journal of Physiology, 586*, 353–366.
118. Rubattu, S., & Volpe, M. (2001). The atrial natriuretic peptide: A changing view. *Journal of Hypertension, 19*, 1923–1931.
119. Nishikimi, T., Maeda, N., & Matsuoka, H. (2006). The role of natriuretic peptides in cardioprotection. *Cardiovascular Research, 69*, 318–328.
120. Intravenous nesiritide vs nitroglycerin for treatment of decompensated congestive heart failure: A randomized controlled trial. (2002). *JAMA, 287*, 1531–1540.
121. Colucci, W. S., Elkayam, U., Horton, D. P., et al. (2000). Intravenous nesiritide, a natriuretic peptide, in the treatment of decompensated congestive heart failure. Nesiritide Study Group. *New England Journal of Medicine, 343*, 246–253.
122. Keating, G. M., & Goa, K. L. (2003). Nesiritide: A review of its use in acute decompensated heart failure. *Drugs, 63*, 47–70.
123. Arora, R. R., Venkatesh, P. K., & Molnar, J. (2006). Short and long-term mortality with nesiritide. *American Heart Journal, 152*, 1084–1090.
124. Sackner-Bernstein, J. D., Kowalski, M., Fox, M., et al. (2005). Short-term risk of death after treatment with nesiritide for decompensated heart failure: A pooled analysis of randomized controlled trials. *JAMA, 293*, 1900–1905.
125. Sackner-Bernstein, J. D., Skopicki, H. A., & Aaronson, K. D. (2005). Risk of worsening renal function with nesiritide in patients with acutely decompensated heart failure. *Circulation, 111*, 1487–1491.
126. Arora, R. R. (2006). Nesiritide: trials and tribulations. *Journal of Cardiovascular Pharmacology and Therapeutics, 11*, 165–169.
127. Hobbs, A., Foster, P., Prescott, C., et al. (2004). Natriuretic peptide receptor-C regulates coronary blood flow and prevents myocardial ischemia/reperfusion injury: novel cardioprotective role for endothelium-derived C-type natriuretic peptide. *Circulation, 110*, 1231–1235.
128. Sandow, S. L., & Tare, M. (2007). C-type natriuretic peptide: A new endothelium-derived hyperpolarizing factor? *Trends in Pharmacological Sciences, 28*, 61–67.
129. Villar, I. C., Panayiotou, C. M., Sheraz, A., et al. (2007). Definitive role for natriuretic peptide receptor-C in mediating the vasorelaxant activity of C-type natriuretic peptide and endothelium-derived hyperpolarising factor. *Cardiovascular Research, 74*, 515–525.
130. Stingo, A. J., Clavell, A. L., Aarhus, L. L., et al. (1992). Cardiovascular and renal actions of C-type natriuretic peptide. *American Journal of Physiology, 262*, H308–H312.
131. Scotland, R. S., Ahluwalia, A., & Hobbs, A. J. (2005). C-type natriuretic peptide in vascular physiology and disease. *Pharmacology & Therapeutics, 105*, 85–93.
132. Bader, M., & Ganten, D. (2008). Update on tissue renin-angiotensin systems. *Journal of Molecular Medicine, 86*, 615–621.
133. Dzau, V. J., Bernstein, K., Celermajer, D., et al. (2002). Pathophysiologic and therapeutic importance of tissue ACE: A consensus report. *Cardiovascular Drugs Therapeutics, 16*, 149–160.
134. Griendling, K. K., & Ushio-Fukai, M. (2000). Reactive oxygen species as mediators of angiotensin II signaling. *Regulatory Peptides, 91*, 21–27.
135. Harrison, D., Griendling, K. K., Landmesser, U., et al. (2003). Role of oxidative stress in atherosclerosis. *American Journal of Cardiology, 91*, 7A–11A.
136. Touyz, R. M. (2005). Reactive oxygen species as mediators of calcium signaling by angiotensin II: Implications in vascular physiology and pathophysiology. *Antioxidants and Redox Signaling, 7*, 1302–1314.
137. Donoghue, M., Hsieh, F., Baronas, E., et al. (2000). A novel angiotensin-converting enzyme-related carboxypeptidase (ACE2) converts angiotensin I to angiotensin 1-9. *Circulation Research*, 87, E1–E9.
138. Tipnis, S. R., Hooper, N. M., Hyde, R., et al. (2000). A human homolog of angiotensin-converting enzyme. Cloning and functional expression as a captopril-insensitive carboxypeptidase. *Journal of Biological Chemistry, 275*, 33238–33243.
139. Raizada, M. K., & Ferreira, A. J. (2007). ACE2: A new target for cardiovascular disease therapeutics. *Journal of Cardiovascular Pharmacology, 50*, 112–119.
140. Madeddu, P., Emanueli, C., & El-Dahr, S. (2007). Mechanisms of disease: the tissue kallikrein-kinin system in hypertension and vascular remodeling. *Nature Clinical Practice Nephrology, 3*, 208–221.
141. Sharma, J. N. (2003). Does the kinin system mediate in cardiovascular abnormalities? An overview. *Journal of Clinical Pharmacology, 43*, 1187–1195.
142. Granger, J. P., & Hall, J. E. (1985). Acute and chronic actions of bradykinin on renal function and arterial pressure. *American Journal of Physiology, 248*, F87–F92.
143. Sharma, J. N. (2005). The kallikrein-kinin system: from mediator of inflammation to modulator of cardioprotection. *Inflammopharmacology, 12*, 591–596.
144. Westermann, D., Schultheiss, H. P., & Tschope, C. (2008). New perspective on the tissue kallikrein-kinin system in myocardial infarction: Role of angiogenesis and cardiac regeneration. *International Immunopharmacology, 8*, 148–154.
145. Sharma, J. N. (2008). Cardiovascular activities of the bradykinin system. *Scientific World Journal, 8*, 384–393.
146. Daull, P., Jeng, A. Y., & Battistini, B. (2007). Towards triple vasopeptidase inhibitors for the treatment of cardiovascular diseases. *Journal of Cardiovascular Pharmacology, 50*, 247–256.
147. Tschope, C., Schultheiss, H. P., & Walther, T. (2002). Multiple interactions between the renin-angiotensin and the kallikrein-kinin systems: Role of ACE inhibition and AT1 receptor blockade. *Journal of Cardiovascular Pharmacology, 39*, 478–487.
148. Schmaier, A. H. (2003). The kallikrein-kinin and the renin-angiotensin systems have a multilayered interaction. *American Journal of Physiology, 285*, R1–R13.
149. Shen, B., & El-Dahr, S. S. (2006). Cross-talk of the renin-angiotensin and kallikrein-kinin systems. *Biological Chemistry, 387*, 145–150.
150. Packer, M., Califf, R. M., Konstam, M. A., et al. (2002). Comparison of omapatrilat and enalapril in patients with chronic heart failure: The Omapatrilat Versus Enalapril Randomized Trial of Utility in Reducing Events (OVERTURE). *Circulation, 106*, 920–926.
151. Messerli, F. H., & Nussberger, J. (2000). Vasopeptidase inhibition and angio-oedema. *Lancet, 356*, 608–609.
152. Esler, M. (1993). Clinical application of noradrenaline spillover methodology: Delineation of regional human sympathetic nervous responses. *Pharmacology Toxicology, 73*, 243–253.
153. Bevan, J. A. (1977). Some functional consequences of variation in adrenergic synaptic cleft width and in nerve density and distribution. *Federation Proceedings, 36*, 2439–2443.
154. Bevan, J. A. (1979). Some bases of differences in vascular response to sympathetic activity. *Circulation Research, 45*, 161–171.
155. Bevan, J. A., & Su, C. (1974). Variation of intra- and perisynaptic adrenergic transmitter concentrations with width of synaptic cleft in vascular tissue. *Journal of Pharmacology and Experimental Therapeutics, 190*, 30–38.
156. Gallagher, D., & O'Rourke, M. (1993). What is the arterial pressure? In M. O'Rourke, M. Safar, V. Dzau (Eds.), *Arterial vasodilation. Mechanisms and therapy* (pp. 134–148). Philadelphia: Lea & Febiger.

157. O'Rourke, M. (1990). What is blood pressure? *American Journal of Hypertension, 3*, 803–810.
158. Agabiti-Rosei, E., Mancia, G., O'Rourke, M. F., et al. (2007). Central blood pressure measurements and antihypertensive therapy: A consensus document. *Hypertension, 50*, 154–160.
159. Hainsworth, R. (1995). The control and physiological importance of heart rate. In M. Malik & A. Camms (Eds.), *Heart rate variability* (pp. 3–19), Armonk, NY: Futura Publishing.
160. Levy, M. N. (1997). Neural control of cardiac function. *Baillieres Clinical Neurology, 6*, 227–244.
161. Spyer, M. (2000). Vagal preganglionic neurons innervating the heart. In E. Page, H. Fozzard, & R. Solaro (Eds.), *Handbook of physiology, section 2: The cardiovascular system, vol I: The heart* (pp. 213–239). Bethesda, MD: American Physiological Society.
162. Monahan, K. D. (2007). Effect of aging on baroreflex function in humans. *American Journal of Physiology–Regulatory, Integrative and Comparative Physiology, 293*, R3–R12.
163. Rea, R. F., & Eckberg, D. L. (1987). Carotid baroreceptor-muscle sympathetic relation in humans. *American Journal of Physiology, 253*, R929–R934.
164. Ponikowski, P., & Banasiak, W. (2001). Chemosensitivity in chronic heart failure. *Heart Failure Monitor, 1*, 126–131.
165. Ponikowski, P., Chua, T. P., Anker, S. D., et al. (2001). Peripheral chemoreceptor hypersensitivity: An ominous sign in patients with chronic heart failure. *Circulation, 104*, 544–549.
166. Eckberg, D. L., & Karemaker, J. M. (2008). Point: Counterpoint "Respiratory sinus arrhythmia is due to a central mechanism vs. the baroreflex mechanism." *Journal of Applied Physiology*. Epub ahead of print.
167. Eckberg, D. L. (2000). Physiological basis for human autonomic rhythms. *Annals of Medicine, 32*, 341–349.
168. Janicki, J., Sheriff, D., Robotham, J., et al. (1996). Cardiac output during exercise: Contributions of the cardiac, circulatory, and respiratory systems. In L. Rowell & J. Sheperd (Eds.), *Handbook of physiology. Exercise: Regulation and integration of multiple systems* (pp. 649–704). Bethesda, MD: Oxford University Press.
169. Sheriff, D., Zhou, X., Scher, A., et al. (1993). Dependence of cardiac filling pressure on cardiac output during rest and dynamic exercise in dogs. *American Journal of Physiology, 265*, H316–H322.
170. Miller, D., Gleason, W., & Whalen, R. (1962). Effect of ventricular rate in the cardiac output in the dog with chronic heart block. *Circulation Research, 10*, 658–663.
171. Rushmer, R. (1959). Constance of stroke volume in ventricular responses to exertion. *American Journal of Physiology, 196*, 745–750.
172. Bevegård, S., Jonsson, B., Karlof, I., et al. (1967). Effect of changes in ventricular rate on cardiac output and central pressures at rest and during exercise in patients with artificial pacemakers. *Cardiovascular Research, 1*, 21–33.
173. Sonnenblick, E. H. (1962). Force-velocity relations in mammalian heart muscle. *American Journal of Physiology, 202*, 931–939.
174. Starling, E. (1918). *The Linacre Lecture on the Law of the Heart, Given at Cambridge, 1915*. London: Longmans, Green.
175. Sarnoff, S. J. (1955). Myocardial contractility as described by ventricular function curves; observations on Starling's Law of the Heart. *Physiology in Review, 35*, 107–122.
176. Weber, K., Janicki, J., Reeves, R., et al. (1974). Determinants of stroke volume in the isolated canine heart. *Journal of Applied Physiology, 37*, 742–747.
177. Hancock, W. O., Martyn, D. A., & Huntsman, L. L. (1993). Ca^{2+} and segment length dependence of isometric force kinetics in intact ferret cardiac muscle. *Circulation Research, 73*, 603–611.
178. Shiels, H. A., & White, E. (2008). The Frank-Starling mechanism in vertebrate cardiac myocytes. *Journal of Experimental Biology, 211*, 2005–2013.
179. Lakatta, E. G. (1987). Starling's law of the heart is explained by an intimate interaction of muscle length and myofilament calcium activation. *Journal of the American College of Cardiology, 10*, 1157–1164.
180. Brady, A. (1991). Mechanical properties of isolated cardiac myocytes. *Physiology in Review, 71*, 413–428.
181. Hedges, J. R. (1983). Preload and afterload revisited. *JEN, 9*, 262–267.
182. Covell, J., & Ross, J. (2002). Systolic and diastolic function (mechanics) of the intact heart. In E. Page, H. Fozzard, & R. Solaro (Eds.), *Handbook of physiology: Section 2. The cardiovascular system* (pp. 741–784). Bethesda, MD: American Physiological Society.
183. Ross, J., Jr. (1976). Afterload mismatch and preload reserve: A conceptual framework for the analysis of ventricular function. *Progress in Cardiovascular Disease, 18*, 255–264.
184. Ross, J., Jr., Franklin, D., & Sasayama, S. (1976). Preload, afterload, and the role of afterload mismatch in the descending limb of cardiac function. *European Journal of Cardiology, 4*(Suppl.), 77–86.
185. Bombardini, T. (2005). Myocardial contractility in the echo lab: Molecular, cellular and pathophysiological basis. *Cardiovascular Ultrasound, 3*, 27.
186. Endoh, M. (2004). Force-frequency relationship in intact mammalian ventricular myocardium: Physiological and pathophysiological relevance. *European Journal of Pharmacology, 500*, 73–86.
187. Ross, J., Jr., Miura, T., Kambayashi M., et al. (1995). Adrenergic control of the force-frequency relation. *Circulation, 92*, 2327–2332.
188. Yamanaka, T., Onishi, K., Tanabe, M., et al. (2006). Force- and relaxation-frequency relations in patients with diastolic heart failure. *American Heart Journal, 152*, 966.e1–966.e7.
189. Kroeker, C. A., Shrive, N. G., Belenkie, I., et al. (2003). Pericardium modulates left and right ventricular stroke volumes to compensate for sudden changes in atrial volume. *American Journal of Physiology, 284*, H2247–H2254.
190. Spodick, D. (1997). *The pericardium. A comprehensive textbook*. New York: Marcel Dekker, Inc.
191. Belenkie, I., Sas, R., Mitchell, J., et al. (2004). Opening the pericardium during pulmonary artery constriction improves cardiac function. *Journal of Applied Physiology, 96*, 917–922.
192. Belenkie, I., Smith, E. R., & Tyberg, J. V. (2001). Ventricular interaction: From bench to bedside. *Annals of Medicine, 33*, 236–241.
193. Horne, S. G., Belenkie, I., Tyberg, J. V., et al. (2000). Pericardial pressure in experimental chronic heart failure. *Canadian Journal of Cardiology, 16*, 607–613.
194. Kardon, D. E., Borczuk, A. C., & Factor, S. M. (2000). Mechanism of pericardial expansion with cardiac enlargement. *Cardiovascular Pathology, 9*, 9–15.
195. Hammond, H., White, F., Bhargava, V., et al. (1992). Heart size and maximal cardiac output are limited by the pericardium. *American Journal of Physiology, 263*, H1675–H1681.
196. De Hert, S. G., ten Broecke, P. W., Rodrigus, I. E., et al. (2001). The effects of the pericardium on length-dependent regulation of left ventricular function in coronary artery surgery patients. *Journal of Cardiothoracic and Vascular Anesthesia, 15*, 300–305.
197. Stray-Gundersen, J., Musch, T., Haidet, G., et al. (1986). The effect of pericardiectomy on maximal oxygen consumption and maximal cardiac output in untrained dogs. *Circulation Research, 58*, 523–530.
198. Hunter, S., Smith, G. H., & Angelini, G. D. (1992). Adverse hemodynamic effects of pericardial closure soon after open heart operation. *Annals of Thoracic Surgery, 53*, 425–429.
199. Rao, V., Komeda, M., Weisel, R. D., et al. (1999). Should the pericardium be closed routinely after heart operations? *Annals of Thoracic Surgery, 67*, 484–488.
200. Cowley, A. J. (1992). Long-term control of arterial blood pressure. *Physiology in Review, 72*, 231–300.
201. Granger, J. P., Alexander, B. T., & Llinas, M. (2002). Mechanisms of pressure natriuresis. *Current Hypertension Report, 4*, 152–159.
202. Guyton, A. C. (1991). Blood pressure control–special role of the kidneys and body fluids. *Science, 252*, 1813–1816.
203. Brooks, V., & Osborn, J. (1995). Hormonal-sympathetic interactions in long-term regulation of arterial pressure: An hypothesis. *American Journal of Physiology, 268*, R1343–R1358.
204. Evans, R. G., Majid, D. S., & Eppel, G. A. (2005). Mechanisms mediating pressure natriuresis: What we know and what we need to find out. *Clinical and Experimental Pharmacology and Physiology, 32*, 400–409.
205. Bie, P., Wamberg, S., & Kjolby, M. (2004). Volume natriuresis vs. pressure natriuresis. *Acta Physiologica Scandinavica, 181*, 495–503.
206. Brooks, V. L., & Sved, A. F. (2005). Pressure to change? Re-evaluating the role of baroreceptors in the long-term control of arterial pressure. *American Journal of Physiology–Regulatory, Integrative and Comparative Physiology, 288*, R815–R818.
207. Joyner, M. J., Charkoudian, N., & Wallin, B. G. (2008). A sympathetic view of the sympathetic nervous system and human blood pressure regulation. *Experimental Physiology, 93*, 715–724.
208. Lohmeier, T. E., Hildebrandt, D. A., Warren, S., et al. (2005). Recent insights into the interactions between the baroreflex and the kidneys in hypertension. *American Journal of Physiology–Regulatory, Integrative and Comparative Physiology, 288*, R828–R836.

209. Thrasher, T. N. (2005). Baroreceptors, baroreceptor unloading, and the long-term control of blood pressure. *American Journal of Physiology—Regulatory, Integrative and Comparative Physiology, 288,* R819–R827.
210. Thrasher, T. N. (2006). Arterial baroreceptor input contributes to long-term control of blood pressure. *Current Hypertension Report, 8,* 249–254.
211. Barrett, C. J., & Malpas, S. C. (2005). Problems, possibilities, and pitfalls in studying the arterial baroreflexes' influence over long-term control of blood pressure. *American Journal of Physiology—Regulatory, Integrative and Comparative Physiology, 288,* R837–R845.
212. Osborn, J. W., Jacob, F., & Guzman, P. (2005). A neural set point for the long-term control of arterial pressure: Beyond the arterial baroreceptor reflex. *American Journal of Physiology—Regulatory, Integrative and Comparative Physiology, 288,* R846–R855.
213. Osborn, J. W. (2005). Hypothesis: Set-points and long-term control of arterial pressure. A theoretical argument for a long-term arterial pressure control system in the brain rather than the kidney. *Clinical and Experimental Pharmacology and Physiology, 32,* 384–393.
214. Mellander, S. (1989). Functional aspects of myogenic vascular control. *Journal of Hypertension, 7*(Suppl. 4), S21–S30.
215. Seddon, M. D., Chowienczyk, P. J., Brett, S. E., et al. (2008). Neuronal nitric oxide synthase regulates basal microvascular tone in humans in vivo. *Circulation, 117,* 1991–1996.
216. Vallance, P., Collier, J., & Moncada, S. (1989). Effects of endothelium-derived nitric oxide on peripheral arteriolar tone in man. *Lancet, 189,* 997–1000.
217. Sugawara, J., Komine, H., Hayashi, K., et al. (2007). Effect of systemic nitric oxide synthase inhibition on arterial stiffness in humans. *Hypertension Research, 30,* 411–415.
218. Wilkinson, I., MacCallum, H., Cockcroft, J., et al. (2002). Inhibition of basal nitric oxide synthesis increases aortic augmentation index and pulse wave velocity *in vivo. British Journal of Clinical Pharmacology, 53,* 189–192.
219. Sugawara, J., Komine, H., Hayashi, K., et al. (2007). Relationship between augmentation index obtained from carotid and radial artery pressure waveforms. *Journal of Hypertension, 25,* 375–381.
220. Celander, O. (1954). The range of control exercised by sympathicoadrenal system. *Acta Physiologica Scandinavia, 32*(Suppl. 116), 1–132.
221. Johanson, B. (1980). Myogenic responses of vascular smooth muscle. In N. Stevens (Ed.), *Smooth muscle contraction* (pp. 457–472). New York: Marcel Dekker.
222. Johnson, P. (1986). Autoregulation of blood flow. *Circulation Research, 59,* 483–495.
223. Renkin, E. (1984). Control of microcirculation and blood-tissue exchange. In E. Renkin & C. Michel (Eds.), *Handbook of physiology* (pp. 627–687). Bethesda, MD: American Physiological Society.
224. Carlson, B. E., Arciero, J. C., & Secomb, T. W. (2008). Theoretical model of blood flow autoregulation: Roles of myogenic, shear-dependent, and metabolic responses. *American Journal of Physiology Heart and Circulatory Physiology, 295,* H1572–H1579.
225. Schubert, R., & Mulvany, M. J. (1999). The myogenic response: Established facts and attractive hypotheses. *Clinical Science, 96,* 313–326.
226. Feigl, E. (1989). The arterial system. In H. Patton, A. Fuchs, B. Hille, et al. (Eds.), *Textbook of physiology* (pp. 849–859). Philadelphia: WB Saunders.
227. Arciero, J. C., Carlson, B. E., & Secomb, T. W. (2008). Theoretical model of metabolic blood flow regulation: Roles of ATP release by red blood cells and conducted responses. *American Journal of Physiology Heart and Circulatory Physiology, 295,* H1562–H1571.
228. Hester, R. L., & Hammer, L. W. (2002). Venular-arteriolar communication in the regulation of blood flow. *American Journal of Physiology, 282,* R1280–R1285.
229. Johnson, P. (1980). The myogenic response. In D. Bohr, A. Somlyo, & H. Sparks (Eds.), *Handbook of physiology, section 2, vol II, vascular smooth muscle* (pp. 409–442). Bethesda, MD: American Physiological Society.
230. Lombard, J., & Duling, B. (1977). Relative importance of tissue oxygenation and vascular smooth muscle hypoxia in determining arteriolar response to occlusion in the hamster cheek pouch. *Circular Research, 41,* 365–373.
231. Rothe, C. (1983). Venous system: Physiology of the capacitance vessels. In J. Shepherd & F. Abboud (Eds.), *Handbook of physiology. The cardiovascular system. Peripheral circulation and organ blood flow* (pp. 397–452). Bethesda, MD: American Physiological Society.
232. Flavahan, N., Linblad, L., Verbeuren, T., et al. (1985). Cooling and alpha-1 and alpha-2 adrenergic response in cutaneous veins: Role of receptor reserve. *American Journal of Physiology, 249,* H950–H955.
233. Hainsworth, R. (1986). Vascular capacitance: Its control and importance. *Reviews of Physiology, Biochemistry & Pharmacology, 105,* 101–173.
234. Rowell, L. (1973). Regulation of splanchnic blood flow in man. *Physiologist, 16,* 127–142.
235. Rothe, C., & Gaddis, M. (1990). Autoregulation of cardiac output by passive elastic characteristics of the vascular capacitance system. *Circulation, 81,* 360–368.
236. Guyton, A. (1955). Determination of cardiac output by equating venous return curves with cardiac response curves. *Physiology in Review, 35,* 123–129.
237. Guyton A., Abernathy B., Langston J., et al. Relative importance of venous and arterial resistances in controlling venous return and cardiac output. *American Journal of Physiology, 196,* 1008–1014, 1959.
238. Guyton, A., Lindsey, A., Abernathy, B., et al. (1957). Venous return at various right atrial pressures and the normal venous return curve. *American Journal of Physiology, 189,* 609–615.
239. Brengelmann, G. L. (2003). A critical analysis of the view that right atrial pressure determines venous return. *Journal of Applied Physiology, 94,* 849–859.
240. Bridges, E. (2005). Hemodynamic monitoring. In S. Woods, E. Sivarajan Froelicher, S. Motzer, et al. (Eds.), Cardiac nursing (pp. 81–108). Philadelphia: Lippincott.
241. Brengelmann, G. L. (2006). Counterpoint: The classical Guyton view that mean systemic pressure, right atrial pressure, and venous resistance govern venous return is not correct. *Journal of Applied Physiology, 101,* 1525–1526; discussion 1526–1527.
242. Brengelmann, G. L. (2008). Learning opportunities in the study of Curran-Everett's exploration of a classic paper on venous return. *Advances in Physiological Education, 32,* 242–243.
243. Magder, S. (2006). Point: The classical Guyton view that mean systemic pressure, right atrial pressure, and venous resistance govern venous return is/is not correct. *Journal of Applied Physiology, 101,* 1523–1525.
244. Rothe, C. F. (1993). Mean circulatory filling pressure: Its meaning and measurement. *Journal of Applied Physiology, 74,* 499–509.
245. Rothe, C. (2006). The classical Guyton view that mean systemic pressure, right atrial pressure, and venous resistance govern venous return is/is not correct. *Journal of Applied Physiology, 101,* 1529.
246. Casey, D. P., & Hart, E. C. (2008). Cardiovascular function in humans during exercise: Role of the muscle pump. *Journal of Physiology, 586,* 5045–5046.
247. Rowland, T. W. (2001). The circulatory response to exercise: Role of the peripheral pump. *International Journal of Sports Medicine, 22,* 558–565.
248. Osada, T., Katsumura, T., Hamaoka, T., et al. (2002). Quantitative effects of respiration on venous return during single knee extension-flexion. *International Journal of Sports Medicine, 23,* 183–190.
249. Miller, J. D., Pegelow, D. F., Jacques, A. J., et al. (2005). Skeletal muscle pump versus respiratory muscle pump: Modulation of venous return from the locomotor limb in humans. *Journal of Physiology, 563,* 925–943.
250. Michard, F., & Teboul, J. L. (2000). Using heart-lung interactions to assess fluid responsiveness during mechanical ventilation. *Critical Care, 4,* 282–289.
251. Krogh, A. (1912). The regulation of the supply of blood to the right heart. *Skandinavisches Archiv fur Physiologie, 27,* 227–248.
252. Hamilton, W., Woodbury, R., & Harper, H. (1936). Physiologic relationships between intrathoracic, intraspinal, and arterial pressures. *JAMA, 107,* 853–856.
253. Hamilton, W., Woodbury, R., & Harper, H. (1944). Arterial, cerebrospinal and venous pressures in man during cough and strain. *American Journal of Physiology, 141,* 42–50.
254. Levin, A. (1966). A simple test of cardiac function based upon the heart rate changes induced by the Valsalva Maneuver. *American Journal of Cardiology, 18,* 90–99.
255. Smith, M., Beightol, L., Fritsch-Yelle, J., et al. (1996). Valsalva's maneuver revisited: A quantitative method yielding insights into human autonomic control. *American Journal of Physiology, 271,* 1240–1249.
256. Junqueira L. F., Jr. (2008). Teaching cardiac autonomic function dynamics employing the Valsalva (Valsalva-Weber) maneuver. *Advantages in Physiological Education, 32,* 100–106.
257. McGuire J., Green R., Hauenstein V., et al. (1950). Bed pan deaths. *American Practitioner, 1,* 23–28.
258. Metzger B., & Therrien B. (1990). Effect of position on cardiovascular response during the Valsalva Maneuver. *Nursing Research, 39,* 198–202.
259. Sharpey-Schafer E. (1955). Effects of Valsalva's manoeuvre on the normal and failing circulation. *BMJ, 1,* 693–695.

260. Eckberg D. L., & Sleight P. (1992). *Human baroreflexes in health and disease.* Oxford, UK.
261. Mancia, G., & Mark, A. (1983). Arterial baroreflexes in humans. In J. Sheperd & F. M. Abboud (Eds.), *Handbook of physiology. The cardiovascular system. Peripheral circulation and organ blood flow* (pp. 755–794). Bethesda, MD: American Physiologic Society.
262. Prakash, E. S., Madanmohan Pal, G. K. (2004). What is the ultimate goal in neural regulation of cardiovascular function? *Advances in Physiology Education, 28*, 100–101.
263. Sagawa, K. (1983). Baroreflex control of systemic arterial pressure and vascular bed. In J. Sheperd & F. M. Abboud (Eds.), *Handbook of physiology. The cardiovascular system. Peripheral circulation and organ blood flow* (pp. 452–496). Bethesda, MD: American Physiologic Society.
264. Toska, K., & Walloe, L. (2002). Dynamic time course of hemodynamic responses after passive head-up tilt and tilt back to supine position. *Journal of Applied Physiology, 92*, 1671–1676.
265. Ogoh, S., Yoshiga, C. C., Secher, N. H., et al. (2006). Carotid-cardiac baroreflex function does not influence blood pressure regulation during head-up tilt in humans. *Journal of Physiologic Science, 56*, 227–233.
266. Rowell, L. B. (1977). Reflex control of the cutaneous vasculature. *Journal of Investigative Dermatology, 69*, 154–166.
267.Scott-Douglas, N. W., Robinson, V. J., Smiseth, O. A., et al. (2002). Effects of acute volume loading and hemorrhage on intestinal vascular capacitance: A mechanism whereby capacitance modulates cardiac output. *Canadian Journal of Cardiology, 18*, 515–522.
268. Halliwill, J. R. (2007). Virtual conductance, real hypotension: What happens when we stand up too fast? *Journal of Applied Physiology, 103*, 421–422.
269. Sheriff, D. D., Nadland, I. H., & Toska, K. (2007). Hemodynamic consequences of rapid changes in posture in humans. *Journal of Applied Physiology, 103*, 452–458.
270. Wray, D. W., Formes, K. J., Weiss, M. S., et al. (2001). Vagal cardiac function and arterial blood pressure stability. *American Journal of Physiology Heart and Circulatory Physiology, 281*, H1870–H1880.
271. Toska, K., Eriksen, M., & Walloe, L. (1994). Short-term cardiovascular responses to a step decrease in peripheral conductance in humans. *American Journal of Physiology, 266*, H199–H211.
272. Heistad, D., & Kontos, H. (1983). Cerebral circulation. In J. Shepherd, F. Abboud, & S. Geiger (Eds.), *Handbook of physiology. The cardiovascular system: Peripheral circulation and organ blood flow* (pp. 137–182). Bethesda, MD: American Physiological Society.
273. Qureshi, A. I. (2008). Acute hypertensive response in patients with stroke: Pathophysiology and management. *Circulation, 118*, 176–187.
274. Jones, P. P., Christou, D. D., Jordan, J., et al. (2003). Baroreflex buffering is reduced with age in healthy men. *Circulation, 107*, 1770–1774.
275. Minaker, K. L., Meneilly, G. S., Youn, G. J., et al. (1991). Blood pressure, pulse, and neurohumoral responses to nitroprusside-induced hypotension in normotensive aging men. *Journal of Gerontology, 46*, M151–M154.
276. Rudas, L., Crossman, A. A., Morillo, C. A., et al. (1999). Human sympathetic and vagal baroreflex responses to sequential nitroprusside and phenylephrine. *American Journal of Physiology, 276*, H1691–H1698.
277. Wood M., Hyman S., & Wood, A. J. (1987). A clinical study of sensitivity to sodium nitroprusside during controlled hypotensive anesthesia in young and elderly patients. *Anesthesia and Analgesia, 66*, 132–136.

PART II Physiologic and Pathologic Responses

CHAPTER 4 Genetics

Bradley E. Aouizerat

Nearly 6 decades ago, Watson and colleagues discovered the secret of life when they published the chemical structure of DNA.[1] The double helical structure made immediately obvious how this molecular archive of life could encode information in the copious quantities necessary to program a living cell. This discovery set into motion a revolution that has continued to unfold to this day, much of it guided by this original discovery.

Research is a slow process, often with years between each sensation, and even today, the DNA revolution remains largely behind laboratory doors, in the form of scientists' ever-increasing understanding of the mechanisms of life. But a few powerful inventions—forensic DNA examination, DNA-based drug discovery, and specific disease susceptibility mutation screening—have enjoyed a significant active contribution to society (see Display 4-1 for definitions).

DNA underlies almost every aspect of human health. Obtaining a detailed picture of how genes and other DNA sequences function together and interact with environmental factors ultimately will lead to the discovery of pathways involved in normal processes and in disease pathogenesis. Such knowledge will have a profound impact on the way disorders are diagnosed, treated, and prevented and will bring about revolutionary changes in clinical and public health practice. Some of these transformative developments are described herein.

How do scientists study and find these genetic mutations? They have available to them a growing battery of tools and technologies to compare a DNA sequence isolated from a healthy person to the same region of DNA extracted from an afflicted person. Advanced computer technologies, combined with the explosion of genetic data that is currently generated from the various whole-genome sequencing projects, enable scientists to use these molecular genetic tools to more accurately diagnose disease and to design new therapeutic interventions. This chapter reviews some common principles that geneticists—scientists who study the inheritance pattern of specific traits—can use to inform clinical practice.

DNA

Molecular genetics is the study of the units, or segments, of DNA that pass information from generation to generation. These molecules, our genes, are long sequences of deoxyribonucleic acid, or DNA. Just four chemical building blocks or bases, deoxyguanine (G), deoxyadenine (A), deoxythymine (T), and deoxycytosine (C), are placed in a unique order to encode for all of the heritable units in all living organisms (Fig. 4-1).

DNA is the chemical responsible for preserving, copying, and transmitting information within cells. DNA, located in the nucleus of every cell, harbors the instructions that provide almost all of the information necessary for a living organism to grow and function. The DNA molecule resembles a twisted ladder, usually described as a double helix. The rungs are repeating units called nucleotides, which are the quantum building blocks of DNA. Nucleotides are composed of one sugar-phosphate molecule (the linear strands or outer rails of the DNA ladder) and one base (Fig. 4-2). DNA in eukaryotic cells consists of two nucleotide strands joined by weak chemical bonds between the two bases, forming base pairs. Therefore, a base pair constitutes a "rung" on the ladder of the DNA. The four bases organize in two fundamental pairs, A with T and C with G. One rail of a DNA ladder is a single strand of DNA that is denoted by a sequence of nucleotides (e.g., ACGTGCTGACCTGACGTAGGGCATA), which has complementary bases on the opposite rail, forming complementary nucleotide strands (e.g., TATGCCCTACGTCAGGTCAGCACGT). Within the regions of DNA that express information, these strings of nucleotides are organized into three unit "words" termed *codons.* These codons are organized into groups called *exons.* Ultimately, these exons form sentences, or *genes.* Genes encode all of the necessary information to produce a messenger molecule composed of ribonucleic acids (RNA), which are composed of four other nucleotides: guanine (G), adenine (A), cytosine (C), and uracil (U). Thus, DNA sentences are *transcribed* into RNA messages, which are single-stranded complementary copies of DNA. Once processed, these messages leave the nucleus and enter another cellular compartment where they are threaded into cellular machinery, which *translates* the information into its final state, the *protein.* Proteins are required for the structure, function, and regulation of the body's cells, tissues, and organs. This process, where DNA is transcribed into RNA and subsequently translated into proteins, represents the central dogma of molecular biology. It is worth noting that a small subset of genes expresses RNA without being translated into proteins. These other forms of RNA play crucial roles in the biology of the cell.

Humans have approximately 3 billion base pairs of DNA in most of their cells. This complete set of genes is called a *genome.* The exact sequence of the bases is different for everyone, which makes

DISPLAY 4-1 Definitions

Amino acids. The building block for proteins. Humans require 20 amino acids as building blocks.

Chromosome. An arrangement of tightly packed and coiled DNA and protein. Diploid cells such as the human body cells have 23 sets of chromosomes; haploid cells such as gametes—sperm or ova—have only a single set of chromosomes.

DNA. Deoxyribonucleic acid, the double helix, which codes for the proteins and other elements necessary to construct an organism.

Exon. Regions of DNA that are expressed, coding for RNA and/or protein.

Gamete. A sex cell, such as egg or sperm, capable of joining with an opposite gamete (egg plus sperm) to make a zygote.

Gene. A gene is a segment of DNA or RNA that performs a specific function; usually, it is a segment of DNA that codes for some molecular product, often a protein. Aside from the nucleotides that code for the protein, a gene also consists of segments that determine the type, quantity, and timing of protein expression. Genes can produce different combinations of proteins under different stimuli.

Genome. The sum total of genetic material in an individual organism.

Genotype. A relative term that can refer to a particular nucleotide position, or even an entire segment of DNA. A genotype has two components, one from the same position on each chromosome.

Intron. In most eukaryotic cells, introns are segments of DNA that are a component of gene structure but do not generally code for proteins. Introns are processed out of transcribed messenger RNA (mRNA), or *spliced* out, before it is threaded into ribosomes for translation into protein.

Mutation. An alteration in a gene or segment of DNA; mutations are largely accidental and unproductive. On rare occasions, mutations can be dangerous and/or even beneficial. Thus, mutations can lead to variation in the phenotype of an organism.

Phenotype. The physical structure and/or composition of an organism, or group of organisms. Genotypes expressed in and operating in the context of a given environment(s) determine phenotype.

Protein. Genes often encode for proteins, which help form and regulate all organisms. Proteins are molecular machines composed of strings of 20 different types of amino acids. Proteins can in turn form complexes, which interact to perform more complex actions and functions.

Ribosomes. Ribosomes are complexes of RNA and protein, which use the information encoded in mRNA to assemble specific proteins out of amino acids via a process termed *translation.*

RNA. Ribonucleic acid; an intermediate, complementary copy of DNA. mRNA is used by ribosomes as templates for the construction of proteins.

Sex chromosomes. In humans, the X and Y chromosomes. Two X chromosomes result in a female gender, while an X chromosome and a Y chromosome result in a male gender. Other species have different types of sex chromosomes.

Synteny. Segments of chromosomes, which contain the same sequence of genes, which are shared between different organisms.

each of us unique. DNA is an exquisitely small yet extremely long molecule that lacks the tensile strength to remain unprotected during cell division. Accordingly, DNA molecules are packaged into tightly coiled units called *chromosomes,* found in the nucleus of every cell. Chromosomes consist of the double helix of DNA wrapped around proteins called histones. DNA in the human genome is arranged into 24 distinct chromosomes (i.e., 22 autosomes and two sex chromosomes), physically separate molecules that range in length from about 50 million to 250 million base pairs. The two sex chromosomes determine gender; two copies of the "X" chromosome result in female gender, while one copy each of the "X" and "Y" chromosomes determines male gender (Fig. 4-3). There are 23 pairs of chromosomes in the normal diploid genome in humans (i.e., 22

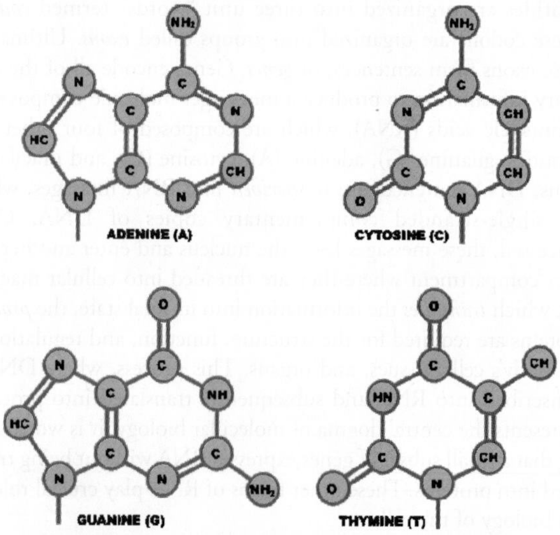

■ **Figure 4-1** The four DNA bases. Each DNA is made up of the sugar 2′-deoxyribose linked to a phosphate group and one of the four bases depicted above.

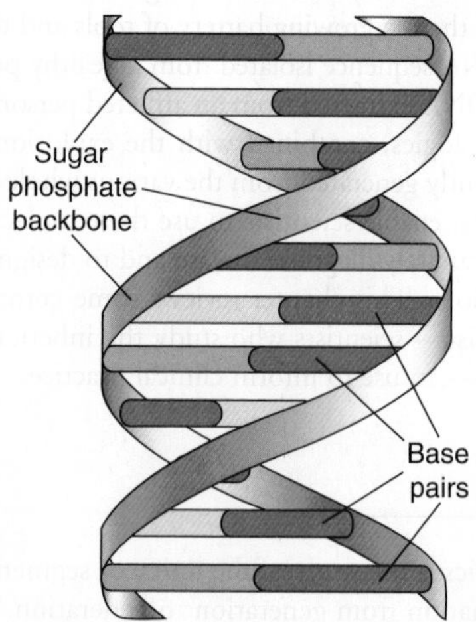

■ **Figure 4-2** The DNA molecule consists of two antiparallel, complementary strands of nucleotides that pair A + T or G + C.

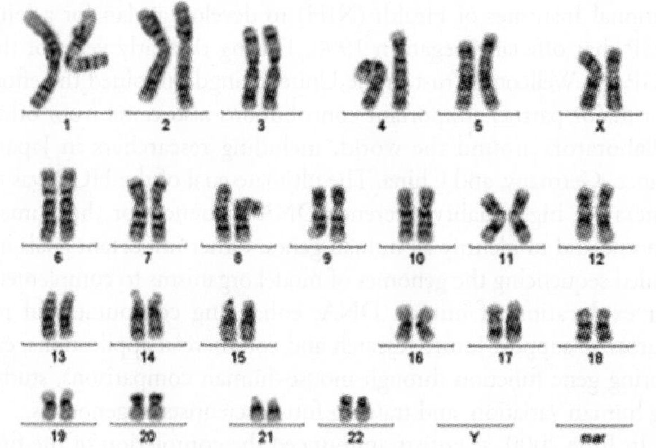

■ **Figure 4-3** An example of the human genome condensed into the 22 chromosome pairs (autosomes) and the two sex chromosomes.

autosome pairs and either two X chromosomes [i.e., female] or an X and a Y chromosomal pair [i.e., male]). A few types of major chromosomal abnormalities, including missing or extra chromosome copies or gross chromosomal breaks that rejoin at another chromosome location (translocations), can be detected by microscopic examination. Most changes in DNA, however, are far subtler and require a much closer analysis of the DNA molecule.

Genes

Each chromosome contains many genes, the basic physical and functional units of heredity in living cells. Genes constitute approximately 2% of the human genome; the remainder consists of noncoding regions, whose functions may include providing chromosomal structural integrity and regulating where, when, and in what quantity proteins are made. Genes consist of a length of DNA that encodes instructions for making a specific RNA or protein. Through these molecular products, our genes influence almost everything about us, including how we grow, process nutrients, reproduce, respond to environmental influences including infections and medicines, and perhaps most important our susceptibility and response to disease.

On cell division, DNA becomes tightly packed into a complex structure called chromatin, which is arranged into chromosomes in each cell nucleus. With a few exceptions, such as red blood cells, platelets, and specialized immune cells and platelets, the DNA in each cell of the human body is complete and identical. The human genome—the complete collection of genetic instructions—is estimated to be composed of approximately 20,000 to 25,000 genes. Genes are defined as the segments of DNA that contain the code for all proteins. Proteins are molecular machines that can perform a vast array of diverse and complex functions. DNA is the template that guides the synthesis of those machines through the direction of DNA's intermediate, messenger ribonucleic acid (mRNA). The mRNA leaves the nucleus to be processed in the cytoplasm. Ribosomes (a complex of protein and RNA) then use the mRNA to translate the original DNA instructions and synthesize proteins. Some genes perform other functions, such as making the RNA constituents of ribosomes.

When DNA is transcribed to RNA, many lengths of nucleotides do not encode for proteins. These segments of RNA are called *introns* and are processed out of the RNA segments. The segments that remain (termed *exons*) are spliced together, forming the mature *mRNA*; these abridged versions of our genes encode for proteins. In some cases, a length of newly transcribed RNA can be processed in different ways; the sequence of exons used can be spliced together in different combinations to make a variety of different proteins. Thus, a single gene can produce or express a diverse series of protein products, depending on the cell type, timing, and ambient activating conditions. This explains in part how identical embryonic cells differentiate to become a variety of different tissues. Similarly, cardiac cells synthesize proteins required for that organ's structure and function, whereas liver cells make proteins important in the metabolic functions of that organ.

DNA AND HUMAN DIVERSITY

Although we all look quite different from one another, we are surprisingly alike at the genetic level. The DNA of most people is 99.9% identical. Only approximately 3 million base pairs are responsible for the differences among us, which is only one tenth of 1% of our genome. Yet these DNA base sequence variations influence most of our physical differences and many other characteristics, also. Gene sequence variations occur in our genes, and a subset of the variations results in different forms of the same gene and are called *alleles*. People can have two identical or two different alleles for a particular gene.

Genes determine hereditary traits such as eye color or hair color. They do this by providing precise instructions for how every activity in every cell of our body should be performed. For example, a gene may guide a liver cell to remove excess cholesterol from our bloodstream. How does a gene do this? It will instruct the cell to make a particular protein and this protein then performs the actual task. In the case of excess blood cholesterol, it is the receptor proteins on the outside of a liver cell that bind to and remove cholesterol from the blood. The cholesterol molecules can then be transported into the cell, where they are further processed by other proteins.

GENETIC VARIATION

A *mutation*, more neutrally referred to as a genetic variation, is a change in the DNA sequence of a gene (e.g., an "A" is altered into a C, G, or T) or even a gross alteration in the chromosomes. Polymorphisms (i.e., *poly* meaning many and *morph* meaning forms) are arbitrarily defined as common differences in the sequence of DNA, occurring in at least 1% of the population. Mutations are less common differences, which occur in less than 1% of the population. Most DNA variation is functionally neutral (neither beneficial nor harmful), but harmful sequence changes do occur. Changes within genes can result in proteins that do not work normally or do not work at all, which can contribute to disease or affect how an individual responds to a medicine. Mutations may be passed down from parent to child (i.e., in the sperm or egg cells), may occur around the time of conception, or may be acquired during a person's lifetime. Mutations can arise spontaneously during normal cell functions, such as when a cell divides, or in response to environmental factors such as toxins, radiation, hormones, and even diet.

Many diseases are caused by mutations or changes in the DNA sequence of a gene. When the information encoded in a gene changes, the resulting protein may not function properly or may not even be made at all. In either case, the cells containing that genetic change may no longer perform as expected. For example, it is now known that mutations in the gene that codes for the cholesterol receptor protein (i.e., the low-density lipoprotein receptor, LDLR) are associated with a disease called familial hypercholesterolemia. The cells of most individuals with this disease exhibit reduced receptor function and, as a result, cannot remove a sufficient amount of low-density lipoprotein (LDL), which carries cholesterol throughout their bloodstream. Such an affected person may then have dangerously high levels of cholesterol, a known risk factor for development of atherosclerosis, putting him or her at increased risk for cardiovascular disease culminating in heart attack and/or stroke.

Genetic variations are differences in DNA sequence among individuals that may underlie differences in health. Genetic variations occurring in more than 1% of a population would be considered useful polymorphisms for population genetic analyses. Polymorphism types include single nucleotide polymorphisms (SNPs), small-scale insertions/deletions, and repetitive elements (satellite DNA). Satellite DNA is common throughout the genome. These groups of variations are segments of DNA that are repeated in tandem and can be used to differentiate individuals with differing numbers of repeats. The most common variations found in genes are SNPs, which can change the protein product, alter the temporal or spatial expression of a gene, or silence its expression altogether. A comprehensive and complex system of repair genes encodes for enzymes that correct nearly all DNA errors. As our bodies change in response to age, illness, and other factors, our DNA repair systems may become less efficient and uncorrected mutations can accumulate, resulting in diseases such as cancer.

GENE TESTING

DNA-based tests are among the first commercial medical applications of the new genetic discoveries. Gene tests can be used to diagnose disease, confirm, and more precisely define a clinical diagnosis, provide prognostic information about the course of a disease, or confirm the existence of a disease in asymptomatic individuals.

Currently, several hundred genetic tests are in clinical use, with a large expansion in available tests expected as a result of the Human Genome Project (HGP). Most current tests detect mutations associated with rare genetic disorders that follow mendelian inheritance patterns. These include cystic fibrosis, sickle cell anemia, and Huntington disease. Recently, tests have been developed to detect mutations for a few more complex conditions such as breast, ovarian, and colon cancers. Although they have limitations, these tests sometimes are used to make risk estimates in asymptomatic individuals with a family history of the disorder. One potential benefit to using such gene tests is that they may provide information to help health care providers and patients and caregivers manage the disease more effectively.

THE HUMAN GENOME PROJECT

HGP traces its roots to an initiative in the United States Department of Energy (DOE), which since 1947 has supported the development of new energy resources and technologies and acquiring a deeper understanding of potential health and environmental risks posed by their production and use. In 1986, the DOE announced the Human Genome Initiative, the result of which would provide a reference human genome sequence. Soon thereafter, the DOE joined with the National Institutes of Health (NIH) to develop a plan for a joint HGP that officially began in 1990. During the early years of the HGP, the Wellcome Trust in the United Kingdom joined the effort as a major partner. Important contributions also came from other collaborators around the world, including researchers in Japan, France, Germany, and China. The ultimate goal of the HGP was to generate a high-quality reference DNA sequence for the human genome and to identify all human genes. Other important goals included sequencing the genomes of model organisms to complement our exploration of human DNA, enhancing computational resources to support future research and commercial applications, exploring gene function through mouse–human comparisons, studying human variation, and training future scientists in genomics.

In June 2000, scientists announced the completion of the first working draft of the entire human genome.[2,3] The high-quality reference sequence was completed 2 years ahead of schedule in April 2003, marking the achievement of the initial goal of the HGP. Available to researchers worldwide, the human genome reference sequence provides an unprecedented biological resource that will accelerate research and discovery, which are expected to seed a myriad of practical applications. The draft sequence has already aided locating genes associated with human disease. Hundreds of other genome sequence projects on microbes, plants, and animals have been completed since the initiation of the HGP, which have enabled detailed comparisons among organisms.

PHARMACOGENOMICS

It is estimated that more than 100,000 people die each year from adverse responses to medications. Another 2.2 million individuals experience serious reactions, while others fail to respond at all. Researchers are beginning to correlate DNA variants with individual responses to medical treatments, permitting identification of particular subgroups of patients, and develop drugs customized for those populations. The discipline that blends pharmacology with genomics is called *pharmacogenomics.*

DNA variants in genes involved in drug metabolism are the focus of much current research in this area. Enzymes encoded by these genes are responsible for metabolizing most drugs used today, including many for treating cardiovascular diseases. Enzyme function affects patient responses to both the drug and its dose response. Future advances will enable rapid testing to determine the patient's genotype and guide treatment with the most effective drugs, in addition to drastically reducing adverse reactions.

Genomic data and technologies also are expected to make drug development faster, cheaper, and more effective. New drugs aimed at specific sites in the body and at particular biochemical events leading to disease will cause fewer side effects than many current medicines. Ideally, the new genomic drugs could be administered earlier in the disease process. As knowledge becomes available to select patients most likely to benefit from a potential drug, pharmacogenomics will hasten the design of clinical trials to bring drugs into clinical use sooner.

BIOCHEMICAL BASIS OF GENETIC DISEASE

Our genetic constitution, the way in which our individual genome interacts with the environment, can impact our health in many ways. An individual can inherit genetic diseases, caused by abnormal groups of genes passed down from one generation to the next. Such heritable disorders are classified into three general classes. The first class is single gene mutations of large effect, which can be readily identified given detailed family history review coupled with appropriate genetic testing (e.g., familial hypercholesterolemia). This class of genetic disorders is commonly referred to as mendelian disorders, named after the founder of the modern principles of genetics, Gregor Mendel.[4] The more common class of heritable disorders is those of multifactorial inheritance, caused by the complex interplay of several genes and environmental factors (e.g., diabetes, hypertension, and atherosclerosis). The last class is chromosomal aberrations, abnormalities of either chromosomal structure or number. Such gross alterations to the genome can result from a cellular "accident" or from a parent who carries a chromosomal aberration (e.g., trisomy 21 or Down syndrome).

Altered gene function can manifest at the molecular level in several ways. Genetic alterations can result in enzyme defects, which result in the synthesis of a defective enzyme with reduced activity or reduce quantity. This can lead to substrate accumulation, a metabolic block with a decreased amount of end product, or the failure to inactivate a tissue-damaging substrate. Another mechanism of disease is malfunctions in receptors and transport systems. For example, in familial hypercholesterolemia, a reduced function of LDL receptor leads to an inability to transport LDL into the cell, which causes elevated levels of plasma cholesterol and accelerates atherosclerosis.[5]

As the science of genetics has matured, research has shifted focus from rare, single gene disorders to common, multifactorial chronic diseases. Chronic disease affects more than 90 million Americans, accounting for 70% of all deaths and 60% of the nation's medical costs. As research progresses, genetics offers the opportunity to target health promotion and disease prevention programs better and the possibility to conserve health care program resources. However, the contribution of genetics to chronic disease is complex, reflecting the interaction of many genes with the environment and with one another.[6]

OVERVIEW: HEART DISEASE

Cardiovascular Disease

According to the Centers for Disease Control and Prevention, cardiovascular disease, principally heart disease and stroke, is the leading cause of death among men and women in all racial and ethnic groups. Cardiovascular disease affects approximately 58 million Americans and costs the nation $274 billion each year, including health expenditures and lost productivity. Research has begun to uncover a number of potential genetic susceptibility genes for heart disease and stroke and their risk factors (e.g., obesity and high blood pressure).[7]

Heart disease has become a major focus of genetic research. In the past decade, the number of publications on genetic contributions to heart disease has risen exponentially. Genetic mutations have been associated with various risk factors for heart disease, including lipid metabolism and transport, hypertension, and elevated plasma homocysteine levels. It is believed that while traditional risk factors including environmental influences explain approximately 50% of the cases of cardiovascular disease, genetics may help explain the remaining disease burden.

Stroke

Studies also have indicated a genetic predisposition to ischemic and hemorrhagic stroke. Although single gene disorders explain a small fraction of strokes, the genetic contribution to stroke most likely will be multifactorial and complex. Recent family studies, including the Framingham Heart Study, have highlighted a significant genetic component to stroke.[8] Twin and family studies provide evidence that genetic factors contribute to the risk of stroke and that their role may be at least as important in stroke as in coronary heart disease. Genetic variation of cystathionine β-synthase or methylenetetrahydrofolate reductase[9] result in markedly elevated plasma homocysteine levels and homocystinuria.[10] Homocysteine is a sulfur-containing amino acid derivative formed during methionine metabolism. Homocystinemia increases the risk of coronary artery disease (CAD), peripheral artery disease, stroke, and venous thrombosis, and it is a risk factor for premature vascular disease.[11] The angiotensin-1-converting enzyme gene harbors a polymorphism, which in some but not all studies is a risk factor for myocardial infarction. Similar studies in stroke patients also show inconsistent results, but most of these studies have been underpowered to detect a small contribution to stroke risk from the ACE gene. Recent meta-analysis suggests that the polymorphism, acting recessively, is a modest but independent risk factor for ischemic stroke onset.[12]

The apolipoprotein E (apoE) ε_4 allele is associated with increased risk of coronary heart disease and is also a major genetic susceptibility locus for Alzheimer disease. This polymorphism is also associated with ischemic stroke and poorer outcomes after stroke. Carriers of the rare ε_4 are more frequent among patients with ischemic cerebrovascular disease compared with control subjects. A recent meta-analysis provides evidence for a role for the apoE genotype in the pathogenesis of some cases of ischemic cerebrovascular disease.[13]

Atherosclerosis

Atherosclerosis is a progressive disease characterized by the accumulation of lipids and fibrous elements in the large arteries (see Chapter 5). The early lesions of atherosclerosis consist of subendothelial accumulations of cholesterol-engorged macrophages called foam cells. Lesions are usually found in the aorta in the first decade of life, the coronary arteries in the second decade, and the cerebral arteries in the third or fourth decade. Because of differences in blood flow dynamics, there are preferred sites of lesion formation within the arteries. Plaques can become increasingly complex, involving calcification, ulceration, and hemorrhage from small vessels within the lesion. Although advanced lesions may encroach and block blood flow, the critical clinical complication is an acute occlusion caused by thrombus formation, resulting in angina, myocardial infarction, or stroke.

Sudden Cardiac Death

Although CAD accounts for the majority of sudden death cases in cardiac arrest, a small proportion (<5%) is attributable to sudden arrhythmia death syndrome. A prolonged Q-T interval is a common thread among the various phenotypes associated with this phenomenon. A number of drugs are known to cause QT prolongation, as well as disorders of potassium, calcium, and magnesium homeostasis, myocarditis, and endocrine and nutritional disorders.

Recently, attention has focused on a group of inherited gene mutations in cardiac ion channels that cause long QT syndrome with an increased risk for sudden death. The age of onset for long QT-related death is the early 30s, with men disproportionately affected. Most cardiac events are precipitated by intense exercise or emotional stress, but they can also occur during sleep. Unfortunately, not all persons with long QT syndrome have previous symptoms or identifiable electrocardiographic abnormalities and may present with sudden death. Antiarrhythmic agents and implantable defibrillators are used for the treatment of long QT syndrome, although identification of the specific gene variants underlying this syndrome will almost certainly better direct prophylactic therapy.[14]

THE GENETICS OF CARDIOVASCULAR DISEASE

Epidemiological studies over the past 50 years have identified many risk factors for atherosclerosis (Table 4-1). Dyslipidemia appears to be of primary importance, because raised levels of atherogenic lipoproteins are a prerequisite for most forms of atherosclerosis. With the exception of gender and the level of lipoprotein(a), each of the genetic risk factors involves multiple genes. An added level of complexity involves the interactions between risk factors that are often not simply additive. For example, the effects of hypertension on CAD are considerably amplified if cholesterol levels are high.[24]

The importance of genetics and environment in human CAD has been examined in family and twin studies.[21] The heritability (the portion attributed to genetic factors and shared environment) of atherosclerosis has been high in most population studies, often in excess of 50%. It is also evident that the environment explains much of the variation in disease incidence between populations. Thus, the common forms of CAD result from the combination of unfavorable genetic and environmental factors and our increased lifespan.[24]

Generally, the manifestation of CAD is caused by the interaction of several genetic and environmental factors, with those patients with the greatest number of risk factors, including genetic and environmental, facing the highest risk at earlier ages. Several biochemical processes are involved in atherosclerosis formation, progression, and culmination as acute coronary syndromes. Lipid and apolipoprotein metabolism, inflammatory response, endothelial function, platelet function, thrombosis, fibrinolysis, homocysteine metabolism, insulin sensitivity, and blood pressure regulation have been demonstrated to influence disease pathophysiology.[28–30] Each of these biochemical processes involves the complex interplay of enzymes, receptors, and ligands encoded by our genes, the expressions of which are also influenced by environmental factors. Genetic variations can modulate the function of these constituents, resulting in altered susceptibility to the development and progression of CAD.[31] Several well-established environmental risk factors that predispose to CAD have also been identified (Table 4-2).

The treatment and prevention of CAD has improved greatly in the past decades; however, it remains the leading cause of death and premature disability in the United States. The cumulative risk for CAD by age 70 is 30% and 15% in men and women, respectively, and increases to 48% and 30% by the age of 90 years.[44] Moreover, it is now clear that disability and mortality from CAD at young ages is particularly devastating to families and has a substantial impact on our economy. Understanding the genetic basis of CAD is expected to improve disease management by providing improved diagnosis, targeted therapies, and prognosis.

Genetic Aspects/Dissection of Atherosclerosis

Although the common forms of atherosclerosis are multifactorial, studies of rare, mendelian forms have contributed vital insights

Table 4-1 ■ GENETIC AND ENVIRONMENTAL FACTORS ASSOCIATED WITH ATHEROSCLEROSIS AND CORONARY HEART DISEASE

Trait	Epidemiologic Studies	Population Genetic Studies	Animal Models of Disease	Clinical Trials	Reference
Factors with a Strong Genetic Component					
↑ LDL/VLDL	•	•	•	•	15
↓ HDL cholesterol	•	•	•		16
↑ Lipoprotein(a)	•	•	•		17
↑ Blood pressure	•			•	15,18
↑ Homocysteine	•	•			19
↑ Triglycerides	•	•		•	20
Family history	•	•			21
Diabetes and obesity	•	•	•		15
↑ Hemostatic factors		•			15
Depression and other behavioral traits		•			18
Gender (male)	•	•			22
Systemic inflammation	•	•		•	23
Metabolic syndrome	•	•			24
Environmental Factors					
High-fat diet	•	•	•		15
Smoking	•			•	15
↓ Antioxidant levels	•		•	•	25
Lack of exercise	•	•			15
Infectious agents	•	•	•		26

Adapted from Lusis, A. J. [2000]. Atherosclerosis. *Nature, 407*[6801], 233–241.[27]

Table 4-2 ■ GENETIC CHANGES RELEVANT TO HEART DISEASE*

Trait	Mendelian Characteristics
↑ LDL/VLDL levels	Familial hypercholesterolemia → LDL receptor gene defects resulting in a dominant disorder resulting in very high LDL cholesterol levels and early CAD[24]
	Familial defective apoB-100 → Dominant disorder caused by apoB mutations that affect binding to LDL receptor[24]; less severe than FH
↓ HDL cholesterol levels	ApoAI deficiency (apoAI)[24]; in the homozygous state, null mutations of apoAI result in the virtual absence of HDL and early CAD
	Tangier disease (ABC1 transporter)[32,33]. This recessive disorder results in the inability of cells to export cholesterol and phospholipids, resulting in very low levels of HDL
Coagulation	Various genetic disorders of genetic hemostasis[24]: unlike rare disorders of lipid metabolism where atherosclerotic disease is a primary manifestation, disorders of hemostasis usually present either as increased risk of bleeding or as thrombosis (usually venous), with no outstanding effect on atherogenesis
Elevated homocysteine	Homocystinuria (cystathionine β-synthase): recessive metabolic disorder resulting in very high levels of homocysteine and severe occlusive vascular disease[19]
Diabetes, type 2	MODY1 (hepatocyte nuclear factor 4a), MODY2 (glucokinase), and MODY3 (hepatocyte nuclear factor 1a)[24]: MODY1, 2, and 3 are characterized by the development of non-insulin-dependent diabetes mellitus in young adults
Hypertension	Glucorticoid-remediable aldosteronism: a dominant disorder with early-onset hypertension and stroke (hybrid gene from cross-over of 11-b-hydroxylase and aldosterone synthase)[34]
	Liddle syndrome (epithelial sodium: dominant disorder with hypertension and metabolic alkalosis channel)[34]
	Mineralocorticoid receptor[35]: early-onset hypertension associated with pregnancy
Common Genetic Variations Contributing to Heart Disease and Its Risk Factors	
LDL/VLDL	ApoE[24]: three common missense alleles explain ~5% of variance in cholesterol levels
HDL levels	Hepatic lipase[36]: promoter polymorphism
	ApoAI-CIII-AIV cluster[36]: multiple polymorphisms
	Cholesteryl ester transfer: common null mutations (Japanese); protein[24] missense polymorphisms
	Lipoprotein lipase[37]: missense polymorphisms
Lipoprotein(a)	Apolipoprotein(a)[17]: many alleles explain >90% variance
Homocysteine	Methylene tetrahydrofolate: missense polymorphism reductase[24]
Coagulation	Fibrinogen B[24]: promoter polymorphism
	Plasminogen activator: promoter polymorphism inhibitor type 1[24]
	Factor VIII[24]: missense polymorphism
Blood pressure	Angiotensinogen[34]: missense and promoter polymorphisms
	β2-Adrenergic receptor[34]: missense polymorphism
	Alpha-adducin[34]: missense polymorphism
CAD	Angiotensin-converting insertion—deletion polymorphism enzyme[38]
	Serum paraoxonase[39,40]: missense polymorphism affecting enzymatic activity
	Hemachromatosis: missense polymorphism-associated gene[41]
	Endothelial nitric oxide: missense polymorphism synthase[42]
	Factor XIII[43]: missense polymorphism

*Only genes exhibiting evidence of linkage or association in two or more studies are cited.

Adapted from Lusis, A. J. [2000]. Atherosclerosis. *Nature, 407*[6801], 233–241.[27]

into disease pathogenesis (see Table 4-2). Studies of familial hypercholesterolemia helped unravel the pathways that regulate plasma cholesterol metabolism, knowledge of which was important for the development of cholesterol-lowering interventions. In contrast to the mendelian disorders, dissecting the genetic contribution of common, complex forms of CAD has proven more difficult. Studies of candidate genes have suggested a number of genes influencing the traits relevant to atherosclerosis, but our understanding remains incomplete (see Table 4-2). Large-scale sequencing is now underway to identify polymorphisms for many other candidate genes for hypertension, diabetes, and other traits relevant to atherosclerosis.[45] In an attempt to identify further atherosclerosis genes, whole-genome scans (a method of fingerprinting the entire genome in attempts to identify genes shared in affected individuals more often than with their relatives) for loci associated with diabetes, hyperlipidemia, low high-density lipoprotein (HDL) levels, and hypertension have been performed,[46] but few loci with significant evidence of linkage have been found, emphasizing the complexity of these traits.

As a result of the genome projects and large-scale sequencing, literally millions of gene variations are being identified and catalogued. Given the rapid development of DNA chip technology, it will soon be possible to genotype large numbers of such polymorphisms in many thousands of individuals. However, appropriate methods to analyze such data are evolving.[47,48]

EVIDENCE FOR A GENETIC BASIS OF CORONARY ARTERY DISEASE

Significant amounts of research support a genetic basis for coronary heart disease and its risk factors. The methods of investigation include family and twin studies, animal models, and gene association studies. Although, historically, single gene mutation was the first to be described as a class, only rarely is susceptibility to atherosclerosis the result of a single gene mutation. The most familiar single gene mutation is familial hypercholesterolemia, which is caused by disruptive mutations of the LDL receptor or apolipoprotein B.[49–51]

Twin Studies

Twins have been useful in studying the genetic contribution to many common diseases. A higher concordance of a trait found in monozygotic twins (who share all of their genes) compared with dizygotic twins (who share only half of their genes) suggests a genetic component.[6,52] Several large twin registries, including the Danish Twin Registry, which includes approximately 8,000 unselected twin pairs, observed a significant difference in concordance of CAD deaths in monozygotic twins compared with dizygotic twins in men and women.[53–59] A common observation in twin studies was the delayed age of onset of CAD in women versus men.

Familial Aggregation

A genetic epidemiologic study analyzing data regarding 19 traditional risk factors from cases with myocardial infarction before age 55 compared with matched controls[60] suggested that the highest odds ratio was associated with a family history of a first-degree relative with CAD before age 55. The risk increased 7.1-fold if the CAD was diagnosed before age 55. These risks were substantially greater than those associated with elevated cholesterol level, smoking, or inactivity. Population studies have shown on average a 2- to 3-fold increase in CAD risk in first-degree relatives of cases,[35,61–64] and prospective studies have shown a 1.5- to 2-fold increase in CAD risk associated with a positive family history.[65–71] The observation of aggregation of CAD-associated risk factors (e.g., dyslipidemia, hypertension, obesity, and diabetes) in families with CAD further suggests a genetic basis for these conditions and explains, in part, the familial aggregation of CAD.[64, 72–78]

Angiography studies have confirmed that family history of CAD is an independent risk factor for angiographically evident CAD.[76,79,80] Many studies of familial aggregation of CAD have indicated that the age of onset of a case is inversely proportional to the risk to relatives and that the risk of disease is typically several times greater in relatives of females with CAD compared with males with CAD.[61,63] The heritability for CAD is estimated at approximately 56%, suggesting that more than half of the cases of premature CAD (diagnosed before age 55) are caused by the contribution of genes. Moreover, in families with CAD onset before age 46, heritability was estimated at 90% to 100%, whereas within families of the oldest cases the heritability ranged from 15% to 30%.[61]

Animal Models

In the past two decades, understanding of the molecular mechanisms in atherogenesis has been revolutionized by studies in genetically engineered animal models.[81] These models include studies in rabbits, pigs, nonhuman primates, and rodents. Mice deficient in apoE or the LDL receptor have advanced lesions and are the models most used in genetic and physiological studies.[82] These have permitted in vivo testing of hypotheses. Caveats to such studies are the limits imposed by species differences compared with humans.

Excellent animal models exist for the study of heart disease and the associated conditions of diabetes, dyslipidemia, hypertension, and obesity. Use of animals eliminates problems caused by genetic heterogeneity (mixed population backgrounds) and environmental influences. Given a controlled environment, trait differences between animal strains are best explained by genetic factors. Gene associations in animal models can result in the identification of candidate genes for study in human families, because conserved chromosomal segments exist between model animals and humans (synteny).[83]

The use of animal models is a potentially powerful way of identifying genes that contribute to common forms of atherosclerosis.[84] Many animal models have common variations in many traits relevant to atherosclerosis, and orthologous genes (i.e., those having an evolutionary counterpart in other species) frequently contribute to a trait in rodents and humans.[85] Mapping and identification of genes contributing to complex traits is easier in animals than in humans. During this decade, it is likely that genome scan approaches and large-scale gene expression studies in animal models of disease will become widely used in atherosclerosis research.

Gene Associations

Many polymorphisms have been associated with atherosclerosis[27,86] (Table 4-3). Because of methodological constraints, these genes were historically identified as a result of their participation in biochemical pathways implicated in the development and progression of atherosclerosis. There are also numerous studies that have found gene associations with related disorders that are indirectly implicated in the development and progression of CAD, diabetes,[87–92] hypertension,[35,46,93,94] and obesity.[95–101] Recent investigations using genome scan approaches, which are unbiased screens of the entire genome that can implicate novel genes, have identified additional genetic loci associated with CAD, hypertension, and diabetes, which might provide additional insight into genetic factors contributing to atherosclerosis.[74,139–146] Genetic factors have been identified that accelerate progression and clinical coronary events by influencing the response to risk factor modification such as diet, alcohol, and use of postmenopausal hormone replacement therapy.[108,118,123] For example, the risk of myocardial infarction is lower in men with an alcohol dehydrogenase variation that is associated with a slower rate of ethanol metabolism, and a significant interaction between this genetic variation and alcohol intake was found.[147] Those who were homozygous for the susceptibility allele and drank at least one drink per day had the greatest reduction in risk for myocardial infarction and the highest HDL cholesterol levels. Genetic variation also plays a role in response to diet.[148–150] A recent study found that 40% of the interindividual variation in LDL cholesterol levels in response to a diet low in saturated fat is a familial trait.[151]

Although genetic association studies have generated a veritable tidal wave of attractive candidate genes, an important caveat to such studies exists. While these studies may provide strong and exciting correlations between particular genetic variations and disease, they must be replicated and generalized to the population (by their study in large epidemiologic studies) before their clinical usefulness can be accepted and realized.

Table 4-3 ■ CANDIDATE GENES IMPLICATED IN RISK FOR HEART DISEASE IN HUMANS

Candidate Genes
Lipid Metabolism
Apolipoprotein(a)[74,102]
Apolipoprotein B[51]
Apolipoprotein E[103–106]
Cholesterol ester transfer protein[107,108]
LDL receptor[49,50]
Lipoprotein lipase[109]
Paraoxonase[110]
Blood Pressure Regulation
Angiotensinogen[111–114]
Angiotensin II receptor, type 1[112,114,115]
Angiotensin-converting enzyme inhibitor[114–117]
Thrombosis
Factor II (Prothrombin)[118]
Factor V (Factor V Leiden)[119,120]
Factor VII[49,121–124]
Fibrinolysis
Fibrinogen[124–127]
Plasminogen activator inhibitor-1b[128]
Platelet function glycoprotein IIIa[129–131]
Endothelial Function/Inflammatory Response
Endothelial leukocyte adhesion molecule-1 (E-selectin)[132]
Endothelial cell nitric oxide synthase[129]
Homocysteine Metabolism
Cystathionine β-synthase[133–135]
Methylene tetrahydrofolate reductase[136–138]

Adapted from Lusis, A. J. [2000]. Atherosclerosis. *Nature, 407*[6801], 233–241.[27]

DIAGNOSIS AND RISK ASSESSMENT: APPLICATION OF GENETIC SUSCEPTIBILITY INFORMATION IN THE PREVENTION OF CORONARY ARTERY DISEASE

CAD is a heterogeneous disorder; logically, no universal path of prevention exists for all patients.[152] In the future, knowledge of a patient's genetic risk factors will identify important biologic differences that could improve disease prevention and management through targeted interventions. Failure to recognize these differences may deny appropriate access to care for those patients who may benefit from alternative prevention and management strategies.

Cardiovascular disease is heterogeneous in manifestation, and the most appropriate therapy will depend on the particular subtype of disease. Therefore, one application of screening may be to distinguish different forms of the disease so that pharmacological intervention can be more effectively targeted. Classification is already used clinically because patients are grouped according to the variety of risk factors they display, but genetic testing will greatly expand the subdivisions of the disease.

Because heart disease and stroke are diseases of adulthood, knowledge of susceptibility to disease could be available years before clinical disease develops, permitting earlier intervention. Testing for elevated LDL cholesterol and decreased HDL cholesterol levels and blood pressure have long been advocated as a way of identifying individuals at increased risk, and other factors have emerged more recently as risk indicators (see Table 4-1). Once the genes contributing to common forms of the disease have been identified, along with their underlying genetic lesions, genetic tests will add greatly to our ability to assess risk.

Cholesterol lowering is a central tenet of primary and secondary prevention of CAD.[153–160] However, despite effective lipid lowering, CAD will develop in a substantial proportion of individuals, or those with CAD will have progression of their disease.[161] Moreover, elevated plasma cholesterol level is not a sensitive predictor of individuals with the greatest genetic susceptibility to CAD.[162] Elevated levels of lipoprotein(a) [Lp(a)], a proinflammatory subpopulation of LDL particles modified by the apolipoprotein(a) protein, are not currently detected with routine cholesterol screening, and only 3% of patients with hyper-Lp(a) had elevated LDL cholesterol values. Epidemiological studies have shown that plasma HDL cholesterol is inversely related to CAD and that there is an inverse relationship between HDL cholesterol and triglyceride levels.[163] Also, hypertriglyceridemia is an independent risk factor for CAD.[20] Fibrates reduce death from CAD and nonfatal myocardial infarction in secondary prevention of CAD in men with low levels of HDL cholesterol. During fibrate treatment, HDL cholesterol levels predicted the magnitude of reduction in risk for CAD events. Supplementation with the cofactors involved in homocysteine metabolism, vitamins B_6, B_{12}, and folate, is effective in reducing homocysteine levels, particularly if there is a vitamin deficiency,[164–166] although the long-term effect of cofactor supplementation on reducing cardiovascular events is still undergoing study. However, data are lacking regarding the efficacy of these agents on reducing cardiovascular events in individuals who have modified novel genetic risk factors contributing to unfavorable homocysteine and Lp(a) levels. Despite this lack of evidence, knowledge of genetic susceptibility to CAD has value in providing risk information and can guide decision making regarding lifestyle modification and participation in disease prevention and management strategies.

Early detection strategies for CAD are generally not recommended for the general population, because many lack adequate sensitivity and specificity whereas others are too invasive and costly. However, use of early detection strategies such as electron beam computed tomography may ultimately prove to be more cost-effective for genetically susceptible persons at high risk. There is consistent evidence that coronary calcification correlates highly with the presence and degree of obstructive and nonobstructive plaque,[167,168] nonfatal infarction, and need for subsequent coronary revascularization in asymptomatic individuals[169–171] and patients undergoing coronary angiography.[172] Once CAD is identified in high-risk individuals with a genetic susceptibility, more aggressive risk factor modification, for example, pharmacological intervention and procedures such as angioplasty or revascularization, can be considered.

Genetic susceptibility to disease can be assessed by direct DNA-based testing, direct measurement of biochemical traits, physical and pathologic characteristics, and personal and family history collection. Physical examination findings can be instrumental in identifying a genetic risk for CAD (e.g., tendon xanthomas and xanthelasma seen in hereditary lipid disorders). However, many hereditary syndromes are rare and account for only a small percentage of cardiovascular disease.[173] Conversely, DNA markers associated with common forms of disease are generally prevalent and of low magnitude, and thus in isolation are not highly predictive of CAD risk.[174] Moreover, modeling the cumulative risk of the multiple low-magnitude genetic risk factors is still evolving and their application to clinical risk assessment is currently premature. Therefore, the systematic collection of family history information currently appears to be the most appropriate screening approach for identification of individuals with a genetic susceptibility to CAD (see Tables 4-1 and 4-2).

In addition to identifying individuals with increased cardiovascular risk, the family history can identify qualitative characteristics of CAD risk, which are important when planning disease prevention and management strategies.[175] Familial aggregation of CAD, dyslipidemia, hypertension, stroke, and type 2 diabetes suggests insulin resistance (commonly referred to as the metabolic syndrome).[176] Altered hemostasis may be suspected in a family that features multiple affected relatives with early onset of CAD and stroke or other thromboembolic events. Recognition of these qualitative features may have important implications for recommending appropriate diagnostic tests as well as individualized surveillance and prevention strategies.

Family history reports of CAD, diabetes, and hypertension are generally accurate, with sensitivity of a case report for CAD ranging from 67% to 85%.[177–179] Specificity values for family history reports of these conditions approach 90%.[177] A positive family history can generally be used with a high degree of confidence for the identification of individuals who may be at increased risk for CAD. Nonetheless, when possible, verification of family history by review of medical records and death certificates is preferable, although not always feasible. Studies of family history validity indicate some underreporting of disease in relatives; thus, a negative report should not be used as an indicator of a minimum or decreased disease risk (less than the general population risk).

An important goal of genetic evaluation for CAD is the development of individualized preventive strategies based on genetic risk assessment and the personal medical history and lifestyle.

Patient participation in the process is vital to the success of the prevention plan. Genetic counseling is an integral component of the genetic evaluation, helping to identify a patient's motivations and understanding of the genetic risk assessment and perceived barriers and benefits to learning of a genetic risk.[180] This communication process ensures the opportunity to provide an informed consent, including discussion of the potential benefits, risks, and limitations regarding genetic risk assessment and testing.[181–184]

Generally, individuals are motivated to participate in genetic risk assessment with the hope that it will clarify the most appropriate plan for disease management and prevention and for the benefit that such genetic information may have for family members. Several studies have shown that family history can influence compliance with lipid screening and other preventive interventions.[185] Common barriers to obtaining genetic risk information for common disease include fear of discrimination in the workplace and by insurers, cost, and uncertainty about the value of interventions.[186–189] The evidence regarding genetic discrimination of otherwise healthy individuals is minimal, although uncertain.[190,191] Yet because of the fear of potential discrimination, individuals may choose to forego genetic risk assessment that may deprive a patient of beneficial surveillance or therapeutic measures to reduce disease risk. The past 15 years have seen escalating interest regarding the use of genetic information by health insurers.[192] In 1996, the Health Insurance Portability and Accountability Act (HIPAA) became the first federal law to limit the use of genetic data by health insurers. It forbids, among other features, health insurers from using genetic predisposition to disease as a "pre-existing" condition that could delay or limit coverage.

ETHICAL CONSIDERATIONS

Sharing information about the risk of future disease can have significant emotional and psychological effects, also. The lack of sufficient privacy and legal protections could lead to discrimination in employment and insurance or other misuse of personal genetic information. Additionally, because genetic tests identify information about individuals and their families, test results can impact family dynamics. Results can also pose risks for population groups if they lead to group stigmatization. Families or individuals who have genetic disorders or who are at risk for these often seek help from medical geneticists and genetic counselors. These professionals can diagnose and explain disorders, review available options for testing, preventive strategies, and treatment, and provide emotional support. Other issues related to genetic tests include their effective introduction into clinical practice, the regulation of laboratory genetic testing quality assurance, the availability of testing, and the education of health care providers and patients about correct interpretation and attendant risks.

SUMMARY

CAD management and prevention can improve with genetic risk assessment. Our genetic profile contributes to susceptibility, development, and progression of cardiovascular diseases and our response to risk factor modification and lifestyle choices. Identification of genetically susceptible individuals through the family history and biochemical and DNA testing is possible, and many inherited cardiovascular risk factors are modifiable. Early detection of CAD may be appropriate for genetically susceptible individuals to guide decision making about risk factor modification. However, data are lacking regarding the efficacy of this approach in preventing clinical events. Research is necessary to investigate the outcome of genetic risk assessment in the management of CAD. Despite the current paucity of evidence, knowledge of genetic CAD susceptibility likely has value in providing risk information and guiding subsequent clinical decision making. Genetics will play an important role in health promotion and prevention and treatment strategies for chronic diseases such as cardiovascular disease. There is a need for informing the public about the significance of genetic discovery and health status. Translational research that takes the discovery of disease susceptibility genes and creates opportunities for better-targeted prevention and treatment strategies is imperative to decrease the effect of cardiovascular morbidity and mortality.

REFERENCES

1. Watson, J. (2000). The double helix revisited. The man who launched the Human Genome Project celebrates its success. *Time, 156*(1), 30.
2. Lander, E. S., Linton, L. M., Birren, B., et al. (2001). Initial sequencing and analysis of the human genome. *Nature, 409*(6822), 860–921.
3. Venter, J. C., Adams, M. D., Myers, E. W., et al. (2001). The sequence of the human genome. *Science, 291*(5507), 1304–1351.
4. Mendel, G. (1965). *Experiments in plant hybridisation.* London: Oliver and Boyd.
5. Soutar, A. K., & Naoumova, R. P. (2007). Mechanisms of disease: Genetic causes of familial hypercholesterolemia. *Nature Clinical Practice. Cardiovascular Medicine, 4*(4), 214–225.
6. Haines, J. L., & Pericak-Vance, M. A. (2006). *Genetic analysis of complex diseases* (2nd ed.). Hoboken, NJ: Wiley-Liss.
7. Kullo, I. J., & Ding, K. (2007). Mechanisms of disease: The genetic basis of coronary heart disease. *Nature Clinical Practice. Cardiovascular Medicine, 4*(10), 558–569.
8. Larson, M. G., Atwood, L. D., Benjamin, E. J., et al. (2007). Framingham Heart Study 100K project: Genome-wide associations for cardiovascular disease outcomes. *BMC Medical Genetics, 8*(Suppl. 1), S5.
9. Kelly, P. J., Rosand, J., Kistler, J. P., et al. (2002). Homocysteine, MTHFR 677C→T polymorphism, and risk of ischemic stroke: Results of a meta-analysis. *Neurology, 59*(4), 529–536.
10. Wald, D. S., Law, M., & Morris, J. K. (2002). Homocysteine and cardiovascular disease: Evidence on causality from a meta-analysis. *BMJ, 325*(7374), 1202.
11. Engman, M. (1998). Homocysteinemia: New information about an old risk factor for vascular disease. *Journal of Insurance Medicine, 30*(4), 231–236.
12. Sharma, P. (1998). Meta-analysis of the ACE gene in ischaemic stroke. *Journal of Neurology Neurosurgery, and Psychiatry, 64*(2), 227–230.
13. McCarron, M. O., Delong, D., & Alberts, M. J. (1999). APOE genotype as a risk factor for ischemic cerebrovascular disease: A meta-analysis. *Neurology, 53*(6), 1308–1311.
14. Meyer, J. S., Mehdirad, A., Salem, B. I., et al. (2003). Sudden arrhythmia death syndrome: Importance of the long QT syndrome. *American Family Physician, 68*(3), 483–488.
15. Assmann, G., Cullen, P., Jossa, F., et al. (1999). Coronary heart disease: Reducing the risk. The scientific background to primary and secondary prevention of coronary heart disease. A worldwide view. International Task force for the Prevention of Coronary Heart disease. *Arteriosclerosis, Thrombosis, and Vascular Biology, 19*(8), 1819–1824.
16. Gordon, D. J., & Rifkind, B. M. (1989). High-density lipoprotein—The clinical implications of recent studies. *New England Journal of Medicine, 321*(19), 1311–1316.
17. Kronenberg, F., Kronenberg, M. F., Kiechl, S., et al. (1999). Role of lipoprotein(a) and apolipoprotein(a) phenotype in atherogenesis: Prospective results from the Bruneck study. *Circulation, 100*(11), 1154–1160.
18. Glassman, A. H., & Shapiro, P. A. (1998). Depression and the course of coronary artery disease. *American Journal of Psychiatry, 155*(1), 4–11.
19. Gerhard, G. T., & Duell, P. B. (1999). Homocysteine and atherosclerosis. *Current Opinion in Lipidology, 10*(5), 417–428.

20. Fruchart, J. C., & Duriez, P. (2002). HDL and triglyceride as therapeutic targets. *Current Opinion in Lipidology, 13*(6), 605–616.
21. Goldbourt, U., & Neufeld, H. N. (1986). Genetic aspects of arteriosclerosis. *Arteriosclerosis, 6*(4), 357–377.
22. Shepard, D. R., Jneid, H., & Thacker, H. L. (2003). Gender, hyperlipidemia, and coronary artery disease. *Comprehensive Therapy, 29*(1), 7–17.
23. Kugiyama, K., Ota, Y., Takazoe, K., et al. Circulating levels of secretory type II phospholipase A(2) predict coronary events in patients with coronary artery disease. *Circulation, 100*(12), 1280–1284.
24. Lusis, A. J., Weinreb, A., & Drake, T. (1998). *Textbook of cardiovascular medicine*. Philadelphia: Lippincott-Raven.
25. Steinberg, D., & Witztum, J. (1999). *Molecular basis of cardiovascular disease*. Philadelphia: Saunders.
26. Hu, H., Pierce, G. N., & Zhong, G. (1993). The atherogenic effects of chlamydia are dependent on serum cholesterol and specific to *Chlamydia pneumoniae. Journal of Clinical Investigations, 103*(5), 747–753.
27. Lusis, A. J. (2000). Atherosclerosis. *Nature, 407*(6801), 233–241.
28. Lefkowitz, R. J., & Willerson, J. T. (2001). Prospects for cardiovascular research. *JAMA, 285*(5), 581–587.
29. Rauch, U., Osende, J. I., Fuster, V., et al. (2001). Thrombus formation on atherosclerotic plaques: Pathogenesis and clinical consequences. *Annals of Internal Medicine, 134*(3), 224–238.
30. Weissberg, P. L. (2000). Atherogenesis: Current understanding of the causes of atheroma. *Heart, 83*(2), 247–252.
31. Scheuner, M. T. (2001). Genetic predisposition to coronary artery disease. *Current Opinion in Cardiology, 16*(4), 251–260.
32. Orso, E., Broccardo, C., Kaminski, W. E., et al. (2000). Transport of lipids from golgi to plasma membrane is defective in tangier disease patients and Abc1-deficient mice. *Natural Genetics, 24*(2), 192–196.
33. Young, S. G., & Fielding, C. J. (1999). The ABCs of cholesterol efflux. *Natural Genetics, 22*(4), 316–318.
34. Luft, F. C. (1998). Molecular genetics of human hypertension. *Journal of Hypertension, 16*(12, Pt. 2), 1871–1878.
35. Geller, D. S., Farhi, A., Pinkerton, N., et al. (2000). Activating mineralocorticoid receptor mutation in hypertension exacerbated by pregnancy. *Science, 289*(5476), 119–123.
36. Cohen, J. C., Wang, Z., Grundy, S. M., et al. (1994). Variation at the hepatic lipase and apolipoprotein AI/CIII/AIV loci is a major cause of genetically determined variation in plasma HDL cholesterol levels. *Journal of Clinical Investigations, 94*(6), 2377–2384.
37. Wittrup, H. H., Tybjaerg-Hansen, A., & Nordestgaard, B. G. (1999). Lipoprotein lipase mutations, plasma lipids and lipoproteins, and risk of ischemic heart disease. A meta-analysis. *Circulation, 99*(22), 2901–2907.
38. Samani, N. J., Thompson, J. R., O'Toole, L., et al. (1996). A meta-analysis of the association of the deletion allele of the angiotensin-converting enzyme gene with myocardial infarction. *Circulation, 94*(4), 708–712.
39. Hegele, R. A. (1999). Paraoxonase genes and disease. *Annals of Medicine, 31*(3), 217–224.
40. Shih, P. T., Brennan, M. L., Vora, D. K., et al. (1999). Blocking very late antigen-4 integrin decreases leukocyte entry and fatty streak formation in mice fed an atherogenic diet. *Circulation Research, 84*(3), 345–351.
41. Tuomainen, T. P., Kontula, K., Nyyssonen, K., et al. Increased risk of acute myocardial infarction in carriers of the hemochromatosis gene Cys282Tyr mutation: A prospective cohort study in men in eastern Finland. *Circulation, 100*(12), 1274–1279.
42. Hingorani, A. D., Liang, C. F., Fatibene, J., et al. (1999). A common variant of the endothelial nitric oxide synthase (Glu298→Asp) is a major risk factor for coronary artery disease in the UK. *Circulation, 100*(14), 1515–1520.
43. Franco, R. F., Pazin-Filho, A., Tavella, M. H., et al. (2000). Factor XIII val34leu and the risk of myocardial infarction. *Haematologica, 85*(1), 67–71.
44. Lloyd-Jones, D. M., Larson, M. G., Beiser, A., et al. (1999). Lifetime risk of developing coronary heart disease. *Lancet, 353*(9147), 89–92.
45. Cargill, M., Altshuler, D., Ireland, J., et al. (1999). Characterization of single-nucleotide polymorphisms in coding regions of human genes. *Natural Genetics, 22*(3), 231–238.
46. Krushkal, J., Xiong, M., Ferrell, R., et al. (1998). Linkage and association of adrenergic and dopamine receptor genes in the distal portion of the long arm of chromosome 5 with systolic blood pressure variation. *Human Molecular Genetics, 7*(9), 1379–1383.
47. Risch, N. J. (2000). Searching for genetic determinants in the new millennium. *Nature, 405*(6788), 847–856.
48. Zhang, H., Liu, L., Wang, X., et al. (2007). Guideline for data analysis of genomewide association studies. *Cancer Genomics Proteomics, 4*(1), 27–34.
49. Day, I. N., Whittall, R. A., O'Dell, S. D., et al. (1997). Spectrum of LDL receptor gene mutations in heterozygous familial hypercholesterolemia. *Human Mutation, 10*(2), 116–127.
50. Hobbs, H. H., Brown, M. S., & Goldstein, J. L. (1992). Molecular genetics of the LDL receptor gene in familial hypercholesterolemia. *Human Mutation, 1*(6), 445–466.
51. Tybjaerg-Hansen, A., Steffensen, R., Meinertz, H., et al. (1998). Association of mutations in the apolipoprotein B gene with hypercholesterolemia and the risk of ischemic heart disease. *New England Journal of Medicine, 338*(22), 1577–1584.
52. Haines, J., & Pericak-Vance, M. (2006). *Genetic analysis of complex diseases*. Hoboken, NJ: Wiley-Liss.
53. Allen, G., Harvald, B., & Shields, J. (1967). Measures of twin concordance. *Acta Genetica et Statistica Medica, 17*(6), 475–481.
54. Berg, K. (1984). Twin studies of coronary heart disease and its risk factors. *Acta Geneticae Medicae et Gemellologiae (Roma), 33*(3), 349–361.
55. Cederlof, R., Friberg, L., & Jonsson, E. (1967). Hereditary factors and "angina pectoris." A study on 5,877 twin-pairs with the aid of mailed questionnaires. *Archives of Environmental Health, 14*(3), 397–400.
56. de Faire, U., Friberg, L., & Lundman, T. (1975). Concordance for mortality with special reference to ischaemic heart disease and cerebrovascular disease. A study on the Swedish Twin Registry. *Preventive Medicine, 4*(4), 509–517.
57. Marenberg, M. E., Risch, N., Berkman, L. F., et al. (1994). Genetic susceptibility to death from coronary heart disease in a study of twins. *New England Journal of Medicine, 330*(15), 1041–1046.
58. Mosteller, M. (1993). A genetic analysis of cardiovascular disease risk factor clustering in adult female twins. *Genetics and Epidemiology, 10*(6), 569–574.
59. Reed, T., Quiroga, J., Selby, J. V., et al. (1991). Concordance of ischemic heart disease in the NHLBI twin study after 14–18 years of follow-up. *Journal of Clinical Epidemiology, 44*(8), 797–805.
60. Nora, J. J., Lortscher, R. H., Spangler, R. D., et al. (1980). Genetic–epidemiologic study of early-onset ischemic heart disease. *Circulation, 61*(3), 503–508.
61. Rissanen, A. M. (1979). Familial occurrence of coronary heart disease: Effect of age at diagnosis. *American Journal of Cardiology, 44*(1), 60–66.
62. Rose, G. (1964). Familial patterns in ischaemic heart disease. *British Journal of Preventive and Social Medicine, 18*, 75–80.
63. Slack, J., & Evans, K. A. (1966). The increased risk of death from ischaemic heart disease in first degree relatives of 121 men and 96 women with ischaemic heart disease. *Journal of Medical Genetics, 3*(4), 239–257.
64. Thomas, C. B., & Cohen, B. H. (1955). The familial occurrence of hypertension and coronary artery disease, with observations concerning obesity and diabetes. *Annals of Internal Medicine, 42*(1), 90–127.
65. Barrett-Connor, E., & Khaw, K. (1984). Family history of heart attack as an independent predictor of death due to cardiovascular disease. *Circulation, 69*(6), 1065–1069.
66. Colditz, G. A., Rimm, E. B., Giovannucci, E., et al. (1991). A prospective study of parental history of myocardial infarction and coronary artery disease in men. *American Journal of Cardiology, 67*(11), 933–938.
67. Colditz, G. A., Stampfer, M. J., Willett, W. C., et al. (1986). A prospective study of parental history of myocardial infarction and coronary heart disease in women. *American Journal of Epidemiology, 123*(1), 48–58.
68. Hopkins, P. N., Williams, R. R., Kuida, H., et al. (1988). Family history as an independent risk factor for incident coronary artery disease in a high-risk cohort in Utah. *American Journal of Cardiology, 62*(10, Pt. 1), 703–707.
69. Phillips, A. N., Shaper, A. G., Pocock, S. J., et al. (1988). Parental death from heart disease and the risk of heart attack. *European Heart Journal, 9*(3), 243–251.
70. Schildkraut, J. M., Myers, R. H., Cupples, L. A., et al. (1989). Coronary risk associated with age and sex of parental heart disease in the Framingham Study. *American Journal of Cardiology, 64*(10), 555–559.
71. Sholtz, R. I., Rosenman, R. H., & Brand, R. J. (1975). The relationship of reported parental history to the incidence of coronary heart disease in the Western Collaborative Group Study. *American Journal of Epidemiology, 102*(4), 350–356.
72. Adlersberg, D., Parets, A. D., & Boas, E. P. (1949). Genetics of atherosclerosis: Studies of families with xanthoma and unselected patients with coronary artery disease under the age of 50 years. *JAMA, 141*(4), 246–254.
73. Becker, D. M., Becker, L. C., Pearson, T. A., et al. (1988). Risk factors in siblings of people with premature coronary heart disease. *Journal of the American College of Cardiology, 12*(5), 1273–1280.

74. Berg, K., Dahlen, G., & Borresen, A. L. (1979). Lp(a) phenotypes, other lipoprotein parameters, and a family history of coronary heart disease in middle-aged males. *Clinical Genetics, 16*(5), 347–352.
75. Blumenthal, S., Jesse, M. J., Hennekens, C. H., et al. (1975). Risk factors for coronary artery disease in children of affected families. *Journal of Pediatrics, 87*(6, Pt. 2), 1187–1192.
76. Hamby, R. I. (1981). Hereditary aspects of coronary artery disease. *American Heart Journal, 101*(5), 639–649.
77. Rissanen, A. M., & Nikkila, E. A. (1977). Coronary artery disease and its risk factors in families of young men with angina pectoris and in controls. *British Heart Journal, 39*(8), 875–883.
78. Rosengren, A., Wilhelmsen, L., Eriksson, E., et al. (1990). Lipoprotein (a) and coronary heart disease: A prospective case-control study in a general population sample of middle aged men. *BMJ, 301*(6763), 1248–1251.
79. Anderson, A. J., Loeffler, R. F., Barboriak, J. J., et al. (1979). Occlusive coronary artery disease and parental history of myocardial infarction. *Preventive Medicine, 8*(3), 419–428.
80. Sharp, S. D., Williams, R. R., Hunt, S. C., et al. (1992). Coronary risk factors and the severity of angiographic coronary artery disease in members of high-risk pedigrees. *American Heart Journal, 123*(2), 279–285.
81. Smithies, O., & Maeda, N. (1995). Gene targeting approaches to complex genetic diseases: Atherosclerosis and essential hypertension. *Proceedings of the National Academy of Science USA, 92*(12), 5266–5272.
82. Tamminen, M., Mottino, G., Qiao, J. H., et al. (1999). Ultrastructure of early lipid accumulation in ApoE-deficient mice. *Arteriosclerosis, Thrombosis, and Vascular Biology, 19*(4), 847–853.
83. Mehrabian, M., & Lusis, A. J. (1992). *Molecular genetics of coronary artery disease. Candidate genes and processes in atherosclerosis.* New York: Karger.
84. Heeneman, S., Lutgens, E., Schapira, K. B., et al. (2008). Control of atherosclerotic plaque vulnerability: Insights from transgenic mice. *Frontiers in Bioscience, 13,* 6289–6313.
85. Stoll, M., Kwitek-Black, A. E., Cowley, A. W., Jr., et al. (2000) New target regions for human hypertension via comparative genomics. *Genome Research, 10*(4), 473–482.
86. Villa-Colinayo, V., Shi, W., Araujo, J., et al. (2000). Genetics of atherosclerosis: The search for genes acting at the level of the vessel wall. *Current Atherosclerosis Reports, 2*(5), 380–389.
87. Altshuler, D., Hirschhorn, J. N., Klannemark, M., et al. (2000). The common PPARgamma Pro12Ala polymorphism is associated with decreased risk of type 2 diabetes. *Natural Genetics, 26*(1), 76–80.
88. Hart, L. M., Stolk, R. P., Dekker, J. M., et al. (1999). Prevalence of variants in candidate genes for type 2 diabetes mellitus in The Netherlands: The Rotterdam study and the Hoorn study. *The Journal of Clinical Endocrinology and Metabolism, 84*(3), 1002–1006.
89. Horikawa, Y., Oda, N., Cox, N. J., et al. (2000). Genetic variation in the gene encoding calpain-10 is associated with type 2 diabetes mellitus. *Natural Genetics, 26*(2), 163–175.
90. Reis, A. F., Ye, W. Z., Dubois-Laforgue, D., et al. (2000). Association of a variant in exon 31 of the sulfonylurea receptor 1 (SUR1) gene with type 2 diabetes mellitus in French Caucasians. *Human Genetics, 107*(2), 138–144.
91. Stone, L. M., Kahn, S. E., Fujimoto, W. Y., et al. (1996). A variation at position -30 of the beta-cell glucokinase gene promoter is associated with reduced beta-cell function in middle-aged Japanese-American men. *Diabetes, 45*(4), 422–428.
92. Vinik, A., & Bell, G. (1988). Mutant insulin syndromes. *Hormone and Metabolic Research, 20*(1), 1–10.
93. Frossard, P. M., Lestringant, G. G., Malloy, M. J., et al. (1999). Human renin gene BglI dimorphism associated with hypertension in two independent populations. *Clinical Genetics, 56*(6), 428–433.
94. Williams, R. R., Hunt, S. C., Hopkins, P. N., et al. (1994). Evidence for single gene contributions to hypertension and lipid disturbances: Definition, genetics, and clinical significance. *Clinical Genetics, 46*(1, Special No.), 80–87.
95. Heinonen, P., Koulu, M., Pesonen, U., et al. (1999). Identification of a three-amino acid deletion in the alpha2B-adrenergic receptor that is associated with reduced basal metabolic rate in obese subjects. *The Journal of Clinical Endocrinology Metabolism, 84*(7), 2429–2433.
96. Large, V., Hellstrom, L., Reynisdottir, S., et al. (1997). Human beta-2 adrenoceptor gene polymorphisms are highly frequent in obesity and associate with altered adipocyte beta-2 adrenoceptor function. *Journal of Clinical Investigations, 100*(12), 3005–3013.
97. Mitchell, B. D., Blangero, J., Comuzzie, A. G., et al. (1998). A paired sibling analysis of the beta-3 adrenergic receptor and obesity in Mexican Americans. *Journal of Clinical Investigations, 101*(3), 584–587.
98. Nagase, T., Aoki, A., Yamamoto, M., et al. (1997). Lack of association between the Trp64 Arg mutation in the beta 3-adrenergic receptor gene and obesity in Japanese men: A longitudinal analysis. *The Journal of Clinical Endocrinology Metabolism, 82*(4), 1284–1287.
99. Ristow, M., Muller-Wieland, D., Pfeiffer, A., et al. (1998). Obesity associated with a mutation in a genetic regulator of adipocyte differentiation. *New England Journal of Medicine, 339*(14), 953–959.
100. Sina, M., Hinney, A., Ziegler, A., et al. (1999). Phenotypes in three pedigrees with autosomal dominant obesity caused by haploinsufficiency mutations in the melanocortin-4 receptor gene. *American Journal of Human Genetics, 65*(6), 1501–1507.
101. Walder, K., Norman, R. A., Hanson, R. L., et al. (1998). Association between uncoupling protein polymorphisms (UCP2-UCP3) and energy metabolism/obesity in Pima Indians. *Human Molecular Genetics, 7*(9), 1431–1435.
102. Kraft, H. G., Lingenhel, A., Kochl, S., et al. (1996). Apolipoprotein(a) kringle IV repeat number predicts risk for coronary heart disease. *Arteriosclerosis, Thrombosis, and Vascular Biology, 16*(6), 713–719.
103. Hixson, J. E. (1991). Apolipoprotein E polymorphisms affect atherosclerosis in young males. Pathobiological Determinants of Atherosclerosis in Youth (PDAY) Research Group. *Arteriosclerosis Thrombosis, 11*(5), 1237–1244.
104. Moore, J. H., Reilly, S. L., Ferrell, R. E., et al. (1997). The role of the apolipoprotein E polymorphism in the prediction of coronary artery disease age of onset. *Clinical Genetics, 51*(1), 22–25.
105. Wang, X. L., McCredie, R. M., & Wilcken, D. E. (1995). Polymorphisms of the apolipoprotein E gene and severity of coronary artery disease defined by angiography. *Arteriosclerosis, Thrombosis, and Vascular Biology, 15*(8), 1030–1034.
106. Wilson, P. W., Schaefer, E. J., Larson, M. G., et al. (1996). Apolipoprotein E alleles and risk of coronary disease. A meta-analysis. *Arteriosclerosis, Thrombosis, and Vascular Biology, 16*(10), 1250–1255.
107. Gudnason, V., Thormar, K., & Humphries, S. E. (1997). Interaction of the cholesteryl ester transfer protein I405V polymorphism with alcohol consumption in smoking and non-smoking healthy men, and the effect on plasma HDL cholesterol and apoAI concentration. *Clinical Genetics, 51*(1), 15–21.
108. Kuivenhoven, J. A., Jukema, J. W., Zwinderman, A. H., et al. (1998). The role of a common variant of the cholesteryl ester transfer protein gene in the progression of coronary atherosclerosis. The Regression Growth Evaluation Statin Study Group. *New England Journal of Medicine, 338*(2), 86–93.
109. Jukema, J. W., van Boven, A. J., Groenemeijer B, et al. (1996). The Asp9 Asn mutation in the lipoprotein lipase gene is associated with increased progression of coronary atherosclerosis. REGRESS Study Group, Interuniversity Cardiology Institute, Utrecht, The Netherlands. Regression Growth Evaluation Statin Study. *Circulation, 94*(8), 1913–1918.
110. Sanghera, D. K., Aston, C. E., Saha, N., et al. (1998). DNA polymorphisms in two paraoxonase genes (PON1 and PON2) are associated with the risk of coronary heart disease. *American Journal of Human Genetics, 62*(1), 36–44.
111. Gardemann, A., Stricker, J., Humme, J., et al. (1999). Angiotensinogen T174M and M235T gene polymorphisms are associated with the extent of coronary atherosclerosis. *Atherosclerosis, 145*(2), 309–314.
112. Wang, J., Liu, Z., & Chen, B. (2000). Association between genetic polymorphism of dopamine transporter gene and susceptibility to Parkinson's disease. *Zhonghua Yi Xue Za Zhi, 80*(5), 346–348.
113. Winkelmann, B. R., Russ, A. P., Nauck, M., et al. (1999). Angiotensinogen M235T polymorphism is associated with plasma angiotensinogen and cardiovascular disease. *American Heart Journal,* 137(4, Pt. 1), 698–705.
114. Wang, J. G., & Staessen, J. A. (2000). Genetic polymorphisms in the renin-angiotensin system: Relevance for susceptibility to cardiovascular disease. *European Journal of Pharmacology, 410*(2/3), 289–302.
115. Tiret, L., Bonnardeaux, A., Poirier, O., et al. (1994). Synergistic effects of angiotensin-converting enzyme and angiotensin-II type 1 receptor gene polymorphisms on risk of myocardial infarction. *Lancet, 344*(8927), 910–913.
116. Cambien, F., Poirier, O., Lecerf, L., et al. (1992). Deletion polymorphism in the gene for angiotensin-converting enzyme is a potent risk factor for myocardial infarction. *Nature, 359*(6396), 641–644.

117. Keavney, B., McKenzie, C., Parish, S., et al. (2000). Large-scale test of hypothesised associations between the angiotensin-converting-enzyme insertion/deletion polymorphism and myocardial infarction in about 5000 cases and 6000 controls. International Studies of Infarct Survival (ISIS) Collaborators. *Lancet, 355*(9202), 434–442.
118. Psaty, B. M., Smith, N. L., Lemaitre, R. N., et al. (2001). Hormone replacement therapy, prothrombotic mutations, and the risk of incident nonfatal myocardial infarction in postmenopausal women. *JAMA, 285*(7), 906–913.
119. Le, W., Yu, J. D., Lu, L., et al. (2000). Association of the R485K polymorphism of the factor V gene with poor response to activated protein C and increased risk of coronary artery disease in the Chinese population. *Clinical Genetics, 57*(4), 296–303.
120. Rosendaal, F. R., Siscovick, D. S., Schwartz, S. M., et al. (1997). Factor V Leiden (resistance to activated protein C) increases the risk of myocardial infarction in young women. *Blood, 89*(8), 2817–2821.
121. Di Castelnuovo, A., D'Orazio, A., Amore, C., et al. (2000). The decanucleotide insertion/deletion polymorphism in the promoter region of the coagulation factor VII gene and the risk of familial myocardial infarction. *Thrombosis Research, 98*(1), 9–17.
122. Feng, D., Tofler, G. H., Larson, M. G., et al. (2000). Factor VII gene polymorphism, factor VII levels, and prevalent cardiovascular disease: The Framingham Heart Study. *Arteriosclerosis, Thrombosis, and Vascular Biology, 20*(2), 593–600.
123. Girelli, D., Russo, C., Ferraresi, P., et al. (2000). Polymorphisms in the factor VII gene and the risk of myocardial infarction in patients with coronary artery disease. *New England Journal of Medicine, 343*(11), 774–780.
124. Green, F., Hamsten, A., Blomback, M., et al. (1993). The role of beta-fibrinogen genotype in determining plasma fibrinogen levels in young survivors of myocardial infarction and healthy controls from Sweden. *Thrombosis and Haemostasis, 70*(6), 915–920.
125. Humphries, S. E., Panahloo, A., Montgomery, H. E., et al. (1997). Gene-environment interaction in the determination of levels of haemostatic variables involved in thrombosis and fibrinolysis. *Thrombosis and Haemostasis, 78*(1), 457–461.
126. Tybjaerg-Hansen, A., Agerholm-Larsen, B., Humphries, S. E., et al. (1997). A common mutation (G-455→A) in the beta-fibrinogen promoter is an independent predictor of plasma fibrinogen, but not of ischemic heart disease. A study of 9,127 individuals based on the Copenhagen City Heart Study. *Journal of Clinical Investigations, 99*(12), 3034–3039.
127. Yu, Q., Safavi, F., Roberts, R., et al. (1996). A variant of beta fibrinogen is a genetic risk factor for coronary artery disease and myocardial infarction. *Journal of Investigative Medicine, 44*(4), 154–159.
128. Pastinen, T., Perola, M., Niini, P., et al. (1998). Array-based multiplex analysis of candidate genes reveals two independent and additive genetic risk factors for myocardial infarction in the Finnish population. *Human Molecular Genetics, 7*(9), 1453–1462.
129. Hooper, W. C., Lally, C., Austin, H., et al. (1999). The relationship between polymorphisms in the endothelial cell nitric oxide synthase gene and the platelet GPIIIa gene with myocardial infarction and venous thromboembolism in African Americans. *Chest, 116*(4), 880–886.
130. Ridker, P. M., Hennekens, C. H., Schmitz, C., et al. (1997). PIA1/A2 polymorphism of platelet glycoprotein IIIa and risks of myocardial infarction, stroke, and venous thrombosis. *Lancet, 349*(9049), 385–388.
131. Weiss, E. J., Bray, P. F., Tayback, M., et al. (1996). A polymorphism of a platelet glycoprotein receptor as an inherited risk factor for coronary thrombosis. *New England Journal of Medicine, 334*(17), 1090–1094.
132. Wenzel, K., Felix, S., Kleber, F. X., et al. (1994). E-selectin polymorphism and atherosclerosis: An association study. *Human Molecular Genetics, 3*(11), 1935–1937.
133. Boers, G. H., Fowler, B., Smals, A. G., et al. (1985). Improved identification of heterozygotes for homocystinuria due to cystathionine synthase deficiency by the combination of methionine loading and enzyme determination in cultured fibroblasts. *Human Genetics, 69*(2), 164–169.
134. Boers, G. H., Smals, A. G., Trijbels, F. J., et al. (1985). Heterozygosity for homocystinuria in premature peripheral and cerebral occlusive arterial disease. *New England Journal of Medicine, 313*(12), 709–715.
135. Franken, D. G., Boers, G. H., Blom, H. J., et al. (1996). Prevalence of familial mild hyperhomocysteinemia. *Atherosclerosis, 125*(1), 71–80.
136. Christensen, B., Frosst, P., Lussier-Cacan, S., et al. (1997). Correlation of a common mutation in the methylenetetrahydrofolate reductase gene with plasma homocysteine in patients with premature coronary artery disease. *Arteriosclerosis, Thrombosis, and Vascular Biology, 17*(3), 569–573.
137. Frosst, P., Blom, H. J., Milos, R., et al. (1995). A candidate genetic risk factor for vascular disease: A common mutation in methylenetetrahydrofolate reductase. *Natural Genetics, 10*(1), 111–113.
138. Kang, S. S., Passen, E. L., Ruggie, N., et al. (1993). Thermolabile defect of methylenetetrahydrofolate reductase in coronary artery disease. *Circulation, 88*(4, Pt. 1), 1463–1469.
139. Aouizerat, B. E., Allayee, H., Cantor, R. M., et al. (1999). A genome scan for familial combined hyperlipidemia reveals evidence of linkage with a locus on chromosome 11. *American Journal of Human Genetics, 65*(2), 397–412.
140. Bray, M. S., Krushkal, J., Li, L., et al. (2000). Positional genomic analysis identifies the beta(2)-adrenergic receptor gene as a susceptibility locus for human hypertension. *Circulation, 101*(25), 2877–2882.
141. Ghosh, S., Watanabe, R. M., Valle, T. T., et al. (2000). The Finland–United States investigation of non-insulin-dependent diabetes mellitus genetics (FUSION) study. I. An autosomal genome scan for genes that predispose to type 2 diabetes. *American Journal of Human Genetics, 67*(5), 1174–1185.
142. Hein, L., Barsh, G. S., Pratt, R. E., et al. (1995). Behavioural and cardiovascular effects of disrupting the angiotensin II type-2 receptor in mice. *Nature, 377*(6551), 744–747.
143. Krushkal, J., Ferrell, R., Mockrin, S. C., et al. (1999). Genome-wide linkage analyses of systolic blood pressure using highly discordant siblings. *Circulation, 99*(11), 1407–1410.
144. Pajukanta, P., Cargill, M., Viitanen, L., et al. (2000). Two loci on chromosomes 2 and X for premature coronary heart disease identified in early- and late-settlement populations of Finland. *American Journal of Human Genetics, 67*(6), 1481–1493.
145. Vionnet, N., Hani, E. H., Dupont, S., et al. (2000). Genomewide search for type 2 diabetes-susceptibility genes in French whites: Evidence for a novel susceptibility locus for early-onset diabetes on chromosome 3q27-qter and independent replication of a type 2-diabetes locus on chromosome 1q21–q24. *American Journal of Human Genetics, 67*(6), 1470–1480.
146. Watanabe, R. M., Ghosh, S., Langefeld, C. D., et al. (2000). The Finland–United States investigation of non-insulin-dependent diabetes mellitus genetics (FUSION) study. II. An autosomal genome scan for diabetes-related quantitative-trait loci. *American Journal of Human Genetics, 67*(5), 1186–1200.
147. Hines, L. M., Stampfer, M. J., Ma, J., et al. (2001). Genetic variation in alcohol dehydrogenase and the beneficial effect of moderate alcohol consumption on myocardial infarction. *New England Journal of Medicine, 344*(8), 549–555.
148. McCombs, R. J., Marcadis, D. E., Ellis, J., et al. (1994). Attenuated hypercholesterolemic response to a high-cholesterol diet in subjects heterozygous for the apolipoprotein A-IV-2 allele. *New England Journal of Medicine, 331*(11), 706–710.
149. Ordovas, J. M. (1999). The genetics of serum lipid responsiveness to dietary interventions. *Proceedings of the Nutrition Society, 58*(1), 171–187.
150. Tall, A., Welch, C., Applebaum-Bowden, D., et al. (1997). Interaction of diet and genes in atherogenesis. Report of an NHLBI working group. *Arteriosclerosis, Thrombosis, and Vascular Biology, 17*(11), 3326–3331.
151. Denke, M. A., Adams-Huet, B., & Nguyen, A. T. (2000). Individual cholesterol variation in response to a margarine- or butter-based diet: A study in families. *JAMA, 284*(21), 2740–2747.
152. Mirvis, D. M., & Chang, C. F. (1997). Managed care, managing uncertainty. *Archives of Internal Medicine, 157*(4), 385–388.
153. Summary of the second report of the National Cholesterol Education Program (NCEP) Expert Panel on Detection, Evaluation, and Treatment of High Blood Cholesterol in Adults (Adult Treatment Panel II). (1993). *JAMA, 269*(23), 3015–3023.
154. Effect of simvastatin on coronary atheroma: The Multicentre Anti-Atheroma Study (MAAS). (1994, September 3) *Lancet, 344*(8923), 633–638.
155. Randomised trial of cholesterol lowering in 4444 patients with coronary heart disease: The Scandinavian Simvastatin Survival Study (4S). (1994). *Lancet, 344*(8934), 1383–1389.
156. Blankenhorn, D. H., Azen, S. P., Kramsch, D. M., et al. (1993). Coronary angiographic changes with lovastatin therapy. The Monitored Atherosclerosis Regression Study (MARS). *Annals of Internal Medicine, 119*(10), 969–976.
157. Blankenhorn, D. H., Nessim, S. A., Johnson, R. L., et al. (1987). Beneficial effects of combined colestipol-niacin therapy on coronary atherosclerosis and coronary venous bypass grafts. *JAMA, 257*(23), 3233–3240.

158. Brown, G., Albers, J. J., Fisher, L. D., et al. (1990). Regression of coronary artery disease as a result of intensive lipid-lowering therapy in men with high levels of apolipoprotein B. *New England Journal of Medicine, 323*(19), 1289–1298.
159. Downs, J. R., Clearfield, M., Weis, S., et al. (1998). Primary prevention of acute coronary events with lovastatin in men and women with average cholesterol levels: Results of AFCAPS/TexCAPS. Air Force/Texas Coronary Atherosclerosis Prevention Study. *JAMA, 279*(20), 1615–1622.
160. Jukema, J. W., Bruschke, A. V., van Boven, A. J., et al. (1995). Effects of lipid lowering by pravastatin on progression and regression of coronary artery disease in symptomatic men with normal to moderately elevated serum cholesterol levels. The Regression Growth Evaluation Statin Study (REGRESS). *Circulation, 91*(10), 2528–2540.
161. Kreisberg, R. A. (1996). Cholesterol-lowering and coronary atherosclerosis: Good news and bad news. *American Journal of Medicine, 101*(5), 455–458.
162. Genest, J. J., Jr., Martin-Munley, S. S., McNamara, J. R., et al. (1992). Familial lipoprotein disorders in patients with premature coronary artery disease. *Circulation, 85*(6), 2025–2033.
163. Szapary, P. O., & Rader, D. J. (2004). The triglyceride-high-density lipoprotein axis: An important target of therapy? *American Heart Journal, 148*(2), 211–221.
164. Brattstrom, L., Israelsson, B., Norrving, B., et al. (1990). Impaired homocysteine metabolism in early-onset cerebral and peripheral occlusive arterial disease. Effects of pyridoxine and folic acid treatment. *Atherosclerosis, 81*(1), 51–60.
165. Brattstrom, L. E., Israelsson, B., Jeppsson, J. O., et al. (1988). Folic acid—An innocuous means to reduce plasma homocysteine. *Scandinavian Journal of Clinical Laboratory Investigations, 48*(3), 215–221.
166. Ubbink, J. B. (1997). The role of vitamins in the pathogenesis and treatment of hyperhomocyst(e)inaemia. *Journal of Inherited Metabolic Disorders, 20*(2), 316–325.
167. Rumberger, J. A., Simons, D. B., Fitzpatrick, L. A., et al. (1995). Coronary artery calcium area by electron-beam computed tomography and coronary atherosclerotic plaque area. A histopathologic correlative study. *Circulation, 92*(8), 2157–2162.
168. Schmermund, A., Baumgart, D., Adamzik, M., et al. (1998). Comparison of electron-beam computed tomography and intracoronary ultrasound in detecting calcified and noncalcified plaques in patients with acute coronary syndromes and no or minimal to moderate angiographic coronary artery disease. *American Journal of Cardiology, 81*(2), 141–146.
169. Arad, Y., Spadaro, L. A., Goodman, K., et al. (1996). Predictive value of electron beam computed tomography of the coronary arteries. 19-month follow-up of 1173 asymptomatic subjects. *Circulation, 93*(11), 1951–1953.
170. Raggi, P., Callister, T. Q., Cooil, B., et al. (2000). Identification of patients at increased risk of first unheralded acute myocardial infarction by electron-beam computed tomography. *Circulation, 101*(8), 850–855.
171. Secci, A., Wong, N., Tang, W., et al. (1997). Electron beam computed tomographic coronary calcium as a predictor of coronary events: Comparison of two protocols. *Circulation, 96*(4), 1122–1129.
172. Detrano, R., Hsiai, T., Wang, S., et al. (1996). Prognostic value of coronary calcification and angiographic stenoses in patients undergoing coronary angiography. *Journal of the American College of Cardiology, 27*(2), 285–290.
173. Iyengar, S. K., & Elston, R. C. (2007). The genetic basis of complex traits: Rare variants or "common gene, common disease"? *Methods in Molecular Biology, 376*, 71–84.
174. Kathiresan, S., Musunuru, K., & Orho-Melander, M. (2008). Defining the spectrum of alleles that contribute to blood lipid concentrations in humans. *Current Opinion in Lipidology, 19*(2), 122–127.
175. Scheuner, M. T., Wang, S. J., Raffel, L. J., et al. (1997). Family history: A comprehensive genetic risk assessment method for the chronic conditions of adulthood. *American Journal of Medical Genetics, 71*(3), 315–324.
176. Reaven, G. M., & Chen, Y. D. (1988). Role of insulin in regulation of lipoprotein metabolism in diabetes. *Diabetes Metabolism Review, 4*(7), 639–652.
177. Bensen, J. T., Liese, A. D., Rushing, J. T., et al. (1999). Accuracy of proband reported family history: The NHLBI Family Heart Study (FHS). *Genetic Epidemiology, 17*(2), 141–150.
178. Kahn, L. B., Marshall, J. A., Baxter, J., et al. (1990). Accuracy of reported family history of diabetes mellitus. Results from San Luis Valley Diabetes Study. *Diabetes Care, 13*(7), 796–798.
179. Kee, F., Tiret, L., Robo, J. Y., et al. (1993). Reliability of reported family history of myocardial infarction. *BMJ, 307*(6918), 1528–1530.
180. Fraser, F. C. (1974). Genetic counseling. *American Journal of Human Genetics, 26*(5), 636–661.
181. Statement on use of DNA testing for presymptomatic identification of cancer risk. National Advisory Council for Human Genome Research (1994). *JAMA, 271*(10), 785.
182. The American Society of Human Genetics. (1996). Statement on informed consent for genetic research. ASHG report. *American Journal of Human Genetics, 59*(2), 471–474.
183. Geller, G., Botkin, J. R., Green, M. J., et al. (1997). Genetic testing for susceptibility to adult-onset cancer. The process and content of informed consent. *JAMA, 277*(18), 1467–1474.
184. McKinnon, W. C., Baty, B. J., Bennett, R. L., et al. (1997). Predisposition genetic testing for late-onset disorders in adults. A position paper of the National Society of Genetic Counselors. *JAMA, 278*(15), 1217–1220.
185. Tamragouri, R. N., Martin, R. W., Cleavenger, R. L., et al. (1986). Cardiovascular risk factors and health knowledge among freshman college students with a family history of cardiovascular disease. *Journal of the American College of Health, 34*(6), 267–270.
186. Croyle, R. T., Smith, K. R., Botkin, J. R., et al. (1997). Psychological responses to BRCA1 mutation testing: Preliminary findings. *Health Psychology, 16*(1), 63–72.
187. Hudson, K. L., Rothenberg, K. H., Andrews, L. B., et al. (1995). Genetic discrimination and health insurance: An urgent need for reform. *Science, 270*(5235), 391–393.
188. Lerman, C., Narod, S., Schulman, K., et al. (1996). BRCA1 testing in families with hereditary breast-ovarian cancer. A prospective study of patient decision making and outcomes. *JAMA, 275*(24), 1885–1892.
189. Rothenberg, K., Fuller, B., Rothstein, M., et al. (1997). Genetic information and the workplace: Legislative approaches and policy changes. *Science, 275*(5307), 1755–1757.
190. Billings, P. R., Kohn, M. A., de Cuevas, M., et al. (1992). Discrimination as a consequence of genetic testing. *American Journal of Human Genetics, 50*(3), 476–482.
191. Geller, L. N., Alper, J. S., Billings, P. R., et al. (1996). Individual, family, and societal dimensions of genetic discrimination: A case study analysis. *Science and Engineering Ethics, 2*(1), 71–88.
192. Reilly, P. R. (1998). Genetic risk assessment and insurance. *Genetic Testing, 2*(1), 1–2.

WEB RESOURCES

International Societies of Nurses in Genetics:
www.globalreferrals.com/isong.html
National Center for Biotechnology Information:
www.ncbi.nlm.nih.gov
Department of Energy/Human Genome Project Information:
www.ornl.gov/TechResources/Human_Genome/publicat/primer/index.html
The International Atherosclerosis Society:
www.athero.org/
The American Heart Association:
www.americanheart.org

CHAPTER 5

Atherosclerosis, Inflammation, and Acute Coronary Syndrome

Bradley E. Aouizerat / Polly E. Gardner / Gaylene Altman

Acute coronary syndrome encompasses the clinical entities of myocardial ischemia and myocardial infarction. The diagnosis of acute coronary syndrome is based on history, risk factors, diagnostic laboratory tests, functional studies, and, to a lesser extent, the electrocardiogram (ECG). This chapter focuses primarily on the incidence, mechanisms, causes, and pathophysiology, including the cellular and metabolic changes of myocardial ischemia and infarction. Hemodynamic mechanisms affecting the balance of oxygen supply and demand are addressed. The role of inflammation in myocardial ischemia and myocardial infarction is also addressed. Clinical manifestations are briefly discussed and are fully detailed in Chapter 22.

INTRODUCTION

Many factors affect the pathophysiologic events that lead to ischemia, infarction, and injury of myocardial muscle. Injury to the myocardium can range from reversible to permanent damage of cellular components in localized tissue. Ischemia occurs from a transient imbalance of blood supply to an area of tissue, with the chief result being tissue hypoxia. Ischemia can be a sudden event or a gradual occurrence from a partial or totally occluded coronary vessel or vessels. The burden of the ischemic event depends on the sensitivity of the tissue to hypoxia, the degree and duration of ischemia, and the ability of the tissue to regenerate when conditions improve.[1,2]

Myocardial ischemia is a condition that results from diminished oxygen supply coupled with inadequate removal of metabolites because of reduced perfusion to the heart muscle.[3,4] Pure anoxia or hypoxia, without metabolic clearance, can occur in patients with congenital heart disease, severe anemia, asphyxiation, carbon monoxide poisoning, or cor pulmonale.[5] Myocardial ischemia can occur as a result of reduced oxygen and nutrient *supply* or increased metabolic *demand* to meet tissue demands[6] (Fig. 5-1). In the presence of coronary artery occlusion, an increase in oxygen demand requirements from exercise or emotional stress can cause a transitory imbalance known as *demand ischemia.* Angina pectoris is a condition characterized by chest pain or discomfort, which results from myocardial ischemia. Patients with chronic stable angina experience this *demand ischemia* when they exert themselves yet obtain relief with rest. An abrupt or acute reduction in blood flow to myocardium is termed *supply ischemia.* This abrupt imbalance is caused by an increase in coronary vascular tone, such as coronary vasospasm, or by a marked reduction or cessation of blood flow caused by thrombi or platelet aggregation. *Supply ischemia* is seen in patients with unstable angina or myocardial infarction.[7] Unstable angina is not relieved with rest. Crescendo angina, a worsening chest pain that may lead to myocardial infarction or preinfarct angina, can develop in some patients with unstable angina.[3,8,9]

The coronary arteries supply blood flow to meet the specific demands of the myocardium under varying workloads such as stress, sleep, or exercise. If oxygen needs are not met, then normal coronary arteries dilate to increase delivery of oxygenated blood to the myocardium.[5] Various pathologic states can affect the endothelium of the epicardial arteries impairing and impacting the normal vasomotor response of vasodilatation when myocardial demand increases. Atherosclerotic plaques (discussed later in this chapter) are the primary cause of endothelial injury and dysfunction, interfering with normal vasomotor response causing a paradoxical response of vasoconstriction.[10–15]

The heart is an aerobic organ that relies on oxidation of substrates for maximal efficiency. The myocardium has a small margin of oxygen debt to maintain normal function. Myocardial oxygen consumption ($M\dot{V}O_2$) is a measure of the heart's total metabolism and is used to determine myocardial oxygen consumption.[16] Factors that determine myocardial oxygen consumption are heart rate, contractility, systolic wall tension, and metabolic and vasomotor regulations of coronary blood flow.[4,16]

Heart rate has a linear relationship with myocardial oxygen consumption. The faster the heart rate, the greater the myocardial oxygen consumption. Myocardial contractility is influenced by different stimuli. Positive inotropes such as epinephrine or dobutamine augment the contractile forces of the myocardium, increasing myocardial oxygen consumption. Researchers believe the increase in $M\dot{V}O_2$ may result from enhanced excitation–contraction coupling or more rapid uptake of calcium by the sarcoplasmic reticulum.[5,16]

Evans and Matsuoka, who concluded that a relationship exists between myocardial tension during systole and metabolism of contractile tissue, described myocardial systolic wall tension in 1915 (as cited in Braunwald, 2000).[16] For every heart beat there is a generated ventricular tension or pressure, as measured in the area under the left ventricular curve. See Chapter 1 for discussion of the Starling mechanism. Increases in myocardial tension or pressure increase myocardial oxygen consumption.

Low blood pressure causing decreased blood return can lead to imbalances of oxygen supply and demand. Examples are hypotension or hypovolemia. Increased oxygen demand is caused by conditions such as hyperthyroidism, anemia, or hyperviscosity of the blood.

MECHANISMS THAT REGULATE CORONARY BLOOD FLOW

Mechanisms that determine coronary blood flow can be divided into mechanical factors and metabolic mediators. *Mechanical*

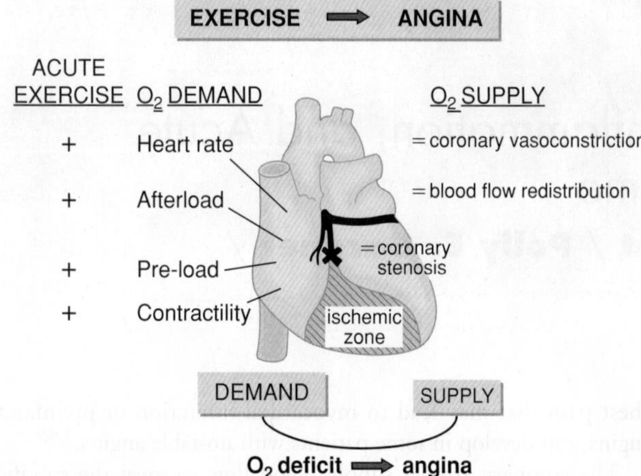

Figure 5-1 Myocardial oxygen balance. The major determinants in the normal heart are heart rate, afterload, preload and contractility. When the myocardial oxygen demand increases and blood flow is not concomitantly increased or even reduced, as in exercising patients with coronary stenosis, the result is the chest pain called angina pectoris. Clinically, the heart rate increase during exercise is one of the major determinants of myocardial oxygen uptake. (From Opie, L. H. [2004]. *Heart physiology: From cell to circulation* [4th ed., p. 526]. New York: Lippincott Williams & Wilkins.)

factors affect blood flow by a driving force or resistance to pressure. Blood flow is directly related to the driving pressure and inversely related to the arteriolar resistance. Driving pressure, the mean arterial pressure less the central venous pressure, is influenced by volume, contractility, heart rate, and, hence, cardiac output. Any clinical state that reduces cardiac output to below the tissue's ability to compensate leads to ischemia. Examples are hypovolemia (reduction in the total vascular volume), decreased pumping efficiency of the heart, or increased vascular space secondary to systemic vasodilatation. Pumping action of the heart is decreased in the presence of ventricular arrhythmias, heart failure, and direct trauma to the myocardium. In addition, the circular events of ischemia to the myocardium, decreased perfusion, and decreased contractility lead to decreased output. Vascular resistance is the result of obstruction of vessels, shunting of blood flow, or increased vascular resistance. Local trauma, vasoconstriction, calcific changes, or thrombus can enhance resistance. Obstruction can result from vasospastic stimuli, such as thermal changes, tissue edema, or injury leading to compression of vessels. Shunting of blood flow is the result of vasoactive substances that cause shunting, congenital malformations, or trauma to vessels. Arteriolar resistance is dependence on the effects of systemic mediators, which are locally released in response to the tissue energy, and oxygen needs.

Metabolic and vasoactive mediators influence the regulation of coronary blood flow. These metabolic mediators include adenosine, serotonin, acetylcholine, carbon dioxide, bradykinin, histamine, substance P, and prostaglandins.[5,13,17] Stimulation of the metabolic mediators induces arterial vasodilatation, thereby increasing coronary blood flow and subsequent increase in myocardial oxygen consumption.[5,17,18] An imbalance of oxygen supply and demand of less than 1 second leads to changes in coronary vascular resistance or tone. When a coronary vessel is occluded and then released, coronary blood flow increases, causing a response called coronary reactive hyperemia.[19] Metabolic mediators are released to relax vasomotor tone and improve blood flow to re-establish homeostasis. The vascular endothelium located between the vascular lumen and smooth muscle cells also releases vasoactive substances that ultimately regulate vascular tone. These substances are known as prostacyclin, nitric oxide, endothelial-derived relaxing factor, and hyperpolarizing factor are potent vasodilators.[6,13,20–23] In addition, endothelin-1, a potent vasoconstrictor, causes a reduction of Na^+-/K^+-ATPase activity. ATPases are impaired by anoxia and produce superoxides and free radicals. Thus, decreased oxygen leads to a production of superoxides and hydrogen peroxide, which are highly diffusible and induce cell damage. Early or chronic atherosclerosis and factors such as dyslipidemia, hypertension, diabetes mellitus, cigarette smoking, menopause, hyperhomocystinemia, and mutations in nitric oxide synthetase, may inhibit mediator effects and impair arterial endothelial function, causing increased permeability of blood lipids and monocytes.[6,17,21,22,24] Further discussion of atherosclerosis is mentioned below.

CAUSES OF MYOCARDIAL ISCHEMIA AND INFARCTION

The leading cause of myocardial ischemia is atherosclerotic plaque or atheroma disease.[7,15,22,25,26] Atherosclerosis is a disease of the large and medium arteries, especially the aorta and arteries supplying the heart, brain, kidneys, and lower extremities.[22] The intima or innermost arterial layer is thickened by the development of fibrous tissue and the accumulation of lipid-forming atheromatous plaques.[27] These plaques or atheromas continue to develop and grow over the years, resulting in a narrowed arterial lumen. Blood flow through the coronary arteries is lessened, and some patients may begin to experience angina.

Atherosclerosis is a thickening or hardening of arteries. It is a progressive disease that evolves from deposits of lipids, cellular debris, calcium, and fibrin (a clotting agent) that accumulate in the lining of large arteries, all of which initiates and is compounded by a progressive inflammatory component. The later stages of these lesions are termed plaques. While atherosclerosis is primarily a disease of the large arteries, medium-size vessels can also be affected, with significant interindividual variation in the sites and rate of plaque formation. Plaques can enlarge to partially or completely impede blood flow through an artery. Some plaques may hemorrhage within the plaque or rupture, initiating thrombus formation at the site with possible embolic consequences. Occlusion of arterial blood flow can lead to angina, myocardial infarction, or stroke.

Deposition of lipids, platelets, cellular debris, and calcium stimulate cells in the locale of the damaged artery wall to produce still other substances that contribute further to the atherosclerotic process. This results in recruitment of immune cells into the lesion as well as proliferation of arterial smooth muscle cells in an attempt to "heal" the lesion. As a result, the innermost layer of the artery, the intima, thickens, enlarges, and eventually encroaches on the vessel lumen, progressively restricting the flow of blood (and thus oxygen) to the vascular bed. Critical reductions in the supply of oxygen to the heart can result in angina or myocardial infarction or ischemic stroke in the brain, often exacerbated by arterial thrombus formation.

Atherosclerosis is a slow progressive disease that may start in childhood. In some persons, this condition may progress rapidly to cause symptoms in their third decade, whereas in others it does not become clinically significant until the fifth or sixth decades. In industrialized nations, it accounts for more than 50% of all cause adult mortality. However, the underlying complexity of the disease has made precise delineation of the cellular and molecular mechanisms involved difficult. Over the past decade, new investigative tools have contributed to a clearer picture of the molecular mechanisms underlying the development of atherosclerotic plaque. It is clear that atherosclerosis is not simply an inevitable consequence of ageing.

American Heart Association Lesion Classification System

More than a decade ago, the American Heart Association (AHA) endeavored to provide an organized system for the categorization of lesions based on histological and morphological data.[28] This system has helped standardize research in atherosclerosis, though modifications have been proposed.[29]

Coronary artery lesions can be grouped into seven major types (I to VII).[28,30–33] Consistent morphologic data would seem to indicate that each lesion type is relatively stable and will not progress to the next lesion type without additional factors or pressures. While the advanced lesions (types IV to VII) can manifest clinically, the early lesions (types I to III) are clinically silent and can be organized temporally. Types I and II are generally found in children, whereas type III tends to occur later and bridges early and advanced lesions. Perhaps the most important observation is that the clinically silent lesions (types I to III) have been shown capable of regression in animal models. Advanced lesions are generally disorganized and lead to thickening and eventual compromise of the vessel wall. Lipid-laden macrophages (termed "foam cells") are the predominant cellular components of type I lesions. In types II and III lesions, intimal smooth muscle cells dominate, with minimal involvement of lymphocytes, plasma cells, and mast cells in the pathological processes. This group of inflammatory cells becomes quite active in advanced (types IV and V) lesions. Figures 5-2 and 5-3 summarize the essential characteristics and temporal occurrence of atherosclerotic lesions.

Type I Lesions

Type I lesions, often termed the "initial lesion," are the earliest detectable lesion type. The lesion can only be observed microscopically and histochemically (by staining for lipid deposits) in the intima. Type I lesions are most often observed in infants and children,[34] although they are readily identifiable in adults with little atherosclerosis or in areas of the vasculature not prone to arteriosclerosis. These lesions occur in regions of the intima that display adaptive intimal thickening caused by the hemodynamic force of blood flow. These regions eventually evolve into types II and III lesions. Although more common in early adulthood, the occurrence of type III lesions has been reported as early as the first year of life.[34,35] The accumulation of intimal foam cells is a consequence and a marker of pathological accumulation of atherogenic lipoproteins.

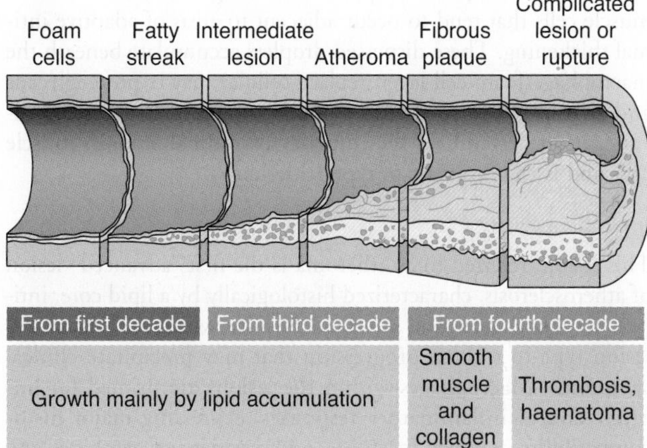

■ **Figure 5-2** Progression of atheromatous plaque from initial lesion to complex and ruptured plaque. (Modified from Grech, E. D. [2003]. ABC of interventional cardiology: Pathophysiology and investigation of coronary artery disease. *BMJ, 326*[7397], 1027–1030.)

Type II Lesions

Type II lesions, also known as fatty streaks that are visible on gross inspection, are yellow spots or streaks on arterial intima. The transmigration of macrophages into the subendothelial space and their subsequent transformation into foam cells produces an adaptive intimal thickening, which may obscure the fatty streak, potentially leading to an underestimate of the extent of these lesions. Recruitment of macrophages to the intima marks one of the defining events in the initiation of the atherosclerotic lesion. Specific adhesion molecules expressed on the surface of vascular endothelial cells mediate leucocyte adhesion. In addition, modified lipoproteins contain oxidized phospholipids that induce the expression of adhesion molecules and cytokines implicated in early atherogenesis.[22]

Progression of atheroma involves accumulation of smooth muscle cells that elaborate extracellular matrix macromolecules. Microscopic examination of type II lesions reveals that the foam cells are more organized, stratifying into layers, and that smooth muscle cells also begin to show signs of intracellular lipid accumulation. The properties of these lesions results in continued recruitment of macrophage and evidence suggests that T-lymphocytes and mast cells (components of the immune system) begin to invade the lesion.[30,36,37] At this stage, the preponderance of the lipid in type II lesions resides in cells, with the majority found in foam cells. A limited amount of extracellular lipid (droplets) can also be detected.

Consistent colocalization of type II lesions to specific portions of the arterial tree is characteristic.[38] Additionally, subgroups of type II lesions can be described dependent on their location and the lipoprotein profile of the individual. Type IIa lesions represent the subset of lesions that may potentially progress to type III lesions over time or with increases in atherogenic (triglyceride- and cholesterol-enriched) lipoproteins. This smaller subgroup of type II lesions occurs in predictable locations in the arterial tree (proximal to bifurcations), where adaptive intimal thickenings occur, and are also termed progression-prone or advanced lesion-prone. Type IIb (progression-resistant or advanced lesion-resistant) lesions consist of the larger subset of type II lesions that are less likely to progress and are located in regions with relatively normal intima with little subendothelial smooth muscle cell invasion or proliferation. Type IIb lesions *do* have the potential to progress, particularly in persons with high plasma levels of atherogenic lipoproteins. Type IIb lesions are further distinguished from IIa by the presence of smooth muscle cells that produce intercellular matrix in the region of adaptive thickening. In type IIb lesions, macrophages without lipid are found mostly near the endothelial surface, foam cells are found deeper within the intima, and the extracellular lipid accumulates even deeper within the adaptive thickening.

The fate of a type II lesion, to become progression-prone or progression-resistant, is dependent not only on the relative atherogenicity of one's plasma lipoprotein profile but also on the direct

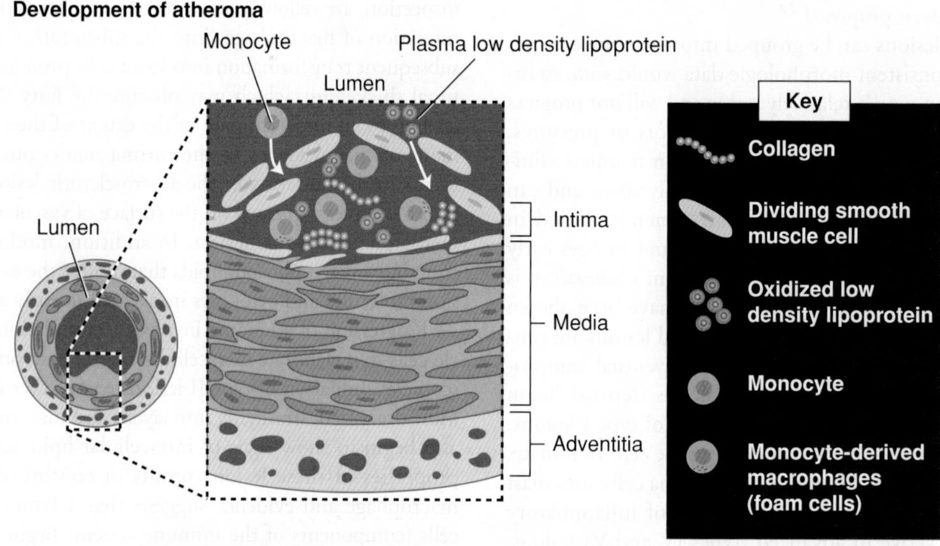

■ **Figure 5-3** Schematic representation of normal coronary artery wall (*top*) and development of atheroma (*bottom*). (Modified from Grech, E. D. [2003]. ABC of interventional cardiology: Pathophysiology and investigation of coronary artery disease. *BMJ,* 326[7397], 1027–1030.)

mechanical forces that act on the vessel wall. The flow of blood through the vasculature causes nonuniform distributions of mechanical force, particularly immediately distal to vessel bifurcations. Lesion-prone regions experience greater shear stress, which increases the opportunity for blood-borne components (e.g., lipids) and the vessel wall to interact, facilitating greater transendothelial diffusion.[39] Clearly, individuals with greater plasma concentrations of atherogenic lipoproteins will provide the opportunity for accelerated influx and early accumulation of lipid in the lesion-prone areas. In individuals with very high plasma levels of atherogenic lipoproteins, such as those with familial hypercholesterolemia, type II lesions rapidly evolve into advanced lesions, even in arterial locations outside the progression-prone zones. It is noteworthy that by middle age, the development of advanced lesions outside the progression-prone areas occurs even in the absence of high plasma cholesterol (i.e., even in individuals free of premature risk factors).

Type III Lesions

Type III lesions are also known as intermediate or transitional lesions or preatheroma. Type III lesions contain more free cholesterol, fatty acid, sphingomyelin, lysolecithin, and triglyceride than type II lesions.[36,40] Fatty acid composition differs between type II and more advanced lesions and may be explained by the overall increase in lipids and the change from intracellular to predominantly extracellular storage. Type III lesions contain extracellular lipid deposits (droplets and particles) among the layers of smooth muscle cells that tend to occur adjacent to areas of adaptive intimal thickening. These dispersed droplets accumulate beneath the macrophage/foam cell layer, replace cellular matrix proteoglycans and fibers, and also divide smooth muscle cells. This lipid-variegation destabilizes the integrity of intimal smooth muscle cells and is characteristic of type III lesions.

Type IV Lesions

This lesion, referred to as atheroma is the first "advanced" lesion of atherosclerosis, characterized histologically by a lipid core, intimal disorganization, and arterial deformity, which predispose this lesion type to sudden progression that may precipitate clinical symptoms. Macrophages within the lesions are primed for immune and/or inflammatory responses, expressing major histocompatibility complex receptors, and a variety of cytokines and growth regulatory molecules. These lesions possess a large, well-defined intimal pool of extracellular lipid known as the lipid core. The type IV lesion is also known as an atheroma. The continued growth of these extracellular lipid pools is a result of continued transmigration from the plasma, encouraged by the areas of decreased local blood flow (called eddies) at lesion-prone sites. Initially, these lesions colocalize with adaptive intimal thickenings. Lipid cores thicken the artery wall and are clearly visible when the luminal surface of the lesion is examined, although thickening usually occurs at the external boundary and contributes little to narrowing of the vessel lumen at this stage.[39]

This lesion type is characterized by the displacement of the intimal smooth muscle cells and the intercellular matrix of the deep intima by accumulating pools of extracellular lipid. The dispersed cells appear attenuated and elongated with thickening of the basement membranes. Calcium particles are often found within the lipid cores and even within the organelles of some of the smooth muscle cells. In addition, capillaries may be readily identified around the lipid core and are most common at the lateral margins and facing the lumen. Macrophages, smooth muscle cells, and even mast cells and lymphocytes, populate the region between the lipid core and the endothelial surface. Coalescence of the lipid core leads to a subsequent increase in fibrous tissue (mainly collagen), which will in turn alter the intima above the lipid core. When the fibrous tissue enrichment of the intima covering the lipid core occurs, the lesion is classified as type V. In either conventional histological sections, or by examination by the unaided eye, the upper intimal layer of a type IV lesion is indistinguishable from the fibrotic cover (also known as the fibrous cap) of a type V lesion. This explains why both types IV and V lesions are referred to as fibrous plaques.

Although this lesion class only minimally contributes to luminal narrowing, type IV lesions have important clinical significance. Enrichment of the region between the lipid core and the lesion surface with proteoglycans, foam cells, and dispersed smooth muscle cells with decreased collagen content renders the lesion susceptible to fissures or ulceration. Ominously, localization and accumulation of macrophages in the periphery of advanced lesions, particularly type IV, makes them vulnerable to sudden rupture.

Type V Lesions

This stage in lesion progression is referred to as a fibroatheroma, because of the intimal accumulation of abundant fibrous connective tissue adjacent to a lipid core. When a type V lesion has both a lipid core and calcification within the lesion, it is referred to as a type Vb lesion. Type Vc lesions are devoid of a lipid core and contain minimal lipid deposition. Type V lesions tend to cause a more noticeable narrowing of arteries than type IV lesions and are particularly clinically relevant given their susceptibility to fissure, hemorrhage, and rupture with hematoma and/or thrombus formation.

Population studies of advanced lesion histology reveal that reparative smooth muscle cells infiltrate regions of the intima in which lipid cores disturb or disrupt the cell and intercellular matrix structure. This fibrous tissue often accounts for more of the thickness of the lesion than its underlying lipid core. The new tissue is composed of both collagen and smooth muscle cells. These new smooth muscle cells are distinct from their older counterparts in that they are enriched in rough-surfaced endoplasmic reticulum. Previous thrombi appear to result in thicker lesions and surrounding tissue as they are incorporated into the growing lesion. Type V lesions also contain large, numerous, and newly formed vessel capillaries at the periphery of the lipid core. The media adjacent to the intima of type V lesions are characterized by depletion and disorganization of smooth muscle cells. The surrounding media and adjacent adventitia are enriched in lymphocytes, macrophages, and macrophage foam cells.

Type Va lesions can form larger compound lesions, composed of irregular intercalating lipid cores separated by thick layers of fibrous connective tissue (variably termed multilayered fibroatheroma). Both hemodynamic and tensile forces may contribute to the formation of such compound lesions; as lesions impinge on the circulation, alterations in blood flow promote asymmetric vascular narrowing and a redistribution of the regions of predisposition to lesion formation.[39] An alternate explanation may be the serial rupture of the lesion surface, hematoma formation, and thrombosis followed by fibrious organization.

Although type Vb lesions are primarily differentiated by calcification, they tend to possess greater fibrous connective tissue compared to earlier lesion types. Mineral deposits may eventually replace a lesion's core (an accumulation of dead cells and extracellular lipid). Such calcified lesions are variably also termed a type VII lesion.[28,31]

The type Vc lesions, being fibrotic and largely devoid of lipid core, often occur in the arteries in the lower extremities[24] and have been referred to as a type VIII lesion by some investigators.[28,33] These lesions may form by one of several mechanisms including thrombus organization, extension of the fibrous component of an adjacent fibroatheroma, or resorption of lipid cores. Although fibrotic lesions rarely possess a lipid core, a positive stain for lipids is not uncommon in this lesion type. It is noteworthy that wall shear stress caused by increased hydrostatic pressure is common in the lower extremities and could conceivably provide another mechanism for this lesion formation.

Type VI Lesions

Lesion types V and VI may undergo disruption of the lesion surface or develop hematoma, hemorrhage, or thrombotic deposits. They account for the majority of atherosclerotic morbidity and mortality. Any one of these complications is sufficient to recategorize type IV or V lesions as type VI lesions; they are also referred to as complicated lesions. Moreover, the particular complicating event permits subdivision of type VI lesions into three subtypes according to (a) disruption, (b) hemorrhage, or (c) thrombosis; although practically, lesions are often complex and rarely conform perfectly to the lesion classification criteria. Indeed, instances of surface disruptions, hematoma, and thrombosis superimposed on other lesions types or even on intima without a noticeable lesion are not uncommon. The composition of blood, the integrity of the intima, the sensitivity of the inflammatory response, and the dynamic range of shear and tensile forces to which the lesion or intima is exposed varies greatly between persons. While physiological and biochemical studies aimed at characterizing both the determinants and mechanisms resulting in the spectrum of lesion types is ongoing, continued innovation in clinical imaging of lesions has contributed much to the more accurate identification of lesion types and their associated clinical syndromes.

In the past, clinical assessment of atherosclerotic lesions was confined to advanced, gross vascular abnormalities, including aneurysms and vascular stenoses. But the integration of newer and emerging technologies has permitted more accurate depiction of lesion morphology, which in turn informs more specific interventions (Table 5-1). Targeting of treatment has been honed further by the growing understanding of the pathophysiology of lesion progression and associated clinical events. This has permitted clinicians to move beyond simple diagnosis to proactive prevention of complicated lesions through detection of earlier lesions and more accurate lesion characterization. Morphological, immunohistochemical, and

Table 5-1 ■ TECHNOLOGIES PERMITTING EARLIER DETECTION AND ESTIMATION OF LESION VOLUME ARE LISTED

Method	Features Detected
B-mode ultrasonography and Doppler flow	Permits measurement of the severity of stenosis in peripheral arteries
Intravascular ultrasound	Produces cross-sectional images of the vascular wall, revealing lesion composition and lumen contour
Magnetic resonance angiography	A noninvasive alternative to angiography, permitting study of major vessels (the aorta and carotid arteries and coronary arteries)
Angioscopy	Direct vascular vascularization detects specific morphological features such as thrombus
Ultrafast computed tomography	A noninvasive method detecting coronary artery calcium

While angiography is the definitive method for evaluation of the vascular lumen, it cannot detail the vascular wall. The sensitivity of coronary angiography for early detection of atherosclerosis may be increased by these methods. Emerging methodologies that may allow noninvasive monitoring of atherosclerosis include magnetic resonance spectroscopy, labeled antiplatelet monoclonal antibody imaging and radiolabeling of low-density lipoproteins and monocytes.

epidemiological data have supported the construction of a lesion classification system, which has helped clinical decision making and research into the underlying pathophysiology and potential therapeutic intervention (Table 5-2).

Vascular Surface Defects and Hematoma

The degree of luminal narrowing by an atheroma has little relation to whether thrombosis will occur. Myocardial infarctions of most patients often result from atheromas of less than 50% luminal narrowing or occlusion.[11,18,41] Fissuring and disruption of atherosclerotic plaque can occur at any time during this chronic process.[12,14] The ability of the plaque to disrupt is a major factor in future ischemic events. Plaque composition, rather than the amount of narrowing, is a major determinant of the vulnerability of the plaque formation. Both mechanical and inflammatory changes affect the vulnerability of the plaque and propensity for thrombosis.[10] Superimposed thrombosis on the ruptured, ulcerated plaque can impede blood flow and the delivery of nutrients to the myocardium.

As lesions progress, disruptions of the lesion surface may present as fissures or even ulcerations and are highly variable in their severity and scope. Fissures of the lesion surface vary in length and depth and most likely reseal, leading to lesion progression by incorporating hematoma and thrombus.[42,43] Ulcerations can range from minor focal loss of a microscopic portion of the endothelial cell layer to deep ulcerations that can expose lipid cores and release lipid and other components that activate the coagulation cascade. Atheromatous lesions (types IV and Va) are particularly prone to intimal disruptions and ultimately thrombosis.[42–45] This susceptibility is caused in part by the presence of activated inflammatory cells within the lesions,[46,47] the release of proteolytic enzymes by macrophages within the lesions,[42,48,49] coronary spasm,[50] structural weakness related to lesion composition,[45] the release of toxic factors from cell death (necrosis), and shear stress.[39,51] In addition to intimal hematoma caused by tearing of the lesion surface, some hemorrhage may begin internally from disruption of newly formed vessels within the lesion.[52]

Thrombosis

Although plaque disruption and thrombosis can be separate processes, they appear to be interrelated. Thrombosis formation may be exacerbated by changes in the endothelium. Contractility, secretory, and mitogenic activities of the vessel wall all are factors that affect ischemia.[10] A dysfunctional endothelium leads to the potential for thrombosis and the development of atherosclerotic lesions. Platelets migrate quickly to the site of plaque rupture and adhere. Platelet aggregation releases metabolic substances that cause vasoconstriction.[53] Thrombin formation is activated by factor XII, and the coagulation pathway results in the formation of fibrin. A fibrin mesh binds with the platelets and leads to formation of a clot.[3,11,25,26,54]

Advanced atherosclerotic lesions containing thrombi or their remnants become common by the fourth decade of life, ranging in size from microscopic to grossly visible deposits, with some consisting of stratified layers of lesions of different ages.[55] Incorporation of recurrent hematomas and thrombi over time (months

Table 5-2 ■ TERMS USED TO DESIGNATE DIFFERENT TYPES OF HUMAN ATHEROSCLEROTIC LESIONS IN PATHOLOGY

Terms for Atherosclerotic Lesions in Histological Classification			Other Terms for the Same Lesions Often Based on Appearance With the Unaided Eye	
Type lesion	I	Initial lesion	Fatty dot or streak	Early lesions
Type lesion	IIa	Progression-prone type II lesion		
	IIb	Progression-resistant type II		
Type lesion	III	Intermediate lesion (preatheroma)		
Type lesion	IV	Atheroma	Atheromatous plaque, fibrolipid plaque, fibrous plaque	
Type lesion	Va	Fibroatheroma (type V lesion)		Advanced lesions, raised lesions
	Vb	Calcific lesion (type VII lesion)	Calcified plaque	
	Vc	Fibrotic lesion (type VIII lesion)	Fibrous plaque	
Type lesion	VI	Lesion with surface defect, and/or hematoma–hemorrhage, and/or thrombotic deposit	Complicated lesion, complicated plaque	

Reproduced from Stary et al. (1995). A report from the Committee on Vascular Lesions of the Council on Arteriosclerosis, American Heart Association. *Arteriosclerosis, Thrombosis, and Vascular Biology,* 15, 1512–1531.

to years) results in the progressive narrowing of the arterial lumen. Thrombus remnants contain increasing numbers of smooth muscle cells derived by ingrowth from the intima. These smooth muscle cells synthesize collagen, providing the stratum for overgrowth of endothelial cells at the lumen. Ultimately, thrombi may continue to enlarge, with the potential to rapidly occlude the lumen of a medium-sized artery (within days or even hours).

Several mechanisms can influence the location, frequency, concentration, and size of thrombi. Shear stress participates in lesion progression, with thrombotic occlusions being common at vessel bifurcations and locations of arterial angulation.[56] Increased levels of low-density lipoproteins (LDLs) (demonstrated to impair platelet function),[57,58] nutrition,[59] contents of cigarette smoke,[60] and elevated lipoprotein(a) levels[61,62] have been associated with greater risk for clinical coronary artery disease. Taken together, systemic factors play a significant role in modulating the development of thrombi.

Atherosclerotic Aneurysms

A common sequela of advanced lesions (types IV, V, and VI) is the development of distensions in the entire vascular wall. These aneurysms are most commonly associated with type VI lesions, when the intimal surface is eroded. Both old and new mural thrombi permeate atherosclerotic aneurysms, and the thrombi become layered in older aneurysms. Whereas the thrombi can form large masses that can fill an aneurysm, the underlying lumen remains generally well preserved and approximates the dimensions of the original vessel. The evolution of atherosclerotic aneurysms is preceded by a series of changes in the locale of the lesion. Matrix fibers are continuously degraded and resynthesized,[63] causing a progressive decay of matrix architecture that results in dilation and potentially rupture.[64] Susceptibility to atherosclerotic aneurysm is modulated by secondary risk factors resulting in increased hemodynamic and/or tensile stress (e.g., hypertension) and by genetic variation. The search for genetic factors predisposing to atherosclerotic aneurysm development is ongoing.

Severity of Stenosis

The severity of lesion stenosis modulates the degree of impaired blood flow. The degree of stenosis is estimated by the ratio of the maximum diameter of a stenosed artery in comparison to an adjacent normal arterial diameter. Coronary artery blood flow begins to decrease to a clinically significant degree with 50% stenosis and blood flow decreases rapidly when stenosis exceeds 70%,[65] and the determination of stenosis is of particular clinical benefit above and below these cutoffs. However, this physiological marker (decrease in blood flow) is technically difficult to measure accurately and fails to account for other factors that can influence the clinical impact of stenosis on a patient (e.g., rate of lesion growth and lesion length and/or geometry).[66] Nevertheless, percent stenosis measured by a variety of means provides a powerful tool with significant clinical usefulness in the evaluation of coronary disease.[67–69]

Cells and Extracellular Matrix of Lesions

A host of changes exist in the cellular compartment and extracellular matrix composition of lesions. Interaction of the apolipoprotein B on LDL with cell surface glycosaminoglycans appears to be a mechanism for trapping LDL in the arterial intima. Moreover, production of glycosaminoglycans increases during the early stages of atherosclerosis, which contribute to more avid cellular lipoprotein recruitment.[70–72] Dermatan sulfate proteoglycans are another surface moiety hypothesized to increase the rate of progression of atherosclerosis.[72] This class of molecules also binds plasma LDL under physiological conditions with increased affinity in comparison with other molecules of this class.[73] In vitro studies of smooth muscle cells exposed to conditioned media from cultured macrophages provides evidence for a role for macrophages in modulating the type and amount of proteoglycans found in the developing lesion.[74] Macrophage accumulation in type II lesions leads to the production of enzymes capable of degrading proteoglycans within the lesion locale. Enzymatic digestion of the chondroitin sulfate proteoglycan, versican, leads to progression of the lesion because of its role in maintaining the viscoelasticity and the integrity of the vessel wall against the passage of plasma materials.

Although there are significant decreases in elastin content in advanced atherosclerotic lesions, few changes are reported in initial and fatty streak lesions. A variety of elastases attack elastic fibers, and the possibility exists for macrophages[75] and smooth muscle cells[76] to produce such proteases. This results in a decrease in structural integrity. Moreover, degradation of elastic fibers may have significant consequences in early lesions, because elastin-derived peptides are extremely chemotactic for macrophages. The component cells and extracellular matrix of the atherosclerotic lesion are reviewed briefly below.

Smooth Muscle Cells

Alterations in the functional properties and amount of smooth muscle cells are a central feature of atherogenesis. Changes result from stimuli, including lipid accumulation, disruption of intimal structure, damage to intimal cells and matrix, and deposits of platelets and fibrinogen. These stimuli activate resident cells to produce mitogenic factors, spurring smooth muscle cell proliferation, and ultimately contributing to lesion progression.

Macrophages

Whereas macrophages are generally located proximal to the lumen, foam cells are trapped within the intima. However, this distribution becomes less obvious in complicated lesions or regions in which the intima is relatively thin. When a lipid core is present, macrophage foam cells are usually most evident along the luminal aspect and at the lateral margins of the core. Macrophage foam cells are more numerous and found closer to the surface of the lesion boarder, largely because of a lack of intimal thickening at the lesion periphery. Foam cells eventually die as the lesion develops, contributing to the growth of what is more appropriately termed a "necrotic" core, being composed of extracellular lipid and necrotizing cells. Unfortunately, there are currently no appropriate biomarkers for defining this type of cellular injury.

An accumulating body of evidence indicates that in addition to lipid accumulation, macrophages contribute to atherogenesis by secretion of a range of factors modulating the formation and modeling of advanced lesions, including monocyte chemotactic protein-1 and tumor necrosis factor (TNF).[77] Lesions laden with monocytes and macrophage foam cells[42,43] are more prone to rupture because of the release of proteolytic enzymes (e.g., collagenase and elastase) by the macrophages. It is not clear yet if macrophages secrete these enzymes throughout lesion formation or only as they die. The capacity of macrophages to express cytokines and growth regulatory molecules was reviewed earlier.[31]

Lymphocytes

Monoclonal antibodies against CD antigens reveal the presence of T (CD4+ T helper and CD8+ T killer) and B lymphocytes in advanced lesions.[78] It is yet unclear to what extent these immune cells participate in the atherogenic process. Macrophage foam cell-derived oxidized lipids constitute a significant but variable component of the core of advanced lesions.[79–81] Autoantibodies that recognize oxidized LDL have been isolated from human sera,[82] and the titers of these antibodies may potentially be diagnostic of advanced atherosclerosis.[83] In addition, viral and bacterial (e.g., chlamydia) antigens have been found in advanced human lesions using molecular and immunocytochemical techniques.[84]

Lipid and Lipoprotein in the Extracellular Matrix

While the transfer of lipoproteins from the plasma into the intima is a physiological process, the concentrations of these particles are particularly elevated in advanced lesions.[33] Definitive identification of the types and amounts of extracellular lipid are difficult and depend largely on methods of tissue preparation and study. More extracellular lipid is observed in lesion types III, IV, Va, and VI. In addition, extracellular lipid accumulates and pools, forming "lipid cores," in lesion types IV, Va, and VI. Lesions contain many lipid-laden cells that die or can be found in various stages of disintegration, evidence that much of the extracellular lipid is derived from cells and lipoproteins originally internalized by cells.[79,80] In addition, intracytoplasmic lipid can also be expelled from intact cells into the extracellular space.[85] Extracellular lipid is also derived in part by direct coalescence of plasma-derived lipoproteins.[86,87]

Fibrinogen

The degree and extent to which fibrinogen accumulates in advanced lesions or parts of advanced lesions varies. Immunohistochemical techniques show that the cores of advanced lesions stain for fibrinogen more than any other part of advanced lesions, except superimposed thrombi. It must be recalled that immunohistochemical staining alone cannot distinguish thrombus-associated fibrinogen from physiological infiltration of fibrinogen from the plasma. However, it is generally accepted that intensely fibrinogen-positive bands found in the majority of advanced lesions constitute evidence of incorporated past thrombi.[55] Fibrinogen contributes directly and indirectly (by promoting smooth muscle cell growth) to the volume of most advanced lesions.

Proteoglycans

Proteoglycans are a class of glycosylated proteins that have covalently linked sulfated glycosaminoglycans, (i.e., chondroitin sulfate, dermatan sulfate, heparan sulfate, heparin). The protein component of proteoglycans is a core protein that is modified by the addition of a complex set of sugar groups. Glycosaminoglycans are sulfated polysaccharides made of repeating disaccharides (40 to 100 repeats, on average). These complex groups endow proteoglycans with unique properties. In contrast to arterial glycosaminoglycans, little is known about qualitative changes in specific proteoglycan molecules in atherosclerotic lesions. Large extracellular proteoglycans, mainly chondroitin sulfate-containing molecules, function in arterial permeability, ion exchange, transport, and deposition of plasma materials such as LDL. Extracellular heparin sulfate proteoglycans possessing particular oligosaccharide or carbohydrate sequences have different functional properties. Functions attributed to specific oligosaccharides include antiproliferative effects on arterial smooth muscle cells,[88] fibroblast growth factor binding,[89,90] lipoprotein lipase binding,[91] and antithrombin III binding.[92] While hypotheses regarding the concentrations, composition, and function of various proteogyclans are currently being evaluated, the lack of clinical studies to inform the clinical relevance of such hypotheses makes discussion of these molecules premature in this venue.

Collagen

Second only to lipids, collagen is the major extracellular component of type V lesions. The increased collagen of atherosclerotic lesions is produced by intimal smooth muscle cells. The major collagen type of advanced lesions is the fibrillar collagen type I. Type I collagen is particularly prevalent in the fibrous cap and in vascularized regions of advanced lesions.[93] A significant and consistent change in the minor collagen types of advanced atherosclerotic lesions includes type V collagen, which increases with advancing fibrosis[94–96] and plays a role in cell migration[97]; and type IV collagen, which is associated with the basement membranes of smooth muscle cells. The exact stimulus for collagen accumulation in atherosclerosis is unknown, although redistribution of mechanical stress has been shown to produce changes in matrix production.

Elastin

The relative concentration and localization of elastin fibers varies with the location and type of lesion. De novo synthesis of subendothelial, medial, and adventitial elastin is common in type V lesions, along with collagen. Whereas the smooth muscle cells of advanced lesions produce elastin, integration of the protein into a functional elastic fiber may be impaired.

Split or frayed elastic fibers tend to associate closely with lipid and calcium deposits. Lipid bound to elastic fibers may change elasticity of tissue by modifying the functionality of the elastin fibers and increase their susceptibility to proteolytic degradation.[98,99] Both calcium and magnesium may increase the degradation of elastin,[100] the degradation products of which have been reported to produce chemotactic derivatives, which recruit macrophages.[101]

Calcium

Mineralization of atherosclerotic lesions is a well-substantiated phenomenon. Accumulation of calcium in the arterial wall in the course of the atherogenic process is considered to be a manifestation of advanced atherosclerosis. Unfortunately, very little is known about the factors controlling the quantity of calcium in the lesions. Vesicles in the extracellular matrix of advanced lesions may serve as sites for calcification.[102] Mineral deposits in atherosclerosis may also be associated with elastic fibers.[103]

Inflammation

Epidemiological research in cohort studies over the past three decades (e.g., the Framingham Heart Study and the Multiple Risk Factor Intervention Trial) has resulted in the elucidation of several risk factors for cardiovascular disease (CVD).[104,105] Such studies have established the following risk factors for CVD: age, male gender, hypertension, diabetes mellitus, dyslipidemia, and smoking. Strong evidence also exists to implicate lack of physical activity, obesity, and alcohol intake. While recognition and control of these risk factors have engendered a substantial reduction in

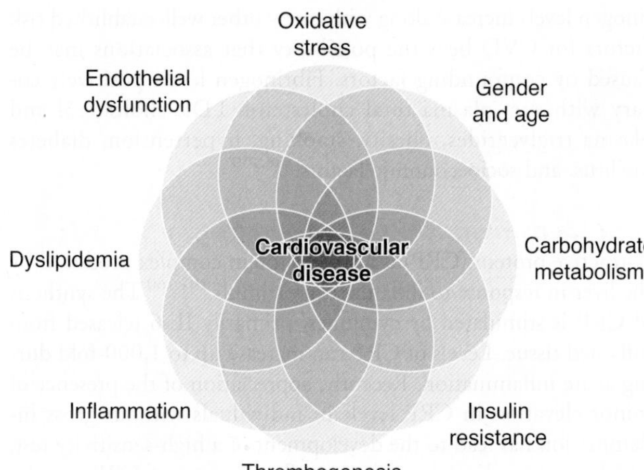

■ **Figure 5-4** Myriad population studies, animal models of disease and biochemical studies have demonstrated the participation and complex interaction of lipid metabolism, endothelial function, carbohydrate metabolism, thrombogenesis, oxidative stress and inflammation in the occurrence of cardiovascular disease.

CVD-related morbidity and mortality, more than 35% of CVD occurs among those without any known risk factors.[106] This observation motivates a large part of the medical research community to identify novel markers of disease, including inflammatory markers of CVD.

It is now abundantly clear that CVD is the result of the interaction of multiple physiological processes. Myriad population studies, animal models of disease, and biochemical studies have demonstrated the participation and interaction of lipid metabolism, endothelial function, carbohydrate metabolism, thrombogenesis, oxidative stress, and inflammation in the occurrence of CVD (Fig. 5-4). Inflammation is the process by which the body responds to injury. Laboratory evidence and findings from clinical and population studies suggest that inflammation plays an important role in all stages of atherosclerosis.[107] The demonstration of the presence of inflammatory cytokines in patients with heart failure immediately sparked interest in the role that these molecules play in regulating cardiac structure and function, particularly with respect to their potential role in the progression of heart failure.

The goal of understanding the role of inflammatory mediators in heart failure derives from the observation that many aspects of the syndrome of heart failure can be explained in large part by the biological effects of proinflammatory cytokines. When expressed in the circulation at sufficiently high concentrations, cytokines are potent enough to recapitulate many facets of heart failure, including progressive left ventricular dysfunction and remodeling, pulmonary edema, and cardiomyopathy.[108–110] Growing experimental evidence suggests that heart failure progresses in part as a result of the deleterious effects of cytokines in the heart and peripheral circulation, thus exacerbating heart failure.[111] What is also clear is that the sustained expression (in clinical terms), caused by high-level production of inflammatory mediators inducing maladaptive effects in the heart or cardiovascular system as a whole.

Appreciation of the pathophysiological consequences of sustained expression of proinflammatory mediators in preclinical and clinical heart failure models has led to a series of multicenter clinical trials in patients with moderate to advanced heart failure. The often contradictory outcomes of these clinical trials underscore the complex participation of proinflammatory mediators in the initiation and progression of CVD.[112]

Inflammation is a key feature of all stages of atherothrombogenesis. This paradigm shift has prompted the search for inflammatory, as well as hemostatic, markers, which may reflect current risk or predict future CVD. Their identification is also tantalizing in their potential to serve as targets for new therapeutic interventions, or provide more appropriate targeting of established therapies. It is critical to note that these serve as potential markers, because, at present, there remains insufficient evidence to support incorporation of any of these risk markers into routine clinical practice. A description of those inflammatory markers with sustained and consistent evidence of a role in CVD is examined below.

Brain Natriuretic Peptide

The heart is an endocrine organ. Natriuretic peptides are neurohormones produced by the heart, which participate in an important counter-regulatory system to balance the effects of sympathetic neurohormones. Brain natriuretic peptide (BNP) is a cardiac neurohormone secreted from the ventricles of the heart in response to ventricular volume expansion and pressure overload.[113] BNP is a diuretic, a natriuretic, and a vasorelaxant.[114] Secreted in a precursor form (ProBNP), it is cleaved into two fragments: physiologically active BNP and a biologically inactive fragment (NTproBNP).[115] NTproBNP has a longer biological half-life than BNP, is more stable in serum and plasma, and is a more specific marker of cardiac activity than BNP.

Epidemiologic studies indicate that BNP and NTproBNP are useful prognostic indicators after the onset of heart failure,[116,117] transmural myocardial infarction,[118,119] and non-ST segment elevation acute coronary syndromes.[120] In addition, they appear to be sensitive diagnostic markers of myocardial diseases: hypertrophy and ventricular dysfunction.[116,121] Therapy that modifies NTproBNP has been shown to not only reduce total cardiovascular events but also delay time to first event.[122] Of particular interest is the mounting evidence that these biomarkers are effective prognostic indicators of mortality in the general population.[117,123]

Circulating Adhesion Molecules

When inflammatory markers come into contact with endothelial cell membranes, they produce a series of proteins termed adhesion molecules. Activation of endothelial cells and platelets is an important mediator of atherothrombosis.[124] Adhesion molecules are specific proteins that regulate the different steps of leukocyte migration from the blood stream into the vessel wall.[125–127] Markers of endothelial cell and platelet activation, such as soluble adhesion molecules, can be measured in plasma. Soluble forms of adhesion molecules occur on enzymatic cleavage of membrane-bound molecules, which serve as markers of endothelial cell activation and inflammation.[128] Intracellular adhesion molecule I (ICAM-I), vascular adhesion molecule I (VCAM-I), and E-selectin are three such proteins that are expressed in response to inflammatory markers such as interleukin 1 (IL-1), TNF-α, and interferon-γ).[129,130] Leukocyte migration is a definitive early event in atherogenesis, and expression of these adhesion molecules can be detected in atherosclerotic plaques.[131–133] Elevated levels of the soluble forms of E-selectin, ICAM-1, and VCAM-1 are found in the plasma of patients with stable angina and acute coronary syndromes.[134]

Circulating adhension molecules are independent of other risk factors.[22] Soluble (s)VCAM-1, sICAM-1, and sE-selectin are currently measured by commercial enzyme-linked immunoabsorbent assay (ELISA); these assays are sensitive (being able to detect less than one 1/100 of the physiological concentration of each adhesion molecule) and 100% specific (no cross-reaction with other serum components occurs).

Data from the Atherosclerosis Risk in Communities studies indicates a five-fold increased risk of coronary heart disease (CHD) and a two-fold increased risk of carotid atherosclerosis between the extreme quartiles of plasma ICAM-1 levels.[135] Analysis of ICAM-1 levels in the Physicians' Health Study (PHS) revealed a 1.6-fold increase risk of myocardial infarction in men with ICAM-1 concentrations in the highest quartile compared with those in the lowest quartile.[136] Evidence from the ARIC study indicates that E-selectin is more closely associated with carotid disease.[135] The fact that no association was demonstrated for VCAM-1 levels in the ARIC cohort[135] is potentially caused by the fact that VCAM-1 production is limited to vascular wall components, whereas ICAM-1 is also expressed by fibroblasts and hemopoietic cells. This suggests that ICAM-1 acts as a more general marker of inflammation. In the secondary preventive setting, all three biomarkers appear to be significantly and independently related to future death from cardiovascular causes in patients with confirmed coronary artery disease.[137] This study also indicated that VCAM-1 levels increased the predictive value of classic risk factors. Taken together, these data suggest that ICAM-1 has predictive usefulness for CVD in healthy people, whereas VCAM-1 is an appropriate biomarker in individuals with established atherosclerotic disease. In a recent population genetic study, several soluble adhesion molecules (soluble P-selectin, soluble intercellular adhesion molecule-1, and soluble vascular cell adhesion molecule-1) were found to be lower in individuals of West African origin (a population with lower risk for CHD) compared with European individuals.[138] Although preliminary evidence supports a role for circulating adhesion molecules as predictors of CVD risk, additional research is necessary before widespread clinical use.

Fibrinogen

Fibrinogen is an acute phase reactant synthesized in the liver and is the substrate of the enzyme thrombin and the precursor to fibrin. Fibrinogen binds platelet glycoproteins, which facilitates platelet aggregation, and plays a central role in the coagulation cascade.[139,140] These properties make fibrinogen an important determinant of thrombogenesis and plasma viscosity, and thus a potentially useful candidate biomarker of CVD risk. While its association with the development of CVD is well established[141,142] evidence of causality has not been demonstrated. Fibrinogen modulates atherothrombosis, in part by binding LDL and homing in on lesions and inducing proliferation of vascular smooth muscle.[143,144] Fibrinogen is involved in the initial stages of plaque formation, where its integration into the artery wall leads to its conversion to fibrin and fibrinogen degradation products. It also binds to high-density lipoprotein (HDL), which sequesters more fibrinogen.[141] Moreover, fibrinogen and fibrinogen degradation products stimulate smooth muscle cell proliferation and migration,[145,146] and may mediate the adhesion of macrophages into the subendothelial space and further migration into the intima.[147]

A host of epidemiological evidence supports a positive correlation between plasma fibrinogen levels and risk of CVD.[148–155] Taken together, there exists an approximate doubling in risk for CHD between individuals from the extreme quartiles for plasma fibrinogen. Plasma fibrinogen levels have been variably correlated with incidence of ischemic stroke.[156,157] The observation that fibrinogen levels increase along with many other well-established risk factors for CVD begs the possibility that associations may be caused by confounding factors. Fibrinogen levels positively covary with age, plasma total cholesterol, LDL cholesterol and plasma triglycerides, obesity, smoking, hypertension, diabetes mellitus, and socioeconomic factors.[158,159]

High Sensitivity C-Reactive Protein

C-reactive protein (CRP) is a small protein complex produced by the liver in response to inflammatory stimuli.[107,160] The synthesis of CRP is stimulated by cytokines, primarily IL-6 released from inflamed tissue. Levels of CRP can increase up to 1,000-fold during acute inflammation. Recently, appreciation of the presence of minor elevation in CRP levels in individuals without gross inflammation has lead to the development of a high-sensitivity test, which permits detection of minor fluctuations of CRP not detectable by conventional assays. Several large epidemiological studies have supported a role for elevated high-sensitivity CRP (hsCRP) predicting future CVD.

The Physicians' Health Study (PHS) consists of a cohort of nearly 15,000 middle-aged to elderly men followed-up prospectively and free of disease at baseline. When participants with baseline levels of hsCRP in the lowest quartile were compared with individuals in the highest quartile, they exhibited a two-fold increase in the risk of subsequent stroke or peripheral vascular disease and a three-fold increase in the risk of myocardial infarction.[136,161,162] These findings have already been consistently supported by six other large population studies: the Air Force/Texas Coronary Atherosclerosis Prevention Study (AFCAPS/TexCAPS),[163] smokers from the Multiple Risk Factor Intervention Trial (MRFIT) study,[164] elderly patients from the Cardiovascular Health Study (CHS),[154,165] postmenopausal women in the Women's Health Study (WHS),[166] the Augsburg cohort of the Monitoring Trends and Determinants in Cardiovascular Disease (MONICA) Study,[167] and the Helinski Heart Study.[168]

hsCRP was the strongest independent risk factor for future myocardial infarction in the PHS and the WHS studies, even considering traditional risk factors or equivalent levels of homocysteine.[136,161,164,166,169] Modeling of risk factors indicated that an absolute risk assessment incorporating the ratio of total cholesterol to HDL cholesterol and hsCRP resulted in the most accurate estimation of overall cardiovascular risk. Moreover, in studies of patients suffering acute coronary syndromes, elevated hsCRP levels were associated with poorer outcomes,[170–172] suggesting prognostic usefulness in secondary preventive settings.

Although no specific treatment currently exists for the modulation of the determinants of elevated CRP, the predictive value of hsCRP measurement in conjunction with other established risk factors appears to more accurately quantify CVD risk. Preliminary studies support the usefulness of incorporating hsCRP in more accurate and informed primary and secondary preventive strategies. Males with the highest baseline hsCRP levels were found to experience the greatest risk reduction after the use of aspirin in the PHS study,[161,163] whereas added benefit of pravastatin treatment was observed in individuals with elevated hsCRP in the Cholesterol and Recurrent Events (CARE) trial.[173] In the AFCAPS/TexCAPS, treatment with lovastatin was also associated with reduction in hsCRP levels.[163]

At the present time, hsCRP represents the most promising of all new risk biomarkers of CVD. The AHA and the Centers for Disease Control and Prevention published a joint scientific statement about using inflammatory markers in clinical and public health practice[174] after systematically reviewing the evidence of association between inflammatory markers (mainly CRP) and CHD and stroke. CRP levels show a consistent dose-dependent and independent association with cardiovascular risk, and it can be measured reliably and relatively cheaply.[175] These preliminary studies suggest that hsCRP may be able to predict response to aspirin and lipid-lowering therapy, although more data are required to confirm if interventions can be reliably targeted to and guided by hsCRP levels. However, limitations in the use of this biomarker exist, namely its lack of specificity and the uncertainty surrounding its etiological roles.[176]

Homocysteine

Homocysteine (Hcy) is a sulfur-containing amino acid that is closely related to the essential amino acid methionine and to cysteine. Hcy is formed during the metabolism of methionine in the methionine cycle and is metabolized through two pathways: remethylation or transsulfuration. The remethylation of homocysteine is performed by the enzyme methionine synthase, which requires vitamin B_{12} and methyltetrahydrofolate. In the liver and kidneys, an alternative pathway for the remethylation of homocysteine exists, but most tissues are entirely dependent on the former mechanism of homocysteine recycling. The remaining homocysteine is converted in the transsulfuration pathway to cysteine in two reactions requiring vitamin B_6. Cysteine is a precursor to glutathione, the major cellular reduction/oxidation (redox) buffer, which in turn regulates various aspects of cellular function. The transsulfuration pathway also directs Hcy to degradation and its ultimate removal as sulfate through the kidneys.

Hcy exists in several forms; the combined measurement is termed total homocysteine (tHcy). Plasma tHcy increases throughout life, being low in childhood and increasing during puberty, with the relative increase being greater in males. It is at this time that population differences start to emerge. On menopause, the gender-related differences in tHcy diminish, but concentrations remain lower in women than in men. The higher tHcy concentrations seen in the elderly may be caused by many factors such as malabsorption, insufficient dietary supply, reduced metabolic activity, reduced kidney function, and other physiological age-related changes. In addition, many drugs affect tHcy levels either by reducing the absorption of cofactors or by increasing their catabolism. Certain diseases also influence homocysteine metabolism.

A role for homocysteine levels in the risk of CVD was first suggested by detection of an association between hyperhomocystinemia and premature vascular disease in individuals with inherited homocystinuria.[156,177] Subsequent studies exploring the potential of modest changes in plasma Hcy levels correlating with risk of CVD yielded mixed results.[178,179] Results have not been consistent but seem to support a continuous positive relationship with risk, in addition to a potential threshold effect. A preliminary meta-analysis indicates a positive association with CVD risk in which every 5 mmol/L increase in Hcy increased the risk of incident coronary disease by 60% in men and 80% in women.[178] However, this report was not corroborated in a subsequent study.[179] Several hypotheses may prove to account for the association of Hcy with risk of CVD. They include the ability of Hcy to stimulate the endothelium directly, thereby increasing proliferation of smooth muscle cells[180] and the tendency toward thrombosis.[178] The correlation of Hcy with renal dysfunction, smoking, fibrinogen levels, and plasma CRP levels suggests the potential for confounding.[181]

That folic acid and vitamins B_6 and B_{12} participate in Hcy metabolism provides a ready target for intervention; several studies have demonstrated dose-dependent reductions in Hcy after supplementation of folic acid, vitamin B_6, and vitamin B_{12}.[182,183] Measurement of Hcy is inexpensive and reliable.[184,185] Because dietary intervention and supplementation could alter CVD risk by lowering plasma Hcy, it makes Hcy an attractive biomarker. The AHA has not yet defined hyperhomocystinemia (high plasma homocysteine levels) as a major risk factor for CVD and does not yet recommend widespread use of folic acid and B vitamin supplements to reduce the risk of heart disease and stroke.

Interleukin 6

IL-6 is a pleiotropic cytokine produced by several cell types and is a central mediator of the acute-phase response. It regulates humoral and cellular responses and plays a central role in inflammation and tissue injury.[186] The effects of IL-6 are mediated through the interaction of IL-6 with its receptor complex, IL-6R. IL-6 is the primary determinant of CRP release from the liver and is produced in response to several factors, including IL-1, interferon-γ, and TNF.[187] This cytokine is the only known biomarker that can induce the synthesis of all acute phase proteins. In addition to its role in inflammatory processes, experimental evidence suggests that IL-6 possesses procoagulant activity.[188] IL-6 is synthesized in the endothelial and smooth muscle cells from normal and aneurysmal arteries.[189,190] Large quantities of IL-6 have been identified in human atherosclerotic plaques.[191] Approximately one third of circulating IL-6 is synthesized from adipose tissue, which suggests that IL-6 and obesity may be interrelated[192,193]; this is particularly relevant given that obesity is a risk factor for CVD. Some cytokines have been demonstrated to inhibit insulin signaling,[194] induce hypertriglyceridemia,[195] and cause endothelial activation.[196] Epidemiological studies suggest that chronic inflammatory states are associated with insulin resistance and endothelial dysfunction.[197]

Whereas the epidemiological evidence demonstrating an association between IL-6 and CVD independent of CRP is mixed and limited, it remains suggestive. After adjustment for CRP and other cardiovascular risk factors, men segregated in the highest quartile of baseline IL-6 levels from the PHS cohort exhibited greater than twice the risk of first myocardial infarction than did those in the lowest quartile.[198] Complimentary results were observed in women with CVD participating in the Women's Health and Ageing Study. Similarly, after adjustment for CRP and other cardiovascular risk factors, women found in the highest tertile of the cohort's IL-6 levels displayed a three-fold increased risk of death compared with members of the lowest tertile.[199] In contrast, the associated risk of mortality and IL-6 and CRP in the elderly was found to be similar for those with and without CVD, although their effects were not assayed independently.[200] In a population-based cross-sectional study, ECG abnormalities were found to be associated independently with elevated IL-6.[201] This biomarker appears to be predictive of future heart disease[200] and is elevated in patients with unstable angina.[202] Patients displaying persistent IL-6 elevation tend to experience a worse in-hospital outcome after admission with unstable angina.[203,204]

IL-6 is a systemic biomarker not specific to CVD, which means routine cardiovascular risk evaluation cannot be based on isolated consideration of IL-6 levels. Taken with the lack of a specific treatment for elevated IL-6 levels, more data are required before the clinical use of this promising biomarker.

Serum Amyloid A

Serum amyloid A (SAA) proteins, a family of inflammatory apolipoproteins, are major acute-phase reactants that are produced in response to various insults.[205] Their concentrations can increase up to 1,000-fold during inflammation.[206,207] They bind HDL with high affinity after their synthesis and participate in modifying cholesterol transport during inflammatory conditions.[205,208] SAA is synthesized primarily in the liver[207] and has been identified in human atherosclerotic plaque.[209]

The exact role of SAA in atherogenesis has not been fully defined. It is complicated by its role in the metabolism of HDL, in which evidence suggests it may act as a signal for redirecting HDL to sites of tissue destruction and cholesterol accumulation.[210] In addition, SAA might influence HDL-mediated cholesterol efflux by displacing apolipoprotein A-I from HDL[211] and by modulating the activity of lecithin cholesterol acyltransferase.[212] SAA may contribute further to atherogenesis by participating in the remodeling of atherosclerotic plaque by inducing the secretion of collagenase from smooth muscle cells.[213,214] This in turn affects thrombus formation by inhibiting platelet aggregation and adhesion at the endothelial cell surface and increasing the oxidation of LDL. This causes adhesion and chemotactic recruitment of inflammatory cells to the sites of inflammation in atherosclerotic coronary arteries.[215–217] SAA concentrations parallel those of CRP; some studies suggest SAA is a more sensitive marker of inflammatory disease.[205] Concentrations of SAA are increased in patients with CHD and seem to have a useful prognostic utility with acute coronary syndromes.[169,218–220] Further epidemiological studies testing the diagnostic and/or prognostic usefulness of SAA are required.

von Willebrand Factor

Factor VIII is one of the plasma proteins important for coagulation. It is a complex of two components, each under independent genetic control and with biochemical function: (1) factor VIIIc, a coagulation protein; and (2) factor VIIIvW, a platelet adhesion protein (also known as von Willebrand factor [vWF]). vWF is a large protein complex necessary for normal platelet adhesion and acts as a bridge between a receptor on the platelet surface and the exposed basement membrane or subendothelial collagen. Factor VIIIc forms a complex with vWF in plasma, with the latter acting as a carrier protein. vWF, a glycoprotein synthesized in endothelial cells and megakaryocytes, promotes thrombus formation by mediating platelet adhesion and aggregation.[221] It is released from endothelial cells and platelets after endothelial damage and is a marker of endothelial dysfunction, which in turn is an indicator of early atherogenesis.[222]

Several epidemiological studies have established an independent positive association between vWF and CHD.[223–225] One compelling report provided evidence of increased risk of reinfarction and mortality in survivors of myocardial infarction with elevated levels of vWF.[226] Initial reports of increased risk of stroke[223] failed to be corroborated in other population studies.[157,223,227]

RISK FACTORS FOR CORONARY ARTERY DISEASE

Epidemiological studies have identified many important genetic and environmental risk factors associated with atherosclerosis (Table 5-3). Cardiac risk factors have been identified that precipitate and exacerbate the development of coronary artery disease.[7,174,228] Some modifiable risk factors can be altered to decrease one's risk of CVD. These factors include hyperlipidemia, hypertriglyceridemia, hypertension, and cigarette smoking. Other modifiable risk factors include diabetes mellitus type 2, obesity, sedentary lifestyle, and ovarian hormone therapy. These factors remain controversial in the role of contributing to coronary artery disease. Nonmodifiable risk factors are variables that cannot be altered and include age, being male and younger than age 70, genetic predisposition, and diabetes mellitus type 1. Nontraditional emerging risk factors include hyperhomocystinemia, hypoalphalipoproteinemia, high lipoprotein A, and high iron levels. See Chapter 32 for a complete overview of coronary risk factors.

Table 5-3 ■ CARDIOVASCULAR RISK FACTORS

Cardiovascular Risk Factors		
Nonmodifiable Risk Factors		
Age	Male Gender	
Modifiable Risk Factors		
Alcohol intake	Hypertension	Overweight and obesity
Diabetes	Lack of exercise	Positive family history
Hypercholesterolemia	Left ventricular hypertrophy	Smoking
Emerging Risk Factors		
C-reactive protein	Hypertriglyceridemia	Renin
Fibrinogen	Hyper-Lp(a)	Uricemia
Hyperhomocysteinuria	Microalbuminuria	

Inheritance of CVD has been a subject of discussion for many years, especially in relation to certain metabolic types and in studies of families. In the past few years, several researchers have identified gene polymorphisms with central obesity and metabolic syndrome in CHD populations. Markers that have been identified include IL-1 gene polymorphism,[229] resistin gene variation,[230] a genomic region on chromosome 2[231,232] and fam5c.[233] In addition, inflammatory markers have been investigated with coronary disease, IL-6,[234] monocyte chemoattractant protein-1, and CRP; albeit controversy still exists regarding the role of inflammatory mediators in coronary syndrome.

Inflammation can be present in coronary vasospasm without significant homodynamic changes associated with coronary artery disease. Another genetic area of research with coronary syndrome is gene therapy in treatment in coronary syndrome and congestive heart failure. A genome scan in acute coronary syndrome has suggested the involvement of the gene encoding the insulin receptor substrate-1 gene. Some genes are likely relevant to the process of atherosclerosis and thrombosis. Preliminary research has lead to targeting the heart with gene therapy-optimized gene delivery. In addition, the 719Arg variant of Trp719Arg (rs20455), a polymorphism in kinesin-like protein 6, is associated with greater risk of coronary events and has been found to have a greater benefit from pravastatin as compared to placebo.[235]

INCIDENCE OF MYOCARDIAL ISCHEMIA

The incidence of myocardial ischemia is difficult to ascertain because patients may have silent ischemia. Ischemic heart disease parallels that of CHD, with approximately 1 in 5 deaths per year.[16,236] More than 16 million Americans had a history of myocardial infarction or experienced angina pectoris in 2000.[3] Approximately every 1 minute, an American dies from a coronary event. In developed countries, the number of coronary events parallels the number of coronary events in the United States.

Racial and gender variations exist in the incidence, prevalence, presentations, and treatment responses.[7,228] Blacks have higher morbidity and mortality rates from myocardial ischemia and they also have a higher incidence of hypertension, obesity, and metabolic syndrome. Their access to medical care often is delayed after a coronary event. Indian-Asians have twice the incidence of CHD than whites in the United States. Asians tend to have higher levels of lipoprotein A. People of Mediterranean descent have a much lower incidence of ischemic heart disease. The incidence of ischemic heart disease is equal in men and postmenopausal women. Older adults experience higher mortality and morbidity from ischemic heart disease and have more complications from multiple therapeutic interventions.

Cellular Mechanisms and Events Caused by Myocardial Ischemia

Myocardial ischemia develops if blood flow containing oxygen-rich nutrients is insufficient in meeting metabolic demands of the myocardial cells. Consequences of myocardial ischemia are depicted in Figure 5-5. Oxygen deprivation of the tissues caused by diminished blood flow can cause ischemia within 10 seconds.[21] Myocardial oxygen reserves are used within 8 seconds. Myocardial function and contractility become profoundly depressed within 1 minute. The myocardium shifts from aerobic metabolism to anaerobic metabolism through the glycolic pathway. Glycolysis can supply only 65% to 70% of the total myocardial energy requirement. Anaerobic glycolysis will generate some ATP but is insufficient in

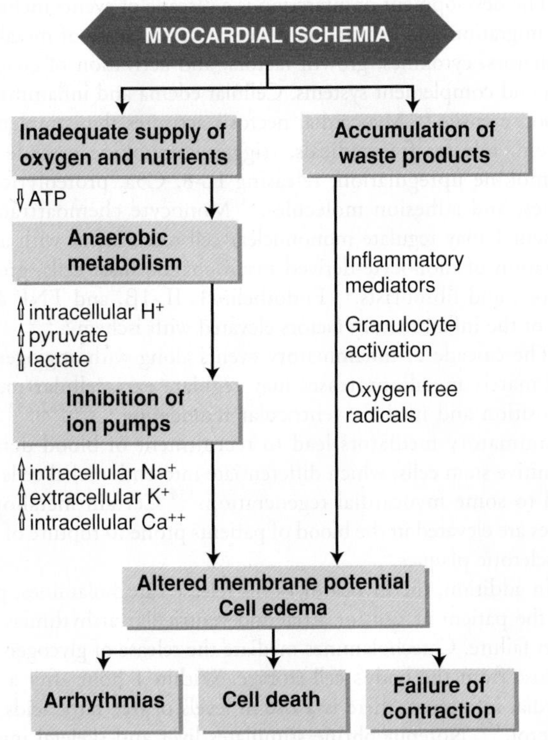

■ **Figure 5-5** Consequences of ischemia.

maintaining homeostasis of myocardial cells. Phosphate production is markedly reduced. Intracellular hydrogen ions and lactic acid accumulate. Within a few minutes, ultrastructural changes can be seen, including cell swelling and depletion of glycolic stores. The combination of hypoxia, reduced energy reserves, and acidosis further hampers left ventricular function.[25] Myocardial cells remain viable for at least 20 minutes. After 20 minutes, irreversible injury begins to occur.[41] The actual events leading to cell death are unknown.[237,238] It has been postulated that calcium overload may be a contributing factor because of the activation of various proteases and phospholipases.[21,22] The integrity of the sarcoplasmic membrane is damaged by these enzymes, leading to eventual cell death. ATPases are impaired by anoxia, which results in the production of superoxides and hydrogen peroxide, both of which are highly diffusible and induce cell damage.[239] In addition, oxidative stress causes a repertoire of cellular defenses to emerge. Ischemia can lead to endogenous antioxidant factors to modulate injury by enzymatic pathways of cellular signals, which may determine the outcome of injury.[240] For example, mitogen-activated protein kinase and nuclear factor-κB inhibit injury and signal ICAM-1 to mediate injury.[241,242]

Ischemic preconditioning, which refers to a state in which tissue is rendered resistant to deleterious prolonged ischemia and reperfusion before exposure of vascular occlusion, may be critical in determining the extent of injury that myocardial cells can sustain. Activation of adenosine receptors and protein kinase is essential to this preconditioning. A cascade of events including postischemic leukocyte rolling, which leads to adhesion and emigration, is dependent on expression of p-selectin on venular endothelium.[243] Another factor affecting endothelium may be the reduction in L-arginine availability, which has been identified with impairment of endothelium-dependent, nitric oxide-mediated vasodilation by ischemia–reperfusion.[244] Downregulation of endothelial nitric oxide synthase may lead to the inability of arginase blockage or L-argine supple mentation to completely restore vasodilatory function. In addition, activation of peroxisome proliferatory-activated receptor α, which regulates genes of myocardial fatty acid oxidation, may exhibit cardioprotection through metabolic mechanisms.[245]

Restoration of oxygenated blood to the previously ischemic myocardium is called reperfusion.[6,8] Occlusion of coronary blood vessel followed by a sudden release is called coronary reactive hyperemia.[246] Reperfusion of a tissue bed results in reversal of ischemia but also releases toxic free radicals and an overabundance of calcium. Although reperfusion is absolutely necessary to restoring cellular homeostasis, there are also detrimental effects that can result.[41] Myocardial stunning is a diminished contractile state in the noninfarcted myocardium from excess production of free radicals.[4,25] Reperfusion arrhythmias are observed and are believed to be caused by myocardial cells that were fatally damaged by the previous ischemic event.

The hemodynamic effects of myocardial ischemia are reduced contractility and abnormal wall motion in the area of ischemia. Changes in wall compliance and stiffness are affected, thereby reducing cardiac output and stroke volume. Because of reduced emptying of the left ventricle, pressures within the heart become elevated. Pulmonary artery wedge pressure and left ventricular end-diastolic pressure rise. Sympathetic compensatory mechanisms respond to the decreased myocardial function. Blood pressure and heart rate increase. A decreased blood pressure indicates a large area of myocardial ischemia or vasovagal response.[3]

The electrocardiographic findings with myocardial ischemia result from cellular changes. These changes may be reflected as ST-segment depression or T-wave inversion. Two conditions, Prinzmetal angina resulting from coronary artery spasm and pericarditis, are associated with ST-segment elevation. Refer to Chapter 15 for electrocardiographic examples of ischemic changes.

Clinical Manifestations of Myocardial Ischemia

Angina pectoris is the clinical description of chest pain or pressure that results from myocardial ischemia. Some patients describe a sensation of heaviness, tightness, or pressure to severe, clutching, griplike pain. The pain or discomfort may be localized or radiate to the shoulder, neck, jaw, or right or left arms. Associated symptoms include lightheadedness, dyspnea, diaphoresis, and fatigue. Anginal pain is probably caused by extracellular accumulation of substances in the area of ischemia.[53] These substances include adenosine, potassium, lactic acid, and bradykinin. Abnormal stretching of the myocardium irritates afferent nerve fibers of the heart. Afferent nerve fibers that enter the spinal column from levels C3 to T4 account for the variety of locations and radiation patterns.[247]

There are three types of angina, including stable angina, unstable angina, and Prinzmetal angina.[236] Stable angina is a condition in which there is chronic stable stenosis of one or more coronary arteries that are inefficient in supplying oxygenated during exertional or emotional stress. When the patient rests, the anginal pain resolves. Unstable angina is a condition characterized by pain that is not relieved with rest. This pain often indicates that there is an acute thrombosis of a coronary artery. Prinzmetal angina is a condition caused by vasospasm of one or more coronary arteries. It can occur at night during sleep and has a cyclical pattern to its occurrence. This condition may result from overstimulation of the sympathetic nervous system, increased flux of calcium in arterial smooth muscle cells, or impaired function of thromboxane or prostaglandins.[13,20]

INCIDENCE OF MYOCARDIAL INFARCTION

Acute myocardial infarction is the leading cause of morbidity and mortality of women and men in the United States. There are 1.3 million reports of patients who experience nonfatal myocardial infarctions each year. For every 100,000 people, there are at least 600 people who experience a coronary event.[8]

Approximately 500,000 to 700,000 deaths occur from coronary artery disease per year in the United States. More than half these deaths occur in the field or prehospital setting because of delay and access to medical treatment. Ten percent of patients die within the hospital setting. Another 10% of patients die within the first year after infarct.[228] Myocardial infarction usually occurs in patients older than 45 years. Certain subpopulations of patients are at risk for myocardial ischemia and infarction, including insulin-dependent diabetic patients, cocaine and amphetamine users, and patients with hypercholesterolemia or a positive family history of early-onset (45 years old or younger) coronary artery disease.

The American College of Cardiology criteria for myocardial infarction are a typical rise and gradual fall of troponin or a rapid rise and fall of creatine kinase-MB, with at least one of the following: symptoms of ischemia, development of pathological Q-waves on the ECG, electrocardiographic changes of ST elevation or depression.[174,248,249] In addition, patients qualify under the definition of myocardial infarction if they have any pathological findings of myocardial necrosis.

Cellular Mechanisms and Events Caused by Myocardial Infarction

Prolonged ischemia of more than 30 minutes will cause irreversible cellular damage of the myocardium and is termed myocardial infarction.[3,41] Sudden occlusion of a coronary artery leads to an ischemic zone with potentially viable tissue that surrounds this zone. The size of this ischemic zone and the degree of blood flow within the area depends on the anatomy of the coronary circulation and the area of occlusion within the blood vessel. Collateral vessels, which form anastomoses or connections between major coronary branches, develop in some patients with long-standing atherosclerosis.[9] When a coronary branch is occluded, pressure changes occur in neighboring arteries that cause rapid recruitment of these collateral vessels to minimize this infarct zone. Ischemia is a major stimulus for angiogenesis, the growth of new capillaries.[20] This revascularization occurs mainly by sprouting or intussusception. Many cytokines stimulate endothelial and smooth muscle cell proliferation with the migration or recruitment of activated monocytes.[12] Once coronary blood flow is interrupted and the delivery of nutrients to the myocardium is blocked, the area of myocardium becomes depressed and hypokinetic. Gradually irreversible cardiac myocyte death occurs within the ischemic zone, leading to necrosis. The endocardial region is the first area of tissue that dies, followed by the midmyocardium or subendocardium. If the ischemia persists, then eventually the infarct will be transmural, the full thickness of the myocardium. Loss of functional myocardium results in reduced left ventricular function affecting the patient's quality of life and morbidity and mortality.[250]

The development of infarction is a cascade of events including the migration and infiltration of leukocytes, release of metabolic mediators, cytokines, growth factors, and activation of coagulation and complement systems. Cellular edema and inflammatory response ensue.[22] Myocardial necrosis activates the complement system, releases free radicals, triggers a cytokine cascade and chemokine upregulation, releasing IL-8, C5a, proteolytic enzymes, and adhesion molecules.[23] Monocyte chemoattractant protein-1 may regulate mononuclear cell recruitment with accumulation of monocyte-derived macrophages, mast cells, growth factors, and fibroblasts.[22] Endothelin-1, IL-1β, and TNF are a few of the inflammatory factors elevated with ischemia.[251]

The cascade of inflammatory events along with angiogenesis and matrix metalloproteases may regulate extracellular matrix deposition and mediate ventricular remodeling.[15,20,252,253] The inflammatory mediators lead to recruitment of blood-derived primitive stem cells, which differentiate into endothelial cells and lead to some myocardial regeneration.[254] Certain metalloproteases are elevated in the blood of patients prone to rupture of atherosclerotic plaques.[255]

In addition, the myocardial cells release catecholamines, placing the patient at risk for atrial and ventricular arrhythmias and heart failure. Catecholamines mediate the release of glycogen and glucose from the body's cell storage. Within 1 hour after a myocardial infarction, there is a rise in levels of free fatty acids and glycerol.[256] Norepinephrine stimulates liver and skeletal muscle cells, elevating blood glucose levels and suppressing insulin production. The infarcted area is further complicated by coronary vasoconstriction and thrombi embolization. Cardiac myocyte cell death may activate the production of free radicals that plug the coronary capillaries causing the "no flow" phenomenon.[237,238] The location of the infarction correlates with disease in a particular area of the coronary circulation. For example, disease in the proximal left anterior descending artery may cause wall motion abnormalities in the anterior or anterior–septal walls of the myocardium. Other common designated infarct areas include inferior, lateral, posterior, or septal sites.

Reperfusion of the infarcted area is necessary to alter the necrotic process. Re-establishment of coronary blood flow can be achieved by thrombolytics or catheter-based procedures.[18] Streptokinase, anistreplase, and tissue plasminogen activator are fibrinolytic agents that act as "clot busters."[257] Percutaneous coronary interventions are performed to place a wire across the blocked or stenosed coronary artery and inflate a balloon within the stenotic portion of the artery. This procedure is called percutaneous transluminal coronary angioplasty (PTCA). More often, a stent is placed in the coronary artery to ensure effective coronary artery blood flow to the myocardium. Some patients may have spontaneous reperfusion when a thrombus disperses naturally. See Chapter 23 for details outlining these interventional cardiology procedures. If patients are not amenable to these interventions, then they may undergo surgical revascularization with coronary artery bypass surgery (see Chapter 25).

Evolution of Myocardial Infarction and Postinfarct Remodeling

The immediate and long-term consequences of acute myocardial infarction are determined by the size of the infarct zone and position of the infarct.[1,258] A large myocardial infarct, more than 40% damage of the myocardium, can cause markedly reduced left ventricular failure and circulatory failure. Cardiogenic shock will eventually occur if blood perfusion to the myocardium is not restored. The infarcted segment undergoes a series of changes during the process of healing and wound repair. Some of these changes can pose further risks to the patients. Initially, the infarct area is bruised and cyanotic from lack of nutrients and blood flow. Cardiac enzymes are released from the cells and can be detected in the blood stream.[22] These biochemical markers of cellular injury include creatinine kinase and creatinine kinase-MB, which are the cardiac muscle enzymes sometimes present in skeletal muscle. They increase within 4 to 6 hours of cellular injury, peak in 18 to 24 hours, and last approximately 2 to 3 days.[249] The cardiac-specific troponins are regulatory proteins that control the calcium-mediated interaction of actin and myosin. Cardiac-specific troponin T and cardiac-specific troponin I elevate 4 to 6 hours after cellular injury, peak at 18 to 24 hours, and persist for at least 10 days.[248] In addition, cardiotrophin-1, a member of the IL-6 family of cytokines, is elevated in ischemic heart disease and thought to have a role in postmyocardial infarction wound healing. Occasionally, elevated troponins are seen in chronic dialysis patients and postcardiac bypass patients.[259] Biomarkers of myocardial injury can be measured and are discussed in Chapter 14. One of the most promising biomarkers is CRP, manufactured in the liver, which increases during inflammatory response to tissue injury.[260]

By the second or third day after myocardial infarction, leukocytes infiltrate the necrotic area and scavenger neutrophils release proteolytic enzymes to break down the necrotic tissue. The necrotic wall is very thin during this phase. Cardiac rupture can occur at any time after an infarction but most commonly within this first week. Rupture of the myocardial wall causes massive hemorrhage into the pericardial space, resulting in cardiac tamponade and pump failure. In the second week of the repair process, insulin secretion increases to mobilize glucose from the wound repairs. The initial phase of the collagen matrix is weak and vulnerable to reinjury.[22] By the third week, scar formation has begun. Postinfarct remodeling of the noninfarcted myocardium also begins.[253] The surviving myocytes hypertrophy because they cannot divide to make up for the loss of pump function of the dead myocytes. Fibrous connective tissue replaces necrotic tissue. There may be excessive deposition of collagen in the hypertrophied myocardium. Collagen is not a contractile protein and fibrosis may lead to a stiff or noncompliant ventricle and impaired contractility of the surviving myocardium. Current research has focused on early metalloproteases activation and decreasing extracellular matrix degradation.[261] After 6 weeks, the necrotic area is completely replaced by scar tissue, which is strong but ineffective in contributing to overall contractility of the myocardium. Myocardial infarction can result in abnormal wall motion abnormality, decreased myocardial function, reduced stroke volume, diminished ejection fraction, elevated ventricular filling pressures, and sinoatrial node dysfunction.

The degree of left ventricular functional impairment after a myocardial infarction depends on the size and location of the infarct, function of noninfarcted myocardium, collateral circulation, and compensatory mechanisms.[258] These compensatory mechanisms operate to optimize cardiac output and peripheral perfusion. Impairment of left ventricular function with subsequent decreased cardiac output activates arterial vasoconstriction, which increases vascular resistance and mean arterial pressure. Venoconstriction increases venous return to the heart and ventricular filling. Higher diastolic filling pressures are necessary to maintain adequate stroke volume to a point. Increased ventricular pressure and volume stretches myocardial fibers to increase the force of contraction, according to the Starling law. Aldosterone is released to stimulate renal retention of sodium and water, thereby further increasing circulatory filling pressures. The depressed myocardium develops temporary left ventricular enlargement caused by cardiac dilatation from these compensatory mechanisms attempting to sustain cardiac output.

The hemodynamic effects of a myocardial infarction depend on the extensiveness and location of myocardial damage and restoration of coronary blood flow.[1,3,250,253,257,258] Heart rate may be normal or borderline normal with mild myocardial depression. Tachycardia is observed in some patients with more extensive myocardial damage and is considered a poor clinical correlate. Blood pressure may be hypertensive in the initial phases of a myocardial ischemia. As myocardial depression worsens, hypotension ensues. Reflex sympathetic stimulation increases heart rate and contractility. Conversely, inferior wall myocardial infarctions may stimulate parasympathetic response of reduced heart rate and blood pressure, further compromising the depressed myocardium. As myocardial function worsens, contractility is reduced, wall compliance is altered, stroke volume is reduced, and filling pressures including left ventricular end-systolic and end-diastolic volumes are elevated resulting in pulmonary edema and circulatory failure. If the cycle is not reversed with restoration of coronary blood flow, then cardiogenic shock, cardiac rupture, and death ensue.

Clinical Manifestations of Myocardial Infarction

Acute myocardial infarction or acute coronary syndrome may present with a sudden onset of severe chest, jaw, back, or arm pain or pressure. The pain is described as heavy, crushing, and like a tight squeeze or elephant on the chest. Sometimes the pain will radiate to the shoulder, neck, and jaw and may be associated with symptoms of fatigue, lightheadedness, nausea, shortness of breath, or diaphoresis. At least 40% to 50% of individuals do not experience pain, especially in diabetic individuals or older adults.[25,54] Some patients may have unrelenting gastric distress. Peripheral vasoconstriction may cause cool, clammy skin. Sometimes a low-grade fever may result from the inflammatory response within the myocardium.

The extent of complications after a myocardial infarction depends on the location and extent of necrosis and ischemia, the physiologic status of the patient before the event, and timing and availability of therapeutic interventions. Myocardial infarction can occur in the various regions of the heart muscle. An ECG is used in the diagnosis to localize the affected area. The zone of infarction and necrosis is surrounded the zone of hypoxia, which is surrounded by the zone of ischemia. Infarcted tissue is electrically silent and is not reflected on the ECG. Transmural infarctions reflect as a Q wave on the ECG in the region of infarction. Nontransmural or non-Q (zone of hypoxia) wave infarctions do not reflect a Q wave. Injured and ischemic tissues (zone of ischemia) are reflected as ST-segment depression or T-wave inversions, or as nonspecific ST-T wave changes. See Chapter 18 for electrocardiographic examples of myocardial infarction.

IMPLICATIONS FOR NURSES

Acute coronary syndrome addresses both myocardial ischemia and myocardial infarction. Myocardial ischemia is a condition that results from reduced supply of oxygen and nutrients to the myocardium or increased demand of the myocardium for oxygen and nutrients. Myocardial infarction is a condition that results from an interruption in the normal coronary blood flow to the myocardium. Changes occur within seconds in the myocardium if ischemia persists, including shifting from aerobic metabolism to anaerobic metabolism through the glycolic pathway. Cell death occurs after 20 minutes if coronary blood flow is not restored. Nurses play a very important role in identifying patients through careful history taking and identifying early signs and symptoms of ischemia. Early intervention of establishing and restoring coronary blood flow will salvage myocardium and save the patient short-term and long-term postinfarction complications. Nurses can help patients identify risk factors that can be modified and promote positive outcomes and responses to lead healthy and productive lives.

REFERENCES

1. Baxter, G. F., Sumeray, M. S., & Walker, J. M. (1996). Infarct size and magnesium: Insights into LIMIT-2 and ISIS-4 from experimental studies. *Lancet, 348*, 1424–1426.
2. Virchow, R. (1858). *Cellular pathology*. London: John Churchill.
3. Boersmas, E., Mercado, N., Poldermans, D., et al. (2003). Acute myocardial infarction. *Lancet, 361*, 847–858.
4. Bolli, R., & Marban, E. (1999). Molecular and cellular mechanisms of myocardial stunning. *Physiology in Review, 79*, 609–634.
5. Feigl, E. O. (1989). Coronary autoregulation. *Journal of Hypertension Supplement, 7*, S55–S58.
6. Opie, L. H. (1989). Reperfusion injury and its pharmacologic modification. *Circulation, 80*, 1049–1062.
7. Hackam, D. G., & Anand, S. S. (2003). Emerging risk factors for atherosclerotic vascular disease: A critical review of the evidence. *Journal of the American Medical Association, 290*, 932–940.
8. Braunwald, E., & Kloner, R. A. (1985). Myocardial reperfusion: A double-edged sword? *Journal of Clinical Investigations, 76*, 1713–1719.
9. Cohen, M. V. (1978). The functional value of coronary collaterals in myocardial ischemia and therapeutic approach to enhance collateral flow. *American Heart Journal, 95*, 396–404.
10. Corti, R., Fuster, V., & Badimon, J. J. (2003). Pathogenetic concepts of acute coronary syndromes. *Journal of the American College of Cardiology, 41*, 7S–14S.
11. Davies, M. J., & Thomas, A. (1984). Thrombosis and acute coronary-artery lesions in sudden cardiac ischemic death. *New England Journal of Medicine, 310*, 1137–1140.
12. Falk, E., Shah, P. K., & Fuster, V. (1995). Coronary plaque disruption. *Circulation, 92*, 657–671.
13. Houston, D. S., Shepherd, J. T., & Vanhoutte, P. M. (1986). Aggregating human platelets cause direct contraction and endothelium-dependent relaxation of isolated canine coronary arteries. Role of serotonin, thromboxane A2, and adenine nucleotides. *Journal of Clinical Investigations, 78*, 539–544.
14. Kullo, I. J., & Ding, K. (2007). Mechanisms of disease: The genetic basis of coronary heart disease. *Nature Clinical Practice Cardiovascular Medicine, 4*, 558–569.
15. Lee, R. T., & Libby, P. (1997). The unstable atheroma. *Arteriosclerosis, Thrombosis, and Vascular Biology, 17*, 1859–1867.
16. Braunwald, E. (2000). 50th anniversary historical article. Myocardial oxygen consumption: the quest for its determinants and some clinical fallout. *Journal of the American College of Cardiology, 35*, 45B–48B.
17. Mombouli, J. V., & Vanhoutte, P. M. (1999). Endothelial dysfunction: From physiology to therapy. *Journal of Molecular and Cellular Cardiology, 31*, 61–74.
18. Gibson, C. M., Dotani, M. I., Murphy, S. A., et al. (2002). Correlates of coronary blood flow before and after percutaneous coronary intervention and their relationship to angiographic and clinical outcomes in the RESTORE trial. Randomized Efficacy Study of Tirofiban for Outcomes and REstenosis. *American Heart Journal, 144*, 130–135.
19. Gorlin, R. (1982). Role of coronary vasospasm in the pathogenesis of myocardial ischemia and angina pectoris. *American Heart Journal, 103*, 598–603.
20. Lee, S. H., Wolf, P. L., Escudero R., et al. (2000). Early expression of angiogenesis factors in acute myocardial ischemia and infarction. *New England Journal of Medicine, 342*, 626–633.
21. Libby, P. (1995). Molecular bases of the acute coronary syndromes. *Circulation, 91*, 2844–2850.
22. Libby, P. (2000). Changing concepts of atherogenesis. *Journal of Internal Medicine, 247*, 349–358.
23. Raines, E. W., Dower, S. K., & Ross, R. (1989). Interleukin-1 mitogenic activity for fibroblasts and smooth muscle cells is due to PDGF-AA. *Science, 243*, 393–396.
24. Ross, R., Wight, T. N., Strandness, E., et al. (1984). Human atherosclerosis. I. Cell constitution and characteristics of advanced lesions of the superficial femoral artery. *American Journal of Pathology, 114*, 79–93.
25. Fuster, V., Badimon, L., Badimon, J. J., et al. (1992). The pathogenesis of coronary artery disease and the acute coronary syndromes (2). *New England Journal of Medicine, 326*, 310–318.
26. Ross, R. (1999). Atherosclerosis—an inflammatory disease. *New England Journal of Medicine, 340*, 115–126.
27. Lendon, C. L., Davies, M. J., Born, G. V., et al. (1991). Atherosclerotic plaque caps are locally weakened when macrophages density is increased. *Atherosclerosis, 87*, 87–90.
28. Stary, H. C. (1992). Composition and classification of human atherosclerotic lesions. *Virchows Archives A Pathology Anatomy and Histopathology, 421*, 277–290.
29. Stary, H. C. (2000). Natural history and histological classification of atherosclerotic lesions: an update. *Arteriosclerosis, Thrombosis, and Vascular Biology, 20*, 1177–1178.
30. Stary, H. C. (1990). The sequence of cell and matrix changes in atherosclerotic lesions of coronary arteries in the first forty years of life. *European Heart Journal, 11*(Suppl. E), 3–19.

31. Stary, H. C. (1994). Changes in components and structure of atherosclerotic lesions developing from childhood to middle age in coronary arteries. *Basic Research in Cardiology, 89*(Suppl. 1), 17–32.
32. Stary, H. C., Blankenhorn, D. H., Chandler, A. B., et al. (1992). A definition of the intima of human arteries and of its atherosclerosis-prone regions. A report from the Committee on Vascular Lesions of the Council on Arteriosclerosis, American Heart Association. *Circulation, 85*, 391–405.
33. Stary, H. C., Chandler, A. B., Glagov, S., et al. (1994). A definition of initial, fatty streak, and intermediate lesions of atherosclerosis. A report from the Committee on Vascular Lesions of the Council on Arteriosclerosis, American Heart Association. *Circulation, 89*, 2462–2478.
34. Stary, H. C. (1987). Macrophages, macrophage foam cells, and eccentric intimal thickening in the coronary arteries of young children. *Atherosclerosis, 64*, 91–108.
35. Stary, H. C. (1989). Evolution and progression of atherosclerotic lesions in coronary arteries of children and young adults. *Arteriosclerosis, 9*, I19–I32.
36. Katsuda, S., Boyd, H. C., Fligner, C., et al. (1992). Human atherosclerosis. III. Immunocytochemical analysis of the cell composition of lesions of young adults. *American Journal of Pathology, 140*, 907–914.
37. Munro, J. M., van der Walt, J. D., Munro, C. S., et al. (1987). An immunohistochemical analysis of human aortic fatty streaks. *Human Pathology, 18*, 375–380.
38. Cornhill, J. F., Herderick, E. E., & Stary, H. C. (1990). Topography of human aortic sudanophilic lesions. *Monographs on Atherosclerosis, 15*, 13–19.
39. Glagov, S., Zarins, C., Giddens, D. P., et al. (1988). Hemodynamics and atherosclerosis. Insights and perspectives gained from studies of human arteries. *Archives of Pathology and Laboratory Medicine, 112*, 1018–1031.
40. Small, D. M. (1988). George Lyman Duff memorial lecture. Progression and regression of atherosclerotic lesions. Insights from lipid physical biochemistry. *Arteriosclerosis, 8*, 103–129.
41. Jennings, R. B., Murry, C. E., Steenbergen, C., Jr., et al. (1990). Development of cell injury in sustained acute ischemia. *Circulation, 82*, II2–I12.
42. Davies, M. J., Gordon, J. L., Gearing, A. J., et al. (1993). The expression of the adhesion molecules ICAM-1, VCAM-1, PECAM, and E-selectin in human atherosclerosis. *Journal of Pathology, 171*, 223–229.
43. Falk, E. (1992). Why do plaques rupture? *Circulation*, 86, III30–III42.
44. Falk, E. (1989). Morphologic features of unstable atherothrombotic plaques underlying acute coronary syndromes. *American Journal of Cardiology, 63*, 114E–120E.
45. Richardson, P. D., Davies, M. J., & Born, G. V. (1989). Influence of plaque configuration and stress distribution on fissuring of coronary atherosclerotic plaques. *Lancet, 2*, 941–944.
46. Tracy, R. E., Devaney, K., & Kissling, G. (1985). Characteristics of the plaque under a coronary thrombus. *Virchows Archives A Pathology Anatomy and Histopathology, 405*, 411–427.
47. van der Wal, A. C., Becker, A. E., van der Loos, C. M., et al. (1994). Site of intimal rupture or erosion of thrombosed coronary atherosclerotic plaques is characterized by an inflammatory process irrespective of the dominant plaque morphology. *Circulation, 89*, 36–44.
48. Henney, A. M., Wakeley, P. R., Davies, M. J., et al. (1991). Localization of stromelysin gene expression in atherosclerotic plaques by in situ hybridization. *Proceedings of the National Academy of Sciences USA, 88*, 8154–8158.
49. Steinberg, D., & Witztum, J. L. (1990). Lipoproteins and atherogenesis. Current concepts. *Journal of the American Medical Association, 264*, 3047–3052.
50. Nobuyoshi, M., Tanaka, M., Nosaka, H., et al. (1991). Progression of coronary atherosclerosis: Is coronary spasm related to progression? *Journal of the American College of Cardiology, 18*, 904–910.
51. Ku, D. N., Giddens, D. P., Zarins, C. K., et al. (1985). Pulsatile flow and atherosclerosis in the human carotid bifurcation. Positive correlation between plaque location and low oscillating shear stress. *Arteriosclerosis, 5*, 293–302.
52. Barger, A. C., Beeuwkes, R., III, Lainey, L. L., et al. (1984). Hypothesis: Vasa vasorum and neovascularization of human coronary arteries. A possible role in the pathophysiology of atherosclerosis. *New England Journal of Medicine, 310*, 175–177.
53. Kullo, I. J., Edwards, W. D., & Schwartz, R. S. (1998). Vulnerable plaque: Pathobiology and clinical implications. *Annals of Internal Medicine, 129*, 1050–1060.
54. Fuster, V., Badimon, L., Badimon, J. J., et al. (1992). The pathogenesis of coronary artery disease and the acute coronary syndromes (1). *New England Journal of Medicine, 326*, 242–250.
55. Bini, A., Fenoglio, J. J., Jr., Mesa-Tejada, R., et al. (1989). Identification and distribution of fibrinogen, fibrin, and fibrin(ogen) degradation products in atherosclerosis. Use of monoclonal antibodies. *Arteriosclerosis, 9*, 109–121.
56. Taeymans, Y., Theroux P., Lesperance J., et al. (1992). Quantitative angiographic morphology of the coronary artery lesions at risk of thrombotic occlusion. *Circulation, 85*, 78–85.
57. Aviram, M., & Brook, J. G. (1987). Platelet activation by plasma lipoproteins. *Progress in Cardiovascular Diseases, 30*, 61–72.
58. Brook, J. G., & Aviram, M. (1988). Platelet lipoprotein interactions. *Seminars in Thrombosis and Hemostasis, 14*, 258–265.
59. Betteridge, J. (1987). Nutrition and platelet function in atherogenesis. *Proceedings of the Nutrition Society, 46*, 345–359.
60. Miller, G. J. (1992). Hemostasis and cardiovascular risk. The British and European experience. *Archives of Pathology and Laboratory Medicine, 116*, 1318–1321.
61. Loscalzo, J. (1990). Lipoprotein(a). A unique risk factor for atherothrombotic disease. *Arteriosclerosis, 10*, 672–679.
62. Scanu, A. M. (1991). Lp(a) as a marker for coronary heart disease risk. *Clinical Cardiology, 14*, I35–I39.
63. Dobrin, P. B., Baker, W. H., & Gley, W. C. (1984). Elastolytic and collagenolytic studies of arteries. Implications for the mechanical properties of aneurysms. *Archives of Surgery, 119*, 405–409.
64. Langille, B. L., & O'Donnell, F. (1986). Reductions in arterial diameter produced by chronic decreases in blood flow are endothelium-dependent. *Science, 231*, 405–407.
65. Gould, K. L., & Lipscomb, K. (1974). Effects of coronary stenoses on coronary flow reserve and resistance. *American Journal of Cardiology, 34*, 48–55.
66. Goldstein, R. A., Kirkeeide, R. L., Demer, L. L., et al. (1987). Relation between geometric dimensions of coronary artery stenoses and myocardial perfusion reserve in man. *Journal of Clinical Investigations, 79*, 1473–1478.
67. Arnett, E. N., Isner, J. M., Redwood, D. R., et al. (1979). Coronary artery narrowing in coronary heart disease: Comparison of cineangiographic and necropsy findings. *Annals of Internal Medicine, 91*, 350–356.
68. Blankenhorn, D. H., & Curry, P. J. (1982). The accuracy of arteriography and ultrasound imaging for atherosclerosis measurement. A review. *Archives of Pathology and Laboratory Medicine, 106*, 483–489.
69. Markis, J. E., Joffe, C. D., Cohn, P. F., et al. (1976). Clinical significance of coronary arterial ectasia. *American Journal of Cardiology, 37*, 217–222.
70. Stevens, R. L., Colombo, M., Gonzales, J. J., et al. (1976). The glycosaminoglycans of the human artery and their changes in atherosclerosis. *Journal of Clinical Investigations, 58*, 470–481.
71. Tammi, M., Seppala, P. O., Lehtonen, A., et al. (1978). Connective tissue components in normal and atherosclerotic human coronary arteries. *Atherosclerosis, 29*, 191–194.
72. Wagner, W. D., & Salisbury, B. G. (1978). Aortic total glycosaminoglycan and dermatan sulfate changes in atherosclerotic rhesus monkeys. *Laboratory Investigations, 39*, 322–328.
73. Iverius, P. H. (1972). The interaction between human plasma lipoproteins and connective tissue glycosaminoglycans. *Journal of Biological Chemistry, 247*, 2607–2613.
74. Edwards, I. J., Wagner, W. D., & Owens, R. T. (1990). Macrophage secretory products selectively stimulate dermatan sulfate proteoglycan production in cultured arterial smooth muscle cells. *American Journal of Pathology, 136*, 609–621.
75. Banda, M. J., & Werb, Z. (1981). Mouse macrophage elastase. Purification and characterization as a metalloproteinase. *Biochemistry Journal, 193*, 589–605.
76. Robert, L., Jacob, M. P., Frances, C., et al. (1984). Interaction between elastin and elastases and its role in the aging of the arterial wall, skin and other connective tissues. A review. *Mechanisms of Ageing and Development, 28*, 155–166.
77. Barath, P., Fishbein, M. C., Cao, J., et al. (1990). Detection and localization of tumor necrosis factor in human atheroma. *American Journal of Cardiology, 65*, 297–302.
78. Jonasson, L., Holm, J., Skalli, O., et al. (1986). Regional accumulations of T cells, macrophages, and smooth muscle cells in the human atherosclerotic plaque. *Arteriosclerosis, 6*, 131–138.

79. Ball, R. Y., Stowers, E. C., Burton, J. H., et al. (1995). Evidence that the death of macrophage foam cells contributes to the lipid core of atheroma. *Atherosclerosis, 114,* 45–54.
80. Mitchinson, M. J., Hothersall, D. C., Brooks, P. N., et al. (1985). The distribution of ceroid in human atherosclerosis. *Journal of Pathology, 145,* 177–183.
81. Rosenfeld, M. E., & Ross, R. (1990). Macrophage and smooth muscle cell proliferation in atherosclerotic lesions of WHHL and comparably hypercholesterolemic fat-fed rabbits. *Arteriosclerosis, 10,* 680–687.
82. Palinski, W., Rosenfeld, M. E., Yla-Herttuala, S., et al. (1989). Low density lipoprotein undergoes oxidative modification in vivo. *Proceedings of the National Academy of Sciences USA, 86,* 1372–1376.
83. Salonen, J. T., Yla-Herttuala, S., Yamamoto, R., et al. (1992). Autoantibody against oxidised LDL and progression of carotid atherosclerosis. *Lancet, 339,* 883–887.
84. Kuo, C. C., Shor, A., Campbell, L. A., et al. (1993). Demonstration of Chlamydia pneumoniae in atherosclerotic lesions of coronary arteries. *Journal of Infectious Diseases, 167,* 841–849.
85. Schmitz, G., & Muller, G. (1991). Structure and function of lamellar bodies, lipid-protein complexes involved in storage and secretion of cellular lipids. *Journal of Lipid Research, 32,* 1539–1570.
86. Guyton, J. R., & Klemp, K. F. (1989). The lipid-rich core region of human atherosclerotic fibrous plaques. Prevalence of small lipid droplets and vesicles by electron microscopy. *American Journal of Pathology, 134,* 705–717.
87. Guyton, J. R., & Klemp, K. F. (1994). Development of the atherosclerotic core region. Chemical and ultrastructural analysis of microdissected atherosclerotic lesions from human aorta. *Arteriosclerosis and Thrombosis, 14,* 1305–1314.
88. Schmidt, A., Yoshida, K., & Buddecke, E. (1992). The antiproliferative activity of arterial heparan sulfate resides in domains enriched with 2-O-sulfated uronic acid residues. *Journal of Biological Chemistry, 267,* 19242–19247.
89. Turnbull, J. E., Fernig, D. G., Ke, Y., et al. (1992). Identification of the basic fibroblast growth factor binding sequence in fibroblast heparan sulfate. *Journal of Biological Chemistry, 267,* 10337–10341.
90. Tyrrell, D. J., Ishihara, M., Rao, N., et al. (1993). Structure and biological activities of a heparin-derived hexasaccharide with high affinity for basic fibroblast growth factor. *Journal of Biological Chemistry, 268,* 4684–4689.
91. Parthasarathy, N., Goldberg, I. J., Sivaram, P., et al. (1994). Oligosaccharide sequences of endothelial cell surface heparan sulfate proteoglycan with affinity for lipoprotein lipase. *Journal of Biological Chemistry, 269,* 22391–22396.
92. Rosenberg, R. D., Jordan, R. E., Favreau, L. V., et al. (1979). Highly active heparin species with multiple binding sites for antithrombin. *Biochemical and Biophysical Research Communications, 86,* 1319–1324.
93. Rekhter, M. D., Zhang, K., Narayanan, A. S., et al. (1993). Type I collagen gene expression in human atherosclerosis. Localization to specific plaque regions. *American Journal of Pathology, 143,* 1634–1648.
94. Morton, L. F., & Barnes, M. J. (1982). Collagen polymorphism in the normal and diseased blood vessel wall. Investigation of collagens types I, III and V. *Atherosclerosis, 42,* 41–51.
95. Murata, K., Motayama, T., & Kotake, C. (1986). Collagen types in various layers of the human aorta and their changes with the atherosclerotic process. *Atherosclerosis, 60,* 251–262.
96. Ooshima, A. (1981). Collagen alpha B chain: Increased proportion in human atherosclerosis. *Science, 213,* 666–668.
97. Stenn, K. S., Madri, J. A., & Roll, F. J. (1979). Migrating epidermis produces AB2 collagen and requires continual collagen synthesis for movement. *Nature, 277,* 229–232.
98. Chaudiere, J., Derouette, J. C., Mendy, F., et al. (1980). In vitro preparation of elastin–triglyceride complexes. Fatty acid uptake and modification of the susceptibility to elastase action. *Atherosclerosis, 36,* 183–194.
99. Guantieri, V., Tamburro, A. M., & Gordini, D. D. (1983). Interactions of human and bovine elastins with lipids: Their proteolysis by elastase. *Connective Tissue Research, 12,* 79–83.
100. Bernier, F., Bakala, H., & Wallach, J. (1981). Effect of Mg2+ and Ca2+ on enzymatic elastolysis of insoluble elastin determined by a conductimetric method. *Connective Tissue Research, 8,* 71–75.
101. Senior, R. M., Griffin, G. L., & Mecham, R. P. (1980). Chemotactic activity of elastin-derived peptides. *Journal of Clinical Investigations, 66,* 859–862.
102. Kim, K. M. (1976). Calcification of matrix vesicles in human aortic valve and aortic media. *Federation Proceedings, 35,* 156–162.
103. Urry, D. W. (1971). Neutral sites for calcium ion binding to elastin and collagen: A charge neutralization theory for calcification and its relationship to atherosclerosis. *Proceedings of the National Academy of Sciences USA, 68,* 810–814.
104. Kannel, W. B. (1997). Cardiovascular risk factors in the elderly. *Coronary Artery Diseases, 8,* 565–575.
105. Kannel, W. B., McGee, D., & Gordon, T. (1976). A general cardiovascular risk profile: The Framingham Study. *American Journal of Cardiology, 38,* 46–51.
106. Koenig, W. (2001). Inflammation and coronary heart disease: An overview. *Cardiology in Review, 9,* 31–35.
107. Libby, P., Ridker, P. M., & Maseri, A. (2002). Inflammation and atherosclerosis. *Circulation, 105,* 1135–1143.
108. Bozkurt, B., Kribbs, S. B., Clubb, F. J., Jr., et al. (1998). Pathophysiologically relevant concentrations of tumor necrosis factor-alpha promote progressive left ventricular dysfunction and remodeling in rats. *Circulation, 97,* 1382–1391.
109. Kubota, T., McTiernan, C. F., Frye, C. S., et al. (1997). Dilated cardiomyopathy in transgenic mice with cardiac-specific overexpression of tumor necrosis factor-alpha. *Circulation Research, 81,* 627–635.
110. Thaik, C. M., Calderone, A., Takahashi, N., et al. (1995). Interleukin-1 beta modulates the growth and phenotype of neonatal rat cardiac myocytes. *Journal of Clinical Investigations, 96,* 1093–1099.
111. Seta, Y., Shan, K., Bozkurt, B., et al. (1996). Basic mechanisms in heart failure: The cytokine hypothesis. *Journal of Cardiac Failure, 2,* 243–249.
112. Alexander, R. W. (1994). Inflammation and coronary artery disease. *New England Journal of Medicine, 331,* 468–469.
113. Tateyama, H., Hino, J., Minamino, N., et al. (1990). Characterization of immunoreactive brain natriuretic peptide in human cardiac atrium. *Biochemical and Biophysical Research Communications, 166,* 1080–1087.
114. MacGregor, A. S., Price, J. F., Hau, C. M., et al. (1999). Role of systolic blood pressure and plasma triglycerides in diabetic peripheral arterial disease. The Edinburgh Artery Study. *Diabetes Care, 22,* 453–458.
115. Hunt, P. J., Richards, A. M., Nicholls, M. G., et al. (1997). Immunoreactive amino-terminal pro-brain natriuretic peptide (NT-PROBNP): A new marker of cardiac impairment. *Clinical Endocrinology (Oxford), 47,* 287–296.
116. Dries, D. L., & Stevenson, L. W. (2000). Brain natriuretic peptide as bridge to therapy for heart failure. *Lancet, 355,* 1112–1113.
117. McDonagh, T. A., Cunningham, A. D., Morrison, C. E., et al. (2001). Left ventricular dysfunction, natriuretic peptides, and mortality in an urban population. *Heart, 86,* 21–26.
118. Richards, A. M., Nicholls, M. G., Yandle, T. G., et al. (1998). Plasma N-terminal pro-brain natriuretic peptide and adrenomedullin: New neurohormonal predictors of left ventricular function and prognosis after myocardial infarction. *Circulation, 97,* 1921–1929.
119. Richards, A. M., Nicholls, M. G., Yandle, T. G., et al. (1999). Neuroendocrine prediction of left ventricular function and heart failure after acute myocardial infarction. The Christchurch Cardioendocrine Research Group. *Heart, 81,* 114–120.
120. de Lemos, J. A., Morrow, D. A., Bentley, J. H., et al. (2001). The prognostic value of B-type natriuretic peptide in patients with acute coronary syndromes. *New England Journal of Medicine, 345,* 1014–1021.
121. McDonagh, T. A., Robb, S. D., Murdoch, D. R., et al. (1998). Biochemical detection of left-ventricular systolic dysfunction. *Lancet, 351,* 9–13.
122. Troughton, R. W., Frampton, C. M., Yandle, T. G., et al. (2000). Treatment of heart failure guided by plasma aminoterminal brain natriuretic peptide (N-BNP) concentrations. *Lancet, 355,* 1126–1130.
123. Wallen, T., Landahl, S., Hedner, T., et al. (1997). Brain natriuretic peptide predicts mortality in the elderly. *Heart, 77,* 264–267.
124. Cherian P., Hankey G. J., Eikelboom J. W., et al. (2003). Endothelial and platelet activation in acute ischemic stroke and its etiological subtypes. Stroke, 34, 2132–2137.
125. Jang, Y., Lincoff, A. M., Plow, E. F., et al. (1994). Cell adhesion molecules in coronary artery disease. *Journal of the American College of Cardiology, 24,* 1591–1601.
126. Luscinskas, F. W., & Gimbrone, M. A., Jr. (1996). Endothelial-dependent mechanisms in chronic inflammatory leukocyte recruitment. *Annual Review of Medicine, 47,* 413–421.
127. Springer, T. A. (1995). Traffic signals on endothelium for lymphocyte recirculation and leukocyte emigration. *Annual Review of Physiology, 57,* 827–872.

128. Blann, A. D., & McCollum, C. N. (1994). Circulating endothelial cell/leukocyte adhesion molecules in atherosclerosis. *Thrombosis and Haemostasis, 72*, 151–154.

129. Fukumoto, Y., Shimokawa, H., Ito, A., et al. (1997). Inflammatory cytokines cause coronary arteriosclerosis-like changes and alterations in the smooth-muscle phenotypes in pigs. *Journal of Cardiovascular Pharmacology, 29*, 222–231.

130. Pober, J. S., Bevilacqua, M. P., Mendrick, D. L., et al. (1986). Two distinct monokines, interleukin 1 and tumor necrosis factor, each independently induce biosynthesis and transient expression of the same antigen on the surface of cultured human vascular endothelial cells. *Journal of Immunology, 136*, 1680–1687.

131. Cybulsky, M. I., Iiyama, K., Li, H., et al. (2001). A major role for VCAM-1, but not ICAM-1, in early atherosclerosis. *Journal of Clinical Investigations, 107*, 1255–1262.

132. Davies, M. J., Richardson, P. D., Woolf, N., et al. (1993). Risk of thrombosis in human atherosclerotic plaques: Role of extracellular lipid, macrophage, and smooth muscle cell content. *British Heart Journal, 69*, 377–381.

133. Li, H., Cybulsky, M. I., Gimbrone, M. A., Jr., et al. (1993). Inducible expression of vascular cell adhesion molecule-1 by vascular smooth muscle cells in vitro and within rabbit atheroma. *American Journal of Pathology, 143*, 1551–1559.

134. Haught, W. H., Mansour, M., Rothlein, R., et al. (1996). Alterations in circulating intercellular adhesion molecule-1 and L-selectin: Further evidence for chronic inflammation in ischemic heart disease. *American Heart Journal, 132*, 1–8.

135. Hwang, S. J., Ballantyne, C. M., Sharrett, A. R., et al. (1997). Circulating adhesion molecules VCAM-1, ICAM-1, and E-selectin in carotid atherosclerosis and incident coronary heart disease cases: The Atherosclerosis Risk In Communities (ARIC) study. *Circulation, 96*, 4219–4225.

136. Ridker, P. M. (1998). C-reactive protein and risks of future myocardial infarction and thrombotic stroke. *European Heart Journal, 19*, 1–3.

137. Blankenberg, S., Rupprecht, H. J., Bickel, C., et al. (2001). Circulating cell adhesion molecules and death in patients with coronary artery disease. *Circulation, 104*, 1336–1342.

138. Miller, M. A., Sagnella, G. A., Kerry, S. M., et al. (2003). Ethnic differences in circulating soluble adhesion molecules: The Wandsworth Heart and Stroke Study. *Clinical Science (London), 104*, 591–598.

139. Lefkovits, J., Plow, E. F., & Topol, E. J. (1995). Platelet glycoprotein IIb/IIIa receptors in cardiovascular medicine. *New England Journal of Medicine, 332*, 1553–1559.

140. Lefkovits, J., & Topol, E. J. (1995). Platelet glycoprotein IIb/IIIa receptor inhibitors in ischemic heart disease. *Current Opinion in Cardiology, 10*, 420–426.

141. Ernst, E., & Resch, K. L. (1993). Fibrinogen as a cardiovascular risk factor: A meta-analysis and review of the literature. *Annals of Internal Medicine, 118*, 956–963.

142. Meade, T. W., Mellows, S., Brozovic, M., et al. (1986). Haemostatic function and ischaemic heart disease: Principal results of the Northwick Park Heart Study. *Lancet, 2*, 533–537.

143. Eber, B., & Schumacher, M. (1993). Fibrinogen: Its role in the hemostatic regulation in atherosclerosis. *Seminars in Thrombosis and Hemostasis, 19*, 104–107.

144. Smith, E. B. (1986). Fibrinogen, fibrin and fibrin degradation products in relation to atherosclerosis. *Clinical Haematology, 15*, 355–370.

145. Smith, E. B., Keen, G. A., Grant, A., et al. (1990). Fate of fibrinogen in human arterial intima. *Arteriosclerosis, 10*, 263–275.

146. Thompson, W. D., & Smith, E. B. (1989). Atherosclerosis and the coagulation system. *Journal of Pathology, 159*, 97–106.

147. Miyao, Y., Yasue, H., Ogawa, H., et al. (1993). Elevated plasma interleukin-6 levels in patients with acute myocardial infarction. *American Heart Journal, 126*, 1299–1304.

148. Danesh, J., Collins, R., Appleby P., et al. (1998). Association of fibrinogen, C-reactive protein, albumin, or leukocyte count with coronary heart disease: Meta-analyses of prospective studies. *Journal of the American Medical Association, 279*, 1477–1482.

149. Folsom, A. R., Aleksic, N., Ahn, C., et al. (2001). Beta-fibrinogen gene-455G/A polymorphism and coronary heart disease incidence: The Atherosclerosis Risk in Communities (ARIC) Study. *Annals of Epidemiology, 11*, 166–170.

150. Lee, A. J., Lowe, G. D., Woodward, M., et al. (1993). Fibrinogen in relation to personal history of prevalent hypertension, diabetes, stroke, intermittent claudication, coronary heart disease, and family history: The Scottish Heart Health Study. *British Heart Journal, 69*, 338–342.

151. Ma, J., Hennekens, C. H., Ridker, P. M., et al. (1999). A prospective study of fibrinogen and risk of myocardial infarction in the Physicians' Health Study. *Journal of the American College of Cardiology, 33*, 1347–1352.

152. Maresca, G., Di Blasio, A., Marchioli, R., et al. (1999). Measuring plasma fibrinogen to predict stroke and myocardial infarction: An update. *Arteriosclerosis, Thrombosis, and Vascular Biology, 19*, 1368–1377.

153. Sato, S., Nakamura, M., Iida, M., et al. (2000). Plasma fibrinogen and coronary heart disease in urban Japanese. *American Journal of Epidemiology, 152*, 420–423.

154. Tracy, R. P., Arnold, A. M., Ettinger, W., et al. (1999). The relationship of fibrinogen and factors VII and VIII to incident cardiovascular disease and death in the elderly: Results from the cardiovascular health study. *Arteriosclerosis, Thrombosis, and Vascular Biology, 19*, 1776–1783.

155. Tracy, R. P., Bovill, E. G., Yanez, D., et al. (1995). Fibrinogen and factor VIII, but not factor VII, are associated with measures of subclinical cardiovascular disease in the elderly. Results from The Cardiovascular Health Study. *Arteriosclerosis, Thrombosis, and Vascular Biology, 15*, 1269–1279.

156. Folsom, A. R., Rosamond, W. D., Shahar, E., et al. (1999). Prospective study of markers of hemostatic function with risk of ischemic stroke. The Atherosclerosis Risk in Communities (ARIC) Study Investigators. *Circulation, 100*, 736–742.

157. Smith, F. B., Lee, A. J., Fowkes, F. G., et al. (1997). Hemostatic factors as predictors of ischemic heart disease and stroke in the Edinburgh Artery Study. *Arteriosclerosis, Thrombosis, and Vascular Biology, 17*, 3321–3325.

158. Genest, J., Jr., & Cohn, J. S. (1995). Clustering of cardiovascular risk factors: Targeting high-risk individuals. *American Journal of Cardiology, 76*, 8A–20A.

159. Muldoon, M. F., Herbert, T. B., Patterson, S. M., et al. (1995). Effects of acute psychological stress on serum lipid levels, hemoconcentration, and blood viscosity. *Archives of Internal Medicine, 155*, 615–620.

160. Pepys, M. (1995). The acute phase response and c-reactive protein. *Oxford Textbook of Medicine*. Oxford, UK: Oxford University Press.

161. Ridker, P. M., Cushman, M., Stampfer, M. J., et al. (1997). Inflammation, aspirin, and the risk of cardiovascular disease in apparently healthy men. *New England Journal of Medicine, 336*, 973–979.

162. Ridker, P. M., Cushman, M., Stampfer, M. J., et al. (1998). Plasma concentration of C-reactive protein and risk of developing peripheral vascular disease. *Circulation, 97*, 425–428.

163. Ridker, P. M., Rifai, N., Clearfield, M., et al. (2001). Measurement of C-reactive protein for the targeting of statin therapy in the primary prevention of acute coronary events. *New England Journal of Medicine, 344*, 1959–1965.

164. Kuller, L. H., Tracy, R. P., Shaten, J., et al. (1996). Relation of C-reactive protein and coronary heart disease in the MRFIT nested case-control study. Multiple Risk Factor Intervention Trial. *American Journal of Epidemiology, 144*, 537–547.

165. Tracy, R. P., Lemaitre, R. N., Psaty, B. M., et al. (1997). Relationship of C-reactive protein to risk of cardiovascular disease in the elderly. Results from the Cardiovascular Health Study and the Rural Health Promotion Project. *Arteriosclerosis, Thrombosis, and Vascular Biology, 17*, 1121–1127.

166. Ridker, P. M., Buring, J. E., Shih, J., et al. (1998). Prospective study of C-reactive protein and the risk of future cardiovascular events among apparently healthy women. *Circulation, 98*, 731–733.

167. Koenig, W., Sund, M., Frohlich, M., et al. (1999). C-Reactive protein, a sensitive marker of inflammation, predicts future risk of coronary heart disease in initially healthy middle-aged men: Results from the MONICA (Monitoring Trends and Determinants in Cardiovascular Disease) Augsburg Cohort Study, 1984 to 1992. *Circulation, 99*, 237–242.

168. Roivainen, M., Viik-Kajander, M., Palosuo, T., et al. (2000). Infections, inflammation, and the risk of coronary heart disease. *Circulation, 101*, 252–257.

169. Ridker, P. M., Hennekens, C. H., Buring, J. E., et al. (2000). C-reactive protein and other markers of inflammation in the prediction of cardiovascular disease in women. *New England Journal of Medicine, 342*, 836–843.

170. Biasucci, L. M., Liuzzo, G., Buffon, A., et al. (1999). The variable role of inflammation in acute coronary syndromes and in restenosis. *Seminars in Interventional Cardiology, 4*, 105–110.

171. de Winter, R. J., Bholasingh, R., Lijmer, J. G., et al. (1999). Independent prognostic value of C-reactive protein and troponin I in patients with unstable angina or non-Q-wave myocardial infarction. *Cardiovascular Research, 42*, 240–245.

172. Liuzzo, G., Biasucci, L. M., Gallimore, J. R., et al. (1994). The prognostic value of C-reactive protein and serum amyloid a protein in severe unstable angina. *New England Journal of Medicine, 331*, 417–424.
173. Sacks, F. M., Pfeffer, M. A., Moye, L. A., et al. (1996). The effect of pravastatin on coronary events after myocardial infarction in patients with average cholesterol levels. Cholesterol and Recurrent Events Trial investigators. *New England Journal of Medicine, 335*, 1001–1009.
174. Pearson, T. A., Mensah, G. A., Alexander, R. W., et al. (2003). Markers of inflammation and cardiovascular disease: Application to clinical and public health practice: A statement for healthcare professionals from the Centers for Disease Control and Prevention and the American Heart Association. *Circulation, 107*, 499–511.
175. Folsom, A. R., Pankow, J. S., Tracy, R. P., et al. (2001). Association of C-reactive protein with markers of prevalent atherosclerotic disease. *American Journal of Cardiology, 88*, 112–117.
176. Yu, H., & Rifai, N. (2000). High-sensitivity C-reactive protein and atherosclerosis: From theory to therapy. *Clinical Biochemistry, 33*, 601–610.
177. McCully, K. S. (1969). Vascular pathology of homocysteinemia: Implications for the pathogenesis of arteriosclerosis. *American Journal of Pathology, 56*, 111–128.
178. Boushey, C. J., Beresford, S. A., Omenn, G. S., et al. (1995). A quantitative assessment of plasma homocysteine as a risk factor for vascular disease. Probable benefits of increasing folic acid intakes. *Journal of the American Medical Association, 274*, 1049–1057.
179. Christen, W. G., Ajani, U. A., Glynn, R. J., et al. (2000). Blood levels of homocysteine and increased risks of cardiovascular disease: Causal or casual? *Archives of Internal Medicine, 160*, 422–434.
180. Tsai, J. C., Perrella, M. A., Yoshizumi, M., et al. (1994). Promotion of vascular smooth muscle cell growth by homocysteine: A link to atherosclerosis. *Proceedings of the National Academy of Sciences USA, 91*, 6369–6373.
181. El-Khairy, L., Ueland, P. M., Nygard, O., et al. (1999). Lifestyle and cardiovascular disease risk factors as determinants of total cysteine in plasma: The Hordaland Homocysteine Study. *American Journal of Clinical Nutrition, 70*, 1016–1024.
182. Lowering blood homocysteine with folic acid based supplements: Meta-analysis of randomised trials. Homocysteine Lowering Trialists' Collaboration. (1998). *BMJ, 316*, 894–898.
183. Eikelboom, J. W., Lonn, E., Genest, J., Jr., et al. (1999). Homocyst(e)ine and cardiovascular disease: A critical review of the epidemiologic evidence. *Annals of Internal Medicine, 131*, 363–375.
184. Shipchandler, M. T., & Moore, E. G. (1995). Rapid, fully automated measurement of plasma homocyst(e)ine with the Abbott IMx analyzer. *Clinical Chemistry, 41*, 991–994.
185. Zighetti, M. L., Chantarangkul, V., Tripodi, A., et al. (2002). Determination of total homocysteine in plasma: Comparison of the Abbott IMx immunoassay with high performance liquid chromatography. *Haematologica, 87*, 89–94.
186. Van Snick, J. (1990). Interleukin-6: An overview. *Annual Review of Immunology, 8*, 253–278.
187. Baumann, H., & Gauldie, J. (1990). Regulation of hepatic acute phase plasma protein genes by hepatocyte stimulating factors and other mediators of inflammation. *Molecular Biology/Medicine, 7*, 147–159.
188. Mestries, J. C., Kruithof, E. K., Gascon, M. P., et al. (1994). In vivo modulation of coagulation and fibrinolysis by recombinant glycosylated human interleukin-6 in baboons. *European Cytokine Network, 5*, 275–281.
189. Loppnow, H., & Libby, P. (1989). Adult human vascular endothelial cells express the IL6 gene differentially in response to LPS or IL1. *Cell Immunology, 122*, 493–503.
190. Loppnow, H., & Libby, P. (1989). Comparative analysis of cytokine induction in human vascular endothelial and smooth muscle cells. *Lymphokine Research, 8*, 293–299.
191. Rus, H. G., Vlaicu, R., & Niculescu, F. (1996). Interleukin-6 and interleukin-8 protein and gene expression in human arterial atherosclerotic wall. *Atherosclerosis, 127*, 263–271.
192. Herity, N. A. (2000). Interleukin 6: A message from the heart. *Heart, 84*, 9–10.
193. Mohamed-Ali, V., Goodrick, S., Rawesh, A., et al. (1997). Subcutaneous adipose tissue releases interleukin-6, but not tumor necrosis factor-alpha, in vivo. *Journal of Clinical Endocrinology & Metabolism, 82*, 4196–4200.
194. Hotamisligil, G. S., Murray, D. L., Choy, L. N., et al. (1994). Tumor necrosis factor alpha inhibits signaling from the insulin receptor. *Proceedings of the National Academy of Sciences USA, 91*, 4854–4858.
195. Hardardottir, I., Moser, A. H., Memon, R., et al. (1994). Effects of TNF, IL-1, and the combination of both cytokines on cholesterol metabolism in Syrian hamsters. *Lymphokine & Cytokine Research, 13*, 161–166.
196. van der Poll, T., van Deventer, S. J., Pasterkamp, G., et al. (1992). Tumor necrosis factor induces von Willebrand factor release in healthy humans. *Thrombosis and Haemostasis, 67*, 623–626.
197. Yudkin, J. S., Kumari, M., Humphries, S. E., et al. (2000). Inflammation, obesity, stress and coronary heart disease: Is interleukin-6 the link? *Atherosclerosis, 148*, 209–214.
198. Ridker, P. M., Rifai, N., Stampfer, M. J., et al. (2000). Plasma concentration of interleukin-6 and the risk of future myocardial infarction among apparently healthy men. *Circulation, 101*, 1767–1772.
199. Volpato, S., Guralnik, J. M., Ferrucci, L., et al. (2001). Cardiovascular disease, interleukin-6, and risk of mortality in older women: The women's health and aging study. *Circulation, 103*, 947–953.
200. Harris, T. B., Ferrucci, L., Tracy, R. P., et al. (1999). Associations of elevated interleukin-6 and C-reactive protein levels with mortality in the elderly. *American Journal of Medicine, 106*, 506–512.
201. Mendall, M. A., Patel, P., Asante, M., et al. (1997). Relation of serum cytokine concentrations to cardiovascular risk factors and coronary heart disease. *Heart, 78*, 273–277.
202. Biasucci, L. M., Vitelli, A., Liuzzo, G., et al. (1996). Elevated levels of interleukin-6 in unstable angina. *Circulation, 94*, 874–877.
203. Biasucci, L. M., Liuzzo, G., Fantuzzi, G., et al. (1999). Increasing levels of interleukin (IL)-1Ra and IL-6 during the first 2 days of hospitalization in unstable angina are associated with increased risk of in-hospital coronary events. *Circulation, 99*, 2079–2084.
204. Biasucci, L. M., Liuzzo, G., Grillo, R. L., et al. (1999). Elevated levels of C-reactive protein at discharge in patients with unstable angina predict recurrent instability. *Circulation, 99*, 855–860.
205. Malle, E., & De Beer, F. C. (1996). Human serum amyloid A (SAA) protein: A prominent acute-phase reactant for clinical practice. *European Journal of Clinical Investigations, 26*, 427–435.
206. Benditt, E. P., Lagunoff, D., Eriksen, N., et al. (1962). Amyloid. Extraction and preliminary characterization of some proteins. *Archives of Pathology, 74*, 323–330.
207. Gabay, C., & Kushner, I. (1999). Acute-phase proteins and other systemic responses to inflammation. *New England Journal of Medicine, 340*, 448–454.
208. Banka, C. L., Yuan, T., de Beer, M. C., et al. (1995). Serum amyloid A (SAA): Influence on HDL-mediated cellular cholesterol efflux. *Journal Lipid Research, 36*, 1058–1065.
209. Yamada, T., Kakihara, T., Kamishima, T., et al. (1996). Both acute phase and constitutive serum amyloid A are present in atherosclerotic lesions. *Pathology International, 46*, 797–800.
210. Kisilevsky, R., & Subrahmanyan, L. (1992). Serum amyloid A changes high density lipoprotein's cellular affinity. A clue to serum amyloid A's principal function. *Laboratory Investment, 66*, 778–785.
211. Coetzee, G. A., Strachan, A. F., van der Westhuyzen, D. R., et al. (1986). Serum amyloid A-containing human high density lipoprotein 3. Density, size, and apolipoprotein composition. *Journal of Biology and Chemistry, 261*, 9644–9651.
212. Steinmetz, A., Hocke, G., Saile, R., et al. (1989). Influence of serum amyloid A on cholesterol esterification in human plasma. *Biochimica Biophysica Acta, 1006*, 173–178.
213. Brinckerhoff, C. E., Mitchell, T. I., Karmilowicz, M. J., et al. (1989). Autocrine induction of collagenase by serum amyloid A-like and beta 2-microglobulin-like proteins. *Science, 243*, 655–657.
214. Migita, K., Kawabe, Y., Tominagam, M., et al. (1998). Serum amyloid A protein induces production of matrix metalloproteinases by human synovial fibroblasts. *Laboratory Investment, 78*, 535–539.
215. Shainkin-Kestenbaum, R., Zimlichman, S., Lis, M., et al. (1996). Modulation of prostaglandin I2 production from bovine aortic endothelial cells by serum amyloid A and its N-terminal tetradecapeptide. *Biomedical Peptides, Proteins and Nucleic Acids, 2*, 101–106.
216. Syversen, P. V., Saeter, U., Cunha-Ribeiro, L., et al. (1994). The effect of serum amyloid protein A fragment-SAA25-76 on blood platelet aggregation. *Thrombosis Research, 76*, 299–305.
217. Zimlichman, S., Danon, A., Nathan, I., et al. (1990). Serum amyloid A, an acute phase protein, inhibits platelet activation. *Journal of Laboratory and Clinical Medicine, 116*, 180–186.
218. Cushman, M., Lemaitre, R. N., Kuller, L. H., et al. (1999). Fibrinolytic activation markers predict myocardial infarction in the elderly. The Cardiovascular Health Study. *Arteriosclerosis, Thrombosis, and Vascular Biology, 19*, 493–498.

219. Haverkate, F., Thompson, S. G., Pyke, S. D., et al. (1997). Production of C-reactive protein and risk of coronary events in stable and unstable angina. European Concerted Action on Thrombosis and Disabilities Angina Pectoris Study Group. *Lancet, 349*, 462–466.
220. Morrow, D. A., Rifai, N., Antman, E. M., et al. (1998). C-reactive protein is a potent predictor of mortality independently of and in combination with troponin T in acute coronary syndromes: A TIMI 11A substudy. Thrombolysis in Myocardial Infarction. *Journal of the American College of Cardiology, 31*, 1460–1465.
221. Ruggeri, Z. M. (1997). von Willebrand factor. *Journal of Clinical Investigations, 99*, 559–564.
222. Ruggeri, Z. M. (1992). von Willebrand factor as a target for antithrombotic intervention. *Circulation, 86*, III26–III29.
223. Folsom, A. R. (2001). Hemostatic risk factors for atherothrombotic disease: An epidemiologic view. *Thrombosis and Haemostasis, 86*, 366–373.
224. Meade, T. W., Cooper, J. A., Stirling, Y., et al. (1994). Factor VIII, ABO blood group and the incidence of ischaemic heart disease. *British Journal of Haematology, 88*, 601–607.
225. Rumley, A., Lowe, G. D., Sweetnam, P. M., et al. (1999). Factor VIII, von Willebrand factor and the risk of major ischaemic heart disease in the Caerphilly Heart Study. *British Journal of Haematology, 105*, 110–116.
226. Jansson, J. H., Nilsson, T. K., & Johnson, O. (1991). von Willebrand factor in plasma: A novel risk factor for recurrent myocardial infarction and death. *British Heart Journal, 66*, 351–355.
227. Thogersen, A. M., Jansson, J. H., Boman, K., et al. (1998). High plasminogen activator inhibitor and tissue plasminogen activator levels in plasma precede a first acute myocardial infarction in both men and women: Evidence for the fibrinolytic system as an independent primary risk factor. *Circulation*, 98, 2241–2247.
228. Dankner, R., Goldbourt, U., Boyko, V., et al. (2003). Predictors of cardiac and noncardiac mortality among 14,697 patients with coronary heart disease. *American Journal of Cardiology, 91*, 121–127.
229. Carter, K. W., Hung, J., Powell, B. L., et al. (2008). Association of Interleukin-1 gene polymorphisms with central obesity and metabolic syndrome in a coronary heart disease population. *Human Genetics, 124*(3), 199–206.
230. Qasim, A. N., Metkus, T. S., Tadesse, M., et al. (2008). Resistin gene variation is associated with systemic inflammation but not plasma adipokine levels, metabolic syndrome or coronary atherosclerosis in non-diabetic Caucasians. *Clinical Endocrinology (Oxford)*. Epub ahead of print.
231. Harrap, S. B., Zammit, K. S., Wong, Z. Y., et al. (2002). Genome-wide linkage analysis of the acute coronary syndrome suggests a locus on chromosome 2. *Arteriosclerosis, Thrombosis, and Vascular Biology, 22*, 874–878.
232. Tang, W., Miller, M. B., Rich, S. S., et al. (2003). Linkage analysis of a composite factor for the multiple metabolic syndrome: The National Heart, Lung, and Blood Institute Family Heart Study. *Diabetes, 52*, 2840–2847.
233. Connelly, J. J., Shah, S. H., Doss, J. F., et al. (2008). Genetic and functional association of FAM5C with myocardial infarction. *BMC Medical Genetics, 9*, 33.
234. Ozdemir, O., Gundogdu, F., Karakelleoglu, S., et al. (2008). Comparison of serum levels of inflammatory markers and allelic variant of interleukin-6 in patients with acute coronary syndrome and stable angina pectoris. *Coronary Artery Diseases, 19*, 15–19.
235. Iakoubova, O. A., Sabatine, M. S., Rowland, C. M., et al. (2008). Polymorphism in KIF6 gene and benefit from statins after acute coronary syndromes: Results from the PROVE IT-TIMI 22 study. *Journal of the American College of Cardiology, 51*, 449–455.
236. Braunwald, E., Antman, E. M., Beasley, J. W., et al. (2000). ACC/AHA guidelines for the management of patients with unstable angina and non-ST-segment elevation myocardial infarction. A report of the American College of Cardiology/American Heart Association Task Force on Practice Guidelines (Committee on the Management of Patients With Unstable Angina). *Journal of the American College of Cardiology, 36*, 970–1062.
237. Dispersyn, G. D., & Borgers, M. (2001). Apoptosis in the heart: About programmed cell death and survival. *News in Physiological Sciences, 16*, 41–47.
238. Isner, J. M., Kearney, M., Bortman, S., et al. (1995). Apoptosis in human atherosclerosis and restenosis. *Circulation, 91*, 2703–2711.
239. Asano, G., Takashi, E., Ishiwata, T., et al. (2003). Pathogenesis and protection of ischemia and reperfusion injury in myocardium. *Journal of Nippon Medical School, 70*, 384–392.
240. Marczin, N., El-Habashi, N., Hoare, G. S., et al. (2003). Antioxidants in myocardial ischemia-reperfusion injury: Therapeutic potential and basic mechanisms. *Archives of Biochemistry and Biophysics, 420*, 222–236.
241. Kaur, J., Woodman, R. C., & Kubes, P. (2003). P38 MAPK: Critical molecule in thrombin-induced NF-kappa B-dependent leukocyte recruitment. *American Journal of Physiology, Heart and Circulatory Physiology, 284*, H1095–H1103.
242. Squadrito, F., Deodato, B., Squadrito, G., et al. (2003). Gene transfer of IkappaBalpha limits infarct size in a mouse model of myocardial ischemia-reperfusion injury. *Laboratory Investment, 83*, 1097–1104.
243. Kubes, P., Payne, D., & Ostrovsky, L. (1998). Preconditioning and adenosine in I/R-induced leukocyte-endothelial cell interactions. *American Journal of Physiology, 274*, H1230–H1238.
244. Hein, T. W., Zhang, C., Wang, W., et al. (2003). Ischemia-reperfusion selectively impairs nitric oxide-mediated dilation in coronary arterioles: Counteracting role of arginase. *FASEB Journal, 17*, 2328–2330.
245. Yue, T. L., Bao, W., Jucker, B. M., et al. (2003). Activation of peroxisome proliferator-activated receptor-alpha protects the heart from ischemia/reperfusion injury. *Circulation, 108*, 2393–2399.
246. Kloner, R. A. (1993). Does reperfusion injury exist in humans? *Journal of the American College of Cardiology, 21*, 537–545.
247. Feigl, E. O. (1998). Neural control of coronary blood flow. *Journal of Vascular Research, 35*, 85–92.
248. Antman, E. M., Tanasijevic, M. J., Thompson, B., et al. (1996). Cardiac-specific troponin I levels to predict the risk of mortality in patients with acute coronary syndromes. *New England Journal of Medicine, 335*, 1342–1349.
249. Brogan, G. X., Jr., Vuori, J., Friedman, S., et al. (1996). Improved specificity of myoglobin plus carbonic anhydrase assay versus that of creatine kinase-MB for early diagnosis of acute myocardial infarction. *Annals of Emergency Medicine, 27*, 22–28.
250. Pierard, L. A. (2003). Assessing perfusion and function in acute myocardial infarction: How and when? *Heart, 89*, 701–703.
251. Namiki, A., Kubota, T., Fukazawa, M., et al. (2003). Endothelin-1 concentrations in pericardial fluid are more elevated in patients with ischemic heart disease than in patients with nonischemic heart disease. *Japan Heart Journal, 44*, 633–644.
252. Jugdutt, B. I. (2003). Ventricular remodeling after infarction and the extracellular collagen matrix: When is enough enough? *Circulation, 108*, 1395–1403.
253. Pfeffer, M. A. (1995). Left ventricular remodeling after acute myocardial infarction. *Annual Review of Medicine, 46*, 455–466.
254. Ren, G., Dewald, O., & Frangogiannis, N. G. (2003). Inflammatory mechanisms in myocardial infarction. *Current Drug Targets – Inflammation and Allergy, 2*, 242–256.
255. Ferroni, P., Basili, S., Martini, F., et al. (2003). Serum metalloproteinase 9 levels in patients with coronary artery disease: A novel marker of inflammation. *Journal of Investigation Medicine, 51*, 295–300.
256. Klein, R. F., Troyer, W. G., Thompson, H. K., et al. (1968). Catecholamine excretion in myocardial infarction. *Archives of Internal Medicine, 122*, 476–482.
257. Gershlick, A. H., & More, R. S. (1998). Treatment of myocardial infarction. *BMJ, 316*, 280–284.
258. Galcera-Tomas, J., Castillo-Soria, F. J., Villegas-Garcia, M. M., et al. (2001). Effects of early use of atenolol or captopril on infarct size and ventricular volume: A double-blind comparison in patients with anterior acute myocardial infarction. *Circulation, 103*, 813–819.
259. McDonough, J. L., Labugger, R., Pickett, W., et al. (2001). Cardiac troponin I is modified in the myocardium of bypass patients. *Circulation, 103*, 58–64.
260. Ishikawa, T., Hatakeyama, K., Imamura, T., et al. (2003). Involvement of C-reactive protein obtained by directional coronary atherectomy in plaque instability and developing restenosis in patients with stable or unstable angina pectoris. *American Journal of Cardiology, 91*, 287–292.
261. Dollery, C. M., McEwan, J. R., & Henney, A. M. (1995). Matrix metalloproteinases and cardiovascular disease. *Circulation Research, 77*, 863–868.

CHAPTER 6 Hematopoiesis, Coagulation, and Bleeding

Nancy Munro

The physiological functions of blood include nutrition, oxygenation, respiration, and excretion. These various components of blood accomplish these functions. Approximately 55% of blood volume is composed of plasma, which is a transport medium for ions, proteins, hormones, and end products of cellular metabolism. The most important ions carried in the plasma are sodium, potassium, chloride, hydrogen, magnesium, and calcium. Examples of proteins transported in the plasma are immunoglobulins and the coagulation proteins. Formed elements or cells including red blood cells (RBC; erythrocytes), white blood cells (WBC; leukocytes), and platelets (thrombocytes) constitute the other 45% of blood volume. Erythrocytes transport oxygen to the tissues and carbon dioxide to the lungs for excretion. Leukocytes protect against infection and play a major role in the inflammatory process. Thrombocytes, along with coagulation proteins, protect against blood loss through the formation of blood clots.[1]

Because these functions are vital, a significant blood loss has devastating consequences for all body tissues. A complex series of events leading to hemostasis achieves protection against such blood losses and potential exsanguination from injuries. The endothelium of the vasculature plays a vital role in the coagulation process and is now considered an organ by the Margaux III Conference on Critical Illness: The Endothelium: An Underrecognized Organ in Critical Illness.[2] The endothelial cell participates by releasing mediators that effect coagulation and the role of the vessel's participation in hemostasis. The equally complex mechanism of fibrinolysis, which dissolves clots, balances this system. Normal blood flow through the vasculature depends partly on the balance of these two systems, hemostasis and fibrinolysis. Recent research has also revealed a link between coagulation and the inflammatory process that has caused the scientific community to re-examine the process of atherosclerosis.[3] Knowledge of these normal processes is important as a basis for understanding the many alterations that may result from disease states or drug administration.

HEMATOPOIETIC CELLS

Hematopoiesis, or the production of blood cells, occurs primarily in the bone marrow. The liver, spleen, lymph nodes, and thymus are involved in hematopoiesis during embryonic life, but after birth extramedullary (outside the bone marrow) hematopoiesis occurs only during abnormal circumstances. If it occurs at all after birth, extramedullary hematopoiesis occurs mainly in the liver and spleen. The hematopoietic stem cell resides mainly in the bone marrow and in small numbers in the peripheral blood. The hematopoietic stem cell is the source of all the types of blood cells: RBC, WBC, and platelets.

The stem cell is an immature (undifferentiated) cell that has the capacity to reproduce itself and to mature (differentiate) into any of the different types of blood cells. As the stem cell divides and matures, it differentiates into one of two committed cell lines: lymphoid or myeloid progenitor cells. The committed lymphoid progenitor cell eventually matures into T and B lymphocytes and natural killer cells. The committed myeloid stem progenitor cell develops into (1) the megakaryocyte–erthrocyte precursors leading to the development of platelets and RBC and (2) the granulocyte–monocyte precursors leading to the development of the granulocyte and monocyte.[4] Maturation of these cell lines is influenced by multiple growth factors such as granulocyte colony-stimulating factor, erythropoietin, thrombopoietin, interleukins, interferon, and many others.[4] As the various types of blood cells mature, they are released into the peripheral circulation. Figure 6-1 shows a model for hematopoietic cell differentiation.

Red Blood Cells

The major role of the RBC is respiration, which is the exchange of gases. The mature RBC is a biconcave disc filled with hemoglobin but it does not have a nucleus. The lack of a nucleus allows the RBC to change shape and facilitates movement through small capillary beds. Heme, the iron-containing pigment, is the actual oxygen-transporting portion of the hemoglobin molecule. Oxygen diffuses from the alveoli into the alveolar capillaries and binds to each of four to five sites on the heme portion of hemoglobin. One gram of hemoglobin can carry 1.34 to 1.36 milliliters of oxygen. The remarkable oxygen-binding capacity of the RBC is influenced by three factors that affect the oxyhemoglobin dissociation curve: pH, temperature, and the amount of 2,3-diphosphogylcerate (see Chapter 2). Tissue metabolism produces carbon dioxide as a waste product that is also transported from the tissues by the RBC. Carbon dioxide diffuses into the RBC and combines with water to form carbonic acid that further dissociates to the hydrogen and bicarbonate ions. The bicarbonate ion is inactivated when combined with hydrogen ions to again form water and carbon dioxide, which is eliminated at the alveoli.

The rate of bone marrow stem cell differentiation into erythrocytes is primarily controlled by erythropoietin. Most of this hormone is produced by the kidney. The creation of RBC is influenced by the oxygen content of the blood as sensed by the kidneys. Production also requires necessary substrates including vitamin B_{12}, vitamin B_6, folic acid, and iron. The vitamins and folic acid are obtained from dietary sources, as is iron. However, most iron is gained through the recycling of the RBC in the spleen. RBC production is increased at times of blood loss, at high altitude, and in pulmonary diseases that affect the transport of oxygen from the lungs to the blood. It takes approximately 3 to 5 days for RBC to

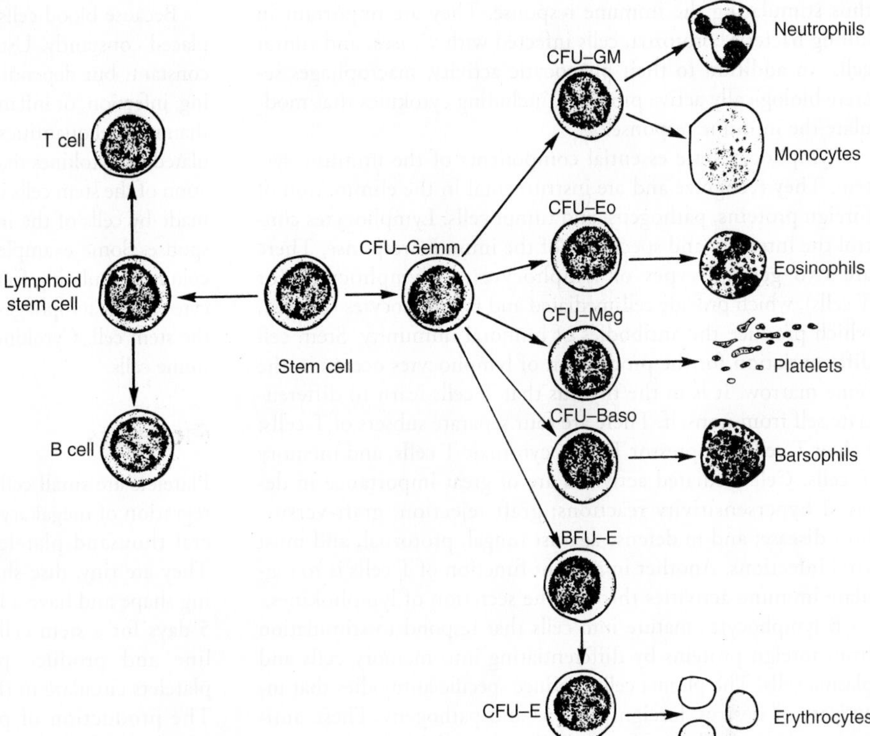

■ **Figure 6-1** The hematopoietic hierarchy. As hematopoietic stem cells divide, they give rise to common lymphoid and common myeloid precursor cells that eventually generate all mature blood lineages of the body. LT-HSC, long-term hematopoietic stem cells; GMP, granulocyte-monocyte precursors; MEP, megakaryocyte–erythrocyte precursors; NK, natural killer; ST-HSC, short-term hematopoietic stem cells. (Reproduced with permission from Hoffman, R., Benz, E., Shattil, S., et al. (2005). *Hematology: Basic principles and practice*. Philadelphia: Elsevier–Churchill-Livingstone.)

mature in the marrow and be released into the peripheral circulation. RBCs live approximately 120 days, at which time they are recycled by the spleen.

White Blood Cells

WBC can be divided into two major categories: phagocytes and lymphocytes. The primary role of phagocytes is to locate and kill invading microorganisms or foreign antigens. The primary role of lymphocytes is to initiate and direct the immune response including the manufacture of antibodies. WBC travel throughout the body and will migrate into different tissues depending on chemical mediators that signal the cells. Phagocytes perform their role primarily out in the tissues, where they travel toward the site of an inflammation (chemotaxis) and kill microbes by engulfing them (phagocytosis). Many substances, including complement fragments and bacterial products, stimulate this chemotactic migration. Phagocytosis is an active process that uses energy derived from anaerobic glycolysis. Phagocytic cells are divided into two subgroups: granulocytes (granular substances within the cell after staining) and monocytes. The granulocytes include neutrophils ("polys"), basophils, and eosinophils. Neutrophils compose 60% to 70% of all WBC. Neutrophil maturation in the marrow takes 7 to 10 days. Their main function is to find and kill bacteria, especially resident microorganisms such as staphylococci and Gram-negative enteric flora.[1] They also play an important role in acute inflammatory processes. Neutrophils are one of the first phagocytic cells to appear at the site of an acute inflammation. During severe inflammatory reactions, neutrophils can actually cause damage to surrounding tissues by releasing proteolytic enzymes and oxygen-free radicals. Once in the bloodstream, some of the neutrophils freely circulate while others linger along the blood vessel wall, which is called margination. Adhesion molecules emanating from an injury or from an organism make the blood vessel wall sticky; so that the marginated neutrophils adhere to the vessel walls. The neutrophil releases substances that allow the endothelial cells to separate and permit the neutrophil to crawl into the connective tissue (diapedesis). The neutrophil migrates to the area of injury through chemotaxis. The migration of neutrophils to the tissues takes place rapidly, within 12 hours on entering the bloodstream. Once in the bloodstream, the neutrophil must be able to differentiate cells or substances that are foreign. Opsonization is a process in which molecules in the plasma coat the microorganism, making it more recognizable to the neutrophil.

Esosinophils and basophils are WBC that have specific functions that are also important in the defense of the body. Eosinophils compose approximately 4% of a normal WBC count. Eosinophils have been postulated to play a defensive role against parasites and allergic reactions. Basophils account for only 0.5% to 1% of the total WBC count. Agranular leukocytes are WBC without granular substances within the cells after staining. Monocytes and lymphocytes are agranular leukocytes. Monocytes constitute 4% to 8% of the total WBC count. Within 24 to 36 hours of entering the circulation, they migrate into the tissues where they undergo further maturation and are called macrophages. Hepatic Kupffer cells, alveolar macrophages, and peritoneal macrophages are examples of tissue macrophages. Once lodged in their target organ, macrophages can live for up to 60 days. In the bloodstream, monocytes have similar functions to the neutrophil. However, in addition, monocytes and macrophages play a crucial role in recognizing foreign invaders and presenting foreign antigens to lymphocytes, thus stimulating the immune response. They are important in killing bacteria, protozoa, cells infected with viruses, and tumor cells. In addition to their phagocytic activity, macrophages secrete biologically active products, including cytokines that modulate the immune response.

Lymphocytes are essential components of the immune system. They recognize and are instrumental in the elimination of foreign proteins, pathogens, and tumor cells. Lymphocytes control the intensity and specificity of the immune response. There are two general types of lymphocytes, T lymphocytes (or T cells), which provide cell-mediated and B lymphocytes (B cells), which produce the antibodies of humoral immunity. Stem cell differentiation for the production of lymphocytes occurs in the bone marrow. It is in the thymus that T cells learn to differentiate self from nonself. There are four separate subsets of T cells: helper T cells, suppressor T cells, cytotoxic T cells, and memory T cells. Cell-mediated activities are of great importance in delayed hypersensitivity reactions; graft rejection; graft-versus-host disease; and in defense against fungal, protozoal, and most viral infections. Another important function of T cells is to regulate immune activities through the secretion of lymphokines.

B lymphocytes mature into cells that respond to stimulation from foreign proteins by differentiating into memory cells and plasma cells. The plasma cells produce specific antibodies that inactivate or destroy foreign proteins and pathogens. These antibodies are particularly effective against bacterial infections, especially encapsulated bacteria, such as pneumococci, streptococci, meningococci, and hemophilus influenzae, as well as certain viruses. The helper cells of the T cells stimulate B cells to produce antibodies. Natural killer cells, another subset of lymphocytes, kill tumor cells and cells infected by viruses. They play an important role in tumor surveillance. The activities of phagocytes and immune cells overlap in numerous mutually beneficial ways. For example, immune cells often participate in chronic inflammatory reactions. Conversely, engulfment of foreign protein by macrophages is a preparatory step leading to antibody production. Table 6-1 summarizes the WBC and their function.

Table 6-1 ■ WHITE BLOOD CELLS

Name	Function
WBC or leukocyte	Combat pathogens and other foreign substances that enter the body
Granular Leukocytes	
Neutrophils	Phagocytosis or the destruction of bacteria with lysozyme, defensins, and strong oxidants
Eosinophils	Combat the effects of histamine in allergic reactions, phagocytize antigen–antibody complexes
Basophils	Liberate heparin, histamine, and serotonin in allergic reactions that intensify the overall inflammatory response
Agranular Leukocytes	
Lymphocytes (T cells, B cells, natural killer cells)	Mediate immune responses including antigen–antibody reactions
Monocytes	Phagocytosis after transforming into macrophages

Adapted from Tortora, G., & Grabowski, S. (2003). *Principles of anatomy and physiology*. New York: John Wiley & Sons, Inc.

Because blood cells have a limited lifespan, they need to be replaced constantly. Usually, the number of cells produced is fairly constant, but depending on environmental stimuli such as bleeding, infection, or inflammation various cells may be needed in larger than normal quantities at times. Thus, each of these cell lines is regulated by cytokines that influence the rate of growth and differentiation of the stem cells in the marrow. Cytokines are proteins that are made by cells of the immune system and regulate the immune response. Some examples of cytokines are granulocyte–macrophage colony-stimulating factor, which stimulates the growth of granulocytes and macrophages, and interleukin-3 (IL-3), which stimulates the stem cell. Cytokines also stimulate the function of mature immune cells.

Platelets

Platelets are small cell fragments that are produced by the disintegration of megakaryocytes in the bone marrow, producing several thousand platelets that are released into the circulation. They are tiny, disc-shaped fragments that are capable of changing shape and have a high metabolic rate. It takes approximately 5 days for a stem cell to differentiate along the megakaryocyte line and produce platelets. Under normal circumstances, platelets circulate in the bloodstream for approximately 10 days. The production of platelets is regulated by thrombopoietin, which is a humoral hormone-like substance. Platelets are also called thrombocytes, which means *clot cell.* They play a major role in hemostasis by adhering to a damaged blood vessel wall and aggregating together to form a mechanical barrier to the flow of blood thereby preventing blood loss. Platelets will then release various mediators to attract other cells and components to the site so that fibrin formation can start. There are three storage granules in the platelets: alpha granules, dense bodies, and lysomes. Alpha granules contain and release fibrinogen. Dense bodies release adenine nucleotides, serotonin, and platelet factor 4 (PF4). Lysomes contain degradative acid hydrolases.[1] Platelets are sequestered in the spleen and are released as needed to combat bleeding. Their function is vital to the coagulation process, so much so that many cardiac interventions are now aimed at disabling platelet function.

Coagulation Factors

The major component of blood, plasma, contains many particles including proteins (clotting factors) that are involved in coagulation. To standardize the identification of these proteins, an international committee assigned a nomenclature for these proteins using Roman numerals listed in order of their discovery. However, the order does not refer to the sequence of reactions in the coagulation cascade. A lowercase "a" is also used to indicate the activated form of a clotting factor. Table 6-2 lists these clotting factors. The liver plays a significant role in maintaining adequate amounts of these clotting factors, because it is the primary site of protein synthesis. Tissue thromboplastin, or tissue factor (III), is an exception that can be found in most body tissues, especially around vessels and organs. Antihemophilic factor (VIII) is a factor that is synthesized in the endothelial cells. It is also important to recognize that there are multiple enzymes and mediators that play key roles in the activation of these clotting factors. Synthesis of factors II, VII, IX, and X requires vitamin K to be present, and these are known as vitamin K-dependent factors. Calcium is also a coagulation factor

Table 6-2 ■ BLOOD COAGULATION PROTEINS

Number	Name(s)
I	Fibrinogen
II	Prothrombin
III	Tissue factor (thromboplastin)
IV	Calcium ions
V	Proaccelerin, labile factor, or accelerator globulin (AcG)
VII	Serum prothrombin conversion accelerator (SPCA), stable factor, or proconvertin
VIII	Antihemophilic factor (AHF), antihemophilic factor A, or antihemophilic globulin (AHG)
IX	Christmas factor, plasma thromboplastin component (PTC), or anthemophilic factor B
X	Stuart factor, prower factor, or thrombokinase
XI	Plasma thromboplastin antecedent (PTA) or antihemophilic factor C
XII	Hageman factor, glass factor, contact factor, or antihemophilic factor D
XIII	Fibrin-stabilizing factor (FSF)

Adapted from Tortora, G., & Grabowski, S. (2003). *Principles of Anatomy and Physiology*. New York: John Wiley & Sons, Inc.

whose role can be underestimated. To balance the coagulation process, there are also a number of proteins and systems that will inhibit coagulation including antithrombin III, proteins C and S, as well as components of the fibrinolytic cascade. The interaction of all these proteins in a chemical sequence will produce a clot to repair blood vessels and then dissolve the clot so that normal flow can be restored.

HEMOSTASIS

The normal hemostatic system is designed to protect against bleeding from injured blood vessels. Hemostasis is usually accomplished by a sequence of interrelated processes involving blood vessels and endothelial activity, platelets, and coagulation proteins. This complex system is highly regulated to ensure that clotting occurs only at a site of injury and only as long as the integrity of the vessel is compromised. The process of hemostasis consists of several components: (1) blood vessel spasm; (2) formation of a platelet plug; (3) contact between damaged blood vessel, blood platelet, and coagulation proteins; (4) development of a blood clot around the injury; and (5) fibrinolytic removal of excess hemostatic material to reestablish vascular integrity.[5] Coagulation proteins make up the coagulation cascade. The coagulation cascade consists of three components: the intrinsic pathway (vascular trauma), the extrinsic pathway (tissue trauma), and the common pathway leading to fibrin formation. The clotting processes are balanced by the complex mechanism of fibrinolysis, which breaks down clots and maintains or re-establishes blood flow once the vessel damage has healed. The balance between these two mechanisms and their activators and inhibitors is vital. An imbalance in one direction leads to excessive bleeding; whereas an imbalance in the other direction leads to excessive clotting. The following sections present the normal sequence of coagulation and fibrinolysis, as well as selected coagulation disorders most commonly associated with the patient experiencing cardiovascular disease.

Vascular Spasm

The sympathetic nervous system is automatically stimulated when a blood vessel is injured. Epinephrine and norepinephrine are released causing contraction of the vascular smooth muscle and vasoconstriction. Endothelin I, which is a peptide produced by the endothelial cell, angiotensin II, and vasoconstrictor prostaglandins are additional agents that contribute to vasoconstriction.[5] The vasoconstriction of arterioles may be sufficient to decrease blood flow and close disrupted capillaries. Larger vessels may require longer periods of more intense vasoconstriction to assist with hemostasis, but may ultimately require surgical intervention.

Role of the Endothelium in Hemostasis

The endothelial cell was once thought to be inert and have no specific role in maintaining vascular integrity. Research over the years has proven this hypothesis to be incorrect. The endothelial cell is a vital component of normal homeostasis. Under normal conditions, the endothelium surface is intact and there is minimal interaction with platelets or the coagulation proteins. The function of the endothelium is to promote blood flow. The endothelial cell inhibits blood coagulation by: (1) expressing thrombomodulin, a clotting enzyme that binds thrombin; (2) changing the specificity of thrombomodulin from fibrin to protein C, which blocks the ability to convert fibrinogen to fibrin; (3) using proteoglycans on their surfaces to bind and potentiate the coagulation inhibitors antithrombin III and tissue factor pathway inhibitor; (4) releasing small amounts of plasminogen activator tissue-type plasminogen activator (tPA); (5) inhibiting platelet aggregation by producing prostacyclin and nitric oxide, which vasodilates the microcirculation; and (6) inhibiting adherence of peripheral blood cells.[6] These interactions maintain the anticoagulant properties of the endothelium by keeping platelets inactive and inhibiting key coagulation proteins such as tissue factor and thrombin.

Once the endothelial surface is disrupted by various factors, including physical injury or circulating mediators, it will develop procoagulant properties. When the endothelium is stimulated by inflammatory cytokines such as ILα-, ILβ-, or tumor necrosis factor α, it is referred to as activated endothelium. Once the subendothelial connective tissue is exposed and activated, it will lose thrombomodulin and heparin sulfate and begin to synthesize tissue factor (factor III). Factor III interacts with factor VII to start the extrinsic pathway. Therefore, protein C is not activated and the action of clotting inhibitor systems will be lost. This activation of the cascade will further incite the endothelial cell to produce more inflammatory mediators (cytokines and chemokines) that will start the expression of adhesion molecules. Leukocytes will adhere to the endothelial cell and become activated by the production of leukocyte agonists such as platelet activating factor.[6] Platelets are now attracted to the site and augment the coagulation process.

Platelet Phase

The platelet phase refers to the formation of a soft mass of aggregated platelets that provides a temporary patch over the injured vessel. Almost immediately after vascular injury, platelets begin to adhere to the exposed subendothelial basement membrane and collagen fibers. Adherent platelets release adenosine diphosphate, which causes platelets to change from their normal disc shape into a spherical form with pseudopods that attach along the surface and allow platelets to clump together.[5] During activation, the platelets become sticky when bridges formed by fibrinogen in the presence of calcium cause platelets to adhere to each other, increasing the size of the platelet plug. Adenosine diphosphate and collagen also trigger formation of arachidonic acid from phospholipids in the platelet membrane. Arachidonic acid leads to the formation of thromboxane A_2, a substance that induces further platelet aggregation. Thromboxane A_2 causes conformational changes in glycoprotein IIb/IIIa, a receptor on the platelet surface, which exposes fibrinogen-binding sites. Fibrinogen builds bridges to adjacent platelets, a process called platelet adhesion, which advances platelet aggregation. When these aggregates are reinforced with fibrin, they are referred to as a thrombus.[5] Ultimately, aggregated platelets plug the injured vessel.

Coagulation Cascade

The final phase of hemostasis is the formation of a fibrin blood clot. The coagulation process is most commonly viewed as a series of enzymatic reactions in which clotting factors are sequentially activated. This process is known as the coagulation cascade. The clotting factors are all present in the circulating blood in their inactive form until a stimulus for clot formation occurs. Twelve different substances have been officially designated as clotting factors (see Table 6-2). As studied in the laboratory, the coagulation process can be initiated by two different pathways: the extrinsic pathway and the intrinsic pathway. Although differentiating between them is helpful for understanding pathologic mechanisms, medication actions, and coagulation tests, these two pathways are functionally inseparable in vivo. The extrinsic pathway, whose major mediators are rapidly inactivated, is the primary initiator of the clotting cascade. The intrinsic pathway, whose major mediators are more slowly degraded, is thought to be important for maintenance and amplification of the clotting cascade. Both extrinsic and intrinsic mechanisms eventually lead to the activation of factor X, with the remaining steps of the coagulation sequence being identical and referred to as the common pathway. The sequence of the coagulation process is shown in Figure 6-2.

Extrinsic Pathway

The extrinsic pathway is initiated by the combination of tissue factor with factor VIIa and ionized calcium, which together convert factor X to its activated form, factor Xa. The function of the extrinsic pathway is tested in the laboratory by the prothrombin time (PT). Tissue factor, also called tissue thromboplastin

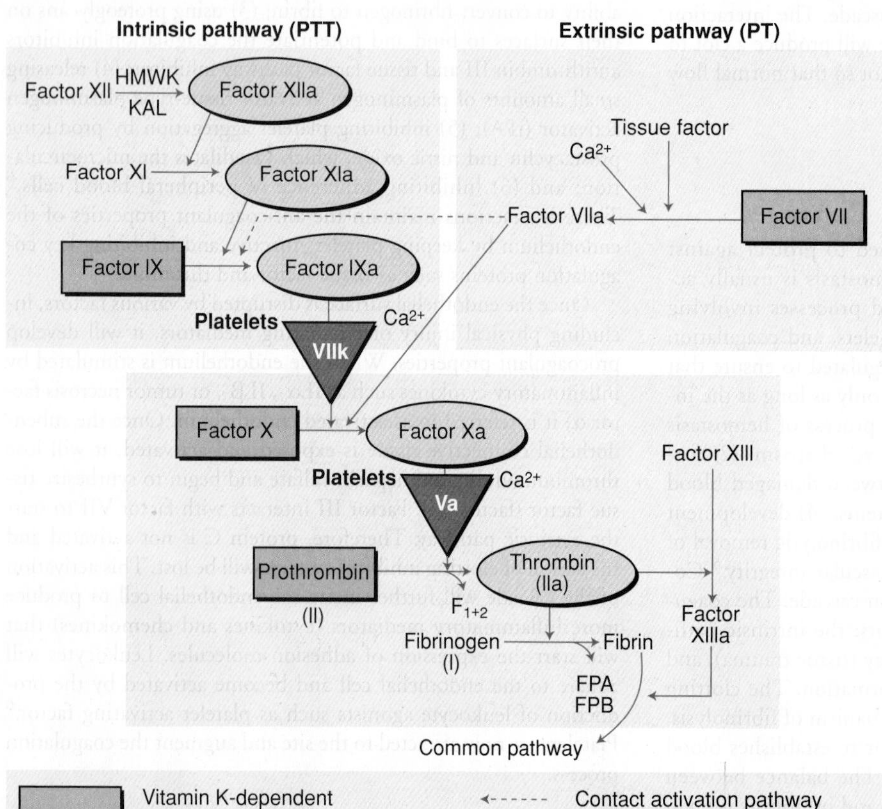

■ **Figure 6-2** The intrinsic, extrinsic, and common coagulation pathways. Lower case "a" denotes an activated factor. The protime (PT) measures the function of the extrinsic and common pathways; the partial thromboplastin time (PTT or aPTT) measures the activity of the intrinsic and common pathways. HMWK, high-molecular-weight kininogen and KAL, kallikrein. (Reproduced with permission from Dipiro, J. T., Talbert, R. L., Yee, G. C., et al. [2006]. *Pharmacotherapy: A pathophysiologic approach* [6th ed.]. New York: McGraw-Hill.)

(formerly factor III), is a membrane glycoprotein that is particularly prevalent in tissues, where it plays a vital role in the prevention of hemorrhage. Tissue factor is exposed to and binds to factor VII, which is activated to factor VIIa. Factor VIIa is a potent enzyme that activates factor X to Xa. The reactions from this step on are referred to as the common pathway. Calcium plays a significant role in each step leading to the formation of thrombin.[5]

Intrinsic Pathway

Because the intrinsic pathway is initiated by a separate set of factors that is not degraded by rapid-acting inhibitors, the process may proceed more slowly and the results may last longer and be more pronounced than those initiated by the extrinsic pathway. The function of the intrinsic pathway is commonly analyzed by the partial thromboplastin time (PTT). Intrinsic activation is initiated when blood is exposed to a negatively charged surface, such as the site of blood vessel injury. The negative charge, along with collagen and endotoxin, attracts factor XII, which binds to the surface and autoactivates to factor XIIa. Factor XIIa converts prekallikrein to kallikrein, which in turn converts circulating factor XII to its activated form, XIIa. Both the activated form of factor XII and kallikrein catalyze the activation of factor XI into XIa. Factor XIa, together with ionized calcium, cleaves factor IX at two sites to produce factor IXa. Factor IXa, together with factor VIII, phospholipid, and ionized calcium convert factor X to its activated form, factor Xa. As discussed previously, factor X can also be activated through the extrinsic pathway. From here, the coagulation process proceeds along the common pathway, regardless of whether initiation was extrinsic or intrinsic.[5]

Common Pathway and Fibrin Formation

The final common sequence involves the combination of factors Xa and V, phospholipid, and ionized calcium into a complex that converts prothrombin to thrombin. The thrombin formed subsequently cleaves the long molecule fibrinogen to fibrin. The fibrin monomer is able to polymerize spontaneously to form a loose web of fibers that is capable of stopping the bleeding in small- and medium-sized arteries and veins. The fibrin clot is eventually stabilized and thickened by the action of factor XIII, which is activated by the presence of ionized calcium and thrombin. Fibrin forms a loose covering over the injured area and reinforces the platelet plug. After a short period of time, the clot begins to retract. This process is thought to be a reaction of the platelets, which send out cytoplasmic processes that attach to the fibrin and pull the fibers closer.[5] Plasminogen and other components of the fibrinolytic mechanism are incorporated into the fibrin clot as it solidifies.

Fibrinolysis

The removal of clots when the site of vessel injury has healed is as important as the formation of the clot itself. Fibrinolysis is the physiological process that removes insoluble fibrin deposits by enzymatic digestion of the stabilized fibrin polymers.[5] The process of fibrinolysis re-establishes blood flow. Plasmin dissolves clots by digesting fibrin and fibrinogen using hydrolysis. Plasminogen is a glycoprotein and an inactive form of plasmin, which is synthesized by the liver. It is activated to plasmin by the activity of proteolytic enzymes, the kinases that cleave a bond on the plasminogen molecule. Activators of plasminogen are found in various tissues, blood, and urine. The best-known endogenous activators are tPA and urokinase, which is a urinary activator of plasminogen. Some exogenous plasminogen activators are related to types of bacteria such as streptokinase and staphylokinase.[5] Drugs have been developed to mimic the activity of these kinases to dissolve clots. Fragments of the fibrin clot, known as fibrin degradation products (FDP), are released into the circulation as the clot is broken down. FDP are potent inhibitors of coagulation. They act by binding to thrombin, thus inhibiting its action, and by interfering with the binding of fibrin threads to form the fibrin clot. Except in some abnormal situations, FDP are present in such small numbers that their anticoagulant effect is not clinically important. Plasminogen is then converted back to plasmin and neutralized by a number of antiplasmin and inhibitor systems. All these reactions that occur in the coagulation cascade and fibrinolytic system are time dependent and can be monitored using laboratory testing as listed in Table 6-3.

Natural Anticoagulant Systems

Coagulation is regulated by three major mechanisms: the elimination of activated clotting factors, the protease inhibitors (inhibitors of coagulation), and the destruction of the fibrin clot. There must be a balance between coagulation and anticoagulation processes in the body to maintain homeostasis. The natural anticoagulant systems include antithrombin III, heparin cofactor II, and protein C and its cofactor, protein S.

Antithrombin III is an α2-globulin glycoprotein, which is considered the major inhibitor of coagulation. It slowly inactivates thrombin as well as factors Xa, IXa, XIa, and XIIa. In the presence of heparin, antithrombin III–thrombin binding is increased significantly. This is thought to be the main mechanism for heparin's anticoagulation ability and its interaction with antithrombin III and tissue factor pathway inhibitor.

Heparin cofactor II is a heparin-dependent thrombin inhibitor whose activity is also accelerated by the presence of heparin. This cofactor not only inhibits thrombin but also thrombin-induced platelet aggregation and release.[5]

Protein C and protein S are major natural anticoagulants in the body and have a powerful role in anticoagulation. Deficiency in either of these proteins can lead to the development of thrombus. Protein C is a vitamin K-dependent protein, which is synthesized in the liver and circulates as a zymogen, an inactive precursor form in the blood. Activation occurs faster when thrombin, in the presence of thrombomodulin, assists with proteolytic cleavage that converts protein C to its active enzymatic form, activated protein C (APC). Protein S must also be present to help APC proteolytically cleave factors Va and VIIIa, which will decrease the conversion of prothrombin to thrombin, and acts as a regulatory feedback loop to balance coagulation. The dual role of thrombin in both coagulation and anticoagulation is exemplified here. Protein C also has a function in promoting fibrinolysis by neutralizing the inhibitors of tPA, which allows the conversion of plasminogen to plasmin. Inactivation of APC is a slower process with a plasma protease inhibitor that has a short half-life intimating that other unidentified direct cell mechanisms.[5] The properties of protein C have been applied clinically with the development of the medication, Drotrecogin alfa. Drotrecogin alfa is a recombinant intravenous (IV) form of APC, which is used in severely ill patients with sepsis to decrease

Table 6-3 ■ COAGULATION LABORATORY TESTS

Test	Normal Value	Coagulation Correlation	Clinical Significance
Activated partial thromboplastin time (aPTT)	<35 seconds	Generation of thrombin and fibrin to via intrinsic and common pathway	**Increased** with heparin or thrombin inhibitor therapy
Prothrombin time (PT)	10 to 13 seconds	Generation of thrombin and fibrin via extrinsic and common pathway	**Increased** with liver disease, extrinsic factor deficiencies, or oral anticoagulants
International normalized ratio (INR)	Therapy goal dependent	Standardized values used to correct for different thromboplastin reagents used in PT calculations	See American College of Chest (ACCP) Guidelines
Thrombin time (TT)	<20 seconds	Rate of thrombin induced cleavage of fibrinogen to fibrin	**Increased** with low fibrinogen levels, DIC, liver disease, increased FDP
Fibrinogen	200 to 400 mg/dL	Deficiencies in fibrinogen and alterations in conversion of fibrinogen to fibrin	**Increased** with inflammatory response **Decreased** with liver disease or consumption of fibrinogen with intravascular clotting
Fibrin degradation products (FDP)	8 to 10 μg/mL	Generation of fibrin fragments upon degeneration	**Increased** in fibrinolysis, DIC
Platelet count	150,000 to 400,000/mm^3	Amount of circulating platelets; does not reflect functional ability	**Increased** in myeloproliferative disorders, inflammation, post splenectomy **Decreased** in consumptive states, DIC, drug reactions, platelet disorders
Bleeding time (BT)	2 to 9 minutes, depending on reagent	Determines platelet adhesion and aggregation	**Increased** with platelet abnormalities, aspirin, severe liver disease
Protein C	4 to 5 μg/mL	Determines activity of natural anticoagulation systems	**Increased** in inflammation **Decreased** in consumptive disorders
D-dimer assay	<400 ng/mL	Determines the level of endogenous thrombolysis; plasmin activity on fibrin	**Increased** with excessive endogenous thrombolysis
Activated clotting time (ACT)	46 to 70 seconds or 1.5 to 2.5 times control	Alternative test that can be performed at the bedside to determine heparin's anticoagulation level	**Increased** with heparin therapy **Decreased** with protamine administration
Functional platelet assessment Thromboelastography (TEG)*	Graph analysis; maximum amplitude (MA) normal 55 to 73 mm	Newer testing that monitors the dynamic process of hemostasis; can determine the number and functional capacity of platelets	Maximum amplitude or width of graph estimates the number of platelets and their functioning capacity

*Sorensen, E., Lorme, T., & Heath, D. (2005). Thromboelastography: A means to transfusion reduction. *Nursing Management, 36*, 27–34.
Modified from Kinney, M., et al. (1998). *AACN Clinical Reference For Critical Care Nursing*. St. Louis: CV Mosby.

microemboli formation and inhibit immune function. Activated protein C has a major role as an agent that suppresses inflammation and prevents microvascular coagulation. Initial studies had shown the efficacy and safety of APC for severe sepsis.[7,8] However, current research has demonstrated variable results and the 2008 Surviving Sepsis guidelines list the use of APC as a weak recommendation.[7]

COAGULATION–INFLAMMATION LINK

The role of the inflammatory process has become a major focus of study in many areas of medicine, especially inflammation's role in the atherosclerotic process. The study of the relationship between coagulation and inflammation is focused on the integrity of the endothelium and the recruitment of leukocytes.[3] Normally, the endothelium does not encourage the binding of WBC to the wall. However, with elevated levels of low-density lipoproteins, the excess low-density lipoproteins molecules will begin to infiltrate the endothelial wall and experience oxidation and glycation.[9] These chemical changes will cause the endothelial cell to express an adhesion molecule, vascular cell adhesion molecule I, which will bind various types of leukocytes, especially monocytes and T lymphocytes. This process occurs especially at arterial branch points where the endothelial cells are exposed to abnormal laminar flow. This abnormal laminar flow decreases the endothelial cells protective ability to secrete nitric oxide and to limit the expression of vascular cell adhesion molecule I.[3]

Once the monocyte is attached to the endothelial wall, it releases monocyte chemoattractant protein-1, which will help the migration of the monocyte into the intima. With the assistance of macrophage colony-stimulating factor, the monocyte starts to ingest the excess lipids and transform itself into a macrophage foam cell. The macrophage foam cells are the trigger for activating the coagulation system. They release proteolytic enzymes that degrade the collagen fibers that compose the fibrous cap, so that it weakens and can rupture. The macrophage foam cell also produces tissue factor (Factor III) and once the plaque cap ruptures and exposes the tissue factor to the circulating blood, coagulation will ensue.[3] The T cells also release cytokines such as tumor necrosis factor β, which stimulates the macrophages, endothelial cells, and the smooth muscles. Peptide growth factors are released that promote the replication of smooth muscle cells into an extracellular matrix, which is characteristic of an atherosclerotic lesion.[3]

However, this link between coagulation and inflammation may not only be limited to the atherosclerosis process. Hypertension may also be linked to inflammation because angiotensin II not only may be a vasoconstrictor but also may cause intimal inflammation by stimulating the smooth muscle and endothelial cells to express proinflammatory cytokines such as IL-6 and monocyte chemoattractant protein-1.[3] Hyperglycemia associated with diabetes can lead to the formation of advance glycation end products that may augment the secretion of proinflammatory cytokines.[3] Even chronic extravascular infections such as gingivitis, prostatitis, bronchitis, etc., can augment extravascular production of inflammatory cytokines, which can accelerate the evolution of atherosclerotic lesions.[3] This new scientific insight into the role of inflammation in the development of atherosclerosis has led to using new markers to determine the degree of inflammation. Findings of a relationship between increased C-reactive protein levels and unfavorable cardiovascular outcomes have led to new therapeutic considerations for acute coronary syndrome.[3]

BLEEDING DISORDERS

Bleeding can occur when the intricate relationship between the various elements of the hemostatic system is disturbed. Bleeding defects in the hemostatic system can be categorized into three areas: vascular issues, platelet dysfunction, or coagulation dysfunction. Vascular issues generally cause endothelial damage by an autoimmune process (allergy induced), endotoxins from infections, or abnormal vascular structure. Platelet dysfunction can present as thrombocytopenia (low platelet count) or thrombocytosis (high platelet count). Thrombocytopenia can result from decreased production, decreased distribution, or increased destruction of platelets. Thrombocytosis can result from either a primary or a secondary cause. Coagulation dysfunction can be either congenital or acquired deficiencies in the coagulation factors (Display 6-1). In each case, bleeding is the primary manifestation. The bleeding may be minor, such as petechiae and easy bruising of the skin, or major, with massive hemorrhage.

The focus of cardiac interventions today emphasizes maintaining blood flow with percutaneous interventions (vascular injury) and anticoagulation to prevent thrombus formation. This intentional disruption of the coagulation system can potentially lead to bleeding disorders or even shock with excessive blood loss from percutaneous interventions and/or thrombolysis. Shock can lead to hypoperfusion and decreased oxygen delivery, which can trigger the intrinsic and extrinsic pathways simultaneously. Disseminated intravascular coagulation (DIC) is a complication of shock. Although DIC is actually a disorder of coagulation, it is discussed as a bleeding disorder because its major manifestation is bleeding.

Disseminated Intravascular Coagulation

DIC is a pathological syndrome resulting in the indiscriminate formation of fibrin clots throughout all or most of the microvasculature. Paradoxically, diffuse bleeding occurs as a result of the consumption of clotting factors and is usually the hallmark sign of the syndrome. It is a disorder in which the coagulation cascade has been "pathologically activated" either by the extrinsic pathway releasing tissue factor or by the intrinsic pathway with endothelial injury.[1] It is considered a complication of many different diseases and is known as a consumptive coagulopathy or defibrination syndrome.[5] Successful treatment of DIC must include treatment of the primary cause of the disorder as well as the hematologic consequences. (See Display 6-2 for diseases associated with disseminated intravascular coagulation.)

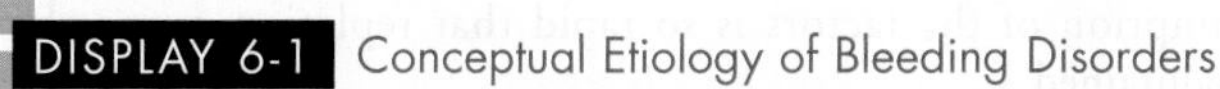

DISPLAY 6-1 Conceptual Etiology of Bleeding Disorders

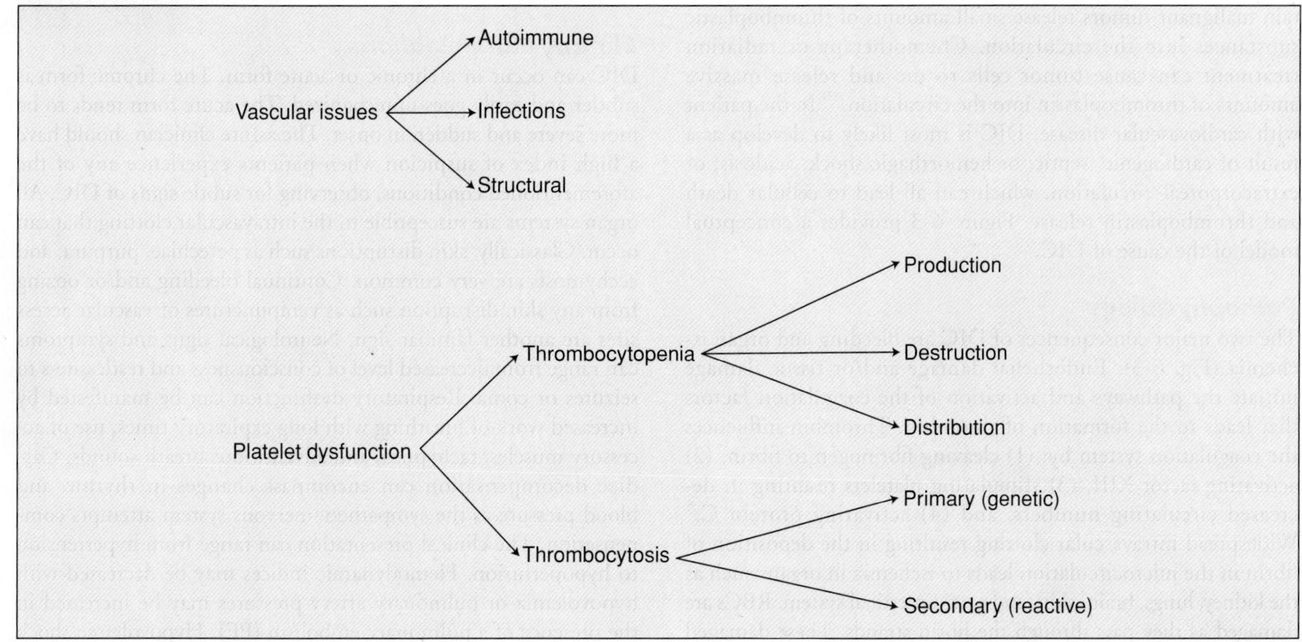

DISPLAY 6-2 Diseases Associated with Disseminated Intravascular Coagulation

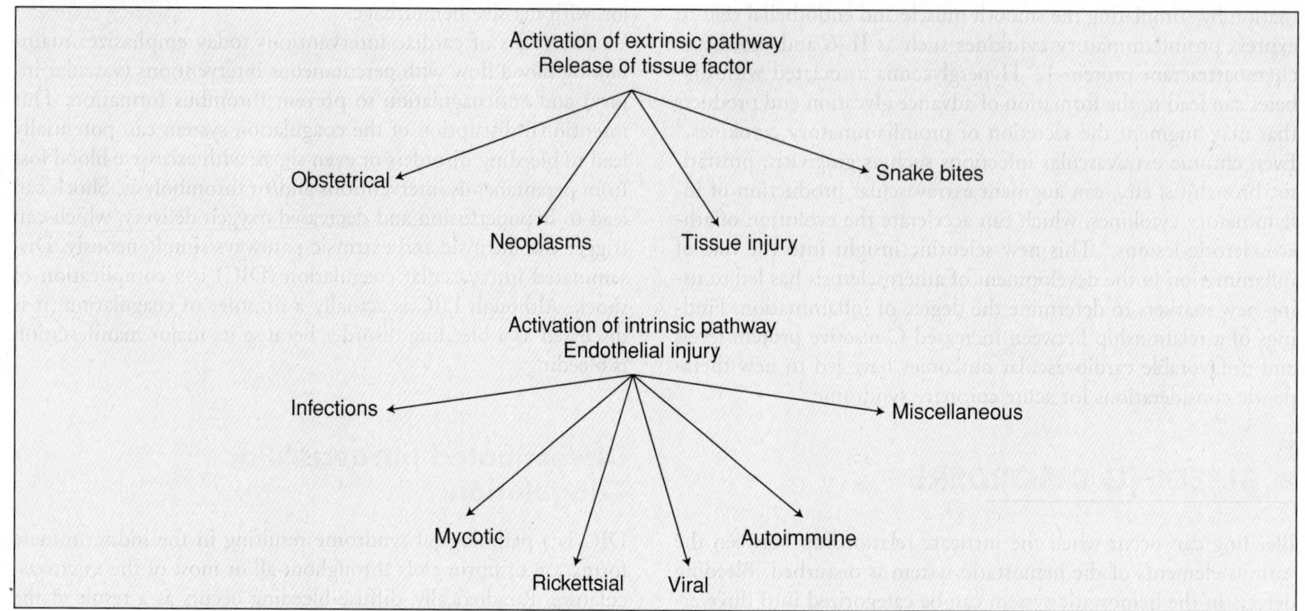

Etiology

Inappropriate coagulation results from the presence of thromboplastic substances in the bloodstream. These thromboplastic substances stimulate clotting despite the lack of actual bleeding. Tissue thromboplastin (tissue factor) is released into the circulation by damaged cells in massive burns, injuries, and systemic infections. DIC is a common complication of serious infections, especially Gram-negative sepsis. The fetus, placenta, and amniotic fluid contain thromboplastic substances that are released into the maternal circulation during obstetric complications such as abruptio placentae and amniotic fluid embolism. Certain malignant tumors release small amounts of thromboplastic substances into the circulation. Chemotherapy or radiation treatment can cause tumor cells to die and release massive amounts of thromboplastin into the circulation.[10] In the patient with cardiovascular disease, DIC is most likely to develop as a result of cardiogenic, septic, or hemorrhagic shock; acidosis; or extracorporeal circulation, which can all lead to cellular death and thromboplastin release. Figure 6-3 provides a conceptual model of the cause of DIC.

Pathophysiology

The two major consequences of DIC are bleeding and organ ischemia (Fig. 6-3). Endothelial damage and/or tissue damage initiate the pathways and activation of the coagulation factors that leads to the formation of thrombin. Thrombin influences the coagulation system by: (1) cleaving fibrinogen to fibrin, (2) activating factor XIII, (3) stimulating platelets resulting in decreased circulating numbers, and (4) activating protein C.[5] Widespread intravascular clotting resulting in the deposition of fibrin in the microcirculation leads to ischemia in organs such as the kidney, lungs, brain, skin, and gastrointestinal system. RBCs are damaged as they pass through the fibrin strands. These damaged RBC are called schistocytes. As the disseminated clotting continues, circulating platelets and clotting factors are consumed and bleeding ensues. Fibrinolysis is activated as a result of the widespread fibrin deposition, converting plasminogen to plasmin, which destroys fibrin and fibrinogen, yielding abnormally large amounts of circulating FDP.[5] In these large numbers, FDPs aggravate bleeding because they: (1) inhibit platelet aggregation by coating receptor sites, (2) act as anticoagulants by competing with thrombin, and (3) impair fibrin polymerization.[5] Consumption of the factors is so rapid that repletion cannot be maintained.

Clinical Manifestations

DIC can occur in a chronic or acute form. The chronic form is subtler and easily goes unrecognized. The acute form tends to be more severe and sudden in onset. The astute clinician should have a high index of suspicion when patients experience any of the aforementioned conditions, observing for subtle signs of DIC. All organ systems are susceptible to the intravascular clotting that can occur. Classically, skin disruptions such as petechiae, purpura, and ecchymosis are very common. Continual bleeding and/or oozing from any skin disruption such as venipunctures or vascular access sites are another familiar sign. Neurological signs and symptoms can range from decreased level of consciousness and restlessness to seizures or coma. Respiratory dysfunction can be manifested by increased work of breathing with long expiratory times, use of accessory muscles, tachypnea, and adventitious breath sounds. Cardiac decompensation can encompass changes in rhythm and blood pressure as the sympathetic nervous system attempts compensation. The clinical presentation can range from hypertension to hypoperfusion. Hemodynamic indices may be decreased with hypovolemia or pulmonary artery pressures may be increased in the presence of a pulmonary embolism (PE). Hypovolemic shock

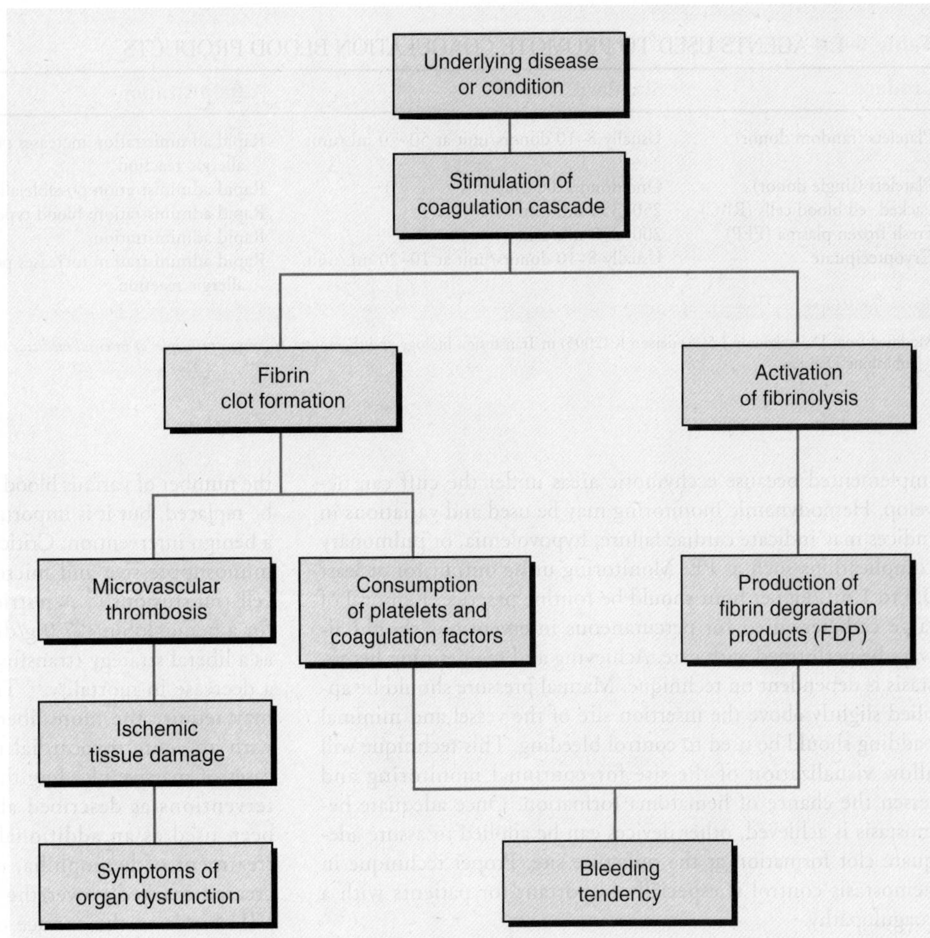

■ **Figure 6-3** Pathophysiology of disseminated intravascular coagulation. (From Kinney, M., Dunbar S. Brooks-Brun, J., et al. [1998]. *AACN's clinical reference for critical care nursing*. St. Louis: CV Mosby.)

may result if blood loss is severe. Potential spaces for bleeding, especially the retroperitoneal space and thighs, need to be closely observed when femoral vascular access devices are in place or are removed. Acute abdominal signs such as distention, tenderness, pain, and decreased or absent bowel sounds may indicate major gastrointestinal dysfunction, Urine output may be decreased and signs of renal failure, such as an increase in creatinine, may occur. It is important to remember that the primary disorder that led to DIC must also be treated to correct DIC.

Medical Management

The diagnosis of DIC should be suspected whenever abnormal bleeding occurs in association with any of the primary disorders described previously. Multiple coagulation test abnormalities are found in DIC. These include prolonged PT, PTT, and thrombin time; decreased fibrinogen and platelet counts; and decreased levels of factors II, V, VIII, and X indicate the consumption of clotting factors. The elevation of FDP and the D-dimer levels confirm fibrinolysis. D-dimer levels indicate the level of activity of plasmin on fibrin, that is, thrombolysis. Schistocytes may also be present.[11] The presence of clotting and fibrinolysis with a suspicious clinical presentation can assist the practitioner in making the diagnosis of DIC. The prognosis of DIC varies markedly depending on the underlying cause and the amount of intravascular clotting. DIC may cease spontaneously, it may respond to prompt and aggressive treatment or it may lead to organ ischemia, bleeding, and potentially death. DIC always occurs as the result of some other underlying abnormality, and thus the treatment of DIC is directed toward improvement of the underlying disorder. For example, infection requires the use of antibiotics. General supportive measures such as fluid and blood replacement, mechanical ventilation, and vasoactive drugs to maintain tissue perfusion are essential.[12] Transfusions of platelets, fresh-frozen plasma, RBC, and cryoprecipitate will be needed to attempt to replace consumed coagulation factors. The use of heparin, a potent anticoagulant that inactivates the intravascular clotting and thus inhibits consumption of the coagulation factors, is very controversial and probably inappropriate in the face of active bleeding.[12]

Nursing Interventions

Perceptive nursing skill can be the pivotal factor in the patient with DIC. Early recognition of the subtle signs could avert further decompensation. If the patient displays any sign of restlessness or agitation, physiological factors such as hypoxemia should be the first consideration. Monitoring oxygenation using pulse oximetry will give some estimate of oxygenation that can be confirmed with an arterial blood gas (ABG). If gas exchange is adequate and restlessness and agitation persist, neurological causes must be considered and sedation should be avoided unless indicated. The patient's heart rate, rhythm, and blood pressure should be continually monitored for any changes. If manual or noninvasive blood pressure monitoring is being used, rotation of the cuff should be

Table 6-4 ■ AGENTS USED TO PROMOTE COAGULATION BLOOD PRODUCTS

Product	Standard Volume	Administration	Factor Replaced
Platelets (random donor)	Usually 8–10 donors/unit at 50–70 mL/unit	Rapid administration increases possible allergic reaction	
Platelets (single donor)	One donor/200–300 mL	Rapid administration possible allergic reaction	
Packed red blood cells (RBC)	250–350 mL/unit	Rapid administration; blood type mismatch	
Fresh frozen plasma (FFP)	200–250 mL/unit	Rapid administration	II, V, VII, IX, X, XI, XII
Cryoprecipitate	Usually 8–10 donors/unit at 10–20 mL/unit	Rapid administration increases possible allergic reaction	I

Modified from Dzieczkowski J & Anderson K (2005) in Transfusion biology and therapy in *Harrison's principles of internal medicine* (16th ed.). New York: McGraw-Hill Medical Publishing Division.

implemented because ecchymotic areas under the cuff can develop. Hemodynamic monitoring may be used and variations in indices may indicate cardiac failure, hypovolemia, or pulmonary complications such as PE. Monitoring urine output for at least 0.5 to 1 mL/kg per hour should be routine practice. Removal of large catheters used for percutaneous interventions should always be performed with care. Achieving and maintaining hemostasis is dependent on technique. Manual pressure should be applied slightly above the insertion site of the vessel and minimal padding should be used to control bleeding. This technique will allow visualization of the site for continual monitoring and lessen the chance of hematoma formation. Once adequate hemostasis is achieved, other devices can be applied to assure adequate clot formation at the puncture site. Proper technique in hemostasis control is especially important for patients with a coagulopathy.

If hemorrhage is present, the priority should be volume resuscitation. Blood products should be replaced depending on estimated blood loss and laboratory values. Aggressive fluid resuscitation should be performed through short, large-bore venous access using pressure bags if the patient is hypotensive to assure fast intravascular volume repletion. While infusing blood products, the nurse should observe for allergic reactions (Tables 6-4 and 6-5). Continual bleeding may require massive blood product replacement, which can cause a "washout" effect of most of the functioning coagulation proteins, and paradoxically cause further coagulopathy. It is also important to keep accurate records as to the number of various blood products received. RBC loss needs to be replaced, but it is important to realize that a transfusion is not a benign intervention. Critically ill patients may be at risk for immunosuppressive and microcirculatory complications with red cell transfusions.[13] A restrictive transfusion strategy (transfuse for a hemoglobin <7.0 g/dL) has been shown to be as effective as a liberal strategy (transfuse for a hemoglobin <10 g/dL) with a decrease in mortality.[13] The only two groups of patients that may require the more liberal transfusion strategy are patients with an acute myocardial infarction or unstable angina.[13] In cases of massive bleeding that is not responsive to the usual interventions as described above, recombinant factor VIIa has been used as an additional intervention. Originally used for treatment of hemophilia, off-label use of factor VIIa has increased markedly over the last 10 years. Recombinant factor VIIa binds to the surface of activated platelets and promotes thrombin formation thereby enhancing clot formation.[1] Dosing of this drug for off-label use varies greatly depending on the setting (surgery, trauma, hemorrhagic stroke, reversal of oral coagulation therapy, or impaired hepatic function).[14] Caution should be used when using factor VIIa due to the risk of thromboembolic adverse events.[14,15] Observation for bleeding should include monitoring of all vascular accesses as well as the area around the site. Vigilant surveys by the nurse of the skin surface and digits are necessary to observe for petechiae, ecchymosis, and other skin disruptions that may provide early warning signs of impending DIC (Display 6-3).

Table 6-5 ■ DRUGS USED TO PROMOTE COAGULATION

Drug	Dose	Side Effects	Mechanism
Protamine	1 mg for every 100 u of IV heparin	Hypotension; possible anaphylaxis if exposed to NPH	Binds heparin to neutralize anticoagulant effect
Desarginine vasopressin (DDAVP)	0.3 μg/kg IV at 12- to 24-h interval	Mild flushing, headache, mild-to-moderate abdominal pain	Temporarily improves platelet function in patient with renal or liver disease; mechanism not clear
Recombinant activated Human factor VII (rFVIIa) (Novo-Seven)*	Dose varies depending on indication; most current use is off-label dose can range from 5 to 300+ mcg/kg in varying number of doses	Thrombotic events	Binds to surface of activated Platelets and promotes Factor X activation and thrombin generation where platelets are localized at a site of injury

*Goodnough, L., & Shander, A. (2007). Recombinant factor VIIa: Safety and efficacy. *Current Opinion in Hematology, 14*, 504–509.
Brunton, L., Lazo, J., & Parker, K. (2006). *Goodman and Gilman's the pharmacological basis of therapeutics*. New York: McGraw-Hill Company.

DISPLAY 6-3 Nursing Interventions with Bleeding Disorders

Non-Emergent Interventions

1. Close observation of skin, mucus membranes, wounds, and intravascular access sites, especially femoral areas.
2. Assess for decreased tissue perfusion.
   a. Cellular: SvO_2, lactate levels, pH
   b. Cerebral: Decreased level of consciousness, restlessness, agitation, apprehension
   c. Myocardial: Chest pain, ECG changes, respiratory distress
   d. Renal: Decreased urine output, rising BUN, and creatinine
3. Test all body secretions for occult blood.
4. Measure and record blood loss.
5. Prevent injury.
   a. Soft toothbrush/swab for oral care
   b. Use electric razor
   c. No IM/SQ injections
   d. Minimize blood drawing and venipunctures
   e. Avoid invasive procedures (i.e., nasogastric tubes, rectal tubes, etc.)

Emergent Interventions

1. Aggressive volume resuscitation through short, large-bore catheters; use warming devices for core temperature <36°C
2. Controlling bleeding at access sites using manual pressure applied slightly above site and minimal dressing to observe site closely
3. Accurate hemodynamic monitoring (see Chapter 21)
4. Supportive ventilatory care

BUN, blood urea nitrogen.

CLOTTING DISORDERS

Excessive or inappropriate coagulation is also of great clinical significance. Venous thrombosis involves the interacting conditions of stasis, vascular damage, and hypercoagulability. The most common life-threatening complication, PE, is a major cause of mortality in hospitalized patients. Recognition of patients likely to have any of these conditions is a nursing responsibility.

Clot Formation

A thrombus is a clot or solid mass formed by blood components. Thrombosis refers to the formation or presence of blood clots in a vessel. A thrombus that breaks loose and travels in the blood vessel is termed an embolus, hence the term thromboembolism. The potential outcome from either thrombosis or embolism is ischemia, leading to infarction with cellular and tissue necrosis. A thrombus develops when the normal process of hemostasis is inappropriately activated. Three factors (vessel injury, stasis, and hypercoagulability) can predispose a patient to thrombosis. These three factors are commonly known as Virchow's triad[16,17] (Fig. 6-4).

First, the vessel involved must have suffered some type of injury, particularly damage to the endothelial layer. Vessel injury may be the result of sustained pressure on the vessel or surrounding tissue, as might occur from prolonged immobility of an extremity or pressure points caused by crossed legs, elastic-topped knee socks, or a bed where the knee gatch is raised too high. Vessel wall injury can also result from direct trauma by surgery or, more commonly, by IV or arterial catheters. Underlying vascular disease also creates vessel wall abnormalities. Chemical irritation may result from IV solutions and drugs. Anything that exposes collagen fibers in the vessel wall of arteries and veins may cause rapid platelet adhesion, aggregation, and thrombus formation. In addition, injury to vessels activates an inflammatory response that can be seen histologically and, in most cases, is seen most vividly in the lower extremities. When an extremity is immobile for any period of time, the pumping action is lost, resulting in venous stasis. For example, during the postoperative period there is a decrease in total limb blood flow because of immobility. Stasis may also result from reduced cardiac output (CO) caused by heart failure or shock. Alteration in blood flow leading to arterial thrombosis may be caused by turbulent flow at points of arterial bifurcation or stenosis, or with aneurysms. Fortunately, the rapid blood flow in arteries tends to discourage thrombus formation. Reduced blood flow in the atria occurs with atrial fibrillation, leading to thrombus formation. When the patient's cardiac rhythm converts to a regular sinus rhythm, these thrombi can be expelled into the lungs or systemic circulation.[16,17]

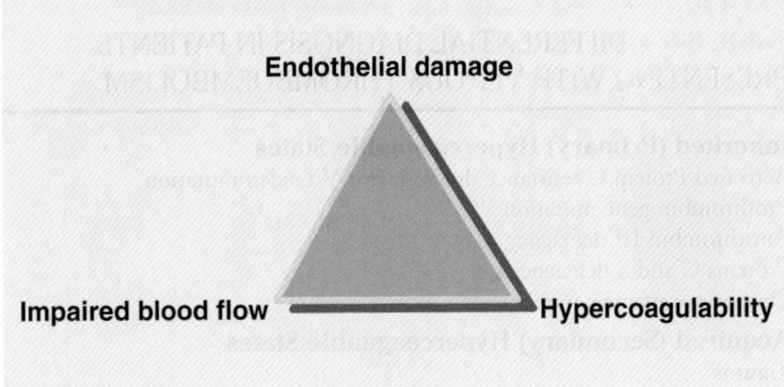

Figure 6-4 Virchow's triad.

The final predisposing factor of Virchow's triad is hypercoagulability of the blood. Changes in blood leading to hypercoagulability may occur during pregnancy or in women using oral contraceptive drugs, which can cause elevated levels of coagulation factors. Changes in blood constituents may also occur in polycythemia, in severe anemia, or with circulating endotoxins from systemic infections. Deficiencies in antithrombin III and decreased hepatic function may be thrombogenic in patients with liver disease and in premature infants. The type of thrombus formed usually differs between arteries and veins. Arterial thrombi usually begin at the site of endothelial injury or turbulence. A venous thrombus is almost always occlusive. In the slower-moving blood of the veins, the thrombus frequently creates a long cast in the lumen of the vessel. No matter what type of clot is present, embolic disorders are a clinical challenge in which tissue perfusion will be compromised and intervention is needed.

Deep Vein Thrombosis

The clinical problems associated with venous thromboembolism (VTE) include deep vein thrombosis (DVT) and pulmonary embolism (PE). One of the most common and potentially life-threatening problems confronting health care professionals is the diagnosis, prophylaxis, and treatment of DVT and PE in both medical and surgical patients. The major risk associated with DVT

Table 6-6 ■ DIFFERENTIAL DIAGNOSIS IN PATIENTS PRESENTING WITH VENOUS THROMBOEMBOLISM

Inherited (Primary) Hypercoaguable States
Activated Protein C resistance due to factor V Leiden mutation
Prothrombin gene mutation
Antithrombin III deficiency
Proteins C and S deficiencies
Dysfibrinogenemias (rare)
Acquired (Secondary) Hypercoaguable States
Trauma
Pregnancy (especially postpartum period)
Immobilization (paralysis, extended bedrest, or sitting)
Advancing age
Postoperative state
Obesity
Prolonged air travel
Malignancy
Estrogens (hormone replacement therapy, oral contraceptives)
Lupus anticoagulant or antiphospholipid antibody syndrome

Modified from Hoffman, R., Benz, E., Shattil, S., et al. (2005). *Hematology: Basic Principles and Practice.* Philadelphia: Elsevier-Churchill-Livingstone.

is that it can lead to PE. Venous thrombosis in the lower extremity can involve superficial leg veins, the deep veins of the calf (calf vein thrombosis), and the more proximal veins, including the popliteal veins, the superficial femoral, common femoral, and iliac veins. In superficial vein thrombosis, sometimes called thrombophlebitis, the thrombosis is the result of inflammation in the venous wall of the superficial venous system and is benign and self-limiting.

Etiology

The risk factors associated with VTE can be divided into two categories: primary and secondary hypercoaguable states. Virchow's triad (see Fig. 6-4) theory can be applied to some of these risk factors (Table 6-6).

Pathophysiology

Thrombi can form because the balance that is maintained in normal homeostasis has been disrupted. Coagulation is enhanced or fibrinolysis is impaired, which can lead to a hypercoaguable state. Primary inherited disorders that cause a hypercoaguable state are usually deficiencies in factors that inhibit coagulation, so there is less counterbalance to the coagulation process. The three main deficiencies are antithrombin III, protein C, and protein S.[5] Secondary hypercoaguable states may result from endothelial activation by cytokines that will lead to loss of normal vessel wall anticoagulant surface functions with conversion to proinflammatory thrombogenic functions.[18] Vascular endothelial damage can expose circulating blood components to subendothelial structures that initiate thrombosis. This process can also lead to vasoconstriction, which causes stasis and makes it easier for platelets to detach from flowing blood. The accumulation of platelets can furnish phospholipid for the intrinsic pathway, promoting thrombin formation by absorbing activated factor X to their surface.[18] Platelets can also undergo alterations in their surface area that can lead to spontaneous aggregation or increased adhesiveness.[18] Increased blood viscosity may also predispose thrombosis. Patients with increased levels of fibrinogen can induce erythrocyte aggregation, increasing viscosity and decreasing blood flow.

Clinical Manifestations

The classic signs and symptoms of pain, edema, warmth, erythema, and tenderness of the leg are common with DVT, but can also be caused by nonthrombotic events. There can also be a palpable cord, discoloration, cyanosis, venous distention, and prominence of the superficial veins.[18] The size of the thrombus, the location of the affected vein, and the adequacy of collateral channels are some of the factors that cause the variability of the clinical presentation.[24] In the past, a positive Homans' sign, which is pain occurring in the affected calf with forceful dorsiflexion of the foot, was thought to be diagnostic for a DVT. However, a positive Homans' sign is not specific for thrombotic disease and could indicate minor muscle injury or other lower leg disorder.[24] Therefore, caution must be used when interpreting Homans' sign because any inflammation near the calf muscles may also elicit similar pain. Asymmetry between two extremities may also be present, with the affected limb being slightly larger because of the congestion and edema associated with the inflammatory process. These signs and symptoms in combination with the presence of the associated risk factors should assist in the diagnostic process. The clinical manifestations of DVT are sometimes elusive and should always be confirmed by objective diagnostic tests.

Medical Management

Objective testing and a careful history and physical examination should be obtained if a DVT is suspected. The patient's history and physical examination are important components of the diagnostic process, because they may reveal an alternative cause of the patient's symptoms. Diagnostic studies for DVT include B-mode or duplex ultrasonography, venography, and impedence plethysmography. Some form of ultrasound, either compression or color duplex, is usually the most common test used for diagnosing DVT because it is more specific and sensitive. Venography is used but is technically difficult to perform and requires experience to execute the test accurately. Impedence plethysmography is also used but is not sensitive to calf vein thrombosis.[19] Once the diagnosis of DVT is confirmed, anticoagulation will be initiated immediately. Prevention is also an important priority to deter further decompensation of the patient's condition. Both these interventions will be discussed and more radical interventions, such as venous filters, will be discussed in the treatment of PE.

Anticoagulation

The main goal of therapy for VTE, of any origin, is anticoagulation to prevent further formation of thrombi. Depending on the severity of the embolism, anticoagulation can be used conservatively or aggressively if thrombolytic therapy is needed to lyse a life-threatening clot. The Seventh American College of Chest Physicians (ACCP) Consensus Conference on Antithrombotic Therapy[20] recommends these drugs to be used for anticoagulation with VTE: the heparins, oral anticoagulants, and thrombolytic agents. The most common and one of the oldest drugs used for anticoagulation is heparin. Heparin is a glycosaminoglycan that binds to and activates antithrombin III and reduces the formation of thrombin and fibrin. The best method of administering heparin is according to a weight-based protocol, which starts with a bolus loading dose of 5,000 units or 75 units/kg intravenously followed by a heparin IV drip at 18 units/kg per hour. The dose is then regulated by aPTT results that are sampled initially every 6 hours, with the aPTT goal of 1.5 to 2 times the normal aPTT. The use of a heparin weight-based protocol has been found to be more efficient in achieving an aPTT above the lower limit of the therapeutic range in 24 hours.[21] The goal for anticoagulation is that the dose of unfractionated heparin should be sufficient to prolong the aPTT to a range that corresponds to a plasma heparin level of 0.2 to 0.4 IU/mL by protamine sulfate or 0.3 to 0.6 IU/mL by an amidolytic anti-Xa assay.[21] Another group of drugs in the same class are the low-molecular-weight heparins (LMWH), which have a reduced ability to catalyze the inhibition of thrombin while retaining the ability to inhibit the activity of factor Xa. The advantage to the LMWH is that they do not bind to most plasma proteins, which contribute to a more predictable anticoagulant dose, and there is no need for laboratory monitoring. Enoxaparin is the more common LMWH used currently and it can be administered either once or twice per day subcutaneously (SC). If prescribed once daily, the dose is 1.5 mg/kg and if prescribed twice daily (BID), the dose is 1.0 mg/kg. Another LMWH is Dalteparin.[21] There are other LMWH agents such as tinzaparin, nadroparin, and reviparin that are used less commonly.

The next drug category used for anticoagulation for VTE is oral anticoagulants. Warfarin is the primary oral drug used. There are other oral agents available, such as dicumarol, which are not used as much because of erratic absorption and gastrointestinal side effects.[3] The major action of oral anticoagulants is that they antagonize vitamin K. The starting dose is usually 5 mg orally (po), which is then adjusted according to PT and international normalized ratio (INR). When prescribing warfarin, it is important to remember that the effect of the dose administered today will not be reflected in the PT/INR until approximately 3 days after that dose is administered. The anticoagulation treatment for VTE is initially heparin, which is administered for 5 days. Oral anticoagulant therapy overlaps with heparin therapy for at least 4 to 5 days until the INR goal of 2.0 to 3.0 is achieved.[20] Once the target for INR is reached and the level remains stable, the heparin can be discontinued and the warfarin dose adjusted further until stable and then followed-up by intermittent INR sampling. Oral anticoagulation is continued for at least 3 months up to as long as 6 months, depending on the reason for the development of VTE.[20]

When a DVT dislodges and becomes a life-threatening PE, thrombolytic agents can be used. Thrombolytic agents can be used in patients with hemodynamically unstable PE or massive iliofemoral thrombosis, and in those who are also at low risk for bleeding.[20] These agents are used as fibrinolytic therapy, which are designed to facilitate thrombolysis and decrease the ischemic damage produced by thrombotic events.[21] The drugs used for this purpose are known as plasminogen activators that bind to or induce a conformational change in plasminogen, proteolytically cleaving plasminogen to plasmin, thereby enhancing the fibrinolytic system.[21] Steptokinase is the oldest plasminogen activator approved for use with DVTs and is administered intravenously with a loading dose of 250,000 IU, followed by a 100,000 IU/h infusion for 24 hours. A limiting factor in the use of streptokinase is that patients can have an allergic reaction to the drug if they have had a recent streptococcal infection that can generate antibodies. Urokinase is another plasminogen activator that is administered intravenously with a loading dose of 2,000 IU followed by an infusion at 2,000 IU/kg per hour for 24 to 48 hours.[21] The disadvantage of both these drugs is that they lack fibrin specificity and will induce a systemic lytic effect.[22] tPA is also approved for use in the treatment of these patients. It is also administered intravenously and for DVT, the dose is 100 mg over the course of 2 hours.[21] Unlike the other two drugs, tPA does have relative fibrin specificity, which may not be as important as once thought, but the lytic state produced by tPA is less pronounced than streptokinase or urokinase.[21] There is no laboratory test that correlates with clinical efficacy of fibrinolytic therapy. However, a fibrinogen level less than 100 mg/dL has been associated with an increased hemorrhagic risk.[21] Table 6-7 summarizes the anticoagulants used for treating DVT and VTE.

The obvious side effect of any type of anticoagulation is bleeding. If the INR goal of 2.0 to 3.0 is attained, the risk of bleeding is minimal.[23] Careful consideration must be given to the patient's situation before starting anticoagulation, especially with the use of fibrinolytic therapy. Absolute contraindications for fibrinolytic therapy include active internal bleeding, hemorrhagic stroke, nonhemorrhagic stroke within the past year, intracranial neoplasm, and suspected aortic dissection. Relative contraindications can include prolonged cardiopulmonary resuscitation, severe hypertension, trauma within the past 4 weeks, surgery within the past 3 weeks, a history of bleeding diathesis, pregnancy, and active peptic ulcer disease.[21] The use of thrombolytic agents in the treatment of VTE should be individualized and careful consideration must be given to the risks and benefits of this type of intervention.[20]

Bleeding associated with anticoagulant therapy can be treated with various reversal agents such as protamine sulfate for heparin and vitamin K for coumadin. Treatment is also directed at correction of coagulopathies, as indicated by abnormal coagulation studies (e.g., PT/PTT). Use of blood products such as fresh-frozen plasma, cryoprecipitate, and platelets may be able to stop or decrease bleeding. Repletion of blood loss may also be necessary. Locating the major site of bleeding is very important but can be a challenging task, especially if the site is more occult in nature. Surgical intervention may be required, and this type of high-risk patient will need to be optimized before surgery.

Prophylaxis

Although treatment for DVT has become more delineated over the years, the key intervention with DVT and possible PE is prevention. The most common and oldest intervention is the use of low-dose unfractionated subcutaneous heparin of 5,000 units every 8 to 12 hours. LMWH has also been shown to be effective in preventing VTE, especially in surgical patients, even with patients undergoing hip and knee surgery.[23] Fondaparinux is a newer agent with selective antifactor Xa activity which is synthesized using no animal products and therefore does not generate allergic reactions such as heparin-induced thrombocytopenia.[21] Because of this unique property, fondaparinux use in prophalaxis is increasing. Oral anticoagulants are not used because of the higher rate of bleeding. Aspirin is also considered ineffective for VTE prophylaxis.[20,23] External pneumatic compression is a nonpharmacologic intervention that has proven valuable in many types of surgical patients including hip procedures. Elastic stockings are also used and found to be useful in nonorthopedic, moderate-risk surgical patient.[23] These prophylactic measures are stratified for use depending on the risk for DVT (Table 6-8).

Nursing Interventions

The primary approach to nursing management of the patient at risk for DVT includes identifying the risk category for a patient and implementing preventive strategies. Such strategies include active or passive leg exercises and early ambulation to increase muscle activity, thereby improving venous blood flow. Frequent turning, coughing, and deep breathing help to improve venous

Table 6-7 ■ DRUGS USED TO PROMOTE ANTICOAGULATION

Drug Category	Mechanism	Dose
Heparin, unfractionated (UFH)	Binds to and activates antithrombin III and reduces the formation of thrombin and fibrin	Load: 5,000 u or 75 u/kg followed by initial infusion 18 units/kg/min; adjust according weight based protocol using aPTT (goal is usually 1.5 to 2.5 times the normal aPTT value ~70 seconds)
Heparin, low-molecular-weight (LMWH), Enoxaparin	Similar to heparin but reduced ability to catalyze the inhibition of thrombin with retained ability to inhibit activity of factor Xa	1.5 mg/kg subcutaneously (SC) if dosed daily or 1.0 mg/kg if dosed q12hr (treatment doses) Prophylaxis dose range 20 to 60 mg q12hr depending on indication
Heparin, low-molecular weight, Dalteparin	Same as enoxaparin	100 units/kg q12hr or 200 u/kg SC daily (treatment dose) 2500 units 1 to 2 h preoperation and daily (prophylaxis)
Antithrombin-dependent anticoagulant, Danaparoid	Indirect inhibition of factor Xa and thrombin activity	750 units SC twice daily (prophylaxis) For HIT: 2250 units followed by 400 u/h × 4 h then 300 u/h × 4 h then 150 to 200 u/h*
Factor Xa inhibitor, Fondaparinux	Inhibits Factor Xa but not thrombin	2.5 mg SC daily
Oral anticoagulants, Warfarin	Antagonist of vitamin K	Dosed according to PT/INR (goal is related to reason for anticoagulation; usual INR goal is 2.0 to 3.0)
Plasminogen activator, Streptokinase	Induce a conformational change in plasminogen by proteolytically cleaving plasminogen to plasmin, enhancing fibrinolysis; no fibrin specificity	250,000 IU IV load followed by infusion 100,000 IU/h for 24 h
Plasminogen activator, Urokinase	Same as streptokinase	2,000 IU IV load followed by infusion 2000 IU/h for 24 to 48 h
Plasminogen activator, t-PA	Same as streptokinase but has relative fibrin specificity	100 mg over 2 h
Thrombin inhibitors, Argatroban	Directly inhibits thrombin formation enhancing fibrinolysis	1 to 2 mcg/kg/min infusion not to exceed 10 mcg/kg/min; adjust for hepatobiliary dysfunction*
Thrombin inhibitors, Lepirudin	Same as argatroban	0.4 mg/kg loading dose followed by 0.15 mg/kg/h infusion For HIT: 0.2 to 0.4 mg/kg bolus (only in case of life threatening thrombosis) followed by infusion at 0.1 mg/kg/h; reduce for renal dysfunction*
Thrombin inhibitors, Bivalirudin	Same as argatroban	1 mg/kg bolus; 2.5 mg/kg/h × 4 h then 0.2 mg/kg/h to 20 h

*Warkentin, T. (2007). Heparin-induced thrombocytopenia. *Hematology/Oncology Clinics of North America, 21*(4), 589–607.
Modified from Francis, C., & Kaplan, K. (2006). *Wilaims's hematology* (7th ed.). New York: McGraw-Hill Medical Publishing Division.

return. Other measures to promote venous return are pneumatic compression stockings, graduated compression stockings, elevating the foot of the bed 6 to 8 inches, and not raising the knee gatch to avoid excessive popliteal pressure. A thorough history of the patient's risk factors along with the vigilant physical assessment of extremities for any evidence of inflammation, such as redness, swelling, asymmetry, and tenderness, are critical. If any signs and symptoms are observed, objective diagnostic testing should be pursued. Bleeding is the most common complication of anticoagulant and fibrinolytic therapy. The patient must be observed for subtle signs of bleeding. Careful monitoring of all puncture sites is mandatory, especially femoral interventional

Table 6-8 ■ LEVELS OF THROMBOEMBOLISM RISK IN SURGICAL PATIENTS WITHOUT PROPHALAXIS

Risk Category	Successful Prevention Strategies
Low Risk	
Minor surgery in patients <40 years old with no additional risks	No specific prophylaxis except early and "aggressive" ambulation
Moderate Risk	
Minor surgery in patients with additional risk factors Surgery in patients aged 40–60 years with no additional risk factors	Low-dose unfractionated heparin (LDUH) q12h Low-molecular-weight heparin (LMWH) ≤3,400 units daily; graduated compression stockings (GCS) or intermittent pneumatic compression
High Risk	
Surgery. >60 years old or age 40–60 years with additional risk factors (prior VTE, cancer, or molecular hypercoagulability)	LDUH q 8 hours; LMWH >3,400 units daily or intermittent pneumatic compression
Highest Risk	
Surgery in patients with multiple risk factors (prior VTE, cancer, age >40 years)	LMWH >3,400 units daily, fondaparinux, oral
Hip or knee arthroplasty, major trauma, spinal cord injury	Vitamin K antagonists (INR 2–3); or intermittent pneumatic compression/GCS + LDUH/LMWH

Modified from Geerts, W., et al. (2004). Prevention of venous thromboembolism: The Seventh ACCP Conference on Antithrombotic and Thrombolytic Therapy. *Chest, 126*(3, Suppl.), 338S–400S.

sites, with special attention to the abdomen and flank areas where large amounts of blood can sequester before the patient becomes symptomatic. Gastrointestinal bleeding is also another mechanism for blood loss. Assessing for symptoms of abdominal discomfort as well as guiac testing of excretions of patients on anticoagulation should be routine nursing interventions. Patient education regarding PT monitoring, anticoagulant medications and their side effects, and interactions with other drugs should be reviewed. Leg elevation while sitting should be emphasized and the importance of physical activity when discharged should be emphasized. Risk factors such as obesity, smoking, and estrogen therapy should be identified and interventions designed to assist the patient to modify them as appropriate.[24] Because embolization is always a threat, special attention to the assessment of cardiopulmonary indicators is paramount. PE may present with sudden onset of dyspnea, chest pain, and tachypnea, accompanied by other symptoms that will be discussed in the next section.

Pulmonary Embolism

Although diagnostic and therapeutic modalities have improved over the years, PE remains a challenging clinical entity. The incidence of symptomatic PE is estimated to occur in more than 600,000 patients annually in the United States and contributes to 50,000 to 200,000 deaths.[17] Two thirds of patients with fatal cases will die within 1 hour of presentation. The mortality rate for hospitalized patients with PE has remained at approximately 15% over the past 40 years.[17] Similar information has been gleaned from the International Cooperative Pulmonary Embolism Registry (ICOPER), which is a collaborative study developed to gather worldwide data about PE. The overall 3-month mortality rate for all PE patients in the ICOPER was 17.4%.[25] An interesting finding of the ICOPER is that postoperative prophylaxis is not instituted in more than half the patients in that database. Concern regarding lack of prophylaxis was echoed in the ACCP Consensus Conference report,[20] which recommended that every hospital develop a formal strategy that addresses the prevention of thromboembolic complications with a written thromboprophylaxis policy, especially for high-risk groups.

PE may be the result of either arterial or venous thrombi. Common sources of PE include deep venous thrombi from the lower legs, right atrial thrombi, septic foci (often related to IV drug abuse or infected vascular access sites), and tumors. Other sources of emboli are amniotic fluid, fat, air, bone marrow, and other foreign bodies. These latter sources have a pathophysiology that is different from the usual venous source and occur less frequently. Many factors predispose patients to PE and are similar to those risk factors for development of DVT discussed earlier. One unique factor that predisposes patients to PE is an inherited predisposition to hypercoagulability caused by a resistance to APC. This inherited predisposition manifests itself as a gene mutation known as factor V Leiden in the factor V gene. Factor V Leiden is the most common of all the other inherited hypercoaguable states.[25]

Pathophysiology

A PE is a mechanical complete or partial obstruction to blood flow from the right to left heart. The physiological response of the patient is dependent on the degree of obstruction and the underlying cardiopulmonary function.[17] A patient with good cardiopulmonary function and a complete obstruction may have the same outcome as a patient with poor cardiopulmonary function and a partial obstruction. Cardiac failure with a massive PE is caused by increased wall stress and ischemia that comprises the right ventricular (RV) function quickly and eventually impacts left ventricular (LV) function.[17] Increased afterload develops due to obstruction of blood flow out of the right ventricle. Additional factors that increase afterload are neural reflexes, the release of humoral factors, mediators that are released by platelets (platelet activating factor and serotonin), and systemic arterial hypoxemia.[17] The CO is initially maintained by increased catecholamine release resulting in an increased heart rate and contractility. The RV will attempt to contract against the resistance presented by the embolism, but will eventually decompensate leading to an increase in RV volume. This increased RV preload leads to increased wall stress and compromised RV coronary blood flow and ischemia. Increased RV volume will also cause a septal shift that will decrease LV distensibility and decrease LV preload. This alteration in preload will lead to a decrease in CO and mean arterial pressure (MAP). RV coronary perfusion pressure is dependent on the gradient between the MAP and the RV subendocardial pressure.[17] The decrease in MAP will aggravate the compromised RV oxygen supply. Further RV ischemia will perpetuate decreased RV performance and the cycle will continue until complete decompensation occurs. This pathophysiological cycle is summarized in Figure 6-5.

The emboli itself can lead to a local aggregation of platelets and the release of vasoactive substances, which increase vasoconstriction. Gas exchange abnormalities are related to the size and type of embolic material, the extent of the occlusion and the underlying cardiopulmonary status and length of time since embolization.[17] With PE, there is initial adequate ventilation coupled with inadequate perfusion (i.e., alveolar deadspace). The persistent obstruction and associated vasoconstriction can lead to bronchoconstriction, which produce shunting, another ventilation–perfusion (VQ) imbalance. Any sustained VQ mismatch results in arterial hypoxemia. The hemodynamic and gas exchange consequences of a massive PE can lead to a dramatic clinical presentation.

Clinical Manifestations

PE may occur with a sudden, abrupt onset, or have an insidious onset that mimics other cardiopulmonary disorders. Dyspnea is the most common symptom associated with PE and tachypnea is the most frequent sign.[26] Other signs such as pleuritic pain, cough, or hemoptysis can be present and may indicate a small PE located near the pleura.[26] Classic cardiac signs such as tachycardia, low-grade fever, and neck vein distention can also be observed on presentation but may also be the function of age, the size of the PE, and the underlying cardiopulmonary status. Younger patients may not have any of these signs whereas older patients may present with several or all of these signs.[26] There may also be vague complaints of chest discomfort, which can also be associated with acute coronary ischemic syndromes.

The presentation of a patient with a massive PE can be very similar to the signs and symptoms mentioned above. The only difference is that the signs and symptoms are a more extreme and exaggerated response to the embolic event. The classic clinical presentation of a massive PE can include syncope, cyanosis, tachycardia (heart rate >120 beats/min), tachypnea (respiratory rate >30 breaths/min), and hepatomegaly.[17] Because symptoms of a massive PE can be so vague, it is important to gather data about patients and continually consider what their risk factors are for having a PE.

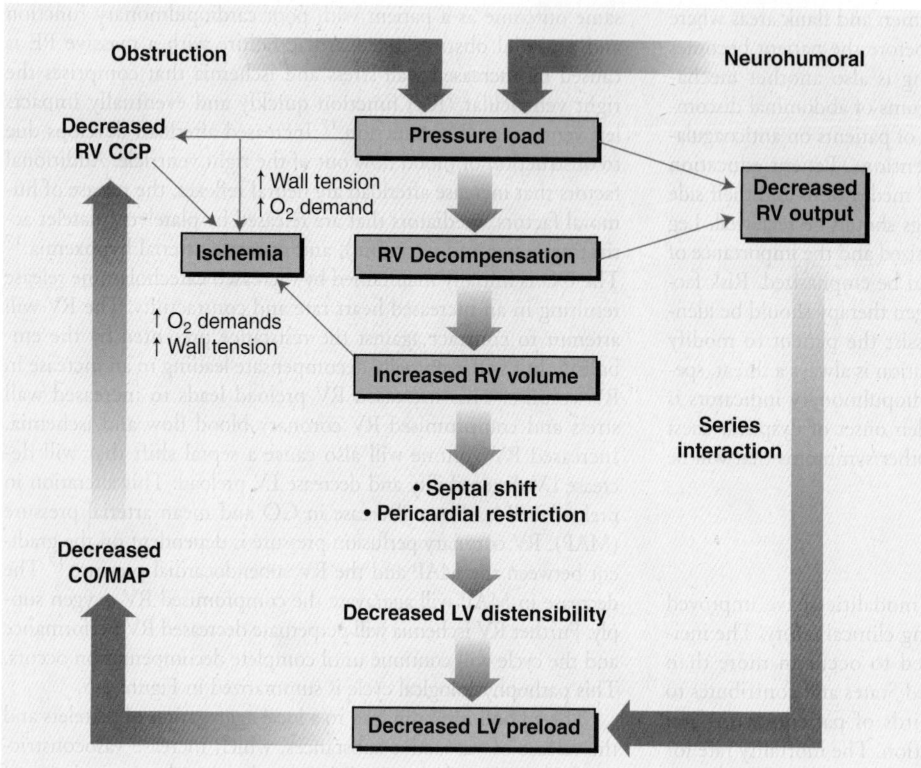

■ **Figure 6-5** Pathophysiology of pulmonary embolism. (From Wood, K. [2002]. Major pulmonary embolism. Review of pathophysiologic approach to the golden hour of hemodynamically significant pulmonary embolism. *Chest, 121*[3], 877–905.)

Medical Management

The diagnosis of PE is challenging, because PE can mimic other cardiorespiratory or musculoskeletal disorders such as myocardial infarction, pneumonia, congestive heart failure, asthma, or costochondritis. The diagnosis of PE should always be confirmed by objective tests. However, there are few tests that are specific for PE. Because the protective mechanism of fibrinolysis is triggered with the formation of a clot, tests reflecting fibrinolysis have been helpful in making the diagnosis of PE. The quantitative plasma D-dimer enzyme-linked immunosorbent assay (ELISA) level is elevated (>500 ng/mL) in more than 90% of patients with PE but is not specific and therefore not useful when considering hospitalized patients.[26] ABG values are not valuable in the diagnosis of PE, which is contrary to classic teaching. The expected hypoxemia associated with PE was not found to be consistently present in patients with documented PE. The ECG may be abnormal with an S wave in lead I, a Q wave in lead III, and inverted T wave in lead III; however, these changes are usually seen in patients with a massive PE. A normal chest radiograph in a dyspneic patient could suggest a possible PE.[26] However, a more definitive diagnosis can be made by means of a noninvasive lung VQ scan. In PE, a defect is evident in the perfusion portion of the scan in conjunction with a normal ventilation scan. An abnormal VQ scan suggests PE. If the VQ scan is normal, the likelihood of PE is low. This test needs to be carefully evaluated since pre-existing cardiopulmonary disease can distort the interpretation and both the ventilation and perfusion portion of the test should be performed.

If the VQ scan is nondiagnostic, a pulmonary angiogram should be performed and is considered the gold standard. A definitive diagnosis of PE is best made by pulmonary angiography because a well-performed pulmonary angiogram excludes the diagnosis of PE. Although the time and costs involved with the invasive pulmonary angiography preclude its routine use in the diagnosis of PE, it remains the most reliable clinical study available.[17] Recent radiological advances now include the spiral chest computed tomography (CT), which is a newer test used in diagnosing PE. The strength of the spiral CT is its ability to detect emboli in the central arteries but it is not as sensitive for finding peripheral emboli in the pulmonary vasculature.[20] Both tests require a significant contrast dye load and this fact should be considered when deciding on the test. Contrast-induced nephropathy may be caused by direct toxic effects on the tubular epithelial cells by the formation of reactive oxygen species or reduced antioxidant activity.[27] Decreased renal function from contrast dye load may also be caused by an alteration in renal hemodynamics resulting in renal vasoconstriction and erythrocyte aggregation.[27] The hallmark intervention for prevention of contrast-induced nephropathy is hydration, usually with normal saline.[27] Hydration with sodium bicarbonate has also been shown to be as effective as hydration with normal saline.[11] Administration of acetylcysteine before and after dye load has been shown to have renal vasodilatory effects as well as antioxidant benefits.[28] However, a meta-analysis did not clearly confirm the efficacy of acetylcysteine.[27]

Once PE is diagnosed, anticoagulation is the first intervention. The previous section on anticoagulation for DVT discusses the usual approach for treatment. If the patient is severely compromised and experiencing cardiopulmonary failure due to a PE, thrombolytic therapy is indicated. Caval interruption or inferior vena cava filter can also be used to treat a PE. This intervention helps prevent passage of emboli to the lung and is used in cases where anticoagulation may not be appropriate. There are two types of filters: bird's nest filter, which is placed infrarenally, and the Greenfield filter, which is placed suprarenally.[26] In rare instances, pulmonary embolectomy may be performed in conjunction with cardiopulmonary bypass. Mortality rates with this procedure can exceed 50% and should be performed only in institutions that can quickly mobilize a cardiac surgery team.[17] With prompt identification and treatment, prognosis is good for patients with PE. Successful treatment results in little long-term morbidity. Sequelae such as pulmonary hypertension and cor pulmonale may be seen in patients with underlying cardiopulmonary disease or those with massive emboli.

Nursing Interventions

Because PE can be a life-threatening event, the emphasis of nursing management is on prevention. As discussed previously, prevention of thrombus formation and early detection of PE is essential. Fifty percent of those patients who die of PE do so within the first hour. Any patient experiencing a sudden onset of dyspnea, tachypnea, and possible chest pain must be evaluated for the possibility of PE. Assessing the character of the patient's chest pain is important because most patients describe their pain as pleuritic. A 12-lead ECG and an ABG also provide useful data. Explaining all procedures and tests helps reassure patients during a time of discomfort and anxiety about the sudden change of their condition. Once the diagnosis of PE has been established, continued nursing management of the patient's cardiopulmonary function is essential.

Because profound arterial hypoxemia can accompany PE, the primary goal is to normalize gas exchange. By normalizing the exchange of gases and minimizing the VQ mismatch, other systemic effects of impaired gas exchange can also be ameliorated. Interventions to support respiratory function by patient positioning and the use of supplemental oxygen may help decrease the degree of hypoxemia accompanying PE. Supplemental oxygen may be administered by face mask or, if necessary, by endotracheal intubation and mechanical ventilation. Positioning the patient with the head of the bed elevated allows for better chest expansion with respiration. Coaching of the patient to promote the best respiratory pattern can be very important and maintaining a calm environment and approach to the patient can make the difference in the patient's course. The administration of prescribed analgesics and sedatives may help relieve the patient's discomfort and anxiety. By reducing discomfort and anxiety, respiratory rate may also decrease, thus reducing the additional vasoconstriction and bronchoconstriction caused by lower Pa_{CO_2} levels. Anticoagulants and thrombolytic agents, as described earlier, are usually ordered by the physician. These agents help decrease the recurrence of emboli and may help lyse the embolus; thus, restoring normal blood flow through the pulmonary vasculature.

Frequent assessment of cardiopulmonary function is also important. Vital signs, particularly respiratory rate, heart rate, and blood pressure should be assessed and documented hourly and as needed. Normal vital signs may indicate improved gas exchange. ABG analysis offers a quantitative assessment of gas exchange. Because of the prolonged duration of anticoagulant therapy, patients require extensive teaching about the administration and follow-up schedules of oral anticoagulants, a medication identification card or band, potential hazards associated with therapy, and the signs and symptoms of bleeding and recurrent VTE. Dietary restrictions and foods that contain large amounts of vitamin K should be reviewed. This is a disease with long-term implications that can be successfully managed with patient participation and education.

Heparin-Induced Thrombocytopenia

Anticoagulation is a key intervention in treating cardiovascular disease. The primary agent that has been used for years is heparin and with an increased use of heparin, a new syndrome has been identified. Heparin-induced thrombocytopenia (HIT) is a challenging immunohematologic issue that was originally described in the early 1960s. Key elements of the syndrome were discovered in the mid 1970s, and the antigen target of the HIT antibody was identified in 1992.[29] However, knowledge about this disease is still in the developmental stages. With more patients being exposed to heparin or related drugs, the occurrence of HIT is increasing. One issue with the disease is that it is difficult to diagnose and unpredictable in incidence but can have some devastating outcomes. Unlike other clotting disorders, HIT is the result of an immunohematologic reaction.

Pathophysiology

The development of the pathogenic IgG is the key to this disorder. The heparin binds with PF4, which leads to the development of a highly reactive antigenic complex. Pathogenic IgG is formed and activates the platelets.[30] The major target antigen is a macromolecular complex comprising heparin or other high-sulfated oligosaccharides and PF4, which binds to the platelet surface.[30]

HIT is an immune-mediated adverse drug reaction that is caused by heparin-dependent, platelet-activating IgG antibodies that recognize complexes of PF4 bound to "heparin."[31(p589)] These antibodies are known as HIT antibodies because once they "see" heparin, the autoimmune response is triggered and they become anti PF4/heparin, platelet-activating IgG antibodies. The activated platelets release procoagulant and PF4 neutralizes heparin that leads to increased thrombin generation.[31] With more thrombin available, a hypercoagulable state develops and can lead to the formation of thrombi (arterial and venous). The HIT antibodies are also thought to activate the endothelium and monocytes leading to the expression of tissue factor at cell surfaces, which can also lead to thrombin formation (see Fig. 6-6). With this immunologic cascade of events, HIT is a potentially devastating thrombotic disorder.

Etiology

The cause of HIT is the exposure to heparin leading to the development of anti-PF4/heparin platelet-activating IgG antibodies, which leads to thrombocytopenia. Patients generally experience a 50% decrease in platelet count, but it is important to note that the postoperative patient's "baseline" platelet count is the highest postoperative count prior to the decrease suspected with HIT.[31]

An immune response requires time for the reaction to develop. Because of this aspect of the disease, HIT can have varying time onsets and is important in diagnosing HIT. The usual onset for 70% of patients is a decrease in platelet count 5 to 10 days after starting heparin (first day of heparin use = day 0).[31] If patients have an exposure to heparin within the past few weeks or months leading to HIT antibody development, a "rapid onset" HIT presentation can occur within 24 hours of subsequent heparin administration.[31] When the platelet count decreases after all heparin has been stopped, this is a "delayed presentation" HIT and thought to be due to high levels of circulating antibodies.[31] Although HIT can develop in any patient who has exposure to heparin, there are certain patient populations that seem to have a higher incidence. These risk factors include: (1) duration of

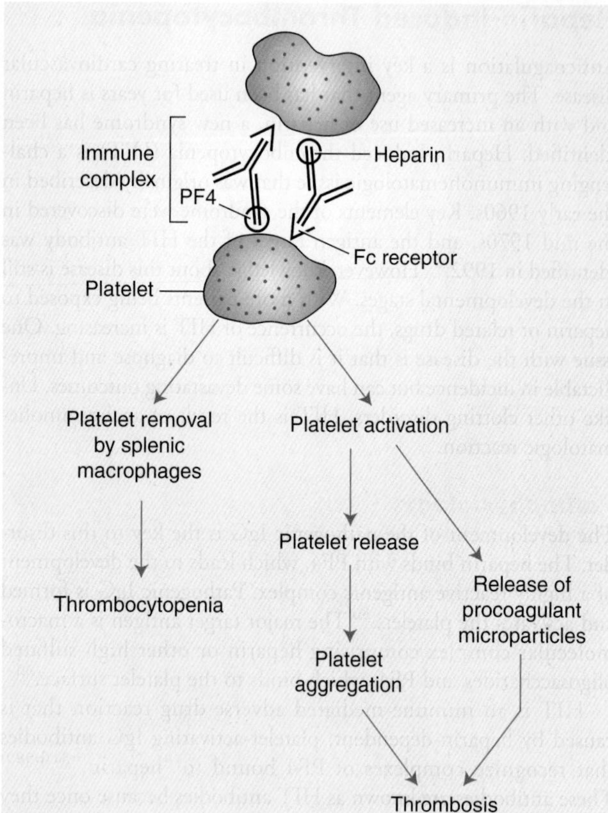

■ **Figure 6-6** Pathophysiology of HIT. Two explanations for thrombosis in HIT. Activation of platelets (plt) by antiplatelet factor 4 (PF4)/heparin IgG antibodies (HIT antibodies), leading to formation of procoagulant, platelet-derived microparticles, and neutralization of heparin by PF4 released from activated platelets, lead to marked increase in thrombin (hypercoagulability state) characterized by an increased risk of venous and arterial thrombosis, as well as increased risk for coumarin-induced venous limb gangrene. However, it is also possible that unique pathogenetic mechanisms operative in HIT explain unusual thromboses, such as arterial "white clots." For example, HIT antibodies have been shown to activate endothelium and monocytes (leading to cell surface tissue factor expression), although this stimulation may be largely "indirect" through poorly defined mechanisms involving platelet activation and, possibly, formation of platelet-derived microparticles. Further, aggregates of platelets and polymorphonuclear leukocytes have been described in HIT. To what extent these cooperative interactions between platelets, platelet-derived microparticles, polymorphonuclear leukocytes, monocytes, and endothelium lead to arterial (or venous) thrombotic events in HIT, either in large or small vessels, remains unclear. HIT, heparin-induced thrombocytopenia. (Reproduced from Warkentin, T. E. [2004]. An overview of the heparin-induced thrombocytopenia syndrome. *Seminars in Thrombosis and Hemostasis, 30*[3], 275.)

heparin use greater than 1 week, (2) exposure to unfractionated heparin has the highest risk, (3) postsurgical thromboprophalaxis; and (4) higher occurrence in women.[31]

Clinical Presentation

The initial presentation of HIT is thrombocytopenia during or after heparin therapy leading to the development of thrombosis. Venous thrombotic complications are most common including DVT (50%) and PE (25%). Venous thrombosis of the adrenal vein occurs and can lead to adrenal hemorrhage.[31] Arterial thrombotic complications include limb artery thrombosis, thrombotic stroke, myocardial infarction, or other arterial thrombosis (mesentery or spinal).[31] Skin necrosis at heparin injection sites is another presentation that can range from painful erythematous papules to dermal necrosis. Warfarin necrosis with HIT is characterized by venous limb gangrene usually with DVT or classic necrosis in nonacral sites (breasts, abdominal wall, thigh, calf, or forearm). Overt DIC is another sequelae of HIT that occurs in 10% to 20% of patients. There has even been anaphylactic reaction to IV heparin 5 to 30 minutes after administration with symptoms ranging from cardiac arrest to an inflammatory presentation, that is, fever, chills, rigors, or flushing.[31]

Arterial thrombosis usually involves the distal portion of the aorta, and the symptoms can vary in degree depending on the thrombus size. Absent pulses indicate total arterial thrombosis occlusion whereas pulses with distal extremity ischemia indicate microvascular occlusion.[31] The classic presentation for acute arterial thrombosis is known as the "6 Ps": pallor, pulselessness, pain, paresthesias, paralysis, and poikilothermy (coolness).[24] Either the arms or the legs can be involved. The pain and paralysis are the result of nerve and skeletal muscle ischemia that can occur as early as 4 to 6 hours after the occlusion. Beyond this time period, the situation can progress to potential compartment syndrome with severe pain, tense swelling, and muscle tenderness of the affected extremity.[24] In HIT, limb amputation is common.

Medical Management

Medical management is challenged with making the diagnosis of HIT. The diagnosis of HIT is based on the patient's exposure to heparin, which can extend to 100 days before the event.[32] The diagnostic process continues with the assessment of the platelet count. Thrombocytopenia after heparin exposure is the hallmark signal to indicate HIT, but other reasons for a decrease in platelets also need to be considered. Because of the complexity of diagnosing HIT, Warkentin[31] has developed a "4Ts" scoring system (thrombocytopenia, timing, thrombosis, and other cause of thrombocytopenia) to help estimate the pretest probability of HIT (Table 6-9). Any source of heparin or LMWH must be discontinued. Even the smallest amounts of heparin such as heparin-coated catheters or heparin flush solutions must be eliminated.

The next step is to pursue laboratory detection of HIT antibodies. Platelet activation assays are the newer tests that test patient serum against donor platelets "washed" in apyrase-containing buffer (potentiator of HIT antibody-induced platelet activation) and have high sensitivity.[31] PF4-dependent enzyme immunoassays (EIA) were one of the original tests developed for HIT and a negative test essentially rules out the diagnosis of HIT.[33] However, the EIAs detect more clinically insignificant antibodies, which can lead to overdiagnosis of HIT.[31,34] A combination of the platelet activation assays and the EIAs should be used in the diagnosis of HIT. Varying laboratory practices in North America may impact the correct detection of the HIT diagnosis.[34] The presence of antibodies may not always confirm the diagnosis of HIT. HIT antibodies develop and can be transient emphasizing the importance to test acute plasma or serum.[31] Clinical as well as laboratory data need to be compiled and interpreted to properly diagnose HIT. This is the reason why Warkentin has described HIT as a "clinicopathologic syndrome."[29]

The major clinical decision will be starting anticoagulation using one of the three nonheparin anticoagulants approved for the

Table 6-9 ■ "4Ts" SCORING SYSTEM FOR ESTIMATING PRETEST PROBABILITY FOR HIT POINTS (0, 1, OR 2 FOR EACH OF FOUR CATEGORIES; MAXIMUM SCORE = 8)

Date	2	1	0
Thrombocytopenia score = ____	>50% platelet decrease to nadir ≥20 × 10^9/L	30% to 50% platelet count decrease (or >50% directly resulting from surgery) or nadir (10 to 19) × 10^9/L	<30% platelet decrease or nadir <10 × 10^9/L
Timing of platelet count decrease, thrombosis, or other sequelae (first day of heparin course = day 0) score = _____	Day 5 to 10 onset or ≤1 day (with recent heparin exposure within 5 to 30 days)	Consistent with day 5 to 10 decrease, but not clear (e.g., missing platelet counts), or ≤1 day (heparin exposure within past 31 to 100 days) or platelet decrease after day 10	Platelet count decrease ≤4 days without recent heparin exposure
Thrombosis (including adrenal infarction) or other sequelae (e.g., skin lesions) score = ___	Proven new thrombosis or skin necrosis (at injection site) or post IV heparin bolus anaphylactoid reaction	Progressive or recurrent thrombosis, or erythematous skin lesions (at injection sites), or suspected thrombosis (not proven)	None
OTher cause for thrombocytopenia score = _____	No explanation for platelet count decrease is evident	Possible other cause is evident	Definite other cause is present
Total score = ____ (pretest probability score: 6 to 8 = high; 4 and 5 = intermediate; 0 to 3 = low)			

Changes to score can occur, based upon new information (e.g., further decrease in platelets, new thrombosis).
Warkentin, T. (2007). Heparin-induced thrombocytopenia. *Hematology/Oncology Clinics of North America, 21*(4): 589–607.

treatment of HIT: danaparoid, lepirudin, and argatroban (see Table 6-7). Bivalirudin and fondaparnux are used for treating HIT but their use is not supported by controlled studies.[31] Danaparoid is an indirect inhibitor of factor Xa and thrombin. Argatroban is a direct thrombin inhibitor. Lepirudin is a recombinant hirudin and has high affinity binding to two sites on thrombin.[31] All three approved nonheparin anticoagulants can be administered intravenously. Hirudin is the most potent natural thrombin inhibitor that is found in the salivary gland of the medicinal leech and lepirudin is a derivative of hirudin using recombinant DNA therapy. Dosing recommendations for these drugs can be found in Table 6-7. A baseline aPTT should be obtained before the start of therapy. Infusion doses of these drugs are maintained to achieve an aPTT 1.5 to 2.5 times the normal value, similar to the goal of heparin therapy. The aPTT is usually sampled every 6 hours, but with lepirudin, the aPTT should be drawn every 4 hours.[31] Danaparoid monitoring utilizes antifactor Xa levels with a therapeutic target range of 0.5 to 0.8 anti-Xa U/mL.[31]

Warkentin[31] summarized the principles of HIT when it is strongly suspected or has been confirmed. It is important to (1) stop all heparin including LMWH and heparin administered as flushes and (2) start alternative nonheparin anticoagulantion. Evidence supports the use of the three approved nonheparin anticoagulants described previously. Warfarin is contraindicated in the acute phase of HIT due to the risk of warfarin necrosis manifested by venous limb gangrene or classic skin necrosis.[31] Warfarin can also prolong the aPTT values, which could lead to underdosing of the direct thrombin inhibitors.[31] Prophylactic platelet transfusions should not be given. Diagnostic laboratory testing should include EIA testing, which can rule in or out the HIT diagnosis in 80% to 90% of cases in the appropriate clinical context. Platelet activation assays should be used with the remaining percentage of patients.[31] Finally, duplex ultrasonography should be performed to investigate for lower limb DVT.[31] For patients with a history of HIT who have an important indication for heparin, it is recommended that sufficient time has elapsed since the episode (more than 2 to 3 months) to ensure that the antibodies are no longer present.[31]

Nursing Interventions

This clinicopathological syndrome requires the most astute observational and correlation skills of a nurse. A high index of suspicion is needed especially with postoperative surgical patients who are receiving prophylactic doses of unfractionated heparin for at least 5 days.[32] A thorough history of the patient's possible exposure to heparin, including 100 days before the event, must be obtained. Platelet count should be measured promptly in these patient populations and monitored closely. ACCP guideline[20] recommend at least every other day platelet count monitoring in high risk patients until day 14 or stopping heparin (whichever comes first). Similar monitoring during the use of therapeutic unfractionated heparin should also be followed.[35]

A decreasing platelet count should cause suspicion and the search for possible thrombosis formation should begin. Vigilant physical assessment of extremities for any evidence of embolic events such as erythema, asymmetrical edema of the extremities, and/or tenderness is critical. The "6 Ps" should provide guidelines for monitoring limb perfusion.[24] Early observation of limb compromise may allow appropriate vascular intervention, which could avert amputation. Further evaluation and observation of all body systems, especially neurological, pulmonary, and cardiac, may reveal early signs and symptoms of embolic events. If the patient displays any sign of restlessness or agitation, physiological factors such as hypoxemia should be the first consideration. Monitoring oxygenation using pulse oximetry will give some estimate of oxygenation that can be confirmed with an ABG. If gas exchange is adequate and restlessness and agitation persist, neurological causes must be considered and sedation should be avoided unless indicated. Respiratory distress with tachypnea, dyspnea on exertion, prolonged expiratory time as well as restlessness, and agitation could be indications of pulmonary emboli. The patient's heart rate, rhythm, and blood pressure should be continually monitored for any changes. Hemodynamic monitoring may be used and variations in indices may indicate cardiac failure, myocardial infarction, or pulmonary complications such as PE depending on the situation and the primary disorder. Gastrointestinal dysfunction can present with a wide range of signs and symptoms from nausea and vomiting to acute abdominal pain. Assessment of the abdomen, as well as monitoring trends in liver function test, should never be omitted and given special attention if HIT is suspected. Any abdominal discomfort should be carefully considered and monitored for any progression. Monitoring urine output for at least 0.5 to 1 mL/kg per hour should be routine practice. The BUN and creatinine trends should also be closely reviewed. If these organ systems are severely compromised, multisystem organ dysfunction may be the end result, with poor outcomes. HIT can be a devastating syndrome.

REFERENCES

1. Lichtman, M., Beutler, E., Kipps, T., et al. (2006). *Williams hematology.* New York: McGraw-Hill.
2. Proceedings of the Third Margaux Conference on Critical Illness: The Endothelium—An Underrecognized Organ in Critical Illness? Sedona, Arizona, USA. November 14–18, 2001. (2002). *Critical Care Medicine, 30,* S179–S348.
3. Libby, P., Ridker, P. M., & Maseri, A. (2002). Inflammation and atherosclerosis. *Circulation, 105,* 1135–1143.
4. Hoffman, R. S., Benz, E., Shattil, S., et al. (2005). *Hematology: Basic physiology and practice.* Philadelphia: Churchill-Livingstone.
5. Turgeon, M. (2005). *Clinical hematology: Theory and procedures.* Philadelphia: Williams & Wilkins.
6. Hack, C. E., & Zeerleder, S. (2001). The endothelium in sepsis: Source of and a target for inflammation. *Critical Care Medicine, 29,* S21–S27.
7. Dellinger, R. P., Levy, M. M., Carlet, J. M., et al. (2008). Surviving Sepsis Campaign: International guidelines for management of severe sepsis and septic shock: 2008. *Critical Care Medicine, 36,* 296–327.
8. Bernard, G. R., Vincent, J. L., Laterre, P. F., et al. (2001). Efficacy and safety of recombinant human activated protein C for severe sepsis. *New England Journal of Medicine, 344,* 699–709.
9. Libby, P. (2002). Atherosclerosis: The new view. *Scientific American, 286,* 46–55.
10. Owen, D., & Webster, J. (1998). *Hematology: Clinical physiology AACN clinical reference for critical care nursing.* St. Louis: CV Mosby.
11. Merten, G. J., Burgess, W. P., Gray, L. V., et al. (2004). Prevention of contrast-induced nephropathy with sodium bicarbonate: A randomized controlled trial. *Journal of the American Medical Association, 291,* 2328–2334.
12. Liebman, H., & Weltz, I. (2005). Disseminated intravascular coagulation. In R. S. Hoffman, E. Benz, S. Shattil, et al. (Eds.), *Williams hematology.* New York: Churchill-Livingstone.
13. Hebert, P. C. (1999). Anemia and red cell transfusion in critical care. Transfusion requirements in Critical Care Investigators and the Canadian Critical Care Trials Group. *Minerva Anestesiologica, 65,* 293–304.
14. Goodnough, L. T., & Shander, A. S. (2007). Recombinant factor VIIa: Safety and efficacy. *Current Opinion in Hematology, 14,* 504–509.
15. O'Connell, K. A., Wood, J. J., Wise, R. P., et al. (2006). Thromboembolic adverse events after use of recombinant human coagulation factor VIIa. *Journal of the American Medical Association, 295,* 293–298.
16. Grenvik, A., Ayres, S., Holbrook, P., et al. (2000). *Textbook of critical care.* Philadelphia: WB Saunders.
17. Wood, K. E. (2002). Major pulmonary embolism: Review of a pathophysiologic approach to the golden hour of hemodynamically significant pulmonary embolism. *Chest, 121,* 877–905.
18. Crowther, M. A. (2005). Venous thromboembolism. In R. S. Hoffman, E. Benz, S. Shattil, et al. (Eds.), New York: Churchill-Livingstone.
19. Hull, R. D., Pineo, G., & Raskob, G. (2000). Diagnosis and treatment of venous thromboembolism. In A. Grenvik, S. Ayres, P. Holbrook, et al. (Eds.), *Textbook of critical care medicine.* Philadelphia: WB Saunders.
20. Geerts, W. H., Pineo, G. F., Heit, J. A., et al. (2004). Prevention of venous thromboembolism: The Seventh ACCP Conference on Antithrombotic and Thrombolytic Therapy. *Chest, 126,* 338S–400S.
21. Francis, C., & Kaplan, K. (2006). Principles of antithrombotic therapy. In M. Lichtman, E. Beutler, T. Kipps, et al. (Eds.), *Williams hematology.* New York: McGraw-Hill.
22. Brunton, L., Lazo, J., & Parker, K. (2006). *Goodman & Gilman's the pharmacologic basis of therapeutics.* New York: McGraw-Hill.
23. Dalen, J. E. (2002). Pulmonary embolism: What have we learned since Virchow? Treatment and prevention. *Chest, 122,* 1801–1817.
24. Fahey, V. (1999). *Vascular nursing.* Philadelphia: WB Saunders.
25. Goldhaber, S. Z., Visani, L., & De Rosa, M. (1999). Acute pulmonary embolism: Clinical outcomes in the International Cooperative Pulmonary Embolism Registry (ICOPER). *Lancet, 353,* 1386–1389.
26. Goldhaber, S. Z. (2005). Deep vein thrombosis and pulmonary thromboembolism. In A. Fauci, E. Braunwald, D. Kasper, et al. (Eds.), *Harrison's principles of internal medicine.* New York: McGraw-Hill.
27. Bartorelli, A. L., & Marenzi, G. (2008). Contrast-induced nephropathy. *Journal of Interventional Cardiology, 21,* 74–85.
28. Tepel, M., van der Giet, M., Schwarzfeld, C., et al. (2000). Prevention of radiographic-contrast-agent-induced reductions in renal function by acetylcysteine. *New England Journal of Medicine, 343,* 180–184.
29. Warkentin, T. E. (1999). Heparin-induced thrombocytopenia: A clinicopathologic syndrome. *Thrombosis and Haemostasis, 82,* 439–447.
30. Warkentin, T. E., Chong, B. H., & Greinacher, A. (1998). Heparin-induced thrombocytopenia: Towards consensus. *Thrombosis and Haemostasis, 79,* 1–7.
31. Warkentin, T. E. (2007). Heparin-induced thrombocytopenia. *Hematology and Oncology Clinics of North America, 21,* 589–607, v.
32. Warkentin, T. E. (2002). Platelet count monitoring and laboratory testing for heparin-induced thrombocytopenia. *Archives of Pathology and Laboratory Medicine, 126,* 1415–1423.
33. Tortora, G., & Grabowski, S. (2003). *Principles of anatomy and physiology.* New York: John Wiley & Sons.
34. Price, E. A., Hayward, C. P., Moffat, K. A., et al. (2007). Laboratory testing for heparin-induced thrombocytopenia is inconsistent in North America: A survey of North American specialized coagulation laboratories. *Thrombosis and Haemostasis, 98,* 1357–1361.
35. Warkentin, T. E., & Greinacher, A. (2004). Heparin-induced thrombocytopenia: Recognition, treatment, and prevention: The Seventh ACCP Conference on Antithrombotic and Thrombolytic Therapy. *Chest, 126,* 311S–337S.

WEBSITES

www.accp.org (especially for guidelines for prophalaxis and treatment of DVT, PE, and HIT)
www.guidelines.gov

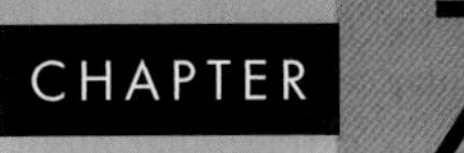

CHAPTER 7 Fluid and Electrolyte and Acid–Base Balance and Imbalance

Linda Felver

PRINCIPLES OF FLUID BALANCE

The fluid in the body serves many vital functions. In addition to being the milieu in which cellular chemistry occurs, it provides the transport medium for oxygen and other nutrients to reach the cells and for carbon dioxide and other metabolic waste products to be removed from the body. Technically, *fluid* is water plus the substances dissolved in it.

With aging, the amount of water in the body decreases. The body ranges from 70% water by weight (newborn infant) to 60% (young or middle-aged adult) to 45% (older adult woman). Women have less water by weight than men because a higher percentage of their weight is fat. Similarly, water is a lower percentage of body weight in obese people. One liter of water weighs 1 kg (2.2 lb). Thus, a standard 70-kg (154-lb) middle-aged man (60% water) has 42 L of body water (70 kg × 0.60 = 42 kg; 42 kg = 42 L).[1]

Body Fluid Compartments

The fluid in the body lies in several compartments. The *extracellular fluid* consists primarily of vascular and interstitial fluids. Some extracellular fluid is located in bone and dense connective tissue; this fluid is not considered accessible for dynamic exchange. *Intracellular fluid*, as the name indicates, lies in the cells. *Transcellular fluid* is fluid that is secreted by epithelial cells. Examples of transcellular fluid are cerebrospinal fluid (CSF), saliva, and intestinal secretions. Many of the transcellular fluids are reabsorbed by the body after they have been secreted.

More water is located inside the cells than outside of them. Clinically, approximately two thirds of body water in adults is considered intracellular and one third extracellular. Thus, the 70-kg man who has 42 L of body water can be considered to have approximately 28 L of water inside the cells and 14 L of extracellular water. This extracellular water is approximately one third vascular and two thirds interstitial. For clinical purposes, the 70-kg man can be considered to have approximately 4.5 L of water in the vascular compartment and approximately 9.5 L in the interstitial compartment.

Osmolality

The relative proportion of water to particles in body fluid is measured as osmolality. Osmolality can be considered to be the degree of concentration. Technically, osmolality is defined as the number of moles of particles per kilogram of water. The normal range of osmolality of the blood is 280 to 300 mOsm/kg (lower in normal pregnancy).[2] Fluids that have osmolality within this normal range are called *isotonic*. Extracellular and intracellular fluids have the same osmolality. If the osmolality of the extracellular fluid is increased or decreased, then the osmolality of the intracellular fluid changes rapidly until intracellular and extracellular fluids again have the same osmolality. This process is discussed later in the "Fluid Distribution" section.

Although the osmolality of intracellular and extracellular fluids is the same, the ion composition of the two fluids differs. Thus, they have the same particle concentration, but the specific kinds of particles are different in the two fluids. Intracellular fluid has a higher concentration of protein and potassium, magnesium, and phosphate ions; extracellular fluid has a higher concentration of sodium, calcium, chloride, and bicarbonate ions.[3] Transcellular fluids are usually hypotonic; their ion composition varies widely depending on their physiologic function.

Processes Involved in Fluid Balance

Fluid balance is the net result of fluid intake, fluid distribution, fluid excretion, and fluid loss by abnormal routes. Fluid balance is maintained when fluid excretion and fluid loss through any abnormal routes are matched by fluid intake and when the fluid is distributed normally into its compartments.[1]

Fluid Intake

The major determinant of fluid intake in a healthy adult is habit. Thirst, another important determinant of fluid intake, can be caused by several physiologic mechanisms.[4] These include dryness of the oral mucous membranes, increase in osmolality of the body fluids (osmoreceptor-mediated thirst), decrease in extracellular fluid volume (ECV) (baroreceptor-mediated thirst), and increased renin secretion (angiotensin-mediated thirst). Osmoreceptor-mediated thirst is the most common cause of thirst in healthy adults. This mechanism becomes less effective with aging. Thus, older adults often have a greater need for water before they become thirsty. Cultural factors have an important influence on fluid intake. For example, intake of certain herbal teas may be considered necessary by some individuals when they become ill. Many people refuse to drink cold water when they have certain illnesses due to their cultural beliefs. In clinical settings, health care professionals often regulate the fluid intake. Routes of fluid intake include oral, rectal, intravenous, and intraosseous, as well as through tubes into body cavities. Oral fluid intake includes liquids and the water contained in food, as well as water made by cellular metabolism of ingested nutrients.

Fluid Distribution

Two types of fluid distribution operate in the body. First, fluid is distributed between the vascular and interstitial spaces, the two subcompartments of the extracellular compartment. Second, fluid is distributed between the extracellular and intracellular compartments. Different processes regulate these two types of fluid distribution.

Fluid distribution between the vascular and interstitial spaces is regulated by filtration. Filtration is the net result of four opposing forces. Two of these forces tend to move fluid out of the capillaries, whereas the other two tend to move fluid into the capillaries. Which direction the fluid moves in any one location depends on which forces are stronger. The two forces that tend to move fluid out of capillaries are the blood hydrostatic pressure (outward force against the capillary walls) and the interstitial fluid osmotic pressure (inward pulling force caused by particles in interstitial fluid). The two forces that tend to move fluid into capillaries are the blood osmotic pressure (inward pulling force caused by particles in blood) and the interstitial fluid hydrostatic pressure.

Usually, the blood hydrostatic pressure is highest at the arterial end of a capillary, and there is filtration from the capillary into the interstitial fluid. This flow of fluid out of the capillaries is useful in carrying oxygen, glucose, amino acids, and other nutrients to the cells that are surrounded by interstitial fluid. Most proteins are too large to cross into the interstitial fluid and remain in the capillary. At the venous end of a capillary, the blood hydrostatic pressure is usually lower and the blood osmotic pressure higher because fluid has left the capillary but the proteins have remained. These changes cause a net flow of fluid from the interstitial space back into the venous end of a capillary. The flow of fluid back into the capillaries is physiologically useful in carrying carbon dioxide, metabolic acids, and other waste products into the blood for further metabolism or excretion.

Changes in any of the four forces that determine the direction of filtration at the capillaries can cause abnormal distribution between the vascular and interstitial compartments. The most common abnormal distribution is edema, which is expansion of the interstitial space. Edema can be caused by increased blood hydrostatic pressure (e.g., venous congestion), increased microvascular permeability that allows proteins to leak into interstitial fluid, increased interstitial fluid osmotic pressure (e.g., inflammation), decreased blood osmotic pressure (e.g., hypoalbuminemia), or blockage of the lymphatic system, which normally removes excess fluid from the interstitial space and returns it to the vascular compartment.

The second type of fluid distribution occurs between the extracellular and intracellular compartments. This process is regulated by osmosis. Cell membranes are freely permeable to water, but the passage of ions and other particles depends on membrane transport processes. Osmotic pressure is an inward-pulling force caused by particles in a fluid. Both the extracellular and intracellular fluids exert osmotic pressure. Because the osmolality of the two compartments normally is the same, the osmotic pressures are the same. Therefore, the force pulling water into the cells balances the force pulling water into the interstitial space, maintaining the normal fluid distribution. If the osmolality of the extracellular fluid changes, however, then osmosis occurs, altering the fluid distribution until the osmolality in the extracellular and intracellular compartments again is the same. For example, if the extracellular fluid becomes more concentrated (increased osmolality), then the osmotic pressure of the extracellular fluid becomes higher than the osmotic pressure of the intracellular fluid. Water leaves the intracellular compartment until the intracellular fluid becomes as concentrated as the extracellular fluid. This process decreases the amount of water that is distributed into the intracellular compartment. Similarly, if the extracellular fluid becomes more dilute (decreased osmolality), then the osmotic pressure of the extracellular fluid becomes lower than the osmotic pressure of the intracellular fluid. Water moves by osmosis into the intracellular compartment until the intracellular fluid becomes as dilute as the extracellular fluid. This process increases the amount of water that is distributed into the intracellular compartment.

In summary, fluid distribution between the vascular and interstitial compartments depends on filtration, the net result of four forces that act on fluid at the capillary level. Fluid distribution between the extracellular and intracellular compartments depends on osmosis, the movement of water across cell membranes to equilibrate particle concentrations.

Fluid Excretion

Normal routes of fluid excretion are respiratory tract, urine, feces, and skin (insensible perspiration and sweat). In a standard adult, approximately 400 mL of water is excreted daily through the respiratory tract, even if the person is fluid-depleted. This amount increases during fever. The urine volume of a healthy adult varies according to the fluid intake, the needs of the body, and the hormonal status. It averages 1,500 mL. Major hormones that regulate urinary excretion of fluid are summarized in Table 7-1. Diuretics, ethanol, and caffeine increase urine volume. Fecal excretion of water averages 200 mL per day in healthy adults who have a normal fluid balance and a fully functioning bowel. Diarrhea causes a dramatic increase in fecal excretion of water.

Insensible perspiration is fluid excretion through the skin that is not visible. It averages 500 mL per day in a healthy adult. Insensible perspiration occurs even if the person is fluid-depleted. It increases during fever. Sweat is visible fluid excretion through the skin. The volume of sweat varies greatly depending primarily on thermoregulatory needs.

Fluid Loss by Abnormal Routes

Examples of abnormal routes of fluid loss are emesis, drains, suction, paracentesis, and hemorrhage. Third-spacing (e.g., ascites) can be considered abnormal fluid loss, even though the fluid remains in the body, because the fluid is not freely available to the normal fluid compartments.

Summary of Fluid Balance

In summary, the processes of fluid intake, fluid distribution, fluid excretion, and fluid loss by abnormal routes act together to determine fluid balance or imbalances. A change in one of these processes must be matched by a change in another to maintain fluid balance. For example, if an increased urine output is matched by an increased fluid intake, then fluid balance can be maintained. If changes in one or more of these processes are not matched by changes in the others, however, then a fluid imbalance occurs. Fluid imbalances may be characterized by altered *volume* of fluid (ECV imbalances), altered *concentration* of fluid (osmolality imbalances), or a combination of both.

EXTRACELLULAR FLUID VOLUME BALANCE

The ECV is the net result of fluid intake, fluid distribution, fluid excretion, and fluid loss by abnormal routes. A normal ECV is maintained when fluid excretion and any fluid loss are balanced

Table 7-1 ■ HORMONES THAT REGULATE RENAL FLUID EXCRETION

Hormone	Physiologic Source	Major Physiologic Actions	Stimuli That Increase Hormone Secretion	Stimuli That Decrease Hormone Secretion
Aldosterone	Adrenal cortex (zona glomerulosa)	Kidneys retain more saline (expands extracellular fluid volume) Kidneys excrete more potassium and hydrogen ions	Angiotensin II (from the renin–angiotensin system; kidneys release more renin during hypovolemia and other causes of decreased blood flow through the renal artery and by stimulation of renal sympathetic nerves) Hypokalemia	Decreased angiotensin II Hyperkalemia
Natriuretic peptides	*A-type natriuretic peptide*: atrial myocardium *B-type natriuretic peptide*: ventricular myocardium *C-type natriuretic peptide*: endothelial cells	Natriuresis (kidneys excrete more saline, which reduces extracellular fluid volume) Vasodilation (suppresses endothelin; arterioles dilate, which reduces peripheral vascular resistance and lowers blood pressure) Suppression of renin–angiotensin system	*A-type natriuretic peptide*: atrial dilation (stretch) *B-type natriuretic peptide*: increased ventricular end-diastolic pressure and volume *C-type natriuretic peptide*: vascular shear stress	*A-type natriuretic peptide*: lack of atrial dilation (decreased stretch) *B-type natriuretic peptide*: normal or decreased ventricular end-diastolic pressure and volume *C-type natriuretic peptide*: reduced vascular shear stress
Antidiuretic hormone (ADH)	Synthesized in preoptic and paraventricular nuclei of hypothalamus Secreted from posterior pituitary gland	Kidneys retain more water (dilutes body fluids, decreasing osmolality)	Increased osmolality of body fluids Hypovolemia Physiologic and psychological stressors, surgery/anesthesia, trauma, pain, nausea	Decreased osmolality of body fluids Hypervolemia Ethanol

by fluid intake and when the fluid distribution is normal. The body's responsiveness to administration of a fluid load has a circadian rhythm (i.e., varies in a cyclic manner over 24 hours). The kidneys can excrete an excess fluid load more efficiently if it is administered during the time that the person is normally active than if it is administered during a person's customary sleeping time.

The blood volume is an important determinant of the work of the heart and provides the medium for oxygen delivery to tissues. Therefore, ECV imbalances can interfere with cardiac function and tissue oxygenation.

Extracellular Fluid Volume Deficit

ECV deficit is caused by removal of sodium-containing fluid from the vascular and interstitial spaces. Usually, the fluid is removed from the body; however, in some cases, fluid is sequestered in the peritoneal cavity, the intestinal lumen, or some other "third space." ECV deficits occur when intake of sodium-containing fluid does not keep pace with increased fluid excretion or loss of fluid through abnormal routes. Clinical causes of ECV deficit are presented in Table 7-2. ECV deficit may develop in people with cardiac disease who use diuretics if the dosage is excessive.

Clinical manifestations of ECV deficit include sudden weight loss (unless there is third-spacing), poor skin turgor, dryness of opposing mucous membranes, hard dry stools, longitudinal furrows in the tongue, absence of tears and sweat, and soft sunken eyeballs. Although weight loss occurs immediately, most of these signs appear only after substantial fluid depletion. Cardiovascular manifestations are among the early signs; these are discussed next.

Many of the clinical manifestations of ECV deficit are evident in the cardiovascular system. Decreased volume in the vascular compartment causes postural blood pressure drop with postural tachycardia, delayed capillary refill, prolonged small vein filling time, flat neck veins when supine (or neck veins that collapse during inspiration), and decreased central venous pressure.

A postural blood pressure drop is assessed by measuring blood pressure and heart rate with the individual supine and then standing or sitting with the legs dependent (not horizontal). If both systolic and diastolic blood pressures decrease substantially and heart rate increases substantially, then these postural changes are due to ECV deficit. The increased heart rate indicates that autonomic reflexes are functioning and rules out autonomic insufficiency, which may cause an upright blood pressure to decrease when the ECV is normal. Postural blood pressure drop is not a reliable assessment for ECV deficit in individuals who have a transplanted heart. The heart rate may not increase in these individuals when their blood pressure drops from ECV deficit.

Small vein filling time is assessed by placing an individual's hand or foot below the level of the heart, occluding a small vein, milking it flat by stroking toward the heart, and then releasing it. If the vein takes longer than 3 to 5 seconds to refill, then the person probably has an ECV deficit (unless occlusive arterial disease is present).

Table 7-2 ■ CAUSES OF EXTRACELLULAR FLUID VOLUME DEFICIT

Category	Clinical Examples
Excessive removal of gastrointestinal fluid	Diarrhea Emesis Gastrointestinal fistula drainage Nasogastric or intestinal tube suctioning or drainage
Excessive renal excretion of saline	Adrenal insufficiency Diuresis due to bed rest Excessive use of diuretics
Excessive removal of sodium-containing fluid by other routes	Hemorrhage Third-space accumulation Burns Excessive diaphoresis

Table 7-3 ■ CAUSES OF EXTRACELLULAR FLUID VOLUME EXCESS

Category	Clinical Examples
Excessive infusion of isotonic, sodium-containing solutions	Excessive normal saline (0.9% NaCl) Excessive Ringer's or lactated Ringer's
Renal retention of saline	Endocrine: Excessive aldosterone (CHF, cirrhosis, hyperaldosteronism); excessive glucocorticoids (Cushing syndrome, pharmacologic doses of glucocorticoids) Renal: Oliguric renal failure

CHF, congestive heart failure.

Table 7-4 ■ CAUSES OF HYPONATREMIA

Category	Clinical Examples
Gain of water relative to salt	Endocrine: Excessive ADH (ectopic production; stimulation by surgery/anesthesia, stressors, pain, nausea) Iatrogenic: Excessive infusion of D5W, tap water enemas, or water ingestion (after poisoning or before ultrasound examination); absorption of water from hypotonic irrigation solution Other: Near-drowning in fresh water; excessive ingestion of low-sodium fluid such as water (psychogenic polydipsia) or beer (beer potomania)
Loss of salt relative to water	Gastrointestinal: Replacement of water but not salt after emesis, diarrhea, or nasogastric suction; removal of sodium with hypotonic irrigation Renal: Diuretics, especially thiazides; salt-wasting renal diseases Other: Replacement of water but not salt after excessive diaphoresis

The decreased preload of ECV deficit leads to decreased cardiac output, with resulting dizziness, syncope, and oliguria. If ECV deficit becomes severe, tachycardia, pallor caused by cutaneous vasoconstriction, and other manifestations of hypovolemic shock occur (see Chapter 24).

Extracellular Fluid Volume Excess

Excess ECV is an overload of fluid in the vascular and interstitial compartments. It is common in individuals with heart failure because their decreased cardiac output activates the renin–angiotensin–aldosterone system.[5] Aldosterone causes renal retention of sodium and water, which expands the extracellular volume. People who have hypertension caused by elevated renin also develop ECV excess. Other causes of ECV excess are listed in Table 7-3. Clinical manifestations of ECV excess include sudden weight gain, peripheral edema, and the cardiovascular effects described next.

Increased vascular volume is manifested by bounding pulse, distended neck veins when upright, and elevated central venous pressure. The crackles, dyspnea, and orthopnea of pulmonary edema may be present. A sudden overload of isotonic fluid increases cardiac work and may cause heart failure, especially in an older adult or an infant.

OSMOLALITY BALANCE

The osmolality of body fluids is determined by the relative proportion of particles and water. The serum sodium concentration usually parallels the osmolality of the blood. When the serum sodium concentration is abnormally low, the osmolality is decreased; in other words, the blood is relatively too dilute. Conversely, when the serum sodium concentration is elevated, the osmolality is increased; in that case, the blood is relatively too concentrated. Antidiuretic hormone (ADH), also called vasopressin, (see Table 7-1) is the major regulator of osmolality.[6]

Hyponatremia

Hyponatremia is a relative excess of water that causes a decreased serum sodium concentration. It is caused by a gain of water relative to salt or a loss of salt relative to water (Table 7-4). ADH increases the reabsorption of water by the renal tubules and thus dilutes body fluids. In people who have had cardiac surgery, hyponatremia may occur in the first few days after surgery if excess free water is administered because the stressors of surgery, anesthesia, pain, and nausea increase the secretion of ADH.[1] Hyponatremia is common in individuals with chronic heart failure because their decreased cardiac output stimulates arterial baroreceptors, triggering nonosmotic release of ADH.[7] Diuretic therapy also contributes to hyponatremia, as discussed below. Hyponatremia in hospitalized heart failure patients is associated with longer hospitalization and increased in-hospital and post-discharge mortality.[8–10] Although clinical trials have shown that vaptans, aquaretic drugs that block vasopressin receptors in the kidney, are capable of correcting hyponatremia in hyponatremic heart failure patients, no improvement in morbidity or mortality have been demonstrated.[11,12] In people with either ST-elevation myocardial infarction (MI) or suspected acute coronary syndrome, non-ST-elevation MI, hyponatremia is associated with adverse outcomes such as death or recurrent MI.[13]

The most common medications used by people with cardiovascular disease that may cause hyponatremia are diuretics, especially the thiazide diuretics and the thiazide-like diuretic indapamide.[14–16] Hyponatremia from thiazide diuretics occurs more frequently in women than men, especially in older women.[17]

The hypo-osmolality of hyponatremia causes water to enter cells by osmosis. The clinical manifestations of hyponatremia are primarily nonspecific markers of cerebral dysfunction: malaise, confusion, lethargy, seizures, and coma. The extent of these manifestations depends on the speed with which hyponatremia develops as well as its severity. Hyponatremia does not have significant clinical effects on cardiac electrophysiology or function.

Hypernatremia

Hypernatremia is a relative deficit of water that causes an increased serum sodium concentration. It is caused by a loss of water relative to salt or a gain of salt relative to water (Table 7-5). The hyperosmolality of hypernatremia causes water to leave cells by osmosis. The clinical manifestations are similar to those of hyponatremia:

Table 7-5 ■ CAUSES OF HYPERNATREMIA

Category	Clinical Examples
Loss of water relative to salt	Endocrine: Lack of ADH (diabetes insipidus) Renal: Osmotic diuresis; renal concentrating disorders Other: Inadequate water replacement after diarrhea or excessive diaphoresis
Gain of salt relative to water	Decreased intake of water: Inability to respond to thirst (coma, aphasia, paralysis, confusion); lack of access to water; difficulty swallowing fluids (advanced Parkinsonism); prolonged nausea Increased intake of salt: Excessive hypertonic NaCl or $NaHCO_3$; near-drowning in salt water; tube feedings without adequate water intake

malaise, confusion, lethargy, seizures, and coma.[3] Thirst (except in some older adults) and oliguria (except in hypernatremia caused by decreased ADH) may also occur. As with hyponatremia, the extent of these manifestations depends on the speed with which hypernatremia develops as well as its severity. Hypernatremia is much less common than hyponatremia in cardiac patients who do not have other pathophysiologies, although it is common in critically ill patients.[18] Hypernatremia also does not have significant clinical effects on cardiac electrophysiology or function.

Mixed ECV and Osmolality Imbalances

ECV and osmolality imbalances may occur at the same time in the same person. For example, in a person who has severe gastroenteritis without proper fluid replacement, concurrent ECV deficit and hypernatremia (clinical dehydration) will develop. The fluid lost in the emesis and diarrhea, plus the usual daily fluid excretion (urine, feces, respiratory, insensible through skin), is hypotonic sodium-containing fluid (analogous to isotonic saline that has extra water added). People who have chronic heart failure frequently develop concurrent ECV excess and hyponatremia, sometimes called a hypervolemic hyponatremia.[12]

The signs and symptoms of such mixed fluid imbalances are a combination of the clinical manifestations of the two separate imbalances. In the example of clinical dehydration, the individual has the sudden weight loss, manifestations of decreased vascular volume, and signs of decreased interstitial volume that result from ECV deficit plus the thirst and nonspecific signs of cerebral dysfunction that result from hypernatremia.[3] In heart failure, the clinical manifestations include the weight gain, distended neck veins, and edema of ECV excess plus the nonspecific signs of cerebral dysfunction of hyponatremia.

PRINCIPLES OF ELECTROLYTE BALANCE

Electrolyte balance is the net result of several concurrent dynamic processes. These processes are electrolyte intake, absorption, distribution, excretion, and loss through abnormal routes[1] (Table 7-6). Electrolyte intake in healthy people is primarily by the oral route; other routes of electrolyte intake include the intravenous and rectal routes, and also through tubes into various body cavities. Electrolytes that are taken into the gastrointestinal tract must be absorbed into the blood. Although some electrolytes (e.g., potassium) are absorbed readily by mechanisms based on gradients, the absorption of other electrolytes (e.g., calcium and magnesium) is more complex and can be impaired by many factors.

Electrolytes are distributed into all body fluids, but their concentrations in the different body fluid compartments vary greatly. Substantial amounts of most electrolytes are located in pools outside the extracellular fluid. For example, the major pool of potassium is inside cells; the major pool of calcium is in the bones.

Electrolyte excretion occurs through the normal routes of urine, feces, and sweat. Any removal of electrolytes through other routes can be considered loss of electrolytes through an abnormal route. Examples of these abnormal routes are emesis, nasogastric suction, fistula drainage, and hemorrhage.

To maintain normal balance of any specific electrolyte, electrolyte intake and absorption must equal electrolyte excretion and electrolyte loss through abnormal routes, and the electrolyte must be distributed properly within the body. Alterations in any of these processes can cause an electrolyte imbalance.[1]

ELECTROLYTE IMBALANCES

Plasma electrolyte imbalances can have profound effects on cardiovascular function. Because cardiac function depends on ion currents across myocardial cell membranes, action potential generation, impulse conduction, and myocardial contraction are all vulnerable to alterations in electrolyte status. In addition to their effects on the myocardium itself, some electrolyte imbalances have vascular effects.

Potassium Balance

Potassium balance is the net result of potassium intake and absorption, distribution, excretion, and abnormal losses. These components are summarized in Table 7-6. Although the plasma potassium concentration describes the status of potassium in the extracellular fluid, it does not necessarily reflect the amount of potassium inside the cells. The plasma potassium concentration has a circadian rhythm, rising during the hours a person is usually active and reaching its trough when a person is usually asleep. A classic study demonstrated that the kidneys handle an intravenous potassium load much less efficiently during the hours a person is customarily asleep, which has implications for potassium administration to ICU patients.[19]

The potassium concentration of the extracellular fluid has a major influence on the function of the myocardium. Specifically, the resting membrane potential of cardiac cells is proportional to the ratio of potassium concentrations in the extracellular and intracellular fluids. The potassium concentration within cardiac cells is approximately 140 mEq/L; the normal potassium concentration of the extracellular fluid is 3.5 to 5 mEq/L. A small change in the extracellular concentration of potassium has a large effect on the extracellular-to-intracellular concentration ratio because the initial extracellular value is relatively small. A similar change in the intracellular potassium concentration has a lesser effect because the initial intracellular value is so large.

Table 7-6 ■ ELECTROLYTE HOMEOSTASIS

Electrolyte	Sources of Intake	Absorption	Electrolyte Pool	Distribution	Excretion
Potassium (K^+)	*Foods:* Almonds Apricots Bananas Cantaloupe Coffee (instant) Dates Molasses Oranges Peaches Potatoes Prunes Raisins Strawberries *Intravenous:* Packed red blood cells or whole blood; penicillin G	Based on gradient between lumen and blood concentrations	Inside cells	*Cause shift into cells:* β-Adrenergic agonists Insulin Alkalosis *Cause shift out of cells:* Acidosis caused by mineral acids Lack of insulin Cell death	*Urinary:* Increased by increased flow in distal nephron, glucocorticoids Aldosterone causes K^+ excretion *Fecal:* Increased with diarrhea *Sweat*
Calcium (Ca^{2+})	*Foods:* Beet greens Broccoli Dairy products Farina Kale Milk chocolate Oranges Salmon (canned) Sardines Tofu	Most efficient in duodenum; increased by vitamin D Decreased by phosphates, phytates, oxalates, increased intestinal pH, undigested fat, diarrhea, glucocorticoids	Physiologically unavailable when bound in blood to proteins and small organic anions	*Cause more binding in blood:* Alkalosis Citrate in blood products Protein plasma expanders Increased free fatty acids	*Urinary:* Decreased by parathyroid hormone Increased by saline diuresis, high protein diet *Fecal:* Increased with undigested fat *Sweat*
			Bones	*Cause shift into bones:* Lack of parathyroid hormone *Cause shift from bones:* Parathyroid hormone High-protein diet Glucocorticoids Immobility	
Magnesium (Mg^{2+})	*Foods:* Cocoa Chocolate Dried beans and peas Green leafy vegetables Hard water Nuts Peanut butter Sea salt Whole grains	Most efficient in terminal ileum Decreased by phosphates, phytate, undigested fat, alcohol, diarrhea Increased by lactose	Physiologically unavailable when bound in blood to proteins and small organic anions	*Cause more binding in blood:* Citrate in blood products Increased free fatty acids	*Urinary:* Increased with extracellular fluid volume expansion, rising blood alcohol, high-protein diet, acidosis *Fecal:* Increased with undigested fat, increased aldosterone *Sweat*
			Bones	*Cause shift from bones:* Parathyroid hormone	
			Inside cells	*Cause shift into cells:* Epinephrine Insulin	
Phosphate (P_i)	*Foods:* Eggs Meat Milk Processed foods Almost all foods have some phosphates	Decreased by aluminum and magnesium antacids, diarrhea	Inside cells	*Cause shift into cells:* Epinephrine Insulin Increased cellular metabolism *Cause shift out of cells:* Ketoacidosis Cell death	*Urinary:* Increased by parathyroid hormone, phosphatonins, extracellular fluid volume expansion *Fecal* *Sweat*
			Bones	*Cause shift out of bones:* Parathyroid hormone Immobility	

From Felver, L. (1995). Fluid and electrolyte balance and imbalances. In S. L. Woods, E. S. Froelicher, C. J. Halpenny et al. (Eds.), *Cardiac nursing* (3rd ed., p. 126). Philadelphia: JB Lippincott.

Hypokalemia

Hypokalemia, a decrease in the plasma potassium concentration, is caused by decreased potassium intake, shift of potassium ions from the extracellular fluid into the cells, increased excretion of potassium, loss of potassium through an abnormal route, or any combination of these factors.[1] Some specific etiologic factors in these categories are listed in Table 7-7. Hypokalemia is common in people with heart failure because of their increased secretion of aldosterone and their diuretic therapy, and it is associated with increased mortality in ambulatory people who have chronic heart failure.[20,21]

Table 7-7 ■ CAUSES OF HYPOKALEMIA

Category	Clinical Examples
Decreased potassium intake	NPO orders
	Anorexia
	Fad diets
	Fasting
	Prolonged IV therapy without K^+
Potassium shift into cells	Alkalosis
	Excessive β_2-adrenergic stimulation (epinephrine, β-agonists)
	Hypothermia (accidental or induced)
	Excessive insulin
	Rapid correction of acidosis during hemodialysis
	Familial periodic paralysis
Increased potassium excretion	Diarrhea (includes laxative overuse)
	Hyperaldosteronism (increases renal excretion of potassium)
	Chronic excessive ingestion of black licorice (contains aldosterone-like compounds)
	Excessive glucocorticoids (Cushing syndrome; glucocorticoid therapy)
	Hypomagnesemia (causes renal potassium wasting)
	Diuretic therapy with loop or thiazide diuretics or mannitol
	Polyuria
	High-dose penicillin therapy (nonreabsorbable anion effect in kidney)
Potassium loss by abnormal route	Emesis
	Nasogastric suction
	Drainage from gastrointestinal fistula
	Dialysis

IV, intravenous.

Catecholamines and β-agonist drugs cause potassium ions to shift into cells by a β_2-adrenergic mechanism. This effect can produce hypokalemia.[22,23] Plasma catecholamines increase rapidly during MI and hypokalemia is common during acute coronary syndromes.[24] This hypokalemic effect is not as strong in people who have diabetic autonomic neuropathy.[24] Transient hypokalemia associated with catecholamine release during an MI may cause further impairment of an already compromised myocardium (see Chapter 5).

The increased potassium excretion caused by many types of diuretics is well known.[21,25] Hypokalemia caused by diuretic therapy occurs most frequently within 2 to 8 weeks, although it may arise after more than 1 year.[26] The necessity of monitoring the plasma potassium concentration in individuals using diuretics, especially older adults, is clear.[27] Individuals with hypokalemia have significantly more ventricular arrhythmias after MI than do normokalemic individuals. The hypokalemic effect of catecholamines is stronger in people who are using thiazide diuretics than it is in those who are not using diuretics.

Because of the cardiac effects of hypokalemia, the National Council on Potassium in Clinical Practice has established guidelines for potassium replacement.[28] For individuals with hypertension, the guideline is to maintain a serum potassium concentration of at least 4.0 mEq/L. Potassium replacement should be considered routinely in people with congestive heart failure, even with a serum potassium level of 4.0 mEq/L. Potassium levels of at least 4.0 mEq/L are necessary in individuals who have cardiac arrhythmias. The guidelines also emphasize the necessity of routine monitoring of serum potassium in people who have congestive heart failure or cardiac arrhythmias.

Clinical manifestations of hypokalemia include diminished bowel sounds, abdominal distention, constipation, polyuria, skeletal muscle weakness, flaccid paralysis, cardiac arrhythmias, and postural hypotension. Cardiac and vascular effects of hypokalemia are discussed next.

Cardiac Effects of Hypokalemia. The cardiac effects of hypokalemia include changes in cell membrane resting potential. When the extracellular potassium concentration decreases, the extracellular/intracellular potassium concentration ratio decreases. This change in ratio causes cardiac muscle cells to hyperpolarize (i.e., the resting membrane potential becomes more negative). In hyperpolarized cells, the distance between resting potential and action potential is increased; hyperpolarized cells are less responsive to stimuli than are normal cells. The hyperpolarizing effect of hypokalemia on cardiac cells does not occur at all levels of hypokalemia. At low plasma potassium concentrations, a *hypopolarizing* effect may be seen. This is probably caused by decreased potassium conductance (analogous to decreased potassium permeability) of the cell membrane. The specific alteration of cardiac cell membrane resting potential thus depends on the degree of hypokalemia. In any case, the normal resting potential is altered, which contributes to the development of arrhythmias.

In addition to its effect on cell membrane resting potential, hypokalemia increases the rate of cardiac cell diastolic depolarization.[29] Diastolic depolarization is the normal mechanism that initiates the depolarization of pacemaker cells (see Chapter 16). Under usual circumstances, diastolic depolarization is fastest in the sinus node cells; consequently, the sinus node serves as the predominant pacemaker. During hypokalemia, however, the rate of diastolic depolarization increases in other myocardial cells, especially in diseased myocardium. Ectopic beats may arise, even from hyperpolarized cells.

Other effects of hypokalemia on the myocardium also predispose to arrhythmias. Hypokalemia decreases conduction velocity, especially in the atrioventricular node. Hypokalemia prolongs the action potential by decreasing the rate of repolarization, at least in part by decreasing cardiac cell membrane permeability to potassium efflux.[30,31] It alters the normal relationship between action potential duration in the epicardium and the endocardium, which may contribute to cardiac arrhythmias, and decreases the ventricular effective refractory period, which predisposes to the development of extrasystoles and reentrant arrhythmias (see Chapter 16).[31–33]

The cardiac alterations of hypokalemia may cause many types of arrhythmias. Hypokalemia-induced arrhythmias include supraventricular premature depolarizations and tachycardias, ventricular ectopic beats, ventricular tachycardia, torsade de pointes, and ventricular fibrillation.[34–39] Hypokalemia potentiates digitalis toxicity. Animal studies indicate that downregulation of gap junction proteins in diabetic cardiomyopathy increases the vulnerability to ventricular fibrillation in hypokalemia.[40]

As might be expected from the previous discussion, electrocardiographic (ECG) changes are seen in individuals with hypokalemia (see Chapter 16). A characteristic change is the development of U waves.[41,42] Other ECG changes include increased amplitude of P waves, prolonged PR interval, prolonged QT interval, flattened or inverted T waves, and ST segment depression.[23,32,35,36,42,43]

Long-standing hypokalemia is associated with selective myocardial cell necrosis. As discussed in Chapter 27, selective myocardial cell necrosis is associated with sudden cardiac death.

Vascular Effects of Hypokalemia. In addition to the multiple cardiac effects discussed previously, hypokalemia has vascular effects. Postural hypotension often occurs in hypokalemia,[3] most likely caused by impaired smooth muscle function.

Classic studies indicate that chronic potassium depletion in humans impairs vasodilation during strenuous exercise.[44] The resulting impaired muscle blood flow decreases oxygen delivery and contributes to the rhabdomyolysis that occurs with whole-body potassium depletion.[45–47]

Hyperkalemia

Hyperkalemia, an increased plasma potassium concentration, results from increased potassium intake, shift of potassium ions from the cells to the extracellular fluid, decreased potassium excretion, or any combination of these factors.[1] Examples of specific etiologic factors in each of these categories are listed in Table 7-8. Hyperkalemia may occur during hemorrhagic or hypovolemic shock and during cardiopulmonary resuscitation.

Several medications commonly administered to individuals with cardiac disease may cause hyperkalemia.[48] *Angiotensin-converting enzyme inhibitors* such as captopril and enalapril, *angiotensin II receptor blockers* such as losartan, *selective aldosterone blockers* such as eplerenone, and *direct renin inhibitors* such as aliskiren decrease the release of aldosterone. Aldosterone normally facilitates renal excretion of potassium. When these drugs decrease the availability of aldosterone, hyperkalemia may occur.[49–52] The *potassium-sparing diuretics* spironolactone, triamterene, and amiloride may cause hyperkalemia, especially if given with potassium supplementation or angiotensin-converting enzyme inhibitors or used by people who have any degree of renal impairment.[50,51,53,54] *Nonselective β-adrenergic blockers* promote the development of hyperkalemia by blocking catecholamine action at β_2 receptors that normally stimulates potassium entry into cells.[49,56] The hyperkalemic effect of β-blockade is especially pronounced during exercise, which has relevance to treadmill stress testing, and is enhanced in people who take digitalis.[48,56,57] Administration of either unfractionated or low-molecular-weight *heparin*, even in low-dose therapy, decreases the synthesis of aldosterone; hyperkalemia is likely to occur in heparinized individuals who have even mild renal insufficiency.[48,58] A massive *digitalis overdose* causes hyperkalemia by allowing intracellular potassium to leak into the extracellular fluid and impairing its movement back into cells.[52]

Table 7-8 ■ CAUSES OF HYPERKALEMIA

Category	Clinical Examples
Increased potassium intake	Excessive IV potassium Insufficiently mixed KCl in flexible plastic IV bag Massive transfusion of blood stored longer than 3 days (K^+ leaves red blood cells) Large doses of IV potassium penicillin G (contains 1.6 mEq K^+/million units) Large oral intake only if decreased renal excretion
Potassium shift out of cells	Acidosis due to mineral acids (not organic acids like ketoacids) Insulin deficiency Massive cell death (crushing injuries, burns, cytotoxic drugs) Large digitalis overdose Familial periodic paralysis
Decreased potassium excretion	Oliguria Extracellular fluid volume depletion Oliguric renal failure Decreased aldosterone from any cause (Addison disease, chronic heparin administration, lead poisoning, ACE inhibitors, angiotensin II receptor antagonists, selective aldosterone blockers, direct renin inhibitors) Potassium-sparing diuretics

IV, intravenous; ACE, angiotensin-converting enzyme.

Another cardiovascular-related source of hyperkalemia is massive blood transfusion. While blood is stored, potassium ions leak from the erythrocytes into the plasma. The longer the storage time, the greater the potassium load contained in a unit of blood.[59,60] A classic study indicates that if the blood has been in storage for more than 3 days, rewarming the blood before administration causes only minimal return of potassium to the cells.[61] Individuals receiving more than 7 or 8 units of stored blood within a few hours are considered at high risk for severe hyperkalemia; however, fatal hyperkalemia has occurred with transfusion of fewer units, especially when they are administered rapidly.[60,62]

Hyperkalemia may be manifested clinically by intestinal cramping and diarrhea, skeletal muscle weakness, flaccid paralysis, cardiac arrhythmias, and cardiac arrest. The cardiac effects of hyperkalemia are potentially fatal; they are discussed in the next section.

Cardiac Effects of Hyperkalemia. Hyperkalemia alters myocardial cell function in several ways. When the plasma potassium concentration increases, the extracellular/intracellular potassium concentration ratio increases. Consequently, the resting membrane potential of cardiac cells becomes partially depolarized (hypopolarized).[48] Initially, the partial depolarization of resting cardiac cells increases their excitability because the resting potential is close to threshold potential (see Chapter 16). As the extracellular potassium concentration increases, however, the cardiac cells depolarize to the extent that they cannot repolarize. Cells in this state are nonexcitable; no further contractile activity occurs. The ability of hyperkalemia to cause asystolic cardiac arrest is exploited by using potassium as a cardioplegic agent during cardiac surgery.[63]

Other effects of hyperkalemia include decreased duration of the action potential at all heart rates and increased rate of repolarization, the latter due to increased permeability of the cardiac cell membrane to potassium efflux.[32] Hyperkalemia lengthens the effective refractory period of atrial muscle and slows diastolic depolarization of pacemaker cells, two antiarrhythmic effects. Cardiac cells vary in their sensitivity to the effects of hyperkalemia. Atrial cells are more sensitive than ventricular cells; the conduction system is the last to be affected.[48]

As the plasma potassium increases, the rate of rise of the action potential decreases. Slow upstroke velocity decreases cell-to-cell conduction velocity (see Chapter 16). Hyperkalemia decreases conduction velocity at all levels of the conduction system: atrial, atrioventricular nodal, and intraventricular.[48,52] In severe hyperkalemia, intraventricular conduction may be completely inhibited. Bundle-branch block or, less frequently, complete heart block may occur.[42,64]

Although some of the cellular effects of hyperkalemia are antiarrhythmogenic, cardiac arrhythmias do occur in hyperkalemia. The differential effects of hyperkalemia on different cell types cause slow and nonhomogeneous conduction to cells with variable degrees of excitability. When intra-atrial conduction is decreased, sinus node impulses may be delayed in exit or may fail to propagate. This situation gives rise to Wenckebach (type I) or Mobitz (type II) sinoatrial block (see Chapter 16). Reentrant ventricular arrhythmias may arise. Ventricular tachycardia may terminate in ventricular fibrillation.[42] Asystolic cardiac arrest also is a potentially fatal event.[39]

The characteristic ECG changes of hyperkalemia arise from the electrophysiologic changes previously described. The initial ECG abnormality is the T waves becoming peaked (tented) with a narrow base and symmetric shape.[65,66] The QRS complex widens; ST depression may occur. Occasionally, ST elevation occurs, mimicking an MI.[67–69] Hyperkalemia also causes decreased amplitude and prolongation of P waves and PR prolongation.[70,71] As the plasma potassium concentration increases to high levels, the P waves disappear. A sine-wave pattern appears in severe, often terminal, hyperkalemia.[39,42,72]

The ECG changes of hyperkalemia are not well correlated with plasma potassium levels.[42,73,74] Although the ECG usually is abnormal with severe hyperkalemia (serum potassium greater than 8 mEq/L), minimal ECG changes have been observed in individuals with serum potassium concentrations greater than 9 mEq/L. The rate of increase of the plasma potassium concentration may contribute more to the ECG changes in hyperkalemia than does the absolute plasma potassium level. Hemodialysis patients may not exhibit the characteristic peaked T wave or other ECG signs when they are severely hyperkalemic. This may be caused in part by concurrent hypercalcemia, which can flatten the T wave.[75] The ECG changes of hyperkalemia also are blunted during hypothermia.[76]

ECG interpretation software may double or triple count the heart rate during severe hyperkalemia[77,78] Individuals who have implantable cardioverter defibrillators have received multiple inappropriate shocks upon developing acute hyperkalemia.[77,79]

During myocardial ischemia, potassium concentration increases quickly in the extracellular spaces of the myocardium and promotes development of lethal ventricular re-entry arrhythmias.[80,81] During exercise, elevated catecholamines counteract the negative cardiac effects of hyperkalemia in normal hearts; this protective effect is diminished in ischemic hearts.

Hyperkalemia also has an indirect cardiac effect in that it stimulates aldosterone secretion. Through its saline-retaining action on the kidneys, aldosterone expands the ECV, which may have a detrimental effect on individuals in heart failure.

Vascular Effects of Hyperkalemia. Hyperkalemia reduces the smooth muscle relaxation normally mediated by endothelium-derived hyperpolarizing factor.[82] In high concentrations, potassium ions cause contraction of smooth muscle of coronary arteries.[83]

Calcium Balance

Calcium balance is the net result of calcium intake and absorption, distribution, excretion, and abnormal losses. These components are summarized in Table 7-6. Calcium in the plasma exists in three forms: protein bound, complexed, and ionized (free). The calcium that is bound to plasma proteins and complexed with small anions (e.g., citrate) is physiologically inactive. Only the ionized calcium is physiologically active. Two laboratory measures for extracellular calcium are available in many settings: total calcium concentration (bound, complexed, and ionized) and ionized calcium concentration.

Calcium ions play crucial roles in the automaticity of the sinus and atrioventricular nodes, in the plateau phase of the Purkinje and ventricular cell action potentials, in excitation–contraction coupling, and in cardiac and vascular muscle contraction (see Chapters 1 and 16). Not unexpectedly, one of the cardiac effects of an abnormal extracellular calcium concentration is altered duration of the plateau phase. Extracellular fluid calcium imbalances are less likely to cause cardiac arrhythmias than are potassium imbalances, but arrhythmias associated with hypercalcemia have been fatal. In addition to their cardiac effects, acute calcium imbalances also affect the vasculature.

Hypocalcemia

Hypocalcemia may be defined as a decreased extracellular *total* calcium concentration or as a decreased extracellular *ionized* calcium concentration. The first definition refers to the commonly measured total calcium value. The second definition of hypocalcemia, however, is used in this chapter because decreases in ionized calcium concentration cause physiologic effects even if the total plasma concentration is within normal limits. Ionized hypocalcemia occurs frequently in intensive care units.[84,85]

Hypocalcemia results from decreased calcium intake or absorption, decreased physiologic availability of calcium, increased calcium excretion, loss of calcium by an abnormal route, or any combination of these factors.[1] Table 7-9 lists specific causative factors for hypocalcemia. Several of these specific factors may cause hypocalcemia in individuals with cardiac disease. The preservative used in storage of blood contains citrate, which complexes with

Table 7-9 ■ CAUSES OF HYPOCALCEMIA

Category	Clinical Examples
Decreased calcium intake or absorption	Diet deficient in calcium Diet deficient in vitamin D Malabsorption syndromes Chronic diarrhea (including laxative overuse) Steatorrhea Pancreatitis
Shift of calcium into physiologically unavailable form or into bones	Alkalosis Massive blood transfusion (citrate binds Ca^{2+}) Rapid infusion of albumin Pancreatitis Lack of PTH (hypoparathyroidism; surgical removal of parathyroid gland during thyroid surgery) Hypomagnesemia Hyperphosphatemia (overuse of phosphate-containing laxatives or enemas; excessive oral or IV phosphate intake; tumor lysis syndrome) Acute fluoride poisoning
Increased calcium excretion	*Gastrointestinal:* Pancreatitis *Renal:* Chronic renal insufficiency

PTH, parathyroid hormone; IV, intravenous.

calcium ions. Large or rapid transfusions of citrated blood cause hypocalcemia by decreasing the physiologic availability of calcium in the blood.[86] The hypocalcemic effect of blood transfusions is greater in critically ill patients.[84] Similarly, rapid administration of proteinaceous plasma expanders such as albumin also decreases the physiologic availability of plasma calcium and may cause symptomatic hypocalcemia.

Hypocalcemia increases neuromuscular excitability. The clinical manifestations of hypocalcemia may include digital and perioral paresthesias, positive Chvostek's sign, positive Trousseau's sign, muscle twitching and cramping, grimacing, hyperactive reflexes, tetany, carpopedal spasm, laryngospasm, seizures, cardiac arrhythmias, cardiac arrest, and hypotension (with acute hypocalcemia).

Cardiac Effects of Hypocalcemia. Hypocalcemia prolongs the plateau phase, thereby increasing the duration of the cardiac action potential. In addition, hypocalcemia slows atrioventricular and intraventricular conduction to a moderate degree.[87]

These hypocalcemia-related changes in the myocardium usually are not great enough to give rise to significant cardiac arrhythmias in clinical settings, although they may occasionally predispose to ventricular arrhythmias, including torsade de pointes.[88] Hypocalcemia does cause characteristic alterations in the ECG. Hypocalcemia prolongs the ST segment.[89] This finding is not unexpected because hypocalcemia prolongs the plateau phase of the action potential. The prolongation of the ST segment causes a prolonged QT interval.[39,90] The degree of prolongation of the QT interval is not a reliable indicator of the degree of hypocalcemia or of the decrease in ionized calcium concentration, but it is influenced by the rate of decrease of the ionized calcium.[86] Concurrent hypomagnesemia magnifies the ECG effects of hypocalcemia. ECG changes in individuals with hypocalcemia and hypomagnesemia may mimic MI.[91]

Hypocalcemia impairs myocardial contractility and thus may cause heart failure.[92–95] People who already have heart failure may decompensate if they become hypocalcemic. Hypocalcemia-associated heart failure may be unresponsive to digitalis until the hypocalcemia is corrected. The role of calcium ions in the regulation of myocardial contraction is clear (see Chapter 16). Although most of the calcium ions that initiate myocardial contraction come from the sarcoplasmic reticulum rather than directly from the extracellular fluid, entry of calcium from the extracellular fluid is necessary to trigger calcium release from the sarcoplasmic reticulum. The depressive effect of hypocalcemia on myocardial contractility may be most important in individuals who have pre-existing downregulation of β-adrenergic receptors.[91] In a normal heart, hypocalcemia reduces stroke work at any particular left ventricular end-diastolic pressure. This impairment is even greater in an ischemic heart. A classic study showed that patients who are administered albumin for resuscitation during hypovolemic shock may also exhibit impaired myocardial contractility when the ionized calcium binds to the albumin and becomes physiologically unavailable.[96]

Vascular Effects of Hypocalcemia. Calcium ions play several important roles in contraction of vascular smooth muscle. They are involved in the action potential, the regulation of cell membrane permeability, and in excitation–contraction coupling. In smooth muscle, as well as in cardiac muscle, contraction is initiated by an increase in cytoplasmic calcium. Most of the calcium ions that initiate the contraction come from the sarcoplasmic reticulum rather than from the extracellular fluid. Any short-term effects of hypocalcemia on the vasculature are more likely to arise from alterations in cell membrane permeability than from alteration in the contractile mechanisms. Acute (but not chronic) hypocalcemia causes hypotension. The mechanisms involved are not completely understood but likely include decreased peripheral vascular resistance and impaired cardiac function.

Table 7-10 ■ CAUSES OF HYPERCALCEMIA

Category	Clinical Examples
Increased calcium intake or absorption	Milk-alkali syndrome Excessive vitamin D
Shift of calcium out of bone	Hyperparathyroidism Prolonged immobility Bone tumors Multiple myeloma Cancers that produce parathyroid hormone-related peptide and other bone-resorbing factors
Decreased calcium excretion	Thiazide diuretics Familial hypocalciuric hypercalcemia

Hypercalcemia

Hypercalcemia results from increased intake or absorption of calcium, the shift of calcium from the bones into the extracellular fluid, decreased calcium excretion, or any combination of these factors.[1] Specific causative factors are listed under these categories in Table 7-10. Note that thiazide diuretics, often administered to people with cardiac disease, decrease the urinary excretion of calcium.[25,97] Another type of diuretic should be substituted if hypercalcemia develops.

The clinical manifestations of hypercalcemia include anorexia, nausea, vomiting, constipation, abdominal pain, polyuria, renal calculi, skeletal muscle weakness, diminished reflexes, confusion, lethargy, possible personality change, frank psychosis, cardiac arrhythmias, and hypertension (with acute hypercalcemia).

Cardiac Effects of Hypercalcemia. Hypercalcemia shortens the plateau phase of the cardiac action potential, thereby decreasing the duration of the action potential. In addition, it increases the rate of diastolic depolarization of sinus node cells and may increase the initial rate of increase and amplitude of the action potential. It may also delay atrioventricular conduction.

Cardiac arrhythmias that have been reported to arise from hypercalcemia include various types of heart block, paroxysmal atrial fibrillation, and severe bradycardia.[98] Hypercalcemia potentiates digitalis toxicity.[39] People using digitalis may acquire heart block if they become hypercalcemic. Sudden death has occurred in severe hypercalcemia, possibly caused by ventricular fibrillation.

The ECG in hypercalcemia reflects the short plateau phase in a shortened ST segment. The QT interval is decreased as a result.[39] The length of the QT interval is a clinically unreliable index of the extent of hypercalcemia. Hypercalcemia has been accompanied by lengthening of the QRS complex and diffuse flattening of T waves.[99]

Vascular Effects of Hypercalcemia. In people who have intact parathyroid glands, acute hypercalcemia causes vasoconstriction and raises systolic blood pressure by impairing the vasodilatory function of the endothelium.[100–102] Increased intracellular calcium in vascular smooth muscle also causes increased vascular resistance. In many people with essential hypertension, increased intracellular calcium occurs with normal plasma calcium levels. Parathyroid hormone and parathyroid hormone-related factor are implicated in transepithelial calcium transport and likely play a role in the hypertensive mechanism.

Magnesium Balance

Magnesium balance is the net result of magnesium intake and absorption, distribution, excretion, and abnormal losses. These components are summarized in Table 7-6. Similar to calcium, magnesium in the plasma exists in three forms: protein-bound, complexed, and ionized (free). Only the ionized magnesium is physiologically active; however, the only widely available clinical laboratory measure for magnesium is the total serum magnesium concentration (bound, complexed, and ionized).

Magnesium, like potassium, is primarily an intracellular ion. For this reason, plasma levels of magnesium do not necessarily reflect the intracellular magnesium content. Total-body magnesium depletion may be present even when the plasma magnesium is normal. Intracellular magnesium is a cofactor for many enzymes, including Na^+–K^+ adenosine triphosphatase (ATPase). Changes in magnesium balance, especially hypomagnesemia, cause alterations in ion transport across membranes. Because the function of cardiac and smooth muscle depends on ion fluxes, magnesium imbalances have myocardial and vascular effects.

Hypomagnesemia and Total-Body Magnesium Depletion

Hypomagnesemia and total-body magnesium depletion are caused by decreased magnesium intake or absorption, decreased physiologic availability of magnesium, increased magnesium excretion, loss of magnesium by an abnormal route, or any combination of these factors.[1] Specific causative factors for hypomagnesemia are listed in Table 7-11. Hypomagnesemia and total-body magnesium depletion are common in chronic alcoholism; therefore, people who have alcoholic cardiomyopathy need assessment for hypomagnesemia.

Table 7-11 ■ CAUSES OF HYPOMAGNESEMIA

Category	Clinical Examples
Decreased magnesium intake or absorption	Prolonged IV therapy without Mg^{2+} Chronic malnutrition Chronic diarrhea Steatorrhea Pancreatitis Malabsorption syndromes Chronic alcoholism Ileal resection
Increased magnesium excretion	*Gastrointestinal*: Steatorrhea *Renal*: Diabetic ketoacidosis; diuretic therapy; increased aldosterone (CHF, cirrhosis, hyperaldosteronism); chronic alcoholism; renal damage from drugs (amphotericin B, aminoglycosides)
Magnesium loss by abnormal route	Emesis Nasogastric suctioning Drainage from GI fistula

IV, intravenous; GI, gastrointestinal.

Diuretics (except for spironolactone, triamterene, and amiloride) cause increased renal excretion of magnesium and can lead to hypomagnesemia.[21] Individuals with heart failure are at high risk for hypomagnesemia or total-body magnesium depletion.[103] In addition to diuretic therapy, people with heart failure often have congestion of the splanchnic vessels, which decreases magnesium absorption. Also, the secondary hyperaldosteronism and elevated catecholamines of heart failure increase urinary excretion of magnesium.[104] Among people with heart failure, those who are hypomagnesemic have more arrhythmias than those who are normomagnesemic and hypomagnesemia is associated with shorter survival.[103,105] Individuals with acute MI often have ionized hypomagnesemia.[106] Hypomagnesemia may be a causative factor for MI as well as a result of pathophysiologic changes immediately after MI.

Hypomagnesemia causes increased neuromuscular excitability. The signs and symptoms of hypomagnesemia include hyperactive reflexes, positive Chvostek's sign, positive Trousseau's sign, leg and foot cramps, muscle twitching, grimacing, tremors, dysphagia, nystagmus, ataxia, tetany, seizures, extreme confusion, cardiac arrhythmias, and hypertension.

Cardiac Effects of Hypomagnesemia and Total-Body Magnesium Depletion. Magnesium is a cofactor for Na^+–K^+ ATPase, the enzyme that plays a major role in the regulation of intracellular potassium concentration in the myocardium. When magnesium is deficient, the decreased intracellular magnesium leads to decreased activity of this enzyme. As a result, the intracellular potassium ion concentration decreases and intracellular sodium concentration increases in myocardial cells. Decreased activity of Na^+–K^+ ATPase interferes with the reentry of potassium ions into depolarized cells and promotes diastolic leak of potassium from cells that are already depolarized. In addition, hypomagnesemia causes increased membrane permeability to potassium, an effect that also tends to decrease intracellular potassium concentration in the myocardium.

In hypomagnesemia, the sinus node has an increased spontaneous firing rate, and there is a rate-dependent decrease in the duration of the cardiac action potential. The absolute refractory period is shortened, and the relative refractory period is lengthened. Hypomagnesemia thus predisposes to arrhythmias, especially tachyarrhythmias. The imbalance is associated with supraventricular tachycardia, supraventricular ectopy, ventricular ectopic beats, ventricular tachycardia, ventricular fibrillation, and torsade de pointes.[106–109] Whether these arrhythmias are caused directly by the hypomagnesemia itself or by hypomagnesemia-induced changes in potassium transport across myocardial membranes is uncertain. What is clear, however, is that both hypomagnesemia and total-body magnesium depletion lead to cardiac arrhythmias that can be corrected only by the administration of magnesium. Clinical studies demonstrate that correction of ionized hypomagnesemia during coronary artery bypass surgery (CABG) leads to fewer postoperative episodes of ventricular tachycardia.[110] Administration of magnesium reduces postoperative arrhythmias in CABG patients and in children having surgery for congenital heart defects, regardless of whether they are initially hypomagnesemic.[111,112] In individuals who are not hypomagnesemic, magnesium has been used pharmacologically to treat arrhythmias, including atrial fibrillation, ventricular tachycardia, and torsade de pointes, and to reduce arrhythmias in acute MI and in heart failure.[113,114]

A classic study demonstrated that heart muscle magnesium content decreases after acute MI.[115] This post-MI magnesium decrease may be caused by leakage of magnesium from necrotic cells and interference with ion transport in hypoxic cells. Another mechanism for the cardiac muscle magnesium decrease after MI may be the action of catecholamines. It is likely that localized decreases of myocardial magnesium after acute MI predispose to the development of cardiac arrhythmias. Animal studies show decreased tolerance to ischemic stress with chronic magnesium deficiency.[116]

Hypomagnesemia potentiates digitalis toxicity. Hypomagnesemia-related digitalis toxicity arises in part from the intracellular potassium deficiency caused by the magnesium imbalance. Digitalis toxicity arrhythmias have been observed in individuals with therapeutic digitalis levels and either decreased serum magnesium levels or normal serum levels with total-body magnesium depletion.

The ECG changes in hypomagnesemia are not easily characterized; rather, they are somewhat nonspecific. Prolongation of the QT interval is frequently observed in hypomagnesemia.[109] This ECG change probably occurs because of altered potassium transport caused by hypomagnesemia. Other ECG changes that have been seen with hypomagnesemia, such as ST segment depression, prolonged PR interval, wide QRS complex, and T-wave abnormalities, may be caused by multiple electrolyte imbalances that occur in conjunction with hypomagnesemia, or by the hypomagnesemia itself.

Vascular Effects of Hypomagnesemia and Total-Body Magnesium Depletion. Hypomagnesemia has important effects on vascular smooth muscle. A decrease in the extracellular magnesium concentration causes arteriolar vasoconstriction, in part by increasing the intracellular calcium concentration in vascular smooth muscle and by reducing endothelial production of the vasodilators nitric oxide and prostacyclin.[117,118] The resulting increased peripheral vascular resistance causes the hypertension that often accompanies acute or chronic hypomagnesemia. In addition to this direct vasoconstrictive effect, hypomagnesemia also decreases the vasodilation response to acetylcholine.[119] Low levels of dietary magnesium and low serum magnesium are associated with increased prevalence of hypertension.[120] Meta-analysis of clinical trials shows that magnesium supplementation has a small blood pressure lowering effect in hypertension.[121]

The vascular actions of hypomagnesemia promote the occurrence of vasospasm.[122] The coronary arteries are extremely sensitive to the effects of hypomagnesemia. Coronary artery spasm may cause acute myocardial ischemia in clinical hypomagnesemia.[123] Sudden-death, associated with a reduced dietary intake of magnesium, may be the result of coronary vasospasm. Plasma free fatty acids bind ionized magnesium, rendering it physiologically inactive. An increase in plasma free fatty acids thus causes a decrease in the amount of ionized magnesium. In individuals who have total-body magnesium depletion, it is possible that epinephrine-induced increases in plasma free fatty acids are a triggering factor for coronary vasospasm (and subsequent sudden death).

Total-body magnesium depletion (with or without hypomagnesemia) appears to play an important role in the development of atherosclerosis and ischemic heart disease.[124] Animal studies show hypertension, endothelial dysfunction, and vascular remodeling with chronic magnesium deficiency.[119] Animal studies also demonstrate plasma elevation of proinflammatory cytokines and neuropeptides that stimulate free radical formation.[116,125] Thus, magnesium deficiency can cause changes that are part of the atherosclerotic process.

Table 7-12 ■ CAUSES OF HYPERMAGNESEMIA

Category	Clinical Examples
Increased magnesium intake or absorption	Excessive use of Mg^{2+}-containing laxatives, antacids, or urologic irrigation solutions Excessive IV infusion of Mg^{2+} Aspiration of sea water
Decreased magnesium excretion	Oliguric renal failure Adrenal insufficiency

IV, intravenous.

In summary, the vascular effects of hypomagnesemia include vasoconstriction, increased peripheral resistance, hypertension, impaired vasodilation, and a tendency to vasospasm. Current evidence relates total-body magnesium depletion, with or without hypomagnesemia, to congestive heart failure, ischemic heart disease, and essential hypertension.

Hypermagnesemia

Hypermagnesemia is caused by increased magnesium intake or absorption, increased physiologic availability of magnesium, decreased magnesium excretion, or any combination of these factors.[1] Specific causative factors for hypermagnesemia are listed in Table 7-12. Older adults who use magnesium-containing antacids and laxatives are at especially high risk for development of hypermagnesemia, in part because they may have unrecognized renal insufficiency.[126,127]

The cardiac effects (bradycardia, arrhythmias, cardiac arrest) and vascular effects (flushing, hypotension) of hypermagnesemia are discussed next. In addition to these effects, hypermagnesemia may cause a subjective sensation of warmth, diaphoresis, drowsiness, lethargy, coma, diminished deep tendon reflexes, flaccid skeletal muscle paralysis, and respiratory depression.

Cardiac Effects of Hypermagnesemia. A plasma excess of magnesium interferes with cardiac conduction throughout the heart. Atrioventricular block or complete heart block may occur at high plasma levels of magnesium.[127] Hypermagnesemia inhibits myocardial contraction and depresses membrane excitability, although intracellular contractile mechanisms remain intact.

Hypermagnesemia suppresses the sinoatrial node and causes sympathetic nervous system blockade.[126] Both of these factors contribute to clinically significant supraventricular bradycardia. Cardiac arrest in asystole may be fatal in severe hypermagnesemia. ECG changes associated with hypermagnesemia include prolonged PR interval and increased duration of the QRS complex.[127,128] These changes are somewhat variable and do not present a classic, easily recognizable picture.

Vascular Effects of Hypermagnesemia. Hypermagnesemia reduces peripheral vascular resistance by inhibiting calcium movement into vascular smooth muscle cells, inhibiting calcium release from intracellular storage, and depressing contractile responses to vasoactive substances such as epinephrine and angiotensin II. The peripheral vasodilation caused by these mechanisms leads to hypotension.[128] Vasodilation of cutaneous vessels in hypermagnesemia causes flushing.

Phosphate Balance

Phosphate balance is the net result of phosphate intake and absorption, distribution, excretion, and abnormal losses. These components are summarized in Table 7-6. Phosphate is necessary for many cell metabolic processes and is a component of ATP, the cellular energy source.

The normal range of serum phosphate concentration is 2.5 to 4.5 mg/dL. Mild or moderate hypophosphatemia (1.0 to 2.4 mg/dL) may be asymptomatic. Severe hypophosphatemia, with a serum phosphate less than 1 mg/dL, usually has dramatic clinical manifestations.

Severe Hypophosphatemia

Hypophosphatemia is caused by decreased intake or absorption of phosphate, shift of phosphate into cells, or increased phosphate excretion.[1] Specific causative factors included in these categories are presented in Table 7-13.

Of importance to people with cardiac disease is the decrease in plasma phosphate concentration that occurs with intravenous glucose administration. Glucose infusion by itself does not usually cause severe hypophosphatemia; however, if glucose infusion is combined with other factors, such as diuretics that increase phosphate excretion, severe hypophosphatemia may occur. Insulin, as well as glucose, promotes the movement of phosphate into cells. Catecholamines and β-adrenergic agonist drugs also shift phosphate into cells and predispose to hypophosphatemia.[129]

Hypophosphatemia is common in chronic alcoholism.[130,131] Individuals with newly diagnosed alcoholic cardiomyopathy need to have their phosphate levels checked. If they undergo alcohol withdrawal, then they will likely be hyperventilating and respiratory alkalosis will develop, which also causes hypophosphatemia; therefore, their phosphate levels will need continued monitoring.

Table 7-13 ■ CAUSES OF HYPOPHOSPHATEMIA

Category	Clinical Examples
Decreased phosphate intake or absorption	Prolonged or excessive antacid use Starvation Malabsorption syndromes Chronic diarrhea Chronic alcoholism
Shift of phosphate into cells	Total parenteral nutrition Rapid cell proliferation (refeeding after starvation or malnutrition; leukemic blast crisis) Respiratory alkalosis (hyperventilation) Insulin Epinephrine, β-adrenergic agonists Infusion of IV glucose, fructose, or lactate
Increased phosphate excretion	Diabetic ketoacidosis Alcohol withdrawal Diuretic phase after severe burns Infusion of IV bicarbonate Renal tubular acidosis Diuretic therapy Glucocorticoid therapy
Phosphate loss by abnormal route	Emesis Hemodialysis

IV, intravenous.

The signs and symptoms of severe hypophosphatemia include anorexia, nausea, malaise, diminished reflexes, paresthesias, muscle aching, muscle weakness, rhabdomyolysis, severe debility, acute respiratory failure, hemolysis (possible hemolytic anemia), confusion, stupor, seizures, coma, and impaired cardiac function. These effects of hypophosphatemia are caused primarily by decreased intracellular ATP and by decreased 2,3-biphosphoglycerate (BPG) in the red blood cells. Decreased erythrocyte BPG causes tissue hypoxia by increasing hemoglobin–oxygen affinity, which reduces oxygen release. Administration of phosphate to hypophosphatemic individuals increases erythrocyte BPG, which decreases hemoglobin–oxygen affinity and allows greater tissue oxygenation.[130]

Cardiac Effects of Severe Hypophosphatemia. Severe hypophosphatemia impairs myocardial function by decreasing cardiac contractility. This cardiac impairment may progress to acute congestive failure or congestive cardiomyopathy.[130,132] The decreased cardiac performance of hypophosphatemia is reversed by the intravenous administration of phosphate.[129,132]

Cardiac arrest can occur from sudden severe hypophosphatemia caused by the refeeding syndrome, a situation that arises when a malnourished person with low phosphate stores begins to receive oral or parenteral nutrition. The plasma phosphate concentration falls rapidly within a few days of beginning nutritional repletion because a sudden increase in cellular metabolism depletes the individual's phosphate stores.[133,134] The sudden phosphate depletion leads to lack of ATP and cellular dysfunction.

The role of severe hypophosphatemia in cardiac arrhythmias is not well understood. Arrhythmias do occur in these individuals. However, many people who have severe hypophosphatemia also have hypokalemia or hypocalcemia or multiple electrolyte imbalances, so it may be difficult to isolate the effect of the decreased phosphate.

Vascular Effects of Severe Hypophosphatemia. Clinically, any vascular effects of severe hypophosphatemia are difficult to separate from the cardiac effects. Mean arterial pressure in hypophosphatemic individuals increases after phosphate repletion.[132] It is possible that this effect is caused by a vascular as well as a myocardial action; however, clearly the cardiac effect predominates in most situations.

SUMMARY OF FLUID AND ELECTROLYTES

Fluid balance is determined by the interplay of fluid intake, distribution, excretion, and fluid loss through abnormal routes. The two types of fluid imbalances are ECV imbalances and osmolality imbalances. ECV imbalances are increases or decreases in the amount of fluid in the vascular and interstitial compartments. Osmolality imbalances are alterations in the concentration of body fluids and result in movement of water into or out of cells caused by osmosis. Extracellular volume and osmolality imbalances may occur concurrently or separately in people with cardiac disease.

A normal plasma electrolyte concentration is necessary for optimal cardiovascular function. Because electrolytes play important roles in the generation of action potentials and the contraction of cardiac and smooth muscle, electrolyte imbalances exert cardiac and vascular effects. The effects of a specific electrolyte imbalance depend on the specific role of that electrolyte in normal cardiovascular function.

People who do not have cardiovascular disease may acquire an electrolyte imbalance that subsequently causes cardiovascular impairment. In addition, people who have pre-existing cardiovascular disease have specific risk factors for electrolyte imbalances. If imbalances develop in these individuals, then the cardiovascular effects of the electrolyte imbalances may cause severe disturbance to an already compromised cardiovascular system. Successful nursing management of these individuals involves careful assessment of risk factors, elimination of those risk factors when possible, surveillance for the manifestations of fluid and electrolyte imbalances, and nursing interventions to protect and support function during the correction of fluid and electrolyte imbalances.[1]

PRINCIPLES OF ACID–BASE BALANCE

The degree of acidity of the body fluids plays an important role in physiology. It influences the structure and function of many enzymes and also modifies the affinity between oxygen and hemoglobin. Deviations of acid–base balance from normal can affect cellular function and tissue oxygenation. In the extreme, these imbalances can be fatal.

Terminology Review

An *acid* is a substance that donates hydrogen ions (H^+) in solution. A *base* is a substance that accepts hydrogen ions. The more hydrogen ions a solution contains, the more acidic it is. The actual number of hydrogen ions in extracellular fluid is small and unwieldy to write (0.00004 mmol/L).[135] Therefore, the degree of acidity of body fluids is reported as the pH. The pH is the negative logarithm of the hydrogen ion concentration. It ranges from 1 (very acidic) to 14 (very alkaline). A pH of 7 is neutral. The blood is normally slightly alkaline. The normal pH range of the blood is 7.35 to 7.45. If the pH of the blood falls below the normal range (i.e., becomes more acidic), the person has *acidemia.* The process that tends to decrease the pH is called *acidosis.*[3] Similarly, if the pH of the blood rises above the normal range (i.e., becomes more alkaline), the person has *alkalemia.* The process that tends to increase the pH is called *alkalosis.*

Processes Involved in Acid–Base Balance

Normal cellular metabolism continually produces acids, which can cause dangerous acidemia without the closely regulated processes by which the body maintains pH within the normal range. After acid production, the processes of acid buffering and acid excretion work to maintain or re-establish a normal pH.

Acid Production

Cellular metabolism produces two types of acids: carbonic acid and metabolic acids. Carbonic acid (H_2CO_3) is produced as carbon dioxide (CO_2); the enzyme carbonic anhydrase combines the CO_2 with water (H_2O) to produce carbonic acid. In a standard adult, approximately 15,000 mmol of carbonic acid are generated per day from metabolism of carbohydrates and fats.[3] Because carbonic acid is excreted as the two gases CO_2 and H_2O, it sometimes is called *volatile acid.*

Metabolic acids are produced primarily from the metabolism of phosphate-containing compounds and amino acids that contain sulfur. These metabolic acids include sulfuric and phosphoric acids. Metabolic acids are handled differently by the body than is carbonic acid. For this reason, they sometimes are called *noncarbonic acids* or *nonvolatile acids.*

Cellular metabolism also produces small amounts of base (bicarbonate ions; HCO_3^-) as a result of oxidation of small organic anions such as citrate. Much more metabolic acid is produced than base. In a standard adult, a net 50 to 100 mEq of hydrogen ions is generated per day from metabolism.[3]

Acid Buffering

Buffers in the body act to minimize changes in pH because of gain of acid or base. They neutralize acids by taking up excess hydrogen ions and neutralize bases by releasing hydrogen ions. Buffers are located in all body fluids; however, the most important buffers are those in the extracellular fluid, intracellular fluid, bone, and urine. Different body fluids contain different buffers, which meet specific needs (Table 7-14).

The major extracellular buffer is the carbonic acid–bicarbonate–carbon dioxide buffer system (commonly termed the *bicarbonate buffer system*). Carbonic acid is a weak acid, which means that it dissociates partially when in solution so that it is in equilibrium with bicarbonate and hydrogen ions. The carbonic acid concentration can be altered by variations in alveolar ventilation (variations in CO_2 excretion). The chemical equation for the bicarbonate buffer system is written as follows:

$$\underset{\text{carbon dioxide}}{CO_2} + \underset{\text{water}}{H_2O} \rightleftharpoons \underset{\text{carbonic acid}}{H_2CO_3} \rightleftharpoons \underset{\text{hydrogen ion}}{H^+} + \underset{\text{bicarbonate ion}}{HCO_3^-}$$

To maintain the pH of the blood within the normal range, there must be 20 bicarbonate ions for every carbonic acid molecule. The Henderson–Hasselbalch equation, a mathematical description of the pH of a buffered solution, shows how this 20:1 ratio is necessary:

$$pH = pKa + \log\frac{[A^-]}{[HA]} \quad \text{(general equation)}$$

$$pH = 6.1 + \log\frac{[HCO_3^-]}{[H_2CO_3]} \quad \text{(substituting values for bicarbonate buffer system)}$$

$$pH = 6.1 + \log\frac{20}{1}$$

$$pH = 6.1 + 1.3$$

$$pH = 7.4$$

Table 7-14 ■ THE MAJOR BUFFERS

Extracellular Fluid	Intracellular Fluid	Bone	Urine
Bicarbonate	Proteins	Carbonates	Inorganic phosphates
Inorganic phosphates	Organic and inorganic phosphates	Phosphates	
Plasma proteins	Hemoglobin (in erythrocytes)		

Table 7-15 ■ ROLE OF BUFFERS WITH RESPECT TO AN ACID OR BASE LOAD

Buffer	Role with Carbonic Acid Load	Role with Metabolic Acid Load	Role with Base (Bicarbonate) Load
Extracellular bicarbonate	Not effective	Major role (immediate action)	Not effective
Other extracellular buffers	Minor role (immediate action)	Minor role (immediate action)	Minor role (immediate action)
Intracellular buffers	Major role (10–30 minutes)	Important role (2–4 hours)	Important role (hours)
Bone buffers	Probably not important	Important role (2–4 hours)	Important role (hours)

A buffer system cannot buffer its own acid. Thus, the bicarbonate buffer system cannot buffer carbonic acid. The carbonic acid that is produced by cells (as CO_2 and H_2O) is buffered primarily by intracellular buffers. The bicarbonate buffer system is a major buffer for metabolic acids. Table 7-15 summarizes the role of buffers with respect to acid or base loads.

Acid Excretion

Even though the buffers minimize pH changes while acid is produced, they have a limited capacity. Therefore, acid excretion mechanisms are necessary to maintain acid–base balance. The body has two acid excretion methods: the lungs excrete carbonic acid and the kidneys excrete metabolic acids.

Role of the Lungs. The lungs excrete carbonic acid in the form of carbon dioxide and water. They cannot excrete metabolic acids. When alveolar ventilation increases (increased rate and depth of ventilation), more carbonic acid is excreted. Conversely, when alveolar ventilation decreases, less carbonic acid is excreted. Because carbonic acid essentially is carbon dioxide and water, the body actually senses and regulates the partial pressure of carbon dioxide (Pa_{CO_2}).

If carbonic acid begins to accumulate (increased Pa_{CO_2}), chemoreceptors in the medulla and carotid and aortic bodies are stimulated by the increased Pa_{CO_2} and decreased pH.[135] The resulting increased alveolar ventilation causes excretion of the excess carbonic acid. Similarly, if too little carbonic acid is present (decreased Pa_{CO_2}), the chemoreceptors are less stimulated, and alveolar ventilation decreases somewhat to retain carbonic acid in the body. Hypoxia, sensed by the carotid chemoreceptors, stimulates alveolar ventilation and may override the suppression of ventilation from decreased Pa_{CO_2}. In a healthy person, alveolar ventilation changes rapidly in response to changes in Pa_{CO_2}, and thus carbonic acid is excreted at a rate effective in maintaining acid–base balance.

Role of the Kidneys. The kidneys excrete metabolic acids. They cannot excrete carbonic acid. The renal epithelial cells that line the proximal tubules secrete hydrogen ions into the renal tubular fluid and reabsorb bicarbonate ions in the process.[136] Bicarbonate is the major extracellular buffer of metabolic acids. Therefore, the bicarbonate ion concentration indicates how much metabolic acid is present. A decreased serum bicarbonate concentration indicates increased amounts of metabolic acid. When the proximal tubular cells secrete hydrogen ions that are eventually excreted in the urine, they reabsorb bicarbonate ions, replenishing the bicarbonate ions that were used in buffering. Hydrogen ions also are secreted into the renal tubular fluid by cells that line the distal tubules and collecting ducts and these cells also can secrete bicarbonate into the tubular fluid or reabsorb it into the blood.[137]

If the urine were to become too acidic, it could damage the cells that line the urinary tract. Fortunately, the urine does not become dangerously acidic because the hydrogen ions in the renal tubules are buffered by the urine buffers or combine chemically with ammonia. Ammonia (NH_3) is produced by renal tubular cells and then diffuses into the tubular fluid.[135] Hydrogen ions combine with ammonia in the tubular fluid to produce ammonium ions (NH_4^+). Because ammonium ions are charged particles, they cannot cross the cell membranes to enter the blood; thus, they are "trapped" in the renal tubular fluid and excreted in the urine. An increase of acid in the body (decreased pH) causes the production of more ammonia, which facilitates renal excretion of acid. This process begins within 2 hours but takes several days to be maximally effective.[3]

Thus, the kidneys have several mechanisms that result in the excretion of metabolic acids produced by cellular metabolism. These mechanisms can be adjusted to excrete more acid or less acid, thereby maintaining the bicarbonate ion concentration within normal limits. Changes in renal function with normal aging cause older adults to excrete an acid load more slowly than younger adults.

Summary of Acid–Base Balance

Cellular metabolism produces carbonic acid and metabolic acids. These acids must be excreted to maintain normal acid–base balance. Buffers in all body fluids act to minimize changes in pH due to an acid load or a bicarbonate (base) load. Carbonic acid is excreted by the lungs; increases or decreases in alveolar ventilation regulate the amount of carbonic acid excretion. The Pa_{CO_2} is the clinical indicator of carbonic acid. Metabolic acids are excreted by the kidneys, which can excrete more or less acid as needed. The plasma bicarbonate ion concentration (or total CO_2) is the clinical indicator of the amount of metabolic acid.[138] Table 7-16 summarizes the physiologic responses that maintain acid–base balance.

ACID–BASE IMBALANCES

Acid–base imbalances occur when the capacity of the buffers to modulate pH changes is exceeded. Two terms are important in understanding the physiologic responses to acid–base imbalances. *Correction* of the imbalance occurs when the original problem is fixed so that the pH, Pa_{CO_2}, and plasma bicarbonate ion concentration can return to normal.[138,139] *Compensation* for an acid–base imbalance restores the pH toward normal, but does not correct the problem that originally caused the imbalance.[139] In many cases, an acid–base imbalance persists long enough that compensatory physiologic processes occur. A *partially compensated* acid–base imbalance

Table 7-16 ■ SUMMARY OF PHYSIOLOGIC RESPONSES THAT MAINTAIN ACID–BASE BALANCE

Physiological Mechanism	Response to Decreased pH (too much acid in blood)	Response to Increased pH (too much bicarbonate in blood)
Buffers	Accept hydrogen ions	Release hydrogen ions
Respiratory system	Excretes carbonic acid by increasing rate and depth of respiration	Retains carbonic acid in the body by decreasing rate and depth of respiration
Kidneys	Excrete more metabolic acid by increasing secretion of H^+ into renal tubular fluid, increasing reabsorption of bicarbonate, and increasing production of NH_3	Excrete less metabolic acid by decreasing secretion of H^+ into renal tubular fluid, decreasing reabsorption of bicarbonate, and decreasing production of NH_3

is characterized by abnormal pH, Pa_{CO_2}, and plasma bicarbonate ion concentration. However, the pH is not as abnormal as it was before the partial compensation. When an acid–base imbalance is *fully compensated,* the pH is in the normal range, but the Pa_{CO_2} and plasma bicarbonate ion concentration both are abnormal. By moving the pH toward normal, compensation for an acid–base imbalance helps to protect cells from death.

Acidosis

An individual who has acidosis has processes that tend to decrease the pH of the blood below normal by creating a relative excess of acid. The resulting acidemia may persist or may be lessened by the body's compensatory response. A pH below 6.9 usually is fatal. Acidosis is classified as respiratory or metabolic, depending on what type of acid initially is relatively excessive.

Respiratory Acidosis

Respiratory acidosis occurs when too much carbonic acid accumulates in the blood. Clinically, the increase of carbonic acid is measured as an increased Pa_{CO_2}. Carbonic acid normally is excreted by the lungs. Thus, any factor that decreases ventilation can cause respiratory acidosis (Table 7-17). People in whom pulmonary heart disease (cor pulmonale) develops because of chronic lung disease commonly have chronic respiratory acidosis.

Carbon dioxide diffuses readily through membranes.[135] Thus, the pH of CSF decreases when respiratory acidosis occurs. As excess CO_2 enters brain cells, intracellular acidosis alters enzyme activity and central nervous system (CNS) depression results. Clinical manifestations of respiratory acidosis are CNS depression (disorientation, lethargy, somnolence), headache, blurred vision, tachycardia, and cardiac arrhythmias.

Respiratory acidosis can be corrected only by restoring lung function because the lungs are the only route of excretion of carbonic acid. If the respiratory acidosis lasts long enough, the kidneys compensate by excreting more than the usual amount of metabolic acids, moving the pH back toward normal, even though the blood chemistry remains abnormal.[140] Excretion of more metabolic acids raises the bicarbonate ion concentration because fewer bicarbonate ions are used in buffering. Thus, renal compensation for respiratory acidosis restores the 20:1 ratio of bicarbonate to carbonic acid, even though the absolute values of both are elevated. Restoring the 20:1 ratio normalizes the pH. Renal compensation for respiratory acidosis takes 3 to 5 days to be fully effective.[3] Compensated respiratory acidosis is characterized by elevated Pa_{CO_2} (the sign of the primary problem), elevated bicarbonate ion concentration (the sign of the renal compensation), and pH that is decreased (partially compensated) or normal (fully compensated).

In respiratory acidosis, excess CO_2 diffuses into cardiac cells. Although intracellular buffering of carbonic acid may protect intracellular pH in cardiac cells more effectively than in many other types of cells, the intracellular pH in cardiac cells does decrease.[141] Respiratory acidosis depresses cardiac contractility.[142] The negative effects of decreased myocardial cell contractility in respiratory acidosis are offset partially by increased sympathetic neural discharge and increased catecholamine levels.[143] Tachycardia and cardiac arrhythmias in individuals who have respiratory acidosis may be caused by the increased circulating catecholamines.

Respiratory acidosis also affects blood vessels, altering both peripheral vascular resistance and distribution of blood flow. Peripheral vasodilation decreases the peripheral vascular resistance.[144] and coronary vasodilation also occurs.[145] The peripheral vasculature becomes less sensitive to α- and β-adrenergic stimulation. Decreased

Table 7-17 ■ CAUSES OF RESPIRATORY ACIDOSIS

Category	Clinical Examples
Decreased gaseous exchange (problem in the airways or alveoli of lungs)	Decreased alveolar ventilation for any reason Acute airway obstruction by foreign body Severe asthma Sleep apnea (obstructive type) Chronic obstructive pulmonary disease (COPD) type A (emphysema) in end-stage Chronic obstructive pulmonary disease (COPD) type B (chronic bronchitis) Atelectasis Pneumonia Adult respiratory distress syndrome (ARDS) Pulmonary edema Hypoventilation with mechanical ventilator
Impaired neuromuscular function of chest (problem in the chest muscles or nerves)	Chest injury Surgical incision in chest or upper abdomen (pain limits chest expansion) Respiratory muscle fatigue Severe hypokalemia Poliomyelitis Guillain–Barré syndrome Myasthenia gravis Kyphoscoliosis Pickwickian syndrome (obesity limits chest expansion)
Suppression of respiratory neurons in brainstem (medulla) (problem in the brainstem)	Opioids Barbiturates Anesthetics Sleep apnea (central type)

peripheral vascular resistance and the decreased cardiac contractility can cause hypotension, which may be diminished by constriction in splanchnic and peripheral venous beds (the venous capacitance beds). This response increases central arterial blood volume.

The decreased pH in the CSF increases the synthesis of nitric oxide, which causes cerebral vasodilation, increasing cerebral blood flow.[146] This is the source of the headache that is experienced by many individuals with respiratory acidosis. Increased cerebral blood flow from cerebral vasodilation may also raise CSF pressure and cause papilledema. In contrast to its effect on other vascular beds, respiratory acidosis causes vasoconstriction in the pulmonary vasculature.[144,147] The resulting increase in pulmonary vascular resistance may worsen the clinical status of people with preexisting right heart failure.

In summary, the major cardiovascular effects of respiratory acidosis are tachycardia, cardiac arrhythmias, decreased cardiac contractility, decreased peripheral vascular resistance, increased pulmonary vascular resistance, and shift of blood flow from the venous capacitance beds into the central and cerebral arterial beds.

Metabolic Acidosis

Metabolic acidosis is caused by relatively too much metabolic acid. It can be due to a gain of acid or a loss of base.[139] Acid can be gained from intake of acids or substances that are converted to acid in the body, from an increased rate of normal metabolism, from production of unusual acids due to altered metabolic processes, or from factors that decrease renal excretion of acid. Bicarbonate ions (base) can be lost in the urine or through the gastrointestinal tract. Table 7-18 lists clinical conditions that cause metabolic acidosis by each of these mechanisms. Cardiogenic shock causes metabolic acidosis by accumulation of lactic acid from anaerobic metabolism and through failure of the decreased circulation to deliver metabolic acids to the kidneys for excretion. No matter what its cause, metabolic acidosis is characterized by a decreased plasma bicarbonate ion concentration. The bicarbonate either is depleted by being used to buffer excess metabolic acids or is lost directly from the body.

Table 7-18 ■ CAUSES OF METABOLIC ACIDOSIS

Category	Clinical Examples
Acid accumulation by ingestion or infusion of acid or acid precursors	Aspirin (acetylsalicylic acid) Boric acid Ammonium chloride (releases H^+) Methanol (converts to formic acid) Antifreeze (ethylene glycol converts to oxalic acid) Paraldehyde (converts to acetic and chloroacetic acids) Elemental sulfur (converts to sulfuric acid)
Acid accumulation by increased production of normal metabolic acids	Hyperthyroidism Hypermetabolic state after burns, trauma, or sepsis Lactic acidosis Shock
Acid accumulation by utilization of abnormal or incomplete metabolic pathways	Alcoholic ketoacidosis Diabetic ketoacidosis Starvation ketoacidosis
Acid accumulation by impaired acid exceration	Prolonged oliguria from any cause Oliguric renal failure Severe hypovolemia Shock Renal tubular acidosis (type 1) Hypoaldosteronism
Loss of base (bicarbonate ions)	Severe diarrhea Intestinal decompression Fistula drainage from pancreas or intestine Vomiting of intestinal contents Ureterosigmoidostomy Renal tubular acidosis (type 2)

Some clinicians use the *anion gap* when evaluating metabolic acidosis.[148] The anion gap is the difference between the concentrations of the major positive and negative ions in plasma or serum:

$$\text{Anion gap} = (Na^+ + K^+) - (Cl^- + HCO_3^-)$$

Some people omit the potassium concentration, a relatively small number, from the calculation to simplify it. The normal range of anion gap varies with the laboratory procedures used for electrolyte measurements, so that it may be reported as 6 to 16 mEq/L, 12 to 20 mEq/L, or another such range.[148–150] If unmeasured anions such as lactate or β-hydroxybutyrate accumulate in the body, the anion gap increases. Calculation of the anion gap is rapid and uses clinically available parameters, but it is less informative for individuals who have hypoalbuminemia unless a correction is used and may be misleading when two primary acid–base imbalances coexist.[150]

Calculating the anion gap enables division of metabolic acidosis into two groups: *high serum anion gap metabolic acidosis* and *normal serum anion gap metabolic acidosis*.[3,148] The anion gap increases when an abnormal metabolic acid accumulates in the body, such as with lactic acidosis or ketoacidosis. Normal anion gap acidosis, also called *hyperchloremic acidosis*, typically occurs with diarrhea or loss of HCO_3^- from the kidneys, which retain NaCl in response. Critically ill patients who have lactic acidosis, a type of high anion gap acidosis, have been shown to have a higher mortality rate than those who have normal anion gap acidosis.[151]

In research and some clinical settings, metabolic acid–base imbalances may be evaluated using a quantitative physical chemistry method often called the *Stewart approach* or the *strong ion gap* (SIG).[151,152] The SIG is the apparent strong ion difference minus the charge on buffer base:

$$\begin{aligned}\text{Strong ion gap} = {} & (Na^+ + K^+ + Ca^{2+} + Mg^{2+} - Cl^- - \text{lactate}) \\ & - (\text{charge on albumin} + \text{charge on phosphate} + HCO_3^-)\end{aligned}$$

One advantage of the SIG over the traditional anion gap is that it enables quantification of the unmeasured anion, but disadvantages are that the calculation is time-consuming and includes clinical parameters such as serum magnesium and lactate concentrations that frequently are not readily available.[153] Whether the SIG is useful in predicting outcomes of metabolic acidosis is controversial.[151–153]

Metabolic acidosis can be corrected physiologically only by the kidneys, which are the sole excretory route for metabolic acids. Renal correction of metabolic acidosis may take several days. Meanwhile, respiratory compensation occurs within hours. The respiratory compensation for metabolic acidosis is hyperventilation. By increasing the excretion of carbonic acid, hyperventilation makes the blood less acid. This makes the blood chemistry more abnormal (decreased Pa_{CO_2}), but tends to restore the 20:1 ratio of bicarbonate to carbonic acid and move the pH toward the normal range, thus helping to preserve cellular function. Compensated metabolic acidosis is characterized by a decreased Pa_{CO_2} (the sign of the respiratory compensation), a decreased bicarbonate ion

Table 7-19 ■ VASCULAR EFFECTS OF ACID–BASE IMBALANCES

Vascular Bed	Respiratory Acidosis	Metabolic Acidosis	Respiratory Alkalosis	Metabolic Alkalosis
Peripheral	Vasodilation	Vasodilation	Vasoconstriction (debatable)	Vasoconstriction (likely)
Coronary	Vasodilation	Vasodilation	Vasoconstriction	Vasoconstriction
Cerebral	Vasodilation	Vasodilation	Vasoconstriction	Vasoconstriction
Pulmonary	Vasoconstriction	Vasoconstriction	Vasodilation	Vasodilation

concentration (the sign of the primary problem), and a pH that is decreased (partially compensated) or normal (fully compensated).

The clinical manifestations of metabolic acidosis include headache, abdominal pain, cardiac arrhythmias, and CNS depression (confusion, drowsiness, lethargy, stupor, and coma). The CNS depression arises from decreased pH of the CSF and resultant intracellular acidosis of brain cells. The exact cause of the abdominal pain is not clearly understood. Tachypnea reflects the compensatory hyperventilation.

Although intracellular pH in myocardial cells is regulated to some extent through the action of H^+ transporters in the sarcolemma, these mechanisms become overwhelmed in metabolic acidosis and intracellular acidosis occurs.[154] Myocardial intracellular acidosis depresses cardiac contractility because it changes the charge on many different proteins. This alters intracellular signaling and delivery of calcium ions to the myofilaments and inhibits myofilament responsiveness to calcium.[142,155] Cardiac arrhythmias may be related to an increase in circulating catecholamine levels caused by metabolic acidosis or other concurrent pathophysiological processes, including inhibiting the transient outward potassium ion current from myocytes.[156,157] The catecholamine increase helps to preserve cardiac output during mild metabolic acidosis, but in more severe metabolic acidosis the decreased myocardial contractility predominates. Coronary artery occlusion causes myocardial acidosis, so that these cardiac effects occur in individuals who have acute MI without the systemic effects of metabolic acidosis.

The action of increased circulating catecholamines on the heart also helps to protect the arterial blood pressure from the peripheral vasodilation caused by acidosis. This peripheral vasodilation is caused by several factors, including increased release of nitric oxide by the vascular endothelium.[158,159] Arterial vascular smooth muscles relax due to activation of ATP-sensitive potassium (K_{ATP}) channels that cause cell membrane hyperpolarization, with less entry of extracellular calcium through voltage-dependent calcium channels.[160] These mechanisms contribute to peripheral, coronary, and cerebral vasodilation.[161] Mild cerebral vasodilation is probably responsible for the headache experienced by some individuals.[159] As acidosis progresses, the peripheral vasculature becomes hyporesponsive to adrenergic vasopressors. Contrary to other arterioles, pulmonary vessels respond to acidosis with vasoconstriction, in part due to suppression of nitric oxide synthesis.[147] Vascular effects of acid–base imbalances are summarized in Table 7-19.

Alkalosis

An individual who has alkalosis has processes that tend to increase the pH of the blood above normal by creating a relative excess of base (a relative deficit of acid). The resulting alkalemia may persist or may be modulated by a compensatory response. A pH above 7.8 usually is fatal. Alkalosis is classified as respiratory or metabolic, depending on what type of acid initially is relatively deficient.

Respiratory Alkalosis

Respiratory alkalosis occurs when there is too little carbonic acid in the blood. Clinically, the decreased carbonic acid is measured as a decreased Pa_{CO_2}. Any factor that causes hyperventilation can cause excretion of too much carbonic acid, leading to respiratory alkalosis (Table 7-20).

Note that hypoxia, as from pulmonary embolism or severe anemia, causes appropriate hyperventilation with resultant respiratory alkalosis. In such cases, the cause of the hypoxia should be the primary focus of treatment rather than the respiratory alkalosis.

Individuals who have respiratory alkalosis may evidence lightheadedness, diaphoresis, paresthesias (digital and circumoral), muscle cramps, carpal and pedal spasms, tetany, syncope, and cardiac arrhythmias. Most of these manifestations are the result of increased neuromuscular excitability. The CSF becomes alkalotic. Chvostek's and Trousseau's signs (nonspecific signs of increased neuromuscular excitability) are positive in many of these individuals.

Respiratory alkalosis can be corrected only by the lungs. If any compensation occurs, it is performed by the kidneys, which increase the urinary excretion of bicarbonate ions to restore the 20:1 ratio of bicarbonate ion to carbonic acid. Renal compensation for a respiratory acid–base imbalance requires several days. Most cases of respiratory alkalosis have a short duration; therefore, the disorder is often uncompensated or partially compensated. Compensated respiratory alkalosis is characterized by a decreased Pa_{CO_2} (the sign of the primary problem), a decreased bicarbonate ion concentration (the sign of the renal compensation), and a pH that is increased (partially compensated) or normal (fully compensated).

Table 7-20 ■ CAUSES OF RESPIRATORY ALKALOSIS

Category	Clinical Examples
Hyperventilation due to hypoxemia	Pulmonary disease that causes decreased Pa_{O_2} Pulmonary embolism High altitude
Hyperventilation due to situational factors	Anxiety or fear Pain Prolonged crying and gasping Hyperventilation with mechanical ventilator
Hyperventilation due to stimulation of respiratory neurons in brainstem (medulla)	High fever Encephalitis Meningitis Salicylate overdose Gram-negative sepsis

Respiratory alkalosis causes increased pH inside myocardial cells and increases cardiac contractility by increasing the calcium sensitivity of myofibrils as shown in classic work by Hunjan et al.[162] The imbalance also increases sympathetic nervous system activity and circulating catecholamines that may cause cardiac arrhythmias. Although respiratory alkalosis may cause a transient peripheral vasodilation, which decreases peripheral vascular resistance, it is most likely to cause peripheral vasoconstriction and increased peripheral vascular resistance.[163,164] Respiratory alkalosis also causes coronary and cerebral vasoconstriction.[164,165] This latter effect reduces intracranial pressure and cerebral blood flow and may be the reason for the light-headedness and syncope experienced by some individuals with respiratory alkalosis. In contrast to its effect on other blood vessels, respiratory alkalosis causes pulmonary vasodilation.[147] This effect is decreased in conditions with chronically increased pulmonary blood flow, such as some congenital heart defects.[166]

Metabolic Alkalosis

Metabolic alkalosis is caused by relatively too little metabolic acid. It can be due to a loss of acid or a gain of base.[139] Acid can be lost through the gastrointestinal tract or in the urine. Acid may also be shifted into cells and thus "lost" from the blood. Base (bicarbonate ions) may be gained from intake of bicarbonate or of substances that are converted to bicarbonate in the body. More commonly, base is gained through renal bicarbonate reabsorption. For example, diuretic therapy often causes a mild "contraction alkalosis," metabolic alkalosis associated with extracellular volume contraction.[3] Contraction alkalosis is especially common with loop and thiazide diuretic therapy for heart failure because a high volume of sodium is delivered to the distal tubules by the diuretic in the presence of excessive stimulation of distal tubule mineralocorticoid receptors from the elevated aldosterone that is a compensatory mechanism in heart failure.[167,168] In an individual with hypovolemic shock from hemorrhage, a metabolic alkalosis may develop if eight or more units of packed red cells or other forms of blood are infused in a short time because the liver metabolizes the citrate in the blood into bicarbonate. Additional causes of metabolic alkalosis are listed in Table 7-21.

Table 7-21 ■ CAUSES OF METABOLIC ALKALOSIS

Category	Clinical Examples
Decrease of acid	Emesis
	Gastric suction
	Hyperaldosteronism (increases renal excretion of acid)
	Chronic excessive ingestion of black licorice (contains aldosterone-like compounds)
	Glucocorticoid excess
	Loop or thiazide diuretics
	Hypokalemia (acid moves into cells)
Increase of base (bicarbonate ions)	Excess ingestion of baking soda or bicarbonate antacids
	Excess infusion of $NaHCO_3$
	Excess administration of lactate or acetate (convert to bicarbonate)
	Massive blood transfusion (citrate converts to bicarbonate)
	Citrate anticoagulation during chronic renal replacement therapy (citrate converts to bicarbonate)
	Extracellular fluid volume deficit (contraction alkalosis)

The initial clinical manifestations of metabolic alkalosis are often milder than those of respiratory alkalosis because bicarbonate ions cross membranes (and thus alter CSF and intracellular pH) less rapidly than does carbon dioxide. These clinical manifestations may include light-headedness, paresthesias, muscle cramps, carpal and pedal spasms, and cardiac arrhythmias. An initial CNS excitation is followed by the CNS depression of severe metabolic alkalosis: confusion, lethargy, and coma. The plasma bicarbonate ion concentration is elevated.

Correction of metabolic alkalosis must be accomplished by the kidneys because they are the excretory organs for bicarbonate ions. Compensation for the disorder, therefore, is the role of the lungs. Because the bicarbonate ion concentration is increased in metabolic alkalosis, the 20:1 ratio of bicarbonate ion to carbonic acid that creates a normal pH can be restored by increasing the amount of carbonic acid in the blood. Thus, the respiratory compensation for metabolic alkalosis is decreased rate and depth of respiration.[169] This compensatory hypoventilation retains carbonic acid (carbon dioxide and water) in the body, which tends to normalize the pH. Compensatory hypoventilation, however, is limited by the body's need for oxygen, so full compensation for metabolic alkalosis is not common. Compensated metabolic alkalosis is characterized by an increased Pa_{CO2} (the sign of the respiratory compensation), an increased bicarbonate ion concentration (the sign of the primary problem), and a pH that is somewhat increased (partially compensated).

Metabolic alkalosis causes increased cardiac contractility by increasing calcium sensitivity, although intracellular pH does not increase in myocardial cells as it does in respiratory alkalosis.[162] Cardiac arrhythmias may occur. Vascular effects are likely to include peripheral vasoconstriction. Other vascular effects of metabolic alkalosis are coronary vasoconstriction, pulmonary vasodilation, and cerebral vasoconstriction with resulting decreased cerebral blood flow and light-headedness.[147]

Principles of Interpreting Arterial Blood Gas Reports

Arterial blood gases are used to assess an individual's acid–base status. The material presented earlier in this chapter provides the basis for understanding and interpreting acid–base aspects of arterial blood gases. The principles are summarized in this section. The Pa_{O2}, a measure of oxygenation, is discussed in Chapter 2.

The first laboratory value to consider is the pH.[170] If the pH is below the normal range (i.e., less than 7.35 or the reported laboratory normal), then the individual has acidosis. If the pH is above the normal range (greater than 7.45 or the reported laboratory normal), then the individual has alkalosis. If the pH is within the normal range, there may be no acid–base imbalance, or the individual may have a fully compensated imbalance. For purposes of interpretation, then, if the pH is less than 7.40, the individual is tentatively considered to have acidosis; if the pH is greater than 7.40, the individual is tentatively considered to have alkalosis.

The next value to consider is the Pa_{CO2}. If the Pa_{CO2} is above the normal range, then the individual has respiratory acidosis. This respiratory acidosis may be the primary problem, or it may be compensatory. On the other hand, if the Pa_{CO2} is below the normal range, then the individual has respiratory alkalosis. This respiratory alkalosis may be the primary problem or it may be compensatory. If the Pa_{CO2} is within the normal range, then the individual does not have a respiratory acid–base disorder.

Table 7-22 ■ MIXED ACID–BASE IMBALANCES

Concurrent Primary Acid–Base Imbalances	Effect on pH	Clinical Examples	Blood Gas Values
Respiratory acidosis plus metabolic alkalosis	Opposing effect on pH	Person with type B COPD (chronic bronchitis) develops repeated emesis	pH possibly near normal Pa_{CO_2} increased HCO_3^- increased
Respiratory alkalosis plus metabolic acidosis	Opposing effect on pH	Person with encephalitis develops circulatory shock	pH possibly near normal Pa_{CO_2} decreased HCO_3^- decreased
Metabolic acidosis plus metabolic alkalosis	Opposing effect on pH	Person with chronic renal failure develops repeated emesis	Vary, depending on severity and duration of imbalances
Respiratory acidosis and metabolic acidosis	Same effect on pH	Person with type B COPD (chronic bronchitis) develops prolonged diarrhea	pH greatly decreased Pa_{CO_2} increased HCO_3^- decreased
Two different types of metabolic acidosis	Same effect on pH	Person with diabetic ketoacidosis becomes dehydrated and develops lactic acidosis from poor tissue perfusion	pH greatly decreased Pa_{CO_2} likely decreased (compensation) HCO_3^- greatly decreased
Metabolic alkalosis and respiratory alkalosis	Same effect on pH	Person who received massive blood transfusion hyperventilates from pain and fear	pH greatly increased Pa_{CO_2} decreased HCO_3^- increased

A basic understanding of acid–base imbalances facilitates differentiating between primary and compensatory respiratory imbalances. If the individual has *primary respiratory acidosis*, then the pH would be expected to be below 7.40. A *compensatory respiratory acidosis* would occur in response to a metabolic alkalosis, so the pH would be above 7.40.

The third laboratory value to consider is the bicarbonate ion concentration.[171] If it is above the normal range, the individual has metabolic alkalosis, which may be the primary problem or may be compensatory. If the bicarbonate ion concentration is below the normal range, then the individual has primary or compensatory metabolic acidosis. A bicarbonate ion concentration within the normal range indicates no metabolic acid–base disorder. The differentiation between primary and compensatory imbalances is made by considering the pH. An individual who has a *primary metabolic acidosis* would be expected to have a pH below 7.40. A *compensatory metabolic acidosis* would be a response to a primary respiratory alkalosis, so the pH would be above 7.40. Following similar logic, with a *primary metabolic alkalosis*, the pH would be above 7.40; with a *compensatory metabolic alkalosis*, the pH would be below that value.

Once the three values have been examined, the final step in interpreting arterial blood gas values is to compare the interpretation with the individual's history and condition to verify that it makes sense. The principles of laboratory value interpretation presented in this section apply to people who have only one primary acid–base imbalance. Mixed acid–base imbalances (more than one concurrent primary imbalance) are presented briefly in the next section.

Mixed Acid–Base Imbalances

Occasionally, an individual may have more than one primary acid–base imbalance at the same time. In this circumstance, coexisting primary acidosis and alkalosis may somewhat neutralize each other so that the pH is near normal while the Pa_{CO_2} and bicarbonate ion concentration are grossly abnormal. Alternatively, two primary disorders that cause the same pH alteration (e.g., types of coexisting alkalosis) can create a pH that rapidly approaches the fatal limit. Examples of mixed acid–base imbalances are presented in Table 7-22.

SUMMARY OF ACID-BASE

Cellular metabolism generates carbonic acid, which the lungs excrete, and metabolic acids, which the kidneys excrete. Respiratory acid–base imbalances are disorders of too much or too little carbonic acid (carbon dioxide and water). Their laboratory marker is an altered Pa_{CO_2}. The body compensates for an ongoing respiratory acid–base disorder by excreting more or fewer metabolic acids in the urine to normalize the pH.

Metabolic acid–base imbalances are disorders of too many or too few metabolic acids. Their laboratory marker is an altered bicarbonate ion concentration. The body compensates for metabolic acid–base disorders by adjusting alveolar ventilation to excrete more or less carbonic acid to normalize the pH. In addition to their other effects, acid–base imbalances alter cardiac contractility and may cause cardiac arrhythmias. They influence the degree of vasoconstriction in various vascular beds. Thus, an understanding of acid–base balance and imbalances is important in the care of people who have heart failure and other cardiovascular pathophysiologies.

REFERENCES

1. Felver, L. (2010). Fluid and electrolyte homeostasis and imbalances. In L. Copstead & J. Banasik (Eds.), *Pathophysiology* (4th ed.) (pp. 592–614). St Louis: Elsevier Saunders.
2. Blackburn, S. (2003). *Maternal, fetal and neonatal physiology.* Philadelphia: WB Saunders.
3. Rose, B. (2009). *Clinical physiology of acid-base and electrolyte disorders.* New York: McGraw-Hill.
4. Johnson, A. K. (2007). The sensory psychobiology of thirst and salt appetite. *Medicine and Science in Sports and Exercise, 39,* 1388–1400.
5. Selektor, Y., & Weber, K. T. (2008). The salt-avid state of congestive heart failure revisited. *American Journal of Medical Science, 335,* 209–218.

6. Ball, S. G. (2007). Vasopressin and disorders of water balance: The physiology and pathophysiology of vasopressin. *Annals of Clinical Biochemistry, 44*, 417–431.
7. LeJemtel, T. H., & Serrano, C. (2007). Vasopressin dysregulation: Hyponatremia, fluid retention and congestive heart failure. *International Journal of Cardiology, 120*, 1–9.
8. Gheorghiade, M., Abraham, W. T., Albert, N. M., et al. (2007). Relationship between admission serum sodium concentration and clinical outcomes in patients hospitalized for heart failure: An analysis from the OPTIMIZE-HF registry. *European Heart Journal, 28*, 980–988.
9. Gheorghiade, M., Rossi, J. S., Cotts, W., et al. (2007). Characterization and prognostic value of persistent hyponatremia in patients with severe heart failure in the ESCAPE Trial. *Archives of Internal Medicine, 167*, 1998–2005.
10. Rossi, J., Bayram, M., Udelson, J. E., et al. (2007). Improvement in hyponatremia during hospitalization for worsening heart failure is associated with improved outcomes: Insights from the Acute and Chronic Therapeutic Impact of a Vasopressin Antagonist in Chronic Heart Failure (ACTIV in CHF) trial. *Acute Cardiac Care, 9*, 82–86.
11. Decaux, G., Soupart, A., & Vassart, G. (2008). Non-peptide arginine-vasopressin antagonists: The vaptans. *Lancet, 371*, 1624–1632.
12. Verbalis, J. G., Goldsmith, S. R., Greenberg, A., et al. (2007). Hyponatremia treatment guidelines 2007: Expert panel recommendations. *American Journal of Medicine, 120*, S1–S21.
13. Singla, I., Zahid, M., Good, C. B., et al. (2007). Effect of hyponatremia (<135 mEq/L) on outcome in patients with non-ST-elevation acute coronary syndrome. *American Journal of Cardiology, 100*, 406–408.
14. Chow, K. M., Szeto, C. C., Kwan, B. C., et al. (2007). Influence of climate on the incidence of thiazide-induced hyponatraemia. *International Journal of Clinical Practice, 61*, 449–452.
15. Liamis, G., Mitrogianni, Z., Liberopoulos, E. N., et al. (2007). Electrolyte disturbances in patients with hyponatremia. *Internal Medicine, 46*, 685–690.
16. Mok, N. S., Tong, C. K., & Yuen, H. C. (2008). Concomitant-acquired long QT and Brugada syndromes associated with indapamide-induced hypokalemia and hyponatremia. *Pacing and Clinical Electrophysiology, 31*, 772–775.
17. Chapman, M., Hanrahan, R., McEwen, J., et al. (2002). Hyponatraemia and hypokalaemia due to indapamide. *Medical Journal of Australia, 176*, 219–222.
18. Hoorn, E. J., Betjes, M. G., Weigel, J., & Zietse, R. (2008). Hypernatraemia in critically ill patients: Too little water and too much salt. *Nephrology Dialysis Transplantation, 23*, 1562–1568.
19. Moore-Ede, M. C., Meguid, M. M., Fitzpatrick, G. F., et al. (1978). Circadian variation in response to potassium infusion. *Clinical Pharmacology and Therapeutics, 23*, 218–227.
20. Ahmed, A., Zannad, F., Love, T. E., et al. (2007). A propensity-matched study of the association of low serum potassium levels and mortality in chronic heart failure. *European Heart Journal, 28*, 1334–1343.
21. Papadopoulos, D. P., & Papademetriou, V. (2007). Metabolic side effects and cardiovascular events of diuretics: Should a diuretic remain the first choice therapy in hypertension treatment? The case of yes. *Clinical and Experimental Hypertension, 29*, 503–516.
22. Beal, A. L., Deuser, W. E., & Beilman, G. J. (2007). A role for epinephrine in post-traumatic hypokalemia. *Shock, 27*, 358–363.
23. Hahn, R. G., & Lofgren, A. (2000). Epinephrine, potassium and the electrocardiogram during regional anaesthesia. *European Journal of Anaesthesiology, 17*, 132–137.
24. Foo, K., Sekhri, N., Deaner, A., et al. (2003). Effect of diabetes on serum potassium concentrations in acute coronary syndromes. *Heart, 89*, 31–35.
25. Ives, H. (2007). Diuretic agents. In B. Katzung (Ed.), *Basics and clinical pharmacology* (pp. 236–254). New York: Lange Medical Books, McGraw-Hill.
26. Blanning, A., Westfall, J. M., & Shaughnessy, A. F. (2001). Clinical inquiries. How soon should serum potassium levels be monitored for patients started on diuretics? *Journal of Family Practice, 50*, 207–208.
27. Zuccala, G., Pedone, C., Cocchi, A., et al. (2000). Older age and in-hospital development of hypokalemia from loop diuretics: Results from a multicenter survey. GIFA Investigators. Multicenter Italian Pharmacoepidemiologic Study Group. *Journals of Gerontology Series A: Biological Sciences and Medical Sciences, 55*, M232–M238.
28. Cohn, J. N., Kowey, P. R., Whelton, P. K., et al. (2000). New guidelines for potassium replacement in clinical practice: A contemporary review by the National Council on Potassium in Clinical Practice. *Archives of Internal Medicine, 160*, 2429–2436.
29. Killeen, M. J., Gurung, I. S., Thomas, G., et al. (2007). Separation of early after depolarizations from arrhythmogenic substrate in the isolated perfused hypokalaemic murine heart through modifiers of calcium homeostasis. *Acta Physiologica (Oxford), 191*, 43–58.
30. Killeen, M. J., Thomas, G., Gurung, I. S., et al. (2007). Arrhythmogenic mechanisms in the isolated perfused hypokalaemic murine heart. *Acta Physiologica (Oxford), 189*, 33–46.
31. Sabir, I. N., Fraser, J. A., Killeen, M. J., et al. (2007). The contribution of refractoriness to arrhythmic substrate in hypokalemic Langendorff-perfused murine hearts. *Pflugers Archives, 454*, 209–222.
32. Yelamanchi, V. P., Molnar, J., Ranade, V., et al. (2001). Influence of electrolyte abnormalities on interlead variability of ventricular repolarization times in 12-lead electrocardiography. *American Journal of Therapeutics, 8*, 117–122.
33. Sabir, I. N., Fraser, J. A., Cass, T. R., et al. (2007). A quantitative analysis of the effect of cycle length on arrhythmogenicity in hypokalaemic Langendorff-perfused murine hearts. *Pflugers Archives, 454*, 925–936.
34. Boccalandro, C., Lopez-Penabad, L., Boccalandro, F., et al. (2003). Ventricular fibrillation in a young Asian man. *Lancet, 361*, 1432.
35. Facchini, M., Sala, L., Malfatto, G., et al. (2006). Low-K^+ dependent QT prolongation and risk for ventricular arrhythmia in anorexia nervosa. *International Journal of Cardiology, 106*, 170–176.
36. Kannankeril, P. J., & Roden, D. M. (2007). Drug-induced long QT and torsade de pointes: Recent advances. *Current Opinion in Cardiology, 22*, 39–43.
37. Maeder, M., Rickli, H., Sticherling, C., et al. (2007). Hypokalaemia and sudden cardiac death–lessons from implantable cardioverter defibrillators. *Emergency Medicine Journal, 24*, 206–208.
38. Notarstefano, P., Pratola, C., Toselli, T., et al. (2005). Atrial fibrillation and recurrent ventricular fibrillation during hypokalemia in Brugada syndrome. *Pacing and Clinical Electrophysiology, 28*, 1350–1353.
39. Slovis, C., & Jenkins, R. (2002). ABC of clinical electrocardiography: Conditions not primarily affecting the heart. *BMJ, 324*, 1320–1323.
40. Okruhlicova, L., Tribulova, N., Misejkova, M., et al. (2002). Gap junction remodelling is involved in the susceptibility of diabetic rats to hypokalemia-induced ventricular fibrillation. *Acta Histochemica, 104*, 387–391.
41. Spodick, D. H. (2008). Hypokalemia. *American Journal of Geriatric Cardiology, 17*, 132.
42. Webster, A., Brady, W., & Morris, F. (2002). Recognising signs of danger: ECG changes resulting from an abnormal serum potassium concentration. *Emergency Medical Journal, 19*, 74–77.
43. Humphreys, M. (2007). Potassium disturbances and associated electrocardiogram changes. *Emergency Nurse, 15*, 28–34.
44. Knochel, J. P., & Schlein, E. M. (1972). On the mechanism of rhabdomyolysis in potassium depletion. *Journal of Clinical Investigations, 51*, 1750–1758.
45. Lane, R., & Phillips, M. (2003). Rhabdomyolysis. *BMJ, 327*, 115–116.
46. Ozgur, B., & Kursat, S. (2002). Hypokalemic rhabdomyolysis aggravated by diuretics complicating Conn's syndrome without acute renal failure. *Clinical Nephrology, 57*, 89–91.
47. Yasue, H., Itoh, T., Mizuno, Y., et al. (2007). Severe hypokalemia, rhabdomyolysis, muscle paralysis, and respiratory impairment in a hypertensive patient taking herbal medicines containing licorice. *Internal Medicine, 46*, 575–578.
48. Evans, K. J., & Greenberg, A. (2005). Hyperkalemia: A review. *Journal of Intensive Care Medicine, 20*, 272–290.
49. Desai, A. S., Swedberg, K., McMurray, J. J., et al. (2007). Incidence and predictors of hyperkalemia in patients with heart failure: An analysis of the CHARM Program. *Journal of the American College of Cardiology, 50*, 1959–1966.
50. Indermitte, J., Burkolter, S., Drewe, J., et al. (2007). Risk factors associated with a high velocity of the development of hyperkalaemia in hospitalised patients. *Drug Safety, 30*, 71–80.
51. Raebel, M. A., McClure, D. L., Simon, S. R., et al. (2007). Laboratory monitoring of potassium and creatinine in ambulatory patients receiving angiotensin converting enzyme inhibitors and angiotensin receptor blockers. *Pharmacoepidemiology and Drug Safety, 16*, 55–64.
52. Schaefer, T. J., & Wolford, R. W. (2005). Disorders of potassium. *Emergency Medicine Clinics of North America, 23*, 723–747.
53. Blaustein, D. A., Babu, K., Reddy, A., et al. (2002). Estimation of glomerular filtration rate to prevent life-threatening hyperkalemia due to combined therapy with spironolactone and angiotensin-converting

enzyme inhibition or angiotensin receptor blockade. *American Journal of Cardiology, 90*, 662–663.
54. Hauben, M., Reich, L., Gerrits, C. M., et al. (2007). Detection of spironolactone-associated hyperkalaemia following the Randomized Aldactone Evaluation Study (RALES). *Drug Safety, 30*, 1143–1149.
55. Raebel, M. A., McClure, D. L., Chan, K. A., et al. (2007). Laboratory evaluation of potassium and creatinine among ambulatory patients prescribed spironolactone: Are we monitoring for hyperkalemia? *The Annals of Pharmacotheraphy, 41*, 193–200.
56. Takaichi, K., Takemoto, F., Ubara, Y., et al. (2007). Analysis of factors causing hyperkalemia. *Internal Medicine, 46*, 823–829.
57. Lucia, A., Hoyos, J., Santalla, A., et al. (2002). Lactic acidosis, potassium, and the heart rate deflection point in professional road cyclists. *British Journal of Sports Medicine, 36*, 113–117.
58. Day, J. R., Chaudhry, A. N., Hunt, I., et al. (2002). Heparin-induced hyperkalemia after cardiac surgery. *Annals of Thoracic Surgery, 74*, 1698–1700.
59. Keidan, I., Amir, G., Mandel, M., et al. The metabolic effects of fresh versus old stored blood in the priming of cardiopulmonary bypass solution for pediatric patients. *Journal of Thoracic and Cardiovascular Surgery, 127*, 949–952.
60. Smith, H. M., Farrow, S. J., Ackerman, J. D., et al. (2008). Cardiac arrests associated with hyperkalemia during red blood cell transfusion: A case series. *Anesthesia and Analgesia, 106*, 1062–1069.
61. Eurenius, S., & Smith, R. M. (1973). The effect of warming on the serum potassium content of stored blood. *Anesthesiology, 38*, 482–484.
62. Aboudara, M. C., Hurst, F. P., Abbott, K. C., et al. (2008). Hyperkalemia after packed red blood cell transfusion in trauma patients. *Journal of Trauma, 64*, S86–S91.
63. Li, H. Y., Wu, S., He, G. W., et al. (2002). Aprikalim reduces the Na+-Ca2+ exchange outward current enhanced by hyperkalemia in rat ventricular myocytes. *Annals of Thoracic Surgery, 73*, 1253–1259.
64. Mirandi, A., Williams, T., Holt, J., et al. (2008). Hyperkalemia secondary to a postobstructive uropathy manifesting as complete heart block in a hypertensive patient receiving multiple atrioventricular nodal blocking agents. *Angiology, 59*, 121–124.
65. Indik, J. H. (2005). A pointed clue. *American Journal of Medicine, 118*, 1221–1222.
66. Somers, M. P., Brady, W. J., Perron, A. D., et al. (2002). The prominant T wave: Electrocardiographic differential diagnosis. *American Journal of Emergency Medicine, 20*, 243–251.
67. Cook, L. K. (2005). An acute myocardial infarction? *American Journal of Critical Care, 14*, 313–315.
68. Sims, D. B., & Sperling, L. S. (2005). Images in cardiovascular medicine. ST-segment elevation resulting from hyperkalemia. *Circulation, 111*, e295–e296.
69. Tatli, E., Buyuklu, M., & Onal, B. (2008). Electrocardiographic abnormality: Hyperkalaemia mimicking isolated acute inferior myocardial infarction. *Journal of Cardiovascular Medicine (Hagerstown), 9*, 210.
70. Littmann, L., Monroe, M. H., Taylor, L., III, et al. (2007). The hyperkalemic Brugada sign. *Journal of Electrocardiology, 40*, 53–59.
71. Petrov, D., & Petrov, M. (2008). Widening of the QRS complex due to severe hyperkalemia as an acute complication of diabetic ketoacidosis. *Journal of Emergency Medicine, 34*, 459–461.
72. Scarabeo, V., Baccillieri, M. S., Di Marco, A., et al. (2007). Sine-wave pattern on the electrocardiogram and hyperkalaemia. *Journal of Cardiovascular Medicine (Hagerstown), 8*, 729–731.
73. Mitra, J. K., Pandia, M. P., Dash, H. H., et al. (2008). Moderate hyperkalaemia without ECG changes in the intraoperative period. *Acta Anaesthesiologica Scandinavica, 52*, 444–445.
74. Montague, B. T., Ouellette, J. R., & Buller, G. K. (2008). Retrospective review of the frequency of ECG changes in hyperkalemia. *Clinical Journal of the American Society of Nephrology, 3*, 324–330.
75. Aslam, S., Friedman, E. A., & Ifudu, O. (2002). Electrocardiography is unreliable in detecting potentially lethal hyperkalaemia in haemodialysis patients. *Nephrology Dialysis Transplantation, 17*, 1639–1642.
76. Mattu, A., Brady, W. J., & Perron, A. D. (2002). Electrocardiographic manifestations of hypothermia. *American Journal of Emergency Medicine, 20*, 314–326.
77. Khan, E., Voudouris, A., Shorofsky, S. R., et al. (2006). Inappropriate ICD discharges due to "triple counting" during normal sinus rhythm. *Journal of Interventional Cardiac Electrophysiology, 17*, 153–155.
78. Littmann, L., Brearley, W. D., Jr., Taylor, L., III, et al. (2007). Double counting of heart rate by interpretation software: A new electrocardiographic sign of severe hyperkalemia. *American Journal of Emergency Medicine, 25*, 584–586.
79. Oudit, G. Y., Cameron, D., & Harris, L. (2008). A case of appropriate inappropriate device therapy: Hyperkalemia-induced ventricular oversensing. *Canadian Journal of Cardiology, 24*, e16–e18.
80. Lin, C., Ke, X., Cvetanovic, I., et al. (2007). The effect of high extracellular potassium on IKr inhibition by anti-arrhythmic agents. *Cardiology, 108*, 18–27.
81. Terkildsen, J. R., Crampin, E. J., & Smith, N. P. (2007). The balance between inactivation and activation of the Na+-K+ pump underlies the triphasic accumulation of extracellular K+ during myocardial ischemia. *American Journal of Physiology – Heart and Circulatory Physiology, 293*, H3036–H3045.
82. Long, C., Li, W., Lin, D. M., et al. (2002). Effect of potassium-channel openers on the release of endothelium-derived hyperpolarizing factor in porcine coronary arteries stored in cold hyperkalemic solution. *Journal of Extracorporeal Technology, 34*, 125–129.
83. Krassoi, I., Pataricza, J., & Papp, J. G. (2003). Thiorphan enhances bradykinin-induced vascular relaxation in hypoxic/hyperkalaemic porcine coronary artery. *Journal of Pharmacy and Pharmacology, 55*, 339–345.
84. Carlstedt, F., & Lind, L. (2001). Hypocalcemic syndromes. *Critical Care Clinics, 17*, 139–153.
85. Sedlacek, M., Schoolwerth, A. C., & Remillard, B. D. (2006). Electrolyte disturbances in the intensive care unit. *Seminars in Dialysis, 19*, 496–501.
86. Zivin, J. R., Gooley, T., Zager, R. A., et al. (2001). Hypocalcemia: A pervasive metabolic abnormality in the critically ill. *American Journal of Kidney Disease, 37*, 689–698.
87. Al-Wahab, S., & Munyard, P. (2001). Functional atrioventricular block in a preterm infant. *Archives of Disease in Childhood Fetal & Neonatal Edition, 85*, F220–F221.
88. RuDusky, B. M. (2001). ECG abnormalities associated with hypocalcemia. *Chest, 119*, 668–669.
89. Keegan, M. T., Bondy, L. R., Blackshear, J. L., et al. (2002). Hypocalcemia-like electrocardiographic changes after administration of intravenous fosphenytoin. *Mayo Clinic Proceedings, 77*, 584–586.
90. Mishra, A., Wong, L., & Jonklaas, J. (2001). Prolonged, symptomatic hypocalcemia with pamidronate administration and subclinical hypoparathyroidism. *Endocrine, 14*, 159–164.
91. Lehmann, G., Deisenhofer, I., Ndrepepa, G., et al. (2000). ECG changes in a 25-year-old woman with hypocalcemia due to hypoparathyroidism. Hypocalcemia mimicking acute myocardial infarction. *Chest, 118*, 260–262.
92. Hurley, K., & Baggs, D. (2005). Hypocalcemic cardiac failure in the emergency department. *Journal of Emergency Medicine, 28*, 155–159.
93. Iwazu, Y., Muto, S., Ikeuchi, S., et al. (2006). Reversible hypocalcemic heart failure with T wave alternans and increased QTc dispersion in a patient with chronic renal failure after parathyroidectomy. *Clinical Nephrology, 65*, 65–70.
94. Kazmi, A. S., & Wall, B. M. (2007). Reversible congestive heart failure related to profound hypocalcemia secondary to hypoparathyroidism. *American Journal of the Medical Sciences, 333*, 226–229.
95. Tsironi, M., Korovesis, K., Farmakis, D., et al. (2006). Hypocalcemic heart failure in thalassemic patients. *International Journal of Hematology, 83*, 314–317.
96. Kovalik, S. G., Ledgerwood, A. M., Lucas, C. E., et al. (1981). The cardiac effect of altered calcium homeostasis after albumin resuscitation. *Journal of Trauma, 21*, 275–279.
97. Sato, K., Hasegawa, Y., Nakae, J., et al. (2002). Hydrochlorothiazide effectively reduces urinary calcium excretion in two Japanese patients with gain-of-function mutations of the calcium-sensing receptor gene. *Journal of Clinical Endocrinology & Metabolism, 87*, 3068–3073.
98. Wolf, M. E., Ranade, V., Molnar, J., et al. (2000). Hypercalcemia, arrhythmia, and mood stabilizers. *Journal of Clinical Psychopharmacology, 20*, 260–264.
99. Ashizawa, N., Arakawa, S., Koide, Y., et al. (2003). Hypercalcemia due to vitamin D intoxication with clinical features mimicking acute myocardial infarction. *Internal Medicine, 42*, 340–344.
100. Kamycheva, E., Jorde, R., Haug, E., et al. (2005). Effects of acute hypercalcaemia on blood pressure in subjects with and without parathyroid hormone secretion. *Acta Physiologica Scandinavica, 184*, 113–119.

101. Nilsson, I. L., Rastad, J., Johansson, K., et al. (2001). Endothelial vasodilatory function and blood pressure response to local and systemic hypercalcemia. *Surgery, 130*, 986–990.
102. Sim, M. T., & Stevenson, F. T. (2008). A fatal case of iatrogenic hypercalcemia after calcium channel blocker overdose. *Journal of Medical Toxicology, 4*, 25–29.
103. Cohen, N., Almoznino-Sarafian, D., Zaidenstein, R., et al. (2003). Serum magnesium aberrations in furosemide (frusemide) treated patients with congestive heart failure: Pathophysiological correlates and prognostic evaluation. *Heart, 89*, 411–416.
104. Gao, X., Peng, L., Adhikari, C. M., et al. (2007). Spironolactone reduced arrhythmia and maintained magnesium homeostasis in patients with congestive heart failure. *Journal of Cardiac Failure, 13*, 170–177.
105. Oladapo, O. O., & Falase, A. O. (2000). Congestive heart failure and ventricular arrhythmias in relation to serum magnesium. *African Journal of Medicine and Medical Sciences, 29*, 265–268.
106. Elming, H., Seibaek, M., Ottesen, M. M., et al. (2000). Serum-ionised magnesium in patients with acute myocardial infarction. Relation to cardiac arrhythmias, left ventricular function and mortality. *Magnesium Research, 13*, 285–292.
107. Klevay, L. M., & Milne, D. B. (2002). Low dietary magnesium increases supraventricular ectopy. *American Journal of Clinical Nutrition, 75*, 550–554.
108. Mela, T., Galvin, J. M., & McGovern, B. A. (2002). Magnesium deficiency during lactation as a precipitant of ventricular tachyarrhythmias. *Pacing and Clinical Electrophysiology, 25*, 231–233.
109. Onagawa, T., Ohkuchi, A., Ohki, R., et al. (2003). Woman with postpartum ventricular tachycardia and hypomagnesemia. *Journal of Obstetrics and Gynaecology Research, 29*, 92–95.
110. Wilkes, N. J., Mallett, S. V., Peachey, T., et al. (2002). Correction of ionized plasma magnesium during cardiopulmonary bypass reduces the risk of postoperative cardiac arrhythmia. *Anesthesia and Analgesia, 95*, 828–834.
111. Dorman, B. H., Sade, R. M., Burnette, J. S., et al. (2000). Magnesium supplementation in the prevention of arrhythmias in pediatric patients undergoing surgery for congenital heart defects. *American Heart Journal, 139*, 522–528.
112. Speziale, G., Ruvolo, G., Fattouch, K., et al. (2000). Arrhythmia prophylaxis after coronary artery bypass grafting: Regimens of magnesium sulfate administration. *Thoracic and Cardiovascular Surgery, 48*, 22–26.
113. Ceremuzynski, L., Gebalska, J., Wolk, R., et al. (2000). Hypomagnesemia in heart failure with ventricular arrhythmias. Beneficial effects of magnesium supplementation. *Journal of Internal Medicine, 247*, 78–86.
114. Kaye, P., & O'Sullivan, I. (2002). The role of magnesium in the emergency department. *Emergency Medicine Journal, 19*, 288–291.
115. Speich, M., Bousquet, B., & Nicolas, G. (1980). Concentrations of magnesium, calcium, potassium, and sodium in human heart muscle after acute myocardial infarction. *Clinical Chemistry, 26*, 1662–1665.
116. Kramer, J. H., Mak, I. T., Phillips, T. M., et al. (2003). Dietary magnesium intake influences circulating pro-inflammatory neuropeptide levels and loss of myocardial tolerance to postischemic stress. *Experimental Biology and Medicine (Maywood), 228*, 665–673.
117. Mubagwa, K., Gwanyanya, A., Zakharov, S., et al. (2007). Regulation of cation channels in cardiac and smooth muscle cells by intracellular magnesium. *Archives of Biochemistry and Biophysics, 458*, 73–89.
118. Sontia, B., & Touyz, R. M. (2007). Role of magnesium in hypertension. *Archives of Biochemistry and Biophysics, 458*, 33–39.
119. Touyz, R. M., Pu, Q., He, G., et al. (2002). Effects of low dietary magnesium intake on development of hypertension in stroke-prone spontaneously hypertensive rats: Role of reactive oxygen species. *Journal of Hypertension, 20*, 2221–2232.
120. Fox, C. H., Mahoney, M. C., Ramsoomair, D., et al. (2003). Magnesium deficiency in African-Americans: Does it contribute to increased cardiovascular risk factors? *Journal of the National Medical Association, 95*, 257–262.
121. Dickinson, H. O., Nicolson, D. J., Campbell, F., et al. (2006). Magnesium supplementation for the management of essential hypertension in adults. *Cochrane Database of Systematic Reviews*, 3: CD004640.
122. Fox, C., Ramsoomair, D., & Carter, C. (2001). Magnesium: Its proven and potential clinical significance. *Southern Medical Journal, 94*, 1195–1201.
123. Ortega-Carnicer, J., de la Nieta, D. S., & Alcazar, R. (2001). Acute myocardial injury caused presumably by coronary spasm after magnesium fluoro-silicate ingestion. *Journal of Electrocardiology, 34*, 335–337.
124. Bo, S., & Pisu, E. (2008). Role of dietary magnesium in cardiovascular disease prevention, insulin sensitivity and diabetes. *Current Opinion in Lipidology, 19*, 50–56.
125. Mazur, A., Maier, J. A., Rock, E., et al. (2007). Magnesium and the inflammatory response: Potential physiopathological implications. *Archives of Biochemistry and Biophysics, 458*, 48–56.
126. Schelling, J. R. (2000). Fatal hypermagnesemia. *Clinical Nephrology, 53*, 61–65.
127. Zaman, F., & Abreo, K. (2003). Severe hypermagnesemia as a result of laxative use in renal insufficiency. *Southern Medical Journal, 96*, 102–103.
128. Birrer, R. B., Shallash, A. J., & Totten, V. (2002). Hypermagnesemia-induced fatality following epsom salt gargles. *Journal of Emergency Medicine, 22*, 185–188.
129. Subramanian, R., & Khardori, R. (2000). Severe hypophosphatemia. Pathophysiologic implications, clinical presentations, and treatment. *Medicine (Baltimore), 79*, 1–8.
130. Miller, D. W., & Slovis, C. M. (2000). Hypophosphatemia in the emergency department therapeutics. *American Journal of Emergency Medicine, 18*, 457–461.
131. Shiber, J. R., & Mattu, A. (2002). Serum phosphate abnormalities in the emergency department. *Journal of Emergency Medicine, 23*, 395–400.
132. Claudius, I., Sachs, C., & Shamji, T. (2002). Hypophosphatemia-induced heart failure. *American Journal of Emergency Medicine, 20*, 369–370.
133. Korbonits, M., Blaine, D., Elia, M., et al. (2007). Metabolic and hormonal changes during the refeeding period of prolonged fasting. *European Journal of Endocrinology, 157*, 157–166.
134. Lin, K. K., Lee, J. J., & Chen, H. C. (2006). Severe refeeding hypophosphatemia in a CAPD patient: A case report. *Renal Failure, 28*, 515–517.
135. Guyton, A., & Hall, J. (2006). *Textbook of medical physiology*. Philadelphia: Elsevier Saunders.
136. Boron, W. F. (2006). Acid-base transport by the renal proximal tubule. *Journal of the American Society of Nephrology, 17*, 2368–2382.
137. Wang, W., Praetorius, J., Li, C., et al. (2007). Vacuolar H+-ATPase expression is increased in acid-secreting intercalated cells in kidneys of rats with hypercalcaemia-induced alkalosis. *Acta Physiologica (Oxford), 189*, 359–368.
138. Schoolwerth, A. C., Kaneko, T. M., Sedlacek, M., et al. (2006). Acid-base disturbances in the intensive care unit: Metabolic acidosis. *Seminars in Dialysis, 19*, 492–495.
139. Felver, L. (2010). Acid-base homeostasis and imbalances. In L. Copstead & J. Banasik (Eds.), *Pathophysiology* (4th ed.) (pp. 615–626). St. Louis: Elsevier.
140. de Seigneux, S., Malte, H., Dimke, H., et al. (2007). Renal compensation to chronic hypoxic hypercapnia: Downregulation of pendrin and adaptation of the proximal tubule. *American Journal of Physiology – Renal Physiology, 292*, F1256–F1266.
141. Kupriyanov, V. V., Xiang, B., Sun, J., et al. (2002). Effects of regional hypoxia and acidosis on Rb(+) uptake and energetics in isolated pig hearts: (87)Rb MRI and (31)P MR spectroscopic study. *Biochimica et Biophysica Acta, 1586*, 57–70.
142. Crampin, E. J., Smith, N. P., Langham, A. E., et al. (2006). Acidosis in models of cardiac ventricular myocytes. *Philosophical Transactions. Series A, Mathematical, Physical and Engineering Science, 364*, 1171–1186.
143. Mizukoshi, Y., Shibata, K., & Yoshida, M. (2001). Left ventricular contractility is reduced by hypercapnic acidosis and thoracolumbar epidural anesthesia in rabbits. *Canadian Journal of Anaesthesiology, 48*, 557–562.
144. Avidan, M. S., Ali, S. Z., Tymkew, H., et al. (2007). Mild hypercapnia after uncomplicated heart surgery is not associated with hemodynamic compromise. *Journal of Cardiothoracic and Vascular Anesthesia, 21*, 371–374.
145. Phillis, J. W., Song, D., & O'Regan, M. H. (2000). Mechanisms involved in coronary artery dilatation during respiratory acidosis in the isolated perfused rat heart. *Basic Research in Cardiology, 95*, 93–97.
146. Najarian, T., Marrache, A. M., Dumont, I., et al. (2000). Prolonged hypercapnia-evoked cerebral hyperemia via K(+) channel- and prostaglandin E(2)-dependent endothelial nitric oxide synthase induction. *Circulation Research, 87*, 1149–1156.
147. Mizuno, S., Demura, Y., Ameshima, S., et al. (2002). Alkalosis stimulates endothelial nitric oxide synthase in cultured human pulmonary arterial endothelial cells. *American Journal of Physiology – Lung Cellular and Molecular Physiology, 283*, L113–L119.
148. Kraut, J. A., & Madias, N. E. (2007). Serum anion gap: Its uses and limitations in clinical medicine. *Clinical Journal of the American Society of Nephrology, 2*, 162–174.

149. Chernecky, C. (2008). *Laboratory tests and diagnostic procedures*. St. Louis: Elsevier Saunders.
150. Emmett, M. (2006). Anion-gap interpretation: The old and the new. *Nature Clinical Practice Nephrology, 2*, 4–5.
151. Gunnerson, K. J., Saul, M., He, S., et al. (2006). Lactate versus non-lactate metabolic acidosis: A retrospective outcome evaluation of critically ill patients. *Critical Care, 10*, R22.
152. Dubin, A., Menises, M. M., Masevicius, F. D., et al. (2007). Comparison of three different methods of evaluation of metabolic acid-base disorders. *Critical Care Medicine, 35*, 1264–1270.
153. Gunnerson, K. J. (2005). Clinical review: The meaning of acid-base abnormalities in the intensive care unit – epidemiology. *Critical Care, 9*, 508–516.
154. Ch'en F. F., Villafuerte, F. C., Swietach, P., et al. (2008). S0859, an N-cyanosulphonamide inhibitor of sodium-bicarbonate cotransport in the heart. *British Journal of Pharmacology, 153*, 972–982.
155. Orchard, C. (2007). Downhill all the way: H(+) gradients within cardiac myocytes. *Biophysical Journal, 92*, 371–372.
156. Du, Z., Chaoqian, X., Shan, H., et al. (2007). Functional impairment of cardiac transient outward K^+ current as a result of abnormally altered cellular environment. *Clinical and Experimental Pharmacology & Physiology, 34*, 148–152.
157. Fichet, J., Genee, O., Pierre, B., et al. (2008). Fatal QT interval. *American Journal of Emergency Medicine, 26*, 739, e735–e736.
158. Hattori, K., Tsuchida, S., Tsukahara, H., et al. (2002). Augmentation of NO-mediated vasodilation in metabolic acidosis. *Life Sciences, 71*, 1439–1447.
159. Horiuchi, T., Dietrich, H. H., Hongo, K., et al. (2002). Role of endothelial nitric oxide and smooth muscle potassium channels in cerebral arteriolar dilation in response to acidosis. *Stroke, 33*, 844–849.
160. Kawano, T., Tanaka, K., Nazari, H., et al. (2007). The effects of extracellular pH on vasopressin inhibition of ATP-sensitive K^+ channels in vascular smooth muscle cells. *Anesthesia and Analgesia, 105*, 1714–1719.
161. Kitakaze, M., Node, K., Takashima, S., et al. (2001). Role of cellular acidosis in production of nitric oxide in canine ischemic myocardium. *Journal of Molecular and Cellular Cardiology, 33*, 1727–1737.
162. Hunjan, S., Mason, R. P., Mehta, V. D., et al. (1998). Simultaneous intracellular and extracellular pH measurement in the heart by 19F NMR of 6-fluoropyridoxol. *Magnetic Resonance in Medicine, 39*, 551–556.
163. Jundi, K., Barrington, K. J., Henderson, C., et al. (2000). The hemodynamic effects of prolonged respiratory alkalosis in anesthetized newborn piglets. *Intensive Care Medicine, 26*, 449–456.
164. Steinback, C. D., & Poulin, M. J. (2008). Cardiovascular and cerebrovascular responses to acute isocapnic and poikilocapnic hypoxia in humans. *Journal of Applied Physiology, 104*, 482–489.
165. Strauss, G. I. (2007). The effect of hyperventilation upon cerebral blood flow and metabolism in patients with fulminant hepatic failure. *Danish Medical Bulletin, 54*, 99–111.
166. Cornfield, D. N., Resnik, E. R., Herron, J. M., et al. (2002). Pulmonary vascular K+ channel expression and vasoreactivity in a model of congenital heart disease. *American Journal of Physiology – Lung Cellular and Molecular Physiology, 283*, L1210–L1219.
167. De Santo, N. G., Cirillo, M., Perna, A., et al. (2005). The kidney in heart failure. *Seminars in Nephrology, 25*, 404–407.
168. Laski, M. E., & Sabatini, S. (2006). Metabolic alkalosis, bedside and bench. *Seminars in Nephrology, 26*, 404–421.
169. Giovannini, I., Greco, F., Chiarla, C., et al. (2005). Exceptional nonfatal metabolic alkalosis (blood base excess +48 mEq/l). *Intensive Care Medicine, 31*, 166–167.
170. Edwards, S. L. (2008). Pathophysiology of acid base balance: The theory practice relationship. *Intensive and Critical Care Nursing, 24*, 28–38.
171. Woodrow, P. (2004). Arterial blood gas analysis. *Nursing Standard, 18*, 45–52.

CHAPTER 8

Sleep

Kathy P. Parker / Rebecca A. Gary / Sandra B. Dunbar

INTRODUCTION

Physiological changes that accompany normal sleep may have adverse effects on patients with cardiovascular disease, and because cardiac patients as a group also have a high prevalence of sleep abnormalities, attention to sleep in overall cardiovascular care has become increasingly important.[1,2] Cardiovascular nurses are well positioned to assess sleep patterns, identify poor sleep quality and quantity, intervene to prevent sleep loss, educate and counsel cardiovascular patients regarding sleep, and work with the interdisciplinary team to assure treatments for sleep and sleep-related problems. To assist nurses in helping patients with cardiovascular disease achieve adequate, restful, and restorative sleep, this chapter reviews normal sleep and sleepiness, changes in cardiopulmonary and other system functions during sleep, sleep problems commonly seen in patients with cardiovascular disease, and appropriate management.

NORMAL SLEEP

Sleep and Sleepiness

The human need for sleep has been recognized throughout the centuries, and few physiological phenomena have received as much attention from scholars, scientists, poets, and other literary figures. Before the twentieth century, sleep was thought to be a simple, passive phenomenon—a state often described as existing between waking and death.[3] Although much remains to be fully understood about the topic, the modern study of sleep has revealed some of its secrets. Sleep is now understood as an active process regulated by a multiplicity of behavioral, neuroendocrine, and central nervous system factors.[4,5] Insufficient and/or poor quality nocturnal sleep and daytime sleepiness adversely affect important clinical outcomes.[6–9] Numerous primary sleep disorders[10] have been recognized, and the field of sleep medicine is now a bona fide, empirically based subspecialty.[11]

The modern definition of sleep is "a reversible behavioral state of perceptual disengagement from and unresponsiveness to the environment."[4] Sleep is further defined according to behavioral and physiological criteria. Behavioral criteria include quiescence, closed eyes, decreased response to external stimuli, recumbent position, and reversible unconsciousness.[4] Physiological criteria are based on recordings from a polysomnogram that includes electroencephalography (EEG), electro-oculography (EOG), and electromyography (EMG)[12] (Figs. 8-1 and 8-2).

Daytime sleepiness refers to the tendency or propensity to fall asleep during the day. In normal individuals, sleepiness typically has a biphasic circadian rhythm,[13] with an increased sleep tendency in the mid-afternoon and, as is well known to nightshift workers, in the early morning hours[13,14] (Fig. 8-3). In fact, a continuum between being very alert and very sleepy (often referred to as *arousal state*) provides a background for all waking endeavors and is a far more important dimension of human function than commonly recognized. Many adults are chronically sleepy in the daytime because of insufficient or disrupted night-time sleep. The problem may initially go unnoticed when masked by stimulating factors such as movement, excitement, high motivation, or hunger. However, daytime sleepiness can be unmasked by situational factors such as boredom, a warm dark room, or a prolonged dull task.[13] Although poor nocturnal sleep can cause sleepiness, abnormal daytime sleep can also adversely affect nocturnal sleep. Thus, a complete assessment includes an examination of nocturnal and daytime sleep/wake patterns.

Stages of Sleep

Typical EEG patterns during wakefulness and sleep are shown in Figure 8-2. During relaxed wakefulness with the eyes open, the EEG consists predominantly of mixed frequency (cycle per second; Hz), low-voltage activity (low amplitude), or *desynchronized* brain-wave activity. Rapid eye movements (REMs) and blinks may occur, and muscle tone is usually at its highest level. With eyes closed, alpha waves are often noted (8 to 12 Hz).[15]

Sleep onset is heralded by a general slowing of the EEG activity and the emergence of delta waves (4 to 7 Hz) during more than 50% of the epoch. Sleep then progresses through several stages of nonrapid eye movement (NREM) and rapid eye movement (REM) sleep and cycles (an NREM/REM cycle) that are well described and form characteristic patterns in individuals and groups. NREM sleep is divided somewhat arbitrarily into three stages based on the EEG pattern. Sleep depth increases from stage 1 to stage 2 to slow wave sleep (SWS; deep sleep; previously defined as stages 3 and 4) based on the fact that the sleeper becomes more difficult to awaken.

In stages 1 and 2, or light sleep, the EEG consists of relatively low-amplitude waves with a predominant frequency of 2 to 7 Hz. High, narrow, vertex, sharp waves may appear late in stage 1. Stage 2 is identified by two sporadic waveforms that stand out from the background EEG: sleep spindles and K complexes. Sleep spindles are waxing–waning bursts of waves in the 12 to 14 Hz range.[4,12] They originate in the thalamus and are thought to reflect impulses that inhibit the relay of sensory information to the cerebral cortex.[16] K complexes consist of a sharp negative wave (upward deflection by EEG) followed by a slower positive wave (downward deflection).[17] They occur spontaneously and in response to mild external stimuli, such as sounds. SWS is differentiated by the percentage of slow (0.5 to 2 Hz), high-amplitude ($>$75 μV) EEG waves (referred to as *synchronized* brain-wave activity). They account for 20% to 50% of the waves in each

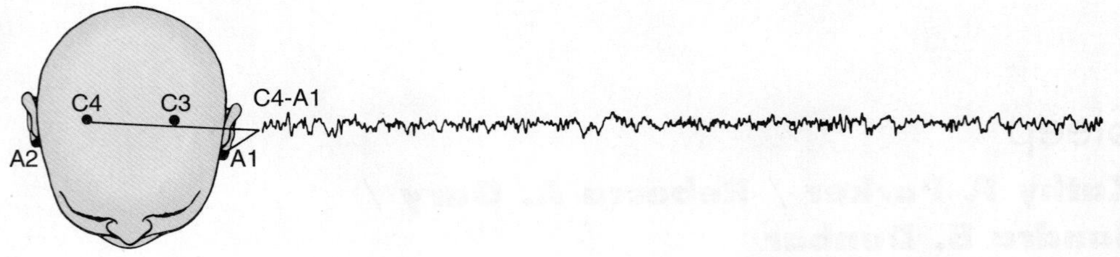

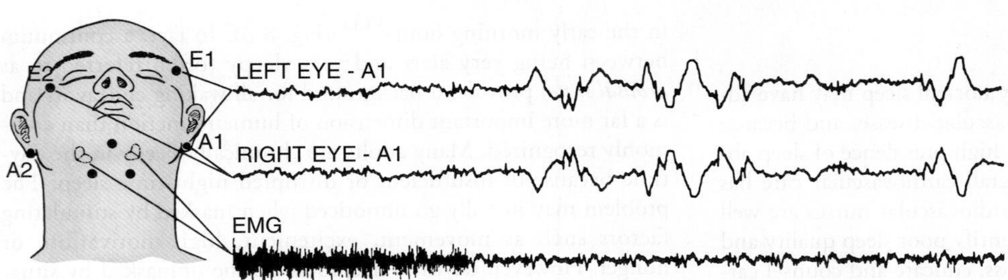

■ **Figure 8-1** Placement of electrodes for (*top*) electroencephalogram and (*bottom*) electro-oculogram and electromyogram in polygraphic sleep recordings. (From Rechtschaffen, A., & Kales, A. [Eds.]. [1968]. *A manual of standardized terminology, techniques and scoring system for sleep stages of human subjects* [p. 15]. Los Angeles, CA: Brain Information Service/Brain Research Institute, University of California, 1968.)

epoch. The eyes are relatively quiet during NREM sleep, except for slow rolling movements that usually occur at the beginning of stage 1 and disappear in stage 2. Muscle tone is moderately reduced from the waking level.[12,15]

There are two types of REM sleep. Similar to waking, *tonic REM sleep* is characterized by desynchronized brain activity—a mixed frequency, relatively low-amplitude EEG. However, in REM sleep there is also a complete loss of postural muscle tone caused by hyperpolarization of brainstem and spinal motorneurons.[18] The sleeper has an active brain in a paralyzed body, with only the diaphragm and extraocular muscles retaining substantial tone. Some suggest that the purpose of this physiological phenomenon is to prevent the enactment of dreams. REM behavior disorder, in which there is loss of this normally occurring paralysis,

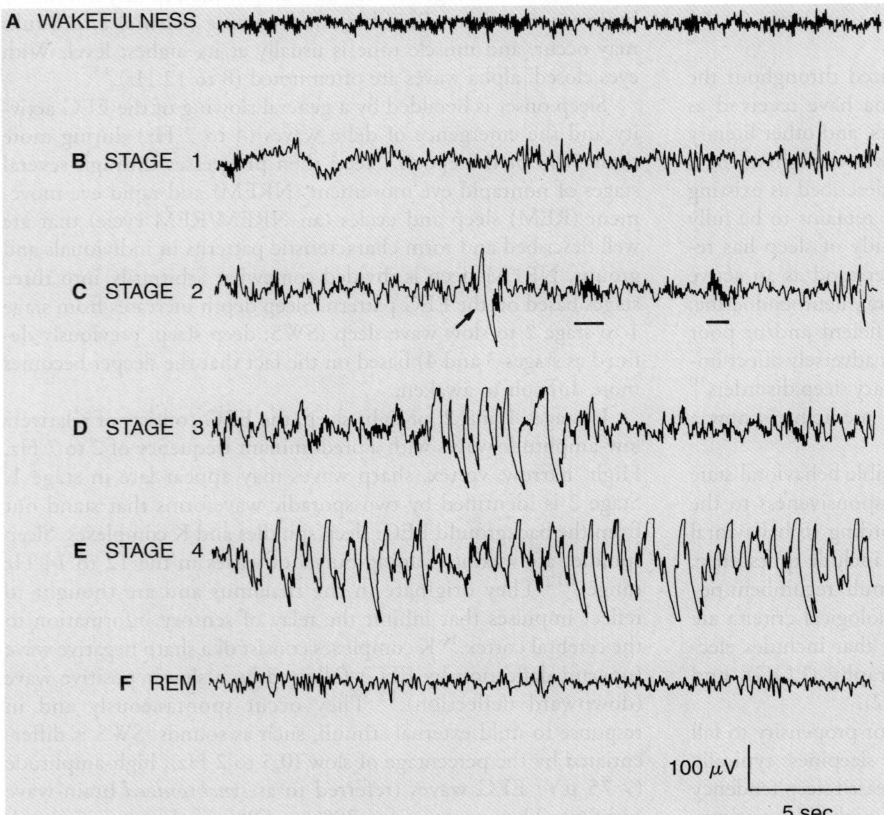

■ **Figure 8-2** Electroencephalogram patterns in wakefulness and sleep in a young adult. **(A)** Rhythmic α-wave activity at 8 to 10 Hz in relaxed wakefulness with the eyes closed. **(B)** Mixed-frequency, relatively low-amplitude waves in nonrapid-eye-movement (REM) stage 1, with a vertex sharp wave toward the end of the tracing. **(C)** K complex (*arrow*) and sleep spindles (*underscored*) begin in stage 2. **(D, E)** Progressively greater percentages of slow, high-amplitude waves in stages 3 and 4. **(F)** Mixed-frequency, relatively low-amplitude waves in rapid-eye-movement sleep, similar to the pattern in stage 1. (From Dement, W., Richardson, G., Prinz, P. et al. [1985]. Changes of sleep and wakefulness with age. In C. E. Finch, & E. L. Schneider [Eds.], *Handbook of the biology of aging,* [2nd ed., p. 694]. New York: Van Nostrand Reinhold.)

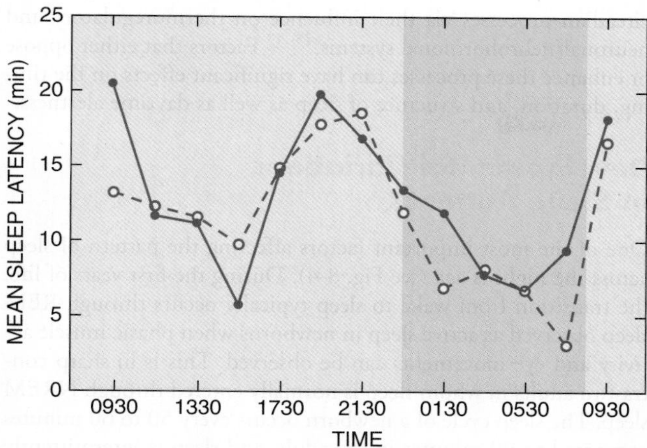

■ **Figure 8-3** Mean sleep latency in minutes in young adults (*open circles*) and old adults (*solid circles*) at different times of day. The shaded area represents the night-time sleep period. A biphasic rhythm exists with maximal sleepiness in the mid-afternoon and early morning, as indicated by shorter latencies. (From Richardson, G. S., Carskadon, M. A., Orav, E. F., et al. [1982]. Circadian variation of sleep tendency in elderly and young adult subjects. *Sleep, 5*[Suppl. 2], S87.)

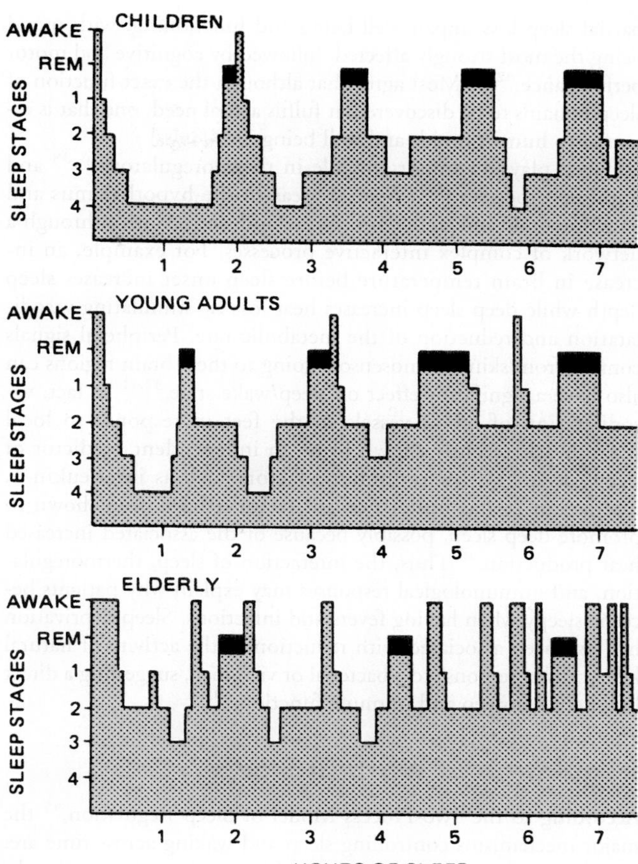

■ **Figure 8-4** Normal sleep cycles in children, young adults, and the elderly. Rapid-eye-movement (REM) sleep (*darkened area*) occurs cyclically throughout the night at intervals of approximately 90 minutes in all age groups and shows little variation in the different age groups, whereas stage 4 non-REM (NREM) sleep decreases with age. In addition, the elderly have frequent awakenings and a marked increase in total wake time. (From Kales, A., & Kales, J. D. [1974]. Sleep disorder. *New England Journal of Medicine, 290*, 488.)

is typified by abnormal movements, behaviors, and dream enactment during REM sleep. *Phasic REM sleep* occurs intermittently and is characterized by bursts of REMs (for which the stage is named), muscle twitches in the face and distal extremities (potent motor excitation briefly overrides the paralysis), and fluctuations in blood pressure, heart rate, and breathing.[18]

Approximately 80% of people awakened from REM sleep and 40% awakened from NREM sleep report having dreams. In NREM sleep, the mental activity tends to have a dull, sketchy quality without much basis in reality. In contrast, dreams recalled from REM sleep are usually vivid, well-formed, story-like narratives. Dreams include more visual imagery and emotional tone as the night progresses in relation to longer REM periods and greater intensity of phasic events.[4] Penile and clitoral erections also often occur during REM sleep.

Sleep Cycles

Most people have their major sleep period at night, organized in a rhythmic sequence of sleep stages (Fig. 8-4). After a short period of relaxed wakefulness, a young adult enters stage 1 sleep, followed by a descent into stage 2 for 10 to 25 minutes and approximately 20 to 40 minutes of SWS. The sleeper then goes through stage 2 and has a brief REM period approximately 90 minutes after sleep onset (the period from sleep onset to the first REM period is referred to as REM latency). The cycle begins again and repeats another four to six times during the night. Slow-wave sleep occupies less of the second cycle and may then disappear, whereas REM periods lengthen across the night. Therefore, most SWS occurs in the first third of the night, and most REM sleep occurs in the last third. If an awakening occurs, the sleep cycle typically starts again with stage 1 sleep. Frequent disruptions of sleep prevent the normal progression into SWS and REM sleep and increase stages 1 and 2 sleep.[4,15]

Adults typically change their body position 40 to 50 times during a normal sleep period; the characteristics and number of movements that occur are relatively stable personal traits.[19–21] Major body shifts often occur at changes from SWS to lighter NREM stages or from REM to NREM sleep. A sudden muscle contraction involving all or part of the body (hypnic jerk, hypnic myoclonus, or sleep start) often accompanied by intense visual imagery occasionally occurs at sleep onset and is normal; however, the frequency of the events may increase with stress or irregular sleep schedules.[4,22]

The Function of Sleep

The function of sleep remains a topic surrounded by controversy. Some have postulated that it is important for mental and physical restoration[23,24] and energy conservation.[25,26] Others propose that the primary function of sleep is the maintenance of synaptic and neuronal network function, information processing, and synaptic plasticity.[27–31] Sleep deprivation studies have shown that total and partial sleep loss impair well being and functioning, with mood being the most strongly affected, followed by cognitive and motor performance.[32–34] Most agree that although the exact function of sleep remains to be discovered, it fulfils a vital need, one that is essential to human health and well being.[35]

Sleep plays an important role in thermoregulatory[36–38] and immune processes.[39,40] Special areas in the hypothalamus and basal forebrain integrate temperature and sleep control through a network of complex interactive processes. For example, an increase in brain temperature before sleep onset increases sleep depth while deep sleep increases heat loss by stimulating vasodilatation and reduction of the metabolic rate. Peripheral signals coming from skin thermosensors going to these brain regions can also have a significant effect on sleep/wake state.[37,41] In fact, vasodilatation of blood vessels in the feet in response to local warmth was recently shown to be an independent predictor of sleep onset.[42,43] Many immune factors such as interleukin-1, interleukin-2, and tumor necrosis factor-α have been shown to promote deep sleep, possibly because of the associated increased heat production.[40] Thus, the interaction of sleep, thermoregulation, and immunological responses may explain why patients become sleepy when having fevers and infections. Sleep deprivation has also been associated with reduction in the activity of natural killer cells in response to a bacterial or viral load, suggesting a direct link between sleep and immune function.[39,44]

Regulation of Normal Sleep

According to the Two-Process Model of Sleep Regulation,[45] the major mechanisms controlling sleep and waking across time are: (a) a homeostatic process determined by previous sleep and waking; and (b) a circadian process that designates periods of high and low sleep propensity. The homeostatic process reflects the physiological need for sleep, which builds across the day and dissipates throughout the night (Fig. 8-5).[10] A key indicator of this process is EEG slow wave activity, which is high during the beginning of a sleep episode but decreases as the night progresses. The circadian process, a sinusoidal rhythm of approximately 24 hours, is controlled by a biologic oscillator (suprachiasmatic nucleus). This process regulated sleep propensity and its effects a least in the early morning hours. The rhythm of core body temperature is a key indicator of the circadian process. The timing and duration of sleep are determined by the combined action of homeostatic and circadian processes via their influence on thermoregulatory and neuronal/neurohormonal systems.[45–47] Factors that either oppose or enhance these processes can have significant effects on the timing, duration, and structure of sleep as well as daytime alertness.

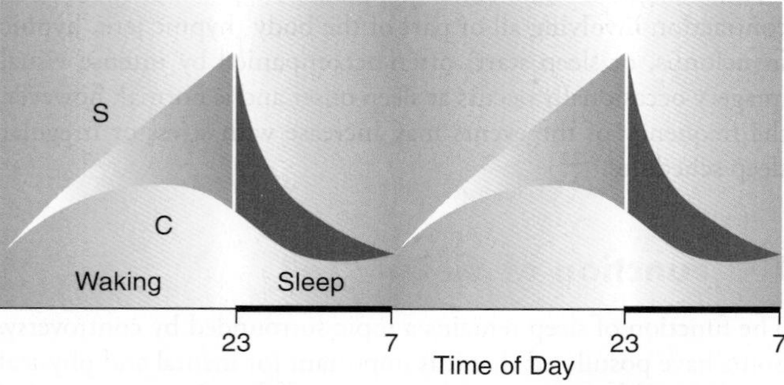

■ **Figure 8-5** The two-process model of sleep regulation. Two primary processes regulate sleep: a homeostatic process determined by prior sleep and waking, and a circadian process that designates periods of high and low sleep propensity.

Developmental Variations in Sleep Patterns

One of the most important factors affecting the pattern of sleep across the night is age (see Fig. 8-4). During the first years of life, the transition from wake to sleep typically occurs through REM sleep observed as active sleep in newborns when phasic muscle activity and eye movements can be observed. This is in sharp contrast to adults in whom sleep is normally entered through NREM sleep. The sleep cycle of a newborn occurs every 50 to 60 minutes compared to 90 minutes in the adult, and sleep is intermittently dispersed across both the day and night. Gradually, over a period of 2 to 6 months, infants develop a consolidated nocturnal sleep period once appropriate brain structures and process have developed.

SWS is at its peak in young children and is much deeper than that of adults. For example, it is not uncommon for a child's clothes to be changed and to be put to bed without awakening. However, a subsequent decrease in SWS occurs across adolescence, a trend that continues to occur with age. REM sleep, as a percentage of total sleep time, is relatively well maintained across the entire life span.[4]

With increasing age, particularly in men, sleep becomes lighter and more fragmented (see Fig. 8-4). In contrast to young adults, older people usually spend more time in bed but less time asleep (reduced sleep efficiency) and are more easily awakened from sleep. The time needed to fall asleep (sleep latency) shows little change with aging, but more night-time awakenings, brief arousals, and stage changes occur.[48] There is a striking reduction in SWS and an increase in stage 1 sleep, with little change in the percentages of stage 2 and REM sleep.[4] Bedtime and wake-up time come earlier (circadian phase advance), daytime sleep tendency may be increased, daytime napping is more common, and tolerance for changes in the sleep–wake schedule is reduced. Sleep apnea (discussed later) and periodic leg movements (involuntary repetitive jerks) are more common in older adults and can contribute to sleep disruption.[49–54] Other factors may include poor sleep habits, a reduced activity level, psychological concerns, physical illness, and medications.[48] Not surprisingly, older people often are dissatisfied with their sleep, complain of taking longer to fall asleep, and have more frequent night-time awakenings—all of which result in an increased using of sleeping medications.[55,56] Insomnia has been associated with increased mortality in the elderly.[57] However, it now appears that sleep duration, whether it be excessively short or long, may not be a mortality risk factor in this population but rather a function of the measurement of sleep close to the time of death and the number of concurrent medical conditions.[58]

■ SLEEP PHYSIOLOGY

The physiological basis of nursing care has rested almost entirely on studies of responses during wakefulness. However, NREM sleep, REM sleep, and wakefulness are very different physiological states associated with state-dependent changes in the function of most body systems.[5] In healthy individuals, these changes are well tolerated; but in patients with cardiovascular disease, the sleep state may make them vulnerable to serious, sometimes fatal, complications.[59]

Cardiovascular Function in Sleep

Cardiovascular control during sleep is primarily determined by variation in autonomic nervous system activity, which causes changes in blood pressure and heart rate, the major determinants of myocardial O_2 demand.[59,60] Increased parasympathetic tone and, to a lesser extent, decreased sympathetic tone, lead to a reduction in heart rate and cardiac output in NREM sleep. Vasodilatation causes a reduction in systemic vascular resistance and a 5% to 15% decrease in blood pressure which can impair blood flow through stenotic coronary blood vessels and trigger myocardial ischemia or infarction.[59] In contrast, pulmonary artery pressure increases slightly.[61,62] Baroreceptor gain is heightened and contributes to the reduction and stability of blood pressure. Brief surges in blood pressure and heart rate occur with K complexes, arousals, and large body movements.[62–64] An age-related decrease in this response has been demonstrated in middle-aged subjects in comparison to younger subjects, possibly reflecting the decline in parasympathetic function that occurs with increasing age.[65] Sharp increases in heart rate and blood pressure occur with morning awakening and beginning the day's activities[66,67] as well as after other periods of sleep, such as afternoon naps.[66]

REM sleep brings an increase in cardiovascular demands. Although blood pressure and heart rate have average levels near those observed in light NREM sleep or quiet wakefulness, their variability increases markedly during phasic REM sleep, with wide erratic fluctuations.[59,68] These changes are related to bursts of increased sympathetic activity and to reduced vagal input to the heart.[59,69] Cardiac efferent vagal tone and baroreceptor regulation are generally suppressed during REM sleep.[59,68]

Respiratory Function in Sleep

Sleep alters breathing patterns, ventilation, and arterial blood gas values. Periodic breathing, a cyclic waxing and waning of tidal volume, sometimes with brief apnea, is common at sleep onset in association with fluctuations between wakefulness and light sleep. Breathing is remarkably regular; however, in stable stage 2 and SWS. The pattern becomes faster and more erratic during phasic REM sleep.[70]

Minute ventilation falls, mainly because of reduced tidal volume, with an average decrease of approximately 0.4 to 1.5 L/min compared with quiet wakefulness.[70] This hypoventilation leads to small changes in arterial blood gases, including a mild hypercapnia (increases of 3 to 7 mm/Hg in carbon dioxide tension), decreases of 0.01 to 0.06 units in pH, and a mild hypoxemia (decreases of 35 to 9.4 mm Hg in Pa_{O2} and 2% or less in Sa_{O2}).[70,71] Data regarding REM sleep are somewhat contradictory but suggest that minute ventilation, tidal volume, and respiratory frequency are similar to those in NREM sleep, with similar or somewhat greater changes in blood gas values.[70,71] Other factors that contribute to hypoventilation in NREM sleep include reduced central drive to breathe caused by loss of the wakefulness stimulus and increased upper airway resistance to airflow due to reduced pharyngeal muscle tone.[70,71] Tone in the intercostal muscles and diaphragm; however, is maintained. In REM sleep, tone is lost in both the intercostal and upper airway muscles, reducing the rib cage contribution to breathing and increasing upper airway resistance; however, the diaphragm is relatively spared from REM-related paralysis. Phasic REM sleep also includes dysrhythmic changes in the stimulation of brainstem respiratory neurons, resulting in an erratic breathing pattern.[70,71]

The arterial blood gas changes stimulate an adaptive increase in ventilation, although the response is less effective in sleep than in wakefulness. In men, the ventilatory responses to both hypercapnia and hypoxemia decrease by approximately half from wakefulness to NREM sleep, with a further reduction in REM sleep. Women respond similarly to hypercapnia but somewhat differently to hypoxemia. Women have a lower ventilatory response than men when awake and little change in NREM sleep, but a similar fall in REM sleep.[72,73]

Arousal from sleep is a second adaptive response to blood gas changes because the change stimulates ventilation and permits voluntary action to cope with the situation, such as moving a pillow that interferes with breathing. Hypercapnia is a relatively effective arousal stimulus, awakening most healthy subjects before carbon dioxide tension rises 15 mm/Hg; concurrent hypoxemia enhances the response. Hypoxemia alone; however, is a poor arousal stimulus; study subjects often fail to awaken despite an Sa_{O2} as low as 70%.[70]

Adaptive responses that protect the airway are less effective during sleep. Respiratory secretions are cleared less readily because of diminished mucociliary clearance,[74] and the tendency to aspirate increases.[75] In addition, sleep suppresses the cough reflex to irritating substances in the airways in both REM and NREM sleep.[71]

Thermoregulation in Sleep

Body temperature is regulated at a lower set point in NREM sleep than in wakefulness. In combination with reduced motor activity, this results in a decrease in temperature at sleep onset.[36,47] The normal temperature-regulating mechanisms are markedly inhibited during REM sleep; during this stage of sleep, body temperature is influenced more by the environment than the hypothalamus. Body temperature also has an independent circadian rhythm that typically peaks in the late afternoon and reaches a minimum in the early morning hours of sleep.[47]

Sleep length depends on the phase of the circadian temperature rhythm at bedtime because the rising phase triggers awakening from sleep. A sleep period that begins when body temperature is low—for example, going to bed at 3:00 AM—is relatively short because temperature soon rises. In contrast, a sleep period that begins when temperature is high is relatively long because temperature drops and a subsequent rise in temperature does not occur for some time.[47] The body temperature rhythm shifts a little earlier (phase advance) with aging, which may partly explain why many older people have an earlier wake-up time than younger adults.[47,48]

Cerebral Blood Flow in Sleep

Brain blood flow decreases in sleep in comparison to waking.[76] Brain imaging studies reveal that there is a small to moderate decrease in brain blood flow in NREM sleep in the brainstem and cortex.[77,78] In contrast, there is an marked increase in brain blood flow in REM sleep in the brain stem and limbic decrease, but a decrease in the frontal cortex.[79] Poor performance on tasks after sleep deprivation is associated with reduced metabolic activity in the frontal lobes, thalamus, and midbrain, which may be associated with the state of reduced alertness.[80,81]

Renal Function in Sleep

Urine flow is reduced and more concentrated during sleep with a decreased excretion of sodium, chloride, potassium, and calcium. The mechanisms involved in these changes are complex and include changes in renal blood flow, glomerular filtration, hormone secretion (vasopressin, aldosterone, prolactin, parathormone), and sympathetic neural stimulation.[82] Because night-time potassium excretion is reduced, potassium infusions given at night may lead to higher serum levels than daytime infusions.[83]

From infancy to old age, males have penile erections (nocturnal penile tumescence) during REM sleep. Total tumescence time is greatest just before and during puberty and then may gradually decline. Sleep-related erectile activity can be monitored to aid in differentiating physical and psychological components of impotence.[84]

Endocrine Function in Sleep

Endocrine hormone secretion is influenced by sleep. For example, growth hormone secretion is highly sleep-dependent and most secretion occurs during the first few hours after sleep onset during SWS. If sleep is advanced or delayed, growth hormone secretion shifts accordingly. In contrast, thyroid hormone and cortisol secretions have independent circadian rhythms. Thyroid hormone secretion increases in the late evening; cortisol concentration increases in the latter half of the night and peaks toward the end of the normal sleep period or soon after awakening.[85]

The hormone melatonin, secreted by the pineal gland, induces sleepiness and has a marked circadian rhythm that is closely linked to the light–dark cycle, temperature, and cortisol rhythms. A late evening surge in melatonin begins at darkness, approximately 2 hours before bedtime, and is considered a marker of the body's circadian timing system. Secretion peaks at approximately 3:00 AM but is suppressed by daylight to levels that are barely detectable. Bright light exposure suppresses melatonin secretion and can be used to help reset a person's circadian clock.[86]

CLINICAL EVALUATION, DIAGNOSIS, AND APPROACHES

There are three primary ways in which sleep and sleepiness are measured: subjectively, behaviorally, and objectively. In health, these measures are often, but not always, congruent; however, they become much less well associated when impaired sleep or other health problems are present.[87–92]

Subjective Measurement

Subjective measures of sleep can be particularly useful for screening, triage, and assessing the effects of treatment.[15,93] Types of information typically obtained include an individual's assessment of sleep latency (time from lights out to the onset of sleep), number of awakenings, depth and length of sleep, refreshing quality of sleep, satisfaction with sleep, and soundness of sleep. This information can be collected through the use of sleep questionnaires, that is, the Pittsburgh Sleep Quality Index,[94–96] St. Mary's Hospital Sleep Questionnaire,[97] Sleep Disorders Questionnaire,[98] sleep diaries, visual analogue scales, Leed's Sleep Evaluation Questionnaire,[99] and interviews.[93,100,101]

Daytime sleepiness can also be measured using subjective measures such as the Epworth Sleepiness Scale, an instrument that has been widely used in the clinical and research settings.[102–105] Test scores greater than 10 or 11 have been reported in patients with sleep disorders that cause excessive daytime sleepiness (EDS); the average score for control subjects is 6 (possible range of scores is 0 to 24; higher score = greater subjective sleepiness).[102,106] Although the results of studies examining the relationship between Epworth Sleepiness Scale scores and sleep apnea severity, for example, have been equivocal,[11,107,108] improvement in scores after treatment of apnea with continuous positive airway pressure (CPAP) has been described.[109,110] Thus, the instrument may be sensitive to and particularly helpful in evaluating clinical responses to interventions designed to improve sleep (Display 8-1).

Behavioral Assessment

Assessment of behaviors related to sleep and sleepiness are an important part of a thorough assessment. In fact, observation is considered the "gold standard" for sleep monitoring in infants.[15] Typically, individuals who are sleepy or sleep-deprived manifest characteristic behaviors including yawning, eye rubbing, head nodding, ptosis of the eyelids, irritability, and slowed movement. Other observable waking behaviors that may be noted include automatic behavior, unintentional sleep episodes, cataplexy (a stereotypical feature of narcolepsy in which there is a sudden decrement in muscle tone and loss of deep tendon reflexes leading to muscle weakness, paralysis, and/or postural collapse), and sleep drunkenness.[10] Although lying quietly in a horizontal position is typical, movements and position changes can occur and are a normal part of sleep behavior. Abnormal sleep-related behaviors include bizarre postures, restless sleep, jerking of the extremities, seizure activity, and dream enactment. Video recordings of these behaviors during polysomnography (PSG) are often made to assist in the assessment and diagnosis of sleep problems. Observations of patients' nocturnal behaviors by health care providers, bed partners, or parents often play an important role in the diagnosis and treatment of sleep disorders.

Objective Measurement

The structure and timing of sleep stages and cycles can be studied objectively using PSG, a procedure involving the simultaneous recording of the EEG, the EMG, and the EOG. At the usual recording speed of 1 cm/s, a standard 30-cm page represents a 30-second period, or *epoch*. Each epoch is assigned a single sleep-stage score based primarily on changes in EEG frequency (in cycles/s, or hertz [Hz]) and amplitude (in microvolts [μV]), with confirmation by the EOG and EMG patterns.[12] In addition to sleep-staging signals, PSG often includes the measurement of other physiological parameters, such as respiratory movements of the chest and abdomen, airflow at the nose and mouth, Sa_{O2}, electrocardiogram and leg movements (anterior tibialis EMG).

Daytime sleepiness (daytime sleep propensity or tendency) can be quantified using the Multiple Sleep Latency Test (MSLT).[105] Beginning 1.5 to 2 hours at the end of a nocturnal polysomnographic recording, four to five 20-minute nap opportunities are typically given in 2-hour intervals. The sleep latency of any given nap

DISPLAY 8-1 Epworth Sleepiness Scale

Name: ______________________________

Today's date: ______________ Your age: ______________

Your sex (male = M; female = F): ______________

How likely are you to doze off or fall asleep in the following situations, in contrast to feeling just tired? This refers to your usual way of life in recent times. Even if you have not done some of these things recently, try to work out how they would have affected you. Use the following scale to choose the *most appropriate number* for each situation:

0 = would *never* doze
1 = *slight* chance of dozing
2 = *moderate* chance of dozing
3 = *high* chance of dozing

Situation	Chance of Dozing
Sitting and reading	______
Watching TV	______
Sitting, inactive in a public place (theater or meeting)	______
As a passenger in a car for an hour without a break	______
Lying down to rest in the afternoon when circumstances permit	______
Sitting and talking to someone	______
Sitting quietly after a lunch without alcohol	______
In a care, while stopped for a few minutes in traffic	______

From Johns, M. W. (1991). A new method for measuring daytime sleepiness: The Epworth sleepiness scale. *Sleep,* 14(6), 540–545.

opportunity is defined as the time from lights out to the first 30-second epoch scored as sleep. The average sleep latency across all naps is calculated and expressed as the mean sleep latency. Possible mean sleep latency scores on the MSLT range from 0 to 20 minutes, with a low score indicating greater sleepiness. An MSLT score less than 5 minutes indicates pathological sleepiness and is a level at which patients often experience marked impairment of social and/or occupational functioning and at which they are generally advised against driving or operating heavy equipment.[15,111] Scores between 5 and 10 minutes are considered to be in the "diagnostic gray zone," whereas scores greater than 10 are considered normal.

Actigraphy is an alternative method sometimes used to objectively measure sleep/wake patterns by monitoring periods of activity and rest.[112,113] Using a battery-operated wristwatch-size microprocessor that senses movement with a piezoelectric beam, continuous motion data can be obtained for long periods. Computer algorithms allow for analysis of activity and non-activity, as well as scoring of sleep and wakefulness.[114] While actigraphy cannot determine sleep stages, information on total sleep time, percent of time spent awake, number of awakenings, time between awakenings, and sleep onset latency can be obtained. Actigraphy data correlate well with PSG data, particularly when sleep is normal.[112,115] Correlations decrease when sleep is disturbed or activity is limited.[114,116,117]

Environmental Assessment

The environment can play an important role in the quantity and quality of sleep obtained. A thermoneutral environment (neither too hot nor too cold) is essential for normal thermoregulatory changes needed to optimize sleep.[41] Excessive noise has also been shown to cause poor subjective and objective sleep measures.[118–121] Too much light exposure alters melatonin production.[86] Nursing interventions themselves can significantly disturb sleep. Comfortable beds/mattresses, pillows, and nightwear facilitate sleep.[122]

IMPAIRED SLEEP, SLEEP DISORDERS, AND EXCESSIVE DAYTIME SLEEPINESS

Impaired sleep can be generally categorized as either sleep deprivation (resulting from inadequate sleep) or sleep disruption (resulting from fragmented sleep during the night)[123] (Fig. 8-6). Sleep deprivation frequently occurs in association with particular lifestyles or stages of development. Sleep disruption is often seen in health-related conditions. Both sleep deprivation and sleep disruption result in sleep loss.[123] Important information has been obtained through sleep deprivation studies that have shown that sleep loss has numerous adverse effects including fatigue, anxiety, increase illness, increased sensitivity to pain, decreased immune response, restlessness, disorientation, decreased alertness/attention during the day, and decreased sense of well being.[124–130] The results of several studies suggest that the duration of self-reported sleep time increases mortality, with those sleeping longer than 9 hours and less than 5 hours per night, had an increased risk of

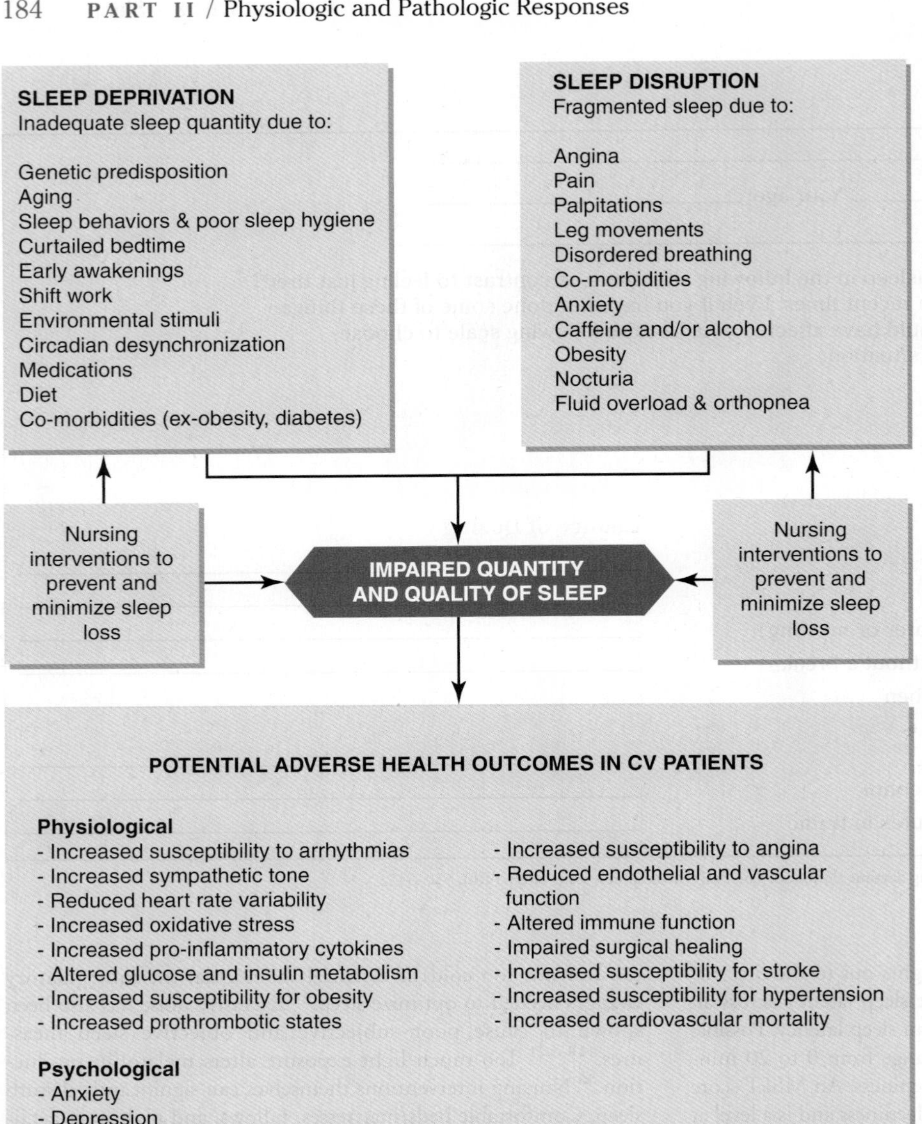

SLEEP DEPRIVATION
Inadequate sleep quantity due to:
Genetic predisposition
Aging
Sleep behaviors & poor sleep hygiene
Curtailed bedtime
Early awakenings
Shift work
Environmental stimuli
Circadian desynchronization
Medications
Diet
Co-morbidities (ex-obesity, diabetes)
SLEEP DISRUPTION
Fragmented sleep due to:
Angina
Pain
Palpitations
Leg movements
Disordered breathing
Co-morbidities
Anxiety
Caffeine and/or alcohol
Obesity
Nocturia
Fluid overload & orthopnea
Nursing interventions to prevent and minimize sleep loss
IMPAIRED QUANTITY AND QUALITY OF SLEEP
Nursing interventions to prevent and minimize sleep loss
POTENTIAL ADVERSE HEALTH OUTCOMES IN CV PATIENTS
Physiological
- Increased susceptibility to arrhythmias
- Increased sympathetic tone
- Reduced heart rate variability
- Increased oxidative stress
- Increased pro-inflammatory cytokines
- Altered glucose and insulin metabolism
- Increased susceptibility for obesity
- Increased prothrombotic states
- Increased susceptibility to angina
- Reduced endothelial and vascular function
- Altered immune function
- Impaired surgical healing
- Increased susceptibility for stroke
- Increased susceptibility for hypertension
- Increased cardiovascular mortality
Psychological
- Anxiety
- Depression
- Mood disturbances
Behavioral/Cognitive
- Altered problem-solving
- Excessive daytime sleepiness
- Fatigue
- Adherence difficulties
- Impaired short-term memory
Social
- Impaired family & social interactions
- Increased susceptibility for accidents
- Impaired work performance
- Increased health care utilization

■ **Figure 8-6** Causes and consequences of impaired sleep and targets of intervention in cardiovascular patients.

mortality.[131–135] However, the extent to which the duration of self-reported sleep is confounded by a number of demographic, behavioral, and psychological factors is unknown and further research is this area is greatly needed.[136]

Sleep disorders, specific diagnostic entities, include a wide array of problems characterized by insomnia (difficulty initiating or maintaining sleep or early morning awakening), EDS, and/or abnormal movements, behaviors, or sensations during sleep (Display 8-2).[10] There are eight groups of primary sleep disorders outlined in the International Classification of Sleep Disorders,[10] including the insomnias, sleep-related breathing disorders, hypersomnias of central origin, circadian rhythm disorders, parasomnias, sleep-related movement disorders, normal sleep variants, and "other" (physiological, nonphysiological, and environmental sleep disorders).

EDS, the inability to maintain the alert awake state, is the most common consequence of sleep disorders and/or insufficient or poor sleep and is the most prevalent symptom of patients seen in sleep disorders centers in the United States.[13] However, because of its often vague and nonspecific clinical presentation, the condition is frequently unrecognized by health care providers. Patients themselves may have very little insight into the nature and severity of the problem and the negative effects that EDS has on their lives. For in its milder forms, EDS may cause only minor, barely perceived decrements in social and occupational functioning. When

DISPLAY 8-2 International Classification of Sleep Disorders

Insomnia

Adjustment insomnia (acute Insomnia)
Psychophysiological insomnia
Paradoxical insomnia
Idiopathic insomnia
Insomnia due to mental disorder
Inadequate sleep hygiene
Behavioral insomnia of childhood
Insomnia due to drug or substance
Insomnia due to medical condition
Insomnia not due to substance or known physiological condition, unspecified (nonorganic insomnia, NOS)
Physiological (organic) insomnia, unspecified

Sleep-Related Breathing Disorders

Central Sleep Apnea Syndromes

Primary central sleep apnea
Central sleep apnea due to Cheyne–Stokes breathing pattern
Central sleep apnea high-altitude periodic breathing
Central sleep apnea due to medical condition not Cheyne–Stokes
Central sleep apnea due to drug or substance
Primary sleep apnea of infancy (formerly primary sleep apnea of newborn)
Obstructive Sleep Apnea Syndromes
Obstructive sleep apnea, adult
Obstructive sleep apnea, pediatric
Sleep-Related Hypoventilation/Hypoxemic Syndromes
Sleep-related nonobstructive Aaveolar hypoventilation, idiopathic
Congenital central alveolar hypoventilation syndrome

Sleep-Related Hypoventilation/Hypoxemia Due to Medical Condition

Sleep-related hypoventilation/hypoxemia due to pulmonary parenchymal or vascular pathology
Sleep-related hypoventilation/hypoxemia due to lower airways obstruction
Sleep-related hypoventilation/hypoxemia due to neuromuscular and chest wall disorders

Other Sleep-Related Breathing Disorder

Sleep apnea/sleep-related breathing disorder, unspecified

Hypersomnias of Central Origin Not Due to a Circidian Rhythm Sleep Disorder, Sleep-Related Breathing Disorder, or Other Cause of Disturbed Nocturnal Sleep

Narcolepsy with cataplexy
Narcolepsy without cataplexy
Narcolepsy due to medical condition
Narcolepsy, unspecified
Recurrent hypersomnia
Kleine–Levin syndrome
Menstrual-related hypersomnia
Idiopathic hypersomnia with long sleep time
Idiopathic hypersomnia without long sleep time
Behaviorally induced insufficient sleep syndrome
Hypersomnia due to medical condition
Hypersomnia due to drug or substance
Hypersomnia not due to substance or known physiological condition (nonorganic hypersomnia, NOS)
Physiological (organic) hypersomnia, unspecified (organic hypersomnia, NOS)

Circadian Rhythm Sleep Disorders

Circadian rhythm sleep disorder, delayed sleep phase type (delayed sleep phase disorder)
Circadian rhythm sleep disorder, advanced sleep phase type (advanced sleep phase disorder)
Circadian rhythm sleep disorder, irregular sleep–wake type (irregular sleep–wake rhythm)
Circadian rhythm sleep disorder, free-running type (nonentrained type)
Circadian rhythm sleep disorder, jet lag type (jet lag disorder)
Circadian rhythm sleep disorder, shift work type (shift work disorder)
Circadian rhythm sleep disorder due to medical condition
Other circadian rhythm sleep disorder (circadian rhythm disorder, NOS)
Other circadian rhythm sleep disorder due to drug or substance

Parasomnias

Disorders of Arousal (From NREM Sleep)

Confusional arousals
Sleepwalking
Sleep terrors

Parasomnias Usually Associated With REM Sleep

REM sleep behavior disorder (including parasomnia overlap disorder and status dissociatus)
Recurrent isolated sleep paralysis
Nightmare disorder

Other Parasomnias

Sleep-related dissociative disorders
Sleep enuresis
Sleep related groaning (catathrenia)
Exploding head syndrome
Sleep-related hallucinations
Sleep-related eating disorder
Parasomnia, unspecified
Parasomnia due to drug or substance
Parasomnia due to medical condition

Sleep-Related Movement Disorders

Restless legs syndrome
Periodic limb movement disorder
Sleep-related leg cramps
Sleep-related bruxism
Sleep-related rhythmic movement disorder
Sleep-related movement disorder, unspecified
Sleep-related movement disorder, due to drug or substance
Sleep-related movement disorder due to medical condition

Isolated Symptoms, Apparently Normal Variants and Unresolved Issues

Long sleeper
Short sleeper
Snoring
Sleep talking
Sleep starts (hypnic Jerks)
Benign sleep myoclonus of infancy
Hypnagogic foot tremor and alternating leg muscle activation during sleep

(display continues on page 186)

DISPLAY 8-2 International Classification of Sleep Disorders (continued)

Propriospinal myoclonus at sleep onset
Excessive fragmentary myoclonus

Other Sleep Disorders

Other physiological (organic) sleep disorder
Other sleep disorder not due to substance or known physiological condition
Environmental sleep disorder

Appendix A: Sleep Disorders Associated With Conditions Classifiable Elsewhere

Fatal familial insomnia
Fibromyalgia
Sleep-related epilepsy
Sleep-related headaches
Sleep-related gastroesophageal reflux disease
Sleep-related coronary artery ischemia
Sleep-related abnormal swallowing, choking, and laryngospasm

Appendix B: Other Psychiatric and Behavioral Disorders Frequently Encountered in the Differential Diagnosis of Sleep Disorders

Mood disorders
Anxiety disorders
Somatoform disorders
Schizophrenia and other psychotic disorders
Disorders usually first diagnosed in infancy, childhood, or adolescence
Personality disorders

From AASM. (2005). *The international classification of sleep disorders.* Westchester, IL: American Academy of Sleep Medicine.

severe; however, it can be debilitating, causing a broad range of neuropsychological deficits affecting daytime functioning and quality of life. EDS can even be life threatening because of associated alterations in alertness and reactivity.[124–130] Increased napping has also been associated with increased mortality in the elderly.[137,138]

SLEEP-RELATED DISORDERED BREATHING

Sleep-related changes in breathing and oxygenation have important cardiovascular consequences. This section focuses on the cardiovascular impact of sleep in obstructive sleep apnea (OSA), central sleep apnea (CSA), and snoring/upper airway resistance syndrome (UARS).

Obstructive Sleep Apnea

Patients with sleep apnea repeatedly stop breathing during sleep for periods of 10 seconds or longer (Fig. 8-7).[10] Apnea can be obstructive (a collapsed upper airway blocks airflow despite effort to breathe), central (no respiratory effort), or mixed (central, then obstructive component). A predominance of obstructive apnea is the most common pattern and can lead to repetitive episodes of hypoxemia that are terminated by brief arousals. Typical patients

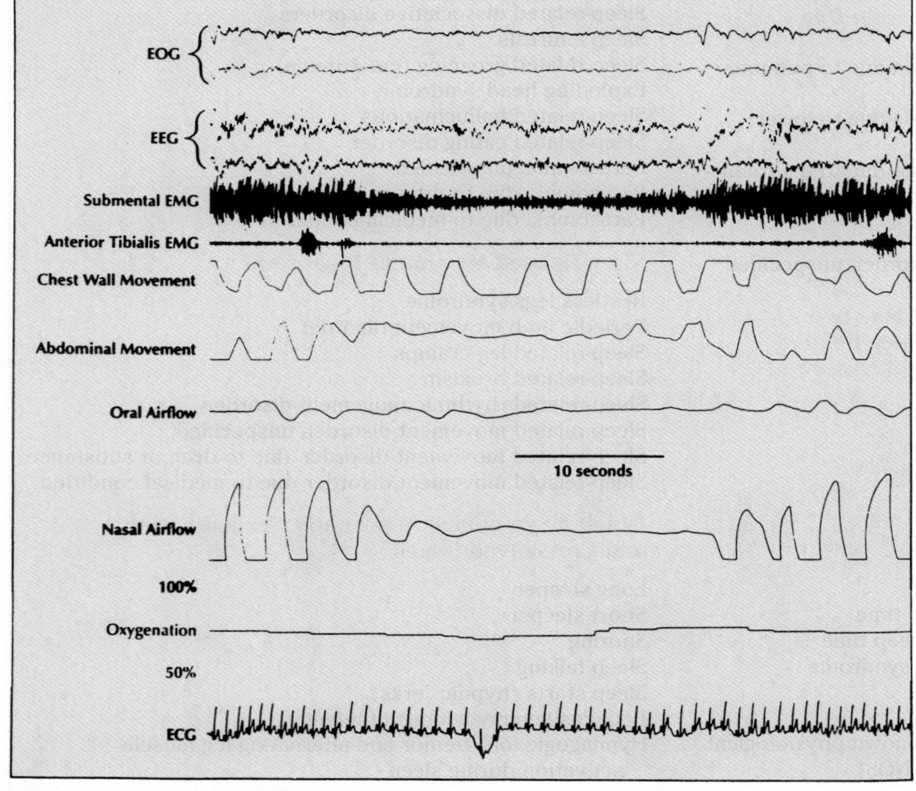

■ **Figure 8-7** Recording of multiple physiologic signals in a formal polysomnographic sleep evaluation. In this example, the patient has an obstructive apnea with cessation of oral and nasal airflow despite effort to breathe. The interrupted breathing is accompanied by a decrease in oxygen saturation and slowing of the heart rate and is followed by an arousal. ECG, electrocardiogram; EEG, electroencephalogram; EMG, electromyogram; EOG, electro-oculogram. (From White, D. [1992]. Obstructive sleep apnea. *Hospital Practice, 27*[5A], 68.)

are middle-aged men who are overweight, snore loudly during sleep, and experience daytime sleepiness that interferes with normal activities; women with sleep apnea are usually post-menopausal. Other risk factors include a positive family history and race (African Americans, Mexican Americans, Pacific Islanders, and East Asians).[139–141] Sleep apnea is likely to be worsened by sleep deprivation,[142–144] alcohol ingestion,[141,145–147] and sedative or hypnotic use.[148]

OSA has significant cardiovascular consequences.[149] Pulmonary arterial pressures increase in a stepwise fashion with repeated apnea.[150–152] Numerous population-based studies have also demonstrated a strong association between systemic hypertension and sleep apnea.[153–157] Whether the hypertension is caused directly by sleep apnea or a related common factor, such as obesity, is unclear. The Wisconsin Sleep Cohort Study prospectively evaluated the clinical course of hypertension in patients with OSA and found that blood pressure increased linearly with apnea severity.[156,157] The Sleep Heart Health Study, the largest prospective performed to date, found that although some of the association was related to body mass index, there was a significant relationship between apnea severity and hypertension.[155]

Cardiac arrhythmias are relatively common and include premature ventricular contractions (PVCs), atrioventricular block, and bradycardia. Apneas are often associated with a progressive sinus bradycardia, sometimes with a prolonged sinus pause, followed by an abrupt increase in heart rate when breathing resumes. A decrease and subsequent increase in cardiac output parallels the heart rate changes.[158]

To minimize possible complications, early diagnosis and treatment are critical. The treatment of choice for OSA is nasally applied CPAP. A soft, firmly fitting nasal mask is held in place by straps and attached to a bedside blower that provides continuous pressure (usually 5 to 15 cm/H_2O) to prevent collapse of the upper airway. Recent improvements in CPAP devices include gradual onset of pressure, separate control of inspiratory and expiratory pressures, and autotitration of the pressure delivered.[159,160] Conservative treatment strategies include weight loss, learning to sleep in a side-lying position (e.g., putting a ball in a pouch on the pajama back), and avoidance of alcohol and sedatives. Oral appliances which move the lower mandible forward in order to increase the posterior airway space are now also available.[161] Pharmacological approaches with purported respiratory stimulants (e.g., acetazolamide, methylprogesterone, and protriptyline) have had variable effectiveness.[162] Occasionally, surgery is performed to enlarge the upper airway (uvulopalatopharyngoplasty) or to bypass it (tracheostomy) when other measures do not alleviate the apnea.[163] If the patient has been receiving antihypertensive medication, the dosage may need to be reduced when the sleep apnea is effectively managed.

Central Sleep Apnea

Patients with severe congestive heart failure (HF) often have a pattern of periodic (Cheyne–Stokes) breathing during light sleep in which periods of central apnea alternate with hyperpnea.[164,165] This breathing pattern causes recurrent episodes of hypoxemia that can further impair the failing heart. Frequent arousals during the hyperpneic phase that disrupt sleep can impair daytime alertness.[166] One mechanism for the abnormal breathing pattern is prolonged circulation time that delays the ventilatory responses to blood gas changes. The resulting hypoxemia sets up a vicious cycle whereby increased ventilation improves oxygenation but decreases carbon dioxide tension below the apneic threshold; the resulting apnea then leads to hypoxemia, which perpetuates the cycle. In addition, cardiac enlargement and pulmonary congestion decrease gas stores in the lungs, which allow wider swings in blood gas values with changes in ventilation. Effective treatment of the HF and low-flow O_2 therapy during sleep help to correct the hypoxemia and stabilize the breathing pattern.[166–168] Use of nasal CPAP has also been shown to decrease the severity of central apneas in patients with HF.[169,170]

Snoring and Upper Airway Resistance

Snoring, present in approximately 40% of the population, occurs because underlying abnormalities cause narrowing of the pharyngeal airway. Snoring is a primarily inspiratory (but may also be expiratory) noise during sleep caused by partial upper airway obstruction and vibration of the soft tissues. Snoring intensifies as NREM sleep deepens and diminishes in REM sleep. Factors that worsen snoring include: obesity, supine position, sleep deprivation, use of alcohol or sedatives, and smoking.[171] UARS is a condition marked by frequent arousals from sleep related to an increase in respiratory effort needed to overcome resistance to air flow resulted in disturbed sleep and EDS.[171,172]

Simple snoring has been associated with a variety of health problems including type II diabetes and headaches, but it is possible that these relationships are coincidental rather than causal.[171] Epidemiologic studies indicate that habitual snoring/UARS is associated with a greater prevalence depression and insomnia.[173,174] As association between snoring/UARS and cardiovascular disease has also been suggested;[175–178] however, others debate this relationship.[179] Treatment options for these conditions include CPAP, posterior pharyngeal airway surgery, or a dental appliance (used to move the lower jaw and tongue forward, thus increasing the posterior pharyngeal airway space).[171]

Restless Legs Syndrome (RLS) and Periodic Limb Movement (PLMD)

RLS is a neurological sensorimotor disorder characterized by disagreeable leg sensations that usually occur prior to sleep onset and accompanied by an almost irresistible urge to move the legs.[10] Vividly described by the English physician Willis in 1671,[180] the disorder was more completely characterized in 1945, when Ekbom described its classic clinical features and made recommendations for treatment.[181] Although, RLS has more recently received significant attention by the scientific and lay communities, it remains poorly understood and under diagnosed.

The four criteria necessary to make the clinical diagnosis of RLS include:

1. an urge to move the limbs usually associated with paresthesias or dysesthesias;
2. motor restless manifested by using different motor strategies to relieve the discomfort such as floor pacing, tossing and turning in bed, and rubbing the legs;
3. symptoms that become worse or are exclusively present at rest with at least partial and temporary relief by activity; and
4. symptoms that are worse in the evening or night (typically between 6:00 PM and 4:00 AM).[10]

Other associated features commonly seen in patients with RLS—but that are not necessary for the diagnosis—are sleep disturbance, daytime fatigue/sleepiness, and involuntary, repetitive, jerking limb movements either during sleep or while awake and at rest.

A related condition, PLMD, was originally termed nocturnal myoclonus by Symonds in 1953.[182] The periodic nature of the movements and their common association with RLS were later described by Lugaresi et al.[183] and Coleman et al.[184] Periodic limb movements (PLMs) usually involve the legs and consist of a sudden extension of the great toe (similar to the Babinski reflex) associated with flexion at the ankle, knee, and hip. Because the arms are sometimes included, many prefer the term PLMs rather than the previously used term, periodic leg movements. Similar to RLS, the expression of PLMs also appears to have a circadian component and is typically worse at night.

RLS is common and its prevalence is estimated to be between 5% and 10% in northern European populations, while the prevalence of the disorder in other groups remains to be determined.[10] The disorder can occur at any age, but symptoms often begin in middle-aged individuals with the mean age of onset being between 27 and 41 years.[185,186] However, recent surveys have reported that approximately 40% of RLS patients experienced their first symptom before the age of 20.[187–190] The disorder is slightly more common in women.[10] PLMD is also very prevalent, occurring in up to 6% of the general population and increasing to over 20% in patients 60 and older.

Both RLS and PLMD occur in idiopathic and secondary forms. The idiopathic form, especially in the case of RLS, is often found in those who have afflicted first-degree relatives.[191] The exact of mode inheritance remains unclear, but the frequency with which offspring of affected individuals develop the condition suggests an autosomal-dominant genetic pattern. RLS and PLMD may also develop in association with several medical, neurological, and metabolic conditions and secondary to conditions characterized by iron deficiency such as anemia, pregnancy,[192,193] and uremia.[194] Recently, RLS and PLMD in children have been associated with attention-deficit/hyperactivity disorder[195–197] and cardiovascular disease.[198,199]

The treatment of RLS and PLMD is symptomatic. Patients with the mild forms of the disorders may respond favorably to nonpharmacological interventions. When symptoms are moderate to severe, pharmacological therapy is also indicated.

Initially, it is important to listen, support, and validate the experiences of both the patient and family, as they may have gone for years with their symptoms and concerns being dismissed by health care providers. Referral to support groups such as those offered through the Restless Legs Syndrome Foundation can help provide additional support and education. The Restless Legs Syndrome Foundation also has a web site with important and relevant patient and professional information (www.RLS.org). Other nonpharmacological interventions that may be beneficial to some patients include hot baths, stretching muscles in the morning and night, delayed sleep time/rise time, massage, vibration, and moderate exercise.[200]

Three reversible forms of RLS, including pregnancy, renal failure, and anemia, are each characterized by iron deficiency (as reflected in low ferritin levels; <50 and treatment with both oral and intravenous iron has been found to improve or resolve RLS symptoms. Two types of dopaminergic medications are beneficial in the treatment of RLS and PLMD. Both decrease symptoms and numbers of limb movements. Dopamine precursors, such as regular or sustained-release carbidopa/levodopa, increase the delivery of levodopa to the brain where it is converted to dopamine. The carbidopa is a dehydroxylase inhibitor, which decreases the peripheral breakdown of the levodopa so more can get to the brain. This medication is excellent for patients with sporadic, infrequent symptoms. However, with chronic use, there is frequent development of *rebound* (return of symptoms) or *augmentation*, the tendency for symptoms to develop earlier in the day and/or to be more severe than prior to treatment. In these situations, it is often best to change to a dopamine agonist, in which case the symptoms of rebound and augmentation usually disappear in a few day or weeks. Although dopamine agonists have been traditionally used for Parkinson's disease, several controlled clinical trials have also demonstrated the efficacy of pergolide,[201] pramipexole,[202] and ropinirole[203] in the treatment of RLS and PLMD. In fact, these agents are currently considered first-line drugs for most patients. Side effects from these medications such as sleepiness, nausea, and hypotension occur infrequently, and can most often be avoided by slowly increasing the dose until symptoms abate. Other medications which can be used include opioids (for painful symptoms), anticonvulsants, and benzodiazepines.[204]

SLEEP IN PATIENTS WITH CARDIOVASCULAR DISEASE

Sleep in Coronary Heart Disease (CHD)

Although more than 16 million Americans are estimated to have CHD,[205] their sleep patterns have only recently been studied. Several recent large studies, such as the Sleep Heart Health Study, have begun to link sleep symptoms and sleep-disordered breathing with risk factors and outcomes of cardiovascular disease.[206] Assessing the independent contribution of sleep to cardiovascular outcomes is often complicated by confounding variations in age, sex, type and severity of cardiovascular impairment, other risk factors, and medications. However, growing evidence consistently links sleep disorders with increased cardiovascular risk and suggests that patients with coronary heart disease often have disturbed sleep. The magnitude of the sleep disturbance may be the key in that sleep hypopneas with oxyhemoglobin desaturation of at least 4% are independently associated with cardiovascular disease, whereas milder episodes are not.[207]

While mechanisms linking sleep with adverse neurobehavioral and cardiovascular outcomes are currently being defined, sleep apnea and sleep-related disorders are known to contribute to increased CHD risk factors such as hypertension, obesity, inflammatory markers, and metabolic changes related to glucose and insulin.[205,207,208] Thus, during any assessment of cardiovascular risk, sleep patterns should be considered and evaluated for contribution to other risk factors. The threshold for sleep duration on risk factors appears to be a habitual sleep time around less than 5 to 6 hours per night, or over 9 hours per night.[208,209]

The relationship is reciprocal in that impaired cardiac function from multiple causes can produce symptoms such as chest pain and dyspnea that interfere with sleep. Even when patients with a variety of diseases are considered, cardiovascular symptoms are a major factor associated with symptoms of reduced total sleep and increased night-time wakefulness. The psychological impact of heart disease also has a major impact on sleep. Acute myocardial infarction (MI), for example, not only affects physical health and comfort but also influences social relationships, living patterns, work options and income, and sense of personal vulnerability.

Fear of death, reinfarction, or inability to resume former living patterns are common as described more fully in Chapter 33. It is not surprising that anxiety and depression, typically accompanied by poor sleep, are common after MI; many patients report troublesome insomnia that lasts for months and sometimes years. This may in fact be due to altered sleep architecture after acute MI due to the infarction itself and its associated physiological and inflammatory changes.[210]

Sleep apnea may increase the risk of CHD via pathways mediated by hypertension and the metabolic consequences of increased oxidative stress, C-reactive protein, and insulin resistance. PSG-verified sleep disruptions and desaturations are associated with adverse changes in coagulation proteins/factors and increased prothrombotic state.[211] Patients with OSA may also be obese and have a greater prevalence of other underlying cardiovascular risk factors suggesting a bidirectional relationship. Poor sleep appears to be a precursor to MI as symptoms of insomnia, habitual short sleep, waking up exhausted, daytime sleepiness, and frequent napping are common in the preceding months. One study of prodromal acute MI symptoms found that sleep disturbance as early as 1 month prior to an acute MI was reported by as many as 47% of women participating in the study.[212] A common link with the period of depression and elevated inflammatory markers that often precedes MI is a possible explanation for these symptoms.[213] An OSA has also been linked to subclinical CHD as measured by coronary artery calcification, and attention to OSA as a modifiable cardiac risk factor is becoming increasingly important.[214]

Sleep in the Coronary Care Unit (CCU)

Specialized CCUs reduce inhospital deaths after MI, but they can be far from optimal environments for sleep. The setting is unfamiliar and frightening to patients, the schedule and bedtime routines differ from those at home, noise and lighting may never be completely suppressed, and interruptions for patient care procedures are frequent. Sedatives and analgesics are routinely used in cardiovascular patients, yet they have the potential for side effects, such as delirium and sleep architecture disruption. These medications are extremely important in providing patient comfort; however, the goals of care must focus on the right balance of sedative and analgesic administration while reducing unnecessary or overzealous use. True sleep versus the appearance of sleep due to sedating side effects of medications is important to assess in the CCU.

In PSG studies, CCU patients typically have a pattern of light, fragmented sleep with reduced slow-wave and REM sleep, frequent stage changes, and considerable night-time wakefulness.[215] Although total sleep time is not necessarily reduced, the normal circadian sleep–wake rhythm is disrupted, with sleep occurring off and on during the 24 hours. REM and slow-wave (deep) sleep may be significantly decreased and disrupted. Sleep is more disturbed as illness severity increases. Sleep patterns may improve over time with improving health status, fewer interruptions for care, and increased adaptation to the CCU environment. Although logic and earlier studies suggested that increased noise in the ICU may be a major contributor to poor sleep, later studies suggested that patient monitoring and pain may play a larger role.[216] Ruggiero and Dziedzic[217] demonstrated that environmental disruptions are not inevitable by implementing a daily, 2-hour, quiet time in intensive care units. Patients were offered earplugs, do not disturb signs were posted, conversations were held in whispered voices, and reduced rounds and procedures were implemented. The changes yielded increased patient and staff satisfaction, actual sleep for patients, and improved outcomes related to length of stay, nosocomial infections, and ventilator days.[217]

Sleep After Cardiac Surgery

Sleep disruption after surgery is related to the magnitude of procedure and associated postoperative care, asynchrony between patient needs and unit procedures, and temporary physiological changes in brain stem and hypothalamus due to circulatory changes. Patients who undergo cardiac surgery experience dramatic sleep pattern disturbances (SPD). Severe sleep deprivation is common in the early postoperative period, with only a few hours of fragmented sleep each 24 hours and virtual absence of slow-wave and REM sleep.[218] One small study comparing preoperative and postoperative PSG recordings in six men who underwent CABG surgery revealed a significant decrease in mean sleep time, mean percentage stages 3 to 4 sleep, and mean REM sleep with reduced sleep time correlated with behavioral and mental changes.[219] Additionally, patient ventilator discordance causes sleep disruption. Proportional assist ventilation (a mode of partial ventilatory support in which the ventilator applies pressure in proportion to the inspiratory effort) may be more efficacious than pressure support ventilation in matching ventilatory requirements with ventilator assistance; therefore, resulting in fewer patient–ventilator asynchronies and better quality of sleep.[220] Another factor is the type of circulatory assist used during the surgery. Off-pump CABG surgical procedures have been advocated to reduce the adverse effects of cardiopulmonary bypass on the brain. An analysis using both objective and subjective measures of sleep and mood disturbance between patients after on-pump and off-pump suggests that off-pump surgery was associated with better objective sleep continuity (decreased percentage of wake time after sleep onset and fewer awakenings) but not longer sleep duration after controlling for age and sex.[221] The patients did not differ overall in subjective sleep characteristics, mood disturbance, or preoperative sleep quality. The authors concluded that off-pump coronary artery bypass surgery may improve sleep continuity during the early postoperative period.[221]

As with the coronary care environment, cardiac surgical patients report sleep disturbances and distress at uninterrupted sleep because of nursing care. Contributing environmental and clinical factors to postoperative sleep problems include persistent interruptions and activity, high noise and lighting levels, anxiety, pain, and medications.[216] Additionally, cardiac surgery patients may be elderly and have pre-existing sleep disorders. Sleep deprivation often is implicated as a risk factor for the postoperative delirium that develops in some cardiac surgical patients.

Although sleep patterns gradually improve after cardiac surgery, slow-wave and REM sleep may be suppressed for several weeks after the patient returns home, with many patients reporting continuing sleep disturbances. The cause of sleeplessness after CABG surgery may be temporary deterioration of circulation in the centers of the brain stem and hypothalamus that control sleep and awakening. Improvement of the circulation in these centers occurs a few months after the operation helps to regain sleep control and reduce sleep disturbances over time.[222] An initial contributing factor for some patients with heart valve replacements is noise generated by the mechanical valve prosthesis, including audible high-frequency closing clicks and low-frequency sounds conducted by body tissues that the patient becomes accustomed to over time. Although very few interventions have been tested for their effects on promoting sleep after cardiac surgery, attention to reducing noxious environmental stimuli is an obvious approach. Examples are found in studies reporting positive effects of structured quiet time, guidelines to reduce noise, and providing patients with earplugs while in intensive care units, use of white noise and music therapy.[217,223] Because sleep disruptions after cardiac surgery are multifactorial and include environmental, treatment-related, and intrinsic factors, a comprehensive approach to management of these problems is essential.

Sleep and HF

SPD are one of the most burdensome and frequently occurring symptoms in patients with HF.[224,225] Insomnia is the most common SPD, and evidence suggests that up to 70% of patients with HF experience at least one sleep complaint, far exceeding the 10% to 15% reported in the general population.[226] Factors that contribute to sleep SPD in persons with HF include increased age, body mass index, comorbidities, fluid overload, medications, and psychological distress, particularly depression.[224,227,228]

Sleep-related breathing disorders (SRBD) have been more widely studied in HF patients than SPDs. Estimates are that SRBD occur in approximately 50% of HF patients compared to 5% in the general population. Both OSA and Cheyne–Stokes respiration (CSR) with CSA or a mix of both are common in patients with HF. The hallmarks of CSR–CSA are higher NYHA class, atrial fibrillation, frequent nocturnal ventricular arrhythmias, lower Pa_{CO_2} and a left ventricular ejection fraction of 20% or less.[229] Patients with CSR–CSA have interrupted sleep, frequent awakenings, and nocturnal O_2 desaturation that results in poor sleep efficiency. Heightened risk for cardiac arrhythmias, poor clinical outcomes, and increased mortality are also associated with CSR–CSA.[230,231]

EDS, poor sleep quality, fatigue, reduced physical function, higher depressive symptoms, and a considerably lower quality of life are reported among HF patients who experience SPD or SRBD.[229,232,233] PLMs are also associated with SRBD, and contribute to more frequent nocturnal arousals, poor sleep quality and daytime sleepiness.[229]

Sleep and Hypertension

SRBD, particularly OSA, is an independent risk factor for hypertension more than any other cardiovascular disease.[234–236] Epidemiological studies show that approximately 40% of hypertensive patients have SRBD, and this number rises to over 80% among drug-resistant hypertension.[237,238] Recent studies have also established a dose–response relationship between severity of SRBD and hypertension, independent of age, body mass index, gender, alcohol consumption, and smoking.[239–241] For example, the Wisconsin Sleep Cohort Study[242] demonstrated that an apnea–hypopnea index (i.e., the average number of apnea and hypopnea events pre hour of sleep) was progressively related to the odds of developing hypertension over the next 4 years compared to age-matched controls.

Elevated nocturnal blood pressure and reduced blood pressure "dipping" during sleep also suggests a higher probability of underlying sleep apnea, even among normotensive individuals.[243] The cumulative effects of excess sympathetic activity, in addition to other vasoactive factors in response to hypoxia (such as endothelin), may result in daytime hypertension. Even without daytime hypertension, patients with SRBD do not often exhibit the normal nocturnal dip in blood pressure during sleep due to apnea-induced sympathetic activation. Higher nocturnal blood pressure, independent of daytime hypertension, places the individual at greater risk for cardiovascular morbidity and mortality.[243,244]

Patients with SRBD and hypertension experience frequent arousals, reduced length and depth of non-REM sleep, and shortened REM latency, all of which lead to EDS, fatigue, and impaired concentration.[245] Sleep duration has also been recently shown to influence the risk of hypertension in patients <60 years of age who sleep <5 hours per night[246] and is supported by findings from the Sleep Heart Health Study, which suggests a median sleep duration of <7 to 8 hours per night increases the prevalence of hypertension.[153] Because hypertension is often associated with other comorbid conditions such HF, obesity, and diabetes, better self-management of these conditions will likely alter the progression of SPD or SRBD, and this is an area for future investigation.[1,236,247]

Sleep and Stroke

Almost every fifth stroke occurs during sleep, yet the data on the relationship between stroke and sleep are conflicting.[248] Some evidence suggests that OSA is an independent risk factor for stroke and transient ischemic attack (TIA). Other studies have shown sleep itself is not a risk factor for stroke because most stroke and TIAs begin between 6:00 AM and noon, while the individual is awake.[249] Some suggest that stroke or TIA is more a cause, rather than consequence of OSA because PSG studies have shown obstructive versus central apneas in stroke and equivalent frequency and severity of apneas when comparing patients with stroke and TIA. Untreated OSA patients have more strokes, stroke morbidity and mortality than those who are treated. Regardless of its role as a risk factor or consequence, assessment and treatment of OSA in patients with stroke and TIA is advocated. Its contribution to hypertension and prothrombosis over time is highly relevant to initial and recurrent stroke. Treating OSA patients with CPAP can prevent or improve hypertension, reduce abnormal elevations of inflammatory cytokines and adhesion molecules, reduce excessive sympathetic tone, avoid increased vascular oxidative stress, reverse coagulation abnormalities, and reduce leptin levels. Grigg-Damberger[249] recommends a polysomnogram should become part of a neurologist's armamentarium for stroke and TIA.

Sleep and Diabetes Mellitus (DM)

Given the high prevalence of DM in patients with cardiac conditions, it is prudent to note that sleep disordered breathing and sleep loss have been associated with glucose intolerance and insulin resistance. More specifically, a habitual sleep duration of 6 hours or less or 9 hours or more is associated with increased prevalence of DM and impaired glucose tolerance.[209] When confounding risk factors are rigorously controlled in studies, sleep-related hypoxemia was also associated with glucose intolerance independent of age, gender, body mass index, and waist circumference and may lead to type 2 DM.[250,251]

While recent epidemiological, biological, and behavioral evidence suggests that sleep disorders may contribute to the development of DM, conversely, diabetes itself may contribute to sleep disorders.[252] In patients with diabetes, sleep loss may contribute to elevations in HgA1c, and symptoms resulting from diabetes, such as nocturia and neuropathic pain, may in turn contribute to sleep disturbance and exacerbate sleep deprivation.[252]

Sleep and Chronic Obstructive Pulmonary Disease (COPD)

Cardiac patients may have COPD as a comorbidity, and approximately 10% to 15% of COPD patients experience sleep apnea. The term "Overlap Syndrome" describes the relationship between COPD and sleep apnea. Patients with overlap syndrome are characterized by having lower Pa_{O_2} during wakefulness, higher Pa_{CO_2}, elevated pulmonary artery pressure, and more significant episodes of nocturnal hypoxemia than sleep apnea patients without COPD. COPD and sleep apnea are each recognized to contribute detrimental influence on the respiratory physiology of patients, overall health status and poor quality of life.[253–261]

Patients with COPD who are hypoxic during wakefulness become more hypoxic during sleep.[259] A strong association exists between nocturnal O_2 saturation and level of daytime hypoxia; with higher daytime hypoxia related to more severe nocturnal desaturation and hypoxia. Desaturation is defined as a drop in Sa_{O_2} of 4 from its baseline level, during quiet breathing and just before an episode of hypoxia. Nocturnal desaturation is more severe during REM sleep and may exceed 15 minutes. However, nocturnal desaturation may also occur during non-REM sleep, especially light sleep (stages I and II) but is not as severe and of shorter duration.[259–261] Studies have established that the most optimal index of sleep-related desaturation is the mean nocturnal Sa_{O_2} or the mean percentage of recording time under a certain percentage level. In patients with mild daytime hypoxia Pa_{O_2} ≥60 mm Hg, or with no hypoxia, significant nocturnal desaturation is defined as a mean Sa_{O_2} <90 mm Hg. The best predictor of nocturnal desaturation in patients with mild to moderate daytime hypoxia is level of diurnal Pa_{O_2}, but daytime Pa_{CO_2} is also an independent predictor of Sa_{O_2} during sleep.[257]

Two mechanisms are primarily responsible for worsening hypoxia during sleep in COPD patients: alveolar hypoventilation and ventilation–perfusion mismatching. Alveolar hypoventilation differs according to non-REM and REM sleep stages. In non-REM sleep, alveolar hypoventilation is associated with a lower basal metabolic rate, reduced ventilatory drive, and an increase in upper airway resistance. In REM sleep, ventilatory drive is markedly lower, and the hypoxic and hypercapneic responses are diminished compared to non-REM sleep or wakefulness. A second important factor related to REM sleep hypoventilation is a reduction in muscle strength of the respiratory muscles, which likely explains the significant relation between mean nocturnal Sa_{O_2} and inspiratory muscle strength; the lower the muscle strength the lower the nocturnal Sa_{O_2}. Worsening ventilation perfusion mismatching during REM sleep in patients with COPD is largely due to reduction in functional residual capacity resulting in closing of small airways in dependent areas of the lung.[259,261]

Many patients with COPD complain of poor sleep quality which often worsens as disease severity increases. In addition, they experience reduced sleep efficiency with delayed time for sleep onset, a reduction in total sleep time and periods of wakefulness often prolonged. Poor sleep quality in patients with COPD is likely multifactoral and includes nocturnal coughing and dyspnea, effects of medications (i.e., theophylline), and aging.[257,261]

The cardiovascular consequences in patients with COPD are associated with the pulmonary hemodynamic alterations that often occur with disease progression. During REM sleep in particular, patients with COPD often have alveolar hypoxia resulting in pulmonary vasoconstriction, pulmonary artery pressure elevation, and over time pulmonary hypertension (cor pulmonale) may develop and result in right ventricular overload and right-sided HF. In addition, there is an increase in PVCs in patients with COPD, although the frequency and clinical relevance of PVCs have not been established in COPD, including whether a low nocturnal Sa_{O_2} is the major underlying mechanism. During periods of nocturnal desaturation, the maximal myocardial O_2 demands are considerably higher and often exceed those required for maximal exercise testing. It is speculated that in patients with more advanced COPD, this differences in O_2 demand may be one of the reasons for higher rates of nocturnal death.[254,256]

The cornerstone of treatment for COPD remains smoking cessation, bronchodilation, and pulmonary rehabilitation. Decreased levels of hypoxia in COPD patients are usually achieved by conventional home O_2 therapy (16 to 18 hours/day). Hypnotics are contraindicated in hypercapnic patients and should be used with caution in hypoxic individuals. Alcohol worsens hypoxia and should be avoided in the evening in particular, since heavy consumption is linked to hypercapnic respiratory failure. Finally, improving sleep quality will likely improve overall health status and enhance quality of life in this population.[258,262] This is especially important in those with overlap syndrome whose 5-year survival is lower than that of patients with sleep apnea alone.[253,260]

Sleep and Depression

Sleep is an essential component of the pathophysiology and treatment of depression.[263] The majority of people with depressive disorders experience SPD, and most diagnostic criteria for depression include sleep disturbances. While the likelihood of developing a mood disorder is not simply a consequence of having a sleep pattern disturbance, longitudinal studies document that insomnia is a risk factor for onset of depressive disorder[264] and may increase the risk for relapse in patients with recurrent illness.[265] More than 90% of depressed patients complain about impairments of sleep quality. Typically, patients suffer from difficulties in falling asleep, frequent nocturnal awakenings, and early morning awakening. Whereas sleep onset problems and frequent awakenings accompany almost any kind of insomnia in the general population, lifetime prevalence of depression is approximately 5% to 10%. However, among patients with cardiovascular disease, these rates of depression are two to three times higher. Major depression affects approximately 15% to 20% of patients with CVD, and minor depression is present in another 20%. Similar prevalence rates are reported for sleep disturbances in CVD.[213,266] Physiologically, the brain stem and thalamic nuclei that regulate sleep and the limbic mechanisms that modulate mood are implicated in pathogenesis of both SPD and depression.[267,268]

Most individuals who are depressed exhibit one or more alterations in sleep neurophysiology. Multiple disturbances in PSG recordings have been reported in depressed patients during sleep, and these changes are more pronounced as depression increases. The most common sleep disturbances in depression include decreased sleep efficiency, nocturnal and early-morning awakening, decreased slow-wave sleep, reduced REM latency, an increased number of eye movements during REM periods, and increased REM intensity.[265,268–270]

Major depression and SRBD, particularly CSR–CSA, are well-established risks for poor clinical outcomes and death in patients with CVD. Multiple mechanisms linking depression, sleep disturbances, and heart disease have been proposed. Depression lowers adherence to prescribed medications and increases unhealthy lifestyle behaviors among cardiac patients. Similar underlying hypothalamic–pituitary–adrenal axis, neuroendocrine, and immune dysregulation have been reported in both depression and sleep disturbances, further leading to a heightened risk for arrhythmias and sudden death.[265,267,268]

CARDIAC EVENTS IN SLEEP

Angina

Anginal chest pain results from myocardial ischemia, an imbalance between coronary blood flow and myocardial requirements. In its classic form, angina is precipitated by physical exertion or other situations that increase myocardial O_2 demand. Blood pressure and heart rate characteristically increase before appearance of ischemic changes in the ECG in daytime and sleep-related anginal episodes (see Chapter 15).

Classic (effort) angina and the full spectrum of cardiac ischemic syndromes including unstable angina, non-Q-wave MI, and variant angina occur more often in the morning hours and early after awakening than at night.[271] Sleep is generally a time of reduced myocardial demand because of decreased blood pressure and heart rate. However, in persons with stable coronary artery disease and normal left ventricular function, REM-induced surges in heart rate can increase metabolic demands in the context of stenotic blood flow, thereby setting up a cascade of events that can lead to plaque disruption and arrhythmias.[59] Patients with known daytime ischemia report relatively few night-time anginal episodes and usually have reduced or unchanged ECG evidence of ischemia. Of all angina attacks, 50% occur within the initial 6 hours after awakening with 74% associated with possible external triggers such as physical activity or anger demonstrating a marked wake time-related circadian variation in the occurrence of angina pectoris attacks.[272]

Variant (Prinzmetal) angina is a less common form of ischemic chest pain. It is caused by coronary artery spasm and is characterized by angina at rest and ST segment elevation. Variant angina has a clear circadian rhythm, with episodes clustering in the early morning hours of sleep. At one time, increased sympathetic activity during REM sleep was believed to be the mechanism for nocturnal coronary spasm; however, more contemporary understandings have emerged from research documenting circadian alterations in endothelial function and reduced nocturnal vagal nerve and cardiac parasympathetic activity.[273]

Arrhythmias

Sinus bradycardia and sinus arrhythmia are the most frequent changes in heart rhythm during sleep in healthy people, consistent with the dominance of parasympathetic activity. Bradycardia during sleep is more common in men than in women, and the difference between daytime and night-time heart rates decreases with age. Although heart rate usually is lowest in slow-wave sleep, little information is available about sleep stage relationships with bradyarrhythmias. REM sleep-related bradyarrhythmia syndrome is a rare problem characterized by asystoles lasting several seconds during REM sleep accompanied by alterations in sympathetic and parasympathetic bursts in otherwise healthy individuals.[274] Bradycardia-dependent changes in atrial repolarization predisposing to intra-atrial re-entry have been suggested to lead to vagally mediated atrial fibrillation during sleep in susceptible patients.[275] Obesity increases the risk for OSA, specifically the magnitude of nocturnal O_2 desaturation, and both are independent risk factors for incident atrial fibrillation in patients under the age of 65 years.[276] Disruptions in sleep, increased night-time activity and restlessness, daytime sleepiness and fatigue are present in atrial fibrillation patients and contribute to a reduced quality of life.[277,278]

PVCs are common after MI and, when frequent or complex, carry a higher mortality risk. Sleep usually suppresses arrhythmogenesis and the frequency of PVCs in healthy people. Night-time PVCs have no consistent relation to sleep stage in that some individuals experience greater numbers during the wake sleep transition and others during REM. The frequency of PVCs; however, may be independently related to heart rate and is increased by factors such as hypoxemia, increased circulating catecholamines, and loss of vagal activity during the night. Hypoxemia is especially important in patients with sleep apnea and COPD, in whom PVCs are clearly more common during sleep than wakefulness.

Patients with implantable cardioverter defibrillators and atrial defibrillators may experience sleep disruption initially after implant due to incisional pain and increased awareness of the device. Sleep disruptions may be due to device activations, appropriate and inappropriate shocks. Atrial defibrillation therapy has not been found to affect sleep; however, atrial fibrillation symptoms and depression may contribute to sleep disruptions.

The impact of sleep disordered breathing in cardiac patients on arrhythmogenesis cannot be overemphasized. In the Sleep Heart Health Study, individuals with severe sleep disordered breathing had two- to four-fold higher odds of complex arrhythmias including atrial fibrillation, ventricular tachycardia, and ventricular ectopy than those without cardiac disease, even after adjusting for potential confounding factors.[279] OSA as a cause of atrial fibrillation is not proven; however, in PSG studies of adults, both obesity and nocturnal O_2 desaturations independently predicted atrial fibrillation in subjects under the age of 65 years.[276] Appropriate treatment with CPAP in OSA patients is associated with lower recurrence of AF.[280]

NURSING CARE GOALS

After evaluating the subjective and objective data related to sleep noted earlier in the chapter, a nursing assessment may indicate that a patient is experiencing sleep difficulties. A nursing diagnosis of impaired sleep is made when patients experience or are at risk of experiencing a change in the quantity or quality of sleep that causes discomfort or interferes with daily life. The general nursing management plan focuses on promoting adequate, restful sleep for patients with cardiovascular disorders. This can be accomplished first by preventing or reducing the factors that are disturbing the patient's sleep. A second goal is to provide bedtime routines, comfort measures, and a setting conducive to sleep. A third goal is to detect alterations in physiological function that are caused by or may accentuate the underlying health problem. A fourth goal is to assist patients to learn behavioral patterns that enhance the quality of their sleep.

SLEEP PROMOTING INTERVENTIONS

Nonpharmacological Outpatient Interventions for the Management of Sleep Disturbances in Patients with Cardiovascular Disease

Nonpharmacological therapies for sleep problems are often effective but underutilized by health care providers. Treatment of sleep disturbances using nonpharmacological methods involves behavioral, cognitive, and physiological interventions. These therapies may be used alone or in combination and typically are more effective for the long-term management of sleep disturbances than medications alone.[281,282]

Relaxation Therapy and Imagery

Anxiety and related thoughts are often detrimental to sleep and may prevent or delay sleep onset. Relaxation training originally designed to reduce anxiety has also been used successfully for the treatment of sleep onset insomnia. Several relaxation techniques are recommended for the treatment of sleep disturbances. These techniques include progressive muscle relaxation, autogenic training, and imagery. Autogenic training focuses on increasing blood flow to the legs and arms. The sensations of warmth and heaviness are used to promote somatic relaxation. Positive imagery may also be used to promote sleep in conjunction with relaxation techniques. Once a selected technique is established, the patient must practice it at least twice per day. Typically, it requires several weeks of practice before the technique is acquired. Relaxation techniques may be best used as a method to extend sleep rather than used as an initial therapy for sleep onset.[282,283]

Stimulus Control

To cope with being awake during the night, many individuals with chronic sleep disturbances engage in behaviors in the bedroom that may further contribute to wakefulness. These may include worrying, reading, and watching television among other behaviors. One report of sleep onset insomniacs found there was an improvement in sleep in 70% of the subjects when they consistently followed the practice of having only 10 minutes to fall asleep (20 minutes in the elderly).[281] Stimulus control is designed to break the relationship between maladaptive behaviors and arousal.[282] Patients using stimulus control are told to:

- Go to bed only if you are sleepy
- Avoid activities in the bedroom that keep you awake, other than sex
- Only sleep in the bedroom
- Leave the bedroom when awake
- Return to the bedroom only when sleepy
- Get up at the same time each morning, regardless of the amount of sleep
- Avoid napping during the day

Sleep Restriction Therapy

Sleep restriction therapy causes sleep deprivation, and consequently increases the sleep drive. Before beginning sleep restriction therapy the individual maintains a sleep log for 2 weeks. This log facilitates estimating the average sleep time versus time spent in bed. The allowed sleep time is the average subjective sleep time, but is never less than 5 hours. The time in bed is adjusted by 15-minute increments or decrements, depending on the sleep efficiency. Sleep efficiency is defined as the average sleep time or time in bed multiplied by 100%. If sleep efficiency is greater than 90%, the time in bed is increased by 15 minutes, and if it is less than 85%, the time is decreased by 15 minutes.[282]

Sleep restriction has been shown in one study to increase total sleep time, improve sleep latency, total wake time, sleep efficiency, and subjective assessment of insomnia. Using this technique, improvement continued to be significant for all sleep parameters at 36 weeks. The efficacy of sleep restriction alone or in combination with other modalities has also been shown in other controlled trials.[162,284,285] However, the use of this technique with cardiovascular patients has not been fully tested and should be used with caution given the vulnerability of the cardiac patient to sleep deprivation.

Sleep Education and Hygiene

Sleep hygiene measures alone are not adequate for the treatment of sleep disturbances; however, they may be beneficial when used in conjunction with other therapies. Sleep hygiene includes health practices, habits, and environmental factors that influence sleep. Health care providers need to educate cardiac patients regarding sleep and its disorders. It is important to emphasize that simple lifestyle changes can help in the treatment of their sleep problems. Some of the sleep-related practices and habits that may impair sleep are listed in Display 8-3. Additionally, some patients with cardiovascular disease or HF may be taking over-the-counter or herbal medications with stimulant properties. Patients may not volunteer this information unless specifically asked. Assessment of these factors and education regarding behavior change may help improve sleep.

Light Therapy

The circadian cycle is responsible for the 24-hour sleep and wake rhythm. Circadian rhythm disorders can cause sleep disturbances as a result of a dysfunctional relationship existing between one's

DISPLAY 8-3 Behaviors and Habits Nonconducive to Sleep

Spending too much time in bed
Frequent daytime napping
Too few daytime activities
Late evening exercise
Inadequate morning light exposure
Excessive caffeine, especially in the later half of the day
Evening alcohol consumption
Smoking in the evening
Late heavy dinner
Anxiety in anticipation of poor sleep
Environmental factors, such as the room being too warm, too noisy, or too bright

internal clock and the external schedule. Delayed sleep phase disorder, when sleep time is delayed in relation to the desired clock time, and advanced sleep phase disorder, when the patient goes to sleep in the early evening and wakes up earlier than desired in the morning are two common circadian sleep-related disturbances.[285,286] Patients with a delayed sleep phase have been reported to benefit from early morning light exposure. This requires bright light exposure to be given in the morning as close to the patient's scheduled arising time as possible. Light therapy delays the shift toward a later phase and may be useful in sustaining a 24-hour circadian period. Evening bright light exposure is useful for treating advance sleep phase disorders by impeding the circadian sleep phase.[287]

Natural sunlight or artificial light, using a light box, can be used to administer light therapy. Artificial light requires using 10,000 lux for 30 to 40 minutes upon awakening. Evening light exposure is decreased to attain positive results in those with delayed phase sleep disorders. Blue-blocking sunglasses may be worn to counter the phase-delaying effect of evening light exposure. Response is usually seen in 2 to 3 weeks and often requires indefinite treatment. Advanced phase disorder patients require a light box in the evenings. The use of sun glasses that block blue light in the morning may also be beneficial.[41,286,288,289]

Complementary and Alternative Therapies

One of the most frequent uses of complementary and alternative medicines (CAM) is in the treatment of sleep disturbances. While the terms are often used synonymously, a more accurate statement is the National Institutes of Health—National Center for Complementary and Alternative Medicine (NCCAM) definition that complementary medicines are "used together with conventional medicine," while alternative medicines are "used in place of conventional medicine." The NCCAM lists five broad categories of CAM therapies including: (1) alternative medical systems. These include acupuncture, Ayurveda, or homeopathy; (2) biologically based practices, such as herbal products; (3) mind-body medicine, meditation, Tai Chi, yoga, and biofeedback; (4) manipulative and body-based practices, massage-based therapies; and (5) energy medicine that focuses on the use of energy fields, including bioelectromagnetic-based therapies.

Melatonin. Melatonin is a hormone produced by the pineal gland that is thought to play an important role in regulating the sleep–wake cycle. During the daytime, circulating levels are low with nocturnal levels becoming elevated, which coincide with the sleep phase. Melatonin can alter the timing of the circadian sleep–wake cycle.[290] Melatonin also has sedative effects, possibly by inhibiting the suprachiasmatic nucleus. Melatonin has exhibited positive effects on the cardiovascular system.[291,292] Studies of the effectiveness of melatonin have been inconsistent using both wrist-worn actigraphy and PSG to document sleep parameters. Melatonin is well tolerated by most individuals in the dose range of 0.1 to 10 mg with few reported adverse events.[293] However, melatonin may reduce the antihypertensive effectiveness of calcium channel blockers to a mild degree. Patients taking nifedipine, who were treated with melatonin, showed a mean increase in systolic blood pressure of 6.5 mm Hg, and in diastolic blood pressure of 4.9 mm Hg.[294]

Manipulative and Body-Based Practices. The manipulative and body-based practices include a wide range of hands-on interventions. Massage therapy studies have primarily been conducted for sleep disorders in infants and children. Studies in adult populations are limited and focus on patients with comorbid medical conditions. One study examined aromatherapy massage for hospice patients using self-report measures of sleep. Although this study reported no benefits in quality of life or pain control, there were statistically significant improvements in self-reports of sleep and depression.[295] Another randomized study compared therapeutic massage and relaxation tapes in the management of stress with both modalities showing improvements in sleep, but no significant benefit of one over the other.[296] Among patients with cardiovascular disease, massage therapy and its effects on sleep have received little attention.

Another form of manipulative therapy is acupressure, a noninvasive technique that involves stimulation of meridian or acupoints on the body using finger pressing movements. It can be administered by nursing staff or by family members of a patient. Acupressure in end-stage renal patients has shown improvements in self-reported sleep quality, sleep latency, and sleep efficiency.[297] Acupressure has had limited use in cardiac patients for sleep, requires further study, and has exhibited little effectiveness for lowering nausea and vomiting following cardiac surgery.[298]

Meditation. While there are several forms of meditation, one of the most commonly studied for insomnia is mindfulness meditation. Stress reduction may be one of the mechanisms by which meditation can exert a beneficial effect on sleep and most of the studies that have demonstrated improved sleep during meditation therapy have been conducted as stress reduction studies. In this regard, it can be used as part of a cognitive therapy approach. In addition to stress reduction, there may also be differences in slow-wave sleep as a result of meditation. Few studies have used meditation as a method to improve sleep in patients with cardiovascular disease but recent data from a yoga intervention, which included posture, breathing, and meditation, suggests it may improve autonomic function.[299]

Yoga. Yoga incorporates the holistic components of physical activity, specific postures, breathing exercises, and a philosophic attitude toward life. It has been shown to reduce anxiety levels and physiological arousal in cardiac patients.[300] A randomized, parallel group study conducted over a 6-month treatment period compared yoga (60-minute session 6 days a week, with a 15-minute evening session), Ayurvedic therapy, and wait-list control in 69 older adults. Self-reported sleep measures were assessed and demonstrated a 1-hour increase in total sleep time relative to pretreatment in the yoga group that was significantly higher than changes in the wait-list or Ayurveda groups.[301]

Tai Chi. Tai chi is a low- to moderate-intensity traditional Chinese exercise that includes a meditational component. Previous findings supports that Tai chi enhances aerobic capacity, muscular strength, endothelial function and psychological wellbeing.[302] A study of the effects of tai chi (three 60-minute sessions for 24 weeks) in older adults, in comparison to low-impact exercise, noted that Tai chi improved self-reported sleep duration by 48 minutes.[303] General health-related quality of life and daytime sleepiness levels also improved. Tai chi appears to be safe and effective for patients with MI and HF, and post-CABG surgery. Yeh et al[304] reported improved sleep time in patients receiving 12 weeks of Tai chi training compared to controls. Therefore, Tai chi may be viewed as an alternative exercise program that may enhance sleep for selected patients with cardiovascular diseases.

Cognitive Behavioral Therapy for Sleep Disturbances

Dysfunctional beliefs and attitudes about sleep contribute to SPD. In particular, cognitive processes such as worry over sleep and its consequences and automatic or altered beliefs are thought to play a critical role in the development and maintenance of SPD. An example of an altered belief system is the belief in need for 8 hours of sleep per night to feel refreshed. Since the amount of sleep varies among individuals, this belief can exacerbate or worsen SPD when this expectation is not met. These cognitive processes increase physiological and emotional arousal and in some individuals lead to a downward and cyclic trajectory that perpetuates the underlying.[305–310]

Nonpharmacologic approaches to management of SPD, particularly those emphasizing cognitive behavioral therapy to directly target faulty beliefs and negative thoughts about sleep, have increased in popularity over the past decade.[306,311] Conceptually, the basis for CBT is that dysfunctional thinking and behaviors associated with SPD are cognitively mediated. The cognitive component of CBT is tailored to the individual needs of the participant to identify, challenge, and change stressful, distorted sleep thoughts that contribute to SPD.[285,305,310,311] The behavioral aspects include sleep restriction therapy, modified stimulus control, and use of relaxation techniques which are described in greater detail in the section "Sleep Education and Hygiene".

Evidence from SPD research suggests that CBT results in short-term improvements that are as effective as pharmacotherapy with sedative-hypnotics. This effect is especially relevant given the adverse events and side effects associated with sedatives and hypnotics, especially among the elderly. The potentially greatest advantage of CBT is over time, since it may be more durable than pharmacotherapy because the beneficial effects persist after therapy has ended. Therefore, although CBT may be a more costly approach than pharmacotherapy in the short run, it becomes cost-effective over 6 months or longer.[312–314]

Previous studies of psychological interventions for insomnia have primarily used behavioral approaches such as stimulus control and sleep restriction, which focused on modifying maladaptive sleep habits.[308] The addition of cognitive restructuring that targets factors known to perpetuate SPDs (i.e., consequences of not falling asleep), or that reduce compliance with behavioral therapy may improve treatment effectiveness for SPDs.[305]

Pharmacological Interventions to Promote Sleep

The consequences and impact of insomnia (difficulty initiating and/or maintaining sleep, early morning awakenings, or unrefreshing sleep) are associated with a significant negative impact on daytime function including increased fatigue, decreased motivation and vigilance, reduced concentration, and impaired psychomotor function. Chronic sleep problems may also increase the risk of psychiatric disorders, such as depression and anxiety. In addition, the effects of poor sleep impact, not only the patient, but on family, friends, and caregivers. In many situations, the judicious use of pharmacologic agents to enhance sleep is indicated—often in conjunction with behavioral therapy. An assessment of the type and duration of the sleep problem within the context of the underlying cardiac disease should dictate which agent is used.[315] However, before initiating pharmacologic therapy, the medications taken by the patient should be carefully examined as many have the potential to disturb sleep (Display 8-4). Simply discontinuing, or advising that the patient take these medications that interfere with sleep in the morning rather (or visa versa) than at bedtime, may improve sleep. There are a number of pharmacologic agents currently used to enhance sleep and specific information regarding dose, action, and side effects appear in Table 8-1. As with all medications, follow-up and further evaluation of patient response to treatment is critical.

DISPLAY 8-4 Medications Associated with Insomnia

Antidepressants

Tricyclics
Amitriptyline
Doxepin
Imipramine
Trimipramine
Desipramine
Nortriptyline
Protriptyline

Selective Serotonin Reuptake Inhibitors
Fluoxetine
Paroxetine
Sertraline
Fluvoxamine

Serotonin and Norepinephrine Reuptake Inhibitors
Venlafaxine

Monoamine Oxidase Inhibitors
Phenelzine
Tranylcypromine

Antihypertensives

β-Blockers (Lipophilic Blockers)
Propranolol
Timolol

Others

Hypolipidemic Drugs
Atorvastatin
Lovastatin
Simvastatin

Nasal Decongestants
Pseudoephedrine
Phenylpropanolamine

Bronchodilators
Theophylline

Antiparkinsonian Medications
Levodopa

Corticosteroids
Prednisone

Adapted from Schweitzer, P. K. (2005). *Drugs that disturb sleep and wakefulness.* In M. H. Kryger, T., Roth, & W. C., Dement (Eds.), *Principles and practice of sleep medicine* (pp. 499–518). Philadelphia: Elsevier Saunders.

Over-the-Counter Medications

The major over the counter medications include antihistamines, melatonin, and herbal therapies, such as valerian. There are insufficient data to documents the effectiveness of the use of these agents.

Table 8-1 ■ PHARMACOLOGIC AGENTS THAT PROMOTE SLEEP

Medication	Dose	Action	Side Effects
Over the counter			
Diphenhydramine	25–50 mg	Histamine antagonist	Dry mouth, urinary retention, daytime drowsiness, fatigue, tinnitus, nausea, constipation, urinary retention
Valerian	400–900 mg	May increase $GABA_a$-like activity	Headache, weakness, hepatic toxicity
Melatonin		Melatonin receptor agonist	Headache, blood pressure alterations
Sedating Antidepressants (not FDA approved for insomnia)			
Trazadone	25–150 mg	Inhibition of serotonin reuptake with antihistaminic effects	Sedation, orthostatic hypotension, premature ventricular contraction, weight gain, priapism
Doxepine	25–150 mg	Inhibition of serotonin and norepinephrine reuptake, antihistaminic effects	Dry mouth, constipation, urinary retention, cardiac conduction delays, ocular crises in those with narrow-angle glaucoma, seizures, and anticholinergic delirium
Amitriptyline	25–150 mg		
Mirtazapine	15–30 mg	Antihistaminic effects	Sedation, dry mouth, increased appetite, weight gain
Antipsychotics			
Quetiapine	25 mg	Antihistaminic effects, serotonin, and dopamine antagonist	Asthenia, weight gain, postural hypotension, tachycardia, anorexia
Olanzapine	10 mg		Weight gain, somnolence, dizziness, headache, nervousness, postural hypotension, tachycardia, akathisia
Melatonin Receptor Agonist			
Ramelteon	8 mg	Synthetic melatonin receptor agonist	Depression, dizziness, fatigue, unpleasant taste, arthralgia
Benzodiazipines			
Temazepam	15–30 mg	Binds to $GABA_a$ type I and type II (nonselective) receptor with sedative, anxiolytic, muscle relaxant, and anticonvulsant effects	Dizziness, lethargy, confusion, headache, anorexia
Quazepam	7.5–15 mg		Drowsiness, headache, fatigue, dizziness, dry mouth
Estazolam	1–2 mg		Headache, dizziness, palpitations, anorexia
Flurazapam	15–30 mg		Lightheadedness, drowsiness, dizziness, nervousness, depression, nausea
Triazolam	0.125–0.25 mg		Drowsiness, headache, ataxia, memory impairment, anterograde amnesia, nausea
Nonbenzodiazepines			
Zolpidem	5–10 mg	Bind to $GABA_a$ type I receptor (selective) with sedative effects	Headache, lethargy, depression, anxiety, nausea
Zolpidem-extended release	7.5–12.5 mg		
Zaleplon	5–10 mg		Amnesia, dizziness, nervousness, nausea
Eszopiclone	2–3 mg		Headache, somnolence, unpleasant taste, tachycardia

Buysse, D. J., Schweitzer, P. K., Moul, D. E. (2005). Clinical pharmacology of other drugs used as hypnotics. In M. H. Kryger, T. Roth, W. C. Dement, (Eds.), *Principles and practice of sleep medicine* (pp. 452–467). Philadelphia: Elsevier Saunders.
Mendelson, W. B. (2005). Pharmacology. In M. H. Kryger, T. Roth, & W. C. Dement, (Eds.), *Principles and practice of sleep medicine* (pp. 444–451). Philadelphia: Elsevier Saunders.

Adverse effect may include residual daytime sedation and decreased cognitive function in the elderly. Antihistamines may also have anticholinergic side effects (dry mouth, blurred vision, urinary retention, constipation, etc.) and may be contraindicated in patients with cardiac disease. Hepatotoxicity following use of valerian has also been reported.[315,316] Lack of regulation by the Food and Drug Administration (FDA) results in variability of the quality of these preparations.[315] The use of melatonin was previously discussed.

Antidepressants

Trazadone is frequently used as a hypnotic and does have some initial sedating properties. However, these effects are not longstanding and research on its efficacy is limited.[317] In fact, the longest study on trazadone has been only 2 weeks in duration.[315] Major side effects include hypotension, lightheadedness, weakness, and abnormal penile erections. Trazadone has also been associated with hepatic failure and death.[317] Tricyclics, such as amitriptyline and doxepin, also have sedating properties but have shown little efficacy in treating insomnia. Both have anticholinergic side effects, the most important of which include hypotension, syncope, increased heart rate, and arrhythmias, making them generally contraindicated in cardiac patients.[317]

Benzodiazepines

Benzodiazepines bind nonselectively to and activate all α-receptor subtypes on the γ-aminobuteric acid (GABA) receptor, accounting for their hypnotic, myorelaxant, anticonvulsant, and amnestic effects. Binding to the GABA receptor opens the chloride channel, resulting in a hyperpolarized cell membrane, preventing further excitation of the cell. Polysomnographic studies of sleep indicate that benzodiazepines decreased sleep latency and wake time and increase total sleep time. Daytime sedation and dependency may become problematic. Worsening of sleep apnea has also been reported.[317] The benzodiazepines approved for use in insomnia differ primarily based on their half-life; triazolam (1.7 to 5 hours), temazepam (8 to

22 hours), estazolam (10 to 24 hours), quazepam (25 to 100 hours), and flurazepam (74 to 160 hour for active metabolite).[317]

Nonbenzodiazepines

The nonbenzodiazepines, recently approved by the FDA for insomnia, possess chemical structures that differ from each other as well as the traditional benzodiazepines.[315,317] These medications bind to the GABA receptor at a selective and limited recognition site, explaining the absence of myorelaxant and anticonvulsant effects. Three nonbenzodiazepine drugs (and their half-lives) are indicated for insomnia—zolpidem (regular formulation 2.5 hour; continued release 2.8 hours), zaleplon (1 hour), and eszopiclone (6 hours in adult; 9 hours in elderly) (see Table 8-1). These medications have demonstrated efficacy in acute management of chronic insomnia. Longer term studies also suggest their efficacy. Potentially serious side effects include nocturnal falls, sleep walking, and sleep eating.[315,318] This class of medications does not appear to adversely affect nocturnal respiration or apnea severity.[315]

THE HEALTH CARE PROVIDERS' SLEEP

Hospital nurses, physicians, and others who work the night shift or rotating schedules often experience irregular sleep–wake schedules and inferior sleep, causing reduced alertness and general fatigue. This reduced alertness and fatigue is accentuated by the pronounced circadian alertness–sleepiness rhythm, with maximal sleepiness and lowest performance at approximately 4:00 to 5:00 AM, at the low point of the body temperature rhythm.[319] Mental tasks that require sustained visual attention, such as monitoring an ECG oscilloscope or driving home from work, are more affected than are physical tasks.[320] Suggested strategies to improve shift worker's sleep/rest include staying on a night schedule on nonwork days (often socially unattractive), scheduling one or more nights off after night duty, reduced work hours (no shift greater than 12 hours) fatigue management, sleep hygiene education for staff, using rotation schedules that move forward around the clock rather than backward, and taking a nap before going to work.[321] Use of melatonin in the evening to help reset the circadian timing system or bright light therapy to suppress natural melatonin secretion from the pineal gland also appear to be promising strategies.[322]

Sleep deprivation among nurses and physicians has been shown to be related to serious medical errors as well as occupational injuries.[320,321] Mandates from the Accreditation Council for Graduate Medical Education (ACGME) were issued several years ago limiting work hours to promote improved sleep–work habits and performance and reduced sleepiness. Parthasarathy et al[323] studied the effect of work-hour reduction on quality of life of residents and fellows and observed minor improvements in sleep time, subjective sleepiness and quality of life during an ICU rotation; however, significant levels of objective sleepiness were retained. Thus, optimal scheduling and further work-hour reduction measures may need to be undertaken to address the persistence of sleepiness in critical care medical and nursing staff.

SUMMARY

Patients with cardiovascular disease often have disturbed sleep, especially in intensive cardiac care settings, and may be at risk for physiological changes during sleep that adversely affect their health status. Sleep disorders contribute to risk for cardiac disease and to other cardiac risk factors. Although beliefs regarding the relationship between sleep and well being are widely shared, hospital practices are rarely designed to encourage optimal sleep. Research is needed to clarify the role of night-time sleep and daytime naps in recovery from cardiovascular disease and surgery (e.g., what are optimal sleep patterns?) and to identify nursing interventions that prevent sleep deprivation, minimize adverse sleep-related physiological changes, and promote good sleep.

REFERENCES

1. Javaheri, S. (2005). Sleep and cardiovascular disease: Present and future. In M. H. Kryger, T. Roth, & W. C. Dement (Eds.), *Principles and practice of sleep medicine* (pp. 1157–1160). Philadelphia: Elsevier Saunders.
2. Somers, V. K., White, D. P., Amin, R., et al. (2008). Sleep apnea and cardiovascular disease. An American Heart Association/American College of Cardiology Foundation Scientific Statement from the American Heart Association Council for High Blood Pressure Research Professional Education Committee, Council on Clinical Cardiology, Stroke Council, and Council on Cardiovascular Nursing Council. *Circulation, 118*, 1080–1111.
3. Thorpy, M. J. (19991). History of sleep and man. In M. J. Thorpy & J. Yager (Eds.), *The encyclopedia of sleep and sleep disorders* (pp. ix–xxxiii). New York: Oxford.
4. Carskadon, M. A., & Dement, W. C. (2005). Normal human sleep: An overview. In M. H. Kryger, T. Roth, & W. C. Dement (Eds.), *Principles and practice of sleep medicine* (pp. 13–23). Philadelphia: WB Saunders Company.
5. Collop, N. A., Salas, R. E., Delayo, M., et al. (2008). Normal sleep and circadian processes. *Critical Care Clinics, 24*, 449–460.
6. Andruskiene, J., Varoneckas, G., Martinkenas, A., et al. (2008). Factors associated with poor sleep and health-related quality of life. *Medicina (Kaunas), 44*, 240–246.
7. Orwelius, L., Nordlund, A., Nordlund, P., et al. (2008). Prevalence of sleep disturbances and long-term reduced health-related quality of life after critical care: A prospective multicenter cohort study. *Critical Care, 12*, R97.
8. Saleh, P., & Shapiro, C. M. (2008). Disturbed sleep and burnout: Implications for long-term health. *Journal of Psychosomatic Research, 65*, 1–3.
9. Trupp, R. J. (2008). Sleep and health. *Progress in Cardiovascular Nursing, 23*, 60–62.
10. American Academy of Sleep Medicine. (2005). *The international classification of sleep disorders*. Westchester, IL: American Academy of Sleep Medicine.
11. Chervin, R. D., & Aldrich, M. S. (1999). The Epworth Sleepiness Scale may not reflect objective measures of sleepiness or sleep apnea. *Neurology, 52*, 125–131.
12. Rechtschaffen, A., & Kales, A. (1968). *A manual of standard terminology: Techniques and scoring system for sleep stages in human subjects*. Washington, DC: U.S. Government Printing Office.
13. Roehrs, T., Carskadon, M. A., Dement, W. C., et al. (2005). Daytime sleepiness and alertness. In M. H. Kryger, T. Roth, & W. C. Dement (Eds.), *Principles and practice of sleep medicine* (pp. 39–50). Philadelphia: Elsevier Saunders.
14. Kaida, K., Takahashi, M., Haratani, T., et al. (2006). Indoor exposure to natural bright light prevents afternoon sleepiness. *Sleep, 29*, 462–469.
15. Carskadon, M. A., & Rechtschaffen, A. (2005). Monitoring and staging of human sleep. In M. H. Kryger, T. Roth, & W. C. Dement (Eds.), *Principles and practice of sleep medicine* (pp. 1359–1378). Philadelphia: WB Saunders Company.
16. Chase, J. M. Brain electrical activity and sensory processing during wakefulness and sleep states. In M. H. Kryger, T. Roth, & W. C. Dement (Eds.), *Principles and practice of sleep medicine* (pp. 101–119). Philadelphia: Elsevier Saunders.
17. Steriade, M. (2005). Brain electrical activity and sensory processing during wakefulness and sleep states. In M. H. Kryger, T. Roth, & W. C. Dement (Eds.), *Principles and practice of sleep medicine* (p. 101). Philadelphia: Elsevier Saunders.
18. Siegel, J. M. (2005). REM sleep. In M. H. Kryger, T. Roth, & W. C. Dement (Eds.), *Principles and practice of sleep medicine* (pp. 120–135). Philadelphia: Elsevier Saunders.

19. Johnson, H., Swan, T., & Weigand, G. (1930). In what positions do healthy people sleep? *Journal of the American Medical Association, 94*, 2058–2062.
20. Kleitman, N., Cooperman, N., & Mullin, F. (1933). Studies on the physiology of sleep IX. Motility and body temperature during sleep. *American Journal of Physiology, 105*, 574–584.
21. Moses, J., Lubin, A., Naitoh P., et al. (1972). Reliability of sleep measures. *Psychophysiology, 9*, 78–82.
22. Walters, A. S. (2007). Clinical identification of the simple sleep-related movement disorders. *Chest, 131*, 1260–1266.
23. Cirelli, C., & Bushey, D. (2008). Sleep and wakefulness in Drosophila melanogaster. *Annals of the New York Academy of Science, 1129*, 323–329.
24. Mackiewicz, M., Naidoo, N., Zimmerman, J. E., et al. (2008). Molecular mechanisms of sleep and wakefulness. *Annals of the New York Academy of Science, 1129*, 335–349.
25. Zepelin, H., & Rechtschaffen, A. (1974). Mammalian sleep, longevity, and energy metabolism. *Brain, Behavior and Evolution, 10*, 425–470.
26. Tobler, I. (2005). Phylogeny of sleep regulation. In M. H. Kryger, T. Roth, & W. C. Dement (Eds.), *Principles and practice of sleep medicine* (pp. 77–90). Philadelphia: Elsevier Saunders.
27. Peirano, P. D., & Algarin, C. R. (2007). Sleep in brain development. *Biological Research, 40*, 471–478.
28. Euston, D. R., Tatsuno, M., & McNaughton, B. L. (2007). Fast-forward playback of recent memory sequences in prefrontal cortex during sleep. *Science, 318*, 1147–1150.
29. Dang-Vu, T. T., Desseilles, M., Peigneux, P., et al. (2006). A role for sleep in brain plasticity. *Pediatric Rehabilitation, 9*, 98–118.
30. Maquet, P. (2001). The role of sleep in learning and memory. *Science, 294*, 1048–1052.
31. Peigneux, P., Laureys, S., Delbeuck, X., et al. (2001). Sleeping brain, learning brain. The role of sleep for memory systems. *Neuroreport, 12*, A111–A124.
32. Banks, S., & Dinges, D. F. (2007). Behavioral and physiological consequences of sleep restriction. *Journal of Clinical Sleep Medicine, 3*, 519–528.
33. Dinges, D. F. (2006). The state of sleep deprivation: From functional biology to functional consequences. *Sleep Medicine Reviews, 10*, 303–305.
34. Lim, J., & Dinges, D. F. (2008). Sleep deprivation and vigilant attention. *Annals of the New York Academy of Sciences, 1129*, 305–322.
35. Mignot, E. (2008). Why we sleep: The temporal organization of recovery. *PLoS Biology, 6*, e106.
36. Heller, H. C. (2005). Temperature, thermoregulation, and sleep. In M. H. Kryger, T. Roth, & W. C. Dement (Eds.), *Principles and practice of sleep medicine* (pp. 292–304). Philadelphia: Elsevier Saunders.
37. Raymann, R. J., Swaab, D. F., & Van Someren, E. J. (2008). Skin deep: Enhanced sleep depth by cutaneous temperature manipulation. *Brain, 131*, 500–513.
38. Krauchi, K. (2007). The human sleep-wake cycle reconsidered from a thermoregulatory point of view. *Physiology and Behavior, 90*, 236–245.
39. Kreuger, J. M., & Majde, J. A. (2005). Host defense. In M. H. Kryger, T. Roth, & W. C. Dement (Eds.), *Principles and practice of sleep medicine* (pp. 256–265). Philadelphia: Elsevier Saunders.
40. Opp, M. R. (2005). Cytokines and sleep. *Sleep Medicine Reviews, 9*, 355–364.
41. Lack, L. C., Gradisar, M., Van Someren, E. J., et al. (2008). The relationship between insomnia and body temperatures. *Sleep Medicine Reviews, 12*, 307–317.
42. Krauchi, K., & Wirz-Justice, A. (2001). Circadian clues to sleep onset mechanisms. *Neuropsychopharmacology, 25*, S92–S96.
43. Krauchi, K., Cajochen, C., Werth, E., et al. (1999). Warm feet promote the rapid onset of sleep. *Nature, 401*, 36–37.
44. Dimitrov, S., Lange, T., Nohroudi, K., et al. (2007). Number and function of circulating human antigen presenting cells regulated by sleep. *Sleep, 30*, 401–411.
45. Borbely, A. A., & Acherman, P. (2005). Sleep homeostasis and models of sleep regulation. In M. H. Kryger, T. Roth, & W. C. Dement (Eds.), *Principles and practice of sleep medicine* (pp. 405–417). Philadelphia: Elsevier Saunders.
46. McCarley, R. W. (2007). Neurobiology of REM and NREM sleep. *Sleep Medicine, 8*, 302–330.
47. Van Someren, E. J. (2006). Mechanisms and functions of coupling between sleep and temperature rhythms. *Progress in Brain Research, 153*, 309–324.
48. Bliwise, D. L. (2005). Normal aging. In M. H. Kryger, T. Roth, & W. C. Dement (Eds.), *Principles and practice of sleep medicine* (pp. 24–38). Philadelphia: WB Saunders.
49. Unruh, M. L., Redline, S., An, M. W., et al. (2008). Subjective and objective sleep quality and aging in the Sleep Heart Health Study. *Journal of the American Geriatric Society, 56*, 1218–1227.
50. Norman, D., & Loredo, J. S. (2008). Obstructive sleep apnea in older adults. *Clinics in Geriatric Medicine, 24*, 151–165.
51. Karatas, M. (2007). Restless legs syndrome and periodic limb movements during sleep: Diagnosis and treatment. *Neurologist, 13*, 294–301.
52. Ferri, R., Manconi, M., Lanuzza, B., et al. (2007). Age-related changes in periodic leg movements during sleep in patients with restless legs syndrome. *Sleep Medicine, 9*, 790–798.
53. Malhotra, A., Huang, Y., Fogel, R., et al. (2006). Aging influences on pharyngeal anatomy and physiology: The predisposition to pharyngeal collapse. *American Journal of Medicine, 119*, 72.e9–72.e14.
54. Spiegelhalder, K., & Hornyak, M. (2008). Restless legs syndrome in older adults. *Clinics in Geriatric Medicine, 24*, 167–180.
55. Harrington, J. J., Lee-Chiong, T., Jr. (2007). Sleep and older patients. *Clinics in Chest Medicine, 28*, 673–684.
56. Wysowski, D. K., & Baum, C. (1991). Outpatient use of prescription sedative-hypnotic drugs in the United States, 1970 through 1989. *Archives of Internal Medicine, 151*, 1779–1783.
57. Manabe, K., Matsui, T., Yamaya, M., et al. (2000). Sleep patterns and mortality among elderly patients in a geriatric hospital. *Gerontology, 46*, 318–322.
58. Gangwisch, J. E., Heymsfield, S. B., Boden-Albala, B., et al. (2008). Sleep duration associated with mortality in elderly, but not middle-aged, adults in a large US sample. *Sleep, 31*, 1087–1096.
59. Verrier, R. L., Harper, R. M., & Hobson, J. A. (2005). Cardiovascular physiology: Central and autonomic regulation. In M. H. Kryger, T. Roth, & W. C. Dement (Eds.), *Principles and practice of sleep medicine* (pp. 192–202). Philadelphia: Elsevier Saunders.
60. Penzel, T., Wessel, N., Riedl, M., et al. (2007). Cardiovascular and respiratory dynamics during normal and pathological sleep. *Chaos, 17*, 015116.
61. Coccagna, G., Mantovani, M., Brignani, F., et al. (1972). Continuous recording of the pulmonary and systemic arterial pressure during sleep in syndromes of hypersomnia with periodic breathing. *Bulletin in Physiopathology Respiration (Nancy), 8*, 1159–1172.
62. Lugaresi, E., Coccagna, G., Cirignotta, F., et al. (1978). Breathing during sleep in man in normal and pathological conditions. *Advances in Experimental Medicine and Biology, 99*, 35–45.
63. Blasi, A., Jo, J., Valladares, E., et al. (2003). Cardiovascular variability after arousal from sleep: Time-varying spectral analysis. *Journal of Applied Physiology, 95*, 1394–1404.
64. Tank, J., Diedrich, A., Hale, N., et al. (2003). Relationship between blood pressure, sleep K-complexes, and muscle sympathetic nerve activity in humans. *American Journal of Physiology—Regulatory, Integrative and Comparative Physiology, 285*, R208–R214.
65. Gosselin, N., Michaud, M., Carrier, J., et al. (2002). Age difference in heart rate changes associated with micro-arousals in humans. *Clinical Neurophysiology, 113*, 1517–1521.
66. Mulcahy, D., Wright, C., Sparrow, J., et al. (1993). Heart rate and blood pressure consequences of an afternoon SIESTA (snooze-induced excitation of sympathetic triggered activity). *American Journal of Cardiology, 71*, 611–614.
67. Floras, J. S., Jones, J. V., Johnston, J. A., et al. (1978). Arousal and the circadian rhythm of blood pressure. *Clinical Science and Molecular Medicine—Supplement, 4*, 395s–397s.
68. Valladares, E. M., Eljammal, S. M., Motivala, S., et al. (2008). Sex differences in cardiac sympathovagal balance and vagal tone during nocturnal sleep. *Sleep Medicine, 9*, 310–316.
69. Monti, A., Medigue, C., Nedelcoux, H., et al. (2002). Autonomic control of the cardiovascular system during sleep in normal subjects. *European Journal of Applied Physiology, 87*, 174–181.
70. Krieger, J. (2005). Respiratory physiology: Breathing in normal subjects. In M. H. Kryger, T. Roth, & W. C. Dement (Eds.), *Principles and practice of sleep medicine* (pp. 232–244). Philadelphia: Elsevier Saunders.
71. Douglas, N. J. (2005). Respiratory physiology: Control of ventilation. In M. H. Kryger, T. Roth, & W. C. Dement (Eds.), *Principles and practice of sleep medicine* (pp. 224–231). Philadelphia: Elsevier Saunders.
72. Jordan, A. S., McEvoy, R. D., Edwards, J. K., et al. (2004). The influence of gender and upper airway resistance on the ventilatory response

to arousal in obstructive sleep apnoea in humans. *Journal of Physiology, 558*, 993–1004.

73. Jordan, A. S., Eckert, D. J., Catcheside, P. G., et al. (2003). Ventilatory response to brief arousal from non-rapid eye movement sleep is greater in men than in women. *American Journal of Respiratory Critical Care Medicine, 168*, 1512–1519.
74. Douglas, N. J. (2005). Asthma and chronic obstructive pulmonary disease. In M. H. Kryger, T. Roth, & W. C. Dement (Eds.), *Principles and practice of sleep medicine* (pp. 1112–1135). Philadelphia: Elsevier Saunders.
75. Gleeson, K., Eggli, D. F., & Maxwell, S. L. (1997). Quantitative aspiration during sleep in normal subjects. *Chest, 111*, 1266–1272.
76. Franzini, C. (2005). Cardiovascular physiology: The peripheral circulation. In M. H. Kryger, T. Roth, & W. C. Dement (Eds.), *Principles and practice of sleep medicine* (pp. 203–212). Philadelphia: Elsevier Saunders.
77. Maquet, P., Degueldre, C., Delfiore, G., et al. (1997). Functional neuroanatomy of human slow wave sleep. *Journal of Neuroscience, 17*, 2807–2812.
78. Maquet, P., & Phillips, C. Functional brain imaging of human sleep. *Journal of Sleep Research, 7*(Suppl. 1), 42–47.
79. Maquet, P., Peters, J., Aerts, J., et al. (1996). Functional neuroanatomy of human rapid-eye-movement sleep and dreaming. *Nature, 383*, 163–166.
80. Maquet, P. (2004). A role for sleep in the processing of memory traces. Contribution of functional neuroimaging in humans. *Bulletin on Member Academy of Royal Medicine of Belgium, 159*, 167–170.
81. Chee, M. W., Chuah, L. Y., Venkatraman, V., et al. (2006). Functional imaging of working memory following normal sleep and after 24 and 35 h of sleep deprivation: Correlations of fronto-parietal activation with performance. *NeuroImage, 31*, 419–428.
82. Buxton, O. M., Spiegel, K., & Van Cauter, E. (2002). Modulation of endocrine function and metabolism by sleep and sleep loss. In T. L. Lee-Chiong, M. J. Sateia, & M. A. Carskadon (Eds.), Sleep medicine (pp. 59–69). Philadelphia: Hanley & Belfus.
83. Moore-Ede, M. C., Meguid, M. M., Fitzpatrick, G. F., et al. (1978). Circadian variation in response to potassium infusion. *Clinical Pharmacology and Therapeutics, 23*, 218–227.
84. Ware, J. C., & Hirshkowitz. (2005). Assessment of sleep-related erections. In M. H. Kryger, T. Roth, & W. C. Dement (Eds.), *Principles and practice of sleep medicine* (pp. 1394–1402). Philadelphia: Elsevier Saunders.
85. Van Cauter, E. (2005). Endocrine physiology. In M. H. Kryger, T. Roth, & W. C. Dement (Eds.), *Principles and practice of sleep medicine* (pp. 266–282). Philadelphia: Elsevier Saunders.
86. Scheer, F. A., Cajochen, C., Turek, F. W., et al. (2005). Melatonin and the regulation of sleep and circadian rhythms. In M. H. Kryger, T. Roth, & W. C. Dement (Eds.), *Principles and practice of sleep medicine* (pp. 395–404). Philadelphia: Elsevier Saunders.
87. Bonnefond, A., Roge, J., & Muzet, A. (2006). Behavioural reactivation and subjective assessment of the state of vigilance—application to simulated car driving. *International Journal of Occupational Safety and Ergonomics, 12*, 221–229.
88. Currie, S. R., Malhotra, S., & Clark, S. (2004). Agreement among subjective, objective, and collateral measures of insomnia in postwithdrawal recovering alcoholics. *Behavioral Sleep Medicine, 2*, 148–161.
89. Hossain, J. L., Ahmad, P., Reinish, L. W., et al. (2005). Subjective fatigue and subjective sleepiness: Two independent consequences of sleep disorders? *Journal of Sleep Research, 14*, 245–253.
90. Richardson, A., Crow, W., Coghill, E., et al. (2007). A comparison of sleep assessment tools by nurses and patients in critical care. *Journal of Clinical Nursing, 16*, 1660–1668.
91. Tworoger, S. S., Davis, S., Vitiello, M. V., et al. (2005). Factors associated with objective (actigraphic) and subjective sleep quality in young adult women. *Journal of Psychosomatic Research, 59*, 11–19.
92. Kushida, C. A., Chang, A., Gadkary, C., et al. (2001). Comparison of actigraphic, polysomnographic, and subjective assessment of sleep parameters in sleep-disordered patients. *Sleep Medicine, 2*, 389–396.
93. Spielman, A. J., & Yang, C. M. (2005). Glovinsky. Assessment techniques for insomnia. In M. H. Kryger, T. Roth, & W. C. Dement (Eds.), *Principles and practice of sleep medicine* (pp. 1403–1416). Philadelphia: Elsevier Saunders.
94. Buysse, D. J., Reynolds, C. F., III, Monk, T. H., et al. (1989). The Pittsburgh Sleep Quality Index: A new instrument for psychiatric practice and research. *Psychiatry Research, 28*, 193–213.
95. Cole, J. C., Motivala, S. J., Buysse, D. J., et al. (2006). Validation of a 3-factor scoring model for the Pittsburgh sleep quality index in older adults. *Sleep, 29*, 112–116.
96. Ehlers, C. L., Kupfer, D. J., Buysse, D. J., et al. (1998). The Pittsburgh study of normal sleep in young adults: Focus on the relationship between waking and sleeping EEG spectral patterns. *Electroencephalogr and Clinical Neurophysiology, 106*, 199–205.
97. Ellis, B. W., Johns, M. W., Lancaster, R., et al. (1981). The St. Mary's Hospital sleep questionnaire: A study of reliability. *Sleep, 4*, 93–97.
98. Douglass, A. B., Carskadon, M. A., & Houser, R. (1990). Historical data base, questionnaries, sleep and life cycle diaries. In L. E. Miles & R. Broughton (Ed.), *Medical monitoring in the home and work environment* (pp. 17–28). New York: Raven Press.
99. Parrott, A. C., & Hindmarch, I. (1980). The Leeds Sleep Evaluation Questionnaire in psychopharmacological investigations—a review. *Psychopharmacology (Berlin), 71*, 173–179.
100. Reuveni, H., Tarasiuk, A., Wainstock, T., et al. (2004). Awareness level of obstructive sleep apnea syndrome during routine unstructured interviews of a standardized patient by primary care physicians. *Sleep, 27*, 1518–1525.
101. Shaver, J. L., & Giblin, E. C. (1989). Sleep. *Annual Review of Nursing Research, 7*, 71–93.
102. Johns, M. W. (1991). A new method for measuring daytime sleepiness: The Epworth sleepiness scale. *Sleep, 14*, 540–545.
103. Johns, M. W. (1992). Reliability and factor analysis of the Epworth Sleepiness Scale. *Sleep, 15*, 376–381.
104. Johns, M. W. (1994). Sleepiness in different situations measured by the Epworth Sleepiness Scale. *Sleep, 17*, 703–710.
105. Mitler, M. M., Carskadon, M. A., & Hirshkowitz, M. (2005). Evaluating sleepiness. In M. H. Kryger, T. Roth, & W. C. Dement (Eds.), *Principles and practice of sleep medicine* (pp. 1417–1423). Philadelphia: Elsevier Saunders.
106. Johns, M. W. (2000). Sensitivity and specificity of the multiple sleep latency test (MSLT), the maintenance of wakefulness test and the epworth sleepiness scale: Failure of the MSLT as a gold standard. *Journal of Sleep Research, 9*, 5–11.
107. Rosenthal, L. D., & Dolan, D. C. (2008). The Epworth sleepiness scale in the identification of obstructive sleep apnea. *Journal of Nervous Mental Disorder, 196*, 429–431.
108. Walter, T. J., Foldvary, N., Mascha, E., et al. (2002). Comparison of Epworth Sleepiness Scale scores by patients with obstructive sleep apnea and their bed partners. *Sleep Medicine, 3*, 29–32.
109. Monasterio, C., Vidal, S., Duran, J., et al. (2001). Effectiveness of continuous positive airway pressure in mild sleep apnea-hypopnea syndrome. *American Journal of Respiratory Critical Care Medicine, 164*, 939–943.
110. Sin, D. D., Mayers, I., Man, G. C., et al. (2002). Long-term compliance rates to continuous positive airway pressure in obstructive sleep apnea: A population-based study. *Chest, 121*, 430–435.
111. Pizza, F., Contardi, S., Mostacci, B., et al. (2004). A driving simulation task: Correlations with Multiple Sleep Latency Test. *Brain Research Bulletin, 63*, 423–426.
112. Ancoli-Israel, S., Cole, R., Alessi, C., et al. (2003). The role of actigraphy in the study of sleep and circadian rhythms. *Sleep, 26*, 342–392.
113. Blackwell, T., Redline, S., Ancoli-Israel S., et al. (2008). Comparison of sleep parameters from actigraphy and polysomnography in older women: The SOF study. *Sleep, 31*, 283–291.
114. Pollak, C. P., Tryon, W. W., Nagaraja, H., et al. (2001). How accurately does wrist actigraphy identify the states of sleep and wakefulness? *Sleep, 24*, 957–965.
115. Jean-Louis, G., von Gizycki, H., Zizi, F., et al. (1996). Determination of sleep and wakefulness with the actigraph data analysis software (ADAS). *Sleep, 19*, 739–743.
116. Sadeh, A., & Acebo, C. (2002). The role of actigraphy in sleep medicine. *Sleep Medicine Reviews, 6*, 113–124.
117. Sadeh, A., Hauri, P. J., Kripke, D. F., et al. (1995). The role of actigraphy in the evaluation of sleep disorders. *Sleep, 18*, 288–302.
118. Aasvang, G. M., Moum, T., & Engdahl, B. (2008). Self-reported sleep disturbances due to railway noise: Exposure-response relationships for nighttime equivalent and maximum noise levels. *Journal of Acoustical Society of America, 124*, 257–268.
119. Basner, M., Glatz, C., Griefahn, B., et al. (2008). Aircraft noise: Effects on macro- and microstructure of sleep. *Sleep Medicine, 9*, 382–387.

120. Basner, M., Muller, U., Elmenhorst, E. M., et al. (2008). Aircraft noise effects on sleep: A systematic comparison of EEG awakenings and automatically detected cardiac activations. *Physiological Measure, 29*, 1089–1103.
121. Muzet, A. (2007). Environmental noise, sleep and health. *Sleep Medicine Reviews, 11*, 135–142.
122. Parker, K. P. (1995). Promoting sleep and rest in critically ill patients. *Critical Care Nursing Clinics of North America, 7*, 337–349.
123. Lee, K. A. (2003). Impaired sleep. In V. Carrieri-Kohlman, A. M. Lindsey, & C. M. West (Eds.), *Pathophysiological phenomena in nursing: Human responses to illness* (pp. 363–385). St. Louis: Saunders.
124. Frey, D. J., Fleshner, M., Wright, K. P., Jr. (2007). The effects of 40 hours of total sleep deprivation on inflammatory markers in healthy young adults. *Brain, Behavior and Immunity, 21*, 1050–1057.
125. Kundermann, B., Hemmeter-Spernal, J., Huber, M. T., et al. (2008). Effects of total sleep deprivation in major depression: Overnight improvement of mood is accompanied by increased pain sensitivity and augmented pain complaints. *Psychosomatic Medicine, 70*, 92–101.
126. Lockley, S. W., Barger, L. K., Ayas, N. T., et al. (2007). Effects of health care provider work hours and sleep deprivation on safety and performance. *Joint Commission Journal on Quality of Patient Safety, 33*, 7–18.
127. McKenna, B. S., Dicjinson, D. L., Orff, H. J., et al. (2007). The effects of one night of sleep deprivation on known-risk and ambiguous-risk decisions. *Journal of Sleep Research, 16*, 245–252.
128. Salas, R. E., & Gamaldo, C. E. (2008). Adverse effects of sleep deprivation in the ICU. *Critical Care Clinics, 24*, 461–476, v–vi.
129. Wisor, J. P., Pasumarthi, R. K., Gerashchenko, D., et al. (2008). Sleep deprivation effects on circadian clock gene expression in the cerebral cortex parallel electroencephalographic differences among mouse strains. *Journal of Neuroscience, 28*, 7193–7201.
130. Zhang, N., & Liu, H. T. (2008). Effects of sleep deprivation on cognitive functions. *Neuroscience Bulletin, 24*, 45–48.
131. Hublin, C., Partinen, M., Koskenvuo, M., et al. (2007). Sleep and mortality: A population-based 22-year follow-up study. *Sleep, 30*, 1245–1253.
132. Ferrie, J. E., Shipley, M. J., Cappuccio, F. P., et al. (2007). A prospective study of change in sleep duration: Associations with mortality in the Whitehall II cohort. *Sleep, 30*, 1659–1666.
133. Hammond, E. C. (1964). Some preliminary findings on physical complaints from a prospective study of 1,064,004 men and women. *American Journal of Public Health Nations Health, 54*, 11–23.
134. Kripke, D. F., Simons, R. N., Garfinkel, L., et al. (1979). Short and long sleep and sleeping pills. Is increased mortality associated? *Archives of General Psychiatry, 36*, 103–116.
135. Youngstedt, S. D., & Kripke, D. F. (2004). Long sleep and mortality: Rationale for sleep restriction. *Sleep Medicine Reviews, 8*, 159–174.
136. Bliwise, D. L., & Young, T. B. (2007). The parable of parabola: What the U-shaped curve can and cannot tell us about sleep. *Sleep, 30*, 1614–1615.
137. Bursztyn, M., Ginsberg, G., Hammerman-Rozenberg, R., et al. (1999). The siesta in the elderly: risk factor for mortality? *Archives of Internal Medicine, 159*, 1582–1586.
138. Bursztyn, M., Ginsberg, G., & Stessman, J. (2002). The siesta and mortality in the elderly: Effect of rest without sleep and daytime sleep duration. *Sleep, 25*, 187–191.
139. Redline, S., Tishler, P. V., Hans, M. G., et al. (1997). Racial differences in sleep-disordered breathing in African-Americans and Caucasians. *American Journal of Respiratory Critical Care Medicine, 155*, 186–192.
140. Schmidt-Nowara, W. W., Coultas, D. B., Wiggins, C., et al. (1990). Snoring in a Hispanic-American population. Risk factors and association with hypertension and other morbidity. *Archives of Internal Medicine, 150*, 597–601.
141. Guilleminault, C., & Bassiri, A. (2005). Clinical features and evaluation of obstructive sleep apnea and upper airway resistance syndrome. In M. H. Kryger, T. Roth, & W. C. Dement (Eds.), *Principles and practice of sleep medicine* (pp. 1043–1053). Philadelphia: Elsevier Saunders.
142. Desai, A. V., Marks, G., & Grunstein, R. (2003). Does sleep deprivation worsen mild obstructive sleep apnea? *Sleep, 26*, 1038–1041.
143. Desai, A. V., Marks, G. B., Jankelson, D., et al. (2006). Do sleep deprivation and time of day interact with mild obstructive sleep apnea to worsen performance and neurobehavioral function? *Journal of Clinical Sleep Medicine, 2*, 63–70.
144. Persson, H. E., & Svanborg, E. (1996). Sleep deprivation worsens obstructive sleep apnea. Comparison between diurnal and nocturnal polysomnography. *Chest, 109*, 645–650.
145. Rains, V. S., Ditzler, T. F., Newsome, R. D., et al. (1991). Alcohol and sleep apnea. *Hawaii Medical Journal, 50*, 282–287.
146. Remmers, J. E. (1984). Obstructive sleep apnea. A common disorder exacerbated by alcohol. *American Review of Respiratory Disease, 130*, 153–155.
147. Peppard, P. E., Austin, D., & Brown, R. L. (2007). Association of alcohol consumption and sleep disordered breathing in men and women. *Journal of Clinical Sleep Medicine, 3*, 265–270.
148. Nunes, J. P. (2008). Usage of antihypertensive drugs and benzodiazepines to estimate apnea/hypopnea index in arterial hypertension. *Clinical and Experimental Hypertension, 30*, 143–150.
149. Young. T., & Javaheri S. (2005). Systemic and pulmonary hypertension in obstructive sleep apnea. In M. H. Kryger, T. Roth, & W. C. Dement (Eds.), *Principles and practice of sleep medicine* (pp. 1192–1202). Philadelphia: Elsevier Saunders.
150. Kessler, R., Chaouat, A., Weitzenblum, E., et al. (1996). Pulmonary hypertension in the obstructive sleep apnoea syndrome: Prevalence, causes and therapeutic consequences. *European Respiratory Journal, 9*, 787–794.
151. Laks, L., Lehrhaft, B., Grunstein, R. R., et al. (1995). Pulmonary hypertension in obstructive sleep apnoea. *European Respiratory Journal, 8*, 537–541.
152. Sanner, B. M., Doberauer, C., Konermann, M., et al. (1997). Pulmonary hypertension in patients with obstructive sleep apnea syndrome. *Archives of Internal Medicine, 157*, 2483–2487.
153. Gottlieb, D. J., Redline, S., Nieto, F. J., et al. (2006). Association of usual sleep duration with hypertension: The Sleep Heart Health Study. *Sleep, 29*, 1009–1014.
154. Haas, D. C., Foster, G. L., Nieto, F. J., et al. (2005). Age-dependent associations between sleep-disordered breathing and hypertension: Importance of discriminating between systolic/diastolic hypertension and isolated systolic hypertension in the Sleep Heart Health Study. *Circulation, 111*, 614–621.
155. Nieto, F. J., Young, T. B., Lind, B. K., et al. (2000). Association of sleep-disordered breathing, sleep apnea, and hypertension in a large community-based study. Sleep Heart Health Study. *Journal of the American Medical Association, 283*, 1829–1836.
156. Peppard, P. E., Young, T., Palta, M., et al. (2000). Longitudinal study of moderate weight change and sleep-disordered breathing. *Journal of the American Medical Association, 284*, 3015–3021.
157. Peppard, P. E., Young, T., Palta, M., et al. (2000). Prospective study of the association between sleep-disordered breathing and hypertension. *New England Journal of Medicine, 342*, 1378–1384.
158. Somers, V. K., & Javaheri, S. (2005). Cardiovascular effects of sleep-related breathing disorder. In M. H. Kryger, T. Roth, & W. C. Dement (Eds.), *Principles and practice of sleep medicine* (pp. 1180–1191). Philadelphia: Elsevier Saunders.
159. Grunstein, R. (2005). Continuous positive airway pressure treatment for obstructive sleep apnea-hypopnea syndrome. In M. H. Kryger, T. Roth, & W. C. Dement (Eds.), *Principles and practice of sleep medicine* (pp. 1066–1080). Philadelphia: Elsevier Saunders.
160. Morgenthaler, T. I., Aurora, R. N., Brown, T., et al. (2008). Practice parameters for the use of autotitrating continuous positive airway pressure devices for titrating pressures and treating adult patients with obstructive sleep apnea syndrome: An update for 2007. An American Academy of Sleep Medicine report. *Sleep, 31*, 141–147.
161. Kushida, C. A., Morgenthaler, T. I., Littner, M. R., et al. (2006). Practice parameters for the treatment of snoring and Obstructive Sleep Apnea with oral appliances: An update for 2005. *Sleep, 29*, 240–243.
162. Morgenthaler, T. I., Kapen, S., Lee-Chiong, T., et al. (2006). Practice parameters for the medical therapy of obstructive sleep apnea. *Sleep, 29*, 1031–1035.
163. Powell, N. B., Riley, R. W., & Guilleminault, C. (2005). Surgical management of sleep-disordered breathing. In M. H. Kryger, T. Roth, & W. C. Dement (Eds.), *Principles and practice of sleep medicine* (pp. 1081–1097). Philadelphia: Elsevier Saunders.
164. Cheyne, J. (1818). A case of apoplexy in which the fleshy part of the heart was converted into fat. *Dublin Hospital Report, 2*, 216–222.
165. Stokes, W. (1854). *The disease of the heart and aorta*. Dublin: Hodges & Smith.
166. White, D. P. (2005). Central sleep apnea. In M. H. Kryger, T. Roth, & W. C. Dement (Eds.), *Principles and practice of sleep medicine* (pp. 969–982). Philadelphia: Elsevier Saunders.

167. Eckert, D. J., Jordan, A. S., Merchia, P., et al. (2007). Central sleep apnea: Pathophysiology and treatment. *Chest, 131*, 595–607.
168. Javaheri, S. (2000). Treatment of central sleep apnea in heart failure. *Sleep, 23*(Suppl. 4), S224–S227.
169. Olson, L. J., & Somers, V. K. (2007). Treating central sleep apnea in heart failure: Outcomes revisited. *Circulation, 115*, 3140–3142.
170. Arzt, M., Floras, J. S., Logan, A. G., et al. (2007). Suppression of central sleep apnea by continuous positive airway pressure and transplant-free survival in heart failure: A post hoc analysis of the Canadian Continuous Positive Airway Pressure for Patients with Central Sleep Apnea and Heart Failure Trial (CANPAP). *Circulation, 115*, 3173–3180.
171. Hoffstein, V. (2005). Snoring and upper airway resistance syndrome. In M. H. Kryger, T. Roth, & W. C. Dement (Eds.), *Principles and practice of sleep medicine* (pp. 1001–1012). Philadelphia: Elsevier.
172. Gold, A. R., Gold, M. S., Harris, K. W., et al. (2008). Hypersomnolence, insomnia and the pathophysiology of upper airway resistance syndrome. *Sleep Medicine, 9*, 675–683.
173. Guilleminault, C., Kirisoglu, C., Poyares, D., et al. (2006). Upper airway resistance syndrome: A long-term outcome study. *Journal of Psychiatric Research, 40*, 273–279.
174. Bao, G., & Guilleminault, C. (2004). Upper airway resistance syndrome–one decade later. *Current Opinion in Pulmonary Medicine, 10*, 461–467.
175. Lugaresi, E. (1975). Snoring. *Electroencephalography and Clinical Neurophysiology, 39*, 59–64.
176. Lugaresi, E., Cirignotta, F., Coccagna, G., et al. (1980). Some epidemiological data on snoring and cardiocirculatory disturbances. *Sleep, 3*, 221–224.
177. Bixler, E. O., Vgontzas, A. N., Lin, H. M., et al. (2000). Association of hypertension and sleep-disordered breathing. *Archives of Internal Medicine, 160*, 2289–2295.
178. Roux, F., D'Ambrosio, C., & Mohsenin, V. (2000). Sleep-related breathing disorders and cardiovascular disease. *American Journal of Medicine, 108*, 396–402.
179. Dart, R. A., Gregoire, J. R., Gutterman, D. D., et al. (2003). The association of hypertension and secondary cardiovascular disease with sleep-disordered breathing. *Chest, 123*, 244–260.
180. Willis, T. (1672). *De animae brutorum*. London: Wells and Scott.
181. Ekbom, K. A. (1945). Restless legs: A clinical study. *Acta Medica Scandinavica*, 1–122.
182. Symonds, C. P. (1953). Nocturnal myoclonus. *Journal of Neurology, Neurosurgery, and Psychiatry, 16*, 166.
183. Lugaresi, E., Coccagna, G., Mantovani, M., et al. (1972). Some periodic phenomena arising during drowsiness and sleep in man. *Electroencephalography and Clinical Neurophysiology, 32*, 701–705.
184. Coleman, R. M., Pollak, C. P., & Weitzman, E. D. (1980). Periodic movements in sleep (nocturnal myoclonus): Relation to sleep disorders. *Annals of Neurology, 8*, 416–421.
185. Ondo, W., & Jankovic, J. (1996). Restless legs syndrome: Clinicoetiologic correlates. *Neurology, 47*, 1435–1441.
186. Tan, E. K., & Ondo, W. (2000). Restless legs syndrome: Clinical features and treatment. *American Journal of Medicine Science, 319*, 397–403.
187. Maheswaran, M., & Kushida, C. A. (2006). Restless legs syndrome in children. *Medscape General Medicine, 8*, 79.
188. Mohri, I., Kato-Nishimura, K., Tachibana, N., et al. (2008). Restless legs syndrome (RLS): An unrecognized cause for bedtime problems and insomnia in children. *Sleep Medicine, 9*, 701–702.
189. Picchietti, D., Allen, R. P., Walters, A. S., et al. (2007). Restless legs syndrome: Prevalence and impact in children and adolescentsis—the Peds REST study. *Pediatrics, 120*, 253–266.
190. Picchietti, M. A., & Picchietti, D. L. (2008). Restless legs syndrome and periodic limb movement disorder in children and adolescents. *Seminars in Pediatric Neurology, 15*, 91–99.
191. Michaud, M., Lavigne, G., Desautels, A., et al. (2002). Effects of immobility on sensory and motor symptoms of restless legs syndrome. *Movement Disorder, 17*, 112–115.
192. Goodman, J. D., Brodie, C., & Ayida, G. A. (1988). Restless leg syndrome in pregnancy. *BMJ, 297*, 1101–1102.
193. Lee, K. A., Zaffke, M. E., & Baratte-Beebe, K. (2001). Restless legs syndrome and sleep disturbance during pregnancy: The role of folate and iron. *Journal of Women's Health and Gender Based Medicine, 10*, 335–341.
194. Enomoto, M., Inoue, Y., Namba, K., et al. (2008). Clinical characteristics of restless legs syndrome in end-stage renal failure and idiopathic RLS patients. *Movement Disorder, 23*, 811–816.
195. Cortese, S., Konofal, E., Lecendreux, M., et al. (2005). Restless legs syndrome and attention-deficit/hyperactivity disorder: A review of the literature. *Sleep, 28*, 1007–1013.
196. Cortese, S., Lecendreux, M., Bernardina, B. D., et al. (2008). Attention-deficit/hyperactivity disorder, Tourette's syndrome, and restless legs syndrome: The iron hypothesis. *Medical Hypotheses, 70*, 1128–1132.
197. Konofal, E., Cortese, S., Marchand, M., et al. (2007). Impact of restless legs syndrome and iron deficiency on attention-deficit/hyperactivity disorder in children. *Sleep Medicine, 8*, 711–715.
198. Kapoor, S. (2008). The relationship between restless legs syndrome and cardiovascular disease. *European Journal of Neurology, 15*, e42.
199. Winkelman, J. W., Shahar, E., Sharief, I., et al. (2008). Association of restless legs syndrome and cardiovascular disease in the Sleep Heart Health Study. *Neurology, 70*, 35–42.
200. Allen, R. P., & Earley, C. J. (2001). Restless legs syndrome: A review of clinical and pathophysiologic features. *Journal of Clinical Neurophysiology, 18*, 128–147.
201. Earley, C. J., Yaffee, J. B., & Allen, R. P. (1998). Randomized, double-blind, placebo-controlled trial of pergolide in restless legs syndrome. *Neurology, 51*, 1599–1602.
202. Becker, P. M., Ondo, W., & Sharon, D. (1998). Encouraging initial response of restless legs syndrome to pramipexole. *Neurology, 51*, 1221–1223.
203. Ondo, W. (1999). Ropinirole for restless legs syndrome. *Movement Disorder, 14*, 138–140.
204. Montplaisir, J., Allen, R. P., Walters, A. S., et al. (2005). Restless legs syndrome and periodic limb movement disorder during sleep. In M. H. Kryger, T. Roth, & W. C. Dement (Eds.), *Principles and practice of sleep medicine* (pp. 839–852). Philadelphia: Elsevier Saunders.
205. American Heart Association. (2008). Heart and stroke statistics 2008 update. *Circulation, 117*, e25–e146.
206. Shahar, E., Whitney, C. W., Redline, S., et al. (2001). Sleep-disordered breathing and cardiovascular disease: Cross-sectional results of the Sleep Heart Health Study. *American Journal of Respiratory Critical Care Medicine, 163*, 19–25.
207. Punjabi, N. M. (2008). The epidemiology of adult obstructive sleep apnea. *Proceedings of the American Thoracic Society, 5*, 136–143.
208. Lopez-Garcia, E., Faubel, R., Leon-Munoz, L., et al. (2008). Sleep duration, general and abdominal obesity, and weight change among the older adult population of Spain. *American Journal of Clinical Nutrition, 87*, 310–316.
209. Gottlieb, D. J., Punjabi, N. M., Newman, A. B., et al. (2005). Association of sleep time with diabetes mellitus and impaired glucose tolerance. *Archives of Internal Medicine, 165*, 863–867.
210. BaHammam, A. (2006). Sleep quality of patients with acute myocardial infarction outside the CCU environment: A preliminary study. *Medical Science Monitor, 12*, CR168–CR172.
211. von Kanel, R., Loredo, J. S., Ancoli-Israel, S., et al. (2007). Association between polysomnographic measures of disrupted sleep and prothrombotic factors. *Chest, 131*, 733–739.
212. McSweeney, J. C., Cody, M., O'Sullivan, P., et al. (2003). Women's early warning symptoms of acute myocardial infarction. *Circulation, 108*, 2619–2623.
213. Carney, R. M., Howells, W. B., Freedland, K. E., et al. (2006). Depression and obstructive sleep apnea in patients with coronary heart disease. *Psychosomatic Medicine, 68*, 443–448.
214. Sorajja, D., Gami, A. S., Somers, V. K., et al. (2008). Independent association between obstructive sleep apnea and subclinical coronary artery disease. *Chest, 133*, 927–933.
215. Richards, K. C., & Bairnsfather, L. (1988). A description of night sleep patterns in the critical care unit. *Heart & Lung, 17*, 35–42.
216. Friese, R. (2008). Sleep and recovery from critical illness and injury: A review of theory, current practice, and future directions. *Critical Care Medicine, 36*, 697–705.
217. Ruggiero, C., & Dziedzic, L. (2004). Promoting a healing environment: Quiet time in the intensive care unit. *Joint Commission Journal on Quality and Safety, 30*, 465–467.
218. Redeker, N. S., & Hedges, C. (2002). Sleep during hospitalization and recovery after cardiac surgery. *Journal of Cardiovascular Nursing, 17*, 56–68.
219. Edell-Gustafsson, U. M., Hetta, J. E., Aren, G. B., et al. (1997). Measurement of sleep and quality of life before and after coronary artery

bypass grafting: A pilot study. *International Journal of Nursing Practice, 3*, 239–246.

220. Bosma, K., Ferreyra, G., Ambrogio, C., et al. (2007). Patient-ventilator interaction and sleep in mechanically ventilated patients: Pressure support versus proportional assist ventilation. *Critical Care Medicine, 35*, 1048–1054.
221. Hedges, C., & Redeker, N. S. (2008). Comparison of sleep and mood in patients after on-pump and off-pump coronary artery bypass surgery. *American Journal of Critical Care, 17*, 133–140.
222. Yilmaz, H., & Iskesen, I. (2007). Follow-up with objective and subjective tests of the sleep characteristics of patients after cardiac surgery. *Circulation Journal, 71*, 1506–1510.
223. Wilkins, M. K., & Moore, M. L. (2004). Music intervention in the intensive care unit: A complementary therapy to improve patient outcomes. *Evidence Based Nursing, 7*, 103–104.
224. Chen, H. M., & Clark, A. P. (2007). Sleep disturbances in people living with heart failure. *Journal of Cardiovascular Nursing, 22*, 177–185.
225. Zambroski, C. H., Moser, D. K., Bhat, G., et al. (2005). Impact of symptom prevalence and symptom burden on quality of life in patients with heart failure. *European Journal of Cardiovascular Nursing, 4*, 198–206.
226. Caples, S. M., Garcia-Touchard, A., & Somers, V. K. (2007). Sleep-disordered breathing and cardiovascular risk. *Sleep, 30*, 291–303.
227. Ng, A. C., & Freedman, S. B. (2008). Sleep disordered breathing in chronic heart failure. *Heart Failure Reviews*. Epub ahead of print.
228. Parker, K. P., & Dunbar, S. B. (2002). Sleep and heart failure. *Journal of Cardiovascular Nursing, 17*, 30–41.
229. Javaheri, S. (2006). Sleep disorders in systolic heart failure: A prospective study of 100 male patients. The final report. *International Journal of Cardiology, 106*, 21–28.
230. Garcia-Touchard, A., Somers, V. K., Olson, L. J., et al. (2008). Central sleep apnea: Implications for congestive heart failure. *Chest, 133*, 1495–1504.
231. Krachman, S. L., D'Alonzo, G. E., Permut, I., et al. (2008). Treatment of sleep disordered breathing in congestive heart failure. *Heart Failure Reviews*. Epub ahead of print.
232. Carmona-Bernal, C., Ruiz-Garcia, A., Villa-Gil, M., et al. (2008). Quality of life in patients with congestive heart failure and central sleep apnea. *Sleep Medicine, 9*, 646–651.
233. Redeker, N. S. (2008). Sleep disturbance in people with heart failure: Implications for self-care. *Journal of Cardiovascular Nursing, 23*, 231–238.
234. Benjamin, J. A., & Lewis, K. E. (2008). Sleep-disordered breathing and cardiovascular disease. *Postgraduate Medicine Journals, 84*, 15–22.
235. Phillips, C. L., & Cistulli, P. A. (2006). Obstructive sleep apnea and hypertension: Epidemiology, mechanisms and treatment effects. *Minerva Medica, 97*, 299–312.
236. Punjabi, N. M., Newman, A. B., Young, T. B., et al. (2008). Sleep-disordered breathing and cardiovascular disease: An outcome-based definition of hypopneas. *American Journal of Respiratory and Critical Care Medicine, 177*, 1150–1155.
237. Budhiraja, R., Sharief, I., & Quan, S. F. (2005). Sleep disordered breathing and hypertension. *Journals of Clinical Sleep Medicine, 1*, 401–404.
238. Calhoun, D. A., Jones, D., Textor, S., et al. (2008). Resistant hypertension: diagnosis, evaluation, and treatment: A scientific statement from the American Heart Association Professional Education Committee of the Council for High Blood Pressure Research. *Circulation, 117*, e510–e526.
239. Drager, L. F., Bortolotto, L. A., Figueiredo, A. C., et al. (2007). Obstructive sleep apnea, hypertension, and their interaction on arterial stiffness and heart remodeling. *Chest, 131*, 1379–1386.
240. Hargens, T. A., Nickols-Richardson, S. M., Gregg, J. M., et al. (2006). Hypertension research in sleep apnea. *The Journal of Clinical Hypertension (Greenwich), 8*, 873–878.
241. Okcay, A., Somers, V. K., & Caples, S. M. (2008). Obstructive sleep apnea and hypertension. *Journal of Clinical Hypertensions (Greenwich), 10*, 549–555.
242. Hla, K. M., Young, T., Finn, L., et al. (2008). Longitudinal association of sleep-disordered breathing and nondipping of nocturnal blood pressure in the Wisconsin Sleep Cohort Study. *Sleep, 31*, 795–800.
243. Kapa, S., Sert Kuniyoshi, F. H., & Somers, V. K. (2008). Sleep apnea and hypertension: Interactions and implications for management. *Hypertension, 51*, 605–608.
244. Weiss, J. W., Liu, M. D., & Huang, J. (2007). Physiological basis for a causal relationship of obstructive sleep apnoea to hypertension. *Experimental Physiology, 92*, 21–26.
245. Parati, G., & Staessen, J. A. (2007). Day-night blood pressure variations: Mechanisms, reproducibility and clinical relevance. *Journal of Hypertension, 25*, 2377–2380.
246. Gangwisch, J. E., Heymsfield, S. B., Boden-Albala, B., et al. (2006). Short sleep duration as a risk factor for hypertension: Analyses of the first National Health and Nutrition Examination Survey. *Hypertension, 47*, 833–839.
247. de Sousa, A. G., Cercato, C., Mancini, M. C., et al. (2008). Obesity and obstructive sleep apnea-hypopnea syndrome. *Obesity in Review, 9*, 340–354.
248. Spengos, K., Tsivgoulis, G., Manios, E., et al. (2005). Stroke etiology is associated with symptom onset during sleep. *Sleep, 28*, 233–238.
249. Grigg-Damberger, M. (2006). Why a polysomnogram should become part of the diagnostic evaluation of stroke and transient ischemic attack. *Journal of Clinical Neurophysiology, 23*, 21–38.
250. Punjabi, N. M., Shahar, E., Redline, S., et al. (2004). Sleep-disordered breathing, glucose intolerance, and insulin resistance: The Sleep Heart Health Study. *American Journal of Epidemiology, 160*, 521–530.
251. Gangwisch, J. E., Heymsfield, S. B., Boden-Albala, B., et al. (2007). Sleep duration as a risk factor for diabetes incidence in a large U.S. sample. *Sleep, 30*, 1667–1673.
252. Taub, L. F., & Redeker, N. S. (2008). Sleep disorders, glucose regulation, and type 2 diabetes. *Biological Research for Nursing, 9*, 231–243.
253. Bhullar, S., & Phillips, B. (2005). Sleep in COPD patients. *COPD, 2*, 355–361.
254. Fanfulla, F., Cascone, L., & Taurino, A. E. (2004). Sleep disordered breathing in patients with chronic obstructive pulmonary disease. *Minerva Medica, 95*, 307–321.
255. Fletcher, E. C., Scott, D., Qian, W., et al. (1991). Evolution of nocturnal oxyhemoglobin desaturation in patients with chronic obstructive pulmonary disease and a daytime Pa_{O_2} above 60 mm Hg. *American Review of Respiratory Disease, 144*, 401–405.
256. Gay, P. C. (2004). Chronic obstructive pulmonary disease and sleep. *Respiratory Care, 49*, 39–51, discussion 51–32.
257. Krachman, S., Minai, O. A., & Scharf, S. M. (2008). Sleep abnormalities and treatment in emphysema. *Proceedings of the American Thoracic Society, 5*, 536–542.
258. Stege, G., Vos, P. J., van den Elshout, F. J., et al. (2008). Sleep, hypnotics and chronic obstructive pulmonary disease. *Respiratory Medicine, 102*, 801–814.
259. Weitzenblum, E., & Chaouat, A. (2004). Sleep and chronic obstructive pulmonary disease. *Sleep Medicine Reviews, 8*, 281–294.
260. Weitzenblum, E., Chaouat, A., Kessler, R., et al. (2008). Overlap syndrome: Obstructive sleep apnea in patients with chronic obstructive pulmonary disease. *Proceedings of the American Thoracic Society, 5*, 237–241.
261. Marrone, O., Salvaggio, A., & Insalaco, G. (2006). Respiratory disorders during sleep in chronic obstructive pulmonary disease. *International Journal of Chronic Obstructive Pulmonary Disease, 1*, 363–372.
262. Mermigkis, C., Kopanakis, A., Foldvary-Schaefer, N., et al. (2007). Health-related quality of life in patients with obstructive sleep apnoea and chronic obstructive pulmonary disease (overlap syndrome). *International Journal of Clinical Practice, 61*, 207–211.
263. Tsuno, N. B. A., & Ritchie, K. (2005). Sleep and depression. *Journal of Clinical Psychiatry, 66*, 1254–1269.
264. Quan, S. F., Katz, R., Olson, J., et al. (2005). Factors associated with incidence and persistence of symptoms of disturbed sleep in an elderly cohort: The Cardiovascular Health Study. *American Journal of Medicine and Science, 329*, 163–172.
265. Thase, M. (2006). Depression and sleep: Pathophysiology and treatment. *Dialogues in Clinical NeuroSciences, 8*, 217–226.
266. Taylor, D. J. (2008). Insomnia and depression. *Sleep, 31*, 447–448.
267. Taylor, D. J., Mallory, L. J., Lichstein, K. L., et al. (2007). Comorbidity of chronic insomnia with medical problems. *Sleep, 30*, 213–218.
268. Thase, M. E. (2005). Correlates and consequences of chronic insomnia. *General Hospital Psychiatry, 27*, 100–112.
269. Ohayon, M. M. (2005). Prevalence and correlates of nonrestorative sleep complaints. *Archives of Internal Medicine, 165*, 35–41.
270. Riemann, D. (2007). Insomnia and comorbid psychiatric disorders. *Sleep Medicine, 8*(Suppl. 4), S15–S20.
271. Libby, P., & Braunwald, E. (2008). *Braunwald's heart disease: A textbook of cardiovascular medicine*. Philadelphia: Saunders/Elsevier.

272. Willich, S. N., Kulig, M., Muller-Nordhorn, J. (2004). European survey on circadian variation of angina pectoris (ESCVA) in treated patients. *Herz, 29,* 665–672.
273. Otto, M., Svatikova, A., Barretto, R., et al. (2004). Early morning attenuation of endothelial function in healthy humans. *Circulation, 109,* 2507–2510.
274. Janssens, W., Willems, R., Pevernagie, D., et al. (2007). REM sleep-related brady-arrhythmia syndrome. *Sleep Breath, 11,* 195–199.
275. Sato, K., Yamasaki, F., Furuno, T., et al. (2003). Rhythm-independent feature of heart rate dynamics common to atrial fibrillation and sinus rhythm in patients with paroxysmal atrial fibrillation. *Journal of Cardiology, 42,* 269–276.
276. Gami, A. S., Hodge, D. O., Herges, R. M., et al. (2007). Obstructive sleep apnea, obesity, and the risk of incident atrial fibrillation. *Journal of the American College of Cardiology, 49,* 565–571.
277. Deaton, C., Dunbar, S. B., Moloney, M., et al. (2003). Patient experiences with atrial fibrillation and treatment with implantable atrial defibrillation therapy. *Heart Lung, 32,* 291–299.
278. Valderrama, A. (2006). Multidimensional factors associated with fatigue in persons with permanent atrial fibrillation. Nell Hodgson Woodruff School of Nursing. Atlanta: Emory University.
279. Mehra, R., Benjamin, E. J., Shahar, E., et al. (2006). Association of nocturnal arrhythmias with sleep-disordered breathing: The Sleep Heart Health Study. *American Journal of Respiratory and Critical Care Medicine, 173,* 910–916.
280. Kanagala, R., Murali, N. S., Friedman, P. A., et al. (2003). Obstructive sleep apnea and the recurrence of atrial fibrillation. *Circulation, 107,* 2589–2594.
281. Bootzin, R. R. (2006). Is brief behavioral treatment for insomnia effective? *Journal of Clinical Sleep Medicine, 2,* 407–408.
282. Joshi, S. (2008). Nonpharmacologic therapy for insomnia in the elderly. *Clinics in Geriatric Medicine, 24,* 107–119.
283. Ernst, E., Pittler, M. H., Wider, B., et al. (2007). Mind–body therapies: Are the trial data getting stronger? *Alternative Therapies in Health and Medicine, 13,* 62–64.
284. McCurry, S. M., Logsdon, R. G., Teri, L., et al. (2007). Evidence-based psychological treatments for insomnia in older adults. *Psychological Aging, 22,* 18–27.
285. Morin, C. M., Vallieres, A., & Ivers, H. (2007). Dysfunctional beliefs and attitudes about sleep (DBAS): Validation of a brief version (DBAS-16). *Sleep, 30,* 1547–1554.
286. Gammack, J. K. (2008). Light therapy for insomnia in older adults. *Clinics in Geriatric Medicine, 24,* 139–149.
287. Bootzin, R. R. (2005). Is bright light exposure an effective therapy for insomnia? *Sleep, 28,* 540–541.
288. Morgenthaler, T., Kramer, M., Alessi, C., et al. (2006). Practice parameters for the psychological and behavioral treatment of insomnia: An update. An American Academy of Sleep Medicine report. *Sleep, 29,* 1415–1419.
289. Terman, M. (2007). Evolving applications of light therapy. *Sleep Medicine Reviews, 11,* 497–507.
290. Lewy, A. J. (2007). Melatonin and human chronobiology. *Cold Spring Harbor Symposia on Quantitative Biology, 72,* 623–636.
291. Pandi-Perumal, S. R., Trakht, I., Srinivasan, V., et al. (2008). The effect of melatonergic and non-melatonergic antidepressants on sleep: Weighing the alternatives. *World Journal of Biology Psychiatry,* 1–13.
292. Sateia, M. J., Kirby-Long, P., & Taylor, J. L. (2008). Efficacy and clinical safety of ramelteon: An evidence-based review. *Sleep Medicine Reviews, 12,* 319–332.
293. Buscemi, N., Vandermeer, B., Friesen, C., et al. (2005). Manifestations and management of chronic insomnia in adults. *Evidence Report on Technology Assessment (Summary),* 1–10.
294. Lusardi, P., Piazza, E., & Fogari, R. (2000). Cardiovascular effects of melatonin in hypertensive patients well controlled by nifedipine: A 24-hour study. *British Journal of Clinical Pharmacology, 49,* 423–427.
295. Soden, K., Vincent, K., Craske, S., et al. (2004). A randomized controlled trial of aromatherapy massage in a hospice setting. *Palliative Medicine, 18,* 87–92.
296. Hanley, J., Stirling, P., & Brown, C. (2003). Randomised controlled trial of therapeutic massage in the management of stress. *British Journal of General Practice, 53,* 20–25.
297. Tsay, S. L. (2004). Acupressure and fatigue in patients with end-stage renal disease—A randomized controlled trial. *International Journal of Nursing Studies, 41,* 99–106.
298. Klein, A. A., Djaiani, G., Karski, J., et al. (2004). Acupressure wristbands for the prevention of postoperative nausea and vomiting in adults undergoing cardiac surgery. *Journal of Cardiothoracic and Vascular Anesthesia, 18,* 68–71.
299. Sathyaprabha, T. N., Satishchandra, P., Pradhan, C., et al. (2008). Modulation of cardiac autonomic balance with adjuvant yoga therapy in patients with refractory epilepsy. *Epilepsy & Behavior, 12,* 245–252.
300. Mamtani, R. (2005). Ayurveda and yoga in cardiovascular diseases. *Cardiology in Review, 13,* 155–162.
301. Manjunath, N. K., & Telles, S. (2005). Influence of Yoga and Ayurveda on self-rated sleep in a geriatric population. *Indian Journal of Medical Research, 121,* 683–690.
302. Lan, C., Chen, S. Y., Wong, M. K., et al. (2008). Tai chi training for patients with coronary heart disease. *Medicine and Sport Science, 52,* 182–194.
303. Li, F., Fisher, K. J., Harmer, P., et al. (2004). Tai chi and self-rated quality of sleep and daytime sleepiness in older adults: A randomized controlled trial. *Journal of the American Geriatric Society, 52,* 892–900.
304. Yeh, G. Y., Wayne, P. M., & Phillips, R. S. (2008). Tai chi exercise in patients with chronic heart failure. *Medicine and Sport Science, 52,* 195–208
305. Carney, C. E., & Edinger, J. D. (2006). Identifying critical beliefs about sleep in primary insomnia. *Sleep, 29,* 444–453.
306. Edinger, J. D., & Means, M. K. (2005). Cognitive-behavioral therapy for primary insomnia. *Clinical Psychology Review, 25,* 539–558.
307. Morin, C. M. (2004). Cognitive-behavioral approaches to the treatment of insomnia. *Journal of Clinical Psychiatry, 65*(Suppl. 16), 33–40.
308. Morin, C. M., Bootzin, R. R., Buysse, D. J., et al. (2006). Psychological and behavioral treatment of insomnia: Update of the recent evidence (1998–2004). *Sleep, 29,* 1398–1414.
309. Smith, M. T., Huang, M. I., & Manber, R. (2005). Cognitive behavior therapy for chronic insomnia occurring within the context of medical and psychiatric disorders. *Clinical Psychology Reviews, 25,* 559–592.
310. Wang, M. Y., Wang, S. Y., & Tsai, P. S. (2005). Cognitive behavioural therapy for primary insomnia: A systematic review. *Journal of Advanced Nursing, 50,* 553–564.
311. Jansson-Frojmark, M., & Linton, S. J. (2008). The role of sleep-related beliefs to improvement in early cognitive behavioral therapy for insomnia. *Cognitive Behaviour Therapy, 37,* 5–13.
312. Jacobs, G. D., Pace-Schott, E. F., Stickgold, R., et al. (2004). Cognitive behavior therapy and pharmacotherapy for insomnia: a randomized controlled trial and direct comparison. *Archives of Internal Medicine, 164,* 1888–1896.
313. Rybarczyk, B., Stepanski, E., Fogg, L., et al. (2005). A placebo-controlled test of cognitive-behavioral therapy for comorbid insomnia in older adults. *Journal of Consulting and Clinical Psychology, 73,* 1164–1174.
314. Verbeek, I. H., Konings, G. M., Aldenkamp, A. P., et al. (2006). Cognitive behavioral treatment in clinically referred chronic insomniacs: Group versus individual treatment. *Behavioral Sleep Medicine, 4,* 135–151.
315. Dolan-Sewell, R. T., Riley, W. T., & Hunt, C. E. (2005). NIH State-of-the-Science Conference on Chronic Insomnia. *Journal of Clinical Sleep Medicine, 1,* 335–336.
316. Dalla Corte, C. L., Fachinetto, R., Colle, D., et al. (2008). Potentially adverse interactions between haloperidol and valerian. *Food and Chemical Toxicology, 46,* 2369–2375.
317. Mendelson, W. B. (2005). Hypnotic medications: Mechanisms of action and pharmacologic effects. In M. H. Kryger, T. Roth, & W. C. Dement (Eds.), *Principles and practice of sleep medicine* (pp. 444–467). Philadelphia: Elsevier Saunders.
318. Tariq, S. H., & Pulisetty, S. (2008). Pharmacotherapy for insomnia. *Clinics in Geriatric Medicine, 24,* 93–105, vii.
319. Akerstedt, T. (2003). Shift work and disturbed sleep/wakefulness. *Occupational Medicine (London), 53,* 89–94.
320. Scott, L. D., Hwang, W.-T., Rogers, A. E., et al. (2007). The relationship between nurse work schedules, sleep duration, and drowsy driving. *Sleep, 30,* 1801–1807.
321. Landrigan, C. P., Czeisler, C. A., Barger, L. K., et al. (2007). Effective implementation of work-hour limits and systemic improvements. *Joint Commission Journal on Quality and Patient Safety, 33,* 19–29.
322. Sharkey, K. M., Fogg, L. F., & Eastman, C. I. (2001). Effects of melatonin administration on daytime sleep after simulated night shift work. *Journal of Sleep Research, 10,* 181–192.
323. Parthasarathy, S., Hettiger, K., Budhiraja, R., et al. (2007). Sleep and well being of ICU housestaff. *Chest, 131,* 1685–1693.

CHAPTER 9

Physiologic Adaptations With Aging

Barbara S. Levine

Aging is a normal developmental process during which physiological and psychosocial changes occur. Wide variation in the aging process exists among individuals as a result of varied environmental exposures, social relationships, genetic endowment, and health status. Whereas maximum lifespan (the age reached by the longest-lived survivors) for humans is 114 to 120 years, the average human lifespan is approximately 75 years. Developmental changes and adaptations continue throughout aging until death.

The lifespan is divided into phases, with the commonly used periods for these phases being infancy (birth to 1 year), early childhood (1 to 6 years), late childhood (7 to 10 years), adolescence (11 to 18 years), young adulthood (19 to 35 years), early middle age (36 to 49 years), late middle age (50 to 64 years), young–old (65 to 74 years), old (75 to 85 years), and old–old (86 years and older). The group of people who are aged 85 years or older is the most rapidly growing segment of the older population (Fig. 9-1). People in this age group typically have a noticeable decline in functional ability and have one or more chronic disorders.

Aging is a multifactorial process with genetic and environmental components. Each system in an organism, each tissue in a system, and each cell type in a tissue appear to have its own trajectory of aging.[1] Theories of the biologic aspects of aging have been developed and studied.[2] The theories can be divided into three groups: organ theories, physiological theories, and genome-based theories. The organ theories examine age changes in the body brought about by the possible initiation from a "master" organ system, such as the immune or neurological system. The physiologic theories analyze cell functioning as related to waste product accumulation or molecular changes. The genome-based theories attribute age changes to the individual's genetic endowment and suggest that a predetermined series of events programmed into cells or random mutations or cell errors are responsible for the process of aging. Probably no one theory can totally explain the aging process, but some or all of these theories may be involved in the complete explanation.

The nurse needs to be aware of several concepts in addressing the health care needs of older adults.

1. Age-related changes are gradual and individual, and different systems age at different rates within an individual. There is more intra-individual variability among older people than there is among younger people.
2. Complex functions that require multisystem coordination show the most obvious decline and require the greatest compensation and support.
3. Vulnerability to disease increases with age.
4. Stressful situations (physiologic or psychosocial) produce a more pronounced reaction in the elderly and require a longer period of time for readjustment.[3]

Although Americans are living longer, they are not necessarily healthier. With increasing age, they are at increased risk for illness. Chronic illnesses, such as arthritis, cardiac and vascular problems, and diabetes, are the major health problems of older people (Fig. 9-2). Chronic illnesses do not occur in isolation; 80% of older Americans have one chronic illness and 50% have two or more. Because of the lifestyle changes in young and middle-aged adults, particularly in the areas of diet and exercise, in the near future, older adults may be sufficiently healthier that definitions and expectations of the aging process may need to be revised. At present, however, heart disease and stroke are the first and third leading cause of death of older adults (Fig. 9-3).

When older people become ill, there is frequently an atypical presentation, such as missing or altered symptoms. Confusion is often one of the earliest indications of a change in health status. Restlessness, confusion, or altered mentation often occur in the presence of illness and should not be confused with dementia, providing that dementia was not present before the illness. Acute onset or unexplained deterioration of health should be carefully evaluated and not accepted as a normal concomitant of aging.

The older person who is ill has many adjustments and adaptations to make. The social supports (family and friends) available to that person may be fewer or less able to be supportive because of their own debilities, such as a spouse who is also ill or an adult child who has other responsibilities. Apprehension, worry, and fear of becoming dependent and helpless may add to the emotional burden of the current illness. Of those older adults between 80 and 84 years of age, 30% require assistance with daily activities, and of those adults who are 85 years and older, 50% require assistance.

Older patients require careful, thorough nursing management during an acute illness and afterward. Discharge planning that begins with the admission process and includes consideration of living arrangements, care providers, and support services is especially important for older patients, who are often adversely affected by the shorter hospitalizations and fewer home nursing care visits that accompany changes in managed care.

GENERAL PHYSIOLOGIC CHANGES

Aging is an integral part of the continuum that begins at conception and ends at death. As contrasted with the developmental growth and maturation of childhood and adolescence, aging is characterized by a decline in function and by changes that are decremental in nature. The inability to maintain homeostasis in a broad range of environments and with a variety of physiologic challenges is central to the decline in function.

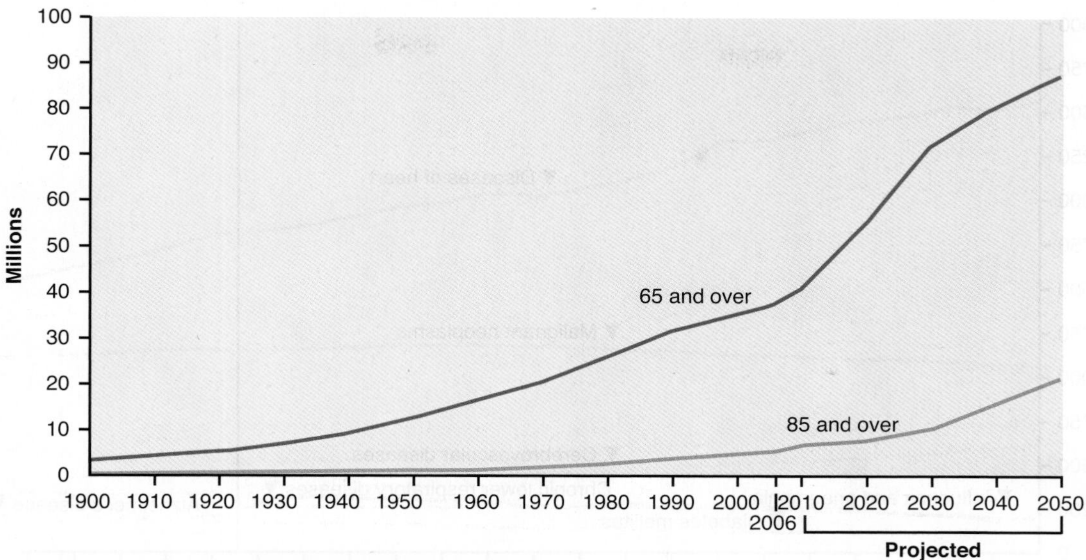

Figure 9-1 Projected growth in population (65 years and older), by age group, in millions, 1900–2050. (From Federal Interagency Forum on Aging-Related Statistics. [2007]. *Older Americans Update 2006: Key Indicators of Well-Being.* Federal Interagency Forum on Aging-Related Statistics, Washington, DC: U.S. Government Printing Office.)

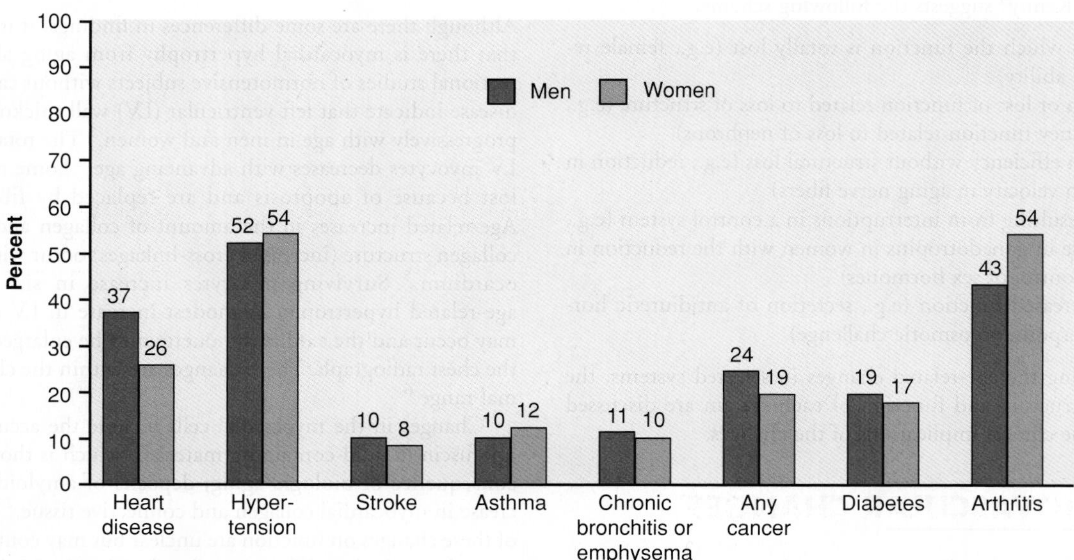

Figure 9-2 The top 10 chronic conditions for people older than 65 years of age, 1996. (From Federal Interagency Forum on Aging-Related Statistics. [2007]. *Older Americans Update 2006: Key Indicators of Well-Being.* Federal Interagency Forum on Aging-Related Statistics, Washington, DC: U.S. Government Printing Office.)

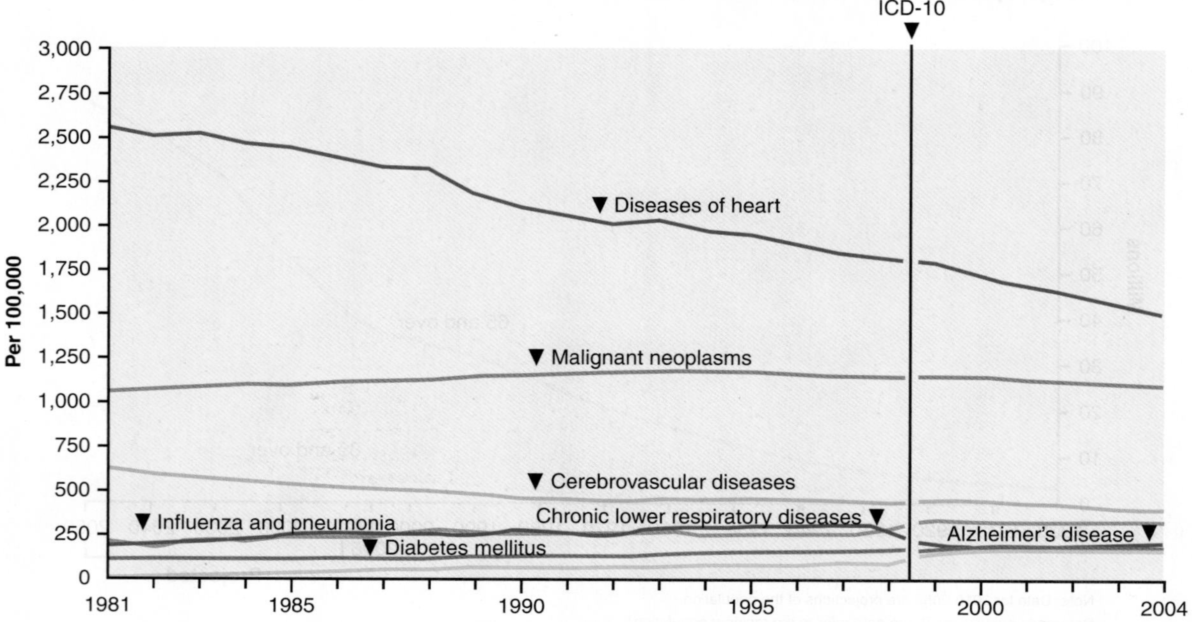
Death rates for selected leading causes of death among people age 65 and over, 1981-2004
ICD-10
Per 100,000
3,000
2,750
2,500
2,250
2,000
1,750
1,500
1,250
1,000
750
500
250
0
Diseases of heart
Malignant neoplasms
Cerebrovascular diseases
Influenza and pneumonia
Chronic lower respiratory diseases
Diabetes mellitus
Alzheimer's disease
1981
1985
1990
1995
2000
2004
Note: Death rates for 1981-1998 are based on the 9th revision of the *International Classification of Diseases* (ICD-9). Starting in 1999, death rates are based on ICD-10, and trends in death rates for some causes may be affected by this change. For the period 1981-1998, causes were coded using ICD-9 codes that are most nearly comparable with the 113 cause list for the ICD-10 and may differ from previously published estimates. Rates are age adjusted using the 2000 standard population.
Reference population : These data refer to the resident population.
Source: Centers for Disease Control and Prevention, National Center for Health Statistics, National Vital Statistics System.

Figure 9-3 The top causes of death among older people, 65 or older. (National Center for Health Statistics [2007]. Health, United States, 2007 with Chartbook on Trends in Health of Americans. Hyattville, MD)

Changes related to aging may be classified or categorized in several ways. Kenny[4] suggests the following scheme:

1. Change in which the function is totally lost (e.g., female reproductive ability)
2. Changes in or loss of function related to loss of structure (e.g., altered kidney function related to loss of nephrons)
3. Changes in efficiency without structural loss (e.g., reduction in conduction velocity in aging nerve fibers)
4. Changes resulting from interruptions in a control system (e.g., the increase in gonadotropins in women with the reduction in feedback control of sex hormones)
5. Rarely, increased function (e.g., secretion of antidiuretic hormone in response to osmotic challenge)

In reviewing the age-related changes in selected systems, the changes in structure and function of each system are discussed along with the clinical implications of the changes.

CARDIOVASCULAR CHANGES

One of the challenges in discussing aging changes in any system is that of separating changes that can be attributed only to age from changes related to disease. This is particularly true in the cardiovascular system. This discussion attempts to identify what is known about changes in cardiovascular structure and function that result from aging changes and, subsequently, increase vulnerability to disease.

Cardiac Structural Changes

Although there are some differences in findings, it is now agreed that there is myocardial hypertrophy from aging alone. Cross-sectional studies of normotensive subjects without cardiovascular disease indicate that left ventricular (LV) wall thickness increases progressively with age in men and women.[5] The total number of LV myocytes decreases with advancing age.[6] Some myocytes are lost because of apoptosis and are replaced by fibrous tissue. Age-related increases in the amount of collagen and changes in collagen structure (increased cross-linkages) occur within the myocardium.[5] Surviving myocytes increase in size, producing age-related hypertrophy. A modest increase in LV cavitary size may occur and the cardiac silhouette may be enlarged slightly on the chest radiograph. These changes are within the clinically normal range.[6]

Changes in the myocardial cells include the accumulation of lipofuscin (a lipid-containing material), which is thought to be a consequence of biologic aging; deposits of amyloid and an increase in myocardial collagen and connective tissue.[2,7] The effects of these changes on function are unclear but may contribute to increased ventricular stiffness associated with aging and with hypertension.

Aging changes in the valves are characterized by increases in fibrosis, collagen degeneration, lipid accumulation, and calcification. Calcifications of the aortic valve ring can contribute to stenosis and valvular incompetence in aging.[7] Mitral annular calcification occurs more commonly in women than men over age

70 years. Mitral annular calcification contributes to mitral stenosis, mitral regurgitation, atrial arrhythmias, and heart block.[8]

Cardiac Functional Changes

Changes in ventricular filling (preload) and diastolic function occur with aging. There is progressive slowing of the early diastolic filling rate coupled with augmented late diastolic filling.[9] Augmentation of late diastolic filling results from vigorous atrial contraction and is accompanied by atrial enlargement. Despite these changes in filling, end-diastolic volume in the sitting or supine position is not usually reduced in women and is slightly increased in men.[9] The change in end-diastolic volume from rest to exercise increases with age.[10] This refutes the previously held belief that LV filling is impaired in the healthy, older heart.

Clinical implications of age-related changes in ventricular filling include greater dependence on atrial contraction, which is lost with atrial fibrillation and greater sensitivity to hypovolemia. The importance of adequate intravascular volume increases further with tachycardia, which limits filling time.

There is no change in resting systolic function, heart rate, or cardiac output during healthy aging.[9] Maximum heart rate during dynamic exercise decreases with age (maximum heart rate = 220 − age). This age-related decrease in maximum heart rate explains the age-related decrease in maximum cardiac output in healthy people. Maximum cardiac output reserve is approximately 3.5-fold in younger and 2.5-fold in older people.[9]

Electrical System

Controversy and conflicting evidence exists about the effects of aging on the cardiac electrical system. In the absence of disease or extreme stress on the cardiac function, the electrical system is adequate for normal conductivity. Limited data support a marked age-associated increase in the prevalence and complexity of ventricular ectopy at rest and during exercise.[9] Ventricular ectopic beats are evident on 24-hour ambulatory electrocardiogram in more than 75% of men and women aged greater than 64 years, with a somewhat higher prevalence in men than women.[11] In 2% to 4% of asymptomatic, healthy older adults, 3 to 5 beat salvos of non-sustained ventricular tachycardia are present; runs of more than 5 beats are rare.

There appears to be a decrease in the number of pacemaker cells in the sinus node and greater irregularity in their shape. By age 75 years, only 10% of original nodal cells remain, although this is compatible with normal pacemaker activity, it also explains the increased incidence of sick sinus syndrome among older patients. The number of conducting cells in the atrioventricular (AV) node and the His bundle decreases in people older than 70 years of age. The decrease in the number of cells in the His bundle begins after age 40, and after age 50 years in the right bundle. Fibrosis of the cardiac conduction system is strongly associated with aging. Idiopathic bundle–branch fibrosis is a common cause of chronic atrioventricular block in people older than 65 years of age. The atrial and AV nodal refractory periods increase with age. It is not clear whether these changes are caused by altered catecholamine or vagal stimulation with age.

The normal electrocardiogram shows little change with age. There may be small increases in the PR, QRS, and QT intervals, along with a small decrease in the amplitude of the QRS complex. When challenged by disease or adverse circumstances, the age-dependent changes in the electrical system increase the potential for conduction abnormalities as well as supraventricular and ventricular dysrhythmias.

Vascular System

Structural Changes

With advancing age, a series of structural changes take place in the vascular system. Central arterial vessel diameter tends to increase and the intimal and medial layers tend to thicken.[12] In the arterial intima, the endothelial cells become irregular in size and shape with an increase in connective tissue. Calcification and lipid deposition also occur. Some scientists argue that intimal media (IM) thickening is an early stage of atherosclerosis. IM thickness predicts the coexistence of silent coronary artery disease in screened subjects.[13] However, IM thickening may be an intrinsic age-related change that provides a foundation for the subsequent development of atherosclerosis.[14] Similar controversy surrounds age-associated endothelial dysfunction, systemic arterial stiffening, and arterial pulse-pressure widening. Whether age-related changes or early atherosclerosis, combinations of these processes occur to varying degrees in older people. Age-associated vascular changes interact with traditional cardiovascular risk factors to produce clinical atherosclerosis.

Functional Changes

Age-associated increase in IM thickness is accompanied by increased arterial stiffness. Arterial stiffness increases the pulse-wave velocity, transmitting the pulse wave faster than the actual movement of blood. When the pulse wave reaches branch points in the arterial tree, the wave is reflected back toward the heart. At distal locations, the reflected waves augment systolic pressure and reduce diastolic pressure.[15] Data from epidemiological studies indicate that increased pulse-wave velocity is seen with age and also in the context of atherosclerosis and diabetes.[16,17]

Age-related changes are also seen in the intravascular environment. Increases in fibrinogen and procoagulant factors are seen without countering increases in anticoagulant factors. Under stress, there is increased binding of platelets to the arterial wall and increased levels of plasminogen activator inhibitor in older people compared to younger people.[8,18] These changes contribute to the age-associated increase in acute coronary syndrome.

Elevation of the blood pressure is not a normal age change; however, it is a change that frequently occurs with the process of aging. Isolated systolic hypertension, in particular, is a distinct pathologic process and accounts for more than 50% of cases of hypertension. It is defined as a systolic pressure greater than 140 mm Hg and diastolic pressure below 90 mm Hg and is probably the result of arterial stiffening and loss of arterial compliance that occur with aging.[19] Treatment of systolic hypertension follows the same principles as treatment of hypertension in general (see Chapter 35).

Autonomic Nervous System Modulation

Optimal cardiovascular function requires communications between the cardiovascular system and autonomic nervous system. Under stress the sympathetic component of the autonomic nervous system prevails, producing arterial vasoconstriction while increasing heart rate and contractility. At rest the parasympathetic nervous system prevails, slowing down the heart rate. The extent of parasympathetic tone is small in older people. Heart rate variability, a reflection of balance between the sympathetic and parasympathetic nervous systems, declines steadily with aging.[5] The decline in heart rate variability is related to decreased parasympathetic activity, because it is the low-frequency component of the variability that is decreased.[7] Decreased heart rate variability has been associated with poor outcomes in people with cardiovascular disease.

The aging cardiovascular system demonstrates decreased response to β-adrenoreceptor stimulation.[15] Decreased responsiveness is not caused by a decreased number of β-receptors, but to a decrease in affinity of β-agonists for the receptors and decreased efficacy of postreceptor intercellular coupling responsible for muscle contraction.[8,9] Stimulation of β_1-receptors in the ventricles increases heart rate and contractility. Increased end-diastolic volume also increases cardiac contractility (Frank–Starling mechanism). If the ventricular response to β_1-receptor stimulation is reduced in the aging heart, the ventricles are more dependent on adequate filling. Consequently, the aging heart is less tolerant of hypoventilation. Decreased β-receptor responsiveness in the vasculature produces less vasodilation and higher resting blood pressure. The combined effect of changes in autonomic function is decreased baroreflex function and response to physiologic stressors.[8]

RESPIRATORY CHANGES

In the absence of disease, the changes that occur in the lungs from maturity through the aging process are so gradual that the lungs are capable of providing normal gas exchange throughout life. However, the lungs are continuously exposed to the external environment and to various internal assaults; hence, it is difficult to separate changes caused solely by aging from those related to injury or disease processes.

Structural Changes

The aging lung undergoes gradual, subtle changes. Host defense mechanisms of airway clearance and immune system function respond less vigorously with age. Studies of bronchoalveolar lavage show more neutrophils and fewer macrophages in fluid from older (70 to 80 years) than from younger subjects (19 to 34 years).[20,21] The activity of the cilia is decreased, producing less ciliary clearance. Decreased cough reflex related to decreased cilia activity together with decreased immune system function increase susceptibility to lower respiratory infection, mechanical irritation, and, possibly, tumor formation.

There is an age-related increase in the ratio of elastin-to-collagen in the lung parenchyma that may contribute to increased lung compliance, reduced expiratory airway diameter, or airflow limitation.[22,23] Increased calcification of the thoracic joints (spine, ribs, and sternum) and reduced intercostal muscle strength produce a decrease in chest wall compliance with aging and an increased anteroposterior diameter of the chest. The resulting reduced mobility of the thorax leads to increased residual air volume and to a breathing pattern that is augmented by the increased use of diaphragmatic and abdominal muscles in breathing.

Functional Changes

The typical changes in lung function with age include decreased lung recoil, increased closing volume, altered lung volumes, and decreased maximum expiratory flow volume.[22] Nonemphysematous enlargement of the alveoli is accepted as a normal change of aging. The effect of this change is decreased efficiency of gas-diffusing capacity and increased residual volume.

During expiration, airways in the dependent lung regions close and no longer participate in respiration. With aging, the lung volume at which these airways close (closing volume) may exceed the functional residual capacity, leading to closure of distal airways before the end of a normal breath.[22] Loss of lung recoil and the effects of gravity on the dependent areas of the lungs allow the airways to close at a higher lung volume and lead to nonuniformity of ventilation (Fig. 9-4).

After adjustment for height, total lung capacity does not change with age.[22,23] There is an increase, however, in residual volume for reasons previously discussed and in the ratio of residual volume-to-total lung capacity. When increased closing capacity closes terminal airways, these airways no longer actively participate in ventilation, resulting in reduced maximal expiratory flow (V_{max}) and in decreased expiratory volume measured in the first second of forced expiration (FEV_1).

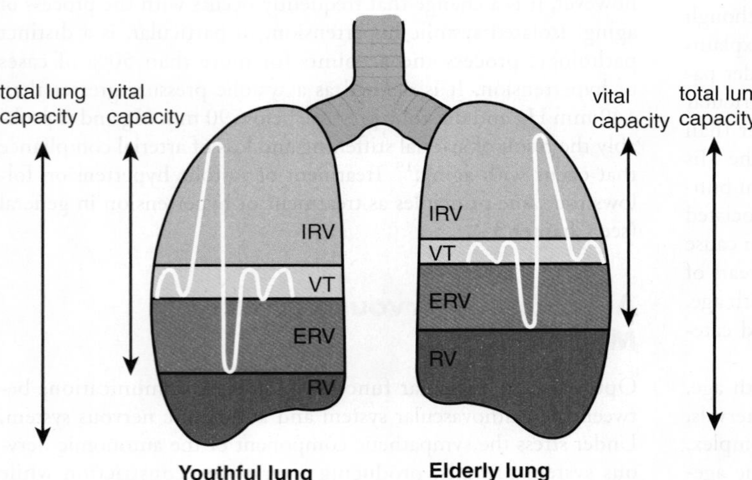

Figure 9-4 Changes in lung volumes with age. With aging note particularly the decrease in vital capacity (VC) and the increase in residual volume (RV). IRV, inspiratory research volume; V_T, tidal volume; ERV, expiratory reserve volume; RV, reserve volume; total lung capacity (TLC) = IRV = V_T + ERV + RV; vital capacity (VC) = IRV + V_T + ERV. (Reproduced from Timiras, P. S. [Ed.]. [2003]. *Physiological basis of aging and geriatrics* [3rd ed., p. 324].)

As a result of changes in airway closure, diffusing capacity, lung volumes, and lung structure, a lower arterial oxygen tension is seen in older adults. The arterial oxygen (Pa_{O2}) decreases and alveolar–arterial oxygen difference ($A-a_{O2}$) widens, whereas arterial carbon dioxide (Pa_{CO2}) and pH remain unchanged.

In summary, although the lung undergoes some structural and functional changes, the nondiseased respiratory system continues to be capable of supporting daily function throughout life. The effect of changes in the respiratory system may become evident under situations of high physiologic demand.

RENAL CHANGES

The kidney is an organ with complex functions that are intimately related with other organ systems, such as the cardiovascular, endocrine, and neurological systems. In discussing the aging kidney, changes are discussed as they relate to intrinsic changes in the kidney as well as those adaptive changes that result from the effects of other systems.

Structural Changes

The volume and weight of the kidney reach maximum in the third decade of life, start to decline during the fourth decade, and continue to decline throughout the remainder of the lifespan. Most of the decline in volume and weight is in the cortex, with a steady decline in the number of nephrons. Renal arteries undergo age-related thickening, producing a decline in renal blood flow and an increase in vascular resistance with age.

Functional Changes

Average renal blood flow decreases approximately 10% per decade, and the majority of older adults lose approximately 10% of glomerular filtration rate (GFR) per decade after the fourth decade. The reduced renal blood flow and decreased number of nephrons contribute to the reduction of GFR. Because of the decrease in muscle mass with aging, increased serum creatinine does not correspond with reduced GFR. Creatinine clearance, not serum creatinine, should be the criterion for assessing renal function in older people. The Cockcroft–Gault equation predicts creatinine clearance from serum creatinine. For men: creatinine clearance = (140 − age) (weight in kg)/(72 × serum creatinine measured in mg/dL). The results are adjusted for women by multiplying by 0.85.

The clinical importance of this formula is apparent when determinations about kidney function and appropriate drug dosage need to be made. The steady decline in renal function impairs the ability of the kidney to excrete a salt or water load and decreases the renal clearance of those medications normally removed by the kidney.[24]

The aging kidney's tendency to lose salt is related to nephron loss, with increased osmotic load per nephron leading to mild osmotic diuresis and the age-related changes in the renin–aldosterone system. Lower levels of renin (decreased by 30% to 50% in older adults) are related to 30% to 50% reductions in plasma concentration of aldosterone. When these lower levels are combined with the decreased GFR, older people are at risk for expansion of extracellular fluid volume when faced with an acute salt load (from diet, drugs, or intravenous fluids).

The limited ability of the kidney to regulate salt balance is compounded by changes in water regulation. The aging kidney exhibits a modest age-related impairment in the ability to dilute urine and excrete a water load. Inability to dilute urine maximally is related to decreased GFR and an inability to suppress antidiuretic hormone. The ability to concentrate urine declines moderately also, with the usual value specific gravity of 1.032 decreasing to 1.024 at age 80 years.[25] Therefore, the older person has more difficulty retaining fluid when it is necessary, as in situations of decreased circulating fluid volume (e.g., dehydration), and in excreting fluid, as in situations of excess circulating fluid volume (e.g., congestive heart failure).

Although baseline homeostasis of fluids and electrolytes is maintained with normal aging, there is a progressive loss of renal reserve. Vitamin D hydroxylation in the kidney is decreased and may contribute to a decreased intestinal absorption of calcium. Decreased renal reserve manifests in older patients' vulnerability to renal failure during acute illness. There are many functions of the kidney (e.g., erythropoietin production, hormone metabolism) that have yet to be thoroughly studied. Of those changes that have been described, the clinical effects on drugs and their excretion and on fluid balance are of primary importance.

HEPATIC CHANGES

Structural Changes

The proportion of liver to body weight remains constant through middle age and decreases gradually after age 70 years.[26] Liver histology in older adults shows more lipofuscin pigment and giant hepatocytes than in younger individuals. In healthy subjects, liver size, blood flow, and perfusion decrease by 30% to 40% between the third and tenth decade.[26]

Functional Changes

There is no change in level of serum bilirubin, aminotransferases, or alkaline phosphatase with aging. Age-related change in liver function is small and, with the exception of some enzymes involved in drug metabolism, is not clinically significant. There is a decrease in the hepatic clearance of drugs, particularly those that have a low-extraction ratio and whose elimination is dependent on the cytochrome P450 system.

EFFECTS OF AGING ON PHARMACOKINETICS

Drug Absorption

Little is known about absorption of oral drugs from the intestines, but it seems to be mildly decreased or unchanged with age. Absorption appears to be the pharmacokinetic parameter least affected by advancing age.

Drug Distribution

Decreased serum albumin concentration is linked to decreased binding capacity of drugs. Drugs that are bound are inactive in terms of therapeutic effect. Unbound, or free, drug is free to exert therapeutic effects. This is one reason why a smaller dosage of drug may exert the same therapeutic effect in an older person as a standard dosage in a younger person.

With aging, lean body mass decreases by approximately 10% and body fat increases by the same amount. This, along with decreased total body water, may also contribute to the retention of fat-soluble drugs, so that they exert effects over a longer period of time because of depot action.

Drug Metabolism and Excretion

The effects of aging on drug metabolism depend on the pathway of metabolism in the liver. There is evidence that first-phase metabolism decreases with age.[2] The liver microsomal drug oxidation/reduction system (P450 system) is responsible for the metabolism of many drugs. Although drug-metabolizing enzymes in the cytochrome P450 system do not decrease with age, most studies show decreases in drug metabolism by this system.[8] Multiple drug and environmental factors affect the P450 system and likely explain the observed decrease in drug metabolism in older patients.

The other route of drug excretion is the kidney. As was previously described, changes in renal plasma flow and GFR may lead to decreased excretion of active drug with consequent prolonged half-lives of drugs and sustained or increased levels of free drug in the serum.

As a result of these changes in absorption, distribution, metabolism, and excretion, greater care must be exercised with drug administration to older patients. Administering drugs in smaller doses and less frequently may accomplish an adequate therapeutic effect. If adverse reactions or side effects occur, it may be more prudent to discontinue a suspected drug rather than add another drug to counteract the effects. Older people are vulnerable to adverse effects from drugs for many reasons (e.g., age changes, chronic conditions, polypharmacy). Consequently, clinical professionals must exercise caution and responsibility when drugs and older adults are concerned.

SUMMARY

Cardiovascular function declines progressively with age, and because of the inter-relatedness of the major systems, it is affected by and affects the other systems as well. Respiratory, renal, and hepatic functions are independent and interconnected with cardiovascular function so that normal age-related changes in any or all of these systems exacerbate changes in other systems. One significant area in which this interconnectedness is exemplified is in drug therapy. The ongoing question and dilemma for the health care provider is differentiating between decline in function that occurs with age and problems resulting from specific cardiovascular diseases.

REFERENCES

1. Cristofalo, V. J., Gerhard, G. S., & Pignolo, R. J. (1994). Molecular biology of aging. *Surgical Clinics of North America, 74*, 1–21.
2. Kane, R. L., Ouslander, J. G., Abrass, I. B., & Kane, R. (2004). *Essentials of clinical geriatrics* (5th ed.). New York: McGraw-Hill.
3. Berry, A. L., & Davignon, D. (1991). Changes with aging. In M. Patrick, S. L. Woods, R. Craven, J. Rokosky, & P. Bruno (Eds.), *Medical-surgical nursing* (2nd ed., pp. 55–70). Philadelphia: Lippincott.
4. Kenny, R. A. (1985). Physiology of aging. *Clinics in Geriatric Medicine, 1*, 37–60.
5. Lakatta, E. G., & Levy, D. (2003). Arterial and cardiac aging: Major shareholders in cardiovascular disease enterprises. Part II: The aging heart in health: Links to heart disease. *Circulation, 107*, 346–354.
6. Lakatta, E. G. (2000). Cardiovascular aging in health. *Clinics in Geriatric Medicine, 16*, 419–444.
7. Taffet, G. E., & Lakatta, E. G. (2003). Aging of the cardiovascular system. In W. R. Hazzard, J. P. Blass, J. B. Halter, J. G. Ouslander, & M. E. Tinetti (Eds.), *Principles of geriatric medicine & gerontology* (5th ed., pp. 403–421). New York: McGraw-Hill.
8. Schwartz, J. B., & Zipes, D. P. (2008). Cardiovascular disease in the elderly. In P. Libby, R. O. Bonow, D. L. Mann, & D. P. Zipes (Eds.), *Braunwald's heart disease: A textbook of cardiovascular medicine* (8th ed., pp. 1923–1952). Philadelphia: Saunders Elsevier.
9. Lakatta, E. G. (2003). Arterial and cardiac aging: Major shareholders in cardiovascular disease enterprises. Part III: Cellular and molecular clues to heart and arterial aging. *Circulation, 107*, 490–497.
10. Cheitlin, M. D. (2003). Cardiovascular physiology – changes with aging. *American Journal of Geriatric Cardiology, 12*(1), 9–13.
11. Rich, M. W., & Curtis A. B. for the PRICE-IV investigators. (2007). Fourth Pivotal Research in Cardiolgy in the Elderly (PRICE-IV) Symposium—Electrophysiology and heart rhythm disorders in the elderly: Mechanisms and management. *American Journal of Geriatric Cardiology, 16*(5), 304–314.
12. Bilato, C., & Crow, M. T. (1996). Atherosclerosis and vascular biology of aging. *Aging, 8*, 221–234.
13. Nagai, J., Metter, E. J., & Earley, C. J., et al. (1998). Increased carotid artery intimal-medial thickness in asymptomatic older subjects with exercise-induced myocardial ischemia. *Circulation, 98*, 1504–1509.
14. Lakatta, E. G., & Levy, D. (2003). Arterial and cardiac aging: Major shareholders in cardiovascular disease enterprises. Part I: Aging arteries: A "set up" for vascular disease. *Circulation, 107*, 139–146.
15. Rooke, G. A. (2000). Autonomic and cardiovascular function in the geriatric patient. *Anesthesiology Clinics of North America, 18*, 31–46.
16. Dart, A. M., & Kingwell, B. A. (2001). Pulse pressure: A review of mechanisms and clinical relevance. *Journal of the American College of Cardiology, 37*, 975–984.
17. Gimbrone, M. A. (1999). Vascular endothelium, hemodynamic forces, and atherogenesis. *American Journal of Pathology, 155*, 1–5.
18. Thompson, A. B., Scholer, S. G., & Daughton, D. M., et al. (1992). Altered epithelial lining fluid parameters in old normal individuals. *Journal of Gerontology, 47*, 171–176.
19. Chobanian, A. V., Bakris, G. L., Black, H. R., et al. (2003). The seventh report of the Joint National Committee on Prevention, Detection, Evaluation, and Treatment of High Blood Pressure: The JNC 7 Report. *JAMA, 289*, 2560–2572.
20. Sharma, G., & Goodwin, J. (2006). Effect of aging on respiratory system physiology and immunology. *Clinical Intervention in Aging, 1*(3), 253–260.
21. McClaran, S. R., Babcock, M. A., & Pegelow, D. F., et al. (1995). Longitudinal effects of aging on lung function at rest and exercise in healthy active fit elderly adults. *Journal of Applied Physiology, 78*, 1957–1968.
22. Zeleznik, J. (2003). Normative aging of the respiratory system. *Clinics in Geriatric Medicine, 19*, 1–18.
23. Pride, N. B. (2005). Ageing and changes in lung mechanics. *European Respiratory Journal, 26*(4), 563–565.
24. Wiggins, J. (2003). Changes in renal function. In W. R. Hazzard, J. P. Blass, & J. B. Halter, et al. (Eds.), *Principles of geriatric medicine & gerontology* (5th ed., pp. 543–549). New York: McGraw-Hill.
25. Miller, M. (2003). Disorders of fluid balance. In W. R. Hazzard, J. P. Blass, & J. B. Halter, et al. (Eds.), *Principles of geriatric medicine & gerontology* (5th ed., pp. 581–592). New York: McGraw-Hill.
26. Hall, K. E. (2003). Effect of aging on gastrointestinal function. In W. R. Hazzard, J. P. Blass, & J. B. Halter, et al. (Eds.), *Principles of geriatric medicine & gerontology* (5th ed., pp. 593–600). New York: McGraw-Hill.

PART III Assessment of Heart Disease

CHAPTER 10 History Taking and Physical Examination

Barbara S. Levine

Assessment data, which are obtained from the patient's history, physical examination, and diagnostic tests, are used to formulate clinical diagnoses, establish patient goals, plan care, and evaluate patient outcomes. A complete history and physical examination includes the same content areas, whether elicited by nurses or physicians. A complete history and physical examination is impractical in most clinical situations. Many hospitals and clinics are using an electronic health record that establishes which data are included. The electronic health record assures systematic assessment but may constrain the kinds of data that are obtained. With freeform records the inclusion of appropriate content areas is determined by the patient's clinical condition and the purpose and context of the clinical encounter. Specific content areas may be investigated in greater detail by clinicians from different disciplines, and the data may be used in different ways. Nurses must be able to incorporate historical data into the nursing assessment so the interdependent nursing and medical responsibilities are completed in the correct priority sequence. Conversely, physicians need to be aware of the data elicited by nurses so the complete database is the foundation for the total plan of care.

The provision of culturally appropriate care requires understanding of and sensitivity to differences in health beliefs and practices that reflect cultures or subcultures. The challenge is to be sensitive to cultural influences that may affect the clinical encounter without stereotyping the patient based on limited knowledge of the culture of origin. Three overarching concepts that are influenced by culture and affect the clinical encounter are perception of illness or explanatory model, patterns of kinship and decision making, and comfort with touch.[1]

This chapter focuses on history taking and physical examination of the patient with heart disease. Emphasis is placed on those sections of the health history and physical examination that are affected by heart disease. General assessment techniques, with their rationale, are described. Competence in obtaining a history and in performing a physical examination cannot be achieved simply by reading the material presented. It is vitally important to become actively involved in clinical assessment, ideally with a qualified preceptor. Many hours of practice are required before the beginning student becomes skilled in assessment techniques.

CARDIOVASCULAR HISTORY

Cardiac patients who are acutely ill require a different initial history than do cardiac patients with stable or chronic conditions. A patient experiencing a myocardial infarction requires immediate, and possibly life-saving, medical and nursing interventions (e.g., relief of chest discomfort and treatment of arrhythmia) rather than an extensive interview. For this patient, asking a few, well-chosen questions regarding chest discomfort using the patient's descriptors are important. In addition, associated symptoms (such as shortness of breath or palpitations), drug allergies and reactions, current medications, history of cardiac and other major illnesses, and smoking history should be determined while assessing vital signs (heart rate and rhythm and blood pressure) and starting an intravenous line. As the patient's condition stabilizes, a more extensive history should be obtained. Cardiac patients who are not acutely ill benefit from a more detailed history and physical examination.

A comprehensive history includes the following areas:

- Identifying information
- Chief complaint or presenting problem
- History of the present illness
- Past history
- Review of systems
- Family history
- Personal and social history
- Perceived health status
- Functional patterns

The responsibility for obtaining particular portions of the health history varies with practice model and setting. In traditional, hospital-based practice models, the first six areas of the history are usually obtained by a physician, some data related to personal and social history are obtained by a physician and some by a nurse, and data related to perceived health status and functional patterns are obtained by a nurse. In collaborative practice models, all data may be obtained by an advanced-practice nurse, or responsibility for all areas of data collection may be shared by the physician, advanced-practice nurse, nurse, and other members of the health care team. The cardiac nurse uses the data to make informed clinical judgments, to monitor change over time, to identify patient and family learning needs, and to coordinate care across settings.

Health History

The health history is the patient's story of his or her diseases, symptoms, illness experiences, and responses to actual and potential health problems. Because concepts of health and healing are rooted in culture, it is essential to elicit information about the

Table 10-1 ■ DIFFERENTIAL DIAGNOSIS OF EPISODIC CHEST PAIN RESEMBLING ANGINA PECTORIS

Diagnosis	Duration	Quality	Provocation	Relief	Location	Comment
Effort angina	5–15 minutes	Visceral (pressure)	During effort or motion	Rest, nitroglycerin	Substernal radiates	First episode vivid
Rest angina	5–15 minutes	Visceral (pressure)	Spontaneous	Nitroglycerin	Substernal radiates	Often nocturnal
Mitral prolapse	Minutes to hours	Superficial (rarely visceral)	Spontaneous (no pattern)	Time	Left anterior	No pattern, variable character
Esophageal reflux	10–60 minutes	Visceral	Recumbency, lack of food	Food, antacid	Substernal epigastric	Rarely radiates
Esophageal spasm	50–60 minutes	Visceral	Spontaneous, cold liquids, exercise	Nitroglycerin	Substernal radiates	Mimics angina
Peptic ulcer	Hours	Visceral (burning)	Lack of food, "acid" foods	Food, antacids	Epigastric substernal	
Biliary disease	Hours	Visceral (wax and wane)	Spontaneous, food	Time, analgesia	Epigastric radiates	Colic
Cervical disc	Variable (gradually subsides)	Superficial	Head and neck movement	Time, analgesia	Arm, neck	Not relieved by rest palpation
Hyperventilation	2–3 minutes	Visceral	Emotion tachypnea	Stimulus removal	Substernal	Facial paresthesia
Musculoskeletal	Variable	Superficial	Movement, palpation	Time, analgesia	Multiple	Tenderness
Pulmonary	30^+ minutes	Visceral (pressure)	Often spontaneous	Rest, time, bronchodilator	Substernal	Dyspneic

From Christie, L. G. Jr., & Conti, C. R. [1981]. Systematic approach to the evaluation of angina-like chest pain. *American Heart Journal, 102,* 899.

person's beliefs about the causes, symptoms, and treatment of illness. Empathy, openness, and interest communicated by the clinician will enable patients to share their perspectives and beliefs.

The history-taking process may be the first phase in establishing a therapeutic relationship. The history is a precise, concise, chronologic description of the patient's current health status. The patient is the primary source of historical data; however, questioning of family members or close friends may provide essential information about symptoms and the impact of heart disease on family members. For example, the bed partner is more likely than the patient to provide a history of periodic respiration or sleep apnea. Review of records from previous encounters is a valuable secondary source of historical data.

The primary symptoms of heart disease include chest discomfort, dyspnea, syncope, palpitations, edema, cough, hemoptysis, and excess fatigue. Heart disease develops slowly, and the patient may have a long period of asymptomatic disease and may present initially with acute collapse. To describe the health history, a sample symptom, chest discomfort, is used throughout this chapter. A systematic approach is useful in differentiating chest discomfort due to serious, life-threatening conditions from those conditions that are less serious or would be treated in a different manner.[2] Table 10-1 summarizes conditions associated with chest discomfort.

Identifying Information

The patient's name, the name by which he or she prefers to be called, his or her age and birth date, and date and time of the interview are all recorded under identification of the patient. Country of origin, religious or cultural group, education, and socioeconomic level constitute optional information that may be included. It is assumed that all data in the history are obtained from the patient; when this is not the case, secondary data sources (e.g., family member, clinical records) should be identified. The use of an interpreter should also be recorded.

Chief Complaint or Presenting Problem

The chief complaint or presenting problem is the reason the person has sought health care and represents his or her priority for treatment. It should be recorded within quotation marks exactly as stated. The chief complaint also should indicate duration, such as "chest discomfort for 2 hours."

An asymptomatic patient may present because of a community screening activity (e.g., "high blood cholesterol discovered on finger-stick last month") or because of a positive diagnostic result (e.g., "positive calcium score on electron beam CT last week").

A patient may have more than one chief complaint. Some complaints are closely related and may be listed together, such as "chest discomfort and weakness for 2 hours." If complaints are unrelated, they should be listed separately in the order of importance to the patient. In general, "the greater the number of symptoms, the less the significance of each."[3]

There are four important points to remember when evaluating chest discomfort.[4]

1. For a patient who has a history of or who is at risk for development of coronary heart disease, always assume that the chest discomfort is secondary to ischemia until proven otherwise. This practice is important because unrelieved myocardial ischemia is immediately life threatening and can extend infarct size, resulting in serious complications such as lethal arrhythmia or cardiogenic shock. Chest discomfort related to other conditions, such as pulmonary emboli, usually is not as immediately life threatening.
2. There may be little correlation between the severity of the chest discomfort and the gravity of its cause. That is, pain is a subjective experience and depends, in part, on a lifetime of learned reactions to it. A stoic person may not admit to having much discomfort and yet may be having a large myocardial infarction. Another person may express extreme pain and yet may be experiencing stable angina rather than an acute myocardial infarction. Stress can increase pain. Taking into account the patient's usual response to pain (often obtained from a family member) may help the nurse interpret the patient's pain response better. In addition, older adults or people with diabetes may have altered sensory perception and little or no discomfort in the presence of severe disease.[5] When present, positive objective signs, such as ST segment shifts on the electrocardiogram, are clear indicators of the significance of the

subjective symptom. It is important to realize that the absence of electrocardiographic criteria for ischemia or infarction does not eliminate the clinical significance of the chest discomfort.

3. There is a poor correlation between the location of chest discomfort and its source because of the concept of "referred pain," which is pain originating in one location but being interpreted by the patient as occurring in another location. Commonly, cardiac discomfort is perceived as being in the arm, jaw, neck, or epigastric area rather than in the chest.
4. The patient may have more than one clinical problem occurring simultaneously, particularly if he or she has delayed seeking medical assistance.

History of the Present Illness

For the symptomatic patient, obtaining the history of the present illness starts with a more detailed discussion of the chief complaint. Begin with an open-ended question, such as "Tell me more about your chest discomfort." There is a wide range in patients' abilities to express thoughts accurately, chronologically, and succinctly. Some patients need guidance more than others. Listen to the patient. It is best to let patients tell their stories in a comfortable manner. However, patients who appear to be rambling need to be redirected by clarifying or leading questions. The information that must be obtained when describing any symptom is the time and manner of onset, frequency and duration, location, quality, quantity, setting, associated symptoms, alleviating or aggravating factors, pertinent negative responses, impact of the symptom on usual or desired activities, and the meaning attributed to the symptom by the patient.

The *time of onset* should be recorded, when possible, with both the date and time (e.g., "9 PM on December 22nd"). When the patient presents with chest discomfort, it is essential to know how long the discomfort has been present and if it has been present continuously since onset. The *manner of onset* is the way in which the symptom began. For example, discomfort may begin suddenly and reach maximum intensity immediately, or there may be a growing awareness of the discomfort over time. *Frequency and duration* should be stated specifically rather than generally (e.g., "once a week," "once a day," or "more than three times a day"). Likewise, patients should be assisted to express the duration of the discomfort, as in "2 minutes," "15 minutes," or "1 hour." For patients with a history of angina, it is also important to determine if there has been any change in frequency or duration of chest discomfort, which suggests worsening of the underlying disease.

Ask the patient to describe the exact *location* of the symptom by pointing to it. Cardiac pain is diffuse, and the patient often rubs a hand over the sternum and precordium. Chest pain that can be precisely located with a fingertip is usually related to chest wall abnormalities.[6] If the pain radiates, the patient should trace its path with a fingertip. The *quality* of a symptom refers to its unique characteristics, such as color, appearance, and texture. Chest discomfort is so subjective that its quality is particularly difficult to describe. Thus, whenever possible, it is important to use the patient's own words (in quotation marks). *Angina* means tightening, and the discomfort associated with angina may be described as "pressing," "squeezing," "tightening," "strangling," or "constricting."[6] The patient's response to the symptom also should be recorded (e.g., "It makes me stop what I'm doing and sit down," or "I can continue my activities without stopping").

Quantity refers to the size, extent, or amount of the symptom. The quantity of the chest discomfort is described in terms of its severity. Again, quantity is extremely subjective and might be rated best on a 10-point scale, ranging from "barely noticeable" (1) to "the worst pain ever" (10). The severity of pain should be recorded as a fraction (e.g., 2/10 or 10/10).

Ask patients to describe the *setting* and if they were alone or with someone when the symptom occurred. If the symptom has occurred before, ascertain if the setting, circumstances, or the presence of another person is consistent during symptom onset. This information may be useful later in counseling or helping a patient gain insight into the development of his or her symptoms. Chest discomfort that is reliably associated with activity (e.g., walking up hill) is a specific indicator of cardiac ischemia.

The patient should be asked to describe any *associated symptoms* that always accompany the chief complaint. For example, palpitations and dizziness might always precede the chest discomfort. If the patient mentions associated symptoms, these should be described in the same manner as the chief complaint (i.e., quality, quantity, onset, duration). It is important to note whether these associated symptoms occur consistently with the chief complaint or occur independently at other times.

Alleviating factors, such as resting, changing position, or taking medication, should be noted. Change in the time it takes for alleviating factors to be effective should be identified. For example, if, in the past, the chest discomfort resolved with 5 minutes of rest and now requires 10 minutes, worsening or a new pathologic process is suggested. *Aggravating factors*, such as eating, exercising, or being in a cold climate, also must be recorded. These factors can provide helpful diagnostic information. To complete the present illness history, it is also important to record any *pertinent negative responses* to the interviewer's questions, such as "The chest discomfort is not made worse by strenuous exercise." The patient should be specifically asked about palpitations, dizziness, syncope, dyspnea, orthopnea, and paroxysmal nocturnal dyspnea, if these symptoms have not already been described.

Impact of the symptom on usual or desired activities should be explored. Some people with recurrent chest discomfort reduce their activity over time to try and prevent chest discomfort. It is essential that clinicians understand how the symptom or disease has affected the patient's activity and perceived quality of life.

Throughout the interview, the nurse observes the patient carefully and may begin to understand the meaning the illness has for the patient. The personal meaning of the illness can amplify or reduce the symptom experience and course of action. When interviewing members of a culture not one's own, ask "Can you tell me what caused your illness?" and about the use of home remedies, foods, or traditional healers.[7]

The results of diagnostic or laboratory testing specifically related to heart disease are included in the *history of present illness*. Prior cardiac events (e.g., coronary artery bypass surgery or myocardial infarction) are included also.

Cardiovascular risk factors and current activity may be added in a separate paragraph to the conventional content of the history of present illness. Risk factors for coronary heart disease are discussed in Chapter 32.

Sample questions that may be used in assessing the patient with acute or recurrent chest discomfort are listed below. Similar questions may be generated to assess patients with other symptoms. However, it is important to phrase the questions according to the appropriateness of the situation and logically to pursue areas where further clarification is necessary.

- When exactly do you get the discomfort? Are you having discomfort now?
- What were you doing when the chest discomfort occurred?

- Exactly how often does the chest discomfort occur?
- How many minutes does it usually last?
- Can you point to the exact location where it starts?
- Does the discomfort move anywhere else?
- If so, can you trace its path with your fingertip?
- What words would you use to describe how the discomfort feels?
- What do you do when you have the chest discomfort?
- Quantify your discomfort on a 1-to-10 scale.
- Where were you when the discomfort occurred?
- If the chest discomfort has occurred before, have you always been in the same place?
- Were you alone at the time or with someone?
- Did you notice any other symptoms that occurred at the same time?
- If yes, does this other symptom ever occur by itself?
- What can you do to make the chest discomfort better?
- What can you do to make it worse?
- Are you taking any medication, botanical medications, supplements, foods or home remedies to improve your chest discomfort?
- If yes, what is the medication, botanical medication, supplement, food, or home remedy?
- Does any medication you are taking affect your chest discomfort?
- If yes, what is the medication?
- What time of day do you prefer to take your medication?
- Are you doing anything else to improve your chest discomfort, for example yoga or meditation?
- What activities have you given up because of your chest discomfort?
- What do you think this chest discomfort means?
- Do you know anyone else who has had this kind of discomfort?

Past History

The past history includes past illnesses and interventions not directly related to the present illness. For a patient with chest discomfort, the history of a previous myocardial infarction, coronary artery bypass surgery, or cholecystectomy belongs in the *history of present illness*, whereas a remote appendectomy does not. Major elements of the *past history* include childhood and adult illnesses, accidents and injuries, current health status, current medications, allergies, and health maintenance. Always ask about major illnesses such as chronic obstructive airway disease, diabetes mellitus, bleeding disorders, and acquired immuno deficiency syndrome (AIDS).

Allergic reactions (e.g., to drugs, food, environmental agents, or animals) also should be noted. Always ask if the patient has an allergy to penicillin or to commonly used emergency drugs, such as lidocaine hydrochloride and morphine sulfate. Allergy to shellfish suggests iodine sensitivity and is important because agents used in cardiac diagnostic tests may contain iodine. Both the allergen and the reaction should always be noted, because some patients confuse an allergic reaction with a drug's side effect.

Medication history includes all prescription and over-the-counter drugs, including botanical medicines, supplements, and home remedies. Over-the-counter preparations, botanical medications, and supplements that increase heart rate or afterload may precipitate or worsen symptoms. If the patient has brought medications with him or her, these should be reviewed by the nurse and then sent home or to the appropriate area for safekeeping.

Family History

The major purpose of the family history is to assess risk factors affecting the patient's current or future health. Notations regarding the age and health status of each first-degree family member are made: living and well, deceased, and the possible or confirmed diagnosis now or at death. Family occurrences of diabetes, kidney disease, tuberculosis, cancer, arthritis, asthma, allergies, mental illness, alcoholism, and drug addiction are included. A family history of coronary heart disease, myocardial infarction, or sudden death would be included in the history of present illness for a patient presenting with chest discomfort.

Personal and Social History

The personal and social history includes important and relevant information about the patient as a person. A person's response to illness is determined in part by his or her cultural background, socioeconomic standing, education, and beliefs about the illness. Major elements include health habits, home situation, and supports and resources. Occupational history may be included here or in the past history. *Health habits* include alcohol, drug, or tobacco use; nutrition; sleep; and physical activity. Use of alcohol and the amount per time period (day, week, year) should be recorded. The use of recreational drugs, especially cocaine and its derivative "crack," should also be assessed. The cigarette smoking history should be recorded as the number of pack-years (packs per day multiplied by the number of years) the patient has smoked. For ex-smokers, approximate quit date should be recorded. Other tobacco use, such as pipe or cigar smoking or chewing tobacco, should be recorded. Special diets, such as low-sodium, low-fat, low-carbohydrate, or high-protein diets, should be identified, and the patient's usual eating pattern should be described. The usual number of hours the patient sleeps and circumstances that impair or facilitate sleep should be assessed.

Current Living Circumstances. These circumstances include marital status, number of children, occupation, financial resources, and hobbies.

Perceived Health and Coping Challenges. The patient's perception of his or her current health status as either good or bad is helpful in assessing how he or she views its effect on daily living. For example, a 42-year-old man with an old anterior myocardial infarction is seen in the clinic. His chief complaint is extreme fatigue that prevents him from working a full day at the office. Initial investigation focuses on ruling out any new process affecting the adequacy of cardiac output, such as a left ventricular aneurysm. Nonpathophysiologic causes for fatigue must be considered also, such as fear of overstressing his heart and sudden death, changes in the work situation, family difficulties, or depression.

Being aware of patients' goals in terms of health and lifestyle is important in determining whether their expectations are realistic. "What do you see yourself doing 3 months from now?" is a good way to ask the patient to define the goal. Another approach is ascertaining what changes the patient would be willing to make in life if the goal could not be achieved.

Assessing the patient's and family's expectations of health care has implications for teaching. For example, is the patient with unstable angina pectoris who has been admitted after "cardiac catheterization" able to explain what the test was and why it resulted in admission? Communication among the health care team members is essential before planning any teaching.

Resources and Support System. It is important to consider the patient's strengths and support system when planning care across the continuum: environmental resources, such as the proximity to the hospital; personal—social support, such as a spouse to provide home care; and economic support, such as adequate insurance, are all examples. Needed resources that are not readily available also must be considered. Knowledge of the patient's health benefits and financial status assists the health care team in designing an affordable therapeutic regimen (e.g., the avoidance of expensive combination or sustained-release medications when other drugs and dosage forms that are as effective and less costly are available).

Review of Systems

To ensure that all important areas have been considered, a systematic review of all body systems is conducted. Lists of major symptoms associated with each body system are included in health assessment textbooks.[8] Some clinicians prefer to conduct the review of systems simultaneously with the physical examination. For the patient with chest discomfort, the review of the cardiac, pulmonary, and gastrointestinal systems is logically included in the history of present illness.

Functional Patterns

Clinical information related to function is collected in the following areas[9]:

- Health perception–health management
- Nutrition–metabolism
- Elimination
- Activity–exercise
- Cognitive–perceptual
- Sleep–rest
- Self-perception–self-concept
- Roles and relationships
- Sexuality
- Coping–stress
- Values–beliefs

Information collected within these functional patterns does not duplicate information collected within other areas of the health history. The sequence of data gathered in the functional assessment is determined by the patient's clinical condition and the purpose of the encounter. Relevant data obtained earlier in the history should not be repeated.

For the acutely ill cardiac patient who is admitted to the hospital, areas that affect the hospital experience are assessed first. As the patient is able, all functional patterns are assessed. To facilitate the gathering of subjective information for the functional assessment, examples of questions, using the sample symptom of chest discomfort, are listed below. Functional assessment is an ongoing process that evaluates the effect of intervention on patient outcome.

Health Perception–Health Management. Collect the following information:

- What concerns do you have about your health or hospitalization?
- What things are important to you while you are hospitalized? How can we make this experience as easy as possible for you?
- What do you think caused this illness (symptom)?
- Compared with others your age, how would you rate your general health?
- What things do you believe are important to maintain your health?

Nutrition–Metabolism. Collect the following information:

- What do you like to eat (including cultural or ethnic favorites)?
- How are your foods prepared (canned or commercially prepared foods versus fresh foods)?
- Do you usually eat in a restaurant, fast-food outlet, or at home?
- Who shops for groceries?
- Who prepares the meals?
- Are you on a special diet?

Elimination. Collect the following information:

- Is the amount that you urinate normal for you?
- Do you ever get up at night to use the bathroom? If so, how many times?
- If there was a change in elimination pattern, when did you notice it?
- Do you sometimes lose urine or find that you cannot quite make it to the bathroom?
- Do you take a diuretic? If so, when do you take it?
- What is your usual frequency of bowel movements? When was your last movement?
- Are there things you do to maintain that pattern?

Activity–Exercise. Collect the following information:

- Have you noticed a change in your usual or desired activity level?
- Do you have sufficient energy for your desired activities?
- What is the most strenuous activity you perform on a regular basis? How often and how long? What stops you?
- What leisure or recreational activities do you enjoy? Are you currently able to participate in these activities? What prevents your participation?
- Are you satisfied with your current level of activity?

Cognitive–Perceptual. Collect the following information:

- Do you have any difficulty with seeing or hearing? Glasses or hearing aid?
- Do you think as fast as you used to? As clearly?
- In general, what is the easiest way for you to learn new material? Any learning difficulties?
- Do you understand why you are in the hospital?
- What does your diagnosis mean to you?
- What is your understanding of the treatment plan?
- Do you understand the risk factors for heart disease and how to modify them?
- Do you understand how long you will be in the hospital and when you can return to your usual activities of daily living?

Sleep–Rest. Collect the following information:

- How many hours do you usually sleep? What hours?
- Do you have difficulty falling asleep or staying asleep? Has this been a change for you or have you always had this difficulty?
- Do you follow a specific bedtime routine or ritual?
- Do you snore loudly?
- Do you feel rested when you wake up in the morning?[10]
- Are you tired and excessively sleepy during daytime hours?[10]

Self-Perception–Self-Concept. Collect the following information:

- How would you describe yourself? Your personality? Your approach to life?

- Most of the time, do you feel good about yourself?
- Have you noticed changes in yourself or your body? Do these changes concern you?

Roles and Relationships. Collect the following information:

- Do you live alone? With whom do you live?
- Do you have a close friend or confidant?
- How do you and those close to you feel about your illness?
- Do you often feel lonely? Do you feel part of the neighborhood in which you live?

Sexuality. Collect the following information:

- Have you experienced any changes in your sexuality? Problems in sexual relationships?
- For women: are you still menstruating? Are you taking hormone replacements? Do you have menopausal symptoms (such as hot flashes and sleep disturbances)?

Coping–Stress. Collect the following information:

- Do you feel tense or anxious much of the time? What helps? Do you use medicines for anxiety?
- When you feel stressed, who is most helpful to you?
- When you have big problems in your life, how do you handle them? Does that usually work for you?

Values–Beliefs. Collect the following information:

- Are you generally satisfied with your life?
- Is religion important to you?
- Do you hold religious or other beliefs that you wish to observe here?

Functional and Therapeutic Classification

After the history is completed, it may be possible to categorize the patient according to the New York Heart Association's Functional and Therapeutic Classification (Table 10-2).[11] This classification may be helpful in assessing symptom severity and monitoring effects of treatment over time. The patient's functional classification may improve as recovery from an acute event, such as myocardial infarction, occurs or as intervention is optimized. Conversely, it may decline with worsening or additional disease.

PHYSICAL ASSESSMENT

Assessment of physical findings confirms or expands data obtained in the health history. Baseline information is obtained at the initial encounter, and frequency of subsequent assessments is based on the clinical encounter. Change in the data over time documents progression of, or recovery from, acute disease; new disease; the effectiveness of current interventions; and the patient's current functional status. The type, degree, and rate of change assist the nurse in identifying or predicting immediate or long-term problems, formulating nursing diagnoses, planning care, and establishing individual patient outcome criteria.

In the acutely ill cardiac patient, segments of the physical examination are performed every 2 to 4 hours or more frequently if indicated. Although some data may be available from monitoring devices, physical examination assists in evaluating the accuracy of those data. As the acutely ill patient improves, assessments are routinely done once per shift or more frequently if indicated. If a rapid change in patient condition occurs, the initial assessment is problem focused and the complete assessment is done at a later time. Because nurses spend 24 hours per day with the hospitalized patient, they are in the best position to identify any changes that occur. It is to the patient's benefit for changes to be detected early, before serious complications develop. Any changes observed in the examination should be documented in the patient's record and reported to the physician. To collect, correlate, and interpret the data accurately, a thorough understanding of the cardiac cycle

Table 10-2 ■ FUNCTIONAL AND THERAPEUTIC CLASSIFICATION OF PATIENTS WITH DISEASES OF THE HEART

Functional Classification		Therapeutic Classification	
Class I	Patients with cardiac disease but without resulting limitations of physical activity. Ordinary physical activity does not cause undue fatigue, palpitation, dyspnea, or anginal pain.	Class A	Patients with cardiac disease whose physical activity need not be restricted in any way.
		Class B	Patients with cardiac disease whose ordinary physical activity need not be restricted, but who should be advised against servere or competitive efforts.
Class II	Patients with cardiac disease resulting in slight limitation of physical activity. They are comfortable at rest. Ordinary physical activity results in fatigue, palpitation, dyspnea, or anginal pain	Class C	Patients with cardiac disease whose ordinary physical activity should be moderately restricted and whose more strenuous efforts should be discontinued.
Class III	Patients with cardiac disease resulting in marked limitation of physical activity. They are comfortable at rest. Less than ordinary physical activity causes fatigue, palpitation, dyspnea, or anginal pain.	Class D	Patients with cardiac disease whose ordinary physical activity should be markedly restricted.
		Class E	Patients with cardiac disease who should be at complete rest, confined to bed or chair.
Class IV	Patients with cardiac disease resulting in inability to carry on any physical activity without discomfort. Symptoms of cardiac insufficiency or of the anginal syndrome may be present even at rest. If any physical activity is undertaken, discomfort is increased.		

From New York Heart Association Criteria Committee [1964]. *Diseases of the heart and blood vessels: Nomenclature and criteria for diagnosis* [6th ed.] Boston, Little, Brown.

(Chapter 1) is essential. A cardiac physical assessment should include an evaluation of:

- The heart as a pump—reduced pulse pressure, cardiac enlargement, and presence of murmurs and gallop rhythms
- Filling volumes and pressures—the degree of jugular venous pressure and the presence or absence of crackles, peripheral edema, and postural changes in blood pressure
- Cardiac output—heart rate, blood pressure, pulse pressure, systemic vascular resistance, urine output, and central nervous system manifestations
- Compensatory mechanisms—increased filling volumes, peripheral vasoconstriction, and elevated heart rate

The order and techniques of examination proceed logically. The precise order may vary with the setting and the condition of the patient. With practice, the focused cardiovascular examination can be done in approximately 10 minutes:

- General appearance
- Head
- Arterial pulse
- Jugular venous pressure
- Blood pressure
- Peripheral vasculature
- Heart
- Lungs
- Abdomen

General Appearance

Observe the general appearance of the patient while the history is being obtained.[6] The patient's appearance and responses provide cues to the cardiovascular status. Note general build, skin color, presence of shortness of breath, and distention of neck veins. Assess the patient's level of distress. If he or she is in pain, the patient's response to it may assist in the differential diagnosis. For example, moving about is a characteristic response to the pain of myocardial infarction, whereas sitting quietly is more characteristic of angina, and leaning forward is more characteristic of pericarditis.[12] Some abnormalities of the arterial pulses may be observed unobtrusively. For example, patients with severe aortic insufficiency may have bounding pulses that cause the head to bob. Note appropriateness of weight; malnutrition and cachexia are associated with chronic, severe heart failure.[6] Skeletal manifestations of Marfan's syndrome, tall stature, and arachnodactyly, may be observed. Level of consciousness should be described. Appropriateness of thought content, reflecting the adequacy of cerebral perfusion, is particularly important to evaluate. Family members who are most familiar with the patient can be of help in alerting the examiner to subtle behavior changes. The nurse also should be aware of the patient's anxiety level, not only to attempt to put the patient more at ease, but to realize its effects on the cardiovascular system.

Height, Weight, and Waist Circumference

Height and weight are best measured using a standing platform scale with a height attachment. Weak, immobile, or critically ill patients may require a bed or chair scale for weighing, and it may be necessary to rely on the patient's self-reported height. Weight is an indicator of nutritional and fluid status; excessive weight indicates increased cardiovascular risk.

Body mass index (BMI) describes relative weight for height. BMI is calculated as weight in kilograms (kg) divided by the square of the height in meters (m^2). In adults, obesity is defined as a BMI of 30 kg/m^2 or more; overweight is a BMI of 25 kg/m^2 or more.[13]

Larger BMI and abdominal fat distribution are associated with increased cardiovascular risk.[14] In overweight people, waist circumference of 102 cm (40 inches) in men or 88 cm (35 inches) in women indicates increased risk of cardiovascular disease, Type II diabetes mellitus, and metabolic syndrome (Chapter 39).

Head

The examination of the head includes assessment of facial characteristics, color, temperature, and eyes. Advanced practice nurses may examine the fundi and retinal vasculature.

Facial Characteristics

Examination of the facial characteristics may aid in the recognition of disorders affecting the cardiovascular system.[6] *Coronary heart disease* is suggested by the presence of an earlobe crease in a person younger than 45 years of age. *Rheumatic heart disease* with severe mitral stenosis is associated with a malar flush, cyanotic lips, and slight jaundice from hepatic congestion. With severe aortic regurgitation, head bobbing with each heartbeat (de Musset's sign) may be present. Infective endocarditis is associated with a "café au lait" complexion. *Constrictive pericarditis* and *tricuspid valve disease* tend to cause facial edema. *Pheochromocytoma* is associated with episodic facial flushing, as well as severe hypertension and tachyarrhythmia.

Systemic conditions may affect or reflect cardiovascular function or treatment.[6] *Systemic lupus erythematosus* may present with a butterfly rash on the face and may suggest inflammatory heart disease. *Myxedema* is characterized by dry, sparse hair; loss of lateral eyebrows; a dull, expressionless face; and periorbital puffiness. Because a myocardial effect of hypothyroidism is reduced cardiac output, heart failure may develop in these patients. *Cushing's syndrome* is characterized by moon facies, hirsutism, acne, and centripetal obesity with thin extremities. High blood pressure frequently occurs with Cushing's syndrome.

Color

Cyanosis is the bluish discoloration seen through the skin and mucous membranes when the concentration of reduced hemoglobin exceeds 5 g/100 mL of blood. *Peripheral cyanosis* implies reduced blood flow to the periphery. Because more time is available for the tissues to extract oxygen from the hemoglobin molecule, the arteriovenous oxygen difference widens. Cyanosis of the nose, lips, and earlobes is considered peripheral. Peripheral cyanosis may occur physiologically with the vasoconstriction associated with anxiety or a cold environment, or pathologically in conditions that reduce blood flow to the periphery, such as cardiogenic shock.

Central cyanosis, as observed in the buccal mucosa, implies serious heart or lung disease and is accompanied by peripheral cyanosis. In severe heart disease, a right-to-left shunt exists in which blood passes through the lungs without being fully oxygenated, as happens in severe heart failure with interstitial pulmonary edema. In severe lung disease, changes produced by chronic obstructive airway disease or fibrosis impede oxygenation. *Pallor* can denote anemia (with concomitant decreased oxygen-carrying capacity) or an increased systemic vascular resistance. *Jaundice* can be associated with hepatic engorgement from right ventricular failure.

Temperature

Temperature reflects the balance of heat production and dissipation in the body. Normal oral temperature is considered to be

37°C (98.6°F). However, there is a diurnal pattern of temperature fluctuation, with temperatures as low as 35.8°C (96.4°F) orally in the early morning to as high as 37.3°C (99.1°F) orally in the late afternoon or evening. Oral temperatures average 0.5°C (1.0°F) lower than rectal temperatures, but this difference is quite variable.[8] Normal body temperature may be less than 37°C in older adults because of reduced heat production (lower metabolic activity, less muscle mass and activity) and conservation (less insulation).[15]

In hospitalized patients, body temperature usually is measured on admission and then every 4 hours or more often if indicated. After cardiac surgery, temperature is measured every 15 to 30 minutes until rewarming is complete, and every 1 to 4 hours until normothermia is achieved. Measure the temperature orally unless the patient is unconscious or unable to close his or her mouth. Body temperatures also may be measured rectally, by means of a pulmonary artery catheter equipped with a thermistor, by means of a thermistor-equipped urinary bladder catheter, or with a device that measures temperature in the insulated auditory meatus close to the tympanic membrane. Pulmonary artery, urinary bladder, tympanic, and rectal temperatures are all considered to be core temperatures; however, they actually measure somewhat different things, and simultaneous measurements may not agree, especially during hypothermia. Pulmonary artery temperature measures the mean blood temperature that results from core thermogenesis and peripheral heat loss or gain. Because urine is a filtrate of blood, urinary bladder temperature also reflects mean blood temperature, but may be falsely low in the setting of low-output renal failure. During hypothermia after cardiac surgery, rectal temperatures reflect peripheral, rather than core, temperatures.[16]

Eyes

The eyes are examined for vision and appearance. A funduscopic examination may be performed.

Vision. Vision is assessed to determine if defects exist that may affect activities of daily living. The examination is as simple as having the patient read a name tag or identify an object.

Appearance. *Corneal arcus,* a thin, grayish-white circle around the iris, may occur normally with aging (Fig. 10-1*A*). When seen in white people younger than age 40 years, corneal arcus suggests hyperlipidemia. *Xanthelasmas* are slightly raised, yellowish plaques of cholesterol in the skin that appear along the nasal side of one or both eyelids (Fig. 10-1*B*). They are associated with hyperlipidemia but also may occur normally. *Ophthalmitis* and *petechial* and *subconjunctival hemorrhages* of the upper and lower eyelids are seen with bacterial endocarditis.

Fundi. Examination of the ocular fundi provides the only opportunity for direct visualization of blood vessels. Vascular changes from high blood pressure and diabetes mellitus can be detected in the arteries and small veins of the retina. In general health care, funduscopic examination is conducted without pharmacologic dilation of the pupils. Physiologic dilation may be maximized by darkening the room and asking the patient to gaze off in the distance. Photographs printed in books are taken through a maximally dilated pupil with a special camera. The view through the ophthalmoscope is only a small portion of the retina. It is necessary to direct the ophthalmoscope in varying directions, following blood vessels and observing the retinal structures and background.

The *funduscopic examination technique* is as follows:[8]

- Darken the room.
- Turn on the ophthalmoscope light; select the large round beam of white light.
- Adjust the lens disc to 0 diopter. Keep your index finger on the lens disc throughout the examination.
- Use your right hand and right eye to examine the patient's right eye; use your left hand and left eye to examine the patient's left eye.
- Place your opposite thumb over the patient's eyebrow to gain proprioceptive guidance as you move closer to the patient.
- Ask the patient to look straight ahead and to fix his or her gaze on a distant point.
- Brace the ophthalmoscope firmly against your face, with your eye directly behind the sight hole.
- Position yourself 15 inches away from the patient and 15 degrees lateral to his or her line of vision. Shine the light beam on the patient's pupil and note the *red reflex.* Absence of a *red reflex* suggests a lens opacity, such as a cataract.
- With both of your eyes open and keeping the light beam focused on the red reflex, move horizontally at a 15-degree angle slowly toward the patient. When you are approximately 1.5 to 2 inches (3 to 5 cm) from the patient, the optic disc or blood vessels should come into view (Fig. 10-2). Rotate lenses with your index finger until fundic structures are as clearly visible as possible.
- To overcome corneal reflection (light reflected back into the examiner's eye), direct the light beam toward the edge of the pupil rather than through its center.
- Examine the *optic disc,* a yellowish-orange to creamy pink oval or round structure. If you do not see the disc, follow a blood vessel centrally (by noting the angles of vessel branching and the progressive enlargement of vessel size toward the disc) until it is visible. Assess disc border clarity (nasal margin may be normally somewhat blurred) and color.

A Corneal Arcus

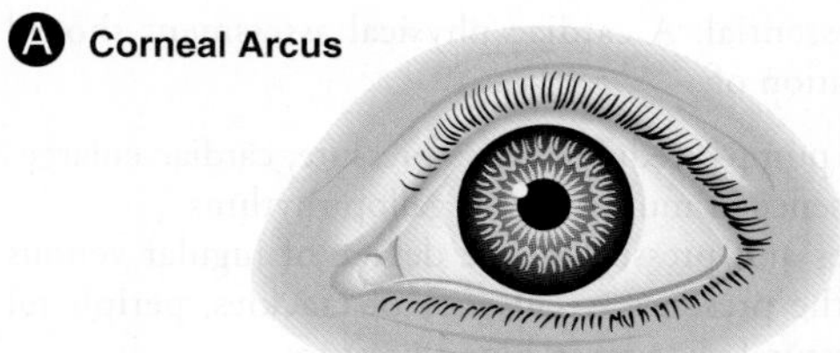

A corneal arcus is a thin grayish white arc or circle not quite at the edge of the cornea. It accompanies normal aging but may also be seen in younger people, especially African Americans. In young people, a corneal arcus suggests the possibility of hyperlipoproteinemia but does not prove it. Some surveys have revealed no relationship.

B Xanthelasmas

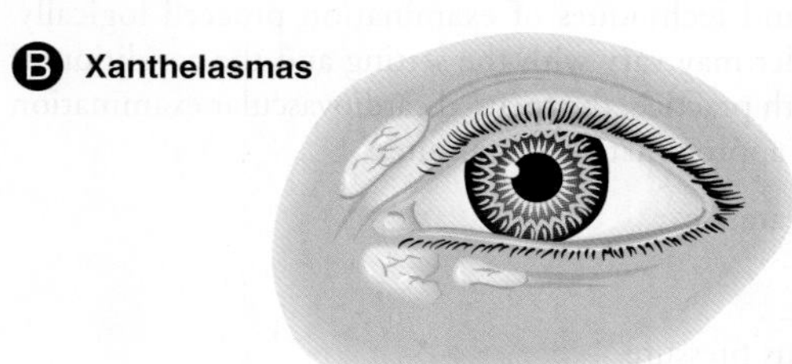

Slightly raised, yellowish, well circumscribed plaques in the skin, xanthelasmas appear along the nasal portions of one or both eyelids. They may accompany lipid disorders (e.g., hypercholesterolemia), but may also occur independently.

Figure 10-1 Eye changes suggestive of hyperlipoproteinemia. (A) Corneal arcus. (B) Xanthelasmas.

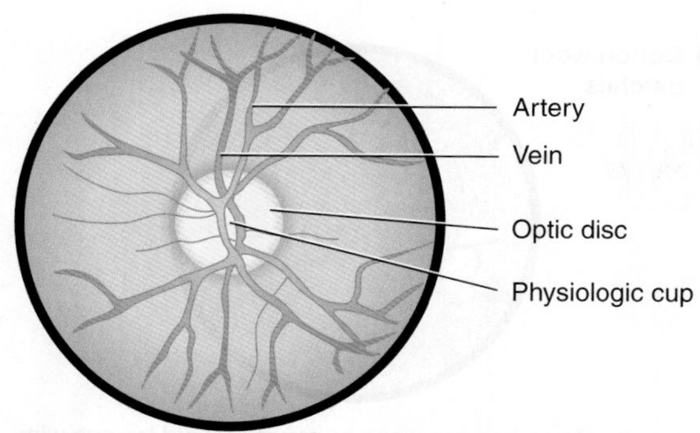

■ **Figure 10-2** Funduscopic examination of retinal structures.

- Identify the *retinal arteries* and *veins* using the differential criteria of color, size, and light reflex (or reflection; Fig. 10-3*A*). Arteries and veins appear to originate from the *physiologic cup*, a small, white depression in the optic disc. Arteries are light red, are two thirds to four fifths the diameter of veins, and have a bright light reflex. Veins are dark red, are larger than arteries, and have an inconspicuous or absent light reflex. Follow the vessels peripherally in all directions, noting the character of the arteriovenous crossings. To examine the extreme periphery, instruct the patient to look up, down, temporally, and nasally.
- Assess the retina for any *lesions,* noting size, shape, color, and distribution. *Optic disc edema* (swollen optic disc with blurred margins) is present in patients with increased intracranial pressure, retinal venous outflow obstruction, inflammation, or ischemia (Fig. 10-4).[8] *Beading* (abnormal constriction) of a retinal vein is common in diabetic retinopathy. With high blood pressure, thickening of the walls and narrowing of the lumen of retinal arteries develop. These changes are observed as *focal narrowing,* a *narrowed column of blood,* and a *narrowed light reflex* (Fig. 10-3*B*). If opacity is such that no blood column is visible, the artery appears as a *silver wire artery* (Fig. 10-3*C*). With increased filling and tortuosity, arteries closest to the optic disc manifest an increased light reflex and are known as *copper wire arteries* (Fig. 10-3*D*). Arteriovenous crossings also are affected by thickening of the artery walls, demonstrated by *tapering* of the vein on either side of the artery (Fig. 10-3*E*), *arteriovenous nicking* (abrupt cessation of the vein on either side of the artery; Fig. 10-3*F*), or *banking* of the vein (venous twisting distal to the artery, forming a dark, wide knuckle; Fig. 10-3*G*).[8,17]

A Normal retinal artery and arteriovenous (A-V) crossing

Arterial wall (invisible)
Column of blood
Light reflex

The normal arterial wall is transparent. Only the column of blood within it can usually be seen. The normal light reflex is narrow–about 1/4 the diameter of the blood column.

Vein
Arterial wall
Artery

Because the arterial wall is transparent, a vein crossing beneath the artery can be seen right up to the column of blood on either side.

B Spasm and thickening of arterial walls

Focal narrowing
Narrowed column of blood
Narrowed light reflex

In hypertension, the arteries may show areas of focal or generalized narrowing. The light reflex is also narrowed. Over many months or years, the arterial wall thickens and becomes less transparent.

C Silver wire arteries

Occasionally a portion of a narrowed artery develops such an opaque wall that no blood is visible within it. It is then called a *silver wire artery.* This change typically occurs in the smallest branches.

D Copper wire arteries

Sometimes the arteries, especially those close to the disc, become full and somewhat tortuous and develop an increased light reflex with a bright coppery luster. Such a vessel is called a *copper wire artery.*

E Tapering

The vein appears to taper down on either side of the artery.

F Concealment or A-V nicking

The vein appears to stop abruptly on either side of the artery.

G Banking

The vein is twisted on the distal side of the artery and forms a dark, wide knuckle.

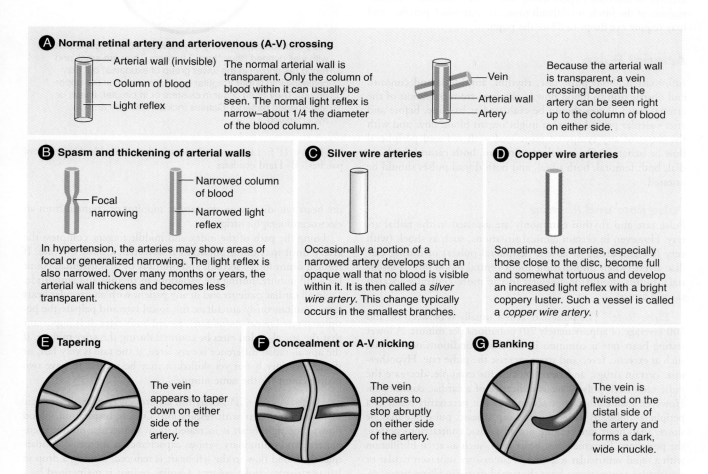

■ **Figure 10-3** Vascular changes associated with high blood pressure. (A) Normal. (B) Spasm and thickening of arteriolar walls. (C) Silver wire arterioles. (D) Copper wire arterioles. (E) Venous tapering. (F) Arteriovenous nicking. (G) Venous banking.

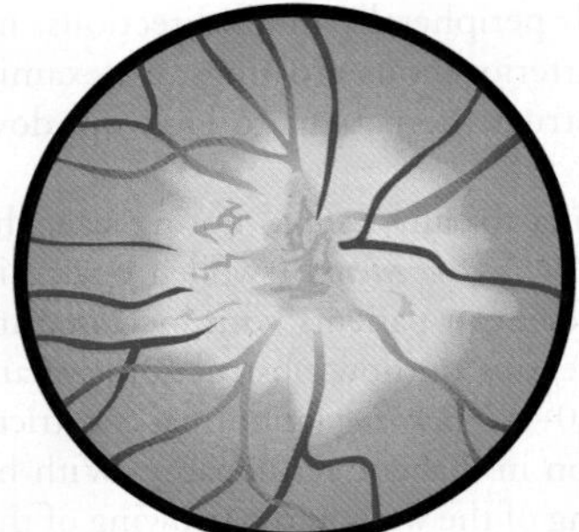

■ **Figure 10-4** Papilledema. The optic disc is swollen, its margins are blurred, and the physiologic cup is not visible.

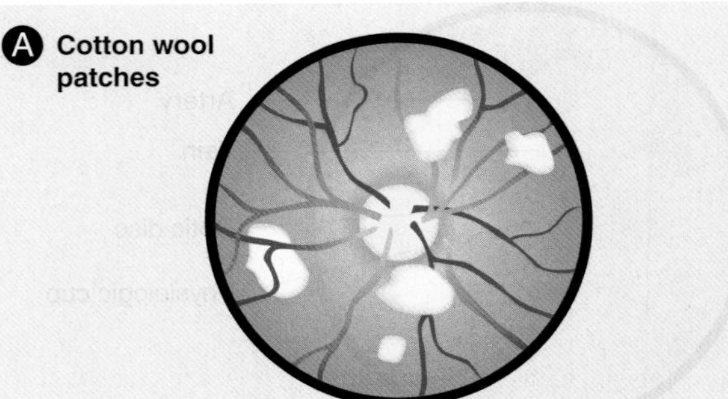

A Cotton wool patches
Cotton wool patches are white or grayish, ovoid lesions with irregular (thus "soft") borders. They are moderate in size but usually smaller than the disc. They result from infarcted nerve fibers and are seen with hypertension and many other conditions.

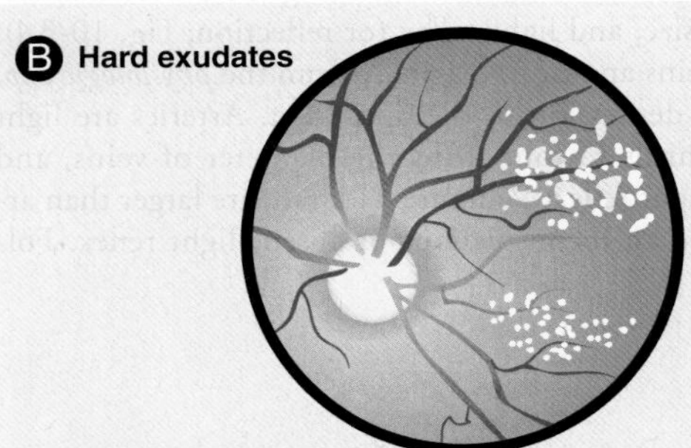

B Hard exudates
Hard exudates are creamy or yellowish, often bright lesions with well defined (thus "hard") borders. Thay are small and round (as shown in the lower group of exudates) but may coalesce into larger irregular spots (as shown in the upper group). They often occur in clusters or in circular, linear, or star-shaped patterns. Causes include diabetes and hypertension.

■ **Figure 10-5** Light-colored spots in the retina. (A) Cotton wool patches. (B) Hard exudates.

Red spots in the retina may be due to hemorrhage or microaneurysms, which can be associated with hypertension, diabetes, or a number of other conditions.[8,17] *Roth's spots,* hemorrhages with white centers, occur with subacute bacterial endocarditis and leukemia.[8,17] *Cotton wool patches* are white or gray and have large irregular shapes and fuzzy borders (Fig. 10-5*A*). They occur with hypertension and are seen frequently in patients with AIDS. *Hard exudates* are small, creamy white or yellow lesions with well-defined borders (Fig. 10-5*B*). They occur frequently in clusters and are indicative of diabetes, hypertension, and other conditions.[8] Abnormalities of the fundi are difficult to see, require much practice, and may require eye drops to dilate the pupil.

Arterial Pulse

Information about pulse rate, rhythm, amplitude and contour, and obstruction to blood flow is obtained from palpation of the arterial pulse. Pulses should be evaluated at baseline, before and after vascular procedures that might impair blood flow, and with the onset of any symptom associated with reduced peripheral flow or ischemia. On initial examination, both carotid, both radial, both femoral, both tibial, and both dorsal pulses should be assessed.

Pulse Rate and Rhythm

Pulse rate and rhythm commonly are assessed in the radial artery. However, in certain clinical situations, such as shock (with very low-amplitude or absent peripheral pulses) or during cardiac arrest (when information about central blood flow is essential), pulses should be assessed in the more centrally located carotid artery.

Pulse Rate. The pulse rate at rest usually is between 60 and 100 (average of approximately 70) pulsations per minute. A lower resting heart rate is common in athletes. Conditions or activities such as exercise, fever, and stress increase the pulse rate. Hypothermia, certain drugs, and heart blocks, for example, decrease the pulse rate. Each pulse wave is indicative of a cardiac contraction. However, each cardiac contraction does not necessarily result in a peripheral pulse. In patients with heart disease, pulse rate may be slower than heart rate because not all cardiac contractions perfuse the periphery. Extremely fast heart rates, such as atrial fibrillation with a rapid ventricular response or premature supraventricular or ventricular contractions, have shortened diastolic filling times, resulting in reduced stroke volume and, therefore, diminished or absent pulses. For this reason, pulse rate should not be recorded from the heart rate display on the cardiac monitor or counted from an electrocardiographic strip.

Using the pads of the index and middle fingers, compress the artery until maximum pulsation is detected. Count the rate. If regular, count for 15 seconds and multiply by 4; if irregular, count for a full minute, noting the variations in rhythm and amplitude.

In all cardiac patients and in any patient with an irregular heart rate, simultaneously auscultate the apical rate and palpate the peripheral rate (*apical–radial rate*); record both rates. It is important that the apical–radial rates be counted during the *same* minute. If the apical–radial difference is very large, if the rate is very fast, or if the examiner is not yet skilled, it may be helpful to have two people count for the same minute.

Pulse Rhythm. Pulse rhythm is normally regular. Physiologic variation can occur with respiration. During inspiration, blood flow to the right heart is increased, right ventricular output is enhanced, and pulmonary venous capacitance is increased. Consequently, blood flow to the left heart is reduced, causing a drop in left ventricular stroke volume. Cardiac output is maintained by a compensatory increase in heart rate (mediated by the baroreceptors). During expiration, the large amount of blood residing in the pulmonary vascular bed during inspiration reaches the left heart. Left ventricular contractility is enhanced by means of the Frank–Starling mechanism, increasing left ventricular stroke volume. Because an increased heart rate is no longer needed to maintain cardiac output, the heart rate returns to baseline. This physiologically irregular rhythm is termed *sinus arrhythmia.* It is common in people younger than 40 years of age. Other irregular rhythms are not normal. The irregularity should be described as regularly irregular (e.g., every other pulse wave is early) or irregularly irregular (e.g., atrial fibrillation). Occasional, early pulsations that are perceived as transient skips or breaks in an otherwise regular rhythm are common and are not necessarily abnormal.

Pulse Amplitude and Contour

Pulses are described in a variety of ways. The simplest classification is absent, present, and bounding. A 0-to-4 scale is often used, and pulses are graded as follows: absent (0), diminished (1+), normal (2+), moderately increased (3+), and markedly increased (4+).[18] This scale is fairly subjective, and, although an individual tends to be internally consistent over time, different people may grade the same pulse differently. There are also other scales in which the numbers are defined differently.

The amplitude of an arterial pulse is a function of the pulse pressure, which is related to stroke volume, elasticity of the arterial tree, and velocity of left ventricular ejection. Increased stroke volume, as occurs with exercise or excitement, results in increased amplitude and a bounding arterial pulse.

Small, weak pulses (Fig. 10-6*B*) have a diminished pulse pressure, which is indicative of a reduced stroke volume and ejection fraction and of increased systemic vascular resistance.

Large, bounding pulses result from an increased pulse pressure (Fig. 10-6*C*). Increased pulse pressure is caused by increased stroke volume and ejection velocity and by diminished peripheral vasoconstriction. *Corrigan's pulse* is a bounding pulse visible in the carotid artery. It occurs with aortic regurgitation.

The amplitude of a pulse contributes to its contour, but contour refers to the rate of rise and the shape of the arterial pulse. Because of the distortion that occurs when the pulse wave is transmitted peripherally, pulse contour is best assessed in the carotid arteries. The *normal pulse contour* has a rapid and smooth upstroke. The dicrotic notch is not palpable (Fig. 10-6*A*), although the dicrotic wave (Fig. 10-6*I*) may be palpable in heart failure and in febrile states.[18] Usually it is palpable only in the peripheral arteries.

Pulsus bisferiens (Fig. 10-6*D*) is characterized by a rapid upstroke and double systolic peak. This pulse may be present in idiopathic hypertrophic subaortic stenosis, aortic stenosis with regurgitation, and pure aortic insufficiency.

Pulsus alternans (Fig. 10-6*E*) is a regular rhythm in which strong pulse waves alternate with weak ones. It is an ominous sign when it occurs at normal heart rates and suggests serious heart disease. The difference in amplitude may be slight and difficult to palpate. The presence of pulsus alternans can be confirmed with a sphygmomanometer. The cuff is inflated above systolic pressure and slowly released until the first heart sound is audible. Cuff pressure is held at this point, and the pulse is palpated to determine if every pulse is audible.

Bigeminal pulses (Fig. 10-6*F*), which should not be confused with pulsus alternans, are caused by a bigeminal, premature ectopic rhythm. Note that every other pulse wave is not only diminished but is early.

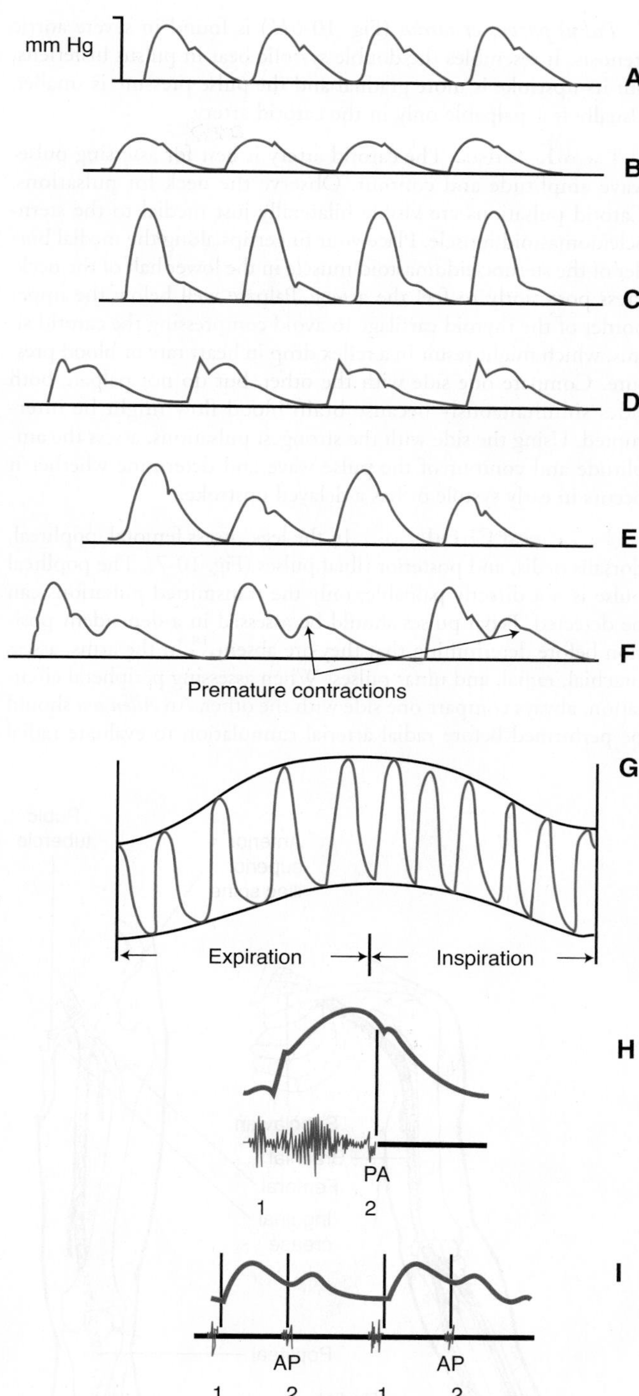

Figure 10-6 Normal and abnormal pulses. (A) Normal. (B) Small and weak. (C) Large and bounding. (D) Bisferiens. (E) Pulsus alternans. (F) Bigeminal. (G) Pulsus paradoxus. (H) Parvus et tardus. (I) Dicrotic.

Pulsus paradoxus (Fig. 10-6*G*) is the reduction in strength of the arterial pulse that can be felt during abnormal inspiratory decline of left ventricular filling. However, it is more apparent and can be quantified if sphygmomanometry is used. (Refer to the discussion of the determination of paradoxical blood pressure below.)

Pulsus parvus et tardus (Fig. 10-6*H*) is found in severe aortic stenosis. It resembles the double systolic beat in pulsus bisferiens, but its upstroke is more gradual and the pulse pressure is smaller. Usually it is palpable only in the carotid artery.

Carotid Pulse. The carotid artery is best for assessing pulse-wave amplitude and contour. Observe the neck for pulsations. Carotid pulsations are visible bilaterally just medial to the sternocleidomastoid muscle. Place your fingertips along the medial border of the sternocleidomastoid muscle in the lower half of the neck. Press posteriorly to feel the artery. Palpate well below the upper border of the thyroid cartilage to avoid compressing the carotid sinus, which might result in a reflex drop in heart rate or blood pressure. Compare one side with the other, but do not palpate both sides simultaneously because brain blood flow might be interrupted. Using the side with the strongest pulsations, assess the amplitude and contour of the pulse wave and determine whether it occurs in early systole or has a delayed upstroke.

Peripheral Circulation. In the legs, assess femoral, popliteal, dorsalis pedis, and posterior tibial pulses (Fig. 10-7). The popliteal pulse is not directly palpable; only the transmitted pulsations can be detected. Pedal pulses should be assessed in a dependent position before determining that they are absent.[18] In the arms, assess brachial, radial, and ulnar pulses. When assessing peripheral circulation, always compare one side with the other. An *Allen test* should be performed before radial arterial cannulation to evaluate radial and ulnar arterial patency. Simultaneously compress the radial and ulnar arteries and ask the patient to make a fist. The hand blanches. Ask the patient to open his or her fist. Release the pressure from the ulnar artery while maintaining pressure on the radial artery. The hand color returns to normal if the ulnar artery is patent. Repeat the process releasing pressure from the radial artery. If dual circulation to the hand is not present, do not attempt radial arterial puncture or cannulation.

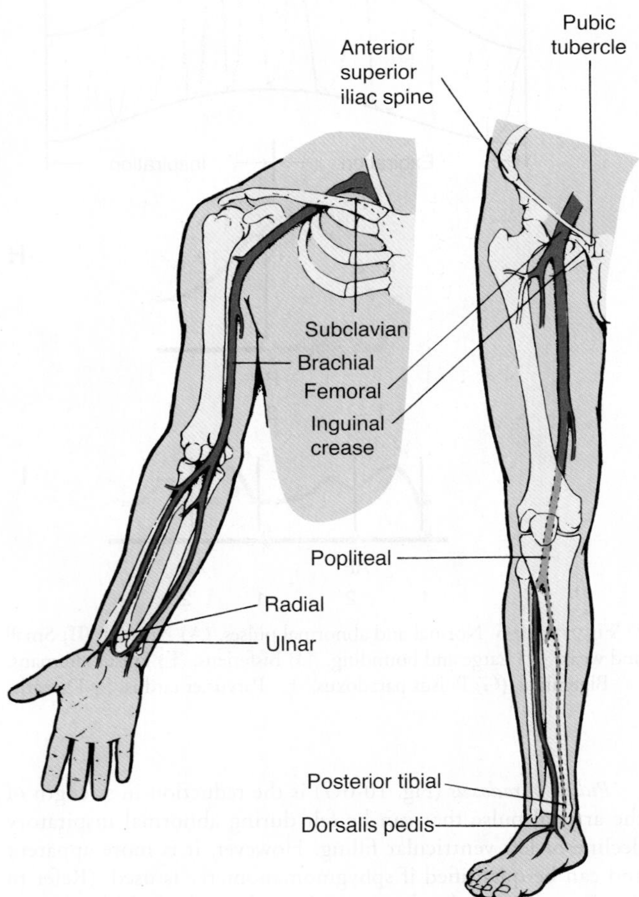

■ **Figure 10-7** Peripheral arteries and their landmarks.

In shock states associated with reduced cardiac output and elevated systemic vascular resistance, or with arterial insufficiency, pulses may not be palpable in the periphery. In this case, *Doppler ultrasound* should be used to evaluate arterial flow. Using light pressure so that the artery is not occluded, place the Doppler probe (with conducting gel) over the general area of the artery to be assessed. Move the probe until the arterial signal is audible. Mark the location of the pulse with indelible ink.

Bruits

Bruits are arterial sounds, similar to cardiac murmurs that occur with turbulence of blood flow. Bruits in the carotid arteries may indicate a partial obstruction to cerebral blood flow, whereas bruits in the femoral arteries suggest partial obstruction to blood flow to the legs. When listening for carotid bruits, instruct the patient to exhale and then hold his or her breath during the examination to prevent bruits from being obscured by respiratory sounds. Auscultate for bruits with the diaphragm of the stethoscope over the carotid, renal, iliac, and femoral arteries.

Jugular Venous Pulse

Inspection of the jugular venous pulse can reveal important information about right heart hemodynamics. The level of the jugular venous pressure reflects the right atrial pressure and, in most instances, reflects the right ventricular diastolic pressure (filling pressure). The pattern of the jugular venous pulse can reveal abnormalities of conduction and abnormal function of the tricuspid valve.[6] Assess the right side of the neck because right heart hemodynamics are transmitted more directly to the right, rather than to the left, jugular vein. It is important to inspect the skin for evidence of previous cannulation of the vessel that may result in thrombosis and affect the accuracy of pressure measurement. Oblique light may assist in visualizing the jugular veins.

Jugular Venous Pressure

Jugular venous pressure reflects filling volume and pressure on the right side of the heart. Jugular veins act like manometers; blood in the jugular veins assumes the level that corresponds to the right atrial (central venous) pressure. The normal jugular venous pressure is less than 9 cm H_2O.[8] The right internal jugular vein provides the most accurate reflection of right heart hemodynamics because it is in an almost straight line with the innominate vein and the superior vena cava.[8] It lies deep to the sternocleidomastoid muscle; however, the pulsations are usually transmitted to the skin. The top level of skin pulsation is recorded as the jugular venous pressure. If the right internal jugular vein is not visible, the right external jugular vein may be used to measure jugular venous pressure, although it is more subject to thrombosis or compression, and the presence of venous valves may make the data less reliable.[19] To measure the jugular venous pressure, follow these below-mentioned steps (Fig. 10-8).

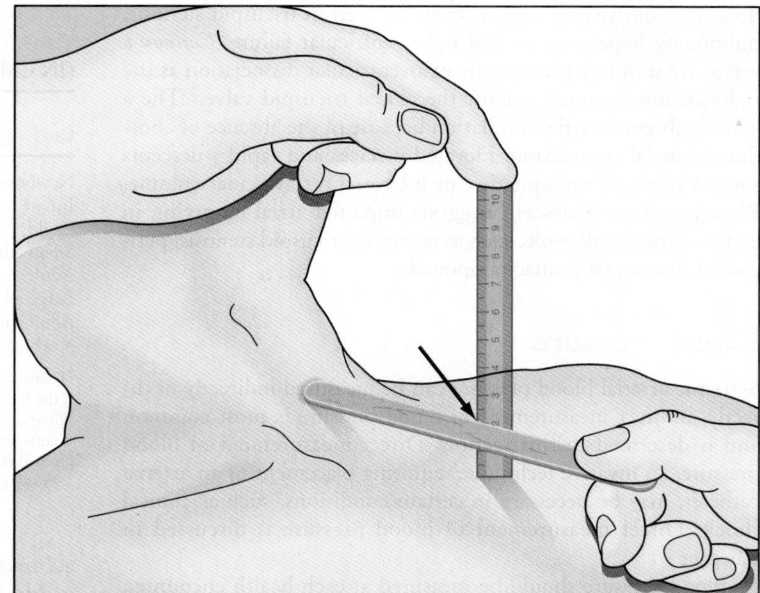

■ **Figure 10-8** Assessment of jugular venous pressure.

- Begin with the patient supine; the head and trunk should be in a straight line without significant flexion of the neck.
- Position the patient's backrest so that the jugular meniscus can be seen in the lower half of the neck. Elevating the backrest 15 to 30 degrees above horizontal is usually sufficient.
- Visualize the right internal jugular vein and identify the level of peak excursion. If the external jugular vein is used, identify the level at which it appears collapsed.
- Place a ruler vertically on the sternal angle (angle of Lewis). Position a straight edge (e.g., tongue blade) horizontally at the highest point of the jugular vein so that it intersects the ruler at a right angle, and measure the vertical distance above the sternal angle.

If the top of the neck veins is more than 3 cm above the sternal angle, venous pressure is abnormally elevated. Elevated venous pressure reflects right ventricular failure (and is a late finding in left ventricular failure), reduced right ventricular compliance, pericardial disease, hypervolemia, tricuspid valve stenosis, and obstruction of the superior vena cava.[18] During inspiration, the jugular venous pressure normally declines, although the amplitude of the *a* wave may increase.[6] With the patient in the horizontal position, if the neck veins collapse on deep inspiration (intrathoracic pressure of −5 cm H_2O), the central venous pressure is less than 5 cm H_2O.

Abdominojugular reflux occurs in right ventricular failure. It can be demonstrated by pressing the periumbilical area firmly for 30 to 60 seconds and observing the jugular venous pressure. If there is a rise in the jugular venous pressure by 1 cm or more that is sustained throughout pressure application, abdominojugular reflux is present.[3] *Kussmaul's sign* is a paradoxical elevation of jugular venous pressure during inspiration and may occur in patients with chronic constrictive pericarditis, heart failure, or tricuspid stenosis.

Patterns of the Venous Pulse

Before evaluating the venous pulse, it is important to discriminate between venous and carotid pulsations. Venous pulse waves are observed more readily than they are palpated. The descents are often more easily seen than the peaks and are inward movements.[3] The carotid pulsation is a brisk, outward movement. Palpation of the jugular vein obliterates the pulsations except in extreme venous hypertension.[19] Palpation of the carotid does not obliterate the observable pulsation in the neck.

Right atrial systole increases right atrial pressure and causes venous distention and the resultant a wave (Fig. 10-9). Atrial emptying and relaxation, and descent of the atrial floor during ventricular systole, result in the *x* descent. The c wave occurs simultaneously with the carotid arterial pulse, interrupting the *x* descent. The c wave may be related to tricuspid valve closure and bulging into the right atrium or it may be an artifact from the adjacent carotid pulse. The v wave reflects the rise in right atrial pressure from atrial filling during ventricular contraction while the tricuspid valve is closed. The *y* descent results from reduction in right atrial volume and pressure when the tricuspid valve opens.[19]

Timing of the venous pulse can be appreciated by auscultating the heart or palpating the carotid artery on the opposite side of the neck. The a wave occurs just before the first heart sound or carotid pulse and has a sharp rise followed by the rapid *x* descent. The v wave occurs immediately after the arterial pulse and has a slower, undulating pattern. The *y* descent is less steep than the *x*

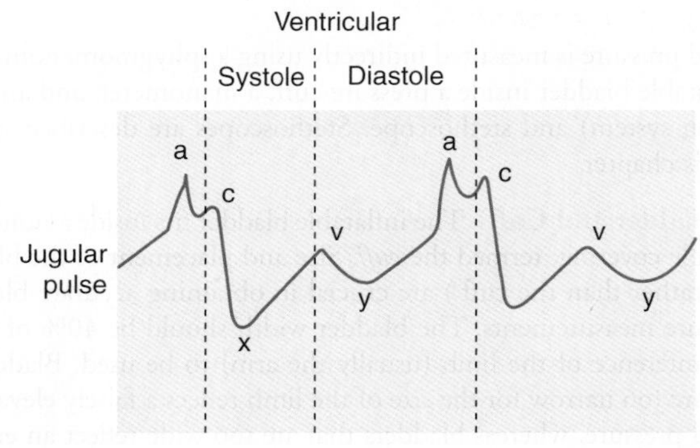

■ **Figure 10-9** Patterns of the venous pulse.

descent. Consistently large a waves are seen in tricuspid stenosis, pulmonary hypertension, and right ventricular failure. *Cannon* a waves are seen in patients with atrioventricular dissociation as the right atrium contracts against the closed tricuspid valve.[3] The a wave is absent in atrial fibrillation because of the absence of coordinated atrial contraction. Elevated v waves and rapid *y* descents suggest tricuspid regurgitation or increased intravascular volume. Blunting of the *y* descent suggests impaired atrial emptying in early ventricular diastole, such as occurs in tricuspid stenosis, pericardial disease, or cardiac tamponade.

Blood Pressure

Systemic arterial blood pressure can be measured indirectly or directly. Indirect measurement of blood pressure is most common and is described in this section. Direct measurement of blood pressure, an invasive technique requiring placement of an arterial catheter, may be necessary in certain conditions, such as clinical shock. Direct measurement of blood pressure is discussed in Chapter 21.

Blood pressure should be measured at each health encounter. The auscultatory method of measurement with a properly calibrated and validated instrument should be used. Patients should be seated quietly in a chair, with feet on the floor and arm supported for at least 5 minutes before measurement.[20]

Evaluate the patient's current blood pressure. If it differs greatly from the usual, immediate intervention may be required. Normal blood pressure in people 18 years of age or older is defined as less than 120/80 mm Hg, and prehypertension is defined as systolic pressure of 120 to 139 mm Hg or diastolic pressure of 80 to 90 mm Hg. Patients with prehypertension are at increased risk for progression to hypertension.[20] Hypertension is defined as systolic blood pressure of 140 mm Hg or greater, diastolic blood pressure of 90 mm Hg or greater, or taking antihypertensive medication.[20] (See Chapter 35 for treatment of hypertension.) In western societies, blood pressure tends to increase with increasing age. This increase is not biologic, and there is clear evidence that lowering blood pressure in older adults reduces the risk of stroke, cardiac disease, and all-cause mortality.[21] The higher the blood pressure, the greater the increase in the heart's work and oxygen consumption. Blood pressures less than 90/60 mm Hg may decrease blood and oxygen delivery to an already compromised myocardium. Taking into account symptoms of myocardial ischemia and adequacy of cerebral and peripheral perfusion may enable the examiner to judge more accurately the clinical significance of blood pressure changes in the cardiac patient.

Sphygmomanometer

Blood pressure is measured indirectly using a sphygmomanometer (inflatable bladder inside a pressure cuff, a manometer, and an inflation system) and stethoscope. Stethoscopes are described later in this chapter.

Bladder and Cuff. The inflatable bladder fits inside a nondistensible covering, termed the *cuff.* Size and placement of the bladder (rather than the cuff) are crucial in obtaining accurate blood pressure measurements. The bladder width should be 40% of the circumference of the limb (usually the arm) to be used. Bladders that are too narrow for the size of the limb reflect a falsely elevated blood pressure, whereas bladders that are too wide reflect an erroneously low blood pressure. Bladder length, which also affects accuracy of measurement, should be approximately twice that of width, or 80% of the limb circumference. Inflatable bladders and cuffs are available in various sizes. Table 10-3 summarizes recommended bladder dimensions for blood pressure cuffs. It is important to remember that cuff size is determined by patient size, not patient age.[22]

Table 10-3 ■ ACCEPTABLE BLADDER DIMENSIONS (IN CM) FOR ARMS OF DIFFERENT SIZES*

Cuff	Bladder Width (cm)	Bladder Length (cm)	Arm Circumference Range at Midpoint (cm)
Newborn	3	6	≤6
Infant	5	15	6–15†
Child	8	21	16–21†
Small adult	10	24	22–26
Adult	13	30	27–34
Large adult	16	38	35–44
Adult thigh	20	42	45–52

*There is some overlapping of the recommended range for arm circumferences to limit the number of cuffs; it is recommended that the larger cuff be used when available.
†To approximate the bladder width:arm circumference ratio of 0.40 more closely in infants and children, additional cuffs are available.
From Perloff, D., Grim, C., Flack, J., et al. (2001). *Human blood pressure determination by sphygmomanometry.* Dallas, TX: American Heart Association.

Manometers. There are two types of manometers: mercury and aneroid. *Mercury manometers,* which are the most reliable, can be mounted either on a portable stand or on the wall above the bed or table. A reservoir of mercury (Hg) is attached to the bottom of the manometer, which is calibrated in millimeters (mm). In response to pressure exerted on the bulb, mercury rises vertically in the manometer. As pressure is released from the bag, the column of mercury falls, and blood pressure can be measured in millimeters of mercury. It is important that the meniscus of the mercury be at eye level when the blood pressure is measured. The blood pressure reading should be taken at the top of the meniscus. If the wall mounting is too high or the portable stand too low, errors in blood pressure determinations will be made.

In response to efforts by the Environmental Protection Agency to reduce potential mercury spills and exposure, many clinical facilities are using aneroid gauges or electronic monitoring devices, To date mercury manometers remain the gold standard. Accurate measurement of blood pressure with non-mercury instruments requires sufficient standards of validation and stringent programs of calibration.[23]

Aneroid manometers have round gauges calibrated in millimeters of mercury, or torr (1 torr = 1 mm Hg), and affixed to the blood pressure cuff. Advantages of the aneroid manometer are that it is easily seen, is conveniently portable, and, with the cuff, composes one unit. Unfortunately, the calibration of the dial frequently becomes inaccurate. It is important before each use to check that the indicator needle is pointing to the zero mark on the dial. If the needle is either below or above this mark, the blood pressure reading will be incorrect and the scale may no longer be linear.

Calibration of an aneroid manometer is performed using a mercury manometer as the reference manometer (Fig. 10-10).[22] The mercury manometer must be functioning correctly to obtain reliable results. Aneroid manometers should be recalibrated by qualified personnel at least yearly or whenever the needle does not point to zero.

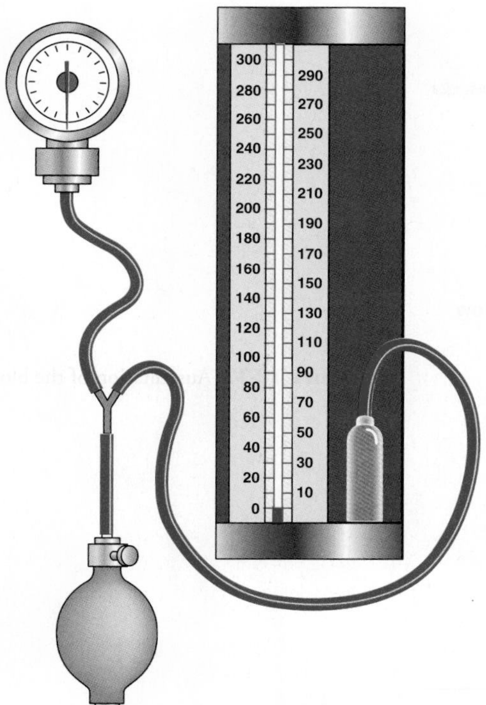

■ **Figure 10-10** Calibration of an aneroid manometer. Disconnect the cuffs from both the aneroid and reference manometers. Attach a bulb to a Y connector and the Y connector to the tubes to each of the manometers. Inflate the bulb and observe the pressure at several points over the entire range on both manometers. The pressures should be equal on both manometers.

The inflation system of aneroid manometers consists of the bulb, exhaust valve, and tubing. The bladder should be able to be inflated and deflated gradually or rapidly. Check frequently for pressure leaks greater than 1 mm Hg per second and for smooth, efficient functioning of the apparatus.

Electronic devices can be used for measuring blood pressure, but the accuracy of these devices and stringent programs of calibration are necessary. Electronic oscillometric devices measure mean pressure (point of maximal oscillation) and use a set of empirically derived algorithms to calculate systolic and diastolic blood pressure.[6] Electronic devices are more sensitive to artifact such as patient movement or muscle contraction than are mercury and aneroid devices. Cardiac arrhythmias and low pulse pressure also reduce the accuracy of electronic devices. Electronic devices do not require use of a stethoscope and may be used by patients for self-monitoring of blood pressure.

Technique

On initial examination, blood pressure should be recorded in both arms and, in infants, in one leg as well. Subsequently, the arm with the higher blood pressure should be used. Indicate whether the blood pressure was taken on the right arm or left arm. Avoid possible development of lymphedema after mastectomy by always taking the patient's blood pressures on the arm *opposite* the affected side. Avoid taking blood pressure on an arm with an arteriovenous shunt or fistula, as well as those with subclavian stenosis.[24]

Differences in blood pressure between the arms or between the arms and the legs have important diagnostic implications. In patients with occlusive arterial disease of the subclavian artery, the blood pressure is lower in the affected arm. In patients with coarctation of the aorta or dissecting aortic aneurysm, depending on the location of the lesion, the blood pressure may be higher in one arm than the other, or in both arms (proximal) compared with the legs (distal).

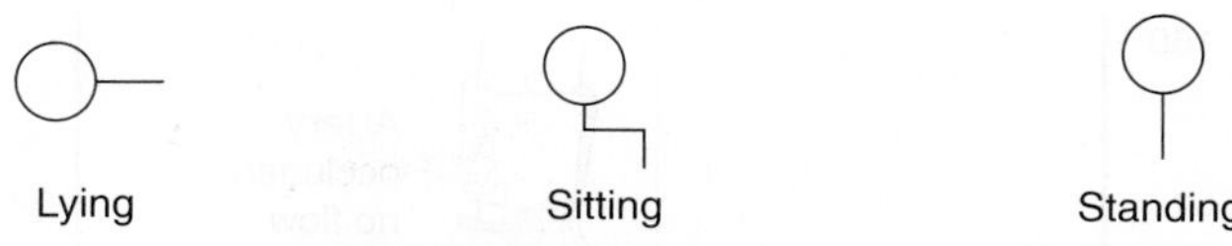

■ **Figure 10-11** Symbols used to record a patient's position during blood pressure determination.

Bladder and Cuff Position. The deflated cuff is placed snugly around the arm, with the bladder covering the inner aspect of the arm and the brachial artery. The lower margin of the cuff should be 2.5 cm above the antecubital space.

Arm Position. As long as the patient's arm is at heart level, the blood pressure can be determined with the patient in any position. Errors up to 10 mm Hg, both systolic and diastolic, can be made if the arm is not at the correct level. Falsely elevated pressures are obtained if the arm is lower than the heart; falsely low pressures are measured if the arm is higher than the heart. The arm must be supported during pressure determination.

Patient Position. The patient's position during blood pressure measurement always should be recorded. Use the symbols or drawings shown in Figure 10-11.

Palpation. After the cuff is in place, the brachial artery is palpated continuously. Once the brachial or radial pulse is obtained, the cuff is inflated rapidly. The pressure at which the pulse disappears should be noted, but the cuff inflation should continue for another 30 mm Hg before the actual measurement of the blood pressure begins. For example, if the brachial pulse disappears when the cuff pressure is 110 mm Hg, the cuff should be pumped to 140 mm Hg before starting. The cuff should not be inflated further than necessary, because high cuff pressures are uncomfortable, create undue anxiety in the patient, and tend to raise the patient's blood pressure. The pressure in the cuff should be reduced gradually by 2 to 3 mm Hg per second. The point at which the brachial pulse is first detected on expiration is the systolic blood pressure. Diastolic blood pressure cannot be determined accurately by palpation. Once measurement is made, the cuff should be deflated rapidly. If possible, allow a minimum of 1 to 2 minutes before the blood pressure is measured again to release venous blood.

Systolic blood pressure is measured by palpation in patients whose blood pressures cannot be heard (e.g., patients in shock). It is also useful when checking blood pressures frequently (e.g., every 1 to 2 minutes). Palpated blood pressures are charted using "P" as diastolic pressure (e.g., 90/P).

Auscultation. Preparation of the patient and use of the blood pressure equipment are identical in the auscultatory method. After the brachial pulse has been located, the stethoscope is applied over the artery using light pressure. Heavy pressure might partially occlude the artery, creating turbulence in the blood flow, prolonging phase IV, and falsely lowering the diastolic blood pressure. Care must be taken to avoid causing extraneous noise, such as from the stethoscope touching the cuff or any other material.

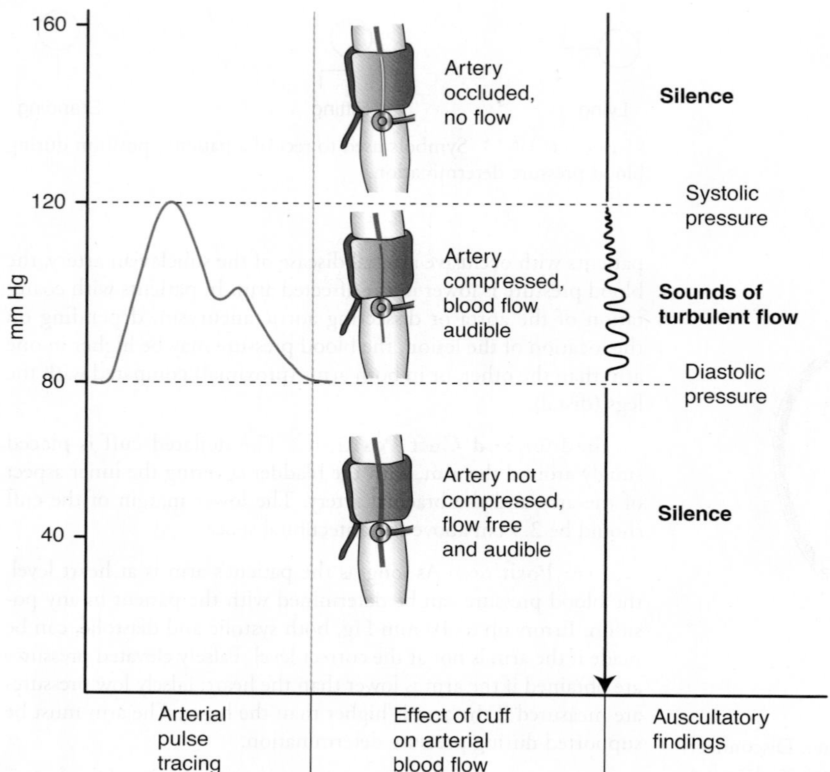

■ **Figure 10-12** Auscultation of the blood pressure.

Korotkoff sounds are the sounds created by turbulence of blood flow within the vessel caused by constriction of the blood pressure cuff (Fig. 10-12). The five Korotkoff sounds are summarized in Table 10-4.

Systolic blood pressure is the highest point at which initial tapping (phase I) is heard in two consecutive beats (to ascertain that the sound is not extraneous) during expiration. Systolic blood pressure is higher in the expiratory phase compared to the inspiratory phase of the respiratory cycle (see "Measurement of Paradoxical Blood Pressure" section). Systolic blood pressure should be read to the nearest 2 mm Hg mark on the manometer.

Diastolic blood pressure is equated with disappearance of Korotkoff sounds (phase V) in adults. Phase V most closely approximates intra-arterial diastolic pressure. Muffling of sounds (phase IV) usually occurs at pressures 5 to 10 mm Hg higher than intra-arterial diastolic pressures and, therefore, is not a good indicator of diastolic blood pressure in adults. However, muffling, rather than disappearance of sounds, is a better index of intra-arterial diastolic pressure in children and in adults with hyperkinetic states. Hyperkinetic conditions, including hyperthyroidism, aortic insufficiency, and exercise, increase the rate of blood flow, resulting in disappearance of sounds (absence of turbulence) far below intra-arterial diastolic pressure. In children and adults with hyperkinetic states, sounds can be detected below muffling for much longer than normal.[22] As with systolic blood pressure, read diastolic pressure to the nearest 2 mm Hg mark on the manometer. If there is a difference of 10 mm Hg or more between disappearance and muffling of sounds, record both diastolic pressures (e.g., 140/56/20 mm Hg).[22]

In some patients, Korotkoff sounds may be soft and could result in falsely low blood pressure values. To augment the loudness of Korotkoff sounds, increase brachial flow by having the patient open and clench a fist; quickly inflate cuff to a value 30 mm above the palpable systolic blood pressure.

Auscultatory gap is a temporary disappearance of sound that occurs during the latter part of phase I and phase II (Fig. 10-13).

Table 10-4 ■ PHASES OF THE KOROTKOFF SOUNDS*

Phase I
The pressure level at which the first faint, consistent tapping sounds are heard. The sounds gradually increase in intensity as the cuff is deflated. The first of at least two of these sounds is defined as the *systolic pressure.*

Phase II
The time during cuff deflation when a murmur of swishing sounds is heard.

Phase III
The period during which sounds are crisper and increase in intensity.

Phase IV
The time when a distinct, abrupt, muffling of sound (usually of a soft blowing quality) is heard. This is defined as the *diastolic pressure* in anyone in whom sounds continue to zero.

Phase V
The pressure level when the last regular blood pressure sound is heard and after which all sound disappears. This is defined as the *diastolic pressure* unless sounds are heard to zero.

*To avoid error, the observer must be prepared to recognize two normal Korotkoff sound variations associated with blood pressure (BP) readings. The auscultatory gap is a period of silence occurring during Korotkoff phases I and II. This disappearance of sound is temporary and is usually short, but the gap can occur over a period of 40 mm Hg. It seems to be associated with higher BP readings. An absent Korotkoff phase V occurs when sounds are heard to zero. When this is the case, phase IV should be recorded along with phase V. In this case, phase IV is the best reference for diastolic pressure.
Grim, C. M., & Grim, C. E. (2003). Blood pressure measurement. In J. L. Izzo & H. R. Black (Eds.), *Hypertension primer* (3rd ed.). Dallas, TX: American Heart Association.

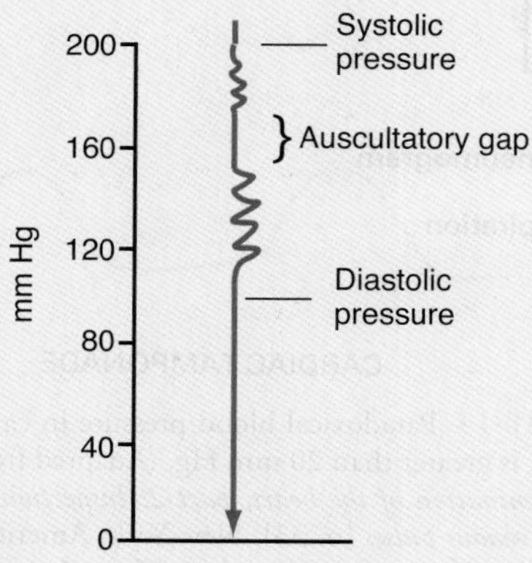
An unrecognized auscultatory gap may lead to serious underestimation of systolic pressure (e.g., 150/98 in the example below) or overestimation of diastolic pressure.
Systolic pressure
Auscultatory gap
Diastolic pressure
mm Hg
200
160
120
80
40
0
If you find an auscultatory gap, record your findings completely (e.g., 200/98 with an auscultatory gap from 170-150).

Figure 10-13 Auscultatory gap.

It is particularly common in patients with high blood pressure, venous distention, or reduced velocity of arterial flow (e.g., severe aortic stenosis).[18] The auscultatory gap can be as wide as 40 mm Hg. Serious errors in blood pressure measurement can be made if the cuff is not inflated high enough to exceed true systolic pressure. Systolic blood pressure would be underestimated if the second appearance of the Korotkoff sounds were recorded as phase I. Diastolic blood pressure would be overestimated if the first muffling of sounds was considered to be phase IV. The auscultatory gap can be avoided if a preliminary palpable blood pressure is obtained before auscultation.

Measurement of Pulse Pressure

Pulse pressure is the difference between the systolic and diastolic blood pressures, expressed in millimeters of mercury. For example, if the blood pressure is 120/80 mm Hg, the pulse pressure is 40 mm Hg. Pulse pressure reflects stroke volume, ejection velocity, and systemic vascular resistance. Use pulse pressure as a noninvasive indicator of the patient's ability to maintain cardiac output.

Pulse pressure is increased in many situations. A widened pulse pressure is seen in sinus bradycardia, complete heart block, aortic regurgitation, anxiety, exercise, and catecholamine infusion, which are examples of situations characterized by increased stroke volume. Examples of conditions that increase pulse pressure by reducing systemic vascular resistance are fever, hot environment, and exercise. Conditions such as atherosclerosis, aging, and high blood pressure widen the pulse pressure because of decreased distensibility of the aorta, arteries, and arterioles. A narrowed pulse pressure also can be caused by many factors: reduced ejection velocity in heart failure, shock, and hypovolemia; mechanical obstruction to systolic outflow in aortic stenosis, mitral stenosis, and mitral insufficiency; peripheral vasoconstriction in shock and with certain drugs; and artifactually from an auscultatory gap.[6,18] If the pulse pressure in the cardiac patient falls below 30 mm Hg, further assessment of the patient's cardiovascular status may be indicated.

Measurement of Postural Blood Pressure

Postural (orthostatic) hypotension occurs when the blood pressure drops after an upright posture is assumed. It usually is accompanied by dizziness, lightheadedness, or syncope. Although there are many causes of postural hypotension, the three most commonly seen in the cardiac patient are (1) intravascular volume depletion, which often results from aggressive diuretic therapy, inadequate intake, or intravascular to extravascular fluid shift; (2) inadequate vasoconstrictor mechanisms, which may be a primary pathologic process but also result from immobility; and (3) autonomic insufficiency, which is often related to the sympathetic blocking drugs used in the cardiac patient. Postural changes in blood pressure, along with the appropriate history, can help the clinician differentiate between them.[25,26] Postural changes in blood pressure and pulse should be measured in patients who are older than 65 years of age, diabetic, receiving antihypertensive therapy, or who complain of dizziness or syncope. Important points to remember are the following:

- Position the patient supine and as flat as symptoms permit for 10 minutes before the initial measurement of blood pressure and heart rate.
- Always check supine measurements before upright measurements.
- Always record both heart rate and blood pressure at each postural change.
- Do not remove the blood pressure cuff between position changes, but do check to see that it remains placed correctly.
- Safety considerations may require assessment of blood pressure and pulse with the patient seated with legs in the dependent position before standing. Measurement of blood pressure and pulse in this position is not sufficient to rule out orthostasis.[26]
- Have the patient assume a standing position. Measure the blood pressure and pulse immediately and after 2 minutes. If orthostasis is strongly suspected and not apparent after 2 minutes, continue to monitor blood pressure and pulse every 2 minutes for 10 minutes. If the purpose of collecting the data is to assess the risk of falling, another approach is to ask the patient to get out of bed as he or she normally does and evaluate the change in pulse rate and blood pressure and associated symptoms at the patient's rate of position change.
- Be alert for any signs or symptoms of patient distress, including dizziness, weakness, blurring of vision, and syncope. When the patient returns to a recumbent position, these symptoms should reverse and the blood pressure and pulse return to normal.
- Record any signs or symptoms that accompany the postural change.

Normal postural responses are a transient increased heart rate of 5 to 20 beats per minute (to offset reduced stroke volume and to maintain cardiac output), a drop in systolic pressure of less than 10 mm Hg, and an increase in diastolic pressure of approximately 5 mm Hg. *Orthostasis* is defined as a drop in systolic pressure of 20 mm Hg or greater or a drop in diastolic pressure of at least 10 mm Hg within 3 minutes of standing,[26] although any drop in diastolic pressure may be cause for concern. The change from lying to sitting position is not sufficient to make a diagnosis of orthostasis; it may be used as a screening test because decreased blood pressure, increased pulse, or symptoms in the sitting position presage similar events in the erect position. Often, the change in blood pressure does not meet the criteria for orthostasis, but it is accompanied by a significant change in heart rate or associated symptoms, or both. These circumstances identify people at risk and should prompt further investigation by the cardiac nurse of the patient's present volume status and vasodilatory or cardioinhibitory drug regimen.

The presence of intravascular volume depletion (such as with diuretic therapy) should be suspected when, in response to sitting or standing, the heart rate increases and the systolic pressure decreases by 15 mm Hg and the diastolic blood pressure drops by 10 mm Hg.[26] It is difficult to differentiate intravascular volume loss from inadequate vasoconstrictor mechanisms solely by changes in vital signs accompanying postural changes. With intravascular volume depletion, reflexes to maintain cardiac output (increased heart rate and peripheral vasoconstriction) function correctly, but, because of reduced intravascular fluid volume, these reflexes are not adequate to maintain systemic arterial pressure and the blood pressure falls. With inadequate vasoconstrictor mechanisms, the heart rate responds appropriately also, but blood pressure drops because of diminished peripheral vasoconstriction. Differentiation, therefore, depends in part on the patient's history. However, intravascular depletion and inadequate vasoconstrictor mechanisms are not mutually exclusive. The following is an example of postural blood pressure recordings showing either saline depletion or inadequate vasoconstrictor mechanisms:

Blood Pressure	Heart Rate	Patient Position
120/70 mm Hg	70 bpm	
100/55 mm Hg	90 bpm	
98/52 mm Hg	94 bpm	

Measurement of Paradoxical Blood Pressure

Paradoxical blood pressure is an exaggerated decrease in the systolic blood pressure during inspiration. The mechanism is complex and controversial. Normally, during inspiration, blood flow into the right heart is increased, right ventricular output is enhanced, and pulmonary venous capacitance is increased. Consequently, less blood reaches the left ventricle, which reduces left ventricular stroke volume and arterial pressure.[27]

During cardiac tamponade, effects of respiration on both right and left ventricular filling appear to be greater than normal, causing a reduction of 10 mm Hg or more in systolic pressure during normal inspiration (Fig. 10-14).[27] In addition, echocardiography has demonstrated a shift of the intraventricular septum to the left, further impairing left ventricular filling and stroke volume. With high intrapericardial pressures, the thin-walled right ventricle may collapse during diastole, further impairing venous return and cardiac output.[27] Chronic obstructive airway disease, constrictive pericarditis, pulmonary emboli, restrictive cardiomyopathy, and cardiogenic shock have also been associated with an abnormal inspiratory decline of blood pressure. Echocardiographic studies of patients with emphysema demonstrate both an augmented inspiratory filling of the right ventricle and an exaggerated inspiratory decline of left ventricular filling.[5]

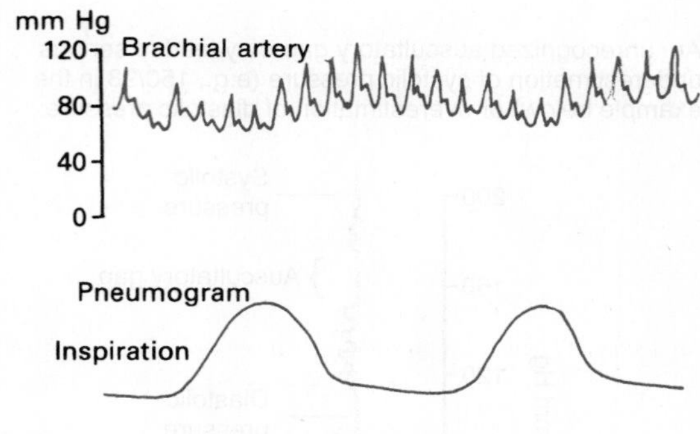

■ **Figure 10-14** Paradoxical blood pressure in cardiac tamponade. The paradox is greater than 20 mm Hg. (Adapted from Fowler, N. O. [1972]. *Examination of the heart, part 2: Inspection and palpation of arterial and venous pulses* [p. 33]. New York: American Heart Association with permission of the American Heart Association, Inc.)

The patient should breathe normally and must not exaggerate respiratory effort during an examination for a paradoxical blood pressure. As before, the nurse should inflate and gradually deflate the cuff until the first systolic sound is heard on expiration and continue slowly releasing the cuff pressure until sounds are heard both on inspiration and expiration. The difference between the two is termed the *paradox*, and it normally is less than 10 mm Hg.[27] For example, if the first systolic sound occurs at 140 mm Hg during expiration and Korotkoff sounds begin appearing with both inspiration and expiration at 120 mm Hg, the paradox is 20 mm Hg. Paradoxical blood pressures should be determined as a baseline in all patients on the cardiac care unit and routinely in all patients with pericarditis or with heart catheters, such as a temporary pacing wire.

Blood Pressure Measurement Under Special Conditions

Arrhythmia. With very irregular rhythms, accurate assessment of blood pressure is difficult because of the beat-to-beat variation in both stroke volume and blood pressure. Systolic blood pressure is related directly to the stroke volume and duration of the preceding cycle. Pulse pressure is related inversely to pulse cycle duration. A short cycle (reduced ventricular filling time) increases the diastolic blood pressure of that cycle and reduces systolic blood pressure during the next cycle. A long pulse cycle (increased ventricular filling time) causes a decreased diastolic blood pressure in that cycle but an increased systolic blood pressure in the next cycle.[3]

Any arrhythmia that alters stroke volume and cardiac output can be detected during blood pressure measurement. Always record the presence of an irregular cardiac rhythm along with the blood pressure.

Premature ectopic beats (either ventricular or supraventricular) have a short cycle followed by a long cycle (post-extrasystolic beat). If they occur only occasionally, they have minimal effects on blood pressure. In *bigeminal rhythms*, as the blood pressure cuff is deflated, Korotkoff sounds of the alternate strong beats are heard first and are half as fast as the heart rate. Further reduction in cuff pressure enables the listener to hear the alternating weaker sounds produced by the ectopic impulses as well.

Pulsus alternans, indicative of severe organic heart disease and left heart failure, also is manifested by alternating strong and weak pulses but with a regular cadence. Pulsus alternans can occur with ectopic bigeminal rhythms that are interpolated rather than premature, but, in this instance, it does not necessarily indicate severe organic heart disease.

Because pulse cycle length changes constantly in *atrial fibrillation,* both systolic and diastolic blood pressures must be approximated.[24] For systolic blood pressure, average a series of readings (three to five) of phase I pressures. For diastolic blood pressure, average the pressure readings obtained in phase IV and phase V.

Atrioventricular dissociation can be detected during auscultation of blood pressure. Examples of rhythms with atrioventricular dissociation include *ventricular tachycardia, high-grade* or *complete atrioventricular block,* and *asynchronous ventricular pacing.* In atrioventricular dissociation, an occasional, well-timed atrial contraction contributes to diastolic ventricular filling. This "atrial kick" augments the stroke volume for that beat. As the cuff bladder is deflated, phase I sounds periodically are increased.

Clinical Shock. In shock states associated with reduced cardiac output and elevated systemic vascular resistance, Korotkoff sounds may not be generated in the periphery. Direct measurement of blood pressure may be required to manage these critically ill patients. When indirect cuff measurements are compared with direct (femoral arterial) pressure measurements, direct pressures are higher than auscultated pressures. In hypotensive states, when direct measurement of blood pressure is not feasible, *Doppler ultrasound* may provide a more reliable indirect measurement of systolic blood pressure than the auscultatory method. Place the Doppler probe (with conducting gel) over the patient's artery. As in auscultatory measurement, inflate the cuff and listen for the arterial signal as the bladder is deflated. Cuff widths of 50% of the arm circumference have been recommended for the Doppler technique.[24]

Obesity. Cuff size and bladder size frequently are too small for use in the obese patient. If a proper-sized cuff cannot be used, apply a standard cuff to the forearm 13 cm from the elbow and auscultate the radial artery to obtain the blood pressure measurement.

Thigh Blood Pressure Measurement. Blood pressures are measured in the thigh if the arms cannot be used or to confirm or rule out certain conditions that alter circulation, such as coarctation of the aorta or dissecting aortic aneurysm.

For thigh blood pressure measurement, use a cuff and bladder that are both longer and wider than an arm cuff. Recommendations for the exact sizes of the thigh cuff and bladder have not been made. With the patient in the prone position, apply the compression bladder over the posterior aspect of the mid-thigh. Place the stethoscope over the artery in the popliteal fossa and auscultate in the same manner as described previously. If the patient is unable to tolerate the prone position, have the patient remain supine with the knee slightly flexed. Apply the stethoscope over the popliteal artery. When cuffs of the correct size are used for both arms and legs, pressures should vary by only a few millimeters of mercury. (The arm cuff, incorrectly used on the thigh, produces a falsely high value.)

Community Blood Pressure Readings. Blood pressures taken in the patient's home may provide a better indication of basal blood pressure than those obtained in an office or clinic setting. However, if the patient takes his or her own blood pressure, readings may be elevated because of the isometric exercise required to inflate the cuff and because of the concentration necessary. Newer devices for home use inflate the cuff automatically and some maintain a record of recent measurements. Many fire stations and hospital auxiliaries provide blood pressure measurement as a community service. Alternately, a fully automated system that measures blood pressure at preset intervals over the 24-hour period may be used.

Pseudohypertension. Misleadingly high systolic blood pressure values may be obtained in older adults because of excessive vascular stiffness.[28] Pseudohypertension should be suspected in the presence of high systolic blood pressure values and the absence of target organ damage. To confirm suspected pseudohypertension, inflate the cuff above systolic pressure and palpate the radial artery. Presence of a palpable, pulseless radial artery provides additional evidence of pseudohypertension.

Peripheral Vascular System

Adequacy of both arterial and venous circulation is assessed when examining the extremities. Always make arm-to-arm and leg-to-leg comparisons. Careful examination of the lower extremities is impossible without removing shoes and stockings.

Inspection and Palpation

Inspection and palpation are the primary techniques used in examining the peripheral vasculature (see "Bruits" section). Observe and compare (right to left) size, temperature, symmetry, swelling, venous pattern, pigmentation, scars, and ulcers. Palpate the superficial lymph nodes, noting their size, consistency, discreteness, and any tenderness.

Clubbing

Clubbing is a pathologic sign that is defined as focal enlargement of the terminal phalanges. Two diagnostic findings are present in clubbing: change in the angle between the base of the nail and the phalangeal skin, and "floating" nails. When viewed from the side, the base angle normally is less than 180 degrees and the distal phalangeal diameter is less than the interphalangeal diameter. In clubbing, the base angle becomes 195 degrees or greater and the distal phalangeal diameter becomes greater than the interphalangeal diameter (Fig. 10-15).[29] Floating nails can be detected by palpating the base of the nail while moving the tip of the nail. Rather than a firm anchor, the base of the nail appears to float or move under the palpating finger. Clubbing may develop in a variety of conditions, including congenital heart disease and lung abscess; its cause is unknown.

Arterial Circulation

Adequacy of peripheral arterial circulation is assessed by arterial pulse; skin color, temperature, and moistness; and capillary refill time. Pulse-wave analysis and skin color are described earlier in this chapter under the "Arterial Pulse" and the "Head" section, respectively.

Temperature and Moistness. Temperature and moistness are controlled by the autonomic nervous system. Normally, hands and feet are warm and dry. Under stress, the periphery may be cool and moist. In cardiogenic shock, skin becomes cold and clammy.

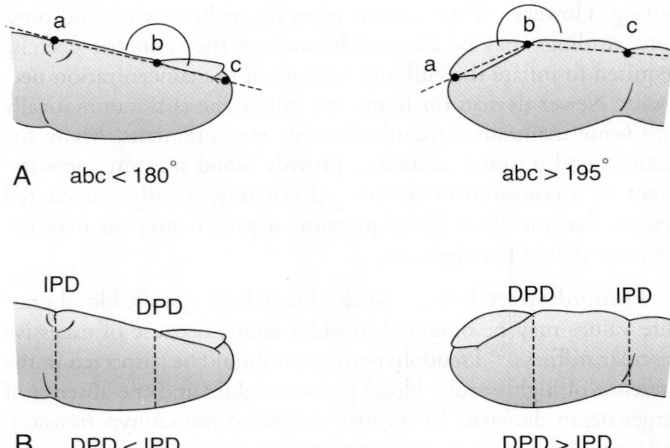

■ **Figure 10-15** Clubbing is diagnosed from the angle between the base of the nail and the skin next to the cuticle and by phalangeal depth. (A) In healthy adults, the hyponychial angle is 180 degrees (*left*); with clubbing, the angle increases above 195 degrees (*right*). (B) The ratio of distal phalangeal depth (DPD) to interphalangeal depth (IPD) is normally less then 1 (*left*). In clubbing, it exceeds 1.0 (*right*). (After Hansen-Flaschen, J. & Nordberg, J. [1987]. Clubbing and hypertrophic osteoarthropathy. *Clinics in Chest Medicine,* 8, 291.)

Capillary Refill Time. Capillary refill time provides an estimate of the rate of peripheral blood flow. When the tip of the fingernail is depressed, the nail bed blanches. When the pressure is released quickly, the area is reperfused and becomes pink. Normally, reperfusion occurs almost instantaneously. More sluggish reperfusion indicates a slower peripheral circulation, such as in heart failure.

Peripheral Atherosclerosis. Risk factors for peripheral atherosclerosis include advancing age, diabetes mellitus, hyperlipidemia, and tobacco use. Peripheral atherosclerosis may present with pain or fatigue in the muscles (intermittent claudication) that occurs with exercise and resolves with rest. Physical findings of chronic arterial insufficiency include decreased or absent pulses, reduced skin temperature, hair loss, thickened nails, smooth shiny skin, and pallor or cyanosis. Elevation of the feet and repeated flexing of the calf muscles may produce pallor of the soles of the feet. Returning the feet to a dependent position may produce rubor secondary to reactive hyperemia. If the ankle–brachial systolic pressure index (calculated by dividing the ankle systolic pressure by the brachial systolic pressure) is less than 0.8, it is highly probable (>95%) that arterial insufficiency is present. When vascular ulcers associated with arterial insufficiency occur, they are more commonly located near the lateral malleolus. Acute arterial occlusion produces sudden cessation of blood flow to an extremity. Severe pain, numbness, and coldness develop in the affected extremity quickly (within 1 hour). Physical findings include loss of pulse distal to the occlusion, decreased skin temperature, loss of sensation, weakness, and absent deep tendon reflexes.[30]

Venous Circulation

Edema. Edema is an abnormal accumulation of fluid in the interstitium. Causes include right-sided heart failure, hypoalbuminemia, excessive renal retention of sodium and water, venous stasis from obstruction or insufficiency, lymphedema, orthostatic edema, or increased capillary permeability.[6] In the cardiac patient, peripheral edema frequently occurs because of sodium and water retention and right-sided heart failure. Bilateral edema of the lower extremities suggests a systemic etiology; unilateral edema is usually the result of a local etiology. A weight gain of 10 lb (indicative of 5 L of extracellular fluid volume) precedes visible edema in most patients. Interstitial edema occurs in the most dependent part of the body, its location varying with the patient's posture. With sitting or standing, edema develops in the lower extremities. With bedrest, edema forms in the sacrum. Because the distribution of edema fluid varies with position, daily weights provide the best serial assessment of edema. *Pitting edema* is a depression in the skin from pressure. To demonstrate the presence of pitting edema, the nurse presses firmly with his or her thumb over a bony surface such as the sacrum, medial malleolus, the dorsum of each foot, and the shins. When the thumb is withdrawn, an indentation persists for a short time. The severity of edema is described on a five-point scale, from none (0) to very marked (4). *Pigmentation, reddening, induration,* and *fibrosis* of the skin and subcutaneous tissues of the lower extremities may result from long-standing edema.[30,31] *Skin mobility* is decreased by edema.

Thrombophlebitis. Thrombophlebitis is inflammation of the vein associated with a clot. Diagnosis is made using subjective and objective data.

In *superficial thrombophlebitis,* the affected vein is hard, red, sensitive to pressure, warm to touch, and engorged. *Deep vein thrombosis* may be asymptomatic or associated with pain, warmth, and mottling of the leg. With severe edema, the leg may be cool and cyanotic. Deep vein thrombosis can cause thromboembolism, resulting in a pulmonary embolus.[32] Among hospitalized patients, hip surgery is the most common precipitant of deep venous thrombosis.[31] Elicitation of pain with dorsiflexion of the foot (*Homans' sign*) is an unreliable diagnostic sign. Noninvasive imaging with duplex venous ultrasonography or plethysmography is required for diagnosis.[32]

Varicose Veins. Varicose veins are tortuous dilations of the superficial veins that result from defective venous valves, intrinsic weakness of the vein wall, high intraluminal pressure, or arteriovenous fistulas. Patients may be concerned about the appearance of their legs or may complain of a dull ache that is present with standing and relieved by elevation. Visual inspection of the legs with the patient in the standing position confirms the presence of varicose veins.

Chronic Venous Insufficiency. Chronic venous insufficiency (incompetence of venous valves) may follow deep venous thrombosis or may occur without previous thrombosis. It may be unilateral, but more commonly is bilateral. Patients complain of a dull ache in the legs that is present with standing and relieved by elevation. Physical examination reveals increased leg circumference, edema, and superficial varicose veins. Erythema, dermatitis, and hyperpigmentation may develop in the distal lower extremity.[30,31] When venous ulcers occur, they are more common near the medial malleolus.

Heart

The precordium should be assessed in an orderly fashion using the techniques of inspection, palpation, and auscultation. Careful inspection and palpation provide better information on heart size than does percussion. Percussion is most useful in the rare instance where dextrocardia is suspected.[6] The room should be quiet and permit privacy. Both the patient and the examiner should be in comfortable positions before beginning the examination.

Topographic Anatomy

Knowledge of the topographic anatomy of the cardiac and vascular structures is essential to understanding the clinical findings. The *left ventricle* is primarily a posterior structure and is evaluated on the anterior chest wall at the cardiac apex, which is normally in the fifth intercostal space (ICS) at, or slightly medial to, the mid-clavicular line (MCL). The *right ventricle* is anterior to the left ventricle and underlies the sternum and the lower left sternal border at the fourth and fifth ICS. The *right atrium* is just lateral to the lower right sternal border. The outflow tracts of both ventricles underlie the third left ICS (Erb's point). The main *pulmonary artery* underlies the second left ICS, and the *ascending aorta* underlies the second right ICS (Fig. 10-16).[8,33]

Inspection

Inspect the precordium with the patient supine, the chest exposed, and the backrest slightly elevated. Stand at the foot or right side of the bed or examining table. Tangential lighting allows the examiner to detect chest wall movements more easily.

Note any *pulsations* (outward movement) or *retractions* (inward movement) and describe the location by ICS and distance in centimeters from the sternum or the MCL. Determine whether it occurs in systole or diastole by timing it with the carotid pulse or the heart sounds. In general, retractions are more easily seen, and pulsations are more easily palpated.

When visible, the normal *apex impulse* can be seen within the fifth ICS at or just medial to the MCL. It is an early systolic pulsation with a rapid upstroke and downstroke. A late systolic retraction, 1 to 2 cm long, in the fourth or fifth ICS may also be normally seen and is produced by ventricular emptying. The apex impulse cannot be seen in every patient. It is easily detected in thin patients, whereas it may not be visible in those who are obese or have large breasts or barrel chests. An apex impulse that is below the fifth ICS, lateral to the MCL, or seen in more than one ICS represents left ventricular enlargement.

Slight movement over the sternum or the epigastrium can be normal in thin people and in those with fever or anemia who may have hyperdynamic heartbeats. A *sternal rise* that is sustained after systole begins usually indicates right ventricular enlargement. Pulsations in other areas are abnormal. For example, pulsation over the second right ICS may represent an aortic aneurysm, and pulsation over the second left ICS can represent increased filling pressure or flow in the pulmonary artery.

Paradoxical movement of the left anterior precordium is suggestive of a left ventricular aneurysm. With paradoxical movement, as the apex contracts, the aneurysmic area bulges. This ectopic impulse usually is seen above the apex impulse. The visibility of abnormal pulsations can be enhanced by balancing a tongue depressor on the chest over the pulsation.

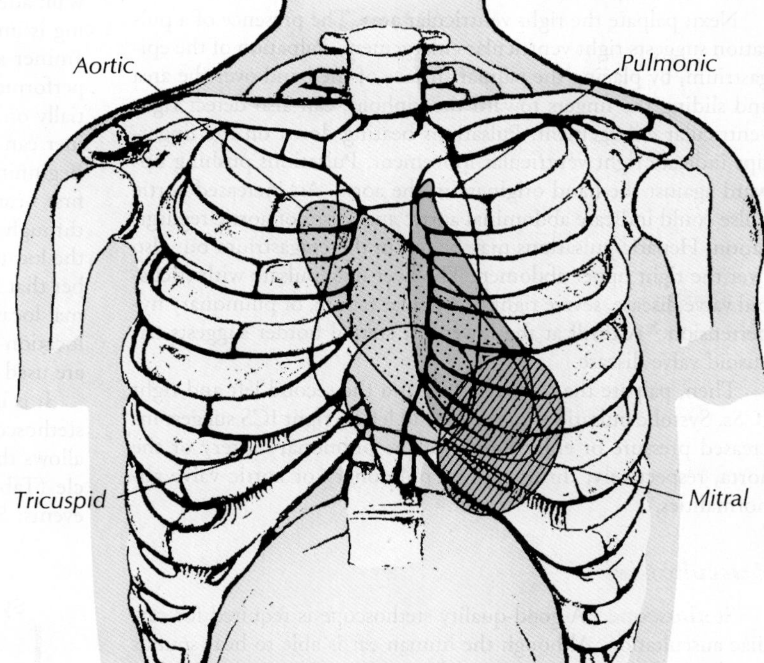

Figure 10-16 Areas to be assessed in the precordial examination. (Drawn from Leatham, A. [1979]. *An introduction to the examination of the cardiovascular system* [2nd ed., p. 20]. Oxford: Oxford University Press.)

Palpation

Movement that was not visible on inspection may be detected by palpation. All areas should be palpated using either the ball of the palm (at the base of the fingers) or the fingertips. In general, the palm surface is more sensitive to *thrills* (vibrations), whereas fingertips are more sensitive to *pulsations.* Thrills indicate turbulence of blood flow and are associated with murmurs. Impulses are described in terms of *location, size, amplitude, duration,* and *time in the cardiac cycle* (systole or diastole). To facilitate measurement of the horizontal location in centimeters from the MCL, or the size of the impulse, it is helpful for the examiner to measure his or her hand and use it as a "ruler." For example, the distance from the tip of the finger to the first joint, the second joint, and the third joint can be used.

Assess the apex impulse for location, size, amplitude, and duration. The apex impulse is, by definition, the furthest point leftward and downward at which a cardiac pulsation can be seen or felt.[3] The normal apex impulse is felt as a light tap, extending over 3 cm or less. The apex impulse is felt immediately after the first heart sound and lasts halfway through systole. An impulse that is diffuse (felt over two ICSs), increased in amplitude, or laterally or inferiorly displaced suggests increased volume load and left ventricular dilatation, such as occurs in mitral insufficiency or left ventricular failure. An impulse that is sustained, enlarged, and, sometimes, laterally displaced suggests obstruction to outflow with increased ventricular pressure load and concentric hypertrophy of the muscle, such as occurs in aortic stenosis or systemic hypertension.[6] If the apex impulse cannot be felt with the patient lying supine, examine the patient in the left lateral position, which brings the apex of the heart against the chest wall; the quality of the apex beat still can be determined even though its size and position may be slightly altered. A diastolic outward pulsation indicates impaired ventricular filling and corresponds to an S_3 (early to mid-diastole) or S_4 (late diastole) heard on auscultation.

Next, palpate the right ventricular area. The presence of a pulsation suggests right ventricular enlargement. Palpation of the epigastrium, by placing the palmar surface of the hand over the area and sliding the fingers toward the xiphoid, can also detect right ventricular enlargement. Pulsations beating down on the fingertips indicate right ventricular movement. Pulsations pushing upward against the hand originate in the aorta. An increased aortic pulse could indicate abdominal aortic aneurysm or aortic regurgitation. Hepatic pulsations may be felt in the epigastrium but also over the right upper abdomen. The liver may pulsate with tricuspid valve disease, severe right ventricular failure, or pulmonary hypertension.[3] A thrill at the lower left sternal border suggests tricuspid valve disease.

Then, palpate the third left ICS and the second left and right ICSs. Systolic pulsations in the second left or right ICS suggest increased pressure or enlargement of the pulmonary artery or the aorta, respectively; thrills suggest pulmonary or aortic valve abnormalities.

Auscultation

Stethoscope. A good-quality stethoscope is required for cardiac auscultation. Although the human ear is able to hear sounds ranging in frequency from 20 cycles per second, or Hertz (Hz), to 20,000 Hz, it is most sensitive to 1,000 to 5,000 Hz. The frequency of most heart sounds is less than 1,000 Hz. The stethoscope must transmit these low-frequency sounds to the ear.

The parts of the stethoscope are the ear pieces, tubing, and chest pieces. The ear pieces should fit comfortably into the ear canal and be snug enough so that extraneous sound cannot enter. They also must be kept free of ear wax. Double tubing with a small internal diameter (3 mm) should extend from the ear pieces to the chest pieces. In addition, the tubing should be reasonably short (25 to 30 cm) so the sound is not diluted and should be thick to minimize room noise.[33]

There are two classic types of chest pieces, the diaphragm and the bell. The *diaphragm,* which brings out higher frequencies and filters out the lower ones, is useful for listening to the first and second heart sounds (S_1 and S_2), high-frequency murmurs, and lung sounds. The diaphragm should be pressed firmly against the chest wall. The *bell* filters out high-frequency sounds and accentuates the low-frequency ones. Diastolic filling sounds and the low-frequency murmurs of mitral and tricuspid stenosis are heard best with the bell.[33] The bell should rest lightly on the chest; if firm pressure is applied, the skin becomes taut and acts like a diaphragm. When auscultating heart sounds, the nurse stands on the patient's right side so that, as he or she places the bell of the stethoscope on the patient's chest, the chest piece is balanced. Because the bell does not have to be held in place, the possibilities of creating extraneous sounds and filtering out low frequencies are reduced. Some stethoscopes have a single chestpiece with tunable diaphragm. Very light skin contact is used to listen to low-frequency sounds and firm pressure is used to listen to high-frequency sounds.

As part of a cardiac examination, all areas identified in Figure 10-17 should be auscultated except the epigastrium. The listener's goals when auscultating the precordium are to identify normal heart sounds, the heart rate, and rhythm; extra diastolic and systolic sounds; murmurs; and pericardial friction rubs.

Technique. The stethoscope is placed directly on the chest wall; adequate auscultation of the heart and lungs through clothing is impossible. The room should be quiet; the patient and examiner should be comfortable. Cardiac auscultation should be performed with the patient in three positions: supine, lying partially on the left side, and sitting up, leaning forward. The examiner can begin listening either at the cardiac apex or at the base. Beginning at the apex allows the examiner to focus initially on the first heart sound, clearly identify systole and diastole, and think through the cardiac cycle while listening at each site. The apex is the location of the apex impulse identified by palpation. Remember that left ventricular enlargement shifts the apex from the normal location. The timing of extra sounds in the cardiac cycle, the location in which they are best heard, and the quality of the sound are used to differentiate one from another.

It is important to proceed in a systematic manner. Inching the stethoscope up and down the chest wall is a useful technique and allows the examiner to focus on specific events in the cardiac cycle (Table 10-5). At each location, listen sequentially to four events: S_1, systole (interval between S_1 and S_2), S_2, and diastole

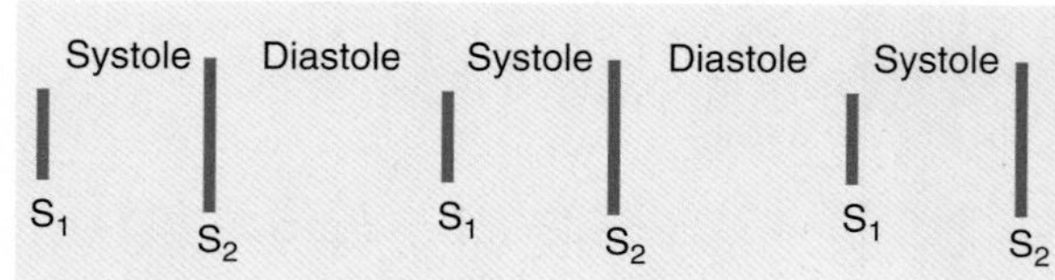

■ **Figure 10-17** Normal heart sounds.

Table 10-5 ■ AUSCULTATORY TECHNIQUE

Location	Chest Piece	Sounds
Apex	Diaphragm	S_1 intensity; opening sounds; murmurs from aortic and mitral valve
	Bell	Left S_3, S_4; murmurs
Left sternal border	Diaphragm	S_2 intensity; split S_1; murmurs from tricuspid and pulmonic valves and from atrial septal defects
	Bell	Right S_3, S_4
Base	Diaphragm	Split S_2; ejection sounds; murmurs from aortic valve
	Bell	Murmurs from aortic valve or dilated aorta

(interval between S_2 and S_1). For example, begin at the apical area with the diaphragm of the stethoscope and focus on S_1 and S_2 (Note, a description of the heart sounds follow.) Normally, S_1 is louder than or equal to S_2 at the apex. Listen carefully during systole and during diastole for clicks, murmurs, or other extra sounds. Inch the stethoscope toward the sternum to the right ventricular area and listen for a split S_1. Continue to move the stethoscope up the left sternal border to the second left ICS and note the change in relative intensity of the heart sounds. Normally, S_2 is louder than S_1 at the base. Continue to listen for splitting of the second heart sound and, if present, determine whether it is physiologic or abnormal. Move the stethoscope to the second right ICS and listen for an ejection sound in early systole after S_1. Listen with the bell along the lower sternal border for right ventricular S_3 and S_4. Move the bell to the apical area and listen for left ventricular S_3 and S_4. An opening sound of the mitral valve (high frequency) can be distinguished from an S_3 by pressing firmly with the bell to stretch the skin. Stretching the skin causes it to act as a diaphragm and filters out low-frequency sounds. When using a stethescope with a tunable diaphragm one can alternate listening with light (bell) and firm (diaphragm) pressure at each site.

Normal Heart Sounds. Normal heart sounds consist of the first and second heart sounds, S_1 and S_2. Both are of relatively high frequency and can, therefore, be heard clearly with the diaphragm of the stethoscope. Systole is normally shorter than diastole; with slow heart rates (less than 100 beats/min), the two sounds are easily distinguished by the cadence of the rhythm (Fig. 10-17). However, in more rapid rhythms, diastole shortens so that systole and diastole are of equal duration or, as the rate increases further, diastole becomes shorter than systole. To identify systole and diastole properly in this instance, the examiner should palpate the carotid artery while listening to the heart; the carotid upstroke immediately follows S_1.

Phonocardiograms or echocardiograms can be used to validate the auscultatory findings. In a phonocardiogram, heart sounds, electrocardiogram, and carotid pulse tracings are recorded simultaneously. Phonocardiograms are most often used for research or teaching. Echocardiograms are used clinically to demonstrate abnormalities of valve structure and cardiac function (Chapter 13).

The *first heart sound* is due primarily to closure of the mitral and tricuspid valves and is, therefore, heard loudest at the apex of the heart. Phonetically, if the heart sounds are "lub-dup," S_1 is the "lub." Mitral and tricuspid closure usually is heard as a single sound.

The intensity of the S_1 depends on leaflet mobility, position of the atrioventricular valves at the onset of systole, and the rate of ventricular upstroke. A loud S_1 is noted clinically in mitral stenosis when the cusps are mobile; with a short PR interval (0.08 to 0.13 second) because the leaflets are wide open when systolic contraction begins; in tachycardia, hyperthyroidism, or exercise because of an increased rate of pressure rise in the ventricle; and in the presence of a mechanical prosthetic mitral valve. Most commonly, a soft S_1 is due to poor conduction of sound through the chest wall, but other causes include a fixed or immobile valve; a long PR interval (0.20 to 0.26 second) or a slow heart rate, which allows the atrioventricular valves to float back into position before the onset of ventricular systole; low flow at the end of diastole; and β-adrenergic or calcium-channel blockers that reduce the rate of rise of ventricular pressure. The intensity of S_1 varies from beat to beat in atrial fibrillation because diastolic filling time is not constant. In a regular rhythm with a variable S_1 intensity, complete heart block should be suspected.[34] Variation in the intensity of S_1 can be evaluated by listening carefully to the relative intensity of S_1 and S_2 at the apex and the base. For example, when the intensity of S_1 is increased, it may be equal to or louder than S_2 at the base.[34] When assessing variation in S_1, it is helpful to have the patient hold his or her breath because respiratory movements may cause variation in the intensity of heart sounds.

Splitting of the first heart sound occurs when tricuspid closure is delayed and is best heard at the lower left sternal border. Pathologic splitting of S_1 results from right bundle-branch block, tricuspid stenosis, and atrial septal defect.[34] Splitting of S_1 helps to differentiate supraventricular from ventricular tachycardia. In supraventricular rhythms, S_1 is normal; in ventricular rhythms, S_1 is split.[3] Unfortunately, when supraventricular rhythms are conducted aberrantly, S_1 is split.

The *second heart sound* results primarily from closure of the aortic and pulmonic valves and is loudest at the base of the heart. Phonetically, the "dup" of the "lub-dup" is the S_2. The intensity of S_2 is determined by the pressure in the receiving vessels, the mobility of the valve leaflets, the degree of apposition of the leaflets, and the size of the aortic root. Intensity is increased with systemic or pulmonary hypertension, ascending aortic aneurysm, and in the presence of a mechanical prosthetic aortic valve. Intensity may be diminished in heart failure, myocardial infarction, pulmonary embolism, clinical shock, and stenosis of the aortic or pulmonic valve.[34]

Physiologic (normal) *splitting* of S_2 occurs during inspiration. During inspiration, an increased amount of blood is returned to the right side of the heart and a decreased amount of blood is returned to the left side of the heart due to trapping in the expanded lung. Pulmonic valve closure (P_2) is delayed because of the extra time needed for the increased blood volume to pass through the pulmonic valve, and aortic valve closure (A_2) occurs slightly early because of the relatively smaller amount of blood ejected from the left ventricle. In addition, the time of closure of P_2 is affected by the "hang out" interval, which is inversely related to pulmonary vascular impedance. During inspiration, the pulmonary vascular impedance decreases and P_2 is delayed; on expiration the opposite occurs.[34] If the two components are fairly close together, it is difficult to appreciate two distinct and separate sounds. A physiologic split S_2 may seem muffled or sound like a short drum roll on inspiration compared with expiration. On expiration, the split sounds merge (Fig. 10-18*A*). Normal splitting should be evaluated during quiet respiration and may be better heard with the patient

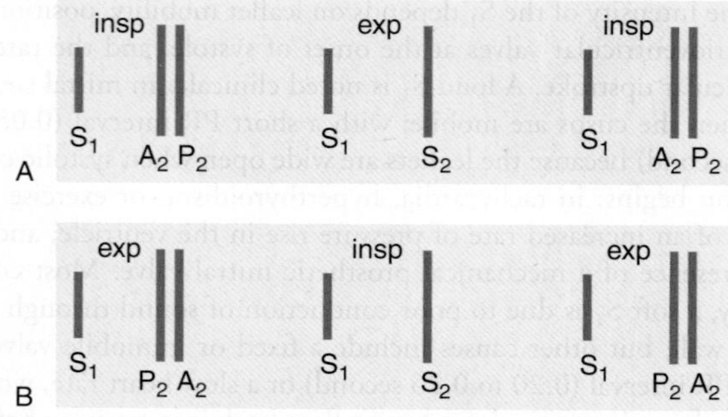

■ **Figure 10-18** Splitting of the S_2. (A) Physiologic splitting. During inspiration (*insp*), the P_2 sound is delayed. (B) Paradoxical splitting. During expiration (*exp*), A_2 is delayed.

sitting.[3] In pathologic splitting of S_2 (wide or fixed splits), the second sound is split during both inspiration and expiration, although there may be some respiratory variation in the amount of the split.

Paradoxical (abnormal) *splitting* of S_2 also can occur. Paradoxical splitting is due to any mechanism that causes late aortic valve closure (A_2), such as electrical delay (left bundle-branch block, right ventricular pacing, or right ventricular ectopy), mechanical obstruction (aortic stenosis or systolic hypertension), or impaired left ventricular contractile function (left ventricular failure or left ventricular ischemia; see Fig. 10-18*B*). Because P_2 is soft and A_2 is comparably loud and easily transmitted, a split S_2 is heard best in the second left ICS (pulmonary outflow tract). In paradoxical splitting, the second component (aortic closure) is louder than the first component (pulmonic closure).

Normally, A_2 is louder than P_2, even in the pulmonic area, and P_2 is not well heard, if at all, in other areas of the precordium. In pulmonary hypertension, the intensity of P_2 increases so that A_2 is less than or equal to P_2. The loud P_2 can be heard in other areas of the precordium, particularly the lower left sternal border and the cardiac apex.[8]

Extra Diastolic Sounds. Extra diastolic sounds consist of diastolic filling sounds and opening snaps. *Diastolic filling sounds* (S_3 and S_4) occur as blood enters a noncompliant ventricle during the two phases of rapid ventricular filling: the end of the early rapid filling phase, as active ventricular relaxation ceases (S_3); and, with atrial contraction, the active, rapid filling phase (S_4). Three theories have been proposed to explain the generation of the third and fourth heart sounds: the mitral valve theory, the chest wall theory, and the ventricular wall vibration theory. The last is the most widely accepted theory. Sound is produced within the ventricle by the abrupt decrease in wall motion (S_3) or with rapid filling of a noncompliant ventricle that causes a rapid deceleration of blood flow.[35] Diastolic filling sounds can arise from either or both ventricles. The cadence suggests the sound of a galloping horse, and these sounds are sometimes called diastolic gallops.

A *physiologic* S_3 can be heard in healthy children or young adults but usually disappears by 40 years of age. Its disappearance with advancing age has been attributed to decreased ventricular wall compliance with reduced early ventricular filling.[3] An S_3 in people older than age 40 years is usually pathologic and signals impaired systolic function.[35] It is one of the first clinical findings associated with cardiac decompensation, such as left ventricular heart failure (left ventricular S_3), primary pulmonary hypertension and cor pulmonale (right ventricular S_3), or insufficiency of the mitral, aortic, or tricuspid valves. An S_3 follows the S_2 in a

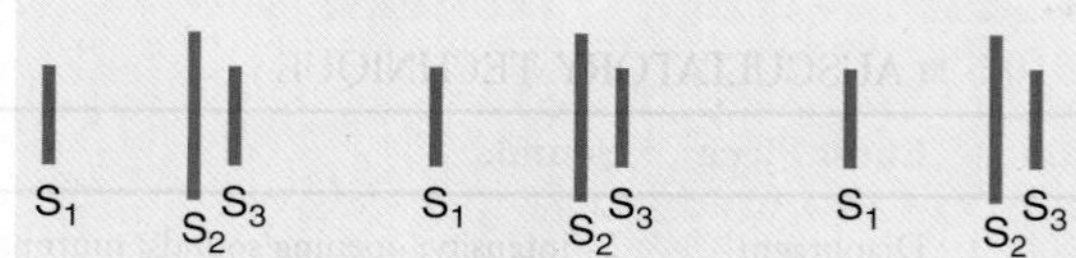

■ **Figure 10-19** An S_3 gallop immediately follows the S_2.

"lub-dup-*ta*" cadence (Fig. 10-19). Using the bell of the stethoscope, listen for a left ventricular S_3 over the apex of the heart; for a right ventricular S_3, listen over the lower left sternal border. By having the patient in the left lateral position, the apex is brought forward against the chest wall, making the left ventricular S_3 louder and, therefore, easier to hear.

The S_4 occurs after atrial contraction as the blood is ejected into a noncompliant ventricle, producing a rapid elevation of ventricular pressure, and signals diastolic dysfunction. Although it is the fourth heart sound, because the S_4 occurs at the end of ventricular diastole, it is heard immediately before S_1 and sounds like "*ta*-lub-dup" (Fig. 10-20). The S_4 is heard in most patients who have had a myocardial infarction, in a large number of patients experiencing angina pectoris, and in patients with coronary heart disease. It is also heard in patients with left ventricular hypertrophy due to hypertension, hypertrophic cardiomyopathy, or aortic stenosis. It is common in older adults because of the decreased compliance of the ventricle that occurs with age and the prevalence of hypertension and aortic stenosis in this population. An S_4 does not necessarily imply cardiac failure in people with ventricular hypertrophy. Because atrial contraction is necessary to produce an S_4, it is not heard in patients with atrial fibrillation. As with the S_3, listen for an S_4 using the bell of the stethoscope. A left ventricular S_4 is heard best at the apex, with the patient lying in the left lateral position; right ventricular S_4 is loudest over the lower left sternal border. Inching the stethoscope from the apex to the lower left sternal border can be helpful in differentiating right- and left-sided sounds. Left-sided sounds fade and right-sided sounds get louder as the stethoscope approaches the sternum.

A *quadruple rhythm* may be heard in patients with severe cardiac failure and both systolic and diastolic dysfunctions. If the heart rate is slow enough, four distinct heart sounds (S_1, S_2, and both S_3 and S_4) can be heard (Fig. 10-21). However, if a patient is ill enough to have a quadruple rhythm, tachycardia also usually is present. In this case, a *summation gallop* is heard, in which the S_3 and S_4 gallops fuse in mid-diastole to one loud diastolic sound. The summation gallop resembles the sound of a galloping horse (Fig. 10-22).

It stands to reason that in a noncompliant ventricle there should be more resistance to active ventricular filling than to passive ventricular filling; therefore, an S_4 gallop should be generated more easily than an S_3 gallop. Therefore, one would expect all patients with normal sinus rhythm who have an S_3 gallop to have an S_4 gallop as well. However, patients with normal sinus rhythm frequently have only an S_3. The cause for this finding is unknown,

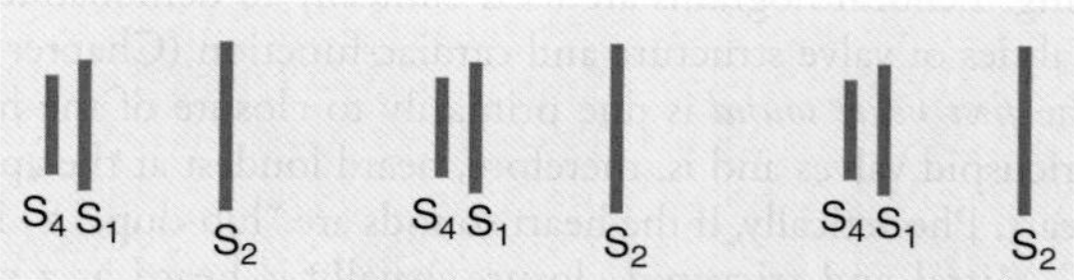

■ **Figure 10-20** An S_4 gallop immediately precedes the S_1.

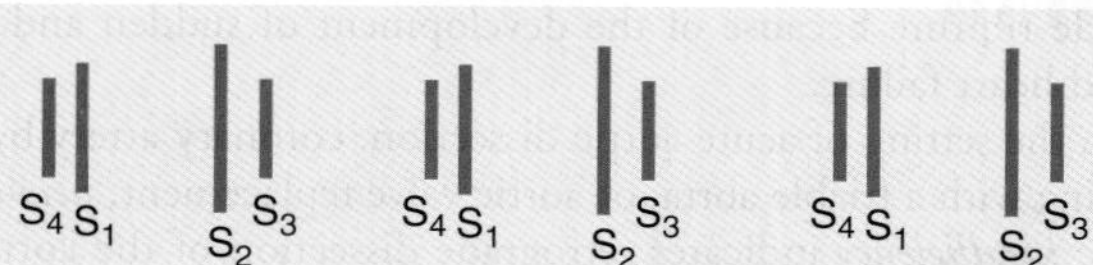

■ **Figure 10-21** Quadruple rhythm.

although one possibility may be an absence of actual mechanical atrial contraction in spite of electrical atrial activity.

Opening snaps are associated with the opening of a stenotic mitral valve. Opening sounds are not heard with normal valves. The sound is heard in very early diastole, medial to the cardiac apex. The sound can be loud and transmitted throughout the precordium (Fig. 10-23). Unlike an S_3, an opening snap has a high-pitched, snapping quality and is heard best with the diaphragm of the stethoscope.[33]

Extra Systolic Sounds. Extra systolic sounds consist of early systolic ejection sounds and systolic clicks. *Early ejection sounds* (Fig. 10-24) coincide with the opening of the aortic and pulmonic valves. They are heard shortly after S_1 and are high-pitched and clicking in quality. An *aortic ejection sound* is heard at the base or apex and accompanies a dilated aorta or aortic stenosis. *Pulmonic ejection sounds* are heard loudest in the second or third left ICSs and occur with pulmonary artery dilatation, pulmonary hypertension, and pulmonary stenosis.[33] *Mid- to late-systolic clicks* are associated with mitral valve prolapse; they occur from tensing of the leaflet or chordae when the limit of excursion is reached, and frequently they are followed by a murmur (Fig. 10-25).

Murmurs. Heart murmurs are sounds produced in the heart or great vessels by turbulent blood flow. Turbulent blood flow can be produced by[33]:

- Increased rate of flow across a normal valve (exercise, pregnancy, anemia)
- Flow across a partial obstruction (valvular stenosis, pulmonary or systemic hypertension)
- Flow across an irregularity without obstruction (bicuspid aortic valve, thickening of aortic cusps with aging)
- Flow into a dilated vessel (dilation of the aortic root)
- Backward flow across an incompetent valve or through a ventricular septal defect

Murmurs are classified according to systolic or diastolic *timing* (Fig. 10-26); *intensity* (Table 10-6); *location* (where the murmur is heard loudest); *radiation,* such as to the back, neck, or axilla; *configuration* (Fig. 10-27); *quality,* such as harsh, rough, rumbling, blowing, squeaking, or musical; and *duration* (Fig. 10-26).[6,33] Murmurs may be organic (due to intrinsic cardiovascular disease), functional (produced by circulatory disturbances such as anemia, pregnancy), or innocent (occur in the absence of disease).[3]

In adults, the most common systolic murmurs are produced by semilunar valve stenosis (ejection murmurs), atrioventricular valve

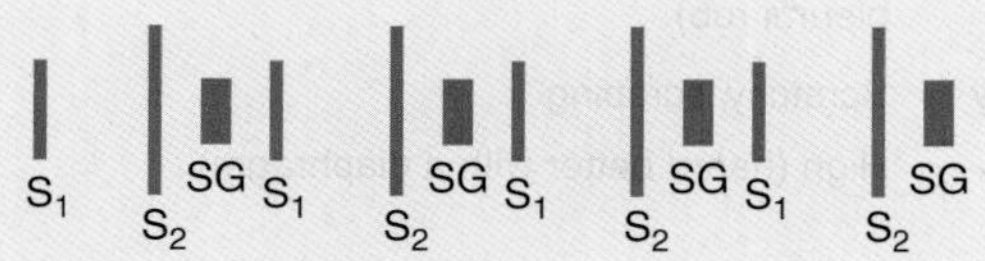

■ **Figure 10-22** Summation gallop.

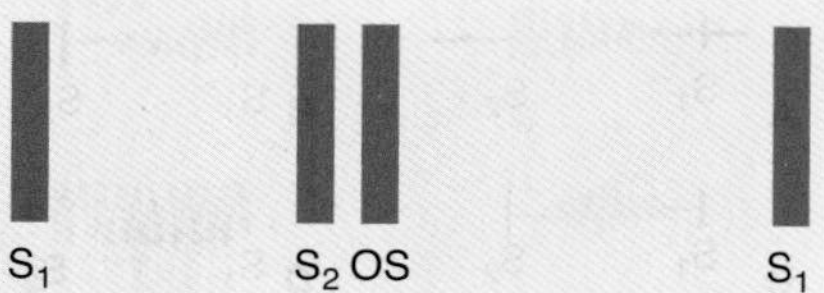

■ **Figure 10-23** Opening snap (OS).

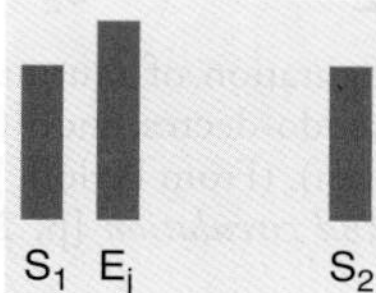

■ **Figure 10-24** Early systolic ejection sound.

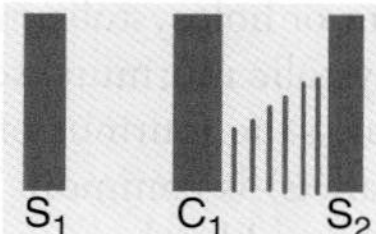

■ **Figure 10-25** Mid- to late-systolic click.

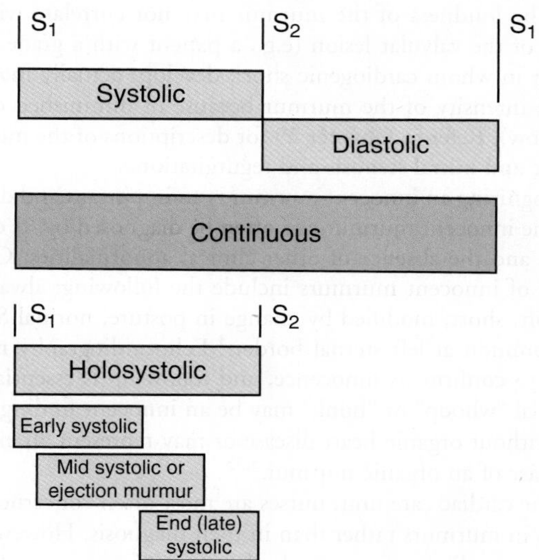

■ **Figure 10-26** Classification of murmurs by timing. (From Tilkian, A. & Conover, M. [1993]. *Understanding heart sounds and murmurs* [3rd ed., p. 99]. Philadelphia: Saunders.)

Table 10-6 ■ GRADATIONS OF MURMURS

Grade	Description
Grade 1	Very faint, heard only after listener has "tuned in"; may not be heard in all positions
Grade 2	Quiet, but heard immediately after placing the stethoscope on the chest
Grade 3	Moderately loud
Grade 4	Loud, with palpable thrill
Grade 5	Very loud, with thrill. May be heard when the stethoscope is partly off the chest
Grade 6	Very loud, with thrill. May be heard with stethoscope entirely off the chest

Bickley, L. S., & Szilagyi, P. G. (2009). *Bates' guide to physical examination and history taking* (10th ed.). Philadelphia: Lippincott Williams & Wilkins.

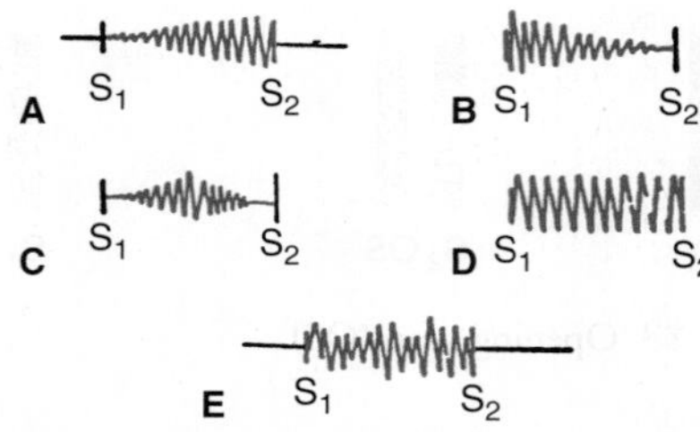

■ **Figure 10-27** Configuration of murmurs. (A) Crescendo. (B) Decrescendo. (C) Crescendo-decrescendo (diamond). (D) Plateau (even). (E) Variable (uneven). (From Perloff, J. K. [1990]. *Physical examination of the heart and circulation* [p. 208]. Philadelphia: WB Saunders.)

insufficiency (regurgitant or holosystolic murmurs), and ventricular septal defect (early systolic murmurs) secondary to myocardial infarction. In older adults, the murmur of aortic sclerosis (thickening of aortic valve leaflets) is common. The most common diastolic murmurs are produced by the reverse set of circumstances: insufficiency of semilunar valves (early regurgitant murmurs) and stenosis of the atrioventricular valves (mid- to late-diastolic rumbles). The loudness of the murmur may not correlate with the severity of the valvular lesion (e.g., a patient with a grade 5 to 6 murmur in whom cardiogenic shock develops actually may have reduced intensity of the murmur because of diminished cardiac blood flow). Refer to Chapter 29 for descriptions of the murmurs of aortic and mitral stenosis and regurgitation.

Recognizing an innocent murmur is an important and difficult skill. The innocent murmur can often be diagnosed by its clinical features and the absence of other clinical abnormalities. Clinical features of innocent murmurs include the following: always systolic, soft, short, modified by change in posture, normal S_2, and most common at left sternal border.[3] Echocardiography may be needed to confirm its innocence, and follow-up is essential. The precordial "whoop" or "honk" may be an innocent finding in patients without organic heart disease or may represent an exaggerated phase of an organic murmur.[3,33]

In the cardiac care unit, nurses are most often concerned with changes in murmurs rather than in their diagnosis. However, it is important to diagnose accurately the onset of murmurs of papillary muscle dysfunction and aortic insufficiency.

Normally, papillary muscle contraction allows for complete closure of the atrioventricular valves. However, when the papillary muscles are ischemic (most often in the left ventricle), they are unable to contract properly, preventing the chordae tendineae from being held tautly and, in turn, from holding the mitral valve leaflets closed during left ventricular contraction. Blood is, therefore, allowed to flow backward through the mitral valve (mitral regurgitation) during systole. The murmur of mitral regurgitation secondary to papillary muscle dysfunction is systolic (occurring in early- to mid-systole) and usually soft, high pitched, and crescendo–decrescendo in configuration. In the presence of heart failure or angina, the murmur may become holosystolic.

A new murmur of *papillary muscle dysfunction* in the patient with acute myocardial infarction must be recognized immediately because interventions must be instituted to relieve the papillary muscle ischemia and prevent progression to papillary muscle infarction. Should the papillary muscles infarct, they also may rupture; there is a high mortality rate associated with papillary muscle rupture because of the development of sudden and profound heart failure.

In the setting of acute aortic dissection, coronary artery bypass grafting with a friable aorta, or aortic valve replacement, *new-onset aortic insufficiency* indicates retrograde dissection of the aorta, or valve dehiscence. The murmur of aortic insufficiency is an early diastolic, decrescendo murmur, heard at the second right or third left ICS that radiates toward the apex. In acute aortic insufficiency, the intensity of S_1 is frequently diminished because of the increase in ventricular volume, and P_2 may be accentuated because of the rapid rise in pulmonary vascular pressure.[33] Acute left ventricular failure may result from volume overload alone or, in the case of continued retrograde dissection, from myocardial infarction secondary to dissection of the coronary arteries.

Pericardial Friction Rubs. Pericardial friction rubs are characteristic of pericarditis, which occurs in more than 15% of patients with acute myocardial infarction. A pericardial friction rub develops in approximately 7% of patients with myocardial infarction, commonly by the fourth day after myocardial infarction. Rubs may be transient, lasting only several hours. The rub occurs with heart movement; each movement creates its own short, scratchy sound (Fig. 10-28). Pericardial friction rubs are classified

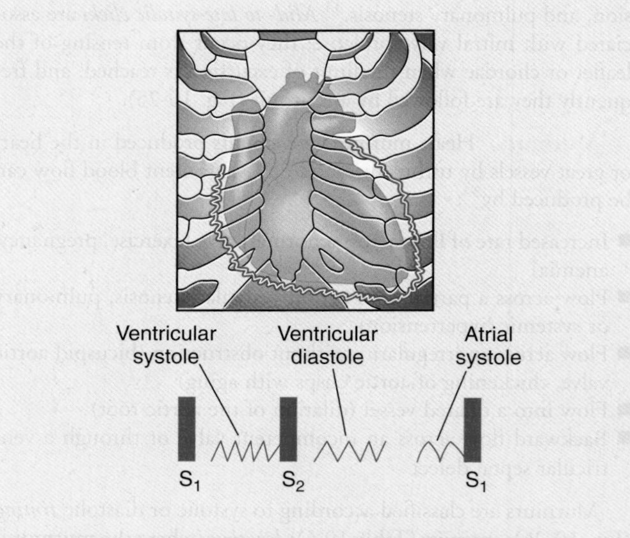

Timing	May have three short components, each associated with cardiac movement: (1) atrial systole, (2) ventricular systole, and (3) ventricular diastole. Usually the first two components are present; all three make diagnosis easy; only one (usually the systolic) invites confusion with a murmur.
Location	Variable, but usually heard best in the 3rd left ICS
Radiation	Little
Intensity	Variable. May increase when the patient leans forward, exhales, and holds breath (in contrast to pleural rub)
Quality	Scratchy, scraping
Pitch	High (heard better with a diaphragm)

■ **Figure 10-28** Pericardial friction rub.

as three-component (atrial systole, ventricular systole, and ventricular diastole), two-component (ventricular systole and diastole), or one-component (ventricular systole) rubs. One-component rubs may be difficult to differentiate from a murmur. Rubs are best heard either with the patient sitting upright and leaning forward with the breath expelled (most appropriate for the patient with an acute myocardial infarction) or with the patient on his or her hands and knees in bed or on the examination table (useful in a nonacute situation). A pericardial friction rub can be heard with or without a pericardial effusion. Pericardial friction rubs can be differentiated from pleural friction rubs by having the patient hold his or her breath.

Pericardial friction rubs are common in postoperative cardiac patients. Also, a respirophasic squeak may be heard that is related to mediastinal or pleural tubes. Air in the mediastinum produces a crunching sound (Hamman's sign) during auscultation of the precordium.

Dynamic Auscultation. Dynamic auscultation can be used to aid in the interpretation of heart sounds and murmurs. A variety of physiologic or pharmacologic maneuvers can be used to alter circulatory dynamics: respiration, postural changes, the Valsalva maneuver, postextrasystolic beats, isometric exercise, and vasoactive agents.[8] Table 10-7 summarizes the auscultatory effects of these maneuvers.

Respiration affects blood flow. *Inspiration* increases venous return to the right heart, increasing right ventricular diastolic pressure, stroke volume, and ejection time. Pulmonary vascular impedance is reduced, with increases in pulmonary vascular capacitance. With a normal respiratory rate, blood return to the left ventricle is reduced, resulting in decreased left ventricular diastolic pressure, stroke volume, and ejection time. Transmission of the augmented right ventricular volume to the left ventricle is delayed by three to four cardiac cycles in the pulmonary vasculature. All of the auscultatory events generated by the right heart are augmented during inspiration.[33] The use of the Müller maneuver (sustained inspiratory effort against a closed glottis) further augments the auscultatory effects of inspiration. *Expiration* increases venous return to the left heart, increasing left ventricular diastolic pressure, stroke volume, and ejection time.[6]

Table 10-7 ■ AUSCULTATORY EFFECTS OF PHYSIOLOGIC AND PHARMACOLOGIC MANEUVERS

Maneuver	Effect	Maneuver	Effect
Inspiration	Physiologically splits S_2 Attenuates left ventricular S_3 and S_4, mitral opening snap, and pulmonic ejection sound	Valsalva maneuver Phase II (strain)	 Attenuates S_3 and S_4 Narrows A_2–P_2 interval
	Accentuates right ventricular S_3 and S_4, tricuspid opening snap, and right heart murmurs	Phase III (release)	Widens A_2–P_2 interval
		Phase IV (overshoot)	Returns to baseline or transiently accentuates S_3 and S_4
	Hastens and accentuates click-murmur of mitral valve prolapse	Postextrasystolic beats	Augments murmurs of aortic and pulmonic stenosis, tricuspid and aortic regurgitation, and hypertrophic obstructive cardiomyopathy
Expiration	Paradoxically splits S_2 Accentuates left ventricular S_3 and S_4, mitral opening snap, and left heart murmurs		Delays click-murmur of mitral valve prolapse
	Attenuates right ventricular S_3 and S_4, and tricuspid opening snap	Isometric exercise	Accentuates left ventricular S_3 and S_4 and murmurs of aortic regurgitation, rheumatic mitral regurgitation
Lying down	Widens split S_2 in all respiratory phases Augments first right, then left, ventricular S_3 and S_4 Augments most systolic murmurs		Ventricular septal defect, mitral stenosis Attenuates murmur of aortic stenosis Delays click-murmur of mitral valve prolapse
	Diminishes systolic murmur of hypertrophic obstructive cardiomyopathy	Amyl nitrate	Augments opening snaps; S_3; and murmurs of aortic, pulmonic, mitral, and tricuspid stenosis, and tricuspid regurgitation
	Delays and attenuates click-murmur of mitral valve prolapse		Diminishes murmurs of mitral and aortic regurgitation, ventricular septal defect, and Austin Flint
Sudden standing	Narrows split S_2 in all respiratory phases Diminishes first right, then left, ventricular S_3 and S_4 Diminishes most systolic murmurs Accentuates systolic murmur of hypertrophic obstructive cardiomyopathy		Hastens click-murmur of mitral valve prolapse
	Hastens and accentuates click-murmur of mitral valve prolapse	Methoxamine and phenylephrine	Accentuates murmurs of aortic and mitral regurgitation, and ventricular septal defect
Squatting	Augments right and left ventricular S_3 and S_4, and most murmurs		Diminishes murmurs of hypertrophic obstructive cardiomyopathy and aortic stenosis
	Delays click-murmur of mitral valve prolapse		Delays click-murmur of mitral valve prolapse

Adapted from Braunwald, E. (1984). The physical examination. In E. Braunwald (Ed.). *Heart disease: A textbook of cardiovascular medicine* (2nd ed., pp. 35—38). Philadelphia: WB Saunders.

The *Valsalva maneuver* (forced expiration against a closed glottis) has variable effects associated with each of its four phases. In *phase I*, the *initial* phase, intrathoracic pressure increases, causing a transient elevation in left ventricular output. In *phase II*, the *straining* phase, venous return is decreased; first right, then left ventricular filling is reduced; stroke volume, mean arterial pressure, and pulse pressure are reduced; and heart rate is increased. In *phase III*, the *release* phase, venous return is increased, with subsequent increases in right, then left, ventricular filling. In *phase IV*, the *overshoot* phase, right ventricular filling and stroke volume return to baseline or may be elevated briefly. The return to baseline of left ventricular hemodynamics is delayed for six to eight beats and also may be elevated briefly.[6,33] During phase II, all murmurs diminish except those of hypertrophic cardiomyopathy and mitral valve prolapse. The Valsalva maneuver should not be held for more than 10 seconds because it reduces cardiac output.

Postural change from sitting or standing to lying down increases venous return first to the right and then to the left ventricle. Recumbence and passive leg raising cause most auscultatory cardiac events to increase except the murmurs of idiopathic hypertrophic

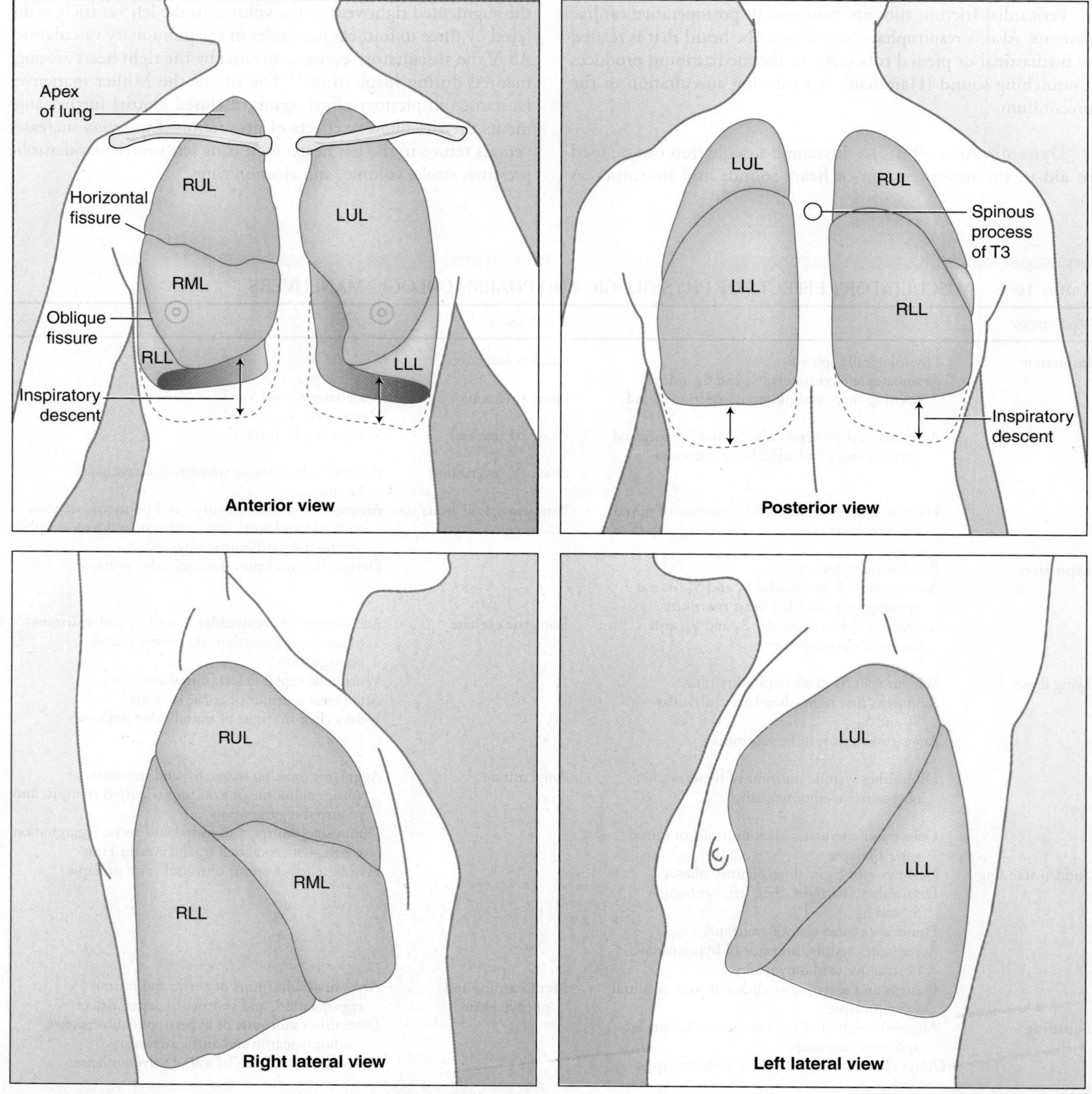

■ **Figure 10-29** Respiratory assessment: Lobar localization. RUL, right upper lobe; RML, right middle lobe; RLL, right lower lobe; LUL, left upper lobe; LLL, left lower lobe.

subaortic stenosis and mitral valve prolapse. Sudden standing has the opposite effect; it reduces venous return and causes most murmurs, except hypertrophic cardiomyopathy and mitral valve prolapse, to decrease. Squatting simultaneously increases venous return and systemic vascular resistance.[6]

Postextrasystolic beats, if followed by a pause, increase ventricular filling and cardiac contractility. Similar hemodynamic changes occur with diastolic pauses in atrial fibrillation and sinus arrhythmia.[6]

Isometric exercise increases systemic vascular resistance, arterial pressure, heart rate, cardiac output, left ventricular filling pressure, and heart size. Using a calibrated handgrip device, the patient sustains the handgrip for 20 to 30 seconds. The handgrip enhances S_3 and S_4 and aortic regurgitant murmurs. Avoid isometric exercise in patients with myocardial ischemia or ventricular arrhythmia. The patient should not perform the Valsalva maneuver simultaneously with isometric exercise.

Pharmacologic agents used in dynamic auscultation are amyl nitrate, methoxamine, and phenylephrine.[6] Inhalation of *amyl nitrate* for 10 to 15 seconds causes marked vasodilatation, reducing systemic arterial pressure and producing a reflex tachycardia, followed by an increase in stroke volume and venous return. *Methoxamine* and *phenylephrine* increase systemic vascular resistance. Both cause a reflex drop in heart rate and decrease contractility and cardiac output. Methoxamine, 3 to 5 mg intravenously, results in blood pressure elevation of 20 to 40 mm Hg, lasting 10 to 20 minutes. Phenylephrine, 0.5 mg intravenously, elevates blood pressure 30 mm Hg for 3 to 5 minutes.

Lungs

The respiratory assessment described in this chapter is elementary and is designed to assist the cardiac nurse in identifying respiratory manifestations seen in patients with heart disease. The room should be quiet and the patient's chest exposed. Proceed in a systematic manner: inspect, palpate, percuss, and auscultate. Always compare one side with the other; always place the stethoscope in direct contact with the chest wall. Begin with examination of the posterior chest, if possible, with the patient sitting upright and arms folded across the chest. Follow with assessment of the anterior chest with the patient lying down. Only the upper and lower lobes of the lung are accessible by posterior chest examination; to assess the right middle lobe, the lateral and anterior chest must be examined (Fig. 10-29).[8]

Inspection

Respiratory Rate, Depth, Rhythm, and Effort. Normally, the respiratory rate is less than 16 breaths per minute and the rhythm is regular (Fig. 10-30*A*). *Tachypnea*, rapid, shallow breathing, may be noted in patients who have heart failure, pain, or anxiety (Fig. 10-30*B*). *Bradypnea,* slow breathing, can be noted during sleep or after administration of respiratory depressant agents, such as morphine sulfate or anesthesia (Fig. 10-30*C*). *Cheyne–Stokes respirations*, characterized by periods of alternating deep breathing and apnea, occur in patients with severe left ventricular failure (Fig. 10-30*D*). Of particular concern is the duration of the apneic period. Use of accessory muscles of respiration, an upright, forward-leaning position, and pursed-lip breathing are visible signs of increased respiratory effort. Retraction of the ICSs is seen in severe asthma or upper airway obstruction.[8] A prolonged expiratory phase is associated with early airway obstruction.

Cough and Sputum. A dry, hacking *cough* from irritation of small airways is common in patients with pulmonary congestion

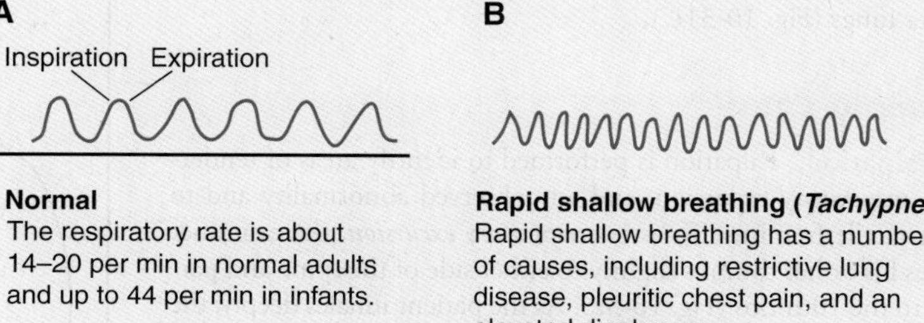

A
Inspiration Expiration
B
Normal
The respiratory rate is about 14–20 per min in normal adults and up to 44 per min in infants.
Rapid shallow breathing (Tachypnea)
Rapid shallow breathing has a number of causes, including restrictive lung disease, pleuritic chest pain, and an elevated diaphragm.

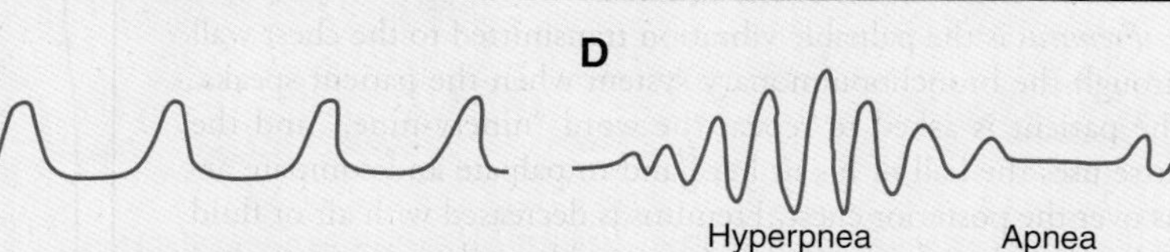

Periods of deep breathing alternate with periods of apnea (no breathing). Children and older adults normally may show this pattern in sleep. Other causes include heart failure, uremia, drug-induced respiratory depression, and brain damage (typically on both sides of the cerebral hemispheres or diencephalon).

Figure 10-30 Respiratory rate and rhythm. (A) Normal. (B) Tachypnea. (C) Bradypnea. (D) Cheyne–Stokes.

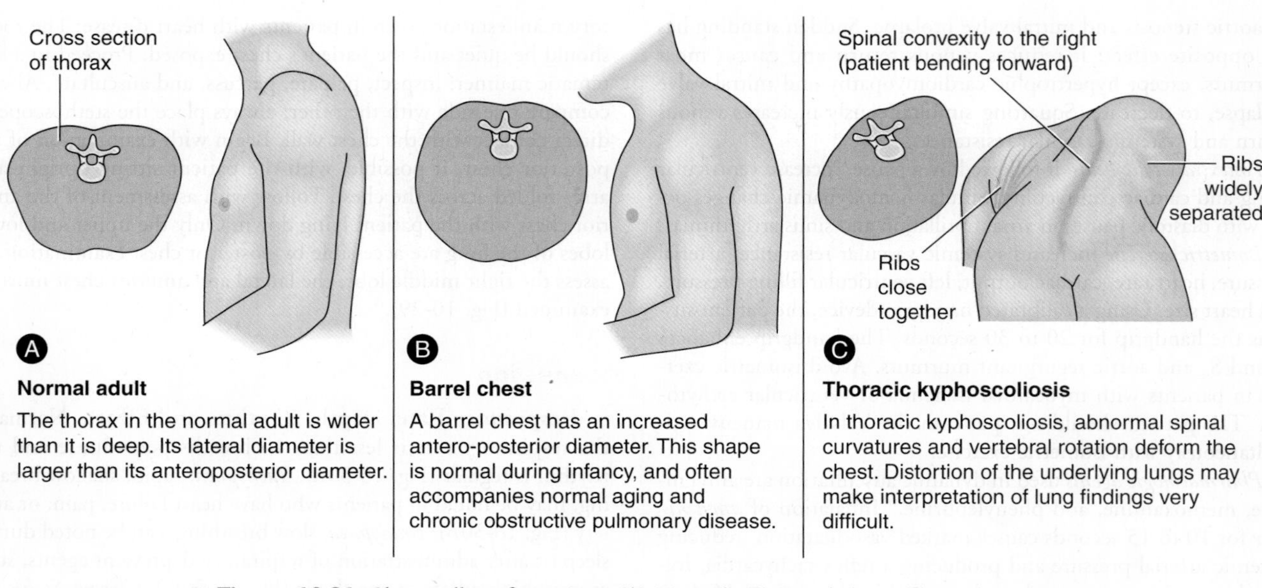
Cross section
of thorax
A
Normal adult
The thorax in the normal adult is wider than it is deep. Its lateral diameter is larger than its anteroposterior diameter.
B
Barrel chest
A barrel chest has an increased antero-posterior diameter. This shape is normal during infancy, and often accompanies normal aging and chronic obstructive pulmonary disease.
Spinal convexity to the right
(patient bending forward)
Ribs
widely
separated
Ribs
close
together
C
Thoracic kyphoscoliosis
In thoracic kyphoscoliosis, abnormal spinal curvatures and vertebral rotation deform the chest. Distortion of the underlying lungs may make interpretation of lung findings very difficult.

■ **Figure 10-31** Chest wall configurations. (A) Normal. (B) Barrel chest. (C) Kyphoscoliosis.

from heart failure or patients taking angiotensin-converting enzyme inhibitors. *Pink, frothy sputum* is indicative of pulmonary edema. Although an occasional cough may be normal, sputum production is always abnormal.

Chest Configuration. With *normal* chest configuration, the anteroposterior to lateral diameter ratio ranges from 1:2 to 5:7 (Fig. 10-31*A*). With a *barrel chest,* associated with pulmonary emphysema and aging, the anteroposterior to lateral diameter ratio increases to 1:1 or more (Fig. 10-31*B*). *Kyphoscoliosis,* an abnormal spinal curvature, may prevent the patient from fully expanding his or her lungs (Fig. 10-31*C*).

Posterior Chest

Palpation. Palpation is performed to identify areas of tenderness, respiratory excursion, and any observed abnormality and to elicit tactile fremitus. To assess *respiratory excursion,* the examiner places his or her thumbs slightly to either side of the spine and parallel to the 10th ribs (Fig. 10-32). As the patient inhales deeply, the examiner evaluates the depth and symmetry of the patient's breath by the movement of his or her thumbs.

Fremitus is the palpable vibration transmitted to the chest wall through the bronchopulmonary system when the patient speaks. The patient is asked to repeat the word "ninety-nine," and the nurse uses the ball of his or her hand to palpate and compare areas over the posterior chest. Fremitus is decreased with air or fluid in the pleural space and by an obstructed bronchus; it is increased by lung consolidation. To estimate the level of the diaphragm bilaterally, the examiner places the ulnar surface of his or her hand parallel to its expected level and progressively moves the hand downward until fremitus is no longer felt. Posteriorly, the diaphragm is located between the 10th and 12th (with deep inspiration) ribs. An abnormally high diaphragm suggests a pleural effusion or atelectasis.

Percussion. Percussion causes vibrations in the underlying tissues, resulting in sounds that indicate if the tissues are solid or filled with fluid or air (Table 10-8). The technique of percussion involves the examiner placing the passive finger firmly over the area to be percussed and striking the distal interphalangeal joint of the middle finger of that hand with the middle finger of the opposite hand (Fig. 10-33). Percuss across both shoulders and then at 5-cm intervals down the back (Fig. 10-34), making side-to-side comparisons. Normal lung tissue (air-filled) produces *resonance. Dullness*

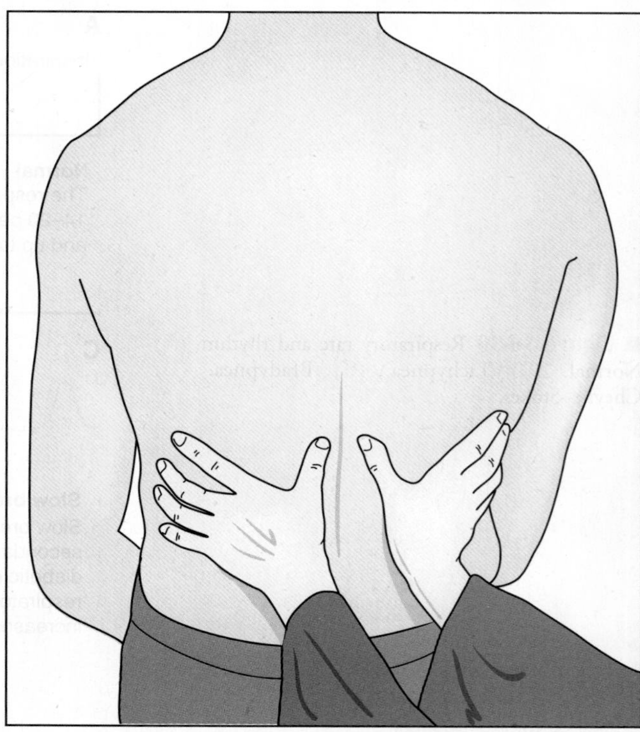

■ **Figure 10-32** Assessment of respiratory excursion.

Table 10-8 ■ PERCUSSION NOTES AND THEIR CHARACTERISTICS

	Relative Intensity	Relative Pitch	Relative Duration	Example of Location
Flatness	Soft	High	Short	Thigh
Dullness	Medium	Medium	Medium	Liver
Resonance	Loud	Low	Long	Normal lung
Hyperresonance	Very loud	Lower	Longer	None normally
Tympany	Loud	High*	*	Gastric air bubble or puffed-out cheek

*Distinguished mainly by its musical timbre.
Bickley, L. S., & Szilagyi, P. G. (2009). *Bates' guide to physical examination and history taking* (10th ed.). Philadelphia: Lippincott Williams & Wilkins.

replaces resonance when fluid or solid tissue replaces air-filled tissue. In patients with emphysema and air trapping, *hyper-resonance* replaces resonance. *Diaphragmatic excursion* can be ascertained by percussion of the border between resonance (lung tissue) and dullness (muscle) in expiration and inspiration. Normal excursion is 5 to 6 cm.

Auscultation. Airflow, obstruction, and the condition of the lungs and pleural space can be assessed with auscultation. Use the diaphragm of the stethoscope pressed firmly on the skin in the sequence illustrated in Figure 10-34. Ask the patient to breathe slowly and deeply through his or her mouth because nose breathing changes the pitch of the sounds. Listen through one full breath in each location for pitch, intensity, and duration of inspiration and expiration.

Normal breath sounds (vesicular) are heard in peripheral lung tissue away from large airways. They are soft, low-pitched, blowing sounds. The inspiratory–expiratory time ratio is 5:2. Normal breath sounds are diminished at the bases. The sounds are decreased in obese patients and with shallow breathing or pleural effusion, and they are increased with exercise.

Bronchovesicular sounds are heard normally in the areas around the mainstem bronchi (below the clavicles and between the scapulae). They have moderate pitch and intensity, with an inspiratory–expiratory time ratio of 1:1. These sounds are abnormal if heard in the lung periphery.

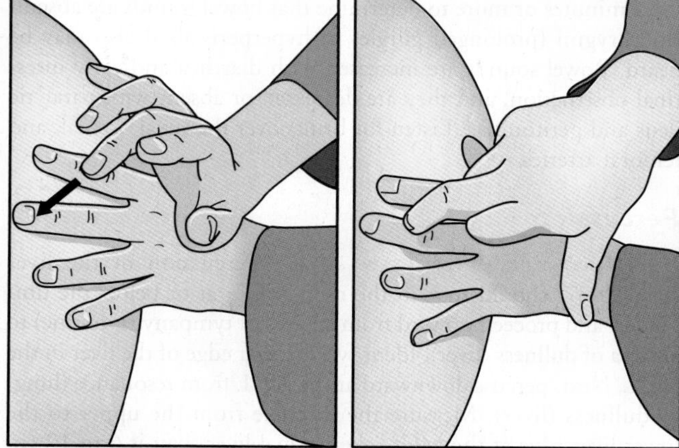

■ **Figure 10-33** The technique of percussion.

Bronchial sounds, heard normally over the bronchial areas, are loud and high pitched. Expiratory time is greater than inspiratory time. If heard in the lung periphery, bronchial sounds are abnormal.

Adventitious breath sounds are superimposed over normal breath sounds. There are two categories of adventitious sounds: discontinuous (crackles) and continuous (wheezes and pleural friction rubs). When adventitious breath sounds are heard, note loudness, pitch, duration, number, timing (phase of respiratory cycle), location on the chest wall, and persistence from breath to breath. Have the patient cough, and note any change in adventitious sounds.

Crackles are discrete, discontinuous sounds that are similar to the sound generated by rubbing hairs together in front of the ears (Fig. 10-35*A*). Crackles are attributed to fluid in the alveoli or to explosive reopening of alveoli. Heart failure or atelectasis associated with bed rest, splinting from ischemic or incisional pain, or the effects of pain medication and sedatives often result in development of crackles. Typically, crackles are noted first at the bases (because of gravity's effect on fluid accumulation and decreased

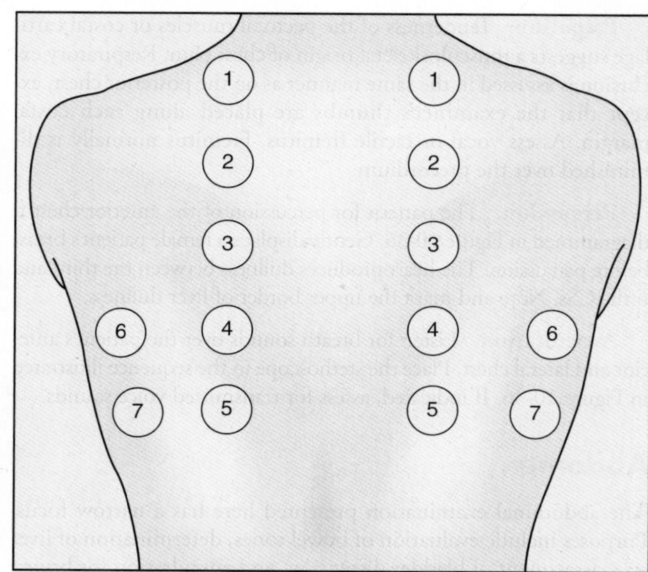

■ **Figure 10-34** Sequence of posterior percussion and auscultation.

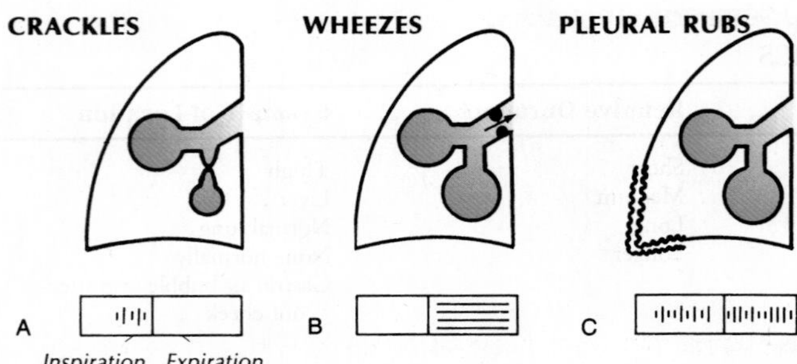

■ **Figure 10-35** Adventitious breath sounds. (A) Crackles. (B) Wheezes. (C) Pleural friction rubs.

ventilation of basilar tissue), but may progress to all portions of the lung fields.

Wheezes are continuous, musical sounds from rapid air movement through constricted airways. They are heard most often on expiration but can be heard during both inspiration and expiration (Fig. 10-35*B*). Although wheezes are characteristic of obstructive lung disease, they can be caused by interstitial pulmonary edema compressing small airways. β-Adrenergic blocking agents, such as propranolol, may precipitate airway narrowing, especially in patients with underlying pulmonary disease. A fixed wheeze is characteristic of an endobronchial mass or tumor.

Transmitted voice sounds may be louder and clearer than normal (bronchophony, whispered pectoriloquy) when heard through the chest wall. The quality of voice sounds may have a nasal or bleating character (egophony). Transmitted voice sounds suggest consolidation of lung tissue.

Pleural friction rubs result from inflamed pleura rubbing together. A pleural friction rub, characteristic of pleuritis, is a coarse, grating sound that can be heard on inspiration and expiration (Fig. 10-35*C*).

Anterior Chest

Palpation. Tenderness of the pectoral muscles or costal cartilage suggests a musculoskeletal origin of chest pain. Respiratory excursion is assessed in the same manner as on the posterior chest, except that the examiner's thumbs are placed along each costal margin. Assess vocal or tactile fremitus. Fremitus normally is diminished over the precordium.

Percussion. The pattern for percussion of the anterior chest is diagrammed in Figure 10-36. Gently displace a female patient's breast before percussion. The heart produces dullness between the third and fifth ICSs. Note and mark the upper border of liver dullness.

Auscultation. Listen for breath sounds over the patient's anterior and lateral chest. Place the stethoscope in the sequence illustrated in Figure 10-36. If indicated, assess for transmitted voice sounds.

Abdomen

The abdominal examination presented here has a narrow focus. Purposes include evaluation of bowel tones, determination of liver size, assessment of bladder distention, and auscultation for bruits. After anesthesia, resumption of bowel tones must be confirmed before initiating a diet. Liver engorgement occurs because of decreased venous return secondary to right ventricular failure. Urine output is an important indicator of cardiac output. In a patient who is unable to void (e.g., secondary to strict bed rest or after atropine sulfate administration) or who has not voided despite adequate fluid intake, always assess for bladder distention before initiating other measures.

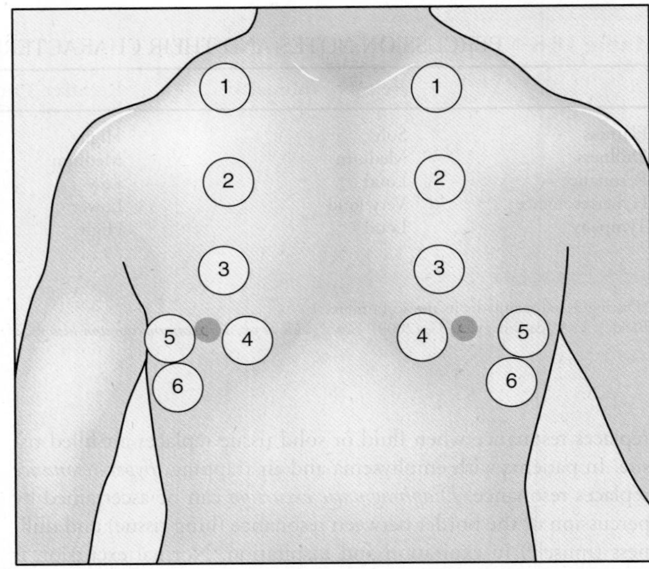

■ **Figure 10-36** Sequence of anterior percussion and auscultation.

Inspection

Observe the abdomen for symmetry and visible peristalsis. Note the presence of abdominal distention. Abdominally localized obesity (waist circumference >35 inches for women or >40 inches for men) is associated with coronary artery disease, adult-onset diabetes mellitus, and metabolic syndrome.

Ausculation

Auscultate the abdomen after observation because palpation and percussion can either increase or diminish bowel sounds. Gently place the diaphragm of the stethoscope on the abdomen. Listen over all quadrants. Normal bowel sounds consist of clicks and gurgles, at a frequency of 5 to 34 per minute. It is necessary to listen for 2 minutes or more to determine that bowel sounds are absent. Borborygmi (prolonged gurgles of hyperperistalsis) also may be heard. Bowel sounds are increased with diarrhea and early intestinal obstruction, and they are decreased or absent with paralytic ileus and peritonitis.[8] Listen for bruits over the renal, ischial, and femoral arteries.

Percussion

Determination of Liver Size. Percussion of the liver (Fig. 10-37) should start in the right MCL, at or below the umbilicus, and proceed upward from an area of tympany (intestine) to an area of dullness (liver). Identify the lower edge of the liver in the MCL. Next, percuss downward at the MCL from resonance (lung) to dullness (liver). Measure the distance from the upper to the lower liver edge at the MCL; the normal liver span is 6 to 12 cm (Fig. 10-38). A right pleural effusion or lung consolidation

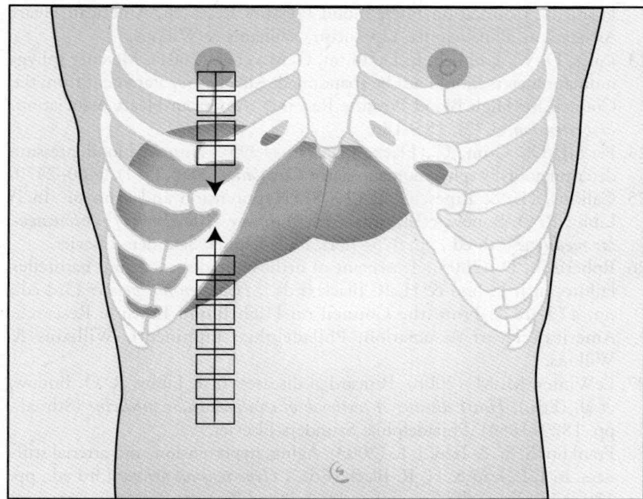

■ **Figure 10-37** Percussion of the liver.

(dullness) may obscure the upper border. Gas in the colon (tympany) may obscure the lower edge.

Assessment of Bladder Distention. Percuss downward from the umbilicus to the symphysis pubis. Suprapubic dullness may indicate a distended urinary bladder. If percussion does not confirm suspicions of a distended urinary bladder, palpate gently above the symphysis pubis. If ascites is present, neither abdominal percussion nor palpation may reveal bladder distention.

Palpation

Determination of Liver Size. Deep palpation is necessary to feel the liver. It is imperative that the patient is relaxed. Place the left hand under the patient's 11th and 12th ribs for support. The liver is easier to palpate if the examiner pushes up with this hand. Place the right hand on the abdomen below the lower edge of dullness, with the fingers pointing toward the right costal margin. As the patient takes a deep abdominal breath and then exhales, gently

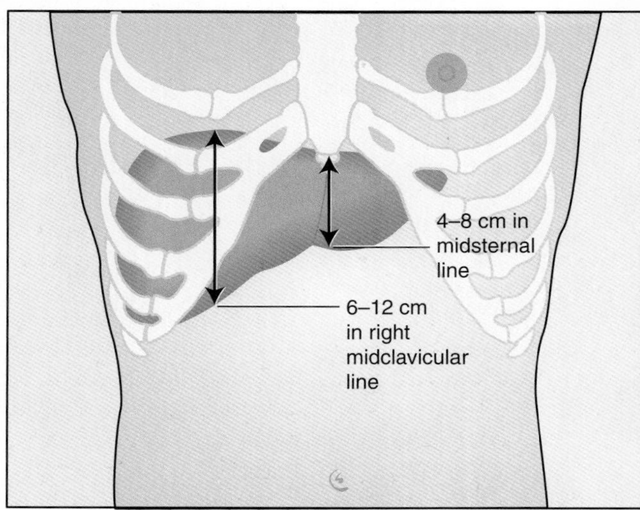

■ **Figure 10-38** Measurement of liver span.

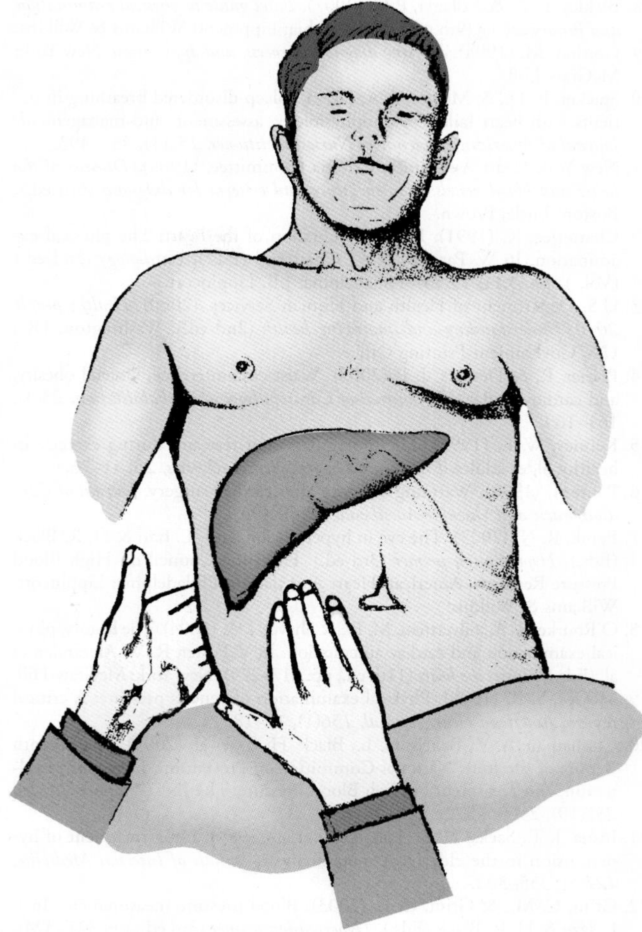

■ **Figure 10-39** Palpation of the liver.

but firmly push in and up with the fingers (Fig. 10-39). With each exhalation, move the hand further toward the liver. The liver edge should come down to meet the fingers. Normally, it feels firm with a smooth edge. It should not be tender. With venous engorgement from right heart failure, the liver is enlarged, firm, tender, and smooth.

REFERENCES

1. Abbott, P. D., Short, E., Dodson, S., et al. (2002). Improving your cultural awareness with culture clues. *Nurse Practitioner, 27*(2), 44–47, 51.
2. Braunwald, E., & Goldman, L. (2002). *Primary cardiology* (2nd ed.). Philadelphia: WB Saunders.
3. Marriott, H. J. L. (1993). *Bedside cardiac diagnosis.* Philadelphia: J.B. Lippincott.
4. Underhill, S. L. (1984). Assessment of cardiovascular function. In L. S. Bruner & D. S. Suddarth (Eds.), *Textbook of medical–surgical nursing* (5th ed., pp. 457–563). Philadelphia: J.B. Lippincott.
5. Chatterjee, K. (1991). The history. In W. Parmley & K. Chatterjee (Eds.), *Cardiology* (2nd ed.) (Vol. 1, pp. 3.2–3.10). Philadelphia: J.B. Lippincott.
6. Fang, J. C., & O'Gara, P. T. (2008). The history and physical examination: An evidence-based approach. In P. Lippy, R. O. Bonow, et al. (Eds.), *Heart disease: A textbook of cardiovascular medicine* (8th ed., pp. 125–148). Philadelphia: Saunders-Elsevier.
7. Staff Development Workgroup, P. a. F. E. C. (1999). Culture cues™: Communicating with your Latino patient: Available from http//depts.washington.edu/pfes/cultureclues.html.

8. Bickley, L. S., & Szilagyi, P. G. (2007). *Bates' guide to physical examination and history taking* (9th ed.). Philadelphia: Lippincott Williams & Wilkins.
9. Gordon, M. (1994). *Nursing diagnosis, process, and application*. New York: McGraw-Hill.
10. Spieker, E. D., & Motzer, S. A. (2003). Sleep-disordered breathing in patients with heart failure: Pathophysiology, assessment, and management. *Journal of American Academic of Nurse Practitioner, 15*(11), 487–493.
11. New York Heart Association Criteria Committee. (1964). *Diseases of the heart and blood vessels: Nomenclature and criteria for diagnosis* (6th ed.). Boston: Little, Brown.
12. Chatterjee, K. (1991). Bedside evaluation of the heart: The physical examination. In W. Parmley & K. Chatterjee (Eds.), *Cardiology* (2nd ed.) (Vol. 1, pp. 3.11–13.53). Philadelphia: J.B. Lippincott.
13. U.S. Department of Health and Human Services. (2000). *Healthy people 2010: Understanding and improving health* (2nd ed.). Washington, DC: U.S. Government Printing Office.
14. Poirier, P., & Despres, J. P. (2003). Waist circumference, visceral obesity, and cardiovascular risk. *Journal of Cardiopulmonary Rehabilitation, 23*(3), 161–169.
15. Kenney, W. L. (1997). Thermoregulation at rest and during exercise in healthy older adults. *Exercise and Sport Sciences Reviews, 25*, 41–76.
16. Ponte, J. (1998). Warming the core after cardiac surgery. *Journal of Cardiothoracic and Vascular Anesthesia, 12*(4), 496.
17. Frank, R. N. (2003). The eye in hypertension. In J. L. Izzo & H. R. Black (Eds.), *Hypertension primer* (3rd ed.). From the Council on High Blood Pressure Research, American Heart Association, Philadelphia: Lippincott, Williams & Wilkins.
18. O'Rourke, R. A., Silverman, M. E., & Shaver, J. A. (2004). The history, physical examination and cardiac auscultation. In V. Fuster, R. W. Alexander, et al. (Eds.), *Hurst's the heart* (11th ed., pp. 217–274). New York: McGraw-Hill.
19. McGee, S. R. (1998). Physical examination of venous pressure: A critical review. *American Heart Journal, 136*(1), 10–18.
20. Chobanian, A. V., Bakris, G. L., Black, H. R., et al. (2003). The Seventh Report of the Joint National Committee on Prevention, Detection, Evaluation, and Treatment of High Blood Pressure: The JNC 7 report. *JAMA, 289*(19), 2560–2572.
21. Insua, J. T., Sacks, H. S., Lau, T. S., et al. (1994). Drug treatment of hypertension in the elderly: A meta-analysis. *Annals of Internal Medicine, 121*(5), 355–362.
22. Grim, C. M., & Grim, C. E. (2003). Blood pressure measurement. In J. L. Izzo & H. R. Black (Eds.), *Hypertension primer* (3rd ed., pp. 321–324). From the Council on High Blood Pressure Research, American Heart Association, Philadelphia: Lippincott, Williams & Wilkins.
23. Jones, D. W., Frohlich, E. D., Grim, C. M., et al. (2001). Mercury sphygmomanometers should not be abandoned: An advisory statement from the Council for High Blood Pressure Research, American Heart Association. *Hypertension, 37*(2), 185–186.
24. Perloff, D., Grim, C., Flack, J., et al. (1993). Human blood pressure determination by sphygmomanometry. *Circulation, 88*(5, Pt. 1), 2460–2470.
25. Calkins, H., & Zipes, D. P. (2008). Hypotension and syncope. In P. Libby, R. O. Bonow, et al. (Eds.), *Heart disease: A textbook of cardiovascular medicine* (8th ed., pp. 975–984). Philadelphia: Saunders-Elsevier.
26. Robertson, D. (2003). Treatment of orthostatic disorders and baroreflex failure. In J. L. Izzo & H. R. Black (Eds.), *Hypertension primer* (3rd ed., pp. 479–482). From the Council on High Blood Pressure Research, American Heart Association, Philadelphia: Lippincott, Williams & Wilkins.
27. LeWinter, M. M. (2008). Pericardial diseases. In P. Libby, R. O. Bonow, et al. (Eds.), *Heart disease: A textbook of cardiovascular medicine* (8th ed., pp. 1829–1854). Philadelphia: Saunders-Elsevier.
28. Franklin, S. S., & Izzo, J. L. (2003). Aging, hypertension, and arterial stiffness. In J. L. Izzo & H. R. Black (Eds.), *Hypertension primer* (3rd ed., pp. 170–175). From the Council on High Blood Pressure Research, American Heart Association, Philadelphia: Lippincott, Williams & Wilkins.
29. Charan, N. B., & Carvalho, P. (1992). Cardinal symptoms and signs in respiratory disease. In D. J. Pierson & R. M. Kacmarek (Eds.), *Foundations of respiratory care* (pp. 672–674). New York: Churchill-Livingston.
30. Fahey, V. A. (2004). Clinical assessment of the vascular system. In V. A. Fahey (Ed.), *Vascular nursing* (4th ed., pp. 49–71). Philadelphia: WB Saunders.
31. Kerr, K. A., Watson, W. C., & Dalsing, M. C. (2004). Chronic venous disease. In V. A. Fahey (Ed.), *Vascular nursing* (4th ed., pp. 399–425). Philadelphia: WB Saunders.
32. Walsh, M. E., & Rice, K. L. (2004). Venous thromboembolic disease. In V. A. Fahey (Ed.), *Vascular nursing* (4th ed., pp. 365–397). Philadelphia: WB Saunders.
33. Tilkian, A., & Conover, M. (2001). *Understanding heart sounds and murmurs with an introduction to lung sounds* (4th ed.). Philadelphia: WB Saunders.
34. Ronan, J. A., Jr. (1992). Cardiac auscultation: The first and second heart sounds. *Heart Disease and Stroke, 1*(3), 113–116.
35. Ronan, J. A., Jr. (1992). Cardiac auscultation: The third and fourth heart sounds. *Heart Disease and Stroke, 1*(5), 267–270 contd.

CHAPTER 11

Laboratory Tests Using Blood

Susan L. Reed

Diagnosis, treatment, and management of patients require a multimodal, multidisciplinary approach. Along with an in-depth history and physical, the clinician frequently depends on test results to complete the assessment picture. One of the most frequently used testing modalities is laboratory testing of blood specimens. Laboratory analysis comprises approximately 43% of the data used by health care workers to make clinical decisions.[1] A host of variables can affect interpretation of blood specimen results. Accurate interpretation starts with proper specimen collection. The nurse has a key role in maximizing the conditions under which specimens are collected, thereby controlling for as many variables as possible.

BLOOD SPECIMEN COLLECTION

Collection of blood specimens is a process that involves three phases: patient preparation, collection of the blood sample, and interpretation of results. The nurse plays an important role during these phases. Tests should not have to be repeated due to errors in any of these three phases.[2]

Patient Preparation

Adequate preparation of patients and their families involves education. Frequently, proper specimen collection and interpretation requires compliance with instructions about food or fluid restrictions, taking or withholding medications, and meeting criteria for proper timing of the blood sample. When the blood sample is taken, patients should receive an explanation about what tests are being drawn, why they have been ordered, and when results will be available. If the sample is being obtained by venipuncture, arterial puncture, or vascular port access, preparation of the patient includes a reminder about pain during the procedure and the importance of complying with instructions to maintain a certain position.[2]

Universal Precautions

All blood is considered a source of potential infection. Universal precautions, as well as organizational policies and procedures, should be followed when collecting and transporting specimens. Universal precautions include proper handwashing, the use of gloves during phlebotomy (or at any time there is risk of exposure to blood or body fluids), complete avoidance of recapping needles, and proper disposal of sharps. When there is the potential that blood or body fluids will splash, protective clothing and eyewear should be worn. Spills should be cleaned with an Environmental Protection Agency (EPA)-approved germicide or a 1:100 solution of household bleach, and soiled linen should be bagged at the location where it was used.[3]

Blood Sample Collection

General guidelines for blood sample collection have been developed that help to ensure patient and clinician safety and maximize interpretation of results. The clinician should consider the policies and procedures of his or her organization with regard to blood specimen collection, as well as the standards for professional, national, and international organizations. Control of variability can be enhanced by use of proper technique during collection and processing of the specimen.

During specimen collection through venipuncture, the use of a tourniquet produces changes within the vein. Once a tourniquet is placed on the arm, veins dilate because of their inability to drain. Cellular injury and hemolysis can be caused by the prolonged use of a tourniquet, described as 3 minutes or longer. Under these conditions, return of fluid and electrolytes to the vein is decreased or prohibited, resulting in a hemoconcentrated specimen. In addition, despite decreased circulation of fresh blood to the tissues, cells continue their metabolic processes, leading to an increased concentration in metabolic waste products, such as lactate. In this more acidic environment, potassium leaks out of cells. In general, the tourniquet should not be left on more than 1 minute.[2] Longer use may be unavoidable during a difficult venipuncture. In such cases, information about a difficult venipuncture should be noted on the laboratory slip to assist with interpretation of results.

Blood specimens can be contaminated in several ways. During collection, contamination may occur from intravenous (IV) fluids. Blood draws should not be done on the same arm as an infusion. If the infusion arm cannot be avoided, a tourniquet may be placed between the IV site and the phlebotomy site. Slowing the IV to a keep-open rate (if not contraindicated) for 3 to 5 minutes before the draw may help to reduce contamination of the blood sample. In any event, it should be noted on the laboratory slip that the sample was obtained under these conditions.

Contamination may also be introduced by improper use of blood tubes. Most specimen collection tubes contain some form of anticoagulant. If blood has been mistakenly collected in one tube containing anticoagulant, it should never be poured into a different tube. Also, blood entering one tube should never be allowed to contaminate remaining blood that will be introduced into another tube.

Another source of contamination is introduced when routine samples are drawn from arterial lines, vascular catheters, or ports. The use of an indwelling intravascular catheter allows access to the patient's blood supply without further invasive procedure. Comfort for the patient, ease, and speed of periodic specimen collection are some of the benefits of using an intravascular line for blood sampling. Intravascular catheters may be kept patent by continuous or intermittent infusion, or by instilling saline or heparin solutions. Sometimes, solutions delivered through the catheter may contain medications. The infusate or any additives may dilute blood constituents. This dilution would have the effect of lowering the concentration of the desired sample.

The diameter and length of the catheter are important determinants when collecting blood specimens. The institution's policy and procedure manual should be consulted for recommended withdrawal and discard from vascular devices. Additional sources, such as professional nursing society standards, may assist in making decisions about recommended discard volumes.

Whether sampling from a pulmonary artery catheter, central venous line, arterial catheter, or other intravascular catheter, attention should be paid to the feasibility of interruption of the system. The pulmonary artery catheter presents particular problems. Both the right atrium (RA) port and venous infusion port (VIP) are useful for the administration of drugs and fluids. Although the RA port allows access to the central circulation, use of this port for thermodilution cardiac output calculations makes it difficult to infuse drugs or fluids (a large amount of the infusate might be delivered during delivery of the cardiac output injectate). Consequently, the VIP is chosen for fluid and drug infusion. In this situation, the use of the RA port may be preferable for blood withdrawal. If vasoactive drugs are not infusing through the VIP, it may also be used for blood sampling. The proximal opening into the RA is upstream of any drugs or fluid infusing through the RA port; therefore, the possibility of contamination of the blood sample by infusates is minimized. Typically, the distal port of the pulmonary artery catheter is only used for blood sampling when measuring a mixed venous blood gas from the pulmonary artery where venous blood mixes after circulating through the superior and inferior vena cavae, coronary sinuses, and the chambers in the right side of the heart.

Many institutions have shifted to the use of saline in lieu of heparin in IV lines and pressure tubing however, questions persist about appropriate discard from vascular catheters (instilled with heparin) when drawing blood for coagulation studies. Inconsistent results may increase the cost to the patient through repeated testing, wasted blood, or erroneous treatment decisions. Again, the nurse may refer to policy and procedure manuals or professional organization standards for guidance. In any event, coordination in obtaining multiple blood specimens decreases the amount of blood that is eventually discarded and the number of times that the sterile system is invaded, thus reducing risk of introducing infection.

Sepsis has been associated with intravascular monitoring equipment including stopcocks and pressure transducers, which may be the most frequent reservoirs for endemic contamination. The incidence of local infection and bacteremia has been reduced by the use of disposable transducers and the percutaneous sheath systems used to introduce pulmonary artery catheters. The withdrawal of blood from an intravascular catheter should be considered a sterile procedure. Once removed, caps used to cover stopcock openings should always be replaced with a sterile cap. The person performing the procedure should be gloved. Syringes, used once, should be discarded.

Types of Specimens

When blood is withdrawn from the body, it eventually clots. The fluid that separates from the clot is called *serum*. Plasma, from unclotted blood, contains fibrinogen, which is eventually converted to fibrin. Most blood tests are done on serum, and therefore require use of a tube that allows blood to clot. Red-top tubes contain no additives; they are used for chemistries, drug monitoring, radioimmunoassays, serology, and blood typing. Lavender-top tubes, which contain ethylenediaminetetraacetic acid (EDTA), are usually used for hematology and certain other chemistries. Green-top tubes contain heparin as the anticoagulant and can be used for chemistries, arterial blood gases, hormone levels, and some immune function studies. Blue-top tubes, used for coagulation studies, contain citrate. Sodium fluoride, found in gray-top tubes, prevents glycolysis and may be used to test blood glucose in its in vivo state.[2]

When multiple blood samples are drawn at the same collection time, the preferred order is as follows: blood culture tubes, tubes with no preservative (red-top); tubes with mild anticoagulants (blue then green); tubes with EDTA (lavender-top); and oxalate/fluoride tubes (gray-top) should be collected last. Blood for coagulation studies should never be drawn first because tissue injury can initiate the clotting process and result in falsely low levels of coagulation factors. Specimens in tubes with additives should be rotated gently to mix the anticoagulant with the blood and should never be shaken.[2]

Hemolysis refers to the lysis of red blood cells (RBCs). When extracellular fluid (plasma) is used for analysis, inaccurate results are produced if the specimen is hemolyzed. Hemolysis may occur in vivo, as in hemolytic disease states such as transfusion reactions. Hemolysis may also occur in some infections and with the use of some drugs. A deficiency of the enzyme glucose-6-phosphate dehydrogenase, responsible for generating chemicals needed for maintenance of normal red cell fragility, contributes to hemolysis.

Hemolysis may also occur as a result of improper specimen collection technique or specimen transport. Hemolysis is the cause for specimen rejection in most nonemergent situations. Specimens may be hemolyzed if they are collected from a poorly flowing venipuncture. The selection of the appropriate size needle and catheter is essential when performing venipuncture. Failure to dry alcohol from the venipuncture site also results in hemolysis. Blood should never be forcibly withdrawn from the venipuncture, nor should it be forcibly entered into the collection tube by pushing on the syringe barrel to fill faster. Specimens should be handled carefully when placed in collection tubes and when transported to the laboratory; rough handling may lead to hemolysis.

Hemolysis increases the laboratory values of creatine kinase (CK), potassium, magnesium, calcium, and phosphorus.[2] Hemolysis invalidates the results of most coagulation tests and can mask hemolyzing antibodies in the antibody screen and crossmatch.[2] If unexpected elevated laboratory values are reported, the blood should be redrawn if hemolysis is suspected.

Nursing research continues to evaluate different techniques and equipment in determining the best method to withdraw blood, obtain accurate results, and reduce hemolysis. Controversy still exists as to whether aspirating blood from an IV catheter or saline lock provides less hemolysis than venipuncture with a needle. Dugan et al.[4] found drawing blood from a size 22-gauge IV catheter caused the most hemolysis in their emergency department. Lowe et al.[5] and Grant[6] found that venipuncture had less hemolysis than IV catheters, Kennedy et al.[7] found larger size IV catheters caused less hemolysis than smaller sized catheters, and Cox et al.[8] found using a 5-ml vacuum collection tube demonstrated better results than 10-ml vacuum tubes. However, Corbo et al.[9] and Sliwa[10] determined aspirating the sample from a saline lock after discarding blood did not result in more hemolysis than venipuncture. Arrants et al.[11] found similar results using 18-gauge saline locks for use with coagulation studies. These studies demonstrate how important technique is to specimen collection.

Proper specimen collection includes accurate identification of the patient and accurate labeling of the specimen at the site of collection. It also includes rapid transport to the laboratory, because cells remain viable after collection and continue their metabolic processes. Specimens that are left to stand unprocessed often yield inaccurate results.

Interpretation of Results

Inherent physiologic variability exists based on patient age, sex, ethnicity, and health status (such as, pregnancy or post-myocardial infarction [MI]). These physiologic differences affect interpretation of results. Physiologic changes associated with the aging process bring concomitant changes in some expected laboratory results. Because men usually have more muscle mass than women, gender differences are seen in substances related to muscle function or metabolism, such as creatinine. There may be significant differences among European, African, and Asian populations in testing for cholesterol, enzymes, and hormones. Various physiologic states, such as pregnancy, stress, obesity, and endurance exercise, also introduce situational changes in expected results.[12]

Cyclic variability produces daily, monthly, or yearly patterns in physiologic states. These cycles are often taken into consideration in the collection or interpretation of laboratory results.[12] As a result, most routine specimens, at least in the hospital setting, are drawn in the early morning to control for any circadian variability.

Blood tests are sometimes affected by the ingestion of food or fluids. Not only are results affected by the absorption of dietary components into the blood after a meal, but hormonal and metabolic changes occur as well. Partial control for the variability introduced by food or fluid ingestion can be achieved either by drawing early morning, pre-meal specimens, or by having the patient fast for 8 to 12 hours. The latter is especially important in lipid testing.[13]

Sometimes, differences based on position are negligible. In other cases, they are significant. Patient position during (and before) sampling can affect results. In the upright position, there may be a shift in extracellular fluid volume into the tissues. With the resulting increased concentration of proteins and protein-bound substances in the vascular space, samples for proteins, enzymes, hematocrit (Hct), hemoglobin (Hb), calcium, iron, hormones, and several drugs may show an average 5% to 8% increase. Redistribution of extracellular fluid volume and electrolytes within the vascular space does not stabilize until a patient has assumed the sitting position for at least 15 minutes (from a standing position), and in some cases 20 to 30 minutes. In some settings, such as the hospital, it is not difficult to stabilize the patient's position and thus reduce variability. In other settings, such as ambulatory care, significant variability is introduced if the patient is not made to sit for at least 15 minutes before the blood draw. Because control over sitting time is not usually feasible or practical, care should be taken in the interpretation of results. Exercising immediately before blood sample collection frequently produces significantly erroneous results, especially with enzyme evaluation. Forearm exercises before blood withdrawal may lead to hemolysis.

The timing of blood sampling should include consideration of the effect of medications on the interpretation of results. Medications affect results of many specimens drawn for chemistry, hematology, coagulation, hormonal, and enzyme studies. Knowledge of the effect of the drug assists in proper timing or subsequent interpretation of the results. Consideration should also be given to the effects of other influences, including over-the-counter medications, caffeine, nicotine, ethanol, home remedies, and herbal therapies.

In therapeutic drug monitoring, blood drug levels are monitored to evaluate the effects of drug therapy, make decisions regarding dosage, prevent toxicity, and monitor patient adherence. Timing of the blood sample usually depends on the half-life of the drug; samples drawn at projected peak level assist in monitoring for toxicity, whereas levels drawn at trough help to verify the minimum satisfactory therapeutic level for that patient. Regardless of the purpose of the blood sample, drugs that may affect interpretation of results should be noted on the laboratory slip. For therapeutic drug monitoring, it is important to note the date and time of the last dose as well.

Different laboratories use different equipment and methods by which to test specimens. Specific reference ranges are usually reported alongside the patient's results on the laboratory report. In an effort to establish a standard for communicating laboratory results, the World Health Organization has recommended that the medical and scientific community throughout the world adopt the use of the International System of Units (ISU). An international unit is defined as the number of moles of substrate converted per second under defined conditions. Thus, many laboratories may report results in different ways, depending on their accepted standard of practice. Most laboratories also report critical (or panic) values. These values should be reported promptly to the provider so that results may be evaluated (and decisions made) in light of the patient condition.

Most reference ranges have been established for venous blood samples. Because arterial blood has higher concentrations of glucose and oxygen and lower concentrations of waste products (i.e., ammonia, potassium, and lactate), an arterial source (instead of venous) should be noted on the laboratory slip. Capillary samples yield results that are closer to arterial blood than venous.

Critical evaluation of laboratory results should take into account how the reference or "normal" values were determined. Patients who have been seen for a long time by the same provider, or those who have been seen within the same health care organization, sometimes establish their own reference range. Reference ranges for a specific disease are sometimes established through large-scale clinical trials.

In most circumstances, each laboratory establishes its own reference values by testing a group that is easy to recruit. It is possible, however, that this technique may not reflect the usual values or range of values of the group that the organization serves. When samples are taken from volunteers, such as those who agree to give a blood sample for reference testing in exchange for a free cholesterol screening, bias may be introduced because those who are likely to volunteer may be those who have or suspect they have illness already. When reference samples are taken from patients who are undergoing routine physical examinations or elective surgery, results may reflect a mix of the surrounding population. Again, these reference values need to be considered in light of who was included or excluded from testing. Usually, those who drink alcohol, smoke, or take certain medications are excluded from reference range testing. However, this exclusion is likely to establish a narrow range of "normal" values, thereby increasing the number of people in the served population who fall outside the established range. Additional care should be taken in interpreting results if the laboratory reports only one set of reference values.

Clinicians who are aware of how reference ranges are obtained are in a better position to interpret laboratory results accurately for their patients. In all situations, interpretation of results should be done in light of all factors that introduce variability, and in light of the clinical condition, remembering that "normal" values do not necessarily indicate absence of disease; just as "abnormal" values do not necessarily establish a pathologic state.

Sensitivity and Specificity of Laboratory Tests

Clinicians should use measures of test performance to judge the quality of a diagnostic test for a particular disease. The ability of a laboratory test to identify a particular disease is quantified by two measurements: sensitivity and specificity.[14]

Sensitivity is the frequency of a positive (abnormal) test result among all patients with a particular disease or the likelihood that a diseased patient has a positive test. If all patients with a given disease have a positive test, the test sensitivity is 100%. Sensitivity is calculated by testing a population of patients who have been found to have a particular disease by some "gold standard" method (a procedure that defines the true disease state of the patient).[14]

Specificity is the frequency of a negative (normal) test among all persons who do not have the disease or the likelihood that a healthy patient has a negative test. If all patients who do not have a particular disease have a negative test, the test specificity is 100%. A test with a high specificity is helpful to confirm a diagnosis, because a highly specific test will have few results that are falsely positive. Specificity is calculated by testing a population of patients who have been found to have a particular disease by some gold standard method.[14]

Under the best of circumstances, no blood test is perfect and results may be misleading. Sensitivity and specificity may be altered by the coexistence of other diseases or complications from the primary disease. The most sensitive tests are used to rule out a suspected disease so that the number of false-negative tests is minimal; thus, a negative test tends to exclude the disease. The most specific tests are used to confirm or exclude a suspected disease and minimize the number of false-positive results.[15]

Point-of-Care Testing

Point-of-care testing (POCT) also known as Bedside Testing or Alternative Site Testing, is the laboratory testing of blood that is performed outside of a central laboratory. The goal of POCT is to reduce the time it takes to diagnose and treat the patient (decision cycle time). Since laboratory analysis of blood comprises approximately 43% of the data used by health care workers to make clinical decisions,[1] POCT provides a decrease in the number of steps required to obtain a blood sample, process the sample, and receive the data, and therefore reduces decision cycle time. POCT is ideal in intensive care units, emergency departments, cardiac catheterization laboratories, and surgical suites where the need for rapid turnaround time of laboratory data is desired. Benefits of POCT include decreased turnaround time, improved patient management, increased patient satisfaction, improved job satisfaction of nurses and physicians, decreased operating room time, decreased mortality and morbidity, and less blood sample volume.

Glucose monitoring has been available for years as POCT to guide dosage of insulin administration. Hospitals have also used portable activated clotting time (ACT) monitors to guide anticoagulation and heparin administration during interventional cardiology procedures and during cardiovascular surgery. In addition to glucose and ACT, POCT assays that are available for care of cardiac patients include Hct, Hb, arterial blood gases (ABGs), electrolytes, blood urea nitrogen (BUN), creatinine, ethanol, drugs of abuse, troponin-I, troponin-T, myoglobin, CK-MB, and Type-B natriuretic peptide (BNP). Use of POCT cardiac biochemical marker testing has increased from 4% in 2001 to 12% in 2004 and is expected to rapidly expand.[16]

To ensure accuracy of data, a POCT system requires that there be up front training of non-laboratory personnel on how to use new equipment, continued proficiency testing of staff, and assurance that electronic quality control requirements are met. It is important that POCT systems are linked to hospital or laboratory systems by radiofrequency and infrared to ensure that information handling, storage, and billing are done properly.

Possible limitations of using a POCT system include its use by personnel with limited training in laboratory technology and the lack of understanding of quality control. POCT is considered to be more expensive than traditional laboratory analysis because the cost of cartridges is more expensive. Cost analysis needs to include the decreased labor by nursing and laboratory personnel plus the ability to make rapid decisions about acutely ill patients that may alter their course of illness.[1]

Administration of a POCT system includes designating someone to be responsible for the POCT service, which would include: knowing who is performing POCT and which test they are performing, maintaining quality control documentation, selecting appropriate equipment, troubleshooting all aspects of POCT, coordinating training, and serving as a liaison between nursing and other services.

Ng et al.[17] and Singer et al.[18] studied use of POCT of cardiac biomarkers in the triaging of patients with chest pain. Cardiac marker POCT reduced length of stay in the emergency department[18] and allowed for accurate triaging of chest pain patients within 90 minutes of presentation to the emergency department.[17]

BIOCHEMICAL MARKERS OF MYOCARDIAL INJURY

The internal environment of the healthy person is in a state of balance with respect to water, electrolytes, energy storage and use, and metabolic end products. Stability is maintained through homeostatic mechanisms that regulate the activities of cells and organs. During periods of critical illness, a disruption in cell membrane stability may cause chemical substances that are responsible for intracellular homeostatic mechanisms to appear in the blood. Frequent evaluation of blood results is a means by which the status of the internal environment and the extent and nature of tissue damage can be monitored. These blood tests can be run expeditiously and require small sample volumes, and provide important information concerning the diagnosis and management of patients.[19]

Certain intracellular enzymes and proteins are rarely found in measurable amounts in the blood of healthy people. However, after an event leading to cellular injury or death, these substances may leak into the blood. A continued question with ongoing research is the extent to which reversible cell damage can cause protein leakage.[20] Because of the importance of the timing of the appearance (and disappearance) of enzymes and proteins in the blood, it is crucial that ordered tests are drawn on time. It is equally important that the date and time of the blood draw are noted on the laboratory slip so that the temporal sequence of the rise and fall can be established by those interpreting the results.

Over the years as more specific biochemical markers of myocardial injury have become available, detecting MI has become more accurate. The original marker, glutamine-oxaloacetic transaminase was replaced by lactate dehydrogenase (LDH) and later by CK and CK-MB. Troponin has now become the preferred laboratory test for diagnosing MI and the other markers are becoming obsolete.[21] Initial diagnosis of MI, reinfarction, or other types of myocardial damage is made through evaluation of clinical signs and symptoms, 12-lead ECG, biochemical markers including myocardial proteins (troponins) and if troponin not available, cardiac enzymes (see Chapter 22).[22] A comparison of the sensitivity and specificity of various tests to detect myocardial injury is in Table 11-1.

Table 11-1 ■ COMPARISON OF SENSITIVITY AND SPECIFICITY OF VARIOUS TESTS FOR MYOCARDIAL INFARCTION

Test	Sensitivity at Peak (%)	Specificity (%)
Electrocardiogram	63–84	100
AST increased	89–97	48–88
CK increased	93–100	57–88
CK-MB increased	94–100	93–100
LDH increased	87	88
Myoglobin	75–95	70
Troponin-I	>98	95
Troponin-T	>98	80

AST, aspartate aminotransferase; CK, creatine kinase; LDH, lactate dehydrogenase. Range of values provided because different studies used various methods, periods after onset of symptoms, serial tests, benchmarks for establishing the diagnosis, and so forth. From Wallach, J. [2007]. Cardiovascular diseases. In *Interpretation of diagnostic tests* [8th ed.]. Philadelphia: Lippincott Williams & Wilkins.

Myocardial Proteins

Troponins

Troponins are protein complexes that regulate the calcium-dependent interaction of myosin with actin in the muscle contractile apparatus of striated muscle. They are found in both cardiac and skeletal muscle. Three isotypes have been identified: troponin-I (cTnI), troponin-T (cTnT), and troponin-C (cTnC). Troponins T and I are both found in the myocardium. Troponin-T binds the troponin complex to tropomyosin, and troponin-I inhibits the muscle contraction in the absence of calcium and troponin-C.[2] Troponin-C lacks cardiac specificity; therefore, it is the least studied of the troponins and has no assay available in the clinical setting.

Because of the high specificity and sensitivity for detecting myocardial injury, troponin has become the most important addition to clinical laboratory testing for assessment of myocardial injury.[12] In patients with acute coronary syndrome, troponin is an enormously useful biochemical marker in the early diagnosis of MI because it is either low or undetectable in healthy people, but in the event of an MI, is detectable as early as 2 to 3 hours after injury.[19] Testing for troponin is typically done at the time of the initial workup for suspected acute coronary syndrome or myocardial damage and then 6 to 9 hours later. An additional sample may be measured between 12 and 24 hours if biochemical markers have not shown elevation and MI is still suspected.[22,23] Because most troponin is so tightly bound to muscle, it is released slowly and may remain detectable for 1 to 2 weeks post-MI.[22] This late-phase presence of troponin represents death of the contractile apparatus. Because troponin remains elevated longer than CK-MB and is more specific than LDH, troponin is now the preferred test for patients who seek medical attention more than 24 to 48 hours after myocardial injury. The appearance of troponin in the blood indicates necrosis or injury to the myocardium and follows a predictable rise and fall over a specified time. See Table 11-2 and Figure 11-1 for the typical appearance, peak, and disappearance of various biochemical markers and enzymes.

In patients with ST-segment elevation MI, percutaneous coronary intervention (PCI) or fibrinolytic therapy should not be delayed waiting for biochemical marker evaluation.[21] For other patients with suspected cardiac symptoms, troponin is used along with clinical signs and symptoms and 12-lead ECG to make

Table 11-2 ■ TIMING OF APPEARANCE AND DISAPPEARANCE OF COMMONLY USED CARDIAC BIOMARKERS AND ENZYMES IN RELATION TO ONSET OF CARDIAC SYMPTOMS

Marker or Enzyme	Starts to Rise (hours)	Peaks (hours)	Returns to Normal (days)
AST	6–12	18–24	7
Total CK	2–6	18–36	3–6
CK-MB	4–8	18–24	3
Myoglobin	2–3	6–9	1–2
Troponin-I	3	10–24	7–10
Troponin-T	3	10–24	10–14

AST, aspartate aminotransferase; CK, creatine kinase
From Chernecky, C. C., & Berger, B. J. [2008] *Laboratory tests and diagnostic procedures* [5th ed.]. St. Louis: Saunders and Pagana, K. D., & Pagana, T. J. [2007], *Mosby's diagnostic and laboratory test reference* [8th ed.]. St. Louis: Mosby.

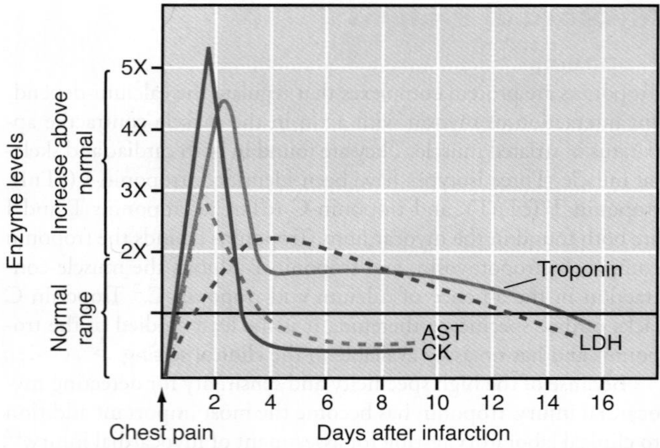

■ **Figure 11-1** Patterns and timing of elevation for aspartate aminotransferase (AST), creatine kinase (CK), lactate dehydrogenase (LDH), and troponin. (From Pagana, K. D., & Pagana, T. J. [2007]. *Mosby's diagnostic and laboratory test reference* [8th ed.]. St. Louis: Mosby Elsevier.)

treatment decisions concerning emergency angiogram versus fibrinolytic therapy.

In the setting of acute coronary syndrome and MI, rapid reperfusion through coronary intervention, a rapid peak or "washout" of troponin-I may be seen indicating reperfusion of the ischemic muscle tissue. This elevation is considered a favorable prognostic indicator.[2,24] Troponin has also been shown to correlate well with estimating myocardial infarct size. Nuclear scintigraphy and/or magnetic resonance imaging have both correlated well with troponin peak levels and infarct size.[25–28]

Between 15% and 48% of patients with unstable angina have an elevated troponin level with normal CK-MB. On coronary angiography, these patients frequently have active, unstable plaques, whereas patients without elevated troponin levels have stable plaques.[29] These patients are considered to have minor myocardial damage. Patients with detectable levels of troponin have a higher in hospital chance of suffering an adverse cardiac event. The risk is correlated with level of troponin: the higher the troponin, the worse the outcome.[24,30]

In patients who have had a recent MI and reinfarction is suspected, troponin is not as helpful since it may still be elevated from the first event.[23] Recurrent MI may be diagnosed if there is a greater than 20% increase in the value in the second sample.[22]

A troponin level (I or T) greater than the 99th percentile of normal reference population (upper reference limit [URL]) is indicative of myocardial necrosis.[22] Troponin rarely exceeds 0.1 ng/mL in healthy individuals.[20] Elevation of troponin reflects myocardial necrosis; however, it does not indicate the mechanism of the injury and may not be from ischemia caused by coronary artery disease.[22] If other clinical evidence of myocardial ischemia is absent, a search for other causes of cardiac damage should be examined.

Elevation of troponin can be detected in a variety of conditions other than coronary ischemia. Other conditions that may release troponin (possibly from myocyte membrane permeability) include tachycardia, pericarditis, heart failure, and strenuous exercise. In addition, a mismatch between myocardial oxygen supply and demand may result in troponin release. Sepsis, hypotension, extracellular fluid volume deficit, atrial fibrillation, and tachycardia may increase the oxygen demand of the heart and cause troponin to leak into the bloodstream in patients with no evidence of coronary artery disease. Patients with critical illness and troponin elevations have been found to have a worse prognosis.[21,31] See Display 11-1 for elevations of troponin in the absence of overt ischemic heart disease.

Troponin elevation may be seen in patients with pulmonary diseases. This elevation is usually associated with right heart strain. Of patients diagnosed with moderate-to-large pulmonary embolism (PE), 30–50% have elevated troponin levels. This elevation may be from the acute right heart overload and has been associated with significant increase in mortality.[21,31]

Assessing for myocardial damage after blunt cardiac trauma may be difficult given the high rate of false-positive and false-negative results when using CK-MB. Troponin-I along with ECG has emerged as an accurate test for confirming presence of myocardial damage after cardiac contusion.[24,32]

As with any test, there are documented incidences of false-positive troponin elevation. These elevations may be caused by heterophilic antibodies, rheumatoid factor, fibrin clots, microparticles, or analyzer malfunction.[21,31] The clinician must always

DISPLAY 11-1 Elevations of Troponin in the Absence of Overt Ischemic Heart Disease

- Trauma (including contusion, ablation, pacing, implantable cardioverter-defibrillator firings including atrial defibrillators, cardioversion, endomyocardial biopsy, cardiac surgery, after interventional closure of atrial septal defects)
- Congestive heart failure, acute and chronic
- Aortic valve disease and hypertrophic obstructive cardiomyopathy with significant left ventricular hypertrophy
- Hypertension
- Hypotension, often with arrhythmias
- Postoperative noncardiac surgery patients who seem to do well
- Renal failure
- Critically ill patients, especially with diabetes, respiratory failure
- Drug toxicity, e.g., adriamycin, 5-fluorouracil, herceptin, snake venoms
- Hypothyroidism
- Apical ballooning syndrome
- Coronary vasospasm
- Inflammatory disease, e.g., myocarditis, Parvovirus B10, Kawasaki disease, sarcoid, smallpox vaccination, or myocardial extension of bacterial endocarditis
- Post-percutaneous coronary intervention patients who seem to have no complications
- Pulmonary embolism, severe pulmonary hypertension
- Sepsis
- Burns, especially if total body surface area is >30%
- Infiltrative disease including amyloidosis, hemachromatosis, sarcoidosis, and scleroderma
- Acute neurological disease, including cerebrovascular accident, subarachnoid bleeds
- Rhabdomyolysis with cardiac injury
- Transplant vasculopathy
- Vital exhaustion

Jaffe, A. S., Babuin, L., & Apple, F. S. [2006]. Biomarkers in acute cardiac disease—The present and the future. *Journal of the American College of Cardiology, 48*(1), 1–11.

evaluate the clinical signs and symptoms and other diagnostic tests to ensure accurate diagnosis and treatment.

Cardiac Enzymes

Enzymes are protein substances that catalyze chemical reactions in cells but do not themselves enter into the reaction. Substrates in the cells bind to the enzymes and form products. After the reaction, the enzyme molecule is free to undergo the same reaction with other substrate molecules. Specific enzymes are responsible for nearly every chemical reaction in the body. Some enzymes are present in almost all cells; others are specific to cells of certain organs.

Creatine Kinase

Creatine kinase is an enzyme specific to cells of the brain, myocardium, and skeletal muscle, but also is found in minimal amounts in other tissues, such as smooth muscle. In these organ systems, the function of CK is primarily that of energy production, where it serves as a catalyst in the phosphorylation of adenosine diphosphate (ADP) to creatine and adenosine triphosphate (ATP). In this manner, CK is responsible for the transfer of an energy-rich bond to ADP. This reaction provides a rapid means of forming ATP for contractile activity in muscle as well as for energy requirements in nonmuscle tissue. The reaction is reversible, and ATP can phosphorylate creatine to form creatine phosphate and ADP during periods of rest.

In an acute MI, inadequate oxygen delivery to the myocardium causes cell injury. An acidic environment promotes the activity of lysosomal enzymes, which are responsible for cell membrane damage or destruction. CK is among the cellular enzymes that diffuse from the damaged cell into the blood. CK is released after irreversible injury. The appearance of CK in the blood indicates cardiac, cerebral, or skeletal muscle necrosis or injury and follows a predictable rise and fall over a specified time (see Fig. 11-1).

Age, sex, race, physical activity, lean body mass, medications, and other unidentified factors are known to affect total CK. A patient's baseline CK level is related to his or her overall muscle mass. Adults have lower values than children. Serum CK declines with age and older adults have very low values. CK values measured in women are lower than those of men; European Americans have lower values than African Americans. Chronic exercise raises serum CK levels; however, there is a training effect, and well-trained athletes have smaller increases in CK after physical exertion. Medications that may increase CK include anticoagulants, aspirin, furosemide, captopril, lidocaine, propranolol, and morphine. In addition, high-intensity lipid-lowering therapy with lipophilic statins (i.e., simvastatin or lovastatin) have been found to increase CK.[33] Early and abnormally high increases in CK are sometimes seen after reperfusion by PCI (Chapter 23) or thrombolytic agents.[2,3]

The importance of monitoring the concentration of serum CK is related to its specificity in the organ in which it functions. Slightly different molecular forms (isoenzymes or *isozymes*) of CK have different tissues of origin. The three CK isoenzymes are combinations of the protein subunits, named for their primary sites of isolation—the muscle (M) and brain (B). CK-MM is the predominant muscle isoenzyme, found in cardiac and skeletal muscle. It also can be detected in normal serum. The myocardium is primarily responsible for the CK-MB form. CK-BB is present in the brain, lung, stomach, prostate, and smooth muscle of the gastrointestinal tract and bladder. Diagnostic precision depends on laboratory analysis of CK isoenzymes and may well be imperative in critically ill patients with multiple organ system involvement.

Because of the wide range in baseline values among "healthy" people, and various enzyme assay techniques, there are no uniform reference values for CK and CK isoenzymes. Consequently, the practice of reporting the isoenzyme as a percentage of the total CK, as well as in U/L has been encouraged.

Creatine Kinase-BB. The brain fraction CK-BB (CK-1) is seen infrequently in serum. Its rare appearance has been associated with brain trauma, cerebral contusions, and cerebrovascular accidents. The presence of CK-BB in association with cancer has been reported. Other causes of serum CK-BB activity include malignant hyperthermia, renal failure, and after central nervous system surgery.[3] With the significant improvement in diagnostic imaging techniques, CK-BB is now rarely evaluated.

Creatine Kinase-MM. CK-MM constitutes almost the entire CK total in healthy people. Skeletal muscle injury or severe muscle exertion is the most frequent source of high serum CK-MM (CK-3) levels. Specific examples include myopathy, vigorous exercise, multiple intramuscular (IM) injections, electroconvulsive therapy, cardioversion, surgery, muscular dystrophy, convulsions, and delirium tremens. Elevations in CK-MM fractions have also been noted in conditions producing less obvious effects on muscle, such as hypokalemia and hypothyroidism.[3]

Creatine Kinase-MB. Prior to the discovery of troponin, CK-MB (CK-2) isoenzyme analysis had been an accepted means for diagnosis of an acute MI. Although troponin has superseded CK-MB in the diagnosis of MI, most institutions continue to evaluate CK, CK-MB, and troponin if MI is suspected.

When CK-MB is released from myocardial tissue, it has a biologic half-life in blood of hours-to-days. Total CK and CK-MB rise within 2 to 8 hours after an acute MI. Peak levels are seen within 18 to 36 hours and are more than six times their normal value. If no additional myocyte necrosis occurs, levels return to normal within 3 to 4 days. See Table 11-2 and Figure 11-1 for the typical appearance, peak, and disappearance of various biomarkers and enzymes.

Elevated CK-MB levels have also been reported after myocardial damage from unstable angina, cardiac surgery, coronary angioplasty, after defibrillation, in vigorous exercise, and after IM injections, trauma, and surgery. Early and abnormally high increases in CK are sometimes seen after reperfusion by PCI or thrombolytic agents. By 6 to 8 hours postangioplasty, 20% of patients have a mild increase in CK-MB. Elevations are occasionally seen in pericarditis, myocarditis, viral myositis, and sustained tachyarrhythmias. An increase in CK-MB may occur after cardioversion, but that time course for increase is different for that of MI, with the mild increase of CK-MB peaking within 4 hours of cardioversion.

Specimens for CK and CK-MB are collected on admission and 8 to 12 hours later. CK and CK isoenzyme results should be evaluated along with troponin, myoglobin, ECG results, and clinical signs and symptoms for the detection of MI. Laboratory slips should be marked with the date and time of any IM injections given to the patient in the prior 24 to 48 hours.

Caution should be exercised in interpretation of CKs drawn in the emergency department. Only 25% to 40% of patients who are having an MI have an abnormal CK at that point. An initial normal CK level should *never* be used to make a decision about discharge from the emergency department, or to withhold thrombolytic therapy.

Myoglobin

Myoglobin is a low-molecular-weight, oxygen-binding protein found in the myocardium and skeletal muscle. Myoglobin is released into the circulation after damage to the heart or skeletal muscle.[2] Because of its release from other muscle tissues, troponin rather than myoglobin is the biomarker of choice for diagnosing MI. After MI, myoglobin levels increase in 2 to 3 hours, peak in 6 to 9 hours, and return to normal (undetectable) as early as 12 hours but more typically after 24 to 36 hours (see Table 11-2).[3]

Elevated myoglobin levels are seen after MI, reinfarction, cocaine use, skeletal muscle injury, trauma, exercise, IM injections, severe burns, electrical shock, polymyositis, alcoholic myopathy, delirium tremens, metabolic disorders (e.g., myxedema), malignant hyperthermia, systemic lupus erythematosus, muscular dystrophy, rhabdomyolysis, and seizures.[2,3] Myoglobin may not be excreted in renal failure, so caution should be used when interpreting results.[2] Further, very high levels of myoglobin are toxic to the kidneys and thus, careful monitoring of renal function is warranted.

Biochemical Marker Activity after PCI

After elective PCI for stable angina, biomarker elevation is fairly common. CK and CK-MB elevation occurs in 5% to 30% of patients. These elevations have been associated with increased risk of death, MI, and need for repeat revascularization.[34] Prasad et al.[35] found that troponin elevation is frequent after elective PCI. Of the patients in their study, 19% had an elevated troponin level. These patients had more complex angiographic characteristics and had undergone multivessel PCI. They found that an elevated troponin level was associated with increased morbidity and mortality. Miller et al.[29] measured troponin before (baseline) and after PCI and found that prognosis was most often related to the baseline troponin level and not the biomarker response after the procedure. Nallamothu et al.[36] analyzed 1,157 patients who underwent elective PCI and found that troponin-I elevation was common after the procedure (29%), and that large troponin elevations, up to eight times normal, were associated with decreased long-term survival. Taken together, these studies demonstrate that continued use and evaluation of biochemical markers is essential after coronary intervention.

Biochemical Marker Activity after Cardiac Surgery

All types of cardiac surgery involve considerable injury to the myocardium. However, differentiating between ischemic alterations associated with surgery and peri-operative MI may be difficult. The evaluation of troponin and cardiac enzymes is common after cardiovascular surgery. Researchers have focused on the prognostic implication of elevated troponin and cardiac enzymes measurements after surgery. Klatte et al.[37] and Costa et al.[38] found that elevated levels of CK-MB in serial measurements after coronary artery bypass graft (CABG) surgery were associated with increased mortality, and that the higher the level of CK-MB, the higher risk of mortality in the immediate to long-term postoperative period. With troponin evaluation becoming more common, Januzzi et al.[39] determined troponin-T levels offered a superior predictor of complications from cardiac surgery than CK-MB. Kathiresan et al.[40] and Croal et al.[41] found similar results, the higher the troponin, I or T, the increased risk of mortality after CABG surgery. These studies demonstrate that biomarker evaluation postoperatively also is important and should not be considered inconsequential.

BLOOD LIPIDS

An accumulation of lipids within the arterial wall is considered a part of the process of atherogenesis. Alteration of blood lipid levels has been identified as a coronary heart disease (CHD) risk factor. Certain lipoproteinemias have been identified as contributing to total plasma cholesterol levels. Plasma normally contains insoluble lipid elements: free fatty acids; exogenous triglycerides; endogenous triglycerides, which are manufactured in the liver; cholesterol; and phospholipids. To be transported, each is attached to a protein. Distinguishing lipoprotein abnormalities is useful because therapy is based on an understanding of the origin of the problem.

Blood Lipid Laboratory Measurement

Elevated lipid levels are considered a risk factor for cardiovascular disease. Cholesterol and the protein components of high-density lipid (HDL), low-density lipid (LDL), and triglycerides are evaluated by electrophoresis when hyperlipoproteinemia is suspected.[42] See Table 11-3 for recommended levels of cholesterol and its components. In most people, the cholesterol values remain constant over 24 hours; a nonfasting blood sample for measurement of total blood cholesterol is acceptable. However, a nonfasting sample for HDL, LDL, and triglyceride levels is of less value. National Cholesterol Education Program 2001 guidelines on cholesterol *screening* recommend everyone over age 20 have a fasting lipoprotein profile (total cholesterol, LDL, HDL, and triglycerides) every 5 years.[13] Lipoprotein electrophoresis is necessary to evaluate serum for hyperlipoproteinemia. LDL is more difficult to isolate and measure. Therefore, if LDL is not measured in a screening lipoprotein test, it may be calculated using the Friedewald formula. The Friedewald formula is inaccurate if the triglycerides are greater than 400 mg/dL (see Display 11-2).[43]

It is recommended that lipid profile tests should be performed after a 12-to-14 hour fast and having a stable diet for 2 to 3 weeks prior to testing. It is also recommended that testing occur in the absence of acute illnesses including stroke, trauma, surgery, acute infection, weight loss, and pregnancy. These conditions often result in values that are not representative of the person's usual level.[13]

Current National Cholesterol Education Program guidelines do recommend patients admitted to the hospital for acute coronary syndromes have lipid measurements taken on admission or within 24 hours.[13] Values obtained during this acute phase may provide guidance for initiating lipid-lowering therapy. LDL cholesterol levels begin to decline in the first few hours after a coronary event and are significantly decreased by 24 to 48 hours and may remain low for many weeks. Thus, the initial LDL cholesterol

Table 11-3 ■ LIPID PROFILE REFERENCE RANGES

Lipid Profile	
Total blood cholesterol	
Desirable	<200 mg/dL
Borderline high	200–239 mg/dL
High	≥240 mg/dL
HDL-C-cholesterol	
Low- A major risk factor for CHD	<40 mg/dL
Better	40–59 mg/dL
High- Considered protective against heart disease	≥60 mg/dL
LDL-C-cholesterol	
Goal for very high risk patients	<70 mg/dL
Optimal	<100 mg/dL
Near or above optimal	100–129 mg/dL
Borderline High	130–159 mg/dL
High	160–189 mg/dL
Very High	>190 mg/dL
LDL-C-cholesterol treatment goals	
No CHD or DM with one or no risk factors	<160 mg/dL
No CHD or DM with two or more risk factors	<130 mg/dL
Very high-risk patients—CHD or DM patients	<70 mg/dL
Triglyceride	
Normal	<150 mg/dL
Borderline High	150–199 mg/dL
High	200–499 g/dL
Very High	≥500 mg/dL

CHD, coronary heart disease; DM, diabetes mellitus.
From Executive Summary of The Third Report of The National Cholesterol Education Program (NCEP). (2001). Expert Panel on Detection, Evaluation, and Treatment of High Blood Cholesterol in Adults (Adult Treatment Panel III), by National Cholesterol Education Program. *JAMA, 285*, 2486–2497 and Grundy, S. M., Cleeman, J. I., Merz, N. B., et al. (2004). Implications of recent clinical trials for the National Cholesterol Education Program Adult Treatment Panel III Guidelines. *Circulation, 110*, 227–239.

level obtained in the hospital may be substantially lower than is usual for the patient.[13] See Chapter 36 for comprehensive evaluation of lipids.

ADDITIONAL LABORATORY TESTS ASSOCIATED WITH CARDIAC DISEASE

Nearly half of all patients with known CHD have no established coronary risk factors (i.e., hypertension, hypercholesterolemia, cigarette smoking, diabetes mellitus, marked obesity, and physical inactivity). Atherosclerosis is now considered an inflammatory disease, with cytokines and other bioactive molecules involved in most steps of the atherogenesis process (see Chapter 5).

With the knowledge that atherosclerosis is an inflammatory disease, researchers are studying different markers to determine if there are other independent risk factors for the disease and if these markers can be used to identify high risk individuals for CHD that may not have traditional risk factors. Markers being studied include but are not limited to adhesion molecules, C-reactive protein (CRP), cytokines, fibrinogen, homocysteine (Hcy), lipoprotein-associated phospholipase A_2, serum amyloid A, tissue-type plasminogen activator, and white blood cell (WBC) count. Hcy is being researched extensively and is utilized as a possible risk factor for CHD. CRP is showing promise from a clinical chemistry perspective and research perspective as a risk factor for CHD.[44]

C-Reactive Protein

CRP is an acute-phase reactant protein that is produced primarily by the liver during the acute inflammatory process. CRP is a nonspecific but sensitive indicator of inflammation, bacterial infection, or

DISPLAY 11-2 Computation Formulas

Computation of LDL Cholesterol
Friedewald Formula*
LDL cholesterol = total cholesterol − HDL cholesterol − (triglycerides divided by 5)

Computation of Ionized Calcium
Serum calcium can be presumed to be normal if:
(4.5 − albumin level) × (0.8) + lab value for total calcium = 8.8 to 11.0 mEq/L
1. Obtain total calcium level (normal = 8.8 to 10.5 mEq/L). If it is less than normal (e.g., <8.8 mEq/L), follow the steps below.
2. Obtain serum albumin level (normal = 4.5 g/dL).
3. If serum albumin level is decreased, subtract the decreased level from normal value for albumin (e.g., albumin level is measured at 3.0; 4.5 [normal] − 3.0 [measured] = 1.5).
4. For every 1.0 decrease in albumin, add 0.8 to calcium level (e.g., for above example, 1.5 × 0.8 = 1.2).
5. Add the calculated figure to the total calcium level (e.g., 7.8 + 1.2 = 9 mEq/L, calcium is within normal range).
6. One-half of this level (9/2) is 4.5, within the normal range for ionized calcium (normal ionized calcium = 4.5 to 5.0).

Computation of Anion Gap
Anion gap = [sodium (140) + potassium (4.0)] − [bicarbonate (24) + chloride (110)] = 10 to 12 mEq/L

Computation of Serum Osmolality
Two times the serum sodium + serum glucose (Glu) divided by 18 + blood urea nitrogen (BUN) divided by 1.8 = serum osmolality ([2 × sodium] + [glucose/18] + [BUN/1.8]) = 280 to 300 mOsm/kg
(e.g., (2 × 122) + (198/2) + (18/1.8) = 265 mOsm (water or intracellular fluid excess); (2 × 155) + (108/2) + (5.4/1.8) = 318 mOsm [water or intracellular fluid deficit])

*Formula valid for estimating LDL cholesterol if the triglyceride level is <400 mg/dL.

acute injury. CRP is a more sensitive indicator of inflammation and responds more rapidly to inflammation than erythrocyte sedimentation rate (ESR). CRP was discovered approximately 70 years ago and has been used for decades to monitor the effectiveness of treatment for patients with lupus erythematosus, rheumatoid arthritis, and other immune-related conditions. Patients with acute MI, sepsis, or post-surgery have elevated CRP levels.

Interest in CRP changed since 1996 due to studies that link elevated CRP levels to increased CHD risk (Fig. 11-2). CRP has been studied to determine its usefulness in detecting a low-level acute-phase response due to chronic atherosclerotic disease. In 1997, Ridker et al.[45] in the Physician's Health Study, established that men who had the highest CRP levels had three times greater risk of MI and two times greater risk of ischemic stroke than the men who had the lowest CRP levels. Rost et al.[46] also found elevated plasma CRP levels to be an independent risk for future ischemic strokes and transient ischemic attack in older adults. Other studies have continued to demonstrate a link between elevated CRP levels and increased risk of CHD in healthy middle-aged men,[47] healthy but high-risk men,[48] women,[49] and older adults.[50] CRP levels have also been shown to be elevated in overweight and obese young adults and adults.[51] Ridker et al.[52] demonstrated that CRP was a stronger predictor of cardiovascular events than LDL level in 15,745 women participants in the Women's Health Study.

Increased body mass index, insulin resistance, hypertension, an intrauterine device, cigarette smoking, chronic infections (e.g., gingivitis, bronchitis), or chronic inflammation (e.g., rheumatoid arthritis) can increase CRP levels.[44] Exogenous hormones may cause an increase in CRP. Increased activity, weight loss, and moderate alcohol consumption decrease CRP levels. Drugs that decrease CRP levels include fibrates, HMG-CoA reductase inhibitors (statins), nicotinic acid (niacin), nonsteroidal anti-inflammatory agents, salicylates, and steroids.[44] Many laboratories offer a routine CRP level or a high-sensitivity CRP (hs-CRP) level.

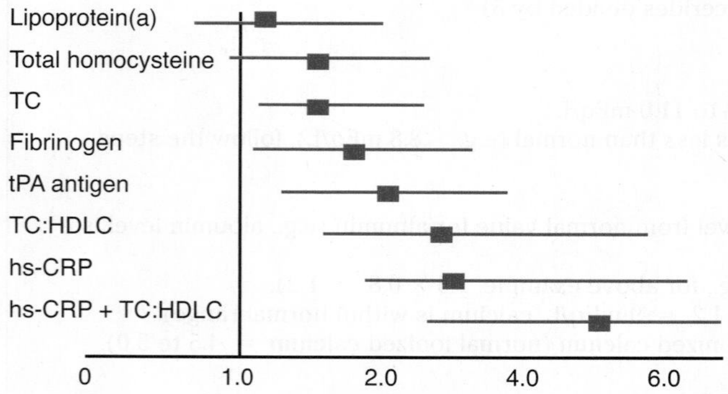

Figure 11-2 Relative risk for future myocardial infarction among apparently healthy middle-aged men in the Physician's Health Study according to baseline levels of lipoprotein(a), total plasma homocysteine, total cholesterol (TC), fibrinogen, tissue-type plasminogen activator (tPA) antigen, the ratio of total cholesterol to high-density lipoprotein cholesterol (HDLC), and high-sensitivity C-reactive protein (hs-CRP). (From Ridker, P. M. [1999]. Evaluating novel cardiovascular risk factors: Can we better predict heart attacks? *Annals of Internal Medicine, 130*, 933–937.)

To evaluate CRP as a risk factor for CHD, the hs-CRP is monitored. In order to classify an individual's risk for atherosclerotic disease, the American Heart Association recommends that two separate hs-CRP measurements be evaluated at least a month apart.[53] Among patients with known CHD, it is suggested that a value greater than 3 mg/L is appropriate for predicting outcomes in patients with stable CHD and that a threshold greater than 10 mg/L may be more predictive in patients with an acute coronary syndrome. A value above 10 mg/L should initiate a search for a source of infection or inflammation. (See Table 11-4 for reference range.) At this point, it is not recommended that all individuals be screened for CRP.[44]

Homocysteine

Hcy is an intermediate amino acid formed during protein catabolism by the conversion of methionine to cysteine. Vitamins B_6, folic acid, B_{12}, and riboflavin, are all required for this metabolism. Epidemiologic studies first showed an association of high levels of Hcy with an increased incidence of atherosclerotic disease.[54] Elevated Hcy is believed to be a part of the process of atherosclerosis by participating in endothelial damage, promoting LDL deposition, decreasing the availability of nitrous oxide, and promoting vascular smooth muscle growth. Research remains controversial that elevated Hcy levels may be an independent risk factor for CHD, carotid and peripheral vascular atherosclerosis.[55] A 2002 meta-analysis of observational studies found Hcy to be only a modest independent predictor of ischemic heart disease and stroke in healthy populations.[56] A meta-analysis on cohort studies showed that elevated Hcy moderately increases the risk of a first cardiovascular event, regardless of age and follow-up duration.[57] Cleophas et al.[58] in their meta-analysis found that elevated Hcy levels may not be as harmful to the heart as first thought, but may indicate an unhealthy lifestyle. Preliminary research suggests treatment of high Hcy levels with B_6, B_{12}, and folic acid improves Hcy and may alter CHD but this approach remains controversial.[59–64]

Elevated Hcy levels can be genetic or acquired. Hyperhomocysteinemia can be caused by a genetic defect in Hcy metabolism. Children with this disease have very premature and accelerated atherosclerosis during childhood. Hcy testing should be performed when there is a strong familial predisposition for atherosclerotic disease or with a progressive or an early-onset of atherosclerotic disease is suspected.

Elevated Hcy levels may also be acquired from a dietary deficiency of vitamins B_6, B_{12}, or folate. Obtaining Hcy levels in the older adults, alcoholics, or drug abusers may be helpful in the diagnosis of nutritional deficiencies. Individuals with megaloblastic anemia may have elevated Hcy levels before anemia and macrocytosis are evident.[2]

Patients with decreased renal function and hypothyroidism have increased Hcy levels. Men tend to have higher levels of Hcy than premenopausal women. Smoking is associated with higher levels of Hcy. Drugs that may increase Hcy levels include carbamazepine, corticosteroids, cyclosporine, methotrexate, nitrous oxide, theophylline, and phenytoin. Drugs that may decrease Hcy levels include folic acid, oral contraceptives, and tamoxifen. A fasting blood sample is recommended when testing Hcy levels. Meat contains elevated levels of Hcy and may alter results.[2] See Table 11-4 for reference range.

Table 11-4 ■ NORMAL REFERENCE RANGES FOR LABORATORY BLOOD TESTS*

Blood Test	Reference Range	Blood Test	Reference Range
Hematologic Studies		SvO_2	60–80%
Red blood cell count		Alkaline phosphatase	35–125 IU/L
Males	4.7–6.1 mil/mm^3	Alanine aminotransferase (ALT)	0–40 IU/L
Females	4.2–5.4 mil/mm^3	Aspartate aminotransferase (AST)	5–40 IU/L
Hematocrit		Bilirubin	
Males	40–50%	Total	0.2–1.3 mg/dL
Females	38–47%	Direct	0–0.4 mg/dL
Hemoglobin		Calcium	
Males	13.5–18.0 g/dl	Total	8.9–10.3 mg/dL
Females	12.0–16.0 g/dl	Free (ionized)	4.6–5.1 mg/dL
Corpuscle indices		Creatinine	
Mean corpuscular volume (MCV)	82–98 fl	Males	0.9–1.4 mg/dL
Mean corpuscular hemoglobin (MCH)	27–31 pg	Females	0.8–1.3 mg/dL
Mean corpuscular hemoglobin concentration (MCHC)	32–36%	Glucose (fasting)	70–99 mg/dL
White blood cell count		LDH	20–200 IU/L
Total	4,500–11,000/mm^3	Magnesium	1.3–2.2 mEq/L
Differential (in number of cells/mm^3 blood)		Phosphorus	2.5–4.5 mg/dL
Total leukocytes	5,000–10,000 (100%)	Protein (total)	6.5–8.5 g/dL
Total neutrophils	3,000–7,000 (60–70%)	Urea nitrogen	8–26 mg/dL
Lymphocytes	1,500–3,000 (20–30%)	Uric acid	
Monocytes	375–500 (2–6%)	Males	4.0–8.5 mg/dL
Eosinophils	50–400 (1–4%)	Females	2.8–7.5 mg/dL
Basophils	0–50 (0.1%)	*Serum Enzymes*	
Sedimentation rate	0–30 mm/hr	CK-MM	95–100%
Coagulation Studies		CK-MB	0–5%
Platelet count	250,000–500,000/mm^3	*Myocardial Proteins*	
Prothrombin time	12–15 s	Troponin-I	0–1.6 ng/mL
Partial thromboplastin time	60–70 s	Troponin-T	0–0.1 ng/mL
Activated partial thromboplastin time	35–45 s	Myoglobin	
Activated clotting time	75–105 s	Males	20–90 ng/mL
Fibrinogen level	160–300 mg/dL	Females	10–75 ng/mL
Blood Chemistries		**High sensitivity-C-reactive protein (hs-CRP)**	
Serum electrolytes		Low	<1.0 mg/L
Sodium	135–145 mEq/L	Average	1.0–3.0 mg/L
Potassium	3.3–4.9 mEq/L	High	>3.0 mg/L
Chloride	97–110 mEq/L	**Homocysteine (Hcy)**	
Carbon dioxide	22–31 mEq/L	Optimal	<12 μmol/L
Blood gases		Borderline	12–15 μmol/L
pH	7.35–7.45	High Risk for cardiovascular disease	>15 μmol/L
$PaCO_2$	35–45 mm Hg	**B-type natriuretic peptide (BNP)**	
PaO_2	80–105 mm Hg	Most diagnostic of heart failure	>100 pg/mL
Bicarbonate	22–29 mEq/L		
Base excess, deficit	0 ± 2.3 mEq/L		

*Examples: Regional laboratory techniques and methods may result in variations.

Lipoprotein-Associated Phospholipase A_2

Lipoprotein-associated phospholipase A_2 also known as platelet-activating factor acetylhydrolase or Lp-PLA_2 is presently being studied as an inflammatory marker of cardiovascular risk. Lp-PLA_2 is an enzyme regulated by inflammatory cytokines and is found predominately on LDL cholesterol. Lp-PLA_2 may contribute directly to atherogenesis by hydrolyzing oxidized phospholipids into pro-atherogenic fragments and by generating lysolecithin, which has proinflammatory properties.[65] Recent studies by Caslake et al.[66] and Packard et al.[67] showed a strong correlation between Lp-PLA_2 levels and risk of CHD in men. By contrast, results from the Women's Health Study showed Lp-PLA_2 was not a strong predictor of future cardiovascular risk in females.[68] Further research is needed to assess Lp-PLA_2 ability to predict cardiovascular risk and establish plasma levels.

Cardiac Natriuretic Peptide Markers

The natriuretic peptide system is part of the neurohormonal system that participates in cardiovascular homeostasis.[69] Investigators have identified three natriuretic peptides; Type-A and Type-B originate in the cardiac myocyte and Type-C originates in the endothelial and renal epithelial cells. A-Type natriuretic peptide (ANP) originates in the atrium and is released into the bloodstream when the atrium is stretched beyond normal capacity. BNP (also known as brain natriuretic peptide because it was first identified in small amounts in the brain) is produced and stored in the ventricles of the heart and is released when ventricular diastolic pressure rises.[70] Researchers believe that ANP is released as an acute response to increased volume in the heart, whereas BNP acts as a backup hormone only activated after prolonged volume overload.[69] Both hormones act in a similar manner to increase the loss of water and sodium through the kidneys. Renin and aldosterone are suppressed by the hormones. Glomerular filtration rate is increased by renal vasculature dilation. ANP and BNP have diuretic and antihypertensive effects.

Although ANP and BNP both have laboratory assays available, BNP has emerged as the laboratory marker of choice for evaluating dyspnea and heart failure since it is synthesized and secreted by the left ventricle. BNP testing is available as a rapid POCT or can be performed in a centralized laboratory. Plasma BNP concentrations can vary with the assay used, age, sex, and body mass index. Normal values tend to increase with age and to be higher in women than in men. BNP levels are often elevated in patients with renal insufficiency and renal failure whether they have heart failure or not. A low BNP level in these patients may be useful to exclude left ventricular dysfunction. Levels may also be elevated in patients with atrial fibrillation, pulmonary hypertension, and sepsis.

McCullough et al.[71] determined that BNP concentrations greater than 100 pg/mL had 90% sensitivity, 73% specificity, and a 90% negative predictive value for diagnosing heart failure. Wieczorek et al.[72] found similar results with a BNP assay of greater than 100 pg/mL having 82% sensitivity and 99% specificity for distinguishing control patients from those patients that had heart failure. Most dyspneic patients with heart failure have a BNP level greater than 400 pg/mL, while values less than 100 pg/mL have a high negative predictive value to rule out heart failure as the cause of the dyspnea. Typically, BNP concentrations are being used in emergency departments to help differentiate heart failure from other causes of dyspnea. Maisel et al.[70] determined that BNP levels were a more accurate tool for diagnosing heart failure than any historical or physical findings in 1586 patients evaluated for dyspnea in the emergency room.

BNP concentrations have been correlated with the New York Heart Association Functional Classification of severity of heart failure, as well as prognosis in heart failure.[69,70,72–74] Fonarow et al.[73] found that admission BNP levels along with elevated troponin levels were independent predictors of in-hospital mortality in patients with acutely decompensated heart failure. The patients with BNP levels greater than 840 pg/mL and increased troponin were at particular risk for mortality.

BNP does not seem to be as useful in the in-hospital management of patients with heart failure. Levitt et al.[75] found that BNP levels did not correlate with invasive hemodynamic measurements, and did not reliably distinguish cardiogenic edema patients from acute lung injury patients in the critical care setting. Research continues to evaluate if serial BNP levels should be monitored.

A newer assay, plasma N-terminal proBNP (NT-proBNP) is more useful than BNP in diagnosing heart failure in patients who have left ventricular dysfunction, are older, and are women NT-proBNP tends to elevate to a greater extent in these patient groups.[76]

BNP cannot be used to monitor therapy in patients being treated for heart failure with the drug nesiritide since the infusion is detected as an increase in BNP; however, NT-proBNP may be used to monitor nesiritide therapy. Other emerging uses of BNP include as a prognostic tool in patients with acute coronary syndrome, stable angina, and chronic mitral regurgitation. It may also be useful in differentiating constrictive pericarditis from restrictive cardiomyopathy. BNP measurements should be used as an adjunct to clinical assessment and treatment of heart failure.[76] See Table 11-4 for reference range.

HEMATOLOGIC STUDIES

Cells in the circulating blood are responsible for oxygen and carbon dioxide transport and the body's immune response. Erythrocytes (RBCs), leukocytes (white blood cells), and platelets are formed in the bone marrow and are suspended in the plasma). Blood is also the transport system for electrolytes, products of metabolism, hormones, and plasma proteins. An appreciation of the roles of erythrocytes, leukocytes, and other hematologic parameters is an important prerequisite to understanding deviations from normal. This approach is helpful in planning care based on an assessment of the demands of daily living. Each of the aspects of a hematologic study has meaning for patients in terms of their ability to withstand the effects of a cardiac event.

Complete Blood Cell Count

A complete blood cell (CBC) count is important for evaluating the oxygen-carrying capacity of the blood and the response of the body to invasion by foreign cells such as bacteria. Because excessive bleeding, bone marrow disease, hemolytic disorders, some drugs, and infections can alter the number of leukocytes, erythrocytes, or platelets in the blood, the CBC of the patient with cardiac disease is closely monitored. A baseline study can be compared with subsequent studies to evaluate bleeding, the effects of treatment, or the presence of infection (see Table 11-4).

Red Blood Cell Count

RBCs are formed in the bone marrow and constitute the majority of peripheral cells. They contain Hb and are responsible for transporting oxygen to the tissues (and carbon dioxide from tissues). The average life span of an RBC is 120 days, after which it is removed from the blood by the liver, spleen, or bone marrow.[2]

When the RBC count is more than 10% below the expected normal value, the patient is said to be anemic. Conditions under which there are a decreased number of RBCs include cirrhosis, hemorrhage, presence of prosthetic valves, renal disease, chronic illnesses, and various malignancies of the bone marrow.[2] Anemia from any cause must be looked for in the patient with cardiac disease because it may precipitate angina, aggravate heart failure, or contribute to a diagnosis of subacute bacterial endocarditis.

An RBC increase is seen in congenital heart disease, severe chronic obstructive pulmonary disease, and polycythemia vera. It is falsely high in extracellular fluid deficit (volume contraction) and falsely low with extracellular fluid excess.[2]

Hematocrit. The Hct is the volume of packed RBCs found in 100 mL of blood, expressed as a percent. As an indirect measure of the RBC count, Hct increases and decreases with the RBC count. Abnormalities in RBC size may alter Hct values.[2] Normal ranges for Hct differ by sex and age group.

Hemoglobin. The RBCs contain a complex protein compound called *hemoglobin.* Hb is the oxygen-carrying protein of the RBC and is an important component of the acid–base buffer system. Insufficient amounts of Hb place a strain on the cardiovascular system, and may cause MI, angina, congestive heart failure, or stroke.

Corpuscular Indices. With the RBC count, the quantity of Hb, and the Hct, the characteristics of individual RBCs can be described in terms of cell size (mean corpuscular volume [MCV]), amount of Hb present in a single cell (mean corpuscular Hb [MCH]), and the proportion of each cell occupied by Hb (mean corpuscular Hb concentration [MCHC]). The indices are calculated by these formulas:

$$\text{MCV} = \text{Hematocrit (as \%)} \times \frac{10}{\text{RBC count}} \text{ (millions/mm}^3\text{)}$$

$$\text{MCH} = \text{Hemoglobin (g/100 mL)} \times \frac{10}{\text{RBC}} \text{ (millions/mm}^3\text{)}$$

$$\text{MCHC} = \text{Hemoglobin (g/dL)} \times \frac{10}{\text{Hematocrit}} \text{ (\%)}$$

White Blood Cell Count

The WBCs, or leukocytes, work to defend against foreign matter and cells in the body. There are five types of WBCs: neutrophils, eosinophils, basophils, monocytes, and lymphocytes. Elevated WBC counts in the patient with cardiac disease may be due to MI, bacterial endocarditis, or Dressler's syndrome. After MI, the elevation may be a result of the body's normal response to stress. After an acute MI, WBCs may be elevated. Leukocytosis occurs as the infarcted site is invaded by leukocytes and macrophages that engulf and phagocytose necrotic tissue.

Although an elevated temperature after MI may be expected, an elevated WBC count should always suggest the possibility of concomitant infection. A urinary or respiratory tract infection or an infection secondary to an invasive procedure is a possibility during an extended illness.

White Cell Differential. The differential count is a descriptive list of the types of WBCs. The differential for each of the five leukocyte types is usually expressed as a percentage of the total leukocyte count; the total should add up to 100 (see Table 11-4).

Erythrocyte Sedimentation Rate

The ESR measures the speed at which anticoagulated erythrocytes settle in a long, narrow tube. The speed depends on the size of the clumps into which the cells aggregate in the presence of blood fibrinogen. The ESR is a nonspecific indicator of inflammatory disease. It may be elevated in MI, pericarditis, and bacterial endocarditis as well as many other diseases but it is usually low in heart failure.[3] The degree of increase of the ESR does not correlate with severity or prognosis.

Laboratory Measurement of Complete Blood Cell Values

The RBC and WBC counts are performed by an automated counter that directly measures all parameters, including Hct, corpuscular indices, and platelets. The precision of the Hct analysis is ±2 points. Consequently, a change in measurement by as much as 4 points may not indicate a change in the true Hct.

Activity and change in position may raise Hct and Hb levels; Hb may be higher by 8% in the morning than in the evening. The usual precautions should be taken to avoid hemolysis and ensure accuracy. The specimen should be rapidly transported to the laboratory to avoid changes in distribution of the cells within the plasma. RBC tests can be done using capillary blood, but massage of the fingertip or earlobe can lead to cell destruction and alter the sample. If difficulty is encountered in locating a vein, the tourniquet should be removed long enough to allow restoration of circulation to avoid a hemoconcentrated sample. A blood smear should also be examined if there is an abnormality in one or more of the CBC parameters to evaluate the size, shape, and color of the RBCs, WBCs, and platelets.[2,3]

Complete Blood Count After Cardiac Surgery

The CBC including the Hb and Hct levels are monitored after cardiac surgery to evaluate bloodloss. Immediately after cardiac surgery, there are rapid shifts in extracellular fluid volume status because of the hemodilutional effects of cardiopulmonary bypass and the rewarming that follows induced hypothermia. This fluid shift may be reflected in a reduced Hb or Hct level. Frequent monitoring of the WBC count helps identify any leukocytosis and infection. Cardiopulmonary bypass results in a period of reduced phagocytic activity that renders the patient more at risk for infection.

COAGULATION STUDIES

Drug-induced anticoagulation is a routine procedure in the cardiac care unit and requires close monitoring of blood coagulation mechanisms. Anticoagulation is used after thrombolytic therapy, during cardiac surgery, to prevent formation of venous thrombus associated with prolonged bed rest and hemostasis, to prevent formation of intracardiac thrombus, and in treatment for established thrombus and embolus (see Chapter 6).

The prevention and treatment of blood coagulation is complex and involves a number of hemostatic functions that play roles in the body's homeostasis. Therapy involves interference with this homeostatic mechanism. An understanding of the laboratory tests used to evaluate the effectiveness of treatment is vital to prevent undesired outcomes of anticoagulation therapy. The normal ranges for the coagulation factors and the methods used depend on the laboratory. Typical reference ranges, however, are listed in Table 11-4.

Platelet Count

Platelets are elements of the blood that promote coagulation and are produced by the bone marrow. They contribute to blood clotting by clumping or sticking to rough surfaces and injured sites. Platelet counts are useful for monitoring the course of a disease or treatment. Thrombocytopenia (low platelet count) is a common cause of abnormal bleeding. There is a serious risk of hemorrhage when the platelet count is less than 30,000 to 50,000/mm^3, and a spontaneous bleed may occur when platelets are less than 20,000/mm^3. Bleeding due to thrombocytopenia is characterized by petechiae, bleeding from the gums or tongue, or epistaxis. Thrombocytopenia may occur by several mechanisms: reduced platelet production, sequestration of platelets, accelerated platelet destruction, loss from hemorrhage, and dilution from massive blood transfusions that contain few platelets.

Specific conditions that may cause a decrease in platelets include hemorrhage, hypersplenism, leukemia, lymphoma, prosthetic heart valves, heparin-induced thrombocytopenia, idiopathic thrombocytopenic purpura, disseminated intravascular coagulation (DIC), systemic lupus erythematosus, hemolytic anemia, and infection. Medications that decrease the platelet count include acetaminophen, aspirin, chemotherapy, histamine-blocking agents, heparin, hydralazine, quinidine, and thiazide diuretics. Nonsteroidal anti-inflammatory drugs may cause a decrease in platelet aggregation. The concurrent use of heparin with antiplatelet agents increases the risk of bleeding. After a large number of blood transfusions (14 units or more) and after extracorporeal circulation, the platelet count is typically low.[2,3]

Aspirin has been incorporated into the treatment plan after MI to prevent hypercoagulability due to platelet aggregation. Antiplatelet agents (clopidogrel and ticlopidine) help prevent platelet aggregation by inhibiting fibrinogen binding and platelet–platelet interaction. Antiplatelet agents are included in most treatment plans to prevent arterial thrombus including post-MI, PCI/stent placement, cardiovascular surgery, and other vascular surgeries. Patients receiving antiplatelet drugs may have a normal platelet count but have increased bleeding due to the drug. The drug alters the platelets for the life of platelets; therefore increased bleeding may be seen for 7 to 14 days after discontinuation of treatment. Glycoprotein (GP) IIb/IIIa agents are also used to decrease platelet aggregation in acute MI and post-PCI/stent placement patients. Patients who receive GPIIb/IIIa agents should be monitored for signs of bleeding and thrombocytopenia.

Increased amounts of platelets may be seen in malignant disorders including, polycythemia vera, postsplenectomy syndrome, and rheumatoid arthritis. Platelet counts may also be increased in those who live at high altitude or exercise strenuously.[2]

Prothrombin Time

The prothrombin time (PT) is used to evaluate the extrinsic system and common pathway in the clotting mechanism. Specifically, it measures the activity of prothrombin, fibrinogen, and factors V, VII, and X. Prothrombin is synthesized by the liver. PT may be prolonged in heart failure, vitamin K deficiency, liver disease, bile duct obstruction, DIC, massive blood transfusion, salicylate intoxication, and alcohol use. Severe liver damage may prolong PT. Drugs that may prolong PT include but are not limited to some antibiotics, allopurinol, amiodarone, warfarin, heparin, many nonsteroidal anti-inflammatory drugs, and aspirin. Decreased PT is seen in thyroid dysfunction, thrombophlebitis, MI, and pulmonary embolus. Medications that may decrease PT include but are not limited to antacids, diuretics, diphenhydramine, and oral contraceptives.[2,3]

The PT is used mainly for monitoring patients on warfarin. Warfarin inhibits vitamin K-dependent synthesis of clotting factors II, VII, IX, and X. Therapeutic prothrombin times are considered to be 1.5 to 2 times normal, or a 15% to 50% change in the normal value. If the PT is allowed to prolong greater than 2.5 times the control value, there is a risk of bleeding.

The international normalized ratio (INR) has been adopted for reporting PT. The INR is calculated from the observed PT ratio. The INR is equivalent to the PT ratio that would have been obtained if the patient's PT had been compared to a PT value obtained using the International Reference Preparation, a standard human brain thromboplastin prepared by the World Health Organization. With the INR, standardized PT results are available for health care providers in different parts of the country and the world. These standardized results are independent of the reagents used and adjust for the type of instrument used. The therapeutic INR in most situations ranges from 2.0 to 3.5. However, different ranges have been established for deep vein thrombosis prophylaxis (1.5 to 2.0), deep vein thrombosis (2.0 to 3.0), prevention of embolus in atrial fibrillation (2.0 to 3.0), PE (2.5 to 3.5), and prosthetic valve prophylaxis (2.5 to 3.5).[2] The INR should not be used to initiate warfarin therapy; it should be used only once the patient is thought to be on a stable dose.

Partial Thromboplastin Time and Activated Partial Thromboplastin Time

The partial thromboplastin time (PTT) and activated partial thromboplastin time (aPTT) measure the intrinsic coagulation system and are used in assessing patients receiving unfractionated heparin. With low-molecular-weight heparin, neither the PTT nor aPTT changes, so laboratory monitoring is not required. The PTT measures deficiencies in all factors except factors VII and XIII, whereas the aPTT measures all coagulation factors except platelet factor III, XIII, and VII. The aPTT is measured by adding test reagents to PTT to shorten clotting time. When clotting time is shortened, minor clotting defects can be detected.

The therapeutic range for both PTT and aPTT is maintained at 1.5 to 2.5 times the patient's baseline value. The PTT and aPTT is usually drawn 30 to 60 minutes before the patient's next dose of heparin. For PTT and aPTT results less than 50 seconds, an increase in the heparin dose should be considered. Conversely, a decrease in dose should be considered for PTT and aPTT values greater than 100 seconds.

The PTT and aPTT are prolonged in heparin administration, congenital clotting factor deficiencies, cirrhosis of the liver, vitamin K deficiency, and DIC. Antihistamines, ascorbic acid, chlorpromazine, and salicylates may also cause an increase.[3]

Activated Clotting Time

The activated clotting time (ACT) is used during cardiac surgery and cardiac catheterization to monitor heparinization. The time it takes whole blood to clot reflects the activity of the intrinsic clotting mechanism. During extracorporeal heparin therapy, the ACT is kept at four to six times the baseline value.

Tests to measure ACT are simple and easy to use at the bedside. The use of ACT rather than aPTT to monitor heparin therapy in patients with unstable angina or acute MI may result in much steadier levels of anticoagulation and prevent ischemic recurrences.[2]

Fibrinogen Level

Fibrinogen is a plasma protein synthesized by the liver. This test measures the conversion of fibrinogen to fibrin by thrombin. Fibrinogen levels are elevated in acute infections, collagen disease, inflammatory diseases, and hepatitis. Decreased levels are seen in severe liver disease, DIC, leukemia, and obstetric complications. Thrombolytic therapy may also affect fibrinogen levels.[3]

Protein C and Protein S

Protein C, with cofactor protein S, is a natural anticoagulant protein whose function is to degrade activated factors V and VIII. Deficiency in either protein C or S can lead to a hypercoagulable state, which may cause venous thrombosis. In order for protein C to be activated, it needs to interact with the thrombin–thrombomodulin complex on the surface of endothelial calls. Protein C is vitamin K-dependent and indirectly promotes fibrinolysis.[2] Hereditary protein C deficiency accounts for approximately 3% to 9% of patients with venous thrombosis. Hereditary protein S deficiency accounts for 2% to 7% of patients with venous thrombosis.[12]

Acquired conditions that cause protein C or protein S deficiency include liver disease, vitamin K deficiency or warfarin use, or consumption of protein C or protein S from thrombosis, DIC, or surgery. Protein S deficiency may also be acquired by use of estrogen, including oral contraceptives or estrogen replacement therapy, or pregnancy. Protein S may also be decreased in nephrotic syndrome, HIV infection, or varicella infection. A rapid fall in protein C or protein S can be caused by initiating warfarin therapy without first reducing other coagulation factors with heparin. This rapid fall in protein C or protein S can cause hypercoagulability and cause warfarin-induced skin necrosis. Warfarin-induced skin necrosis causes thrombosis of skin vessels, which can lead to infarction and necrosis. Treatment requires discontinuation of warfarin and vitamin K administration.[2,3,12]

Warfarin should be discontinued for at least 10 days prior to testing for protein C or protein S. Reference range for protein C or protein S is reported as a percentage of the amount expected in normal plasma. The reference range is approximately 70% to 140%.[12]

D-Dimer (Fibrin Degradation Fragment)

D-dimer is an assay used to measure the amount of clot breakdown products specific for cross-linked fragments derived from fibrin. A positive test indicates that thrombus is forming. This test is most useful in the inpatient and outpatient setting, along with compression ultrasound and chest computed tomography for the diagnosis of deep vein thrombosis or PE. D-dimer may also be used along with fibrin degradation products in the diagnosis of DIC.[2]

For the diagnosis of PE, D-dimer has a good sensitivity and negative predictive value, but poor specificity. D-dimer levels are abnormal in 95% of patients with PE; however, they are abnormal in only 50% of patients with subsegmental PE.[3] Patients with normal D-dimer levels have a 95% likelihood of not having PE, and therefore the test offers an excellent negative predictive value. In the outpatient setting when deep vein thrombosis is suspected, if the D-dimer test is negative, compression ultrasound of the legs is not necessary.[2,77] D-dimer levels are normal in only 25% of patients without PE and so have low specificity. Among patients without PE, D-dimer levels are commonly abnormal in hospitalized patients, particularly those with malignancy or recent surgery.

A normal D-dimer level can exclude recurrent PE in patients with prior venous thrombosis and/or PE. However, fewer patients with prior events will have a normal D-dimer level, thus limiting the test's usefulness. D-dimer testing has been studied to help determine the length of time needed for anticoagulation therapy. Palareti et al.[78] found that patients with an abnormal D-dimer level one month after discontinuing anticoagulation therapy had a significantly higher risk of recurrent venous thromboembolism than patients who continued anticoagulation since they had an abnormal D-dimer level.

ARTERIAL BLOOD GASES

Arterial blood gases are frequently assessed in the patient with cardiac disease. Tissue oxygenation, carbon dioxide removal, and acid–base status are analyzed through the assay of arterial blood gases. Arterial blood gas results guide treatment decisions in ventilated patients and critically ill, nonventilated patients. Knowledge of the normal blood gas values and the meaning of deviation from normal are essential to treatment decisions. A complete discussion of these parameters can be found in Chapter 7.

The arterial oxygen saturation (SaO_2) and the mixed venous oxygen saturation (SvO_2) reflect the relation between oxygen supply and demand and the extent of overall tissue utilization of O_2. Continuous monitoring of SaO_2 (oxygen supply) can be achieved through pulse oximetry; laboratory analysis, however, is useful in distinguishing the SaO_2 at PaO_2 levels above 65 mmHg. A fiberoptic pulmonary artery catheter is capable of evaluating SvO_2 levels continuously. This information is useful in determining the ideal mode of respiratory intervention, the effect of nursing care on tissue O_2 demands, physiologic alterations requiring increased supply of O_2, and the reflection of physiologic changes on cardiac output. Calibration of the SvO_2 catheter oximeter should be performed every 24 hours by laboratory co-oximeter saturation analysis. Table 11-4 provides normal values for SaO_2 and SvO_2. Chapter 21 describes hemodynamic monitoring.

BLOOD CHEMISTRIES

The body's homeostatic mechanisms are responsible for a stable internal environment. The chemical regulation of cellular and plasma metabolites is among the most precise mechanisms in the body. During periods of critical illness, these mechanisms may be inadequate or dramatically altered. The functional alterations that result from altered values are sometimes life threatening. An awareness of the factors affecting blood chemistry homeostasis, as well as the consequences of elevated or decreased levels, aids the nurse in making appropriate patient care decisions.

Some blood chemistry tests are drawn routinely on admission to the hospital to establish the patient's baseline. Other tests are performed frequently over a day and may indicate the need for intervention in the form of altered therapy and treatment modalities. "Normal" or reference values may differ between laboratories or among populations. Typical reference ranges for selected blood chemistry values can be found in Table 11-4.

Serum Electrolytes

Sodium

Sodium is the major cation in the extracellular space. It has several major functions: maintenance of osmotic pressure, regulation of acid–base balance (by combining with chloride or bicarbonate ions), and transmission of nerve impulses by the sodium pump. Sodium balance is regulated by aldosterone, atrial natriuretic hormone, and antidiuretic hormone (ADH). Aldosterone causes sodium conservation (and water retention) by stimulating the kidneys to reabsorb sodium. Aldosterone is secreted in response to low extracellular sodium levels, an increase in intracellular potassium, low blood volume or cardiac output, and physical or emotional stress. When serum sodium levels are too high, atrial natriuretic hormone is secreted from the atrium and acts as an antagonist to renin and aldosterone. ADH, secreted by the posterior pituitary gland, controls serum sodium by regulation of the amount of intracellular fluid reabsorbed at the distal tubules.[2,3]

Potassium

Potassium is the major intracellular cation in concentrations of approximately 150 mEq/L. It is regulated in a very tight range in the extracellular fluid. Potassium plays a crucial role in initiating and sustaining cardiac and skeletal muscle contraction. It is also important for acid—base balance and maintenance of oncotic pressure.

Maintenance of potassium within the normal range is crucial in the care of a patient with cardiac disease. Failure to do so results in dangerous sequelae for the patient. In general, potassium levels in patients with cardiac disease are maintained above 4.0 mEq/L. Special care should be taken in patients with cardiac disease receiving potassium-sparing diuretics or angiotensin-converting enzyme inhibitors, especially in light of decreased renal blood flow. Potassium levels are falsely elevated by analysis of hemolyzed specimens. Prolonged use of a tourniquet, having the patient clench and unclench a fist before blood draw, or delayed processing of the specimen all may cause hemolysis.[2,3]

Chloride

Chloride is the major extracellular anion. It helps to maintain electrical neutrality and acts as an acid–base buffer. The rise and fall of chloride levels follows sodium and bicarbonate shifts. When carbon dioxide increases, chloride shifts to the intracellular space as bicarbonate goes extracellular. Along with sodium, chloride also helps to maintain osmotic pressure. Found primarily in hydrochloric acid in stomach secretions, chloride also provides the acid medium for digestion and enzyme activation.[2,3]

Calcium

Calcium is found mainly in the bones and teeth, with only approximately 10% found in the blood. Calcium is essential for the formation of bones and for blood coagulation. Calcium ions affect neuromuscular excitability and cellular and capillary permeability. It is essential for nerve transmission and cardiac and skeletal muscle contraction. Calcium also contributes to anion–cation balance. Calcium can be found ionized (free) in the serum or bound to serum albumin. The ionized calcium, which is approximately one-half of the total calcium, is the fraction important to cardiac and neuromuscular excitability. In acidosis, more calcium appears in the ionized form; in alkalotic environments, most of the calcium remains protein bound.

Calcium levels in the blood follow a diurnal variation, with the lowest values occurring in the early morning, and highest values occurring at mid-evening. Ionized calcium is difficult to measure, so total calcium is reported in most hospitals. In some situations, the measured calcium level may be low, but by estimating the amount bound to protein, the ionized calcium may be found to be normal. The formula for the computation of ionized calcium is shown in Display 11-2. Decreased serum sodium (<120 mEq/L) increases protein-bound calcium and consequently increases the total calcium; the opposite is true of increased serum sodium.[2,3]

Magnesium

Magnesium is essential for over 300 enzymatic activities involving lipid, carbohydrate, and protein metabolism. It is the second most predominant intracellular cation. Most of the body's magnesium is stored in the bones in an insoluble state; one third is bound to protein, and approximately 1% is found in the serum. Because of its importance in phosphorylation of ATP, magnesium is seen as a critical component of almost all metabolic processes. Its importance in the care of patients with cardiac disease stems from its role in neuromuscular regulation.[2,3]

Ventricular arrhythmias after MI have been associated with magnesium deficiency. Magnesium sulfate 1 to 2 g IV should be considered in ventricular fibrillation or ventricular tachycardia for patients who have alcoholism or malnutrition with suspected low levels of magnesium (hypomagnesemia). It is recommended that magnesium sulfate should be administered to patients with ventricular fibrillation or ventricular tachycardia with a torsades de pointes pattern.[79]

Hypomagnesemia may precipitate cardiac arrhythmias, including atrial fibrillation, because of enhanced myocardium excitability. Hypomagnesemia is very common after cardiovascular surgery and has been found to be an independent risk factor for atrial fibrillation following cardiac surgery, most likely due to hemodilution, elevated epinephrine levels, increased loss through the urine, or due to the use of diuretics. Atrial fibrillation is a common complication after cardiovascular surgery occurring in approximately 20% to 50% of cases.[80] Research on the administration of magnesium sulfate before and/or after cardiovascular surgery has shown mixed results. However, a recent meta-analysis[81] demonstrated a significant reduction in postoperative atrial fibrillation from 28% in the control group to 18% in the treatment group without a significant change in length of hospital stay. Administration of magnesium sulfate after CABG surgery is considered a frontline strategy in the prevention of atrial fibrillation according to the American College of Cardiology/American Heart Association 2004 Guidelines.[82]

Hypermagnesemia results in depressed neuromuscular conduction, and consequent slowing of conduction in the heart. The most common cause of hypermagnesemia is renal failure.

Carbon Dioxide

Measurement of carbon dioxide assists the clinician in evaluation of electrolyte status and acid–base balance. Because approximately 80% of carbon dioxide is found as bicarbonate, it is a good reflection of the bicarbonate level. The carbon dioxide level should not be confused with the $P\text{CO}_2$ obtained from blood gas readings.[2,3]

Anion Gap

The anion gap measures the normal balance between positive and negative electrolytes in the serum. It describes the relation between serum sodium (a cation) and bicarbonate and chloride (anions). A normal anion gap is 12 mEq/L. A value greater than 12 mEq/L is considered abnormal. This test is useful in determining whether an acid–base imbalance is due to an increase in organic acid (increased lactic acid or ketoacids, or ingestion of acid such as salicylic acid). In this case, the anion gap increases. With mineral acid problems (decreased bicarbonate or increased hydrochloric acid), the anion gap is normal.[2,3] A formula for computation of the anion gap is given in Display 11-2.

Serum Osmolality

Serum osmolality reflects the osmotic property of the blood. It is an important parameter in determining whether water excess or deficit exists. Either of these problems can present in the cardiac care unit, where fluid management is often a problem (see Chapter 7). The osmolality can be measured in the laboratory or calculated with a simple formula (see Display 11-2).

Serum Electrolytes After Cardiac Surgery

Fluid volume shifts and changes in electrolytes and serum osmolality is common after cardiac surgery. The examination of serum electrolytes frequently during the first 24 hours after surgery has been recommended. Potassium changes may be rapid, sodium may be increased, total calcium and magnesium may be decreased, and total circulating volume may be increased. The hemodilutional effects of cardiopulmonary bypass are responsible for these changes as well as changes in renal function that, in turn, may affect fluid volume and electrolyte status. During and after cardiac surgery, changes in plasma potassium concentration may develop. There appears to be a decrease in potassium during hypothermia and an increase during rewarming, which has been attributed to washout of ischemic areas or to a direct effect of temperature on the transmembrane distribution of potassium. Serum sodium does fall after surgery if large amounts of glucose-containing fluids have been infused. In this situation, glucose is metabolized slowly and draws fluid from the cells by its osmotic effect. Consequently, the sodium is diluted.

Errors in measurement can be costly to the patient in terms of safety, health status, and cost-effective practice. Changes in potassium and other electrolytes must be closely monitored and treatment initiated to keep levels within a very narrow range. Potassium replacement during rewarming must be handled cautiously.

SELECTED CHEMISTRIES

Alkaline Phosphatase

Alkaline phosphatase is an enzyme released in liver and bone disease. An increased serum level suggests an abnormality in the liver or bones, but can be associated with chronic therapeutic use of anticonvulsant drugs such as phenobarbital or phenytoin. In addition, lipid-lowering agents such as bile acid resins, HMG-CoA reductase inhibitors (statins), and nicotinic acid can alter alkaline phosphatase and other liver tests.[2] Alkaline phosphatase along with other liver enzymes (i.e., alanine aminotransferase [ALT], aspartate aminotransferase [AST]) is typically measured before initiation of lipid-lowering therapy, every 4 to 6 weeks at the start of therapy, every 6 to 12 weeks for the first year of therapy, and then every 6 months throughout treatment.

Alanine Aminotransferase

Alanine aminotransferase (ALT), formerly known as serum glutamic-pyruvic transaminase (SGPT) is found predominately in liver tissue but is also present in kidneys, heart, and skeletal muscle tissue. This hepatocellular enzyme is released into the bloodstream when there is injury or disease affecting liver parenchyma making ALT a specific and sensitive laboratory test. In hepatocellular disease other than viral hepatitis, the ALT/AST ratio is less than 1. In viral hepatitis, the ratio is greater than 1.[2]

ALT may be elevated with hepatitis, hepatic necrosis, hepatic ischemia, cholestasis, hepatic tumor, hepatotoxic drugs, obstructive jaundice, severe burns, myositis, pancreatitis, infectious mononucleosis, and shock. Drugs that may increase ALT levels include acetaminophen, allopurinol, ampillicin, cephalosporins, chlordiazepoxide, clofibrate, codeine, nicotinic acid, nonsteroidal anti-inflammatory drugs, oral contraceptives, phenytoin, procainamide, propranolol, and salicylates.[2] In addition, high-intensity lipid-lowering therapy with hydrophilic statins (i.e., pravastatin or atorvastatin) have been shown to increase ALT.[33] The reference range for normal ALT is listed in Table 11-4.

Aspartate Aminotransferase

Aspartate aminotransferase (AST), formerly known as serum glutamic-oxaloacetic transaminase (SGOT), is located in the cell cytoplasm and in the mitochondria, where it catalyzes amino acid activity. This enzyme, although not specific to myocardial tissue, was the first to be used extensively to confirm an MI.[83] The enzyme is widely distributed, with high concentrations in the liver, skeletal muscle, kidneys, RBCs, and myocardium. It is found in lesser amounts in the lungs, pancreas, and brain. The presence of AST in so many organ systems reduces its specificity for MI. With its reduced specificity and newer, more specific and sensitive tests, AST is no longer used to diagnosis MI. AST is now used to evaluate, diagnose, and monitor hepatocellular diseases.[2]

AST may be elevated with cardiac surgery, cardiac catheterization and angioplasty, severe angina, acute pulmonary embolus, renal infarction, acute pancreatitis, musculoskeletal diseases, trauma, and strenuous exercise. In alcoholic hepatitis, AST is usually elevated but rarely greater than 300 u/L, but AST is almost invariably twice as high as ALT. Drugs that may increase AST levels include antihypertensives, digitalis preparations, salicylates, verapamil, theophylline, and lipid-lowering agents such as bile acid resins and nicotinic acid (niacin). In addition, high-intensity lipid-lowering therapy with hydrophilic statins (i.e., pravastatin or atorvastatin) have been shown to increase AST.[33] False elevations are seen in pyridoxine deficiency (beriberi, pregnancy), uremia, or diabetic ketoacidosis. Levels are slightly increased in older adults. In chronic conditions, such as severe, long-standing liver disease, the elevation is usually persistent.[2,3] The reference range for normal AST is listed in Table 11-4.

Bilirubin

Bilirubin is a product of Hb breakdown and is removed from the body by the liver. Elevated direct bilirubin is the result of obstructive jaundice due to extrahepatic (stones or tumor) or intrahepatic (damaged liver cells) causes. Increases in indirect bilirubin occur with hepatocellular dysfunction or an increase in RBC destruction (e.g., transfusion reaction or hemolytic anemia). Care should be taken not to hemolyze the sample. The sample should also be protected from bright light because bilirubin levels are reduced after 1 hour of such exposure.[2,3]

Catecholamines

Epinephrine and norepinephrine are elevated in pheochromocytoma, a tumor of the adrenal medulla. Pheochromocytoma is a cause of high blood pressure.

Creatinine

Creatinine is a waste product formed during muscle protein metabolism. Serum creatinine is a reflection of the excretory function of the kidneys. It is evaluated in conjunction with BUN, but is a more sensitive indicator of renal function. People with large muscle mass have higher serum creatinine levels than do those with less muscle, such as older adults, amputees, and patients with muscle disease.[2,3]

Glucose

Glucose is elevated whenever endogenous epinephrine is mobilized. Hyperglycemia in the hospital setting is common and may result from a variety of reasons including stress, administration of glucocorticoids and vasopressors, decompensation of diabetes mellitus types 1 and 2, chronic renal failure, acute pancreatitis, acute MI, congestive heart failure, extensive surgery, and infections.

Bedside glucose monitoring is the most common POCT available in the hospital. It is recommended that diabetic patients who are eating have glucose testing before their meals and at bedtime. Diabetic patients who are not eating should be tested every 4 to 6 hours unless they are controlled with IV insulin, which typically requires testing every hour until levels are stable and then every 2 hours.[84]

Studies have shown an association between hyperglycemia and increased mortality in hospitalized patients with and without diabetes mellitus. A variety of populations, including medical and surgical patients, acute MI patients, and cardiac surgery patients, have been studied demonstrating more intensive glucose control decreased mortality, reduced length of stay, and decreased infection rates.[85–91] These studies have led to changes in protocols for the monitoring and treatment of glucose while in the hospital (see Chapter 39).[84]

Glycated Hemoglobin or HbA_{1C}

Glycated hemoglobin (GHb), also referred to as glycohemoglobin, glycosylated hemoglobin, HbA_{1C}, or HbA_1 are terms used to describe a series of stable minor Hb components formed slowly and nonenzymatically from Hb and glucose.[92] The rate at which GHb is formed is proportional to the concentration of blood glucose.[93] Because RBCs survive an average of 120 days, the measurement of GHb provides an index of a person's average blood glucose concentration during a 2- to 3-month period.[84]

GHb comprises a chemically heterogeneous group of substances formed by the reaction between sugars and hemoglobin. In adults, approximately 98% of the Hb in the RBC is hemoglobin A. About 7% of hemoglobin A consists of a type called HbA_1 that can combine strongly with glucose in a process called "glycosylation." Once glycosylation occurs, it is not easily reversible. HbA_{1C} is one of three components of HbA_1 and combines most strongly with glucose. HbA_{1C} is a specific form of GHb that has become the most accurate laboratory blood test in assessing long-term glycemic control in diabetics.[84]

Multiple laboratory methods are used to measure the many components of GHb. Some assays measure all GHb components in a sample, while other assays measure only one or two components. International efforts are being made to standardize the measurement of GHb and now most assays measure HbA_{1C} or are calibrated to produce a result equivalent to that measurement. The American Diabetes Association[94] recommends that laboratories use only methods certified as traceable to the Diabetes Control and Complications Trial (DCCT) reference method. Regardless of the assay method type and specific analyte quantified, all results should be reported as "% HbA_{1C}" or "% HbA_{1C} equivalents."

The American Diabetes Association does not recommend using HbA_{1C} for the diagnosis of diabetes mellitus but for long-term management of the disease.[84] The advantage of testing HbA_{1C} over plasma glucose testing for long-term diabetes mellitus management is that the sample can be drawn at any time because it is not affected by short-term variations (e.g., food intake, exercise, stress, hypoglycemic agents). HbA_{1C} testing is beneficial for evaluating the success and patient compliance of diabetic treatment, determining the duration of hyperglycemia in patients with newly diagnosed diabetes mellitus, individualizing diabetic control regimens, evaluating the diabetic patient whose glucose levels change significantly day to day, and in the hospital, differentiating short-term hyperglycemia in patients who do not have diabetes mellitus (e.g., recent stress from illness or MI) from those that do have diabetes mellitus (where the glucose has been persistently elevated).[84]

In nondiabetic patients, increased levels of HbA_{1C} may be seen with an acute stress response, Cushing's syndrome, pheochromocytoma, corticosteroid therapy, and acromegaly. HbA_{1C} levels may be decreased in patients with hemolytic anemia, chronic blood loss, and chronic renal failure.[2]

Prospective randomized clinical trials such as the U.K. Prospective Diabetes Study[95] and the DCCT[96] have shown that treatment regimens that reduced average HbA_{1C} to approximately 7% (about 1% above the upper limits of normal) were associated with fewer long-term microvascular complications, including rates of retinopathy, nephropathy, and neuropathy. However, in these trials, intensive control was found to increase the risk of severe hypoglycemia and weight gain.

Rohlfing et al.[93] analyzed DCCT data to determine the relation between HbA_{1C} and plasma glucose levels in patients with type 1 diabetes mellitus. Approximate levels of plasma glucose and corresponding HbA_{1C} levels are shown in Table 11-5. The 2007 guidelines from the American Diabetes Association[84] recommend that HbA_{1C} testing be performed at least two times a year in patients who are meeting treatment goals (and who have stable glycemic control) and quarterly in patients whose therapy has changed or who are not meeting glycemic goals (see Chapter 39).

Lactate Dehydrogenase

LDH is an enzyme that catalyzes the reversible conversion of lactate to pyruvate, providing ATP for energy during periods of anaerobic metabolism. LDH is present in nearly all metabolizing

Table 11-5 ■ COMPARISON BETWEEN SPECIFIC HBA_{1C} LEVELS AND SPECIFIC MEAN PLASMA GLUCOSE LEVELS

	Mean Plasma Glucose	
HbA_{1C} (%)	mg/dL	mmol/L
6	135	7.5
7	170	9.5
8	205	11.5
9	240	13.5
10	275	15.5
11	310	17.5
12	345	19.5

From Rohlfing, C. L., Wiedmeyer, H. M., Little, R. R., et al. (2002). Defining the relationship between plasma glucose and HbA_{1C}: Analysis of glucose profiles and HbA_{1C} in the diabetes control and complications trial. *Diabetes Care, 25*, 276.

cells and is released during tissue injury. LDH is widely distributed in the body. It can be found in skeletal muscle, RBCs, kidneys, liver, pancreas, lungs, and brain. Because of its presence in multiple organs throughout the body, evaluation of LDH is used to help establish many diagnoses. LDH has become obsolete in its use as a diagnostic aid in MI due to the more specific and sensitive troponin markers. Drugs that may cause an elevated LDH include clofibrate, codeine, meperidine, morphine, procainamide, and lipid-lowering agents such as HMG-CoA reductase inhibitors (statins) and nicotinic acid.[2,3] The normal reference range for LDH is listed in Table 11-4.

Protein

Total protein measurement includes albumin (53%) and globulin (15% α, 12% β, and 20% γ). These protein components can be quantified with the use of protein electrophoresis. Albumin (4 to 5.5 g/dL) contributes to the balance of osmotic pressure between blood and tissues. Globulins (2 to 3 g/dL) influence osmotic pressure and include the immunoglobulins (antibodies). Because albumin is produced in the liver, a low serum albumin level is seen in liver disease. Low serum albumin also reflects poor nutritional status, and the finding should prompt a complete nutritional assessment. The half-life of albumin is 18 days. If albumin is reduced, edema results because albumin accounts for 90% of the serum colloid osmotic pressure. Albumin is reduced in heart failure because of hypervolemic dilution. The α- and β-globulins tend to decrease with abnormal liver function. The γ-globulins, the body's antibodies, increase with chronic disease.[2,3]

Urea Nitrogen

Urea nitrogen is the end product of protein metabolism. It is produced by the liver and excreted by the kidneys. BUN is used with creatinine to evaluate renal function. Increases in BUN are referred to as *azotemia*. Prerenal azotemia occurs whenever a disease or condition affects urea nitrogen before the kidneys are actually damaged or diseased including congestive heart failure, salt and water depletion from vomiting, diarrhea, diuresis, sweating, or shock.[2] Postrenal azotemia is the result of any condition that affects BUN after it has cleared the kidneys, such as in ureteral and urethral obstruction. BUN levels in older adults may be slightly higher because the number of nephrons tends to decrease in the aging process. The BUN may be higher in hospitalized patients because of their increased catabolic state.[97]

Uric Acid

Uric acid is synthesized in the liver and intestinal mucosa and is the end product of purine metabolism. Uric acid may be increased in a variety of conditions but the most common cause in an increase in blood levels is gout. Levels are monitored during the diagnosis and treatment of gout. Levels may also be increased in patients with atherosclerosis, hypertension, and elevated triglycerides. Severe renal disease results in a high level of serum uric acid because excretion is reduced. Levels are very labile and show day-to-day and seasonal variation within the same person. Levels are also increased by emotional stress, total fasting, and increased body weight. Large doses of salicylates may interfere with accurate test results.[97]

BLOOD CULTURES

Blood cultures are indicated when a fever of unknown origin is present. Blood cultures aid in identifying specific bacterial organisms in the blood (bacteremia), and when combined with antibiotic sensitivity tests, can provide information to clinicians about which antibiotic works best against that particular species of bacteria. Policies differ with regard to the number and timing of cultures considered adequate for diagnosis; the policy and procedure of the institution should be followed. Regardless of the number of cultures recommended and the timing between them, collection of blood cultures requires meticulous technique to protect the specimen from contamination. Sampling should be done while the patient's temperature is still elevated and before treatment with antibiotics. Both Beutz et al.[98] and Martinez et al.[99] determined that, although blood cultures may be obtained from a central IV catheter, they are considered less sensitive than through venipuncture but offer an excellent negative predictive value in diagnosing bacteremia. With either method of blood draw, the blood is placed into a specialized culture media. Preliminary results should be available within 24 hours, but final results may not be available for a week or more.[2,3]

SERUM CONCENTRATION OF SELECTED DRUGS

Serum levels of cardiac drugs may be obtained for multiple reasons including determining the effectiveness of drug therapy, especially for drugs with narrow therapeutic ranges or with wide variabilities in metabolism between patients, and confirming cause of organ toxicity. Usual ranges of therapeutic and toxic serum concentrations of selected cardiac drugs are given in Table 11-6.

The serum concentrations must always be interpreted in the context of the clinical data. For example, digitalis intoxication may occur within the usual range of therapeutic serum concentrations if the patient has hypokalemia, hypercalcemia, hypomagnesemia, acid–base imbalances, increased adrenergic tone, hypothyroidism, hypoxemia, or myocardial ischemia.[100]

Table 11-6 ■ THERAPEUTIC REFERENCE RANGES AND TOXIC LEVELS OF COMMON CARDIAC DRUGS

Drug	Therapeutic Range	Toxic Level
Amiodarone	1.5–2.5 mg/L	> 3.5 mg/L
Digitoxin	9–25 ng/ml	> 30 ng/ml
Digoxin	0.5–2.0 ng/ml	>2.5 ng/ml
Diltiazem	40–200 ng/ml	
Flecainide	0.2–1.0 mg/L	>1.0 mg/L
Lidocaine	1.4–6.0 mg/L	≥6.0 mg/L
N-Acetylprocainamide (NAPA)	<30 mg/L	>30 mg/L
Nifedipine	25–100 ng/ml	
Phenytoin	10–20 μg/ml (total)	>20 μg/ml (total)
	1-2 mg/L (free)	≥2.0 mg/L (free)
Procainamide	4.0–8.0 mg/L	>12 mg/L
Propafenone	64–1044 ng/ml	
Propranolol	50–100 ng/ml	>1000ng/mL
Quinidine	2.0–5.0 mg/L	>7.0 mg/L
Theophylline	10–20 mg/ml	>20 mg/ml
Verapamil	50–200 ng/ml	≥400 ng/ml

From Wallach, J. (2007). Therapeutic drug monitoring and drug effects. In *Interpretation of diagnostic tests*. Philadelphia: Lippincott Williams & Wilkins

Serum concentrations of drugs can be altered by many mechanisms including influences on pharmacokinetics such as half-life, time to peak, time to steady state, protein binding, and excretion. For example, a number of factors are known to alter digoxin concentration when the dosage is kept constant, including altered absorption, impaired renal excretion, drug interaction, and impaired metabolism. Theophylline concentration is increased in neonates, in older adults, with obesity, with high carbohydrate diets, and with some comorbid conditions. Theophylline concentration is reduced in children, with a low carbohydrate diet, with eating charcoal-cooked meats, and with some drugs. There is as much as a 50-fold difference in plasma concentration of phenytoin among patients taking the same dosage; altered metabolism and altered protein binding account for the large individual variation in the disposition of phenytoin.

The blood specimen to determine serum concentration of a drug usually is drawn 1 to 2 hours after an oral drug is given because absorption and distribution are usually complete by this time; however, blood should be drawn at a time specified by that laboratory (e.g., 1 hour before the next dose is due to be administered). The route of administration and sampling time after last dose of drug must be known for proper interpretation.[100]

REFERENCES

1. Giuliano, K. K., & Grant, M. E. (2002). Blood analysis at the point of care: Issues in application for use in critically ill patients. *AACN Clinical Issues, 13*(2), 204–220.
2. Pagana, K. D., & Pagana, T. J. (2007). *Mosby's diagnostic and laboratory test reference* (8th ed.). St. Louis: Mosby Elsevier.
3. Chernecky, C. C., & Berger, B. J. (2008). *Laboratory tests and diagnostic procedures* (5th ed.). Philadelphia: Saunders Elsevier.
4. Dugan, L., Leech, L., Speroni, K. G., et al. (2005). Factors affecting hemolysis rates in blood samples drawn from newly placed IV sites in the emergency department. *Journal of Emergency Nursing, 31*(4), 338–345.
5. Lowe, G., Stike, R., Pollack, M., et al. (2008). Nursing blood specimen collection techniques and hemolysis rates in an emergency department: Analysis of venipuncture versus intravenous catheter collection techniques. *Journal of Emergency Nursing, 34*(1), 26–32.
6. Grant, M. S. (2003). The effect of blood drawing techniques and equipment on the hemolysis of ED laboratory blood samples. *Journal of Emergency Nursing, 29*(2), 116–121.
7. Kennedy, C., Angermuller, S., King, R., et al. (1996). A comparison of hemolysis rates using intravenous catheters versus venipuncture tubes for obtaining blood samples. *Journal of Emergency Nursing, 22*(6), 566–569.
8. Cox, S. R., Dages, J. H., Jarjoura, D., et al. (2004). Blood samples drawn from IV catheters have less hemolysis when 5-mL (vs 10-mL) collection tubes are used. *Journal of Emergency Nursing, 30*(6), 529–533.
9. Corbo, J., Fu, L., Silver, M., et al. (2007). Comparison of laboratory values obtained by phlebotomy versus saline lock devices. *Academic Emergency Medicine, 14*(1), 23–27.
10. Sliwa, C. M. Jr. (1997). A comparative study of hematocrits drawn from a standard venipuncture and those drawn from a saline lock device. *Journal of Emergency Nursing, 23*(3), 228–231.
11. Arrants, J., Willis, M. E., Stevens, B., et al. (1999). Reliability of an intravenous intermittent access port (saline lock) for obtaining blood samples for coagulation studies. *American Journal of Critical Care, 8*(5), 344–348.
12. Jacobs, D. S., & DeMott, W. R. (2001). *Laboratory test handbook* (5th ed.) Hudson, OH: Lexi-Comp/NC.
13. National Cholesterol Education Program. (2001). Executive summary of the third report of the National Cholesterol Education Program (NCEP) Expert Panel on detection, evaluation, and treatment of high blood cholesterol in adults (Adult Treatment Panel III). *Journal of the American Medical Association, 285*(19), 2486–2497.
14. Oxley, D. K., Garg, U., & Olsowka, E. S. (2001). Maximizing the information from laboratory tests—The Ulysses syndrome: Tests in search of disease. In D. S. Jacobs & W. R. DeMott (Eds.), *Laboratory test handbook* (pp. 15–23). Hudson, OH: Lexi-Comp/NC.
15. Wallach, J. (2007). Introduction to normal values (reference ranges). In *Interpretation of diagnostic tests*. Philadelphia: Lippincott Williams & Wilkins.
16. Kost, G. J., & Tran, N. K. (2005). Point-of-care testing and cardiac biomarkers: The standard of care and vision for chest pain centers. *Cardiology Clinics, 23*, 467–490.
17. Ng, S. M., Krishnaswamy, P., Morissey, R., et al. (2001). Coronary artery disease: Accelerated pathway for chest pain evaluation. *American Journal of Cardiology, 88*, 611–617.
18. Singer, A. J., Ardise, J., Gulla, J., et al. (2005). Point-of-care testing reduces length of stay in emergency department chest pain patients. *Annals of Emergency Medicine, 45*(6), 587–591.
19. Saenger, A. K., & Jaffe, A. S. (2007). The use of biomarkers for the evaluation and treatment of patients with acute coronary syndromes. *Medical Clinics of North America, 91*, 657–681.
20. McPherson, R. A., & Pincus, M. R. (2007). Markers of myocardial damage. In *Henry's clinical diagnosis and management by laboratory methods*. Philadelphia: WB Saunders Company.
21. Jaffe, A. S., Babuin, L., & Apple, F. S. (2006). Biomarkers in acute cardiac disease: The present and the future. *Journal of the American College of Cardiology, 48*(1), 1–11.
22. Thygesen, K., Alpert, J., White, H. D., et al. (2007). Universal definition of myocardial infarction. *Circulation, 116*, 2634–2653.
23. Alpert, J. S., Thygesen, K., Antman, E., et al. (2000). Myocardial infarction redefined—A consensus document of The Joint European Society of Cardiology/American College of Cardiology Committee for the redefinition of myocardial infarction. *American Journal of Cardiology, 36*, 959–969.
24. Sarko, J., & Pollack, C. V., Jr. (2002). Cardiac troponins. *Journal of Emergency Medicine, 23*(1), 57–65.
25. Giannitsis, E., Steen, H., Kurz, K., et al. (2008). Cardiac magnetic resonance imaging study for quantification of infarct size comparing directly serial versus single time-point measurements of cardiac troponin T. *Journal of the American College of Cardiology, 51*, 307–314.
26. Licka, M., Zimmermann, J., Zehelein, J., et al. (2002). Troponin T concentrations 72 hours after myocardial infarction as a serological estimate of infarct size. *Heart, 87*, 520–524.
27. Panteghini, M., Cuccia, C., Bonetti, G., et al. (2002). Single-point cardiac troponin T at coronary care unit discharge after myocardial infarction correlates with infarct size and ejection fraction. *Clinical Chemistry, 48*(9), 1432–1436.
28. Steen, H., Giannitsis, E., Futterer, S., et al. (2006). Cardiac troponin T at 96 hours after acute myocardial infarction correlates with infarct

size and cardiac function. *Journal of the American College of Cardiology, 48*(11), 2192–2194.

29. Miller, W. L., Garratt, K. N., Burritt, M. F., et al. (2006). Baseline troponin level: Key to understanding the importance of post-PCI troponin elevation. *European Heart Journal, 27*, 1061–1069.
30. Kontos, M. C., Shah, R., Fritz, L. M., et al. (2004). Implication of different cardiac troponin I levels for clinical outcomes and prognosis of acute chest pain patients. *Journal of the American College of Cardiology, 43*, 958–965.
31. Roongsritong, C., Warraich, I., & Bradley, C. (2004). Common causes of troponin elevations in the absence of acute myocardial infarction: Incidence and clinical significance. *Chest, 125*, 1877–1884.
32. Velmahos, G. C., Karaiskakis, M., Salim, A., et al. (2003). Normal electrocardiography and serum troponin I levels preclude the presence of clinically significant blunt cardiac injury. *Journal of Trauma: Injury, Infection and Critical Care, 54*, 45–51.
33. Dale, K. M., White, C. M., Henyan, N. N., et al. (2007). Impact of statin dosing intensity on transaminase and creatine kinase. *American Journal of Medicine, 120*, 706–712.
34. Califf, R. M., Abdelmeguid, A. E., Kuntz, R. E., et al. (1998). Myonecrosis after revascularization procedures. *Journal of the American College of Cardiology, 31*(2), 241–251.
35. Prasad, A., Singh, M., Lerman, A., et al. (2006). Isolated elevation in troponin T after percutaneous coronary intervention is associated with higher long-term mortality. *Journal of the American College of Cardiology, 48*(9), 1765–1770.
36. Nallamothu, B. K., Chetcuti, S., Mukherjee, D., et al. (2003). Prognostic implication of troponin I elevation after percutaneous coronary intervention. *American Journal of Cardiology, 91*, 1272–1274.
37. Klatte, K., Chaitman, B. R., Theroux, P., et al. (2001). Increased mortality after coronary artery bypass graft surgery is associated with increased levels of postoperative creatine kinase-myocardial band isoenzyme release. *Journal of the American College of Cardiology, 38*, 1070–1077.
38. Costa, M. A., Carere, R. G., Lichtenstein, S. V., et al. (2001). Incidence, predictors, and significance of abnormal cardiac enyzme rise in patients treated with bypass surgery in the arterial revascularization therapies study (ARTS). *Circulation, 104*, 2689–2693.
39. Januzzi, J. L., Lewandrowski, K., MacGillivray, T. E., et al. (2002). A comparison of cardiac troponin T and creatine kinase-MB for patient evaluation after cardiac surgery. *Journal of the American College of Cardiology, 39*, 1518–1523.
40. Kathiresan, S., Servoss, S. J., Newell, J. B., et al. (2004). Cardiac troponin T elevation after coronary artery bypass grafting is associated with increased one-year mortality. *American Journal of Cardiology, 94*, 879–881.
41. Croal, B. L., Hillis, G. S., Gibson, P. H., et al. (2006). Relationship between postoperative cardiac troponin I levels and outcome of cardiac surgery. *Circulation, 114*, 1468–1475.
42. Grundy, S. M., Cleeman, J. I., Merz, N. B., et al. (2004). Implications of recent clinical trials for the National Cholesterol Education Program Adult Treatment Panel III Guidelines. *Circulation, 110*, 227–239.
43. Wallach, J. (2007). Cardiovascular diseases. In *Interpretation of diagnostic tests*. Philadelphia: Lippincott Williams & Wilkins.
44. Pearson, T. A., Mensah, G. A., Alexander, R. W., et al. (2003). Markers of inflammation and cardiovascular disease: Application to clinical and public health practice. *Circulation, 107*, 499–511.
45. Ridker, P. M., Cushman, M., Stampfer, M. J., et al. (1997). Inflammation, aspirin, and the risk of cardiovascular disease in apparently healthy men. *New England Journal of Medicine, 336*, 973–979.
46. Rost, N. S., Wolf, P. A., Kase, C. S., et al. (2001). Plasma concentration of c-reactive protein and risk of ischemic stroke and transient ischemic attack. *Stroke, 32*, 2575–2579.
47. Koenig, W., Sund, M., Frohlich, M., et al. (1999). C-reactive protein, a sensitive marker for inflammation, predicts future risk of coronary heart disease in initially healthy middle-aged men. *Circulation, 99*, 237–242.
48. Kuller, L. H., Tracy, R. P., Shaten, J., et al. (1996). Relation of C-reactive protein and coronary heart disease in the MRFIT nested case-control study. *American Journal of Epidemiology, 144*, 537–547.
49. Ridker, P. M., Hennekens, C. H., Buring, J. E., et al. (2000). C-reactive protein and other markers of inflammation in the prediction of cardiovascular disease in women. *New England Journal of Medicine, 342*, 836–843.
50. Tracy, R. P., Lemaitre, R. N., Psaty, B. M., et al. (1997). Relationship of C-reactive protein to risk of cardiovascular disease in the elderly. *Arteriosclerosis, Thrombosis, and Vascular Biology, 17*, 1121–1127.
51. Visser, M., Bouter, L. M., McQuillan, G. M. et al. (1999). Elevated C-reactive protein levels in overweight and obese adults. *Journal of the American Medical Association, 282*, 2131–2135.
52. Ridker, P. M., Rifai, N., Rose, L., et al. (2002). Comparison of C-reactive protein and low-density lipoprotein cholesterol levels in the prediction of first cardiovascular events. *New England Journal of Medicine, 347*, 1557–1565.
53. Myers, G. L., Rifai, N., Tracy, R. P., et al. (2004). CDC/AHA workshop on markers of inflammation and cardiovascular disease. *Circulation, 110*, e545–e549.
54. Lily, L. S. (2001). Ischemic heart disease. In J. Noble (Ed.), *Textbook of primary care medicine* (pp. 545–570). St. Louis: Mosby.
55. Ridker, P. M. (1999). Evaluating novel cardiovascular risk factors: Can we better predict heart attacks? *Annals of Internal Medicine, 130*, 933–937.
56. Homocysteine Studies Collaboration, Homocysteine and risk of ischemic heart disease and stroke. *Journal of the American Medical Association, 16*, 2015–2022.
57. Bautista, L. E., Arenas, I. A., Penuela, A., et al. (2002). Total plasma homocysteine level and risk of cardiovascular disease: A meta-analysis of prospective cohort studies. *Journal of Clinical Epidemiology, 55*(9), 882–887.
58. Cleophas, T. J., Hornstra, N., van Hoogstraten, B., et al. (2000). Homocysteine, a risk factor for coronary artery disease or not? A meta-analysis. *American Journal of Cardiology, 86*(9), 1005–1009.
59. Chambers, J. C., Ueland, P. M., Obeid, O. A., et al. (2000). Improved vascular endothelial function after oral B vitamins: An effect mediated through reduced concentrations of free plasma homocysteine. *Circulation, 102*(20), 2479–2483.
60. de Bree, A., Verschuren, W. M., Blom, H. J., et al. (2003). Coronary heart disease mortality, plasma homocysteine, and B-vitamins: a prospective study. *Atherosclerosis, 166*(2), 369–377.
61. Doshi, S. N., McDowell, I. F., Moat, S. J., et al. (2002). Folic acid improves endothelial function in coronary artery disease via mechanisms largely independent of homocysteine lowering. *Circulation, 105*(1), 22–26.
62. Schnyder, G., Roffi, M., Pin, R., et al. (2001). Decreased rate of coronary restenosis after lowering of plasma homocysteine levels. *New England Journal of Medicine, 345*(22), 1593–1600.
63. Title, L. M., Cummings, P. M., Giddens, K., et al. (2000). Effect of folic acid and antioxidant vitamins on endothelial dysfunction in patients with coronary artery disease. *Journal of the American College of Cardiology, 36*(3), 758–765.
64. Wald, D. S., Bishop, L., Wald, N. J., et al. (2001). Randomized trial of folic acid supplementation and serum homocysteine levels. *Archives of Internal Medicine, 161*(5), 695–700.
65. Rader, D. J. (2000). Inflammatory markers of coronary risk. *New England Journal of Medicine, 343*(16), 1179–1182.
66. Caslake, M. J., Packard, C. J., Suckling, K. E., et al. (2000). Lipoprotein-associated phospholipase A(2), platelet-activating factor acetylhydrolase: A potential new risk factor for coronary artery disease. *Atherosclerosis, 150*(2), 413–419.
67. Packard, C. J., O'Reilly, D. S., Caslake, M. J., et al. (2000). Lipoprotein-associated phospholipase A2 as an independent predictor of coronary heart disease. West of Scotland Coronary Prevention Study Group. *New England Journal of Medicine, 343*(16), 1148–1155.
68. Blake, G. J., Dada, N., Fox, J. C., et al. (2001). A prospective evaluation of lipoprotein-associated phospholipase A(2) levels and the risk of future cardiovascular events in women. *American Journal of Cardiology, 38*(5), 1302–1306.
69. Grantham, J. A., & Burnett, J. C. (1997). BNP: Increasing importance in the pathophysiology and diagnosis of congestive heart failure. *Circulation, 96*, 388–390.
70. Maisel, A. S., Krishnaswamy, P., Nowak, R. M., et al. (2002). Rapid measurement of B-type natriuretic peptide in the emergency diagnosis of heart failure. *New England Journal of Medicine, 347*(3), 161–167.
71. McCullough, P. A., Nowak, R. M., McCord, J., et al. (2002). B-type natriuretic peptide and clinical judgment in emergency diagnosis of heart failure. *Circulation, 106*, 416–422.
72. Wieczorek, S. J., Wu, A. H., Christenson, R., et al. (2002). A rapid B-type natriuretic peptide assay accurately diagnoses left ventricular dysfunction and heart failure: A multicenter evaluation. *American Heart Journal, 144*, 834–839.
73. Fonarow, G. C., Peacock, W. F., Horwich, T. B., et al. (2008). Usefulness of B-type natriuretic peptide and cardiac troponin levels to predict

in-hospital mortality from ADHERE. *American Journal of Cardiology, 101*, 231–237.
74. Berger, R., Huelsman, M., Strecker, K., et al. (2002). B-type natriuretic peptide predicts sudden death in patients with chronic heart failure. *Circulation, 105*, 2392–2397.
75. Levitt, J. E., Vinayak, A. G., Gehlbach, B., et al. (2008). Diagnostic utility of B-type natriuretic peptide in critically ill patients with pulmonary edema: A prospective cohort study. *Critical Care, 12*(1), R3.
76. Colucci, W. S., & Chen, H. H. (2007). Brain natriuretic peptide measurement in left ventricular dysfunction and other cardiac diseases. Retrieved April 26, 2008, from www.uptodate.com
77. Kearon, C., Ginsberg, J. S., Douketis, J., et al. (2006). An evaluation of D-dimer in the diagnosis of pulmonary embolism. *Annals of Internal Medicine, 144*, 812–821.
78. Palareti, G., Cosmi, B., Legnani, C., et al. (2006). D-dimer testing to determine the duration of anticoagulation therapy. *New England Journal of Medicine, 355*, 1780–1790.
79. American Heart Association. (2005). Part 7.2: Management of cardiac arrest. *Circulation, 112*, IV-58–IV-66.
80. Echahidi, N., Pibarot, P., O'Hara, G., et al. (2008). Mechanisms, prevention, and treatment of atrial fibrillation after cardiac surgery. *Journal of the American College of Cardiology, 51*, 793–801.
81. Miller, S., Crystal, E., Garfinkle, M., et al. (2005). Effects of magnesium on atrial fibrillation after cardiac surgery: A meta analysis. *Heart, 91*, 618–623.
82. Eagle, K., Guyton, R., Davidoff, R., et al. (2004). ACC/AHA 2004 guideline update for coronary artery bypass graft surgery: A report of the American College of Cardiology/American Heart Association Task Force on Practice Guidelines (Committee to Update the 1999 Guidelines for Coronary Artery Bypass Graft Surgery). *Circulation, 110*, e340–e437.
83. LaDue, J. S., Wroblewski, F., & Karmen, A. (1954). Serum glutamic oxaloacetic transaminase activity in human acute transmural myocardial infarction. *Science, 120*, 497–499.
84. American Diabetes Association. (2007). Standards of medical care in diabetes-2007. *Diabetes Care: American Diabetes Association: Clinical Practice, 30*, S4–S41.
85. Van den Berghe, G., Wouters, P., Bouillon, R., et al. (2003). Outcome benefit of intensive insulin therapy in the critically ill: Insulin dose versus glycemic control. *Critical Care Medicine, 31*, 359–366.
86. Van den Berghe, G., Wilmer, A., Hermans, G., et al. (2006). Intensive insulin therapy in the critically ill: Insulin dose versus glycemic control. *New England Journal of Medicine, 354*, 449–461.
87. Zerr, K. J., Furnary, A. P., Grunkemeier, G. L., et al. (1997). Glucose control lowers the risk of wound infection in diabetes after open heart operations. *Annals of Thoracic Surgery, 63*, 356–361.
88. Furnary, A. P., Gao, G., Grunkemeier, G. L., et al. (2003). Continuous insulin infusion reduces mortality in patient with diabetes undergoing coronary artery bypass surgery. *Journal of Thoracic and Cardiovascular Surgery, 125*, 1007–1021.
89. Malmberg, K., Ryden, L., Wedel, H., et al. (2005). Intense metabolic control by means of insulin in patients with diabetes mellitus and acute myocardial infarction (DIGAMI 2): Effects on mortality and morbidity. *European Heart Journal, 26*, 650–661.
90. Mehta, S. R., Yusuf, S., Diaz, R., et al. (2005). Effect of glucose-insulin-potassium infusion on mortality in patients with acute ST-segment elevation myocardial infarction: The CREATE-ECLA randomized controlled trial. *Journal of the American Medical Association, 293*, 437–446.
91. Furnary, A. P., Zerr, K. J., Grunkemeier, G. L., et al. (1999). Continuous intravenous insulin infusion reduces the incidence of deep sternal wound infection in diabetic patients after cardiac surgical procedures. *Annals of Thoracic Surgery, 67*, 352–360.
92. American Diabetes Association. (2003). Standards of medical care for patients with diabetes mellitus. *Diabetes Care, 26*(90001), 33S–50S.
93. Rohlfing, C. L., Wiedmeyer, H. M., Little, R. R., et al. (2002). Defining the relationship between plasma glucose and HbA1c: Analysis of glucose profiles and HbA1c in the Diabetes Control and Complications Trial. *Diabetes Care, 25*(2), 275–278.
94. American Diabetes Association. (2003). Tests of glycemia in diabetes. *Diabetes Care, 26*(90001), 106S–108S.
95. UK Prospective Diabetes Study (UKPDS) Group. (1998). Intensive blood-glucose control with sulphonylureas or insulin compared with conventional treatment and risk of complications in patients with type 2 diabetes (UKPDS 33). *Lancet, 352*(9131), 837–853.
96. The Diabetes Control and Complications Trial Research Group. (1993). The effect of intensive treatment of diabetes on the development and progression of long-term complications in insulin-dependent diabetes mellitus. *New England Journal of Medicine, 329*(14), 977–986.
97. Wallach, J. (2007). Core blood analytes: Alterations by diseases. In *Interpretation of diagnostic tests*. Philadelphia: Lippincott Williams & Wilkins.
98. Beutz, M., Sherman, G., Mayfield, J., et al. (2003). Clinical utility of blood cultures drawn from central vein catheters and peripheral venipuncture in critically ill medical patients. *Chest, 123*, 854–861.
99. Martinez, J. A., DesJardin, J. A., Aronoff, M., et al. (2002). Clinical utility of blood cultures drawn from central venous or arterial catheters in critically ill surgical patients. *Critical Care Medicine, 30*, 7–13.
100. Wallach, J. (2007). Therapeutic drug monitoring and drug effects. In *Interpretation of diagnostic tests*. Philadelphia: Lippincott Williams & Wilkins.

CHAPTER 12

Radiologic Examination of the Chest

Jon S. Huseby / Denise LeDoux

The chest radiography is one of the most common diagnostic tools used in the evaluation of cardiovascular disease and the critically ill. Although a variety of other imaging modalities are available, chest radiography remains fundamental because of its ready availability in most settings, relatively low cost, and the ability to interpret films by a wide variety of health care providers. The most recent advancement in chest radiology has been the rapid conversion from film-based to digital radiographic images.[1]

The cardiac care nurse may be the first health care professional to see the chest radiograph of a patient in acute distress. Valuable time may be saved if the nurse is able to recognize the presence of an abnormality. Knowledge of chest radiograph interpretation and the disease processes that an abnormal film indicate can help the nurse in understanding disease pathophysiology, thereby allowing for better patient care; dual reading of radiographs significantly increases diagnostic accuracy and decreases the incidence of missed abnormalities.

This chapter is divided into four sections: (1) How x-rays work; (2) Interpretation of chest radiographs; (3) Chest film findings in acute care determining line placement; and (4) Chest film findings in cardiovascular disease and acute care.

HOW X-RAYS WORK

X-rays are radiant energy, like light, except that these waves are shorter and can pass through opaque objects. They are produced by bombarding a tungsten target with an electron beam and are channeled so that a narrow but diverging beam is emitted from the tube. When an x-ray exposure is taken, the tube is usually aimed so that the rays pass through the subject to the x-ray film in either a posterior to anterior (posteroanterior) or anterior to posterior (anteroposterior) direction. Because the x-rays are diverging and subject to reflection (scatter), structures more distant from the film are magnified and less distinctly outlined. In general, chest radiographs are taken in the posteroanterior direction because this places the heart, an anterior structure, closer to the film, resulting in less magnification and allowing the cardiac outline to be seen clearly.

When using conventional radiology methods, the chest x-ray image is recorded on a film that is chemically processed. Computerized digital chest radiology utilizes a special phosphor plate instead of traditional film. The digital x-ray image is produced by scanning the phosphor plate with a laser beam that causes light to be released from the phosphor plate. This image is then digitized and converted to an image by computer.[2] The computer image is then viewed from monitors and can also be converted to radiographic film providing a hard copy. Digital images afford many advantages over traditional chest x-rays. Digital images are easily stored and transferred making them more accessible from a variety of remote viewing stations. Digital images can be easily manipulated by changing magnification or relative density, which may add substantial information to the examination without exposing the patient to repeated imaging.[3]

Anteroposterior chest radiographs are often taken in cardiac care units (CCU) because it is difficult to put the x-ray tube behind the patient. The x-ray film is therefore placed behind the patient. Because the heart is relatively far away from the x-ray film, its outline is somewhat less distinct and the heart size is magnified. Moreover, the distance between the tube and the patient in CCU is shorter than usual to cut-down x-ray scatter, which also results in greater magnification.

The degree of darkness of the x-ray film depends on how much x-ray energy traverses the patient and exposes the film. This depends on the density of the material through which the x-ray beam passes. The chest has four major types of tissue densities through which rays must pass: bone, water, fat, and air. Because bone is the densest of these tissues, fewer and less energetic x-rays pass through bone. Thus, the shadow on the x-ray film cast by bone is light. (An x-ray image is like a photographic negative, with white color indicating lack of exposure and black color indicating intense exposure.) The lung, which is largely air, is least dense; therefore, it appears black on a chest radiograph. Soft tissues and blood are largely water, with similar densities, between those of bone and air. Fat is usually visibly less dense than other soft tissues. Thus, a chest radiograph is actually a shadowgraph.

The reason a structure can be outlined is that the shadow of one density contrasts with that of an adjacent density. If two structures are of equal density and adjacent to each other, then a single combined shadow results. If two structures of similar density are in different planes or are separated by a structure of a different density, then the two structures are seen on x-ray film separately. This property of the x-ray shadowgraph is helpful in determining where a certain density lies. For example, if a density on a posteroanterior chest radiograph is inseparable from and therefore adjacent to the descending thoracic aorta, then the observer knows that this abnormal density is in the posterior chest; if the density is inseparable from the right heart border, then the density is in an anterior position, because the heart is an anterior structure.

INTERPRETATION OF CHEST RADIOGRAPHS

The chest radiograph is read as though the reader were looking at the patient. Traditionally, the x-ray film is placed on a view box or light box that allows the radiograph to be backlit so it can be viewed and interpreted. More recently, digital imaging technology is used increasingly in radiology allowing for rapid viewing of films on monitors rather than on light boxes. Computerized radiographs can be viewed immediately on monitors on the CCU and stored images allow the provider to readily compare current films with previous images.[4] To ensure that all anatomic structures are seen, radiographs are read according to a certain pattern. This method is called the directed search method. It is common practice to look at soft tissues, bones, and diaphragms first, then at the lungs from apex to base, and finally at the outline of the heart and the aorta. Except for the heart, most structures in the chest are bilateral. Thus, if an abnormality is found on one side of the chest, the other side should be observed to ensure that this "abnormality" is not present there. Even if an obvious abnormality is present, a directed search should be completed so that additional disease is not missed. Figure 12-1*A* is a normal posteroanterior chest radiograph; Figure 12-1*B* is a normal lateral chest radiograph. Figure 12-2*A* shows the location of the lung lobes on the frontal chest radiograph. Because some lobes are anterior and some are posterior, an abnormality in a certain area on a frontal chest radiograph can be in one of two lobes. Obtaining a lateral film or noticing whether an anterior or posterior structure is obliterated by an abnormal density can help with localization. Figure 12-2*B* shows the location of the lung lobes on a lateral radiograph. Abnormalities of the right middle lobe and lingula would go undetected with posterior chest auscultation.

CHEST FILM FINDINGS IN ACUTE CARE DETERMINING LINE, TUBE, AND CATHETER PLACEMENT

Bedside radiographs are used not only to assess for cardiopulmonary abnormalities, but also to evaluate placement of lines, tubes, and devices used in acute care. In addition to providing valuable information regarding the patient's cardiopulmonary status, the chest radiograph allows for early recognition of complications related to line placement as well as to evaluate therapeutic result after interventions such as drainage of a pleural effusion by chest tube placement. Table 12-1 lists invasive lines, tubes, and devices commonly used in acute cardiovascular care and describes radiologic findings. Figures 12-3 through 12-10 demonstrate radiologic appearance of a variety of invasive lines and devices.

CHEST FILM FINDINGS IN CARDIOVASCULAR DISEASE

The chest radiograph provides useful data that aid in the complete assessment of the patient with acute chest pain and suspected acute coronary syndrome in the CCU and/or emergency department. Chest radiography aids in evaluating other etiologies of

(text continues on page 273)

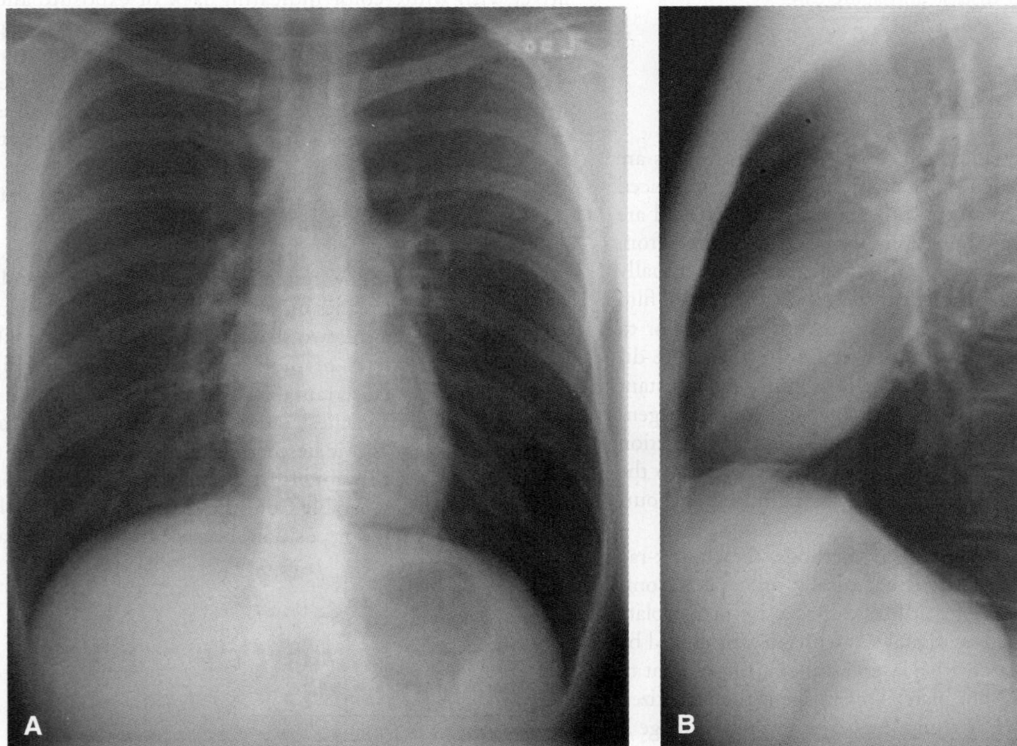

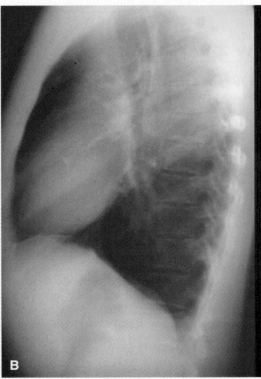

Figure 12-1 (A) Normal posteroanterior chest radiograph. (B) Normal lateral chest radiograph. The spine is posterior and the heart is anterior.

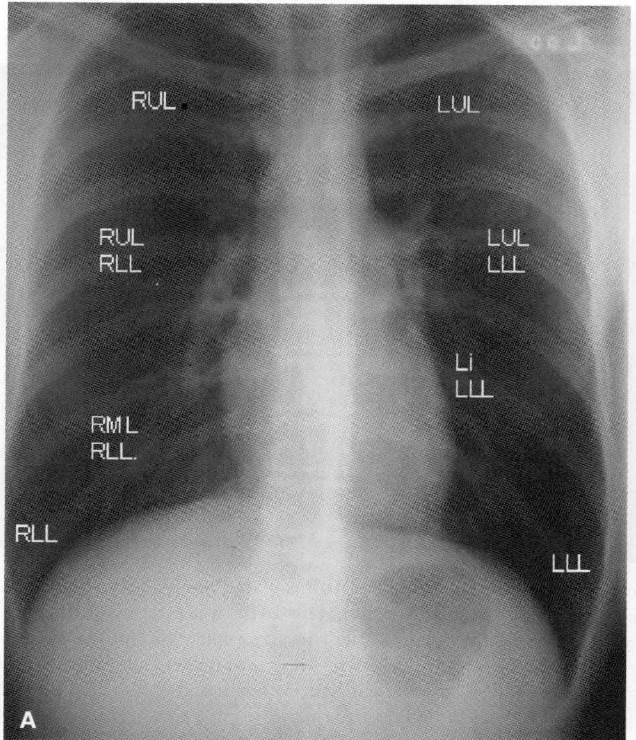

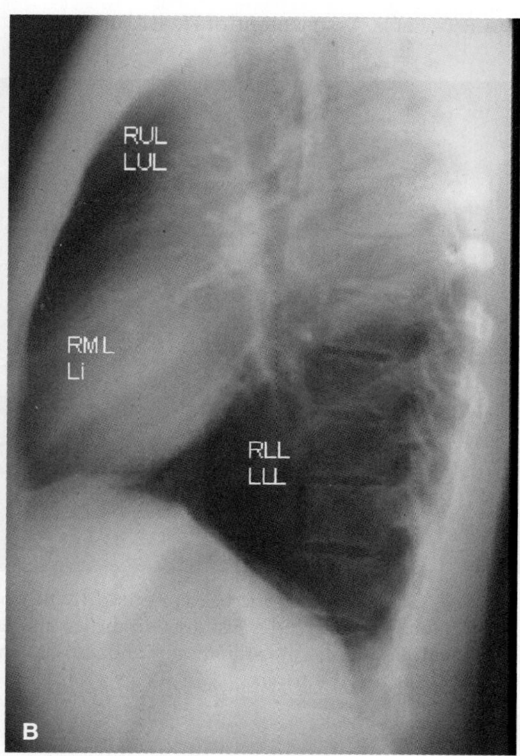

■ **Figure 12-2** (A) Location of the lung lobes on the frontal chest radiograph. Because some lobes are anterior and some are posterior, an abnormality in a certain area on a frontal chest radiograph can be in one of two lobes. Obtaining a lateral film or noticing whether an anterior or posterior structure is obliterated by an abnormal density can help with localization. RUL, right upper lobe; RLL, right lower lobe; LLL, left lower lobe; RML, right middle lobe; LUL, left upper lobe; Li, lingula. (B) Location of the lung lobes on a lateral radiograph. Abnormalities of the right middle lobe and lingula would go undetected with posterior chest auscultation.

Table 12-1 ■ RADIOLOGIC APPEARANCE OF INVASIVE LINES AND DEVICES IN CARDIOVASCULAR CARE

Invasive Line or Device	Description of Radiologic Appearance for Correct Position
Central venous pressure catheter (CVP) or peripherally inserted central catheter (PICC)	Ideal position is in the superior vena cava. The CVP line tip should always be above the level of the right atrium or the catheter tip may slip into the right atrium or ventricle and produce arrhythmias, or rarely, cardiac perforation. Central lines can be misplaced into the subclavian artery or misdirected up into the internal jugular vein. Trace the central line from its point of vascular entry to the tip to insure appropriate placement.
Pulmonary artery catheter (PAC)	The PAC tip should be within the main right or left pulmonary arteries and should extend no more than 2–4 cm beyond the vertebral midline. If the catheter tip is beyond this point there is increased risk of pulmonary artery occlusion, infarction, and rupture. The course of the PAC should be traced from its entry point to ensure that there is no looping in the ventricle. If the catheter tip is in the right ventricle, ventricular tachycardia may result from endocardial irritation.
Endotracheal tube (ETT)	The ETT should be visible as a radiopaque line within the trachea. The distal tip of the ETT should be a minimum of 4 cm above the main carina to avoid accidental right or left mainstem intubation. The ETT distal tip should be no higher than the level of the clavicles to avoid accidental extubation. Position of the head affects the location of the ETT tip. Flexion of the head toward the chest pulls the ETT up the trachea, while extension pushes the tube tip further into the trachea.
Chest tube	Chest tubes are used to drain air or fluid from the pleural cavity. Chest tubes inserted for pneumothorax are inserted toward the apex where gas or air collects and chest tubes inserted to drain fluid are inserted toward dependent areas around the base of the lungs. All of the islets that promote drainage (positioned along the proximal portion of the chest tube) need to be projected within the chest wall.
Intra-aortic balloon pump (IABP)	The tip of the IABP should be located in the distal aortic arch, just below the aortic knob and distal to the left subclavian artery. The oblong radiopaque IABP tip has the appearance of a large grain of rice.
Transvenous pacer (TVP)	Pacemaker leads extend from their point of entry in the right or left brachiocephalic veins into the right atrium (atrial lead) and the trabeculae of the right ventricle (ventricular lead). If the pacer is malfunctioning, the chest x-ray (CXR) may show fractured or misplaced leads.
Feeding tube (FT)	The entire FT is radiopaque. One should be able to trace the FT through the esophagus, stomach, and into the duodenum.
Tracheostomy tube	The tracheostomy tube should be midline within the trachea with the tip several cm above the main carina.

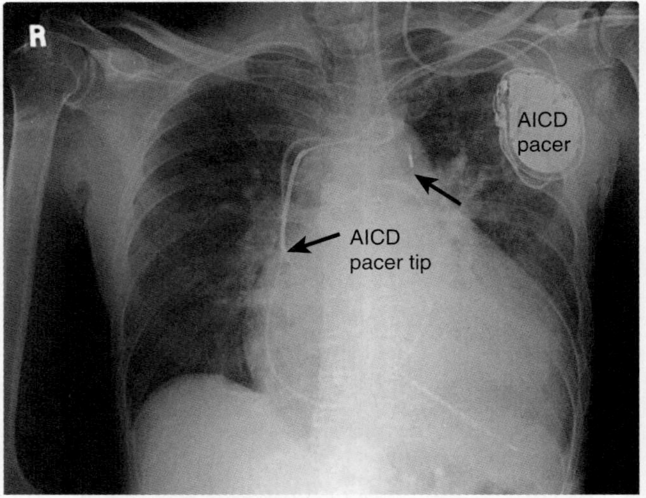

■ **Figure 12-3** Correct intra-aortic balloon pump (IABP) placement in aortic knob. The IABP tip is just distal to the left subclavian artery. The patient has significant cardiomegaly and also has an implantable defibrillator (AICD) pacer.

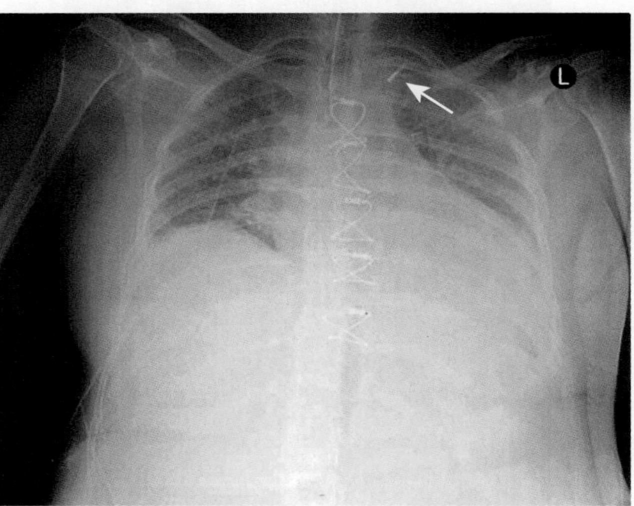

■ **Figure 12-4** The IABP is placed too high into the left subclavian artery (see white arrow). This IABP was inserted at the bedside for a cardiac transplant patient in acute rejection and cardiogenic shock. The tip is above the aortic knob into the left subclavian artery. On examination, the patient had no left radial or brachial pulse until the IABP was pulled back 4 cm.

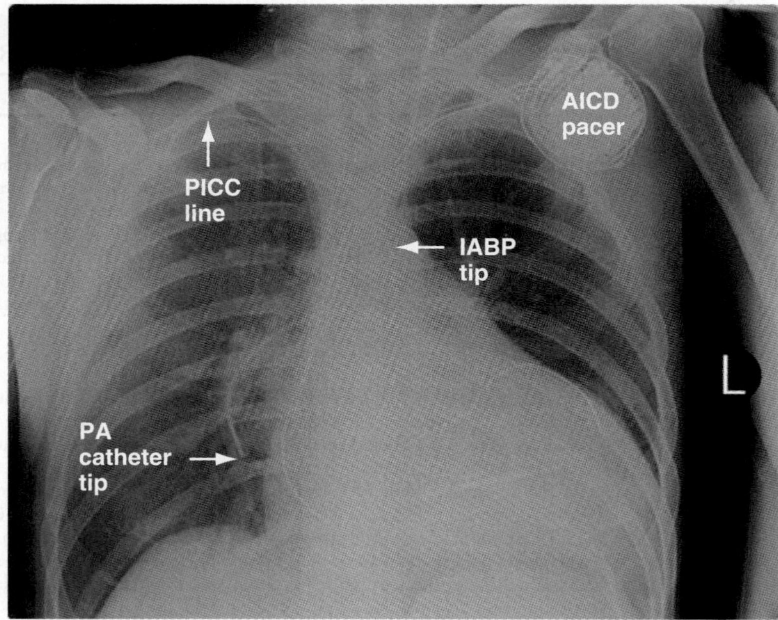

■ **Figure 12-5** The pulmonary artery (PA) catheter tip is out too far. The tip of the PA catheter lies several centimeters beyond the hilum and is at risk for spontaneous wedge and pulmonary infarction. The patient also has an automatic implantable cardioverter defibrillator (AICD), peripherally inserted central catheter (PICC) line, and IABP.

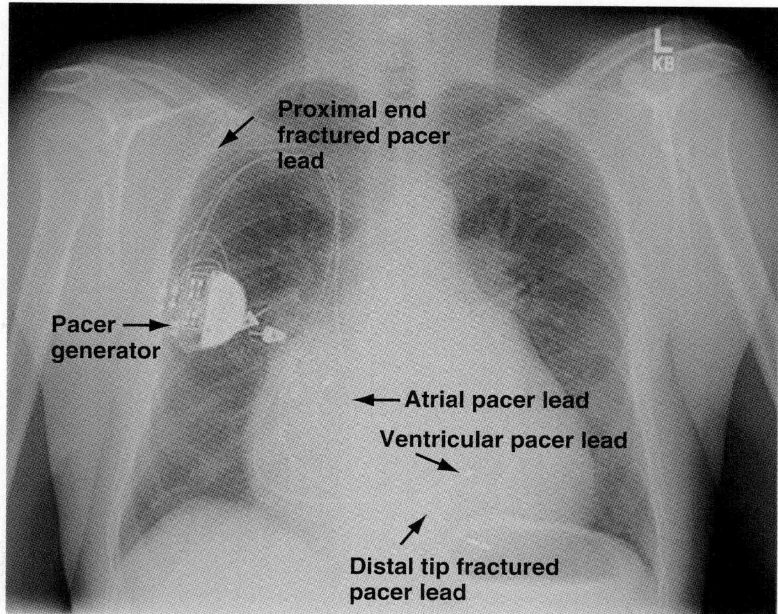

■ **Figure 12-6** Pacemaker in a patient with cardiomegaly. Patient is a 27-year-old man with congenital heart disease. He had a previous pacer, but his original leads fractured and a new device and leads were placed. New leads can be seen in both the right atrium and right ventricle. A second ventricular lead can be seen in the right ventricle; if you trace this lead back, you will find it is fractured at the proximal end.

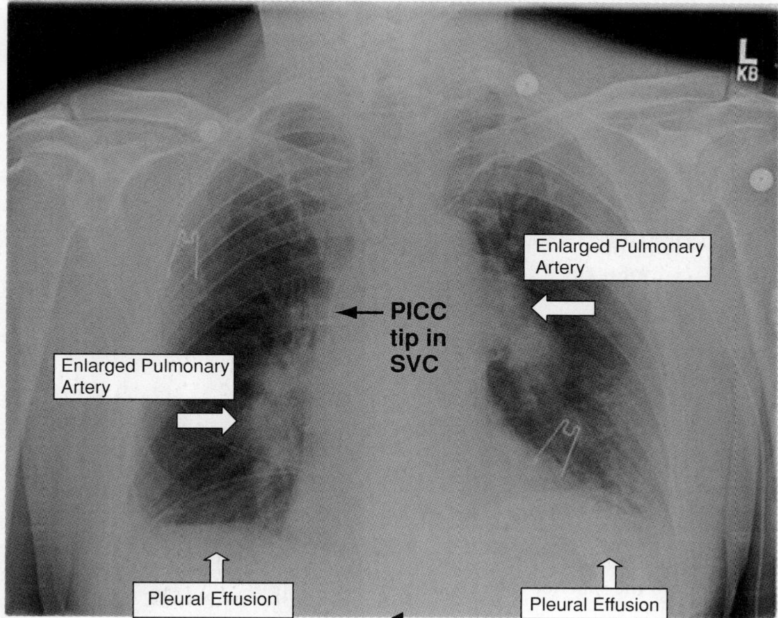

■ **Figure 12-7** PICC line placement in a 56-year-old man with history of severe pulmonary hypertension secondary to chronic thromboembolic disease. He was postoperative after a pulmonary thromboendarterectomy. The tip of the PICC inserted into his left antecubital vein is correctly positioned in the superior vena cava (SVC). Note that, in addition to bilateral pleural effusions (see blunted costal phrenic angles), this individual also has very large pulmonary arteries extending from his hilum.

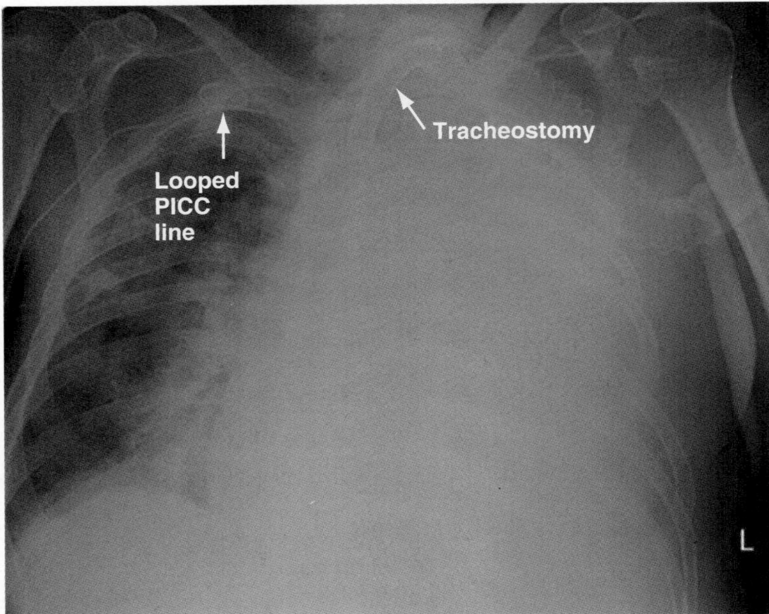

■ **Figure 12-8** The PICC is looped in the right subclavian vein. Patient is a 55-year-old man who had multiple complications after emergency repair of a ruptured descending aortic aneurysm. The white-out on the patient's left is a massive hemothorax, which is pushing the mediastinum including the tracheostomy tube to the right.

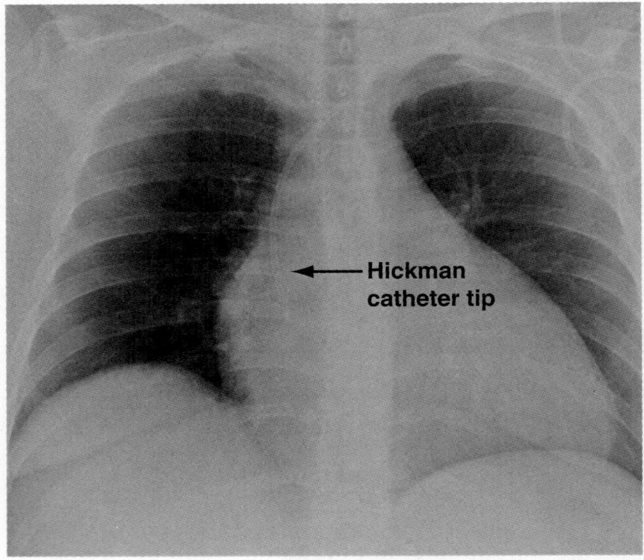

■ **Figure 12-9** Hickman central line placement. There is a tunneled central line with correct position into the superior vena cava.

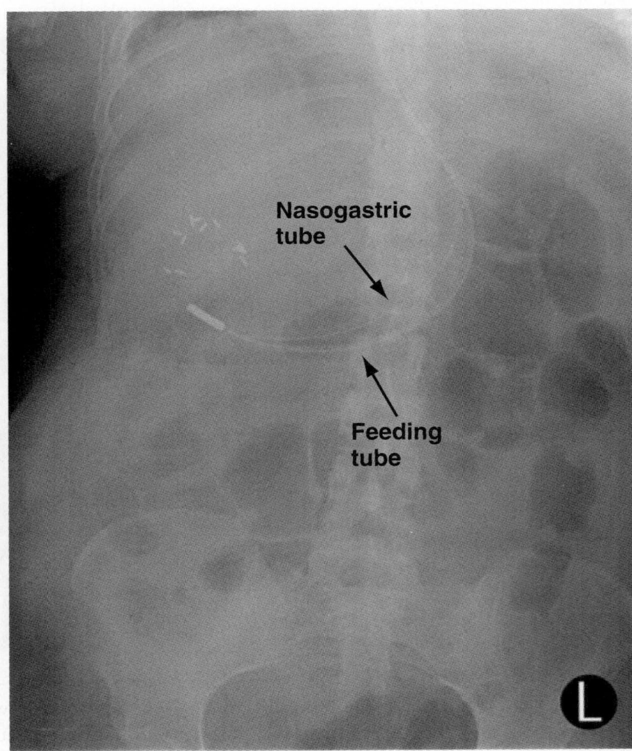

■ **Figure 12-10** Feeding tube placement. The abdominal radiograph shows both the feeding tube and the nasogastric tube in the duodenum.

Table 12-2 ■ COMMON CLINICAL PRESENTATIONS IN ACUTE CARE AND RADIOLOGIC FINDINGS

Clinical Diagnosis	Radiologic Findings
Pericardial effusion	Enlarged cardiac silhouette with a "water bottle" appearance. May look very similar to cardiomegaly. Diagnosis of pericardial effusion should be verified with echocardiography.
Congestive heart failure (CHF)	In chronic CHF the heart is usually enlarged; in acute heart failure the heart may be of normal size. May have cephalization of blood vessels (increased size and number of blood vessels near the lung apices). May have interstitial fluid that begins at the lung bases and extends upwards. Frank pulmonary edema and pleural effusions may develop.
Aortic aneurysm	Ascending and/or descending aorta are enlarged. Widened mediastinum. New pleural effusion if leak or rupture.
Pneumothorax	Frontal, full upright CXR shows the visceral pleura as a thin white line. There is a hyperlucent area where there are no bronchovascular or lung markings. Pneumothorax is more difficult to see in supine film.
Pleural effusion	Fluid moves to dependent areas of pleural space and is best seen on upright or decubitus (side lying) CXR views. At least 200 to 300 cc must be present in the pleural space to cause costophrenic blunting. By doing decubitus views (side lying), one may determine if the effusion is free flowing and amenable to thoracentesis.
Pneumonia	Alveolar or interstitial pattern of white opacity. May be localized to a single lobe or be more diffused. Air bronchograms are frequently present in lobar pneumonia.
Acute respiratory distress syndrome (ARDS)	Diffuse bilateral patchy infiltrates, "ground glass" appearance. May be confused with CHF.

chest pain including pneumothorax, rib fractures, pneumonia, and aortic dissection.[5] Computerized axial tomography angiography is used for the diagnosis of aortic dissection and pulmonary embolism. Table 12-2 lists common cardiovascular clinical diagnoses and their associated radiologic findings. Figures 12-11 through 12-21 illustrate a variety of radiologic findings associated with cardiovascular pathophysiology.

In the past, "routine" daily chest x-rays were frequently taken in critical care, but this practice has been largely abandoned due to low diagnostic efficacy.[6] Chest x-rays should be ordered on the basis of clinical evaluation. Early diagnosis of complications and improperly placed invasive lines improves patient care, and knowledge of the radiographic findings in disease processes augments the nurse's understanding of cardiopulmonary pathophysiology.

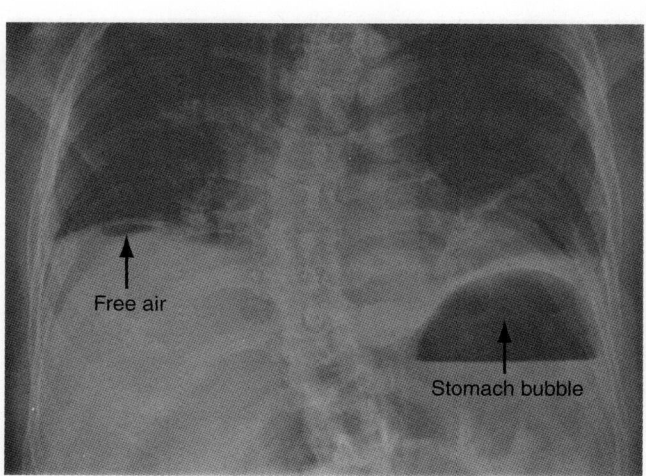

■ **Figure 12-11** Free air under the diaphragm. This patient had epigastric pain and diaphoresis. The admission radiograph showed free air under the diaphragm consistent with a perforated viscus. (Film courtesy of Julie Takasugi, MD)

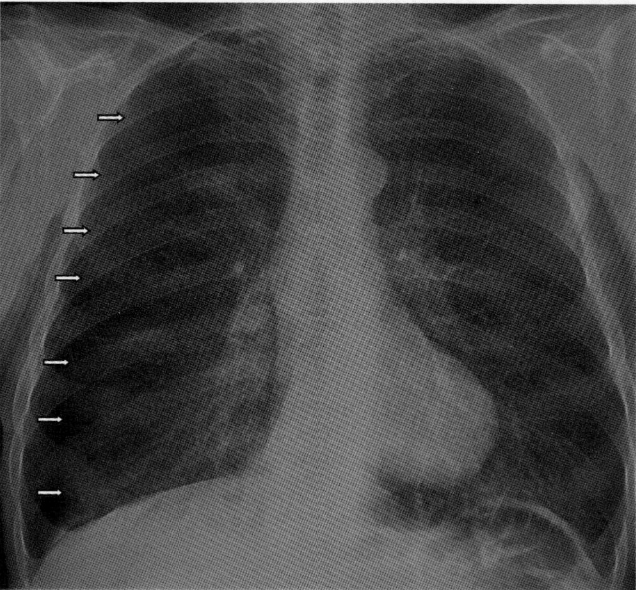

■ **Figure 12-12** Pneumothorax. The patient may have acute chest pain and shortness of breath. Physical findings include absent or reduced breath sounds on the side of the pneumothorax and tympany or a hollow sound on chest percussion, with possibly a shift of the trachea to the side away from the pneumothorax. The *arrows* indicate the outer border of the right lung. The remainder of the right chest cavity is filled with air in the pleural space. (Film courtesy of Julie Takasugi, MD)

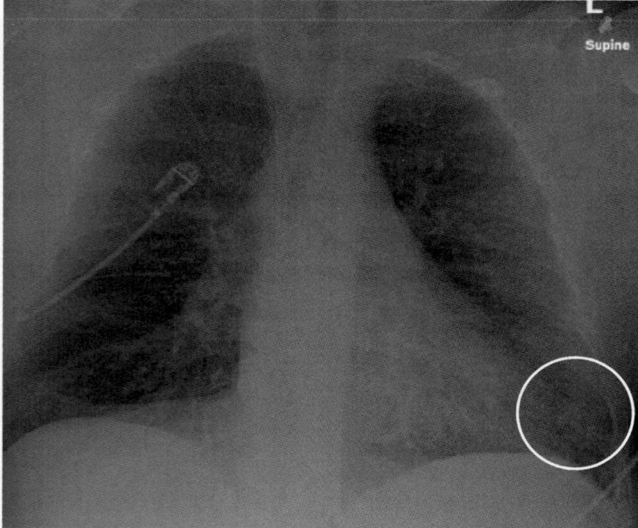

■ **Figure 12-13** Cardiogenic pulmonary edema with cardiomegaly. In this radiograph, Kerley B lines are seen as tiny horizontal lines in the lung periphery. These lines represent dilated pulmonary lymph vessels, which facilitate pulmonary edema removal from the alveolar spaces. (Film courtesy of Julie Takasugi, MD)

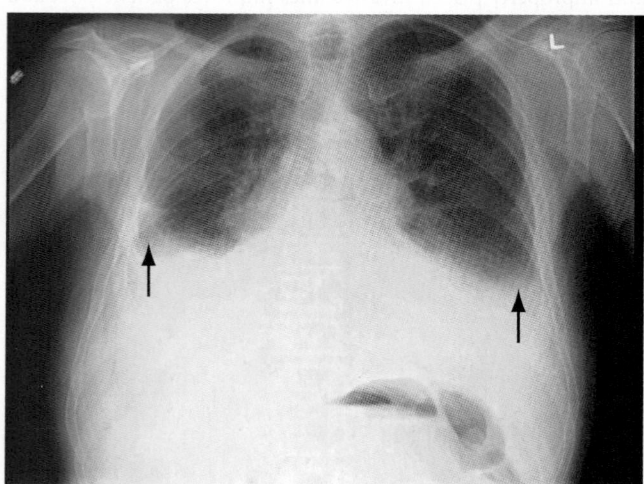

■ **Figure 12-14** Congestive heart failure with bilateral pleural effusions. The arrows show that the normal diaphragmatic contour is obliterated. This 88-year-old man with severe aortic stenosis was admitted with severe shortness of breath and worsening heart failure.

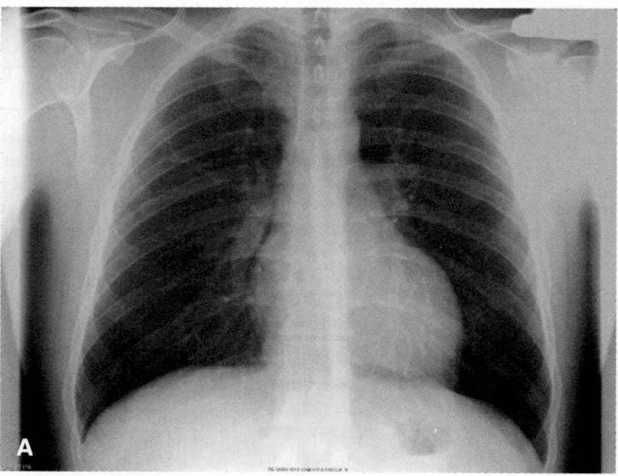

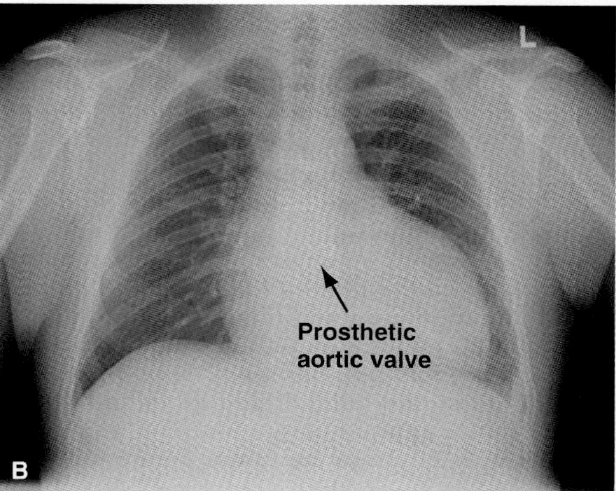

■ **Figure 12-15** (A) Preoperative patient with aortic regurgitation. (B) Same patient 3 weeks after aortic valve replacement. Patient now has a large pericardial effusion (note enlarged cardiac silhouette) creating tamponade physiology.

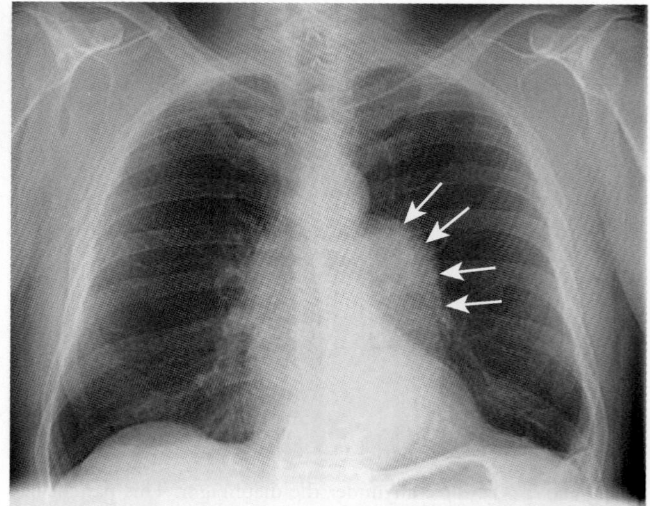

■ **Figure 12-16** Descending thoracic aortic aneurysm. "Bulging" of the descending aorta noted by *arrows* in a 57-year-old man with history of blunt trauma to chest as well as hypertension.

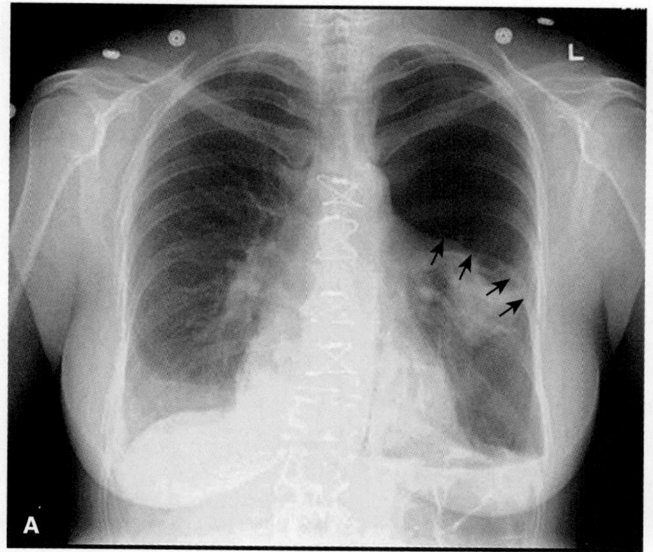

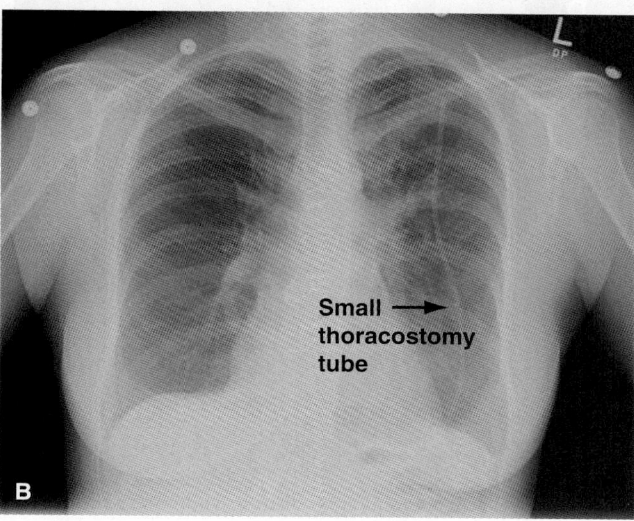

■ **Figure 12-17** (A) Large left pneumothorax after surgical repair of a patent foramen ovale. The arrows indicate the border of the collapsed lung. (B) Re-expansion of left lung after placement of small thoracostomy tube in interventional radiology department.

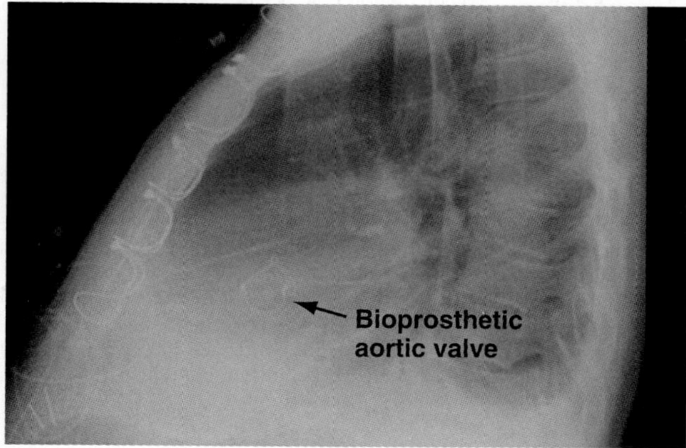

■ **Figure 12-18** Radiologic appearance of stented bioprosthetic aortic valve replacement in lateral chest x-ray (CXR) view. Stents point toward blood flow.

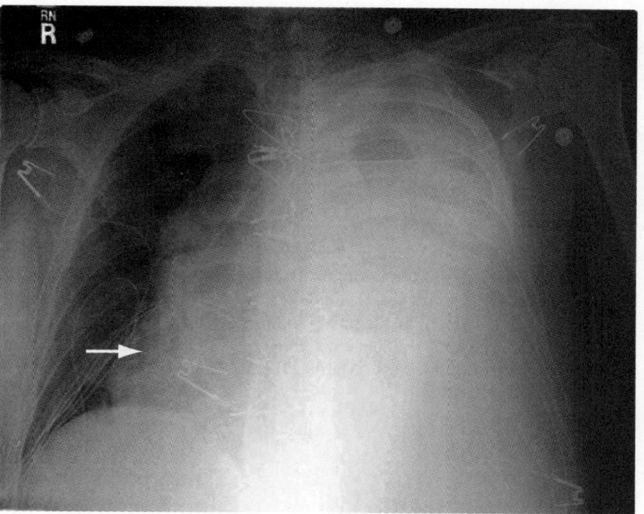

■ **Figure 12-19** Massive left pleural effusion (the patient's left side of chest is whited out) with mediastinal shift, where the right heart border is shifted into the patient's right chest (arrow). This 62-year-old man had massive left pleural effusion causing severe orthopnea and shortness of breath. Patient underwent thoracentesis three times in a 24-hour period to drain a total of 3,500 cc of serosanguineous fluid.

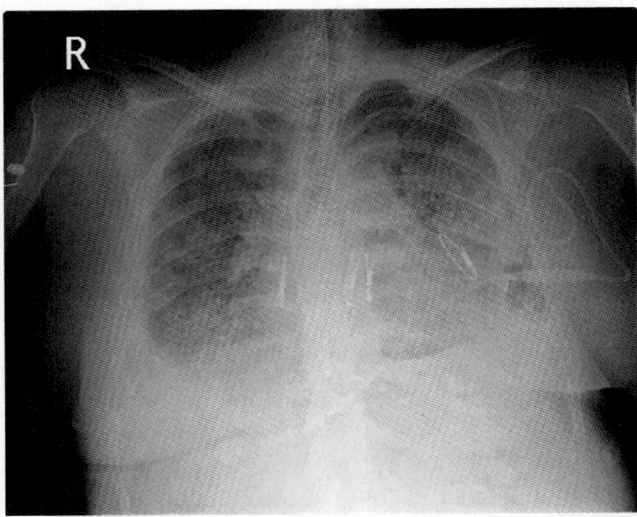

■ **Figure 12-20** Acute respiratory distress syndrome, as evidenced by diffuse bilateral opacities in patient postoperatively after bilateral lung transplantation.

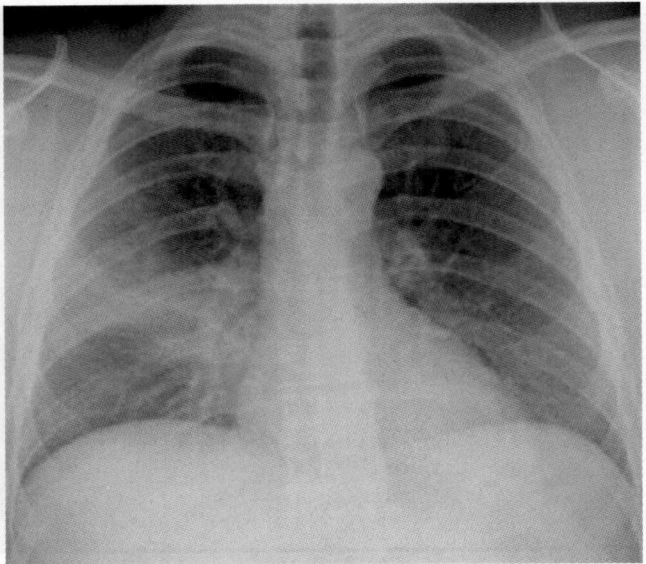

■ **Figure 12-21** Right lower lobe pneumonia. Signs of consolidation (bronchial breathing, crackles, and dullness to percussion) are heard over the right lower chest. In pneumonia, egophony is heard over areas of consolidated lung. The patient is instructed to say the letter "e," and the lung is auscultated to demonstrate this finding. Normally the "e" sound is heard, but consolidated lung changes the "e" to an "a" that sounds like the "bleating of a goat." This sign is also known as "an e-to-a change." (Film courtesy of Julie Takasugi, MD)

REFERENCES

1. McAdams, H. P., Samei, E., Dobbins, J., et al. (2006). Recent advances in chest radiology. *Radiology, 241*(3), 663–683.
2. Erkonen, W. E. (2005). Radiography, computerized tomography, magnetic resonance imaging, and ultrasonography: Principles and indications. In W. E. Erkonen & W. L. Smith (Eds.), *Radiology 101. The basics and fundamentals of imaging* (pp. 3–15). Philadelphia: Lippincott Williams & Wilkins.
3. Bettman, M. A. (2008). The chest radiograph in cardiovascular disease. In P. Libby, R. O. Bonow, D. L. Mann, D. P. Zipes, & E. Braunwald (Eds.), *Braunwald's heart disease* (8th ed., pp. 327–343). Philadelphia: Saunders Elsevier.
4. Connolly, M. A. (2001). Black, white, and shades of gray: Common abnormalities in chest radiographs. *AACN Clinical Issues, 12*(2), 259–269.
5. Stanford, W. (2007). Radiologic evaluation of acute chest pain-suspected myocardial ischemia. *American Family Physician, 76*(4), 533–537.
6. Hendrikse, K. A., Gratama, J. W., Hove, W., et al. (2007). Low value of routine chest radiographs in a mixed medical-surgical ICU. *Chest, 132*(3), 823–828.

CHAPTER 13

Echocardiography

Peter J. Cawley

Echocardiography (echo) is ultrasound technology as applied to imaging the heart and the associated great vessels.[1] As cardiac catheterization and invasive angiography transformed our understanding of the structure and function of the heart, echo allowed clinicians the same opportunities noninvasively. Our clinical experience utilizing echo for patient care is vast and spans many decades. Echo is one of the most widely used imaging modalities today within cardiology because of the following attributes: safe, fast, lacks exposure to ionizing radiation, noninvasive, and portable.

In the United States, the acquisition of echo images is most commonly performed by sonographers (individuals who have completed specialized training programs in ultrasound), echocardiographers (cardiologists with training in echo), or cardiovascular anesthesiologists. As the field has expanded, other physicians including those who practice emergency medicine, primary care, or critical care have received training in image acquisition.

This chapter will focus on three general topics: (1) principles and techniques of echo, (2) echo examination, and (3) special applications of echo.

PRINCIPLES AND TECHNIQUES OF ECHO

Sound Waves

Ultrasound is sound with a frequency above 20,000 Hz (cycles per second) or 20 kHz. This sound is outside of the range of the human ear. Diagnostic ultrasound for cardiovascular imaging uses frequencies ranging from 2 to 30 MHz: adult transthoracic frequencies range from 2 to 4 MHz, transesophageal frequencies from 5 to 7 MHz, and intravascular ultrasound frequencies (coronary artery) from 20 to 30 MHz.

Sound waves are generated at the transducer, the hand-held probe that is applied to the body part of interest. Today, transducers contain a piezoelectric crystal, which when applied to an electric current, will cause the crystal to deform. This deformation results in the generation of a sound wave, which is transmitted to the body. Returning sound waves can also deform the crystal and thus be detected by the transducer.[2] The transducer receives sound waves that are generated from the interaction of the transmitted sound waves and the tissues of the body. The transducer generates and receives reflected sound waves. Interestingly, the time the transducer is in receiver mode (i.e., listening mode) is far greater than when in transmitting mode (i.e., generating sound waves) with one exception—continuous wave Doppler, which will be explained further (See Doppler).

Sound moves through media in the form of waves and may interact with the tissues in different ways. This chapter presents two of the more common interactions, reflection and attenuation. Reflection occurs when a transmitted sound wave interacts with tissues of different density within the body. For example, there is a different density of the blood than of the myocardium. The boundary between the two tissues causes reflection of the transmitted sound wave, which is then detected by the transducer. Depending upon the time it took for the transducer to emit the sound wave and detect the reflected sound wave, it will place that object at a certain distance (depth) on the image.[2]

Attenuation is degradation of the sound wave as it propagates from the transducer. Sound waves pass through tissues and attenuate with greater distances from the transducer. This attenuation results in a finite ability of the transducer to capture reflected sound waves from greater depths. The greater the distance the transducer is from the heart, the greater the number of sound waves that will be attenuated, and the result will be poor image quality. Examples of sound wave attenuation for echo caused by greater depth (distance) include obesity and breast tissue. But depth is not the only cause of sound wave attenuation in echo. Bone and air also result in considerable attenuation. Because the heart is surrounded by the sternum and ribs, imaging can be performed only in the rib spaces. In patients with smaller ribs spaces, imaging can be particularly challenging. Because the heart is in close proximity to the lungs and trachea, these structures must also be avoided. In patients with enlarged lung spaces (i.e., chronic obstructive pulmonary disease), imaging can be difficult. Pneumomediastinum, pneumothorax, and subcutaneous air will all result in signal attenuation.

Experienced echocardiographers and sonographers should possess a thorough understanding of the impact of image artifacts. Inability to recognize artifacts could lead to false interpretation, some with significant consequences. Ultrasound can cause several different types of artifacts and an explanation of each is beyond the scope of this chapter. To reduce misdiagnosing artifacts, abnormalities should be visualized in more than one imaging window, thus reducing the likelihood of false interpretation.

M-Mode

M-mode (motion) echo displays a narrow ultrasound beam of information within the heart along the *y*-axis (vertical axis) and displays it according to time on the *x*-axis (horizontal axis). Heart structures are displayed with respect to motion and time. M-mode echo provides high temporal resolution and provides information regarding both the structure and function of the heart. M-mode echo predated the existence of two-dimensional (2-D) echo and although it is not as commonly used as in the past, M-mode can still be useful to describe motion of structures of the heart with respect to the cardiac cycle (Fig. 13-1).

2-D

2-D echo was developed from similar concepts of M-mode. Because M-mode only allowed a very narrow and focused area of

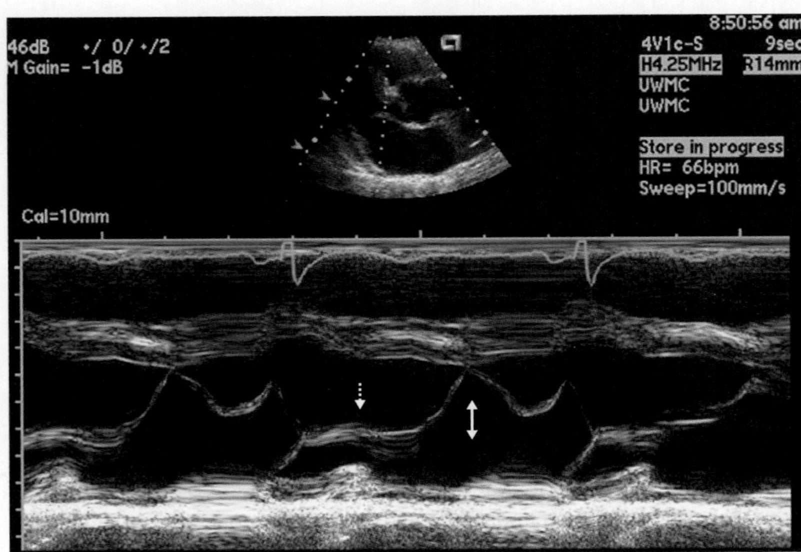

■ **Figure 13-1** Example of 2-D guide M-mode. At the center, top of the image, there is a 2-D image of the heart in still frame. The dashed line going through the center of the 2-D image represents the narrow beam of ultrasound. Motion of the heart structures as they move through this beam is displayed in the bottom of the image. The *x*-axis represents time, which is associated with the ECG tracing. The *y*-axis represents motion of the structures with respect to time. The specific structure of most interest in this image is the motion of the mitral leaflets during the cardiac cycle. The *arrowhead* represents the two mitral leaflets in the closed position as is appropriate in systole. The *double-headed arrow* represents the separation of the two leaflets in diastole. Notice how there are two distinct waves of mitral valve opening: the first wave (E) represents **e**arly, passive filling of the left ventricle; the second wave (A) represents **a**trial contraction. (Echo courtesy of University of Washington Medical Center, Seattle, Washington.)

interrogation of the heart, it was limited. 2-D echo provided a wider area investigation into the structure and function of the heart within a 90-degree scanning sector.[1] Thus, 2-D echo provides a more complete investigation of the entire structure and function of the heart (Figs. 13-2 through 13-6).

Doppler

Doppler affords clinicians a powerful and integral tool for assessing heart function. This is based on the Doppler principle, first described by Christian Johann Doppler in the 19th century.

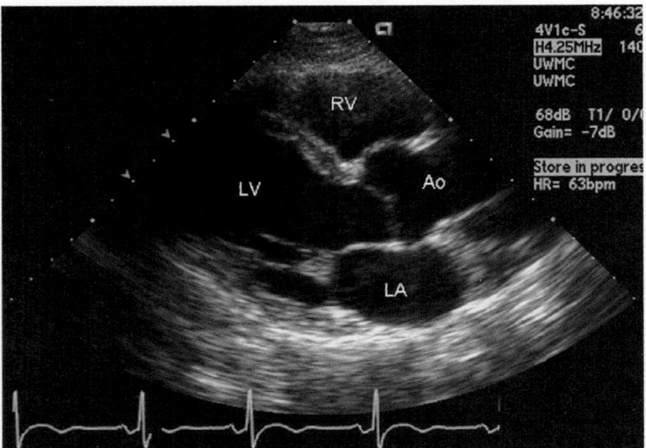

■ **Figure 13-2** 2-D image of the heart. The image is displayed so that the top of the image represents structures closest to the transducer (i.e., closest to the chest wall in this case) and the bottom of the image represents structures farthest away from the transducer. The image displays structures within a 90-degree scanning sector. This image nicely demonstrates that the right ventricle is an anterior structure. LV, left ventricle; RV, right ventricle; Ao, aorta; LA, left atrium. (Echo courtesy of University of Washington Medical Center, Seattle, Washington.)

It describes the change in reflected sound wave frequency compared with the transmitted sound wave frequencies generated from the transducer. These sound waves are reflected off of moving red blood cells. This change in frequency (transmitted to reflected sound waves) is related to the velocity of moving red blood cells through the heart, which can be used to describe the hemodynamics of blood flow through the heart.

One important feature of Doppler interrogation is the angle of the transmitted frequency as compared to blood flow. To achieve the most accurate estimate of the velocity of blood flow, the angle of interrogation (angle of the transmitted sound wave) should be parallel to blood flow. As the angle increases, so does the error, which results in underestimation (never overestimation) of blood flow velocity. Because air (lung) and bones (ribs and sternum) limit the number of imaging spaces that can be used to interrogate blood flow through the heart, Doppler interrogation should be performed from multiple locations to minimize this error. The highest velocity obtained should be interpreted then as the sound wave most parallel to blood flow.[1–3]

There are three types of Doppler techniques: pulse wave, continuous wave, and color. Pulse wave Doppler is used for the assessment of blood flow at specific locations and is useful for velocities less than 2 m/s (Fig. 13-7). Continuous wave Doppler is used for assessing velocities along the entire pathway of the sound wave and is used for velocities up to 8 m/s (Figs. 13-8 and 13-9). Continuous wave Doppler as its name suggests is continuously transmitting and receiving sound waves using separate crystals. This technique is unlike all other echo techniques, such as 2-D echo, pulse wave Doppler, and color Doppler, which all use the same crystal to transmit and receive sound waves and predominantly spend the majority of time receiving sound waves.

Color Doppler is a pulse wave technique in which multiple points in a specified sector are sampled. Depending upon the direction and turbulence of blood flow, a color is encoded upon a 2-D image (Fig. 13-10). This technique is useful for visualizing the presence of blood flow, the presence of turbulent blood flow, and shunts.

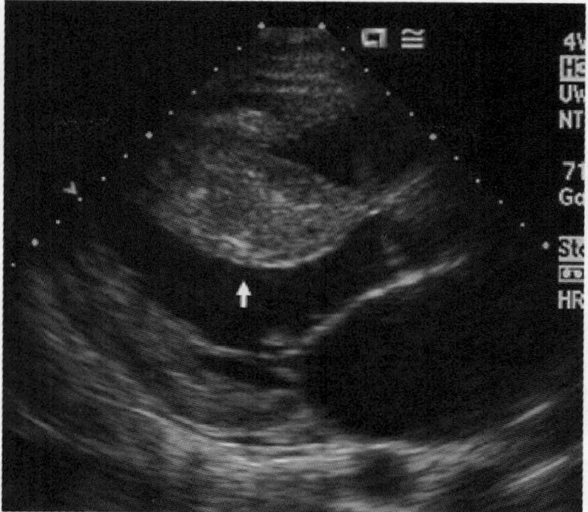

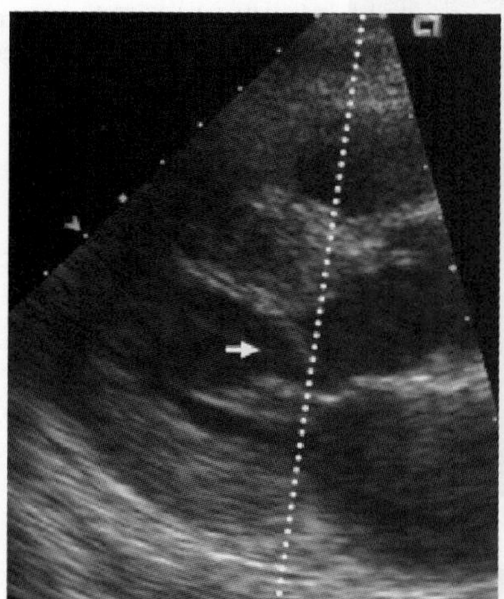

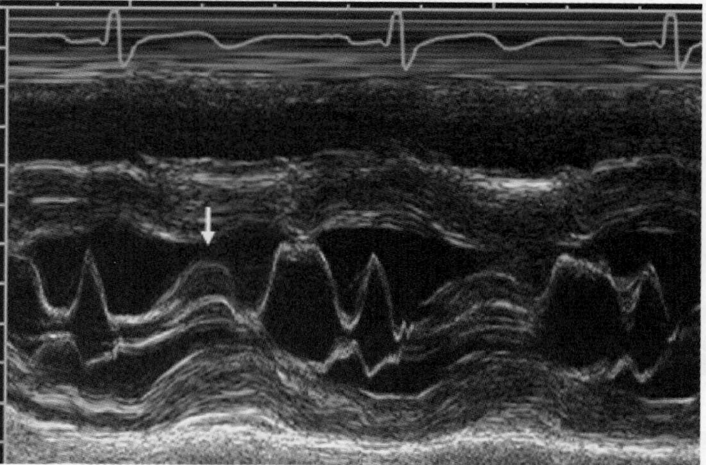

■ **Figure 13-3** *Top:* 2-D image in a patient with hypertrophic cardiomyopathy showing significant asymmetric hypertrophy of the anterior septum (*arrow*). Evidence of systolic anterior motion of the mitral valve apparatus (*arrow*) with 2-D echo (*bottom, left*). In this same 2-D image, the dashed line represents the area of the narrow beam of ultrasound with M-mode echo and that information is displayed in the next image (*bottom, right*) with time (cardiac cycle) on the *x*-axis and motion on the *y*-axis. The arrow represents systolic anterior motion of the mitral valve apparatus resulting in obstruction of blood flow in the left ventricular outflow tract. (Echo courtesy of University of Washington Medical Center, Seattle, Washington.)

ECHO EXAMINATION

Patient Preparation

Imaging is most ideally performed on special examination beds that have a removable section of the mattress to allow placement of the imaging transducer along the patient's left side. This simple feature improves the quality of the examination. However, there are circumstances where the patient cannot be transported safely to the echo laboratory (i.e., ICU level of care, emergency) and in that case, the ultrasound machine can be brought to the patient's bedside. The portability of echo is unique among cardiovascular imaging modalities.

Transthoracic echo is performed by placing an ultrasound transducer on the patient's chest and images are obtained through the chest wall. The patient is positioned in the left lateral decubitus position for the first part of the examination and then is moved to the supine position to complete the image set. Occasionally, the patient is positioned in the right lateral decubitus position. Electrocardiogram (ECG) electrodes are placed on the patient's skin to acquire a continuous ECG rhythm. The timing of events to the cardiac cycle is important. The blood pressure and heart rate should always be recorded at the time of the examination as these measurements affect cardiovascular hemodynamics.

The transducer is the part of the echo machine that is placed on the patient's skin to acquire images. Because ultrasound waves have significant attenuation through air, a coupling gel is used between the transducer and the patient's skin to eliminate any air.

Axis of the Heart

The heart is situated obliquely in the chest with the apex toward the left. Imaging is not therefore performed in a straight

(text continues on page 282)

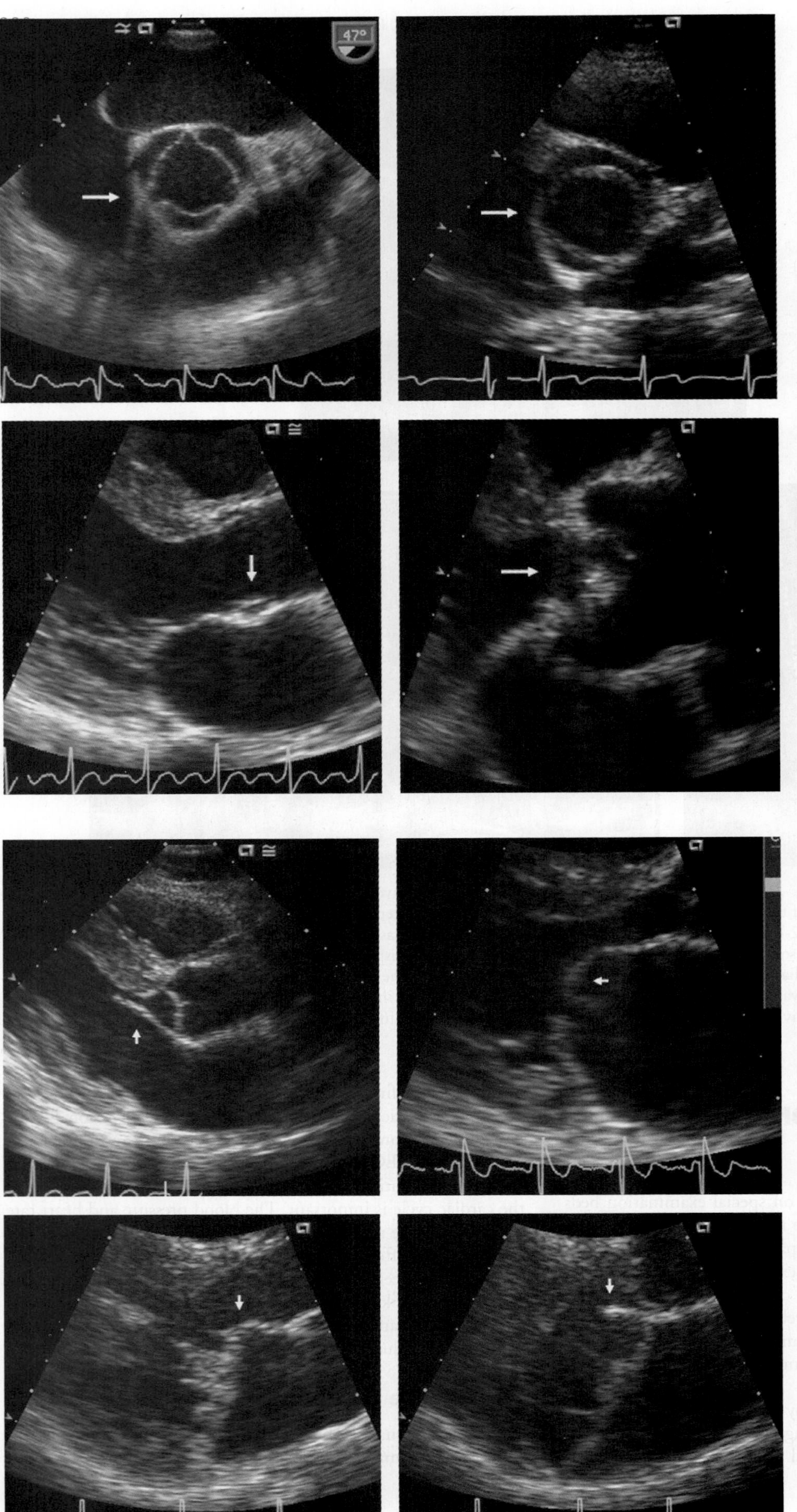

■ **Figure 13-4** 2-D images can also be used for imaging valve leaflets. *Top:* Systolic frame of a normal trileaflet aortic valve (*left*) and a bicuspid aortic valve (*right*). *Bottom:* Normal trileaflet aortic valve in systole with the leaflets fully opened (*left*); a comparison image of a patient with calcific aortic stenosis showing reduced aortic valve leaflet opening in systole (*right*). (Echo courtesy of University of Washington Medical Center, Seattle, Washington.)

■ **Figure 13-5** *Top:* Normal mitral valve in diastole with the leaflets fully open (*left*); a comparison image of a patient with rheumatic mitral stenosis demonstrates significant reduction in leaflet opening in diastole (*right*). *Bottom:* Myxomatous mitral valve disease. In early systole, the valve leaflets are thickened and redundant (*left*). In late systole, there is bileaflet mitral valve prolapse (*right*). The arrow marks the mitral valve annulus. Notice the difference of the leaflets to the annulus compared with early and late systole. (Echo courtesy of University of Washington Medical Center, Seattle, Washington.)

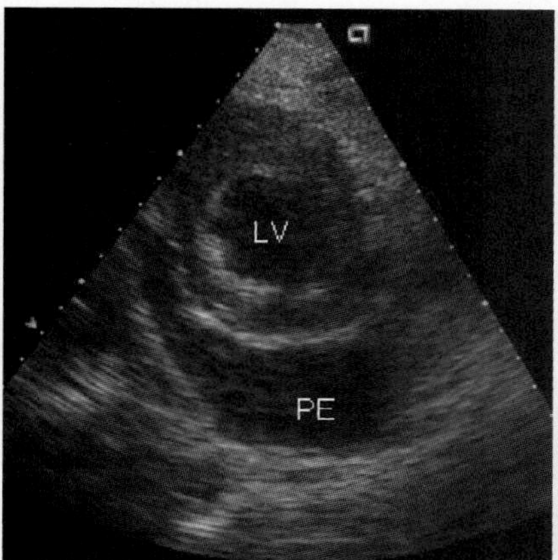

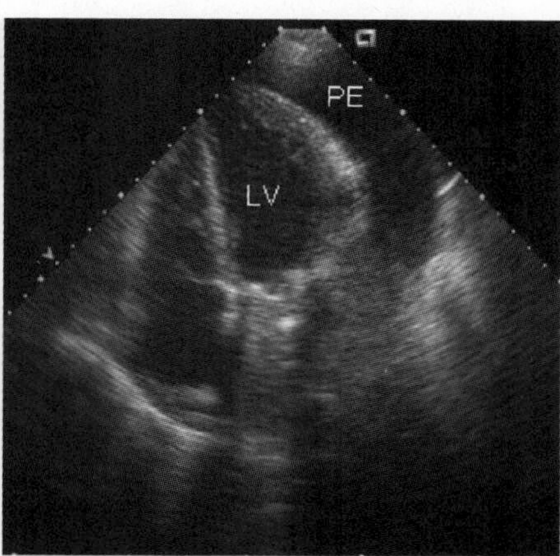

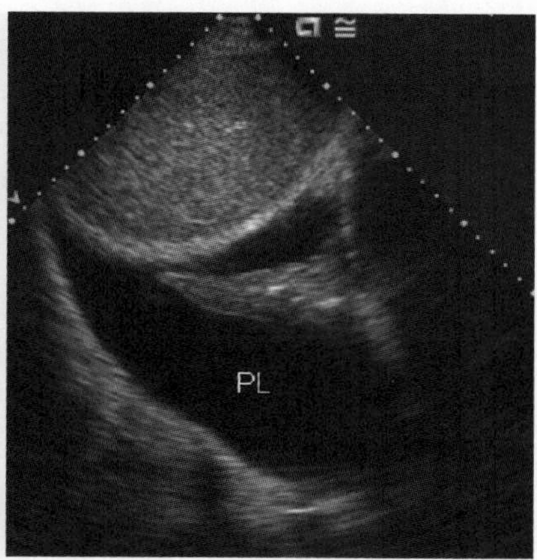

■ **Figure 13-6** Echolucent (black) spaces within the pericardial space (*left and middle*) represent pericardial effusions. Echolucent spaces (*right*) outside of the pericardium but within the pleural space represent a right-sided pleural effusion. LV, left ventricle; PE, pericardial effusion; PL, pleural effusion. (Echo courtesy of University of Washington Medical Center, Seattle, Washington.)

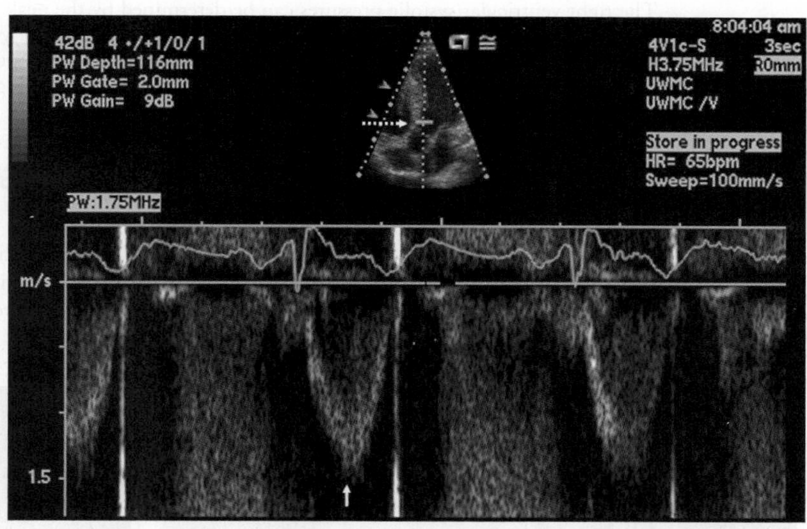

■ **Figure 13-7** With pulse wave Doppler, a 2-D image (*top*) is used to localize the specific area (*dashed arrow*) of the heart in which velocity is measured. Time (cardiac cycle) is displayed on the *x*-axis and velocities on the *y*-axis (m/s). Systole and diastole can be distinguished based on the ECG signal. The *arrow* represents the peak velocity seen in the left ventricular outflow tract in this patient. (Echo courtesy of University of Washington Medical Center, Seattle, Washington.)

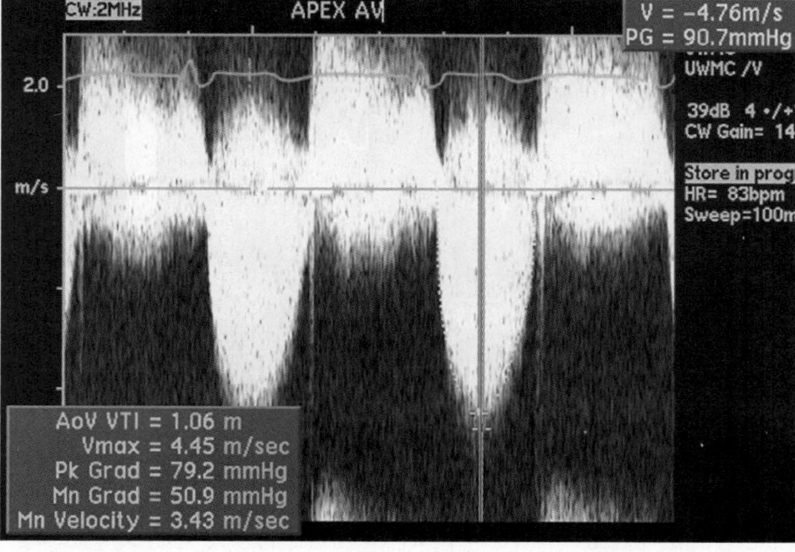

■ **Figure 13-8** Continuous wave Doppler image acquired from the apical window in a patient with severe aortic stenosis. The white signal below the baseline (marked m/s) represents blood away from the transducer, which is located at the apex of the heart. The white signal during systole (see ECG tracing) represents the velocities of red blood cells along the entire wave pathway. In this example, the peak velocity is very high at 4.5 m/s, which translates into a peak gradient of 79 mm Hg. This is interpreted as the velocity of red blood cells which are crossing the aortic valve. By integrating the velocities under the entire spectral curve during systole, one can obtain the mean gradient, which in this case is 51 mm Hg. (Echo courtesy of University of Washington Medical Center, Seattle, Washington.)

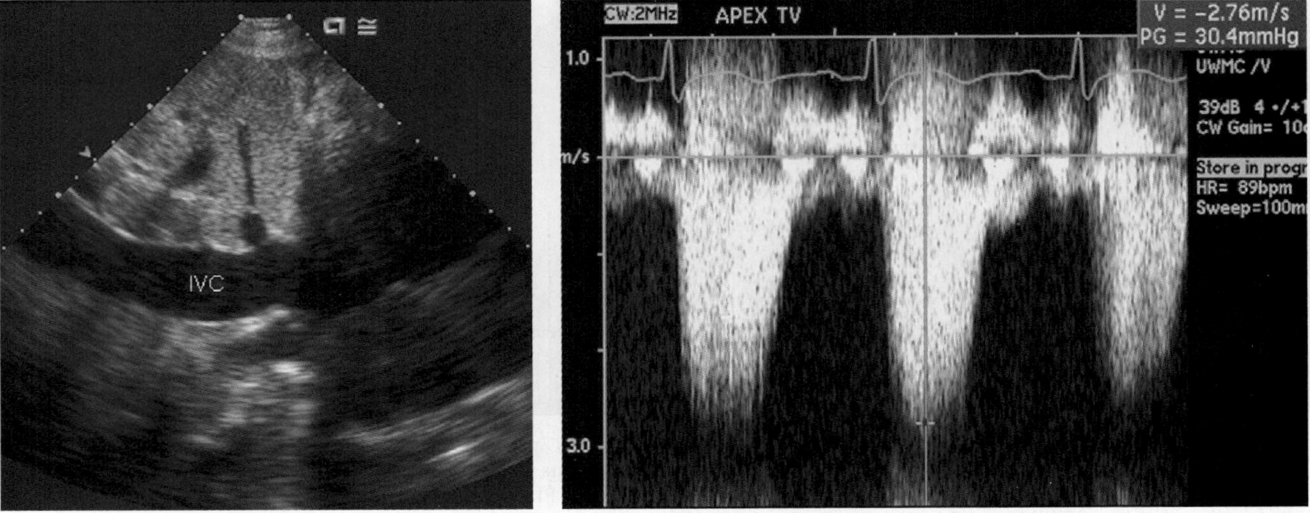

■ **Figure 13-9** The right atrial pressures can be determined noninvasively by imaging the inferior vena cava (IVC) (*left*). The degree of dilatation and collapse of the IVC are used to determine the right atrial pressures. The right ventricular systolic pressures can be determined by the peak velocity of tricuspid valve regurgitation jet with continuous wave Doppler (*right*). In the absence of pulmonary stenosis, the addition of the right atrial pressures plus the right ventricular systolic pressure should equal the pulmonary artery systolic pressure. (Echo courtesy of University of Washington Medical Center, Seattle, Washington.)

axial or sagittal orientation. Instead, most of the cardiovascular imaging is performed along the axis of the heart and not the axis of the body. There are two standard axes of the heart: long and short. In the long axis views, the heart is imaged from the base to the apex. The short axis of the heart is perpendicular to this axis.

Imaging Windows

Ultrasound waves have significant attenuation through air and bone and therefore, care must be taken to avoid the areas over the sternum, ribs, and lungs. Imaging is thereby limited to the spaces between the ribs. There are four standardized anatomic

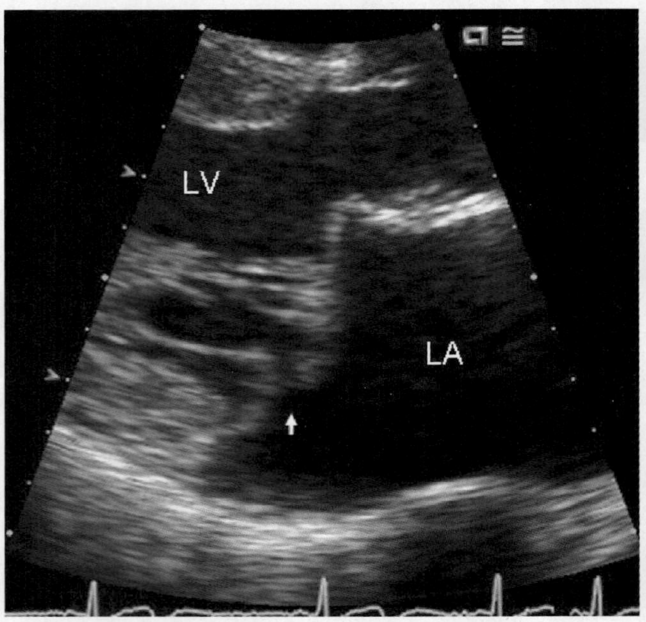

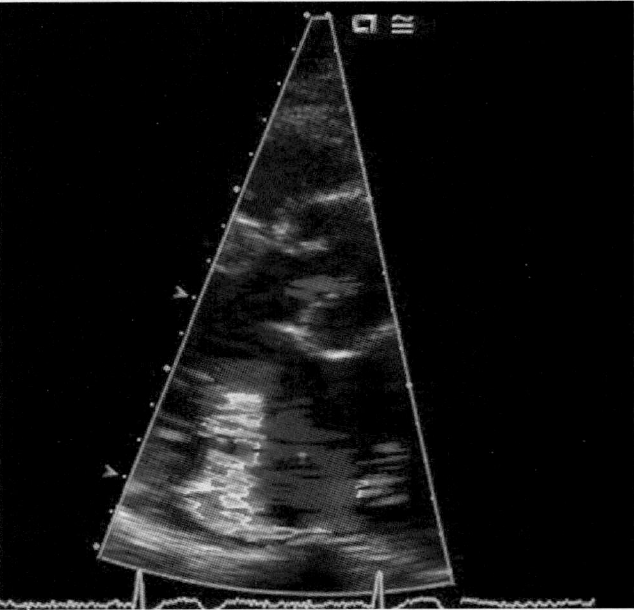

■ **Figure 13-10** 2-D image of an abnormal mitral valve. A chordae tendineae to the anterior mitral leaflet is no longer attached to the valve leaflet, which results in the anterior leaflet prolapsing into the left atrium in systole (*left*). The posterior and anterior leaflets do not completely oppose each other, which results in a regurgitant orifice area. Color Doppler superimposed on a 2-D image (*right*) shows the regurgitation of blood flow through this area in systole. (Echo courtesy of University of Washington Medical Center, Seattle, Washington.)

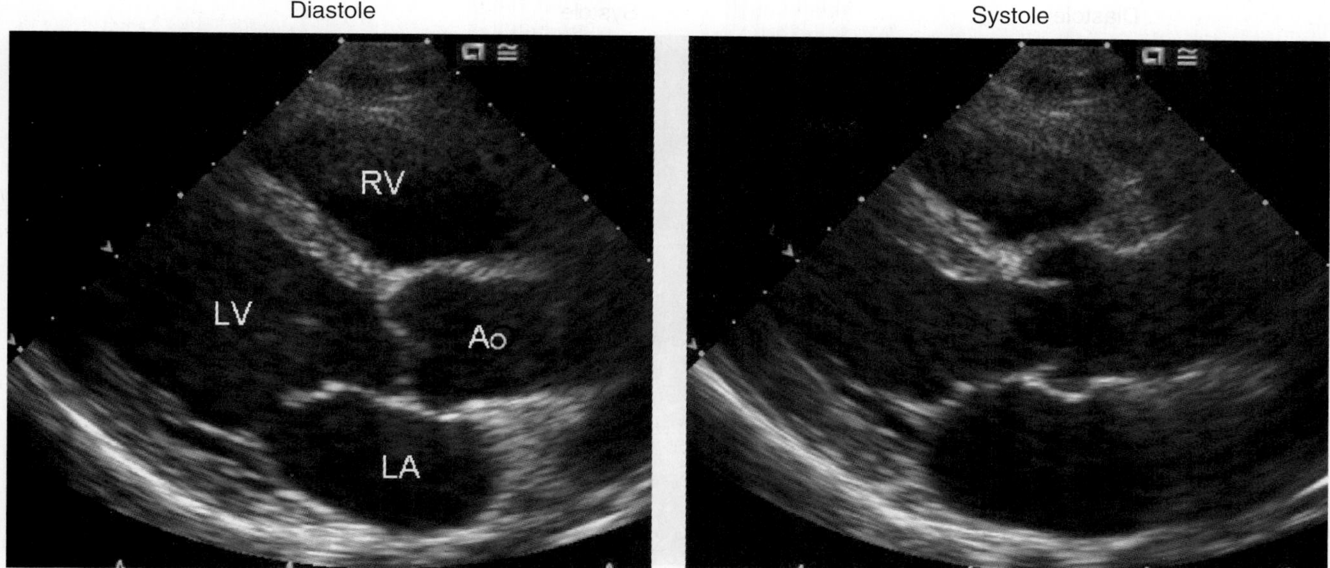

■ **Figure 13-11** 2-D images in the parasternal long axis in diastole and systole in a patient with normal ventricular function. LV, left ventricle; RV, right ventricle; LA, left atrium; AO, aorta. (Echo courtesy of University of Washington Medical Center, Washington.)

windows for the echo examination and are usually acquired in the following order: parasternal, apical, subcostal, and suprasternal. Standard nomenclature used in echo is to first identify the window in which the images were obtained and then whether the long or short axis is used. Multiple windows are used to maximize imaging of heart structures, likewise attempts are made to image most structures from at least two windows. For a standard and complete echo examination, all four windows should be utilized. 2-D echo and Doppler (pulse wave, continuous wave, and color) are typically performed in each window.

Parasternal Window

The patient is positioned in the left lateral decubitus position and imaging is performed in the rib spaces left of the sternum. Imaging is performed in the long axis and short axis (Figs. 13-11 and 13-12). The short axis can be obtained at multiple levels of the heart from base to apex (Fig. 13-13).

Apical Window

The patient is positioned in the left lateral decubitus position and imaging is performed in the rib spaces overlying the apex of the heart. In this window, imaging is performed only along the long

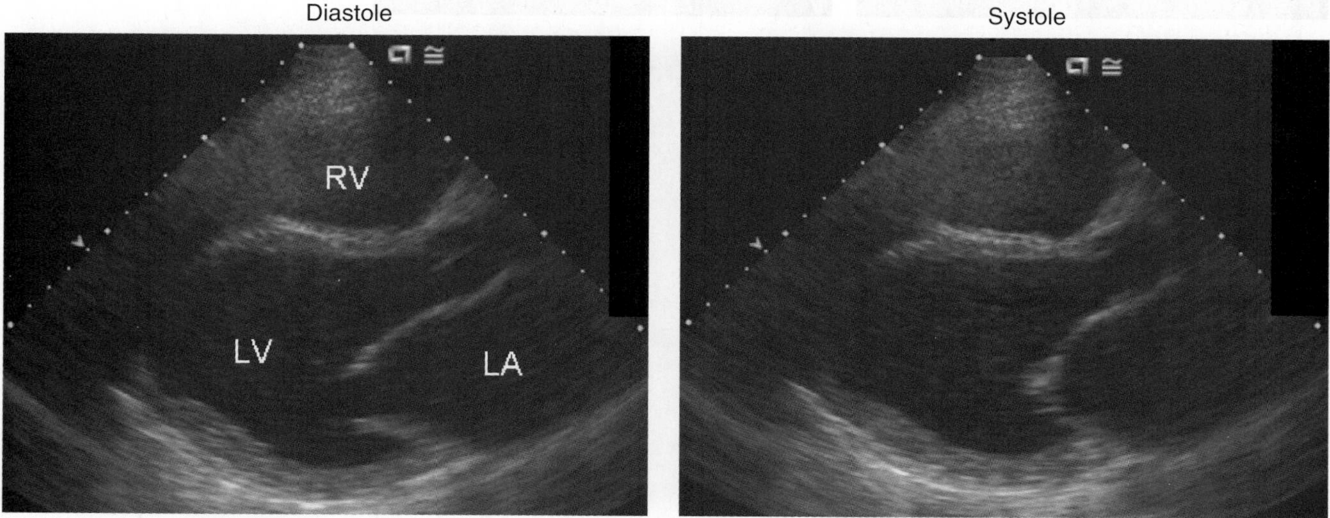

■ **Figure 13-12** Parasternal long axis images in diastole and systole in a patient with a severe dilated cardiomyopathy. There is not much difference in the size of the left ventricle between diastole and systole, indicating poor systolic function. RV, right ventricle; LV, left ventricle; LA, left atrium. (Echo courtesy of University of Washington Medical Center, Seattle, Washington.)

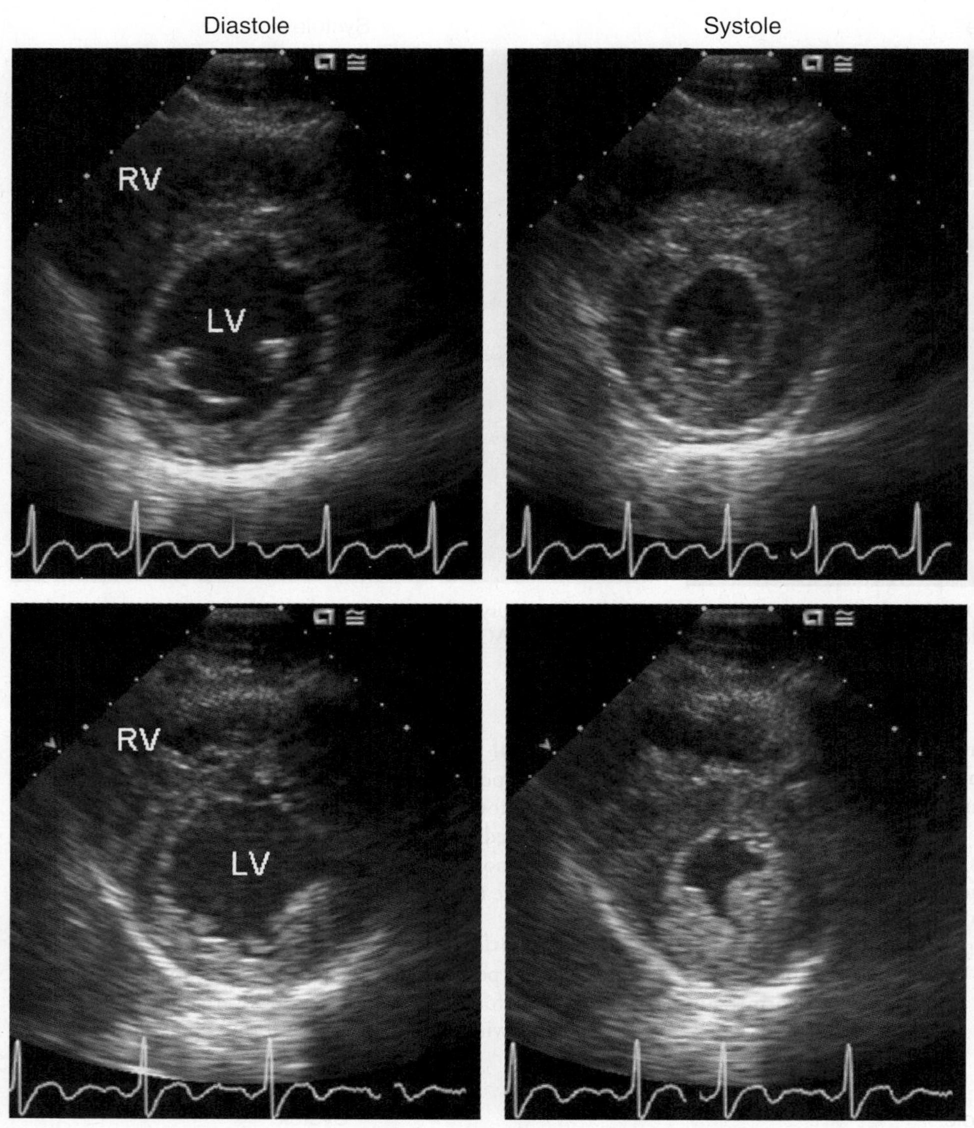

■ **Figure 13-13** *Top:* Parasternal basal short axis at the level of the mitral annulus. *Bottom:* Parasternal mid short axis at the level of papillary muscles. RV, right ventricle; LV, left ventricle. (Echo courtesy of University of Washington Medical Center, Seattle, Washington.)

axis of the heart. By rotating the transducer, multiple different orientations of the long axis of the heart are produced so that each wall of the left ventricle can be visualized (Fig. 13-14).

Subcostal Window

The patient is positioned in the supine position with the knees bent. The transducer is placed just below the xiphoid process of the sternum and images are obtained through the diaphragm. In this window, imaging is performed in the long and short axis of the heart (Fig. 13-15).

Suprasternal Window

The patient is positioned in the supine position with the chin tilted upward and rightward. In this window, imaging is performed in the long and short axis (Fig. 13-16).

SPECIAL ECHO TECHNIQUES

Transesophageal Echo

Transesophageal echo (TEE) uses an imaging crystal placed on the end of a flexible probe that is inserted into the esophagus and stomach to image the heart. Because the distance between the transducer and the heart is reduced, the spatial resolution of TEE is much improved for some (but not all) structures of the heart, resulting in superior image quality. Image quality with transthoracic echo is not always of diagnostic quality and TEE can improve it. For certain clinical circumstances, transthoracic echo cannot provide the diagnostic accuracy needed and TEE is recommended. The specific clinical circumstances may suggest whether TEE is needed but some indications include aortic dissection, valvular endocarditis, prosthetic valve malfunction, left atrial appendage thrombus, interatrial septal defect, and patent foramen ovale (Figs. 13-17 through 13-19).

TEE is usually performed by physicians (cardiologists or anesthesiologists) with the help of sonographers who aid in image acquisition. Depending upon the risk of conscious sedation, a nurse or anesthesiologist is also present to monitor the patient during the procedure (see below).

A detailed patient history should be obtained as there are contraindications (absolute and relative) to TEE. Dysphagia, esophageal strictures or webs, esophageal or gastric cancer, upper gastrointestinal bleeding, cervical neck trauma, thrombocytopenia,

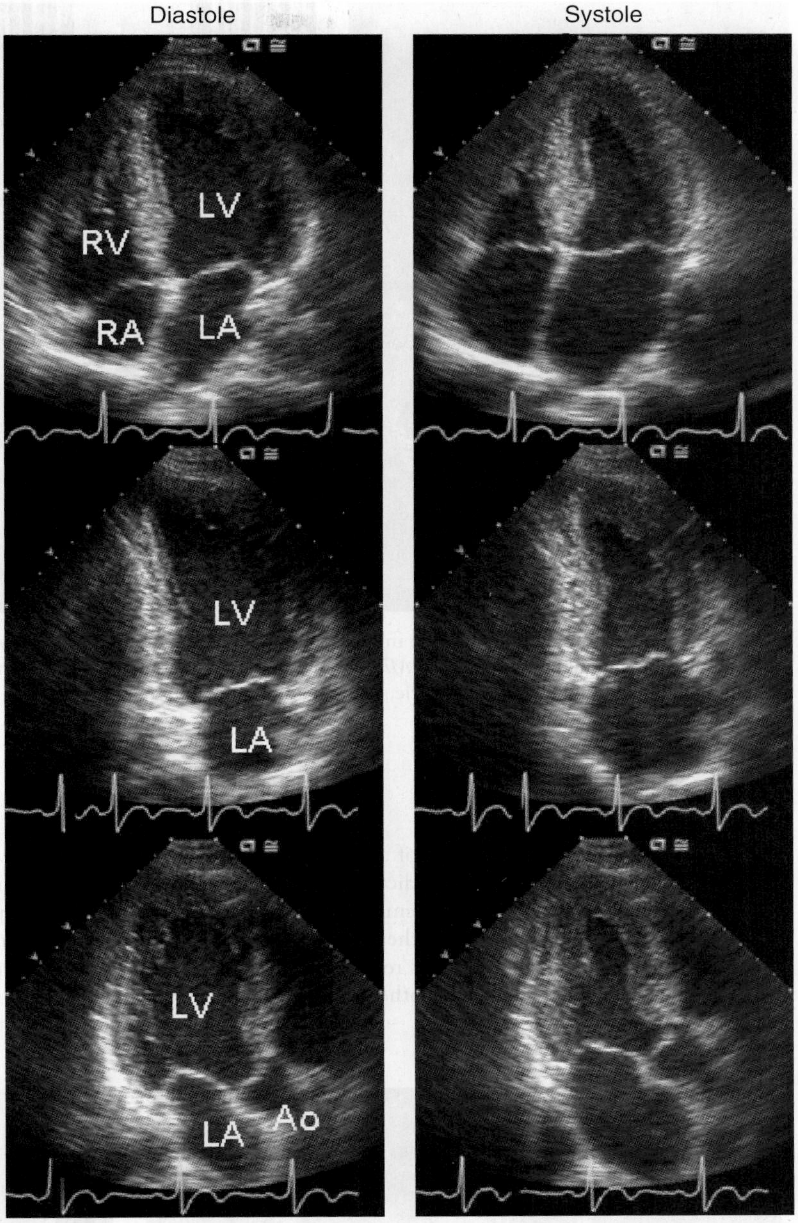

■ **Figure 13-14** *Top:* Apical four-chamber view. *Middle:* Apical two-chamber view. *Bottom:* Apical long axis view. RV, right ventricle; LV, left ventricle; RA, right atrium; LA, left atrium; Ao, aorta. (Echo courtesy of University of Washington Medical Center, Seattle, Washington.)

or coagulopathy are some contraindications that may require consultations with a gastroenterologist first. Anticoagulation with warfarin or heparin is not an absolute contraindication but the internationalized normalized ratio and partial thromboplastin time should be checked beforehand to ensure that supratherapeutic levels are not present. The patient should be fasting for 6 hours and the patient should remain fasting postprocedure until there is an appropriate level of consciousness and the local anesthetic of the posterior pharynx has dissipated.

For the procedure, the patient is positioned in the left lateral decubitus position to minimize the risk of aspiration. A topical anesthetic agent is used on the posterior pharynx to suppress the gag reflex, allowing easier passage of the probe into the esophagus. Typically, TEEs are performed under conscious sedation. Therefore, supervision by nurses with experience and training in sedative and analgesic administration, and in oral airway management is necessary. Conscious sedation requires that heart rate, blood pressure, respiration, and arterial oxygen saturation are monitored throughout the procedure. This monitoring is routinely performed by the nurse. However, clinical circumstances may exist where an anesthesiologist should be present during the procedure. An intravenous catheter is needed to administer analgesics and sedatives. Medicines to reverse analgesics (naloxone for opioids) and sedatives (flumazenil for benzodiazepines) should be readily available. Suctioning should always be available to manage excess oral secretions.

Risks of TEE include, but are not limited to, aspiration, bronchospasm, respiratory depression, or hypotension from sedation, bleeding, and trauma to the teeth, esophagus or stomach such as perforation.[2]

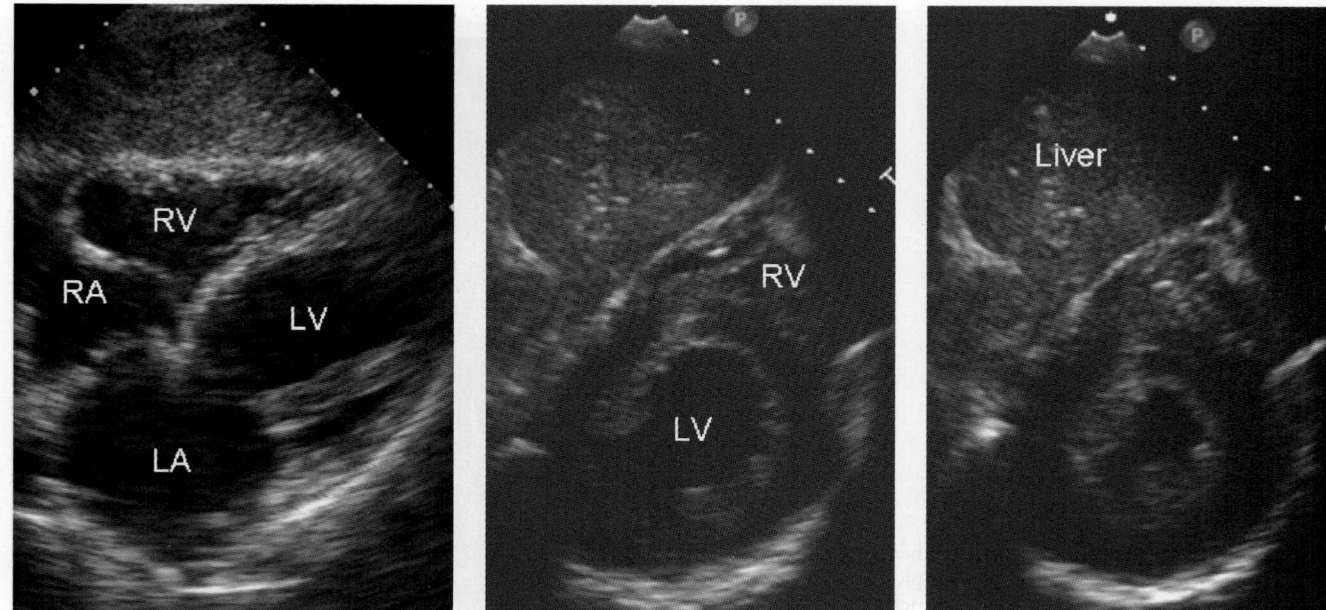

■ **Figure 13-15** These images are from the subcostal window as evidenced by the liver at the top of images. *Left:* Subcostal long axis. *Middle:* Subcostal short axis in diastole. *Right:* Subcostal short axis in systole. RA, right atrium; RV, right ventricle; LA, left atrium; LV, left ventricle. (Echo courtesy of Harborview Medical Center, Seattle, Washington.)

Contrast Echo

There are several purposes for the use of contrast in echocardiography. The diagnostic indication will dictate the specific type of contrast. One simple classification system of echo contrast agents is whether the contrast agent crosses the pulmonary vasculature microcirculation. Some contrast agents remain in the venous circulation (right heart structures) while others will be in the venous and arterial circulation (right and left heart structures). Echo contrast agents are composed of bubbles. The size of the bubbles determines whether they will cross the pulmonary vasculature microcirculation. Red blood cells cross the pulmonary capillaries and are 6 to 8 μm in diameter.

Saline microbubbles (agitated saline) are commonly used for detection of shunts, primarily because the bubbles are too large to cross the pulmonary vasculature microcirculation (Fig. 13-20).

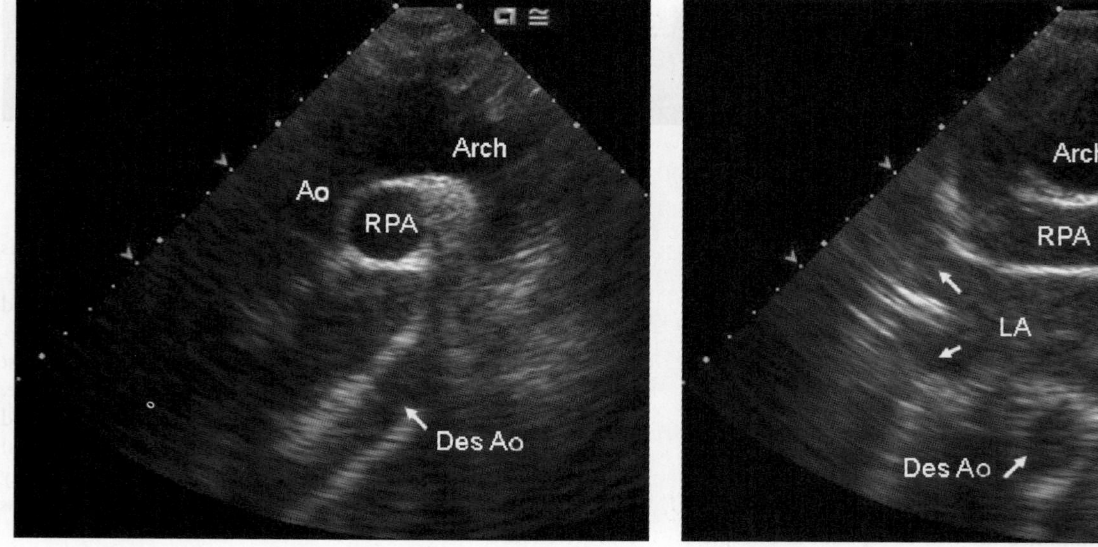

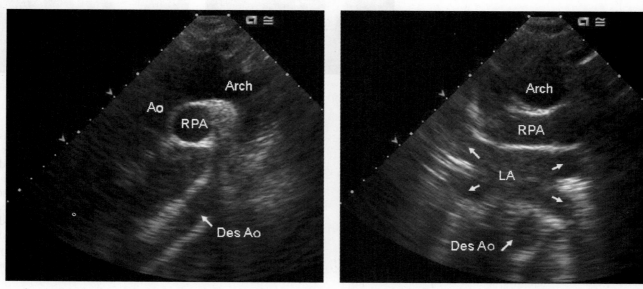

■ **Figure 13-16** *Left:* Suprasternal long axis. *Right:* Suprasternal short axis. Ao, aorta; RPA, right pulmonary artery; Des Ao, descending thoracic aorta; LA, left atrium. Four arrows in left atrium identify each pulmonary vein. (Echo courtesy of University of Washington Medical Center, Seattle, Washington.)

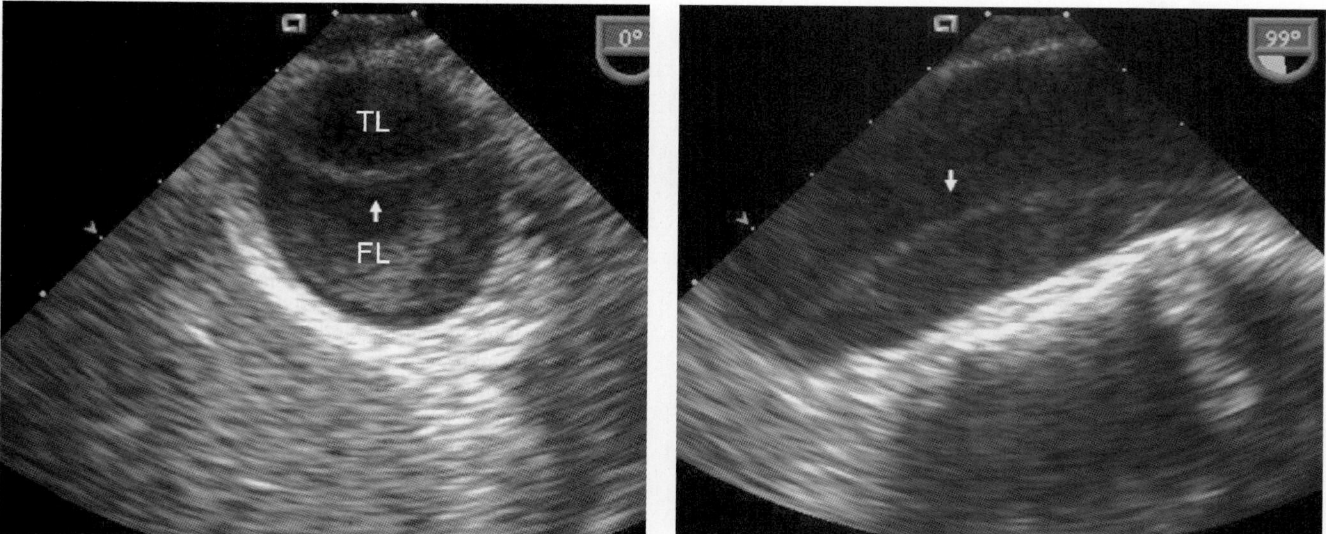

Figure 13-17 Transesophageal echo image of the descending thoracic aorta demonstrating a dissection flap (*arrow*), which creates a true lumen (TL) and false lumen (FL) in the short axis (*left*) and long axis (*right*). (Echo courtesy of University of Washington Medical Center, Seattle, Washington.)

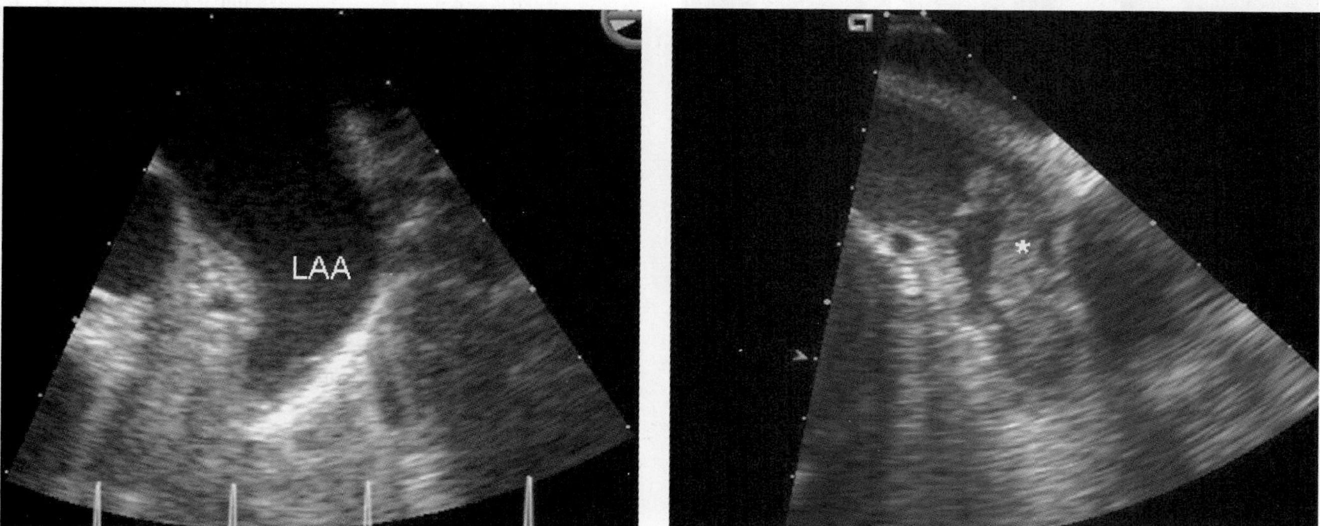

Figure 13-18 *Left:* A normal left atrial appendage (LAA) is a pouch-like structure arising from the left atrium. This LAA does not contain thrombus. Mitral stenosis and atrial fibrillation are risk factors for thrombus formation in the LAA. *Right:* Large thrombus (*) within the LAA. This patient had atrial fibrillation. (Echo courtesy of University of Washington Medical Center, Seattle, Washington.)

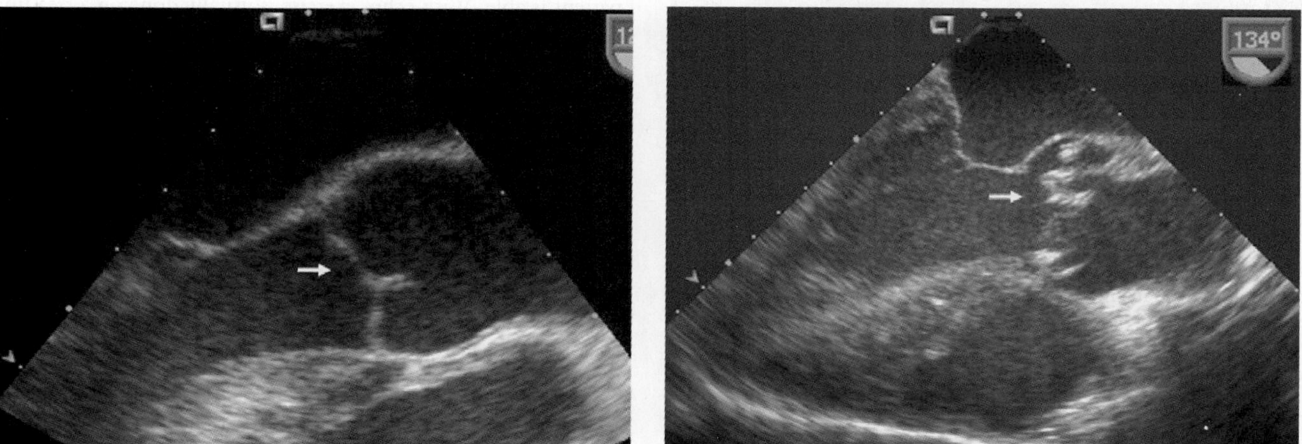

Figure 13-19 *Left:* Transesophageal echo image demonstrating normal aortic valve leaflets (*arrow*) in diastole. *Right:* Thickened aortic valve leaflets with masses attached, all consistent with infectious endocarditis. (Echo courtesy of University of Washington Medical Center, Seattle, Washington.)

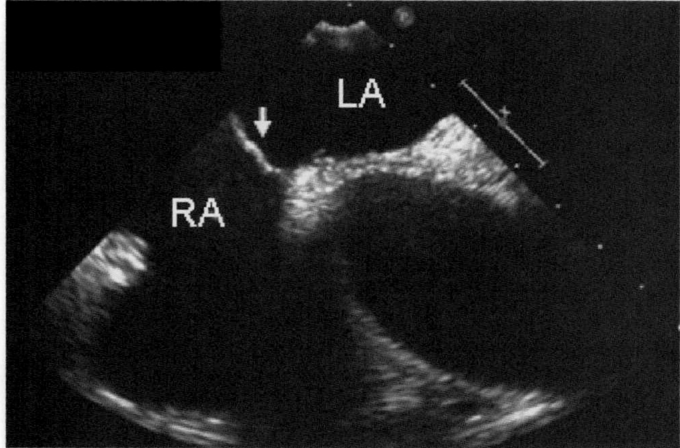

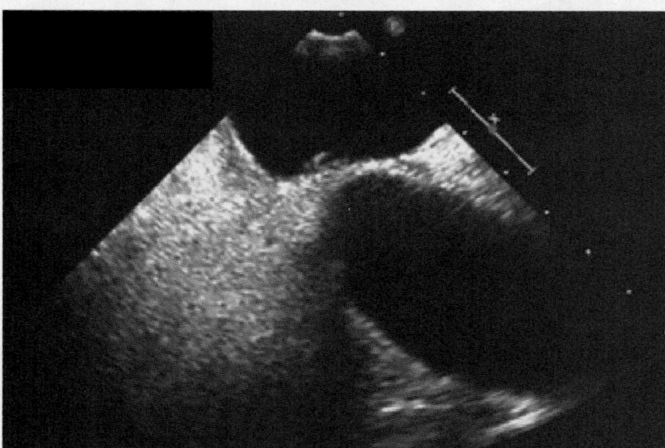

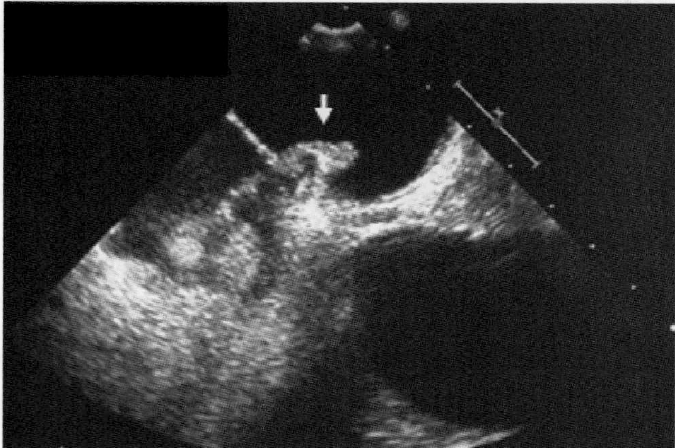

■ **Figure 13-20** *Top:* Transesophageal echo image demonstrating the right atrium (RA), left atrium (LA) and the interatrial septum (*arrow*). *Middle:* Same view as described above during the injection of saline microbubbles via an intravenous catheter. Notice that the right atrium is filled with the bubbles (*white*). *Bottom:* The next cardiac cycle demonstrates shunting of the microbubbles (*arrow*) through the interatrial septum into the left atrium, consistent with a patent foramen ovale. (Echo courtesy of Harborview Medical Center, Seattle, Washington.)

Saline microbubbles are injected into an intravenous catheter and opacify the right side of the heart. Because the microbubbles are larger (>8 µm) than red blood cells, they cannot cross the pulmonary vasculature and are absorbed by the lungs. Therefore, they should not opacify the left heart structures. Saline microbubbles that do appear in the left side of the heart are indicative of a right-to-left shunt (i.e., atrial septal defect, patent foramen ovale, pulmonary arterial venous malformation). Saline microbubbles are created by connecting a two-way stopcock to an intravenous catheter with two 10-cc syringes. One syringe is filled with 9 cc of normal saline and 1 cc of air and then transferred to the empty syringe back and forth. This action makes bubbles of air throughout the saline. The full 10 cc is then *quickly* injected into the intravenous catheter. Emphasis is placed on quickly so as to achieve bolus opacification of contrast and not streaming of contrast of the right heart structures.

Lipid (Definity) or albumin (Optison) microspheres are commercially available contrast agents. They have a diameter of 1.1 to 4.5 µm and contain a gas (perfluoropropane) within their shell,[4,5] permitting opacification of the left ventricle because the microspheres are small enough to cross the pulmonary capillaries (Fig. 13-21). Opacification of the left ventricle allows improved endocardial definition, which enhances the diagnostic accuracy of global and regional wall motion assessment. Contraindications to the use of these contrast agents include: cardiac shunts, unstable congestive heart failure, acute myocardial infarction, ventricular arrhythmias, respiratory failure, pulmonary hypertension, intra-arterial injection, hypersensitivity to perflutren, or hypersensitivity to albumin (Optison).[4,5] Adverse effects are uncommon but can include back/chest pain, headache, dizziness, nausea, flushing, altered taste sensation, palpitations, urticaria, or anaphylaxis.[4,5]

Stress Echo

Stress echo is performed in combination with continuous 12-lead ECG monitoring to improve the diagnostic accuracy of coronary artery detection or risk stratification of patients with known coronary artery disease. Image acquisition is performed in the same standard views, as described previously and optimal endocardial definition is necessary. Sometimes, contrast is needed to provide endocardial definition to visualize wall motion. Global and regional wall motion is compared from rest to stress periods. A normal finding: a myocardial segment has normal function at rest and hyperdynamic function at stress. An abnormal finding suggestive of obstructive coronary artery disease: a myocardial segment has normal function at rest and becomes hypokinetic or akinetic at stress (Fig. 13-22).

The preferred method of stress testing is exercise, provided the patient is able. With echo, exercise is usually done on a treadmill or supine bicycle. For treadmill exercise, rest images are performed while the patient is lying on the examination bed. The patient then exercises on the treadmill with continuous ECG monitoring. When peak exercise is achieved, the patient is quickly moved from the treadmill back to the examination bed and imaging is repeated. This sequencing requires practice and coordination. The longer it takes to perform the imaging after peak exercise, the heart rate decreases and so does the sensitivity of the test. Image acquisition should occur within 60 seconds of the termination of peak exercise. With supine bicycle stress, imaging can be performed *throughout* the exercise period. With treadmill stress, imaging can only be performed *after* exercise is complete. However, the physiological workload with bicycle stress is not the same as treadmill. Some studies have shown that patients are more apt to achieve their peak aerobic capacity with treadmill stress as opposed to bicycle stress.[6] During exercise stress, a physician, nurse practitioner, or physician's assistant is

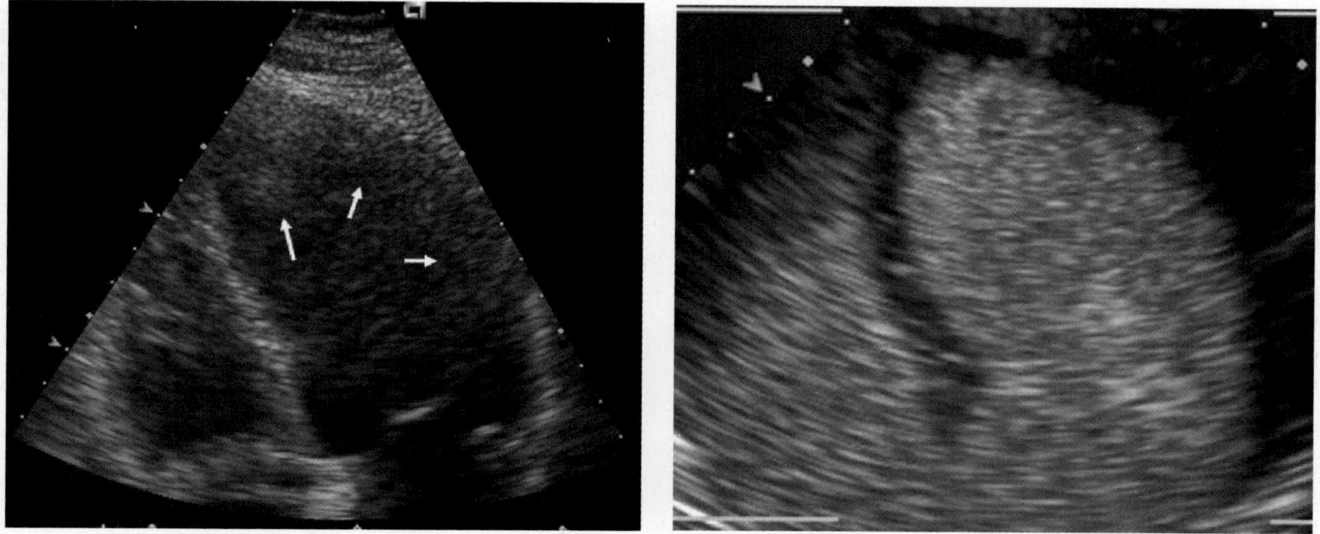

■ **Figure 13-21** *Left:* Apical four-chamber view in a patient with poor endocardial definition and thus suboptimal image quality. *Right:* The same patient with improved image quality with the administration of a transpulmonary contrast agent (Definity). Notice the endocardial definition is now of diagnostic quality. (Echo courtesy of University of Washington Medical Center, Seattle, Washington.)

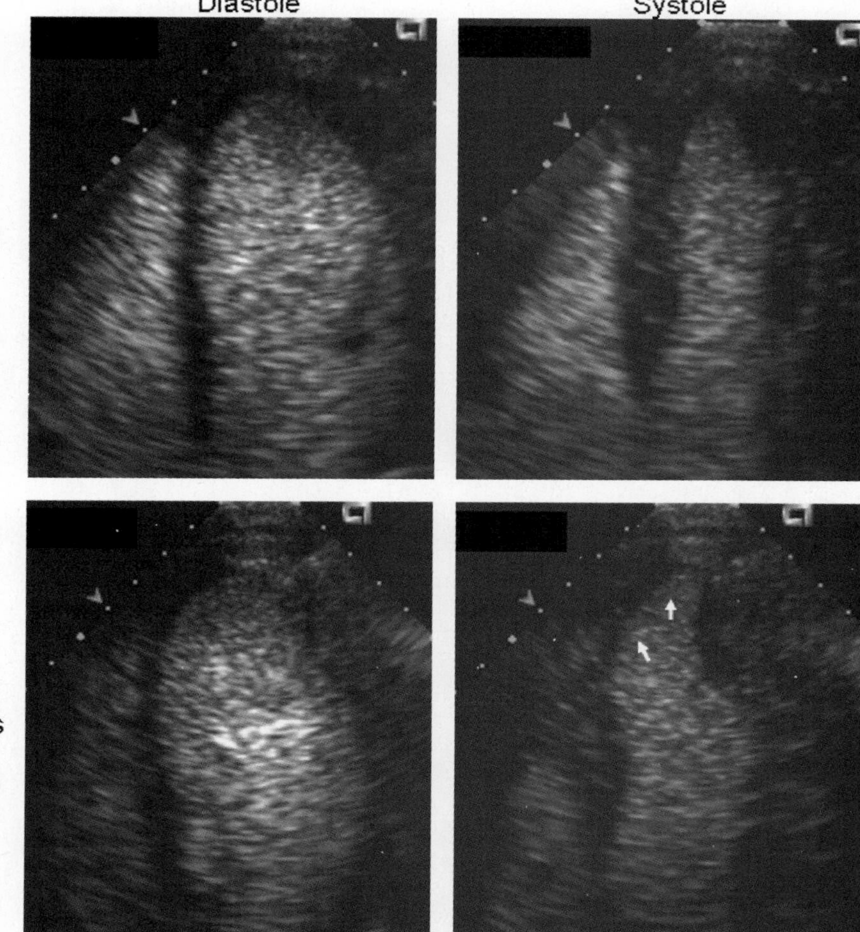

■ **Figure 13-22** Apical four-chamber view of patient undergoing a dobutamine stress echo. *Top:* At rest, there is normal wall motion and the left ventricular cavity is noticeably smaller in systole. *Bottom:* During peak stress, the left ventricular cavity is smaller in systole but there is a noticeable wall motion abnormality in the apical septum and apex (*arrows*), which would be consistent with obstructive epicardial disease in the left anterior descending coronary artery. (Echo courtesy of Harborview Medical Center, Seattle, Washington.)

usually present and responsible for supervising the test (i.e., taking blood pressures, examining the ECG). A sonographer is present for image acquisition; an ECG technician may also be present.

For those patients who cannot exercise, dobutamine is the most common stress agent used; however, it should be understood that dobutamine does not completely simulate the physiological state of exercise. A nurse should be present during dobutamine infusion since medications need to be given intravenously. Starting doses are between 5 and 10 mcg/kg/min, increasing by 10 mcg/kg/min increments every 3 minutes to a peak of 40 mcg/kg/min. Doses of atropine can be given and physical maneuvers can be performed in addition to dobutamine infusion to achieve 85% of the maximally predicted heart rate.

3-D

3-dimensional echo displays a volume of data within 3 spatial orientations.[2] This field is in much flux and clinical applications of this technique are being investigated. Some applications that may hold promise include (but are not limited too) improved assessment of ventricular volumes, improved assessment of the valvular apparatus, and improved detection of thrombus within the left atrial appendage. It is important to remember though that the same artifacts and limitations that apply to 2-D echo also apply to 3-D echo.

REFERENCES

1. Feigenbaum, H., Armstrong, W. F., & Ryan, T. (Eds.). (2005). *Feigenbaum's echocardiography* (6th ed.). Philadelphia: Lippincott Williams & Wilkins.
2. Otto, C. M. (2004). *Textbook of clinical echocardiography* (3rd ed.). Philadelphia: W.B. Saunders.
3. Weyman, A. E. (1994). *Principles and practice of echocardiography* (2nd ed.). Philadelphia: Lea & Febiger.
4. Definity® (2007). Perflutren Lipid Microsphere [Package Insert]. Billerica, MA: Bristol-Myers Squibb Medical Imaging.
5. Optison™ (2003). Perflutren Protein-Type A Microspheres [Package Insert]. Princeton, NJ: Amersham Health.
6. Ellestad, M. H. (1996). *Stress testing: Principles and practice* (4th ed.). New York: Oxford University Press.

CHAPTER 14

Nuclear, Magnetic Resonance, and Computed Tomography Imaging

Laurie A. Soine / Peter J. Cawley

Many advances have been made in noninvasive cardiovascular imaging over the last 20 years. Fueled by scientific advances in the fields of computer technology, processing and storing images, physics, biochemistry, and engineering noninvasive cardiovascular imaging has become a widely available clinical tool. Nuclear cardiology, magnetic resonance imaging (MRI), computed tomography (CT), and ultrasound (echocardiography, or echo) are different imaging modalities able to create tomographic images of cardiovascular structures. A tomogram is an imaging "section" or "slice" of an object created by an imaging modality.

NUCLEAR CARDIOLOGY

Radionuclides, substances that emit radioactivity, have been used as a tracer in the body for more than 65 years. Since the development of the γ-ray camera by Anger some 30 years ago and the introduction of radioactive potassium analogs, the use of radionuclides (radiotracers) to study the heart has been the subject of increasing clinical application. The introduction of new and improved radioisotopes and imaging techniques in the 1980s led to widespread clinical application.

Radioisotope Pharmaceuticals

Radionuclides are atoms in an unstable form. They have a finite probability of spontaneously converting to a more stable configuration. When they do so, small amounts of energy in the form of rays are emitted. The rate at which atoms in a given sample undergo this conversion is denoted by the half-life, the time required for one half of the sample to undergo the conversion. Half-lives of radioactive substances vary from a fraction of a second to a millennia; the half-life for any given radionuclide is always the same. The characteristics of an ideal radiotracer to assess myocardial blood flow would include: a half-life long enough to allow for convenient imaging, easy combination with biologic substances, 100% myocardial extraction across the entire spectrum of achievable or inducible coronary blood flow states, instantaneous intracellular binding, low extraction and clearance by organs adjacent to the heart, and extraction by only viable cells. Unfortunately, to date, no commercially available radiotracer of myocardial perfusion meets all of these criteria.

Single-photon emission computed tomography (SPECT) and positron emission tomography (PET) are the two most common nuclear cardiovascular imaging modalities. The three most common radiotracers used in SPECT imaging are thallium 201 (^{201}Tl) and the two technetium 99m-labeled tracers: ^{99m}Tc-sestamibi (Cardiolite) and ^{99m}Tc-tetrofosmin (Myoview). Nitrogen-13-ammonia, oxygen-15 labeled water, and rubidium-82 are the most common tracers used in PET imaging to assess blood flow; fluorine-18-2-fluoro-2-deoxyglucose is used in PET imaging to assess myocardial metabolism.

Injection and detection of these radiotracers allow for the measurement of relative myocardial blood flow. The radiotracers follow blood flow and are extracted from the blood pool by myocytes in proportion to blood flow. The mechanism by which the various radiotracers, used in SPECT and PET imaging, are extracted from the blood stream and taken up by myocytes varies. In SPECT imaging, the radioactive decay of tracer is detected outside the body as scintillation (flash of light) by a gamma scintillation camera. The camera functions as a scanning device (large Geiger counter) to detect the distribution of radioactivity emitting from the myocardium through the chest wall, allowing examination of myocardial structure and function. ^{201}Tl is a potassium analog. Because of the dynamic equilibrium of potassium between cells and the blood pool, potassium and therefore ^{201}Tl, distributes in the myocardium in proportion to the blood flow. Myocytes with an intact sodium–potassium pump take up ^{201}Tl. However, the relatively low energy (60 keV) emitted by ^{201}Tl makes imaging of this tracer suboptimal in large patients. The technetium 99m-labeled radiotracers passively distribute across sarcolemmal and mitochondrial membranes and remain intracellularly bound. The relatively higher energy (140 keV) emitted by this group of tracers allows for improved transmission through the chest tissue resulting in improved image quality, particularly in large patients.

PET imaging likewise allows for quantitative and tomographic imaging of myocardial perfusion and metabolism without intrinsically altering these processes. A positron-emitting radiotracer travels only a short distance in tissue prior to encountering an electron. This interaction causes annihilation of both particles, producing two high-energy photons that depart at an angle of 180 degrees from each other. PET imaging systems are designed to detect the two photons, which travel in opposite directions at essentially the speed of light (511 keV). By measuring the time that it takes for each photon to encounter the circumferential ring of detectors, localization of the event can be mathematically derived.

Diagnostic Indications for Nuclear Imaging

Table 14-1 summarizes the diagnostic uses of the imaging modalities discussed in this chapter. Stress myocardial perfusion with SPECT and PET imaging is useful clinically for the detection of flow-limiting coronary artery disease and risk stratification for patients with known coronary heart disease.[1] The clinical aim of these studies is to evaluate the physiology of coronary blood flow. Myocardial perfusion images provide the clinician and patient

Table 14-1 ■ CLINICAL APPLICATION OF TOMOGRAPHIC IMAGING MODALITIES

	Nuclear (SPECT/PET)	MRI	CT	Echo
Anatomy				
Chambers	+++	++++	++++	++++
Valves	–	++	++	++++
Large vessels	–	++++	++++	++
Coronary arteries	–	++	++++	+
Pericardium	–	++++	++++	+
Physiology				
Myocardial perfusion (ischemia)	++++	+++	–	++
Global & regional ventricular function	++++	++++	+	++++
Ventricular volumes	++++	++++	–	+++
Valve function	–	+++	+	++++
Tissue Characterization				
Myocardial viability / infarction	++++	++++	–	+++
Masses	++++	++++	++++	++
Larger vessel wall atherosclerosis atherosclerosis	++	++	++	–

++++ Indicates most useful, – Indicates not useful.

with important predictive and prognostic information, including left ventricular (LV) chamber size, and global and regional LV function; location, size, and extent of impairment of coronary flow reserve (myocardial ischemia); and location, size, and extent of myocardial infarction.[2]

Stress myocardial perfusion imaging involves comparing the pattern of myocardial blood flow, as reflected by myocyte uptake of radiotracer, in a resting state and in the hyperemic or stress state. The goals of stress perfusion imaging are creating heterogeneity of myocardial blood flow, marking this effect with a radiotracer, and applying SPECT or PET to obtain images of myocardial uptake.

The most common stress myocardial perfusion study using SPECT imaging is the "dual" (two) isotope imaging protocol. This protocol uses ^{201}Tl to evaluate the pattern of myocardial blood flow at rest and a technetium 99m-labeled product (sestamibi or tetrofosmin) to obtain the stress images. However, increasingly low doses of technetium 99m-labeled products are injected at rest followed by higher doses at peak stress. Regardless of the radiotracer used, the premise remains the same—obtaining images of myocardial blood flow at rest and comparing these images to a pattern of radiotracer myocardial uptake in the stressed state. Thus, all patients receive an intravenous (IV) injection of radiotracer while sitting quietly at rest. A gated set of SPECT or PET myocardial perfusion images are then immediately acquired. After acquisition of the images at rest, the patient is "stressed," or rather a hyperemic state of coronary blood flow is created, and this state is marked with a second radiotracer injection. A patient reaches the stress state by exercising on the treadmill, and achieving 85% of the maximal predicted heart rate for age (220 − patient's age × 0.85). In patients with normal coronary arteries, as the heart rate and blood pressure rise in response to exercise, normal coronary arteries dilate. Coronary flow reserve is maintained in arteries with less than 70% stenosis.[3] In contrast, a region of the myocardium supplied by a diseased artery is unable to appropriately dilate in response to increasing myocardial work resulting in a relative reduction in blood flow/radiotracer uptake compared with normal coronary arteries. Studies of myocardial blood flow have demonstrated that at a heart rate of 85% of maximal predicted for age, blood flow through a normal coronary artery increases approximately two-fold. Therefore, at peak exercise, regions of the myocardium supplied by normal coronary arteries receive two-fold the amount of radiotracer compared with regions of the myocardium supplied by diseased vessels, unable to dilate. In patients unable to exercise adequately, an IV infusion of dipyridamole (0.57 mg/kg infused over 4 minutes) or adenosine (140 mcg/kg/min) reproduce this hyperemic state. The vasodilator agents do not stress the myocardium but rather dilate normal coronary arteries, having little effect on diseased vessels. At the standard infusion doses and rates, these agents dilate normal coronary arteries four- to five-fold.[4] Following the stress study, a second set of gated SPECT or PET images are acquired.

The rest and post-stress gated SPECT images when processed and reconstructed, reflect the pattern of myocardial blood flow in the two states. The images are reconstructed in standardized views (short, vertical, and horizontal long axis). Patterns of radiotracer uptake are compared between the two datasets. A segmental scoring system has become a widely applied quantitative tool to integrate the extent and severity of perfusion abnormalities.[5] Summed stress score is a quantitative tool used to evaluate the extent and severity of myocardium at risk.[6] The score is determined by dividing the myocardium into 17 segments, scoring the percent reduction in radiotracer uptake, and adding the segments. The 17-segment representation of the myocardium is a standard format used in most myocardial imaging modalities.

A segment or region of the myocardium that has reduced radiotracer uptake on the images obtained at stress state that appears more uniform (improved) on the images obtained at rest is consistent with myocardial ischemia. The severity of the impairment of coronary flow reserve can be qualitatively estimated by the degree of reduction of radiotracer uptake (i.e., mildly reduced, moderately reduced, or severely reduced uptake). A segment or region of the myocardium with a fixed (i.e., present on both rest and stress) reduction in radiotracer uptake on both stress and rest images is most consistent with myocardial injury or infarction. An alternative explanation of an apparent fixed region of reduced radiotracer uptake that thickens and moves normally on gated cines may be attenuation artifact. The most common attenuating structures include breast tissue (anterior wall) and diaphragm (inferior wall). A reversible abnormality (present on stress, not on rest) is consistent with myocardial ischemia (Fig. 14-1).

The summed stress score (extent and severity of ischemia and infarction) when combined with Duke Treadmill Score has been shown to be an independent predictor of cardiac death[7] (Fig. 14-2). In addition to increasing the identification and quantification of coronary artery disease, stress myocardial perfusion data have been shown to be an independent additional predictor of serious cardiac events in the ensuing year in men and women of all ages, as well as patients with diabetes.[2,7–11]

Stress myocardial perfusion using PET imaging provides a more quantitative measurement of coronary blood flow. By comparing absolute blood flow at rest with absolute flow in a hyperemic state created by a vasodilator infusion, impairment of coronary flow reserve can be more precisely measured. PET imaging allows for precise detection of global impairment in coronary flow reserve and therefore may increasingly be useful

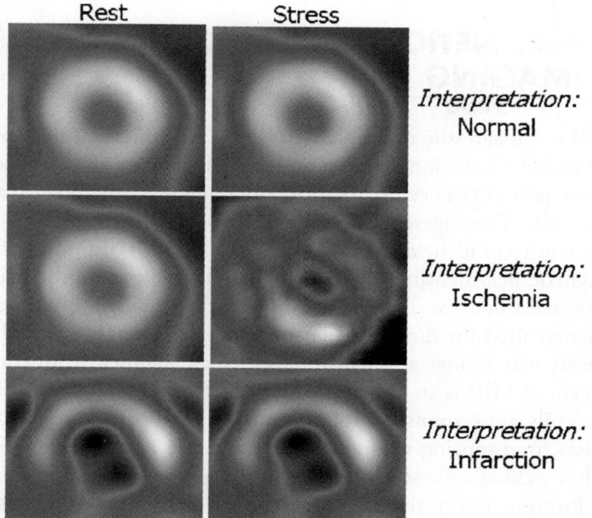

Figure 14-1 Stress and rest SPECT myocardial perfusion images. Top panel demonstrates no abnormalities in radiotracer uptake on either stress or rest image and are normal. Middle panel demonstrates a defect at stress but none at rest, consistent with myocardial ischemia. Lower panel demonstrates a defect at stress and rest, consistent with myocardial infarction. (Images obtained from University of Washington Medical Center, Department of Radiology, Division of Nuclear Medicine, Seattle, Washington.)

in the diagnosis of microvascular disease. Several of the radiotracers used in PET imaging require an on-site cyclotron for radiotracer generation. Thus, widespread application of PET imaging is currently limited by the cost associated with generating the radiotracers.

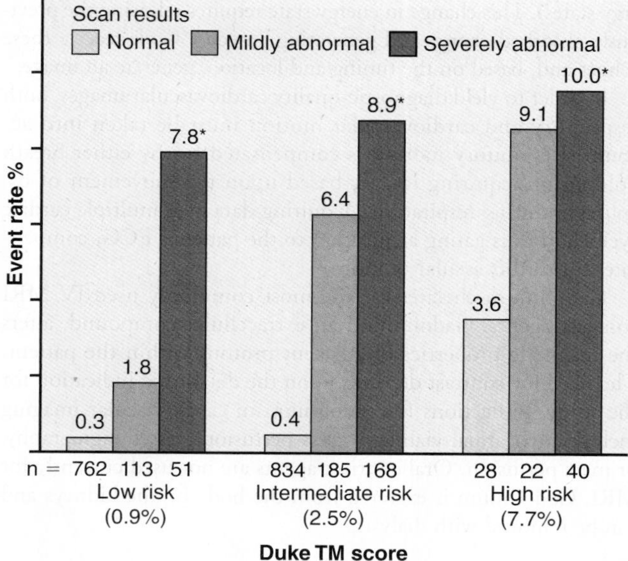

Figure 14-2 SPECT myocardial perfusion scan results add incremental prognostic data when combined with Duke Treadmill (TM) score. Event rates for myocardial infarction or cardiac death are shown in parentheses under Duke TM subgroups. $^{*}p < .05$ across scan results. (Adapted from Hachamovitch, R., Berman, D. S., Kiat, H., et al. [1996]. Exercise myocardial perfusion SPECT in patients without known coronary artery disease: incremental prognostic value and use in risk stratification. *Circulation, 93*, 905.)

Myocardial Viability

LV dysfunction and associated heart failure is increasing in both incidence and prevalence in the United States. The mortality and morbidity associated with LV dysfunction and heart failure are high.[12] While dramatic advances in medical therapy have resulted in improved survival and functional capacity, the best and most definitive therapy, when appropriate, is revascularization. Coronary artery disease accounts for approximately two thirds of cases of heart failure in the United States.[13] Imaging studies to assess myocardial viability help identify patients who may benefit from revascularization. Myocardial viability is described as a condition of chronic sustained abnormal contraction of the myocardium secondary to chronic underperfusion, in patients with known coronary artery disease and in whom revascularization results in recovery of LV function.[14] LV dysfunction may not be the result of irreversible scar but rather caused by impairment in function and energy use of viable myocytes—myocytes that if fueled with adequate blood flow would demonstrate improved function. Chronic myocardial ischemia is associated with a severe reduction in contractile function. Patients with LV dysfunction who have viable myocardium are at highest risk of cardiac death, but at the same time benefit most from revascularization.[15–18] In contrast to infarct-related scar, dysfunctional but viable myocardium has the potential to regain function.[19]

^{201}Tl combined with SPECT imaging has historically been the most common radionuclide used for distinguishing viable or hibernating myocardium from scar. ^{201}Tl is injected in the resting state; gated SPECT images immediately acquired reflect myocardial perfusion. Delayed images acquired 4 to 24 hours later represent tissue metabolism. A region of the myocardium with reduced perfusion (resting thallium uptake) but preserved metabolism (improved thallium uptake on delay images), defines myocardial viability.[20] Myocardial viability studies with ^{201}Tl are clinically helpful in patients with multivessel coronary artery disease and LV dysfunction. Potential reversibility of LV dysfunction is an important clinical consideration in these patients. Multiple studies have demonstrated that patients with viable myocardium benefit from revascularization versus augmented medical therapy. Alternatively, patients without evidence of viability do not show this same improvement after revascularization.[21,22]

PET imaging is emerging as a precise method for the detection of myocardial viability. The use of fluorine-18-2-fluoro-2-deoxyglucose (FDG) to assess myocardial metabolism and nitrogen-13-ammonia to assess perfusion, result in a highly sensitive study for differentiating viable myocardium from scar.[23,24] A perfusion–metabolism mismatch pattern has become synonymous with reversible contractile dysfunction and thus prediction of improvement in LV function after revascularization.[25]

Patient Preparation for Myocardial Perfusion Studies

It is recommended that patients fast for 6 hours before injection of radionuclides. This preparation minimizes gastrointestinal blood flow, resulting in reduced gastric uptake of radionuclides. Consider holding cardiac medications, particularly nitrates, β-blockers, and calcium-channel blockers, before stress studies, because these agents have been shown to reduce the sensitivity of the study for the detection of myocardial ischemia.[26] However, medication administration prior to the study depends upon the clinical question at hand. If a provider is attempting to establish the diagnosis of coronary artery disease, then it is recommended that cardiac medications be held. In a patient with known disease undergoing risk stratification, continuing medications is a reasonable option. Patients should be warned that they may activate radiation detectors (e.g., at the U.S. border crossings and airports) in the days following injection of radiotracers. A letter is commonly given to a patient planning a trip in the days following SPECT or PET imaging.

Radionuclide Ventriculogram

A radionuclide ventriculogram (RNVG), also known as an MUGA (multiple gated acquisition) study, is a procedure in which a small amount of the patient's blood is withdrawn, labeled with a technetium 99m-labeled radionuclide, and then reinjected. Using the electrocardiogram (ECG) signal for timing (gating), images are acquired throughout the cardiac cycle. Radioactive scintillation counts from corresponding time segments are summed to augment image clarity. In this way, the manner in which the radioactivity (and hence the blood pool) changes over the cardiac cycle is demonstrated.[27] This summed cardiac cycle can be played back as a cine loop video display of a normally recurring cardiac cycle. LV ejection fraction (EF), right ventricular (RV) EF, and segmental wall motion can be precisely calculated. The video display resembles a contrast LV or RV angiogram. Variation in radioactive counts over time is analyzed to provide information about systolic function. Rhythm disturbances, such as atrial fibrillation or frequent premature contractions altering beat-to-beat filling and cycle length, may decrease quantitative accuracy. RNVG is commonly used to evaluate cardiac function in patients with heart failure and valvular heart disease or to monitor the potential cardiotoxic effects of the commonly used chemotherapeutic agents.

Patient Preparation for RNVG

There is no special patient preparation for an RNVG study. The patient may continue to take all medications. The entire study usually takes approximately 30 minutes. Patients should be warned that they may activate radiation detectors (e.g., at U.S. border crossings and airports) in the days following injection of radiotracers. A letter is commonly given to a patient planning a trip in the days following an RNVG.

Risks of Radionuclides

In contrast to radioactive substances used for therapeutic (tissue ablation) purposes, radiopharmaceuticals used for imaging have short half-lives (minutes to several hours), contributing to their relatively rapid decay in the body. They are used in very small amounts. Thus, there is no need to isolate patients who have had these studies, and no particular precautions are needed for disposal of body substances (including blood, urine, or stool). The risk to a fetus is small, but it is recommended that patients who are pregnant or breast-feeding not undergo injection of radionuclides. Personnel should remember that radioactivity decreases dramatically with distance from the source. Personnel who work in nuclear medicine departments wear detection badges like those worn by radiology personnel to monitor their exposure.

MAGNETIC RESONANCE IMAGING

MRI is a diagnostic noninvasive imaging modality that does not use ionizing radiation like CT or nuclear imaging. It is composed of two parts: (1) an external superconducting magnet, and (2) various coils. The superconducting magnet is described in terms of the density of its field strength. Tesla (T) is a unit of measure for magnetic field density: the higher the tesla, the greater the magnetic field density. The most common field density of clinical magnets used for cardiovascular imaging is 1.5 T. However, this density may change as the field progresses. The other major component of MRI is an array of several different types of coils. Various coils are responsible for transmitting radiofrequency (RF) pulses, transmitting magnetic gradient pulses, and receiving RF pulses (echoes). These echoes are then processed into an image.

Protons, the positively charged nucleus of atoms, possess a concept known as "spin." "Spin" is the movement of the positive charge around the nucleus and possesses magnetic fields. These protons are oriented randomly in nature. When protons of the object to be imaged are exposed to the environment of a superconducting magnet, randomly oriented magnetic fields become oriented in one of two ways: a higher energy state or a lower energy state. To recap, the object that is placed into the bore of the magnet now contains protons that are no longer oriented randomly but are oriented in one of two energy states.

Coils transmit RF pulses and magnetic gradient pulses to the object within the bore of the magnet. This energy is used to change the direction of the magnetic fields of the protons to assume different energy levels in different imaging axes (x, y, z). After the transmitted pulses are turned off, the protons reassume their energy state prior to the transmission of the RF pulse (the higher or lower energy states). This change in energy state requires releasing the previously absorbed energy and generating an echo. Coils receive these echoes and, based on the timing and location, generate an image.

In order to yield diagnostic-quality cardiovascular images, both respiratory and cardiovascular motion must be taken into account. Respiratory motion is compensated for by either breath holding or acquiring images based upon the movement of diaphragm during respiration. Acquiring data over multiple cardiac cycles and thus gating acquisition to the patient's ECG, compensates for cardiovascular motion.

Gadolinium chelates are the most commonly used IV MRI contrast agents. Gadolinium, an extracellular compound, alters the magnetic properties of adjacent protons within the patient. The need for contrast depends upon the diagnostic indication for the study. Indications for gadolinium in cardiovascular imaging include myocardial viability, stress perfusion, vessel angiography, or mass perfusion. Oral contrast agents are not used currently for MRI. Gadolinium is excreted from the body by the kidneys and can be removed with dialysis.

Diagnostic Indications for Cariovascular MRI

Cardiovascular MRI provides diagnostic information on anatomy, physiology, and tissue characterization (Table 14-1). MRI provides anatomical descriptions of the size, location, and connection of all four cardiac chambers and valves (Fig. 14-3), which is

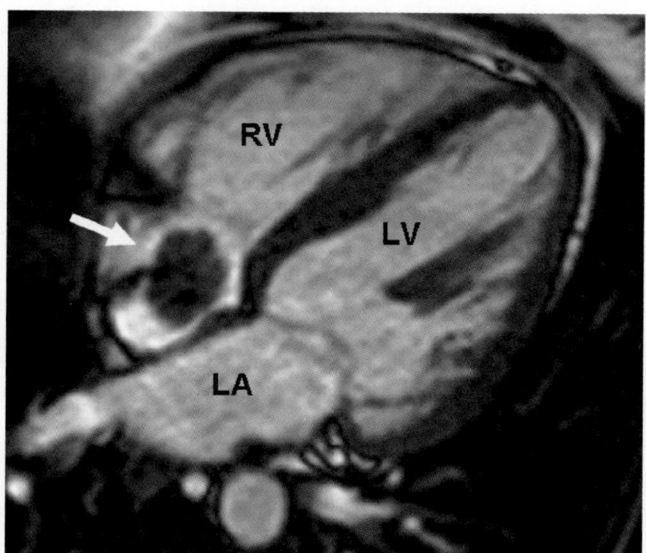

■ **Figure 14-3** Cardiac MRI demonstrating a large mass (arrow) located within the right atrium. RV, right ventricle; LV, left ventricle LA, left atrium. (Images obtained from University of Washington Medical Center, Department of Radiology, Seattle, Washington.)

important and useful information in congenital heart disease. In contrast to echocardiography (echo), MRI can easily provide anatomical information about the right ventricle. The right ventricle's anterior location within the thorax makes it especially difficult to visualize with echo. Furthermore, the utility of echo is limited in adult patients with congenital heart disease because of the smaller field of view and limited acoustic ultrasound windows due to scar tissue from prior surgeries.

Aneurysms and aberrant vascular connections can be easily assessed via MRI. Although MRI descriptions of coronary artery stenoses have been performed in research studies, MRI is not commonly performed clinically for that purpose. However, MRI allows descriptions of anomalous coronary artery origins and courses of the arteries near the great vessels. The pericardium can be visualized by MRI, and thus descriptions of pericardial thickness and locations of pericardial effusions can be provided. Ventricular volumes and function can be obtained by MRI because of the excellent visualization of endocardial borders.[28–31] The right ventricle is seen in limited views with echo and most commonly, the function is described qualitatively. As opposed to echo, quantitation of RV function can be performed in terms of RV volumes and EFs. Trans-valvular velocities, trans-valvular pressure gradients, and valve areas are all measures of the severity of valvular stenosis.[32–35] Typically, these measures are obtained by echo but can also be evaluated by MRI. Quantitation of the amount of valvular regurgitation (regurgitant volumes) can also be performed.[36,37]

Myocardial perfusion can be used to assess the presence or absence of flow-limited coronary artery disease.[38,39] Exercise testing is not performed. Instead, perfusion at stress can be assessed with vasodilator agents such as adenosine.

The ability of MRI to characterize tissues of the human body is a very important and powerful technique by MRI. Independent of wall motion, MRI can depict whether myocardial tissue is viable or scar (infarction)[40,41] (Fig. 14-4). The differential diagnosis of any intracardiac mass includes tumor and thrombus. MRI can help differentiate the two. Much of atherosclerosis imaging has been focused on the degree of luminal stenosis by conventional x-ray angiography. Imaging of the actual disease (wall) can be performed in larger vessels such as the carotid artery or aorta with correlations to histology.[42–46]

Patient Preparation for Magnetic Resonance Imaging

External magnetic fields can cause ferromagnetic metal (metals such as iron, which becomes magnetized when exposed to magnets)

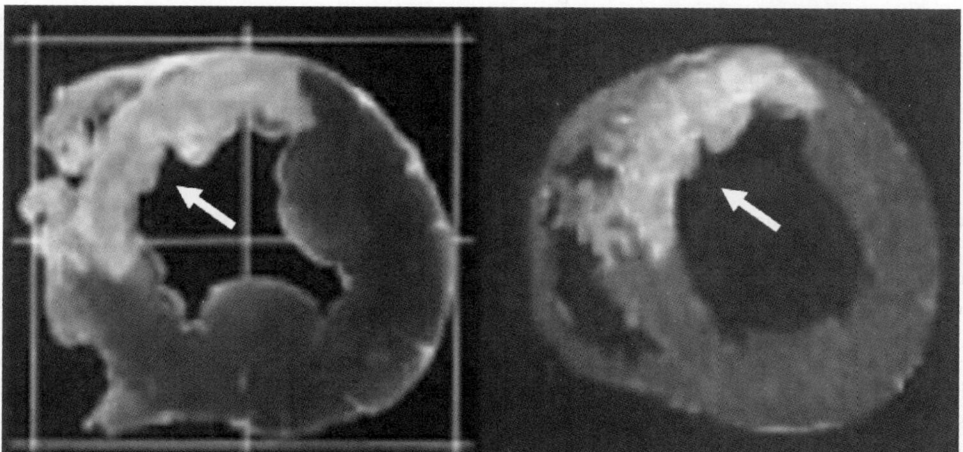

■ **Figure 14-4** *(Left)* Short axis photograph of gross pathology of canine heart stained with triphenyltetrazolium (TTC) to identify the area of myocardial infarction (white area marked by arrow). *(Right) Ex vivo* MRI with gadolinium obtained of that same gross specimen demonstrating a close correlation. In the MRI, the white area marked by the arrow is the area of myocardial infarction. (Adapted from Kim, R. J., Fieno, D. S., Parrish, T. B., et al. [1999]. Relationship of MRI delayed contrast enhancement to irreversible injury, infarct age, and contractile function. *Circulation, 100,* 1992–2002.)

to move or conduct energy into heat, either of which can cause serious bodily injury. Therefore, all patients undergoing an MRI should first undergo a formalized written screening process by a knowledgeable provider, nurse, or certified technician. Resources are available regarding the safety of various external and internal objects. One such Web site is http://www.mrisafety.com.[47]

While most patients tolerate MRI procedures well, some may experience claustrophobia and require sedation. Positioning a family member or friend in the same room as the patient may reduce anxiety. The family member or friend must also undergo MRI prescreening because they also are exposed to the external magnet. During imaging, loud noises are typically emitted from the magnet, so ear protection is required for safety. In order to minimize artifact, patients should not move inside of the MRI and may be asked to hold their breath for short periods. Blood pressure, heart rate, respirations, pulse oximetry, and an ECG rhythm strip are monitored.

If IV contrast is anticipated, an IV will need to be placed. Most contrast injections are performed via a power injector. Specialized, MRI-safe power injectors, IV pumps, and vital sign monitoring equipment must be used since all of this equipment is usually within the same room as the magnet.

Gadolinium chelates are safe and generally well tolerated. However, minor adverse reactions include headache, nausea, abdominal pain, flushing, or transient metallic taste. Recently, the Food and Drug Administration warned of an increased risk of nephrogenic systemic fibrosis in patients with acute or chronic renal insufficiency when exposed to gadolinium. This reaction may be delayed. Clinicians and patients should be informed of this risk when gadolinium use is anticipated; risks and benefits should be weighed on an individual basis.

COMPUTED TOMOGRAPHY

Modern day CT scanners are composed of a moving table and a circulating gantry surrounding the table, containing x-ray tubes (x-ray source) and detector arrays. The table moves through the center of the circulating gantry to expose the body to x-rays. Tubes within the gantry generate x-rays, and detector arrays measure the transmission of x-rays through the body. CT is performed in a 360-degree radius around the patient, as the table is moving. Complex mathematical and computer algorithms analyze the data from the detector arrays assimilating timing and localization to produce an image.

CT scanner technology has advanced significantly in recent years. The latest 64-detector scanners are faster with improved spatial and temporal resolution.[48] It is this improvement in resolution that has allowed for greater clinical use in cardiovascular imaging.

As with MRI, compensation for respiratory and cardiovascular motion is required to yield diagnostic quality images. Respiratory motion is compensated for by asking patients to hold their breath. Cardiovascular motion is compensated for by acquiring the data during the cardiac cycle by triggering acquisition to the patient's ECG.

Contrast is a pharmaceutical agent given during a CT study to highlight vascular structures. Contrast agents increase the absorption of x-rays. Areas with contrast uptake are usually depicted as white (bright). For cardiovascular imaging, IV contrast is used. There are several different types of iodinated IV contrast agents. Many of the contrast agents differ by the osmolality of the preparation that is injected: hyper-, hypo, iso-osmolal in comparison to human serum osmolality.

Diagnostic Indications for CT

Cardiovascular CT is most commonly used for anatomical imaging[49–51] (Table 14-1). It provides excellent descriptions of vascular structures (arteries and veins), chambers within the heart, and the pericardium.[52] CT is commonly used for the localization and characterization of cardiac masses and tumors. Although myocardial perfusion and ventricular and valvular function can be evaluated by CT,[53] CT is not routinely done as the first test of choice for these functions.

CT is playing an increasingly important clinical role in the visualization of coronary arteries. Calcification of coronary arteries is indicative of coronary atherosclerosis; both the presence and quantity of coronary calcification strongly predict future cardiac events.[54–58] While not all coronary plaque is calcified, coronary calcium is a measure of overall plaque burden. Most patients presenting with acute coronary syndromes will have detectable coronary calcification in amounts substantially higher than matched controls.[59] Thus, studies to evaluate the utility of coronary CT in the evaluation of patients presenting with acute chest pain syndromes are underway.

A 64-detector CT with IV contrast injection (CT angiography) results in images in which the lumen of a coronary artery can be visualized (Fig. 14-5). Reconstruction of the images is rendered and allow for visualization and detection of significant stenoses.[60] Although improvements in scanner technology have occurred in the last 5 years, temporal resolution is still a limiting factor. Heart rate and rhythm dramatically affect the resolution of images. At low, regular rates resolution is reasonable.[61] Therefore, most patients are given β-blockers prior to imaging. Patients who have rhythm disturbances, such as atrial fibrillation, or contraindications to β-blockers provide great challenges to coronary CT imaging.

CT provides an accurate anatomical description of the size, location, and connection of all four cardiac chambers and valves. Similar to MRI, CT is of increasing importance in patients with congenital heart disease.[62] CT with three-dimensional reconstructions provides accurate and detailed descriptions of bypass graphs and large vessels including the aorta. CT with contrast injections clearly show LV and RV geometry, wall thickness, and function.[63]

Patient Preparation for CT

Significant renal insufficiency is a contraindication to contrasted cardiovascular CT imaging. Although there is not necessarily a specific glomerular filtration rate at which a study is contraindicated, the risks of worsening renal insufficiency versus the benefits of the diagnostic information must be weighed on an individual basis by the provider ordering the procedure. Before any IV contrast injection is given, the patient's creatinine clearance should be calculated.

To minimize the effects of contrast on renal function, administer IV fluids before and after exposure. The contrast is eliminated from the body mainly via the kidney. Some research has suggested that use of acetylcysteine for 24 hours before and after exposure to contrast minimizes the deleterious effects on renal function.

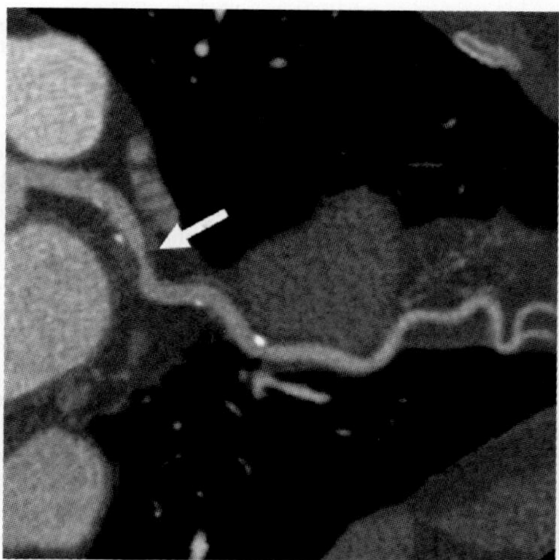
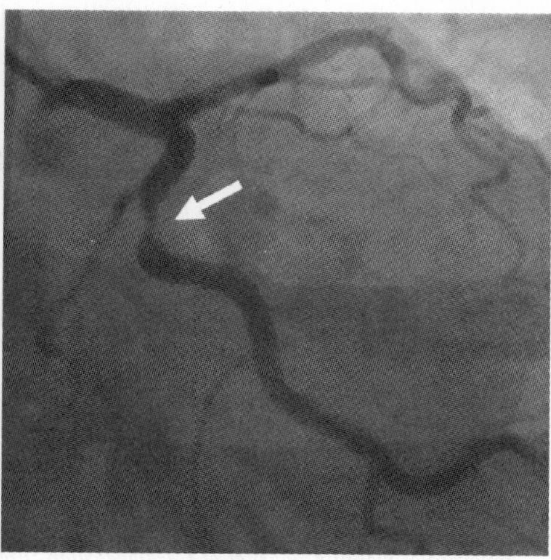

Figure 14-5 *(Left)* CT of the left circumflex coronary artery with a significant stenosis (arrow). *(Right)* The corresponding invasive coronary angiogram of the same artery confirms a significant stenosis (arrow). (Images obtained from University of Washington Medical Center, Department of Radiology and Division of Cardiology, Seattle, Washington.)

Hypersensitivity reactions to contrast occur and cannot always be predicted. In general, reactions occur within minutes to days, with severity ranging from urticaria to angioedema to anaphylaxis. Therefore, a thorough history of prior exposure to contrast agents, asthma, or other allergic or atopic illnesses is required. Premedicate with steroids and antihistamines in patients with a history of a previous hypersensitivity reaction, regardless of the severity. The risk of a contrast reaction versus the benefits of the diagnostic information must be weighted by the provider ordering the procedure on an individual basis. It is important to remember that premedication prior to exposure to a contrast agent does not eliminate completely the risk of a hypersensitivity reaction but does reduce it.

Minor, usually transient, reactions to contrast include but are not limited to flushing, metallic taste, nausea, or bradycardia, and are not usually hypersensitivity reactions. Depending on the diagnostic indication, the patient is exposed to ionizing radiation. The provider ordering the procedure must likewise weigh radiation exposure as a patient risk. Pregnancy is a contraindication.

CONCLUSION

The assessment of cardiovascular structures and function through nuclear cardiology, MRI, and CT has become an integrated element of diagnosis and prognosis in patients with heart disease. The work before the health care community is to continue to evaluate how best to apply these modalities individually to improve the detection and treatment of patient with cardiovascular disease.

REFERENCES

1. Beller, G. A., & Zaret, B. L. (2000). Contributions of nuclear cardiology to diagnosis and prognosis of patients with coronary artery disease. *Circulation, 101*(12), 1465–1478.
2. Hachamovitch, R., Berman, D. S., Kiat, H., et al. (2002). Value of stress myocardial perfusion single photon emission computed tomography in patients with normal resting electrocardiograms: An evaluation of incremental prognostic value and cost-effectiveness. *Circulation, 105*(7), 823–829.
3. Gould, K., & Lipscomb, K. (1974). Effects of coronary stenoses on coronary flow reserve and resistance. *American Journal of Cardiology, 34*, 48–55.
4. Iskandrian, A. S., Verani, M. S., & Heo, J. (1994). Pharmacologic stress testing: Mechanism of action, hemodynamic responses, and results in detection of coronary artery disease. *Journal of Nuclear Cardiology, 1*(1), 94–111.
5. Cerqueira, M. D., Weissman, N. J., Dilsizian, V., et al. (2002). Standardized myocardial segmentation and nomenclature for tomographic imaging of the heart: A statement for healthcare professionals from the Cardiac Imaging Committee of the Council on Clinical Cardiology of the American Heart Association. *Circulation, 105*(4), 539–542.
6. Germano, G., Kavanagh, P. B., Waechter, P., et al. (2000). A new algorithm for the quantitation of myocardial perfusion SPECT. I: Technical principles and reproducibility. *Journal of Nuclear Medicine, 41*(4), 712–719.
7. Hachamovitch, R., Berman, D. S., Kiat, H., et al. (1996). Effective risk stratification using exercise myocardial perfusion SPECT in women: Gender-related differences in prognostic nuclear testing. *Journal of the American College of Cardiology, 28*(1), 34–44.
8. Kang, X., Berman, D. S., Lewin, H., et al. (1999). Comparative ability of myocardial perfusion single-photon emission computed tomography to detect coronary artery disease in patients with and without diabetes mellitus. *American Heart Journal, 137*(5), 949–957.
9. Hachamovitch, R., Berman, D. S., Kiat, H., et al. (1997). Incremental prognostic value of adenosine stress myocardial perfusion single-photon emission computed tomography and impact on subsequent management in patients with or suspected of having myocardial ischemia. *American Journal of Cardiology, 80*(4), 426–433.
10. Giri, S., Shaw, L. J., Murthy, D. R., et al. (2002). Impact of diabetes on the risk stratification using stress single-photon emission computed tomography myocardial perfusion imaging in patients with symptoms suggestive of coronary artery disease. *Circulation, 105*(1), 32–40.
11. Schinkel, A. F. L., Elhendy, A., van Domburg, R. T., et al. (2003). Incremental value of exercise technetium-99m tetrofosmin myocardial perfusion single-photon emission computed tomography for the prediction of cardiac events. *American Journal of Cardiology, 91*(4), 408–411.
12. Levy, D., Kenchaiah, S., Larson, M. G. (2002). Long-term trends in the incidence of and survival with heart failure. *New England Journal of Medicine, 347*(18), 1397–1402.
13. Gheorghiade, M., & Bonow, R. O. (1998). Chronic heart failure in the United States: A manifestation of coronary artery disease. *Circulation, 97*(3), 282–289.
14. Ferrari, R., Ferrari, F., Benigno, M., et al. (1998). Hibernating myocardium: Its pathophysiology and clinical role. *Molecular and Cellular Biochemistry, 186*(1/2), 195–199.
15. Castro, P. F., Bourge, R. C., & Foster, R. E. (1998). Evaluation of hibernating myocardium in patients with ischemic heart disease. *American Journal of Medicine, 104*(1), 69–77.
16. Schinkel, A. F. L., Poldermans, D., Elhendy, A., et al. (2007). Assessment of myocardial viability in patients with heart failure. *Journal of Nuclear Medicine, 48*(7), 1135–1146.
17. Slart, R. H. J. A., Bax, J. J., van Veldhuisen, D. J., et al. (2006). Prediction of functional recovery after revascularization in patients with coronary

artery disease and left ventricular dysfunction by gated FDG-PET. *Journal of Nuclear Cardiology, 13*(2), 210–219.
18. Klein, C., Nekolla, S. G., Bengel, F. M., et al. (2002). Assessment of myocardial viability with contrast-enhanced magnetic resonance imaging: Comparison with positron emission tomography. *Circulation, 105*(2), 162–167.
19. Alderman, E. L., Fisher, L. D., Litwin, P. (1983). Results of coronary artery surgery in patients with poor left ventricular function (CASS). *Circulation, 68*(4), 785–795.
20. Ragosta, M., Beller, G. A., Watson, D. D., et al. (1993). Quantitative planar rest-redistribution 201Tl imaging in detection of myocardial viability and prediction of improvement in left ventricular function after coronary bypass surgery in patients with severely depressed left ventricular function. *Circulation, 87*(5), 1630–1641.
21. Pagley, P. R., Beller, G. A., Watson, D. D., et al. (1997). Improved outcome after coronary bypass surgery in patients with ischemic cardiomyopathy and residual myocardial viability. *Circulation, 96*(3), 793–800.
22. Imamaki, M., Maeda, T., Tanaka, S., et al. (2002). Prediction of improvement in regional left ventricular function after coronary artery bypass grafting: Quantitative stress-redistribution 201Tl imaging in detection of myocardial viability. *Journal of Cardiovascular Surgery (Torino), 43*(5), 603–607.
23. Hamdan, A., Zafrir, N., Sagie, A., et al. (2006). Modalities to assess myocardial viability in the modern cardiology era. *Coronary Artery Disease, 17*(6), 567–576.
24. Wu, Y. W., Tadamura, E., Kanao, S., et al. (2007). Myocardial viability by contrast-enhanced cardiovascular magnetic resonance in patients with coronary artery disease: Comparison with gated single-photon emission tomography and FDG position emission tomography. *International Journal of Cardiovascular Imaging, 23*(6), 757–765.
25. Allman, K. C., Shaw, L. J., Hachamovitch, R., et al. (2002). Myocardial viability testing and impact of revascularization on prognosis in patients with coronary artery disease and left ventricular dysfunction: A meta-analysis. *Journal of the American College of Cardiology, 39*(7), 1151–1158.
26. Sharir, T., Rabinowitz, B., Livschitz, S., et al. (1998). Underestimation of extent and severity of coronary artery disease by dipyridamole stress thallium-201 single-photon emission computed tomographic myocardial perfusion imaging in patients taking antianginal drugs. *Journal of the American College of Cardiology, 31*(7), 1540–1546.
27. Kostuk, W. J., Ehsani, A. A., Karliner, J. S., et al. (1973). Left ventricular performance after myocardial infarction assessed by radioisotope angiocardiography. *Circulation, 47*(2), 242–249.
28. Longmore, D. B., Klipstein, R. H., Underwood, S. R., et al. (1985). Dimensional accuracy of magnetic resonance in studies of the heart. *Lancet, 1*(8442), 1360–1362.
29. Rehr, R. B., Malloy, C. R., Filipchuk, N. G., et al. (1985). Left ventricular volumes measured by MR imaging. *Radiology, 156*(3), 717—719.
30. Sechtem, U., Pflugfelder, P. W., Gould, R. G., et al. (1987). Measurement of right and left ventricular volumes in healthy individuals with cine MR imaging. *Radiology, 163*(3), 697–702.
31. Jauhiainen, T., Jarvinen, V. M., Hekali, P. E., et al. (1998). MR gradient echo volumetric analysis of human cardiac casts: Focus on the right ventricle. *Journal of Computer Assisted Tomography, 22*(6), 899–903.
32. John, A. S., Dill, T., Brandt, R. R., (2003). Magnetic resonance to assess the aortic valve area in aortic stenosis: How does it compare to current diagnostic standards? *Journal of the American College of Cardiology, 42*(3), 519–526.
33. Lin, S. J., Brown, P. A., Watkins, M. P., et al. (2004). Quantification of stenotic mitral valve area with magnetic resonance imaging and comparison with Doppler ultrasound. *Journal of the American College of Cardiology, 44*(1), 133–137.
34. Caruthers, S. D., Lin, S. J., Brown, P., et al. (2003). Practical value of cardiac magnetic resonance imaging for clinical quantification of aortic valve stenosis: Comparison with echocardiography. *Circulation, 108*(18), 2236–2243.
35. Djavidani, B., Debl, K., Lenhart, M., et al. (2005). Planimetry of mitral valve stenosis by magnetic resonance imaging. *Journal of the American College of Cardiology, 45*(12), 2048–2053.
36. Hundley, W. G., Li, H. F., Willard, J. E., et al. (1995). Magnetic resonance imaging assessment of the severity of mitral regurgitation. Comparison with invasive techniques. *Circulation, 92*(5), 1151–1158.
37. Ley, S., Eichhorn, J., Ley-Zaporozhan, J., et al. (2007). Evaluation of aortic regurgitation in congenital heart disease: Value of MR imaging in comparison to echocardiography. *Pediatric Radiology, 37*(5), 426–436.
38. Klem, I., Heitner, J. F., Shah, D. J., et al. (2006). Improved detection of coronary artery disease by stress perfusion cardiovascular magnetic resonance with the use of delayed enhancement infarction imaging. *Journal of the American College of Cardiology, 47*(8), 1630–1638.
39. Nagel, E., Klein, C., Paetsch, I., et al. (2003). Magnetic resonance perfusion measurements for the noninvasive detection of coronary artery disease. *Circulation, 108*(4), 432–437.
40. Kim, R. J., Fieno, D. S., Parrish, T. B., et al. (1999). Relationship of MRI delayed contrast enhancement to irreversible injury, infarct age, and contractile function. *Circulation, 100*(19), 1992–2002.
41. Wagner, A., Mahrholdt, H., Holly, T. A., et al. (2003). Contrast-enhanced MRI and routine single photon emission computed tomography (SPECT) perfusion imaging for detection of subendocardial myocardial infarcts: An imaging study. *Lancet, 361*(9355), 374–379.
42. Yuan, C., Beach, K. W., Smith, L. H., Jr., et al. (1998). Measurement of atherosclerotic carotid plaque size in vivo using high resolution magnetic resonance imaging. *Circulation, 98*(24), 2666–2671.
43. Hatsukami, T. S., Ross, R., Polissar, N. L., et al. (2000). Visualization of fibrous cap thickness and rupture in human atherosclerotic carotid plaque in vivo with high-resolution magnetic resonance imaging. *Circulation, 102*(9), 959–964.
44. Yuan, C., Mitsumori, L. M., Ferguson, M. S., et al. (2001). In vivo accuracy of multispectral magnetic resonance imaging for identifying lipid-rich necrotic cores and intraplaque hemorrhage in advanced human carotid plaques. *Circulation, 104*(17), 2051–2056.
45. Yuan, C., Zhang, S. X., Polissar, N. L., et al. (2002). Identification of fibrous cap rupture with magnetic resonance imaging is highly associated with recent transient ischemic attack or stroke. *Circulation, 105*(2), 181–185.
46. Takaya, N., Yuan, C., Chu, B., et al. (2005). Presence of intraplaque hemorrhage stimulates progression of carotid atherosclerotic plaques: A high-resolution magnetic resonance imaging study. *Circulation, 111*(21), 2768–2775.
47. Shellock, F. G. (2008) from http://www.mrisafety.com.
48. Achenbach, S., Ropers, D., Pohle, F. K., et al. (2005). Detection of coronary artery stenoses using multi-detector CT with 16 × 0.75 collimation and 375 ms rotation. *European Heart Journal, 26*(19), 1978–1986.
49. Chartrand-Lefebvre, C., Cadrin-Chênevert, A., Bordeleau, E., et al. (2007). Coronary computed tomography angiography: Overview of technical aspects, current concepts, and perspectives. *Canadian Association of Radiologists Journal, 58*(2), 92.
50. Cury, R. C., Nieman, K., Shapiro, M. D. (2007). Comprehensive cardiac CT study: Evaluation of coronary arteries, left ventricular function, and myocardial perfusion—Is it possible? *Journal of Nuclear Cardiology, 14*(2), 229–243.
51. Leber, A. W., Knez, A., von Ziegler, F., et al. (2005). Quantification of obstructive and nonobstructive coronary lesions by 64-slice computed tomography: A comparative study with quantitative coronary angiography and intravascular ultrasound. *Journal of the American College of Cardiology, 46*(1), 147–154.
52. Van Mieghem, C. A., McFadden, E. P., de Feyter, P. J., et al. (2006). Non-invasive detection of subclinical coronary atherosclerosis coupled with assessment of changes in plaque characteristics using novel invasive imaging modalities: The Integrated Biomarker and Imaging Study (IBIS). *Journal of the American College of Cardiology, 47*(6), 1134–1142.
53. Butler, J., Shapiro, M., Reiber, J., et al. (2007). Extent and distribution of coronary artery disease: A comparative study of invasive versus noninvasive angiography with computed angiography. *American Heart Journal, 153*(3), 378–384.
54. O'Rourke, R. A., Brundage, B. H., Froelicher, V. F., et al. (2000). American College of Cardiology/American Heart Association Expert Consensus Document on electron-beam computed tomography for the diagnosis and prognosis of coronary artery disease. *Journal of the American College of Cardiology, 36*(1), 326–340.
55. Pohle, K., Ropers, D., Maffert, R., et al. (2003). Coronary calcifications in young patients with first, unheralded myocardial infarction: A risk factor matched analysis by electron beam tomography. *Heart, 89*(6), 625–628.
56. Raggi, P., Callister, T. Q., Cooil, B., et al. (2000). Identification of patients at increased risk of first unheralded acute myocardial infarction by electron-beam computed tomography. *Circulation, 101*(8), 850–855.
57. Schmermund, A., Mohlenkamp, S., Berenbein, S., et al. (2006). Population-based assessment of subclinical coronary atherosclerosis using electron-beam computed tomography. *Atherosclerosis, 185*(1), 177–182.

58. Arad, Y., Spadaro, L. A., Goodman, K., et al. (2000). Prediction of coronary events with electron beam computed tomography. *Journal of the American College of Cardiology, 36*(4), 1253–1260.
59. Schmermund, A., Schwartz, R. S., Adamzik, M., et al. (2001). Coronary atherosclerosis in unheralded sudden coronary death under age 50: Histopathologic comparison with 'healthy' subjects dying out of hospital. *Atherosclerosis, 155*(2), 499–508.
60. Achenbach, S. (2005). Current and future status on cardiac computed tomography imaging for diagnosis and risk stratification. *Journal of Nuclear Cardiology, 12*(6), 703–713.
61. Gilard, M., Cornily, J. C., Pennec, P. Y., et al. (2006). Accuracy of multislice computed tomography in the preoperative assessment of coronary disease in patients with aortic valve stenosis. *Journal of the American College of Cardiology, 47*(10), 2020–2024.
62. Gilkeson, R. C., Markowitz, A. H., & Ciancibello, L. (2003). Multisection CT evaluation of the reoperative cardiac surgery patient. *Radiographics, 23,* S3–S17.
63. Juergens, K. U., Grude, M., Maintz, D., et al. (2004). Multi-detector row CT of left ventricular function with dedicated analysis software versus MR imaging: Initial experience. *Radiology, 230*(2), 403–410.

CHAPTER 15

Electrocardiography

Carol Jacobson

Electrocardiography is the graphic display of the changing potentials of the electrical field generated by the heart as recorded by electrodes placed on the body surface. Recording of the 12-lead electrocardiogram (ECG) is the most frequently used procedure for the diagnosis of heart disease. It is noninvasive, safe, simple to perform, reproducible, and relatively inexpensive. The 12-lead ECG can record changes indicative of primary myocardial disease such as coronary artery disease, cardiomyopathy, hypertension, or infiltrative diseases. It can also reflect changes associated with electrolyte abnormalities, metabolic disorders, drug effect, and other disease processes such as pulmonary embolism or pulmonary hypertension, renal failure, and central nervous system disease. The ECG is the gold standard for noninvasive diagnosis of cardiac arrhythmias and conduction abnormalities (see Chapter 16) and is a useful tool in evaluating function of implanted devices such as pacemakers and implantable cardioverter defibrillators.[1]

This chapter discusses the electrocardiographic features of various cardiac conditions and other disease processes that may cause changes on the ECG. Specific information on the pathophysiology and treatment of cardiac disease and other medical conditions that may affect the ECG can be found in other chapters in this book or in medical textbooks.

ELECTRICAL CONDUCTION THROUGH THE HEART

The electrical impulse of the heart is the stimulus for cardiac contraction. The conduction system (Fig. 15-1) is responsible for the initiation of the electrical impulse and its sequential spread through the atria, atrioventricular (AV) junction, and ventricles.

The Cardiac Conduction System

The conduction system of the heart consists of the following structures.

Sinus Node

The sinus or sinoatrial (SA) node is a small group of cells in the high right atrium that functions as the normal pacemaker of the heart because it has the fastest rate of automaticity. The SA node normally depolarizes between 60 and 100 times per minute.

AV Node

The AV node is a small group of cells in the low right atrium near the tricuspid valve. The AV node has three main functions:

1. Its major job is to slow conduction of the impulse from the atria to the ventricles to allow time for the atria to contract and empty their blood into the ventricles.
2. The area around the AV node (junction) has automaticity at an impulse rate of 40 to 60 beats per minute and can function as a backup pacemaker if the SA node fails.
3. It screens out rapid atrial impulses to protect the ventricles from dangerously fast rates when the atrial rate is very rapid.

Bundle of His

The bundle of His is a short bundle of fibers at the bottom of the AV node leading to the bundle branches. Conduction velocity accelerates in the bundle of His, and the impulse is transmitted to both bundle branches.

Bundle Branches

The bundle branches are bundles of fibers that rapidly conduct the impulse into the right and left ventricles. The *right bundle* branch travels along the right side of the interventricular septum and carries the impulse into the right ventricle. The *left bundle branch* has two main divisions, the anterior fascicle and the posterior fascicle, which carry the impulse into the left ventricle.

Purkinje Fibers

The Purkinje fibers are hairlike fibers that spread out from the bundle branches along the endocardial surface of both ventricles and rapidly conduct the impulse to the ventricular muscle cells. Cells in the Purkinje system have automaticity at a rate of 20 to 40 beats per minute and can function as a backup pacemaker if all other pacemakers fail.

Origin and Spread of the Electrical Impulse Through the Heart

The impulse normally begins in the SA node, located in the high right atrium, because the SA node has the fastest rate of automaticity of all potential pacemaker cells in the heart. The impulse spreads from the SA node through both atria in an inferior and leftward direction, resulting in depolarization of the atrial muscle. When the impulse reaches the AV node, its conduction velocity is slowed before it continues into the ventricles. The slowing in the AV node is necessary to allow time for the atria to contract and empty their blood into the ventricles before the ventricles contract. The atrium's contribution to ventricular filling is referred to as "atrial kick." When the impulse emerges from the AV node, it travels rapidly through the bundle of His and down the right and left bundle branches into the Purkinje network of both ventricles, and results in depolarization of the ventricular muscle. The spread of this wave of depolarization through the heart produces the classic surface ECG, which can be recorded by an electrocardiograph (ECG machine) or monitored continuously on a bedside cardiac monitor.

Waves, Complexes, and Intervals of the Cardiac Cycle

The ECG waves, complexes, and intervals are illustrated in Figure 15-2.

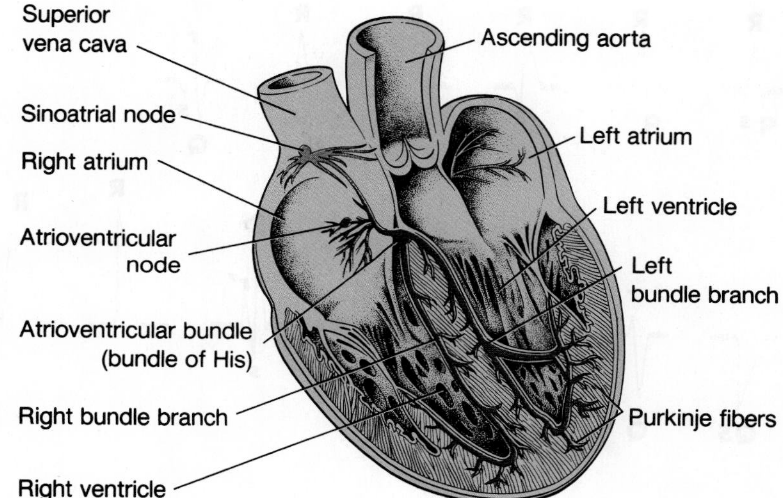

■ **Figure 15-1** Cardiac conduction system. (From Jacobson, C. [1991]. Cardiac arrhythmias and conduction abnormalities. In M. L. Patrick, S. L. Woods, R. F. Craven, et al. [Eds.], *Medical-surgical nursing* [2nd ed., pp. 648–693]. Philadelphia: J. B. Lippincott)

P Wave

The P wave represents atrial muscle depolarization. It is normally small, smoothly rounded, and no taller than 2.5 mm or wider than 0.11 second.

QRS Complex

The QRS complex represents ventricular muscle depolarization. The shape of the QRS complex depends on the lead being recorded and the ventricular activation sequence; not all leads record all waves of the QRS complex. A Q wave is an initial negative deflection from baseline and should be less than 0.03 second in duration and less than 25% of the R-wave amplitude. An R wave is the first positive deflection from baseline. An S wave is a negative deflection that follows an R wave. When a complex is all positive, it is just an R wave; when it is all negative, it is called a QS. Regardless of the shape of the complex, ventricular depolarization waves are called QRS complexes (Fig. 15-3). The width of the QRS complex represents intraventricular conduction time and is measured from the point at which it first leaves the baseline to the end of the last appearing wave. Normal QRS width is 0.04 to 0.10 second.

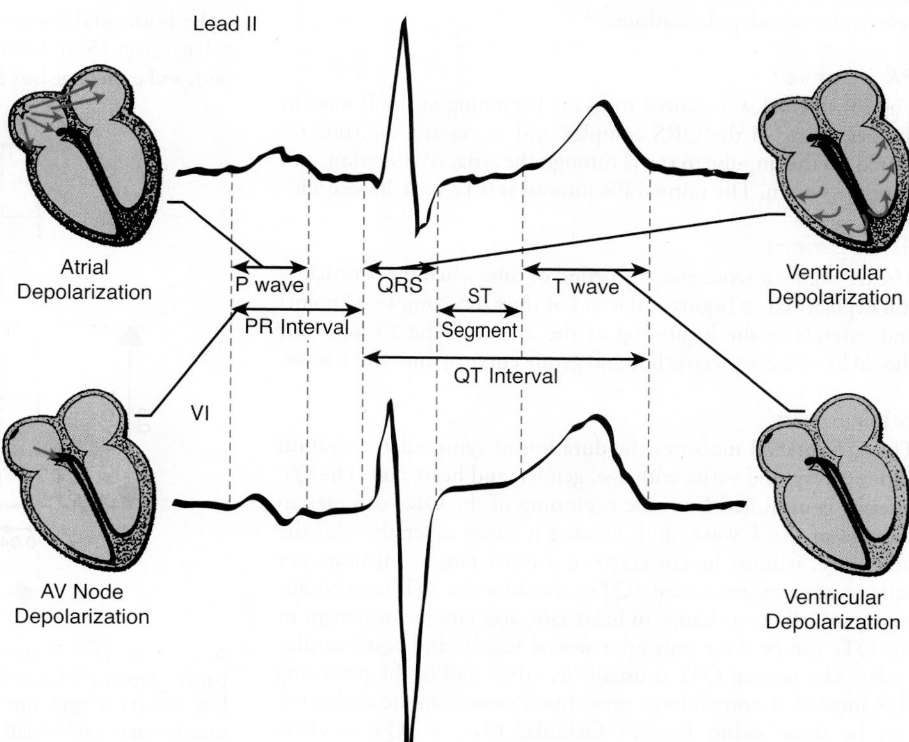

■ **Figure 15-2** Waves, complexes, and intervals of the cardiac cycle in leads II and V_1.

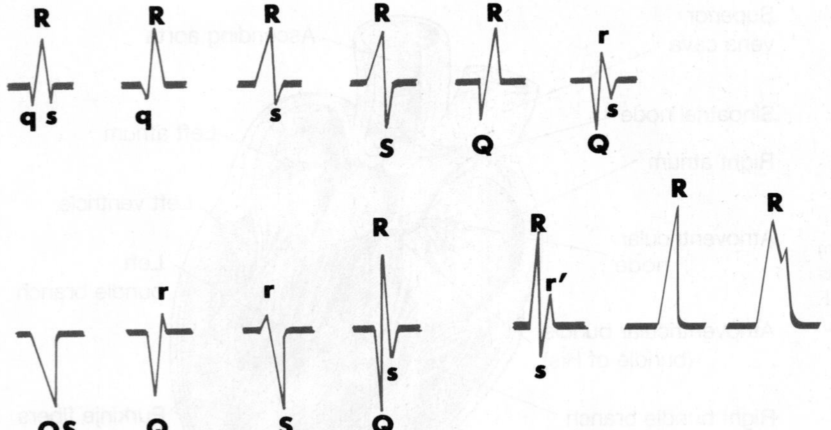

■ **Figure 15-3** Examples of various QRS complexes.

T Wave

The T wave represents ventricular muscle repolarization. It follows the QRS complex and is normally in the same direction as the QRS complex. The T wave is usually rounded and slightly asymmetric, rising more slowly than it descends. T waves are not normally taller than 5 mm in any limb lead or 10 mm in any precordial lead.

U Wave

The U wave is a small, rounded wave that sometimes follows the T wave and is most prominent in leads V_2–V_4. The U wave is normally in the same direction as the T wave but is only approximately 10% of its amplitude. The U wave is thought to be part of the ventricular repolarization process and may represent repolarization of the Purkinje network or certain cells in the deep subepicardial layer of the ventricle (M cells), or summation of ventricular afterdepolarizations.[2,3]

PR Interval

The PR interval is measured from the beginning of the P wave to the beginning of the QRS complex and represents the time required for the impulse to travel through the atria, AV junction, and Purkinje system. The normal PR interval is 0.12 to 0.20 second.

ST Segment

The ST segment represents the period of time when the ventricle is still depolarized. It begins at the end of the QRS complex (J point) and extends to the beginning of the T wave. The ST segment should be at the isoelectric line and gently curve up into the T wave.

QT Interval

The QT interval measures the duration of ventricular activation and recovery, and varies with age, gender, and heart rate. The QT interval is measured from the beginning of the QRS complex to the end of the T wave, and, because it varies inversely with the heart rate, it must be corrected to a heart rate of 60 beats per minute after measurement (QTc). Because the QT interval adjusts gradually to a change in heart rate, accurate measurement of the QTc can be done only after several regular and equal cardiac cycles. The normal QTc is usually less than half of the preceding R-R interval at normal heart rates, but a more accurate evaluation can be done using Bazett's formula: $QTc = QT / \sqrt{R\text{-}R}$ interval, where QT and R-R intervals are in seconds.[4] The upper limit of normal QTc is generally considered to be <0.44 second in adult men and <0.45 second in adult women.[2,3,5]

BASIC ELECTROCARDIOGRAPHY

The ECG is the graphic record of the electrical activity of the heart. The spread of the electrical impulse through the heart produces weak electrical currents through the entire body, which can be detected and amplified by the ECG machine and recorded on calibrated graph paper. These amplified signals form the ECG tracing, consisting of the waveforms and intervals described previously, and are inscribed onto grid paper that moves beneath the recording stylus (pen) at a standard speed of 25 mm/s. The grid on the paper consists of a series of small and large boxes, both horizontally and vertically; horizontal boxes measure time, and vertical boxes measure voltage (Fig. 15-4). Each small box horizontally is equal to 0.04 second, and each large box horizontally is equal to 0.20 second. On the

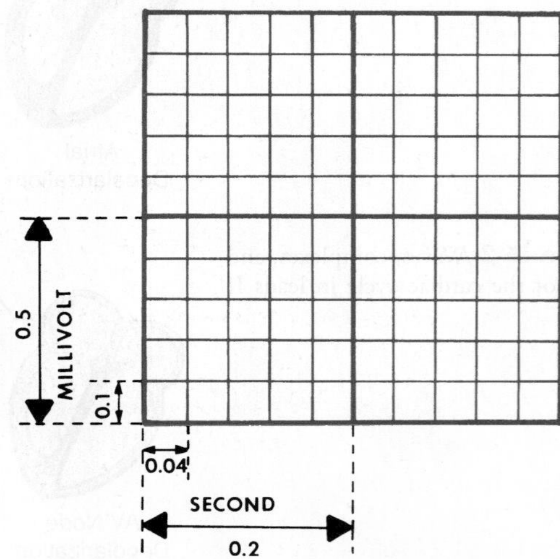

■ **Figure 15-4** Time and voltage lines on ECG paper at standard paper speed of 25 mm/s. Horizontal axis measures time: each small box = 0.04 second, one large box = 0.20 second. Vertical axis measures voltage: each small box = 1 mm or 0.1 mV, one large box = 5 mm or 0.5 mV.

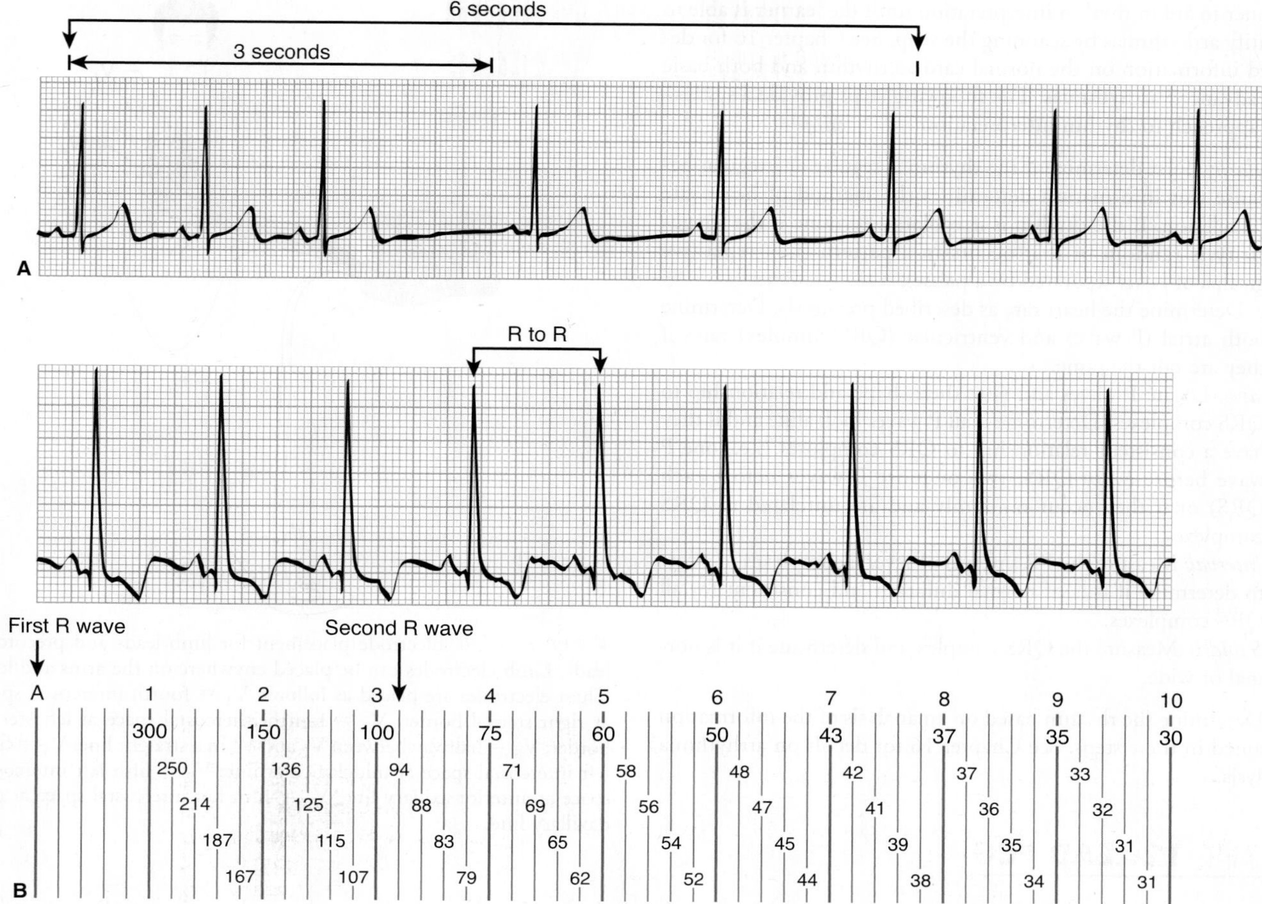

■ **Figure 15-5** (A) Heart rate determination for an irregular rhythm. Count the number or R-R intervals in a 6-second strip and multiply by 10. In (A) there are five complete R-R intervals in a 6-second strip; the heart rate is about 50 beats per minute. (B) Heart rate determination for a regular rhythm using the rate ruler. Count the number of large and small boxes between R waves on the rhythm strip. In (B) there are three large boxes and one small box between the R waves marked on the strip. On the rate ruler, the first R wave is represented by the thick line marked "A." Each large box on the ECG paper is represented by a thick line on the rate ruler and is numbered at the top; each small box on the strip is represented by a thin line on the ruler. The number on the line on the ruler that corresponds to the second R wave on the strip represents the heart rate. In (B), count three large boxes at the top of the ruler and then one small box; the heart rate is 94 beats per minute. (Rate ruler in B from Marriott, H. J. L. [1988]. *Practical electrocardiography* [8th ed., p. 15]. Baltimore: Williams & Wilkins.)

vertical axis, each small box measures 1 mm and is equal to 0.1 mV; each large box measures 5 mm and is equal to 0.5 mV. In addition to the grid, most ECG paper places a vertical line in the top margin at 3-second intervals or places a mark at 1-second intervals.

The waveforms of the cardiac cycle can be recorded by a bedside cardiac monitor and displayed continuously on an oscilloscope or recorded on a rhythm strip, which consists of the same grid as described previously. The standard 12-lead ECG simultaneously records 12 different views of electrical activity as it travels through the heart and displays all 12 views on a full-page layout, which consists of the same grid. The 12 leads of the ECG are described in detail in following sections.

Determining Heart Rate on the ECG

Heart rate can be determined from the ECG strip by several methods. An easy method that can be used for both regular and irregular rhythms is to count the number of R-R intervals (not R waves) in a 6-second strip and multiply that number by 10, because there are ten 6-second intervals in 1 minute (Fig. 15-5*A*).

Another method that can be used only if the rhythm is regular is to count the number of large boxes between two R waves and divide that number into 300, because there are 300 large boxes in a 1-minute strip. The most accurate method to use for a regular rhythm is to count the number of small boxes between two R waves and divide that number into 1,500, because there are 1,500 small boxes in a 1-minute strip. The easiest way to do either of these methods is to use the rate ruler in Figure 15-5*B*.

Determining the Cardiac Rhythm on the ECG

The first step in interpreting a 12-lead ECG is to determine the cardiac rhythm. A rhythm strip should be analyzed in a systematic manner to aid in rhythm interpretation until the learner is able to identify arrhythmias by scanning the strip. See Chapter 16 for detailed information on the normal cardiac rhythm and both basic and advanced arrhythmias. The following steps provide a systematic approach to rhythm interpretation:

Regularity: First determine if the rhythm is regular or irregular because this information determines the method of heart rate calculation. If the rhythm is irregular, determine if the irregularity is random or if it occurs in a pattern (i.e., repetitive groups of beats separated by a pause).

Rate: Determine the heart rate as described previously. Determine both atrial (P wave) and ventricular (QRS complex) rates if they are not the same.

P waves: Locate P waves and note their shape and relationship to QRS complexes. Determine if all P waves look alike and if they have a consistent relationship to QRS complexes (i.e., one P wave before every QRS, two or more P waves before each QRS) or if they occur randomly and are unrelated to QRS complexes.

PR interval: Measure the PR interval of several complexes in a row to determine if it is of normal duration and consistent for all QRS complexes.

QRS width: Measure the QRS complex and determine if it is normal or wide.

Determine the rhythm based on an analysis of the information obtained in these steps. See Chapter 16 for details on arrhythmia analysis.

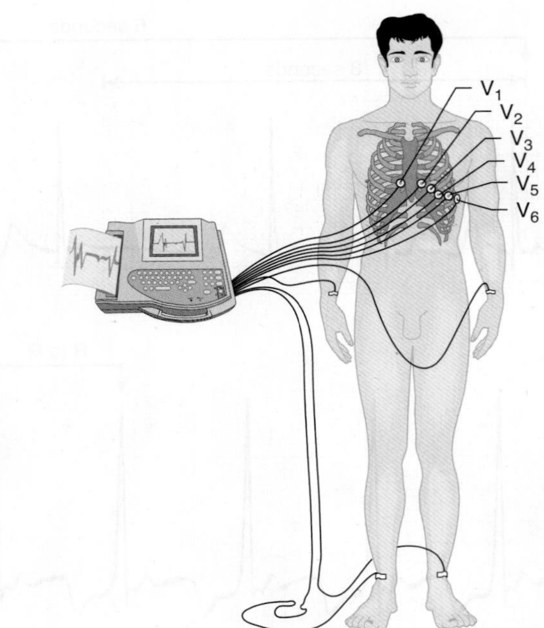

Figure 15-6 Electrode placement for limb leads and precordial leads. Limb electrodes can be placed anywhere on the arms and legs. Chest electrodes are placed as follows: V_1 = fourth intercostal space at right sternal border; V_2 = fourth intercostal space at left sternal border; V_3 = halfway between V_2 and V_4 in a straight line; V_4 = fifth left intercostal space at midclavicular line; V_5 = fifth left intercostal space at anterior axillary line; V_6 = fifth left intercostal space at midaxillary line.

THE 12-LEAD ECG

The 12-lead ECG records electrical activity as it spreads through the heart from 12 different leads that are recorded through electrodes placed on the arms, legs, and specific spots on the chest. Each lead represents a different view of the heart and consists of two electrodes with opposite polarity (bipolar), or one electrode and a reference point (unipolar). A *bipolar* lead has a positive pole and a negative pole, with each contributing equally to the recording. A *unipolar* lead has one positive pole and a reference pole in the center of the chest that is algebraically determined by the ECG machine. The reference pole represents the center of the electrical field of the heart and has a zero potential, so only the positive pole of a unipolar lead contributes to the tracing.

The standard 12-lead ECG consists of six limb leads that record electrical activity in the frontal plane—traveling up/down and right/left in the heart—and six precordial leads that record electrical activity in the horizontal plane—traveling anterior/posterior and right/left. Limb leads are recorded by electrodes placed on the arms and legs, whereas precordial leads are recorded by electrodes placed on the chest (Fig. 15-6). For convenience in continuous bedside monitoring, arm electrodes can be placed on the shoulders and leg electrodes on the lower part of the rib cage rather than on the limbs without significantly altering the signals recorded.

A camera analogy makes the 12-lead ECG easier to understand. Each lead of the ECG represents a picture of the electrical activity in the heart taken by the camera. In any lead, the positive electrode is the recording electrode or the camera lens. The negative electrode tells the camera which way to "shoot" its picture and determines the direction in which the positive electrode records. When the positive electrode detects electrical activity traveling toward it, it records an upright deflection on the ECG. When the positive electrode detects electrical activity traveling away from it, it records a negative deflection (Fig. 15-7). If a positive electrode is positioned where electrical activity travels toward it and then away from it, a diphasic deflection is recorded. If the electrical activity travels perpendicular to a positive electrode, no activity is recorded. The 12-lead ECG records three bipolar frontal plane leads—lead I, lead II, and lead III; three unipolar frontal plane leads—aVR, aVL, and aVF; and six unipolar precordial leads: V_1, V_2, V_3, V_4, V_5, and V_6.

Bipolar Leads

Figure 15-8*A* illustrates the three bipolar frontal plane leads. In each lead, the camera represents the positive pole of the lead. In lead I, the positive electrode is on the left arm and the negative electrode is on the right arm. Any electrical activity in the heart that travels toward the positive electrode (camera lens) on the left arm is recorded as an upright deflection and any traveling away from it is recorded as a negative deflection. In lead II, the positive electrode is on the left leg and the negative electrode is on the right arm. Any electrical activity traveling toward the left leg electrode (camera lens) is recorded as an upright deflection and any traveling away from it toward the right arm electrode is recorded as a negative deflection. In lead III, the positive electrode is on the left leg and the negative electrode is on the left arm. Any electrical activity coming toward the left leg electrode (camera lens) is recorded as an upright deflection and any traveling away from it

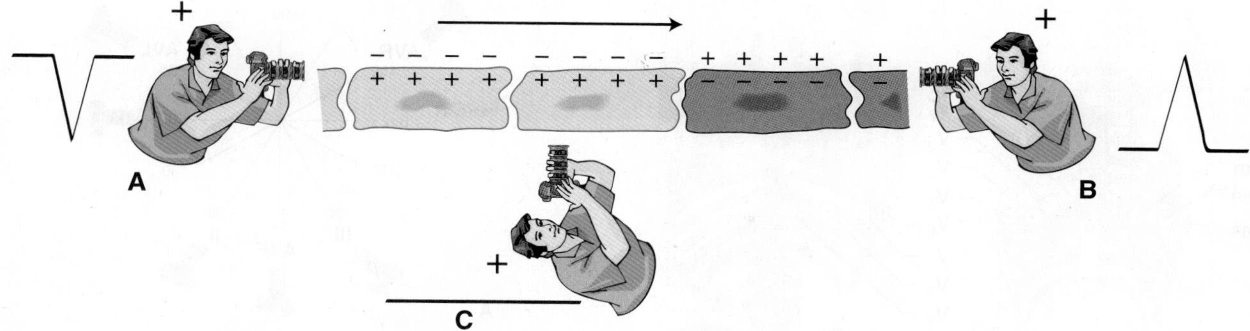

■ **Figure 15-7** A strip of cardiac muscle depolarizing in the direction of the arrow. A positive electrode at B sees depolarization coming toward it and records an upright deflection. A positive electrode at A sees depolarization going away from it and records a negative deflection. A positive electrode at C records a flat line because depolarization is traveling perpendicular to the electrode's view.

toward the left arm is recorded as a negative deflection. The right leg electrode serves as a ground and does not contribute to the signals recorded. The electrical sum of the voltages in the three bipolar frontal plane leads equals zero potential and forms a virtual ground in the center of the triangle used by the unipolar leads as their reference point.

Unipolar Leads

Figure 15-8*B* illustrates the three unipolar frontal plane leads, aVR, aVL, and aVF. The camera represents the location of the positive electrode: on the right shoulder for aVR, on the left shoulder for aVL, and at the foot (left leg) for aVF. The "negative

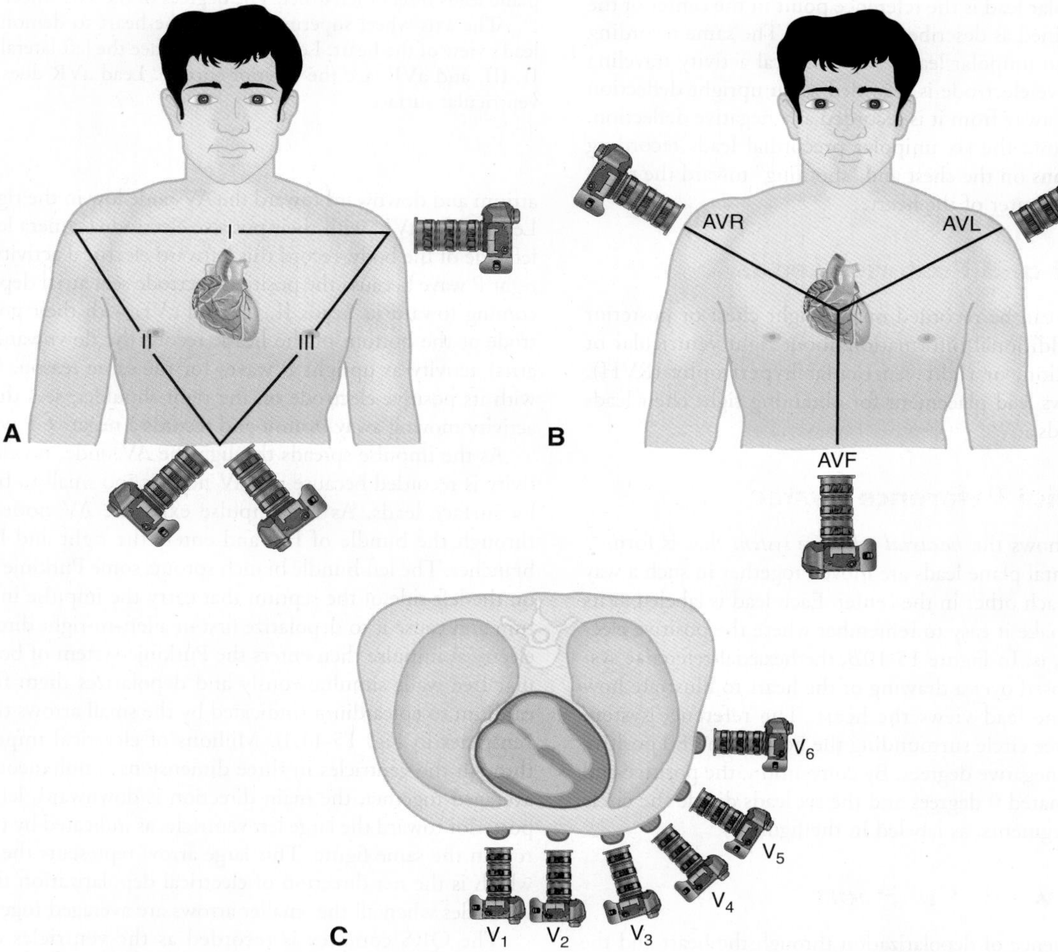

■ **Figure 15-8** The 12 leads of the ECG. The camera represents the location of the positive, or recording, electrode in each lead. (A) Bipolar frontal plane leads I, II, and III. (B) Unipolar frontal plane leads aVR, aVL, and aVF. (C) Unipolar precordial leads V_1–V_6.

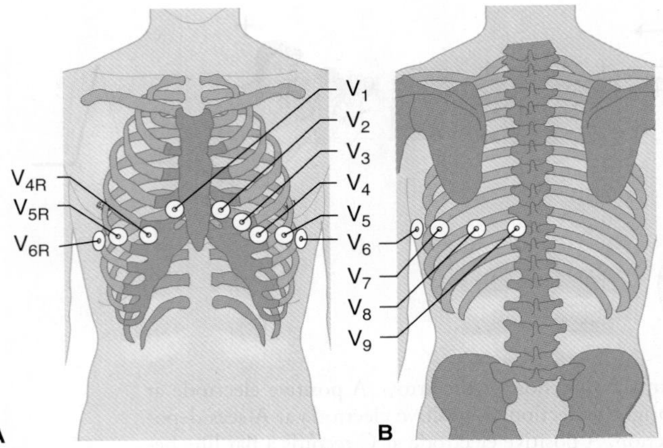

■ **Figure 15-9** (A) Electrode placement for standard precordial and right precordial leads. Only three right-sided leads are needed: V_{4R}, right fifth intercostal space at midclavicular line; V_{5R}, right fifth intercostal space at anterior axillary line; V_{6R}, right fifth intercostal space at midaxillary line. (B) Electrode placement for posterior leads: V_7, left posterior axillary line; V_8, tip of left scapula; V_9, left border of spine. All three are in the same horizontal plane of V_4 to V_6.

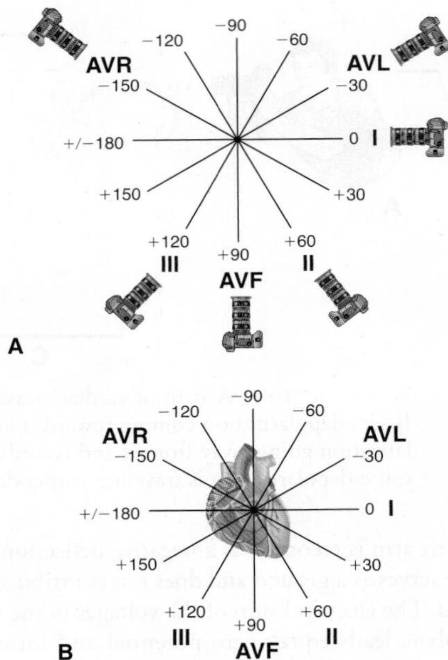

■ **Figure 15-10** Hexaxial reference system (or axis wheel). Each lead is labeled at its positive end in both examples. (A) All six frontal plane leads bisect each other. The degrees of the axis wheel are shown. (B) The axis wheel superimposed on the heart to demonstrate each lead's view of the heart. Leads I and aVL face the left lateral wall, leads II, III, and aVF face the inferior surface. Lead aVR does not face a ventricular surface.

end" of the unipolar lead is the reference point in the center of the chest that is obtained as described previously. The same recording principles apply to unipolar leads: any electrical activity traveling toward the positive electrode is recorded as an upright deflection and any traveling away from it is recorded as a negative deflection. Figure 15-8*C* shows the six unipolar precordial leads recording from their locations on the chest and "shooting" toward the reference point in the center of the heart.

Right Chest and Posterior Leads

Additional leads can be recorded on the right chest or posterior thorax to gain additional information about right ventricular or posterior infarction, or right ventricular hypertrophy (RVH). Figure 15-9 shows lead placement for obtaining right chest leads and posterior leads.

The Hexaxial Reference System

Figure 15-10*A* shows the *hexaxial reference system* that is formed when the six frontal plane leads are moved together in such a way that they bisect each other in the center. Each lead is labeled at its positive end to make it easy to remember where the positive electrode, or camera, is. In Figure 15-10*B*, the hexaxial reference system is superimposed over a drawing of the heart to illustrate how each frontal plane lead views the heart. The reference system forms a 360-degree circle surrounding the heart with 180 positive degrees and 180 negative degrees. By convention, the positive end of lead I is designated 0 degrees and the six leads divide the circle into 30-degree segments, as labeled in the figure.

The 12 Views of the Heart

The normal sequence of depolarization through the heart and the resulting P, QRS, and T waves for each frontal plane lead are illustrated in Figure 15-11*A*. The impulse normally originates in the SA node high in the right atrium and spreads leftward through the left atrium and downward toward the AV node low in the right atrium. Leads I and aVL, with their positive electrode (camera lens) on the left side of the body, record this leftward electrical activity as an upright P wave because the positive electrode sees atrial depolarization coming toward it. Leads II, III, and aVF, with their positive electrode at the bottom of the heart, record the downward spread of atrial activity as upright P waves for the same reason. Lead aVR, with its positive electrode on the right shoulder, sees the electrical activity moving away from it and records a negative P wave.

As the impulse spreads through the AV node, no electrical activity is recorded because the AV node is too small to be recorded by surface leads. As the impulse exits the AV node, it moves through the bundle of His and enters the right and left bundle branches. The left bundle branch sprouts some Purkinje fibers high on the left side of the septum that carry the impulse into the septum and cause it to depolarize first in a left-to-right direction. The electrical impulse then enters the Purkinje system of both ventricular free walls simultaneously and depolarizes them from endocardium to epicardium (indicated by the small arrows through the ventricles in Fig. 15-11*A*). Millions of electrical impulses travel through the ventricles in three dimensions simultaneously, but, if averaged together, the main direction is downward, leftward, and posterior toward the large left ventricle, as indicated by the large arrow in the same figure. This large arrow represents the *mean axis*, which is the net direction of electrical depolarization through the ventricles when all the smaller arrows are averaged together.

The QRS complex is recorded as the ventricles depolarize. Leads I and aVL, with their positive electrodes on the left side of the body, see the septum depolarizing away from them in a left-to-right direction and record a small negative deflection (Q wave).

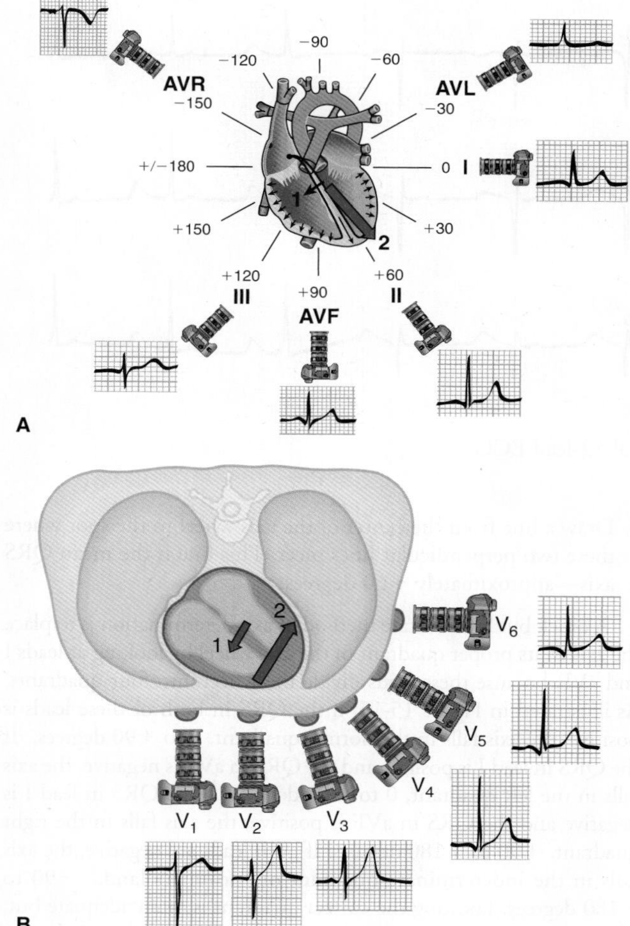

■ **Figure 15-11** (A) Normal sequence of depolarization through the heart as recorded by each of the frontal plane leads. (B) Cross section of the thorax illustrating how the six precordial leads record the normal ECG. In both examples, the small arrow (1) shows the initial direction of depolarization through the septum, followed by the mean direction of ventricular free wall depolarization, larger arrow (2).

They then see the large left ventricular free wall depolarizing toward them and record an upright deflection (R wave). Leads II, III, and aVF, with their positive electrodes at the bottom of the heart may not record septal activity at all. If these leads see septal activity coming slightly toward them, they record a positive deflection. They then see the forces moving downward through the left ventricle toward them and record an upright deflection (R wave). Lead aVR, positive on the right shoulder, sees all activity moving away from it and records a negative deflection (QS complex).

The six precordial leads record electrical activity traveling in the horizontal plane. Figure 15-11*B* illustrates the position of the precordial leads and how they record electrical activity as it spreads through the ventricles in the horizontal plane. Lead V_1 is located on the front of the chest and records a small R wave as the septum depolarizes toward it from left to right. It then records a deep S wave as depolarization spreads away from it through the thick left ventricle. As the positive electrode is moved across the precordium from the V_1 to the V_6 position, it records progressively more left ventricular forces and the R wave gets progressively larger. Lead V_6 is located on the left side of the chest and usually records a small Q wave as the septum depolarizes from left to right away from the positive electrode, and a large R wave as electrical activity spreads toward the positive electrode through the thick left ventricle. Normal R-wave progression means that the R wave gets progressively larger from V_1 to V_6, or that V_6 is predominantly an R wave compared with V_1, which is predominantly an S wave. Often the largest precordial R wave is recorded in lead V_4 or V_5.

Many variations of the above patterns exist among individuals and represent normal variants in the ECG. Leads III and aVR may record larger Q waves because of their rightward orientation (Fig. 15-11*A*)[6,7], lead III may record a large S wave if the heart sits horizontally in the chest, and lead aVL may record a large S wave if the heart sits more vertically in the chest.[8] Variations in P-wave and T-wave morphology can also be normal variants depending on how the heart physically sits in the chest.

The Normal Adult 12-Lead ECG

Figure 15-12 shows a normal 12-lead ECG. Normal sinus rhythm is present at a rate of 70 beats per minute, and the axis is approximately +60 degrees. P waves are normal (they are flat in aVL, but this finding is a normal variant), and T waves are normal (flat or slightly inverted in lead aVL and V_1 is a normal variant). The QRS complex is normal (0.08 second wide), there are no abnormal Q waves, and R-wave progression is normal across the precordium. The ST segment is at baseline in all leads. This ECG can be used for comparison as abnormalities are discussed throughout this chapter.

AXIS DETERMINATION

Conduction of a wave of depolarization through the myocardium results in propagation of thousands of electrical potentials in multiple directions. More than 80% of these potentials are balanced by similar instantaneous charges moving in opposite directions. Balanced alterations in electrical potentials result in an algebraic "canceling out" of these instantaneous vectors. What remains as the detected and amplified ECG tracing is the net vector, which reveals the magnitude, direction, and polarity of the mean electrical force as it travels through the myocardium. Frontal plane axis can be determined for P waves, QRS complexes, and T waves. This section deals only with QRS axis determination.

The normal QRS axis is defined as −30 to +90 degrees because most of the electrical forces in a normal heart are directed downward and leftward toward the large left ventricle. Left axis deviation (LAD) is defined as −31 to −90 degrees and occurs when most of the forces move in a leftward and superior direction, as can happen in left ventricular hypertrophy (LVH), left anterior fascicular block (LAFB), inferior myocardial infarction (MI), left bundle-branch block (LBBB), several congenital defects, and some arrhythmias, especially ventricular tachycardia and Wolff–Parkinson–White syndrome. Right axis deviation (RAD) is defined as +91 to +180 degrees and occurs when most of the forces move rightward, as can happen in RVH, left posterior fascicular block (LPFB), right bundle-branch block (RBBB), dextrocardia, ventricular tachycardia, and Wolff–Parkinson–White syndrome. When most of the forces are directed superior and rightward between −91 and −180 degrees, the term *indeterminate axis* or *extreme axis* is used. This axis can occur with ventricular tachycardia and occasionally with bifascicular block.

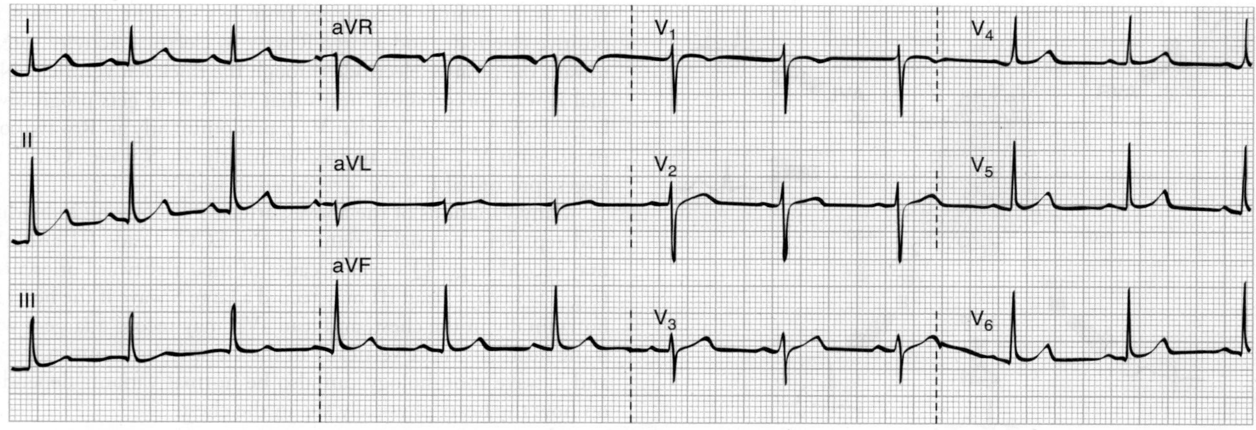

■ **Figure 15-12** Normal 12-lead ECG.

Figure 15-13 shows the axis wheel divided into its normal, left deviation, right deviation, and indeterminate sections.

The mean frontal plane QRS axis can be determined in a number of ways. The most accurate method is to average the forces moving right and left with those moving up and down because this method represents the frontal plane. Because lead I is the most direct right/left lead and lead aVF is the most direct up/down lead, it is easiest to use these two perpendicular leads to calculate the mean axis. Figure 15-14*A* shows the frontal plane leads of a 12-lead ECG. In Figure 15-14*B*, leads I and aVF are shown enlarged along with the axis wheel with small hash marks along the axes of lead I and lead aVF. These hash marks represent the small 1-mV boxes on the ECG paper. To determine the mean QRS axis, follow these steps:

1. Look at the QRS complex in lead I and count the number of positive and negative boxes. Mark the net vector along the appropriate end of lead I on the axis wheel. In Figure 15-14*B*, the QRS complex in lead I is eight boxes positive with no significant negative deflections. Count eight hash marks toward the positive end of lead I and put a mark on the axis wheel at that spot.
2. Look at the QRS complex in aVF and follow the same procedure as before. In this example, the QRS complex in aVF is 14 boxes positive with no significant negative deflections. Count 14 hash marks along the positive end of the aVF axis and place a mark at that spot.
3. Draw a perpendicular line down from the mark on the lead I axis and a perpendicular line across from the mark on the aVF axis.

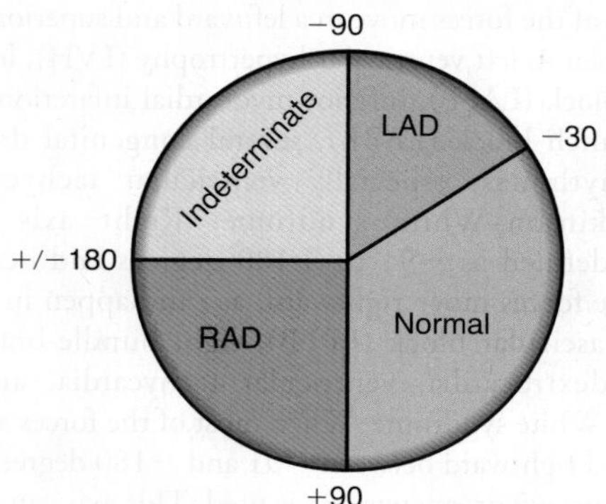

■ **Figure 15-13** Normal axis = −30° to +90°, LAD = −31° to −90°, RAD = +91° to +180°, indeterminate axis = −91° to −180°.

4. Draw a line from the center of the axis wheel to the spot where these two perpendicular lines meet. This line is the mean QRS axis—approximately +60 degrees.

A quick but less accurate method of axis determination is to place the axis in its proper quadrant of the axis wheel by looking at leads I and aVF, because these leads divide the wheel into four quadrants. As illustrated in Figure 15-15, if the QRS in both of these leads is positive, the axis falls in the normal quadrant, 0 to +90 degrees. If the QRS in lead I is positive and the QRS in aVF is negative, the axis falls in the left quadrant, 0 to −90 degrees. If the QRS in lead I is negative and the QRS in aVF is positive, the axis falls in the right quadrant, +90 to +180 degrees. If both leads are negative, the axis falls in the indeterminate quadrant or "no-man's land," −90 to −180 degrees. Locating the correct quadrant is often adequate but, because the portion of the left quadrant between 0 and −30 degrees is considered normal, it is necessary to determine more precisely whether the axis is less than or greater than −30 degrees. To do this quickly, look at Lead II: if the QRS in lead II is positive, the axis is less than −30 degrees; if the QRS in Lead II is negative, the axis is more negative than −30 degrees indicating LAD.

Using the ECG in Figure 15-16*A*, first place the axis in the appropriate quadrant by using leads I and aVF. Lead I is upright and aVF is negative, placing the axis in the left quadrant. However, because 30 degrees of the left quadrant is considered normal, we need to fine-tune the axis to determine where in the left quadrant it actually falls. Look at lead II: the QRS in lead II is mostly negative indicating that the axis is left of −30 degrees and that LAD is present. The axis wheel shows how to count boxes to get a more precise axis. The QRS in lead I is six boxes positive with no negative deflections; count six hashmarks along the positive end of lead I axis and place a mark. The QRS in aVF has an R wave 4 boxes positive and an S wave 16 boxes negative, for a net direction of −12 boxes; count 12 hashmarks along the negative end of aVF and place a mark. The axis is about −70 degrees, indicating LAD.

Using the ECG in Figure 15-16*B*, place the axis in the appropriate quadrant. Because lead I is negative and aVF is positive, the axis is in the right quadrant. The axis wheel shows how to count boxes to obtain a more precise axis. The QRS in lead I is two boxes positive and five boxes negative for a net of three boxes negative; mark this spot on the negative end of lead I on the axis wheel. The QRS in aVF is two boxes negative and 12 boxes positive for a net of +10 boxes; mark this spot on the positive end of lead aVF on the axis wheel. The axis is about +110 degrees, indicating RAD.

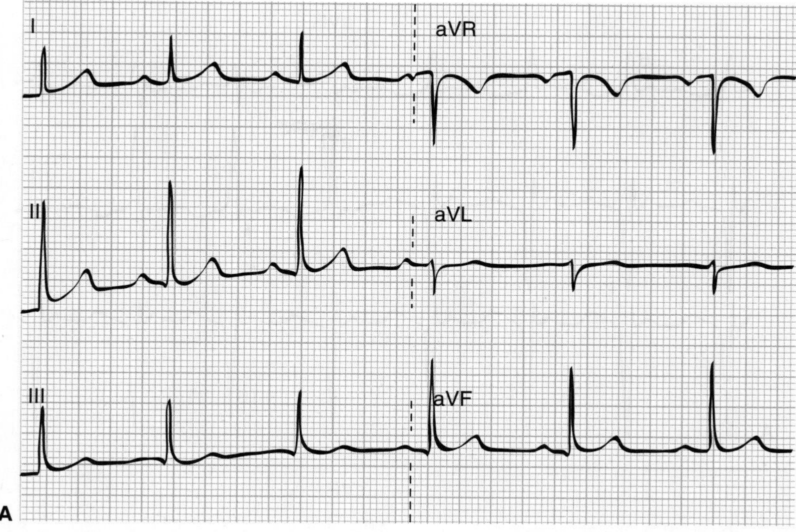

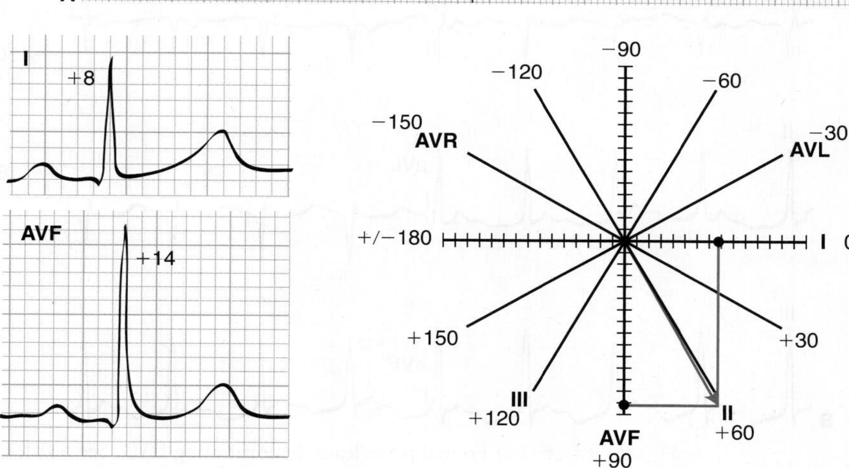

■ **Figure 15-14** Calculating the mean QRS axis. (A) The six frontal plane leads of an ECG. (B) Lead I and lead aVF enlarged. See text for instructions on calculating the axis using leads I and aVF on the axis wheel.

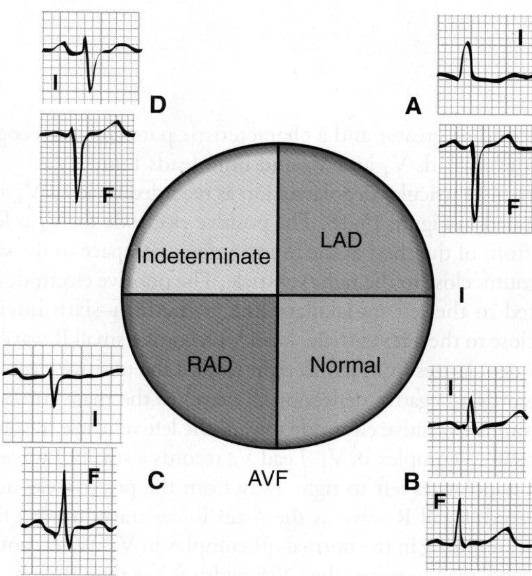

■ **Figure 15-15** The four quadrants of the axis wheel. (A) If the QRS in lead I is positive and the QRS in aVF is negative, the axis is in the left quadrant. (B) If the QRS is positive in both leads I and aVF, the axis is normal. (C) If the QRS in lead I is negative and the QRS in aVF is positive, the axis is in the right quadrant. (D) If the QRS is negative in both leads I and aVF, the axis is indeterminate.

INTRAVENTRICULAR CONDUCTION ABNORMALITIES

The intraventricular conduction system consists of the right bundle branch and the left main bundle branch, which fans out into septal fascicles, an anterior fascicle, and a posterior fascicle. There are numerous individual anatomic variations, but the intraventricular conduction system is generally regarded to consist of three major fascicles that diverge from the bundle of His: (1) the right bundle branch, (2) the anterior division of the left bundle branch (left anterior fascicle), and (3) the posterior division of the left bundle branch (left posterior fascicle[9]; Fig. 15-17). Block may occur in any part of this conduction system. Monofascicular block involves block in only one of the three major fascicles. The term bifascicular block is most commonly used to describe the combination of RBBB and either LAFB or LPFB. Trifascicular block means block in all three major divisions.

Bundle-Branch Block

When one of the bundle branches is blocked, the ventricles depolarize asynchronously. Bundle-branch block is characterized by a delay of excitation to one ventricle and abnormal spread of electrical activity through the ventricle whose bundle is blocked. This delayed conduction results in widening of the QRS complex to

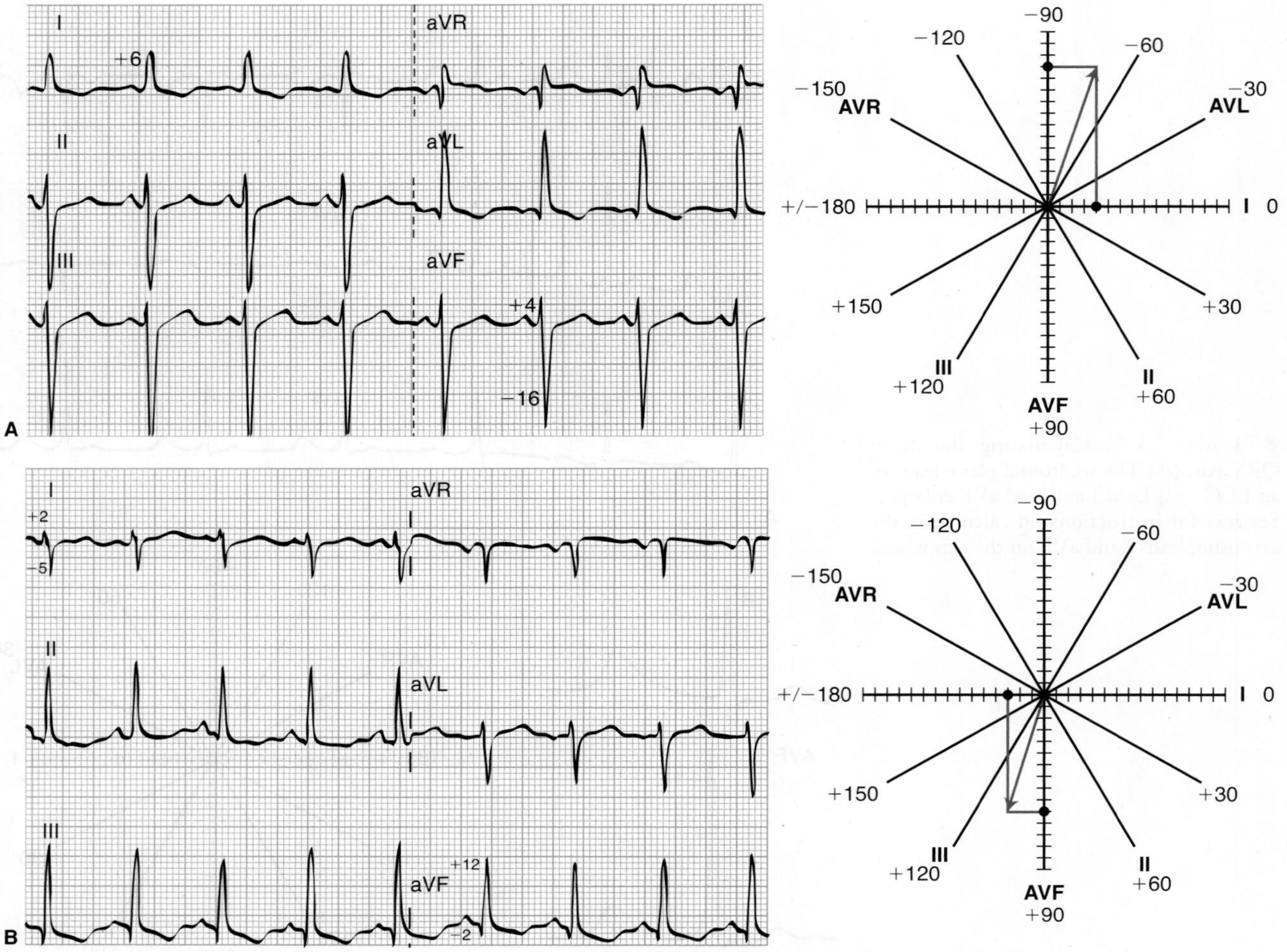

■ **Figure 15-16** (A) Frontal plane leads demonstrating LAD. See text for explanation. This is an example of LAFB. (B) Frontal plane leads demonstrating RAD. See text for explanation. This is an example of LPFB.

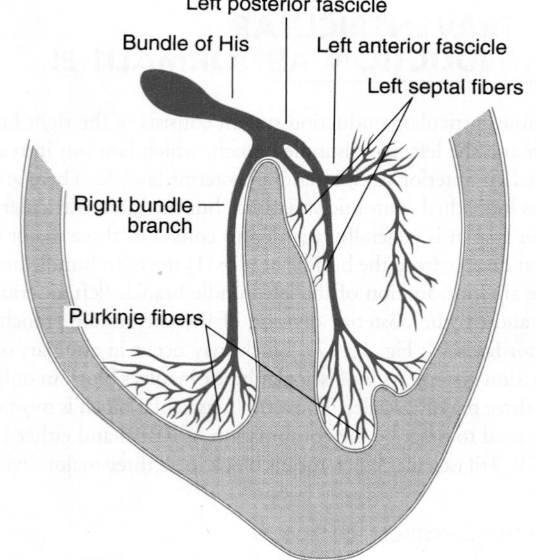

■ **Figure 15-17** Intraventricular conduction system. Right bundle branch carries impulse into right ventricle. Left main bundle branch divides into anterior and posterior fascicles, which carry impulse into left ventricle.

0.12 second or greater and a characteristic pattern best recognized in precordial leads V_1 and V_6 and limb leads I and aVL.

Normal ventricular depolarization as recorded by leads V_1 and V_6 is illustrated in Figure 15-18. The positive electrode for V_1 is located on the front of the chest at the fourth intercostal space to the right of the sternum, close to the right ventricle. The positive electrode for V_6 is located in the left midaxillary line at the fifth–sixth intercostal space, close to the left ventricle. Lead V_1 records a small R wave as the septum depolarizes from left to right toward the positive electrode. It then records a negative deflection (S wave) as the main forces travel away from the positive electrode toward the left ventricle, resulting in the normal rS complex in V_1. Lead V_6 records a small Q wave as the septum depolarizes left to right away from the positive electrode. It then records a tall R wave as the main forces travel toward the left ventricle, resulting in the normal qR complex in V_6. When both ventricles depolarize together, the QRS width is less than 0.12 second.

Right Bundle-Branch Block

Figure 15-19*A* illustrates the spread of electrical forces in the ventricles when the right bundle branch is blocked. Three separate forces occur:

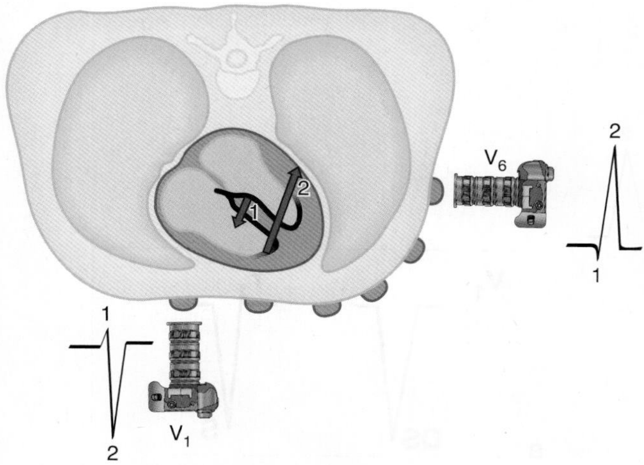

■ **Figure 15-18** Normal ventricular activation as recorded by leads V_1 and V_6.

1. Septal activation occurs first from left to right, resulting in the normal small R wave in V_1 and small Q wave in V_6.
2. The left ventricle is activated next through the normally functioning left bundle branch. Depolarization spreads normally through the Purkinje fibers in the left ventricle, causing an S wave in V_1 as the impulse travels away from its positive electrode and an R wave in V_6 as the impulse travels toward the positive electrode in V_6.
3. The right ventricle depolarizes late and abnormally as the impulse spreads by cell-to-cell conduction through the right ventricle. This abnormal activation causes a wide second R wave (called Rprime) in V_1 as it travels toward the positive electrode in V_1, and a wide S wave in V_6 as it travels away from the positive electrode in V_6. Because muscle cell-to-cell conduction is much slower than conduction through the Purkinje system, the QRS complex widens to 0.12 second or greater.

Typical uncomplicated RBBB can be recognized by a wide rSR prime pattern in V_1 and a wide qRs pattern in V_6 and in leads I and aVL, because the positive electrode in these two limb leads is located on the left side of the body. Figure 15-20*B* illustrates three

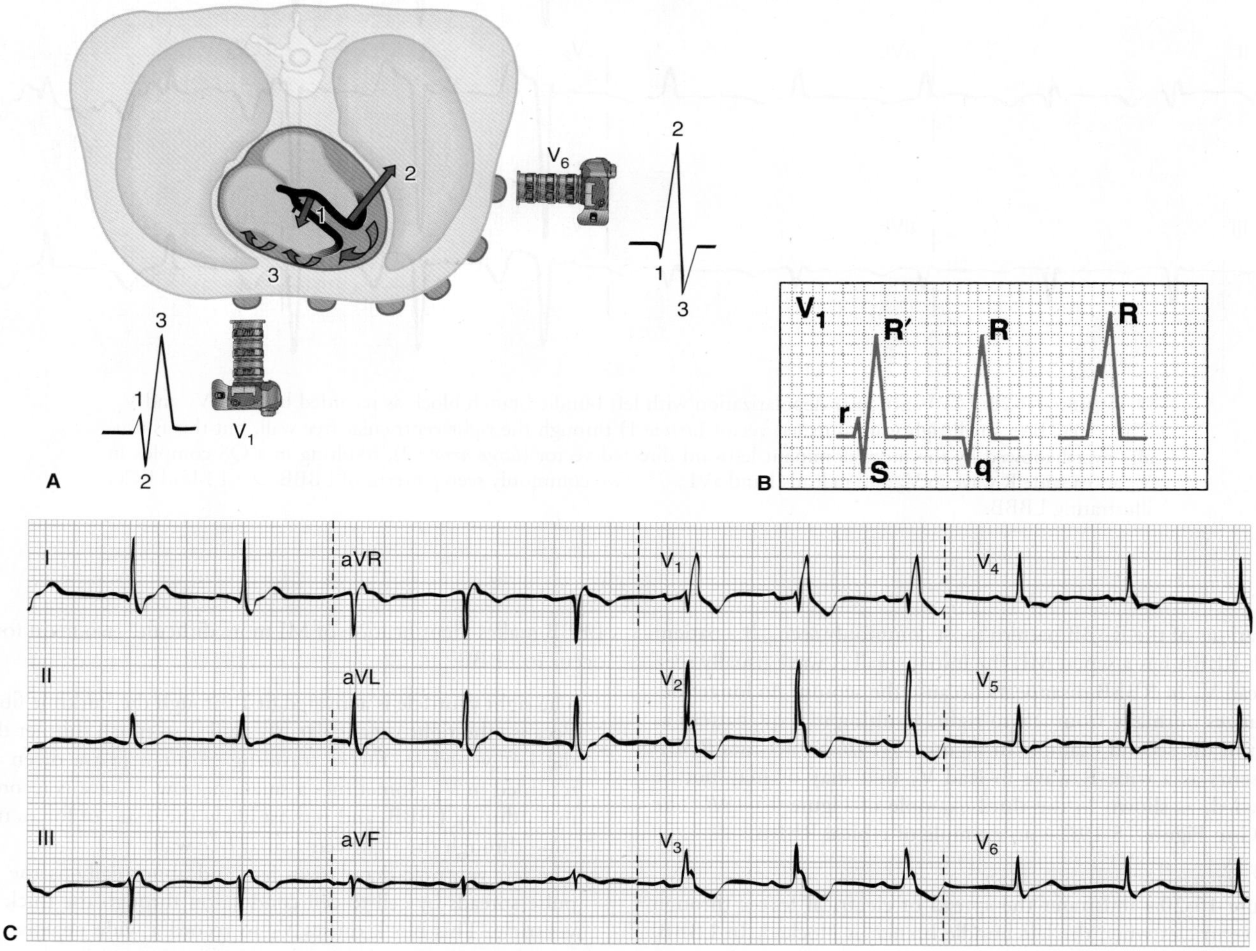

■ **Figure 15-19** (A) Ventricular depolarization with right bundle branch block as recorded by leads V_1 and V_6. Septal activation occurs first (*arrow* 1) causing an R wave in V_1 and Q wave in V_6; left ventricular activation occurs second (*large arrow* 2) causing an S wave in V_1 and an R wave in V_6; right ventricular activation occurs last and slowly (*curved arrows* 3) causing an R' in V_1 and a wide S wave in V_6. (B) Three commonly seen variations of RBBB pattern. (C) 12-lead ECG illustrating RBBB.

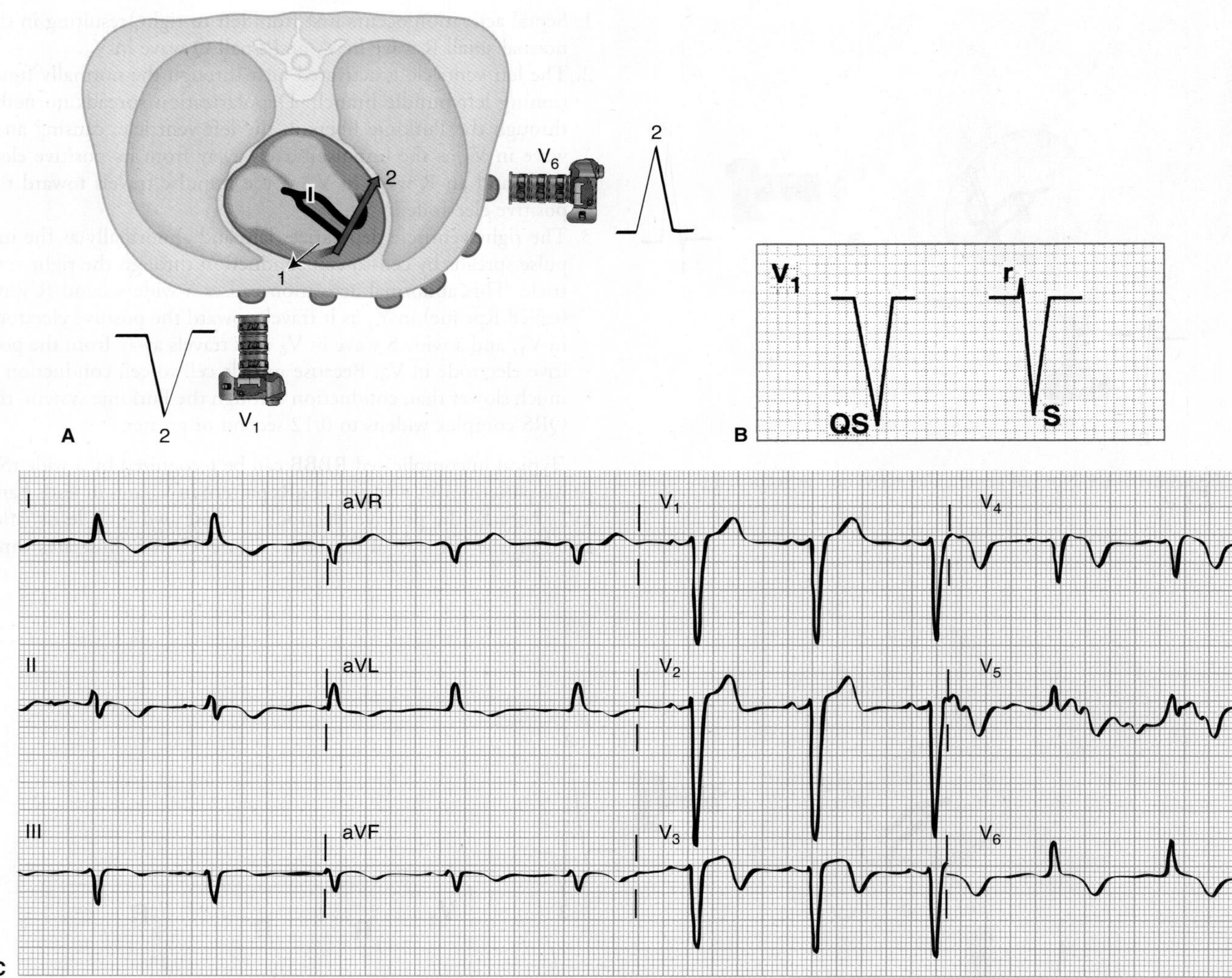

■ **Figure 15-20** (A) Ventricular depolarization with left bundle branch block as recorded by leads V_1 and V_6. There may be a small rightward directed vector (*arrow* 1) through the right ventricular free wall, but this is usually overshadowed by the more dominant leftward directed vector (*large arrow* 2), resulting in a QS complex in V_1 and a wide R wave in V_6 and in leads I and aVL. (B) Two commonly seen patterns of LBBB. (C) 12-lead ECG illustrating LBBB.

variations of the RBBB pattern most commonly seen. If a patient with RBBB has a septal MI, the initial small R wave usually seen in lead V_1 in RBBB disappears because the septum no longer depolarizes normally from left to right, resulting in a qR pattern as seen in the second example in Figure 15-19*B*. Sometimes RBBB presents as a wide R wave in lead V_1 that may or may not be notched, as shown in the third example of Figure 15-19*B*. The ECG in Figure 15-19*C* is an example of typical RBBB.

Left Bundle-Branch Block

Figure 15-20*A* illustrates the spread of electrical forces through the ventricles when the left bundle branch is blocked. In LBBB, the septum does not depolarize in its normal left-to-right direction because the block occurs above the Purkinje fibers that normally activate the left side of the septum. This block causes the loss of the normal small R wave in V_1 and loss of the Q wave in V_6, lead I, and aVL. The loss of normal initial QRS forces in LBBB makes identification of MI more difficult. Two main forces occur in LBBB.

1. The right ventricle is activated first through the Purkinje fibers. Because the right ventricular free wall is so much thinner than the left ventricle, forces traveling through it are often not recorded in V_1. Sometimes a small, narrow R wave is recorded in V_1 during LBBB, and is most likely the result of forces traveling through the right ventricular free wall.
2. The left ventricle depolarizes late and abnormally as the impulse spreads by cell-to-cell conduction through the thick left ventricle. This block causes V_1 to record a wide negative QS complex as the impulse travels away from its positive electrode. The lateral leads V_6, I, and aVL record a wide R wave as the impulse travels through the large left ventricle toward their positive electrodes. The QRS widens to 0.12 second or greater due to the slow cell-to-cell conduction in the left ventricle.

LBBB is recognized by a wide QS complex in V_1 and wide R waves with no Q waves in V_6, lead I, or aVL. Figure 15-20*B* shows two commonly seen LBBB patterns, the most common being the wide QS in lead V_1, and a less common rS complex in V_1. The ECG in Figure 15-20*C* illustrates LBBB.

Fascicular Blocks

The term *fascicular block* or *hemiblock* is used to describe block in either division of the left bundle branch. In fascicular block, both ventricles depolarize simultaneously so the QRS remains narrow, but the direction of left ventricular depolarization is altered. The most useful ECG leads for recognizing fascicular block are leads I and aVF for the QRS axis, and leads I and III for the typical pattern of fascicular block.

Figure 15-17*A* illustrates the normal intraventricular conduction system and the relationship between the anterior and posterior divisions of the left bundle. When the left ventricular free wall is activated normally, the anterior fascicle carries the electrical impulse in a superior and leftward direction, and the posterior fascicle carries it downward and rightward. Because free wall activation proceeds in both directions simultaneously, most of the forces cancel each other and result in the normal QRS shape seen in leads I and III and a normal QRS axis as the combined forces proceed downward and leftward through the left ventricle (Fig. 15-21*A*). When fascicular block occurs, left ventricular activation proceeds from one site instead of both simultaneously, removing the cancellation and altering the shape of the QRS in leads I and III. Because the left ventricle is depolarized in an abnormal direction, an axis deviation always results from fascicular block, but the QRS duration remains normal or is very slightly prolonged.

Left Anterior Fascicular Block

In LAFB (also called *anterior hemiblock*), the impulse conducts through the posterior fascicle and begins depolarizing the ventricle in an inferior and rightward direction. It then travels through the left ventricular free wall in a superior and leftward direction, resulting in an LAD (Fig. 15-21*B*). The degree of LAD required to diagnose LAFB is at least −45 degrees.[9] The initial forces are directed inferiorly and rightward, causing a small Q wave in lead I and a small R wave in lead III. The forces then travel superiorly and leftward, causing a normal R wave in lead I and an abnormally deep S wave in lead III. There may or may not be a Q wave in lead I, depending on whether initial septal activation is directed to the left or to the right. Figure 15-16*A* is an example of LAFB. The ECG characteristics of LAFB are:

1. LAD (−45 degrees or more)
2. Small Q in lead I, large S in lead III (QI, SIII), or an rS pattern in leads II, III, and aVF
3. QRS duration not prolonged more than 0.11 second
4. Increased QRS voltage in limb leads due to loss of cancellation of forces in left ventricle

Left Posterior Fascicular Block

In LPFB (also called *posterior hemiblock*), the impulse conducts through the anterior fascicle and begins depolarizing the ventricle in a superior and leftward direction. It then travels through the left ventricular free wall in an inferior and rightward direction, resulting in an RAD (Fig. 15-21*C*). The initial forces are directed superiorly and leftward, causing a small R wave in lead I and a small Q wave in lead III. The forces then travel inferiorly and rightward, causing a deep S wave in lead I and a tall R wave in lead III. Before diagnosing LPFB, the clinician must rule out RVH because RVH can cause the identical frontal plane picture. Figure 15-16*B* is an example of LPFB. The ECG characteristics of LPFB are:

1. RAD (≥+100 degrees)
2. Small R in leads I and aVL, small Q in leads II, III, and aVF (SI, QIII), or an rS pattern in leads I and aVL
3. Normal QRS duration (not >0.11 second)
4. Increased QRS voltage in limb leads due to loss of cancellation of QRS forces
5. No evidence of RVH

Bifascicular Block

Bifascicular block means that two of the three major fascicles are blocked. Because block in both divisions of the left bundle branch presents as complete LBBB, the term *bifascicular block* is usually used to refer to block in the right bundle branch along with block in either the anterior or posterior divisions of the left bundle branch. The ECG displays the typical RBBB morphology (wide QRS and rSR′ pattern, or one of its variants) along with an axis deviation consistent with the fascicular block. Figure 15-22 is an example of RBBB and LAFB. Figure 15-23 shows RBBB and LPFB.

ACUTE CORONARY SYNDROME

Myocardial ischemia is the result of an imbalance between myocardial O_2 supply and demand and is a reversible process if blood flow is restored before permanent cellular damage occurs. Ischemia can result from increased myocardial O_2 demands or from decreased myocardial O_2 supply. If ischemia is severe and blood flow is not restored relatively soon, cellular injury and eventually necrosis (cell death) result.

The term *acute coronary syndrome* (ACS) is used to refer to the pathophysiologic continuum that begins with plaque rupture in a coronary artery and ultimately results in permanent cell damage (infarction) if the process is not arrested (see Chapter 22). ACS encompasses three distinct phases of this continuum: (1) unstable angina (UA), (2) non-ST elevation MI (NSTEMI), and (3) ST elevation MI (STEMI). Once an infarction has occurred, as indicated by elevated biochemical cardiac markers, it is classified electrocardiographically as either a Q-wave or a non–Q-wave MI based on the presence or absence of Q waves on the ECG.

MI can occur because of blockage of a coronary artery with thrombus or from severe and prolonged ischemia due to coronary artery spasm or unrelieved obstruction of a coronary artery. When infarction does occur, there are varying degrees of damage to cells involved in the process, ranging from ischemia to injury to cell death. MI has traditionally been described as having three "zones" of tissue damage, each of which produces characteristic changes on the ECG (Fig. 15-24). Although this drawing is an oversimplification of what actually happens, the concept is still useful in understanding the ECG changes that occur with MI.

Myocardial ischemia can result in several changes on the ECG (Fig. 15-25). The most familiar pattern of ischemia is T-wave inversion, although T-wave inversion is often a nonspecific finding

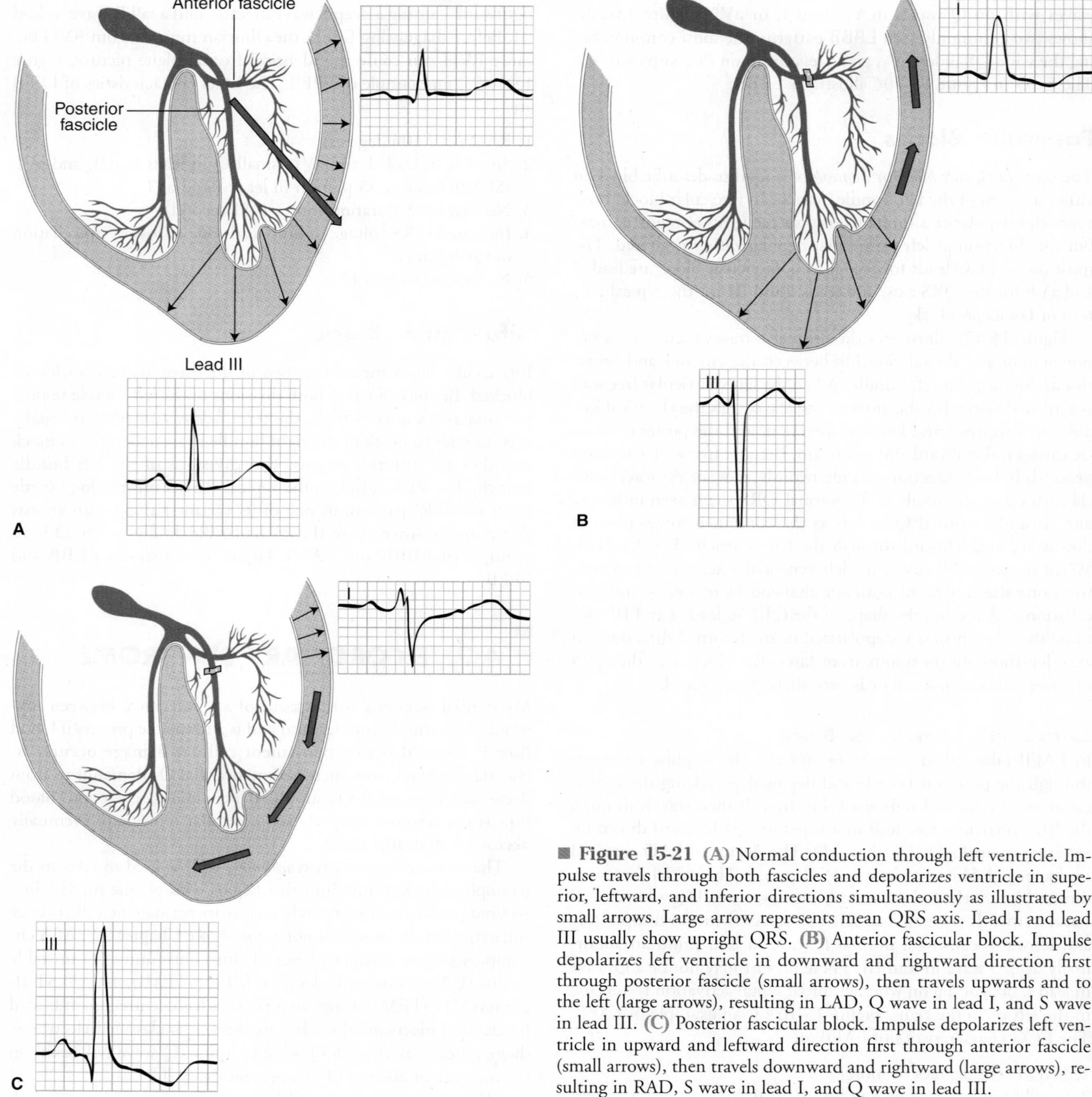

■ **Figure 15-21** (A) Normal conduction through left ventricle. Impulse travels through both fascicles and depolarizes ventricle in superior, leftward, and inferior directions simultaneously as illustrated by small arrows. Large arrow represents mean QRS axis. Lead I and lead III usually show upright QRS. (B) Anterior fascicular block. Impulse depolarizes left ventricle in downward and rightward direction first through posterior fascicle (small arrows), then travels upwards and to the left (large arrows), resulting in LAD, Q wave in lead I, and S wave in lead III. (C) Posterior fascicular block. Impulse depolarizes left ventricle in upward and leftward direction first through anterior fascicle (small arrows), then travels downward and rightward (large arrows), resulting in RAD, S wave in lead I, and Q wave in lead III.

and can be due to a variety of causes other than ischemia. Other indicators of ischemia include horizontal or downsloping ST-segment depression of 0.5 mm or more; an ST segment that remains on the baseline longer than 0.12 second; an ST segment that forms a sharp angle with the upright T wave; tall, wide-based T waves; and inverted U waves.[5–8,10–13] Display 15-1 lists several causes of ST-segment and T-wave changes.

Myocardial injury is most often indicated by ST-segment elevation of 1 mm or more above the baseline in leads with positive electrodes facing the infracted area. Other signs of acute injury include a straightening of the ST segment that slopes up to the peak of the T wave without spending any time on the baseline; tall, peaked T waves; and symmetric T-wave inversion[5–8,12–14] (Fig. 15-26).

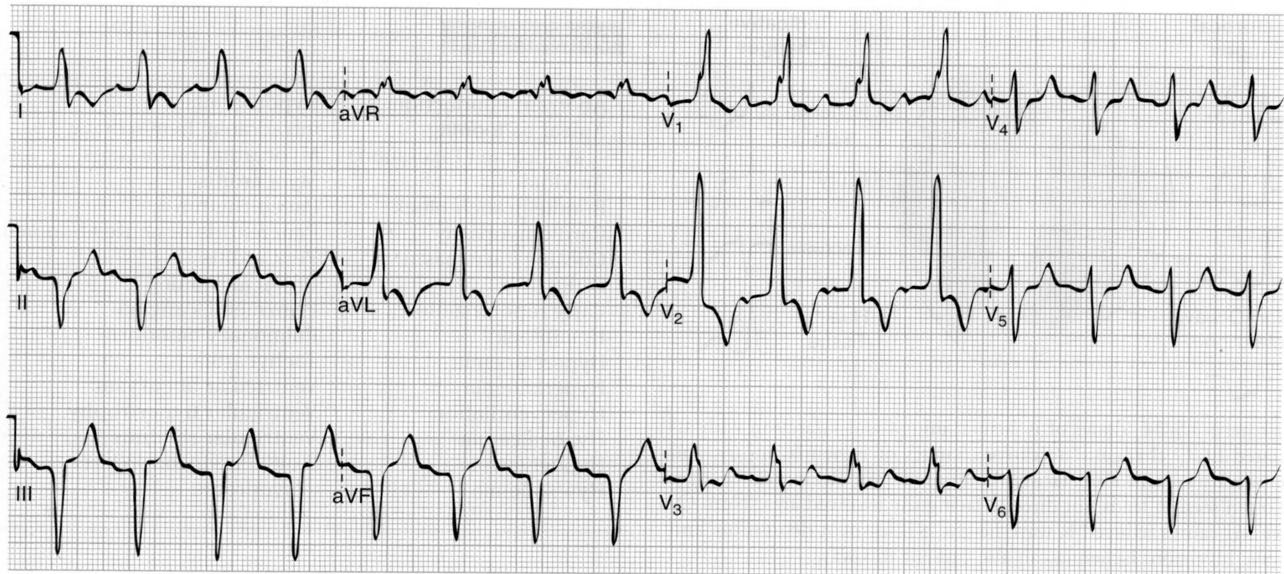

■ **Figure 15-22** ECG of RBBB and LAFB. Rhythm is sinus, QRS width is 0.14 second, there is LAD (–70°) due to LAFB, and V_1 shows the wide notched R-wave variation of RBBB.

Necrosis or death of myocardial tissue is indicated on the ECG by development of new Q waves or deepening of preexisting Q waves. Abnormal Q waves are greater than 0.03 second wide or 25% of the ensuing R-wave amplitude. (See Figs. 15-11 and 15-12 for examples of normal Q waves; Figs. 15-28 through 15-30 show examples of abnormal Q waves.) Display 15-2 lists conditions other than MI that can result in development of Q waves. Traditionally, it was taught that the presence of Q waves indicates transmural MI extending through the entire thickness of the muscle, and that nontransmural (subendocardial) infarction involving less than the entire thickness of the muscle does not produce Q waves. It is now known that Q waves can develop transiently with severe ischemia and with nontransmural MI, and that transmural infarction can occur without the development of Q waves.[7,10–12] Therefore, the newer terms *Q-wave* and *non–Q-wave* MI are preferred over the older terms *transmural* and *nontransmural or subendocaridal* infarction. In any case, the presence of abnormal Q waves is still considered to be ECG evidence of myocardial necrosis.

The ECG reflects the progression of the MI from the acute stage through the fully evolved stage. Very early MI often causes peaking and widening of the T waves followed within minutes by ST-segment elevation. ST-segment elevation can persist for hours to several days but resolves more quickly with successful reperfusion. Once the ST segment has returned to baseline, ECG evidence of the acute stage is lost. Q waves appear within hours of pain onset and usually remain forever, although sometimes Q waves disappear over the years after infarction. T-wave inversion occurs within hours after infarction and can last for months. T waves often return to their previous upright position within a few months after acute MI. Thus, an *evolving infarct* is one in which serial ECGs show ST segments returning toward baseline, the development of Q waves, and T-wave inversion. The term *old infarction* or *infarct of undetermined age* is used when the first ECG recorded shows Q waves, ST segment at baseline, and T waves either inverted or upright, indicating that an MI occurred at some point in the past.

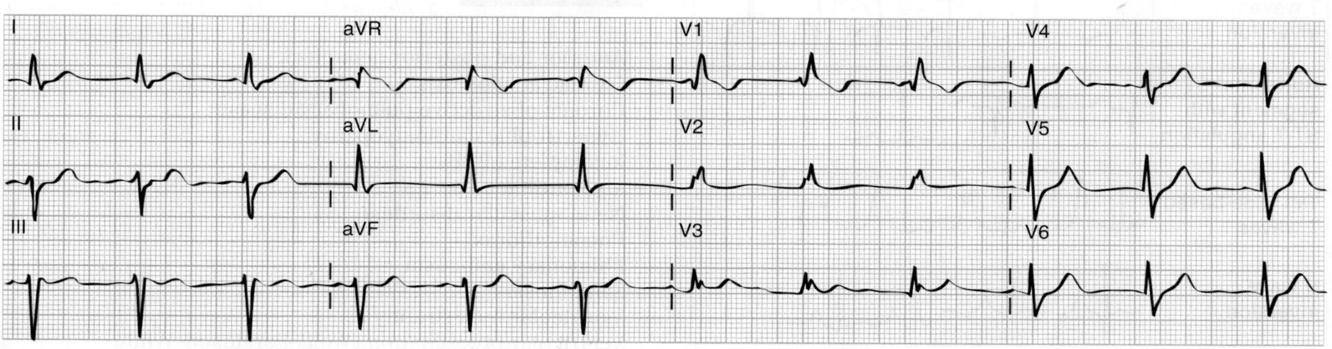

■ **Figure 15-23** ECG of RBBB and LPFB. Rhythm is atrial fibrillation, QRS width is 0.12 second, there is RAD (about +150°) due to LPFB, and V_1 shows the wide R wave variation of RBBB.

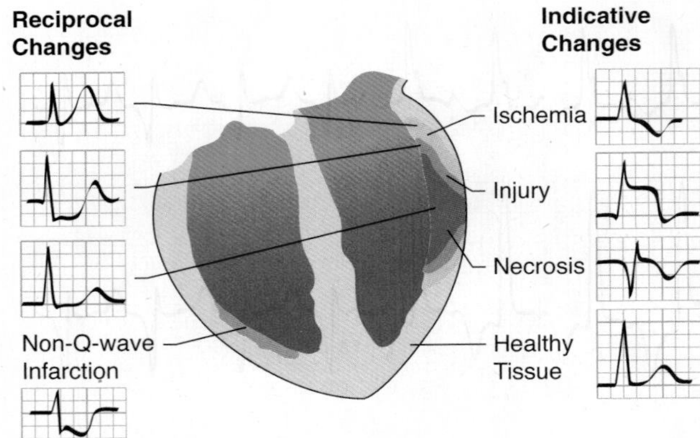

■ **Figure 15-24** Zones of ischemia, injury, and infarction with associated ECG changes. Indicative changes of ischemia, injury, and necrosis are seen in leads facing the injured area. Reciprocal changes are often seen in leads not directly facing the involved area. Non–Q-wave MI causes reduced R wave height, ST segment depression, and T-wave inversion. Ischemia can also present this way.

DISPLAY 15-1 Causes of St-Segment and T-Wave Changes[2,3,5–7,10–12,14–16]

Aberrant conduction	Hypothermia
Apical ballooning syndrome (Takotsubo)	Intracranial hemorrhage
Amyloidosis	Myocardial metastases
Bundle-branch block	Myocarditis
Cardiomyopathy	Paced rhythm
Cocaine vasospasm	Pancreatitis or acute abdomen
Drugs	Pericarditis
Early repolarization	Physical training
Hemiblock	Prinzmetal's angina
Hypercalcemia	Pulmonary embolism
Hyperkalemia	Tachycardia
Hyperventilation	Ventricular aneurysm
Hypocalcemia	Ventricular hypertrophy
Hypoglycemia	Ventricular rhythms
Hypokalemia	Wolff–Parkinson–White syndrome

ECG Diagnosis of STEMI

ST-segment elevation, Q waves, and T-wave inversion are recorded in leads where the positive electrode facing the damaged myocardium and are called the *indicative changes* of infarction. Other leads not facing the involved tissue are often affected by the loss of electrical forces in damaged tissue and record mirror-image changes called *reciprocal changes.* Figure 15-24 illustrates indicative and reciprocal changes associated with MI, and Table 15-1 lists leads in which indicative and reciprocal changes are found in each of the major types of MI. Figure 15-27 illustrates how to localize ischemia, injury, and infarction using the 12-lead ECG.

Anterior MI

Anterior wall MI (see Fig. 15-28) is due to occlusion of the left anterior descending coronary artery and is recognized by indicative changes in leads facing the anterior wall (V_{1-4}). Reciprocal changes are often recorded in the lateral leads I and aVL and the inferior leads II, III, and aVF. Loss of normal R-wave progression or development of Q waves and ST elevation in V_{1-4} are seen in anterior infarction. If only the septum is infarcted, changes occur only in leads V_{1-2}, but, if the entire anterior wall is involved, changes are seen in V_{1-4}. Anterior wall infarction that extends laterally and involves leads I and aVL is often referred to as *extensive anterior* or *anterolateral* infarction (see Fig. 15-31).

Inferior MI

Inferior wall MI (see Fig. 15-29) is usually due to occlusion of the right coronary artery and is diagnosed by indicative changes in leads II, III, and aVF. Reciprocal changes are often seen in leads I, aVL, or the V leads. When inferior MI is due to right coronary artery occlusion, there is usually ST depression in lead I and ST elevation in lead III, which is higher than that in lead II.[7,10] In people with left dominant coronary circulation, the circumflex artery supplies the inferior surface of the heart and circumflex occlusion

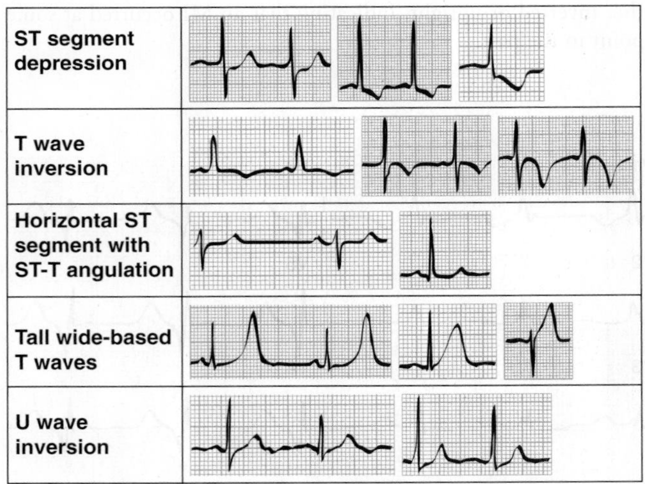

■ **Figure 15-25** ECG patterns associated with myocardial ischemia.

DISPLAY 15-2 Causes of Noninfarction Q Waves[2,3,5–7,10–12,14–16]

- Anterior and posterior hemiblock
- Cardiac amyloidosis
- Chronic obstructive pulmonary disease
- Hypertrophic cardiomyopathy
- Incomplete LBBB
- Myocarditis
- Neuromuscular disorders
- Pneumothorax
- Pulmonary embolism
- Sarcoidosis
- Ventricular hypertrophy
- Ventricular preexcitation (Wolff–Parkinson–White syndrome)

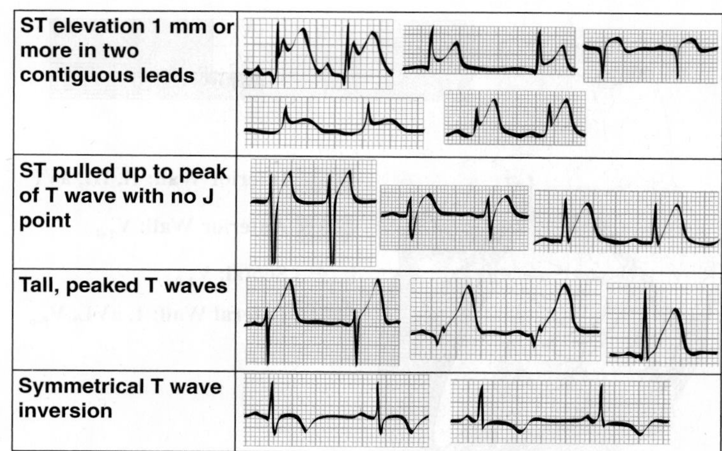

ST elevation 1 mm or more in two contiguous leads
ST pulled up to peak of T wave with no J point
Tall, peaked T waves
Symmetrical T wave inversion

■ **Figure 15-26** ECG patterns associated with acute myocardial injury.

is the cause of inferior MI, resulting in ST elevation in lead II greater than that in lead III, and the ST in lead I is either isoelectric or elevated.[10] Approximately 30% of inferior MIs involve the right ventricle[7,17] (see Fig. 15-32).

Lateral MI

Lateral wall MI is due to circumflex artery occlusion and presents with indicative changes in leads I, aVL, and sometimes V_{5-6}, with reciprocal changes in inferior or anterior leads (see Fig. 15-30). Lateral wall MI does not often occur alone but commonly accompanies anterior MI, as it does in Figure 15-31.

Right Ventricular MI

Right ventricular MI (RVMI; see Fig. 15-32) occurs in up to 45% of inferior MIs, and, therefore, it usually is associated with indicative changes in the inferior leads II, III, and aVF.[7,10,11,17] In addition, it is not uncommon to see ST-segment elevation in V_1 as well, because V_1 is the chest lead that is closest to the right ventricle. ST-segment elevation in V_1 together with ST-segment elevation in the inferior leads is suspect for RVMI. Another clue is discordance between the ST segment in V_1 and the ST segment in V_2. Discordance means that the ST segments do not point in the same direction—V_1 shows ST-segment elevation, whereas V_2 is either normal or shows ST-segment depression. This finding is highly likely to indicate RVMI, although rarely the ST segment will be elevated in V_1–V_4 in RVMI. When RVMI is suspected, right-sided chest leads should be obtained as soon as possible because the changes seen in right-sided leads may disappear within 24 hours (see Fig. 15-9). Leads V_{4R} through V_{6R} develop ST-segment elevation when acute RVMI is present. Lead V_{4R} is the most sensitive and specific lead for recognition of RVMI.[7,10,17] The recording of V_4R in patients with inferior MI and hemodynamic instability is a class I recommendation from the 2004 ACC/AHA Task Force.[18] Some facilities have a policy that directs ECG technicians to obtain automatically right-sided and posterior leads in all patients with ST elevation in the inferior leads.

Posterior MI

Posterior wall MI (Fig. 15-33) is due to occlusion of the posterior descending artery, which is usually a branch of the right coronary artery. In left dominant circulations the posterior descending is a branch of the circumflex artery. Isolated posterior wall MI is uncommon; it usually accompanies inferior or lateral wall MI,[2,6,7,11] as seen in Figure 15-33*B*. ECG changes of posterior MI are less obvious because in the standard 12-lead ECG there are no leads those face the posterior wall, and, therefore, no indicative changes are recorded. The diagnosis is made by observing reciprocal changes in the anterior leads, especially V_1 and V_2, but often all the way to V_4. Reciprocal changes seen in these leads include a taller R wave than normal (mirror image of the Q wave that would be recorded over the posterior wall), ST-segment depression (mirror image of the ST-segment elevation from the posterior wall), and upright, tall T waves (mirror image of the T-wave inversion from the posterior wall). The diagnosis can be confirmed by recording posterior leads (see Fig. 15-9) and observing ST elevation and Q waves. Another way to verify the presence of posterior MI is to flip the ECG over vertically and hold it up to a light, looking at leads V_1 and V_2, which will now show Q waves and ST elevation that would be recorded in posterior leads (Fig. 15-33*C*).

Table 15-1 ■ ELECTROCARDIOGRAPHIC CHANGES ASSOCIATED WITH STEMI

Location of MI	Indicative Changes: ST Elevation, Q Waves, T Wave Inversion	Reciprocal Changes: ST Depression, Tall R Waves, Upright T Waves
Anterior	V_1 to V_4	I, aVL, II, III, aVF
Septal	V_1, V_2	I, aVL
Inferior	II, III, aVF	I, aVL, If seen in V_1 to V_3 suspect posterior MI
Posterior	None in standard 12 leads Posterior leads V_7–V_9	V_1 to V_4
Lateral	I, aVL, V_5, V_6	II, III, aVF If seen in V_1, V_3 suspect posterior MI
Right ventricle	II, III, aVF (inferior MI) Right chest leads V_4R–V_6R	

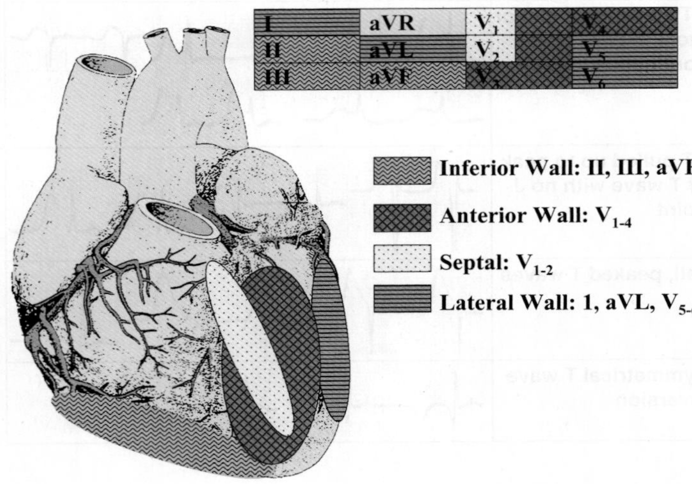

■ **Figure 15-27** Localizing myocardial ischemia, injury, or infarction using the 12-lead ECG. The different areas of the heart are pattern-coded. Standard 12-lead ECG format is illustrated at upper right with leads pattern-coded to correspond to the area of the heart that each lead faces. (Adapted from Cummins, R. O. [2000]. *ACLS provider manual* [p. 129]. Dallas, TX: American Heart Association.)

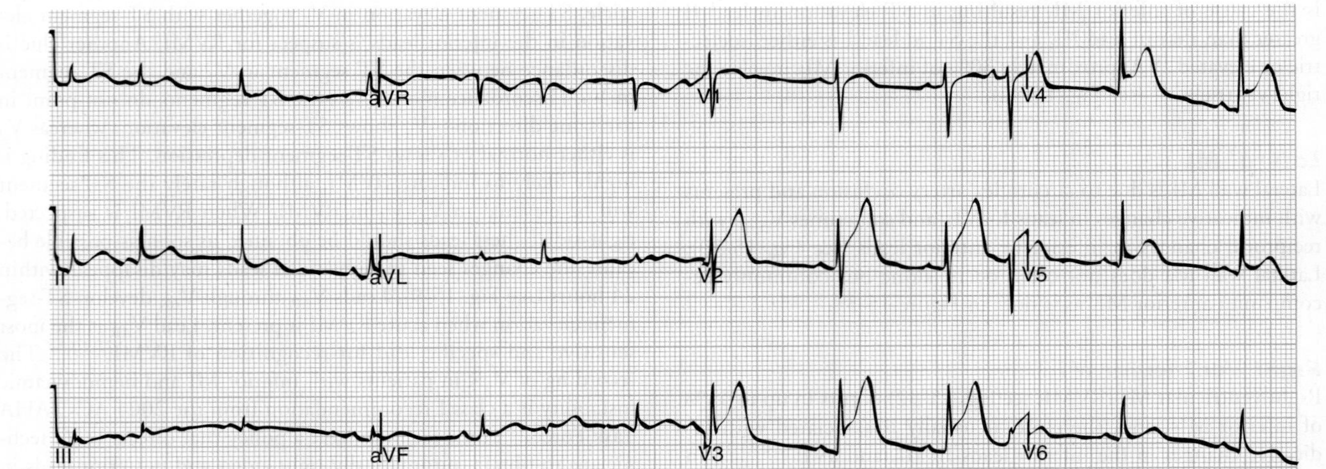

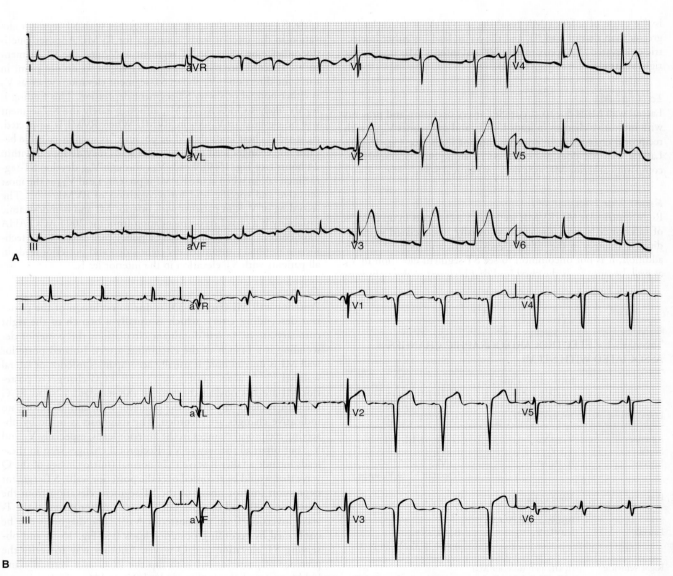

■ **Figure 15-28** (A) Early acute anterior wall MI. Note ST elevation most pronounced in leads V_2–V_5 indicating acute injury and intact R-wave progression in the V leads indicating that no necrosis has yet occurred. (B) Anterior wall MI. ST elevation is present in V_1–V_4 and there is a loss of R-wave progression across the precordium resulting in Q waves in V_1–V_3. The QRS axis is about −50 degrees indicating probable LAFB. *(continued)*

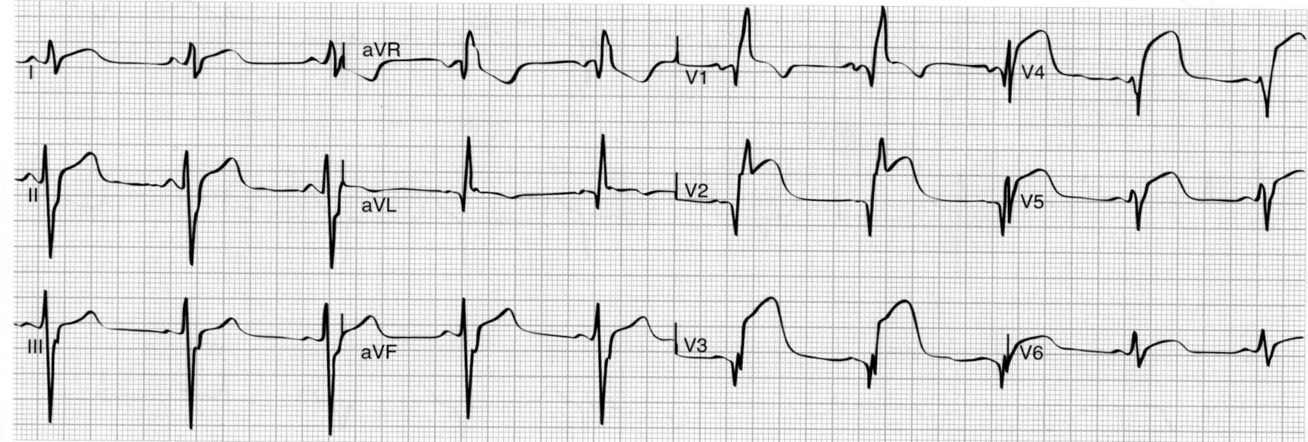

■ **Figure 15-28** *(continued)* (C) Same patient as in (B) an hour later. Now there is RBBB and the axis is further left at about −80 degrees: bifascicular block. ST elevation is now present in the lateral leads I, and V_4–V_6 indicating extension to the lateral wall.

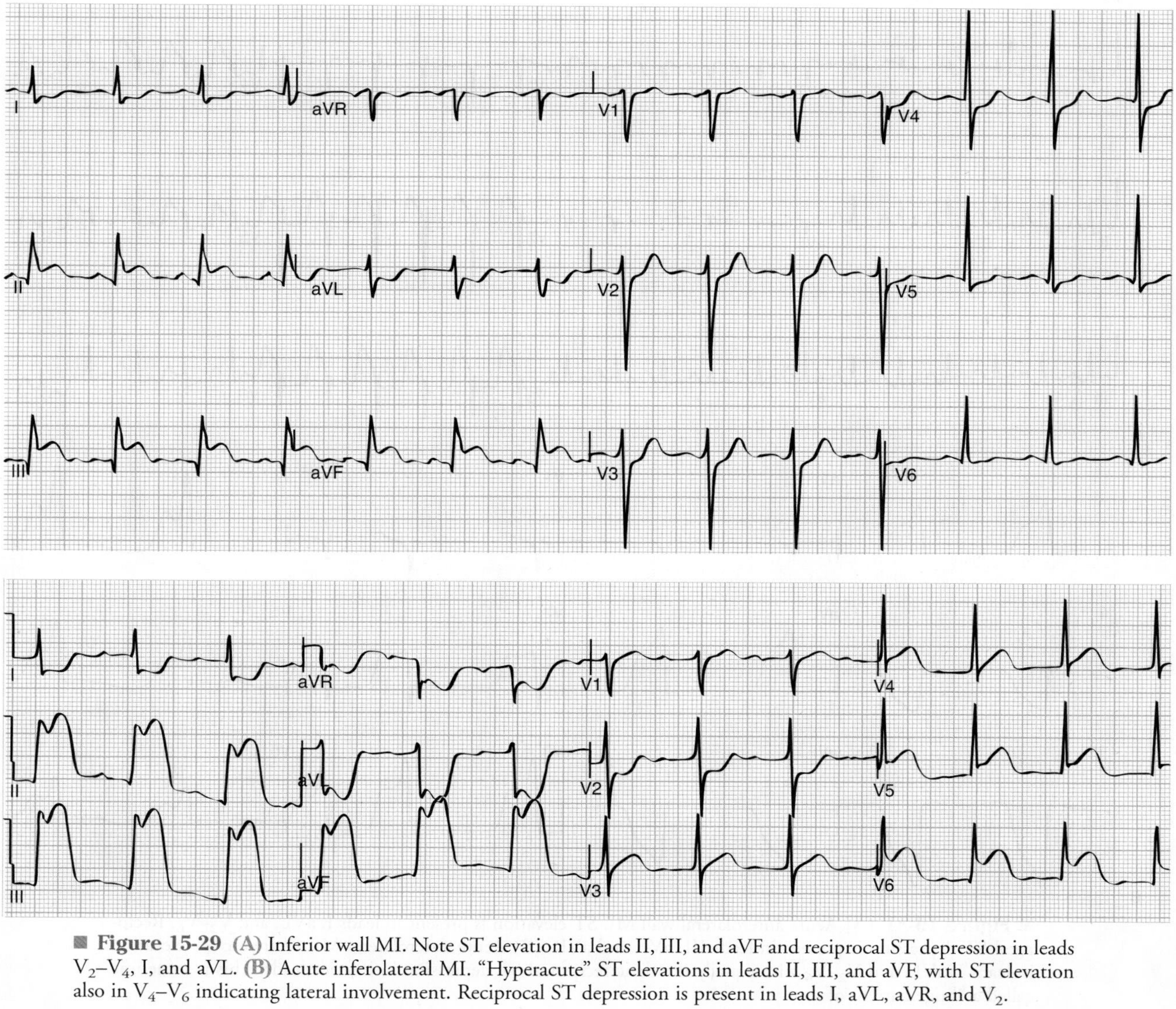

■ **Figure 15-29** (A) Inferior wall MI. Note ST elevation in leads II, III, and aVF and reciprocal ST depression in leads V_2–V_4, I, and aVL. (B) Acute inferolateral MI. "Hyperacute" ST elevations in leads II, III, and aVF, with ST elevation also in V_4–V_6 indicating lateral involvement. Reciprocal ST depression is present in leads I, aVL, aVR, and V_2.

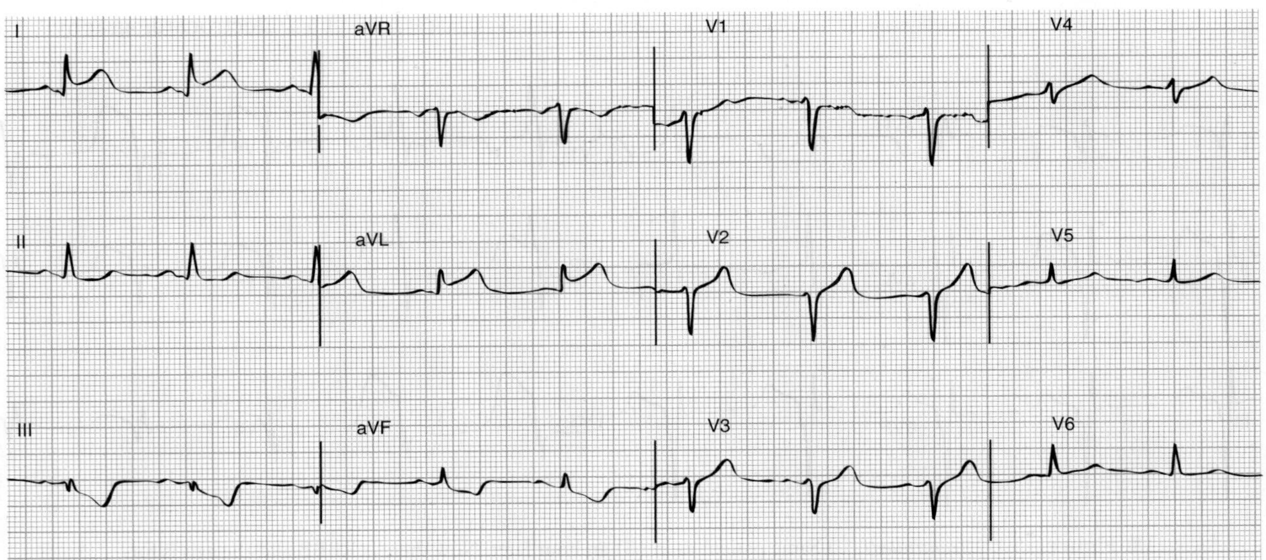

■ **Figure 15-30** Lateral wall infarction. ST elevation is present in leads I and aVL with reciprocal depression in inferior leads. The absence of ST elevation in V_4 and V_5 indicates that the high lateral wall is involved but not the lower portion. R-wave progression is not normal in V_1–V_3, indicating potential anterior involvement.

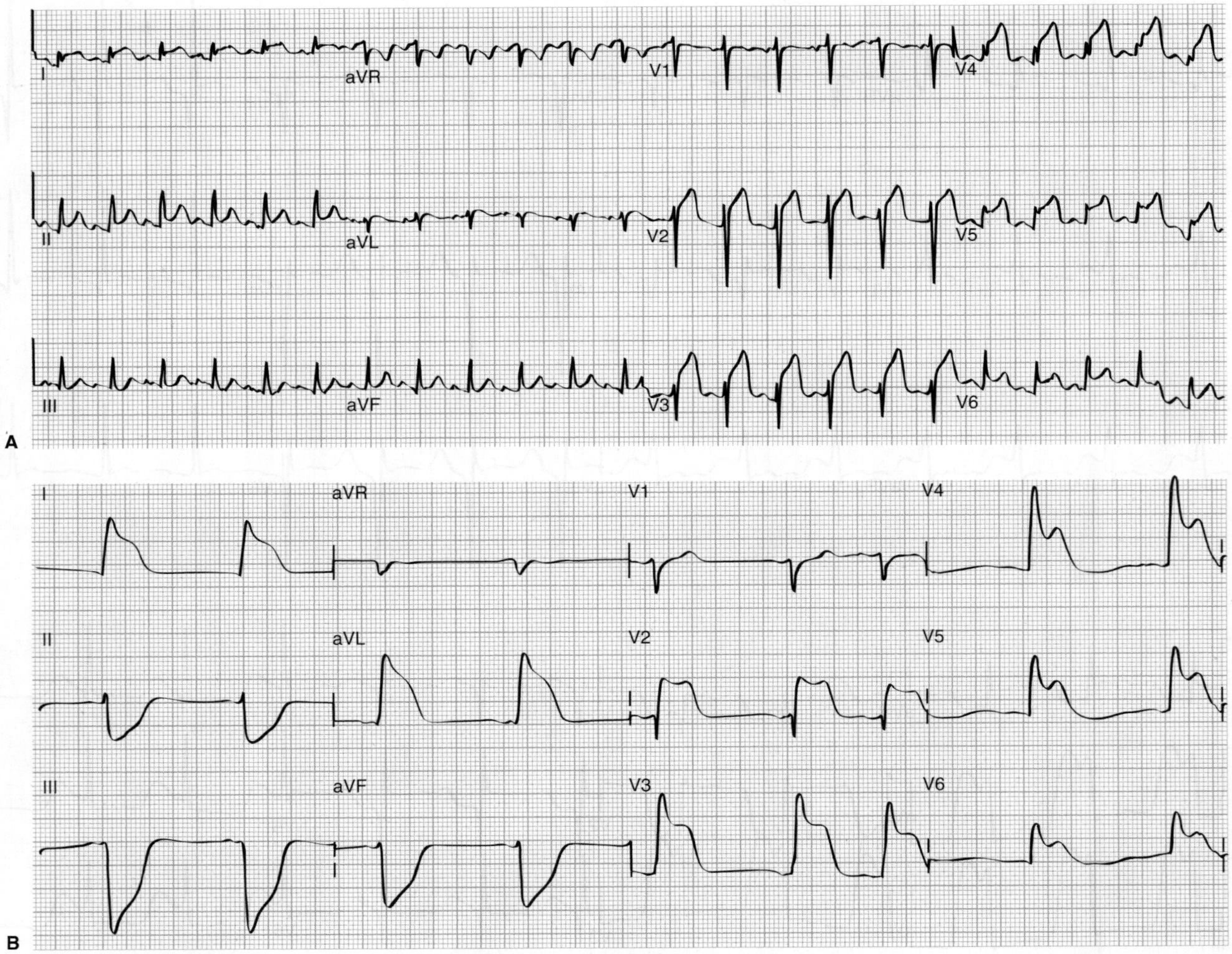

■ **Figure 15-31** (A) Acute anterolateral wall MI. ST elevation is present in leads I, aVL, and V_2–V_6. Reciprocal ST depression is present in leads III, aVF, and aVR. (B) Acute anterolateral MI. Dramatic ST elevation in leads I, aVL, and V_2–V_6 with equally dramatic reciprocal ST depression in inferior leads. This is sometime called a "huge current of injury."

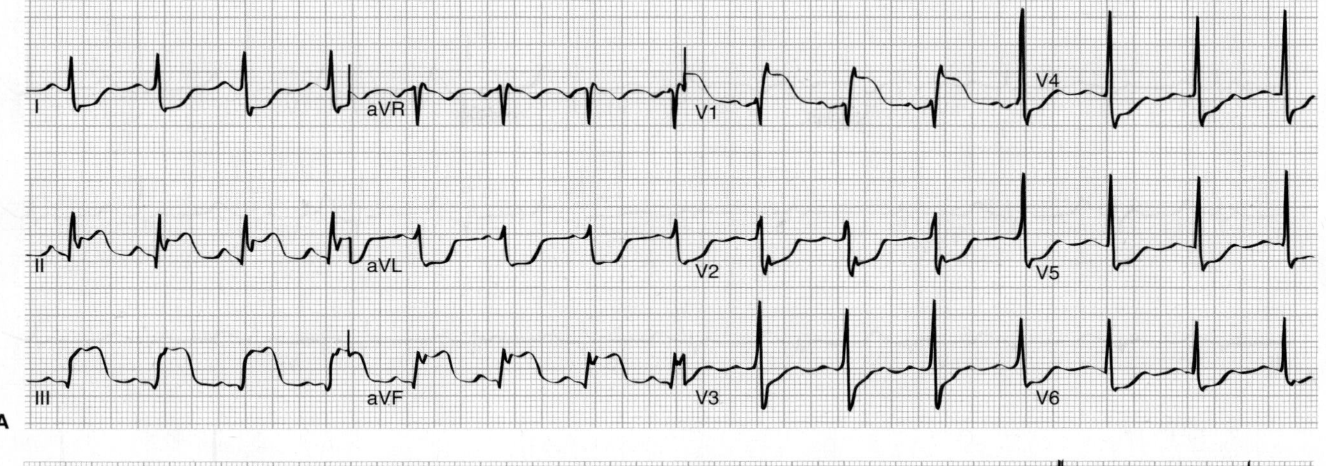

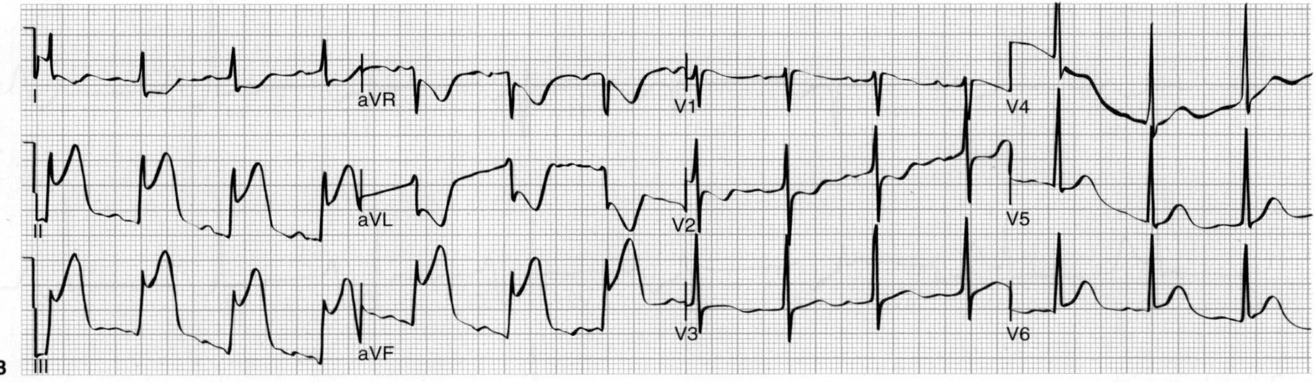

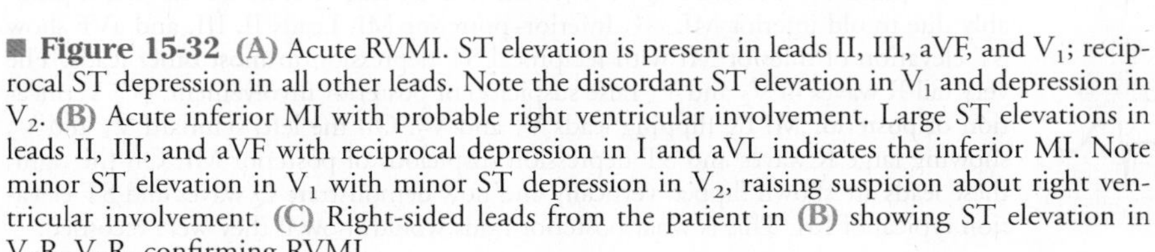

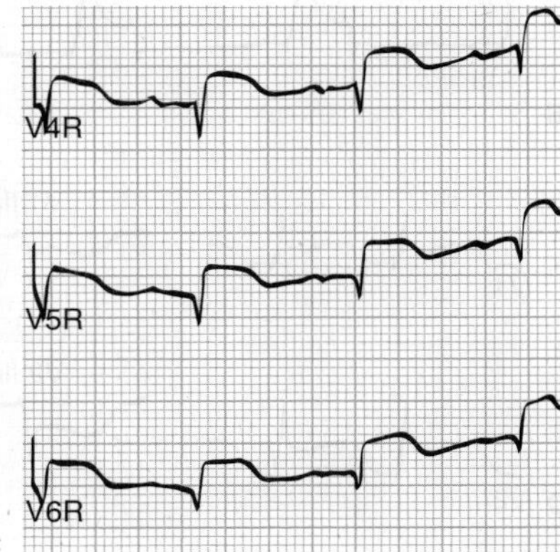

■ **Figure 15-32** (A) Acute RVMI. ST elevation is present in leads II, III, aVF, and V_1; reciprocal ST depression in all other leads. Note the discordant ST elevation in V_1 and depression in V_2. (B) Acute inferior MI with probable right ventricular involvement. Large ST elevations in leads II, III, and aVF with reciprocal depression in I and aVL indicates the inferior MI. Note minor ST elevation in V_1 with minor ST depression in V_2, raising suspicion about right ventricular involvement. (C) Right-sided leads from the patient in (B) showing ST elevation in V_4R–V_6R, confirming RVMI.

ECG Diagnosis of UA/NSTEMI

UA and NSTEMI are subsets of ACS and are diagnosed when the ECG shows ST depression or prominent T-wave inversion without the presence of ST elevation in patients with chest pain typical of ACS.[10,19] The differential diagnosis is made based on the presence or absence of cardiac biomarkers, specifically troponin and/or creatine kinase MB isoenzyme (CK-MB). If ischemia is present without resulting myocardial injury, biomarkers are negative and the diagnosis is UA. If ischemia is severe enough to result in injury with biomarker release, the diagnosis is NSTEMI. The two conditions share the same pathophysiology and differ only in degree of severity, and they appear identical on the ECG.

The terms *Q-wave MI* and *non–Q-wave MI* are used to describe the presence or absence of Q waves on the ECG when the diagnosis of MI has been established. Non–Q-wave MI has traditionally been considered to involve necrosis of the subendocardial layer of the ventricle and not the entire thickness of the ventricular wall. Necrosis of sufficient myocardium can lead to loss of R-wave amplitude rather than to development of Q waves in leads facing the infarcted area (see Fig. 15-24). Most patients who present with

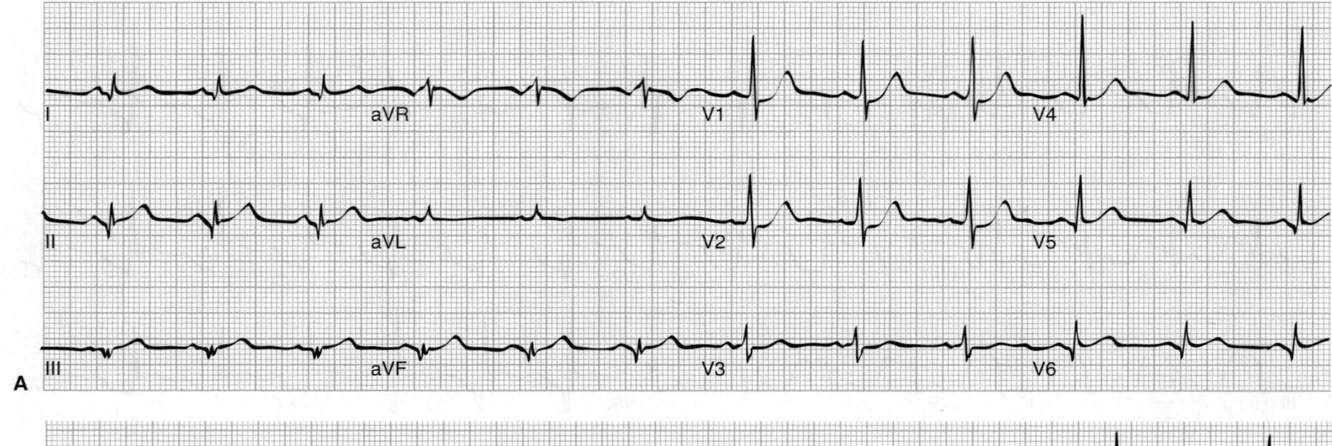

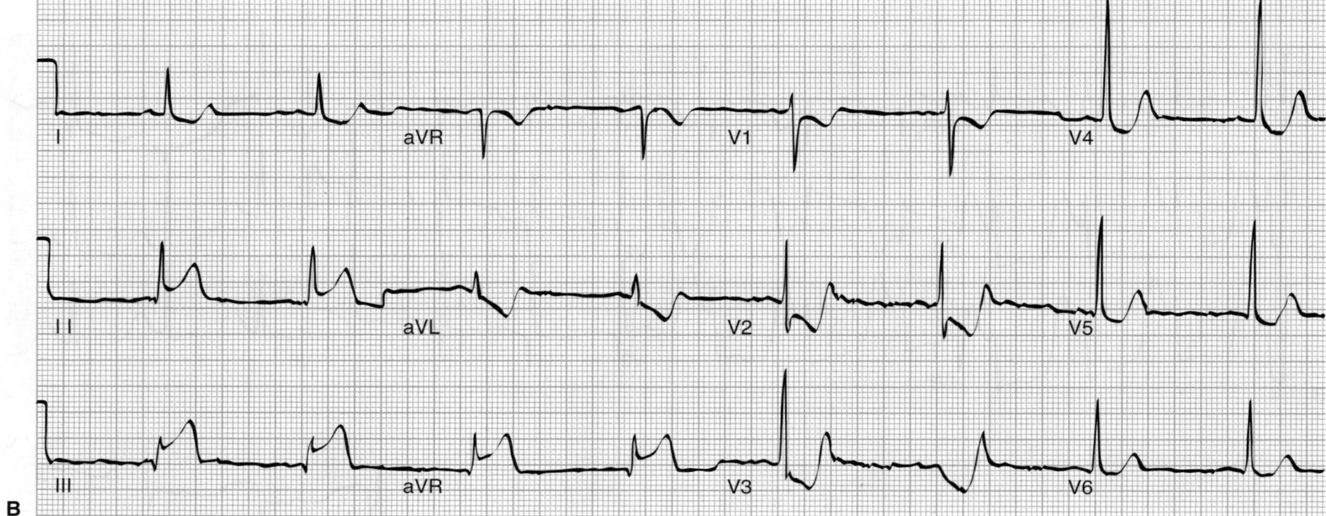

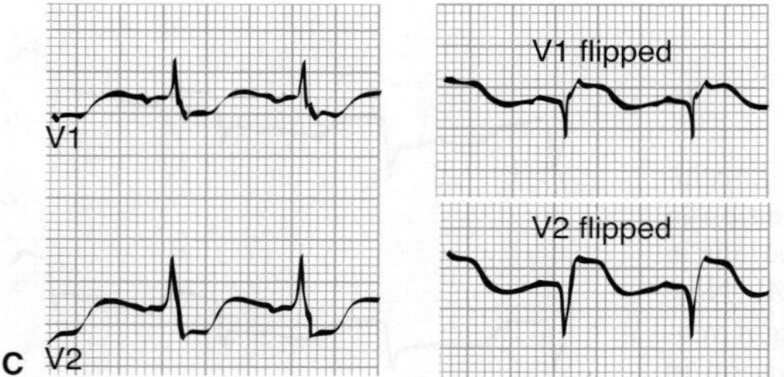

■ **Figure 15-33** (A) Posterior wall MI. Large R waves and ST depression are present in V_1 and V_2. There are Q waves in the inferior leads but no ST elevation, probably due to old inferior MI. (B) Inferior–posterior MI. Leads II, III, and aVF show ST elevation of inferior MI with reciprocal ST depression in most other leads. The very tall R waves in V_2 and V_3 raise suspicion of posterior involvement. (C) Verification of posterior MI by flipping leads V_1 and V_2. On the left, standard V_1 and V_2 showing large R waves and ST depression suspicious of posterior MI. On the right, these leads are shown flipped vertically and now demonstrate Q waves and ST elevation typical of MI. This is what posterior leads would show if they were recorded.

ischemic chest pain and ST elevation ultimately develop a Q-wave MI unless the culprit artery is reperfused quickly. Patients with ST depression or T wave inversion, no ST elevation, and positive biomarkers do not necessarily develop Q waves even though they have had an MI.

Figure 15-34 shows two ECGs obtained in patients with chest pain typical of acute myocardial infarction but without ST elevation on the ECG. ST depression and T wave inversion, often present in multiple leads, are the hallmarks of UA and NSTEMI. The more leads that show ST depression, the greater the extent and severity of coronary artery disease and the more likely the patient will benefit from early invasive therapy.[3,10] The presence of the following ECG findings is an indicator of left main coronary artery disease or significant triple-vessel disease[3,10]: (1) ST depression in at least eight leads; (2) ST elevation in aVR and V_1; (3) deep ST depression in precordial leads, most prominent in V_4; (4) ST elevation in lead III not present in lead II. Many of these features are present in Figure 15-34*A*.

ATRIAL AND VENTRICULAR ENLARGEMENT

Each of the four heart chambers can enlarge because of increased pressure or volume overload. The thin-walled atria usually respond

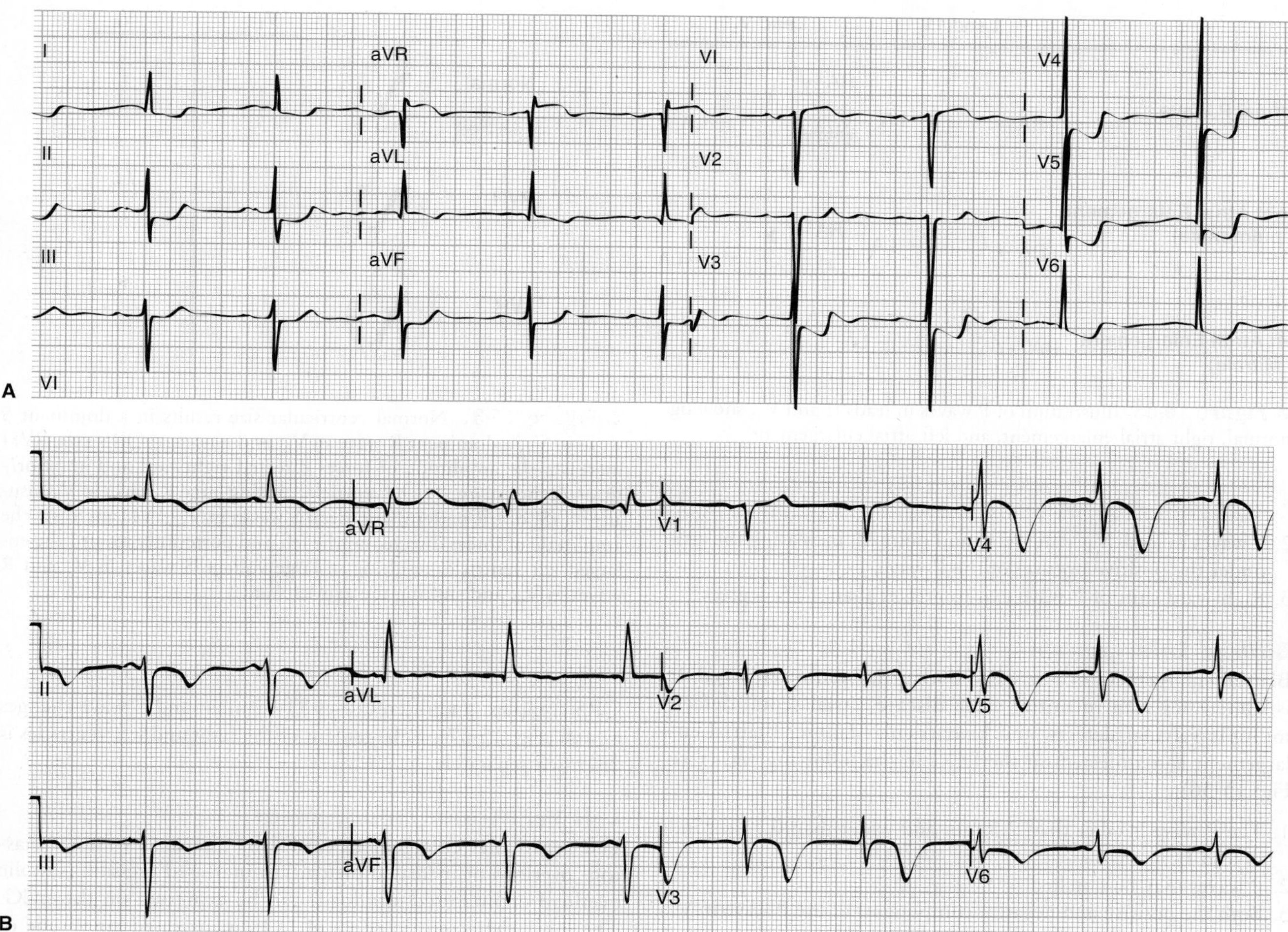

■ **Figure 15-34** (A) NSTEMI. Note widespread ST depression in leads I, II, III, aVF, and V_{2-6}. The ST segment elevation in aVR and V_1 along with ischemic changes in all other leads is suggestive of left main or significant triple vessel coronary artery disease. This patient's troponin and CK-MB were elevated, leading to the diagnosis of NSTEMI. (B) NSTEMI. There is T-wave inversion in several leads, especially deep in V_3–V_5, but no significant Q waves in any lead. Cardiac biomarkers were elevated.

to both pressure and volume overload by dilating, whereas the thicker-walled ventricles tend to dilate with volume overload and hypertrophy (increase wall thickness) with pressure overload.[6]

Atrial Enlargement

Atrial enlargement is reflected on the ECG as changes in P wave size and morphology. Normal P waves are no wider than 0.11 second or taller than 2.5 mm. They are usually upright in leads I, II, and V_{4-6} and diphasic with the initial portion upright and the terminal portion negative in V_1. Right atrial depolarization forms the first half of the P wave, and left atrial depolarization forms the second half (Fig. 15-35). Atrial enlargement usually accompanies ventricular enlargement, so the presence of ECG signs of atrial enlargement is suggestive of ventricular enlargement as well.

Left Atrial Enlargement

Left atrial enlargement is caused by conditions that increase pressure or volume in the left atrium, such as mitral stenosis, mitral regurgitation, systemic hypertension, and left heart failure. Left atrial enlargement can be manifested on the ECG in the following ways (Fig. 15-36):

1. The P wave is wider than 0.12 second and often notched in leads I, II, aVL, and V_{4-6} (termed *P mitrale*). The interval between the notches is >0.04 second, and the P wave may encroach into the PR segment, making the PR segment appear shorter than normal.
2. Increased width and depth of the terminal negative component of the P wave in lead V_1 or V_2.
3. Leftward shift of P wave axis to between −30 and +45 degrees.

Right Atrial Enlargement

Right atrial enlargement is commonly caused by conditions that increase the work of the right atrium, such as pulmonary hypertension, pulmonary or tricuspid stenosis or regurgitation, and congenital heart disease. Right atrial enlargement can be manifested on the ECG in the following ways (see Fig. 15-36):

1. The P waves are tall and peaked (>2.5 mm) in leads II, III, and aVF (termed *P pulmonale*).

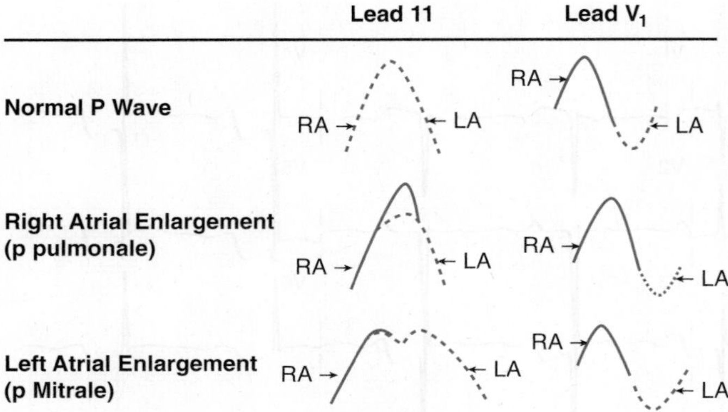

■ **Figure 15-35** Illustration of P waves in leads II and V_1, showing normal, right atrial enlargement, and left atrial enlargement.

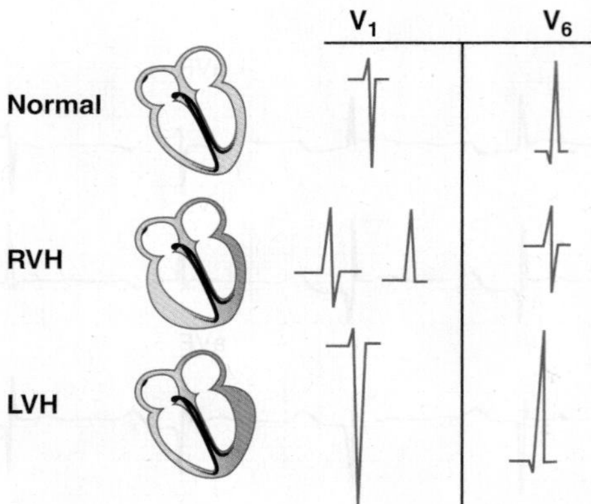

■ **Figure 15-37** Normal ventricular size results in a dominant S wave in V_1, a dominant R wave in V_6, and a normal QRS axis. RVH increases the amplitude of forces directed rightward and anteriorly through the enlarged right ventricle, causing large R waves in V_1 (usually R, rS, or qR pattern) and deep S waves in V_6. LVH increases the amplitude of forces directed to the left and posteriorly toward the enlarged left ventricle, resulting in large voltage S waves in V_1 and R waves in V_6, and shifting the axis leftward.

2. P waves in leads V_{1-3} are sharp and pointed, increasing the area under the positive portion of the P wave.
3. Rightward shift of P wave axis to greater than +75 degrees.

Biatrial Enlargement

Biatrial enlargement occurs when both atria become enlarged. It is sometimes seen in mitral valve disease, atrial septal defect, multiple valvular defects, and biventricular failure. Biatrial enlargement is manifested on the ECG in the following ways (see Fig. 15-36):

1. The P wave is taller than 2.5 mm and wider than 0.11 second in lead II.
2. P waves may be notched.
3. Both the positive and negative components of the P wave in V_1 may be enlarged.

Ventricular Enlargement

The ventricles can enlarge because of increased pressure or volume in the chamber. Ventricular enlargement affects the size of the QRS complex, and often causes ST segment and T wave changes as well (Fig. 15-37). Enlargement of the right and left ventricles is discussed separately.

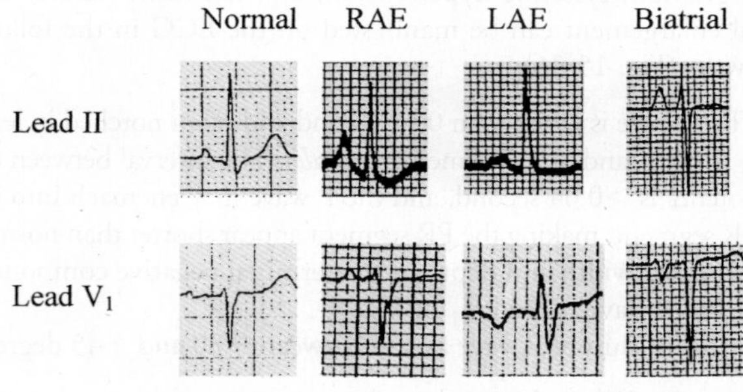

■ **Figure 15-36** Normal P waves compared to those of left atrial enlargement, right atrial enlargement, and biatrial enlargement in leads II and V_1. Left atrial enlargement causes widening and notching of P waves in many leads, and enlargement of the terminal negative portion of the P wave in V_1. Right atrial enlargement causes tall peaked P waves in many leads and enlargement of the initial upright portion of the P wave in V_1. Biatrial enlargement can make the entire P wave wider and taller than normal and vary its configuration in many leads.

Left Ventricular Enlargement

Left ventricular enlargement caused by increased volume (diastolic overload or increased preload) or increased pressure (systolic overload or increased afterload) can be expressed on the ECG. The most characteristic effect of LVH is increased amplitude of the R wave in leads facing the left ventricle (leads I, aVL, V_5, and V_6) as more forces travel through the enlarged left ventricle. There is a concurrent decrease in R-wave amplitude and increase in S-wave amplitude in leads facing the right ventricle (leads V_1 and V_2). The intrinsicoid deflection (the time from the beginning of the QRS complex to the peak of the R wave) is slightly delayed in leads facing the left ventricle, and the QRS width approaches the upper limit of normal because of the increased time required for electrical forces to travel through the thick left ventricular muscle. Figure 15-38 is an example of LVH.

The ST–T-wave changes that occur reflect repolarization abnormalities and may be due to hypertrophy or may be secondary consequences of dilation or ischemia. The term *strain* is often used to describe the ST–T-wave changes that commonly occur with LVH. ST-segment depression, often downsloping, with T-wave inversion commonly develops in left chest leads. Increased T-wave amplitude may be found in leads that show large R waves, and ST segments may be elevated in leads that show deep S waves. A variety of methods have been proposed to help diagnose LVH on the ECG, and Table 15-2 lists several of these methods.

Right Ventricular Enlargement

RVH may be caused by any condition that produces a sufficient load on the right ventricle, such as pulmonary disease or congenital or acquired heart disease, particularly mitral valve disease. The electrical events of the right ventricle are normally masked by the events taking place nearly simultaneously in the dominant left

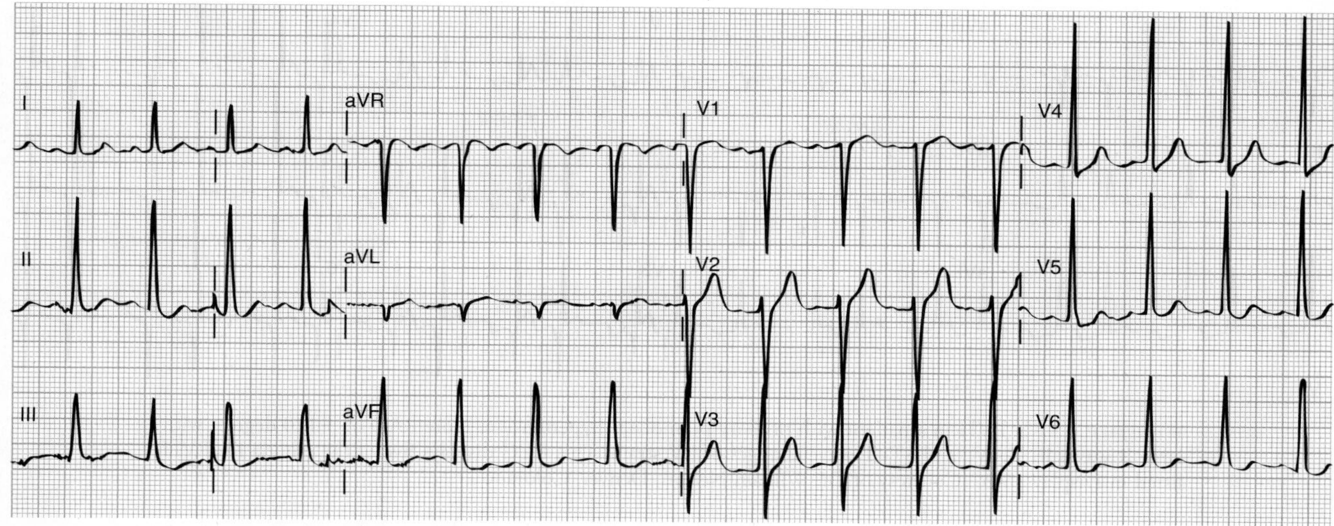

Figure 15-38 LVH with deep S waves in V_{1-2} and large voltage R waves in V_{4-6}. ST depression and T-wave inversion (strain pattern) are seen in V_{4-6}.

ventricle. As the right ventricle enlarges, these right-sided (or anterior) forces are revealed and may become the dominant forces if the right ventricle becomes as large or larger than the left. The normal sequence of depolarization is altered, resulting in ECG changes in axis, QRS morphology and voltage, and ST–T waves (Fig. 15-39).

The most obvious ECG change with RVH is a reversal of normal R-wave progression in precordial leads. R waves become dominant and the S wave shrinks in right chest leads, whereas R waves shrink and S waves dominate in left-sided leads. The same "strain" pattern described previously with ST-segment depression

Table 15-2 ■ METHODS TO DIAGNOSE LEFT VENTRICULAR ENLARGEMENT ON THE ECG

Author/Method	ECG Criteria Favoring Left Ventricular Enlargement	
Dubin, 1988	R wave in lead I + S wave in lead III > 26 mm	
	S wave in lead V_1 + R wave in lead V_5 or V_6 > 35 mm	
Sokolow and Lyon, 1949	R wave in VL ≥ 11 mm	
	S wave in lead V_1 + R wave in lead V_5 or V_6 > 35 mm	
	R wave in V_5 or V_6 > 26 mm	
Estes' Scorecard	*Criteria*	Points*
	1. R or S wave in limb lead 20 mm or more	
	S wave in lead V_1, V_2, or V_3 25 mm or more	
	R wave in lead V_4, V_5, or V_6 25 mm or more	3
	2. Any ST shift (without digitalis)	3
	Typical ST strain (with digitalis)	1
	3. LAD −30 degrees or more	2
	4. QRS interval 0.09 second or more	1
	5. Intrinsicoid deflection in V_5 and V_6 0.05 second or more	1
	6. P-wave terminal force in V_1 > 0.04 second	3
	Total possible	14
Scott's Criteria	Limb leads	
	R in 1 + S in 3 > 25 mm	
	R in aVL > 7.5 mm	
	R in aVF > 20 mm	
	S in aVR > 14 mm	
	Chest leads	
	S in V_1 or V_2 + R in V_5 or V_6 > 35 mm	
	R in V_5 or V_6 > 26 mm	
	R + S in any V lead > 45 mm	
Cornell Index	Women: R in aVL + S in V_3 > 20 mm	
	Men: R in aVL + S in V_3 > 28 mm	

*5 = Left ventricular enlargement; 4 = probable left ventricular enlargement.

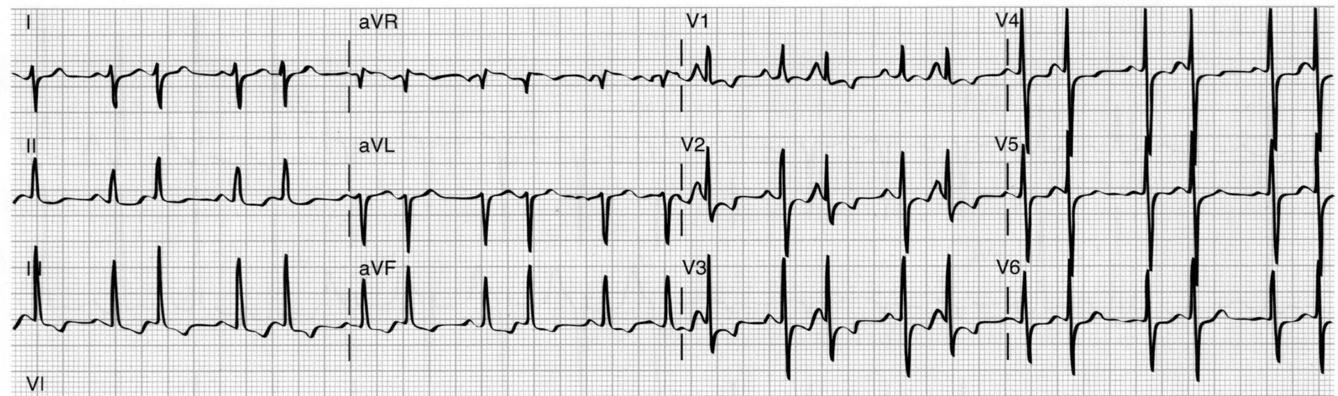

■ **Figure 15-39** RVH in a patient with primary pulmonary hypertension. Note RAD of +120 degrees with large R waves in V_1–V_3 and ST–T wave changes of RV strain. This ECG displays five of the criteria for RVH listed in Display 15-3. (Courtesy of Dr. William Nelson, Denver, Colorado.)

and T-wave inversion occurs in right chest leads and in leads II, III, and aVF. ECG features commonly seen with RVH are listed in Display 15-3. The presence of one of the criteria listed is highly indicative of RVH.

ELECTROLYTE IMBALANCES

Hypokalemia (serum potassium <3.5 mEq/L) may produce ECG changes involving the ST segment, T waves, and U waves (Fig. 15-40). As potassium levels decreases, the ST segment becomes progressively more depressed, T waves flatten, and prominent U waves develop. With advanced hypokalemia, the T and U waves often merge together and the U wave becomes larger than the T wave. These ST–T and U-wave changes relate fairly well with serum potassium levels but are not specific for hypokalemia because they can result from administration of certain drugs and from ventricular hypertrophy. P waves usually widen, and the PR interval may prolong. Hypokalemia promotes atrial and ventricular ectopy and rhythms commonly seen in digitalis toxicity, such as atrial tachycardia with block and AV dissociation (see Chapter 16).

DISPLAY 15-3 Diagnostic Criteria for Right Ventricular Enlargement[3,5,7]

Lead V_1	R/S ratio in $V_1 \geq 1$
	R wave in $V_1 \geq 7$ mm
	QR
	S < 2 mm
	Intrinsicoid deflection ≥ 0.35 second
Lead V_5–V_6	R < 5 mm with S in V_1 < 2 mm
	S wave ≥ 7 mm
	R/S ratio < 1
Lead $V_1 + V_6$	R in V_1 + S in V_6 > 10.5 mm
QRS axis	RAD ≥ + 110 degrees
Other criteria	S_1, S_2, S_3 pattern
	P pulmonale

Severe hypokalemia can cause ventricular tachycardia, torsades de pointes, and ventricular fibrillation.

Hyperkalemia (serum potassium >5.5 mEq/L) produces characteristic ECG changes involving the T wave and QRS complexes (Fig. 15-41). When the serum K^+ level is about 5.5 mEq/L, T waves become tall and peaked with a narrow base (tented) and the QT interval shortens. As the potassium level increases, the QRS complex widens and ST-segment elevation may occur, simulating the injury current seen in acute MI. First-degree AV block often occurs, and, as K^+ levels increase above 7 mEq/L, P waves flatten, and eventually may disappear. With severe hyperkalemia, the QRS complex becomes broad and bizarre with a sine wave formation, and, when K^+ levels reach 12 mEq/L, ventricular fibrillation or asystole often occurs. These ECG changes are typical of hyperkalemia but do not relate well with the actual serum potassium level. Some people do not show ECG changes until serum levels are quite high, whereas others show changes at lower potassium levels.

Hypocalcemia (serum calcium <8.5 mg/dL) prolongs the ST segment and the QT interval (Fig. 15-42). The prolonged QT interval is due to the abnormally long ST segment rather than to widening of the T wave as is seen with abnormal repolarization due to drugs. T waves are usually unchanged, but they may become flat or sharply inverted. With the possible exception of hypothermia, there is nothing other than hypocalcemia that prolongs the duration of the ST segment without changing T-wave duration.[3,12] Arrhythmias are uncommon in hypocalcemia.

Hypercalcemia (serum calcium >12 mg/dL) shortens the QT interval, especially the distance from the beginning of the QRS to the peak of the T wave (Fig. 15-43). The ST segment practically disappears, and the proximal limb of the T wave takes off from the end of the QRS complex. P waves, T waves, and U waves are usually unchanged, and arrhythmias are uncommon in hypercalcemia.[3]

Magnesium imbalances do not produce specific ECG changes. However, hypomagnesemia may contribute to arrhythmias caused by digitalis toxicity, ischemia, drugs, or potassium imbalances. Severe hypermagnesemia has been associated with AV block and intraventricular conduction disturbances.[12,13,15]

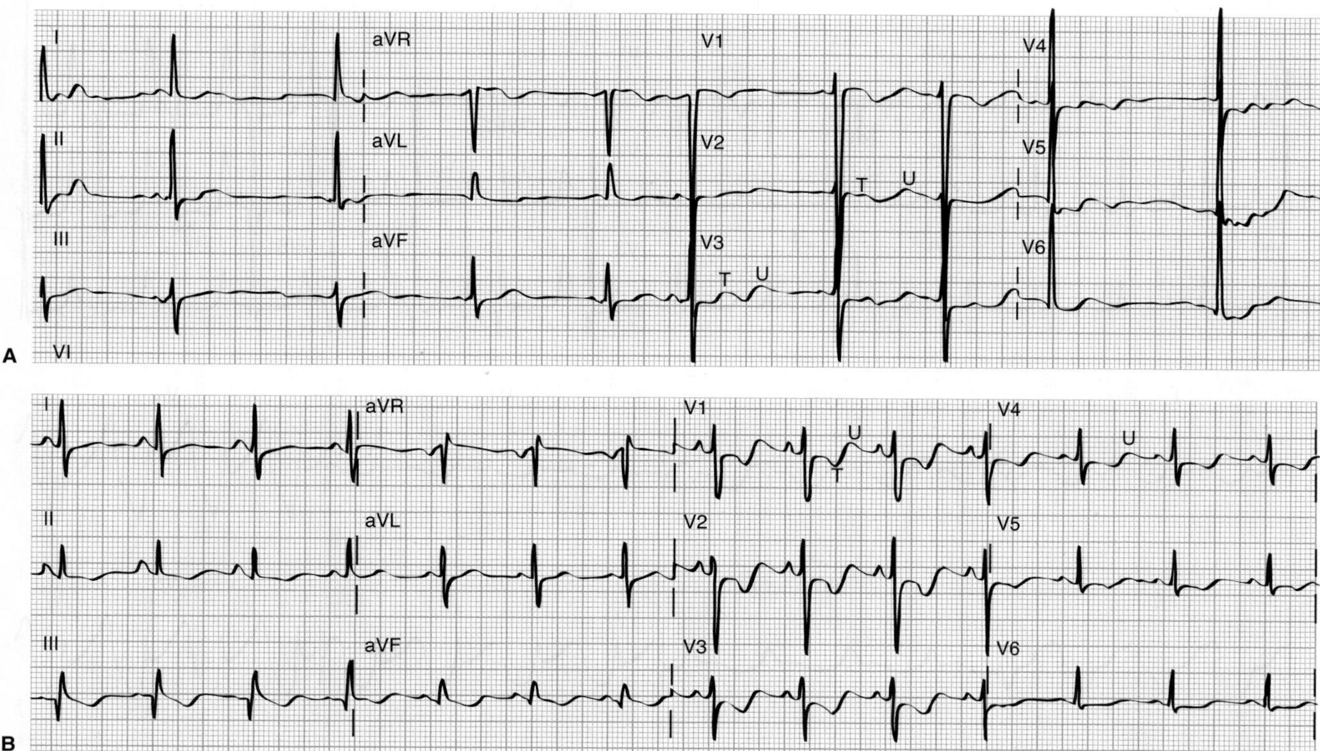

■ **Figure 15-40** ECG effects of hypokalemia. **(A)** T waves are flattened in many leads; large U waves are best seen in the V leads. **(B)** Large U waves of hypokalemia. This ECG also shows the typical pattern of acute cor pulmonale with S wave in lead I, Q-wave and T-wave inversion in lead III (the S1, Q3, and T3 pattern of cor pulmonale). (Courtesy of Dr. William Nelson, Denver, Colorado.)

DRUG EFFECTS

Many drugs can affect the ECG by altering ST segments, T waves, U waves, QT interval, and by causing various arrhythmias such as bradycardia, AV block, and torsades de pointes. The effects of drugs on the ECG are not specific because similar changes can result from cardiac diseases or electrolyte imbalances. The presence of ECG changes does not necessarily indicate toxic levels of the drug but rather represents the effects of the drug on myocardial depolarization and repolarization. Some common drug effects are discussed here.

Digitalis

Therapeutic doses of digitalis cause several changes on the ECG including: (1) flattening of the T wave or T-wave inversion, (2) concave depression of the ST segment, often described as "sagging" or "scooped," (3) shortening of the QT interval, (4) development or enlargement of U waves, and (5) PR interval prolongation.[2,7,10] Figure 15-44 is an example of digitalis effect. Digitalis toxicity causes arrhythmias including sinus bradycardia or SA block, AV block, atrial tachycardia and atrial tachycardia with block, junctional tachycardia, and several ventricular arrhythmias. See Chapter 16 for discussion of arrhythmias.

Drugs That Prolong the QT Interval

Many drugs can prolong the QT interval and lead to arrhythmias, specifically polymorphic ventricular tachycardia called torsades de pointes (see Chapter 16). It is beyond the scope of this chapter to list all of these drugs, but among the more common drugs known to prolong the QT interval are: (1) class IA antiarrhythmics (quinidine, procainamide), (2) class III antiarrhythmics (amiodarone, ibutilide, dofetilide, sotalol), (3) many antipsychotic and antidepressant drugs, (4) some antibiotics, (5) some sedatives and anesthetic agents, and (6) some histamine blockers, and many others. See Elizari et al.[9] or go to www.torsades.org for a more complete list of these drugs. Figures 15-45 and 15-46 show ECG changes commonly due to drugs.

LONG QT SYNDROMES (LQTS)

A long QT interval can be inherited or it can be acquired because of drug therapy, hypokalemia, or hypomagnesemia.[20–22] Seven types of congenital LQTS have so far been identified involving gene mutations that disrupt the function of various ion channels in the cardiac membrane, leading to repolarization abnormalities that manifest as a long QT interval on the ECG.[21–23] Patients with LQTS have an increased risk of sudden cardiac death and are at risk for developing torsades de pointes, a polymorphic ventricular

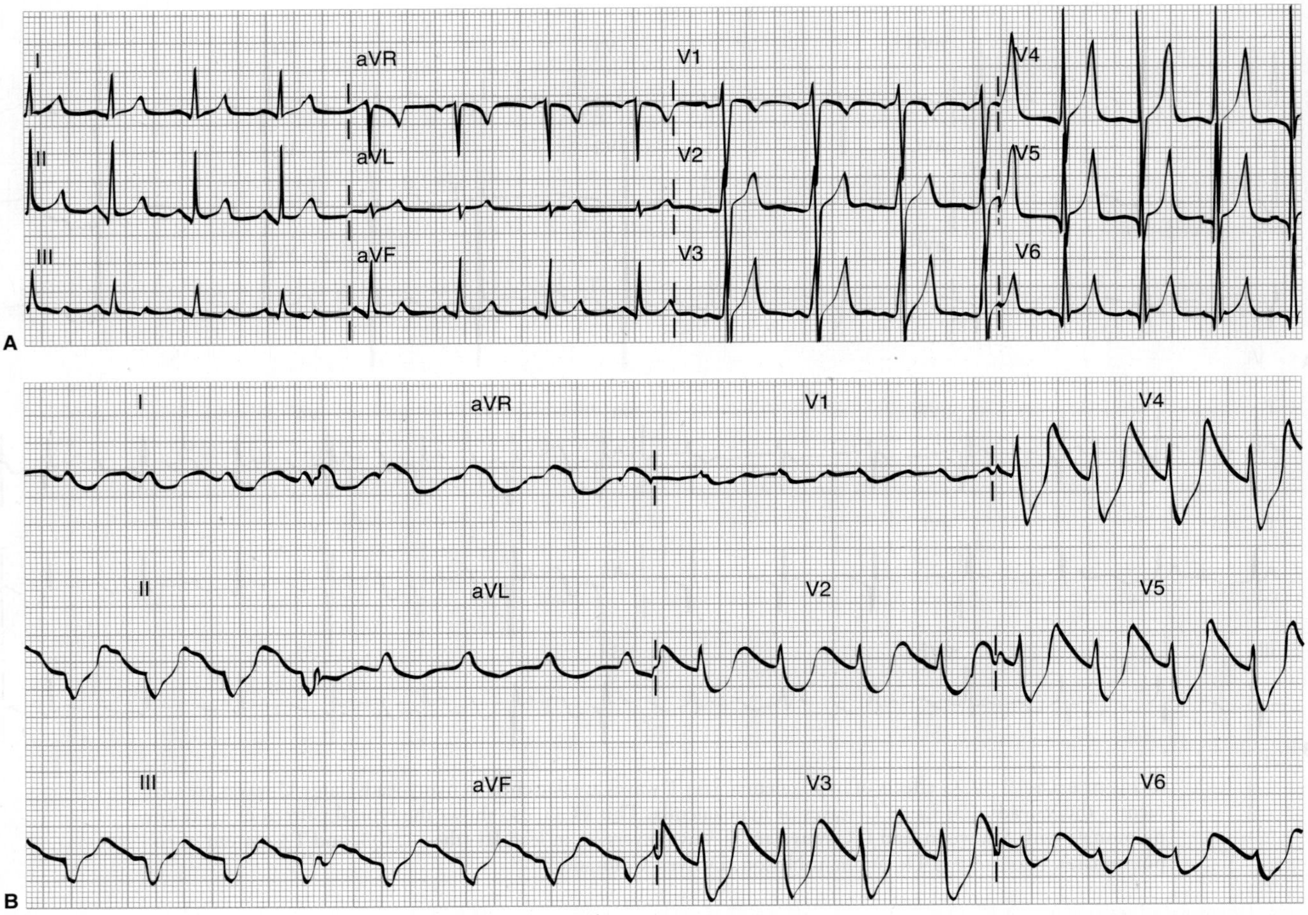

■ **Figure 15-41** ECG effects of hyperkalemia. (A) Tall, peaked, narrow-based T waves typical of hyperkalemia. (B) Advanced hyperkalemia (K = 9.2 mEq/L). Note very wide QRS and almost sine-wave look in leads I and aVR.

tachycardia associated with a long QT interval. ECG characteristics of congenital LQTS include a prolonged QT interval and a variety of T-wave alterations, including T-wave alternans, bifid or notched T waves, wide T waves, and relatively normal T waves following a very prolonged ST segment.[7,10,23] Figure 15-47 is recorded from a patient with congenital LQTS.

BRUGADA SYNDROME

In 1992, Brugada and Brugada described eight cases of aborted sudden cardiac death in patients with the following ECG findings[24]:

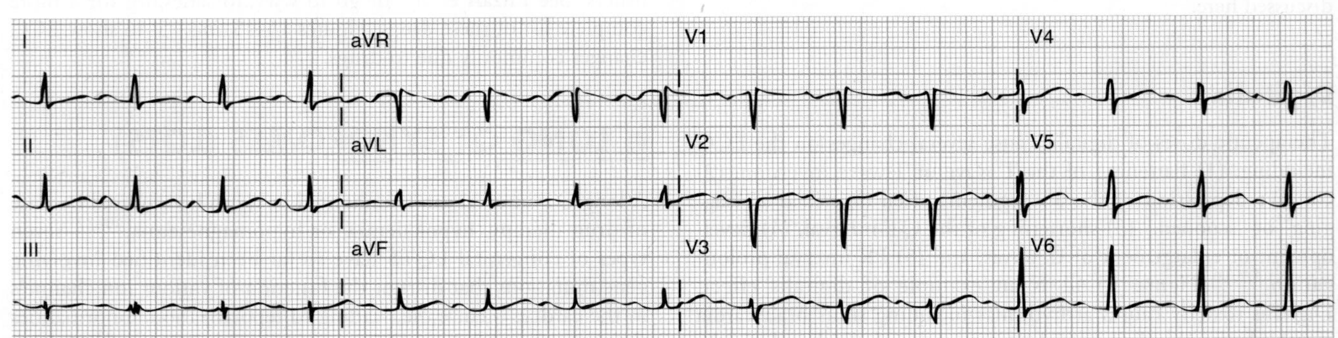

■ **Figure 15-42** ECG effects of hypocalcemia. Note the long ST segment that contributes to a prolonged QT interval.

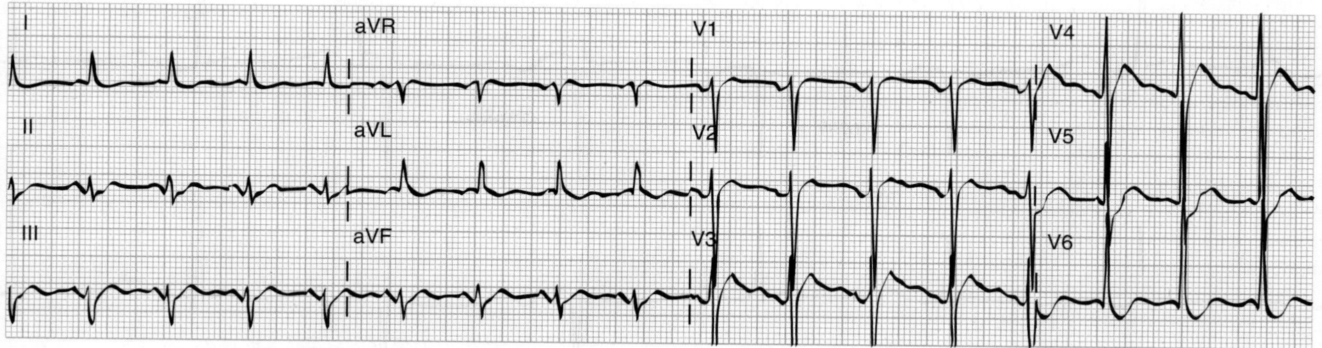

Figure 15-43 ECG effects of hypercalcemia. Note the short QT interval and how the T wave seems to take off from the end of the QRS in the V leads, especially V_3 and V_4.

1. Pattern of RBBB in V_1 to V_3: a late R wave (frequently small and called an "epsilon" wave), often without the corresponding deep S wave in left ventricular leads that is seen with true RBBB.
2. J point elevation in V_1 to V_3.
3. ST elevation in V_1 to V_3 that is unrelated to ischemia, electrolyte abnormalities, or structural heart disease.
4. Normal QT interval.

The ECG can be transiently normal, but patients with Brugada syndrome are prone to develop life-threatening ventricular arrhythmias leading to sudden death. It is now known that Brugada syndrome is an autosomal dominant inherited disease involving a genetic defect that causes abnormal cardiac sodium channel function, but it is also thought that other genetic mutations yet undiscovered may also play a role.[23] Figure 15-48 illustrates an example of Brugada syndrome.

VENTRICULAR PREEXCITATION SYNDROMES

Ventricular preexcitation occurs when a portion of the ventricle is depolarized early via an accessory pathway that bypasses the AV node. Normal AV conduction occurs through the AV node; patients with preexcitation syndromes have alternative tracts or connections (also called bypass tracts) between the atria and ventricles that allow the electrical impulse to bypass the AV node and enter the ventricle early. If the accessory connection conducts the impulse from the atria directly into the normal conduction system below the AV node, the result is a short PR interval (because the normal delay in the AV node does not occur in the accessory pathway), and a normal QRS complex (because the ventricles depolarize via the normal intraventricular conduction system). This type of preexcitation syndrome has been termed Lown–Ganong–Levine syndrome or "short PR-normal QRS syndrome."

Wolff–Parkinson–White Syndrome

The most common type of ventricular preexcitation is called Wolff–Parkinson–White syndrome, which is due to an accessory pathway that connects the atrium directly to the ventricular myocardium. Because the electrical impulse travels more quickly through the bypass tract than through the AV node it enters the ventricle early and begins to depolarize it via muscle cell-to-cell conduction, which creates an initial slurring of the QRS complex called a delta wave. Depending on the location of the bypass tract, the delta wave may be positive or negative in different leads on the ECG. The last part of the QRS complex is usually normal because the bulk of the ventricle is then activated via the normal His–Purkinje system. If most of the ventricle is activated abnormally via the accessory pathway, the entire QRS can be wide. The PR interval is short because the normal delay through the AV node is bypassed. Figure 15-49 shows two examples of Wolff–Parkinson–White syndrome. See Chapter 16 for more information on Wolff–Parkinson–White syndrome and the arrhythmias associated with it.

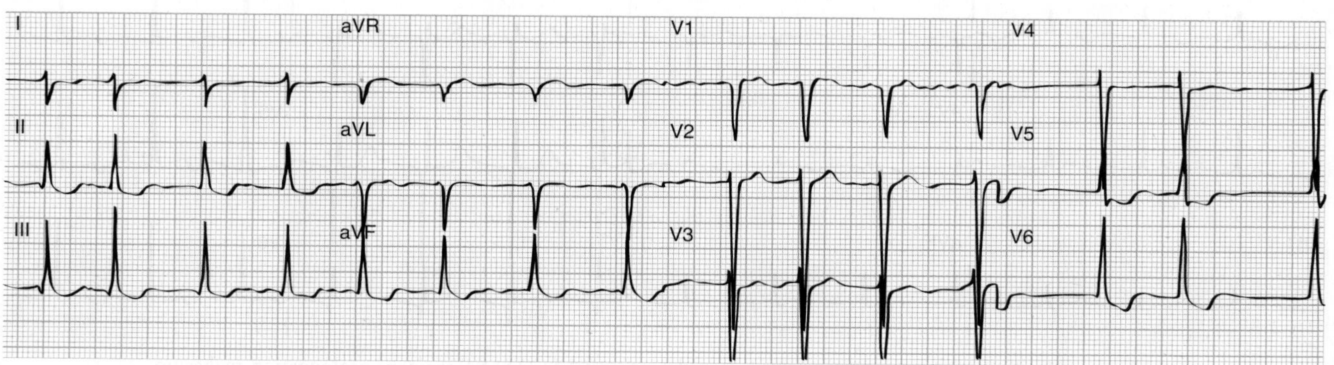

Figure 15-44 ECG effects of digitalis. Note sagging type ST depression in inferior leads and in V_5 and V_6.

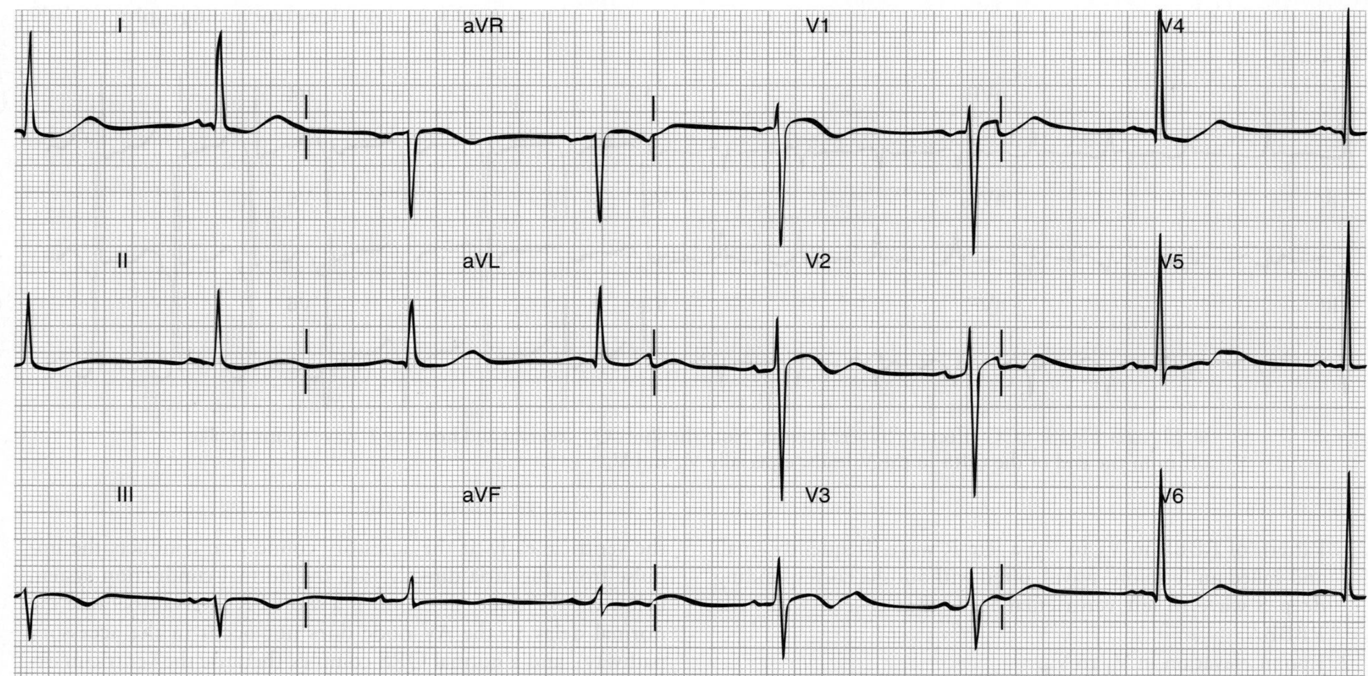

■ **Figure 15-45** ECG effects shown here are typical of many drugs and can also be due to hypokalemia. This is an example of combined quinidine and digitalis therapy causing a "roller coaster" type ST–T–U wave pattern, especially in V_1–V_3, combining to prolong the QT interval. Quinidine is rarely used these days because it is highly proarrhythmic in causing torsades de pointes.

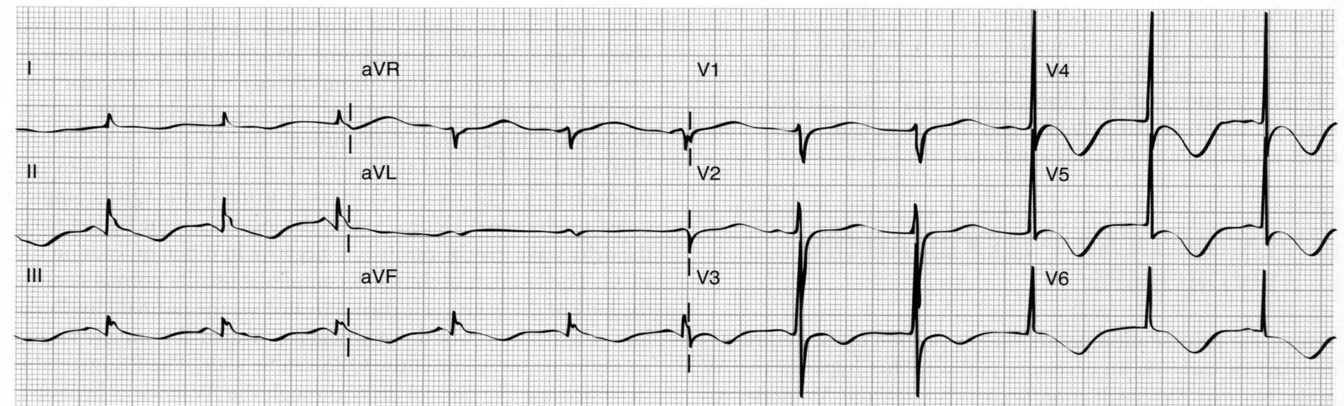

■ **Figure 15-46** ECG showing marked QT interval prolongation and wide bizarre T waves typical of many drugs, especially class III antiarrhythmics.

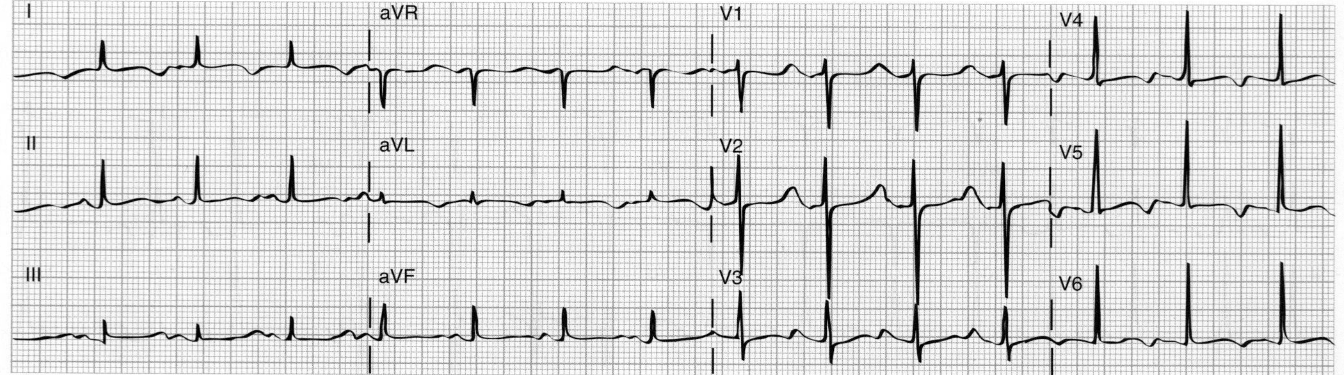

■ **Figure 15-47** ECG recorded from a patient with congenital LQTS. ST segment prolongation makes up most of the length of the QT interval, with a relatively normal width T wave.

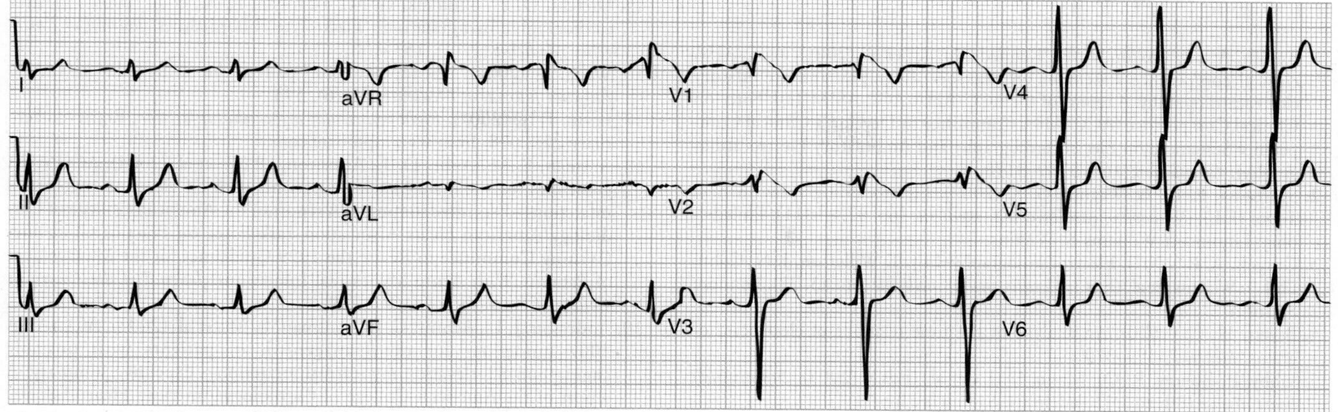

■ **Figure 15-48** Brugada syndrome.

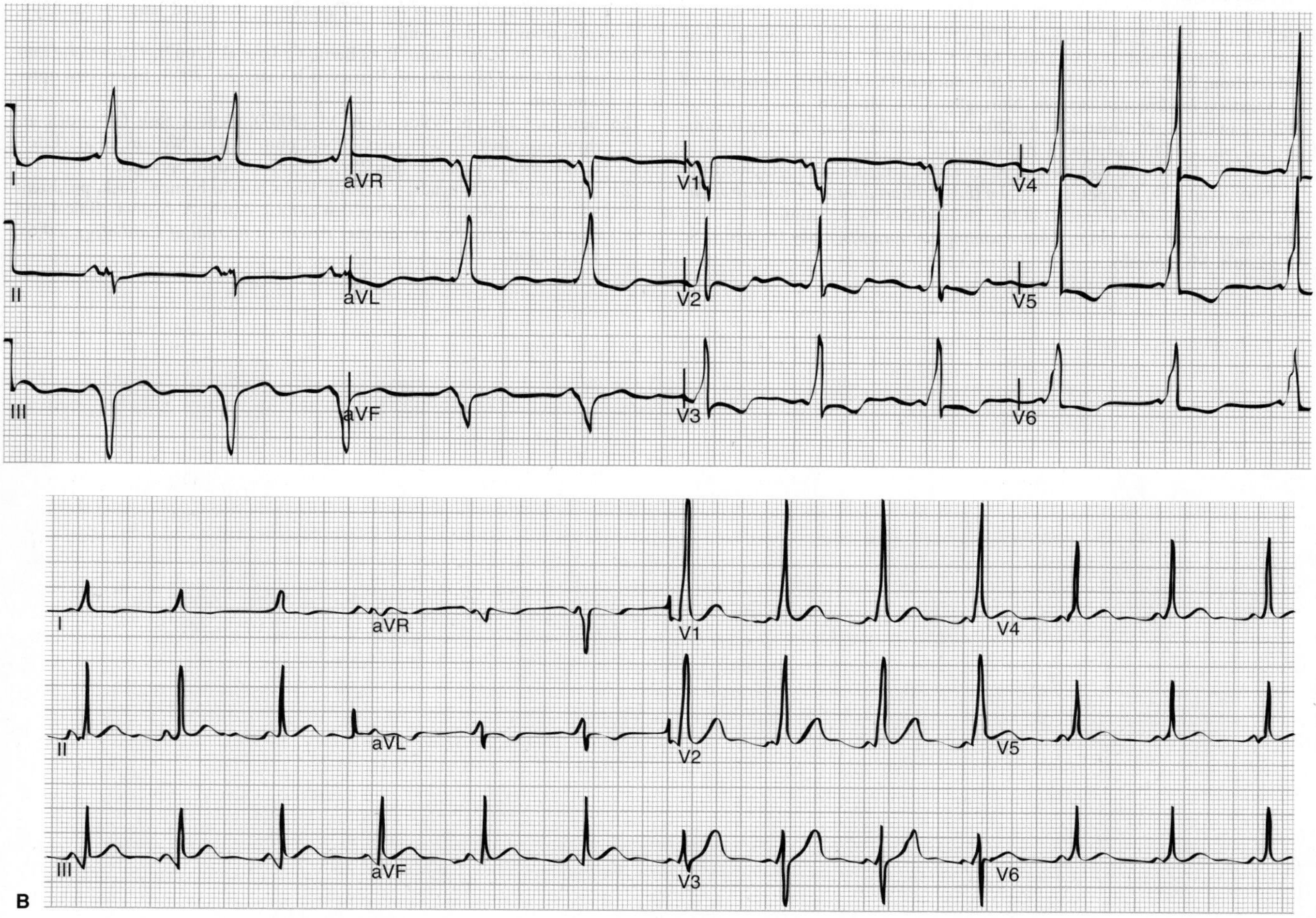

B

■ **Figure 15-49** Wolff–Parkinson–White syndrome. (A) The PR interval is very short and prominent delta waves are present. Delta waves are positive in all leads except aVR and V_1 where they are negative. (B) The PR interval is short and there are positive delta waves in all leads except III and aVF where they are negative and lead II where it is isoelectric. Note how the negative delta waves in III and aVF simulate Q waves of MI.

REFERENCES

1. Kadish, A. H., Buxton, A. E., Kennedy, H. L., et al. (2001). ACC/AHA clinical competence statement on electrocardiography and ambulatory electrocardiography. A report of the ACC/AHA/ACP-ASIM Task Force on Clinical Competence (ACC/AHA Committee to Develop a Clinical Competence Statement on Electrocardiography and Ambulatory Electrocardiography). *Circulation, 104*, 3169–3178.
2. Sgarbossa, E. B., & Wagner, G. S. (2007). Electrocardiography. In E. J. Topol (Ed.), *Textbook of cardiovascular medicine* (pp. 977–1011). Philadelphia: Lippincott Williams & Wilkins.
3. Gorgels, A. P. (2007). Electrocardiography. In J. T. Willerson, J. N. Cohn, H. J. J. Wellens, et al. (Eds.), *Cardiovascular medicine* (pp. 43–77). London: Springer.
4. Bazett, H. C. (1920). An analysis of the time relations of electrocardiograms. *Heart, 7*, 353–370.
5. Libby, P., Bonow, R. O., Mann, D. L., et al. (Eds.). (2008). *Braunwald's heart disease* (8th ed.). Philadelphia: Saunders Elsevier.
6. Wagner, G. S. (2001). *Marriott's practical electrocardiography* (10th ed.). Philadelphia: Lippincott Williams & Wilkins.
7. Chan, T. C., Brady, W. J., Harrigan, R. A., et al. (2005). *ECG in emergency medicine and acute care*. Philadelphia: Elsevier/Mosby.
8. Goldschlager, N., & Goldman, M. J. (1989). *Principles of clinical electrocardiography*. Norwalk: Appleton & Lange.
9. Elizari, M., Acunzo, R. S., & Ferreiro, M. (2006). Hemiblocks revisited. *Circulation, 115*, 1154–1163.
10. Wellens, H. J. J., & Conover, M. B. (2006). *The ECG in emergency decision making* (2nd ed.). St. Louis, MO: Saunders.
11. Nelson, W. P., Marriott, H. J. L., & Schocken, D. D. (2007). *Concepts and cautions in electrocardiography.* Northglen, CO: MedInfo.
12. Surawicz, B., & Knilans, T. K. (2001). *Chou's electrocardiography in clinical practice.* Philadelphia: W.B. Saunders.
13. Mirvis, D. M., & Goldberger, A. L. (2001). Electrocardiography. In E. Braunwald, D. P. Zipes, & P. Libby (Eds.), *Heart disease: A textbook of cardiovascular medicine* (pp. 82–128). Philadelphia: W.B. Saunders.
14. Conover, M. B. (2003). *Understanding electrocardiography* (8th ed.). St. Louis, MO: Mosby.
15. Diercks, D. B., Shumaik, G. M., Harrigan, R. A., et al. (2004). Electrocardiographic manifestations: Electrolyte abnormalities. *Journal of Emergency Medicine, 27*(2), 153–160.
16. Wang, K. (2004). "Pseudoinfarction" pattern due to hyperkalemia. *New England Journal of Medicine, 351*(6), 593.
17. Levin, T. N. (2007). *Right ventricular myocardial infarction.* Retrieved February 22, 2008, from www.uptodate.com.
18. Antman, E. M., Anbe, D. T., Armstrong, P. W., et al. (2004). ACC/AHA guidelines for the management of patients with ST-elevation myocardial infarction—Executive summary: A report of the American College of Cardiology/American Heart Association Task Force on Practice Guidelines (Writing Committee to Revise the 1999 Guidelines for the Management of Patients With Acute Myocardial Infarction). *Journal of the American College of Cardiology, 44*, 671–719.
19. Anderson, J. L., Adams, C. D., Antman, E. M., et al. (2007). ACC/AHA 2007 guidelines for the management of patients with unstable angina/non-ST-elevation myocardial infarction—Executive summary: A report of the American College of Cardiology/American Heart Association Task Force on practice guidelines (Writing Committee to Revise the 2002 Guidelines for the Management of Patients With Unstable Angina/Non-ST-Elevation Myocardial Infarction). *Circulation, 116*, 803–877.
20. Berul, C. I., Seslar, S. P., Zimetbaum, P. J., et al. (2007). *Acquired long QT syndrome.* Retrieved January 22, 2008, from www.uptodate.com.
21. Zimetbaum, P. J., Josephson, M. E., & Kwaku, K. F. (2006). *Genetics of congenital and acquired long QT syndrome.* Retrieved January 22, 2008, from www.uptodate.com.
22. Seslar, S. P., Zimetbaum, P. J., Berul, C. I., et al. (2007). *Diagnosis of congenital long QT syndrome.* Retrieved January 22, 2008, from www.uptodate.com.
23. Bezzina, C. R., & Wilde, A. A. M. (2007). Genetic basis for cardiac arrhythmias. In J. T. Willerson, J. N. Cohn, H. J. J. Wellens, et al. (Eds.), *Cardiovascular medicine* (pp. 2577–2598). London: Springer.
24. Brugada, P., & Brugada, J. (1992). Right bundle branch block, persistent ST segment elevation and sudden cardiac death: A distinct clinical and electrocardiographic syndrome. *American Journal of Cardiology, 20*(6), 1391–1396.

CHAPTER 16

Arrhythmias and Conduction Disturbances

Carol Jacobson

MECHANISMS OF ARRHYTHMIAS

Cardiac arrhythmias result from abnormal impulse initiation, abnormal impulse conduction, or both mechanisms together. Abnormal impulse initiation includes enhanced normal automaticity, abnormal automaticity, and triggered activity resulting from afterdepolarizations; abnormal impulse conduction includes conduction block and reentry.[1–5] Although all of these mechanisms have been shown to cause arrhythmias in the laboratory, it is not possible to prove which mechanism is responsible for a particular arrhythmia using currently available diagnostic tools in the clinical setting. However, it is possible to postulate the mechanism of many clinical arrhythmias based on their characteristics and behavior and to list rhythms most consistent with known electrophysiologic mechanisms.[3–6] Some arrhythmias, such as atrioventricular nodal reentry tachycardia (AVNRT), atrial flutter, some ventricular tachycardias (VTs), and reentry tachycardias involving accessory pathways, have been proven to be caused by reentry. This section describes the major mechanisms of arrhythmias and lists arrhythmias suggested or proven to be caused by each mechanism whenever possible. Knowledge of the cardiac action potential is essential in understanding concepts presented here (see Chapter 1).

Abnormal Impulse Initiation

Abnormal impulse initiation can be due to enhanced normal automaticity, abnormal automaticity, or afterdepolarizations. It is important to understand the property of normal automaticity before considering these other mechanisms.

Automaticity

Automaticity is the ability of certain cardiac cells to spontaneously depolarize and initiate an electrical impulse without external stimulation. The sinus node (or sinoatrial [SA] node) is the normal pacemaker of the heart because it has the fastest rate of automaticity. Other cells in the heart also have the property of automaticity, including cells in several areas of the atria, coronary sinus, pulmonary veins, atrioventricular (AV) junction, AV valves, and Purkinje system. The rates of these other pacemakers are slower than the rate of the SA node; therefore, they are suppressed by the SA node under normal conditions, a phenomenon known as *overdrive suppression.* The site of fastest impulse initiation is referred to as the *dominant pacemaker*, whereas sites of impulse formation that are suppressed by the dominant site are called *subsidiary* or *latent pacemakers.*

Enhanced Normal Automaticity. Impulse initiation can be shifted from the SA node to other parts of the heart if the rate of the SA node drops below that of a subsidiary pacemaker or if the automatic rate of a subsidiary pacemaker rises above that of the SA node. Increased vagal tone, drugs, electrolyte abnormalities, or disease of the SA node can decrease its rate of automaticity or can cause exit block of its impulse, thus allowing subsidiary pacemakers to assume control of the heart. Examples of clinical arrhythmias due to shifting of the pacemaker from the SA node include atrial, junctional, or ventricular escape rhythms that occur due to sinus bradycardia or AV block. Such "escape" pacemaker activity cannot be considered abnormal because it is a manifestation of the normal automaticity of these cells. Sinus tachycardia is due to enhanced normal automaticity, and accelerated ventricular rhythm following myocardial infarction (MI) may be due to enhanced automaticity.[1,3]

Subsidiary pacemaker activity can be enhanced by factors that decrease the transmembrane resting potential (TRP), decrease the threshold potential, or increase the rate of diastolic phase 4 depolarization of the subsidiary pacemaker cells. Figure 16-1 illustrates how these mechanisms can change the rate of firing of pacemaker cells.[7]

Enhanced normal automaticity can occur with enhanced sympathetic activity; drugs such as digitalis and sympathomimetic agents; ischemia; stretch that occurs in heart failure (HF), cardiomyopathy, and ventricular aneurysms; and with genetic mutations that alter the function of ion channels in the cardiac membrane.[3–5,8,9] Clinical arrhythmias that may be due to enhanced normal automaticity include sinus tachycardia, some atrial tachycardias (ATs), junctional tachycardia, accelerated ventricular rhythm, and ventricular parasystole. Automaticity is not the mechanism of most rapid tachycardias but it can precipitate or trigger reentrant tachycardias that can occur at very rapid rates.[4]

Abnormal Automaticity. Atrial and ventricular myocardial cells that do not normally have automaticity can develop abnormal automaticity when their TRP is reduced and is referred to as depolarization-induced automaticity.[1,4] Subsidiary pacemakers like those in the Purkinje system that are normally overdrive suppressed by the faster SA node can also develop abnormal automaticity when their TRP is reduced. This abnormal automaticity is thought to be mediated by the slow inward current carried mainly by calcium (slow channels) because the normal fast sodium channels are inactivated at reduced membrane potentials.[1,3,4] However, both sodium and calcium channels may play a role in the development of abnormal automaticity. Abnormal automaticity that develops at more negative diastolic potentials, between −70 and −50 mV, can be suppressed by sodium channel blockers, indicating that a sodium current is involved, whereas automaticity that develops at less negative diastolic potentials, from −50 to −30 mV, can be suppressed by calcium channel blockers.[2,4]

The resting potential of a cell can be reduced (e.g., from −90 to −70 mV) and the cell partially depolarized by anything that increases the extracellular potassium concentration, decreases the intracellular potassium concentration, increases the permeability of the membrane to sodium, or decreases the membrane permeability

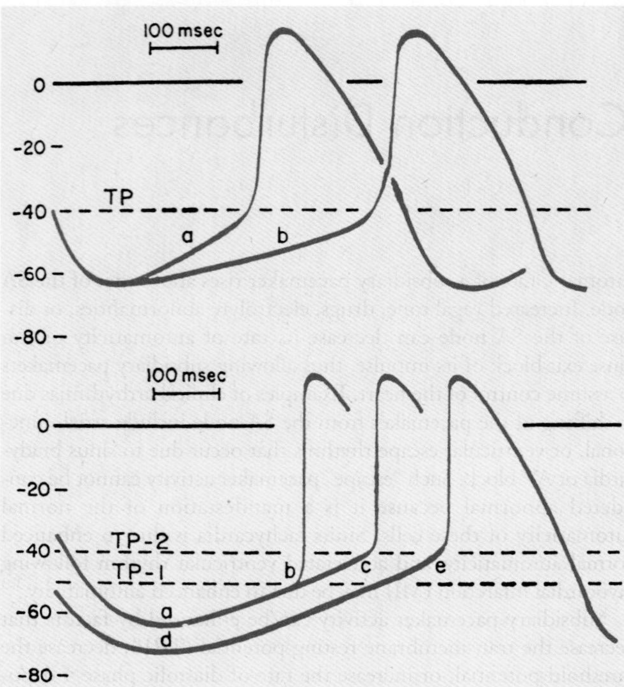

■ **Figure 16-1** Diagram illustrating the principal mechanisms underlying changes in the frequency of discharge of a pacemaker fiber. The upper diagram shows a reduction in rate caused by a decrease in the slope of diastolic, or pacemaker, depolarization from a to b, and thus an increase in the time required for the membrane potential to decline to the threshold potential (TP) level. The lower diagram shows the reduction in the rate associated with a shift in the level of the threshold potential from TP-1 to TP-2, and a corresponding increase in cycle length (b to c); also illustrated is a further reduction in rate due to an increase in the maximal diastolic potential level (Compare a with c and d with e). (From Hoffman, B. F., & Cranefield, P. F. [1960]. *Electrophysiology of the heart.* New York: McGraw-Hill. Used with permission of the McGraw-Hill Book Company.)

to potassium.[1–4] Ischemia, hypoxia, acidosis, hyperkalemia, digitalis toxicity, chamber enlargement or dilation, stretch, and other metabolic abnormalities or drugs can reduce the resting potential and result in abnormal automaticity. Hypoxia and ischemia affect the TRP by decreasing the amount of oxygen available to supply adenosine triphosphate in amounts sufficient to operate the sodium—potassium pump efficiently. Anything that interferes with proper operation of this pump, such as digitalis, reduces normal resting ionic gradients across the cell membrane and results in reduction of the resting potential. When the TRP is reduced at rest, the cell is partially depolarized and the time required for spontaneous diastolic depolarization to reach threshold is reduced, thus increasing pacemaker activity (see Fig. 16-1). For the same reason, automaticity is increased when the threshold potential is reduced (e.g., from −40 to −50 mV) by ischemia or drug effects because less time is required for phase 4 depolarization to reach the lower threshold. The rate of phase 4 depolarization can be increased by several factors, including local norepinephrine release at ischemic sites, systemic catecholamine release, reduced vagal tone, and drugs.

Clinical arrhythmias that may be due to abnormal automaticity include some ATs, accelerated junctional or ventricular rhythm, parasystole, and some VTs associated with acute MI.[1–4] The rate of a rhythm due to abnormal automaticity is related to the membrane potential from which it arose: the less negative the membrane potential (i.e., the greater the depolarization), the faster the rate. Rhythms due to abnormal automaticity tend to occur at faster rates than rhythms due to normal automaticity.[1,2]

Triggered Activity Due to Afterdepolarizations

Afterdepolarization is a transient depolarization of the cell membrane that occurs at some time during or right after repolarization of an action potential. Early afterdepolarizations (EAD) occur during the repolarization of an action potential. Delayed afterdepolarizations (DADs) occur after repolarization is complete but before the next action potential is due to occur. Figure 16-2 shows both EAD and DAD.[10]

Early Afterdepolarizations. EADs that occur early in phase 2 at potentials positive to −30 mV are called phase 2 EADs; those that occur at more negative potentials are called phase 3 EADs.[4] EADs are thought to be due primarily to a calcium current, although sodium channel activity during the plateau phase of the action potential may also play an important role in inducing EADs.[4] If an EAD is large enough to reach threshold, a second upstroke occurs, causing an "early" beat. This second upstroke is called a *triggered beat* because it depends on and arises as a result of the preceding action potential. The triggered beat may be followed by its own afterdepolarization, which initiates yet another upstroke. This activity may be sustained for several beats and may terminate only when the membrane finally repolarizes to a high enough level to extinguish the rhythmic activity. This mechanism of abnormal impulse formation differs from abnormal automaticity in that automatic beats result from spontaneous initiation of each impulse, whereas beats due to afterdepolarizations depend on a preceding impulse.

EADs have been shown to occur most often in Purkinje fibers and midmyocardial M cells in the ventricles.[4] EADs are caused by conditions that delay repolarization of the action potential and occur in the presence of hypoxia, acidosis, hypokalemia,

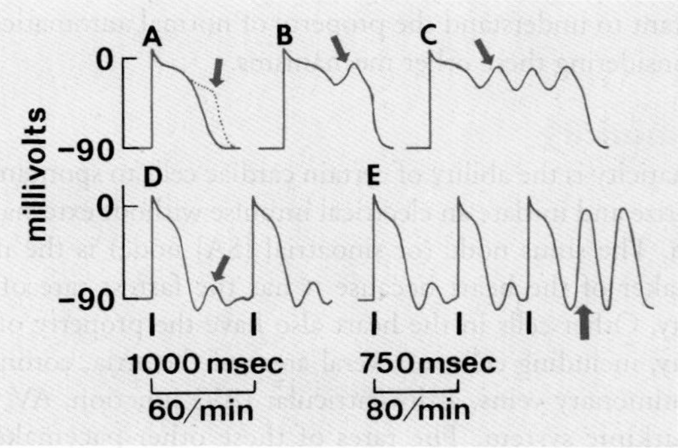

■ **Figure 16-2** **(A)** An early afterpolarization (*arrow*). **(B)** A single triggered action potential caused by this afterdepolarization (*arrow*). **(C)** A train of triggered action potentials (*arrow*). **(D,E)** Action potentials caused by propagating impulses (indicated by *vertical lines*), followed by DAD (arrow in *D*). (*E*) Triggered activity caused by the afterdepolarization (*arrow*). (From Wit, A. L., & Rosen, M. R. [1981]. Cellular electrophysiology of cardiac arrhythmias: Part I. Arrhythmias caused by abnormal impulse generation. *Modern Concepts in Cardiovascular Disease, 50*, 5. Used with permission of the American Heart Association.)

hypomagnesemia, hypothermia, high P_{CO_2}, catecholamines, many drugs, and in ventricular hypertrophy and HF.[2,4] Gene mutations that alter sodium and potassium ion channel activity and result in prolonged action potential duration have been identified and shown to cause EADs. The congenital long QT syndrome (LQTS) associated with torsades de pointes (TdP), a polymorphic VT (PVT) associated with sudden cardiac death (SCD), has been shown to be due to genetic mutations that affect ion channel function and prolong repolarization, thus leading to EAD formation. Triggered activity due to EADs occurs at slow heart rates, and arrhythmias thought to be due to EAD often occur during bradycardia or after a pause in rhythm. The proarrhythmic effects of many drugs, especially class IA and class III antiarrhythmics, are due to their ability to prolong repolarization in cardiac cells and cause EADs. Clinical arrhythmias thought to be due to EAD include both the acquired and congenital types of TdP, and many arrhythmias that occur with hypertrophy and HF.

Delayed Afterdepolarizations. DADs occur after the membrane has repolarized to its original level after an action potential but before the next propagated impulse. Subthreshold afterdepolarizations do not result in triggered activity, but, if the DAD is large enough to reach threshold, a triggered impulse arises. This triggered impulse may also be followed by its own afterdepolarization, leading to trains of triggered beats. Again, the mechanism differs from automaticity in that afterdepolarizations depend on and arise as a result of preceding action potentials. DADs occur in association with increased intracellular calcium levels. There is a direct relation between amplitude of DAD and heart rate: as the heart rate increases, so does afterdepolarization amplitude. Thus, triggered activity tends to occur after premature beats or at rapid heart rates. Factors that increase DAD amplitude and contribute to triggered arrhythmias include high concentrations of catecholamines and digitalis and hypokalemia.[1–4] Clinical arrhythmias that may be due to DAD include digitalis toxic rhythms like accelerated junctional rhythm and AT, idiopathic VT originating in the right ventricular outflow tract (RVOT), accelerated idioventricular rhythm after MI, and tachycardias originating in the coronary sinus.

Abnormal Impulse Conduction

Abnormal impulse conduction can result in bradyarrhythmias or aberrancy when impulses are blocked, or premature beats and tachyarrhythmias when reentrant excitation occurs.

Conduction Block

The electrical impulse can be prevented from propagating through the heart for a variety of reasons. If the propagating impulse is not strong enough to excite the tissue ahead of it, conduction will fail (see section below titled "Decremental Conduction"). If an impulse arrives at an area where the tissue is still refractory after a previous depolarization, it will not be able to conduct further (see section below titled "Phase 3 Block"). If an impulse reaches tissue that is abnormally depolarized due to ischemia, disease, or drugs, it may not be able to conduct at all or will conduct with delay (see section below titled "Phase 4 Block"). Scar tissue from previous MI, surgery, or catheter ablation also prevents conduction.

Decremental Conduction. Decremental conduction is the progressive decrease in conduction velocity of an impulse as it travels through a region of myocardium and occurs when an action potential loses its ability to stimulate the tissue ahead of it. Decremental conduction is a normal function of the AV node, delaying the impulse in the AV node long enough for atrial contraction to contribute to ventricular filling. Decremental conduction normally occurs in areas of the heart where resting potentials are low and action potentials depend on slow channels, such as the AV and SA nodes. It can also occur in areas where resting potentials are low due to ischemia, disease, or drugs. Under such circumstances, conduction velocity is slow because of the slower rate of rise of the action potential that occurs when cells are stimulated at reduced resting potentials. At times, decremental conduction can be so pronounced that the impulse fails to conduct, thus leading to block. This failure of conduction can occur in the SA node, leading to sinus exit block; in the AV node, leading to AV block; or in the bundle-branch system, causing bundle-branch block.

Phase 3 Block. When a cell is stimulated during phase 3 of the action potential, conduction is impaired because the membrane has not yet returned to its resting level. Whenever a cell is stimulated at a less negative membrane potential, the rate of rise of the action potential, and thus conduction velocity, is slow because most sodium channels are inactivated at reduced membrane potentials. Figure 16-3 illustrates phase 3 block occurring in the right bundle branch, resulting in aberrant conduction of the impulse with a right bundle-branch block (RBBB) pattern.

Phase 3 block, also called short-cycle aberrancy[11] or tachycardia-dependent block,[3] can occur in normal hearts if impulses are premature enough to reach fibers during their normal refractory period, resulting in aberrant conduction of premature beats. It is also responsible for rate-dependent bundle-branch blocks and for the aberration that commonly occurs when cycle lengths are very irregular, as in atrial fibrillation (AF). Phase 3 block can occur pathologically if the refractory period is abnormally prolonged by drugs or disease.

Phase 4 Block. Phase 4 block, also called long-cycle aberrancy[11] or bradycardia-dependent block,[3] occurs late in diastole when fibers are stimulated at reduced membrane potentials secondary to spontaneous phase 4 depolarization. In this case, the membrane has begun to depolarize spontaneously during its normal phase 4. By the time a stimulus arrives, the resting potential has been reduced enough to cause slow conduction. Again, whenever a cell is stimulated at a reduced membrane potential, only some of the sodium channels are available, and slow conduction results. Figure 16-4 shows a normal right bundle-branch action potential followed by spontaneous phase 4 depolarization. By the time the second impulse arrives in that bundle, membrane potential has been reduced enough to cause slow conduction and RBBB.

Phase 4 block is responsible for abnormal conduction that occurs only at the end of long cycles or for so-called bradycardia-dependent bundle-branch block. Phase 4 block is uncommon and is considered pathologic when it occurs.

Reentry

Reentry is a type of conduction abnormality that leads to the occurrence of premature beats or sustained tachycardias rather than to a block. Reentry can occur in areas of the heart where conduction velocity is abnormally slow because of ischemia, electrolyte abnormalities, drugs, or disease. *Reentry* means that an impulse can travel through an area of myocardium, depolarize it, and then reenter the same area to depolarize it again. For anatomic reentry to occur, there must be an area of unidirectional block in which an impulse can conduct in one direction but not in the opposite

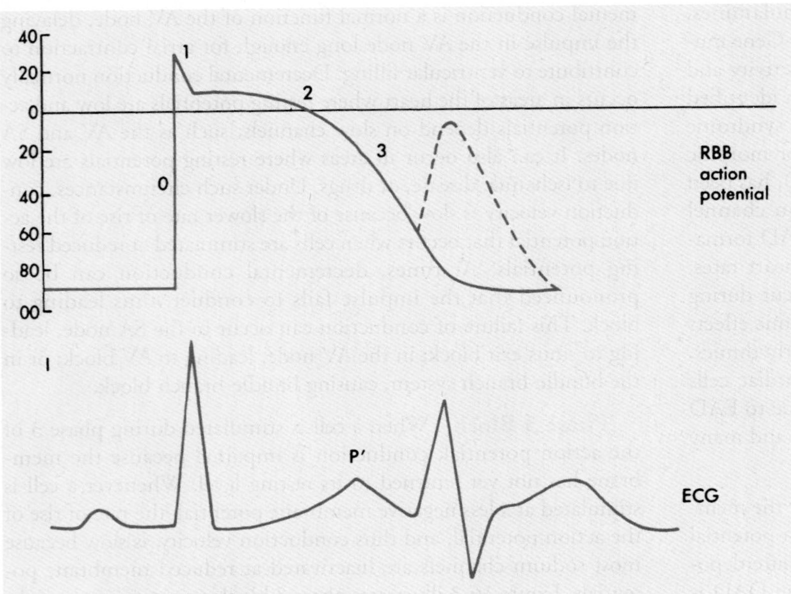

■ **Figure 16-3** Phase 3 block. The ECG on the bottom shows a normal beat followed by a premature atrial beat that conducts with RBBB. The action potentials on top illustrate that the early beat entered the right bundle during phase 3, when the membrane potential was still reduced. The resulting action potential is a slow channel response and conduction fails. (From Conover, M. [2003]. *Understanding electrocardiography* [8th ed., p. 172]. St. Louis, MO: CV Mosby.)

direction. In addition, conduction velocity must be slow enough relative to tissue refractoriness and circuit length to allow the impulse to continue propagating in a circular manner.[3–5] Figure 16-5*A* illustrates normal conduction of an impulse through an area of myocardium, and Figure 16-5*B* shows reentry occurring as a result of an area of unidirectional block and slow conduction.[12]

For reentry to occur, an area of unidirectional block is necessary to allow an impulse to conduct in one direction and to provide a return pathway by which the original stimulus can reenter a previously depolarized area. Conduction velocity must be slow enough and the refractory period short enough to allow time for the previously stimulated area to recover its ability to conduct. If the refractory period of the previously stimulated tissue is long or conduction velocity is fast, the impulse dies out because it encounters tissue that is unable to conduct.

Based on these general concepts, three main types of reentry have been described.[3–5,13] *Anatomic reentry* (see Fig. 16-5) involves an anatomic obstacle around which the circulating wave of

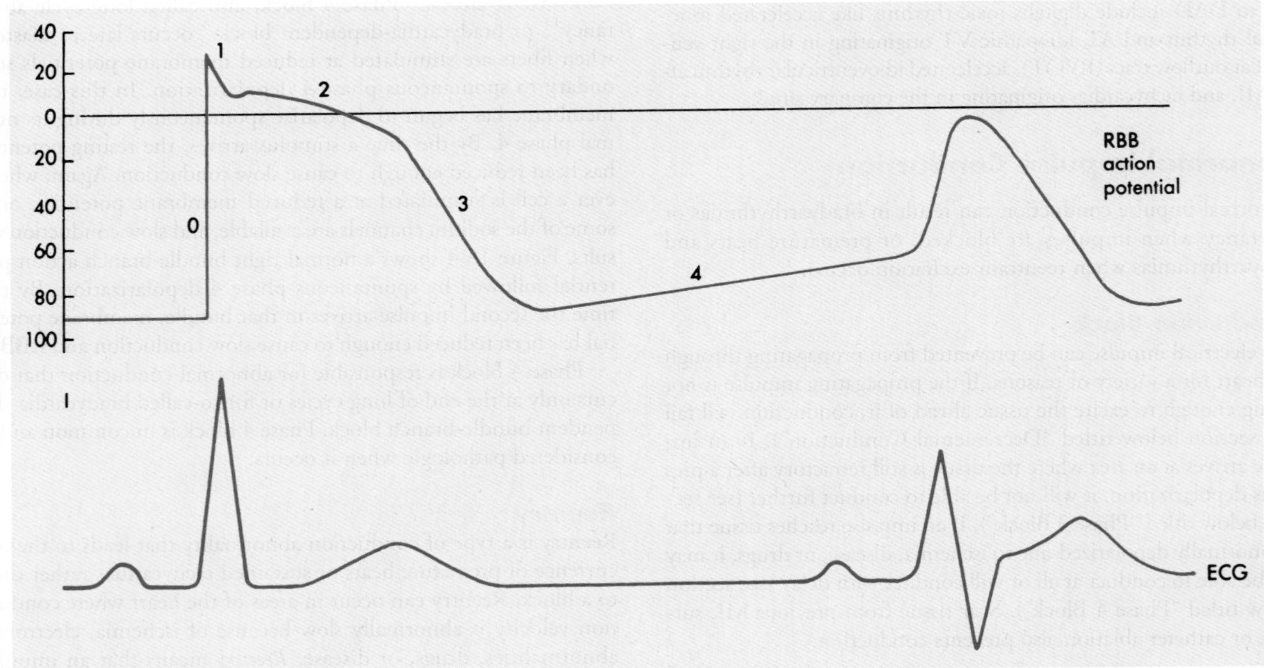

■ **Figure 16-4** Phase 4 block. The ECG on the bottom shows a normal beat followed by a pause and a second beat that conducts with RBBB. The action potential on top illustrates that the pause after the first normal action potential allowed sufficient time for spontaneous phase 4 depolarization to occur in the RBBB. The impulse after the pause enters the RBBB at a time when its membrane potential is reduced, resulting in conduction failure. (From Conover, M. [2003]. *Understanding electrocardiography* [8th ed., p. 173]. St. Louis, MO: CV Mosby.)

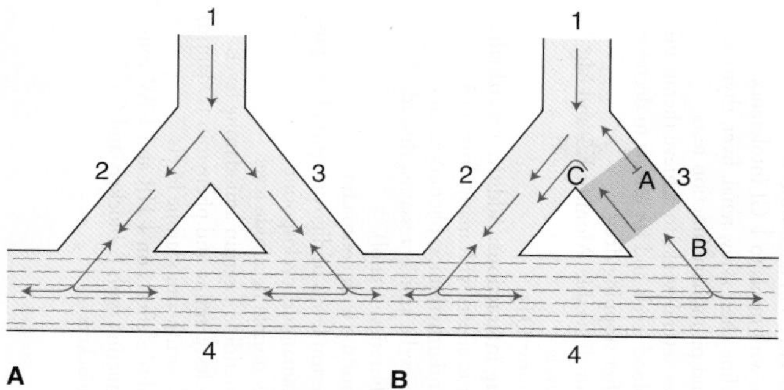

■ **Figure 16-5** (A) Normal conduction of an impulse through Purkinje fibers and ventricular muscle. A Purkinje fiber (1) dividing into two branches (2 and 3) and carrying the impulse into ventricular muscle (4). Normally, impulses from all Purkinje fibers "collide" in the ventricle and extinguish themselves, resulting in one ventricular depolarization. (B) Reentry due to an area of unidirectional block and slow retrograde conduction (shaded area). The impulse enters through Purkinje fiber 1 and depolarizes fiber 2 normally but is blocked from stimulating fiber 3 at point A. It continues down fiber 2 to depolarize ventricular muscle (4) and enters fiber 3 from the area below unidirectional block. The impulse is able to conduct slowly backward through the depressed segment (dashed arrow) and reenter fiber 2 at point C to stimulate it again. (Adapted from Rosen, M. R., & Danilo, P. [1979]. Electrophysiological basis for cardiac arrhythmias. In O. S. Narula [Ed.], *Cardiac arrhythmias: Electrophysiology, diagnosis, management* [p. 9]. Baltimore: Williams & Wilkins.)

depolarization can travel. *Functional reentry* does not require an anatomic obstacle but depends on local differences in conduction velocity and refractoriness among neighboring fibers that allow an impulse to circulate repeatedly around the area. *Anisotropic reentry* is caused by structural differences among adjacent fibers that cause variations in conduction velocity and repolarization between these fibers. An impulse conducts more rapidly when it travels along the length of fibers than it does when it travels in the transverse direction across fibers. These differences in conduction velocity can result in unidirectional block and slow conduction, leading to reentry.

When an impulse travels the reentry loop only once, a single premature beat results. If conduction velocity is slow enough and the refractory period of normal tissue is short enough, a single impulse could travel the loop numerous times, resulting in a run of premature beats or in a sustained tachycardia. Reentry that occurs in small loops of tissue, such as the AV node or Purkinje tissue, is called *microreentry*. If the reentry loop involves large tracts of tissue, such as AV bypass tracts or the bundle-branch system in the ventricles, it is called *macroreentry*.

Many clinical arrhythmias are thought to be due to reentry, including most VT, AF, atrial flutter, and some AT. Arrhythmias that are known to involve discrete reentry circuits are atrial flutter, AVNRT, circus movement tachycardia (CMT) using an accessory pathway in Wolff–Parkinson–White (WPW) syndrome, and bundle-branch reentry VT.

BASIC ARRHYTHMIAS AND CONDUCTION DISTURBANCES

An *arrhythmia* is any cardiac rhythm that is not normal sinus rhythm at a normal rate. The debate continues regarding whether the term *dysrhythmia* should be used instead of *arrhythmia*, because many believe that *arrhythmia* means total absence of rhythm whereas *dysrhythmia* means a disturbance in rhythm. In this chapter, arrhythmia will be used because it is a more commonly used term and continues to be used in the most recent medical textbooks on the subject.

Arrhythmias can be due to abnormal impulse initiation, either at an abnormal rate or from a site other than the SA node, or abnormal impulse conduction through any part of the heart. This section focuses on arrhythmias that originate in the SA node, atria, AV junction, and ventricles, as well as basic AV conduction disturbances. Refer to Tables 16-1 and 16-2 for information related to antiarrhythmic drugs, and Tables 16-3 through 16-5 for current guidelines for the management of specific arrhythmias. The Advanced Cardiac Life Support (ACLS) algorithms for current recommendations for the acute treatment of arrhythmias can be found in Chapter 27.

Table 16-1 ■ CLASSIFICATION OF ANTIARRHYTHMIC DRUGS

Class	Action	ECG Effect	Examples
IA	Sodium channel blockade Prolong repolarization time Slow conduction velocity Suppress automaticity	↑ QRS, ↑ QT	Quinidine Procainamide Disopyramide
IB	Sodium channel blockade Accelerate repolarization	↓ QT	Lidocaine Mexiletine
IC	Sodium channel blockade Marked slowing of conduction No effect on repolarization	↑↑ QRS	Flecainide Propafenone Moricizine (has IA and IB effects too)
II	β-Blockade	↓ HR, ↑ PR	Acebutolol, atenolol, esmolol, metoprolol, propranolol, timolol Sotalol (Other β-blockers are available but not usually used as antiarrhythmics)
III	Potassium channel blockade Prolong repolarization time	↑ QT, ↓ HR, ↑ QRS	Amiodarone Sotalol Ibutilide Dofetilide
IV	Calcium channel blockade	↓ HR, ↑ PR	Verapamil Diltiazem (Other calcium channel blockers are available but not usually used as antiarrhythmics)

↑ = increased, ↓ = decreased, HR = heart rate, PR = PR interval, QRS = QRS width, QT = QT interval.

Rhythms Originating in the SA Node

The SA node is the normal pacemaker of the heart because it has the highest rate of automaticity of all potential pacemaker sites. The arrhythmias that originate in the SA node are sinus bradycardia, sinus tachycardia, sinus arrhythmia, sinus arrest, sinus exit block, and sick sinus syndrome.

(text continues on page 346)

Table 16-2 ■ DRUGS USED FOR HEART RATE AND RHYTHM CONTROL

Drug (Class)	Indication	Dose/Administration Therapeutic Level/Half-Life	Side Effects	Comments
Adenosine (Adenocard)	First-line therapy to terminate AV nodal active SVT (AVNRT, CMT) Can be diagnostic in AV nodal passive rhythms by causing AV block and revealing underlying atrial mechanism, and in wide complex tachycardias of uncertain origin VT arising in the RVOT that is due to after depolarizations may respond to adenosine	6 mg given very rapidly IV followed by rapid saline flush May follow with 12 mg if needed and repeat 12 mg if no effect Half-life = 9 seconds	Acute onset of AV block usually lasting a few seconds. May result in brief period of asystole or bradycardia that is not responsive to atropine Torsades can occur in patients who are susceptible to bradycardia-dependent arrhythmias Flushing, hot flash, acute dyspnea lasting a few seconds, chest pressure Can precipitate bronchoconstriction in asthmatic patients	Very short half-life so side effects are transient Warn patients about side effects before giving drug—especially dyspnea. It may be helpful to have patient take a deep breath while injecting drug to ↓ dyspneic sensation Should not be used when arrhythmia is known to be atrial fib or flutter Monitor ECG during administration and be prepared for cardioversion May accelerate accessory pathway conduction and should not be used when antegrade conduction is occurring over accessory pathway May rarely accelerate ventricular rate in atrial flutter **Drug interactions:** Theophylline (and related drugs) and caffeine antagonize effects of adenosine and make it ineffective Dipyridamole and carbamazepine potentiate effects of adenosine
Amiodarone (Cordarone) (Classified as a class III antiarrhythmic but has powerful class I sodium channel blocking effects, moderate class II β-blocking effects, and weak class IV calcium channel blocking effects)	Life-threatening ventricular arrhythmias: recurrent VF, recurrent hemodynamically unstable VT Also widely used for: Conversion of atrial fib to sinus rhythm and maintenance of NSR Slowing conduction through accessory pathways in atrial fib or CMT	**PO:** 800–1,600 mg q.d. for 1–3 weeks, then 400–800 mg q.d. for 1–3 weeks Maintenance: 100–400 mg/day May be given as single daily dose or bid if GI intolerance occurs **IV:** 1,000 mg over first 24 hours given as follows: **First rapid infusion:** 150 mg over first 10 minutes (15 mg/min) (Add 3 mL [150 mg] to 100 mL D5W) Infuse 100 mL over 10 minutes **Followed by slow infusion:** 360 mg over next 6 hours (1 mg/min) (Add 18 mL [900 mg] to 500 mL D5W) Infuse at 33.6 mL/h **Maintenance infusion:** 540 mg over next 18 hours (0.5 mg/min) (Decrease rate of slow loading infusion to 0.5 mg/min) Infuse at 16.8 mL/h May continue with 0.5 mg/min for 2–3 weeks if needed. Central line recommended for long-term infusions If breakthrough VT occurs, may give supplemental doses of 150 mg over 10 min. (150 mg added to 100 mL D5W)	Bradycardia, heart block Proarrhythmia (VF, incessant VT, torsades) Hypotension with IV form Pulmonary fibrosis, corneal microdeposits, photosensitivity, blue skin, thyroid dysfunction (hypo and hyper), liver dysfunction Tremor, malaise, fatigue, GI upsets, dizziness, poor coordination, peripheral neuropathy, involuntary movements Liver enzyme elevations are common but occur in patients with MI, HF, shock, multiple defibrillations, and so forth. It is unknown if elevations in liver enzymes are due to amiodarone or to associated conditions commonly present in these patients Hepatocellular necrosis has occurred in patients who received IV amiodarone at rates higher than recommended	Give with meals to ↓ GI intolerance Baseline chest x-ray, renal, liver, thyroid, and pulmonary function tests Takes several weeks to achieve therapeutic blood levels and for effects to decrease after stopping drug Is not dialyzable. Monitor K^+ and Mg^{2+} levels Monitor QTc **Drug interactions:** Additive proarrhythmic effects with many drugs (1A antiarrhythmics, phenothiazines, tricyclic antidepressants, thiazide diuretics, sotalol) ↑ Protime with coumadin ↑ Serum levels of digoxin, quinidine, procainamide, cyclosporine May double flecainide level Cimetidine ↑ serum amiodarone levels Cholestyramine and phenytoin (Dilantin) ↓ serum amiodarone levels Additive effects on ↓ HR and ↓ AV conduction with β-blockers and Ca^{2+} blockers

		IV to PO transition: Duration of IV — PO dose <1 week — 800–1600 mg q.d. 1–3 weeks — 600–800 mg q.d. >3 weeks — 400 mg q.d. Therapeutic level = 0.5–2 mcg/mL Very long half-life (26–107 days; average 53 days)		**Special precautions with IV form:** Physically incompatible with aminophylline, heparin, cefamandole, cefazolin, mezlocillin, sodium bicarbonate Must be delivered using a *volumetric pump* (not drop counter) because drop size is altered by drug
Atenolol (Tenormin) (Cardioselective β-blocker)	Ventricular rate control in atrial fib/flutter Slow conduction through AV node in AVNRT and CMT	Initial dose: 12.5–25 mg PO q.d. Maintenance dose: 50–100 mg PO q.d. IV: 5 mg over 5 minutes, may repeat in 5 minutes Half-life = 6–7 hours	Hypotension, bradycardia, AV block. Diarrhea, wheezing, HF	Cardioselective β-blocker used primarily for hypertension and angina **Drug interactions:** Additive effects on HR, AV conduction, BP, and ↑ potential for HF when given with negative inotropic drugs, Ca^{2+} blockers, digoxin
Atropine (Anticholinergic, parasympatholytic)	Treatment of symptomatic bradycardia (sinus, junctional, AV block) and asystole	Symptomatic bradycardia: 0.5 mg IV. May repeat q 3–5 minutes to a total of 3 mg Asystole: 1 mg IV, repeat q 3–5 minutes to a total vagolytic dose of 0.04 mg/kg May be given down ET tube during cardiac arrest if no IV available: use 2–2.5 mg Half-life = 2–5 hours	CV: tachycardia, chest pain, VT/fibrillation (rare) CNS: drowsiness, confusion, dizziness, insomnia, nervousness GI: dry mouth, ↓ GI motility, constipation, nausea Other: urinary retention, hot flushed skin, rash	Doses (0.5 mg may cause paradoxical bradycardia Causes pupils to dilate (significant when checking pupils during cardiac arrest situation) **Drug interactions:** Incompatible with aminophylline, metaraminol, norepinephrine, pentobarbitol, sodium bicarbonate
Digoxin	Ventricular rate control in atrial fib/flutter Rarely used as an antiarrhythmic anymore Used as an inotropic agent in HF	PO loading dose: 0.5–1 mg divided into three or four doses at 6–8-hour intervals PO maintenance dose: 0.125–0.5 mg q.d. IV loading dose: 0.5–1 mg divided into three or four doses given at 4–8-hour intervals Therapeutic level = 0.8–2 ng/mL Half-life = 36–48 hours	CV: bradycardia, AV block Digoxin toxicity: sinus exit block, AV block, AT with block, bidirectional VT, fascicular tachycardia, accelerated junctional rhythm, regularization of ventricular response to atrial fib Visual disturbances (halo vision), anorexia, nausea, vomiting, malaise, headache, weakness, disorientation, seizures	Contraindicated in patients with WPW Digoxin toxicity is more common in the presence of hypokalemia, renal failure, pulmonary or thyroid disease, and in older people **Drug interactions:** The following drugs ↓ digoxin levels: cholestyramine, antacids, kaopectate, neomycin, sulfasalazine, *para*-aminosalicylate The following drugs ↑ digoxin levels: Erythromycin, tetracycline, quinidine, amiodarone, verapamil, spironolactone, nicardipine, indomethacin
Diltiazem (Cardizem) (Calcium channel blocker: nondihydropyridine, "heart rate lowering" Ca^{2+} blocker)	Ventricular rate control in atrial fib/flutter Slow conduction through AV node in AVNRT and CMT	120–360 mg/day in divided doses IV: 0.25 mg/kg bolus over 2 minutes If needed, repeat with 0.35 mg/kg over 2 minutes IV infusion: 5–15 mg/h Therapeutic level = 50–200 ng/mL Half-life = 4–6 hours	Bradycardia, heart block, HF, hypotension, flushing, angina, syncope, insomnia, ringing ears, edema, headache, nausea Less depression of contractility than with verapamil but watch for HF	Contraindicated in patients with accessory pathways (WPW, short PR syndrome) **Drug interactions:** Additive effects on HR, AV conduction, BP, and ↑ potential for HF when given with negative inotropic drugs, β-blockers, digoxin
Disopyramide (Norpace) (Class IA antiarrhythmic)	Used to prevent recurrence of VT or VF Effective in preventing atrial fib and flutter Slows conduction through accessory pathways	Total daily dose = 400–800 mg in divided doses, usually 150 mg q 6 hours SR form = 300 mg q 12 hours Therapeutic level = 3–6 mcg/mL Half-life = 4–10 hours	Anticholinergic effects: dry mouth, urinary retention, constipation, precipitation or exacerbation of glaucoma CV: marked negative inotropic effects, HF, prolongs QT interval, proarrhythmic (less than quinidine or procainamide), ↑ SVR	Monitor QT interval and watch for torsades **Drug Interactions:** May potentiate effect of coumadin Additive negative inotropic effects with β-blockers or Ca^{2+} blockers. Phenobarbitol, dilantin, rifampin ↓ disopyramide levels. Quinidine ↑ disopyramide level

(table continues on page 340)

Table 16-2 ■ DRUGS USED FOR HEART RATE AND RHYTHM CONTROL (continued)

Drug (Class)	Indication	Dose/Administration Therapeutic Level/Half-Life	Side Effects	Comments
Dofetilide (Tikosyn) (Class III antiarrhythmic)	Conversion of atrial fibrillation or flutter to NSR and maintenance of NSR after conversion	Dose based on creatinine clearance: if normal renal function, 500 mcg b.i.d. If abnormal renal function, 250 mcg b.i.d. Do not give if creatinine clearance <20 mL/min Half-life = 9.5 hours	TdP (up to 3% incidence), usually occurs within 3 days after initiating therapy Has no negative inotropic effects and does not lower BP	Patient must be on telemetry during initiation of therapy or with increase in dosage (recommendation is for 3 days monitoring) Monitor QT interval every 2–3 hours: if QTc increases >15% or if QTc is >500 milliseconds, reduce dose. If QTc after second dose is >500 milliseconds, drug should be discontinued **Drug Interactions:** Drugs that increase dofetilide levels include verapamil, ketoconazole, cimetidine, macrolide antibiotics, ritonavir, prochlorperazine, megestrol Maintain normal K^+ and Mg^{2+} levels
Epinephrine (Adrenalin)	Treatment of any cardiac arrest situation requiring CPR: VF, pulseless VT, asystole, PEA	1 mg IV bolus every 3–5 minutes during resuscitation efforts May be given by way of ET tube if IV access not available: use 2–2.5 mg May be infused at 2–10 mcg/min to maintain BP during symptomatic bradycardia	CV: tachycardia, hypertension, arrhythmias, angina CNS: restlessness, headache, tremor, stroke Other: nausea, ↓ urine output, transient tachypnea	**Drug Interactions:** Has potential to cause arrhythmias when given with digoxin, other sympathomimetic agents Physically incompatible with aminophylline, ampicillin, cephapirin, sodium bicarbonate, and other alkaline solutions
Esmolol (Brevibloc) (Cardioselective β-blocker)	Rapid control of ventricular rate in atrial fib/flutter	Loading infusion: 500 mcg/kg/min for 1 minute Maintenance infusion: 50–100 mcg/kg/min Use dosing chart that comes with drug. β-Blocking plasma concentration = 0.15–1 mcg/mL Half-life = 9 minutes	Hypotension, dizziness, diaphoresis, nausea	Short half-life so effects reversed within 10–20 minutes after stopping drug
Flecainide (Tambocor) (Class IC antiarrhythmic)	In absence of structural heart disease: Conversion of atrial fib to sinus rhythm and maintenance of NSR Treatment of SVT: AVNRT, CMT Slow conduction through accessory pathways in atrial fib or CMT Life-threatening ventricular arrhythmias (sustained VT)	100–200 mg PO q 12 hours Therapeutic level = 0.2–1 mcg/mL (Plasma levels do not correlate with efficacy, but incidence of CV toxicity greater when levels >1 mcg/mL) Half-life = 12–27 hours	CV: marked proarrhythmia, marked negative inotropic effects (HF), bradycardia, heart block CNS: blurred vision, dizziness, flushing, ringing ears, drowsiness, headache. Other: bad taste, constipation, edema, abdominal pain	**Drug interactions:** May increase digoxin level Additive effects on HR, AV conduction, BP, and ↑ potential for HF when given with negative inotropic drugs, Ca^{2+} blockers, digoxin Incompatible with sodium bicarbonate, Lasix, Valium, thiopental Higher mortality rate in post-MI patients when studied in CAST. Safest in patients with normal LV function Should not be used in patients with recent MI Prolongs QT interval, potential for proarrhythmia (TdP) Monitor for HF

				Full therapeutic effect may take up to 5 days **Drug Interactions:** ↑ digoxin levels. Cimetidine, amiodarone, propranolol increase flecainide levels Additive negative inotropic effects with β-blockers, Ca^{2+} blockers, disopyramide
Ibutilide (Corvert) (Class III antiarrhythmic)	Conversion of atrial fib or flutter to sinus	IV infusion of 1 mg over 10 minutes May repeat same dose in 10 minutes if needed In patients <60 kg: 0.01 mg/kg Half-life = 6 hours	Hypotension, VT, torsades, bundle-branch block, AV block, nausea, headache	Prolongs QT interval: up to 6% incidence of torsades. Proarrhythmia usually occurs within 40 minutes. Monitor ECG continuously during administration and at least 4 hours after Conversion to NSR usually occurs within 20–30 minutes of infusion **Drug interactions:** Do not give other class I or class III agents within 4 hours
Lidocaine (Xylocaine) (Class IB antiarrhythmic)	Treatment of ventricular arrhythmias: VT, VF Effective for PVC suppression but PVC suppression not usually recommended	For VT: 1 mg/kg IV bolus over 3 minutes followed by infusion at 2–4 mg/min. Repeat bolus of 0.5–0.75 mg/kg in 10 minutes to maintain therapeutic level. May repeat to total of 3 mg/kg For VF or pulseless VT: 1.5 mg/kg IV bolus. May repeat with same amount and follow with infusion at 2–4 mg/min May be given down ET tube during cardiac arrest if no IV available. Therapeutic level = 1.4–5 mcg/mL Half-life of bolus = 10 minutes Half-life once therapeutic level reached = 1.5–2 hours	Side effects relatively rare CNS: lightheadedness, dizziness, tremor, agitation, tinnitus, blurred vision, convulsions, respiratory depression and arrest CV: bradycardia, asystole, hypotension, shock	↓ Dose to half if liver disease or low liver blood flow (shock) **Drug Interactions:** β-Blockers and cimetidine increase lidocaine levels Glucagon and isoproterenol may increase liver blood flow and ↓ lidocaine levels
Magnesium	May be useful for treatment or prevention of both supraventricular and ventricular arrhythmias after MI or cardiac surgery. Treatment of choice for TdP and may be useful in VF or pulseless VT refractory to other drugs	1–2 g diluted in 10 mL D_5W over 1–2 minutes. May be given IV push for VF or torsades Infusion of 0.5–1 g/h for up to 24 hours	CV: hypotension, bradycardia, heart block, cardiac arrest CNS: weakness, drowsiness, peripheral neuromuscular blockade, absent deep tendon reflexes Other: ↓ respiratory rate, respiratory paralysis	**Drug Interactions:** CNS depression when used with general anesthetics, barbiturates, opiate analgesics Additive effects with neuromuscular blocking agents Incompatible with calcium, sodium bicarbonate, ciprofloxacin
Metoprolol (Lopressor) (Cardioselective β-blocker)	Ventricular rate control in atrial fib/flutter Slow conduction through AV node in AVNRT and CMT	PO: 100–450 mg q.d. in divided doses IV: 5 mg q 2–5 minutes for three doses (used in acute MI) β-Blocking plasma concentration = 50–100 ng/mL Half-life = 3–7 hours	Hypotension, bradycardia, AV block	**Drug interactions:** Additive effects on HR, AV conduction, BP, and ↑ potential for HF when given with negative inotropic drugs, Ca^{2+} blockers, digoxin
Mexiletine (Mexitil) (Class IB antiarrhythmic)	Acute and chronic treatment of symptomatic VT Sometimes used in combination with Quinidine or sotalol to increase efficacy May be useful in congenital LQTS	PO loading dose = 400 mg Maintenance dose = 100–300 mg q 8 hours. Up to 400 mg q 8 hours if needed and no intolerable side effects Therapeutic level = 0.5–2 mcg/mL Half-life = 10–17 hours	GI: nausea, vomiting, heartburn, anorexia, diarrhea CNS: tremor, dizziness, ataxia, slurred speech, paresthesias, seizures, hallucinations, emotional instability, insomnia, memory impairment CV: bradycardia, hypotension, HF, proarrhythmia (rare compared to other agents) Other: thrombocytopenia, fever, rash, positive antinuclear antibody	Often given in combination with other antiarrhythmics with increased effectiveness (quinidine, disopyramide, propafenone, amiodarone) **Drug interactions:** Phenobarbitol, dilantin, rifampin ↓ mexiletine levels Cimetidine ↑ mexiletine levels Mexiletine ↑ theophylline levels

(table continues on page 342)

Table 16-2 ■ DRUGS USED FOR HEART RATE AND RHYTHM CONTROL (continued)

Drug (Class)	Indication	Dose/Administration Therapeutic Level/Half-Life	Side Effects	Comments
Procainamide (Pronestyl) (Class IA antiarrhythmic)	Conversion of atrial fib to sinus and maintenance of NSR Treatment of AT, atrial flutter and fib Slows conduction through accessory pathways in WPW Treatment of monomorphic VT	PO dose (regular release form): loading dose of 1,000–1,200 mg; maintenance dose 50 mg/kg/day in divided doses three to four times a day (never more than 6 hour between doses) SR forms: 750–1,500 mg q 6 hours IV loading dose: 17 mg/kg at 20 mg/min. If rapid loading is needed, give 100-mg doses over 5 minutes to total of 1g IV drip 2–4 mg/min Therapeutic level = 4–10 mcg/mL (may be as high as 5–32 mg/L to prevent sustained VT) Half-life = about 3.5 hours Active metabolite is NAPA: therapeutic level = 9–12 mg/L	GI: nausea, vomiting, anorexia CV: bradycardia, heart block, proarrhythmia (less than that with quinidine). Prolongs QT interval Hypotension. With IV use CNS: headache, insomnia, dizziness, psychosis, hallucinations, depression Lupus-like syndrome with long-term use (15%–25% of patients who take drug >1 year) Other: rash, fever, swollen joints, agranulocytosis, pancytopenia	Monitor QT interval, QRS width, PR. Monitor NAPA level (active metabolite) Watch for hypotension with IV use **Drug Interactions:** Amiodarone, cimetidine, ranitidine increase procainamide levels Alcohol ↓ procainamide levels Additive effects on conduction system disease when given with other class IA, class IC, tricyclic antidepressants, or Ca^{2+} blockers
Propafenone (Rythmol) (Class IC antiarrhythmic, also has β-blocker effects)	Conversion of atrial fib to sinus and maintenance of NSR Slow conduction through accessory pathways Life-threatening ventricular arrhythmias (sustained VT)	150–300 mg t.i.d. Therapeutic level = 0.2–3 mcg/mL Half-life = 2–10 hours in normal metabolizers, up to 32 hours in slow metabolizers	GI: nausea, anorexia, constipation, metallic taste CNS: dizziness, headache, blurred vision CV: HF, bradycardia, AV block, bundle-branch block, proarrhythmia	Was not included in CAST but is same class as drugs shown to cause higher mortality post-MI Watch for proarrhythmia **Drug interactions:** ↑ digoxin levels. Potentiates coumadin Has mild β-blocker and Ca^{2+} blocker effects ↑ Cyclosporin levels Quinidine and cimetidine increase propafenone levels
Propranolol (Inderal) (Noncardioselective β-blocker)	Ventricular rate control in atrial fib/flutter Treatment of SVT (slow AV node conduction): AVNRT, CMT Effective in some types of VT: exercise induced, digitalis induced Effective in reducing incidence of VF and sudden death post-MI	PO: 10–30 mg three to four times a day IV: 1–3 mg at rate of 1 mg/min β-Blocking plasma concentration = 50–100 ng/mL Half-life = 3–5 hours	GI: nausea, vomiting, stomach discomfort, constipation, diarrhea CNS: dreams, hallucinations, insomnia, depression Other: bronchospasm, exacerbation of peripheral vascular disease, fatigue, hypoglycemia, impotence	**Drug interactions:** Additive effects on HR, AV conduction, BP, and ↑ potential for HF when given with negative inotropic drugs, Ca^{2+} blockers, digoxin

Quinidine (Class IA antiarrhythmic)	Not used much anymore due to high incidence of proarrhythmia Conversion of atrial fib to NSR and maintenance of NSR May be used for other SVTs: AT, AVNRT, accessory pathways Has been used for VT	Sulfate: 200–400 mg q 6–8 hours Gluconate: 324 mg SR tabs, 1–2 q 8–12 hours Therapeutic level = 2–6 mcg/mL Half-life = 7–9 hours	GI: nausea, diarrhea, abdominal pain CV: hypotension, bradycardia, tachycardias, TdP, HF prolongs QTc interval, proarrhythmia CNS: cinchonism (tinnitus, hearing loss, confusion, delirium, visual disturbances, psychosis) Other: fever, headache, rashes, leukopenia, thrombocytopenia	Give with food. Monitor QT interval, QRS width, PR Watch for proarrhythmia (torsades) IV use rare (hypotension) **Drug Interactions:** ↑ Digoxin levels Increased bleeding when used with coumadin Dilantin, phenobarbital, rifampin, nifedipine, sodium bicarbonate, thiazide diuretics all ↓ quinidine levels Cimetidine, amiodarone, verapamil all increase quinidine levels
Sotalol (Betapace) (Class III antiarrhythmic; and noncardioselective β-blocker)	Maintenance of NSR after conversion from atrial fib/flutter. Not recommended for pharmacological conversion of atrial fib/flutter Treatment of SVT Slow conduction through accessory pathways Life-threatening VT, VF	Should be used only in patients without heart disease or bradycardia when serum electrolytes are normal Contraindicated if baseline QTc >450 milliseconds or CrCl <40 mL/min. 80 mg b.i.d. × 3 days, then 160 mg b.i.d. × 3 days. Decrease dose or discontinue if QT prolongs to 500 milliseconds or more Maximum recommended dose is 160 mg b.i.d Therapeutic level = 1–4 mcg/mL (not clinically useful) Half-life = 8–17 hours with normal renal function; up to 6 days with severe renal failure	CV: bradycardia, heart block, HF, proarrhythmia Other: bronchospasm, fatigue, weakness, GI symptoms, dizziness, dyspnea, hypotension	Prolongs QT interval, potential for proarrhythmia. Monitor QT 2–4 hours after each dose when initiating therapy Watch for bradycardia, AV block, and new or worsening HF
Verapamil (Calan) (Calcium channel blocker: nondihydropyridine "heart rate lowering" Ca^{2+} blocker)	Ventricular rate control in atrial fib/flutter Slow conduction through AV node in AVNRT and CMT	PO: 80–120 mg t.i.d. or q.i.d. IV: 2.5–5 mg over 2 minutes May repeat with 5–10 mg if needed Therapeutic level = 80–400 ng/mL Half-life = 3–7 hours	Bradycardia, heart block, HF, hypotension, fatigue, headache, edema, constipation	Contraindicated in patients with accessory pathways (WPW, short PR syndrome) **Drug interactions:** Additive effects on HR, AV conduction, BP, and ↑ potential for HF when given with negative inotropic drugs, Ca^{2+} blockers, digoxin

CAST, Cardiac Arrhythmia Suppression Trial; CMT, circus movement tachycardia using an accessory pathway; ET, endotracheal, NAPA, *N*-acetylprocainamide; NSR, normal sinus rhythm, PEA, pulseless electrical activity, SVR, systemic vascular resistance, SR, sustained release.
↑ = increases, ↓ = decreases.

Table 16-3 ■ GUIDELINES FOR MANAGEMENT OF AF AND ATRIAL FLUTTER

Pharmacological Rate Control During AF

Class I:
1. Control of rate using either a β-blocker or nondihydropyridine CCB (in most cases) for patients with persistent or permanent AF. (Level B)
2. Administration of AV nodal blocking agents is recommended to achieve rate control in patients who develop postoperative AF. (Level B)
3. In the absence of preexcitation, IV administration of β-blockers (esmolol, metoprolol, or propranolol) or nondihydropyridine CCBs (verapamil, diltiazem) to slow ventricular response to AF in the acute setting, exercising caution in patients with hypotension or HF. (Level B)
4. IV administration of digoxin or amiodarone to control heart rate in patients with AF and HF who do not have an accessory pathway. (Level B)
5. Oral digoxin is effective to control heart rate at rest and is indicated for patients with HF, LV dysfunction, or for sedentary individuals. (Level C)
6. IV amiodarone is recommended to slow a rapid ventricular response to AF and improve LV function in patients with acute MI. (Level C)
7. IV β-blockers and nondihydropyridine CCBs are recommended to slow a rapid ventricular response to AF in patients with acute MI who do not have clinical LV dysfunction, bronchospasm, or AV block. (Level C)

Class IIa
1. A combination of digoxin and either a β-blocker or nondihydropyridine CCB to control heart rate at rest and during exercise in patients with AF. Choice of medication should be individualized and the dose modulated to avoid bradycardia. (Level B)
2. It is reasonable to use ablation of the AV node or accessory pathway to control heart rate when pharmacological therapy is insufficient or associated with side effects. (Level B)
3. IV amiodarone can be useful to control heart rate when other measures are unsuccessful or contraindicated. (Level C)
4. In patients with an accessory pathway, when electrical cardioversion is not necessary, IV procainamide or ibutilide is a reasonable alternative. (Level C)
5. IV digitalis is reasonable to slow a rapid ventricular response and improve LV function in patients with acute MI and severe LV dysfunction and HF. (Level C)

Class IIb
1. Oral amiodarone may be used to control heart rate when ventricular rate cannot be adequately controlled using a β-blocker, nondihydropyridine CCB, or digoxin, alone or in combination. (Level C)
2. IV procainamide, disopyramide, ibutilide, or amiodarone may be considered for hemodynamically stable patients with AF involving conduction over an accessory pathway. (Level B)
3. Catheter ablation of the AV node may be considered when the rate cannot be controlled with pharmacological agents or when tachycardia-mediated cardiomyopathy is suspected. (Level C)

Preventing Thromboembolism

Class I
1. Antithrombotic therapy is recommended for all patients with AF except those with lone AF or contraindications. (Level A)
2. For patients without mechanical heart valves at high risk of stroke (prior stroke, TIA, or systemic embolism; rheumatic mitral stenosis), chronic oral anticoagulant therapy with a vitamin K antagonist is recommended in a dose to achieve the target INR of 2.0 to 3.0 unless contraindicated. (Level A)
3. Anticoagulation with a vitamin K antagonist is recommended for patients with more than one moderate risk factor (age ≥ 75 years, hypertension, HF, LVEF < 35%, diabetes). (Level A)
4. INR should be determined at least weekly during initiation of therapy and monthly when anticoagulation is stable. (Level A)
5. Aspirin 81–325 mg daily is an alternative to vitamin K antagonists in low-risk patients or those with contraindications to anticoagulation. (Level A)
6. For patients with mechanical heart valves, the target intensity of anticoagulation should be based on the type of prosthesis, maintaining an INR of at least 2.5. (Level B)
7. For patients with AF of ≥48 hours duration, or when the duration is unknown, anticoagulation (INR 2.0 to 3.0) is recommended for at least 3 weeks prior to and 4 weeks after cardioversion (electrical or pharmacological). (Level B)
8. For patients with AF of more than 48 hours duration requiring immediate cardioversion, heparin should be administered concurrently (unless contraindicated) by an initial IV bolus followed by a continuous infusion in a dose adjusted to prolong the aPTT to 1.5 to 2 times the reference control value. Oral anticoagulation (INR 2.0 to 3.0) should be given for at least 4 weeks after cardioversion. Limited data support SQ administration of LMWH in this indication. (Level C)
9. For patients with AF of less than 48 hours duration and hemodynamic instability (angina, MI, shock, or pulmonary edema), cardioversion should be performed immediately without delay for prior anticoagulation. (Level C)

Class IIa
1. For primary prevention in patients with nonvalvular AF who have just one of the following risk factors (age ≥ 75 years, HTN, HF, impaired LV function, diabetes), therapy with ASA or a vitamin K antagonist is reasonable. (Level A)
2. For patients with nonvalvular AF who have one or more of the following less well-validated risk factors (age 65–74 years, female, or CAD), therapy with either ASA or a vitamin K antagonist is reasonable. (Level B)
3. As an alternative to anticoagulation prior to cardioversion, it is reasonable to perform TEE in search of thrombus in the left atrium or left atrial appendage. If no thrombus is identified, cardioversion is reasonable immediately after anticoagulation with UFH (aPTT 1.5 to 2 times control), followed by continuation of oral anticoagulation for at least 4 weeks. (Level B) Limited evidence to support use of SQ LMWH in this indication. (Level C)
4. If thrombus is identified by TEE, oral anticoagulation is reasonable for at least 3 weeks prior to and 4 weeks after restoration of sinus rhythm. A longer period of anticoagulation may be appropriate after successful cardioversion because the risk of thromboembolism remains elevated. (Level C)
5. It is reasonable to administer antithrombotic medication in patients who develop postoperative AF, as for nonsurgical patients. (Level B)
6. For patients with AF who do not have mechanical prosthetic heart valves, it is reasonable to interrupt anticoagulation for up to 1 week without substituting heparin for surgical or diagnostic procedures that carry a risk of bleeding. (Level C)

Class IIb
1. In patients ≥ 75 years of age at increased risk of bleeding but without frank contraindications to oral anticoagulant therapy, and in other patients with moderate risk factors for thromboembolism who are unable to safely tolerate an INR 2.0–3.0, a lower INR target of 2.0 (range 1.6 to 2.5) may be considered. (Level C)
2. When surgical procedures require interruption of oral anticoagulant therapy for longer than one week in high-risk patients, UFH may be administered or LMWH given by SQ injection. (Level C)
3. Following PCI or revascularization surgery in patients with AF, low-dose ASA and/or clopidogrel may be given concurrently with anticoagulation to prevent myocardial ischemic events. (Level C)

Table 16-3 ■ GUIDELINES FOR MANAGEMENT OF AF AND ATRIAL FLUTTER (continued)

Cardioversion of AF

Class I
1. Administration of flecainide, dofetilide, propafenone, or ibutilide is recommended for pharmacological cardioversion. (Level A)
2. Immediate electrical (direct-current) cardioversion is recommended for patients with AF involving preexcitation when very rapid tachycardia or hemodynamic instability occurs. (Level B)
3. When a rapid ventricular response does not respond promptly to pharmacological measures in patients with myocardial ischemia, symptomatic hypotension, angina, or HF, immediate r-wave synchronized cardioversion is recommended. (Level C)
4. Electrical cardioversion is recommended in patients without hemodynamic instability when symptoms of AF are unacceptable to the patient. In case of early relapse of AF after cardioversion, repeated electrical cardioversion attempts may be made following administration of antiarrhythmic medication. (Level C)
5. Electrical cardioversion is recommended for patients with acute MI and severe hemodynamic compromise, intractable ischemia, or inadequate rate control with drugs. (Level C)

Class IIa **Pharmacological Cardioversion:**
1. Amiodarone is a reasonable option for pharmacological cardioversion of AF. (Level A)
2. A single oral bolus dose of propafenone or flecainide ("pill-it-the-pocket") can be administered to terminate persistent AF outside the hospital once treatment has proved safe in hospital for selected patients without sinus or AV node dysfunction, BBB, QT-interval prolongation, Brugada syndrome, or structural heart disease. Before antiarrhythmic medication is initiated, a β-blocker or nondihydropyridine CCB should be given to prevent rapid AV conduction in the event atrial flutter occurs. (Level C)
3. Amiodarone can be beneficial on an outpatient basis in patients with paroxysmal or persistent AF when rapid restoration of sinus rhythm is not deemed necessary. (Level C)
4. It is reasonable to restore sinus rhythm by pharmacological cardioversion with ibutilide or electrical cardioversion in patients who develop postoperative AF. (Level B)

Electrical Cardioversion:

5. Electrical cardioversion can be useful to restore sinus rhythm as part of a long-term management strategy. (Level B)
6. Patient preference is a reasonable consideration in the selection of infrequently repeated electrical cardioversions for the management of symptomatic or recurrent AF. (Level C)

Pharmacological Enhancement of Electrical Cardioversion:

7. Pretreatment with amiodarone, flecainide, ibutilide, propafenone, or sotalol can be useful to enhance the success of electrical cardioversion and prevent recurrent AF. (Level B)
8. In patients who relapse to AF after successful cardioversion, it can be useful to repeat the procedure following prophylactic administration of antiarrhythmic medication. (Level C)

Class IIb
1. Quinidine or procainamide might be considered for pharmacological cardioversion, but the usefulness of these agents is not well established. (Level C)
2. For patients with persistent AF, administration of β-blockers, disopyramide, diltiazem, dofetilide, procainamide, or verapamil may be considered, although the efficacy of these agents to enhance the success of electrical cardioversion or to prevent early recurrence of AF is uncertain. (Level C)
3. Out-of-hospital initiation of antiarrhythmic medications may be considered to enhance the success of electrical cardioversion in patients without heart disease or in patients with certain forms of heart disease once the safety of the drug has been verified for the patient. (Level C)

Maintenance of Sinus Rhythm

Class I
1. An oral β-blocker to prevent postoperative AF is recommended for patients undergoing cardiac surgery (unless contraindicated). (Level A)
2. Before initiating antiarrhythmic drug therapy, treatment of precipitating or reversible causes of AF is recommended. (Level C)

Class IIa
1. Preoperative administration of amiodarone reduces the incidence of AF in patients undergoing cardiac surgery and is appropriate prophylactic therapy for patients at high risk for postoperative AF. (Level A)
2. In patients with lone AF without structural heart disease, initiation of propafenone or flecainide can be beneficial on an outpatient basis in patients with paroxysmal AF who are in sinus rhythm at the time of drug initiation. (Level B)
3. Drug therapy can be useful to maintain sinus rhythm and prevent tachycardia-induced cardiomyopathy. (Level C)
4. Infrequent, well-tolerated recurrence of AF is reasonable as a successful outcome of antiarrhythmic drug therapy. (Level C)
5. Outpatient initiation of antiarrhythmic drug therapy is reasonable in patients who have no associated heart disease when the agent is well tolerated. (Level C)
6. Sotalol can be beneficial in outpatients in sinus rhythm with little or no heart disease, prone to paroxysmal AF, if the baseline uncorrected QT interval is less than 460 milliseconds. Serum electrolytes are normal, and risk factors associated with class III drug-related proarrhythmia are not present. (Level C)
7. Catheter ablation is a reasonable alternative to drug therapy to prevent recurrent AF in symptomatic patients with little or no left atrial enlargement. (Level C)

Class IIb
1. Prophylactic administration of sotalol may be considered for patients at risk of developing AF following cardiac surgery. (Level B)

Classification of Recommendations:
Class I: Benefit >>> risk, procedure/treatment *should be* performed/administered
Class IIa: Benefit >> risk, *it is reasonable* to perform procedure/ administer treatment
Class IIb: Benefit ≥ Risk, Procedure/treatment *may be considered*

Level of Evidence Definitions:
Level A: Data derived from multiple randomized clinical trials or meta-analyses
Level B: Data derived from a single randomized trial or nonrandomized studies
Level C: Only consensus opinion of experts, case studies, or standard of care

aPTT, activated partial thromboplastin time; ASA, aspirin; BBB, bundle-branch block; CAD, coronary artery disease; CCB, calcium channel blocker; HTN, hypertension; INR, international normalized ratio; LMWH, low molecular weight heparin; LV, left ventricular; LVEF, left ventricular ejection fraction; PCI, percutaneous coronary interventions; SQ, subcutaneous; TEE, transesophageal echocardiography; TIA, transient ischemic attack; UFH: unfractionated heparin.

Adapted from Fuster, V., Ryden, L. E., Asinger, R. W., et al. (2006). ACC/AHA/ESC guidelines for the management of patients with atrial fibrillation: Executive summary: A report of the American College of Cardiology/American Heart Association Task Force on Practice Guidelines and the European Society of Cardiology Committee for Practice Guidelines (Writing Committee to Revise the 2001 Guidelines for the Management of Patients with Atrial Fibrillation). *Circulation, 114*, 700–752.

Table 16-4 ■ GUIDELINES FOR MANAGEMENT OF SUPRAVENTRICULAR ARRHYTHMIAS

Acute Management of Hemodynamically Stable and Regular Tachycardia

Class I: **Narrow QRS (SVT) and SVT with BBB:**
1. Vagal maneuvers (Valsalva, CSM) (Level B)
2. Adenosine (Level A)
3. Verapamil, diltiazem (Level A)

Preexcited SVT/AF
1. Flecainide (Level B)
2. Ibutilide (Level B)
3. Procainamide (Level B)
4. Electrical cardioversion (Level C)

Wide QRS Tachycardia of Unknown Origin:
1. Procainamide (Level B)
2. Sotalol (Level B)
3. Amiodarone (Level B)
4. Electrical cardioversion (Level B)

Wide QRS Tachycardia of Unknown Origin in Patients with Poor LV Function:
1. Amiodarone (Level B)
2. Lidocaine (Level B)
3. Electrical cardioversion (Level B)

Class IIb **Narrow QRS (SVT) and SVT with BBB:**
1. β-Blockers (Level C)
2. Amiodarone (Level C)
3. Digoxin (Level C)

Wide QRS Tachycardia of Unknown Origin:
1. Lidocaine (Level B)
2. Adenosine (Level C)

Long-Term Treatment of Recurrent AVNRT

Class I:
1. Catheter ablation (Level B)
2. Verapamil for recurrent symptomatic AVNRT (Level B)
3. Diltiazem or β-blockers for recurrent symptomatic AVNRT (Level C)

Infrequent, well-tolerated episodes of AVNRT:
1. Vagal maneuvers (Level B)
2. Pill-in-the-pocket (single dose oral diltiazem plus propranolol) (Level B)
3. Verapamil, diltiazem, β-blockers, catheter ablation (Level B)

Class IIa
1. Verapamil, diltiazem, β-blockers, sotalol, amiodarone (Level C)
2. Flecainide, propafenone in patients with no coronary artery disease, LV dysfunction, or other significant heart disease (Level C)

Class IIb
1. Digoxin (Level C)
2. Amiodarone (Level C)

Focal and Nonparoxysmal Junctional Tachycardia Syndromes

Class I: **Nonparoxysmal junctional tachycardia:**
1. Reverse digitalis toxicity (Level C)
2. Correct hypokalemia (Level C)
3. Treat myocardial ischemia (Level C)

Class IIa
1. β-Blockers, flecainide, catheter ablation (Level C)
2. Propafenone, sotalol, amiodarone in pediatric patients (Level C)

Long-Term Therapy of Accessory Pathway–Mediated Arrhythmias

Class I:
1. Catheter ablation for WPW syndrome (preexcitation and symptomatic arrhythmias) that are well tolerated; or with AF and rapid conduction or poorly tolerated CMT (Level B)
2. Vagal maneuvers for single or infrequent episodes (Level B)
3. Pill-in-the-pocket (verapamil, diltiazem, β-blockers) for single or infrequent episodes (Level B)
   Contraindicated: verapamil, diltiazem, digoxin

Class IIa
1. Flecainide, propafenone, sotalol, amiodarone, β-blockers (Level C)
2. Catheter ablation for single or infrequent episodes, or asymptomatic preexcitation (Level B)

Class IIb
1. β-Blockers in poorly tolerated episodes (Level C)
2. Sotalol, amiodarone for single or infrequent episodes (Level B)
3. Flecainide, propafenone for single or infrequent episodes (Level C)

Treatment of Focal AT

Class I: **Acute Treatment:**
1. Electrical cardioversion if hemodynamically unstable (Level B)
2. β-Blockers, verapamil, diltiazem for rate control (in absence of digitalis therapy) (Level C)

Prophylactic Therapy:
1. Catheter ablation for recurrent symptomatic or incessant AT (Level B)
2. β-Blockers, verapamil, diltiazem (Level C)

Class IIa **Acute Treatment:**
1. Adenosine, β-blockers, verapamil, diltiazem, procainamide, flecainide, propafenone, amiodarone, sotalol for hemodynamically stable patients (Level C)

Prophylactic Therapy:
1. Disopyramide, flecainide, propafenone for recurrent symptomatic AT (these drugs should be combined with an AV nodal blocking agent to prevent rapid ventricular rate if atrial fib or flutter should occur) (Level C)
2. Sotalol, amiodarone for recurrent symptomatic AT (Level C)

Class IIb 1. Digoxin for rate control (Level C)

Classification of Recommendations:

Class I: Benefit >>> Risk, procedure/treatment *should be* performed/administered.

Class IIa: Benefit >> risk, *it is reasonable* to perform procedure/administer treatment.

Class IIb: Benefit ≥ risk, procedure/*treatment may be considered.*

Level of Evidence Definitions:

Level A: Data derived from multiple randomized clinical trials or meta-analyses.

Level B: Data derived from a single randomized trial or nonrandomized studies.

Level C: Only consensus opinion of experts, case studies, or standard of care.

BBB, bundle-branch block; LV, left ventricular.

Adapted from Blomstrom-Lundqvist, C., Scheinman, M. M., Aliot, E. M., et al. (2003). ACC/AHA/ESC guidelines for the management of patients with supraventricular arrhythmias—Executive summary. A report of the American College of Cardiology/American Heart Association Task Force on Practice Guidelines and the European Society of Cardiology Committee for Practice Guidelines (Writing Committee to Develop Guidelines for the Management of Patients With Supraventricular Arrhythmias). *Circulation, 108,* 1871–1909.

Normal Sinus Rhythm

The SA node normally fires at a regular rate of 60 to 100 beats per minute. The impulse spreads from the SA node through the atria and to the AV node, where it encounters a slight delay before it travels through the bundle of His, right and left bundle branches, and Purkinje fibers into the ventricles. The spread of this wave of depolarization through the heart gives rise to the classic surface electrocardiogram (ECG), which can be monitored at the bedside. Chapter 15 presents information on the origin of the waves and intervals of the cardiac cycle.

The characteristics of normal sinus rhythm include the following:

Rate: 60 to 100 beats per minute
Rhythm: Regular
P waves: Precede every QRS complex and are consistent in shape
PR interval: 0.12 to 0.20 second
QRS complex: 0.04 to 0.10 second

Table 16-5 ■ GUIDELINES FOR MANAGEMENT OF VENTRICULAR ARRHYTHMIAS

Sustained Monomorphic VT	
Class I:	1. Wide QRS tachycardia should be presumed to be VT if the diagnosis is unclear. (Level C)
	2. Electrical cardioversion with sedation is recommended with hemodynamically unstable sustained monomorphic VT. (Level C) CONTRAINDICATED: Calcium channel blockers (verapamil, diltiazem) should not be used to terminate wide QRS tachycardia of unknown origin, especially with history of myocardial dysfunction.
Class IIa	1. IV procainamide is reasonable for initial treatment of patients with stable VT. (Level B)
	2. IV amiodarone is reasonable for VT that is hemodynamically unstable, refractory to conversion with countershock, or recurrent despite procainamide or other agents. (Level C)
	3. Transvenous catheter pace termination can be useful for VT that is refractory to cardioversion or is frequently recurrent despite antiarrhythmic medication. (Level C)
Class IIb	1. IV lidocaine might be reasonable for initial treatment of monomorphic VT associated with acute myocardial ischemia or infarction. (Level C)
Repetitive Monomorphic VT	
Class IIa	1. IV amiodarone, β-blockers, and IV procainamide (or IV sotalol or ajmaline in Europe) can be useful for repetitive monomorphic VT in the context of coronary disease and idiopathic VT. (Level C)
PVT	
Class I:	1. Electrical cardioversion with sedation is recommended for sustained PVT with hemodynamic compromise. (Level B)
	2. IV β-blockers are useful if ischemia is suspected or cannot be excluded. (Level B)
	3. IV amiodarone is useful for recurrent PVT in the absence of QT prolongation (congenital or acquired). Level C
	4. Urgent angiography and revascularization should be considered with PVT when myocardial ischemia cannot be excluded. (Level C)
Class IIb	1. IV lidocaine may be reasonable for PVT associated with acute myocardial ischemia or infarction (Level C)
TdP	
Class I:	1. Withdrawal of any offending drugs and correction of electrolyte abnormalities are recommended for TdP. (Level A)
	2. Acute and long-term pacing is recommended for TdP due to heart block and symptomatic bradycardia. (Level A)
Class IIa	1. IV magnesium sulfate is reasonable for patients who present with LQTS and few episodes of TdP. (Level B)
	2. Acute and long-term pacing is reasonable for recurrent pause-dependent TdP. (Level B)
	3. β-Blockade combined with pacing is reasonable acute therapy for TdP and sinus bradycardia. (Level C)
	4. Isoproterenol is reasonable as temporary acute treatment for recurrent pause-dependent TdP who do not have congenital LQTS. (Level B)
Class IIb	1. Potassium repletion to 4.5–5 mM/L may be considered for TdP. (Level B)
	2. IV lidocaine or oral mexiletine may be considered for LQT3 and TdP. (Level C)
Incessant VT	
Class I:	1. Revascularization and β-blockade followed by IV antiarrhythmic drugs such as procainamide or amiodarone are recommended for recurrent or incessant PVT. (Level B)
Class IIa	1. IV amiodarone or procainamide followed by VT ablation can be effective in recurrent or incessant monomorphic VT. (Level B)
Class IIb	1. IV amiodarone and IV β-blockers separately or together may be reasonable for VT storm. (Level C)
	2. Overdrive pacing or general anesthesia may be considered for frequently recurring or incessant VT. (Level C)
	3. Spinal cord modulation may be considered for some patients with frequently recurring or incessant VT. (Level C)

Classification of Recommendations:
Class I: Benefit >>> Risk, Procedure/Treatment *should be* performed/administered.
Class IIa: Benefit >> Risk, *it is reasonable* to perform procedure/administer treatment.
Class IIb: Benefit ≥ Risk, Procedure/treatment *may be considered.*
Level of Evidence Definitions:
Level A: Data derived from multiple randomized clinical trials or meta-analyses.
Level B: Data derived from a single randomized trial or nonrandomized studies.
Level C: Only consensus opinion of experts, case studies, or standard-of-care.

This table covers pharmacological and electrical cardioversion for treatment of VT. Guidelines for ICD implantation are covered in Chapter 28, and guidelines for catheter ablation are presented in Chapter 18.

Adapted from Zipes, D. P., Camm, J. A., Borggrefe, M., et al. (2006). ACC/AHA/ESC 2006 guidelines for management of patients with ventricular arrhythmias and the prevention of sudden cardiac death—Executive summary: A report of the American College of Cardiology/American Heart Association Task Force and the European Society of Cardiology Committee for Practice Guidelines. *Circulation, 114*, 1088–1132.

Example: Normal sinus rhythm. Rate, 65 beats per minute; PR interval, 0.14 second; QRS interval, 0.06 second

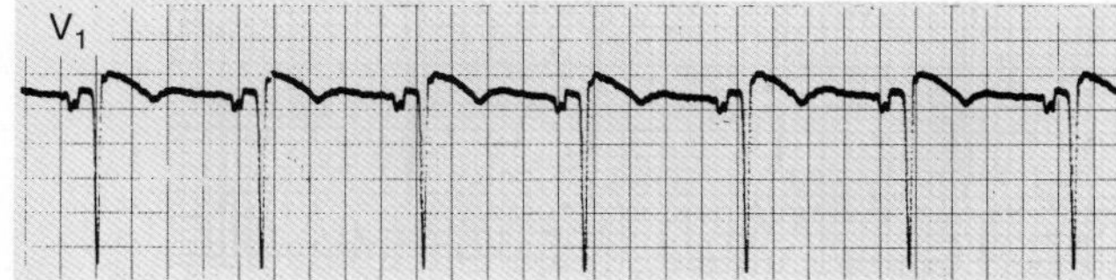

Sinus Bradycardia

Sinus bradycardia is discharge of the SA node at a rate slower than 60 beats per minute. It can be a normal variant, especially in athletes and during sleep. Sinus bradycardia may be a response to vagal stimulation, such as carotid sinus massage (CSM), ocular pressure, coughing, or vomiting. Pathological sinus bradycardia can occur with inferior wall MI, hypothyroidism, hypothermia, sleep apnea, increased intracranial pressure, glaucoma, myxedema, hypoxia, infections, and sick sinus syndrome.[5,14,15] Sinus bradycardia can be a response to several medications, including digitalis, β-blockers, calcium channel blockers, and antiarrhythmics.

The following are ECG characteristics of sinus bradycardia:

Rate: Less than 60 beats per minute
Rhythm: Regular
P waves: Precede every QRS, consistent shape
PR interval: Usually normal (0.12 to 0.20 second)
QRS complex: Usually normal (0.04 to 0.10 second)
Conduction: Normal through atria, AV node, bundle branches, and ventricles
Example: Sinus bradycardia, rate 40 beats per minute

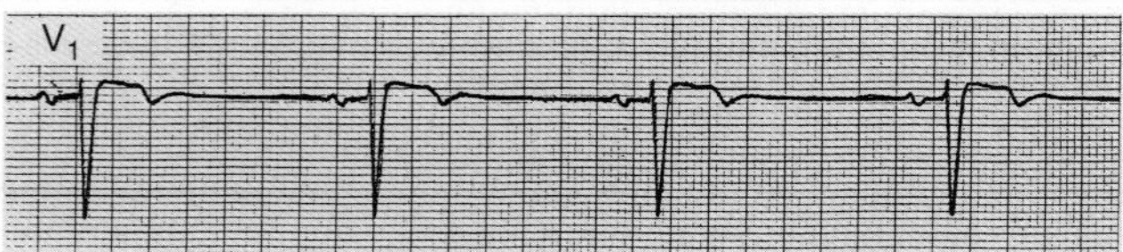

Sinus bradycardia does not require treatment unless the patient is symptomatic. If the arrhythmia is accompanied by hypotension, restlessness, diaphoresis, chest pain, or other signs of hemodynamic compromise or by ventricular ectopy, atropine 0.5 mg intravenously (IV) is the treatment of choice. Attempts should be made to decrease vagal stimulation, and, if bradycardia is due to medications, they should be held until their need has been reevaluated. See Chapter 27 for the ACLS algorithm for treatment of symptomatic bradycardia.

Sinus Tachycardia

Sinus tachycardia is sinus rhythm at a rate faster than 100 beats per minute. It is a normal response to anything that stimulates the sympathetic nervous system, including sympathomimetic drugs, exercise, and emotion. Sinus tachycardia that persists at rest usually indicates some underlying problem, such as fever, blood loss, anxiety, pain, HF, hypermetabolic states, or anemia. Sinus tachycardia is a normal physiologic response to a decrease in cardiac output. Drugs that can cause sinus tachycardia include atropine, isoproterenol, epinephrine, dopamine, dobutamine, norepinephrine, nitroprusside, and caffeine.

The rate of sinus tachycardia should not exceed 220 minus the patient's age. For example, a 40-year-old patient can have sinus tachycardia up to a rate of 180 beats per minute, but a 70-year-old patient should not have sinus tachycardia at a rate faster than 150 beats per minute. If the heart rate exceeds these upper limits, some other mechanism of tachycardia should be suspected.

The ECG characteristics of sinus tachycardia include the following:

Rate: Greater than 100 beats per minute
Rhythm: Regular
P waves: Precede every QRS; have consistent shape; may be buried in the preceding T wave
PR interval: Usually normal, may be difficult to measure if P waves are buried in T waves
QRS complex: Usually normal
Conduction: Normal through atria, AV node, bundle branches, and ventricles
Example: Sinus tachycardia rate, 107 beats per minute

Treatment of sinus tachycardia is directed at the cause. Because this arrhythmia is a physiologic response to a decrease in cardiac output, it should never be ignored, especially in the cardiac patient. Because the ventricles fill with blood and the coronary arteries perfuse during diastole, persistent tachycardia can cause decreased stroke volume, decreased cardiac output, and decreased coronary perfusion secondary to the decreased diastolic time that occurs with rapid heart rates. Carotid sinus pressure may slow the heart rate temporarily and thereby help in ruling out other arrhythmias. β-Blockers are used to treat tachycardia in patients with acute MI without signs of HF or contraindications to β-blocker therapy.

Sinus Arrhythmia

Sinus arrhythmia occurs when the SA node discharges irregularly. It occurs as a normal phenomenon, especially in the young, and decreases with age. Sinus arrhythmia is commonly associated with the phases of respiration: during inspiration, the SA node fires faster; during expiration, it slows. Other than this phasic increase and decrease in rate, sinus arrhythmia looks like normal sinus rhythm and it does not require treatment. The following characteristics are typical of sinus arrhythmia:

Rate: 60 to 100 beats per minute
Rhythm: Irregular; phasic increase and decrease in rate, which may be related to respiration
P waves: Precede every QRS; have consistent shape
PR interval: Usually normal
QRS complex: Usually normal
Conduction: Normal through atria, AV node, bundle branches, ventricles
Example: Sinus arrhythmia

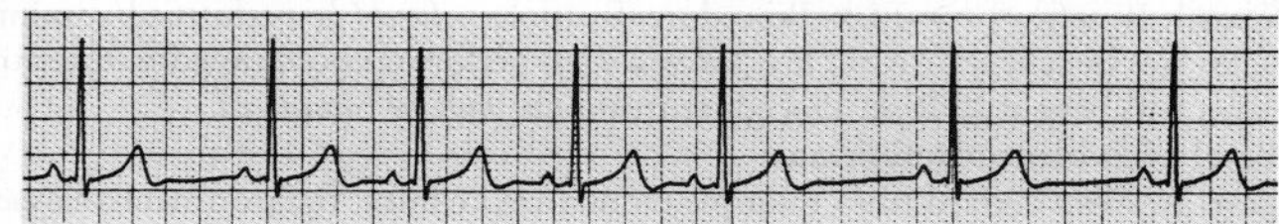

Sinus Arrest

Sinus arrest occurs when the SA node automaticity is depressed and impulses are not formed when expected. This delay results in the absence of a P wave at the time it is expected to occur, and unless there is escape of a junctional or ventricular pacemaker, the QRS

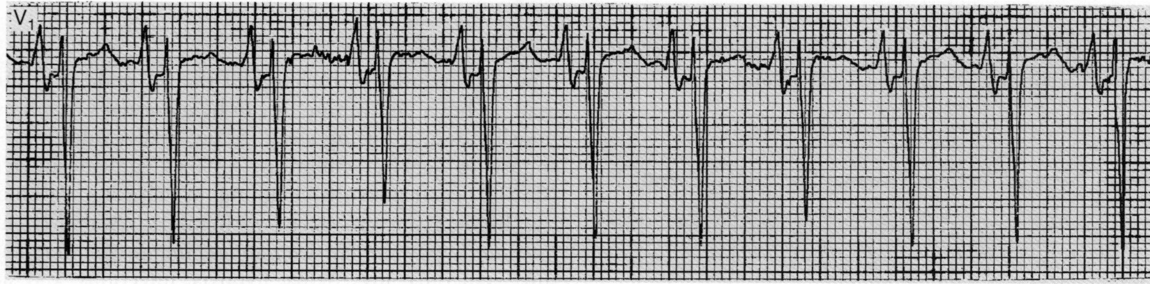

Example of sinus tachycardia

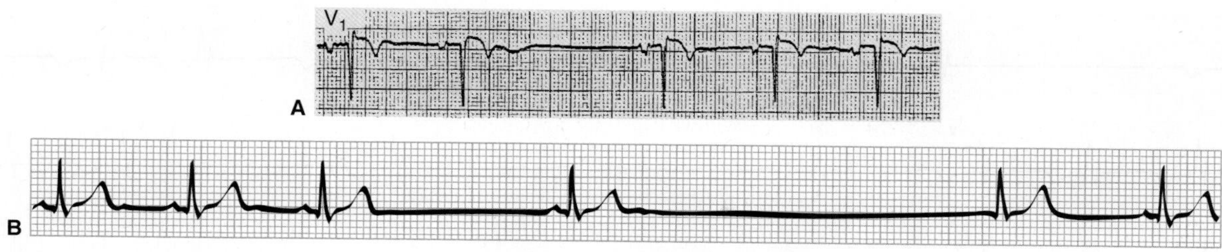

Example of sinus arrest

complex is also missing. If only one sinus impulse fails to form, the term *sinus pause* is usually used, whereas if more than one sinus impulse in a row fails to form, sinus arrest has occurred. Because the SA node has depressed automaticity and does not form impulses regularly as expected, the P-P interval in sinus arrest is not an exact multiple of the sinus cycle. Causes of sinus arrest include vagal stimulation, carotid sinus sensitivity, MI interrupting the blood supply to the SA node, and drugs such as digitalis, β-blockers, and calcium channel blockers. Sinus arrest is characterized by the following ECG changes.

Rate: Atrial—usually within normal range but may be in bradycardic range if several sinus impulses fail to form. Ventricular—usually within normal range but may be in bradycardic range if several sinus impulses fail to form and there are no junctional or ventricular escape beats. Occasionally, the ventricular rate may be faster than the atrial rate because of junctional or ventricular escape beats that occur during the period of sinus arrest.

Rhythm: Irregular due to the absence of SA node discharge

P waves: Present when SA node is firing and absent during periods of sinus arrest. When present, they precede every QRS complex and are consistent in shape. If junctional escape beats occur, P waves may be inverted either before or after the junctional QRS.

PR interval: Usually normal when P waves are present. If junctional escape beats occur, the PR interval is short when the P wave precedes the QRS.

QRS complex: Usually normal when SA node is functioning and absent during periods of sinus arrest unless escape beats occur. If ventricular escape beats occur, QRS complex is wide.

Conduction: Normal through atria, AV node, bundle branches, and ventricles when SA node is firing. When the SA node fails to form impulses, there is no conduction through the atria. If a junctional escape beat occurs, ventricular conduction is usually normal, whereas if a ventricular escape beat occurs, conduction through the ventricles is abnormally slow.

Example: (A) Sinus pause and (B) sinus arrest with a junctional escape beat (5th beat)

Treatment of sinus arrest is aimed at the cause and at increasing ventricular rate if the patient is symptomatic. Any offending drugs should be discontinued, and vagal stimulation should be minimized. If periods of sinus arrest are frequent and cause hemodynamic compromise, atropine 0.5 mg IV may increase the ventricular rate. Pacemaker therapy may be necessary if all other forms of management fail.

Sinus Exit Block

Sinus exit block occurs when the impulse is formed in the SA node normally but fails to exit the node to excite atrial tissue. Sinus exit block can be type I, type II, or complete. The section in this chapter titled "Complex Arrhythmias and Conduction Disturbances" contains a discussion of sinus Wenckebach, which is type I sinus exit block. Type II sinus exit block looks exactly like sinus arrest except for the P-P intervals, which are multiples of the basic sinus cycle length. Complete sinus exit block exists when no impulses reach the atria from the SA node and no P waves occur. In this case, either a junctional or ventricular pacemaker emerges to take over pacing duties, or asystole occurs.

Rate: Atrial—usually within normal range but may be in bradycardic range if several sinus impulses fail to exit the SA node. Ventricular—usually in normal range but may be in bradycardic range if no junctional or ventricular escape beats occur during periods of sinus exit block.

Rhythm: Irregular due to pauses caused by sinus exit block

P waves: Present except when impulse fails to exit SA node. When present, they precede every QRS and are consistent in shape. The P-P interval is an exact multiple of the sinus cycle because impulses are formed regularly but occasionally fail to exit the SA node.

PR interval: Usually normal when P waves are present but may be prolonged if AV node conduction is slow.

QRS complexes: Usually normal when sinus impulse conducts and absent when exit block occurs. If ventricular escape beats occur, QRS is wide.

Conduction: Normal through atria, AV node, bundle branches, and ventricles when impulse exits SA node normally.

Example: Sinus exit block. The length of the pause is exactly double the sinus rate

Treatment of sinus exit block depends on the resulting ventricular rate and its hemodynamic significance. Atropine may cause an increase in rate if bradycardia is symptomatic. Pacing may be necessary, especially with complete sinus exit block. Otherwise, the treatment is similar to that of sinus arrest.

Sick Sinus Syndrome

The term *sick sinus syndrome* is used to describe rhythms in which there is marked sinus bradycardia, sinus pauses, or periods of sinus arrest alternating with paroxysms of rapid atrial arrhythmias, especially atrial flutter or AF. The term *brady-tachy syndrome* is

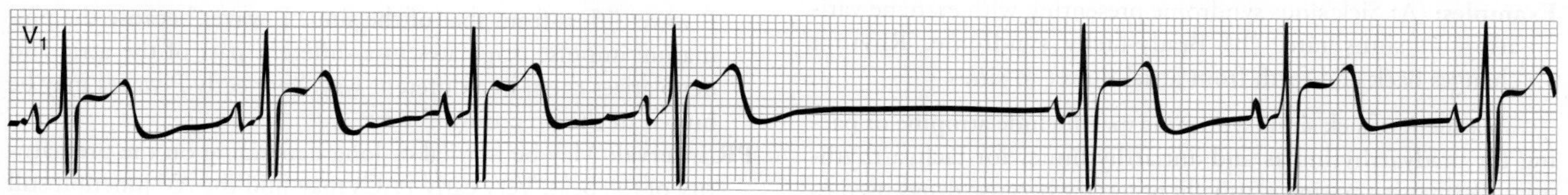

Example of sinus exit block

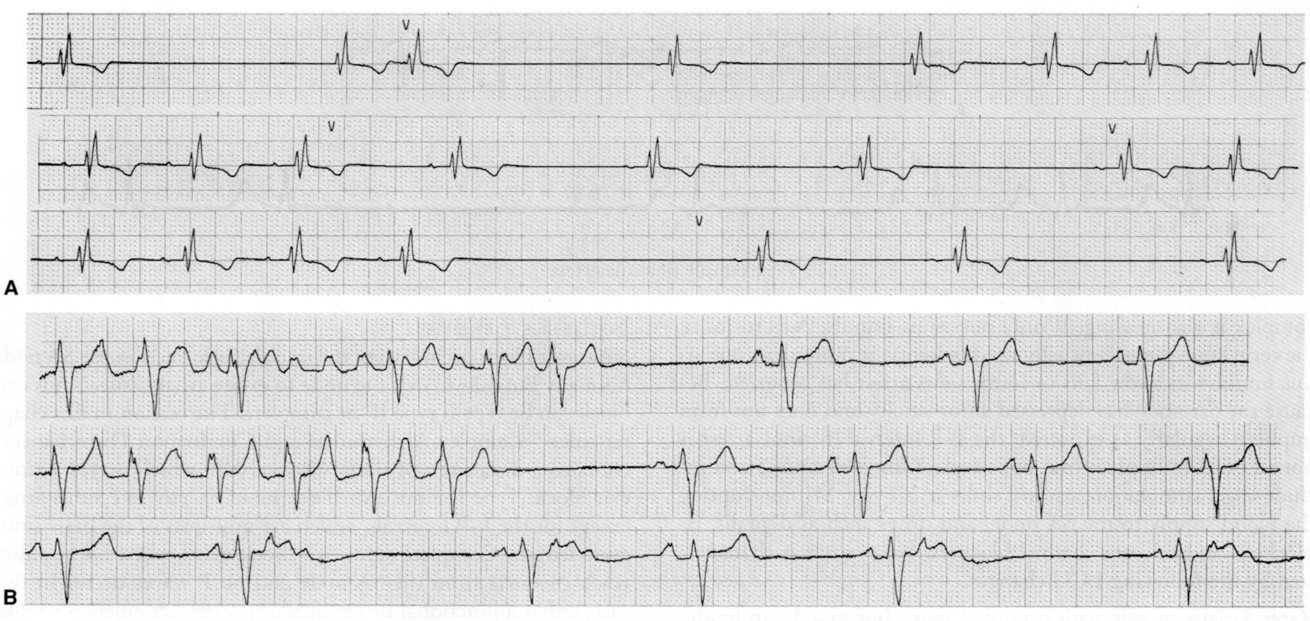

Examples of sick sinus syndrome (A) and brady-tachy syndrome (B).

commonly used to describe the same arrhythmias. During periods of sinus bradycardia or arrest, junctional escape rhythms commonly occur, and AV block is also often associated with the SA node dysfunction that causes sick sinus syndrome. Causes of sick sinus syndrome include coronary artery disease, inflammatory or infiltrative cardiac disease, cardiomyopathy, sclerodegenerative processes involving both the SA and AV nodes, and drugs such as β-blockers, calcium channel blockers, digitalis, amiodarone, propafenone, and adenosine.[5,15,16] ECG characteristics of sick sinus syndrome include the following:

Rate: Varies from bradycardic to tachycardic rates depending on SA node function, rate of escape pacemakers, and presence of atrial tachyarrhythmias

Rhythm: Irregular; pauses of 3 seconds or more can occur during periods of sinus arrest. Regularity of rhythm depends on reliability of SA node and escape pacemakers, and on the type of tachyarrhythmia present (e.g., AF is very irregular).

P waves: Usually normal during periods of sinus rhythm. Absent during periods of sinus arrest or AF, inverted with junctional rhythms. Flutter waves are present during periods of atrial flutter.

PR interval: May be normal or prolonged depending on state of AV conduction

QRS complex: Usually normal unless there is associated bundle-branch block or ventricular escape rhythms

Conduction: Normal through the atria when the SA node is in control; abnormal through atria during periods of atrial tachyarrhythmias. AV conduction may be normal or abnormal depending on the degree of AV node disease. Conduction through ventricles is normal unless bundle-branch block is present or a ventricular escape rhythm occurs.

Examples: (A) Sick sinus syndrome presenting with extreme variation in sinus rate. (B) Brady-tachy syndrome. Rhythm changes back and forth from atrial flutter to sinus.

Treatment of sick sinus syndrome may include atropine or pacing for bradyarrhythmias and antiarrhythmics for tachyarrhythmias. Permanent pacing is usually necessary because drugs used to treat the tachyarrhythmias aggravate bradycardia and often further depress SA node function.

Rhythms Originating in the Atria

Ectopic impulses or reentry circuits can occur in the atrial myocardium, resulting in several atrial arrhythmias: premature atrial complexes (PACs), wandering atrial pacemaker (WAP), AT, multifocal atrial tachycardia (MAT), atrial flutter, and AF. See Chapter 27 for the ACLS algorithm for treatment of tachycardias, Table 16-3 for guidelines for management of AF and flutter, and Table 16-4 for guidelines for management of supraventricular tachycardias (SVT).

PACs (Also Called Atrial Premature Depolarizations)

A PAC occurs when an irritable focus in the atria fires before the next sinus impulse is due. PACs can be caused by caffeine, alcohol, nicotine, stretch on the atria (as in HF or pulmonary disease), interruption of atrial blood supply by myocardial ischemia or MI, anxiety, and hypermetabolic states.[17] PACs often occur in normal hearts and are not considered an abnormal finding.

The ECG characteristics of PACs include the following:

Rate: Usually within normal range

Rhythm: Usually regular except when PACs occur, resulting in early beats. PACs often have a noncompensatory pause (interval between the complex before and that after the PAC is less than two normal R-R intervals) because premature depolarization of the atria by the PAC also causes premature depolarization of the SA node, thus causing the SA node to "reset" itself.

P waves: Precede every QRS. The configuration of the premature P wave differs from that of the sinus P waves because the premature impulse originates in a different part of the atria and depolarizes them in a different way. Very early P waves may be buried in the preceding T wave.

PR interval: May be normal or long depending on the prematurity of the beat. Very early PACs may find the AV junction still partially refractory and unable to conduct at a normal rate, resulting in a prolonged PR interval.

QRS complex: May be normal, aberrant (wide), or absent, depending on the prematurity of the beat. If the bundle branches have repolarized completely, they are able to conduct the early impulse normally, resulting in a normal QRS. If the PAC occurs during the relative refractory period of the bundle branches or ventricles, the impulse conducts aberrantly and the QRS is wide. If the PAC occurs very early during the complete refractory period of the AV node or both bundle branches, the impulse does not conduct to the ventricles and the QRS is absent.

Conduction: PACs travel through the atria differently from sinus impulses because they originate from a different spot. Conduction through the AV node, bundle branches, and ventricles is usually normal unless the PAC is very early (see previous discussion of PR interval and QRS complex).

Examples: (A) Sinus rhythm with PAC. (B) Sinus rhythm with a nonconducted PAC.

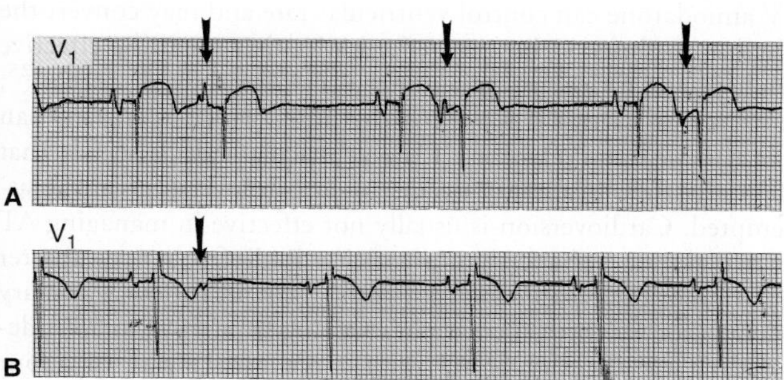

Treatment of PACs is rarely necessary because they do not cause hemodynamic compromise. If they result in symptoms such as "skipped beats" that are bothersome, the patient should be advised to avoid precipitating factors such as smoking, alcohol intake, and coffee consumption. Frequent PACs may precede more serious arrhythmias such as AF and can initiate SVT, especially AV nodal reentry or tachycardias associated with accessory pathways. Drugs such as β-blockers; or type IA, IB, or III antiarrhythmics can be used to suppress atrial activity if necessary.

Wandering Atrial Pacemaker (WAP)

WAP refers to rhythms that exhibit varying P-wave morphology as the site of impulse formation shifts from the SA node to various sites in the atria to the AV junction and back.[18] This arrhythmia occurs when two (usually sinus and junctional) or more supraventricular pacemakers compete with each other for control of the heart. Because the rates of these competing pacemakers are almost identical, it is common to have atrial fusion occur as the atria are activated by more than one wave of depolarization at a time, resulting in varying P-wave morphology. WAP can be due to increased vagal tone that slows the sinus pacemaker or due to enhanced automaticity in atrial or junctional pacemaker cells, causing them to compete with the SA node for control.

WAP is characterized as follows:

Rate: 60 to 100 beats per minute

Rhythm: May be slightly irregular

P waves: Exhibit varying shapes (upright, flat, inverted, notched) as impulses originate in different parts of the atria or junction and as atrial fusion occurs. At least three different P-wave configurations should be seen.

PR interval: May vary depending on proximity of the pacemaker to the AV node

QRS complex: Usually normal

Conduction: Conduction through the atria varies as it is depolarized from different spots. Conduction through the bundle branches and ventricles is usually normal.

Example: WAP

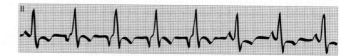

Treatment of WAP is not usually necessary. If the heart rate is slow enough to be symptomatic, atropine can be given.

Multifocal Atrial Tachycardia (MAT)

MAT (also known as chaotic AT) is rapid firing of several ectopic atrial foci at a rate faster than 100 beats per minute. MAT is most commonly seen in elderly patients and is associated with chronic pulmonary disease but can also occur in the presence of HF, hypokalemia, hypomagnesemia, hypoxia, acute MI, and mitral stenosis.[5,18,19] MAT is often misdiagnosed as AF because it shares many of the ECG features of AF.

The ECG characteristics of MAT include the following:

Rate: Usually 100 to 130 beats per minute

Rhythm: Usually irregular

P waves: Vary in shape because they originate in different spots in the atria. At least three different P waves are seen. They usually precede each QRS complex, but some may be blocked in the AV node.

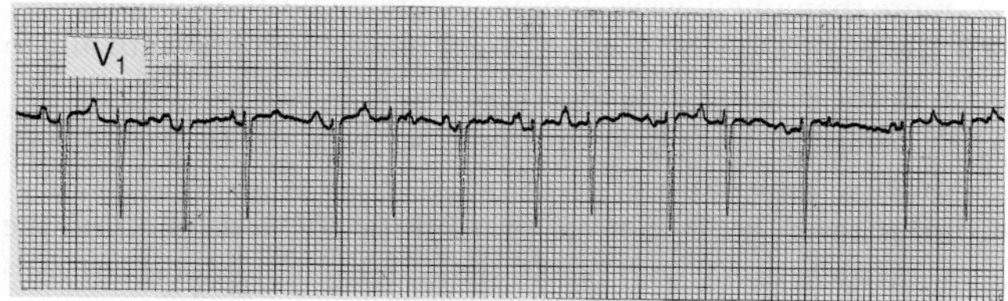

PR interval: May vary depending on proximity of each ectopic atrial focus to the AV node and the prematurity of atrial impulses

QRS complex: Usually normal

Conduction: Usually normal through the AV node and ventricles. Aberrant ventricular conduction may occur if an impulse is conducted into the ventricles while they are partially refractory.

Example: MAT

Treatment of MAT is directed toward eliminating the causes, including hypoxia and electrolyte imbalances. Antiarrhythmic therapy is often ineffective. β-Blockers, verapamil, flecainide, amiodarone, and magnesium have been reported to be successful in the treatment of MAT.[5,18,19] β-Blockers seem to work best but must be used with caution because pulmonary disease is usually associated with MAT. Theophylline may need to be discontinued. If MAT is chronic and unresponsive to drug therapy, radiofrequency ablation of the AV node and insertion of a permanent pacemaker may be necessary to control the ventricular rate.[20]

Atrial Tachycardia (AT)

AT is a rapid atrial rhythm at a rate of 100 to 250 beats per minute that arises from a single site within the right or left atrium. This rhythm may be due to rapid firing of an ectopic atrial focus (automaticity), an atrial microreentry circuit that allows an impulse to travel rapidly and repeatedly around a pathway in the atria, or to afterdepolarizations resulting in a triggered AT.[20–23] The term *paroxysmal atrial tachycardia* is used to describe AT that begins and ends suddenly and can occur in short bursts of several beats or be sustained for longer periods of time. Incessant AT is less common and lasts for more than half a day, sometimes being present more than 90% of the time.[23] AT has been associated with caffeine, tobacco, alcohol, mitral valve disease, rheumatic heart disease, chronic obstructive pulmonary disease, acute MI, theophylline administration, hypokalemia, and digitalis toxicity.

If the atrial rate is very rapid, the AV node begins to block some of the impulses attempting to travel through it to protect the ventricles from excessively rapid rates. In normal, healthy hearts, the AV node can usually conduct each atrial impulse up to rates of 180 beats per minute or more. In patients with cardiac disease or in those who take drugs that slow AV conduction, the AV node cannot conduct each impulse, and AT with block occurs. The presence of AT with block should arouse suspicion of digitalis toxicity, which must be ruled out.

The ECG characteristics of AT include the following:

Rate: Atrial rate is 100 to 250 beats per minute (quite often in the range of 140 to 180 beats per minute). The ventricular rate depends on the amount of block at the AV node and may be the same as the atrial rate or slower.

Rhythm: Regular unless there is variable block at the AV node

P waves: Differ in configuration from sinus P waves because they are ectopic. Precede each QRS complex and usually appear in the second half of the tachycardia cycle (R-R interval) but may be hidden in the preceding T wave. When block is present, more than one P wave appears before each QRS complex.

PR interval: Usually in the normal range but often difficult to measure because of hidden P waves.

QRS complex: Usually normal but may be wide if aberrant conduction is present

Conduction: Usually normal through the AV node and into the ventricles. In AT with block, some atrial impulses do not conduct into the ventricles. Aberrant ventricular conduction may occur if atrial impulses are conducted into the ventricles while the bundle branches are still partially refractory.

Examples: AT. Both strips are from the same patient. (A) AT at a rate of 187 beats per minute. (B) AT with block, occurring after administration of propranolol.

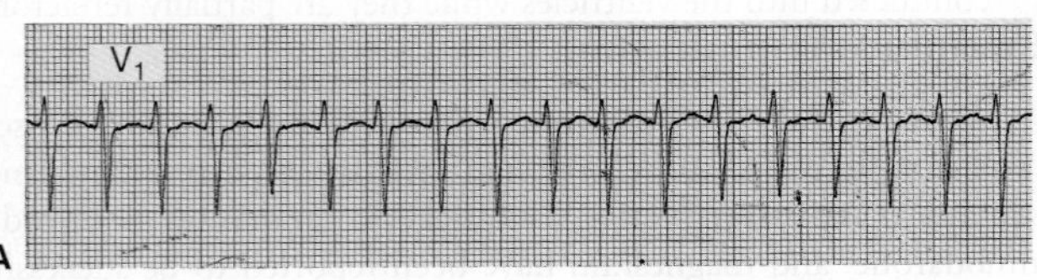

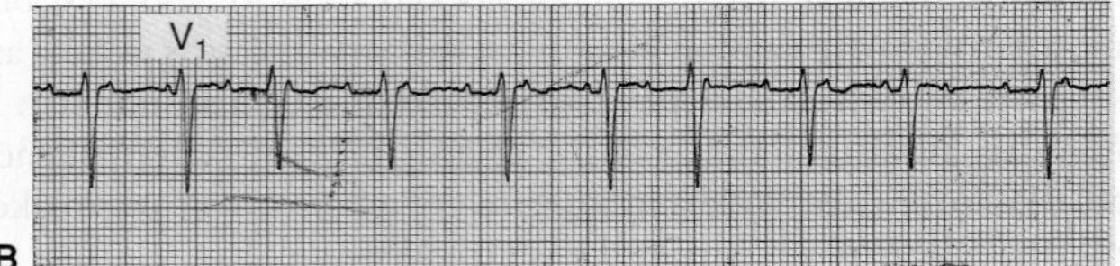

In addition to the potential hemodynamic instability resulting from the rapid ventricular rate, AT, and other SVTs that result in rapid ventricular rates for long periods of time can cause tachycardia-mediated cardiomyopathy.[24] Chronic tachycardia produces complex structural changes and "remodeling" of both the atria and the ventricles. Left ventricular dilation can lead to dilated cardiomyopathy and systolic dysfunction. For this reason, chronic tachycardia needs to be treated to avoid development of cardiomyopathy.

Treatment of AT is directed toward eliminating the cause, decreasing the ventricular rate, and ultimately preventing recurrences of tachycardia. Sedation alone may terminate the rhythm or slow the rate. Vagal stimulation, either through CSM or Valsalva maneuver, or adenosine may terminate some episodes of AT. β-Blockers, verapamil, and diltiazem increase block at the AV node and may slow ventricular response or sometimes terminate the tachycardia. Digitalis slows ventricular rate by increasing block at the AV node, but it can also be the cause of AT with block and should be discontinued if that is the case. If the patient cannot tolerate β-blockers or calcium channel blocker, IV amiodarone can control ventricular rate and may convert the rhythm to sinus. Other antiarrhythmics that might be effective include flecainide, propafenone, procainamide, or sotalol[25]; however, all carry a risk of proarrhythmia, which is greater than the risk with amiodarone. If the ventricular rate is so fast that hemodynamic instability occurs, then cardioversion can be attempted. Cardioversion is usually not effective in managing AT that is due to enhanced automaticity. Radiofrequency catheter ablation of the ectopic focus or reentry circuit is now a primary therapy for AT, with success rates varying from 52% to 98% depending on the site of AT; and a recurrence rate of about 8%.[21,25,26]

Atrial Flutter

Atrial flutter is an organized atrial rhythm in which the atria are depolarized at rates of 250 to 440 times per minute. Classic or typical atrial flutter (type I) is due to a fixed reentry circuit in the right atrium around which the impulse circulates in a counterclockwise direction, resulting in negative flutter waves in leads II and III and an atrial rate between 250 and 350 beats per minute (most commonly 300 beats per minute).[25,27,28] Occasionally, the impulse reverses direction and circulates in a clockwise direction, resulting in positive flutter waves in leads II and III, and is called "atypical" or "reverse typical" flutter.[27,28] Atrial flutter can also result from reentry around surgically created scars within the atria and is still considered to be type I flutter. Less is known about type II flutter, which is more rapid (with atrial rates of 340 to 440 beats per minute), less stable than type I, and more likely to revert to AF.[28,29] About 90% of atrial flutters are considered to be a version of type I flutter.[28]

At such rapid atrial rates, the AV node usually blocks at least half of the impulses to protect the ventricles from excessive rates. Because atrial flutter most often occurs at a rate of 300 beats per minute, and because the AV node usually blocks half of those impulses, a ventricular rate of 150 beats per minute is common. Therefore, whenever a ventricular rate of 150 beats per minute is seen, the diagnosis of atrial flutter with 2:1 conduction should be suspected until proved otherwise. Atrial flutter is seen in left ventricular dysfunction, rheumatic heart disease, mitral valve disease, atherosclerotic heart disease, thyrotoxicosis, HF, cardiac surgery, and myocardial ischemia or MI.[30]

Atrial flutter is characterized on the ECG as follows:

Rate: Atrial rate varies between 250 and 450 beats per minute, most commonly 300 beats per minute. Ventricular rate varies depending on the amount of block at the AV node, most commonly 150 beats per minute and rarely 300 beats per minute. Ventricular rates can be within the normal range when atrial flutter is treated with appropriate drugs. Rarely, 1:1 conduction results in a ventricular rate of 300 beats per minute.

Rhythm: Atrial rhythm is regular. Ventricular rhythm may be regular or irregular because of varying AV block.

P waves: F waves (flutter waves) are seen, characterized by a regular, biphasic sawtooth pattern with no isoelectric segment between waves. One F wave is usually hidden in the QRS complex, and when 2:1 conduction occurs, F waves may not be readily apparent. Flutter waves are best seen in the inferior leads (II, III, and aVF) and may appear more like individual P waves in lead V_1.

PR interval: May be consistent or may vary in a Wenckebach-type pattern.

QRS complex: Usually normal; aberration can occur

Conduction: Usually normal through the AV node and ventricles

Examples: Atrial flutter. All strips are from the same patient. (A) Atrial flutter with 2:1 conduction. (B) Ventricular rate slows momentarily, and flutter waves are clearly visible at a rate of 300 beats per minute. (C) Atrial flutter with variable conduction.

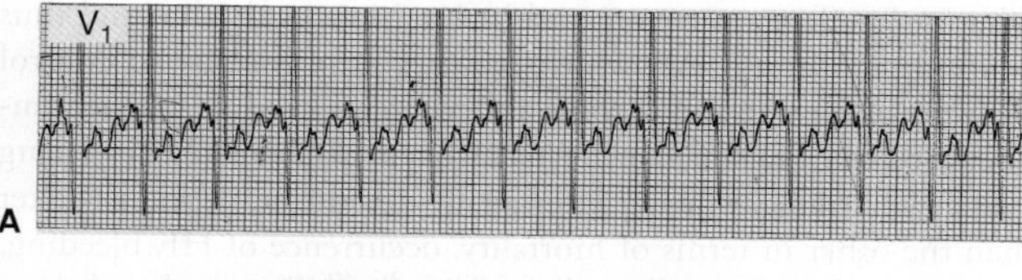

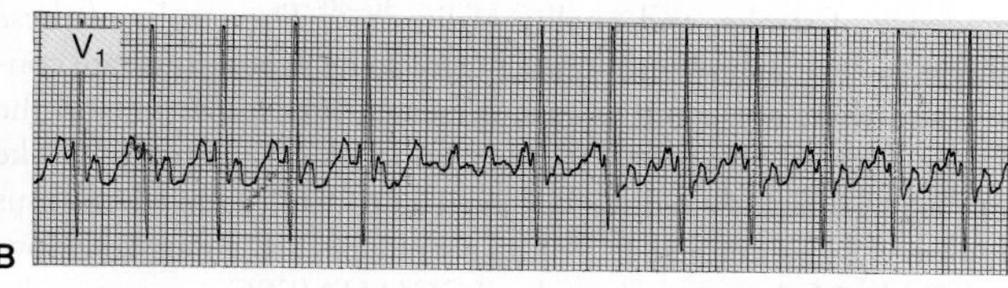

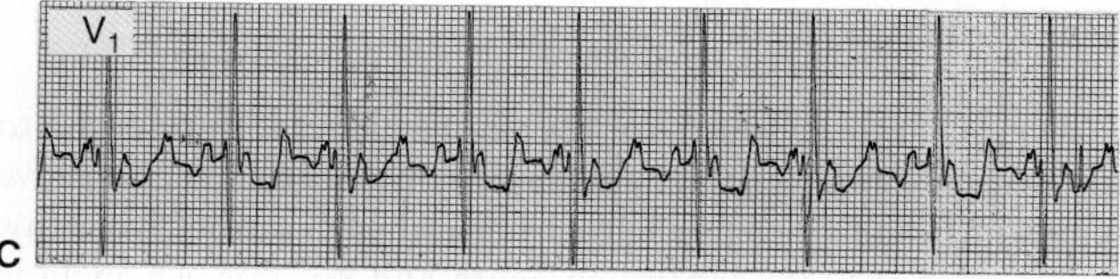

Because the ventricular rate in atrial flutter can be rapid, symptoms associated with decreased cardiac output can occur. Mural thrombi may form in the atria because there is no strong atrial contraction and blood stasis occurs, leading to a risk of systemic or pulmonary emboli. Persistent atrial flutter is uncommon; it usually converts to either sinus rhythm or AF spontaneously or as a result of drug therapy.

The treatment of acute atrial flutter depends on the hemodynamic consequences of the arrhythmia. Ventricular rate control is the immediate goal of therapy if cardiac output is significantly compromised due to rapid ventricular rates. Electrical (direct current) cardioversion may be necessary as an immediate treatment, especially if 1:1 conduction occurs. IV calcium channel blockers (verapamil or diltiazem) or β-blockers can be used for ventricular rate control. If rapid conversion to sinus rhythm is needed, electrical cardioversion is most reliable; overdrive atrial pacing can be attempted if atrial epicardial pacing wires are present following cardiac surgery. Newer type III antiarrhythmic agents, ibutilide (Corvert) and dofetilide (Tikosyn) can be given IV and are often successful in converting atrial flutter to sinus rhythm if flutter is recent in onset. Drug therapy for conversion takes longer than electrical cardioversion and is not recommended in an acute situation.

Class IA (quinidine, disopyramide, and procainamide), type IC (flecainide, propafenone), or type III antiarrhythmics (ibutilide, dofetilide, amiodarone, and sotalol) may convert flutter to sinus rhythm. Some of these agents, especially amiodarone, sotalol, flecainide, and propafenone, are also useful in maintaining sinus rhythm after conversion. Drugs that slow the atrial rate, like class IA or IC drugs, should not be used unless the ventricular rate has been controlled with an AV nodal blocking agent (i.e., calcium channel blocker, β-blocker, or digitalis). The danger of giving class IA or IC agents alone is that, as atrial rate slows from 300 to 200 beats per minute, for example, it is possible for the AV node to conduct each impulse rather than block impulses, thus leading to even faster ventricular rates. Class III antiarrhythmics can prolong the QT interval and result in TdP.

Anticoagulation is needed prior to electrical or chemical cardioversion if atrial flutter has been present for 48 hours or more. Recommendations for anticoagulation are the same for flutter as for AF, and are discussed in the section on atrial fibrillation and in Table 16-3.

Radiofrequency catheter ablation of the flutter reentry circuit has become the treatment of choice for chronic or recurrent atrial flutter and is an alternative to chronic drug therapy.[31] See Chapter 18 for more information on the use of radiofrequency ablation for arrhythmia management.

Atrial Fibrillation

AF is an extremely rapid and disorganized pattern of depolarization in the atria. Several mechanisms for AF have been proposed: (1) Rapid firing of ectopic impulses in the atria, (2) single reentry circuit with variable rate and conduction in the atria or pulmonary veins, and (3) multiple reentry circuits within the atria.[32–34] AF occurs in the presence of atherosclerotic or rheumatic heart disease, thyrotoxicosis, HF, cardiomyopathy, valve disease, pulmonary disease, MI, congenital heart disease, with electrolyte imbalances, and after cardiac surgery.

AF is the most common arrhythmia seen in clinical practice and occurs more frequently with aging. AF is typically classified according to the "three Ps" as follows.[5,32–35]: *Paroxysmal* refers to AF that starts and stops spontaneously, terminating spontaneously in sinus rhythm in less than 7 days. Episodes can last for minutes to hours or days and can recur with varying frequency among individuals. *Persistent* refers to AF that fails to convert spontaneously within 7 days. It can be terminated medically, either by electrical or chemical cardioversion. *Permanent* refers to AF that is present longer than 1 year and cardioversion has either not been attempted or has failed to restore or maintain sinus rhythm. Patients may start out with paroxysmal AF that then becomes persistent or permanent. The term *lone AF* applies to people younger than 60 years who develop AF without any evidence of structural heart disease, pulmonary disease, or hypertension.[34,35] These people are at low risk for thromboembolism and generally have a good prognosis but may be at risk for developing tachycardia-mediated cardiomyopathy.

AF is characterized on the ECG as follows:

Rate: Atrial rate is 400 to 600 beats per minute or faster. Ventricular rate varies depending on the amount of block at the AV node. In new-onset AF, the ventricular response is usually rapid, 110 to 160 beats per minute; in treated AF, the ventricular rate is controlled in the normal range of 60 to 100 beats per minute.

Rhythm: Irregular. One of the distinguishing features of AF is the marked irregularity of the ventricular response because of concealed conduction in the AV junction. If the ventricular response is ever regular in the presence of AF, AV dissociation should be suspected.

P waves: Not present. Atrial activity is chaotic, with no formed atrial impulses visible. Irregular F waves are often seen and vary in size from coarse to very fine.

PR interval: Not measurable because there are no P waves

QRS complex: Usually normal; aberration is common, especially at faster ventricular rates

Conduction: Intra-atrial conduction is disorganized and irregular. Most of the atrial impulses are blocked in the AV junction; those impulses that are conducted through the AV junction are usually conducted normally through the ventricles. If an atrial impulse reaches the bundle-branch system during its refractory period, aberrant intraventricular conduction can occur.

Examples: (A) AF. (B) Alternating coarse and fine AF (sometimes called *atrial fib-flutter*). (C) Fine AF. (D) AF with a slow and regular ventricular response, most likely due to complete AV block.

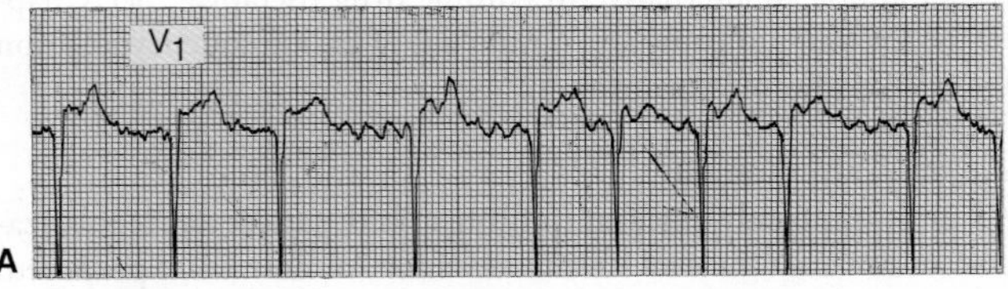

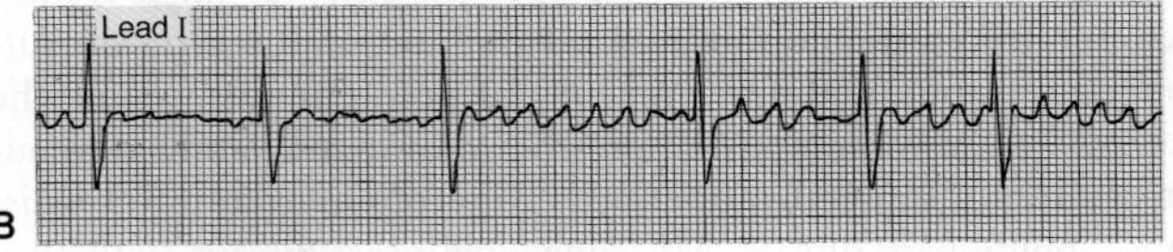

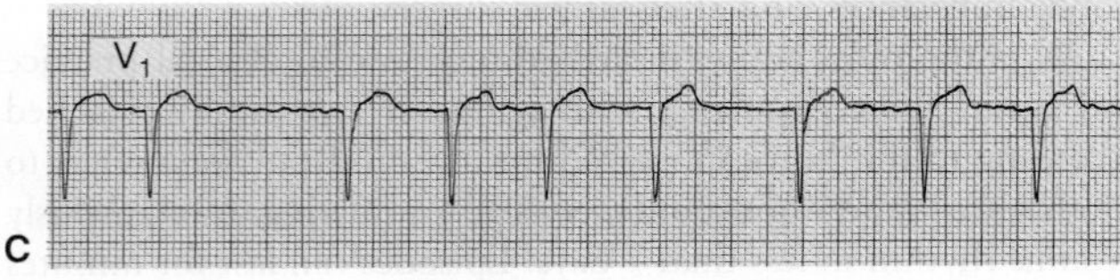

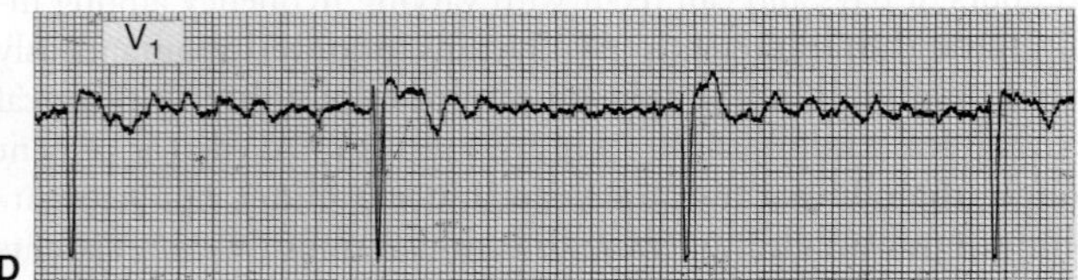

If the ventricular response to AF is rapid, cardiac output can be reduced secondary to decreased diastolic filling time in the ventricles; and coronary blood flow can be impaired because of decreased diastolic coronary perfusion time. Because the atria quiver rather than contract, atrial kick is lost, which can also reduce cardiac output. Another possible complication is mural thrombus formation in the atria due to stasis of blood, leading to pulmonary or systemic embolization if clots dislodge spontaneously or with conversion to sinus rhythm. Any tachyarrhythmia that is sustained for long periods of time can lead to tachycardia-mediated (or tachycardia induced) cardiomyopathy with ventricular dilation and reduced LV function. The mechanism of this cardiomyopathy is not well understood, but improvement in left ventricular function is seen with ventricular rate control or restoration of sinus rhythm.[24]

Treatment of AF is directed toward eliminating the cause, controlling ventricular rate, restoring and maintaining sinus rhythm if possible, and preventing thromboembolism. Emergent or urgent electrical cardioversion may be necessary if the patient is hemodynamically unstable because of a rapid ventricular rate. Cardioversion is more likely to be successful if AF has been present for less than 24 hours.

Two management strategies are available for patients in AF: rate control or rhythm control. Rate control means that ventricular rate is controlled with drug therapy with no intent to restore sinus rhythm. Rhythm control means that treatment is aimed at restoring and maintaining sinus rhythm. Traditionally it has been thought that restoration of sinus rhythm would result in better outcomes because atrial kick would be restored, hemodynamics would improve, the incidence of stroke and of bleeding would be reduced, and quality of life would be better. Many patients are refractory to efforts to restore and maintain sinus rhythm and thus continue in chronic AF, which requires drug therapy to control the ventricular rate and chronic anticoagulation to prevent thromboembolism. Several studies have been performed comparing these two strategies in an attempt to determine if one is better than the other in terms of mortality, occurrence of HF, bleeding, incidence of stroke, and quality of life.[36–40] The results of these studies have not shown rhythm control to be superior to rate control, and there is a trend toward increased hospitalizations in the rhythm control group.[36,38,39] In addition, the incidence of stroke was not significantly reduced by rhythm control, even when sinus rhythm was maintained.[37–39] These strategies are discussed below, and Table 16-3 summarizes the ACC/AHA/ESC recommendations for therapy of AF.[34]

Rate Control. Control of the ventricular rate in response to AF is important to prevent hemocynamic instability, improve symptoms, and prevent tachycardia induced cardiomyopathy. Drugs used for rate control in acute and chronic AF include β-blockers and the nondihydropyridine calcium channel blockers (verapamil, diltiazem), or digoxin if the patient also has HF. For acute ventricular rate control in the absence of preexcitation via an accessory pathway, IV administration of a β-blocker (esmolol, metoprolol, or propranolol) or a calcium channel blocker (verapamil or diltiazem) is indicated. IV digoxin or amiodarone can be used for acute rate control in patients who have HF. Chronic therapy for rate control can include β-blockers, nondihydropyridine calcium channel blockers, digoxin, and amiodarone alone or in combination. Side effects associated with all these rate-control drugs include bradycardia and AV block. β-Blockers and calcium channel blockers can decrease contractility, although β-blockers are indicated in the treatment of HF for a variety of reasons. Amiodarone has little negative inotropic effect, and digoxin increases contractility; both can be safely used in patients with HF. Amiodarone may restore sinus rhythm as well, but it can also be proarrhythmic in some patients.

Radiofrequency ablation of the AV node with insertion of a ventricular pacemaker can be used in patients who are refractory to or intolerant of drug therapy. In this case, AF continues but AV node ablation causes complete heart block and prevents the atrial impulses from reaching the ventricles, thus, the need for a ventricular pacemaker. Ablation of the accessory pathway in patients with WPW syndrome who develop AF is often necessary to prevent an extremely rapid ventricular rate when AF conducts to the ventricle via the accessory pathway.

Rhythm Control. Restoration of sinus rhythm should improve hemodynamics, relieve symptoms associated with AF, and was previously thought to prevent embolization. Until recently, medical therapy for AF was aimed at restoring and maintaining sinus rhythm using aggressive drug therapy and repeated electrical cardioversions. The expected advantages of rhythm control were not confirmed in trials comparing rate control to rhythm control,[37,38] and currently there is a general preference for rate control unless it is a first episode of AF, or the patient prefers rhythm control or remains very symptomatic with rate control.

Elective cardioversion can be performed in patients for whom rhythm control is considered the therapy of choice, in patients who are intolerant of drug therapy, or in whom drug therapy has been unsuccessful. Cardioversion to sinus rhythm can be done pharmacologically or electrically. The ACC/AHA guidelines recommend the following drugs for pharmacological cardioversion: flecainide, dofetilide, propafenone, ibutilide, or amiodarone.[34] The use of class IC antiarrhythmics (flecainide, propafenone) is not recommended in patients with acute MI. In patients with HF, amiodarone and dofetilide are recommended to maintain sinus rhythm. Hospitalization is recommended for patients started on antiarrhythmic drug therapy for restoration or maintenance of sinus rhythm due to a 10% to 15% incidence of adverse cardiac events during initiation of therapy.[41] The side effects of greatest concern are bradycardia and proarrhythmia due to QT interval prolongation.

Nonpharmacologic therapies used for the treatment of AF include implantable atrial defibrillators and radiofrequency catheter ablation. Atrial defibrillators detect the onset of AF and deliver a shock between two intracardiac leads to terminate AF.[42] Ablation to create linear lesions within the atria (similar to the surgical Maze procedure) has been reported to be successful, as well as focal ablations around the orifice of the pulmonary veins in the left atrium to isolate the pulmonary veins form the left atrium.[43,44] See Chapter 18 for more on the use of ablation in managing arrhythmias. A new procedure called PLAATO (percutaneous left atrial appendage transcatheter occlusion) is being used in an effort to prevent embolic stroke in patients with nonrheumatic AF.[45] The PLAATO procedure is performed in a cardiac catheterization laboratory by way of a right heart catheterization and transseptal puncture to place an occluder device into the left atrial appendage to seal it off and prevent embolization of clots that tend to form in the appendage.

Anticoagulation. Anticoagulation is needed prior to electrical or chemical cardioversion in patients who have been in atrial flutter or fibrillation longer than 48 hours due to the risk of embolization when sinus rhythm is restored and the atria begin contracting again. If the duration of fibrillation is not known or is known to be greater than 48 hours, anticoagulation with warfarin to an International Normalized Ratio between 2 and 3 (target is 2.5) for at least 3 weeks should be done prior to electrical or chemical cardioversion and continued for another 4 weeks. If immediate cardioversion due to hemodynamic instability is needed and the duration of flutter is more than 48 hours, a transesophageal echocardiography should be performed to determine if clots are present in the atria. Unfractionated heparin should be given concurrently with cardioversion (unless contraindicated) to keep the activated partial thromboplastin time at 1.5 to 2 times control. Heparin should be continued until oral anticoagulation results in International Normalized Ratio of 2 to 3; and oral anticoagulation should be continued for at least 4 weeks.[34]

Supraventricular Tachycardia

The term SVT could be applied to any rhythm at a rate faster than 100 beats per minute that originates above the ventricle. Technically, sinus tachycardia, AT, atrial flutter, AF, junctional tachycardia, AVNRT, and CMT utilizing an accessory pathway in WPW syndrome can all be called SVT. The other commonly used term to describe the reentrant tachycardia associated with WPW is AV reciprocating (or reentrant) tachycardia; in this chapter the term CMT is used to avoid confusion between the terms AVNRT and AV reciprocating (or reentrant) tachycardia. If the type of tachycardia is clear from the ECG, then it should be called by its appropriate name and the term SVT should be reserved for regular, narrow QRS tachycardias in which the exact mechanism cannot be identified from the ECG. For example, rhythms like sinus tachycardia, atrial flutter, AF, and some ATs are easily recognized by seeing atrial activity that is characteristic of the rhythm on the ECG. However, some ATs, AVNRT, and CMT often appear as regular narrow QRS tachycardias in which atrial activity cannot be seen, making identification of the correct mechanism difficult or impossible from the ECG. Thus, the term SVT is an umbrella term for rhythms that originate above the ventricle (resulting in a narrow QRS complex) but whose exact mechanism cannot be determined from the surface ECG.

SVT is characterized on the ECG by the following:

Rate: Greater than 100 beats per minute; can be as fast as 280 beats per minute

Rhythm: Regular

P waves: Usually not visible, making the exact mechanism of the tachycardia uncertain

PR interval: Not measurable if P waves cannot be seen

QRS complex: Usually narrow; may be wide if aberrant ventricular conduction occurs

Conduction: Conduction through the atria varies depending on the mechanism of tachycardia. Atria may depolarize in a retrograde direction when the mechanism is AVNRT or CMT. Conduction through ventricles is normal unless bundle-branch block is present or there is anterograde conduction through an accessory pathway.

Examples: Two examples of SVT. (A) SVT at a rate of 187, found to be AVNRT during electrophysiology study. (B) Narrow QRS tachycardia at a rate of 187, mechanism is unknown.

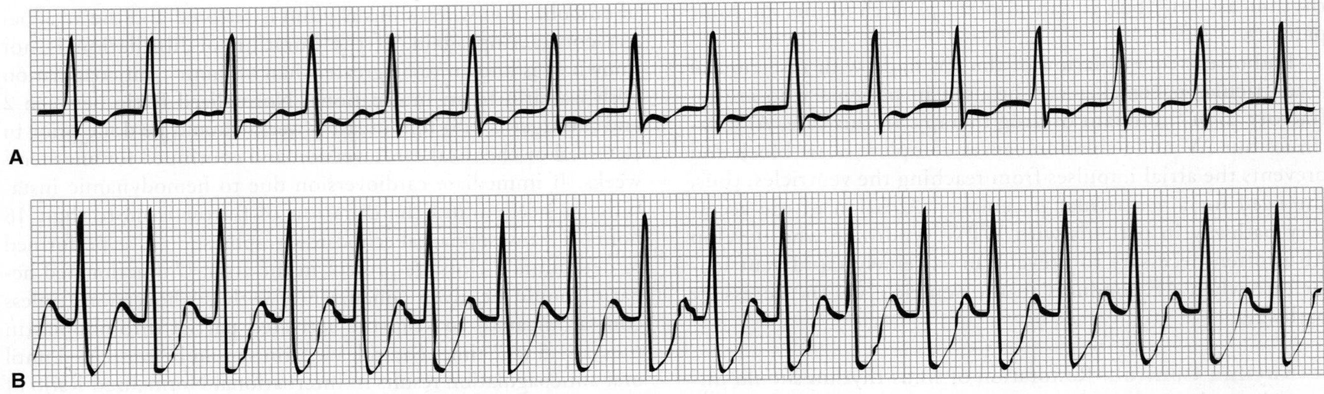

Examples of SVT

Treatment of SVT depends on the patient's tolerance of the arrhythmia. If the ventricular rate is fast enough to cause hemodynamic instability, cardioversion is the treatment of choice. Drugs such as adenosine, β-blockers, or calcium channel blockers (verapamil and diltiazem), can slow the ventricular rate or terminate many SVTs. (See section titled "Complex Arrhythmias and Conduction Disturbances" for more detailed information on SVT.)

Rhythms Originating in the AV Junction

Cells surrounding the AV node in the AV junctional area have automaticity and are capable of initiating impulses and controlling the heart rhythm. Junctional arrhythmias include premature junctional complex (PJC), junctional rhythm, and junctional tachycardia.

Junctional beats and junctional rhythms can appear any of three ways on the ECG depending on the location of the junctional pacemaker and the speed of conduction of the impulse into the atria and ventricles:

1. When a junctional focus fires, the wave of depolarization spreads backward (retrograde) into the atria as well as forward (anterograde) into the ventricles. If the impulse arrives in the atria before it arrives in the ventricles, the ECG shows a P wave (inverted in inferior leads because the atria are depolarized from bottom to top) followed immediately by a QRS complex as the impulse reaches the ventricles. In this case, the PR interval is short, usually 0.10 second or less.
2. If the junctional impulse reaches both the atria and the ventricles at the same time, only a QRS is seen on the ECG because the ventricles are much larger than the atria, and only ventricular depolarization is seen, even though the atria are also depolarizing.
3. If the junctional impulse reaches the ventricles before it reaches the atria, the QRS precedes the P wave on the ECG. Again, the P wave is inverted in inferior leads because of retrograde atrial depolarization, and the RP interval (distance from the beginning of the QRS to the beginning of the following P wave) is short, 0.10 second or less.

Premature Junctional Complexes

PJCs are due to an irritable focus in the AV junction. Irritability can be due to coronary artery disease or MI disrupting blood flow to the AV junction, nicotine, caffeine, catecholamines, or drugs such as digitalis.

PJCs have the following ECG characteristics:

Rate: 60 to 100 beats per minute or the rate of the basic rhythm
Rhythm: Irregular because of the early beats
P waves: May occur before, during, or after the QRS complex and are inverted in the inferior leads (II, III, aVF)
PR interval: Short, 0.10 second or less when P waves precede the QRS
QRS complex: Usually normal but may be aberrant if the PJC occurs very early and conducts into the ventricles during the refractory period of a bundle branch
Conduction: Retrograde through the atria, usually normal through the ventricles
Example: Sinus rhythm with two PJCs

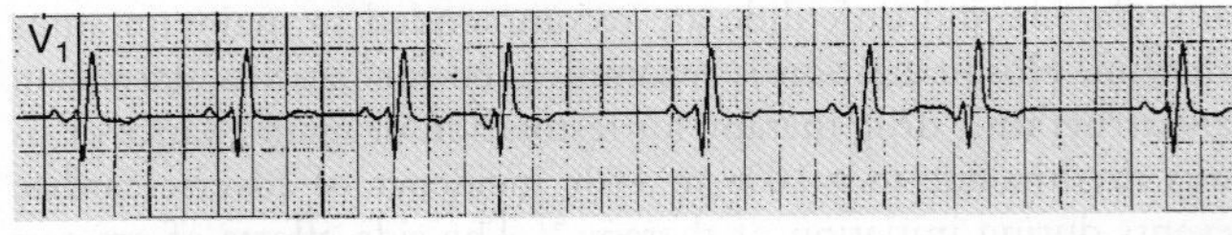

No treatment is necessary for PJC.

Junctional Rhythm and Junctional Tachycardia

Junctional rhythm can occur if the SA node rate falls below the automatic rate of an AV junctional pacemaker, or in the presence of digitalis toxicity. Junctional rhythms commonly occur after inferior wall MI because the blood supply to the SA node and the AV junction is disrupted, and junctional tachycardia is common in children undergoing surgical repair of congenital defects. The rhythms are classified according to their rate; junctional rhythm usually occurs at a rate of 40 to 60 beats per minute, accelerated junctional rhythm occurs at a rate of 60 to 100 beats per minute, and junctional tachycardia occurs at a rate of 100 to 250 beats per minute. In adults, junctional rhythms are usually seen as escape rhythms as a result of sinus bradycardia or AV block; junctional tachycardia is rare and when it occurs digitalis toxicity should be ruled out.

Junctional rhythm has the following ECG characteristics:

Rate: Usually 40 to 60 beats per minute; accelerated junctional rhythm, 60 to 100 beats per minute; junctional tachycardia, 100 to 250 beats per minute

Rhythm: Regular
P waves: May precede or follow QRS
PR interval: Short, 0.10 second or less
QRS complex: Usually normal
Conduction: Retrograde through the atria, normal through the ventricles
Examples: (A) Junctional rhythm (rate, 43 beats per minute). (B) Accelerated junctional rhythm (rate, 84 beats per minute).

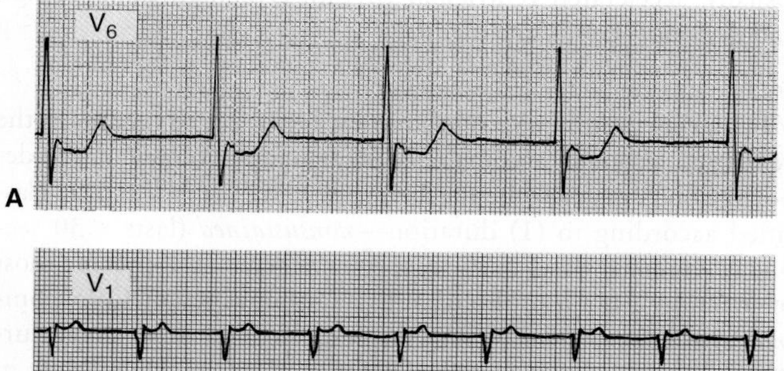

Junctional rhythm rarely requires treatment unless the rate is too slow or too fast to maintain cardiac output. If the rate is slow, atropine can be given to increase the sinus rate and override the junctional focus or increase the rate of firing of the junctional pacemaker. If the rate is fast, drugs such as verapamil, β-blockers, propafenone, flecainide, and amiodarone may be effective in slowing the rate or terminating the arrhythmia. Cardioversion may be necessary if the rate is so rapid that cardiac output is severely limited. Because digitalis toxicity is a common cause of junctional rhythms, the drug should be held until serum levels return to normal and the arrhythmia stops.

Rhythms Originating in the Ventricles

Ventricular arrhythmias originate in the ventricular muscle or Purkinje system and are considered to be more dangerous than other arrhythmias because of their potential to limit cardiac output severely. However, as with any arrhythmia, ventricular rate is a key determinant of how well a patient can tolerate a ventricular rhythm. Ventricular arrhythmias include premature ventricular complex (PVC), accelerated ventricular rhythm, VT, ventricular flutter, ventricular fibrillation (VF), and ventricular asystole. See Chapter 27 for the ACLS algorithm for treatment of VF and pulseless VT and Table 16-5 for guidelines for management of ventricular arrhythmias.

Premature Ventricular Complexes

PVCs (ventricular premature depolarizations) are caused by premature depolarization of cells in the ventricular myocardium or Purkinje system due to enhanced normal automaticity or abnormal automaticity, reentry in the ventricles, or afterdepolarizations.[5,46] PVCs can be caused by hypoxia, myocardial ischemia, hypokalemia, acidosis, exercise, increased levels of circulating catecholamines, digitalis toxicity, caffeine, alcohol, and other causes. PVCs increase with aging and are more common in people with coronary heart disease, valve disease, hypertension, cardiomyopathy, and other forms of heart disease. PVCs are not dangerous in people with normal hearts but are associated with higher mortality rates in patients with structural heart disease or acute MI, especially if left ventricular function is reduced. PVCs are considered potentially malignant when they occur more frequently than 10 per hour or are repetitive (i.e., occur in pairs, triplets, or more than three in a row) in patients with coronary disease, previous MI, cardiomyopathy, and with reduced ejection fraction.[47,48]

PVCs have the following ECG characteristics:

Rate: 60 to 100 beats per minute or the rate of the basic rhythm
Rhythm: Irregular because of the early beats
P waves: Not related to the PVC. Sinus rhythm is often not interrupted, so sinus P waves can frequently be seen occurring regularly throughout the rhythm. P waves may follow a PVC because of retrograde conduction from the ventricle backward through the atria; these P waves are inverted in the inferior leads (II, III, aVF).
PR interval: Not present before most PVC. If a P wave happens, by coincidence, to precede a PVC, the PR interval is short.
QRS complex: Wide and bizarre, usually greater than 0.12 second in duration. May vary in morphology if PVCs originate from more than one focus in the ventricles. T waves are usually in the opposite direction from the QRS complex.
Conduction: Impulses originating in the ventricles conduct through the ventricular myocardium from muscle cell to muscle cell rather than through Purkinje fibers, resulting in wide QRS complexes. Some PVCs may conduct retrograde into the atria, resulting in inverted P waves that follow the PVC.

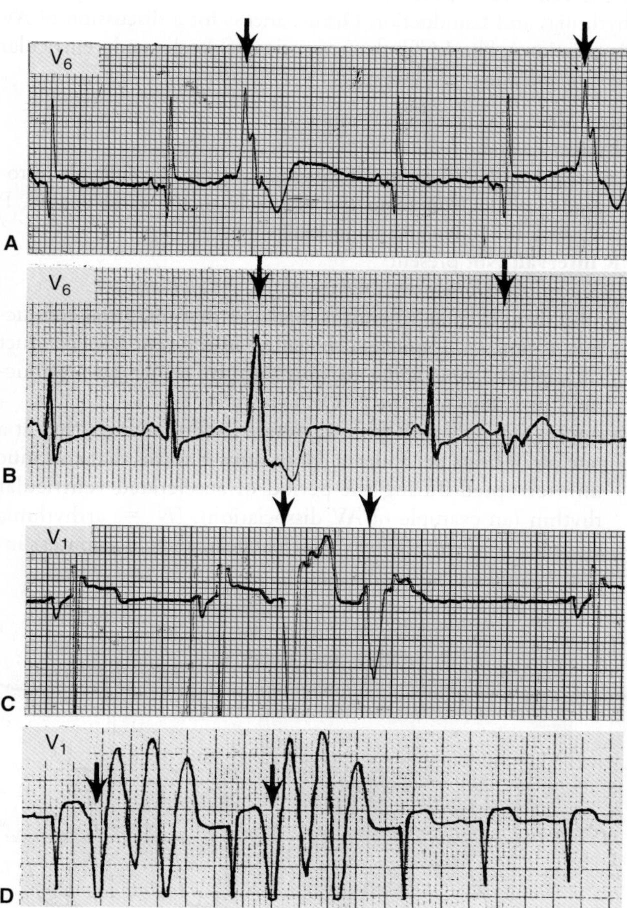

Examples of PVCs

When the sinus rhythm is undisturbed by PVCs, the atria depolarize normally.

Examples: (A) Normal sinus rhythm with a PVC. (B) Sinus rhythm with multifocal PVC. (C) Paired PVC. (D) R-on-T PVC, resulting in short runs of VT.

The significance of PVCs depends on the clinical setting in which they occur. Many people have chronic PVCs that do not need to be treated, and most of these people are asymptomatic. There is no evidence that suppression of PVCs reduces mortality, especially in patients with no structural heart disease. If PVCs cause bothersome palpitations, patients should be told to avoid caffeine, tobacco, other stimulants, and try stress reduction techniques. Low-dose β-blockers may reduce PVC frequency and the perception of palpitations and can be used for symptom relief. In the setting of an acute MI or myocardial ischemia, PVCs may be precursors of more dangerous ventricular arrhythmias, especially when they occur near the apex of the T wave (R-on-T PVC). Prophylactic treatment of asymptomatic nonsustained ventricular arrhythmias is not recommended.[49]

Accelerated Idioventricular Rhythm

Accelerated idioventricular rhythm occurs when an ectopic focus in the ventricles fires at a rate of 50 to 100 beats per minute. Accelerated idioventricular rhythm commonly occurs in the presence of inferior MI and during reperfusion with thrombolytic therapy, when the rate of the SA node slows below the rate of the latent ventricular pacemaker. (See section titled "Complex Arrhythmias and Conduction Disturbances" for a discussion of AV dissociation.) The ECG characteristics of accelerated ventricular rhythm include the following:

Rate: 50 to 100 beats per minute
Rhythm: Usually regular
P waves: May be seen but are dissociated from the QRS. If retrograde conduction from the ventricle to the atria occurs, P waves follow the QRS complex.
PR interval: Not present
QRS complex: Wide and bizarre
Conduction: If sinus rhythm is the basic rhythm, atrial conduction is normal. Impulses originating in the ventricles conduct through the ventricular myocardium by cell-to-cell conduction, resulting in the wide QRS complex.
Example: Sinus rhythm with accelerated ventricular rhythm at a rate of 70 beats per minute. Note sinus P waves that continue uninterrupted during the period of accelerated ventricular rhythm (an example of AV dissociation). (*N* = arrhythmia computer's interpretation of normal beat, *V* = computer's interpretation of ventricular beat.)

The treatment of accelerated ventricular rhythm depends on its cause and how well it is tolerated by the patient. This arrhythmia alone is usually not harmful because the ventricular rate is within normal limits and usually adequate to maintain cardiac output. If the patient is symptomatic because of the loss of atrial kick during long episodes of AV dissociation, atropine can be used to increase the rate of the SA node and overdrive the ventricular rhythm. Suppressive therapy is rarely used because abolishing the ventricular rhythm may leave an even less desirable heart rate. Usually, accelerated ventricular rhythm is transient and benign and does not require treatment.

Ventricular Tachycardia

VT is a rapid ventricular rhythm most likely due to reentry in the ventricles, although automaticity of an ectopic focus and afterdepolarizations may also be mechanisms of VT.[5,22] VT can be classified according to (1) duration—*nonsustained* (lasts <30 seconds), *sustained* (lasts >30 seconds), *incessant* (VT present most of the time); (2) morphology (ECG appearance of QRS complexes)—*monomorphic* (QRS complexes have the same shape during tachycardia), *polymorphic* (QRS complexes vary randomly in shape), *bidirectional* (alternating upright and negative QRS complexes during tachycardia). The terms *salvos* and *bursts* are often used to describe short runs of VT (i.e., 5 to 10 or more beats in a row). See section titled "Complex Arrhythmias and Conduction Disturbances" later in this chapter for more information on monomorphic and PVT.

The most common cause of VT is CHD, including acute ischemia and MI, prior MI, and chronic coronary disease. The next most common cause is cardiomyopathy, both dilated and hypertrophic. Other causes include valvular heart disease, congenital heart disease, arrhythmogenic right ventricular dysplasia, inherited ion channel abnormalities, cardiac surgery, and the proarrhythmic effects of many drugs.[22,48,50,51] VT that occurs in the presence of left ventricular dysfunction and reduced ejection fraction is associated with a higher incidence of adverse cardiac events, including an increased risk of SCD.

Idiopathic VT is VT that occurs in patients with no known structural heart disease.[22,48,52] This type of VT is discussed in more detail later in the section titled "Complex Arrhythmias and Conduction Disturbances".

ECG characteristics of monomorphic VT include the following:

Rate: Ventricular rate is usually 100 to 220 beats per minute
Rhythm: Usually regular but may be slightly irregular
P waves: Often dissociated from QRS complexes. If sinus rhythm is the underlying basic rhythm, regular P waves may be seen but are not related to QRS complexes. P waves are often buried

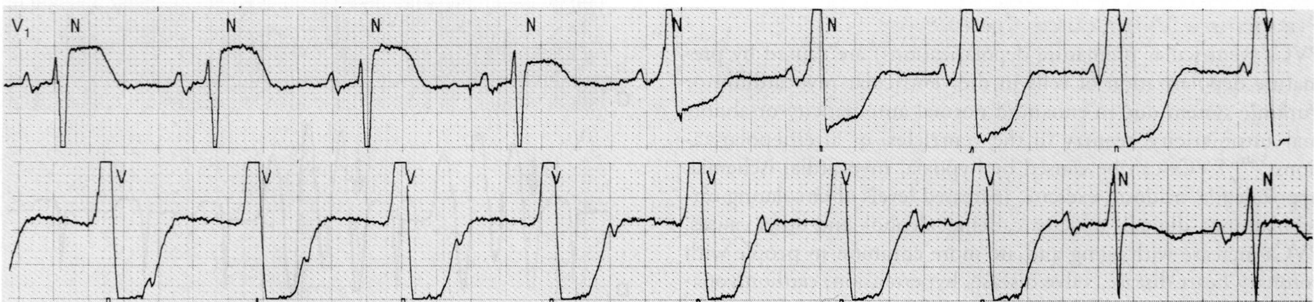

Example of accelerated ventricular rhythm

in QRS complexes or T waves. VT may conduct retrograde to the atria with P waves visible after each QRS.

PR interval: Not measurable because of dissociation of P waves from QRS complexes

QRS complex: Wide and bizarre, greater than 0.12 second in duration

Conduction: Impulse originates in one ventricle and spreads by muscle cell-to-cell conduction through both ventricles. There may be retrograde conduction through the atria, but often the SA node continues to fire regularly and depolarizes the atria normally. Rarely, one of these sinus impulses may conduct normally through the AV node and into the ventricle before the next ectopic ventricular impulse fires, resulting in a normal QRS complex, called a *capture beat.* Occasionally, a *fusion beat* may occur as the ventricles are depolarized by a descending sinus impulse and the ventricular ectopic impulse simultaneously, resulting in a QRS complex that looks different from both the normal beats and the ventricular beats.

Examples: (A) Sinus rhythm with a PVC and a run of monomorphic VT. (B) AV dissociation is evidenced by independently occurring P waves. (C) VT with a fusion beat (fourth complex).

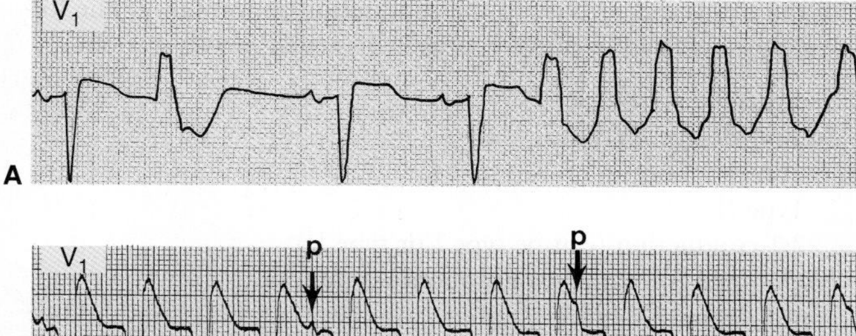

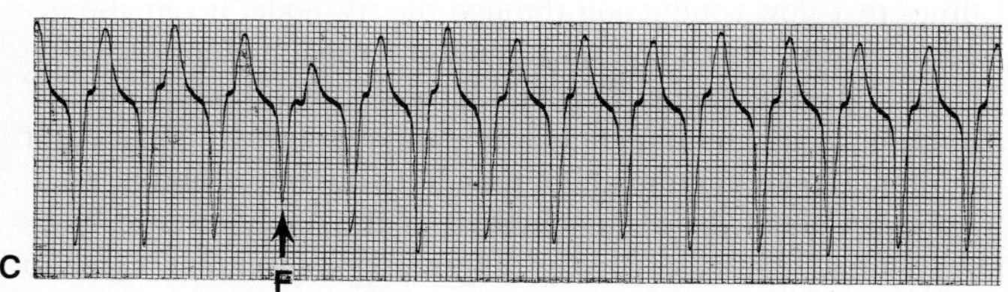

Immediate treatment of VT depends on how well the rhythm is tolerated by the patient. The two main determinants of patient tolerance of any tachycardia are ventricular rate and underlying left ventricular function. VT can be an emergency if cardiac output is severely decreased because of a very rapid rate or poor left ventricular function. Defibrillation is the immediate treatment of pulseless VT. Synchronized electrical cardioversion is the immediate treatment for hemodynamically unstable VT with a pulse present. In stable VT with a pulse, the ACLS recommendation for treatment is administration of amiodarone.[53] See Chapter 27 for the ACLS algorithm for treatment of VT. The ACC/AHA/ESC practice guidelines for managing ventricular arrhythmias recommends procainamide as initial drug treatment of stable sustained VT, and amiodarone for hemodynamically unstable VT or VT that is refractory to cardioversion or recurrent despite procainamide.[49] Lidocaine is reasonable for the initial treatment of stable sustained monomorphic VT associated with acute myocardial ischemia or infarction.[49]

Long-term drug therapy for ventricular arrhythmias includes β-blockers because they are effective in suppressing ventricular arrhythmias and reducing SCD in patients post-MI, those with HF, and cardiomyopathy. Amiodarone and sotalol are effective in suppressing ventricular arrhythmias but most studies show no long-term survival benefit. Nonpharmacologic therapy for recurrent VT includes radiofrequency catheter ablation and the implantable cardioverter defibrillator (ICD) (see Chapters 18 and 28).

Ventricular Flutter

Ventricular flutter is similar to VT, but the rate is faster. Hemodynamically, ventricular flutter is more dangerous because there is virtually no cardiac output. ECG characteristics of ventricular flutter are as follows:

Rate: Ventricular rate is usually 220 to 400 beats per minute
Rhythm: Usually regular
P waves: None seen
PR interval: None measurable
QRS complex: Very wide, regular, sine-wave type of pattern
Conduction: Originates in the ventricle and spreads through muscle cell-to-cell conduction, resulting in very wide, bizarre complexes
Example: Ventricular flutter

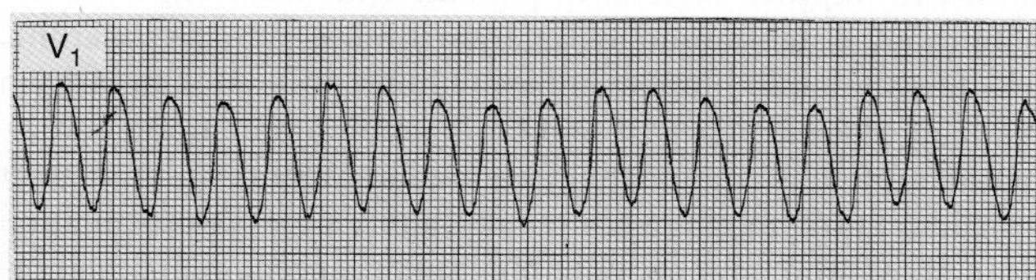

Ventricular flutter is fatal unless treated immediately by defibrillation. If a defibrillator is not immediately available, cardiopulmonary resuscitation (CPR) should be started. After the rhythm is converted, antiarrhythmic drug therapy should be initiated to prevent recurrence. Drug therapy is similar to that used for VT.

Ventricular Fibrillation

VF is rapid, ineffective quivering of the ventricles; is fatal without immediate treatment; and is the most frequent cause of SCD. Electrical activity originates in the ventricles and spreads in a chaotic, irregular pattern throughout both ventricles. There is no cardiac output or palpable pulse with VF. ECG characteristics of VF include the following:

Rate: Rapid, uncoordinated, ineffective
Rhythm: Chaotic, irregular
P waves: None seen
PR interval: None
QRS complex: No formed QRS complexes seen; rapid, irregular undulations without any specific pattern. This erratic electrical activity can be coarse or fine.
Conduction: Random electrical activity in ventricles depolarizes them irregularly and without any organized pattern. There is no organized conduction and the ventricles do not contract.
Examples: Two examples of VF

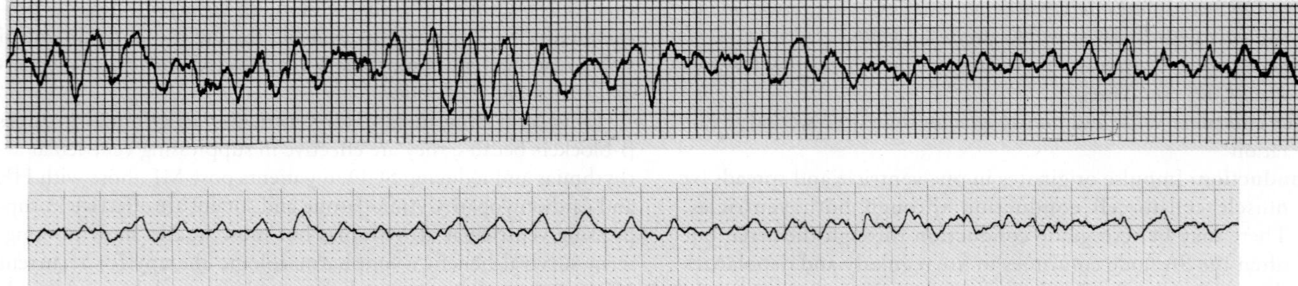

VF requires immediate defibrillation. Synchronized cardioversion is not possible because there are no formed QRS complexes on which to synchronize the shock. CPR must be performed if a defibrillator is not immediately available. The American Heart Association guidelines for VF and pulseless VT call for CPR until a defibrillator is available, then immediate defibrillation using and automatic external defibrillator; or manual defibrillation with 360 J if using a monophasic defibrillator or device-specific energy recommendation (200 J if this is not known) if using a biphasic defibrillator.[53] Immediate CPR for 2 minutes is recommended following the first shock. See Chapter 27 for more information on management of cardiac arrest.

Amiodarone is the drug recommended for antiarrhythmic therapy in VF following defibrillation. Lidocaine is an alternative (but not the preferred drug) according to the ACLS manual and is still used clinically in many hospitals. Drugs have not been shown to improve survival in patients with recurrent hemodynamically unstable ventricular arrhythmias; even amiodarone, which is the most effective antiarrhythmic, is inferior to ICD in reducing the incidence of SCD. However, amiodarone and β-blockers, often in combination, are used in patients with recurrent ventricular arrhythmias who are not eligible for ICD implantation or in those who have an ICD but have recurrent ventricular arrhythmias that cause frequent ICD shocks. Sotalol is also effective in suppressing ventricular arrhythmias in many patients.

Ventricular Asystole

Ventricular asystole is the absence of any ventricular rhythm; there is no QRS complex, no pulse, and no cardiac output. The term "ventricular standstill" is sometimes used when atrial activity is still present but no ventricular activity occurs. Both situations are fatal unless treated immediately. Ventricular asystole has the following characteristics:

Rate: None
Rhythm: None
P waves: May be present if the SA node is functioning
PR interval: None
QRS complex: None
Conduction: Atrial conduction may be normal if the SA node is functioning. There is no conduction into the ventricles.
Example: Ventricular asystole. Two P waves are seen at the beginning of the strip.

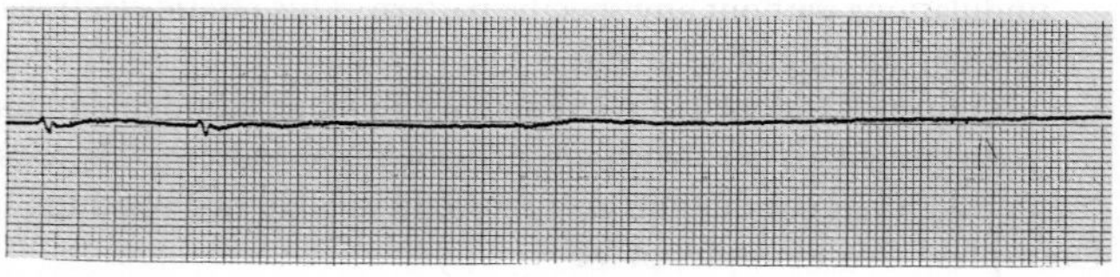

CPR must be initiated immediately if the patient is to survive. IV epinephrine and atropine may be given in an effort to stimulate a rhythm; vasopressin can be used instead of epinephrine as a vasopressor. Asystole has a very poor prognosis despite the best resuscitation efforts because it usually represents extensive myocardial ischemia or severe underlying metabolic problems. See Chapter 27 for the ACLS algorithm for treatment of asystole.

Conduction Abnormalities

The term *AV block* is used to describe arrhythmias in which there is delayed or failed conduction of supraventricular impulses into the ventricles. AV blocks have been classified according to location of the block and severity of the conduction abnormality. The following classification of AV blocks is discussed in this section:

First-degree AV block
Second-degree AV block
  Type I
  Type II
  2:1 conduction (can be type I or type II)
High-grade AV block (or advanced AV block)
Third-degree AV block

AV block can be caused by disease processes that either interrupt the blood supply to structures in the conduction system or otherwise interfere with the function of these structures, or by drugs that slow conduction through the AV node. It can also occur in normal hearts and be a result of normal physiologic variations (e.g., vagal tone) that affect conduction through the AV node, or in athletes or people who exercise regularly; it can occur during sleep when sympathetic tone is reduced or vagal tone is enhanced. One of the main functions of the AV node is to block rapid atrial impulses to prevent dangerously fast ventricular rates in response to rapid atrial rhythms such as rapid AT, atrial flutter, or AF. In this case, the block is physiologic and must not be confused with pathologic block due to abnormal AV node function. For example, a sinus rate of 80 should be conducted through a normally functioning AV conduction system in a 1:1 fashion, so, if any of those sinus impulses are blocked, that is abnormal AV node function and the term *block* appropriately applies. However, atrial flutter with an atrial rate of 300 will result in block of some of those impulses in the AV node in an attempt to keep ventricular rate reasonable, in which case the conduction failure is physiologic and not due to abnormal AV node function. In such a case, the term *conduction* might be a better one to use than *block* (i.e., "atrial flutter with variable conduction" rather than "atrial flutter with block").

Myocardial ischemia and infarction can cause AV block by disrupting the blood supply to the AV node (common with inferior MI) or to the bundle of His or bundle branches (more common with anterior MI). Rheumatic heart disease, inflammatory diseases, infectious diseases (Lyme disease, endocarditis, myocarditis), collagen diseases, idiopathic fibrosis of the conduction system (Lev's disease or Lenègre's disease), valve disease (usually aortic or mitral), atrial septal defects, congenital heart disease, and infiltrative cardiomyopathies (amyloidosis, sarcoidosis) can all cause varying degrees of AV.[54–56] Drugs that slow conduction through the AV node and are often associated with development of intranodal block include digitalis, β-blockers, verapamil, diltiazem, and amiodarone. AV block can also be a temporary or permanent result of cardiac surgery (especially aortic valve surgery) and can occur with AV node ablation, either intentionally (i.e., ablation of the AV node in chronic AF) or as a complication of ablation for SVT.

First-Degree AV Block

First-degree AV block is defined as prolonged AV conduction time of supraventricular impulses into the ventricles. This delay usually occurs in the AV node, and all impulses conduct to the ventricles, but with delayed conduction times. First-degree AV block can be recognized by the following ECG characteristics:

Rate: Can occur at any sinus rate, usually 60 to 100 beats per minute
Rhythm: Regular
P waves: Normal, precede every QRS
PR interval: Greater than 0.20 second. PR intervals as long as 1 second or more have been reported[22,57]
QRS complex: Usually normal unless bundle-branch block exists
Conduction: Normal through the atria, delayed through the AV node, normal through the ventricles
Example: First-degree AV block (PR interval, 0.44 second)

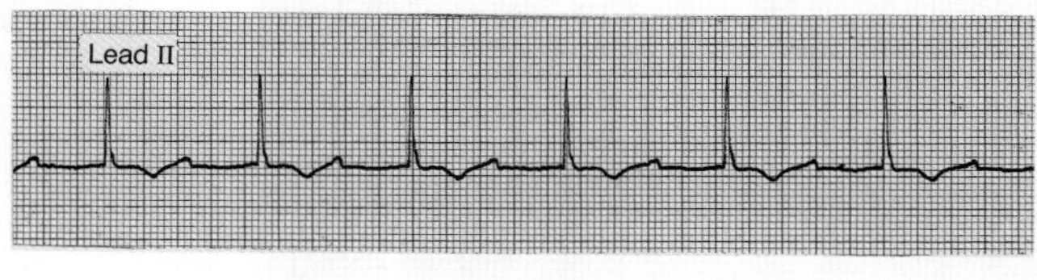

First-degree AV block does not require any specific treatment, but it should be observed for progression to more serious block.

Second-Degree AV Block

Second-degree AV block occurs when one atrial impulse at a time fails to be conducted to the ventricles. Second-degree AV block is divided into two categories: type I block, usually occurring in the AV node, and type II block, occurring below the AV node in the bundle of His or bundle-branch system.

Type I (Wenckebach). Type I second-degree AV block, often referred to as *Wenckebach* or *Mobitz I*, is a progressive increase in conduction times of consecutive atrial impulses into the ventricles until one impulse fails to conduct, or is "dropped." This appears on the ECG as gradually lengthening PR intervals until one P wave fails to conduct and is not followed by a QRS complex, resulting in a pause, after which the cycle repeats itself.

Type I second-degree AV block can be recognized by the following ECG characteristics:

Rate: Can occur at any sinus or atrial rate
Rhythm: Irregular unless 2:1 conduction is present. Overall appearance of the rhythm demonstrates group beating (i.e., groups of beats separated by pauses).
P waves: Normal. Some P waves are not conducted to the ventricles, but only one at a time fails to conduct.
PR interval: Gradually lengthens in consecutive beats. The PR interval preceding the pause is longer than that following the pause. When 2:1 conduction is present, PR intervals are constant.
QRS complex: Usually normal unless there is associated bundle-branch block
Conduction: Normal through the atria, progressively delayed through the AV node until an impulse fails to conduct. Ventricular conduction is normal. Wenckebach conduction ratios describe the number of P waves to QRS complexes: 6:5 conduction means six P waves resulted in five QRS complexes, or every sixth P wave is blocked. Conduction ratios can vary from low (e.g., 2:1, 3:2) to high (e.g., 12:11, 15:14).
Examples: (A) Second-degree AV block, type I (Wenckebach) with 3:2 conduction. (B) Second-degree AV block, type I. Note that the PR interval preceding the pause is longer than the PR interval after the pause.

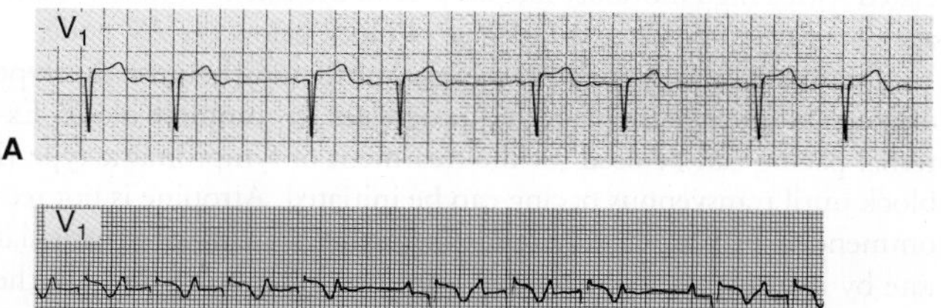

The treatment of type I second-degree AV block depends on the conduction ratio, the resulting ventricular rate, and, most important, the patient's tolerance for the rhythm. If the ventricular rate is slow enough to decrease cardiac output, the treatment is atropine to increase the sinus rate and speed conduction through the AV node. At higher conduction ratios, where the ventricular rate is within a normal range, no treatment is necessary. If the block is due to drug therapy, the drug dose may need to be decreased or a pacemaker implanted to control the drug-induced bradycardia while drug therapy continues. This type of block is usually temporary and benign and seldom requires pacing, although temporary pacing may be needed when the ventricular rate is slow.

Type II. Type II second-degree AV block, also called *Mobitz II*, is sudden failure of conduction of an atrial impulse to the ventricles without progressive increases in conduction time of consecutive P waves. Type II block occurs below the AV node and is usually associated with bundle-branch block; therefore, the dropped beats are usually a manifestation of bilateral bundle-branch block. In this form of block, there is no progressive increase in PR intervals before the blocked P waves. Type II block is less common but more serious than type I block. Type II second-degree AV block can be recognized by the following ECG characteristics:

Rate: Can occur at any basic rate
Rhythm: Irregular due to blocked beats unless 2:1 conduction is present

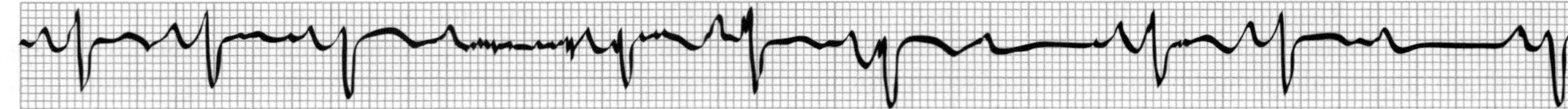

Example of second-degree AV block, type II

P waves: Usually regular and precede each QRS. Periodically, a P wave is not followed by a QRS complex.

PR interval: Constant before all conducted beats. The PR interval preceding the pause is the same as that after the pause.

QRS complex: Almost always wide because of associated bundle-branch block; can be narrow when block occurs in the bundle of His.

Conduction: Normal through the atria and through the AV node but intermittently blocked in the bundle-branch system and fails to reach the ventricles. Conduction through the ventricles is abnormally slow because of associated bundle-branch block. Conduction ratios can vary from 2:1 to only occasional blocked beats.

Example: Second-degree AV block, type II. All PR intervals are constant.

Type II block is more dangerous than type I because of a higher incidence of associated symptoms and progression to complete AV block. When it occurs in the presence of anterior wall MI, it is associated with a high mortality rate because of the extent of muscle damage necessary to produce this degree of block below the AV node.

Treatment usually includes pacemaker therapy because this type of block is often permanent and progresses to complete block. External pacing can be used for the treatment of symptomatic type II block until transvenous pacing can be initiated. Atropine is not recommended because it may result in further slowing of ventricular rate by increasing the number of impulses conducting through the AV node and bombarding the diseased bundles with more impulses than they can handle, resulting in further conduction failure.

2:1 Conduction. The 2:1 conduction ratio deserves special mention because it continues to be the source of much confusion and disagreement among electrocardiographers. The 2:1 block is failure of conduction of every other atrial impulse. Because only one P wave at a time is blocked, it is by definition a second-degree block. If the lesion causing conduction failure is in the AV node, it is type I block; if it is below the AV node, it is type II block. One source of confusion is the lack of progressive prolongation in PR intervals in type I block with 2:1 conduction, which has led educators for years to teach that all 2:1 block was "Mobitz II" block. Type I block with 2:1 conduction does not present with progressively prolonging PR intervals because there are no *consecutively conducted* beats in 2:1 block. The progressive prolongation of PR interval that characterizes Wenckebach conduction occurs on consecutively conducted P waves in type I block; so, when there is block of every other P wave, this typical behavior is not seen. However, the location of the lesion does not change; so, if the lesion is in the AV node, it is type I block regardless of the conduction ratio.

When a patient presents with a 2:1 conduction ratio, it is sometimes impossible to determine whether the block is type I or II without intracardiac recordings. However, an educated guess can be made depending on the length of the PR interval, the QRS width, and the clinical situation. The following ECG findings can be very helpful in determining the type of block in 2:1 conduction in the absence of intracardiac recordings:

PR interval: Often longer than normal (more than 0.20 second) in type I and normal in type II. Sometimes, the PR in

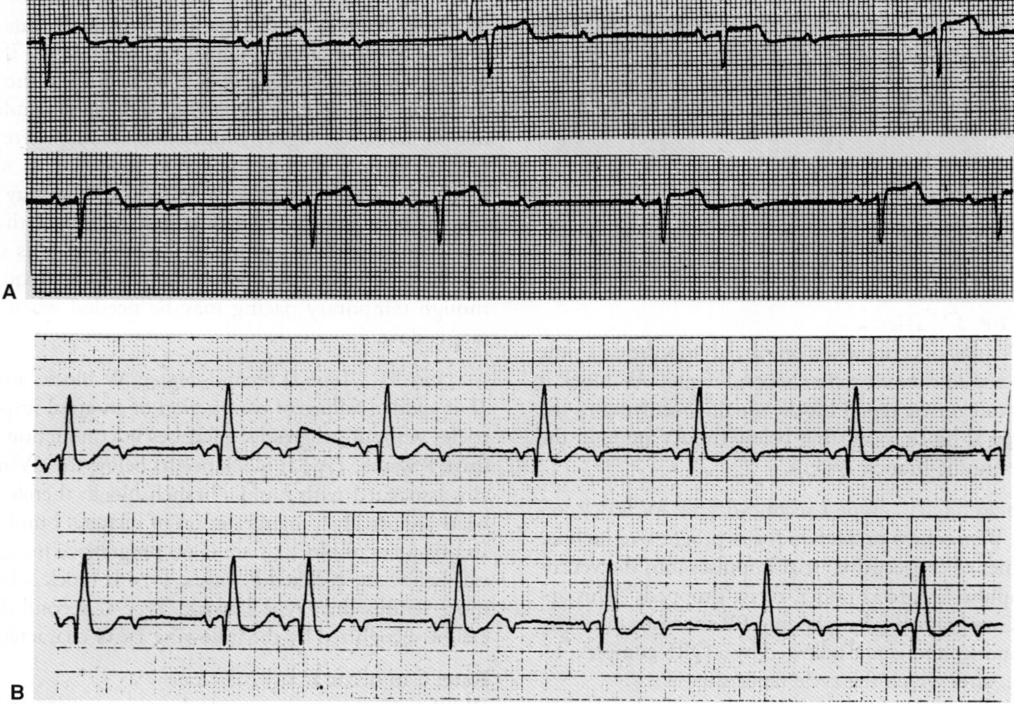

Examples of 2:1 conduction

type I is normal on conducted beats because the blocked P wave allows enough time for the AV node to recover so that it is able to conduct every other P wave with a normal PR interval. If there are any periods of typical Wenckebach conduction with progressive lengthening of the PR interval on consecutively conducted P waves (even if it only happens once), it is type I block.

QRS complex: Usually narrow in type I and almost always wide in type II. Exceptions can occur in type I when there is a coincidental bundle-branch block that widens the QRS, and in type II when the block is in the His bundle (still below the AV node, thus type II), resulting in a narrow QRS. Type II block is rare compared with type I, and intra-His type II block is even more rare, so the odds are greatly in favor of type I block when the QRS is narrow.

Examples: (A) Top strip shows 2:1 conduction that can be assumed to be type I because of the narrow QRS complex. Second strip proves that it is type I when consecutive P waves conduct with increasing PR intervals. (B) Top strip shows 2:1 conduction that can be assumed to be type II because of wide QRS. Second strip proves that it is type II when consecutively conducted PR intervals remain constant.

High-Grade AV Block

High-grade AV block (also called advanced AV block) is present when two or more consecutive atrial impulses are blocked, the atrial rate is reasonable (less than 135 beats per minute), and conduction fails because of the block itself and not because of interference from an escape pacemaker.[58] If the atrial rate is very fast, as in atrial flutter with atrial rates of 300 beats per minute, physiologic AV block occurs as a normal function of the AV node and, therefore, cannot be called high-grade block; hence, the arbitrary atrial rate limit of 135 beats per minute. If a junctional or ventricular escape beat or rhythm occurs as a result of failed conduction of impulses into the ventricles and interferes with the ability of atrial impulses to conduct by causing refractoriness in the AV node or ventricles, high-grade block cannot be diagnosed; the mere presence of the escape beat or rhythm may be the cause of failed conduction, rather than a true block in the AV node or bundle-branch system.

High-grade AV block can occur in the AV node or below the AV node. High-grade block can be recognized by these ECG characteristics:

Rate: Atrial rate less than 135 beats per minute

Rhythm: Regular or irregular, depending on conduction pattern

P waves: Normal, present before every conducted QRS, but several P waves may not be followed by QRS complexes

PR interval: Constant before conducted beats; may be normal or prolonged

QRS complex: Normal unless bundle-branch block is present.

Conduction: Normal through the atria. Two or more consecutive atrial impulses fail to conduct to the ventricles. Conduction through the ventricles is normal if block occurs in the AV node and slow if block occurs in the bundle branches.

Example: High-grade (advanced) AV block. There are three blocked P waves in a row and the ventricular rate is about 25 beats per minute. PR intervals before conducted QRS complexes are constant at 0.32 second.

The significance of high-grade block depends on the conduction ratio and the resulting ventricular rate. Because ventricular rates tend to be slow, this arrhythmia is frequently symptomatic and requires treatment. Atropine can be given and is usually more effective when block occurs in the AV node. External cardiac pacing may be necessary until a temporary transvenous pacemaker can be inserted, and permanent pacing is usually necessary when block is below the AV node.

Third-Degree AV Block (Complete Block)

Third-degree AV block is complete failure of conduction of all atrial impulses to the ventricles. In third-degree AV block, there is complete AV dissociation; the atria are usually under the control of the SA node, although complete block can occur with any atrial arrhythmia; and either a junctional or ventricular pacemaker controls the ventricles. The ventricular rate is usually less than 45 beats per minute; a faster rate could indicate an accelerated junctional or ventricular rhythm that interferes with conduction from the atria into the ventricles by causing physiologic refractoriness in the conduction system, thus causing a physiologic failure of conduction that must be differentiated from the abnormal conduction system function of complete AV block. Third-degree AV block can be recognized from the following ECG criteria:

Rate: Atrial rate is normal when sinus rhythm is present; ventricular rate is usually less than 45 beats per minute

Rhythm: Regular

P waves: Normal but dissociated from QRS complexes

PR interval: No consistent PR intervals because there is no relation between P waves and QRS complexes

QRS complex: Normal if ventricles controlled by a junctional pacemaker, wide if controlled by a ventricular pacemaker

Conduction: Normal through the atria. All impulses are blocked at the AV node or in the bundle branches, so there is no conduction to the ventricles. Conduction through the ventricles is normal if a junctional escape rhythm occurs and is abnormally slow if a ventricular escape rhythm occurs.

Examples: (A) Third-degree AV block with most likely a junctional pacemaker at a rate of 36 beats per minute. (B) Third-degree AV block with a ventricular pacemaker at a rate of 32 beats per minute. (C) AF with third-degree block and ventricular escape pacemaker at rate of 25 beats per minute.

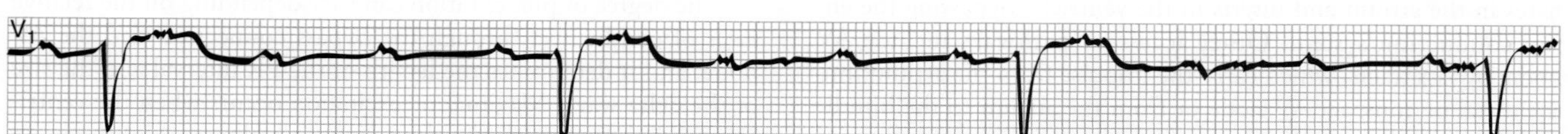

Example of high-grade AV block

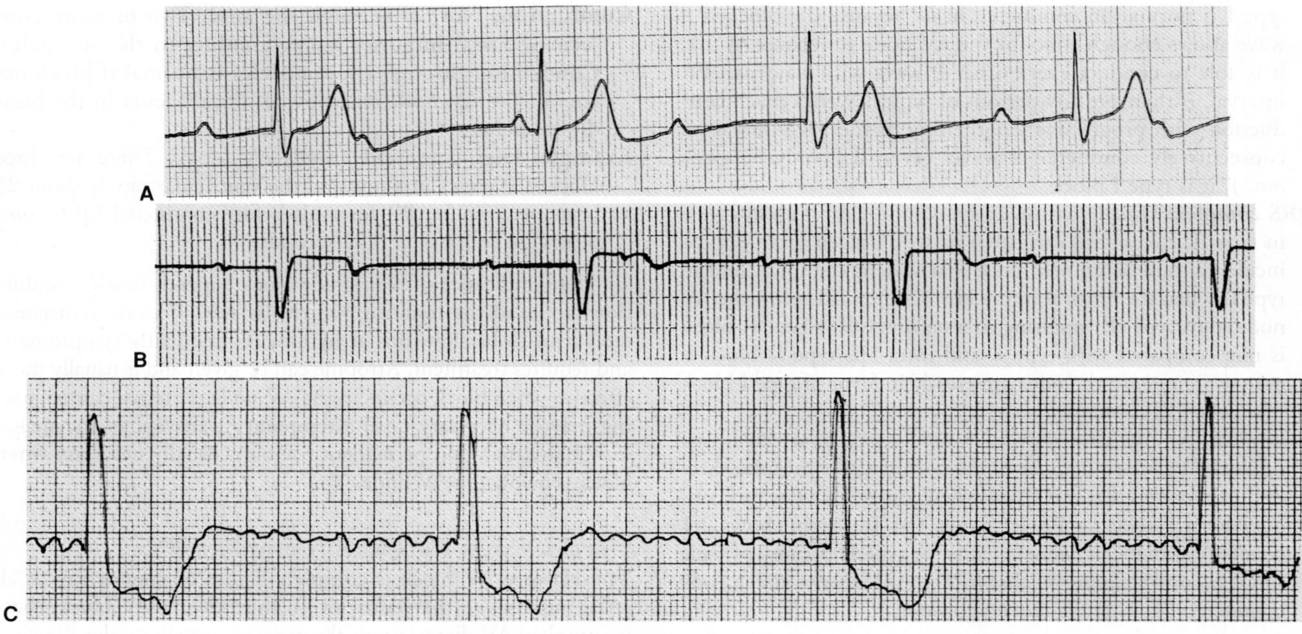

Examples of third-degree AV block

Third-degree AV block can occur without significant symptoms if it is of gradual onset and the heart has time to compensate for the slow ventricular rate. If it occurs suddenly in the presence of acute MI, its significance depends on the resulting ventricular rate and the patient's tolerance. If symptoms of decreased cardiac output occur, external cardiac pacing can be used to maintain a ventricular rate until transvenous pacing can be initiated. Dopamine or epinephrine infusions can be used to maintain blood pressure and CPR should be performed until pacing can be initiated.

COMPLEX ARRHYTHMIAS AND CONDUCTION DISTURBANCES

Abnormalities of cardiac rhythm can range from simple to advanced to complex. Disorders of the heartbeat provide a constant challenge to those interested in the study of arrhythmias. This section discusses advanced concepts in arrhythmia interpretation and provides clues to aid in the recognition of selected advanced arrhythmias.

Preexcitation Syndromes

Preexcitation refers to early activation of the ventricular myocardium by supraventricular impulses entering the ventricles through accessory pathways. These pathways are capable of carrying the impulse directly into the ventricle, bypassing all or part of the normal AV conduction system. The most common accessory pathway is an AV bypass tract, the bundle of Kent, which originates in the atrium and inserts in the ventricle, bypassing the entire conduction system. Other accessory pathways include AV nodal bypass tracts, which carry the impulse from the atrium into the distal or compact AV node or from the atrium to the bundle of His (sometimes called *James fibers* or *atriohisian fibers*), and nodoventricular connections, which originate in or below the AV node and carry the impulse directly into the ventricular myocardium (*Mahaim fibers.*)[5,59–61] Other authors state that these latter fibers have been shown to originate in the right atrial free wall and insert into the right bundle branch and refer to them as atriofascicular fibers.[60] In any case, all of these bypass tracts have the potential to cause tachycardia.

The most common type of preexcitation syndrome is WPW syndrome, in which the impulse is transmitted down the bundle of Kent directly from the atrium into the ventricles, bypassing the AV node.

WPW Syndrome

In WPW syndrome, during sinus rhythm, the ventricle is stimulated prematurely through the Kent bundle while the impulse is simultaneously conducted through the normal His–Purkinje conduction system. Impulses travel faster down the accessory pathway because they bypass the normal AV node delay. Part of the ventricle receives the impulse early through the accessory pathway and begins to depolarize before the rest of the ventricle is activated through the His–Purkinje system. Early stimulation of the ventricle results in a short PR interval and a widened QRS complex as the impulse begins to depolarize the ventricle through muscle cell-to-cell conduction. Premature ventricular stimulation forms a characteristic slurring of the initial portion of the QRS complex, called a *delta wave*. The remainder of the QRS complex is normal because the rest of the ventricle is then activated normally through the Purkinje system. This type of preexcitation results in fusion beats in the ventricles, as they are depolarized simultaneously by the impulse coming through the accessory pathway and through the AV node.

The degree of preexcitation can vary depending on the relative rates of conduction through the bypass connection and the AV node, and it determines the length of the PR interval and the size of the delta wave. Maximal preexcitation occurs when the ventricles are activated totally by the accessory pathway, resulting in an extremely short PR interval and uniformly wide QRS complex.

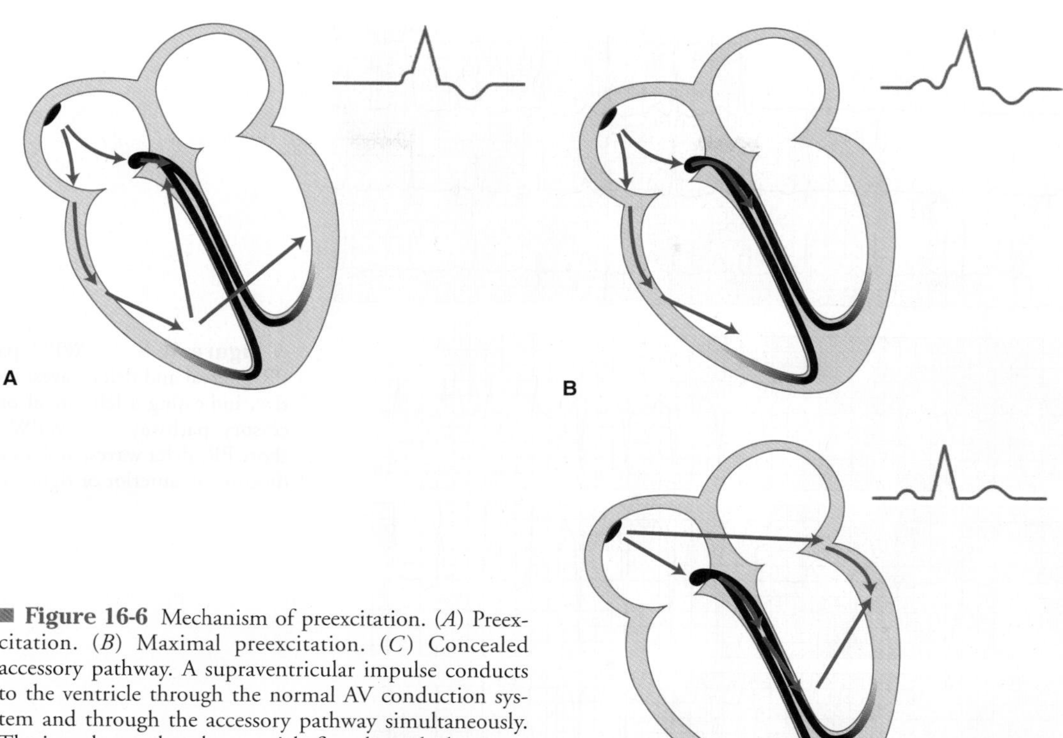

■ **Figure 16-6** Mechanism of preexcitation. (*A*) Preexcitation. (*B*) Maximal preexcitation. (*C*) Concealed accessory pathway. A supraventricular impulse conducts to the ventricle through the normal AV conduction system and through the accessory pathway simultaneously. The impulse reaches the ventricle first through the accessory pathway and preexcites it, causing a delta wave and short PR interval on the ECG.

Less than maximal preexcitation occurs when the impulse enters the ventricle through both pathways simultaneously, and the length of the PR interval and size of delta wave depend on how much of the ventricle is depolarized through the bypass connection. Figure 16-6 illustrates the mechanism of preexcitation and the characteristic short PR interval and delta waves that occur. A concealed pathway is present when the ventricles are depolarized exclusively through the normal conduction system even though a bypass tract exists. In this case, the PR interval and QRS complex are normal because the accessory pathway is not being used for anterograde conduction.

Accessory pathways can be located in multiple places around the valve rings, the septum, and the free walls of both ventricles (Fig. 16-7). The ECG can be helpful in identifying location of accessory pathways: atrial origin can be deduced from polarity of the P waves during orthodromic tachycardia, and the ventricular insertion site can be inferred from the polarity of delta waves during sinus rhythm.[5,62,63] Approximately 50% to 60% are in left free wall, 20% to 30% posteroseptal, 10% to 20% right free wall, and less than 10% are anteroseptal and mid-septal close to the bundle of His.[60] Figure 16-8 illustrates two examples of preexcitation during sinus rhythm.

WPW is clinically significant because the presence of two pathways provides the opportunity for reentry of the impulse and may result in rapid reentrant tachycardias. When tachycardias accompany the WPW pattern described above, the term *WPW syndrome* is used. The most commonly occurring tachyarrhythmia in WPW is CMT, which accounts for up to 95% of tachycardias in patients with WPW syndrome.[59] The incidence of AF occurring in the presence of WPW is estimated to be around 40%, which is

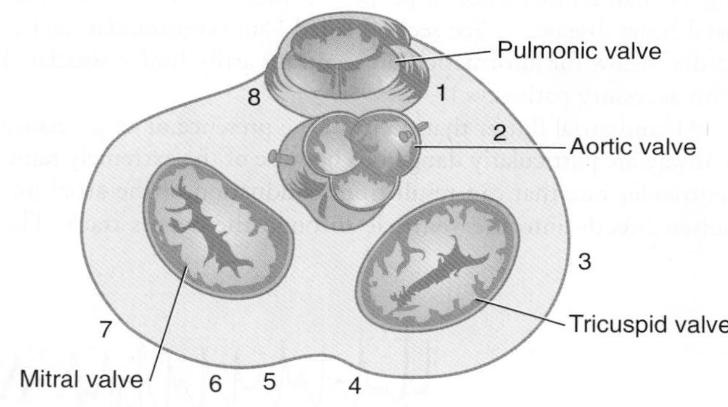

Delta wave polarity

	I	II	III	aV_R	aV_L	aV_R	V_1	V_2	V_3	V_4	V_5	V_6
1	+	+	+	−		+			+	+	+	+
2	+	+	−	−	+	−		+	+	+	+	+
3	+		−	−	+			+	+	+	+	+
4	+	−	−	−	+	−		+	+	+	+	+
5	+	−	−	−	+	−	+	+	+	+	+	+
6	+	+		−		+	+	+	+	+	+	+
7	−		+		−	+	+	+	+	+	+	+
8	−	+	+	−	−	+	+	+	+	+	+	+

■ **Figure 16-7** Locating the accessory pathway from delta wave polarity on the ECG. Numbers on the diagram at top indicate potential sites of accessory pathways. The table at the bottom shows delta wave polarity (+ = positive; − = negative) in each lead of the ECG for each site. (From Conover, M. [2003]. *Understanding electrocardiography* [8th ed., p. 278]. St. Louis, MO: Mosby.)

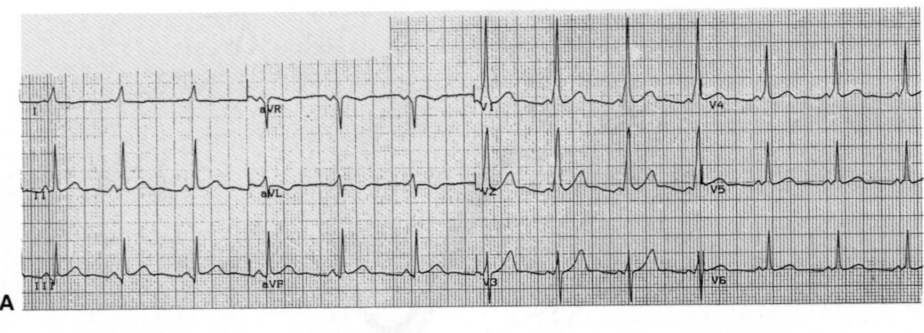

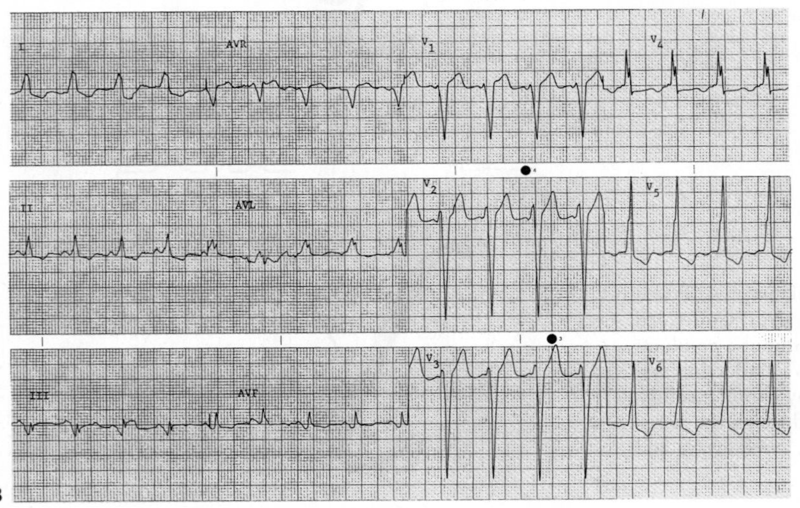

■ Figure 16-8 (A) WPW pattern of short PR interval and delta waves. Lead V_1 is positive, indicating a left lateral or posterior accessory pathway. (B) WPW pattern with short PR, delta waves, and a negative V_1, indicating an anterior or right-sided pathway.

higher than its incidence in people without WPW and no structural heart disease.[59] (See section titled "Supraventricular Tachycardia" below for information on reentrant arrhythmias associated with accessory pathways.)

AF and atrial flutter that occur in the presence of an accessory pathway are particularly dangerous because of the extremely rapid ventricular rate that can result from conduction of the atrial impulses directly into the ventricle through the bypass track. The ventricular rate can be as fast as 250 to 300 beats per minute and can deteriorate into VF, resulting in sudden death. AF with anterograde conduction over an accessory pathway presents on the ECG as a very rapid, irregular, wide QRS rhythm. The irregularity of the ventricular response helps to differentiate this rhythm from other wide QRS tachycardias.

The ECG characteristics of AF with anterograde conduction through an accessory pathway are as follows (Fig. 16-9):

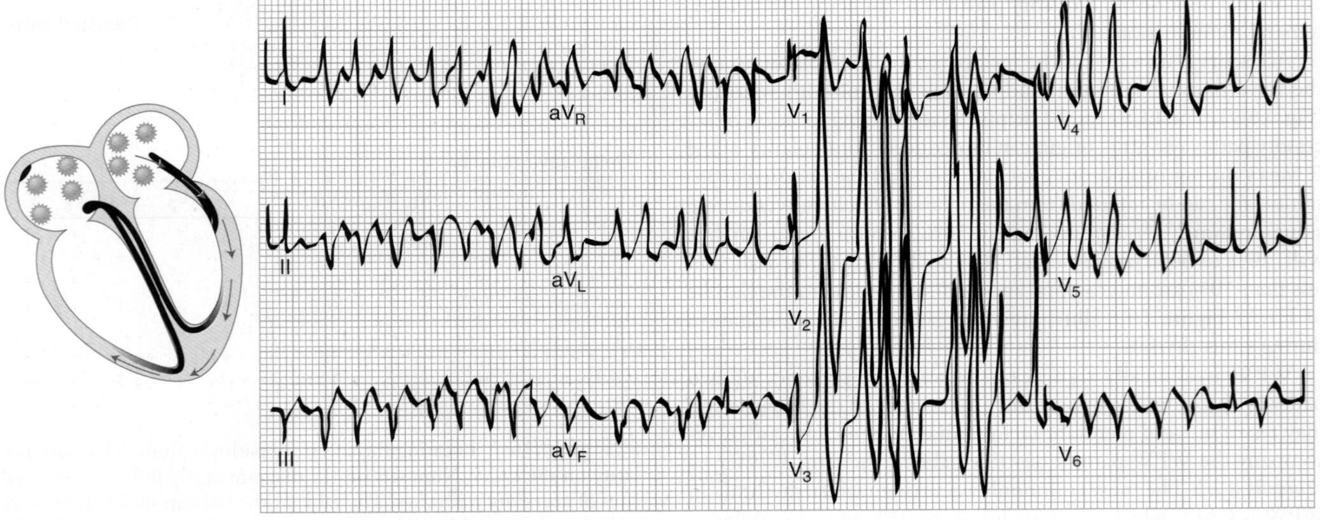

■ Figure 16-9 AF conducting anterograde through an accessory pathway. Note the extremely short R-R intervals in leads V_1 to V_3. QRS is fast, wide, and irregular.

Rate: Ventricular rates up to 300 beats per minute

Rhythm: Irregular. Often appears as groups of very short R-R intervals alternating with groups of longer R-R intervals. The longest R-R intervals are often more than twice the shortest R-R intervals.

P waves: None, because atria are fibrillating

PR interval: None

QRS complex: Wide, bizarre due to abnormal depolarization of ventricles through accessory pathway

Conduction: Disorganized and chaotic through atria. Atrial impulses conduct into ventricles through accessory pathway, resulting in muscle cell-to-cell conduction through ventricles.

Immediate treatment of AF with anterograde conduction through an accessory pathway depends on ventricular rate and the patient's tolerance of the arrhythmia. Cardioversion is the treatment of choice when severe hemodynamic impairment occurs. Drug treatment is directed at slowing conduction through the accessory pathway and restoring and maintaining sinus rhythm. Drugs that increase the refractory period and depress conduction in the bypass tract include procainamide, flecainide, propafenone, amiodarone, and sotalol. Many of these drugs are also effective in preventing recurrences of AF. Digoxin and calcium channel blockers, commonly used to treat AF that conducts through the AV node, are contraindicated whenever the tachycardia is due to anterograde conduction through an accessory pathway because they can accelerate conduction through the bypass tract or depress ventricular contractility, leading to hemodynamic deterioration.[22,61,64]

WPW syndrome can resemble other conditions usually diagnosed by ECG. The presence of anteriorly directed delta waves can simulate RBBB, posterior or inferior MI, right ventricular hypertrophy, or posterior fascicular block. Posteriorly directed delta waves can simulate left bundle-branch block (LBBB), anterior MI, anterior fascicular block, and left ventricular hypertrophy.[22,62,65,66]

Variants of Preexcitation Syndromes

In addition to the Kent bundle described above, which is responsible for WPW syndrome, other anatomical connections exist that can bypass the normal AV node delay or create connections between different parts of the conduction system and the ventricles and cause variations of the preexcitation pattern. Fibers originating in the atria and inserting into the His bundle (atriohisian fibers) have been demonstrated anatomically and can result in a short PR interval and normal QRS complex. This pattern used to be called Lown–Ganong–Levine syndrome (Fig. 16-10), but evidence does not support a specific syndrome consisting of short PR, normal QRS, and tachycardias that can be proven to be related to these fibers.[22]

Another variant of preexcitation involves conduction over a pathway that originates in either the atrium or the AV node and inserts into the right bundle branch (atriofascicular or nodofascicular fibers, also called Mahaim fibers), resulting in a wide QRS (usually LBBB morphology). In these variants, the PR interval may be normal or short. Reentrant tachycardias can occur with any of these variations in anatomy, and the QRS may be normal or wide during tachycardia, depending on the location of the accessory pathways responsible.

Treatment

Preexcitation does not require treatment unless it is associated with symptomatic tachyarrhythmias. Ideally, specific therapy should be based on a known mechanism of the arrhythmia and knowledge of a drug's effect on that mechanism in both conduction pathways. This knowledge is best gained through electrophysiologic study,

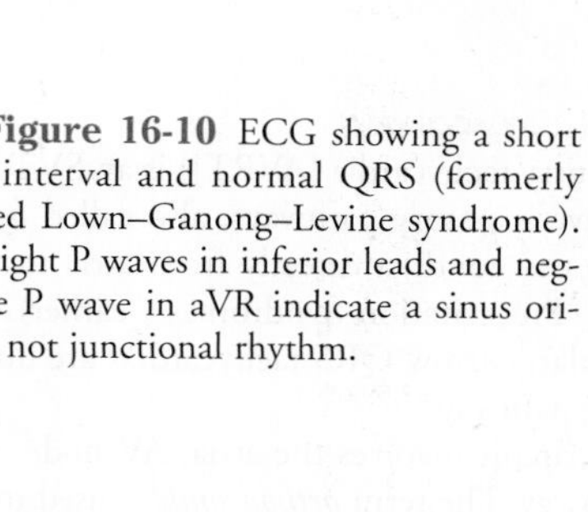

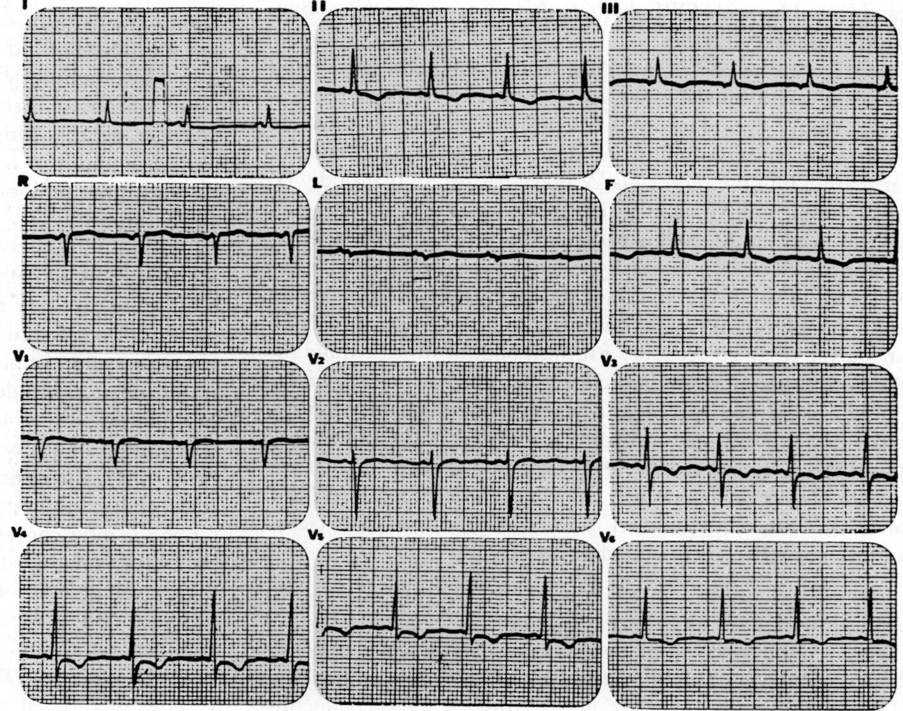

■ **Figure 16-10** ECG showing a short PR interval and normal QRS (formerly called Lown–Ganong–Levine syndrome). Upright P waves in inferior leads and negative P wave in aVR indicate a sinus origin, not junctional rhythm.

which is done to (1) confirm the presence of preexcitation, (2) identify the mechanism of the associated tachyarrhythmia, (3) localize the site of the accessory pathway, (4) confirm participation of the accessory pathway in maintenance of the tachycardia, (5) determine the functional behavior of the accessory pathway, and (6) determine the effects of different drugs on conduction velocity and refractoriness in both pathways. If the arrhythmia is due to reentry, therapy is directed toward changing the conduction time or the refractory period in the AV node or in the accessory pathway, or both, so that reentry is abolished. Prolonging the refractory period in the AV node or in the bypass tract or inducing block in either of these pathways can interrupt reentry and stop the tachycardia. If AF is the mechanism, treatment is aimed at preventing the occurrence of the arrhythmia and slowing conduction through the accessory pathway. Radiofrequency catheter ablation of the bypass tract offers a cure for tachycardias associated with accessory pathways and has become the therapy of choice. The reported success rate for accessory pathway ablation is >95%.[67,68] (See Chapter 18 for more information about electrophysiology studies and ablation in management of arrhythmias. The section below on supraventricular tachycardias covers drug therapy of specific tachycardias in more detail.)

Supraventricular Tachycardia

The term *SVT* is used for all tachycardias that either originate from supraventricular tissue (i.e., SA node reentry, atrial flutter, junctional tachycardia) or incorporate supraventricular tissue in a reentry circuit (i.e., AVNRT and CMT using an accessory pathway).[69] Usually, SVT is used to describe narrow QRS tachycardias because the narrow QRS denotes normal intraventricular conduction through the His–Purkinje system from a supraventricular focus. It is possible for an SVT to conduct with bundle-branch block, which would result in a wide QRS but would not change the fact that the rhythm is supraventricular in origin. Thus, SVT can be used for wide QRS rhythms that are known to be coming from above the ventricles.

SVT can be classified into those that are AV nodal passive and those that are AV nodal active. AV nodal passive SVTs are those in which the AV node does not play a part in the maintenance of the tachycardia but serves only to conduct passively the supraventricular rhythm into the ventricles. AV nodal passive SVTs include AT, atrial flutter, and AF, all of which arise from within the atria and do not need the AV node's participation to sustain the atrial arrhythmia. AV nodal active tachycardias require participation of the AV node in the maintenance of the tachycardia. The two most common causes of a regular, narrow QRS tachycardia are AVNRT and CMT using an accessory pathway, both of which require the AV node as part of the reentry circuit that sustains the tachycardia.

AF is usually easily recognized owing to its irregularity, but AT, atrial flutter, junctional tachycardia, AVNRT, and CMT can all present as a regular, narrow QRS tachycardia whose mechanism cannot always be determined from the ECG. Because AVNRT and CMT are responsible for most regular, narrow QRS tachycardias, these two are discussed in detail here.

AV Nodal Reentry Tachycardia

AVNRT is the most common mechanism of SVT and is responsible for up to two thirds of regular, narrow QRS tachycardias.[69–71] This rhythm involves dual AV nodal pathways: a fast-conducting pathway with a long refractory period and a slow-conducting pathway with a short refractory period. In AVNRT, a reentry circuit is set up in the AV node, using one pathway (usually the slow pathway) for the anterograde limb and the other pathway (usually the fast pathway) as the retrograde limb (Fig. 16-11).

Normally, the sinus impulse conducts down the fast pathway into the ventricles, resulting in a normal PR interval of 0.12 to 0.20 second. If a PAC occurs before the fast pathway with its long refractory period has recovered, the impulse conducts down the slow pathway because of its shorter refractory period, resulting in a PAC with a long PR interval. The long conduction time through the slow pathway allows the fast pathway time to recover, making it possible for the impulse to conduct backward into the fast pathway. The returning impulse can then reenter the slow pathway and initiate a circuit in the AV node, resulting in AVNRT. Figure 16-11 illustrates the most common mechanism of AVNRT. The resulting rhythm is usually a narrow QRS tachycardia because the ventricles are activated through the normal His–Purkinje system. P waves are either not visible at all or are seen peeking out at the end of the QRS complex because the atria are activated in a retrograde direction at the same time as the ventricles are being depolarized in an anterograde direction (Fig. 16-12). In the presence of preexisting bundle-branch block or rate-dependent bundle-branch block, the QRS in AVNRT is wide.

In approximately 10% of cases of AVNRT, the fast pathway is used as the anterograde limb and the slow pathway is used as the retrograde limb of the circuit.[22,69] This results in a long R-P tachycardia in which the P wave appears in front of the QRS because atrial activation is delayed owing to slow conduction backward through the slow pathway. These P waves are inverted in inferior leads because the atria are depolarized in a retrograde direction.

AVNRT is an AV nodal active SVT because the AV node's participation is required to maintain the tachycardia. Therefore, anything that blocks the AV node, such as vagal stimulation or drugs like adenosine, β-blockers, or calcium channel blockers, can terminate the rhythm. AVNRT is usually well tolerated unless the rate is extremely rapid. Many people with this arrhythmia learn to stop it by coughing or breath holding, which stimulates the vagus nerve. Adenosine is the preferred agent for terminating AVNRT except in patients with asthma, but it does not prevent its recurrence.[25] Radiofrequency ablation of the slow pathway has become the treatment of choice for all forms of AVNRT, with almost 100% success.[68,69,72]

Circus Movement Tachycardia

CMT (also called AV reentry tachycardia [AVRT]) is an SVT that occurs in people who have accessory pathways, also called *bypass tracts*, that allow impulses to conduct directly from atria to ventricles (see section titled "Preexcitation Syndromes", earlier). Approximately 30% of regular, narrow QRS tachycardias are due to CMT using an accessory pathway.[22,59,69]

In CMT, the reentry circuit involves the atria, AV node, ventricle, and accessory pathway. The term *orthodromic* is used to describe the most common type of CMT, in which the AV node is used as the anterograde limb and the accessory pathway is used as the retrograde limb of the circuit. This results in a narrow QRS tachycardia because the ventricles are depolarized through the His–Purkinje system. If bundle-branch block is present, the QRS is wide. Because the atria and ventricles depolarize separately, the P waves in CMT, if visible, are often seen in the ST segment or

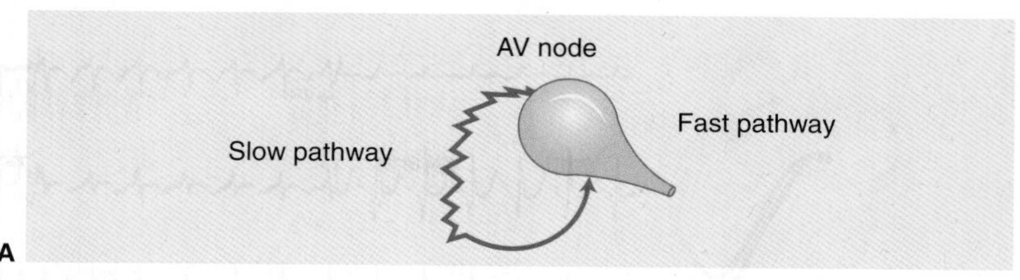

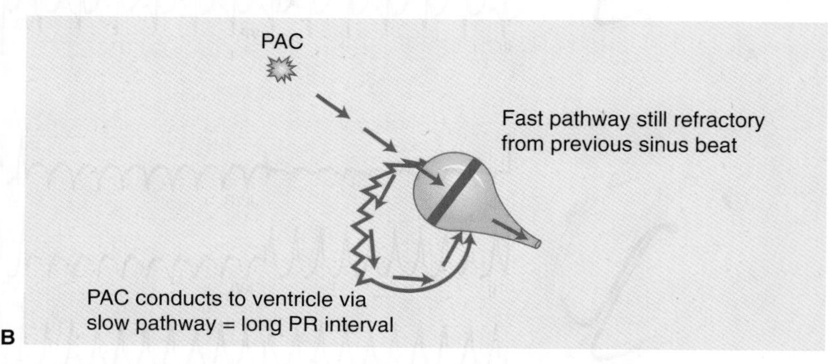

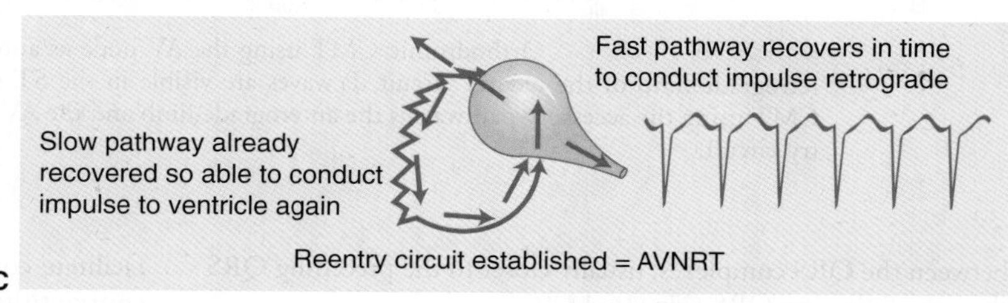

■ **Figure 16-11** Mechanism of AVNRT. (A) The dual AV nodal pathways responsible for AVNRT. The normal AV node is the fast conducting pathway with a long refractory period; the slow conducting pathway lies outside the AV node and has a shorter refractory period. (B) A PAC finds the fast pathway still refractory but is able to conduct through the slow pathway. (C) When the impulse arrives at the end of the slow pathway it finds the AV node recovered and ready to conduct retrograde to the atria. The slow pathway has already recovered due to its short refractory period and is able to conduct the same impulse back into the ventricle. This sets up the reentry circuit and causes AVNRT.

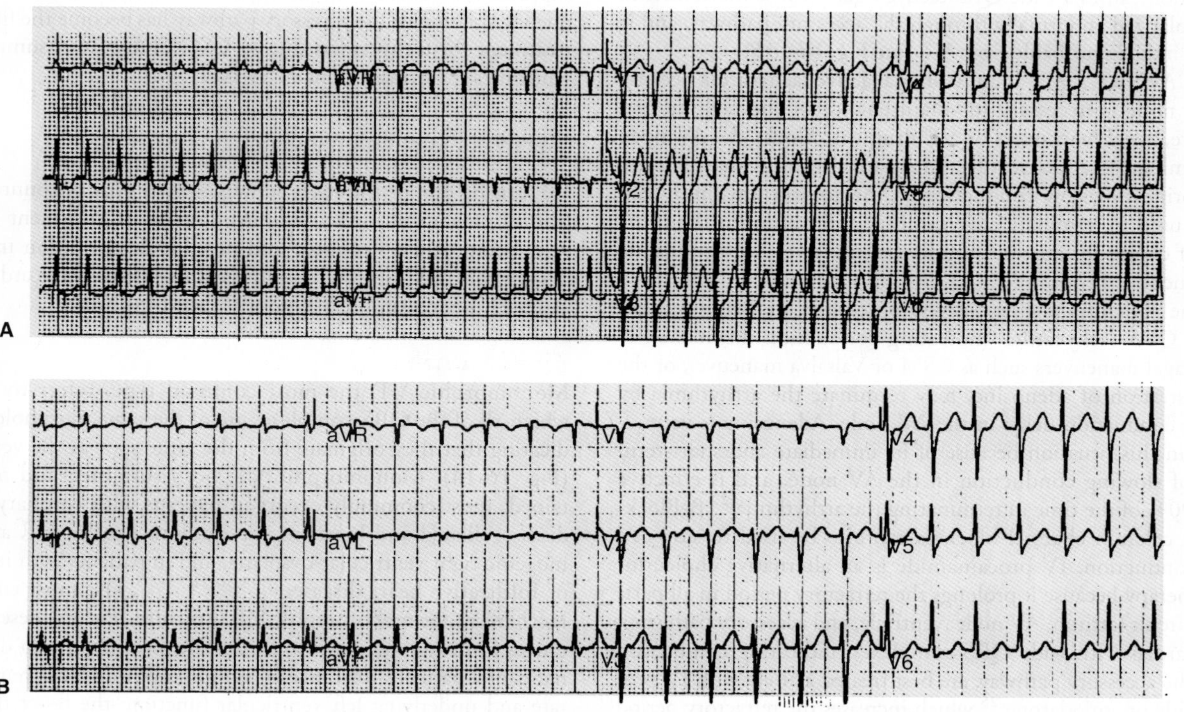

■ **Figure 16-12** (A) AVNRT; rate—214 beats per minute. No P waves are visible. (B) AVNRT; rate—150 beats per minute. P waves distort the end of the QRS complex in leads II, III, aVF, and V_{1-3}.

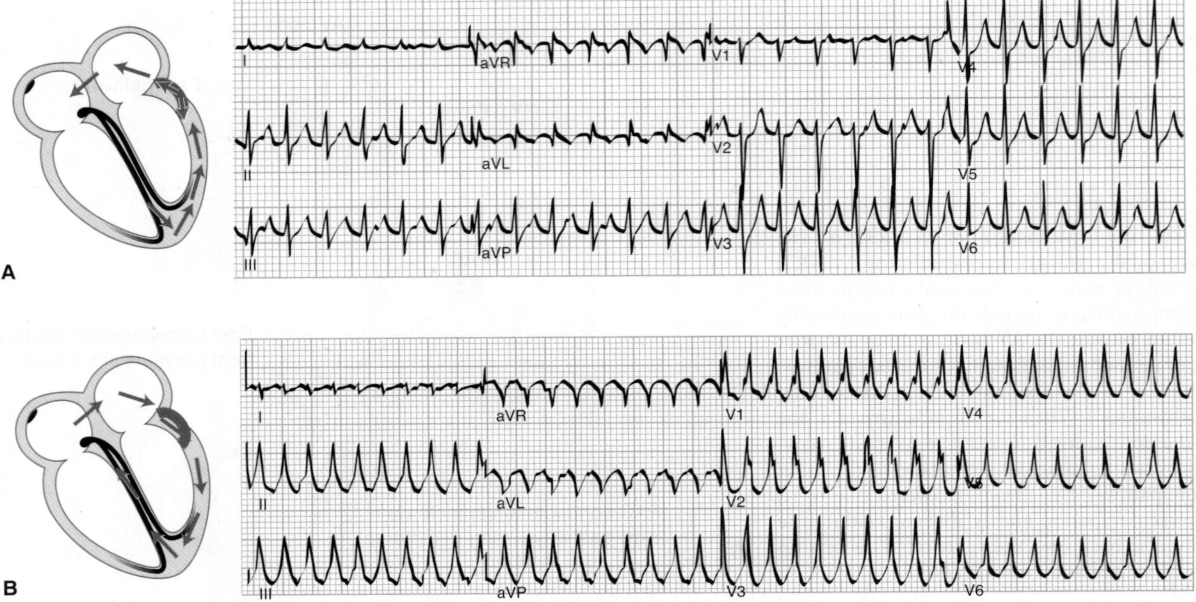

■ **Figure 16-13** (A) Orthodromic CMT using the AV node as anterograde limb and accessory pathway as retrograde limb of the reentry circuit. P waves are visible in the ST segment in most leads. (B) Antidromic CMT using the accessory pathway as the anterograde limb and the AV node as the retrograde limb of the reentry circuit.

between the QRS complexes, usually closer to the preceding QRS than the following QRS (Fig. 16-13*A*).

The term *antidromic* is used to describe a rare form of CMT in which the accessory pathway is used as the anterograde limb of the circuit and the AV node is used as the retrograde limb. This conduction causes a wide QRS tachycardia because the ventricles are depolarized abnormally through the accessory pathway, and it is often indistinguishable from VT (see Fig. 16-13*B*).

Like AVNRT, CMT is an AV nodal active tachycardia because the AV node is necessary for maintenance of the tachycardia; therefore, vagal maneuvers or any drug that blocks the AV node can terminate the tachycardia. Alternatively, drugs that increase refractoriness or slow conduction in the accessory pathway can also be used to terminate tachycardia. Cardioversion is the treatment of choice for any tachycardia causing severe hemodynamic impairment.

If the patient is not seriously symptomatic and has a regular, narrow QRS tachycardia, indicating conduction down the AV node, vagal maneuvers such as CSM or Valsalva maneuver, or the administration of adenosine, may terminate the arrhythmia by causing conduction delay in the AV node. Adenosine is very effective in this situation because of its immediate and short-term effect of slowing conduction in the AV node, and is effective about 90% of the time in terminating the arrhythmia.[22] β-Blockers and calcium channel blockers can also be used to slow AV node conduction. IV procainamide is an alternative choice for acute therapy because it prolongs the refractory period in all parts of the circuit (atrium, AV node, ventricle, and accessory pathway). Tachycardias with wide QRS complexes, indicating conduction down the accessory pathway, are best treated acutely with IV procainamide or amiodarone,[25] which increases the refractory period and depresses conduction in the bypass tract. Digitalis, verapamil, and diltiazem are contraindicated in this setting because they may facilitate conduction through the accessory pathway and depress contractility. Chronic therapy with class IA antiarrhythmics (procainamide, disopyramide), IC drugs flecainide, propafenone), or class III antiarrhythmics (amiodarone, sotalol) can be used to slow conduction through the accessory pathway, and may also suppress PAC and PVC that initiate the tachycardia.[25] Radiofrequency ablation of the accessory pathway has become the first-line treatment for tachycardias due to CMT. Table 16-4 summarizes guidelines for management of SVTs.

Ventricular Tachycardia

VT can be one of the most serious arrhythmias encountered in cardiac patients and often requires immediate treatment to prevent hemodynamic collapse and possible deterioration into VF. Three types of VT are commonly seen in patients with cardiac disease: (1) monomorphic VT, (2) PVT, and (3) TdP.

Monomorphic VT

Monomorphic VT, the most common type, refers to VT in which all of the QRS complexes are of the same morphology, indicating that they originate from the same spot in the ventricles (Fig. 16-14). Monomorphic VT, both sustained and nonsustained, most commonly occurs in patients with coronary artery disease, dilated and hypertrophic cardiomyopathy, HF, arrhythmogenic right ventricular dysplasia, and in patients with infective or infiltrative heart disease.[22,48,50,51,73–75] The most common mechanism for monomorphic VT is reentry, and its presentation ranges from asymptomatic to SCD. The most important determinants of a patient's tolerance of monomorphic VT are ventricular rate and underlying left ventricular function: the faster the ventricular rate and the lower the ejection fraction, the more symptomatic is the VT.

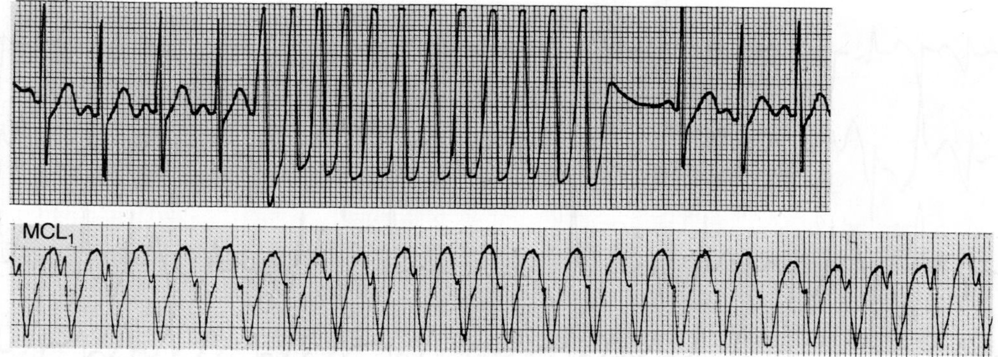

■ **Figure 16-14** Monomorphic VT. Tracings show two different examples, each with QRS complexes of one morphology.

Management of monomorphic VT is discussed earlier in this chapter under the section titled "Ventricular Tachycardia".

The term *idiopathic VT* refers to VT that occurs in people with no structural heart disease. The most common type of idiopathic VT arises in the RVOT, and is seen in 60% to 80% of patients with VT and no structural heart disease.[22,48,52] RVOT tachycardia presents with LBBB morphology and inferior axis, and occurs in two forms: (1) nonsustained, repetitive monomorphic VT characterized by frequent repetitive salvos of VT or (2) paroxysmal, sustained monomorphic VT induced by exercise. Both types can be terminated by adenosine, supporting the hypothesis that the mechanism is triggered activity due to DADs.[52] Although most adenosine-sensitive VTs originate from the RVOT, about 10% to 15% come from the left ventricular outflow tract. The ACC/AHA/ESC practice guidelines for managing ventricular arrhythmias[49] recommend using β-blockers, calcium channel blockers, and/or class IC antiarrhythmics if drug therapy is to be used for managing RVOT tachycardia; and catheter ablation in those who are drug intolerant or do not desire long-term drug therapy.

Idiopathic left VT (also called fascicular tachycardia or verapamil-sensitive VT) originates near the left posterior fascicle in the left ventricle and presents with RBBB morphology, superior axis, and relatively narrow QRS complex (<0.14 second).[22,48,52] The mechanism is thought to be reentry around the distal Purkinje network of the posterior fascicle. This is the one type of VT for which IV verapamil is effective therapy; normally verapamil is not recommended in VT due to its ability to depress contractility and lead to further hemodynamic deterioration. The ACC/AHA/ESC practice guidelines for managing ventricular arrhythmias states that β-blockers or calcium channel blockers may be effective drug therapy, and that catheter ablation is useful in patients who are drug refractory/intolerant or in those who do not desire long-term drug therapy.[49] Table 16-5 summarizes the guidelines for the management of VTs.

Polymorphic VT

PVT refers to VT with unstable, continuously varying QRS morphology often occurring at rates of approximately 200 beats per minute. It can occur in short repetitive salvos, longer sustained runs, or can degenerate into VF and cause SCD. PVT can be classified on the basis of whether it is associated with normal or prolonged QT intervals. Catecholaminergic PVT and short QT syndrome (SQTS) are two types of PVT in which the QT interval is normal or short. TdP is PVT that occurs in the presence of a long QT interval.

PVT with a normal QT interval can occur in the presence of ventricular ischemia during acute coronary syndrome or following MI, although it is not a common arrhythmia.[76] Figure 16-15 shows PVT in a patient during acute anterior wall MI. Therapy for PVT associated with ischemia should be directed toward relieving the ischemia by via either surgery or angioplasty. The ACC/AHA/ESC practice guidelines for managing ventricular arrhythmias[49] recommend IV β-blockers for PVT if ischemia is suspected. For recurrent PVT in the absence of a long QT interval, IV amiodarone is useful and lidocaine may be helpful. Electrical cardioversion is necessary for sustained PVT with hemodynamic compromise, and if the rhythm degenerates to VF, defibrillation is required.

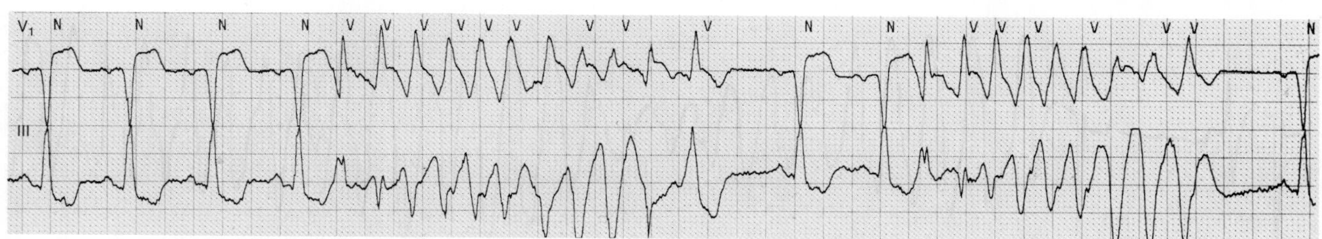

■ **Figure 16-15** PVT recorded in two leads (V$_1$ and III). Note the normal QT interval and the ST elevation in lead V$_1$ with reciprocal ST depression in lead III due to anterior MI. (N = arrhythmia computer's determination of a normal beat; V = computer determination of ventricular beat.)

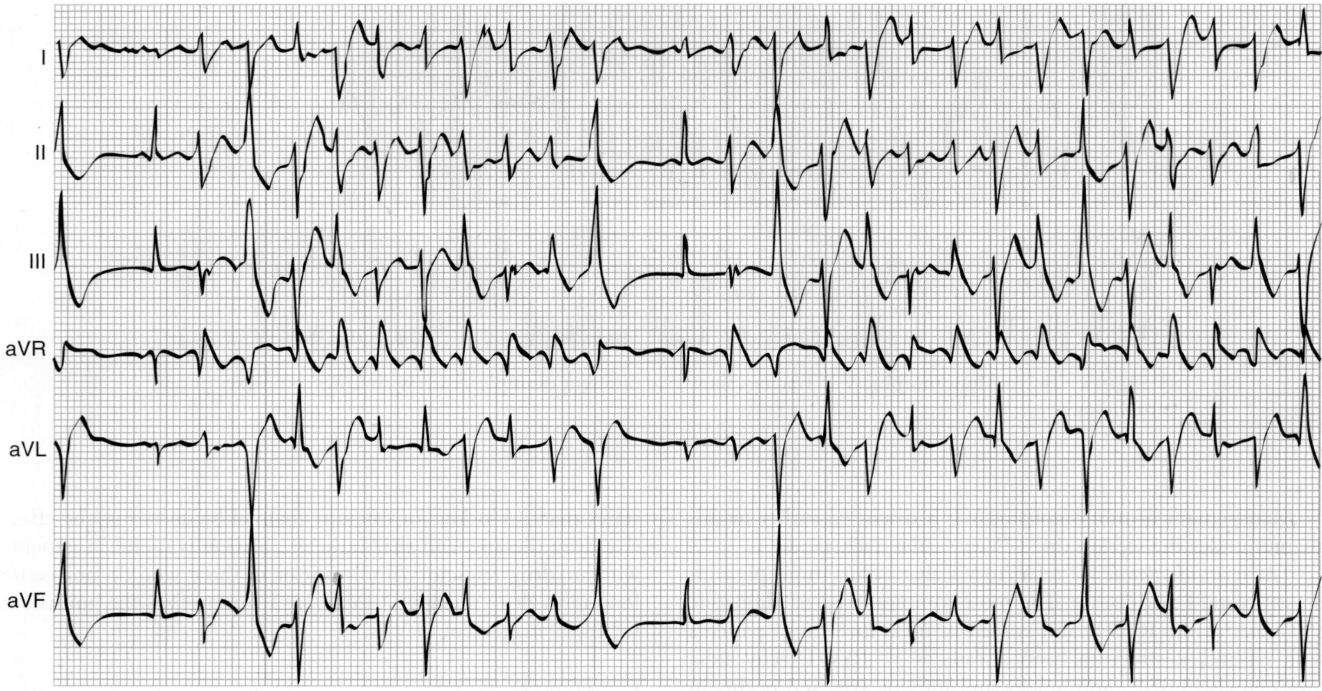

■ **Figure 16-16** Catecholaminergic PVT in a 12-year-old patient during exercise. (From Wellens, H. J. J., & Conover. M. [2006]. *The ECG in emergency decision making* [2nd ed., p. 224]. St. Louis, MO: Saunders.)

Catecholaminergic PVT. Catecholaminergic PVT is a genetic disorder that causes adrenergic-dependent PVT and sudden death in otherwise healthy people.[22,76–78] It usually occurs in children or adolescents who have normal ECG at rest and presents as life-threatening PVT or VF associated with exercise or emotional stress. The VT is typically bidirectional (one QRS pointing up, the next pointing down in alternating fashion) or polymorphic, and begins as isolated PVCs that progress to nonsustained PVT as exercise progresses. Runs of VT get progressively longer as the patient continues to exercise and can become sustained and degenerate to VF.[77] Sudden adrenergic stimulation due to emotional stress can trigger runs of PVT or VF. β-Blockers are the drugs of choice for treatment; and ICD implantation is indicated for patients with sustained, poorly tolerated VT. Figure 16-16 is an example of catecholaminergic PVT.

Short QT Syndrome. SQTS (also called short-coupled TdP) is a cause of SCD in otherwise healthy children and young adults, and is characterized by the onset of malignant PVT with a short coupling interval to the preceding beat.[78–81] This arrhythmia is in contrast to typical TdP that begins with a long coupling interval and occurs in the presence of a long QT interval (see discussion below). SQTS is a genetic disorder in which patients have a corrected QT interval ≤340 milliseconds, sometimes with a measured QT interval as short as 210 milliseconds.[80] The most common presentation is cardiac arrest, which can be seen as early as the first year of life, indicating that SQTS may be one cause of sudden infant death syndrome. Syncope can also be a presenting symptom and is thought to be due to self-terminating runs of PVT. AF is seen at an early age in SQTS and is thought to be due to a very short refractory period in the atria. So far the only reliable treatment to prevent SCD in patients with SQTS is ICD implantation. Quinidine can prolong the refractory period and has been useful in some patients.[80,82] Since this arrhythmia is a relatively newly described syndrome there is much that remains unknown about it, including its prevalence in the general population. Figure 16-17 shows a short-coupled PVT.

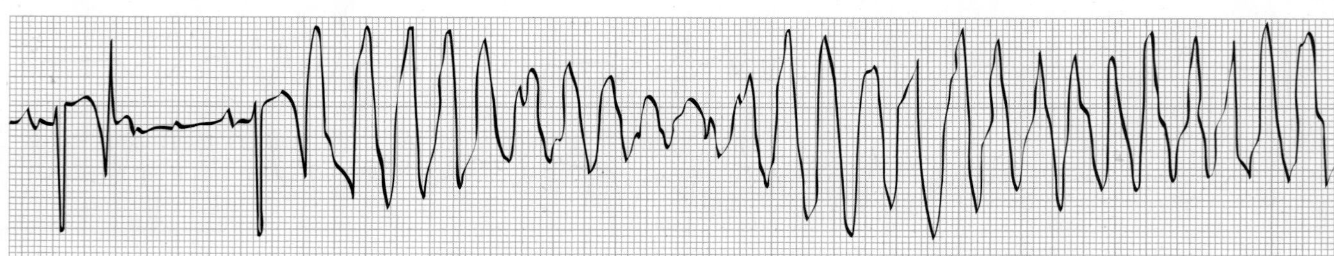

■ **Figure 16-17** Short-coupled PVT. Note the very short coupling interval of about 240 milliseconds between the normal beat and the first beat of VT. This PVT has characteristics of TdP but the QT interval is short.

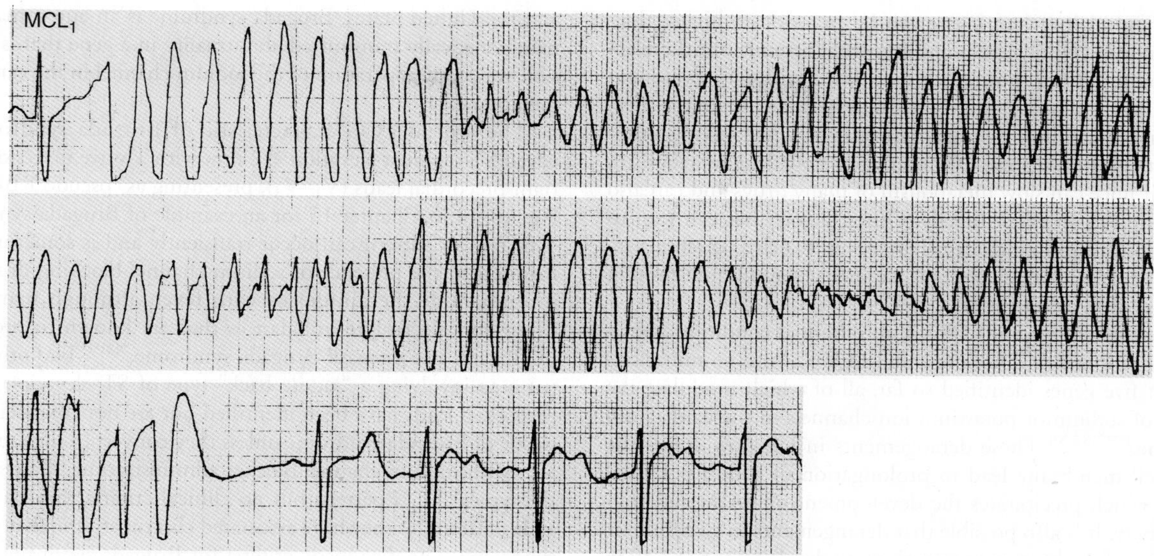

■ **Figure 16-18** TdP. Note characteristic features: (1) multiform QRS complexes that twist and around the baseline, (2) initiation by a PVC with a long coupling interval, and (3) associated long QT interval and wide TU waves during sinus rhythm.

Torsades de Pointes. *TdP* means "twisting of the points" and describes a special type of PVT in which the QRS complexes display continuously changing morphologies and seem to twist around an imaginary line, often resembling VF (Figs. 16-18 and 16-19). The underlying cause of this type of VT is delayed ventricular repolarization, which is manifested on the ECG as an abnormally prolonged QT or QTU interval; a large U wave after the T wave or merging with the T wave; wide, notched, or biphasic T waves; and often associated with T wave alternans.[22,83,84] The proposed electrophysiologic mechanisms of TdP include: (1) dispersion of repolarization due to unequal refractory periods between different cell types in the ventricles and (2) EADs, which arise during the prolonged phase 2 of the cardiac action potential, leading to triggered beats and runs of TdP.[5,83–85] The notch commonly seen on the T wave of patients with TdP and long QT intervals may be a manifestation of EADs arising during the repolarization phase of the action potential.

QT prolongation can be acquired or congenital. The acquired type is most often due to repolarization abnormalities induced by drugs, including class IA and class III antiarrhythmics, macrolide antibiotics, antifungals, antipsychotic and antidepressant drugs, some antihistamines, some gastric motility agents, and many others. Recently the Food and Drug Administration released an alert regarding the risk of QT prolongation and TdP with haloperidol

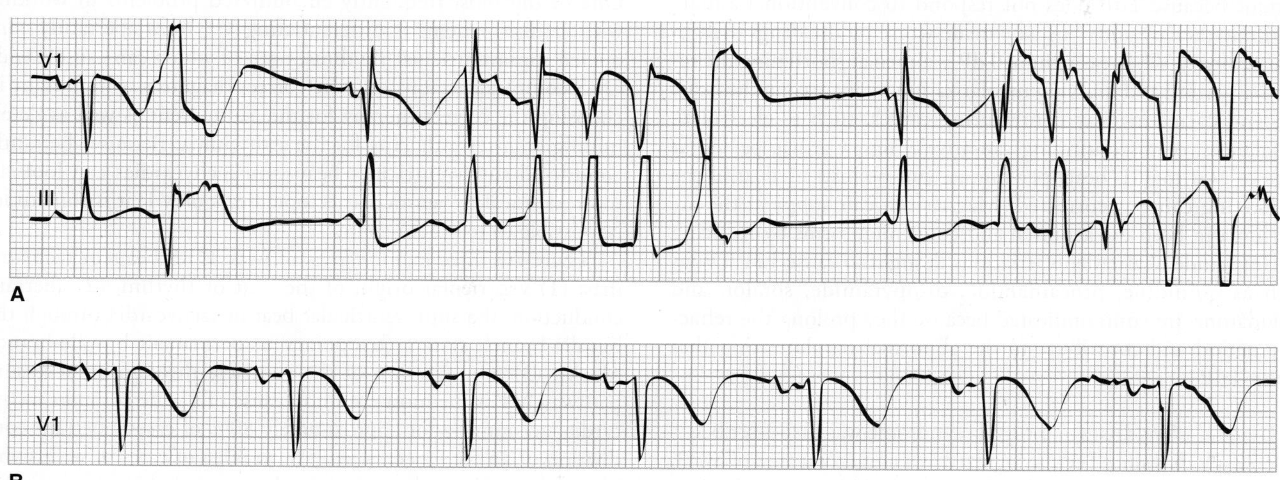

■ **Figure 16-19** **(A)** Short runs of TdP. Note that the episodes of TdP occur following a pause: the first pause follows a PVC; the second pause is due to termination of the first TdP episode and initiates the next episode. **(B)** Same patient in normal sinus rhythm. Note: prolonged QT interval measuring about 520 milliseconds.

(Haldol), especially when it is given IV or in doses higher than recommended. Hypokalemia and hypomagnesemia are the electrolyte abnormalities most often associated with QT prolongation. The risk of developing TdP from drugs increases in the presence of hypokalemia, hypomagnesemia, or when taking other drugs that also prolong the QT interval or slow drug metabolism. Grapefruit juice can slow metabolism of many drugs and can also increase the QT interval directly. Other factors that can lead to delayed repolarization include cerebral events such as cerebral vascular accidents and subarachnoid hemorrhage and liquid protein weight loss diets or starvation.[22,83,84,86]

The congenital type of LQTS is an inherited condition associated with TdP and SCD. Congenital LQTS is due to mutations of at least five genes identified so far, all of which modulate the function of sodium or potassium ion channels in the cardiac cell membrane.[9,77,87,88] These derangements in ion flow across the cardiac cell membrane lead to prolongation of action potential duration which precipitates the development of EADs and triggered activity. It is also possible that derangements in sympathetic innervation of the heart may contribute to development of TdP in congenital LQTS.[85] (See Chapter 4 for more detailed information on genetics related to cardiac diseases.)

Characteristic ECG findings of TdP include (1) markedly prolonged QT intervals with wide TU waves; (2) initiation of the arrhythmia by an R-on-T PVC with a long coupling interval; and (3) wide, bizarre, multiform QRS complexes that change direction frequently, appearing to twist around the isoelectric line (see Figs. 16-18 and 16-19). The acquired type of TdP is usually associated with bradycardia and is "pause dependent," meaning that it tends to occur after pauses produced by a PVC or sudden slowing of the heart rate. TdP is often initiated by a "long–short" cycle sequence in which episodes begin on the T wave of a beat that terminates a long cycle. The congenital type of TdP frequently occurs with a sudden surge in sympathetic tone, such as with loud noises, emotional stress, or physical activity. In this case TdP occurs without a change in preceding cycle length and is not pause dependent or bradycardia dependent. Ventricular rate during TdP is commonly 200 to 250 beats per minute. TdP is usually self-terminating and occurs in repeated episodes, but it can deteriorate into VF.

The differentiation of TdP from PVT and VF is extremely important because TdP does not respond to conventional antiarrhythmic therapy and is usually made worse by the drugs used to treat ordinary VT. Treatment of TdP is aimed at shortening the refractory period and unifying repolarization by increasing the heart rate and correcting any contributing causes, such as electrolyte imbalances, or discontinuing causative drugs. Cardiac pacing at rates of 100 to 110 beats per minute can be instituted until the underlying cause is corrected. Magnesium can suppress the arrhythmia in both the acquired and congenital forms by reducing the amplitude of afterdepolarizations thought to cause TdP. Drugs such as quinidine, procainamide, disopyramide, sotalol, and amiodarone are contraindicated because they prolong the refractory period and contribute to the abnormal repolarization that causes TdP.

Brugada Syndrome. Brugada syndrome was first described[89] in 1992 and has since been recognized as a common cause of SCD, accounting for up to 20% of SCD in people with structurally normal hearts.[90] It was first discovered in young men in Southeast Asia and is most commonly found there, although now that it is a clinically defined syndrome it is seen with increasing frequency in Europe and the United States. Brugada syndrome is an autosomal dominant genetically transmitted abnormality in a gene that is responsible for proper operation of the sodium channel in the cardiac cell membrane.[8,77,90,91]

The typical ECG characteristic of Brugada syndrome is a coved ST segment elevation ≥2 mm with T-wave inversion in the right precordial leads (V_1–V_3), presenting as "pseudo RBBB" (see Fig. 15-48 in Chapter 15 for an example of Brugada syndrome). This typical pattern can occur transiently and is sometimes only manifest in the presence of sodium channel blocking drugs (e.g., procainamide, flecainide) or with fever, although many other drugs and electrolyte imbalances that are known to precipitate LQTS can also unmask Brugada syndrome.[90,91] Two other ECG patterns involving a "saddle back" type of ST elevation in right precordial leads have been identified but are not considered diagnostic of Brugada syndrome unless they convert to the typical pattern with sodium channel blocker administration. If a person has the typical ECG pattern but no clinical criteria they have "Brugada pattern." If they have associated clinical criteria they have the syndrome. The diagnostic criteria for Brugada syndrome include the typical ECG pattern of coved ST elevation in more than one right precordial lead (V_1–V_3) in the presence or absence of a sodium channel blocking agent in conjunction with one of the following: documented VF or PVT, a family history of SCD at an age <45 years, similar ECG patterns in family members, syncope, nocturnal agonal respiration, or inducibility of VT with programmed stimulation during electrophysiology study.[90]

The clinical significance of Brugada syndrome is its association with lethal ventricular arrhythmias and SCD. Often cardiac arrest is the initial presentation, although patients may present with unexplained syncope that is most likely due to self-terminating episodes of PVT. Arrhythmias are more likely to occur at night and during sleep. The only effective therapy for preventing SCD in patients with Brugada syndrome is ICD implantation. Most antiarrhythmic drugs are contraindicated with the possible exception of quinidine, which has been effective in some paients.[90,91]

Differential Diagnosis of Wide QRS Beats and Tachycardias

One of the most frequently encountered problems in working with cardiac patients is differentiating VT from aberrantly conducted supraventricular rhythms, both of which can cause a wide QRS complex. Establishing the correct diagnosis is important in choosing the correct therapy for the acute event as well as determining long-term therapy for the arrhythmia. Because aberrantly conducted supraventricular beats and tachycardias can look almost identical to ventricular ectopic beats or VT, it is sometimes impossible to tell them apart.

There are three major causes of wide QRS beats or tachycardias: (1) ventricular origin of the beat or rhythm, (2) aberrant conduction of a supraventricular beat or tachycardia through the bundle-branch system (temporary or permanent bundle-branch block), (3) preexcitation of the ventricle through an accessory pathway. VT is the most common cause of a wide complex tachycardia, accounting for approximately 80% of cases; aberrant conduction of an SVT occurs in 15% to 30% of cases of wide complex tachycardia; and accessory pathway conduction accounts for 1% to 5% of cases.[92] Other conditions that can also cause the QRS to widen include antiarrhythmic drugs; electrolyte abnormalities, especially hyperkalemia; and ventricular paced rhythms.

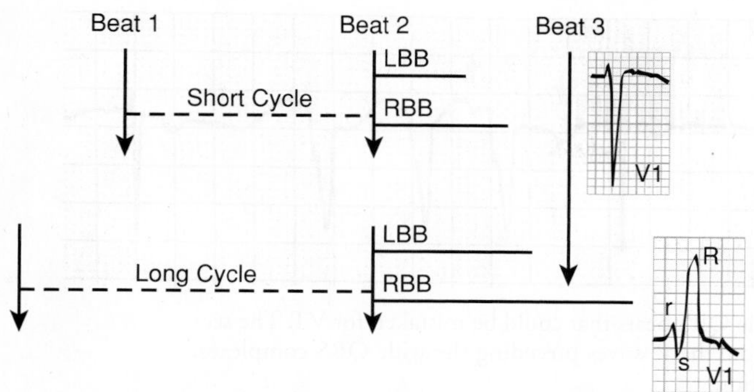

■ **Figure 16-20** Diagram of the effect of cycle length on conduction. Beats 1, 2, and 3 are consecutive beats. The refractory periods of the left bundle branch (LBB) and the right bundle branch (RBB) are shown following beat 2 (note the longer refractory period in the RBB). In the top panel, the basic cycle length from beat 1 to beat 2 is short, resulting in short refractory periods after beat 2 and allowing beat 3 to conduct normally even though it is premature. In the bottom panel the basic cycle lengthens, resulting in longer refractory periods. Beat 3 is no earlier here than it was in the top panel, but it now conducts with RBBB because of the longer refractory periods following the longer cycle. The QRS complexes are recorded in lead V_1 and illustrate normal conduction (top) and RBBB (bottom).

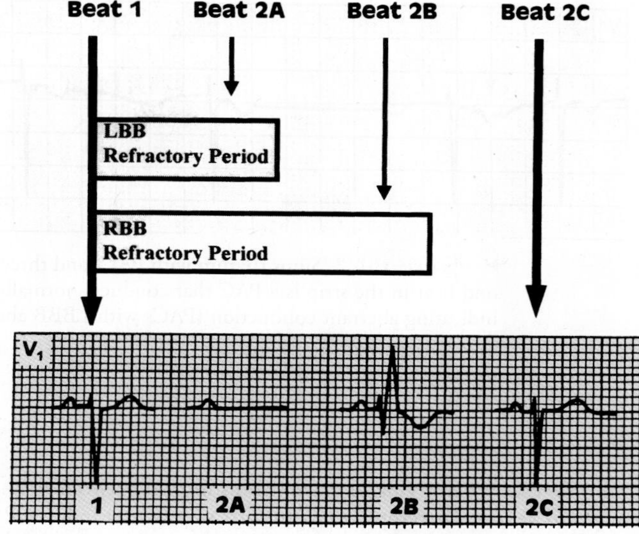

■ **Figure 16-21** Diagram of refractory periods in the bundle branches and the effect of prematurity on conduction. The right bundle has a longer refractory period than the left. Beat 2A occurs so early that it cannot conduct through either bundle branch, resulting in the blocked P wave illustrated in the strip below. Beat 2B encounters a refractory right bundle and conducts with RBBB. Beat 2C falls outside the refractory period of both bundles and is able to conduct normally.

Although many criteria have been proposed to aid in differentiating wide QRS beats and rhythms, this section concentrates only on selected criteria that seem to be the most helpful in the everyday clinical situation. Table 16-6 lists the ECG clues most helpful for differentiating wide QRS rhythms.

Mechanisms of Aberration

Aberrancy can occur whenever the His–Purkinje system is still partly or completely refractory when a supraventricular impulse attempts to traverse it. The refractory period of the conduction system is directly proportional to preceding cycle length. Long cycles (slow heart rates) are followed by long refractory periods, whereas short cycles (fast heart rates) are followed by short refractory periods. Supraventricular beats that occur early in the cycle, like a PAC, may enter the conduction system during its refractory period and be conducted aberrantly. Similarly, beats that follow a sudden lengthening of the cycle may be conducted aberrantly because of the increased length of the refractory period that occurs when the cycle lengthens. There are three situations in which aberration is likely to occur: (1) early supraventricular beats (e.g., PAC), (2) rapid heart rates where the supraventricular focus conducts into the intraventricular conduction system so rapidly that the bundles do not have time to repolarize completely, and (3) irregular rhythms where cycle lengths are constantly changing (e.g., AF). Because the right bundle branch has a longer refractory period than the left, aberrant beats tend to be conducted most often with an RBBB pattern. Figures 16-20 and 16-21 illustrate these principles of refractory periods and cycle lengths.

Table 16-6 ■ ELECTROCARDIOGRAPHIC CLUES FOR DIFFERENTIATING WIDE QRS RHYTHMS

ECG Feature	Aberrancy	Ventricular Ectopy
P waves	Precede QRS complexes (may be hidden in T waves)	Dissociated from QRS or occur at rate slower than that of QRS. If 1:1 ventriculoatrial conduction is present, retrograde P waves follow every QRS
RBBB QRS morphology	Triphasic rSR′ in V_1 Triphasic qRs in V_6	Monophasic r wave or diphasic qR complex in V_1
LBBB QRS morphology	Narrow r wave (<0.04 second) in V_1 Straight downstroke of S wave in V_1 (often slurs or notches on upstroke) Usually no Q wave in V_6	Left "rabbit ear" taller in V_1 Monophasic QS or diphasic rS in V_6 Wide r wave (>0.03 s) in V_1 Slurring or notching on downstroke of S wave in V_1 Delay of >0.06 s to nadir of S wave in V_1 Any Q wave in V_6
Precordial QRS concordance	Positive concordance may occur with WPW	Negative concordance favors VT Positive concordance favors VT if WPW ruled out
Fusion or capture beats	Often normal	Strong evidence in favor of VT
QRS axis	May be deviated to right or left	Indeterminate axis favors VT Often deviated to left or right
QRS width	Usually <0.14 s unless preexisting bundle-branch block	QRS >0.16 second favors VT

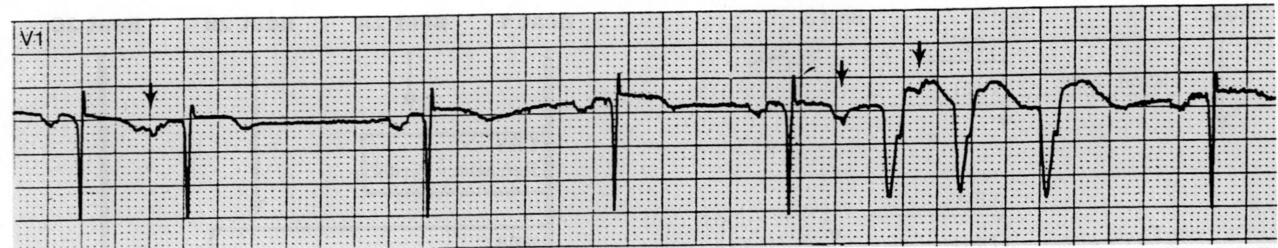

■ **Figure 16-22** Sinus rhythm with PACs and three wide QRS beats that could be mistaken for VT. The second beat in the strip is a PAC that conducts normally. Note the P waves preceding the wide QRS complexes, indicating aberrant conduction (PACs with LBBB aberration).

Electrocardiographic Criteria

P Waves. When trying to make the distinction between aberrancy and ventricular ectopy, a helpful first step is to search for P waves and note their relation to QRS complexes. Atrial activity (represented by a P wave) preceding a wide beat or a run of tachycardia strongly favors a supraventricular origin of that beat or tachycardia. Figure 16-22 illustrates an early ectopic P wave initiating three beats of a wide QRS rhythm that could easily be mistaken for PVCs.

An exception to the preceding P wave rule is the case of end-diastolic PVCs that occur after the sinus P wave has occurred. Figure 16-23 shows sinus rhythm with an end-diastolic PVC occurring immediately after the sinus P wave. In this case, the P wave preceding the wide QRS is merely a coincidence and does not represent aberrant conduction; the PR interval is much too short to have conducted that beat. In addition, the P wave preceding the wide QRS is not early; it is the regularly scheduled sinus beat coming on time. Thus, early P waves that precede early wide QRS complexes are usually related to those QRS, whereas "on time" P waves in front of end-diastolic PVCs are not early and do not cause the wide QRS, although they may result in ventricular fusion beats.

P waves seen during a wide-complex tachycardia can be very helpful in making the differential diagnosis between SVT with aberration and VT. It is common for the SA node to continue to fire regularly and independent of the ventricular focus when VT occurs. By noting the relationship between P waves and QRS complexes, it is sometimes possible to demonstrate AV dissociation, which means that the atria and ventricles are under the control of separate pacemakers (Fig. 16-24). Therefore, the presence of independent P waves in a wide QRS tachycardia indicates AV dissociation and is diagnostic of VT, whereas P waves seen before each QRS complex indicate a supraventricular origin of the rhythm. Figure 16-25 illustrates how P waves can be useful in differentiating two similar wide QRS tachycardias due to two different mechanisms.

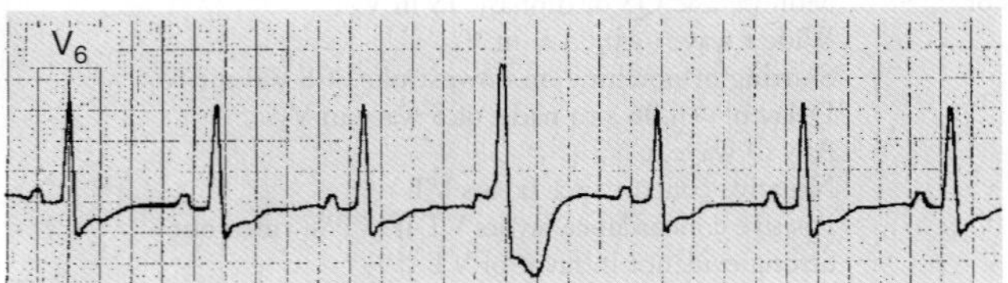

■ **Figure 16-23** Sinus rhythm with one end-diastolic PVC. The P wave preceding the PVC is the sinus P wave that coincidentally occurred just before the PVC.

QRS Morphology. The shape of the QRS complexes in a wide QRS tachycardia can be helpful in determining the mechanism of the arrhythmia. The following sections discuss the morphologic clues for wide complex tachycardias with RBBB and LBBB morphologies.

RBBB Pattern (QRS Wide and Upright in V_1). Because the right bundle has a longer refractory period than the left, an impulse entering the conduction system early or at very rapid rates is more likely to encounter a still-refractory right bundle branch; therefore, most (80% to 85%) aberrantly conducted beats conduct with RBBB. However, approximately 60% of ventricular ectopic beats simulate an RBBB pattern.[93] During normal ventricular depolarization, the septum depolarizes from left to right and creates a small initial r wave in V_1 (see Chapter 15). In the absence of septal infarction, the initial forces remain undisturbed during RBBB and beats that conduct with RBBB aberration have the same initial r wave in V_1 as during normal intraventricular conduction. Studies have shown that, of those beats presenting with an RBBB pattern in lead V_1, most aberrantly conducted supraventricular beats show a triphasic rSR' pattern, whereas almost all ectopic ventricular beats show a monophasic (R) or biphasic (qR) pattern in V_1.[61,92,93] Therefore, a wide QRS complex with a triphasic pattern of RBBB in lead V_1 strongly favors aberrancy, whereas a monophasic or biphasic complex of RBBB type favors ventricular ectopy.

Other morphologic clues are presented in Figure 16-26. A monophasic or biphasic complex of RBBB type in lead V_1 with a taller left "rabbit ear" favors ectopy, whereas a taller right "rabbit ear" favors neither. Often V_6 is as helpful as V_1; a triphasic qRs complex in V_6 favors RBBB aberrancy, whereas a monophasic QS complex or a biphasic rS complex favors ventricular ectopy. Figure 16-27*A* shows VT with RBBB morphology.

LBBB Pattern (QRS Negative in V_1). Leads V_1 or V_2 and V_6 also offer morphologic clues for tachycardias with LBBB morphology)[92,94] (see Fig. 16-26). Three characteristics of the QRS complex in V_1 or V_2 favor a ventricular origin: a wide initial r wave of greater than 0.03 second, slurring or notching on the downstroke of the S wave, and a delay of 0.06 second or more from the beginning of the QRS to the nadir (deepest part) of the S wave. In addition, any q wave (qR or QS) in V_6 favors a ventricular origin. Figure 16-27*B* shows VT with LBBB morphology.

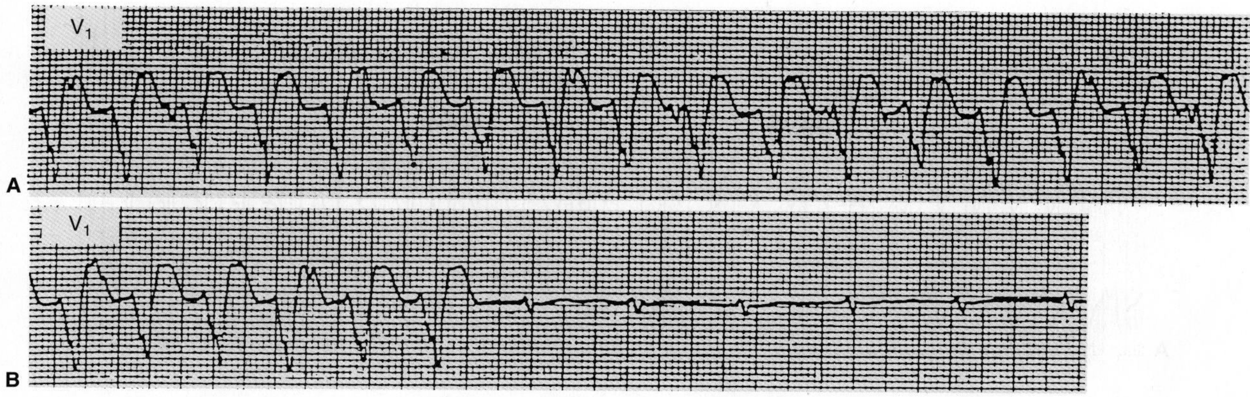

■ **Figure 16-24** (A) VT at a rate of 136 beats per minute. Independent P waves can be seen throughout the strip. (B) Sudden termination of VT, revealing the underlying sinus rhythm at a rate of 94 beats per minute.

Brugada et al.[95] suggest that additional morphologic clues in the precordial leads V_1 through V_6 can also be helpful. They suggest that a helpful first step in diagnosing a wide QRS rhythm is to scan the precordial leads to see if any lead shows an rS complex. If no precordial lead shows an rS pattern, VT is the likely diagnosis. If any precordial lead displays an rS pattern in which the measurement from onset of the r wave to nadir of the S wave exceeds 100 milliseconds (0.10 second), it favors the diagnosis of VT. They also emphasize that the presence of AV dissociation or any of the morphologic clues found in leads V_1, V_2, or V_6 discussed previously favor the diagnosis of VT (Fig. 16-28).

Lead V_6 or MCL_6 can be useful in differentiating supraventricular rhythms with aberrancy from ventricular ectopy.[96,97] In wide QRS rhythms of either RBBB or LBBB pattern, an interval of 50 milliseconds (0.05 second) or less from the onset of the QRS to the tallest peak of the r wave or nadir of the S wave favors a supraventricular origin, whereas an interval of 70 milliseconds (0.07 second) or more favors a ventricular origin (Fig. 16-29).

Fusion and Capture Beats. Ventricular fusion beats are produced when a supraventricular impulse and an ectopic ventricular impulse both contribute to ventricular depolarization. The resulting QRS complex does not look like a normally conducted beat or like the pure ventricular ectopic beat because it is formed by a combination of both depolarization waves (e.g., a "hybrid" morphology). The shape and width of fusion beats vary depending on the relative contributions of both the supraventricular and the ventricular impulses. The presence of fusion beats indicates AV dissociation; the atria and the ventricles are under the control of

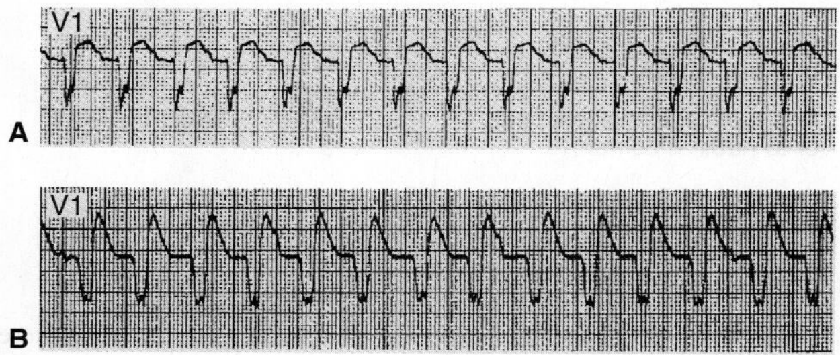

■ **Figure 16-25** Two similar wide QRS tachycardias. (A) Sinus tachycardia; rate—115 beats per minute. P waves can be seen preceding each QRS, indicating a supraventricular origin of the tachycardia. (B) P waves are independent of QRS complexes, indicating AV dissociation that favors VT.

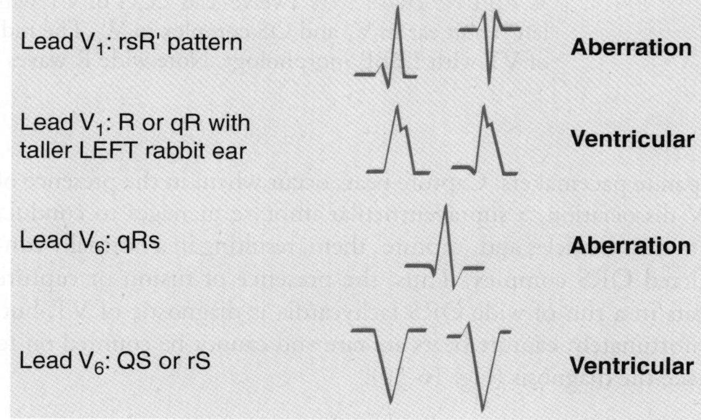

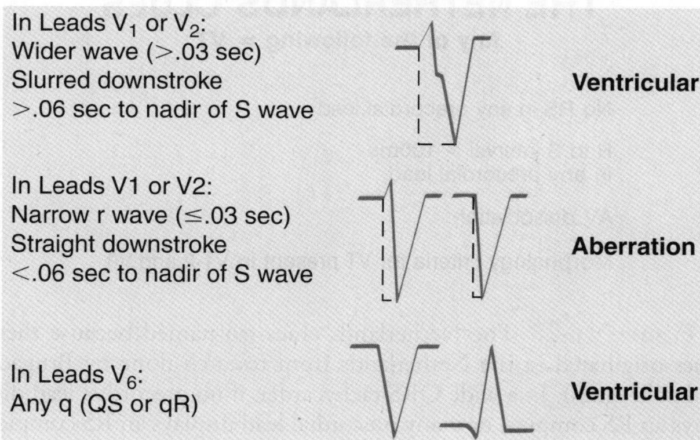

■ **Figure 16-26** Morphology clues for wide QRS beats and rhythms with RBBB morphology and LBBB morphology.

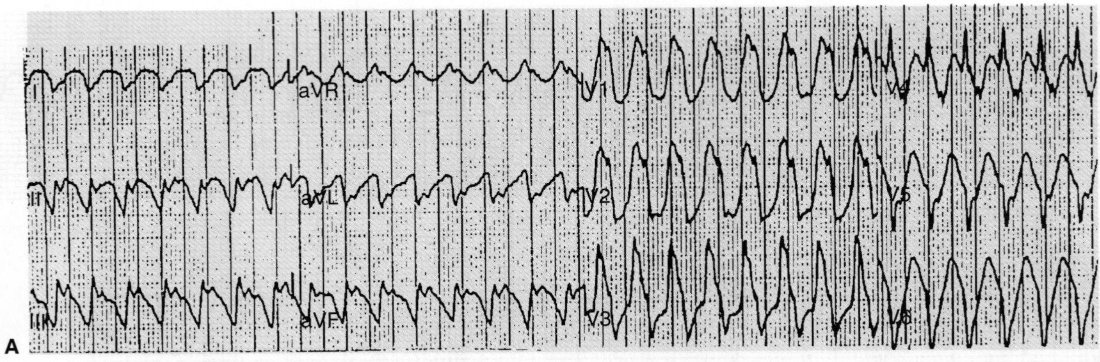

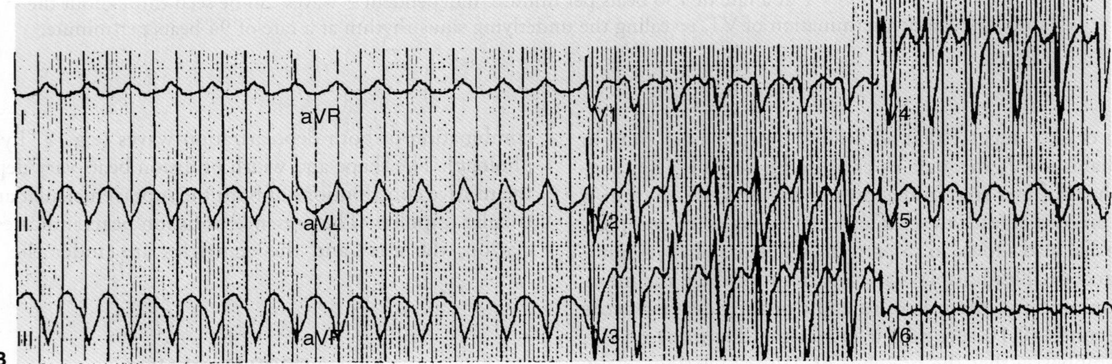

■ **Figure 16-27** (A) Twelve-lead ECG of VT with RBBB morphology. Note monophasic r wave with taller left rabbit ear in V_1 and QS complex in V_6. The indeterminate QRS axis also favors VT. (B) Twelve-lead ECG of VT with LBBB morphology. Note wide R waves in V_1 and V_2, and qR pattern in V_6.

separate pacemakers. Capture beats occur when, in the presence of AV dissociation, a supraventricular impulse manages to conduct into the ventricles and "capture" them, resulting in a normally conducted QRS complex. Thus, the presence of fusion or capture beats in a run of wide QRS tachycardia is diagnostic of VT, but, unfortunately, capture beats are rare and cannot be counted on to make the diagnosis (Fig. 16-30).

THE NETHERLANDS CLUES

Any of the following = VT

No RS in any precordial lead

R to S interval > 100ms in any precordial lead

AV dissociation

Morphology criteria for VT present in V1-2 and V6

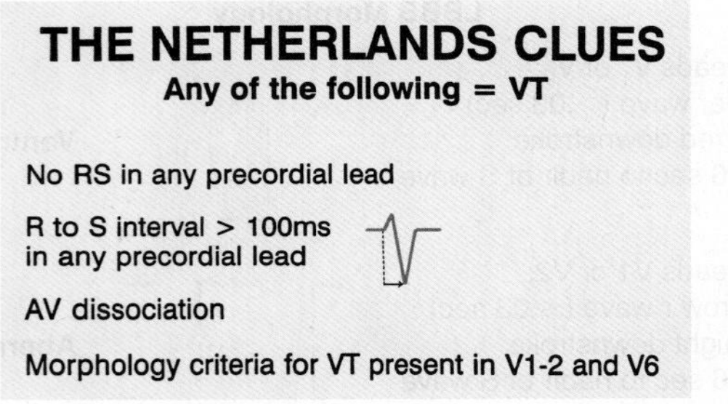

■ **Figure 16-28** The Netherlands clues (so named because these clues originated in the Netherlands from research done by Brugada and colleagues). In a wide QRS tachycardia, if no precordial lead displays an RS complex, or if any precordial lead displays an RS complex that measures greater than 100 milliseconds from onset to nadir, VT is the favored diagnosis. AV dissociation and the morphology clues favoring VT in V_{1-2} and V_6 are also helpful.

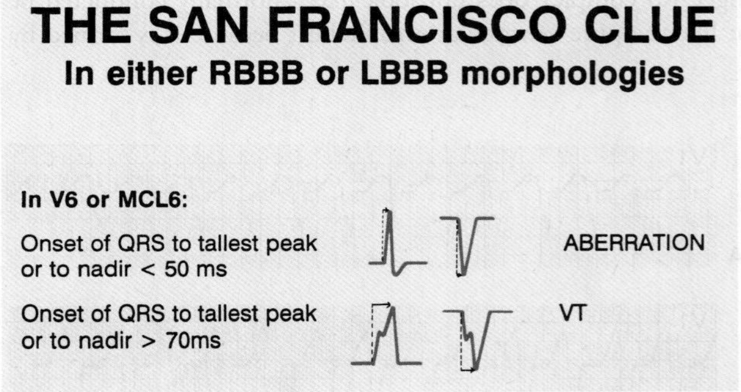

Cycle Length Variations. Ashman's phenomenon states that a beat that terminates a short cycle after a long cycle tends to be aberrantly conducted. Because the refractory period of the conduction system varies with preceding cycle length, a beat that terminates a long cycle has a long refractory period, causing the next

THE SAN FRANCISCO CLUE

In either RBBB or LBBB morphologies

In V6 or MCL6:

Onset of QRS to tallest peak or to nadir < 50 ms	ABERRATION
Onset of QRS to tallest peak or to nadir > 70ms	VT

■ **Figure 16-29** The San Francisco clue (so named because these clues originated from research done in San Francisco by Drew and Scheinman). In wide QRS tachycardias of either right or LBBB morphology, if measurement from beginning of QRS to tallest peak or to nadir of S wave is less than 50 milliseconds in V_6 or MCL_6, aberration is favored. If the measurement is more than 70 milliseconds, VT is favored.

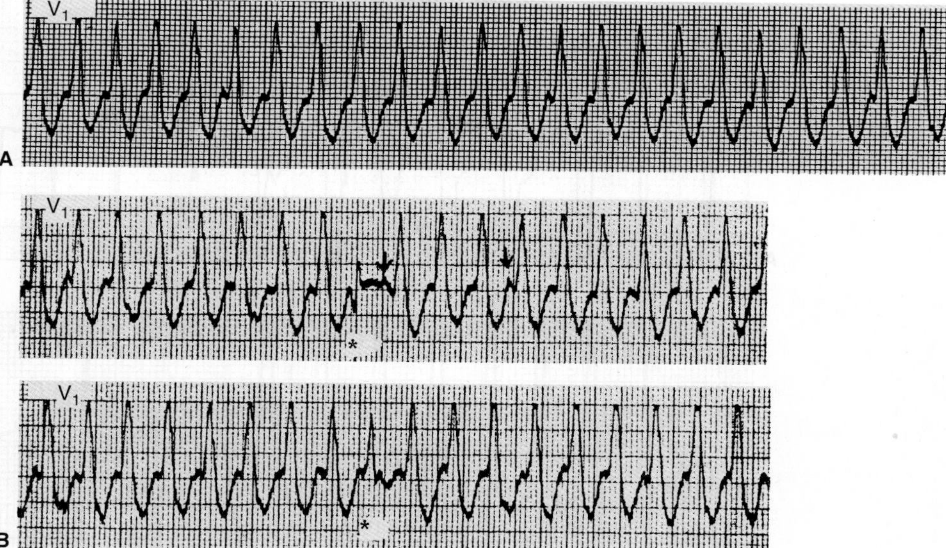

■ **Figure 16-30** (A) Wide QRS tachycardia at a rate of approximately 200 beats per minute. P waves are not easily recognizable, but the monophasic upright qRs morphology in V_1 favors VT. (B) Same patient with fusion beats among the wide QRS complexes (*asterisks*). *Arrows* point to P waves occurring independently of QRS complexes. Fusion beats and independent P waves are diagnostic of VT.

beat to conduct aberrantly if it occurs early (i.e., terminates a short cycle). This aberrant conduction usually occurs with RBBB because the right bundle branch has a longer refractory period than that of the left bundle branch. Thus, aberration tends to occur in early beats that cause a shortening of the cycle, such as PAC, or only in the first beat of a run of SVT. Ashman's phenomenon does not prove aberration, it merely explains it if it occurs. Therefore, the presence of a beat that meets Ashman criteria (i.e., terminates a short cycle that follows a long cycle) does not prove that the wide beat is aberrant, because a PVC could just as easily have occurred in the same spot.

Depending only on cycle lengths to aid in the differentiation of aberration from ectopy is unreliable for another reason as well. By the "rule of bigeminy," a long cycle can also precipitate a PVC.[98] The mechanism responsible for this seems to be that the area of unidirectional block that allows the reentry of the impulse in the ventricular myocardium is able to conduct the impulse in a retrograde direction only after a certain period of rest (i.e., a long cycle). Once a PVC has occurred, the pause that follows results in another long cycle, which allows another PVC; thus, ventricular bigeminy tends to perpetuate itself. Because a long preceding cycle can occur in both aberration and ectopy, it alone cannot be used with certainty in differentiating the two mechanisms. However, the absence of a long preceding cycle favors ectopy and is evidence against aberration.

AF presents special difficulties in the differentiation of wide QRS complexes. The absence of P waves prevents the use of P-wave clues, and the variations in cycle length that are common in AF or atrial flutter provide a perfect setup for both aberrant conduction and ventricular reentry. It is necessary to rely heavily on QRS morphology and it is helpful to compare cycle lengths. When comparing cycle sequences in AF or flutter, it is important to look at several sequences and not only at the sequence containing the beat with the wide QRS. Figure 16-31*A* shows atrial

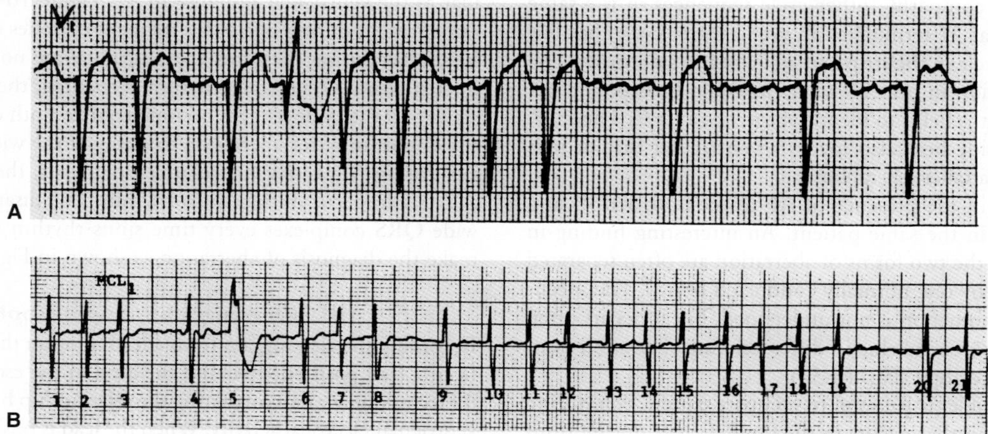

■ **Figure 16-31** (A) Atrial flutter with one aberrantly conducted beat. Note the triphasic rSR' complex of RBBB in V_1. (B) AF with a PVC (beat no. 5). The monophasic QRS with taller left "rabbit ear" favors a ventricular origin. Comparison of cycle lengths indicates that if any beat in this strip should be conducted aberrantly, it is beat no. 21, which terminates a short cycle after the longest cycle in the strip. If the heart can conduct beat 21 normally, there is no reason why it would conduct beat no. 5 aberrantly.

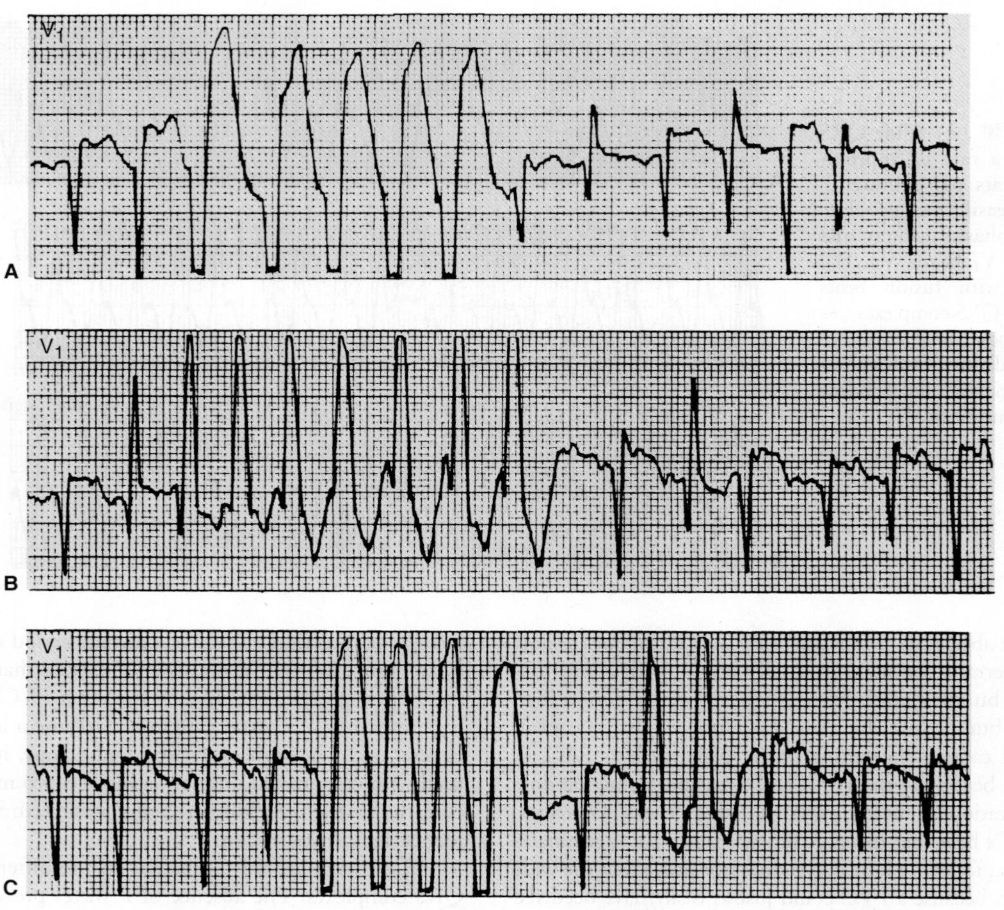

■ **Figure 16-32** AF with both (A) left and (B) right bundle-branch block aberration. (C) LBBB aberration and RBBB aberration are separated by a single normal beat. Note the irregularity of the wide QRS beats.

flutter with an aberrantly conducted beat that terminates a short cycle after a long cycle (i.e., Ashman's phenomenon). In Figure 16-31*B*, beat 5 terminates a cycle that is shorter than the preceding cycle, but, in comparing other cycle sequences in the same strip, note that beat 21 terminates an even shorter cycle that follows the longest cycle in the strip and still conducts normally. The absence of aberration in beat 21 where it would be expected because of cycle lengths helps to identify beat 5 as a PVC. The morphology of the wide beat also favors a ventricular origin: it is monophasic with a taller left rabbit ear.

It is common in the presence of AF to see both RBBB and LBBB aberration in the same patient. An interesting finding in many cases is that the two forms of aberration are often separated from one another by one normally conducted beat.[99] The mechanism of this phenomenon is not understood, but it occurs often enough to make it a useful clue in differentiating aberration from bifocal ventricular ectopy (Fig. 16-32).

Whenever possible, it is useful to compare conduction during AF with conduction that occurs in the same patient during sinus rhythm. Figure 16-33*A* is from a patient in AF with many episodes of LBBB aberration resembling VT. Note that whenever the ventricular response to AF slows even slightly, normal conduction resumes. Also note that the aberrantly conducted beats occur in an irregular pattern, just as the ventricular response to AF typically occurs, and that the morphology favors LBBB rather than VT. The irregularity is a helpful observation because VT, although it does not have to be perfectly regular, is seldom as irregular as the ventricular response to AF. Figure 16-33*B* is from the same patient during one of his frequent episodes of sinus rhythm. Note that during the sinus rhythm, there are no aberrantly conducted beats. When sinus rhythm is restored, the ventricular rate slows and the cycle lengths become regular, both of which remove the opportunity for aberration to occur. If the wide beats that occur during AF were ventricular ectopic beats, they would be just as likely to occur during sinus rhythm. The disappearance of the wide QRS complexes every time sinus rhythm is restored helps make the diagnosis of aberration as shown in Figure 16-33*A*.

Intra-atrial Electrograms and Esophageal Leads. Recording the electrogram from a lead in or on the right atrium or from a lead positioned behind the atria in the esophagus is a useful technique for demonstrating the relationship between atrial and ventricular electrical activity. When the lead is positioned in or very near the atria, atrial activity records as a large deflection and ventricular activity records as a smaller deflection, making it easier to see if P waves are associated with or dissociated from the QRS complexes. Figure 16-34 shows an intra-atrial recording from a patient with a wide QRS tachycardia in whom the diagnosis was uncertain.

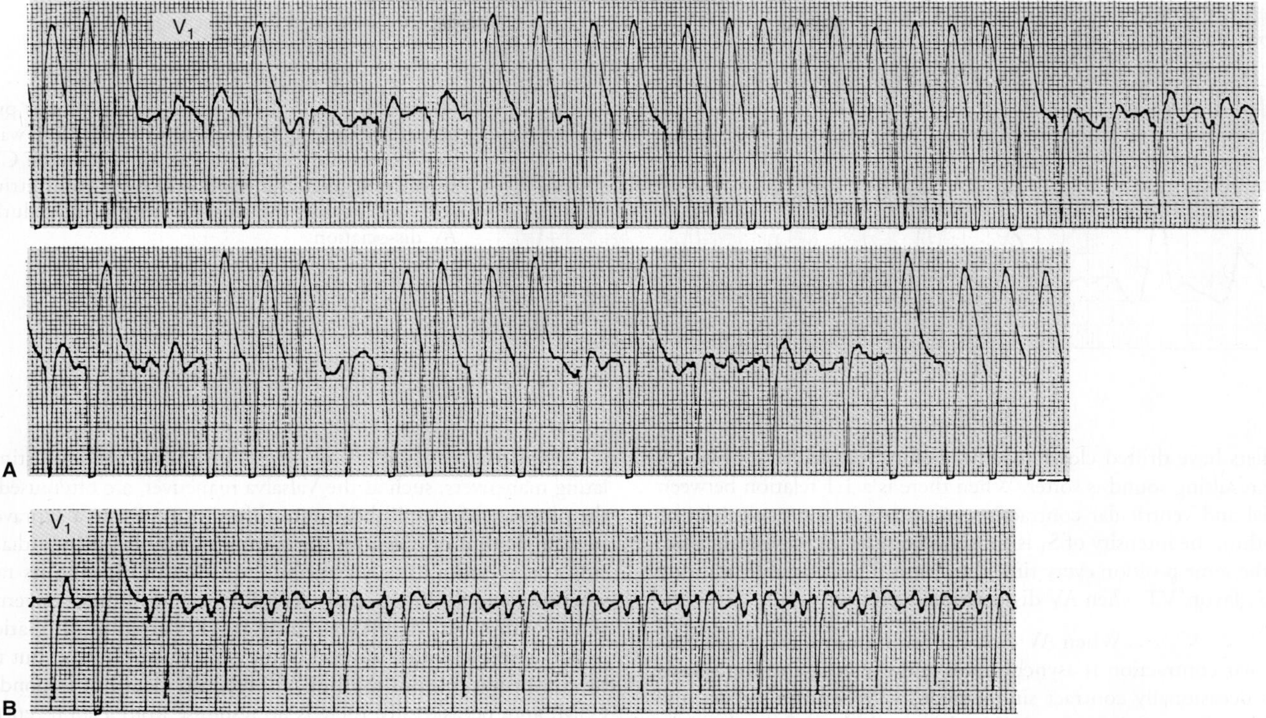

■ **Figure 16-33** (A) AF with frequent LBBB resembling VT. Normal conduction resumes whenever the ventricular rate slows even slightly. (B) Same patient during one of his frequent episodes of sinus tachycardia, restored after the second beat. During sinus tachycardia, no aberration occurs because the rate is slower and cycle lengths are regular, removing the opportunity for aberration.

AV dissociation is clearly present, as demonstrated by very large "P" waves and smaller QRS deflections. When recording an atrial electrogram, the recorder should be run at double the normal paper speed (i.e., at 50 mm/s instead of the usual 25 mm/s) to make it easier to differentiate atrial and ventricular activity.

Clinical Criteria

Several clinical criteria can be used to aid in the differentiation of aberration from ectopy.

Heart Sounds. Varying intensity of the S_1 heart sound occurs whenever the atrial activity is dissociated from ventricular activity, as frequently occurs in VT. The S_1 sound is produced by the closure of the AV valves, and its intensity depends on the proximity of the valve leaflets to one another at the time of ventricular systole. When atrial activity and ventricular activity are dissociated, the atria contract in variable relationship to the ventricles and the valve leaflets are at times wide open when ventricular systole occurs, causing a loud sound when they close. At other times, the

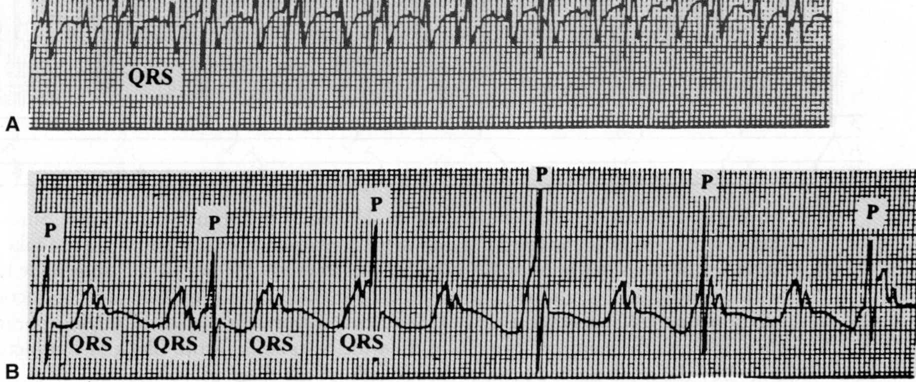

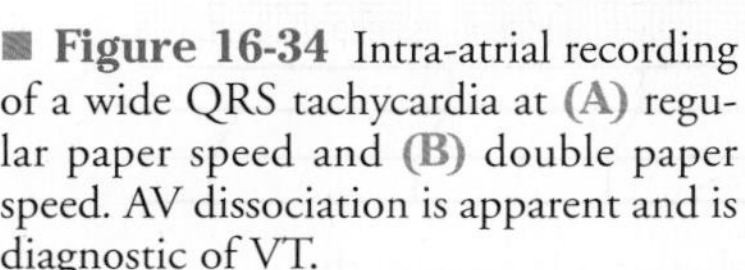

■ **Figure 16-34** Intra-atrial recording of a wide QRS tachycardia at (A) regular paper speed and (B) double paper speed. AV dissociation is apparent and is diagnostic of VT.

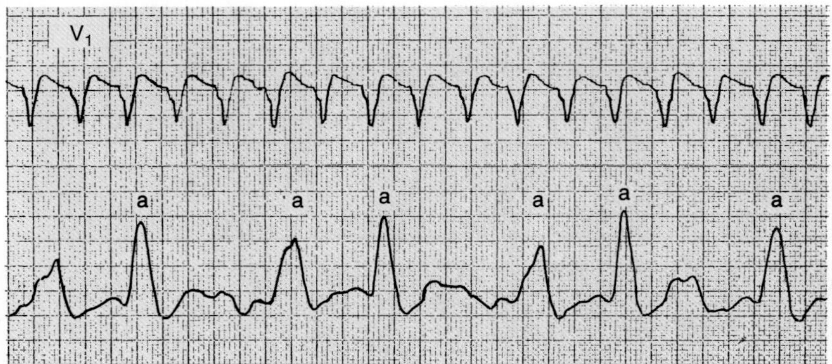

■ **Figure 16-35** ECG and a central venous pressure (CVP) tracing of a patient with VT. No P waves can be seen for certain in the ECG, but the CVP shows exaggerated a waves when the right atrium contracts against the closed tricuspid valve during AV dissociation.

leaflets have drifted closer together before ventricular systole and the resulting sound is softer. When there is a 1:1 relation between atrial and ventricular contraction, as occurs in a supraventricular rhythm, the intensity of S_1 is constant because the valve leaflets are in the same position every time they close. Thus, variable intensity of S_1 favors VT when AV dissociation is present.

Neck Veins. When AV dissociation is present, atrial and ventricular contraction is asynchronous and the atria and the ventricles occasionally contract simultaneously. When this occurs, the atria contract against closed AV valves, and blood from the right atrium has no place to go except back up into the neck veins. Observation of the patient's neck veins during AV dissociation reveals irregularly occurring "cannon a waves," which are large pulsations seen in the neck veins as blood is forced backward during atrial contraction. When atrial activity precedes ventricular activity, as it does in some SVT (e.g., sinus or AT), cannon a waves are not seen. When atrial activity occurs simultaneously with or after ventricular activity in a 1:1 relationship (as it may in junctional tachycardia or VT with retrograde conduction, AVNRT, or in CMT due to an accessory pathway), cannon a waves are often seen with each beat. No a waves at all occur in the presence of AF because the atria do not contract. Therefore, the presence of *irregularly occurring* cannon a waves in the jugular pulse or in the central venous pressure or pulmonary wedge pressure tracing in the presence of a wide QRS tachycardia favors VT (Fig. 16-35).

Response to Vagal Maneuvers. CSM or other vagal stimulating maneuvers, such as the Valsalva maneuver, are often used in the presence of a rapid heart rate either to terminate a supraventricular rhythm or diagnose the mechanism of the tachycardia. A sinus tachycardia usually responds to CSM by slowing its rate, whereas some SVT (especially AVNRT or CMT) may convert to sinus rhythm. Atrial rhythms, such as AT, flutter, or fibrillation, usually respond with a slowing of the ventricular response but not by conversion to sinus rhythm. VT typically does not respond to CSM, and, occasionally, there is no response from a supraventricular rhythm. Therefore, if the rate of the tachycardia slows in response to CSM or the rhythm converts to sinus rhythm, a supraventricular origin of the tachycardia is favored; if there is no response, neither aberration nor VT is favored.

AV Dissociation

AV dissociation means that the atria and ventricles are under the control of separate pacemakers and are beating independent of each other. Usually, the atria are controlled by the SA node, but they can also be under the control of an atrial focus, as in AT, flutter, or fibrillation. The ventricles can be under the control of a junctional pacemaker or a ventricular pacemaker. AV dissociation is not a primary arrhythmia but is always secondary to some other disturbance that results in dissociation. Complete AV dissociation

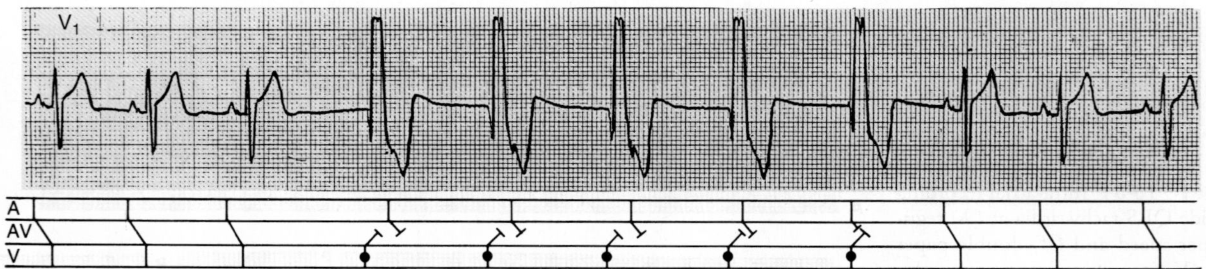

■ **Figure 16-36** AV dissociation due to slowing of the primary pacemaker. Sinus arrhythmia is present; the sinus rate slows after the third beat, allowing a ventricular escape pacemaker to take control of the ventricles at a rate of 60 beats per minute. AV dissociation lasts until the rate of the sinus node becomes faster than the rate of the ventricular pacemaker. The ladder diagram below the strip illustrates conduction through the atrium (A), AV junction (AV), and ventricle (V). Solid circles represent the site of origin of beats: the circles in the V level here indicate the ventricular origin of the wide beats in the strip. Block of conduction in the AV node is indicated by the small slashed lines in the AV level of the diagram.

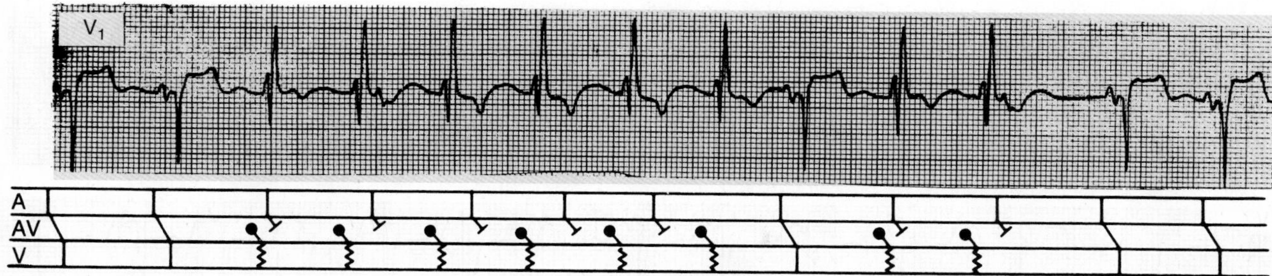

■ **Figure 16-37** AV dissociation due to acceleration of a subsidiary pacemaker. An accelerated junctional pacemaker assumes control of the ventricles and conducts aberrantly (RBBB) at a rate of 88 beats per minute. Sinus arrhythmia is present at a rate that is in the 70s. See the legend of Figure 16-36 for explanation of the ladder diagram below the strip. Vertical wavy lines in the V level indicate aberrant conduction through the ventricles.

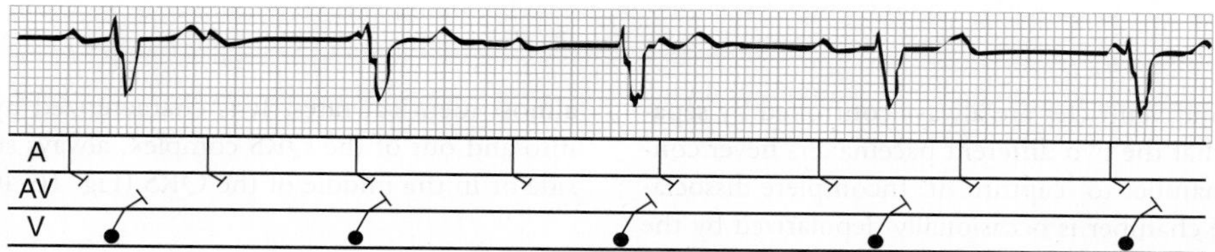

■ **Figure 16-38** AV dissociation due to complete AV block. Sinus rhythm at a rate of 65 beats per minute with third-degree AV block and a ventricular pacemaker controlling the ventricles at a rate of 38 beats per minute. See the legend of Figure 16-36 for explanation of the ladder diagram below the strip.

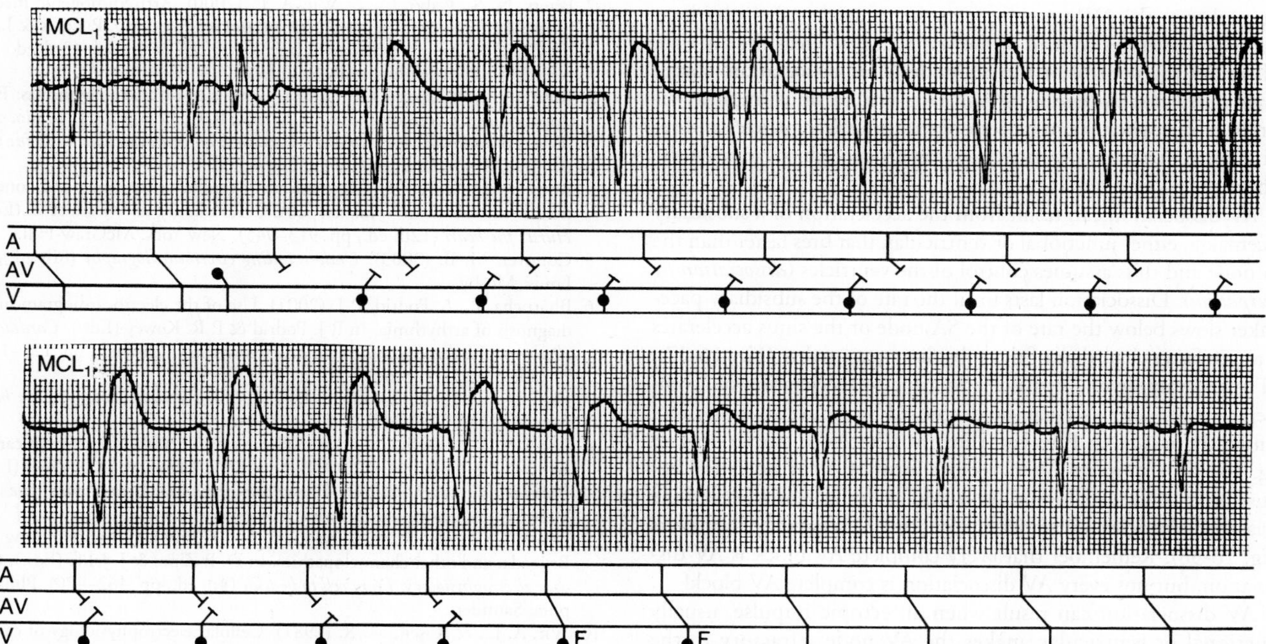

■ **Figure 16-39** AV dissociation due to interference. Strips are continuous. Sinus rhythm is present at a rate of 68 beats per minute. The third beat in the top strip is a PJC that causes refractoriness in the AV junction (gray area in AV level of ladder diagram). The refractory period created by the early beat interferes with conduction of the next sinus impulse, which is blocked in the AV node. The resulting pause allows a ventricular rhythm to emerge at a rate of 65 beats per minute. The bottom strip shows the slightly faster sinus P waves emerging in front of the QRS until ventricular capture occurs in the seventh beat. See the legend of Figure 16-36 for explanation of the ladder diagram drawn below the strips. The vertical wavy line under the PJC indicates aberrant conduction of that beat through the ventricles. F = fusion beats.

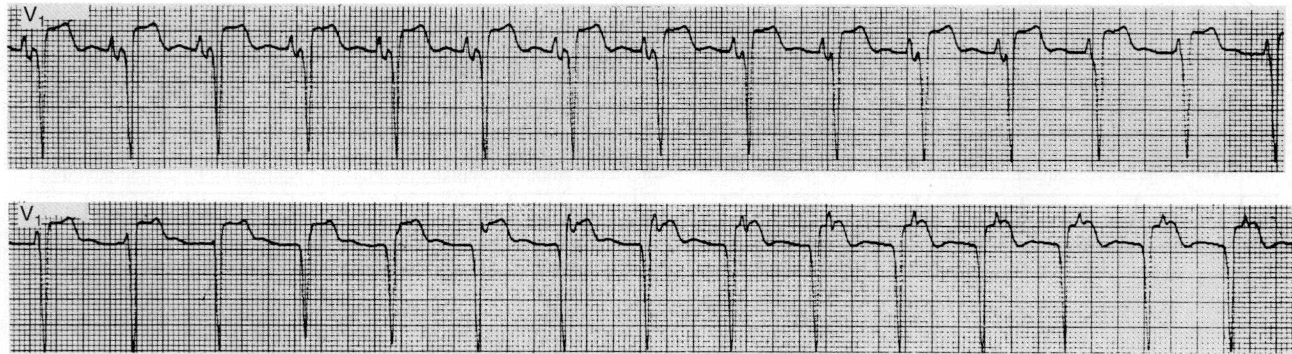

■ **Figure 16-40** Isorhythmic dissociation. There is dissociation between a sinus rhythm and a junctional rhythm, both at a rate of approximately 88 beats per minute. P waves disappear into the QRS complex toward the end of the top strip and emerge on the other side of the QRS in the bottom strip, always staying close to the QRS or in the middle of it.

means that the atria and ventricles are always controlled by separate pacemakers and that the two different pacemakers never conduct into the other chamber to "capture" it. Incomplete dissociation occurs when one chamber is occasionally depolarized by the other chamber's pacemaker.

AV dissociation can be secondary to (1) slowing of the primary pacemaker (SA node), (2) acceleration of a subsidiary pacemaker (AV junction or ventricle), (3) AV block, or (4) interference, or can result from a combination of these causes.[5,56,58]

If the rate of the SA node slows below the rate of a subsidiary pacemaker in the AV junction or in the ventricles, the subsidiary pacemaker assumes control of the ventricles, whereas the atria are still under the control of the SA node. This dissociation, sometimes called *dissociation by default*, lasts until a sinus impulse occurs at a time when it can be conducted into the ventricles and regain control of them or until it speeds up enough to override the subsidiary pacemaker (Fig. 16-36).

AV dissociation can result from the acceleration of a subsidiary pacemaker, either junctional or ventricular, that fires faster than the SA node and thus assumes control of the ventricles (*dissociation by usurpation*). Dissociation lasts until the rate of the subsidiary pacemaker slows below the rate of the SA node or the sinus accelerates to a rate faster than that of the subsidiary pacemaker (Fig. 16-37). VT is an example of AV dissociation due to acceleration of a ventricular pacemaker; VT can be diagnosed by demonstrating independently occurring P waves, thus proving AV dissociation (see Fig. 16-24). Complete AV block is a form of AV dissociation because none of the atrial impulses conducts to the ventricles and the atria and ventricles are under the control of separate pacemakers (Fig. 16-38). Remember that every complete AV block is AV dissociation, but not every AV dissociation is complete AV block!

AV dissociation can result when an ectopic impulse, usually junctional or ventricular, makes the AV node refractory to the next sinus impulse, interfering with the conduction of the sinus impulse and allowing another pacemaker to control the ventricles (Fig. 16-39). Anything that causes a pause in the rhythm, like a premature beat, a blocked P wave, or sudden termination of a tachycardia can allow the escape of a subsidiary pacemaker and result in AV dissociation.

The term *isorhythmic dissociation* refers to AV dissociation with the atrial focus and the focus that controls the ventricles firing at almost identical rates. It is characterized by P waves that move into and out of the QRS complex, always staying close on either side or in the middle of the QRS (Fig. 16-40).

REFERENCES

1. Antzelevitch, C., & Burashinikov, A. (2001). Mechanisms of arrhythmogenesis. In P. J. Podrid & P. R. Kowey (Eds.), *Cardiac arrhythmia: Mechanisms, diagnosis, and management* (2nd ed., pp. 51–79). Philadelphia: Lippincott Williams & Wilkins.
2. Peters, N. S., Cabo, C., & Wit, A. L. (2000). Arrhythmogenic mechanisms: Automaticity, triggered activity, and reentry. In D. P. Zipes & J. Jalife (Eds.), *Cardiac electrophysiology: From cell to bedside* (3rd ed., pp. 340–355). Philadelphia: W.B. Saunders.
3. Rubart, M., & Zipes, D. P. (2008). Genesis of cardiac arrhythmias: Electrophysiological considerations. In P. Libby, R. O. Bonow, D. L. Mann, et al. (Eds.), *Braunwald's heart disease: A textbook of cardiovascular medicine* (8th ed., pp. 727–762). Philadelphia: Elsevier Saunders.
4. Antzelevitch, C. (2008). Mechanisms of cardiac arrhythmias and conduction disturbances. In V. Fuster, R. A. O'Rourke, R. A. Walsh, et al. (Eds.), *Hurst's the heart* (12th ed., pp. 913–945). New York: McGraw-Hill.
5. Conover, M. B. (2003). *Understanding electrocardiography* (8th ed.). St. Louis: Mosby.
6. Bharucha, B., & Podrid, P. J. (2001). Use of the electrocardiogram in the diagnosis of arrhythmia. In P. J. Podrid & P. R. Kowey (Eds.), *Cardiac arrhythmia: Mechanisms, diagnosis and management* (2nd ed., pp. 127–164). Philadelphia: Lippincott Williams & Wilkins.
7. Hoffman, B. F., & Cranefield, P. F. (1960). *Electrophysiology of the heart.* New York: McGraw-Hill.
8. Priori, S. G., Napolitano, C., & Schwartz, P. J. (2008). Genetics of cardiac arrhythmias. In P. Libby, R. O. Bonow, D. L. Mann, & D. P. Zipes (Eds.), *Braunwald's heart disease: A textbook of cardiovascular medicine* (pp. 101–110). Philadelphia: Elsevier Saunders.
9. Priori, S. G., Rivolta, I., & Napolitano, C. (2004). Genetics of long QT, Brugada, and other channelopathies. In D. P. Zipes & J. Jalife (Eds.), *Cardiac electrophysiology: From cell to bedside* (4th ed., pp. 462–470). Philadelphia: Saunders.
10. Wit, A. L., & Rosen, M. R. (1981). Cellular electrophysiology of cardiac arrhythmias. Part I: Arrhythmias caused by abnormal impulse generation. *Modern Concepts in Cardiovascular Disease, 50*, 1–6.
11. Singer, D. H., & Cohen, H. C. (1995). Aberrancy: Electrophysiologic mechanisms and electrocardiographic correlates. In W. J. Mandel (Ed.), *Cardiac arrhythmias* (3rd ed., pp. 461–503). Philadelphia: J. B. Lippincott.
12. Rosen, M. R., & Danilo, P. (1979). Electrophysiological basis for cardiac arrhythmias. In O. S. Narula (Ed.), *Cardiac arrhythmias: Electrophysiology, diagnosis, management* (pp. 9–13). Baltimore: Williams & Wilkins.
13. Gadsby, D. C., Karagueuzian, H. S., & Wit, A. L. (1995). Normal and abnormal electrical activity in cardiac cells. In W. J. Mandel (Ed.), *Cardiac*

arrhythmias: Their mechanisms, diagnosis and management (3rd ed., pp. 55–82). Philadelphia: J. B. Lippincott.

14. Arnsdorf, M. F., & Ganz, L. I. (2006, February 2). *Sinus bradycardia.* Retrieved March 13, 2008, from www.uptodate.com.
15. Reiffel, J. A. (2001). Sinus node function and dysfunction. In P. J. Podrid & P. R. Kowey (Eds.), *Cardiac arrhythmia: Mechanisms, diagnosis, and management* (2nd ed., pp. 653–670). Philadelphia: Lippincott Williams & Wilkins.
16. Arnsdorf, M. F. (2006). Manifestations and causes of the sick sinus syndrome. *UpToDate.* Retrieved March 13, 2008, from www.uptodate.com
17. Podrid, P. J. (2005). Supraventricular premature beats. *UpToDate.* Retrieved March 13, 2008, from www.uptodate.com
18. Olgin, J. E., & Zipes, D. P. (2001). Specific arrhythmias: Diagnosis and treatment. In E. Braunwald, D. P. Zipes, & P. Libby (Eds.), *Heart disease* (6th ed., pp. 659–699). Philadelphia: W. B. Saunders.
19. Arnsdorf, M. F. (2007). Clinical characteristics of multifocal atrial tachycardia. *UpToDate.* Retrieved March 13, 2008, from www.uptodate.com.
20. Goldberger, J. J., & Kadish, A. H. (2001). Sinoartrial/atrial tachyarrhythmias. In P. J. Podrid & P. R. Kowey (Eds.), *Cardiac arrhythmia: Mechanisms, diagnosis, and management* (2nd ed., pp. 411–431). Philadelphia: Lippincott Williams & Wilkins.
21. Prystowsky, E. N., & Waldo, A. L. (2008). Atrial fibrillation, atrial flutter, and atrial tachycardia. In V. Fuster, R. A. O'Rourke, R. A. Walsh, et al. (Eds.), *Hurst's the heart* (12th ed., pp. 953–982). New York: McGraw-Hill.
22. Olgin, J. E., & Zipes, D. P. (2008). Specific arrhythmias: Diagnosis and treatment. In P. Libby, R. O. Bonow, D. L. Mann, et al. (Eds.), *Braunwald's heart disease: A textbook of cardiovascular medicine* (8th ed., pp. 863–932). Philadelphia: Saunders.
23. Arnsdorf, M. F. (2007). Focal atrial tachycardia. *UpToDate.* Retrieved March 13, 2008, from www.uptodate.com.
24. Tracy, C. (2007). Tachycardia-mediated cardiomyopathy. *UpToDate.* Retrieved March, 2008, from www.uptodate.com.
25. Blomstrom-Lundqvist, C., Scheinman, M. M., Aliot, E. M., et al. (2003). ACC/AHA/ESC guidelines for the management of patients with supraventricular arrhythmias—Executive summary. A report of the American College of Cardiology/American Heart Association Task Force on Practice Guidelines and the European Society of Cardiology Committee for Practice Guidelines (Writing Committee to Develop Guidelines for the Management of Patients With Supraventricular Arrhythmias). *Circulation, 108,* 1871–1909.
26. Ganz, L. I. (2006). Catheter ablation of atrial tachycardia. *UpToDate.* Retrieved March, 2008, from www.uptodate.com.
27. Arnsdorf, M. F. (2006). Electrocardiographic and electrophysiologic features of type I (typical) atrial flutter. *UpToDate.* Retrieved March 2008, from www.uptodate.com.
28. Waldo, A. L. (2004). Atrial flutter: Mechanisms, clinical features, and management. In D. P. Zipes & J. Jalife (Eds.), *Cardiac electrophysiology: From cell to bedside* (4th ed., pp. 490–499). Philadelphia: Saunders.
29. Arnsdorf, M. F. (2003). Electrocardiographic and electrophysiologic features of type II (atypical) atrial flutter. *UpToDate.* Retrieved March 2008, from www.uptodate.com.
30. Arnsdorf, M. F., & Ganz, L. I. (2005). Causes of atrial flutter. *UpToDate.* Retrieved March 2008, from www.uptodate.com.
31. Cheng, J., & Arnsdorf, M. F. (2007). Maintenance of sinus rhythm after cardioversion in atrial flutter. *UpToDate* Retrieved March 2008, from www.uptodate.com
32. Jahangir, A., Munger, T. M., & Packer, D. L. (2001). Atrial fibrillation. In P. J. Podrid & P. R. Kowey (Eds.), *Cardiac arrhythmia: Mechanisms, diagnosis, and management* (2nd ed., pp. 457–499). Philadelphia: Lippincott Williams & Wilkins.
33. Nattel, S., & Ehrlich, J. R. (2004). Atrial fibrillation. In D. P. Zipes & J. Jalife (Eds.), *Cardiac electrophysiology: From cell to bedside* (4th ed., pp. 512–522). Philadelphia: Saunders.
34. Fuster, V., Ryden, L. E., Asinger, R. W., et al. (2006). ACC/AHA/ESC guidelines for the management of patients with atrial fibrillation: Executive summary: A report of the American College of Cardiology/American Heart Association Task Force on Practice Guidelines and the European Society of Cardiology Committee for Practice Guidelines (Writing Committee to Revise the 2001 Guidelines for the Management of Patients with Atrial Fibrillation). *Circulation, 114,* 700–752.
35. Arnsdorf, M. F., & Podrid, P. J. (2006). Overview of the presentation and management of atrial fibrillation. *UpToDate* Retrieved March 2008, from www.uptodate.com.
36. Hohnloser, S. H., Kuck, K.-H., & Lilenthal, J. (2000). Rhythm or rate control in atrial fibrillation—Pharmacological intervention in atrial fibrillation (PIAF): A randomised trial. *Lancet, 356,* 1789–1794.
37. Van Gelder, I. C., Hagens, V. E., Bosker, H. A., et al. (2002). A comparison of rate control and rhythm control in patients with recurrent persistent atrial fibrillation. *New England Journal of Medicine, 347*(23), 1834–1840.
38. Wyse, G. D., Waldo, A. L., DiMarco, J., et al. (2002). A comparison of rate control and rhythm control in patients with atrial fibrillation. *New England Journal of Medicine, 347*(23), 1825–1833.
39. Carlsson, J., Miketic, S., Windeler, J., et al. (2003). Randomized trial of rate-control versus rhythm-control in persistent atrial fibrillation. *Journal of the American College of Cardiology, 41*(10), 1690–1696.
40. Opolski, G., Torbicki, A., Kosior, D., et al. (2004). Rate control vs rhythm control in patients with nonvalvular persistent atrial fibrillation. *Chest, 126,* 476–486.
41. Maisel, W., Kuntz, K., Reimold, S., et al. (1997). Risk of initiating antiarrhythmic drug therapy for atrial fibrillation in patients admitted to a university hospital. *Annals of Internal Medicine, 127,* 281–284.
42. Levy, S. (2004). Implantable atrial defibrillators for atrial fibrillation. In D. P. Zipes & J. Jalife (Eds.), *Cardiac electrophysiology: From cell to bedside* (4th ed., pp. 995–999). Philadelphia: Saunders.
43. Haissaguerre, M., Sanders, P., Jais, P., et al. (2004). Catheter ablation of atrial fibrillation: Triggers and substrate. In D. P. Zipes & J. Jalife (Eds.), *Cardiac electrophysiology: From cell to bedside* (4th ed., pp. 1028–1038). Philadelphia: Saunders.
44. Pappone, C., & Rosanio, S. (2004). Pulmonary vein isolation for atrial fibrillation. In D. P. Zipes & J. Jalife (Eds.), *Cardiac electrophysiology: From cell to bedside* (4th ed., pp. 1039–1052). Philadelphia: Saunders.
45. Ussia, G., Mangiafico, S., Privitera, A., et al. (2006). Percutaneous left atrial appendage transcatheter occlusion in patients with chronic nonvalvular atrial fibrillation: Early institutional experience. *Journal of Cardiovascular Medicine, 7*(8), 569–572.
46. Buxton, A. E., & Duc, J. (2001). Ventricular premature depolarizations and nonsustained ventricular tachycardia. In P. J. Podrid & P. R. Kowey (Eds.), *Cardiac arrhythmia: Mechanisms, diagnosis, and treatment* (2nd ed., pp. 549–572). Philadelphia: Lippincott Williams & Wilkins.
47. Bigger, J. T. (1983). Definition of benign versus malignant ventricular arrhythmias: Targets for treatment. *American Journal of Cardiology, 52,* 47C–54C.
48. Rho, R. W., & Page, R. L. (2008). Ventricular arrhythmias. In V. Fuster, R. A. O'Rourke, R. A. Walsh, & P. Poole-Wilson (Eds.), *Hurst's the heart* (12th ed., pp. 1003–1019). New York: McGraw-Hill.
49. Zipes, D. P., Camm, J. A., Borggrefe, M., et al. (2006). ACC/AHA/ESC 2006 guidelines for management of patients with ventricular arrhythmias and the prevention of sudden cardiac death—Executive summary: A report of the American College of Cardiology/American Heart Association Task Force and the European Society of Cardiology Committee for Practice Guidelines. *Circulation, 114,* 1088–1132.
50. Vos, M. A., & Crijns, H. J. (2004). Ventricular tachycardia in patients with hypertrophy and heart failure. In D. P. Zipes & J. Jalife (Eds.), *Cardiac electrophysiology: From cell to bedside* (4th ed., pp. 608–617). Philadelphia: Saunders.
51. Callans, D. J., & Josephson, M. E. (2004). Ventricular tachycardia in patients with coronary artery disease. In D. P. Zipes & J. Jalife (Eds.), *Cardiac electrophysiology: From cell to bedside* (4th ed., pp. 569–574). Philadelphia: Saunders.
52. Lerman, B. B., Stein, K. M., Markowitz, S. M., et al. (2004). Ventricular tachycardia in patients with structurally normal hearts. In D. P. Zipes & J. Jalife (Eds.), *Cardiac electrophysiology: From cell to bedside* (4th ed., pp. 668–682). Philadelphia: Saunders.
53. Field, J. M. (Ed.). (2005). *Advanced cardiovascular life support provider manual.* Dallas, TX: American Heart Association.
54. Arnsdorf, M. F., & Verdino, R. (2001). Atrioventricular nodal conduction abnormalities. In P. J. Podrid & P. R. Kowey (Eds.), *Cardiac arrhythmias: Mechanisms, diagnosis, and management* (2nd ed., pp. 671–691). Philadelphia: Lippincott Williams & Wilkins.
55. Vijayaraman, P., & Ellenbogen, K. A. (2008). Bradyarrhythmias and pacemakers. In V. Fuster, R. A. O'Rourke, R. A. Walsh, & P. Poole-Wilson (Eds.), *Hurst's the heart* (12th ed., pp. 1020–1054). New York: McGraw-Hill.
56. Schwartzman, D. (2004). Atrioventricular block and atrioventricular dissociation. In D. P. Zipes & J. Jalife (Eds.), *Cardiac electrophysiology: From cell to bedside* (4th ed., pp. 485–489). Philadelphia: Saunders.

57. Rusterholz, A. P., & Marriott, H. J. L. (1994). How long can the P-R interval be? *American Journal of Noninvasive Cardiology, 8*, 11–13.
58. Marriott, H. J. L. (1988). *Practical electrocardiography* (8th ed.). Baltimore: Williams & Wilkins.
59. Marinchak, R. A., & Rials, S. J. (2001). Tachycardias in Wolff–Parkinson–White syndrome. In P. J. Podrid & P. R. Kowey (Eds.), *Cardiac arrhythmia: Mechanisms, diagnosis, and management* (2nd ed., pp. 517–548). Philadelphia: Lippincott Williams & Wilkins.
60. Prystowsky, E. N., Yee, R., & Klein, G. (2004). Wolff–Parkinson–White syndrome. In D. P. Zipes & J. Jalife (Eds.), *Cardiac electrophysiology: From cell to bedside* (4th ed., pp. 869–883). Philadelphia: Saunders.
61. Wellens, H. J., & Conover, M. B. (2006). *The ECG in emergency decision making* (2nd ed.). St. Louis, MO: Elsevier Saunders.
62. Gallagher, J. J., Pritchett, E. C., Sealy, W. C., et al. (1978). The preexcitation syndromes. *Progress in Cardiovascular Diseases, 20*, 285–327.
63. Lindsay, B. D., Crossen, K. J., & Cain, M. E. (1987). Concordance of distinguishing electrocardiographic features during sinus rhythm with the location of accessory pathways in the Wolff–Parkinson–White syndrome. *American Journal of Cardiology, 59*, 1093–1102.
64. Opie, L. H., & Gersh, B. J. (2005). *Drugs for the heart* (6th ed.). Philadelphia: Elsevier Saunders.
65. Wagner, G. S. (2001). *Marriott's practical electrocardiography* (10th ed.). Philadelphia: Lippincott Williams & Wilkins.
66. Nelson, W. P., Marriott, H. J. L., & Schocken, D. D. (2007). *Concepts and cautions in electrocardiography*. Northglenn, CO: MedInfo.
67. Ernst, S., Ouyang, F., Antz, M., et al. (2004). Catheter ablation of atrioventricular reentry. In D. P. Zipes & J. Jalife (Eds.), *Cardiac electrophysiology: From cell to bedside* (4th ed.). Philadelphia: Saunders.
68. Miller, J. M., & Zipes, D. P. (2008). Therapy for cardiac arrhythmias. In P. Libby, R. O. Bonow, D. L. Mann, & D. P. Zipes (Eds.), *Braunwald's heart disease: A textbook of cardiovascular medicine* (pp. 779–830). Philadelphia: Elsevier Saunders.
69. Calkins, H. (2008). Supraventricular tachycardia: AV nodal reentry and Wolff–Parkinson–White syndrome. In V. Fuster, R. A. O'Rourke, R. A. Walsh, & P. Poole-Wilson (Eds.), *Hurst's the heart* (12th ed., pp. 983–1002). New York: McGraw-Hill.
70. Lockwood, D., Otomo, K., Wang, Z., et al. (2004). Electrophysiologic characteristics of atrioventricular nodal reentrant tachycardia: Implications for the reentrant circuits. In D. P. Zipes & J. Jalife (Eds.), *Cardiac electrophysiology: From cell to bedside* (4th ed., pp. 537–557). Philadelphia: Saunders.
71. Fogel, R. I., & Prystowsky, E. N. (2001). Atrioventricular nodal reentry. In P. J. Podrid & P. R. Kowey (Eds.), *Cardiac arrhythmia: Mechanisms, diagnosis, and management* (2nd ed., pp. 433–456). Philadelphia: Lippincott Williams & Wilkins.
72. Kalman, J. M. (2004). Catheter ablation of atrioventricular nodal reentrant tachycardia. In D. P. Zipes & J. Jalife (Eds.), *Cardiac electrophysiology: From cell to bedside* (4th ed., pp. 1069–1077). Philadelphia: Saunders.
73. Galvin, J. M., & Ruskin, J. N. (2004). Ventricular tachycardia in patients with dilated cardiomyopathy. In D. P. Zipes & J. Jalife (Eds.), *Cardiac electrophysiology: From cell to bedside* (4th ed., pp. 575–587). Philadelphia: Saunders.
74. Maron, B. F. (2004). Ventricular arrhythmias in hypertrophic cardiomyopathy. In D. P. Zipes & J. Jalife (Eds.), *Cardiac electrophysiology: From cell to bedside* (4th ed., pp. 601–607). Philadelphia: Saunders.
75. Fontaine, G., Fornes, P., Hebert, J.-L., et al. (2004). Ventricular tachycardia in arrhythmogenic right ventricular cardiomyopathies. In D. P. Zipes & J. Jalife (Eds.), *Cardiac electrophysiology: From cell to bedside* (4th ed., pp. 588–607). Philadelphia: Saunders.
76. Podrid, P. J. (2008). Polymorphic ventricular tachycardia in association with a normal QT interval. *UpToDate* Retrieved March 2008, from http://www.uptodateonline.com.
77. Priori, S. G., & Napolitano, C. (2008). Genetics of channelopathies and clinical implications. In V. Fuster, R. A. O'Rourke, R. A. Walsh, & P. Poole-Wilson (Eds.), *Hurst's the heart* (12th ed., pp. 885–897). New York: McGraw-Hill.
78. Napolitano, C., & Priori, S. G. (2004). Catecholaminergic polymorphic ventricular tachycardia and short-coupled torsades de pointes. In D. P. Zipes & J. Jalife (Eds.), *Cardiac electrophysiology: From cell to bedside* (4th ed., pp. 633–639). Philadelphia: Saunders.
79. Leenhardt, A., Glaser, E., Burguera, M., et al. (1994). Short-coupled variant of torsade de pointes: A new electrocardiographic entity in the spectrum of idiopathic ventricular tachyarrhythmias. *Circulation, 89*, 206–215.
80. Giusetto, C., Wolpert, C., Borggrefe, M., et al. (2006). Short QT syndrome: Clinical findings and diagnostic-therapeutic implications. *European Heart Journal, 27*(20), 2440–2447.
81. Pinto, D. S., & Josephson, M. (2008). Sudden cardiac death in the absence of apparent structural heart disease. *UpToDate*. Retrieved March 2008, from www.uptodate.com/online.
82. Gaita, F., Giusetto, C., Bianchi, F., et al. (2004). Short QT syndrome: Pharmacological treatment. *Journal of the American College of Cardiology, 43*, 1494–1499.
83. El-Sherif, N., & Turitto, G. (2004). Torsade de pointes. In D. P. Zipes & J. Jalife (Eds.), *Cardiac electrophysiology: From cell to bedside* (4th ed., pp. 687–699). Philadelphia: Saunders.
84. Hohnloser, S. H. (2001). Polymorphous ventricular tachycardia, including torsades de pointes. In P. J. Podrid & P. R. Kowey (Eds.), *Cardiac arrhythmia: Mechanisms, diagnosis, and management* (2nd ed., pp. 603–619). Philadelphia: Lippincott Williams & Wilkins.
85. Zimetbaum, P., & Josephson, M. E. (2008). Pathophysiology of the long QT syndrome. *UpToDate*. Retrieved April 2008, from www.uptodate.com/online.
86. Berul, C. I., Seslar, S. P., Zimetbaum, P., et al. (2007). Acquired long QT syndrome. *UpToDate*. Retrieved March 2008, from www.uptodate.com/online.
87. Schwartz, P. J., & Priori, S. G. (2004). Long QT syndrome: Genotype-phenotype considerations. In D. P. Zipes & J. Jalife (Eds.), *Cardiac electrophysiology: From cell to bedside* (4th ed., pp. 651–659). Philadelphia: Saunders.
88. Seslar, S. P., Zimetbaum, P., Berul, C. I., et al. (2007). Clinical features of congenital long QT syndrome. *UpToDate*. Retrieved March 2008, from www.uptodate.com/online.
89. Brugada, P., & Brugada, J. (1992). Right bundle branch block, persistent ST segment elevation and sudden cardiac death: A distinct clinical and electrocardiographic syndrome. *Journal of the American College of Cardiology, 20*, 1391–1396.
90. Antzelevitch, C., Brugada, P., Borggrefe, M., et al. (2005). Brugada syndrome: A report of the Second Consensus Conference. *Circulation, 111*, 659–670.
91. Wylie, J. V., Pinto, D. S., & Josephson, M. E. (2007). Brugada syndrome and sudden cardiac death. *UptoDate*. Retrieved April 2008, from www.uptodate.com/online.
92. Miller, J. M., Das, M., Arora, R., et al. (2004). Differential diagnosis of wide QRS complex tachycardia. In D. P. Zipes & J. Jalife (Eds.), *Cardiac electrophysiology: From cell to bedside* (4th ed., pp. 747–757). Philadelphia: Saunders.
93. Marriott, H. J. L., & Sandler, I. A. (1966). Criteria, old and new, for differentiating between ectopic ventricular beats and aberrant ventricular conduction in the presence of atrial fibrillation. *Progress in Cardiovascular Diseases, 9*(1), 18–28.
94. Kindwall, K., Brown, J., & Josephson, M. (1988). Electrocardiographic criteria for ventricular tachycardia in wide complex left bundle branch block morphology tachycardias. *American Journal of Cardiology, 61*, 1279–1283.
95. Brugada, P., Brugada, J., & Mont, L. (1991). A new approach to the differential diagnosis of a regular tachycardia with a wide QRS complex. *Circulation, 83*(5), 1649–1659.
96. Drew, B. J., Scheinman, M. M., & Dracup, K. (1991). MCL1 and MCL6 compared to V1 and V6 in distinguishing aberrant supraventricular from ventricular ectopic beats. *Pacing and Clinical Electrophysiology, 14*, 1375–1383.
97. Drew, B. J., & Scheinman, M. M. (1991). Value of electrocardiographic leads MCL1, MCL6, and other selected leads in the diagnosis of wide QRS complex tachycardia. *Journal of the American College of Cardiology, 18*, 1025–1033.
98. Langendorf, R., Pick, A., & Winternitz, M. (1955). Mechanisms of intermittent ventricular bigeminy: I. Appearance of ectopic beats dependent upon length of the ventricular cycle, the "rule of bigeminy." *Circulation, 11*, 422.
99. Marriott, H. J. L., & Conover, M. B. (1998). *Advanced concepts in arrhythmias* (3rd ed.). St. Louis, MO: Mosby.

DRUG INFORMATION REFERENCES

DiMarco, J. P. (2004). Adenosine and digoxin. In D. P. Zipes & J. Jalife (Eds.), *Cardiac electrophysiology: From cell to bedside* (4th ed., pp. 942–949). Philadelphia: Saunders.

Gillis, A. M. (2004). Class I antiarrhythmic drugs: Quinidine, procainamide, disopyramide, lidocaine, mexiletine, flecainide, and propafenone. In D. P. Zipes & J. Jalife (Eds.), *Cardiac electrophysiology: From cell to bedside* (4th ed., pp. 911–917). Philadelphia: Saunders.

Miller, J. M., & Zipes, D. P. (2008). Therapy for cardiac arrhythmias. In P. Libby, R. O. Bonow, D. L. Mann, et al. (Eds.), *Braunwald's heart disease: A textbook of cardiovascular medicine* (pp. 779–830). Philadelphia: Saunders.

Naccarelli, G. V., Sager, P. T., & Singh, B. N. (2001). Antiarrhythmic agents. In P. J. Podrid & P. R. Kowey (Eds.), *Cardiac arrhythmia: Mechanisms, diagnosis, and management* (2nd ed., pp. 265–301). Philadelphia: Lippincott Williams & Wilkins.

Opie, L. H., & Gersh, B. J. (2005). *Drugs for the heart* (6th ed.). Philadelphia: Elsevier Saunders.

Roden, D. M. (2006). Antiarrhythmics. In L. L. Brunton (Ed.), *Goodman and Gilman's the pharmacological basis of therapeutics* (11th ed., pp. 899–932). New York: McGraw-Hill.

Singh, B. N. (2004). Beta blockers and calcium channel blockers as antiarrhythmic drugs. In D. P. Zipes & J. Jalife (Eds.), *Cardiac electrophysiology: From cell to bedside* (4th ed., pp. 918–931). Philadelphia: Saunders.

Smith, T. W., & Cain, M. E. (2004). Class III antiarrhythmic drugs: Amiodarone, ibutilide, and sotalol. In D. P. Zipes & J. Jalife (Eds.), *Cardiac electrophysiology: From cell to bedside* (4th ed., pp. 932–941). Philadelphia: Saunders.

CHAPTER 17

Heart Rate Variability

Diana E. McMillan / Robert L. Burr

Heart rate variability (HRV) is the beat-to-beat variation of the cardiac cycle that results, in large part, from the interaction of sympathetic and parasympathetic inputs to the sinus node. The term "arrhythmia" often carries negative connotations, and many serious disturbances of heart rhythm and waveform morphology are malignant. However, some variation in the time between successive beats is normal, reflecting a healthy heart and healthy autonomic nervous system (ANS). A moderate amount of respiratory sinus arrhythmia (RSA), for example, is viewed as evidence of good cardiovascular health. In addition to short-term or beat-to-beat variation, a healthy individual also exhibits a marked circadian or 24-hour variation in heart rate.

Measures of HRV provide clinicians and researchers with a noninvasive, practical, reproducible, sensitive, and dynamic insight into the autonomic neural regulation of the heart. These measures are increasingly popular in cardiac care and are recognized as important diagnostic tools for risk identification in a wide range of cardiovascular conditions and health conditions that predispose cardiac complications.

This chapter provides a basic overview of the mechanisms of HRV, the approaches used in measuring HRV, and guidance for the interpretations of these measurements. Current research related to HRV patterns in common cardiovascular conditions and in health conditions predisposing cardiac complications is presented. General health history factors that can influence HRV patterns are discussed. The chapter concludes with a brief review of pharmacological and nonpharmacological interventions and their impact on HRV patterns.

MECHANISMS OF HRV

The beat-to-beat variation of the cardiac electrical signal expressed in normal sinus rhythm is termed HRV and is considered to be an index of ANS balance and imbalance. The time between successive beats is governed by the intrinsic firing rate of the sinoatrial (SA) node and the modulation of the SA node firing rate by input from the ANS. The input of the ANS is based on the relative contributions of the two ANS branches: the sympathetic nervous system (SNS) and the parasympathetic nervous system (PSNS). Thus, HRV does not reflect absolute sympathovagal input, but rather the relative dominance and interaction of these two ANS branches. PSNS activity normally dominates under conditions of rest and restoration. SNS activity predominance is associated with increased physiological arousal.

Complicating the interpretation of HRV indices aimed at identification of these respective ANS inputs are neural and nonneural factors that can modify the SA node firing rate. These factors include the central nervous system integration of cardiac neural input, positive feedback from sympathetic afferents, and negative feedback from baroreceptors and vagal afferents.[1] Despite our incomplete understanding of the physiological mechanisms associated with specific HRV measures, analysis of HRV provides significant clinical predictive usefulness within cardiac care.

HRV MEASUREMENT

HRV measures are statistical or mathematical summaries of within-subject variation in beat-to-beat heart period or instantaneous heart rate.[2] This section summarizes the principles behind some of the more common HRV measures.

General Considerations

The current diversity of HRV measures and nomenclature is partially caused by the relative novelty and rapid proliferation of these methods. It also reflects simultaneous independent development in several distinct disciplines by clinical researchers with very different purposes and very different typical sources of heart rhythm information. Most HRV measures are so strongly correlated with each other that they are nearly redundant. However, no one subset of HRV measures so consistently outperforms all the others, in all circumstances, that clear choices can be made. There have been several attempts at standardization of HRV measures and nomenclature,[3] but the recommendations have not been universally accepted, particularly in the interdisciplinary literature relevant to nursing.

Practically, the instantaneous heart period must be defined from a series of discrete events corresponding to the beating of the heart. This discrete event series itself is usually derived from fiducial features of the raw electrocardiograph (ECG) waveform. The arrival time of a beat, in particular the time interval from the previous beat, provides us with somewhat irregularly spaced information about short-term fluctuations in heart rhythm, and by inference, the dynamic autonomic control of the heart.[4,5]

Despite the variety of purposes motivating HRV analysis, the primary goal is usually to compute some within-subject or within-condition indices of heart rhythm variation to make some qualified inferences, not about the heart organ itself, but about the sympathetic and parasympathetic neural traffic impinging on the SA node of the heart. Thus it would be ideal to base the definition of the interbeat heart period on the interval between adjacent P waves to reflect as closely as possible the statistics of the firing of the SA pacemaker node.[6,7] However, the P-P interval is much harder to empirically define than the R-R interval, particularly from noisy low-frequency Holter recordings of ambulatory subjects. Most HRV studies, and essentially all of those performed using ambulatory ECG monitoring technology, use the R-R interval as the fundamental metric. Although it is conventional to speak of heart period as specific to a particular beat, an R-R interval is actually a measurement of the time interval between the R waves of

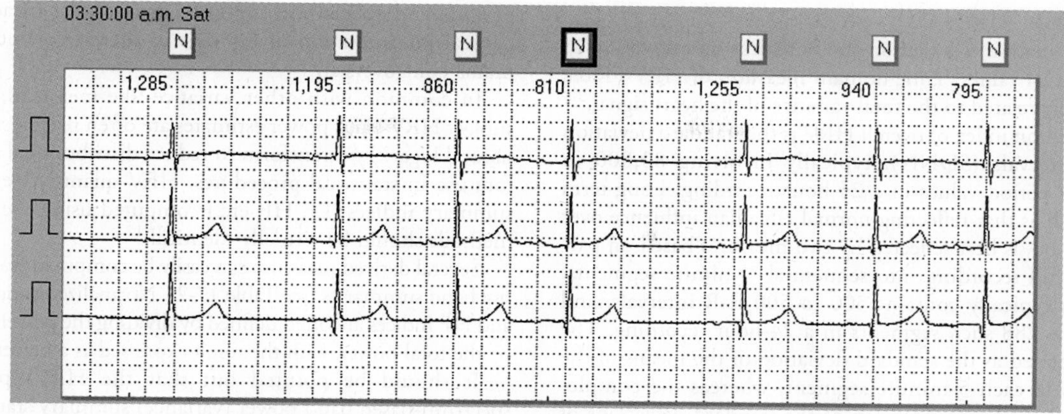

Figure 17-1 Example strip of ambulatory Holter ECG recorded during sleep. The beats are coded as Normal ("N"), and the R-R intervals (in milliseconds) for each overlapping pair of beats are displayed above and slightly to the left of the R wave that terminates the interval. Two respiratory cycles of probable RSA are visually apparent in the strip. Note that the measured sequential R-R intervals vary considerably within a few seconds for this high HRV subject.

two successive normal beats, sometimes called an NN doublet (Fig. 17-1).

The quality of HRV indices is ultimately dependent on the consistency of the basic measurement of each R-R interval. In modern digital applications, the R-R interval is partially determined by the sampling rate of the raw ECG, and also by characteristics of the R-wave location finding algorithm. Typical sampling rates may vary from approximately 100 Hz (samples per second), still common in long time scale ambulatory monitoring, to 1,000 Hz or faster in laboratory studies. In general, a higher digital waveform sampling rate allows proportionally more precision in the estimation of the location of the R waves at the cost of greater processing and memory requirements. However, the resulting apparent gain in precision may be illusory in ambulatory ECG recordings that contain noise and morphologies that vary slightly with posture and activity.

The R-R intervals thus decoded from the raw ECG can be placed into an ordered temporal sequence to form a time series, in which the continuous length of each cardiac cycle is an interval measure of time, usually reported in units of milliseconds(ms). Each R-R interval may be inverted to a beat-specific instantaneous equivalent heart rate, which can be considered the heart rate in beats per minute that would have been observed if all the heart beats in a 60-second period had exactly the length of that specific individual interval.[5]

HRV Measures

Although there are a variety of approaches used to analyze HRV, the two major procedures are time domain analysis and frequency domain analysis. Definitions for HRV measures based on these approaches are presented in Tables 17-1 and 17-2, respectively.

Table 17-1 ■ DESCRIPTION OF TIME DOMAIN MEASURES OF HRV

Measure	Units	Description
Mean RR	ms	Mean of all NN intervals
SDNN	ms	Standard deviation of all NN intervals
CoV		Coefficient of variation, equal to 100 × SDNN/(mean RR)
SDANN	ms	Standard deviation of the averages of NN intervals in all 5-minute segments of the recording
SDNN index	ms	Mean of the standard deviations of all NN intervals in all 5-minute segments of the recording
rmsSD	ms	Square root of the mean squared differences between successive NN intervals
pNN50	%	Number of successive NN intervals differing by more than 50 ms divided by the total number of successive NN intervals, expressed as a percentage

ms, milliseconds.

Table 17-2 ■ DESCRIPTION OF FREQUENCY DOMAIN MEASURES OF HRV

Measure	Units	Description
PSD plot	ms^2/Hz	Plot of power spectral density (PSD) versus frequency; frequency range is generally less than 0.4 Hz
Total power	ms^2	Area under PSD curve, equal to the variance of the segment; segment length can be short (5 minutes) or entire recording
LF	ms^2	Power in the LF band between 0.04 and 0.15 Hz; it reflects both sympathetic and parasympathetic activity
HF	ms^2	Power in the HF band between 0.15 and 0.4 Hz; it predominantly reflects parasympathetic activity
LF:HF		Ratio of LF power to HF power; a higher number indicates increased sympathetic activity or reduced parasympathetic activity
LFnu	%	Low-frequency power in normalized units, LF/(LF + HF), expressed as a percentage
HFnu	%	High-frequency power in normalized units, HF/(LF + HF), expressed as a percentage

LF, low frequency; HF, high frequency.

Time Domain Analysis

Time domain analysis is based on the statistical interpretation of R-R time interval values. Time domain measures of HRV (Table 17-1) are closely related to the total variance of the heart signal.[3,8] The most common index of overall HRV is the standard deviation of all R-R intervals (SDNN), typically involving 80,000 to 150,000 heart period values in a 24-hour recording. Long-term variability, such as that reflecting normal circadian influence over a 24-hour period, is best reflected by two measures based on partitioning the full recording into sequential 5-minute segments. Each segment typically contains 300 to 500 R-R intervals, and there would be 288 such segments in a 24-hour recording. The SDANN is defined as the standard deviation of the means of the R-R intervals in each 5-minute segment, whereas the complementary SDNN index is the mean of the standard deviations of the R-R intervals in each 5-minute segment.

Short-term time domain measures of HRV are derived from the differences of successive normal R-R intervals. They are highly correlated and are considered to provide good estimates of PSNS activity.[3] Short-term measures include the square root of the mean squared difference of successive normal R-R intervals (rmsSD) and the percentage of successive normal R-R intervals that change by more than 50 milliseconds compared with the total number of R-R intervals (pNN50).

Frequency Domain Analysis

Frequency domain analysis, or spectral analysis, is an elegant method for studying the rhythmic components in an R-R interval sequence and presents intriguing possibilities for disentangling PSNS and SNS influences on the heart.[9] A plot of the power spectral density of HRV versus frequency describes how the variances of the frequency components of the heart signal are distributed.[3]

Both parametric and nonparametric methods common to time series analysis have been used to estimate the power spectral density. The most common methods are the discrete Fourier transform (DFT) (nonparametric) and autoregressive (AR) (parametric) time series models. The AR model-based spectrum is usually less computationally efficient than the DFT, but it can be applied to data sequences of arbitrary length, including very short segments. The AR approach tends to produce a spectrum that is statistically more stable than that produced by the DFT but requires assumptions about the time series model.[3]

The total area under the curve of the power spectral density versus frequency plot is equal to the total statistical variance, or the power of the signal. These power (variance) distributions are calculated for defined frequency bands and are interpreted as an estimate of the variance of the HRV signal within that band (Table 17-2). There are two major spectral components seen in HRV data: the high-frequency (HF) (0.15–0.40 Hz) component and the low-frequency (LF) (0.04–0.15 Hz) component (Fig. 17-2). The HF component is associated with respiration[8,10] and is considered to reflect the relative input of the PSNS. The basis of the LF component is more controversial and may be the result of both SNS and PSNS activity input.[11] The LF to HF ratio (LF:HF) has been regarded as reflecting the balance between the mixed PSNS and SNS activity input to the PSNS activity input.[3] The spectral HF and the LF:HF are often reported together in nursing research studies seeking to explore the joint contribution of the SNS and the PSNS branches to HRV phenomena. Studies of very low-frequency and ultra-low-frequency ranges have also been conducted but require long uninterrupted sampling periods and specialized methods of analysis. In addition, the clinical interpretation of findings in these frequency ranges remains controversial.[3]

In common with other variance-like measures, the within-subject HRV band power estimates are often reexpressed using the natural logarithm transform to reduce distributional skewness before use in statistical procedures. HRV quantitative band power summary indices (LF, HF, etc.) computed using the AR or DFT methods should be virtually identical.[12]

Several derived measures can easily be computed from these spectral band summaries (see Table 17-2). Normalized variants of the LF and HF indices are often defined by dividing the power in each band by the total power, with the result expressed as a percentage.[13]

It should be pointed out that the HRV spectrum and spectrum-based band power (variance) summary statistics, like all HRV measures, are defined over blocks of R-R intervals; thus, their meaning is not localized to a particular instant in time or to a particular beat. Typical block window lengths in clinical and research applications range from 2 minutes to 24 hours. Spectra derived from shorter blocks are more localized in time and are more likely to be internally stationary but may have less frequency resolution, especially with respect to slower rhythm patterns. HRV spectra based on very long individual blocks (e.g., 24 hours) will have the ability to resolve very slow rhythmic patterns but will almost certainly span nonstationary data segments and heterogeneous latent autonomic states.

HRV PATTERNS IN COMMON CARDIOVASCULAR CONDITIONS

The following section provides a summary of HRV research findings in myocardial infarction (MI); arrhythmias and sudden death; angina; hypertension (HTN); heart failure; and cardiac surgery, heart transplant, and other invasive procedures. The reader should refer to related chapters for more detailed descriptions of these conditions and interventions.

Myocardial Infarction

It is well established that HRV patterns are disturbed in patients who have experienced MI.[14–17] In post-MI patients, those with restrictive left ventricular filling have been reported to have especially reduced HRV patterns compared with those without this disorder.[18]

Decreased HRV after MI is viewed as a significant risk factor for cardiac death[16,17] or subsequent nonfatal MI within 12 months.[19] HRV measures of total variability, such as SDNN and SDANN, are viewed as the most useful predictors of mortality.[3,16] Erratic sinus rhythms (sinus arrhythmia of nonrespiratory origin) as identified by abnormal Poincaré plots in post-MI patients are significant risk markers for increased mortality at follow-up.[17] Results from a landmark study, the Multicenter Post-Infarction Project, indicate that patients with an SDNN of less than 50 milliseconds (24-hour recording), measured within 11 days of the MI, have a risk of mortality at 1 year that is 5.3 times higher than do patients with an SDNN greater than 100 milliseconds.[20] Predicted risk is also increased for patients with below-normal SDNN and SDANN values in the chronic phase after MI. Reported normal lower limits measured in patients, at least 3 months after MI,

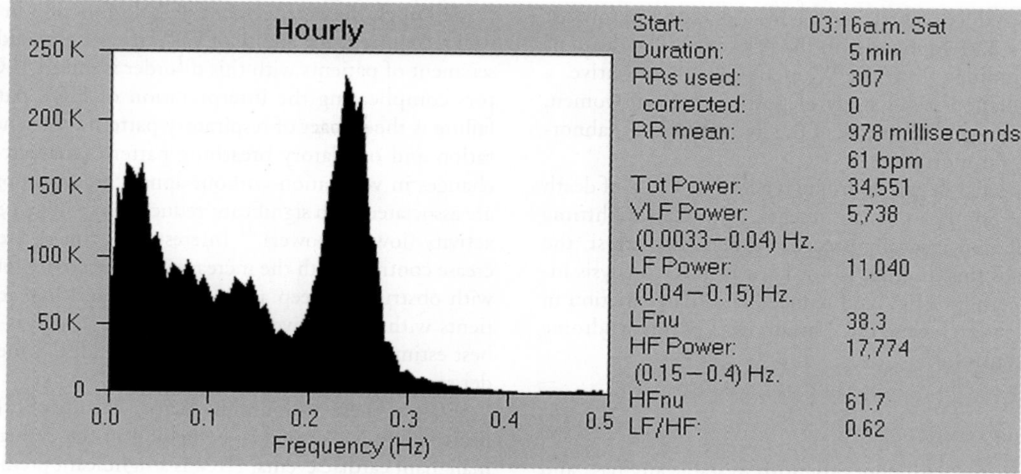

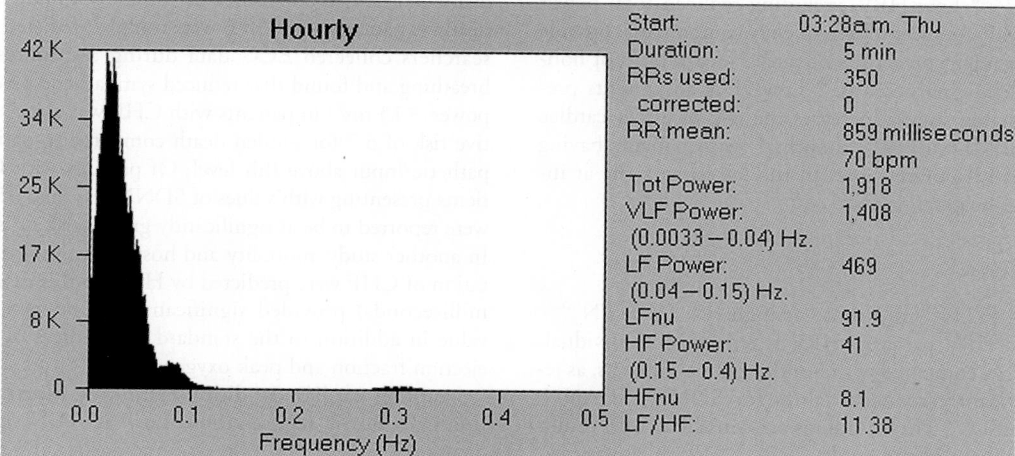

■ **Figure 17-2** Two 5-minute HRV power/variance spectra based on data collected on a single male subject with diabetes during sleep between 3 and 4 a.m. The top figure is based on data collected in 1992 when the subject was 42 years of age. The average heart rate of the analysis segment is 61 beats per minute, and the HRV spectrum demonstrates high total power/variance with a well-developed mid-frequency peak at 0.25 Hz, probably reflective of vagally mediated RSA. The lower figure is based on data collected from the same subject a decade later in 2002, when he was 52 years old. The average heart rate of the nocturnal analysis segment is 70 beats per minute. The total power of the HRV spectrum is an order of magnitude less, and while the low frequency peak has diminished, the high frequency peak is significantly attenuated. The quantitative band power and derived measure summaries appear in the table to the right of each figure, and document that the HF power is lower and the LF:HF much increased in the lower figure. The changes over time may reflect the joint influence of aging and diabetes. VLF, very low frequency.

range between 63 and 89 milliseconds for SDNN and between 57 and 79 milliseconds for SDANN.[16,21] Reduced circadian variation in the cardiac signal, reduced total power, and a shift toward sympathetic predominance as reflected by an increased LF:HF are also seen after MI.[3]

While HRV measures can provide independent risk prediction, the combination of HRV indices with other cardiovascular risk factors can enhance prediction of cardiac events. In a prospective study of 304 patients with acute coronary syndrome without ST-segment elevation, a combination of risk factors including clinical data, troponin T concentrations, ST-segment monitoring, and HRV provided a prediction of risk for ischemic death or nonfatal MI of 40% in the first 30 days and of 46.9% in the first 12 months.[19]

Arrhythmias and Sudden Death

HRV studies indicate autonomic disturbance before arrhythmia, although the pattern of disturbance varies. Clinical research supports that reduced parasympathetic tone and increased sympathetic tone predisposes ventricular fibrillation and ventricular tachycardia.[22] The onset of paroxysmal atrial fibrillation has been reported to follow autonomic changes characterized by an initial steady increase in SNS activity and a subsequent sharp predominance in PSNS activity.[23]

Reduced HRV is a consistent finding in a review of studies monitoring sudden death or sudden death and malignant arrhythmias.[24] In a prospective study ($N = 1071$) of post-MI patients, reduced HRV independently contributed to the risk of sudden death and or sustained ventricular tachycardia.[22] The combination of low HRV, nonsustained ventricular tachycardia, and baroreflex sensitivity led to a 22-fold increase in the risk for sudden death or sustained VT. Findings from the Women's Health Initiative, a prospective, population-based study of postmenopausal women, identify a reduction in HRV as one of the five major ECG abnormality predictors for mortality.[25]

Sudden unexpected death syndrome is a leading cause of death in young men of Southeast Asian descent. Although nighttime ventricular fibrillation typically precedes the cardiac arrest, the pathophysiology of this disorder is not known. HRV analysis indicates reduced 24-hour HRV and reduced circadian variation in HRV, with very low-nighttime HRV in survivors of this syndrome compared with controls.[26]

Angina

Low HRV is associated with poor prognosis in stable angina[27] and unstable angina.[19,28] Low HRV, including reduced total power and reduced HF, LF, and very low-frequency components, provide strong and independent predictors of cardiac death but not nonfatal MI in stable angina pectoris.[27] Low HRV in patients presenting with unstable angina increases the risk of either cardiac death or nonfatal MI within 12 months,[19] with patients having SDNN, HF, and LF power values in the lowest quartile at increased risk for in-hospital death.[28]

Hypertension

Individuals with HTN[29] and those at high risk for HTN[30,31] exhibit abnormal HRV patterns. HRV is reduced in individuals with essential HTN compared with healthy control subjects, as reflected in significantly reduced values for SDNN, SDANN, pNN50, and rmsSD.[32] These findings are consistent with results from the Framingham Heart Study ($N = 1{,}919$), a prospective epidemiological study of coronary risk factors. Singh et al.[31] found significant reductions in time domain measures of HRV in men and women with HTN compared with normotensive subjects. Hypertensive patients also exhibit a lower than normal vagal tone (low HF).[31,32]

Some HTN studies indicate a significant increase in mixed SNS and PSNS activity, reflected by increased resting LF power.[32,33] However, results from the Framingham Heart Study indicate reduced LF activity in patients with HTN and suggest that low vagal tone is a strong risk factor for the development of HTN in men.[31] Methodological differences in covariate adjustment may have contributed to inconsistent study findings.

The normal circadian pattern of HRV is disturbed in patients with HTN. In normotensive individuals, the nighttime fall in blood pressure is paralleled by a corresponding reduction in the mixed PSNS and SNS activity marker LF. This nocturnal drop in LF power is not as great in subjects with HTN.[29]

Heart Failure

Patients with congestive heart failure (CHF) have reduced HRV.[34] The most consistently reported finding is a reduction in SDNN.[35–38] Some researchers report a significant early increase in sympathetic predominance (high LF:HF) using a paced canine model of CHF.[39] This initial SNS surge appears to be lost as the condition worsens.[34] Reduced vagal activity (low HF) and reduced total power have also been reported in patients with CHF.[34]

Although the derangement of ANS function in heart failure is well recognized, the ability of HRV measures to aid in the risk assessment of patients with this disorder is mixed.[40] One of the factors complicating the interpretation of HRV patterns in heart failure is the impact of respiratory patterns. Cheyne–Stokes respiration and oscillatory breathing pattern (characterized by cyclic changes in ventilation without apnea) are common in CHF and are associated with significant reductions in mixed SNS and PSNS activity (low LF power).[41] Interestingly, this severe LF power decrease contrasts with the increase in SNS activity found in patients with obstructive sleep apnea, hypoxia, and hypercapnia. For patients with obstructive sleep apnea, the LF:HF is considered the best estimator of the apnea/hypopnea index, a measure of disorder severity.[42]

Despite these confounding factors, the use of HRV measures in heart failure is reported to be helpful in the evaluation of risk for malignant cardiac events. HRV is a significant predictor for sudden death.[35–38] Based on a multivariate survival model, risk of sudden death in patients with CHF was strongly predicted by HRV.[37] Researchers collected ECG data during 8 minutes of controlled breathing and found that reduced sympathetic predominance (LF power $\leq 13\ ms^2$) in patients with CHF was associated with a relative risk of 3.7 for sudden death compared to patients with sympathetic input above this level. Of patients with CHF, those patients presenting with values of SDNN less than 65.3 milliseconds were reported to be at significantly greater risk for sudden death.[35] In another study, mortality and hospitalization caused by deterioration of CHF were predicted by HRV. In this case, SDNN (<75 milliseconds) provided significant and independent predictive value in addition to the standard risk indices of left ventricular ejection fraction and peak oxygen intake.[36]

Another cardiac condition exhibiting disturbed ANS functioning is aortic regurgitation. Low SDANN significantly predicted risk of death or progression to aortic valve repair in a study of 50 asymptomatic or minimally symptomatic patients with chronic severe aortic regurgitation.[43]

Cardiac Surgery, Heart Transplantation, and Other Invasive Procedures

Cardiovascular surgery has been shown to have an impact on HRV patterns. Results from the Cardiac Arrhythmia Suppression Trial indicate that HRV is significantly reduced in post-MI patients after coronary artery bypass graft (CABG) surgery and that this reduction in HRV is not associated with increased mortality.[44] This finding contrasts with the increased risk of mortality seen in post-MI Cardiac Arrhythmia Suppression Trial patients who did not undergo CABG surgery but who did exhibit reduced HRV, specifically reduced SDANN. This important finding may help to explain the lower than predicted mortality rates seen in some post-CABG surgery patients. Similar reductions in HRV were reported in a Danish study of CABG patients without a recent MI and with ejection fractions of 0.36 ± 0.07.[45] These researchers found significantly reduced HRV immediately post-CABG and at the 6-month follow-up. Furthermore, improvement in myocardial function seen after surgery was not associated with post-CABG measures of HRV.

Heart transplant patients exhibit significantly reduced HRV immediately after surgery.[34] This reduction continues to be significantly reduced 2 years after surgery despite evidence of a return to near-normal cardiac-specific sympathetic nerve firing. This finding suggests insufficient or dysfunctional reinnervation of the cardiac muscle, and particularly the SA node with respect to ANS nerve fiber communication.[34]

Biventricular pacing enhanced ANS functioning in a study of 13 patients with heart failure and ventricular conduction disturbances.[46] In this surgical procedure, chronic cardiac resynchronization is achieved through the permanent implanting of a pacemaker. Significant increases were found in several measures of HRV, although not in LF power. Larger samples and survival impact analysis are needed to confirm these early but positive findings.

Other cardiac procedures have been explored with respect to HRV. Transmyocardial laser revascularization[47] and percutaneous transluminal angioplasty[48] are not associated with a significant change in HRV after procedure, but left ventricular reduction is associated with significant reduction in HRV.[47]

Noncardiac surgeries can also have an impact on postoperative HRV patterns. Reduced 24-hour HRV is found in the postoperative period after major abdominal surgery.[49] Significantly improved HRV has been noted in patients receiving kidney transplants and for those patients with kidney–pancreas transplants.[50] Measures of HRV may provide an indication of recovery in transplantation associated with disorders of autonomic neuropathy.

FACTORS INFLUENCING HRV

Several factors have been found to influence HRV and are important considerations for HRV interpretation. The following section provides a summary of the influences of age, sex, genetics, sleep and wake, body position, general health, and acute and chronic disorders on HRV. Readers should refer to Chapter 8 for a detailed review of sleep.

Age

HRV tends to decrease with increasing age.[51–54] This decline is caused by decreases in absolute PSNS and SNS activity and by reductions in their relative dominance.[9,55] Premature very low-birthweight infants have a better developed SNS but an underdeveloped PSNS.[56]

Stimulus challenge tests, such as active standing, are frequently included in assessments of ANS function. Test results should be interpreted within the context of the patient's age because responses to sympatho-excitatory (i.e., active standing) and sympatho-inhibitory (i.e., cold face challenge) stimuli decrease with age.[57]

Sex and Sex Hormones

Sex and the interaction of sex and age appear to influence HRV. Healthy women typically have higher heart rates and less HRV than healthy men.[53,58,59] Young men are reported to exhibit particularly high values in vagal-related indices (rmsSD, SDNN).[58] Other studies support that lower sympathetic predominance (low LF) and higher vagal activity (high HF) are seen in middle-aged women.[55,60] Sex disparities in HRV values diminish with increasing age,[58] disappearing entirely by 60 years of age,[59,60] and possibly as early as 40 years of age.[21]

The impact of endogenous sex hormones on ANS activity has been explored. HRV is not significantly different across menstrual phases, although heart rate is increased at ovulation. Positive correlations between peak estrogen levels at ovulation and LF power ($p = .05$), HF power ($p = .05$), and total power ($p = .05$) lend modest support for the claim that estrogen has cardioprotective effects.[61]

Genetics

Genetic factors influence many aspects of health, including HRV.[62–64] Genetic components are estimated to contribute 13% to 23% of the variance in HRV measures.[63] Genetic testing provides suggestive but nonsignificant evidence linking LF power to chromosome 2 at 153 cM and linking very low-frequency power to chromosome 15 at 62 cM.[64] Increased HRV is also associated with the genotype factor described as polymorphisms in angiotensin-converting enzyme gene.[62]

Sleep and Wake

Significant autonomic activity differences between wake and sleep and within different sleep states have been identified. HRV is normally characterized by greater variability during sleep than wake in adults[65] and children.[66] This sleep-associated increase in variability persists even after controlling for behavioral rhythms,[67] daytime physical activity, posture,[68] and shift work.[69]

Sleep is characterized by two major states: nonrapid eye movement (NREM) sleep and rapid eye movement (REM) sleep. NREM sleep is further divided into three stages, generally characterized by progressively lower-frequency and higher-amplitude brain wave activity.[70] Low-voltage, mixed-frequency brain wave activity, rapid saccadic eye movements, and CNS-invoked low skeletal muscle tone denote REM sleep. Individuals typically cycle between NREM and REM sleep approximately five times over the course of the night, with the proportion of REM sleep increasing across the night.

Not surprisingly, HRV patterns differ between NREM and REM sleep. NREM sleep is characterized by a low LF:HF, interpreted to reflect PSNS predominance.[71] Researchers report a progressive increase in vagal activity across NREM sleep stages.[72] The higher LF:HF seen during REM sleep is similar to that of wakefulness and reflects a higher sympathetic tone.[71,73,74] During periods of acute psychophysiological stress, the normal increase in PSNS across NREM is blunted and SNS power is higher and this increase in sympathetic activity during NREM is associated with greater difficulties in sleep maintenance.[75]

Sleep is scored in terms of discrete stages in 30-second epochs, but there is a range in the amount of delta (slow wave) activity present within these stages. Findings suggest that mixed SNS and PSNS activity (LF:HF) is negatively dependent on the amount of delta activity, whereas PSNS activity (HF) is independent of delta activity.[76]

A final consideration for HRV patterns in sleep is arousal activity. Electroencephalography-defined arousals occur with a movement to a lower sleep stage or to wake. These arousals are associated with increased LF power in the cardiac signal.[77] Although more subtle, NREM sleep is also characterized by two arousal rhythms. These NREM rhythms include a state of sustained arousal instability known as cyclic alternating pattern (CAP) and a stable arousal condition known as non-CAP. The percentage of LF power is greater in CAP, and HF power is greater in non-CAP within NREM stage 2 sleep and NREM slow-wave sleep.[78] Periodic leg movements in sleep are frequently associated with arousals in sleep. Based on measures of HRV and electroencephalography, it appears that periodic leg movements in sleep are caused by changes in sympathetic activity rather than leading to it.[79]

Body Position

Body position and the frequency of positional change are closely related to whether the person is awake or asleep. During sleep, an individual usually exhibits fewer and less dramatic changes in body position. Whether the patient is asleep or awake, body position should be considered in the interpretation of HRV. Comparative evaluations for treatment or intervention should be based on assessment that is consistent for positioning.

In terms of vertical positioning, HRV is significantly reduced from supine to sitting and further decreased from sitting to standing positions.[80] In healthy subjects, change from supine to standing positions also reduces vagal input (low HF), increases the LF:HF, and reduces LF power.[59] Postural changes evoke a greater HRV response in women than in men,[81] although this difference was not found elsewhere.[59] ANS postural change responses are blunted with increased age.[59,81]

Recumbent positioning that enhances vagal tone in the cardiac care patient could promote recovery by reducing cardiac demand and, subsequently, the risk of malignant cardiac events. The right lateral position is associated with a higher vagal tone (higher HF) than either the left lateral or the supine positions. This position-based vagal enhancement is consistently found in individuals with coronary artery disease,[82] in patients during the acute phase of an MI,[83] and in patients with CHF.[84] Healthy individuals also show vagal predominance with the right lateral position,[82] although this observation is not reported consistently.[84]

Position-related differences in HRV may be an important factor in sudden infant death syndrome. Compared with sleeping in the supine position, sleeping prone is recognized as a significant risk factor for sudden infant death syndrome and is associated with lower HRV in term infants at 1 and 3 months of age.[85] Preterm infants are especially at risk for sudden infant death syndrome. HRV assessment of these high-risk patients measured during a daytime nap showed significantly reduced HRV and reduced PSNS activity in the prone versus supine position at 1 and 3 months of corrected age.[86] These results lend support for promoting sleep in the supine position.

General Health

Results from the Atherosclerosis Risk in Communities (ARIC) Study, a large population-based study of middle-aged men and women, support that low HRV is associated with increased mortality rates that are not attributable to cardiovascular risk factors or to other disease conditions.[87] This suggests that low HRV may be a sensitive indicator for poor general health in addition to an index of cardiovascular risk.

A major contributor to general health is lifestyle. Many aspects of lifestyle have been explored with respect to impact on HRV patterns. These include physical activity, obesity and diet, smoking, and alcohol and coffee consumption.

Physical Activity

Physically active individuals tend to have lower heart rates and increased HRV compared to those with a sedentary lifestyle.[88] The difference in HRV between active and inactive individuals is particularly large in older individuals.[88] Also, type and intensity of activity is important. Resistance (weight) training does not significantly increase HRV[89] but endurance (aerobic) training alone[89] or in combination with stress management can significantly increase HRV.[90] Moderate (8 kcal/kg/week) or high (12 kcal/kg/week) intensity levels of cardiovascular exercise appear to be required for significant HRV improvement.[91]

Obesity and Diet

Obese individuals, as measured by body mass index, are characterized by increased resting sympathetic tone: faster heart rates, higher LF power, and lower HF power.[81] Other researchers have not found significant associations between body mass index and HRV in healthy adolescents[92] or between body mass index and SNS activity markers in mild to moderately obese healthy adults.[93] Rabbia et al.[94] suggest that ANS function is dependent on duration of obesity. Specifically, compared with lean adolescents, measures of SNS activity were increased in subjects with recent (<4 years) obesity but not chronic obesity. HRV reduced significantly with duration of obesity. Orthostatic (lying to standing) stress testing indicates a blunted autonomic response in obese individuals.[81]

The relationship of diet to HRV is gaining attention. Levels of total cholesterol and low-density lipoprotein cholesterol are significant predictors of reduced HRV in "healthy" individuals with hypercholesterolemia.[95] Omega-3 fatty acid supplementation and fish-based oils in particular, are associated with increased HRV.[96,97] Compared with low salt diets (1 mmol/kg sodium, 1 mmol/kg potassium), high salt diets (4 mmol/kg sodium, 1 mmol/kg potassium) significantly increase HF power.[98] Individuals who are chronically underweight and undernourished show reduced total power, LF power, and HF power compared with underweight well-nourished or normal-weight well-nourished individuals.[99]

Smoking and Environmental Exposures

Smoking has an immediate impact on HRV, characterized by an acute decrease in cardiac PSNS activity and a surge in systemic SNS activity, including increased heart rate.[100,101] The long-term and dose-related effects of smoking on HRV are less clear. Some researchers report that smoking, including passive smoke exposure[102] and especially chronic heavy smoking (>25 cigarettes per day), reduces HRV and vagal activity.[100] However, a significant association is not found consistently.[59,81,93]

Exposure to metals (i.e., iron, manganese, aluminum, copper, zinc, chromium, lead, nickel) in the form of particulate matter has been associated with decreased nighttime HRV (rMSSD) in boiler-maker workers.[103,104] Short-term exposure to sulfur dioxin has also been found to lead to a reduction in vagal activity.[105] More studies related to environmental exposures, and lead exposure in particular, are needed to confirm trends for negative impact on HRV.[106]

Alcohol

HRV is one approach used to explore the cardioprotective and cardioputative effects of alcohol. Although population-based study results indicate that alcohol is not a significant lifestyle factor affecting HRV in healthy adults,[59,93] other research supports that the relationship is more complex. In one study involving a randomized crossover design, findings suggest that moderate regular alcohol consumption in healthy individuals enhances vagal activity (increased HF, reduced LF, increased HF:LF).[107]

Alcohol restriction also impacts HRV patterns. Compared with their usual drinking patterns (70.1 ± 4.6 mL/day), 3 weeks of alcohol restriction (19.1 ± 2.5 mL/day) in habitual drinkers led to reduced heart rate, increased HRV, and increased indices of PSNS activity.[108] Findings support ANS activity recovery even after chronic high alcohol consumption.

Caffeine

Caffeine causes an acute increase in systemic vascular resistance through the blocking of central antiadrenergic adenosine receptors. This acute increase in blood pressure is compensated for by a brief reduction in heart rate and a probable increase in vagal predominance. This prediction is in keeping with findings of a sympathetic rebound (higher LF:HF) in people who consume coffee after at least 2 hours of abstinence from caffeine compared with individuals who do not consume caffeine regularly.[81] In patients with Type 1 diabetes, 2 weeks of moderate (500 mg/day) caffeine intake enhanced parasympathetic activity, potentiating reduced cardiovascular risk.[109] More work is needed to fully determine the short-term and long-term impact of caffeine on HRV.

Acute and Chronic Conditions

Pain

Acute pain is clinically seen to increase heart rate and decrease HRV. Interventions that foster good pain management are expected to enhance HRV and reflect a decreased activation of the SNS. Exploration of HRV patterns related to chronic pain is limited and frequently confounded by cardiac pathology. HRV patterns across sleep cycles are not different between patients with chronic low back pain and healthy controls.[110] Standard measures of HRV are not significantly different for patients characterized by either successful or unsuccessful pain reduction after treatment of a herniated disc.[111] These findings suggest that pain is not a modifying factor for HRV. More work is needed, however, before conclusions regarding the relationship between HRV patterns and chronic pain can be drawn.

Brain Injury

The ability to perform continuous and noninvasive assessments of ANS function with HRV has made this a valued additional approach for neurological injury assessment and prognosis.

Traumatic brain injury is associated with ANS dysfunction marked by reduced HRV and reduced LF and HF power.[112] Biswas et al.[113] studied children with brain injury. Factors that predicted poorer outcome, such as a low Glasgow Coma Scale score (3–4 versus 5–8), higher intracranial pressure (>30 mm Hg), and decreased cerebral perfusion pressure (<40 mm Hg), were associated with PSNS dominance as reflected by low LF:HF. Profound vagal dominance is characteristic of patients with brain injury who progress to brain death.[113,114]

Stroke patients exhibit cardiovascular regulatory impairment in both ANS branches. Total power, LF power, and HF power are all reduced,[115–117] although an increase in the LF:HF supports relative sympathetic dominance.[117] Injury in the region of the insula (especially the right) is strongly associated with ANS instability and sudden death.[117] Within the brainstem, only medullary stroke injury is associated with depressed ANS activity (reduced LF and HF power).[116]

Depression

Depression is a significant risk factor for the development of cardiovascular disease and for the increased risk of cardiac mortality and morbidity in those with existing cardiovascular conditions (see reviews by Carney et al.[118] and Musselman et al.[119]) One possible explanation is that depressive disorders may stimulate harmful influences on the ANS by increasing SNS activity and/or reducing vagal tone.[118] Consistent with this hypothesis, lower HRV and reduced vagal tone (low HF) are found in depressed compared with nondepressed individuals with CHD[120] and those with acute coronary syndrome.[121] The severity of depression in cardiac patients is negatively associated with HRV.[120,122–124] The Enhancing Recovery in Coronary Heart Disease study found that low HRV was a statistically significant mediator of the effect of depression on survival after acute MI.[124] Cardiac care patients successfully treated for severe depression exhibit enhanced HRV and reduced heart rate.[121,122] Collectively, these findings underscore the need for prompt assessment and treatment of depression in cardiac care.

Diabetes

Autonomic neuropathy is a common and serious complication of diabetes. Measures of HRV can aid in the early diagnosis and treatment of this ANS dysfunction and are recommended as components of standard diabetic care. Findings from the Framingham Heart Study indicate that individuals with diabetes mellitus have significantly lower HRV (SDNN), LF and HF power, and LF:HF compared to those with normal fasting glucose ($p < .005$).[125] Results also show a strong negative association between these HRV measurements and the level of fasting blood glucose across all subjects. These findings support a blunting of ANS activity and a relative SNS dominance in patients with diabetes and in those with impaired blood glucose regulation.

Not surprisingly, patients with diabetes exhibiting low HRV have an increased risk for CHD.[126] Based on a 9-year follow-up, subjects with diabetes with impaired autonomic function have nearly double the risk of mortality than do the general population[127] although others have reported only trends toward increased mortality risk in patients with diabetes with low HRV as measured by time domain approaches (minimum–maximum RR difference; SDANN, CV).[128]

Lowered HRV has been linked to inflammation, and specifically, increased plasma concentrations of C-reactive protein in the general population[129] and with both C-reactive protein[130] and interleukin-6[131] in patients with Type 1 diabetes.

Overall, diabetes and poor glucose regulation and accompanying inflammatory factors appear to signal serious risk for the development and/or exacerbation of cardiovascular conditions.

Chronic Obstructive Pulmonary Disease

Individuals with COPD exhibit ANS disturbance as measured by HRV, although the nature of the dysfunction reported is not consistent.[132–134] Stein et al.[132] studied young PiZ α_1-antitrypsin-deficient COPD patients and found significant decreases in almost all HRV parameters. Severity of ANS disturbance was directly related to clinical severity as measured by forced expiratory volume in one second (FEV_1). Vagal activity was significantly reduced during the daytime only. Other researchers report that compared with control subjects, COPD patients exhibit increased HF activity during the daytime[134] or abnormally reduced nocturnal vagal activity.[133] Stein et al.[132] studied younger patients with more severe cases and, unlike the two other studies cited, did not wean them from any medications complicating interpretation.

Huntington and Parkinson Diseases

Analysis of HRV indicates disturbed ANS function in Huntington disease.[135] Compared with matched healthy controls, genetically and symptomatically positive patients at the mid-stage of Huntington disease progression exhibit significantly reduced vagal tone (low HF) and a shift toward sympathetic predominance (high LF). Degree of disturbance is significantly related to the severity of clinical symptoms.

Little research has been conducted to explore autonomic activity in patients with Parkinson disease. Further research is needed to determine the representativeness of reported trends of increased SNS tone and reduced HRV.[136]

IMPACT OF INTERVENTIONS ON HRV

Although decreased HRV is strongly linked with poor prognosis, the increase of HRV does not directly appear to improve health outcomes.[24] Still, there is support for improved health outcomes for pharmacologic and nonpharmacologic interventions that are also associated with increased HRV.

Several pharmacologic therapies are known to increase HRV and reduce mortality. These include β-blockers after MI (primarily through the enhancement of vagal tone),[137] angiotensin-converting enzyme inhibitors and carvedilol (a nonselective β-blocker) in CHF, sotalol (a class III antiarrhythmic agent and β-blocker) in the treatment of ventricular arrhythmias, and estrogen replacement therapy in postmenopausal women.[24,61]

Nonpharmacologic interventions, such as physical training,[89,91] psychosocial therapy,[122] and combination therapies involving exercise and stress reduction[90] or exercise, diet, and weight loss,[2,138] increase HRV and improve cardiovascular status. One nursing study combined approaches in a randomized controlled trial of a psychosocial therapy targeting survivors of sudden cardiac arrest (N = 129).[139] Therapy included three components: physiologic relaxation with biofeedback; cognitive behavioral therapy aimed at enhancing mental health; and health education targeting cardiovascular risk factors. Based on a 2-year follow-up period, this comprehensive psychosocial therapy significantly reduced cardiovascular death.

SUMMARY

HRV is disturbed in a number of cardiovascular disorders and health conditions that predispose cardiac complications. Clinicians and researchers who have knowledge of these HRV pattern anomalies and the factors that shape them will be able to include this approach in their work, strengthening their assessment and evaluation of the cardiovascular patient.

REFERENCES

1. Lewis, M. J. (2005). Heart rate variability analysis: A tool to assess cardiac autonomic function. *Computers, Informatics, Nursing, 23*(6), 335–341.
2. Appel, M. L., Berger, R. D., Saul, J. P., et al. (1989). Beat to beat variability in cardiovascular variables: Noise or music? *Journal of American College of Cardiology, 14*(5), 1139–1148.
3. Task Force of the European Society of Cardiology and the North American Society of Pacing and Electrophysiology. (1996). Heart rate variability: Standards of measurement, physiological interpretation and clinical use. *Circulation, 93*(5), 1043–1065.
4. Coenen, A. J., Rompelman, O., & Kitney, R. I. (1977). Measurement of heart-rate variability: Part 2-Hardware digital devices for the assessment of heart-rate variability. *Medical & Biological Engineering & Computing, 15*(4), 423–430.
5. Rompelman, O., Coenen, A. J., & Kitney, R. I. (1977). Measurement of heart-rate variability: Part 1-Comparative study of heart-rate variability analysis methods. *Medical & Biological Engineering & Computing, 15*(3), 233–239.
6. Leffler, C. T., Saul, J. P., & Cohen, R. J. (1994). Rate-related and autonomic effects on atrioventricular conduction assessed through beat-to-beat PR interval and cycle length variability. *Journal of Cardiovascular Electrophysiology, 5*(1), 2–15.
7. Takei, Y. (1992). Relationship between power spectral densities of P-P and R-R intervals. *Annals of Physiological Anthropology, 113*, 325–332.
8. Berntson, G. G., Bigger, J. T., Jr., Eckberg, D. L., et al. (1997). Heart rate variability: Origins, methods, and interpretive caveats. *Psychophysiology, 34*(6), 623–648.
9. Öri, Z., Monir, G., Weiss, J., et al. (1992). Heart rate variability. Frequency domain analysis. *Cardiology Clinics, 10*(3), 499–537.
10. Pagani, M., Lombardi, F., Guzzetti, S., et al. (1986). Power spectral analysis of heart rate and arterial pressure variabilities as a marker of sympatho-vagal interaction in man and conscious dog. *Circulation Research, 58*, 178–193.
11. Akselrod, S., Gordon, D., Ubel, F. A., et al. (1981). Power spectrum analysis of heart rate fluctuations: A quantitative probe of beat-to-beat cardiovascular control. *Science, 213*, 220–222.
12. Cowan, M. J., Burr, R. L., Narayanan, S. B., et al. (1992). Comparison of autoregression and fast Fourier transform techniques for power spectral analysis of heart period variability of persons with sudden cardiac arrest before and after therapy to increase heart period variability. *Journal of Electrocardiology, 25*(Suppl.), 234–239.
13. Burr, R. L. (2007). Interpretation of normalized spectral heart rate variability indices in sleep research: A critical review. *Sleep, 30*(7), 913–919.
14. Bigger, J. T., Jr., Fleiss, J. L., Steinman, R. C., et al. (1995). RR variability in healthy, middle-aged persons compared with patients with chronic coronary heart disease or recent acute myocardial infarction. *Circulation, 91*, 1936–1943.
15. Liao, D., Evans, G. W., Chambless, L. E., et al. (1996). Population-based study of heart rate variability and prevalent myocardial infarction. The Atherosclerosis Risk in Communities Study. *Journal of Electrocardiology, 29*(3), 189–198.
16. Sosnowski, M., MacFarlane, P. W., Czyz, Z., et al. (2002). Age-adjustment of HRV measures and its prognostic value for risk assessment in patients late after myocardial infarction. *International Journal of Cardiology, 86*, 249–258.
17. Stein, P. K., Le, Q., & Domitrovich, P. P. (2008). Development of more erratic heart rate patterns is associated with mortality post-myocardial infarction. *Journal of Electrocardiology, 41*(2), 110–115.
18. Poulsen, S. H., Jensen, S. E., Moller, J. E., et al. (2001). Prognostic value of left ventricular diastolic function and association with heart rate variability after a first acute myocardial infarction. *Heart, 86*(4), 376–380.
19. Kennon, S., Price, C. P., MacCallum, P. K., et al. (2003). Cumulative risk assessment in unstable angina: Clinical, electrocardiographic, autonomic, and biochemical markers. *Heart, 89*, 36–41.
20. Kleiger, R. E., Miller, J. P., Bigger, J. T., et al. (1987). Decreased heart rate variability and its association with increased mortality after acute myocardial infarction. *American Journal of Cardiology, 59*, 256–262.
21. Ramaekers, D., Ector, H., Aubert, A. E., et al. (1998). Heart rate variability and heart rate in healthy volunteers. Is the female autonomic nervous system cardioprotective? *European Heart Journal, 19*, 1334–1341.
22. La Rovere, M. T., Pinna, G. D., Hohnloser, S. H., et al. (2001). Baroreflex sensitivity and heart rate variability in the identification of patients at risk for life-threatening arrhythmias. *Circulation, 103*, 2072–2077.
23. Bettoni, M., & Zimmermann, M. (2002). Autonomic tone variations before the onset of paroxysmal atrial fibrillation. *Circulation, 105*, 2753–2759.
24. Stein, P. K., & Kleiger, R. E. (1999). Insights from the study of heart rate variability. *Annual Review of Medicine, 50*, 249–261.

25. Rautaharju, P. M., Kooperberg, C., Larson, J. C., et al. (2006). Electrocardiographic abnormalities that predict coronary heart disease events and mortality in postmenopausal women: The Women's Health Initiative. *Circulation, 113*(4), 473–480.
26. Krittayaphong, R., Veerakul, G., Bhuripanyo, K., et al. (2003). Heart rate variability in patients with sudden unexpected cardiac arrest in Thailand. *American Journal of Cardiology, 91*, 77–81.
27. Forslund, L., Björkander, I., Ericson, M., et al. (2002). Prognostic implications of autonomic function assessed by analyses of catecholamines and heart rate variability in stable angina pectoris. *Heart, 87*, 415–422.
28. Lanza, G. A., Cianflone, D., Rebuzzi, A. G., et al. (2006). Prognostic value of ventricular arrhythmias and heart rate variability in patients with unstable angina. *Heart, 92*(8), 1055–1063.
29. Lucini, D., Porta, A., & Pagani, M. (2003). Assessing autonomic disturbances of hypertension in the general practitioner's office: A transtelephonic approach to spectral analysis of heart rate variability. *Journal of Hypertension, 21*, 755–760.
30. Lucini, D., Melas, G. S., Malliani, A., et al. (2002). Impairment in cardiac autonomic regulation preceding arterial hypertension in humans: Insights from spectral analysis of beat-by-beat cardiovascular variability. *Circulation, 106*(21), 2673–2679.
31. Singh, J. P., Larson, M. G., Tsuji, H., et al. (1998). Reduced heart rate variability and new-onset hypertension. Insights into pathogenesis of hypertension: The Framingham Heart Study. *Hypertension, 32*, 293–297.
32. Kaftan, A. H., & Kaftan, O. (2000). QT intervals and heart rate variability in hypertensive patients. *Japanese Heart Journal, 41*(2), 173–182.
33. Guzzetti, S., Dassi, S., Balsama, M., et al. (1994). Altered dynamics of the circadian relationship between systematic arterial pressure and cardiac sympathetic drive early on in mild hypertension. *Clinical Science (London), 86*(2), 209–215.
34. Kingwell, B. A., Thompson, J. M., Kaye, D. M., et al. (1994). Congestive heart failure/hypertension/hypertrophy: Heart rate spectral analysis, cardiac norepinephrine spillover, and muscle sympathetic nerve activity during human sympathetic nervous activation and failure. *Circulation, 90*(1), 234–240.
35. Bilchick, K. C., Fetics, B., Djoukeng, R., et al. (2002). Prognostic value of heart rate variability in chronic congestive heart failure Veterans Affairs' Survival Trial of Antiarrhythmic Therapy in Congestive Heart Failure. *American Journal of Cardiology, 90*(1), 24–28.
36. Krüger, C., Lahm, T., Zugck, C., et al. (2002). Heart rate variability enhances the prognostic value of established parameters in patients with congestive heart failure. *Zeitschrift für Kardiolgie, 91*, 1003–1012.
37. La Rovere, M. T., Pinna, G. D., Maestri, R., et al. (2003). Short-term heart rate variability strongly predicts sudden cardiac death in chronic heart failure patients. *Circulation, 107*, 565–570.
38. Nolan, J., Batin, P., Andrews, R., et al. (1998). Prospective study of heart rate variability and mortality in chronic heart failure: Results of the United Kingdom Heart Failure Evaluation and Assessment of Risk Trial UK-Heart. *Circulation, 98*(15), 1510–1516.
39. Eaton, G. M., Cody, R. J., Nunziata, E., et al. (1995). Early left ventricular dysfunction elicits activation of sympathetic drive and attenuation of parasympathetic tone in the paced canine model of congestive heart failure. *Circulation, 92*, 555–561.
40. Notarius, C. F., & Floras, J. S. (2001). Limitations of use of spectral analysis of heart rate variability for the estimation of cardiac sympathetic activity in heart failure. *Europace, 3*, 29–38.
41. Ponikowski, P., Anker, S. D., Chua, T. P., et al. (1999). Oscillatory breathing patterns during wakefulness in patients with chronic heart failure: Clinical implications and role of augmented peripheral chemosensitivity. *Circulation, 100*(24), 2418–2424.
42. Park, D. H., Shin, C. J., Hong, S. C., et al. (2008). Correlation between the severity of obstructive sleep apnea and heart rate variability indices. *Journal of Korean Medical Science, 23*(2), 226–231.
43. Freed, L. A., Stein, K., Borer, J. S., et al. (1997). Relation of ultra-low frequency heart rate variability to the clinical course of chronic aortic regurgitation. *American Journal of Cardiology, 7911*, 1482–1487.
44. Stein, P. K., Domitrovich, P. P., Kleiger, R. E., et al. (2000). Clinical and demographic determinants of heart rate variability in patients post myocardial infarction: Insights from the cardiac arrhythmia suppression trial CAST. *Clinical Cardiology, 23*(3), 187–194.
45. Wiggers, H., Bøtker, H. E., Egeblad, H., et al. (2002). Coronary artery bypass surgery in heart failure patients with chronic reversible and irreversible myocardial dysfunction: Effect on heart rate variability. *Cardiology, 98*, 181–185.
46. Livanis, E. G., Flevari, P., Theodorakis, G. N., et al. (2003). Effect of biventricular pacing on heart rate variability in patients with chronic heart failure. *European Journal of Heart Failure, 5*, 175–178.
47. Brunner, M., Hess, B., Lutter, G., et al. (2002). Transmyocardial laser revascularization and left ventricular reduction surgery affect ventricular arrhythmias and heart rate variability. *American Heart Journal, 143*, 1012–1016.
48. Osterhues, H., Kochs, M., & Hombach, V. (1998). Time-dependent changes of heart rate variability after percutaneous transluminal angioplasty. *American Heart Journal, 135*, 755–761.
49. Gogenur, I., Rosenburg-Adamsen, S., Lie, C., et al. (2002). Lack of circadian variation in the activity of the autonomic nervous system after major abdominal operations. *European Journal Surgery, 168*(4), 242–246.
50. Cashion, A. K., Hathaway, D. K., Milstead, E. J., et al. (1999). Changes in patterns of 24-hr heart rate variability after kidney and kidney-pancreas transplant. *Transplantation, 68*, 1846–1850.
51. Cowan, M. J., Pike, K., & Burr, R. L. (1994). Effects of gender and age on heart rate variability in healthy individuals and in persons after sudden cardiac arrest. *Journal of Electrocardiology, 27*(Suppl.), 1–9.
52. Jensen-Urstad, K., Storck, N., Bouvier, F., et al. (1997). Heart rate variability in healthy subjects is related to age and gender. *Acta Physiologica Scandinavica, 160*(3), 235–241.
53. Stein, P. K., Kleiger, R. E., & Rottman, J. N. (1997). Differing effects of age on heart rate variability in men and women. *American Journal of Cardiology, 80*(3), 302–305.
54. Umetani, K., Singer, D. H., McCraty, R., et al. (1998). Twenty-four hour time domain heart rate variability and heart rate: Relations to age and gender over nine decades. *Journal of American College of Cardiology, 31*(3), 593–601.
55. Liao, D., Barnes, R. W., Chambless, L. E., et al. (1995). Age, race, and sex differences in autonomic cardiac function measured by spectral analysis of heart rate variability—The ARIC study. Atherosclerosis risk in communities. *American Journal of Cardiology, 76*(12), 906–912.
56. Smith, S. L., Doig, A. K., & Dudley, W. N. (2005). Impaired parasympathetic response to feeding in ventilated preterm babies. *Archives of Disease in Childhood. Fetal and Neonatal Edition, 90*(6), F505–F508.
57. Lucini, D., Bertoni, L., Pitto, G., et al. (1993). Reduced response with ageing to sympatho-excitatory and sympatho-inhibitory stimuli in humans. *Journal of Hypertension. Supplement, 11*(Suppl. 5), S170–S171.
58. Bonnemeier, H., Richardt, G., & Potratz, J. (2003). Circadian profile of cardiac autonomic nervous modulation in healthy subjects. *Journal of Cardiovascular Electrophysiology, 14*(8), 791–799.
59. Fagard, R. H., Pardaens, K., & Staessen, J. A. (1999). Influence of demographic, anthropometric and lifestyle characteristics on heart rate and its variability in the population. *Journal of Hypertension, 17*(11), 1589–1599.
60. Kuo, T. B., Lin, T., Yang, C. C., et al. (1999). Effect of aging on gender differences in neural control of heart rate. *American Journal of Physiology, 277*(6, Pt. 2), H2233–H2239.
61. Leicht, A. S., Hirning, D. A., & Allen, G. D. (2003). Heart rate variability and endogenous sex hormones during the menstrual cycle in young women. *Experimental Physiology, 88*(3), 441–446.
62. Busjahn, A., Voss, A., Knoblauch, H., et al. (1998). Angiotensin-converting enzyme and angiotensinogen gene polymorphisms and heart rate variability in twins. *American Journal of Cardiology, 81*(6), 755–760.
63. Singh, J. P., Larson, M. G., O'Donnell, C. J., et al. (2001). Genetic factors contribute to the variance in frequency domain measures of heart rate variability. *Autonomic Neuroscience, 90*(1–2), 122–126.
64. Singh, J. P., Larson, M. G., O'Donnell, C. J., et al. (2002). Genome scan linkage results for heart rate variability: The Framingham Heart Study. *American Journal of Cardiology, 90*, 1290–1293.
65. Malpas, S. C., & Purdie, G. L. (1990). Circadian variation of heart rate variability. *Cardiovascular Research, 24*(3), 210–213.
66. Massin, M. M., Maeyns, K., Withofs, N., et al. (2000). Circadian rhythm of heart rate and heart rate variability. *Archives of Disease in Childhood, 83*, 179–182.
67. Aoyagi, N., Ohashi, K., Tomono, S., et al. (2000). Temporal contribution of body movement to very long-term heart rate variability in humans. *American Journal of Physiology. Heart and Circulatory Physiology, 278*(4), H1035–H1041.
68. Van de Borne, P., Nguyen, H., Biston, P., et al. (1994). Effects of wake and sleep stages on the 24-h autonomic control of blood pressure and heart rate in recumbent men. *American Journal of Physiology, 266*(2, Pt. 2), H548–H554.

69. Ito, H., Nozaki, M., Maruyama, T., et al. (2001). Shift work modifies the circadian patterns of heart rate variability in nurses. *International Journal of Cardiology, 79*, 231–236.
70. Iber, C., Ancoli-Israel, S., Chesson, A., et al. (2007). *The AASM manual for the scoring of sleep and associated events: Rules, terminology and technical specifications* (1st ed.). Westchester, IL: American Academy of Sleep Medicine.
71. Elsenbruch, S., Harnish, M. J., & Orr, W. C. (1999). Heart rate variability during waking and sleep in healthy males and females. *Sleep, 22*(8), 1067–1071.
72. Toscani, L., Gangemi, P. F., Parigi, A., et al. (1996). Human heart rate variability and sleep stages. *Italian Journal of Neurological Science, 17*, 437–439.
73. Scholz, U. J., Bianchi, A. M., Cerutti, S., et al. (1997). Vegetative background of sleep: Spectral analysis of the heart rate variability. *Physiology & Behavior, 62*(5), 1037–1043.
74. Vanoli, E., Adamson, P. B., Ba, L., et al. (1995). Heart rate variability during specific sleep stages. A comparison of healthy subjects with patients after myocardial infarction. *Circulation, 91*, 1918–1922.
75. Hall, M., Vasko, R., Buysse, D., et al. (2004). Acute stress affects heart rate variability during sleep. *Psychosomatic Medicine, 66*(1), 56–62.
76. Yang, C. C. H., Lai, C., Lai, H. Y., et al. (2002). Relationship between electroencephalogram slow-wave magnitude and heart rate variability during sleep in humans. *Neuroscience Letter, 329*, 213–216.
77. Bonnet, M. H., & Arand, D. L. (1997). Heart rate variability: Sleep stages, time of night, and arousal influences. *Electroencephalography and Clinical Neurophysiology, 102*(5), 390–396.
78. Ferri, R., Parrino, L., Smerieri, A., et al. (2000). Cyclic alternating pattern and spectral analysis of heart rate variability during sleep. *Journal of Sleep Research, 9*, 13–18.
79. Guggisberg, A. G., Hess, C. W., & Mathis, J. (2007). The significance of the sympathetic nervous system in the pathophysiology of periodic leg movements in sleep. *Sleep, 30*(6), 755–766.
80. Brguljan, J., Fagard, R., Macor, F., et al. (1993). The sympathetic response to different orthostatic challenges and its daytime variation, assessed by power spectral analysis of heart rate. *Journal of Hypertension Supplement, 11*(Suppl. 5), S150–S151.
81. Stolarz, K., Staessen, J. A., Kuznetsova, T., et al. (2003). Host and environmental determinants of heart rate and heart rate variability in four European populations. *Journal of Hypertension, 21*, 525–535.
82. Kuo, C. D., & Chen, G. Y. (1998). Comparison of three recumbent positions on vagal and sympathetic modulation using spectral heart rate variability in patients with coronary artery disease. *American Journal of Cardiology, 81*, 392–396.
83. Kuo, C. D., Chen, G. Y., & Lo, H. M. (2002). Effect of different recumbent positions on spectral indices of autonomic modulation of the heart during the acute phase of myocardial infarction. *Critical Care Medicine, 28*, 1283–1289.
84. Fujita, M., Miyamoto, S., Sekiguchi, H., et al. (2000). Effects of posture on sympathetic nervous modulation in patients with chronic heart failure. *Lancet, 356*, 1822–1823.
85. Galland, B. C., Reeves, G., Taylor, B. J., et al. (1998). Sleep position, autonomic function, and arousal. *Archives of Disease in Childhood. Fetal Neonatal Edition, 78*, F189–F194.
86. Ariagno, R. L., Mirmiran, M., Adams, M. M., et al. (2003). Effect of position on sleep, heart rate variability, and QT interval in preterm infants at 1 and 3 months' corrected age. *Pediatrics, 111*(3), 622–625.
87. Dekker, J. M., Crow, R. S., Folsom, A. R., et al. (2000). Low heart rate variability in a 2-minute rhythm strip predicts risk of coronary heart disease and mortality from several causes: The ARIC study. *Circulation, 102*, 1239–1244.
88. Ueno, L. M., & Moritani, T. (2003). Effects of long-term exercise training on cardiac autonomic nervous activities and baroreflex sensitivity. *European Journal of Applied Physiology, 89*, 109–114.
89. Grund, A., Krause, H., Kraus, M., et al. (2001). Association between different attributes of physical activity and fat mass in untrained, endurance- and resistance-trained men. *European Journal of Applied Physiology, 84*, 310–320.
90. Blumenthal, J. A., Sherwood, A., Babyak, M. A., et al. (2005). Effects of exercise and stress management training on markers of cardiovascular risk in patients with ischemic heart disease: A randomized controlled trial. *JAMA, 293*(13), 1626–1634.
91. Earnest, C. P., Lavie, C. J., Blair, S. N., et al. (2008). Heart rate variability characteristics in sedentary postmenopausal women following six months of exercise training: The DREW study. *PLoS ONE, 3*(6), e2288.
92. Faulkner, M. S., Hathaway, D., & Tolley, B. (2003). Cardiovascular autonomic function in healthy adolescents. *Heart & Lung, 32*, 10–22.
93. Kageyama, T., Nishikido, N., Honda, Y., et al. (1997). Effects of obesity, current smoking status, and alcohol consumption on heart rate variability in male white-collar workers. *International Archives of Occupational and Environmental Health, 69*, 447–454.
94. Rabbia, F., Silke, B., Conterno, A., et al. (2003). Assessment of cardiac autonomic modulation during adolescent obesity. *Obesity Research, 11*(4), 541–548.
95. Danev, S., Nikolova, R., Kerekovska, M., et al. (1997). Relationship between heart rate variability and hypercholesterolaemia. *Central European Journal of Public Health, 5*(3), 143–146.
96. Holguin, F., Tellez-Rojo, M. M., Lazo, M., et al. (2005). Cardiac autonomic changes associated with fish oil vs soy oil supplementation in the elderly. *Chest, 127*(4), 1102–1107.
97. von Schacky, C. (2006). A review of omega-3 ethyl esters for cardiovascular prevention and treatment of increased blood triglyceride levels. *Vascular Health and Risk Management, 2*(3), 251–262.
98. McNeely, J. D., Windham, B. G., & Anderson, D. E. (2008). Dietary sodium effects on heart rate variability in salt sensitivity of blood pressure. *Psychophysiology, 45*(3), 405–411.
99. Vaz, M., Bharathi, A. V., Sucharita, S., et al. (2003). Heart rate variability and baroreflex sensitivity are reduced in chronically undernourished, but otherwise healthy, human subjects. *Clinical Science (London), 104*(3), 295–302.
100. Hayano, J., Yamada, M., Sakakibara, Y., et al. (1990). Short- and long-term effects of cigarette smoking on heart rate variability. *American Journal of Cardiology, 65*(1), 84–88.
101. Zhang, J., & Kesteloot, H. (1999). Anthropometric, lifestyle and metabolic determinants of resting heart rate. *European Heart Journal, 20*, 103–110.
102. Felber Dietrich, D., Schwartz, J., Schindler, C., et al. (2007). Effects of passive smoking on heart rate variability, heart rate and blood pressure: An observational study. *International Journal of Epidemiology, 36*(4), 834–840.
103. Cavallari, J. M., Eisen, E. A., Fang, S. C., et al. (2008). PM2.5 metal exposures and nocturnal heart rate variability: A panel study of boilermaker construction workers. *Environmental Health, 7*, 36.
104. Cavallari, J. M., Fang, S. C., Eisen, E. A., et al. (2008). Time course of heart rate variability decline following particulate matter exposures in an occupational cohort. *Inhalation Toxicology, 20*(4), 415–422.
105. Routledge, H. C., Manney, S., Harrison, R. M., et al. (2006). Effect of inhaled sulphur dioxide and carbon particles on heart rate variability and markers of inflammation and coagulation in human subjects. *Heart, 92*(2), 220–227.
106. Navas-Acien, A., Guallar, E., Silbergeld, E. K., et al. (2007). Lead exposure and cardiovascular disease—A systematic review. *Environmental Health Perspectives, 115*(3), 472–482.
107. Flanagan, D. E. H., Pratt, E., Murphy, J., et al. (2002). Alcohol consumption alters insulin secretion and cardiac autonomic activity. *European Journal of Clinical Investigation, 32*, 187–192.
108. Minami, J., Yoshii, M., Todoroki, M., et al. (2002). Effects of alcohol restriction on ambulatory blood pressure, heart rate, and heart rate variability in Japanese men. *American Journal of Hypertension, 15*, 125–129.
109. Richardson, T., Rozkovec, A., Thomas, P., et al. (2004). Influence of caffeine on heart rate variability in patients with long-standing type 1 diabetes. *Diabetes Care, 27*(5), 1127–1131.
110. Pivik, R. T., Haman, K., & Matsunga, L. (1997). *Variations in heart rate across sleep cycles in chronic low back pain subjects: Implications for nonrestorative sleep complaints*. San Francisco, CA: APSS.
111. Storella, R. J., Shi, Y., O'Connor, D. M., et al. (1999). Relief of chronic pain may be accompanied by an increase in a measure of heart rate variability. *Anesthesia Analgesia, 89*(2), 448–450.
112. King, M. L., Lichtman, S. W., Seliger, G., et al. (1997). Heart-rate variability in chronic traumatic brain injury. *Brain Injury, 11*(6), 445–453.
113. Biswas, A. K., Scott, W. A., Sommerauer, J. F., et al. (2000). Heart rate variability after acute traumatic brain injury in children. *Critical Care Medicine, 28*(12), 3907–3912.
114. Baillard, C., Vivien, B., Mansier, P., et al. (2002). Brain death assessment using instant spectral analysis of heart rate variability. *Critical Care Medicine, 30*, 306–310.
115. Arad, M., Abboud, S., Radai, M. M., et al. (2002). Heart rate variability parameters correlate with functional independence measures in ischemic stroke patients. *Journal of Electrocardiology, 35*, 243–246.

116. Meglic, B., Kobal, J., Osredkar, J., et al. (2001). Autonomic nervous system function in patients with acute brainstem stroke. *Cerebrovascular Disease, 11*(1), 2–8.
117. Tokgözoglu, S. L., Batur, M. K., Topçuoglu, M. A., et al. (1999). Effects of stroke localization on cardiac autonomic balance and sudden death. *Stroke, 30,* 1307–1311.
118. Carney, R. M., Freedland, K. E., Miller, G. E., et al. (2002). Depression as a risk factor for cardiac mortality and morbidity. A review of potential mechanisms. *Journal of Psychosomatic Research, 53,* 897–902.
119. Musselman, D. L., Evans, D. L., & Nemeroff, C. B. (1998). The relationship of depression to cardiovascular disease. *Archives of General Psychiatry, 55,* 580–592.
120. Stein, P. K., Carney, R. M., Freeland, K. E., et al. (2000). Severe depression is associated with markedly reduced heart rate variability in patients with stable coronary heart disease. *Journal of Psychosomatic Research, 48,* 493–500.
121. Glassman, A. H., Bigger, J. T., Gaffney, M., et al. (2007). Heart rate variability in acute coronary syndrome patients with major depression: Influence of sertraline and mood improvement. *Archives of General Psychiatry, 64*(9), 1025–1031.
122. Carney, R. M., Freedland, K. E., Stein, P. K., et al. (2000). Change in heart rate and heart rate variability during treatment for depression in patients with coronary heart disease. *Psychosomatic Medicine, 62,* 639–647.
123. Hallas, C. N., Thornton, E. W., Fabri, B. M., et al. (2003). Predicting blood pressure reactivity and heart rate variability from mood state following coronary artery bypass surgery. *International Journal of Psychophysiology, 47,* 43–55.
124. Carney, R. M., Blumenthal, J. A., Freedland, K. E., et al. (2005). Low heart rate variability and the effect of depression on post-myocardial infarction mortality. *Archives of Internal Medicine, 165*(13), 1486–1491.
125. Singh, J. P., Larson, M. G., O'Donnell, C. J., et al. (2000). Association of hyperglycemia with reduced heart rate variability (The Framingham Heart Study). *American Journal of Cardiology, 86,* 309–312.
126. Liao, D., Carnethon, M., Evans, G. W., et al. (2002). Lower heart rate variability is associated with the development of coronary heart disease in individuals with diabetes: The atherosclerosis risk in communities (ARIC) study. *Diabetes, 51*(12), 3524–3531.
127. Gerritsen, J., Dekker, J. M., TenVoorde, B. J., et al. (2001). Impaired autonomic function is associated with increased mortality, especially in subjects with diabetes, hypertension, or a history of cardiovascular disease. *Diabetes Care, 24*(10), 1793–1798.
128. Ziegler, D., Zentai, C. P., Perz, S., et al. (2008). Prediction of mortality using measures of cardiac autonomic dysfunction in the diabetic and nondiabetic population: The MONICA/KORA Augsburg Cohort Study. *Diabetes Care, 31*(3), 556–561.
129. Kon, H., Nagano, M., Tanaka, F., et al. (2006). Association of decreased variation of R-R interval and elevated serum C-reactive protein level in a general population in Japan. *International Heart Journal, 47*(6), 867–876.
130. Lanza, G. A., Pitocco, D., Navarese, E. P., et al. (2007). Association between cardiac autonomic dysfunction and inflammation in type 1 diabetic patients: Effect of beta-blockade. *European Heart Journal, 28*(7), 814–820.
131. Gonzalez-Clemente, J. M., Vilardell, C., Broch, M., et al. (2007). Lower heart rate variability is associated with higher plasma concentrations of IL-6 in type 1 diabetes. *European Journal of Endocrinology, 157*(1), 31–38.
132. Stein, P. K., Nelson, P., Rottman, J. N., et al. (1998). Heart rate variability reflects severity of COPD in PiZ alpha1-antitrypsin deficiency. *Chest, 113*(2), 327–333.
133. Tükek, T., Yildiz, P., Atilgan, D., et al. (2003). Effect of diurnal variability of heart rate on development of arrhythmia in patients with chronic obstructive pulmonary disease. *International Journal of Cardiology, 88,* 199–206.
134. Volterrani, M., Scalvini, S., Mazzuero, G., et al. (1994). Decreased heart rate variability in patients with chronic obstructive pulmonary disease. *Chest, 106,* 1432–1437.
135. Andrich, J., Schmitz, T., Saft, C., et al. (2002). Autonomic nervous system function in Huntington's disease. *Journal of Neurology Neurosurgery, and Psychiatry, 72*(6), 726–731.
136. Akincioglu, C., Unlu, M., & Tunc, T. (2003). Cardiac innervation and clinical correlates in idiopathic Parkinson's disease. *Nuclear Medicine Communications, 24*(3), 267–271.
137. Lampert, R., Ickovics, J. R., Viscoli, C. J., et al. (2003). Effects of propranolol on recovery of heart rate variability following acute myocardial infarction and relation to outcome in the beta-blocker heart attack trial. *American Journal of Cardiology, 91,* 137–142.
138. Carnethon, M. R., Prineas, R. J., Temprosa, M., et al. (2006). The association among autonomic nervous system function, incident diabetes, and intervention arm in the Diabetes Prevention Program. *Diabetes Care, 29*(4), 914–919.
139. Cowan, M. J., Pike, K. C., & Budzynski, H. K. (2001). Psychosocial nursing therapy following sudden cardiac arrest: Impact on two-year survival. *Nursing Research, 50*(2), 68–76.

CHAPTER 18

Cardiac Electrophysiology Procedures

Susan Blancher

The use of cardiac electrophysiology (EP) procedures includes diagnostic testing and interventional treatment procedures. In general, diagnostic EP studies are performed to determine an arrhythmia diagnosis or EP mechanism of a known arrhythmia. Interventional or therapeutic EP studies consist of endocardial catheter ablation of supraventricular and ventricular arrhythmias. The placement of implantable cardioverter defibrillators (ICDs) for the management of ventricular tachycardia (VT) and ventricular fibrillation (VF) is also an interventional EP procedure and is discussed in Chapter 32. Knowledge of electrocardiography (see Chapter 15), normal cardiac activation (see Chapter 1), and cardiac activation during arrhythmias (see Chapter 16) is needed to understand EP studies.

DIAGNOSTIC EP STUDIES

Before an EP study, a patient needs to be prepared for the procedure. This preparation and the techniques, complications, and indications of EP studies are presented here.

Patient Preparation

Preparation for EP procedures is similar to that for cardiac catheterization (see Chapter 20). Patients are kept fasting and usually sedated during EP studies. The degree of sedation depends on the type of study being performed and the preferences of the center performing the procedures. A peripheral intravenous line is required for administration of medicine. Systemic anticoagulation may be used during EP studies to decrease the incidence of thromboembolic complications.[1] Appropriate emergency and resuscitation equipment is required for all EP procedures.

Techniques

During invasive EP testing, spontaneous and pacing-induced intracardiac and surface electrical signals are recorded. The normal timing and sequence of electrical activation can be observed and measured during a normal or baseline rhythm. Abnormal timing and electrical activation sequences are recorded and studied during tachyarrhythmias. Programmed electrical stimulation may also be used to induce and analyze paroxysmal arrhythmias that are the same as or similar to a patient's clinical arrhythmia.[2]

Flexible catheters with at least 2 and up to 10 electrodes are introduced percutaneously. The catheters are advanced using fluoroscopy into the heart. The right and left femoral, subclavian, internal jugular, and median cephalic veins are the most commonly used venous access sites. One to several catheters may be placed depending on the type of study to be performed (Fig. 18-1). The usual intracardiac recording sites include the high right atrium, right atrial appendage, right ventricular apex, right ventricular outflow tract, coronary sinus, the His bundle region, and occasionally the left atrium. In addition, a roving catheter can be used to map intracardiac electrograms arising from different regions of the heart during tachycardia. Occasionally, the left ventricle is used during a diagnostic study for programmed electrical stimulation if VT cannot be induced from the right ventricle.

After the catheters are in place and connected to the physiologic recording equipment, intervals are measured from both the 12-lead electrocardiogram (ECG) and the intracardiac electrograms in the baseline state (Fig. 18-2). The AH interval is a measurement of conduction time from the low right atrium through the atrioventricular (AV) node to the His bundle and is an approximation of AV node conduction time. The AH interval can vary a great deal depending on the patient's autonomic state and measures approximately 55 to 120 milliseconds.[2] The HV interval represents conduction time from the onset of His bundle depolarization to the onset of ventricular activity. The normal HV interval measurement is 35 to 55 milliseconds.[3] After baseline recordings, various pacing techniques may be performed to assess the patient's electrical conduction system. Refractory periods for the atrium, AV node, and ventricle are recorded. The presence of retrograde or ventricular–atrial conduction is noted, as is the activation sequence. Attempts to induce and document the arrhythmia using the introduction of extrastimuli in either the atrium or the ventricle are then made. Intravenous isoproterenol or epinephrine may be used to help induce arrhythmias or reveal accessory pathway (AP) or slow pathway conduction.

The patient must be adequately prepared before the study and should understand that arrhythmia induction is often one of the primary goals of the study. The electrophysiologist attempts to gather as much information as possible depending on the type of arrhythmia induced and how well it is hemodynamically tolerated. Special physiologic recording equipment is able to document simultaneously every beat in 12-lead ECG and intracardiac electrogram format. Induced arrhythmias can then be reviewed and analyzed after they are terminated. It is important to note the method of arrhythmia termination. Tachycardias may be self-terminating or require antitachycardia pacing to stop them. Occasionally, it is necessary to cardiovert or defibrillate the patient to stop the arrhythmia. It is usually necessary to wait until the patient loses consciousness before defibrillation to prevent painful shock in an awake state.

If the patient is hemodynamically stable during a ventricular arrhythmia, attempts to map its origin can be performed, particularly if ablation is planned (see the section titled "Interventional EP and Catheter Ablation"). Atrial arrhythmias are usually well tolerated and allow for extensive mapping. Recordings are made at various locations in the heart and compared with a reference signal, either a surface ECG lead or a stable intracardiac electrogram. The site of earliest activation is closest to the site where the arrhythmia originates. Occasionally, the clinical arrhythmia cannot be induced or is not sustained long enough for adequate mapping.

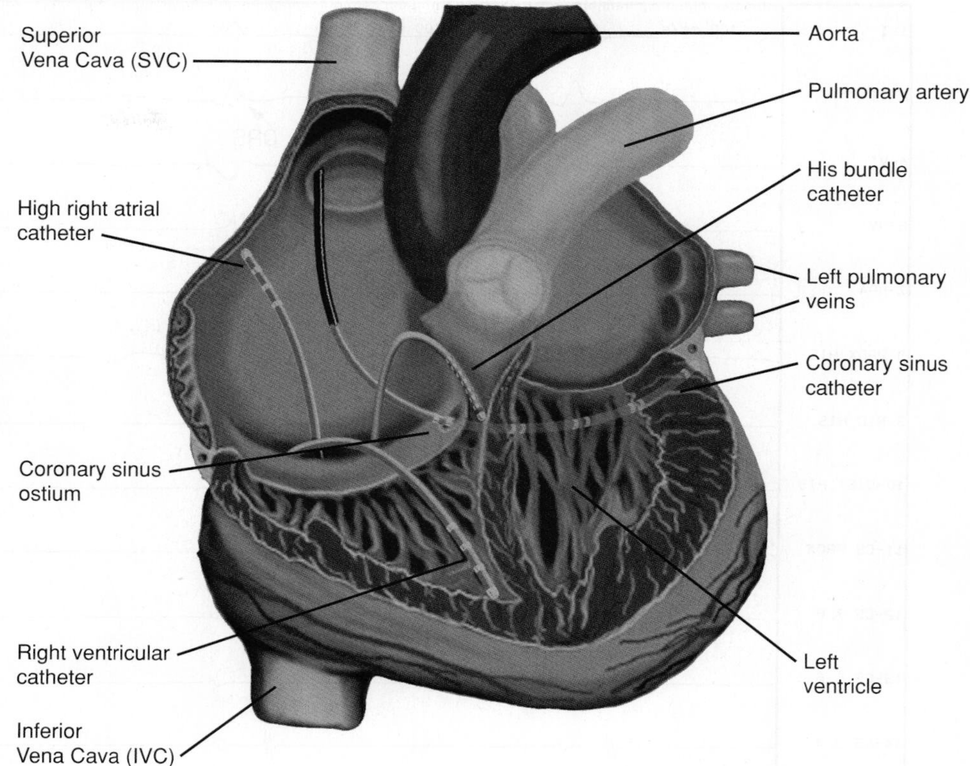

■ **Figure 18-1** Diagram of intracardiac placement of catheters. 1, right atrial recording catheter; 2, right ventricular recording catheter; 3, His recording catheter; 4, coronary sinus catheter.

Complications

Horowitz reviewed the experience of his EP laboratory and the laboratories of five others. During a 4-year period, 8,545 EP studies were performed on 4,015 patients. Five deaths (0.12%) occurred, all caused by intractable VF. The complications that occurred most frequently after EP studies were cardiac perforation (0.5%) and major venous thrombosis (0.5%). Cardiac perforation and pericardial effusion resolved without treatment in most patients; five patients required pericardial drainage or open repair. The femoral catheter site was the location of thrombosis for 95% of the 20 patients with venous thrombosis. Pulmonary emboli followed venous thrombosis in nine patients (0.2%).[1] A slightly higher incidence of venous thrombosis (1.1%) and pulmonary emboli (1.6%) was found in a study by DiMarco et al. including 359 patients during 1,062 EP studies.[4] They reported a 10% incidence of the use of countershock to terminate unstable VT; all patients returned to their original rhythms without complications. Systemic or catheter site infections were reported in 1.7% of patients in the study by DiMarco et al. but were not reported in Horowitz's study. Major hemorrhage and arterial injury are uncommon complications of EP studies and are substantially less than those with standard cardiac catheterization. In general, the actual risk of death from electrophysiological study procedures approaches zero because reentrant VT or fibrillation induced under controlled conditions can be quickly terminated.[5]

Indications

A list of indications for EP testing is provided in Display 18-1. Specific clinical indications are discussed in the subsequent sections. Indications for testing supraventricular tachyarrhythmias are discussed in the section titled "Interventional EP and Catheter Ablation."

Cardiac Arrest Survivors

People who survive a cardiac arrest not associated with an acute transmural myocardial infarction are at high risk for recurrence. The 2-year recurrence rate has been reported at 47%.[6] VF was the rhythm most commonly found at the time of cardiac arrest.[7,8] VT and VF were induced during EP testing in a baseline, antiarrhythmic, drug-free state in 70% to 80% of patients resuscitated from cardiac arrest.[9,10] A full discussion of sudden cardiac death can be found in Chapter 27.

Serial, EP-guided, antiarrhythmic drug testing was once common practice in EP laboratories. The goal was to identify a drug that was effective in suppressing inducible VT or VF and subsequent recurrent cardiac arrest. VT or VF suppression with EP-guided antiarrhythmic drug therapy has been reported in 26% to 80% of cardiac arrest survivors.[9,10] Antiarrhythmic medications may also provoke or exacerbate arrhythmias; this situation is referred to as proarrhythmic effect.

In recent years, several studies have shown ICD therapy as superior to EP-guided antiarrhythmic drugs in reducing all-cause mortality.[11–16] Therefore, ICD therapy is usually recommended as first-line therapy for patients with inducible VT or survivors of cardiac arrest.

EP testing is often recommended for patients who receive nonpharmacologic drug therapy. Implantation of combination antitachycardia pacemakers and ICDs usually requires a baseline EP test and may require testing after implantation to allow for correct

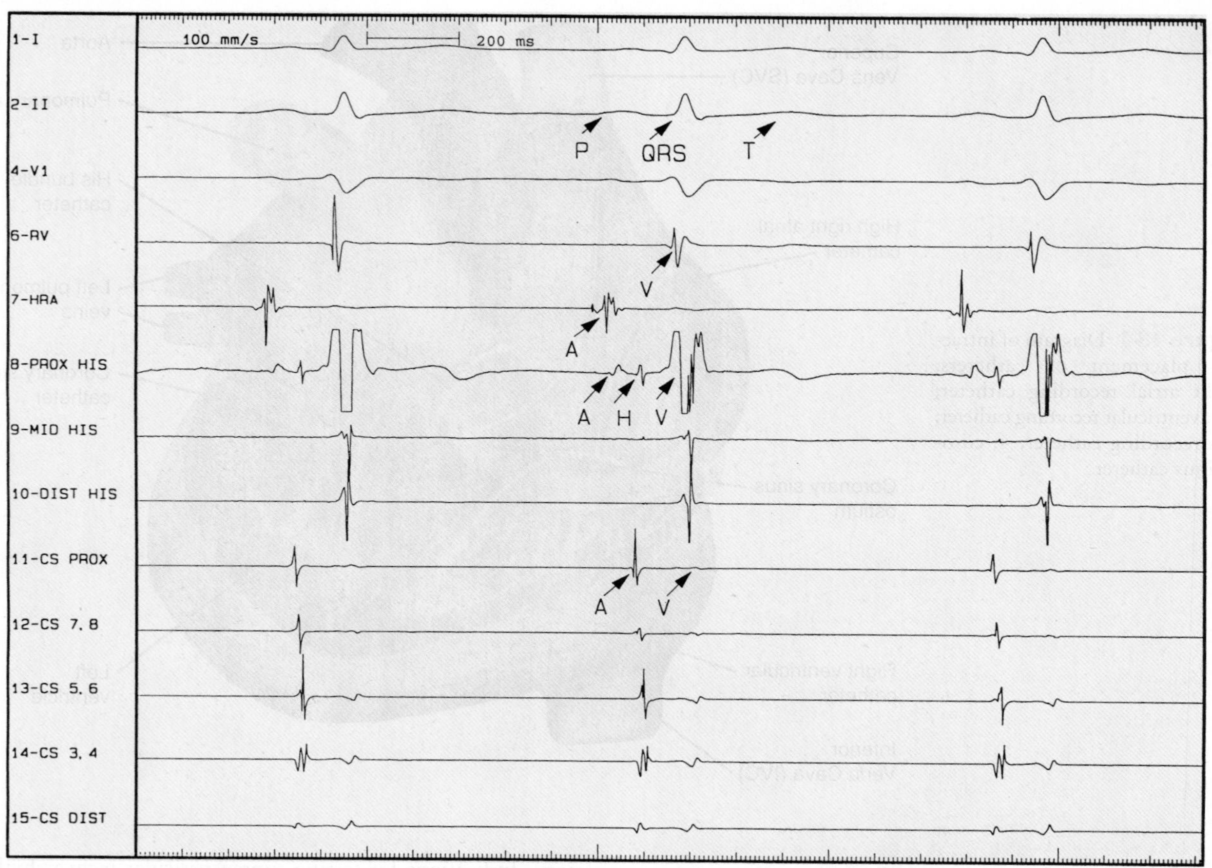

■ **Figure 18-2** Basic intervals. Channel 1-I is lead I; channel 2-II is lead II; channel 4-V1 is lead V_1; channel 6-RV is a right ventricular tracing (V); channel 7-RA is a right atrial tracing (A); channel 8-HIS PROX is a tracing from the proximal portion of the His bundle; channel 9-HIS MID is a tracing from the middle portion of the His bundle; channel 10-HIS DIST is a tracing from the distal portion of the His bundle. On channel 8-HIS PROX, the first waveform represents atrial depolarization (A) and occurs slightly later than the P wave on lead II. The next waveform is the His bundle deflection (H). The last waveform represents ventricular depolarization (V), corresponding to the QRS complex. Atrial and ventricular tracings are also recorded on channels 11–15-CS and reflect proximal to distal coronary sinus electrograms.

programming of the device. Knowledge of baseline conduction and the presence of concurrent atrial arrhythmias are also helpful for appropriate device selection (see Chapter 28). Patients with ischemic or nonischemic cardiomyopathy and reduced left ventricular function may be eligible to undergo prophylactic ICD implantation for primary prevention of cardiac arrest without undergoing prior EP evaluation.[16,17]

Wide-Complex Tachycardias

Wide-complex tachycardias can be caused by VT, supraventricular tachycardia with aberration, or preexcitation syndromes such as antidromic reciprocating tachycardia, in which an accessory bypass tract is the antegrade limb and the AV node is the retrograde limb of the tachycardia. Although guidelines and criteria have been established to help practitioners diagnose wide-complex tachycardias using the 12-lead ECG, necessary criteria may be difficult to identify, and the diagnosis may not be certain.[18,19] In these cases, EP studies are necessary to confirm or establish a diagnosis so that proper safe treatment can be initiated.[20]

During invasive EP testing for wide-complex arrhythmias, the timing and sequence of atrial activation in relation to ventricular activation are recorded. Although it may be difficult to distinguish the various preexcitation syndromes from VT, the presence of AV dissociation favors a diagnosis of VT.

Syncope

Syncope is defined as a sudden, transient loss of consciousness accompanied by loss of postural tone (Display 18-2).[21] It is a common medical problem that is frequently benign, but has a high rate of mortality in patients with underlying heart disease, transient myocardial ischemia, and other cardiac abnormalities. The 1-year mortality rate for presumed cardiac causes of syncope has been reported to be 20% to 30%.[22] Therefore, the principal objective when evaluating a patient with syncope, is to rule out any life-threatening etiology.

Although patients are routinely referred to EP centers for syncope evaluation, invasive EP testing is not always indicated. A thorough history, physical examination, and noninvasive testing can frequently uncover the mechanism and direct treatment. The

DISPLAY 18-1 Electrophysiology Testing in Patients with Coronary Heart Disease, Syncope, and Nonischemic Cardiomyopathy

Coronary Heart Disease

Class I:
1. Recommended for diagnostic evaluation in patients with remote MI with symptoms suggestive of VT, including palpitations, presyncope, and syncope
2. To guide and assess efficacy of VT ablation
3. Evaluation of wide QRS complex tachycardias of unclear mechanism

Class IIa:
1. Reasonable for risk stratification in patients with remote MI, NSVT, and LVEF $<40\%$

Class IIb:
1. Patients with congenital heart disease and ventricular couplets or NSVT to determine risk of ventricular arrhythmia

Syncope

Class I:
1. Syncope of unknown cause with impaired left ventricular function or structural heart disease

Class IIa:
1. Syncope with suspected brady or tachyarrhythmia in whom noninvasive diagnostic studies are not conclusive

Nonischemic Cardiomyopathy

Class I:
1. Diagnose bundle-branch reentrant tachycardia and to guide ablation sustained palpitations, wide QRS complex tachycardia, syncope, or presyncope

Classification

Class I: Conditions for which there is evidence and/or general agreement that a given procedure or treatment is useful and effective.
Class II: Conditions for which there is conflicting evidence and/or a divergence of opinion about the usefulness/efficacy of a procedure or treatment.
Class IIa: Weight of evidence/opinion is in favor of usefulness/efficacy
Class IIb: Usefulness/efficacy is less well established by evidence or opinion
Class III: Conditions for which there is evidence and/or general agreement that the procedure/treatment is not useful or effective and in some cases may be harmful.

MI, myocardial infarction; NSVT, nonsustained ventricular tachycardia; LVEF, left ventricular ejection fraction.
Adapted from Zipes, D., Camm, A., Borggrefe, M., et al. (2006). ACC/AHA/ESC 2006 guidelines for management of patients with ventricular arrhythmias and the prevention of sudden cardiac death: A Report of the American College of Cardiology/American Heart Association Task Force and the European Society of Cardiology Committee for Practice Guidelines (Writing Committee to Develop Guidelines for Management of Patients With Ventricular Arrhythmias and the Prevention of Sudden Cardiac Death). *Journal of the American College of Cardiology, 48*(5), e247–e346.

most common cause of syncope is vasodepressor syncope (otherwise known as neurally mediated syncope (NMS), neurocardiogenic syncope, or vasovagal syncope) followed by primary arrhythmias.

The history, including observers' statements describing the onset and recovery can provide clues for the cause. For example, sudden onset of syncope without any warning signs or symptoms suggests a cardiac arrhythmia. Recovery from syncope caused by a cardiac event is usually rapid, without neurologic sequelae, whereas recovery from a seizure is usually associated with a period of drowsiness and confusion. Transient ischemic attacks rarely result in syncope. Syncope precipitated by neck turning may be due to carotid sinus hypersensitivity. Medications taken that may be associated with proarrhythmia or orthostasis should be identified. Finally, a family history of unexpected sudden cardiac death should be ascertained.[23]

The physical examination should include orthostatic vital signs and carotid sinus pressure in patients who do not have cerebrovascular disease or carotid bruits.[24] Orthostatic vital signs can reveal a dehydrated patient. The presence of carotid bruits suggest impaired cerebral blood flow and underlying coronary artery disease. A positive carotid sinus test is documented by recording a pause of 3 seconds or longer or a blood pressure decrease greater than 50 mm Hg without symptoms. A blood pressure decrease of 30 mm Hg with symptoms is also considered an abnormal test result.[25] Reproduction of symptoms may suggest the cause of syncope, especially if other causes are ruled out. Assessment for abnormalities of visual fields, motor strength, sensation, tremor, cognition and speech, and gait disturbance may point to a neurological etiology.

Once the practitioner determines that a cardiac cause is most likely, a series of noninvasive tests may be indicated. The 12-lead ECG should be evaluated for arrhythmias, long QT syndrome, Brugada syndrome, left ventricular hypertrophy, preexcitation, conduction abnormalities, and ischemia or infarction. An echocardiogram helps to rule out or confirm the presence of structural heart disease, including valvular or obstructive disease and to evaluate left ventricular function. EP study outcomes suggest that an arrhythmia is more likely to be the cause of syncope in patients who have structural heart disease and reduced left ventricular

DISPLAY 18-2 Classification of Syncope

Cardiovascular

Reflex
Vasovagal
Vagovagal (situational)
- Micturition
- Deglutition
- Defecation
- Glossopharyngeal neuralgia
- Postprandial
- Tussive
- Supine hypotensive syndrome of near-term pregnancy
- Valsalva
- Oculovagal
- Sneeze
- Instrumentation
- Diving
- Jacuzzi
- Weight lifting
- Trumpet playing

Orthostatic
- Hyperadrenergic (e.g., volume depletion)
- Hypoadrenergic
  - Primary autonomic insufficiency
  - Secondary autonomic insufficiency (e.g., neurologic disorders or drugs)

Carotid sinus syncope
- Cardioinhibitory
- Vasodepressor
- Mixed
- Central

Cardiac
Mechanical (obstructive)
- Aortic stenosis
- Hypertrophic cardiomyopathy
- Pulmonary embolism
- Aortic dissection
- Myocardial infarction
- Mitral stenosis
- Left atrial myxoma

Cardiovascular ***(continued)***
- Pulmonic stenosis
- Cardiac tamponade
- Prosthetic valve malfunction
- Global myocardial ischemia
- Tetralogy of Fallot
- Pulmonary hypertension

Electrical (dysrhythmic)
- AV block
- Sick sinus syndrome
- Supraventricular or ventricular arrhythmias
- Long QT syndrome
- Pacemaker related

Noncardiovascular

Neurologic
Vertebrobasilar transient ischemic attack
- Atherosclerosis
- Mechanical

Subclavian steal syndrome
Takayasu disease
Normal pressure hydrocephalus
Unwitnessed seizure
Orthostatic syncope

Metabolic
Hypoxia
Hypoglycemia
Hyperventilation

Psychiatric
Panic disorders
Major depression
Hysteria

Unexplained

From Manolis, A. S., Linzer, M., Salem, D., et al. (1990). Syncope: Current diagnostic evaluation and management. *Annals of Internal Medicine, 112,* 850–863.

function. Therefore, when ventricular arrhythmias are suspected, hospitalization with immediate EP testing is indicated because these patients are presumed to be at high risk for sudden cardiac death until proven otherwise.[5] Ambulatory monitoring for 24 to 48 hours may be helpful if the patient is having frequent symptoms and is not considered to be at high risk for ventricular arrhythmias. If symptoms are not frequent enough, patient-activated transtelephonic event recorder[26] or a subcutaneously implanted loop recorder system (Medtronic, Bedford, NH) may be helpful in documenting the presence or absence of arrhythmia during symptoms of presyncope or syncope.[27]

Noninvasive risk stratification tools such as the signal-averaged ECG, T-wave alternans, heart rate variability, and baroreceptor sensitivity may prove helpful in identifying candidates with syncope at risk for VT events or sudden cardiac death. The signal-averaged ECG involves recording, amplifying, and filtering the surface ECG. Low-amplitude, high-frequency signals called late potentials are detected at the terminal portion of the QRS.[28,29] Delayed myocardial activation in areas of scar tissue represented by late potentials is thought to be the cause of ventricular arrhythmias. While the signal-averaged ECG is most accurate in patients with cardiomyopathy or previous myocardial infarction, it is associated with a low positive predictive value.[30] Microvolt T-wave alternans is a test where high-resolution chest electrodes detect tiny beat-to-beat changes in the ECG T-wave morphology during a period of controlled exercise. Spectral analysis, a mathematical method of measuring and comparing time and the electrical signals, is then used to calculate minute voltage changes. The presence of these changes has been associated with an increased risk of ventricular arrhythmias in patients with a history of myocardial infarction or cardiomyopathy. Studies show that the test has good positive and negative predictive accuracy.[31]

There is a growing body of evidence that supports T-wave alternans as the more powerful predictor for future arrhythmic events when compared with the signal-averaged ECG.[31,32] However, to date, no prospective clinical trials have demonstrated enough evidence to support the widespread use of any of these tests for high-risk screening and further research is still needed.[30,33]

The head-upright tilt test is a noninvasive, provocative test used to reproduce and diagnose NMS otherwise known as vasodepressor, neurocardiogenic, or vasovagal syncope. NMS is manifested by a combination of vasodilation and bradycardia, which occurs when the feedback mechanisms between the parasympathetic nervous system and sympathetic nervous system break down. Both systems are thought to activate alternately or simultaneously. Normal circulatory function is interrupted when both systems discharge rapidly. Vagal stimulation becomes exaggerated and causes bradycardia, vasodilation, or both in the presence of sympathetic nervous system stimulation.[34,35] During the head-upright tilt test, the patient is positioned on a tilt table with a footboard. There are various protocols for inducing NMS. Basically, an upright tilt at 60 to 70 degrees for 20 to 45 minutes is performed. If syncope is not induced, isoproterenol is administered in increasing doses for 15 to 20 minutes or until a positive result occurs. A positive response reproduces the patient's syncope along with documentation of bradycardia, hypotension, or both.[36–38] Indiscriminate use of tilt table testing in patients with clear-cut vasovagal syncope should be avoided as 25% to 30% of these patients will have a "false negative" result, which may confuse the diagnosis. The tilt test is most appropriately used in patients with histories suggestive of vasovagal syncope, but when the diagnosis is uncertain.[23,30]

Invasive EP studies are indicated when a noninvasive evaluation for syncope is negative and the suspicion for a cardiac cause remains high.[39–41] Sinus node function is evaluated by measuring the sinus node recovery time. Overdrive pacing is performed in the high right atrium for 30 to 60 seconds.[42] A prolonged sinus node recovery time may be an indication of sick sinus syndrome. The His–Purkinje system is evaluated by measuring the HV interval during sinus rhythm, and during incremental atrial pacing and atrial refractory period determinations. A prolonged HV interval is an indication of infrahisian disease.[5] AV node function is also evaluated by incremental atrial pacing and refractory period determinations. The Wenckebach point is recorded during incremental pacing, whereas the effective refractory periods of the atrium and AV node are recorded with the introduction of atrial extrastimuli. The atrium is refractory when the atrial extrastimuli fail to capture the atrium. The AV node is refractory when the atrial extrastimuli capture the atrium but fail to result in a His bundle depolarization (AV block). Permanent pacing may be indicated if abnormalities are found. Attempts are also made to induce ventricular and supraventricular tachycardia during EP testing for syncope.

In all cases, the findings of the EP study along with reproduction of the patient's symptoms and other findings in the work-up must be evaluated carefully to determine the appropriate course of therapy. The mechanism for syncope remains unexplained in approximately 40% of episodes.[43] The prognosis for this latter group of patients is good.[4]

INTERVENTIONAL EP AND CATHETER ABLATION

This interventional procedure includes a diagnostic EP study and catheter ablation. The mechanism of the arrhythmia is confirmed during the first part of the procedure, and the ablation takes place during the second part. Most centers combine the diagnostic and therapeutic segments of the study into one procedure.[44]

Radiofrequency Catheter Ablation

Catheter ablation techniques have been used for more than 20 years. Originally, high-energy, direct-current shocks were delivered through catheters, using a standard defibrillator, to the endocardial ablation site.[45,46] The technique was not widely used, however, because of the high complication rate, including cardiac tamponade and immediate and late sudden death.[47,48] As a result, efforts to find a safer energy source were pursued. In 1986, radiofrequency (RF) energy was applied through catheters to create endocardial lesions.[49,50] RF energy is a form of electrical energy that is produced by high-frequency alternating current. As the current passes through tissue, heat is generated. RF current is used in the operating room to coagulate blood vessels and to ablate abnormal tissue during neurosurgery. RF current used during endocardial catheter ablation is alternating current with a 500,000 to 750,000-Hz frequency range. The current passes from the electrode tip to a large-surface-area skin patch. The current is typically applied for 10 to 60 seconds at a time using 45 to 55 W. Catheter delivery of RF energy causes tissue heating in a small area around the electrode. The typical lesion is 3 mm × 4 mm × 5 mm.[48] Alternate forms of energy for lesion generation are currently under development, including cryoablation, ultrasound, laser, and microwave energy sources.

Techniques

The first part of the procedure, the diagnostic phase, was described previously. After a diagnosis is made, an ablating catheter is positioned at the targeted area. The ablating catheter can be steered and has four to six electrodes 2 to 5 mm apart. The catheter tip is 4 to 8 mm long and serves as the electrode through which RF current is applied. The targeted area is located using fluoroscopy and by observing the electrogram patterns recorded by the distal mapping electrode pair. Recently developed three-dimensional (3-D) mapping systems have vastly improved the precision and efficiency of mapping.[51]

Complications

Two of the most common complications associated with catheter ablation are inadvertent complete heart block when ablating in close proximity to the conduction system and cardiac perforation with tamponade when ablating within the atria, coronary sinus or other cardiac veins, or right ventricle. Fewer than 1% to 2% of the occurrences of these complications have been reported. Rare complications include creating inadvertent arrhythmogenic foci, producing mitral or tricuspid regurgitation when ablating at or near valves, systemic embolization and stroke (particularly when ablating in the left heart), and the creation of fixed lesions in coronary arteries when RF is applied in an adjacent area.[5,52] Specific complications related to ablation within the left atrium are addressed under the section on atrial fibrillation.

Indications

Combination EP study and catheter ablation procedures are indicated for patients with supraventricular tachycardias caused

DISPLAY 18-3 Indications for Combined Electrophysiology and Catheter Ablation in Patients with SVT

Class I:
1. Recurrent AVNRT:
   a. Poorly tolerated with hemodynamic intolerance
   b. Recurrent symptomatic
   c. Infrequent or single episode in those who desire complete control of arrhythmia
   d. Documented paroxysmal supraventricular tachycardia with only dual AV node pathways or single echo beats on electrophysiological study and no other identified cause of arrhythmia
   e. Infrequent well-tolerated AVNRT
2. AP-mediated arrhythmias:
   a. WPW syndrome, well tolerated
   b. WPW syndrome with rapid conduction or poorly tolerated AF
   c. AVRT (concealed AP), poorly tolerated
   d. AVRT (concealed AP), single or infrequent episodes
3. Focal atrial tachycardias (AT)
   a. Prophylactic therapy for recurrent symptomatic AT
   b. Incessant symptomatic or asymptomatic
4. Atrial flutter (if catheter ablation *cure* not possible, consider AV Node ablation and pacemaker):
   a. First episode, well tolerated
   b. Recurrent, well tolerated
   c. Poorly tolerated
   d. Atrial Flutter after IC antiarrhythmic drug (AAD) or amiodarone for AF
   e. Symptomatic nonisthmus-dependent atrial flutter after failed AAD therapy

Class IIa:
1. AP-mediated arrhythmias:
   a. Preexcitation, asymptomatic (no documented SVT)
2. Focal junctional tachycardia

Class IIb:
1. Inappropriate sinus tachycardia:
   a. Sinus node modification/elimination (as a last resort)

Classification system:
Class I: Conditions for which there is evidence and/or general agreement that a given procedure or treatment is useful and effective.
Class II: Conditions for which there is conflicting evidence and/or a divergence of opinion about the usefulness/efficacy of a procedure or treatment.
Class IIa: Weight of evidence/opinion is in favor of usefulness/efficacy.
Class IIb: Usefulness/efficacy is less well established by evidence or opinion.
Class III: Conditions for which there is evidence and/or general agreement that the procedure/treatment is not useful or effective and in some cases may be harmful.

Adapted from Blomstrom-Lundqvist, C., Scheinman, M. M., Aliot, E. M., et al. (2003). ACC/AHA/ESC guidelines for the management of patients with supraventricular arrhythmias—Executive summary. *European Heart Journal, 24*(20), 1857–1897; doi: 10.1016.

by APs, AV nodal reentry tachycardia, intra-atrial tachycardias caused by either automatic or reentrant mechanism, atrial fibrillation (AF), and atrial flutter. These procedures are also indicated for some patients with certain types of VT (Display 18-3).

AV Nodal Reentrant Tachycardia

Dual AV nodal pathways are the substrate for AV nodal reentrant tachycardia (AVNRT). This arrhythmia is responsible for 60% to 70% of paroxysmal supraventricular tachycardias.[44] The fast pathway has a longer effective refractory period and the slow pathway has a shorter refractory period. The typical form of AVNRT is initiated when a premature beat from the atrium is blocked in the fast pathway. The early beat conducts down the slow pathway and then reenters back into the atrium through the fast pathway. This impulse continues to conduct down the slow pathway and up the fast pathway, thus perpetuating the reentry circuit and the tachycardia. Uncommon or atypical forms of AVNRT can be found and consist of antegrade fast and retrograde slow pathway conduction, or antegrade and retrograde conduction over multiple slow pathway fibers. Ablation of all forms of AVNRT is generally the same and is accomplished by mapping the slow pathway region, which extends from the posterior/inferior interatrial septum near the coronary sinus ostium up to the anterior/superior interatrial septum. After characteristic electrograms are recorded, RF energy is applied through the distal ablating electrode (Fig. 18-3). Repeat programmed stimulation is performed after the ablation in an attempt to induce the tachycardia. The procedure is considered successful when AVNRT cannot be induced and/or when there is no evidence of slow pathway conduction. Complete heart block is a potentially serious complication because of the close proximity of the slow pathway to the compact AV node and has been

DISPLAY 18-3 Indications for Catheter Ablation in Patients with Ventricular Arrhythmias (continued)

Class I:
1. Low risk of SCD, sustained MMVT, drug resistant or intolerant, or do not want long-term drug therapy
2. Bundle-branch reentrant VT
3. Adjunctive therapy in patients with ICDs who are receiving multiple shocks as a result of sustained VT not manageable by reprogramming ICD or changing drug therapy, or do not want long-term drug therapy
4. WPW syndrome resuscitated from SCD due to AF and rapid conduction over AP causing VF

Class IIa:
1. Low risk of SCD, symptomatic nonsustained MMVT that is drug resistant or intolerant, or do not want long-term drug therapy
2. Low risk of SCD, frequent, symptomatic monomorphic PVCs that are drug resistant or intolerant, or do not want long-term therapy
3. Symptomatic WPW syndrome with AP refractory periods less than 240 milllliseconds in duration
4. Recurring or incessant MMVT can be ablated after treatment with IV amiodarone or procainamide

Class IIb:
1. Ablation of Purkinje fiber potentials may be considered in patient with VT storm consistently provoked by PVCs or similar morphology
2. Ablation of very frequent asymptomatic PVCs to avoid or treat tachycardia-induced CM
3. Curative ablation may be considered in lieu of ICD therapy to improve symptoms in patients with left ventricular dysfunction due to prior MI, LVEF >40%, and recurrent hemodynamically stable VT.

Class III:
1. Ablation of asymptomatic, relatively infrequent PVCs is not indicated.

Classification system:
Class I: Conditions for which there is evidence and/or general agreement that a given procedure or treatment is useful and effective.
Class II: Conditions for which there is conflicting evidence and/or a divergence of opinion about the usefulness/efficacy of a procedure or treatment.
Class IIa: Weight of evidence/opinion is in favor of usefulness/efficacy
Class IIb: Usefulness/efficacy is less well established by evidence or opinion
Class III: Conditions for which there is evidence and/or general agreement that the procedure/treatment is not useful or effective and in some cases may be harmful

MMVT, monomorphic ventricular tachycardia; PVC, premature ventricular contraction; SCD, sudden cardiac death; CM, cardiomyopathy; ERP, effective refractory period; IV, intravenous; MI, myocardial infarction; LVEF, left ventricular ejection fraction.
Adapted from Zipes, D., Camm, A., Borggrefe, M. (2006). ACC/AHA/ESC 2006 guidelines for management of patients with ventricular arrhythmias and the prevention of sudden cardiac death: A report of the American College of Cardiology/American Heart Association Task Force and the European Society of Cardiology Committee for Practice Guidelines (Writing Committee to Develop Guidelines for Management of Patients With Ventricular Arrhythmias and the Prevention of Sudden Cardiac Death) *Journal of American College of Cardiology, 48*(5), e247–e346.

reported 1.3% to 3% of the time. The success rate is reported between 96% and 100%.[53,54]

AV Reentrant Tachycardia

Both Wolff–Parkinson–White (WPW) syndrome and concealed AV bypass tracts are responsible for 30% to 40% of paroxysmal supraventricular tachycardias.[55] The anatomy is basically the same. The AP is a small bundle of muscle fibers that crosses the AV groove on either the right or left side of the heart, creating an extra electrical connection that can conduct in one or both directions. When the AP conducts in an anterograde direction, a delta wave can be observed on the ECG and is characteristic of WPW syndrome. Paroxysmal supraventricular tachycardia is initiated in the same manner as described for AVNRT. The AV node serves as the antegrade limb of the tachycardia and the AP serves as the retrograde limb of the tachycardia. This conduction pattern results in a narrow QRS complex and is known as orthodromic reciprocating tachycardia. If conduction travels antegrade over the AP and retrograde up the AV node, then a wide QRS complex is observed and is known as antidromic reciprocating tachycardia. If AF occurs in a patient with WPW syndrome, then a life-threatening situation may develop if conduction over the AP is rapid enough to induce VF. Less common forms of APs are the Mahaim fiber, which slowly conducts only antegrade and is found on the right side of the heart, and the permanent form of junctional reciprocating tachycardia, which slowly conducts only retrograde and is located very near or within the coronary sinus ostium.[54,55]

Catheter ablation of AV bypass tracts on the left side of the heart involves one of two techniques. The mapping and ablating catheter can be advanced from the femoral artery retrograde across the aortic valve. The catheter is then positioned under or on the mitral valve annulus. When the catheter is positioned properly, the AP activation can be recorded and appears as a discrete high-frequency potential.[44,58] RF current is then applied. If the patient has WPW syndrome, the delta wave on the ECG disappears during RF energy application (Fig. 18-4). It is necessary to ablate so that both antegrade and retrograde conduction over the bypass tract are abolished. Testing is performed after ablating to assess for retrograde conduction and to try to induce tachycardia. Another

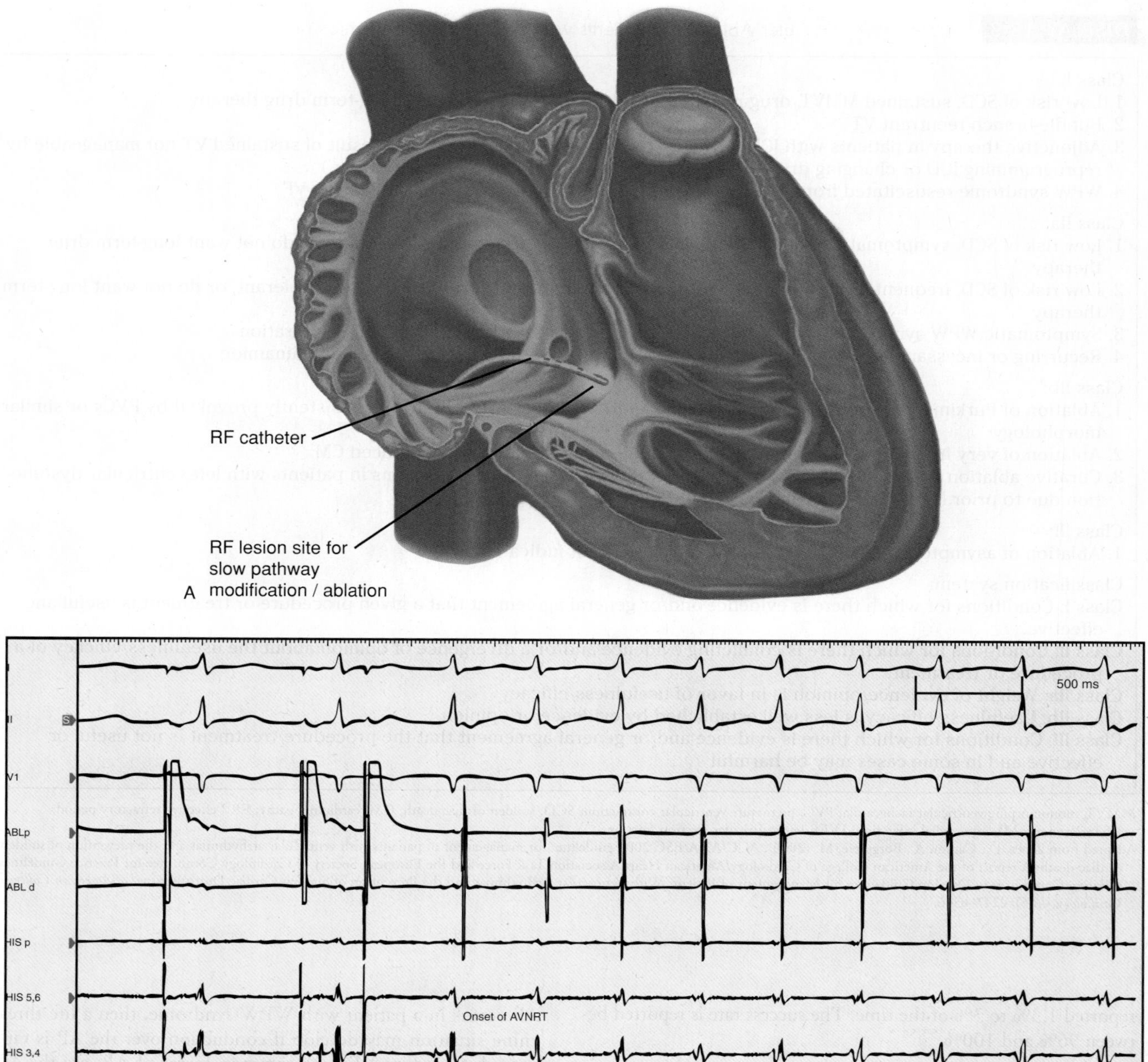

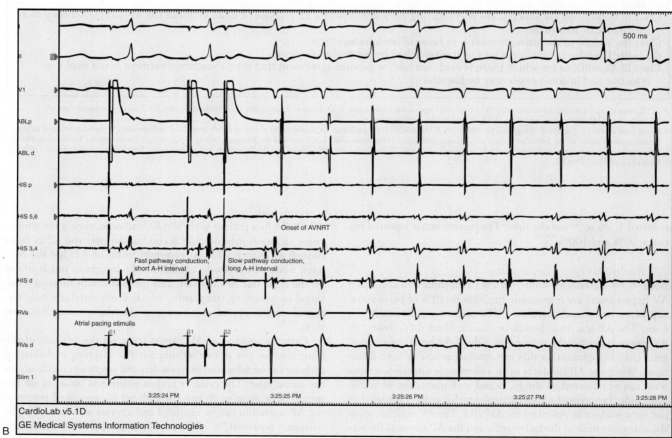

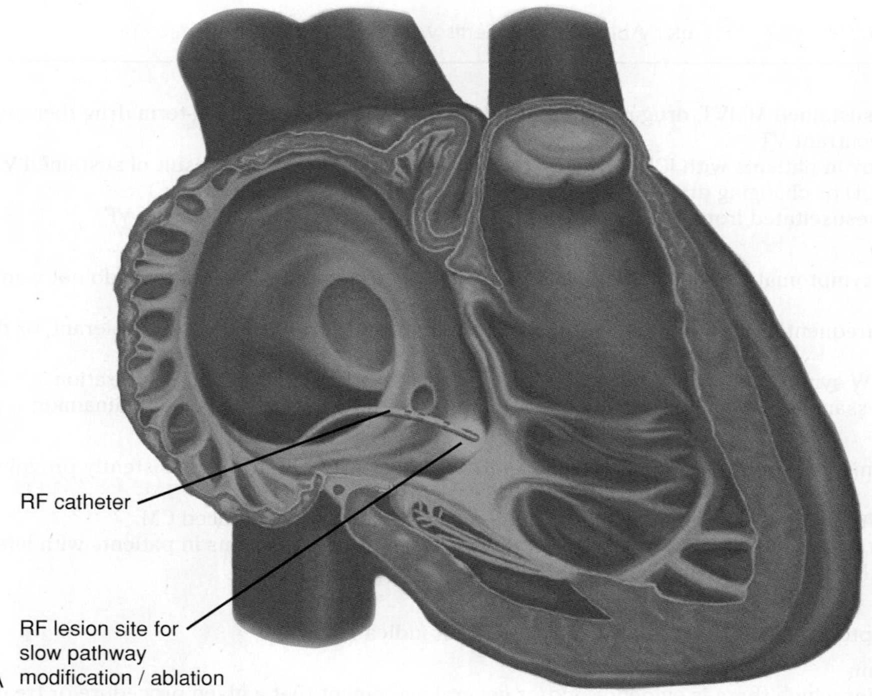

■ **Figure 18-3** (A) Diagram of slow pathway catheter ablation for treatment of AVNRT. (B) Intracardiac electrograms show atrial pacing with AV conduction jumping from fast pathway to slow pathway followed by onset of AVNRT.

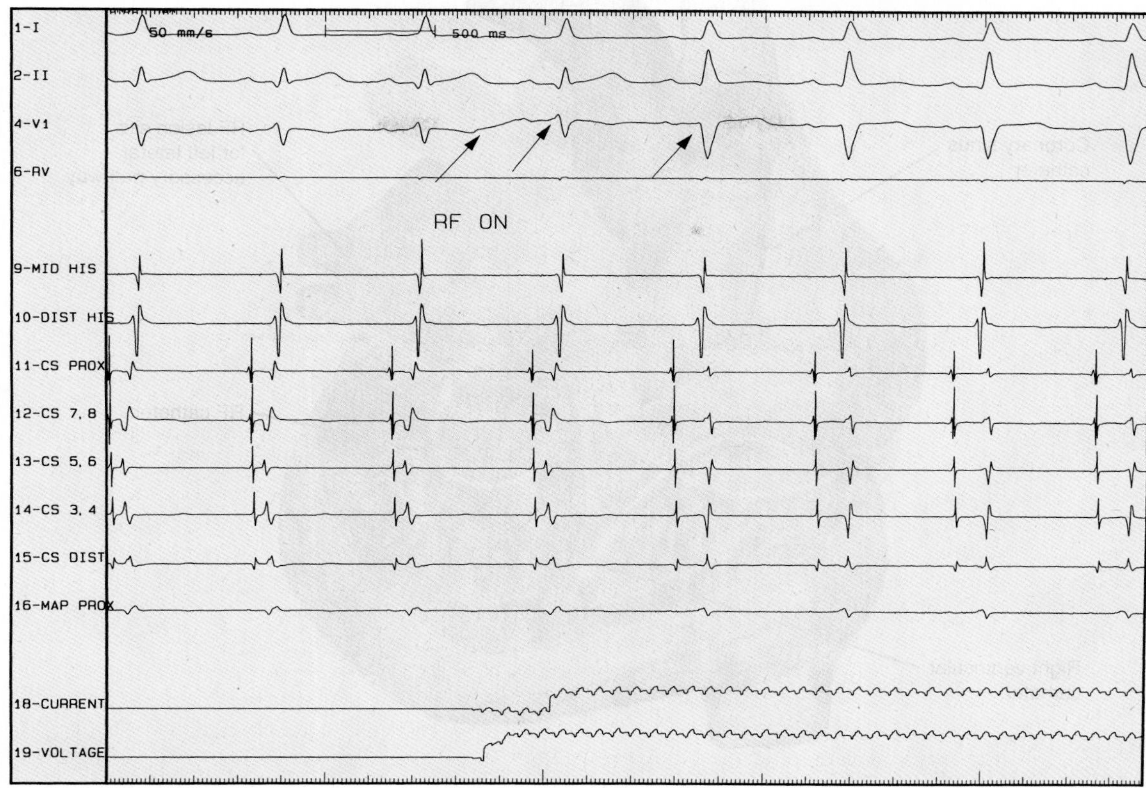

■ **Figure 18-4** Loss of delta wave after onset of RF energy application. Channel 1, lead I; channel 2, lead II; channel 4, lead V_1; channel 6, right ventricular tracing; channels 9 and 10, His bundle electrograms; channels 11–15, coronary sinus (CS) electrograms. Notice that before RF energy is applied, the earliest ventricular depolarization occurs on the CS electrogram labeled CS 5, 6, corresponding to the left posterior septal position. This location is where the mapping and ablating catheter was positioned under the mitral valve annulus. After RF energy application, the delta wave disappears (leads I, II_1, V_1), and the ventricular activation sequence changes to normal on all coronary sinus electrograms. (Fellows, C. L., Brett, C., & Main, C. C. [1992]. Radiofrequency catheter ablation of Wolff-Parkinson-White syndrome. *Virginia Mason Clinic Bulletin, 46,* 45–51.)

approach to the mitral annulus is by means of transseptal catheterization. In this approach, the ablating and mapping catheter is advanced to the left atrium through the right heart using a special sheath assembly to cross the interatrial septum (Fig. 18-5). Both approaches have an 85% success rate.[59] Catheter ablation of right-sided and septal APs are somewhat more difficult because there is no structure analogous to the coronary sinus to aid in mapping the atrial–ventricular groove. Specialized multielectrode, steerable catheters, and long guiding sheaths have proven useful in providing catheter stability for mapping and ablating on the right side of the heart.

Atrial Flutter

Primary ablation of classic right atrial isthmus–dependent flutter is being performed in most centers and can be offered as a first-line therapy in patients with atrial flutter who are not interested in drug therapy.[60] This procedure involves ablation of a discrete anatomic region in the low right atrium thought to be responsible for the macroreentrant circuit. Ablation of the right atrial isthmus between the inferior vena cava and tricuspid valve creates a line of block that prevents perpetuation of the arrhythmia (see Fig. 18-7). Success rates in an experienced center were reported to be 90% ($n = 200$). Although the procedure is safe, with an extremely low complication rate, the recurrence of atrial flutter was 10% to 15%. Repeat ablation was successful in most cases.[61]

Atypical forms of atrial flutter are less common and can arise from the right or left atria. Mapping and ablation of these circuits can be performed but the success rate is lower than that for typical atrial flutter.

Atrial Fibrillation

Complete AV node ablation is indicated for patients who have chronic or paroxysmal AF or flutter with a rapid ventricular response. This procedure should be performed only in patients for whom conventional antiarrhythmic drug therapy has failed or for whom the side effects from effective doses of medication are intolerable. This procedure is performed by advancing the ablating catheter from the right femoral vein to the area of the AV node (Fig. 18-6). Complete heart block with or without a junctional escape rhythm is the result. Permanent, rate-responsive pacing is indicated after AV node ablation, and the patient may discontinue all antiarrhythmic medications.[49,62] Continuous anticoagulation is recommended because the underlying arrhythmia is still present. Left ventricular dysfunction caused by chronic, rapid heart rates in AF has been reported to improve after AV node ablation.[63] In addition, more than 80% of the patients report improved quality of life with increased exercise tolerance after this procedure.[64]

Recent ablation techniques for AF have focused on the ablation of triggers or ectopic beats that arise from the pulmonary

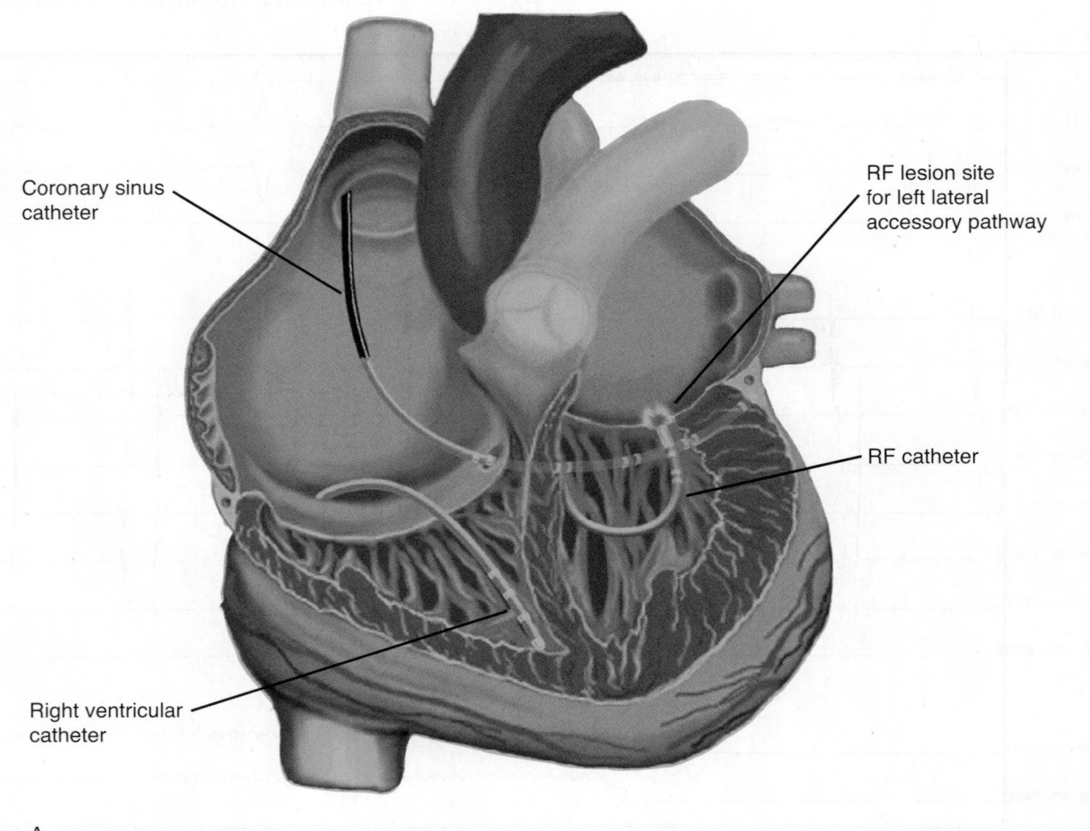

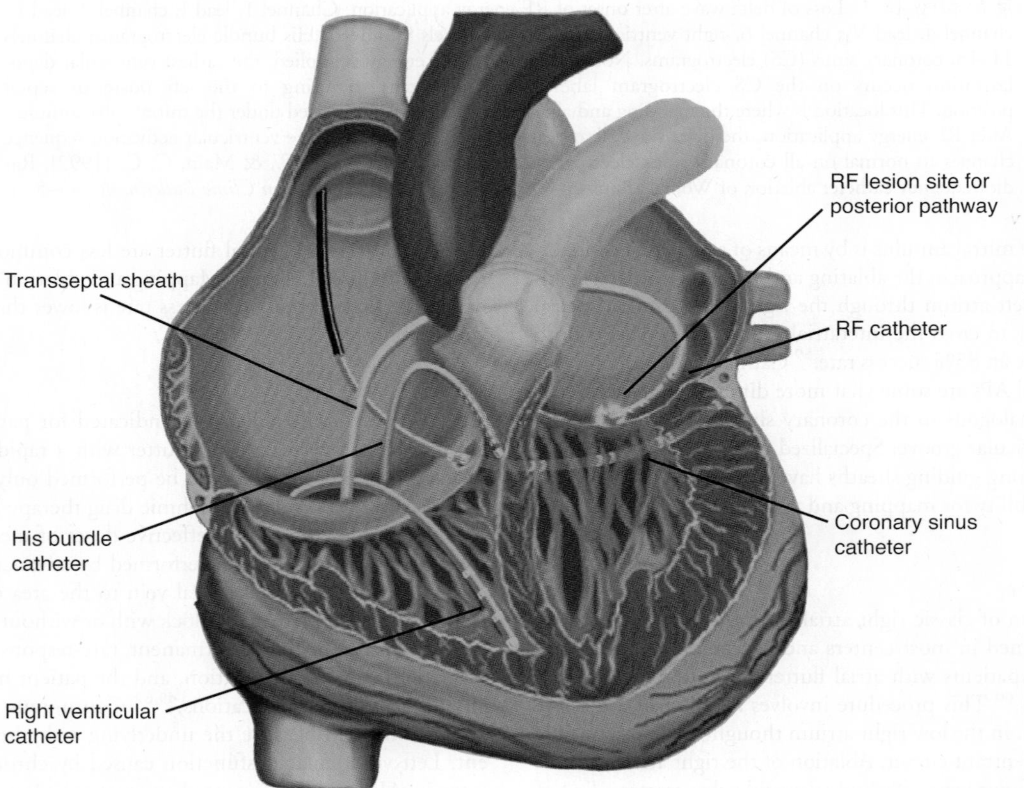

■ **Figure 18-5** Diagram of catheter ablation of **(A)** left lateral AP using aortic approach associated radiograph in the left anterior oblique view and **(B)** left posterior lateral AP using transseptal approach. Intracardiac electrograms show (1) retrograde conduction over a left lateral AP during ventricular pacing and (2) retrograde conduction up AV node during ventricular pacing after successful ablation of pathway.

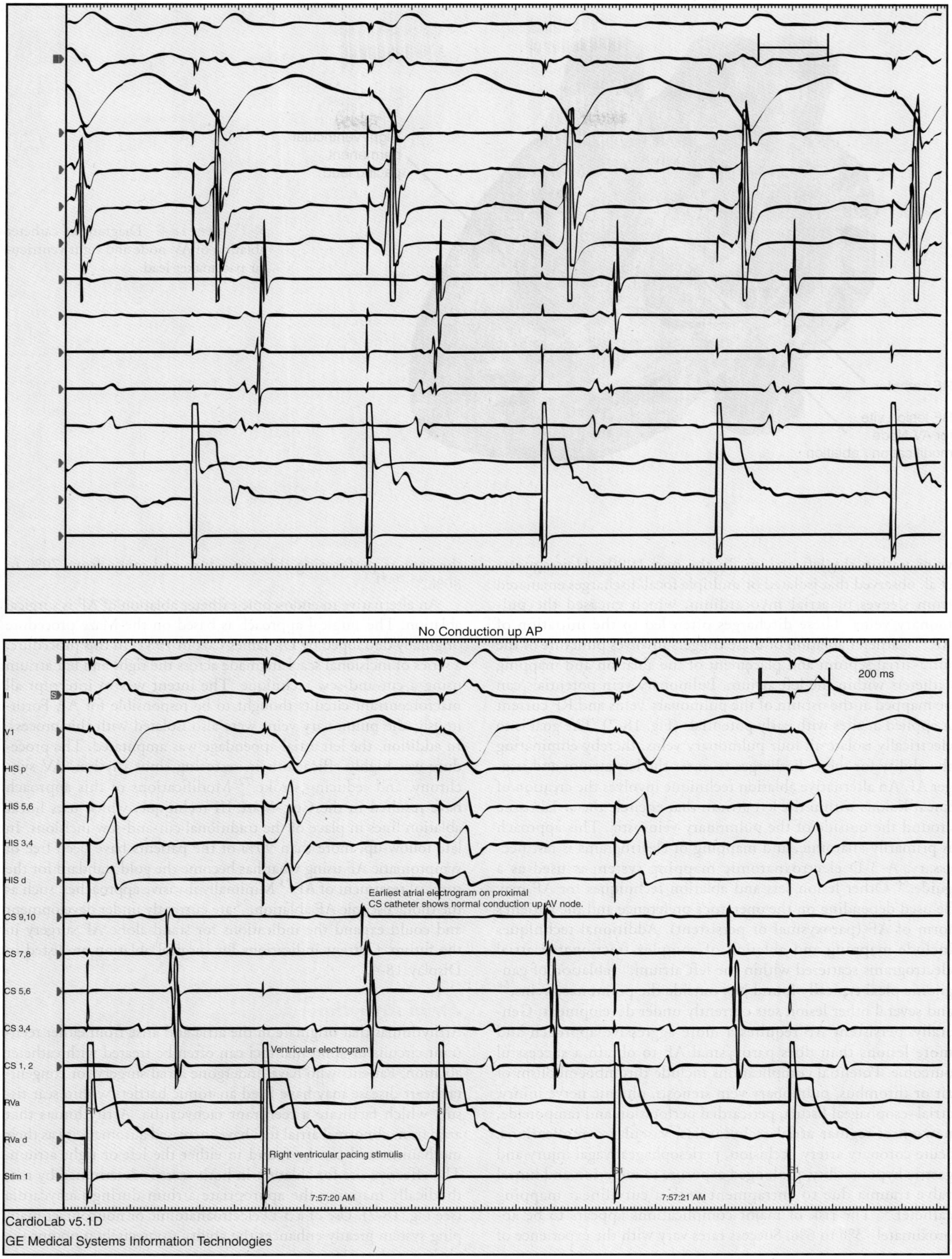

No Conduction up AP

200 ms

II

V1

HIS p

HIS 5,6

HIS 3,4

HIS d

Earliest atrial electrogram on proximal
CS catheter shows normal conduction up AV node.

CS 9,10

CS 7,8

CS 5,6

CS 3,4

Ventricular electrogram

CS 1, 2

RVa

RVa d

Right ventricular pacing stimulis

Stim 1

7:57:20 AM

7:57:21 AM

CardioLab v5.1D

GE Medical Systems Information Technologies

■ **Figure 18-5** *(continued)* Post Ablation: ventricular pacing with retrograde conduction up AV node post successful ablation of left lateral accessory pathway.

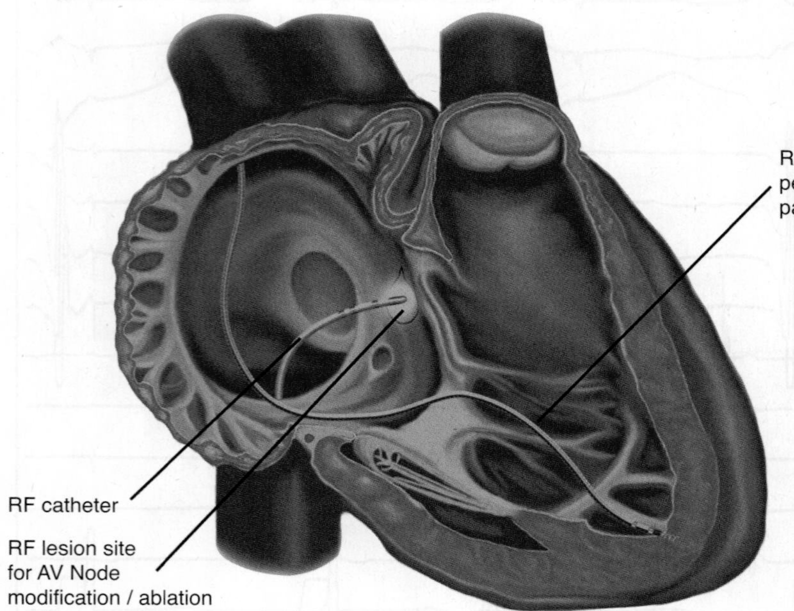

■ **Figure 18-6** Diagram of catheter ablation of AV node and right ventricular pacemaker lead.

veins within the left atrium. In the mid 1990s, Haissaguerre et al. observed that isolated or multiple focal discharges emanated from sleeves of atrial myocardium, which encased the pulmonary veins. These discharges often led to the initiation of AF.[65] Catheter ablation of these triggers involves puncture of the intra-atrial septum and placement of the ablation and mapping catheters within the left atrium. Pulmonary vein potentials can be mapped at the ostium of the pulmonary veins and RF current is applied at sites with early potentials (Fig. 18-7). The goal is to electrically isolate all four pulmonary veins, thereby eliminating the ability for these discharges to enter the left atrium and trigger AF. An alternative ablation technique involves the creation of linear lesions within the left atrium that encircle the atrial tissue around the outside of the pulmonary vein ostia. This approach is primarily anatomic, and mapping of electrograms is not necessary. A 3-D electroanatomic mapping system is used as a guide.[66] Other lesion sets and ablation techniques for AF may be used depending on the operator's preference and the patient's form of AF (paroxysmal or persistent). Additional techniques include mapping and ablation of complex fractionated atrial electrograms scattered within the left atrium,[67] ablation of ganglionic plexi typically found just outside the pulmonary veins,[68] and several other lesion sets currently under development. Generally, persistent AF requires a more aggressive approach and more lesions than does paroxysmal AF to obtain a successful outcome. Potential complications include thromboembolism of air or thrombus, pulmonary vein stenosis, phrenic nerve injury, atrial–esophageal fistula, pericardial perforation and tamponade, new-onset regular atrial tachycardias, vascular complications, acute coronary artery occlusion, periesophageal vagal injury and gastric hypomotility, prolonged exposure to radiation and mitral valve trauma due to entrapment with a curvilinear mapping catheter.[69] The risk of major complications appears to be approximately 3% to 6%. Success rates vary with the experience of the centers performing this procedure and range from 70% to 80%.[66,70,71]

An alternative to endoscopic catheter ablation of AF is surgical ablation. The surgical approach is based on the Maze procedure originally developed by Dr. James Cox in 1987. In this procedure, a series of incisional scars are made across the right and left atrium using a cut-and-sew technique. The intent was to interrupt all macroreentrant circuits thought to be responsible for AF. Fortuitously, the pulmonary veins were also isolated with this process. In addition, the left atrial appendage was amputated. The procedure was highly efficacious in restoring sinus rhythm, AV synchrony, and reducing stroke.[72] Modifications of this approach have resulted in the Cox–Maze III technique, which uses linear ablation lines in place of the traditional cut-and-sew incisions. In late follow-up, more than 90% of the patients have been free of symptomatic AF using what has become the gold standard for the surgical treatment of AF.[73] Minimally invasive approaches, such as the thoracoscopic AF ablation,[74] are currently under development and could expand the indications for stand-alone AF surgery in the future. Current indications for surgical ablation are listed in Display 18-4.

Atrial Arrhythmias

Arrhythmias that originate in the atria and arise from either reentrant circuits or abnormal foci can often be treated with catheter ablation. Patients who have undergone atrial surgery for congenital heart disease may have fixed anatomic barriers within scar tissue, which facilitate a reentrant tachycardia. Arrhythmias that arise from abnormal atrial foci have increased automaticity as their mechanism and can be found in either the left or right atrium. The effective site for ablation in both cases is determined by methodically mapping the appropriate atrium during tachycardia (see Fig. 18-7). Use of a 3-D electroanatomic or noncontact mapping system greatly enhances the ability to precisely pinpoint the

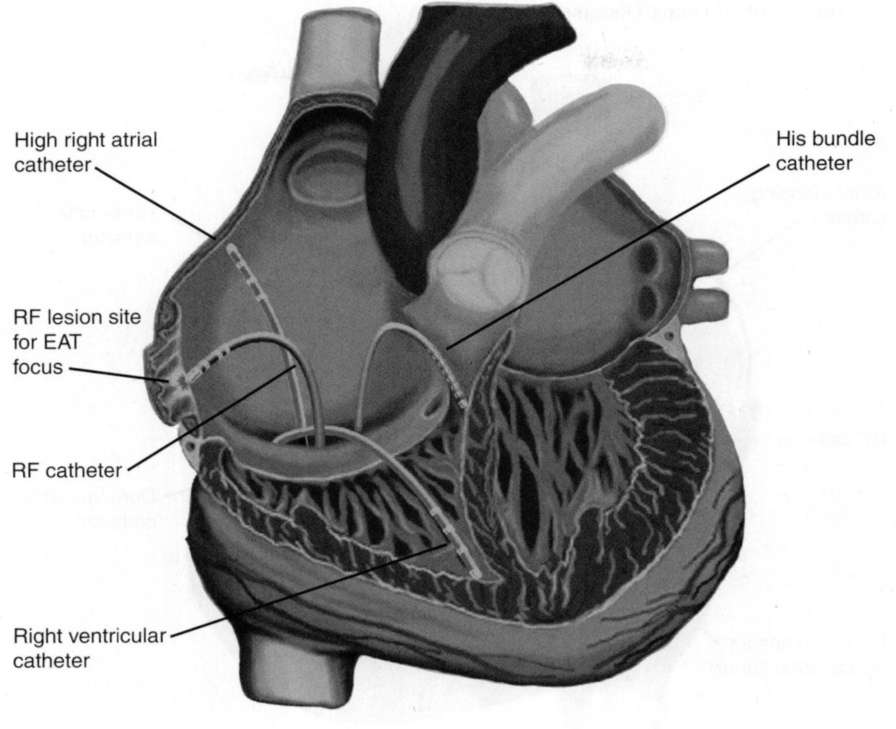

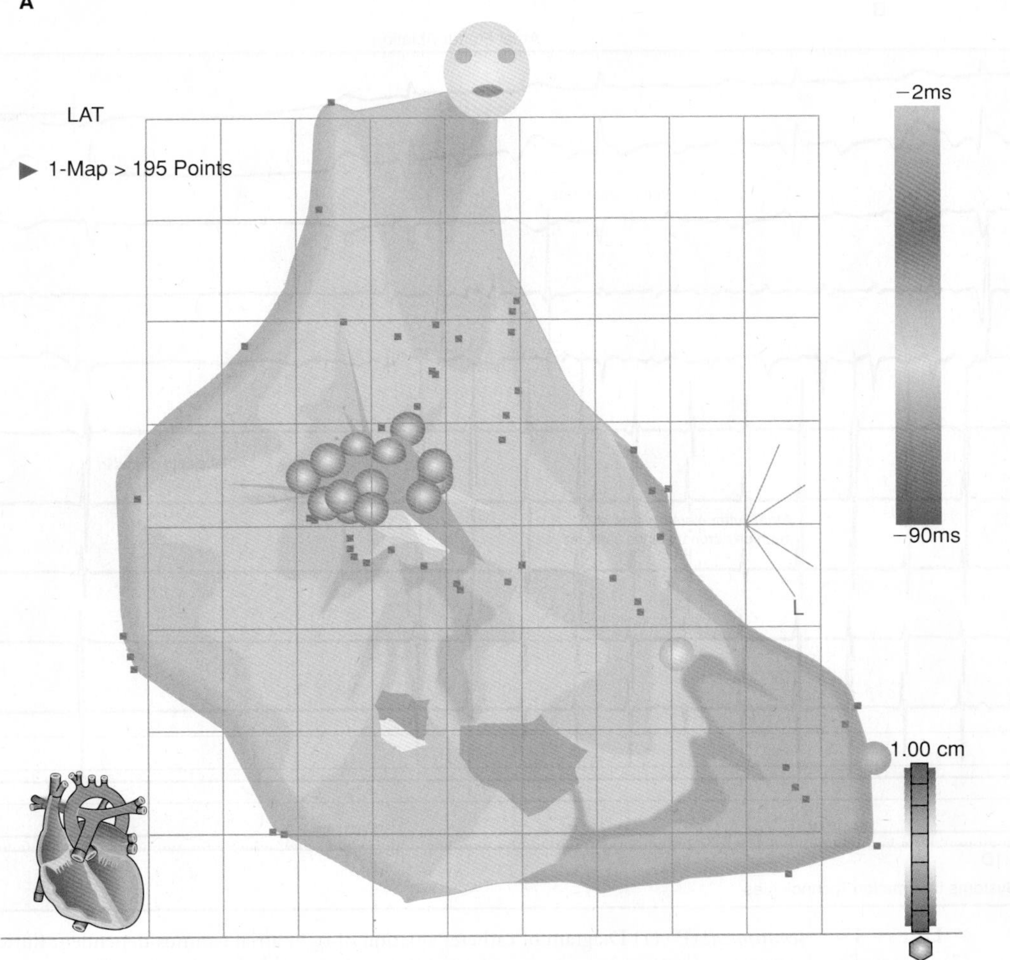

Figure 18-7 **(A)** (1) Diagram of catheter ablation of ectopic atrial tachycardia with focus on lateral wall of right atrium. Red balls show site of ablation where the atrial tachycardia originates. (2) Image of ectopic atrial focus obtained from 3-D mapping system (Biosense-Webster) *(continued)*

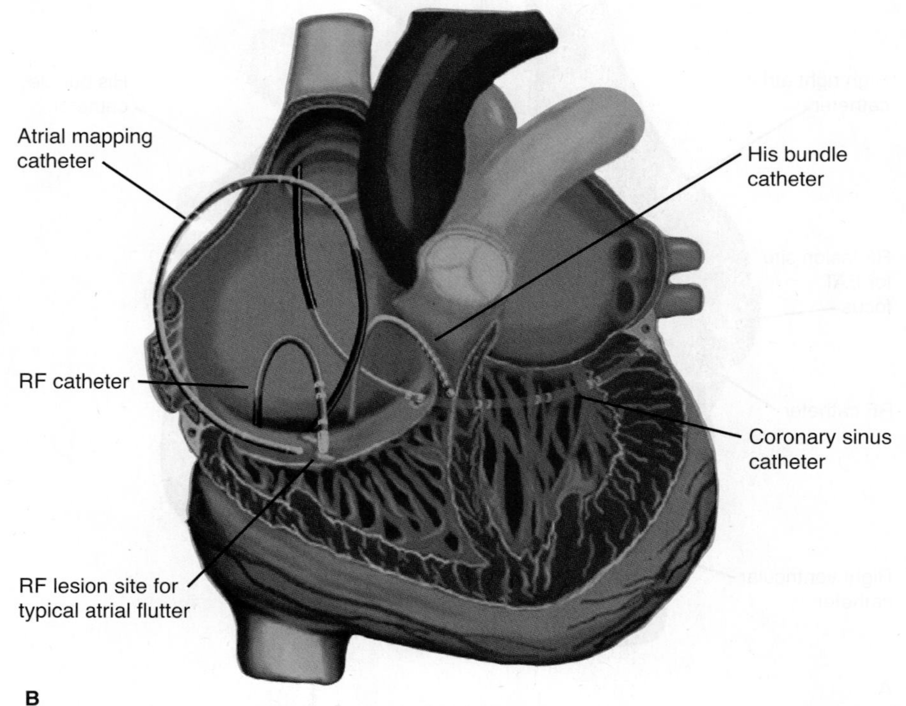

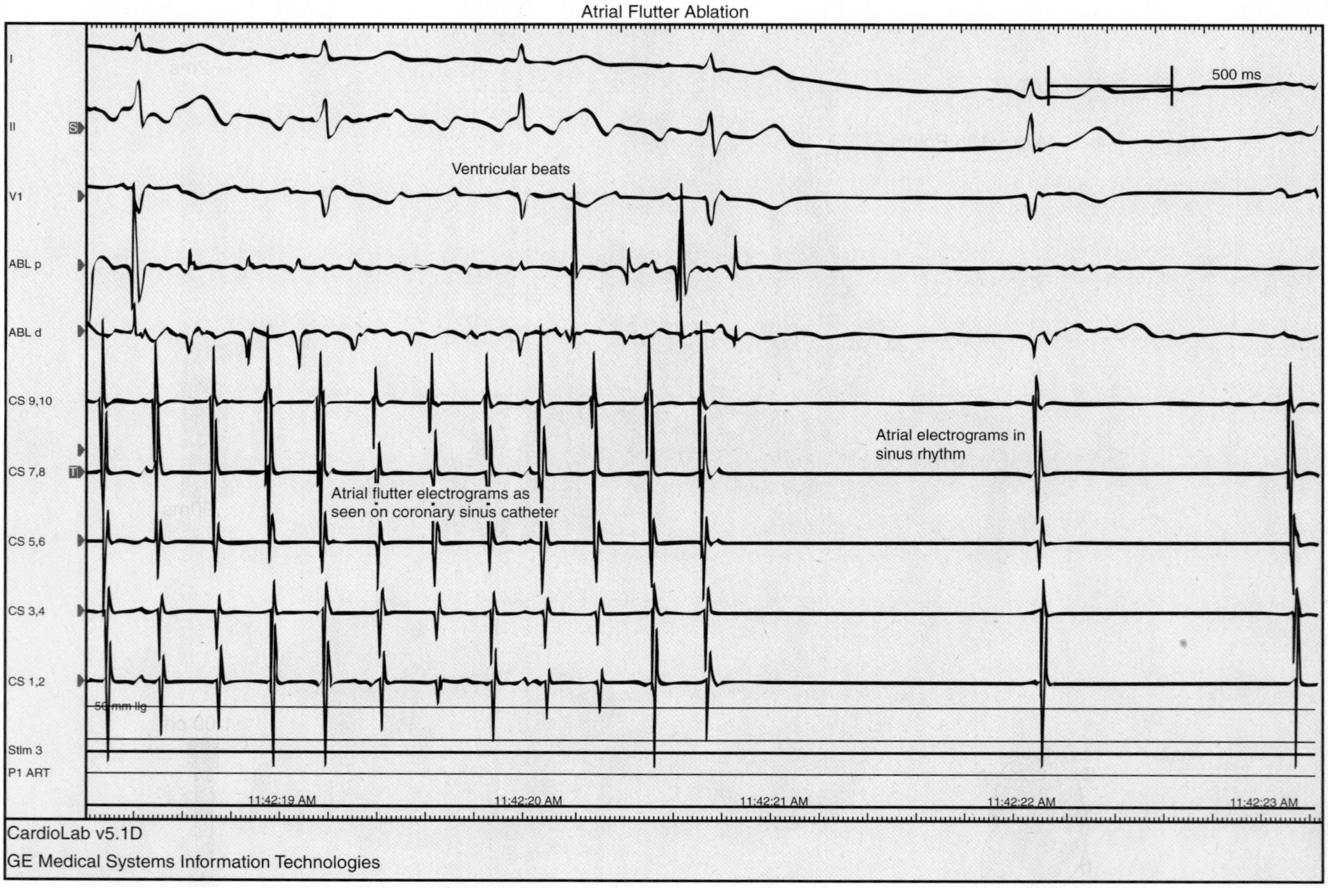

■ **Figure 18-7** *(continued)* **(B)** (1) Diagram of catheter ablation of right atrial isthmus-dependent flutter and (2) intracardiac electrograms showing termination of atrial flutter during ablation. *(continued)*

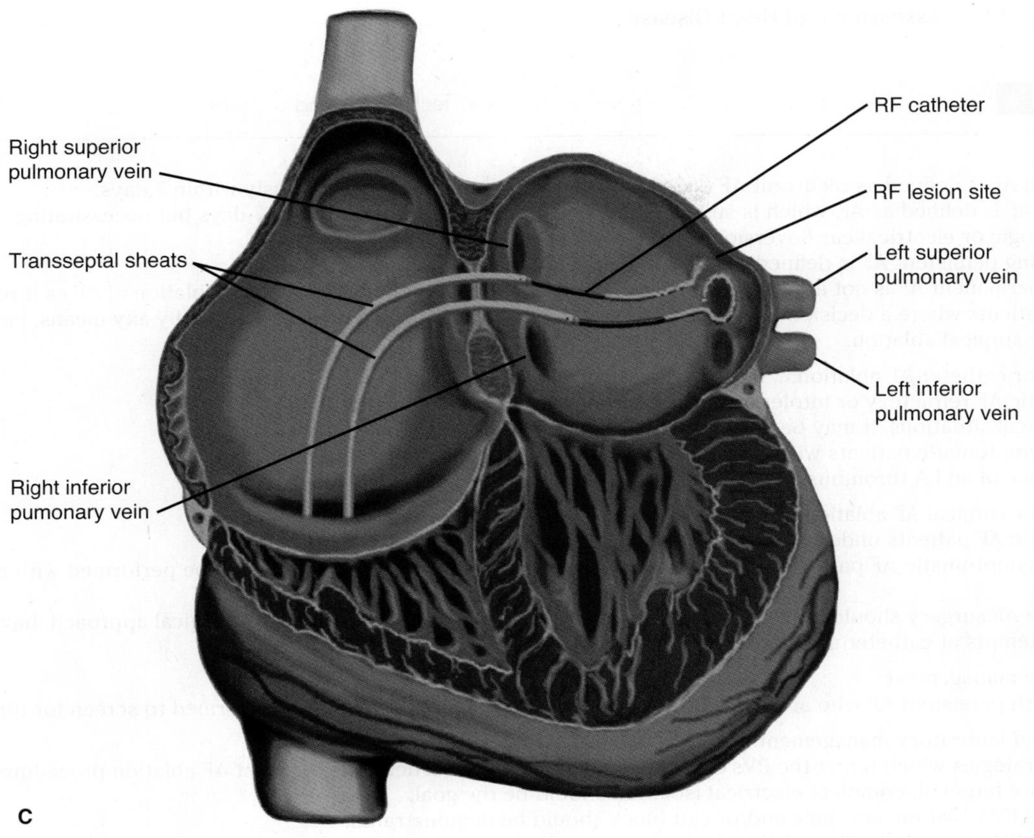

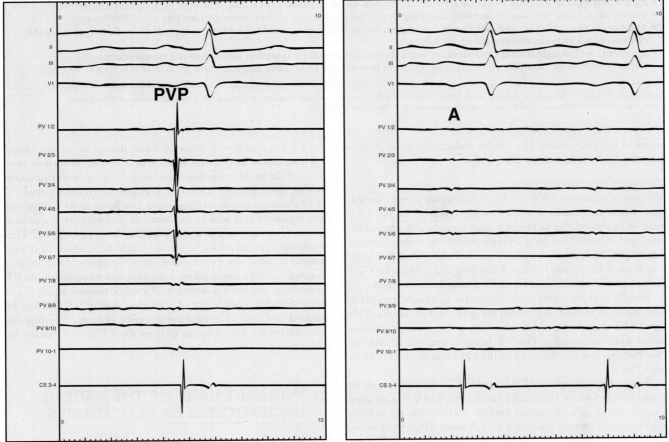

■ **Figure 18-7** *(continued)* **(C)** Diagram of AF ablation. (1) Intracardiac electrograms showing pulmonary vein potentials prior to ablation and (2) loss of pulmonary vein potentials (electrical isolation) after ablation. A, far field atrial electrogram; EAT, ectopic atrial tachycardia; LAT, left atrial tachycardia; PVP, pulmonary vein potential.

DISPLAY 18-4 Atrial Fibrillation Ablation: Definitions, Indications, Technique, and Laboratory Management

AF definition:
- Paroxysmal AF is defined as recurrent AF (>2 episodes) that terminates spontaneously within 7 days.
- Persistent AF is defined as AF, which is sustained beyond 7 days, or lasting less than 7 days but necessitating pharmacologic or electrical cardioversion.
- Longstanding persistent AF is defined as continuous AF of greater than 1-year duration.
- The term permanent AF is not appropriate in the context of patients undergoing catheter ablation of AF as it refers to a group of patients where a decision has been made not to pursue restoration of sinus rhythm by any means, including catheter or surgical ablation.

Indications for catheter AF ablation:
- Symptomatic AF refractory or intolerant to at least one Class 1 or 3 antiarrhythmic medication.
- In rare clinical situations, it may be appropriate to perform AF ablation as a first-line therapy.
- Selected symptomatic patients with heart failure and/or reduced ejection fraction.
- The presence of an LA thrombus is a contraindication to catheter ablation of AF.

Indications for surgical AF ablation:
- Symptomatic AF patients undergoing other cardiac surgery.
- Selected asymptomatic AF patients undergoing cardiac surgery in whom the ablation can be performed with minimal risk.
- Stand-alone AF surgery should be considered for symptomatic AF patients who prefer a surgical approach, have failed one or more attempts at catheter ablation or are not candidates for catheter ablation.

Preprocedure management
- Patients with persistent AF who are in AF at the time of ablation should have a TEE performed to screen for thrombus.

Technique and laboratory management:
- Ablation strategies which target the PVs and/or PV antrum are the cornerstone for most AF ablation procedures.
- If the PVs are targeted, complete electrical isolation should be the goal.
- For surgical PV isolation, entrance and/or exit block should be demonstrated.
- Careful identification of the PV ostia is mandatory to avoid ablation within the PVs.
- If a focal trigger is identified outside a PV at the time of an AF ablation procedure, it should be targeted if possible.
- If additional linear lesions are applied, mapping or pacing maneuvers should demonstrate line completeness.
- Ablation of the cavotricuspid isthmus is recommended only in patients with a history of typical atrial flutter or inducible cavotricuspid isthmus dependent atrial flutter.
- If patients with longstanding persistent AF are approached, ostial PV isolation alone may not be sufficient.
- Heparin should be administered during AF ablation procedures to achieve and maintain an ACT of 300 to 400 seconds.

Adapted from Calkins, H., Brugada, J., Packer, F., et al. (2007). HRS/EHRA/ECAS expert consensus statement on catheter and surgical ablation of atrial fibrillation: Recommendations for personnel, policy, procedures and follow-up. *Heart Rhythm, 4*(6), 816–861.

origin of the tachycardia. The earliest endocardial atrial electrogram marks the origin of the tachycardia.[75]

Ventricular Tachycardia

Ablation of paroxysmal VT can be a challenging therapy for patients whose tachycardia is suited to study and ablation. For a VT focus to be ablated, the tachycardia must be inducible, monomorphic, and tolerated for long enough periods to enable accurate mapping. The advent of electroanatomic and noncontact 3-D mapping systems has greatly facilitated mapping and ablation of VT.[76] For a successful ablation, the type of VT must be determined.

Bundle-branch reentrant tachycardia conducts antegrade over the right bundle and retrograde over the left bundle. This type of VT occurs in patients who have severe ischemic or idiopathic cardiomyopathy. The VT is rapid because it uses the His–Purkinje system. Ablation of the right bundle usually abolishes this VT.[77]

Benign monomorphic VT (idiopathic VT) typically occurs in young people with no structural heart disease. The VT most often arises from the right ventricular outflow tract or from the inferior left ventricular septum (fascicular VT). Various EP techniques are used to map the presumed site of origin before ablating. RF ablation is most often successful in this group of patients.

VT associated with coronary heart disease is usually caused by a reentrant mechanism in an area of patchy fibrosis or scar. One of the problems encountered with ablating in this situation is that these patients may have multiple tachycardia circuits.[59] 3-D electroanatomic voltage maps can be used to reconstruct the region of scar within the ventricle and identify the critical zones of conduction delay responsible for reentrant VT. This technique is known as "substrate mapping." Ablation is employed to eliminate potential reentrant circuits and can be performed during sinus rhythm. Induction and mapping of the VT is not required prior to ablation. If a single monomorphic VT is identified, the earliest site of activation during VT also can be located and ablated using these mapping systems.[76] Techniques to identify the best ablation strategy for VT are still under development.

NURSING CARE OF THE PATIENT UNDERGOING EP PROCEDURES

Health care professionals caring for arrhythmia patients play a pivotal role for the patient undergoing an EP procedure, catheter ablation procedure, or both. The need for patient education during all phases of the arrhythmia experience has been well documented.[78–80] Teaching before the study must include discussions about the nature of the test, a description of the procedure, procedure length, success rates, and complication rates. Nurses must also include postprocedure instructions and discharge instructions. After the procedure, the patient must keep the affected leg(s) straight for 3 to 4 hours to allow the venous puncture site to heal and for 4 to 6 hours if the femoral artery was punctured. The preliminary results of the procedure should be shared immediately with the patient and family. Frequent explanations may be required at first if the patient is recovering from heavy sedation. After a successful ablation, patients have no restrictions and antiarrhythmic medications are usually discontinued.

Most of the intraprocedure and postprocedure nursing care is centered on monitoring the patient for potential complications related to the procedure. In most instances, patients are anxious before and during EP procedures. Adequate sedation to allow for patient comfort should be provided. Oversedation must be prevented. Nurses must be alert for major complications directly related to placement of catheters inside the heart. Bleeding from catheter insertion sites, tamponade from perforation, and tachyarrhythmias and bradyarrhythmias can all occur during and after the EP procedure. Nurses who care for patients with arrhythmias in any setting should be prepared to handle any emergency that may arise. Other potential problems to be monitored include thrombophlebitis, thromboembolism, and infection.

The Heart Rhythm Society, formerly known as the North American Society of Pacing and Electrophysiology, has developed standards of professional practice for allied professionals (nurses, nurse practitioners, physician assistants, technicians) caring for patients with cardiac rhythm disorders. The standards for EP procedures are three-fold and include: (1) the application of scientific principles related to clinical EP to provide technical support and patient care services; (2) the demonstration of technical knowledge and clinical skills to operate laboratory equipment and troubleshoot equipment malfunction; and (3) the integration of cardiovascular and electrical knowledge to effectively monitor the patient throughout the procedure.[81]

Acknowledgment: *The cardiac images were created by Claude Rickerd of St. Jude Medical.*

REFERENCES

1. Horowitz, L. H. (1986). Safety of electrophysiologic studies. *Circulation, 73*, II-28–II-30.
2. Josephson, M. E. (1993). Electrophysiologic investigation: General concepts. In M. E. Josephson (Ed.), *Clinical cardiac electrophysiology techniques and interpretations* (2nd ed., pp. 22–70). Philadelphia: Lea & Febiger.
3. Hammill, S. C., Sugrue, D. D., Gersh, B. J., et al. Clinical intracardiac electrophysiologic testing: Technique, diagnostic indications, and therapeutic uses. *Mayo Clinic Proceedings, 61*, 478–503.
4. DiMarco, J. P., Garan, H., & Ruskin, J. N. (1982). Complications in patients undergoing electrophysiologic procedures. *Annals of Internal Medicine, 97*, 490–493.
5. Fogors, R. N. (2006). The electrophysiologic study in the evaluation of the SA node, AV node and His-Purkinje system. *Electrophysiology Testing* (4th ed., pp. 35–57). Blackwell Publishing.
6. Schaffer, W. A., & Cobb, L. A. (1975). Recurrent ventricular fibrillation and modes of death in survivors of out-of-hospital ventricular fibrillation. *New England Journal of Medicine, 293*, 259–262.
7. Cobb, L., & Hallstrom, A. P. (1977). Clinical predictors and characteristics of the sudden cardiac death syndrome. *Proceedings USA/USSR First Joint Symposium on Sudden Death*. DHEW Publication no. (NIH) 78–1470. Washington, DC: National Institutes of Health.
8. Greene, H. L. (1990). Sudden arrhythmic cardiac death: Mechanisms, resuscitation, and classification. *American Journal of Cardiology, 65*, 4B–12B.
9. Skale, B. T., Miles, W. M., Heger, J. J., et al. (1986). Survivors of cardiac arrest: Prevention of recurrence by drug therapy as predicted by electrophysiologic testing or electrocardiographic monitoring. *American Journal of Cardiology, 57*, 113–119.
10. Wilber, D. J., Garan, H., Finkelstein, D., et al. (1988). Use of electrophysiologic testing in the prediction of long-term outcome. *New England Journal of Medicine, 318*, 19–24.
11. AVID Investigators. (1997). A comparison of antiarrhythmic drug therapy with implantable defibrillators in patients resuscitated from near-fatal ventricular arrhythmias. *New England Journal of Medicine, 337*, 1576–1583.
12. Buxton, A. E., Lee, K. L., Fisher, J. D., et al. (1999). A randomized study of prevention of sudden death in patients with coronary artery disease: Multicenter Unsustained Tachycardia Trial Investigators. *New England Journal of Medicine, 341*, 1882–1890.
13. Connolly, S. J., Gent, M., Roberts, R. S., et al. (2000). Canadian implantable defibrillator study (CIDS): A randomized trial of the implantable cardioverter defibrillator against amiodarone. *Circulation, 101*, 1297–1302.
14. Kuck, K., Cappato, R., Siebels, J., et al. (2000). Randomized comparison of antiarrhythmic drug therapy with implantable defibrillators in patients resuscitated from cardiac arrest: The Cardiac Arrest Study Hamburg (CASH). *Circulation, 102*, 748–754.
15. Moss, A. J., Hall, W. J., Cannom, D. S., et al., for the Madit Investigators. (1996). Improved survival with an implantable defibrillator in patients with coronary artery disease at high risk of ventricular arrhythmia. *New England Journal of Medicine, 335*, 1933–1940.
16. Moss, A. J., Zareba, W., Hall, J., et al. (2002). Prophylactic implantation of a defibrillator in patients with myocardial infarction and reduced ejection fraction. *New England Journal of Medicine, 346*, 877–883.
17. Bardy, G. H., Lee, K. L., Mark, D. B., et al. (2005). Sudden cardiac death in heart failure trial (SCD-HeFT). *New England Journal of Medicine, 352*, 225–237.
18. Dongas, J., Lehman, M. H., Mahmud, R., et al. (1985). Value of preexisting bundle branch block in the ECG differentiation of supraventricular from ventricular origin of wide QRS tachycardia. *American Journal of Cardiology, 55*, 717–721.
19. Wellens, H. J. J., Brugada, P., & Heddle, W. F. (1984). The value of the 12 lead ECG in diagnosis type and mechanism of a tachycardia: A survey among 22 cardiologists. *Journal of the American College of Cardiology, 4*, 176–179.
20. Zipes, D. P., Camm, A. J., Borggrefe, M. (2006). ACC/AHA/ESC 2006 Guidelines for the management of patients with ventricular arrhythmias and the prevention of sudden cardiac death: Executive summary. *Journal of the American College of Cardiology, 9*, 539–548.
21. Hess, D. S., Morady, F., & Scheinman, M. M. (1982). Electrophysiologic testing in the evaluation of patients with syncope of undetermined origin. *American Journal of Cardiology, 50*, 1309–1315.
22. Kapoor, W. N. (2000). Syncope. *New England Journal of Medicine, 343*, 1856–1862.
23. Strickberger, S. A., Benson, D. W., Biaggioni, I. (2006). AHA/ACCF scientific statement on the evaluation of syncope. *Journal of American College of Cardiology, 47*, 473–484.
24. Nelson, S. D., Kou, W. H., De Buitleir, M., et al. (1987). Value of programmed ventricular stimulation in presumed carotid sinus syndrome. *American Journal of Cardiology, 60*, 1073–1077.
25. Sugrue, D. D., Wood, D. L., & McGoon, M. D. (1984). Carotid sinus hypersensitivity and syncope. *Mayo Clinic Proceedings, 59*, 637–640.
26. Linzer, M., Prystowsky, E. N., Brunetti, L. L., et al. (1988). Recurrent syncope of unknown origin diagnosed by ambulatory continuous loop ECG recording. *American Heart Journal, 116*, 1632–1634.
27. Krahn, A. D., Klein, G. J., Norris, C., et al. (1995). The etiology of syncope in patients with negative tilt table and electrophysiology testing. *Circulation, 92*, 1819–1824.
28. Berbari, E. J., & Lazzara, R. (1988). An introduction to high resolution ECG recordings of cardiac late potentials. *Archives of Internal Medicine, 148*, 1859–1863.
29. Hall, P. A., Atwood, J. E., Myers, J., et al. (1989). The signal averaged surface electrocardiogram and the identification of late potentials. *Progress in Cardiovascular Disease, 31*, 295–317.

30. Brignole, M., Alboni, O., Benditt, D., et al. (2004). Guidelines on management (diagnosis and treatment) of syncope—Updated 2004. *Europace, 6*(6), 467–537.
31. Bloomfield, D. M., Bigger, J. T., Steinman, R. C., et al. (2006). Microvolt T-wave alternans and the risk of death or sustained ventricular arrhythmias in patients with left ventricular dysfunction. *Journal of the American College of Cardiology, 47*(2), 456–463.
32. Gold, M. R., Bloomfield, F. M., Anderson, K. P., et al. (2000). A comparison of T-wave alternans, signal-averaged electrocardiography and programmed ventricular stimulation for risk stratification. *Journal of the American College of Cardiology, 36*, 2247–2253.
33. Engel, G., Beckerman, J. G., Froelicher, V. F., et al. (2004). Electrocardiographic arrhythmia risk testing. *Current Problems in Cardiology, 29*(7), 365–432.
34. Clutter, C. (1991). Neurally mediated syncope. *Journal of Cardiovascular Nursing, 5*, 65–73.
35. Purcell, J. A. (1992). Provoking vasodepressor syncope with head-up tilt-table testing. *Progress in Cardiovascular Nursing, 7*, 15–18.
36. Almquist, A., Goldenberg, I. F., & Milstein, S., et al. (1989). Provocation of bradycardia and hypotension by isoproterenol and upright posture in patients with unexplained syncope. *New England Journal of Medicine, 320*, 346–351.
37. Fitzpatrick, A. P., Theodorakis, G., Vardas, P., et al. (1991). Methodology of head-up tilt testing in patients with unexplained syncope. *Journal of the American College of Cardiology, 17*, 125–130.
38. Sheldon, R., & Killam, S. (1992). Methodology of isoproterenol-tilt table testing in patients with syncope. *Journal of the American College of Cardiology, 19*, 773–779.
39. Bass, E. B., Elson, J. J., Fogoros, R. N., et al. (1988). Long-term prognosis of patients undergoing electrophysiology studies for syncope of unknown origin. *American Journal of Cardiology, 62*, 1186–1191.
40. Denes, P., Uretz, E., Ezri, M. D., et al. (1988). Clinical predictors of electrophysiologic testing in patients with syncope of unknown origin. *Archives of Internal Medicine, 148*, 1922–1928.
41. Teichman, S. L., Felder, S. D., Matos, J. A., et al. (1985). The value of electrophysiologic studies in syncope of undetermined origin: Report of 150 cases. *American Heart Journal, 110*, 469–479.
42. Yee R., & Strauss H. C. (1987). Electrophysiologic mechanisms: Sinus node dysfunction. *Circulation, 75*(Suppl. III), 12–18.
43. Kapoor, W. N. (2002). Current evaluation and management of syncope. *Circulation, 106*, 1606–1609.
44. Calkins, H., Kim, Y. N., Schmaltz, S., et al. (1992). Electrogram criteria for identification of appropriate target sites for radiofrequency catheter ablation of accessory connections. *Circulation, 85*, 565–573.
45. Gallagher, J. J., Svenson, R. H., Kasell, J. H., et al. (1982). Catheter technique for closed-chest ablation of the atrioventricular conduction system. *New England Journal of Medicine, 306*, 194–200.
46. Evans, G. J., Scheinman, M. M., Zipes, D. P., et al. (1989). The percutaneous cardiac mapping and ablation registry: Final summary of results. *Journal of Pacing and Clinical Electrophysiology, 11*, 1621–1626.
47. Scheinman, M. M., Morady, F., Hess, D., et al. (1982). Catheter induced ablation of the atrioventricular junction to control refractory supraventricular arrhythmias. *Journal of the American Medical Association, 248*, 851–855.
48. Hauer, R., Straks, W., Borst, C., et al. (1988). Electrical catheter ablation in the left and right ventricular wall in dogs: Relation between delivered energy and histopathologic changes. *Journal of the American College of Cardiology, 8*, 637–643.
49. Langberg, J. J., Chin, M. C., Rosenqvist, M., et al. (1989). Catheter ablation of the atrioventricular junction with radiofrequency energy. *Circulation, 80*, 1527–1535.
50. Huang, S., Bharati, S., Graham, A., et al. (1987). Closed chest catheter desiccation of the atrioventricular junction using radiofrequency energy: A new method of catheter ablation. *Journal of the American College of Cardiology, 9*, 349–358.
51. Fisher, W. G., & Swartz, J. F. (1992). Three-dimensional electrogram mapping improves ablation of left sided accessory pathway. *Journal of Pacing and Clinical Electrophysiology, 15*, 2344–2356.
52. Robbins, I. M., Colvin, E. V., Doyle, T. P., et al. (1998). Pulmonary vein stenosis after catheter ablation of atrial fibrillation. *Circulation, 98*, 1769–1775.
53. Scheinman, M. M. (1994). Patterns of catheter ablation practice in the United States: Results of 1992 NASPE survey. *Journal of Pacing and Clinical Electrophysiology, 17*, 873–875.
54. Jackman, W. M., Beckman, K. J., McClelland, J. H., et al. (1992). Treatment of supraventricular tachycardia due to atrioventricular nodal reentry, by radiofrequency catheter ablation of slow-pathway conduction. *New England Journal of Medicine, 327*, 313–318.
55. Calkins, H., Sousa, J., El-Atassi, R., et al. (1991). Diagnosis and cure of the Wolff-Parkinson-White syndrome or paroxysmal supraventricular tachycardias during a single electrophysiologic test. *New England Journal of Medicine, 324*, 1612–1618.
56. McClelland, J. H., Wang, K., Beckman, K. J., et al. (1994). Radiofrequency catheter ablation of right atriofascicular (Mahaim) accessory pathways guided by accessory pathway activation potentials. *Circulation, 89*, 2655–2666.
57. Ticho, B. S., Saul, J. P., Hulse, J. E., et al. (1992). Variable location of accessory pathways associated with PJRT and confirmation with radiofrequency ablation. *American Journal of Cardiology, 70*, 1559–1564.
58. Jackman, W. M., Wang, X., Friday, K. J., et al. (1991). Catheter ablation of atrioventricular pathways (Wolff-Parkinson-White syndrome) by radiofrequency current. *New England Journal of Medicine, 324*, 1605–1611.
59. Lesh, M. D. (1993). Interventional electrophysiology: State-of-the-art 1993. *American Heart Journal, 126*, 686–698.
60. Fuster, V., Ryden, L. E., Cannom, D. S., et al. ACC/AHA/ESC 2006 guidelines for the management of patients with atrial fibrillation: A report of the American College of Cardiology/American Heart Association Task Force on Practice Guidelines (Writing Committee to Revise the 2001 Guidelines for the Management of Patients with Atrial Fibrillation). *Journal of American College of Cardiology, 48*, e149–e246.
61. Fischer, B., Jais, P., Shah, D., et al. (1996). Radiofrequency catheter ablation of common atrial flutter in 200 patients. *Journal of Cardiovascular Electrophysiology, 7*, 1225.
62. Jackman, W. M., Wang, X., Friday, K. J., et al. (1991). Catheter ablation of atrioventricular junction using radiofrequency current in 17 patients. *Circulation, 83*, 1562–1576.
63. Rodriguez, L. M., Smeets, J. L. R. M., Xie, B., et al. (1993). Improvement of left ventricular function by ablation of atrioventricular nodal conduction in selected patients with lone atrial fibrillation. *American Journal of Cardiology, 72*, 1137–1141.
64. Fitzpatrick, A. P., Kourouyan, H. D., Siu, A., et al. (1996). Quality of life and outcomes after radiofrequency His-bundle ablation and permanent pacemaker implantation: Impact of treatment in paroxysmal and established atrial fibrillation. *American Heart Journal, 121*, 499–507.
65. Haissaguerre, M., Jais, P., Shah, D. C., et al. (1998). A focal source of atrial fibrillation by ectopic beats originating in the pulmonary veins. *New England Journal of Medicine, 339*, 659–666.
66. Pappone, C., Rosanio, S., Oreto, G., et al. (2000). Circumferential radiofrequency ablation of pulmonary vein ostia: A new anatomic approach for curing atrial fibrillation. *Circulation, 104*, 2539–2544.
67. Nademanee, K., McKenzie, J., Kosar, E., et al. (2004). A new approach for catheter ablation of atrial fibrillation: Mapping of the electrophysiologic substrate. *Journal of the American College of Cardiology, 43*, 2044–2053.
68. Scherlag B. J., Nakagawa, H., Jackman, W. M., et al. (2005). Electrical stimulation to identify neural elements on the heart: Their role in atrial fibrillation. *Journal of Interventional Cardiac Electrophysiology, 13*(Suppl. 1), 37–42.
69. Calkins, H., Brugada, J., Packer, F., et al. (2007). HRS/EHRA/ECAS expert consensus statement on catheter and surgical ablation of atrial fibrillation: Recommendations for personnel, policy, procedures and follow-up. *Heart Rhythm, 4*(6), 816–861.
70. Haissaguerre, M., Jais, P., Shah, D. C., et al. (2000). Electrophysiological end point for catheter ablation of atrial fibrillation initiated from multiple pulmonary venous foci. *Circulation, 101*, 1409–1417.
71. Chen, S. A., Hsieh, M. H., Tai, C. T., et al. (1999). Initiation of atrial fibrillation by ectopic beats originating from the pulmonary veins: Electrophysiological characteristics, pharmacological responses, and effects of radiofrequency ablation. *Circulation, 100*, 1879–1886.
72. Schaff, H. V., Dearani, J. A., Daly, R. C., et al. (2000). Cox-Maze procedure for atrial fibrillation: Mayo Clinic experience. *Seminar Thoracic and Cardiovascular Surgery, 12*, 30–37.
73. Prasad, S. M., Maniar, H. S., Camillo, C. J., et al. (2003). The Cox maze III procedure for atrial fibrillation: Long-term efficacy in patients undergoing lone versus concomitant procedures. *Journal of Thoracic Cardiovascular Surgery, 126*, 1822–1828.

74. Koistinen, J., Valtonen, M., Savola, J., et al. (2007). Thoracoscopic microwave ablation of atrial fibrillation. *Interactive Cardiovascular and Thoracic Surgery, 6*, 695.
75. Lesh, M. D., Van Hare, G. F., Epstein, L. M., et al. (1994). Radiofrequency catheter ablation of atrial arrhythmias results and mechanisms. *Circulation, 89*, 1074–1089.
76. Kautzner, J., Cihak, R., Peichl, P., et al. (2003). Catheter ablation of ventricular tachycardia following MI using 3-dimensional electroanatomic mapping. *Journal of Pacing and Clinical Electrophysiology, 26*(1), 342–347.
77. Cohen, T. J., Chien, W. U., Lurie, K. G., et al. (1991). Radiofrequency catheter ablation for treatment of bundle branch reentrant VT: Results and long-term follow-up. *Journal of the American College of Cardiology, 18*, 1767–1773.
78. Berry, V. A. (1993). Wolff-Parkinson-White syndrome and the use of radiofrequency catheter ablation. *Heart & Lung, 22*, 15–25.
79. Connelly, A. G. (1992). An examination of stressors in the patient undergoing cardiac electrophysiologic studies. *Heart & Lung, 21*, 335–342.
80. Moulton, L., Grant, J., Miller, B., et al. (1993). Radiofrequency catheter ablation for supraventricular tachycardia. *Heart & Lung, 22*, 3–14.
81. Gure, M. T., Bubien, R. S., Belco, K. M., et al. (2003). Policy statement: North American Society of Pacing and Electrophysiology: Standards of professional practice for the allied professional in pacing and electrophysiology. *Journal of Pacing and Clinical Electrophysiology, 26*(1), 127–131.

CHAPTER 19

Exercise Testing

Jonathan Myers

Exercise testing is a widely used, noninvasive procedure that provides diagnostic, prognostic, and functional information for a wide spectrum of patients with cardiovascular, pulmonary, and other disorders. Graded exercise tests are used to assess a patient's ability to tolerate increased physical activity, while electrocardiographic, hemodynamic, and symptomatic responses are monitored in a controlled environment. Graded, progressive exercise can produce abnormalities that are not present at rest, the most important of which are manifestations of myocardial ischemia, including ST-segment changes on the electrocardiogram, symptoms, and electrical instability. The test is also commonly used to evaluate other system disorders, such as gas exchange abnormalities in patients with pulmonary disease or chronic heart failure, symptoms associated with peripheral vascular disease, and even neurologic disorders.

In cardiovascular medicine, the exercise test is commonly used for evaluating the efficacy of medical therapy, for the assessment of interventions, and as a first-choice diagnostic tool in patients with suspected coronary artery disease (CAD), a role in which it functions as a "gatekeeper" to more expensive and invasive procedures.[1,2] In the latter role, the test has become even more important in the current era of health care cost containment. Although originally developed as a diagnostic tool, recent studies have established the role of the exercise test in the selection of patients for cardiac transplantation, risk stratification after a myocardial infarction (MI), and the assessment of disability.[3–7]

Because of the need to standardize the implementation and interpretation of the exercise test, professional organizations such as the American Heart Association (AHA), the American College of Cardiology (ACC),[4] the American College of Sports Medicine (ACSM),[8] the American Thoracic Society,[3] and the European Society of Cardiology[9] have developed guidelines designed to optimize the safety, methodology, and objectives of the test. The ACSM has developed certification programs for professional competency in exercise testing[8,10]; ACSM certification has been strongly recommended for nurses, technicians, or physiologists who oversee exercise testing in clinical settings.[10–12] This chapter describes the applications, methodology, and principles of exercise testing for the cardiovascular nurse and the professional standards for exercise testing described in the aforementioned guidelines.

INDICATIONS AND OBJECTIVES

The exercise test has numerous indications. Surveys have shown that the most common reason patients are referred for exercise testing is for the evaluation of chest pain[13,14] or, more generally, to assess signs and symptoms of coronary disease. Other common clinical objectives include the following:

1. Physiologic response of post-MI and postrevascularization patients to exercise
2. Functional capacity for the purpose of exercise prescription
3. Exercise capacity for the purpose of work classification (disability evaluation) and risk stratification (prognosis)
4. The efficacy of medical, surgical, or pharmacologic treatment
5. The presence and severity of arrhythmias
6. Preoperative physiologic status
7. Intermittent claudication

SAFETY AND PERSONNEL

Provided that contraindications to exercise testing are considered and patients who undergo exercise testing are appropriate, the test has been shown to be extremely safe. Widely cited data from the Cooper Clinic in Dallas[15] suggest that an event serious enough to require hospitalization (e.g., sustained arrhythmia, heart attack, or death) occurs at a rate of 0.8 per 10,000 tests. More recent studies have confirmed the low event rate associated with exercise testing. In a survey of 71 medical centers within the Veterans Affairs Health Care System, an event rate of 1.2 per 10,000 tests was reported.[14] Earlier surveys conducted in the 1970s suggested a somewhat higher event rate, ranging from 1 to 4 per 10,000.[16,17] It has been suggested that the apparent improvement in the safety of the test reflected in the more recent surveys is due to a significantly better understanding of when to and when not to perform the test, when to terminate the test, and better preparation for any emergency that may arise.[4,16]

Clinical judgment is the most important consideration when deciding which patients should undergo exercise testing. Contraindications to testing usually describe conditions of cardiovascular instability, such as unstable angina, uncontrolled heart failure, and arrhythmias. A listing of the absolute and relative contraindications to testing is provided in Display 19-1.

Historically, professional guidelines have suggested that physician supervision was necessary for all exercise testing in the clinical setting. Given the remarkable safety record of exercise testing, particularly in recent years,[14–17] there is now some debate regarding the need for physician supervision for exercise testing.[16] This has important implications for nursing because the nurse is frequently the person who prepares the patient and serves as the technician conducting the test, and in many centers the nurse may supervise the test as a surrogate for the physician. Although the most recent AHA/ACC guidelines[4] continue to recommend physician supervision when testing patients with heart disease in a clinical setting, the guidelines also state that ". . . exercise testing in selected patients can be safely performed by properly trained nurses, exercise physiologists, physical therapists, or medical technicians working directly under the supervision of a physician, who should be in the immediate vicinity and available for emergencies." The ACSM has outlined general guidelines regarding when physician supervision is recommended.[8] The nurse, physiologist,

DISPLAY 19-1 Contraindications to Exercise Testing

Absolute

1. A recent change in the resting electrocardiogram suggesting infarction or other acute cardiac event
2. Recent complicated MI
3. Unstable angina
4. Uncontrolled ventricular arrhythmia
5. Uncontrolled atrial arrhythmia that compromises cardiac function
6. Third-degree atrioventricular heart block without pacemaker
7. Acute congestive heart failure
8. Severe aortic stenosis
9. Suspected or known dissecting aneurysm
10. Active or suspected myocarditis or pericarditis
11. Thrombophlebitis or intracardiac thrombi
12. Recent systemic or pulmonary embolus
13. Acute infections
14. Significant emotional distress (psychosis)

Relative

1. Resting diastolic blood pressure >115 mm Hg or resting systolic blood pressure >200 mm Hg
2. Moderate valvular heart disease
3. Known electrolyte abnormalities (hypokalemia, hypomagnesemia)
4. Fixed-rate pacemaker
5. Frequent or complex ectopy
6. Ventricular aneurysm
7. Uncontrolled metabolic disease (e.g., diabetes, thyrotoxicosis, or myxedema)
8. Chronic infectious disease (e.g., mononucleosis or myxedema)
9. Neuromuscular, musculoskeletal, or rheumatoid disorders exacerbated by exercise
10. Advanced or complicated pregnancy

Modified from Gibbons, R. J., Balady, G. J., Bricker, J. T., et al. (2002). ACC/AHA 2002 guideline update for exercise testing. A report of the ACC/AHA Task Force on Practice Guidelines (Committee on Exercise Testing). *Journal of the American College of Cardiology, 40*, 1531–1540.

or technician conducting the test should have a comprehensive knowledge of the indications, contraindications, equipment, physiologic responses to exercise, and clinical condition of the patient to optimize the information yield and conduct the test safely.

A joint statement by the American College of Physicians, the ACC, and the AHA regarding clinical competence in exercise testing outlined the cognitive skills needed to perform exercise testing.[11] These include knowledge of indications and contraindications to testing, basic exercise physiology, principles of interpretation, and emergency procedures. The committee suggested that at least 50 procedures were required during training to achieve these skills. ACSM certification[8,10] is widely used to establish competency for technicians, nurses, or physiologists who oversee exercise testing and training.

PRETEST CONSIDERATIONS

Before an exercise test, all patients should undergo a complete medical evaluation and a physical examination to identify contraindications to exercise testing.[4,17] If the reason the patient was referred for the test in unclear, it should be postponed until this is clarified. The medical history should include any remote or recent medical problems, symptoms, medication use, and findings from previous examinations and tests. Major CAD risk factors and signs and symptoms suggesting cardiopulmonary disease should be identified. Physical activity patterns, vocational requirements, and family history of cardiopulmonary and metabolic disorders should also be assessed. Identification of absolute contraindications (see Display 19-1) should result in cancellation of the test and referral of the patient to the primary physician for further medical management. Patients with relative contraindications may be tested only after careful evaluation of the risk-to-benefit ratio.

Detailed verbal and written instructions, provided to the patient in advance, should include a request that the patient refrain from ingesting food, alcohol, and caffeine or using tobacco products within 3 hours of testing. Patients should be well rested and avoid vigorous activity the day of the test. Clothing should be comfortable and provide freedom of movement as well as allow access for electrode and blood pressure cuff placement. Properly fitting shoes with rubber soles should be worn to ensure good traction, particularly if a treadmill is the mode of testing. A thorough explanation of the potential risks and discomforts associated with exercise testing should be provided. Written informed consent has important ethical and legal implications and ensures the patient knows and understands the purposes and risks associated with the exercise test. There is sufficient case law to suggest that informed consent should always be obtained before beginning a test, although this issue has also been debated.[12] A demonstration of how to get on and off the testing apparatus should be given, what is expected of the patient should be described (reporting of symptoms, level of exertion, testing endpoints), and any questions the patient has should be answered.

Whether patients should remain on all cardiovascular medicines for exercise testing has been the source of some debate. Many commonly used drugs can influence hemodynamic and electrocardiographic responses to exercise[4,17] (Table 19-1), but removing patients from their usual medicines can cause instability of symptoms, rhythm, blood pressure, and other problems. Recent versions of the aforementioned exercise testing guidelines[4,8] suggest that most patients can remain on their medical regimen for testing without greatly compromising the diagnostic performance of the test. Tapering β-blockers over several days or discontinuing antianginal medications for a particular number of hours before testing should be reserved for particular patients in whom diagnostic sensitivity is paramount, and the tapering process should be carefully supervised by a physician.

Preparation for Electrocardiogram

Diagnostically, the electrocardiographic response is the cornerstone of the clinical exercise test. Thus, reliable test interpretation and patient safety mandate a high-quality exercise electrocardiogram. Proper skin preparation and precise electrode placement are critical to obtaining a high-quality electrocardiogram tracing. The goal of skin preparation is to decrease resistance at the skin–electrode interface and thus improve the signal-to-noise ratio. After removing hair from the general areas of placement, each site should be vigorously rubbed with an alcohol pad to remove skin oil. To further reduce resistance, the skin should be lightly

Table 19-1 ■ COMMON DRUGS AND THEIR IMPACT ON EXERCISE TESTING

Drug	Indications	Heart Rate	Blood Pressure	Electrocardiogram	Exercise Capacity
β-Blockers	Angina, hypertension, MI, arrhythmias, tremors, migraine headache	Rest: ↓, exercise: ↓	Rest: ↓, exercise: ↓	↓ Signs of ischemia	↑ In those with angina, ↓ in those without angina
Calcium channel blockers	Angina, coronary artery spasm, hypertension	Rest: ↓, exercise: ↓	Rest: ↓, exercise: ↓	↓ Signs of ischemia	↑ In those with angina, minimal effect in those without angina
Digoxin	CHF, arrhythmias	No change	Rest: ↓, Exercise: ↓	Will cause false-positive responses	↑ In those with CHF
Nitrates	Angina	No change	Rest: ↓, Exercise: ↓	Delayed signs of ischemia	↑ In those with angina (and CHF)

abraded using an abrasive pad or other product designed for this purpose. Finally, each electrode should be carefully placed in the proper location to ensure good skin contact with both the conducting gel and adhesive surfaces of the electrode.

The Mason–Likar limb lead placement[18] (Fig. 19-1) is the standard clinical configuration because it provides a 12-lead electrocardiogram with less artifact and less restriction to movement than does the standard limb placement. However, the Mason–Likar placement can result in differences in electrocardiographic amplitude and axis compared with the standard limb placement.[19–21] Because these shifts may be misinterpreted as diagnostic changes, it is often recommended that a resting supine electrocardiogram be recorded using the standard limb lead placement. It is also important to note that position changes may alter the electrocardiogram. For this reason, diagnostic ST-segment changes should always be made relative to the resting baseline position (i.e., upright rather than supine position for treadmill and cycle ergometry).

EXERCISE TEST SELECTION

The purpose of the test, the health and fitness of the patient, the exercise modality, and the exercise protocol are fundamental considerations when selecting the appropriate test for a given patient. In many exercise testing laboratories, these issues are determined by custom and the availability of equipment, but each can have a profound effect on the response to the exercise test. For example,

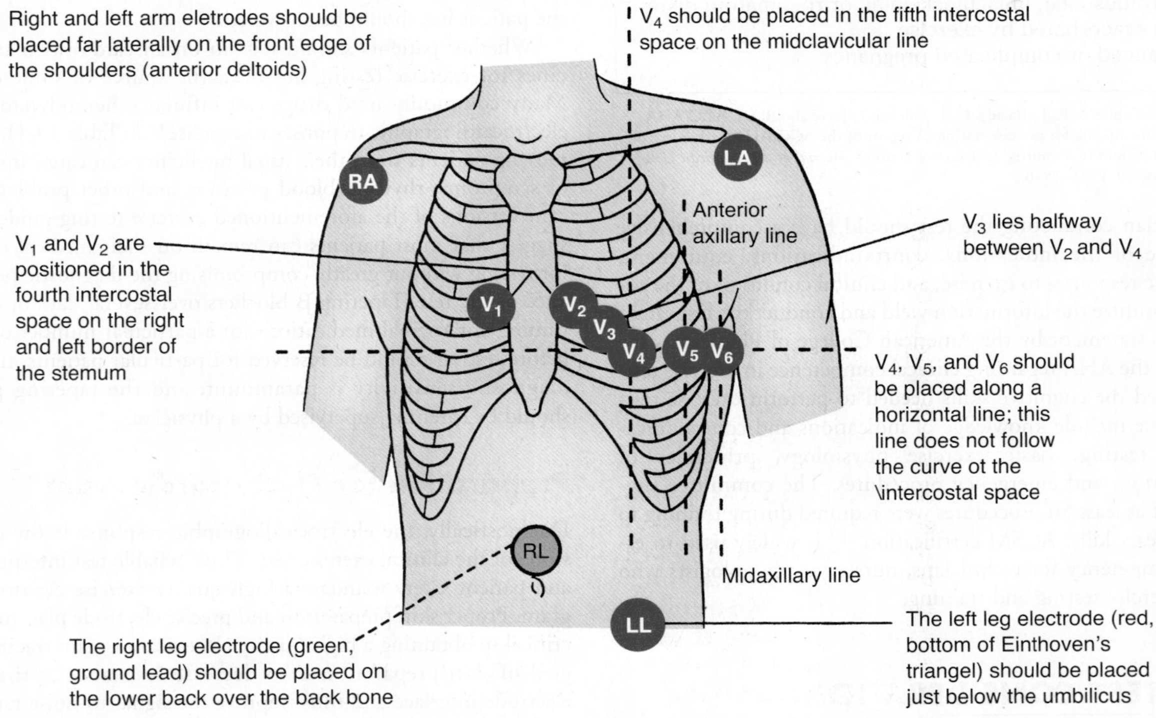
Right and left arm eletrodes should be placed far laterally on the front edge of the shoulders (anterior deltoids)
V_4 should be placed in the fifth intercostal space on the midclavicular line
RA
LA
Anterior axillary line
V_3 lies halfway between V_2 and V_4
V_1 and V_2 are positioned in the fourth intercostal space on the right and left border of the stemum
V_1
V_2
V_3
V_4
V_5
V_6
V_4, V_5, and V_6 should be placed along a horizontal line; this line does not follow the curve ot the \intercostal space
RL
Midaxillary line
LL
The right leg electrode (green, ground lead) should be placed on the lower back over the back bone
The left leg electrode (red, bottom of Einthoven's triangel) should be placed just below the umbilicus

■ **Figure 19-1** The Mason–Likar simulated 12-lead electrocardiogram electrode placement for exercise testing. (With permission from Froelicher, V. F., & Myers, J. [2006]. *Exercise and the heart* [5th ed.]. Philadelphia: W.B. Saunders.)

a treadmill test may be inappropriate for a patient who has difficulty with balance or gait, such as someone who has had a stroke or is otherwise neurologically impaired, or someone who has severe peripheral vascular disease, which causes difficulty in walking. A bicycle ergometer would be a more appropriate choice for such patients. Test specificity should also be considered. For example, it would be more appropriate to use a cycle ergometer to assess physiologic responses to a cycling program. Likewise, if a person is being assessed for readiness for return to work that requires arm strength, an arm ergometer test may provide more appropriate information than will a treadmill test.

Modalities

An ideal exercise mode increases total body and myocardial oxygen demand to its highest level safely and in moderate, continuous, and equal increments. This requires a dynamic exercise device that uses major muscle groups, permitting large increases in cardiac output, oxygen delivery, and gas exchange. Many modalities have been used for diagnostic testing, including cycle ergometers, treadmills, arm ergometers, steps, and, more recently, pharmacologic agents. Isometric exercise, or static exercise, which involves muscle contraction without movement of the corresponding joint, causes a greater increase in systolic blood pressure and heart rate in relation to total body oxygen uptake and therefore a greater pressure load on the heart compared with dynamic exercise. Thus, it is not preferred for diagnostic exercise testing. However, isometric exercise has been used to provide occupation-specific information for patients whose job requires an extensive amount of isometric activity.

The bicycle ergometer and the treadmill are the most commonly used dynamic exercise devices. Bicycle ergometer testing is more commonly used in Europe, whereas the treadmill is more often used in the United States. The bicycle is usually less expensive, occupies less space, and is quieter. Upper body motion is decreased, making blood pressure and electrocardiographic recordings easier. The workload administered by simple, mechanically braked bicycle ergometers is not always accurate and depends on pedaling speed, causing variations in the work performed. These have largely been replaced by electronically braked bicycle ergometers, which maintain the workload at a specified level over a wide range of pedaling speeds, and are therefore more accurate. Bicycle ergometer work is commonly expressed in kilogram-meters per minute (kg · m/min) or watts. The treadmill is usually more expensive than the cycle ergometer, is relatively immobile, and makes more noise. Studies comparing treadmill and bicycle ergometer exercise tests have reported the maximal oxygen uptake to be approximately 10% to 20% higher and maximal heart rate 5% to 20% higher on the treadmill.[22–26] Significant ST-segment changes have been reported to be more frequent and angina is elicited more frequently during treadmill testing compared with the cycle ergometer.[25,26] In addition, exercise-induced myocardial ischemia by thallium scintigraphy was reported to be greater after treadmill testing than after cycle ergometry.[23] Although most of these differences are minor, if assessing the functional limits of the patient and eliciting subjective or objective signs of ischemia are important goals of the test, the treadmill may be preferable.

Protocols

The purpose of the test and the person tested are important considerations in selecting the protocol. Exercise testing may be performed for diagnostic purposes, for functional assessment, or for risk stratification. An often ignored but nevertheless consistent recommendation in the recent exercise testing guidelines is that the protocol be individualized for the patient being tested.[4,8,27,28] For example, a maximal, symptom-limited test on a relatively demanding protocol would not be appropriate (or very informative) for a patient with severe limitations. Likewise, a very gradual protocol might not be useful for an apparently healthy, active person. Use of submaximal testing, gas exchange techniques, the presence of a physician, and the exercise mode and protocol should be determined by considering the person being tested and the goals of the test.

Commonly used exercise protocols, their stages, and the metabolic equivalent task (MET) level (metabolic equivalents; an estimated value representing a multiple of the resting metabolic rate) for each stage are outlined in Figure 19-2. The most suitable protocols for clinical testing should include a low-intensity warm-up phase followed by progressive, continuous exercise in which the demand is elevated to a patient's maximal level within a total duration of 8 to 12 minutes.[3,4,8,22,25,27] In the absence of gas exchange techniques, it is important to report exercise capacity in METs rather than exercise time, so that exercise capacity can be compared uniformly between protocols. METs can be estimated from any protocol using standardized equations that have been put into tabular form.[4,8,29] In general, 1 MET represents an increment on the treadmill of approximately 1.0 mph or 2.5% grade. On a cycle ergometer, 1 MET represents an increment of approximately 20 W (120 kg · m/min) for a person weighing 70 kg. The assumptions necessary for predicting MET levels from treadmill or cycle ergometer work rates (including not holding the handrails, that oxygen uptake is constant [i.e., steady-state exercise is performed], that the subject is healthy, and that all people are similar in their walking efficiency) raise uncertainties as to the accuracy of estimating the work performed for an individual patient. For example, the steady-state requirement is rarely met for most patients on most exercise protocols; most clinical testing is performed among patients with varying degrees of cardiovascular or pulmonary disease; and people vary widely in their walking efficiency.[29] It has therefore been recommended that a patient be ascribed an MET level only for stages in which all or most of a given stage duration has been completed.[30]

Bruce Treadmill Protocol

Surveys have shown that the Bruce protocol is the most widely used in North America.[14,31] An advantage of using this test is that a great deal of functional and prognostic data have been generated over several decades using the Bruce protocol, and many published normative values have been derived from it. For example, some of the most robust databases on the use of the exercise test for assessing prognosis, such as those from the Coronary Artery Surgery Study (CASS)[32] and the Duke Treadmill Score,[33] were generated from patients who underwent exercise testing using the Bruce test. Numerous studies have shown that patients who are unable to complete the first stage of this protocol (approximately 5 METs) have an extremely poor prognosis.[32,34,35] However, the disadvantages of the Bruce protocol include its large and unequal increments in work, which have been shown to result in less accurate estimates of exercise capacity, particularly for patients with cardiac disease. Investigations have demonstrated that work rate increments that are too large or rapid result in a tendency to overestimate exercise capacity, less reliability for studying the effects of

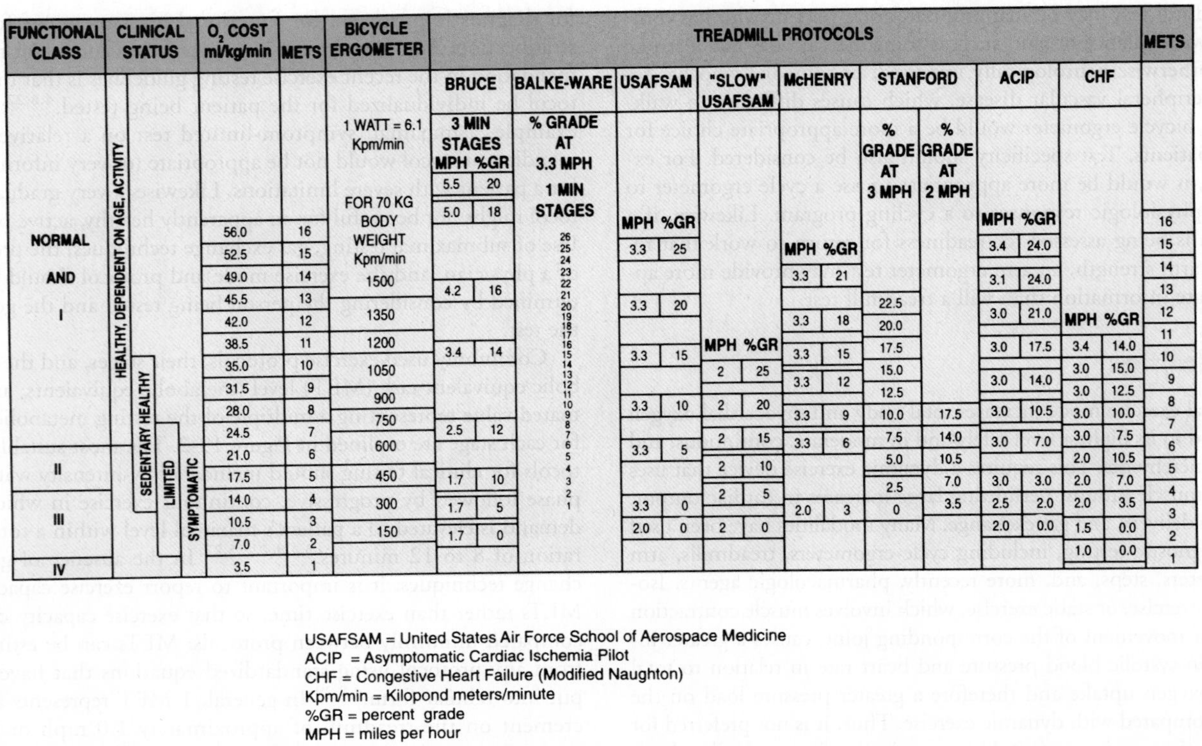

FUNCTIONAL CLASS	CLINICAL STATUS	O_2 COST ml/kg/min	METS	BICYCLE ERGOMETER (1 WATT = 6.1 Kpm/min; FOR 70 KG BODY WEIGHT Kpm/min)
NORMAL AND I	HEALTHY, DEPENDENT ON AGE, ACTIVITY	56.0	16	
		52.5	15	
		49.0	14	1500
		45.5	13	
		42.0	12	1350
		38.5	11	1200
	SEDENTARY HEALTHY	35.0	10	1050
		31.5	9	900
		28.0	8	750
	LIMITED	24.5	7	600
II	SYMPTOMATIC	21.0	6	
		17.5	5	450
III		14.0	4	300
		10.5	3	150
		7.0	2	
IV		3.5	1	

TREADMILL PROTOCOLS

BRUCE — 3 MIN STAGES

MPH	%GR
5.5	20
5.0	18
4.2	16
3.4	14
2.5	12
1.7	10
1.7	5
1.7	0

BALKE-WARE — % GRADE AT 3.3 MPH, 1 MIN STAGES: 26, 25, 24, 23, 22, 21, 20, 19, 18, 17, 16, 15, 14, 13, 12, 11, 10, 9, 8, 7, 6, 5, 4, 3, 2, 1

USAFSAM MPH	USAFSAM %GR	"SLOW" USAFSAM MPH	"SLOW" USAFSAM %GR	McHENRY MPH	McHENRY %GR
3.3	25	2	25	3.3	21
3.3	20	2	20	3.3	18
3.3	15	2	15	3.3	15
3.3	10	2	10	3.3	12
3.3	5	2	5	3.3	9
3.3	0	2	0	3.3	6
2.0	0			2.0	3

STANFORD % GRADE AT 3 MPH	STANFORD % GRADE AT 2 MPH
22.5	
20.0	
17.5	
15.0	
12.5	
10.0	17.5
7.5	14.0
5.0	10.5
2.5	7.0
0	3.5

ACIP MPH	ACIP %GR	CHF MPH	CHF %GR
3.4	24.0	3.4	14.0
3.1	24.0	3.0	15.0
3.0	21.0	3.0	12.5
3.0	17.5	3.0	10.0
3.0	14.0	3.0	7.5
3.0	10.5	2.0	10.5
3.0	7.0	2.0	7.0
3.0	3.0	2.0	3.5
2.5	2.0	1.5	0.0
2.0	0.0	1.0	0.0

METS: 16, 15, 14, 13, 12, 11, 10, 9, 8, 7, 6, 5, 4, 3, 2, 1

USAFSAM = United States Air Force School of Aerospace Medicine
ACIP = Asymptomatic Cardiac Ischemia Pilot
CHF = Congestive Heart Failure (Modified Naughton)
Kpm/min = Kilopond meters/minute
%GR = percent grade
MPH = miles per hour

■ **Figure 19-2** Stages, workloads, and oxygen cost per stage of some commonly used protocols. USAFSAM, United States Air force School of Aerospace Medicine; ACIP, Asyptomatic Cardiac Ischemia Pilot; CHF, congestive heart failure (modified Naughton); kpm/min, kilopond meters/minute; %GR, percent grade; MPH, miles per hour.

therapy, and possibly even lowered sensitivity for detecting coronary disease.[22,25,27,36,37]

Balke Treadmill Protocol

The Balke protocol, and modifications of it, has been widely used for clinical exercise testing. It uses constant walking speeds (2.0 or 3.0 mph) and modest increments in grade (2.5% or 5.0%), and it has been used particularly often in studies assessing angina responses. Modifications of the original Balke treadmill protocol have become widespread. One modification, developed by the United States School of Aerospace Medicine (Balke–Ware)[38] consists of 5% grade increases every 2 minutes and a constant brisk walking speed of 3.3 mph (after an initial warm-up of 2.0 mph), which has been considered the most efficient speed for walking. The constant speed is advantageous in that it requires only an initial adaptation in stride.

Naughton Treadmill Protocol

The Naughton treadmill protocol[39] is a low-level test that has become common for multicenter trials in patients with chronic heart failure. The test begins with 2-minute stages at 1 and 2 mph and 0% grade, then continually increases grade in approximately 1-MET increments at a constant speed of 2 mph for the next 8 minutes. Speed then increases to 3 mph with a slight decrease in grade, followed by increases in grade equivalent to approximately 1 MET. The Naughton protocol provides reasonable and gradual work rate increases for patients with more advanced heart disease. Because this protocol has been used extensively in patients with chronic heart failure, it provides a substantial amount of functional and prognostic comparative data. The Naughton test, however, can result in tests of excessive duration among more fit subjects.

Cycle Ergometer Protocols

Although there are specific bicycle protocols named after early researchers in Europe, such as Astrand and Rodahl,[40] bicycle ergometer protocols tend to be more generalized than those for the treadmill. For example, 15- to 25-W increments per 2-minute stage are commonly used for patients with cardiovascular disease, whereas for apparently healthy adults or athletic individuals, appropriate work rate increments might typically be between 40 and 50 W per stage. Most modern, electronically braked cycle ergometers have controllers that permit ramp testing in which the work rate increments can be individualized in continuous fashion (see next section).

Ramp Testing

An approach to exercise testing that has gained interest in recent years is the ramp protocol, in which work increases constantly and continuously. In 1981, Whipp et al.[41] first described cardiopulmonary responses to a ramp test on a cycle ergometer, and many of the gas exchange equipment manufacturers now include ramp software. Treadmills have also been adapted to conduct ramp tests.[25,42,43] The ramp protocol uses a constant and continuous increase in metabolic demand that replaces the "staging" used in conventional exercise tests. The uniform increase in work allows for a steady increase in cardiopulmonary responses and permits a more accurate estimation of oxygen uptake.[25] The recent call for "optimizing" exercise testing[4,22,27,30] would appear to be facilitated by the ramp approach, because large work increments are avoided and increases in work are individualized, permitting test duration to be targeted. Because there are no stages per se, the numbers of errors associated with predicting exercise capacity alluded to previously are lessened.[4,8,25]

Submaximal Testing

In general, maximal, symptom-limited tests are not considered appropriate until 1 month after MI or surgery. Thus, submaximal exercise testing has an important role clinically for predischarge, post-MI, or postbypass surgery evaluations. Submaximal tests have been shown to be important in risk stratification[44–46] for making appropriate activity recommendations, for recognizing the need for modification of the medical regimen, or for further interventions in patients who have sustained a cardiac event. A submaximal, predischarge test appears to be as predictive for future events as a symptom-limited test among patients less than 1 month after MI. Submaximal testing is also appropriate for patients with a high probability of serious arrhythmias. The testing endpoints for submaximal testing have traditionally been arbitrary but should always be based on clinical judgment. A heart rate limit of 140 beats/min and an MET level of 7 are often used for patients younger than 40 years, and limits of 130 beats/min and an MET level of 5 are often used for patients older than 40 years. For those using β-blockers, a Borg perceived exertion level in the range of 7 to 8 (1 to 10 scale) or 15 to 16 (6 to 20 scale) are conservative endpoints. The initial onset of symptoms, including fatigue, shortness of breath, or angina, is also indication to stop the test. A low-level protocol should be used, that is, one that uses no more than 1-MET increments per stage. The Naughton protocol[39,47] is commonly used for submaximal testing. Ramp testing is also ideal for this purpose because the ramp rate (such as 5 METs achieved over a 10-minute duration) can be individualized depending on the patient tested.[25]

INTERPRETATION OF EXERCISE TEST RESPONSES

The important exercise test responses that should be monitored and recorded are heart rate, blood pressure, electrocardiographic changes, exercise capacity, and subjective responses, including chest discomfort, undue fatigue, shortness of breath, leg pain, and rating of perceived exertion. Each of these responses should be described in a comprehensive test report. Useful programs have been developed that automatically summarize the test responses and apply published regression equations that report pretest and posttest risks of coronary disease, and some provide mortality estimates.[48] An example of one such report is presented in Display 19-2.

Heart Rate

Heart rate increases linearly with oxygen uptake during exercise. Of the two major components of cardiac output, heart rate and stroke volume, heart rate is responsible for most of the increase in cardiac output during exercise, particularly at higher levels. Thus, maximal heart rate achieved is a major determinant of exercise capacity.[17,49,50] The inability to appropriately increase heart rate during exercise (chronotropic incompetence) has been associated with the presence of heart disease and a worse prognosis.[49–51] Although maximal heart rate has been difficult to explain physiologically,[52] it is affected by age, gender, health, type of exercise, body position, blood volume, and environment. Of these factors, age is the most important. There is an inverse relationship between maximal heart rate and age, with correlation coefficients typically in the order of −0.40. However, the scatter around the regression line is quite large, with standard deviations ranging from 10 to 15 beats/min (Fig. 19-3). Thus, age-predicted "target" maximal heart rate is a limited measurement for clinical purposes and should not be used as an endpoint for exercise testing.[4,8,17,50]

Blood Pressure

Assessment of systolic and diastolic blood pressure at rest and during the exercise test is important for patient safety and can provide important diagnostic and prognostic information. Properly trained personnel can obtain accurate and reliable blood pressures using noninvasive auscultatory techniques, and guidelines have been developed for this purpose.[53,54] Blood pressure should be measured at rest before the test in the supine and standing positions. Blood pressure at rest, when measured before an exercise test, may be elevated compared with normal resting conditions because of pretest anxiety. Uncontrolled hypertension is a relative contraindication to exercise testing.[4,8] However, if blood pressure is elevated because of anxiety, it is not uncommon or of concern to observe a slight decrease in blood pressure during the initial stage of an exercise test when the workloads are light.

The increase in systolic blood pressure during exercise reflects the inotropic reserve of the left ventricle. Systolic and diastolic blood pressure should be assessed during the last minute of each exercise stage and more frequently if hypotensive or hypertensive responses are observed. Normally, systolic blood pressure increases in parallel with an increase in work rate, and it is not uncommon in healthy people to exceed 200 mm Hg. In general, a value above 250 mm Hg is an indication to terminate the exercise test.[4,8] Diastolic pressure normally stays the same or increases slightly during exercise. The fifth Korotkov sound, however, can be frequently heard all the way to zero in a young, healthy person. A diastolic blood pressure exceeding 115 mm Hg is an indication to terminate the exercise test.[4,8] A decrease in systolic blood pressure with progressive exercise suggests that cardiac output is unable to increase in accordance with the work rate and is usually a reflection of severe ischemia. If systolic blood pressure appears to decrease, it should be remeasured immediately, and if the decrease is confirmed, the test should be terminated. The clinical consequences of abnormal blood pressure responses to exercise range from modest[45,55] to severe, in which decreases in systolic blood pressure have been associated with ventricular fibrillation in the laboratory.[56] Dubach et al.[57] have observed that systolic blood pressure must drop below the standing resting value to be prognostically valuable, whereas others have suggested that more modest decreases, in the order of 10 to 20 mm Hg, are associated with severe ischemia, left ventricular impairment, a high incidence of future cardiac events, or all three.[58,59]

Exercise Capacity

Exercise capacity can be an extremely important test response to document because it has important implications concerning the efficacy of current therapies, the assessment of disability, and risk stratification. A patient's exercise capacity says a great deal about overall cardiovascular health. The most accurate method of measuring exercise capacity is with the use of ventilatory gas

DISPLAY 19-2 Example of an Automated Exercise Test Summary Report with Diagnostic and Prognostic Probabilities Generated from A Computer Program

Pretest Information

This patient is a 74-year-old active, White, male outpatient 70 in. tall, weighing 180 lb, who underwent a treadmill test on April 12, 2001. This exercise test was performed to evaluate symptoms/signs of possible heart disease or elevated risk factors.

Current Cardiac Medications

The patient is not taking any cardiac medications.

Medical History

The patient has the following symptoms: uncertain chest pain. The patient has no history of dysrhythmias.

Risk Factors

The patient is currently not smoking but has 15 pack-years of smoking. The patient is 8 lb over the average appropriate body mass index. Other risk factors include low high-density lipoprotein level (31 mg/dL) and non-insulin-dependent diabetes mellitus.

History of Cardiac Events

No previous MI. No bypass surgery performed. No percutaneous transluminal coronary angioplasty performed. No catheterization performed.

Resting ECG

The resting ECG is abnormal because of the following: left ventricular hypertrophy. The ejection fraction is approximately 45% based on the resting ECG.

Pulmonary Function

Forced vital capacity was 3.4 L (90.4% of expected), and the forced expiratory volume in 1 second was 76.2% of expected (normal is >75%).

Exercise Test Information

Exercise Capacity

The patient achieved 4.3 estimated METs and 4.1 measured METs at a perceived exertion level of 18 of 20 on the Borg scale. The test was terminated because of ST changes.

Hemodynamic Data	*Heart Rate (bpm)*	*Blood Pressure (mm Hg)*	*Double Product (×1,000)*
Resting:	65	146/70	9.5
At Max Exercise:	116	122/70	14.1

Chest Pain

Typical angina occurred during exercise.

Exercise ECG Response

The resting ECG shows no ST depression in V_5.

At maximal exercise, the ST-segments showed 3.0 mm of downsloping depression in the lateral and inferior leads. In recovery, the ST segments showed 3.0 mm of downsloping depression in the lateral and inferior leads. No significant dysrhythmias occurred in response to exercise. No bundle-branch blocks or conduction defects were present at rest or developed during exercise.

Conclusions

ST segments exhibited abnormal depression during exercise and abnormal depression in recovery (abnormal ST response).
Exertional hypotension occurred (systolic blood pressure dropped below pretest standing SBP).
The exertional hypotension could be due to ischemia (ST depression).
The patient achieved 66% of normal exercise capacity for age and 80% of normal maximal heart rate for age.
The patient has a high probability of having severe CAD.
Estimated prognosis from treadmill scores may be worse than expected for age, sex, and race.

Prognostic Addendum

Cardiovascular Mortality Prediction

The Framingham score (age, sex, cholesterol, diabetes, smoking, left ventricular hypertrophy, SBP) estimates a 5-year incidence of cardiovascular events (angina, MI, or death) of 11% (as expected for age and gender). For comparison with the treadmill scores, the age-expected annual mortality rate from any cause is 5.1% (National Center for Health Statistics, 1990).

The Duke score (METs, ST depression, and angina) estimates an annual cardiovascular mortality of 9.5% (approximately two times the age-expected mortality). The VA score (METs, congestive heart failure, SBP rise, and ST depression) estimates an annual cardiovascular mortality of 15.7% (three times the age-expected mortality).

DISPLAY 19-2 Example of an Automated Exercise Test Summary Report with Diagnostic and Prognostic Probabilities Generated from A Computer Program (continued)

Angiographic CAD Prediction

The patient has no recorded history of coronary disease. Pretest probabilities for any significant coronary disease are 50% (CASS, 1981 [chest pain, age, gender]), 71% (Morise, 1992), and 51% (Do/Froelicher, 1997,1998). Pretest probabilities for severe coronary disease are 22% (Pryor, 1993), 52% (Morise, 1992), and 17% (Do/Froelicher, 1997,1998).

The posttest probabilities for any clinically significant CAD are 99% (Detrano, 1992), 98% (Morise, 1992), and 94% (Do/Froelicher, 1997,1998) due to age, diabetes mellitus, symptoms, and abnormal ST depression.

The probabilities of having severe CAD are 75% (Detrano, 1992) due to abnormal ST depression, 91% (Morise, 1992) due to age abnormal ST depression, and 74% (Do/Froelicher, 1997,1998) due to abnormal ST depression.

Operative Mortality Prediction

If the patient would be selected for nonemergent bypass surgery and no renal dysfunction was present, the estimated operative morality rates are 9% (Parsonnet, 1989), 2% (NY State Department of Health, 1992), and 3% (VA, 1993). This is partially based on an estimated EF of 45%, so compare with measured EF.

Disclaimer: This report was computer generated and the results are dependent on rules and correct data entry. It must be overread by a physician.

EF, ejection fraction; ECG, electrocardiographic; METs, metabolic equivalents; SBP, systolic blood pressure.

From Froelicher, V. F. (1996). *Exercise test reporting aid (EXTRA) software.* St. Louis, MO: Mosby-Year Book.

Morise, A. P., Detrano, R., Bobbio, M., et al. (1993). Development and validation of a logistic regression-derived algorithm for estimating the incremental probability of coronary artery disease before and after exercise testing. *Journal of the American College of Cardiology 22*(1), 340–341.

Do, D., West, J. A., Morise, A., et al. (1997). An agreement approach to predict severe angiographic coronary artery disease with clinical and exercise test data. *American Heart Journal 134*(4),672–679.

Do, D., Marcus, R., Froelicher, V., et al. (1998). Predicting severe angiographic coronary artery disease using computerization of clinical and exercise test data. Chest *114*(5),1437–1445.

Pryor, D. B., Shaw, L., McCants, C.B., et al. (1993). Value of the history and physical in identifying patients at increased risk for coronary artery disease. *Annals of Internal Medicine 118*(2),81–90.

Detrano, R., Janosi, A., Steinbrunn, W., et al. (1991). Algorithm to predict triple-vessel/left main coronary artery disease in patients without myocardial infarction. An international cross validation. *Circulation 83*(5 Suppl),III89–96.

Parsonnet, V., Dean, D., Bernstein A. D. (1989). A method of uniform stratification of risk for evaluating the results of surgery in acquired adult heart disease. *Circulation 79*(6 Pt 2),I3–I12.

exchange techniques, but this requires specialized equipment and is not available in many clinical laboratories. Exercise capacity is therefore usually expressed as exercise duration, watts achieved (on a bicycle ergometer), maximal exercise stage, or METs. In the absence of gas exchange techniques, it is preferable to express exercise capacity in METs rather than exercise time. This is because an MET value can be ascribed to any speed and grade on a treadmill or workload achieved on a cycle ergometer; therefore, exercise capacity can be compared uniformly between protocols.

Figure 19-3 The relationship between maximal heart rate and age among patients referred for exercise testing. Inner lines represent the standard error; outer lines represent 95% confidence limits. (With permission from Morris, C. K., Myers, J., Froelicher, V. F., et al. [1994]. Nomogram based on metabolic equivalents and age for assessing aerobic exercise capacity in men. *Journal of the American College of Cardiology, 22,* 175–182.)

As mentioned previously in the discussion on protocols, there can be a great deal of uncertainty in predicting a person's energy cost from the treadmill or cycle ergometer workload. How accurately an MET level predicts a person's true oxygen uptake depends on several factors. For most patients with cardiovascular or pulmonary disease, there is a substantial overprediction of the MET level.[8,25,29,60] The error associated with this prediction is accentuated when rapidly incremented protocols are used, when patients are unaccustomed to walking on a treadmill or pedaling a cycle ergometer, and when patients are allowed to use handrail support.[8,29,60]

Exercise capacity should be expressed as both an absolute value and as a relative percentage of normal reference values for age and gender. The latter can be important because exercise capacity declines with increasing age and higher values are observed in men. Thus, when measuring or estimating oxygen uptake or MET levels, it is useful to have reference values for comparison. Normal reference values can facilitate communication with patients and between physicians regarding levels of exercise capacity in relation to a given patient's peers. Figures 19-4 and 19-5 are illustrations of nomograms for male patients referred for exercise testing. Expressing relative exercise capacity using a nomogram is advantageous because it offers a simple visual method of classifying a patient's response, without having to make cumbersome calculations from a particular regression equation. However, there are numerous available regression equations for "normal." All are population-specific, and numerous factors affect a person's exercise tolerance other than age and gender, including height, weight, body composition, activity status, and exercise test mode used, in addition to many clinical factors such as smoking history, heart disease, and medications.[10,29]

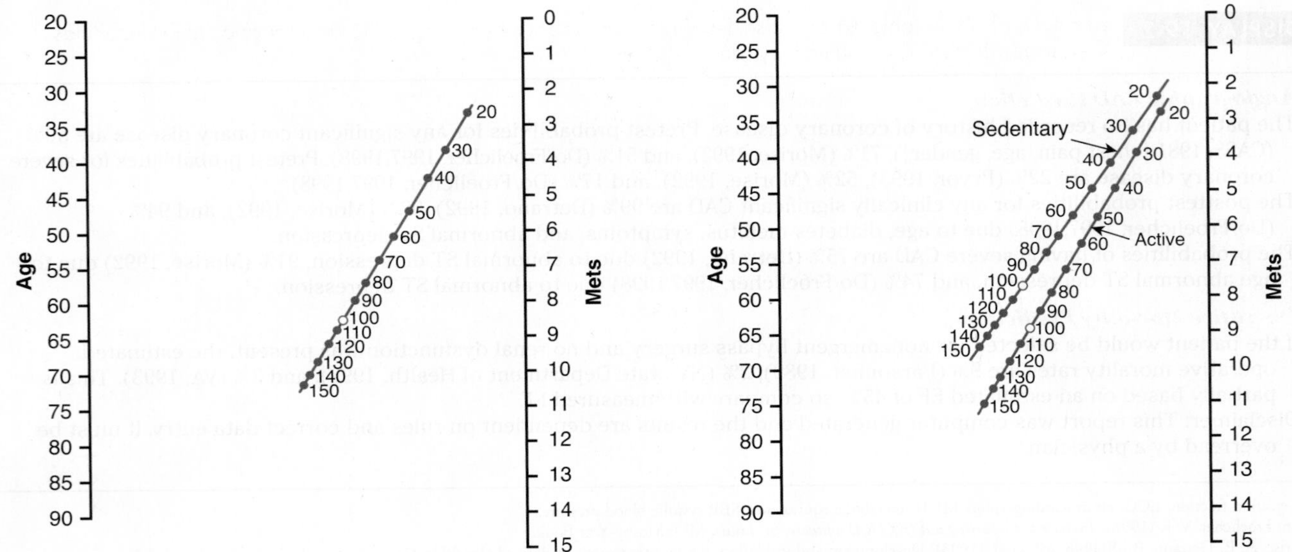

■ **Figure 19-4** Nomogram of percentage normal exercise capacity for age in 1,388 male veterans referred for exercise testing (based on metabolic task equivalents [METs]). (With permission from Morris, C. K., Myers, J., Froelicher, V. F., et al. [1994]. Nomogram based on metabolic equivalents and age for assessing aerobic exercise capacity in men. *Journal of the American College of Cardiology, 22*, 175–182.)

■ **Figure 19-5** Nomogram of percentage normal exercise capacity for age among active and sedentary men referred for exercise testing (based on metabolic equivalents [METs]). (With permission from Morris, C. K., Myers, J., Froelicher, V. F., et al. [1994]. Nomogram based on metabolic equivalents and age for assessing aerobic exercise capacity in men. *Journal of the American College of Cardiology, 22*, 175–182.)

Electrocardiographic Responses

In patients with CAD, exercise can cause an imbalance between myocardial oxygen supply and demand (ischemia), which can result in an alteration (decrease or elevation relative to the baseline) in the ST segment of the electrocardiogram. These changes are the foundation of the exercise test clinically. Normal and abnormal ST-segment responses to exercise are illustrated in Figure 19-6. Ever since electrocardiographic changes were first associated with myocardial ischemia in the 1920s, the diagnostic electrocardiographic criteria and leads that exhibit abnormalities during exercise have been the source of significant debate. Numerous electrocardiographic criteria, including complex mathematical constructs, combined scores, and ST areas during exercise and recovery, have been proposed to optimally diagnose the presence of CAD. Few of these studies, however, have followed accepted rules for evaluating a diagnostic test.[61] Virtually every edition of exercise testing guidelines that has been published suggests the application of a traditional diagnostic criterion: 1.0 mm or greater ST-segment depression that is horizontal or downsloping 60 to 80 milliseconds after the J-point (a "positive" response). ST-segment depression greater than 1.0 mm that is downsloping is generally indicative of more severe CAD. Most (probably 90%) ischemic ST changes occur in the lateral precordial leads.[4] Although it has historically been thought that the diagnostic performance of the test was incomplete without all 12 leads, some evidence suggests that ST-segment changes isolated to the inferior leads may frequently be false-positive responses.[62]

The significance of ST-segment elevation depends on the presence or absence of Q waves. When ST elevation occurs in the presence of a normal resting electrocardiogram, it is usually indicative of

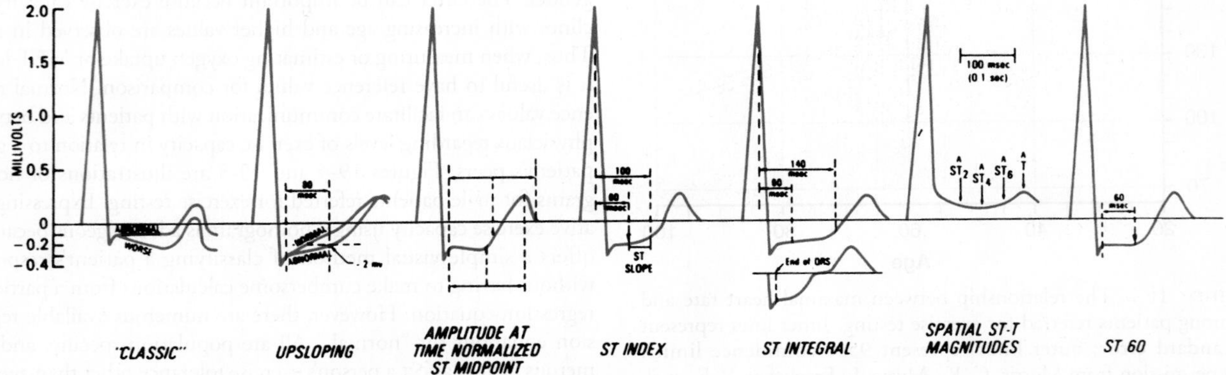

■ **Figure 19-6** Normal and abnormal ST-segment responses to exercise and the various criteria for ST-segment depression. (With permission from Froelicher, V. F., & Myers, J. [2006]. *Exercise and the heart* [5th ed.]. Philadelphia: W.B. Saunders.)

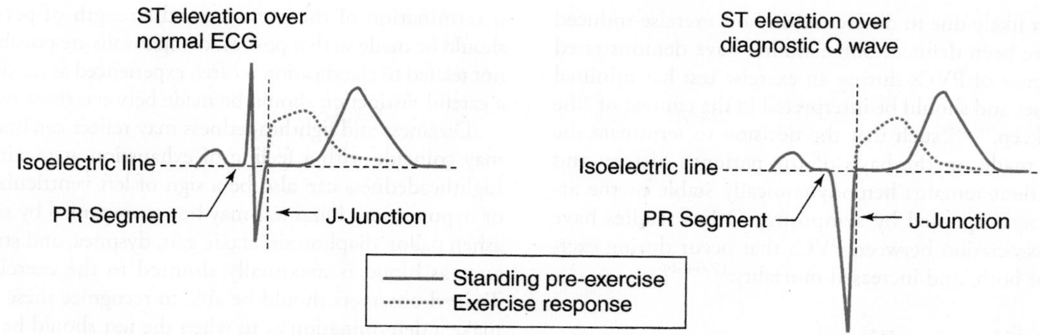

■ **Figure 19-7** Example of exercise-induced ST-segment elevation when the resting electrocardiogram is normal (*left*) and when the resting ECG has a diagnostic Q wave (*right*).

severe transmural ischemia, it can be arrhythmogenic, and it localizes the ischemia. Conversely, exercise-induced ST-segment elevation occurring in leads with Q waves is more common and is related to the presence of dyskinetic areas. This response is relatively common in patients after an MI and is of much less concern. Examples of these two responses are illustrated in Figure 19-7.

There are several important nuances concerning the proper measurement of exercise-induced ST-segment changes. ST-segment depression is measured as a change from the isoelectric line (PR segment) and is considered abnormal if the next 60 to 80 milliseconds after the J-point are flat or downsloping (see Fig. 19-6). However, in patients who exhibit ST-segment depression at rest, exercise-induced ST-segment depression is measured from the baseline (resting) level (Fig. 19-8). In contrast, ST-segment elevation is measured from the level at which the ST segment starts, and slope is not considered. The significance of upsloping or horizontal ST-segment depression with T-wave inversion has been debated. Infarction, ventricular aneurysm, bundle-branch block, hypokalemia, ventricular hypertrophy, abnormal oxygen-carrying capacity of blood caused by anemia, pulmonary disease, and drugs such as digoxin and quinidine may all influence the ST-segment response; these and other conditions may cause exercise-induced ST-segment depression that is not caused by CAD (see section titled "False-Positive and False-Negative Responses").

Arrhythmias During Exercise Testing

Arrhythmias can occur during the exercise test or recovery period and can range in severity from life threatening to benign. There has been a great deal of debate about the importance of arrhythmias during exercise. The occurrence of "serious" arrhythmias during exercise, although rare, is an indication to terminate the exercise test. Arrhythmias may be overt, such as ventricular tachycardia, or subtle, such as unifocal premature ventricular complexes (PVCs) increasing in frequency, or a period of supraventricular tachycardia. Arrhythmias for which there should be no debate about stopping the test include second- or third-degree heart block and ventricular tachycardia of any duration. Other arrhythmias that have been generally classified as "significant" or "complex" include R-on-T PVCs, frequent unifocal or multifocal PVCs (constituting 30% or more of the beats per minute), and coupling of PVCs (two in succession).[4,8] On rare occasion, any of these complex arrhythmias can be a precursor to a life-threatening sustained rhythm disturbance. When there is doubt as to the nature or origin of the arrhythmia, the test should be stopped. Electrophysiologic testing is commonly used to more fully evaluate complex arrhythmias and direct appropriate treatment.

The prognostic significance of exercise-induced PVCs, even when they occur frequently, has varied widely in the literature. This

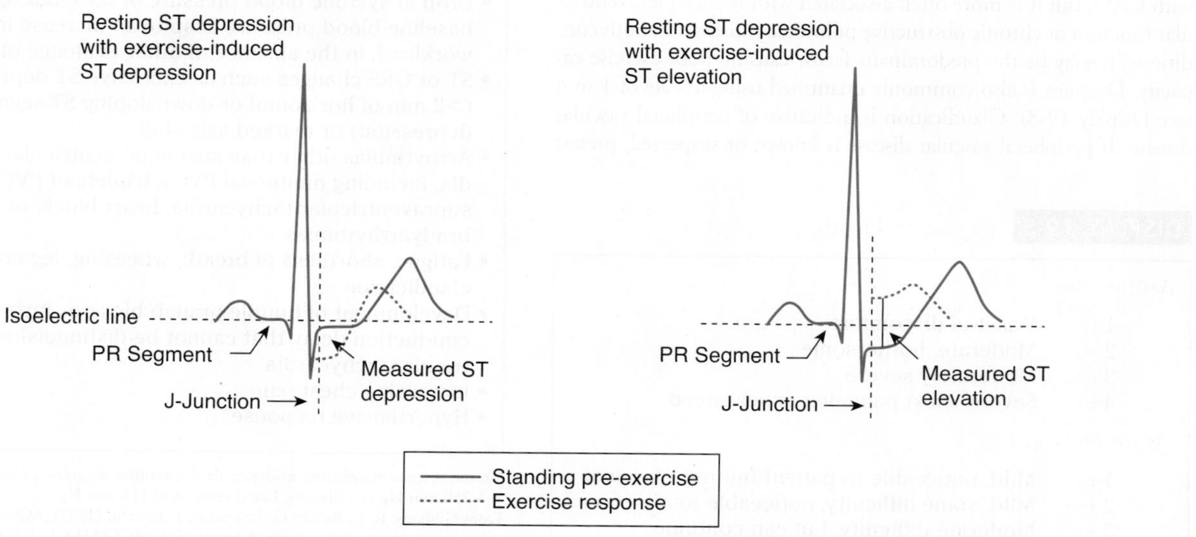

■ **Figure 19-8** Example of how exercise-induced ST-segment depression (*left*) and elevation (*right*) are measured when the electrocardiogram shows ST depression at rest.

variation is most likely due to differences in how exercise-induced arrhythmias have been defined. Some studies have demonstrated that the occurrence of PVCs during an exercise test has minimal prognostic impact and should be interpreted in the context of "the company they keep,"[4,63] such that the decision to terminate the test should be made on the basis of the patient's history and whether the patient remains hemodynamically stable or the arrhythmias are accompanied by symptoms. Other studies have shown a clear association between PVCs that occur during exercise, recovery, or both, and increased mortality.[17,64–66]

Subjective Responses

Assessment of symptoms and perception of effort during the exercise test are important to maximize safety, and these subjective measures yield valuable diagnostic information. Obtaining careful assessments of subjective measures during the exercise test requires thorough explanations to ensure that the patient understands what is expected and how to communicate these responses to those conducting the test. Angina and dyspnea are the most common cardiopulmonary symptoms elicited during exercise and each is typically evaluated using a four-point scale[8,67] (Display 19-3). These scales should be carefully explained to the patient before the exercise test. Patients should be encouraged to report any and all symptoms during exercise.

It is important to distinguish between typical and atypical angina, because they have quite different diagnostic implications. Typical angina tends to be consistent in its presentation and location, is brought on by physical or emotional stress, and is relieved by rest or nitroglycerin. Atypical angina refers to pain that has an unusual location, prolonged duration, or inconsistent precipitating factors that are unresponsive to nitroglycerin. Exercise-induced chest discomfort that has the characteristics of stable, typical angina provides better confirmation of the presence of significant CAD than any other test response. A patient exhibiting the combination of typical angina and an abnormal ST response has a 98% probability of having significant CAD. An important indication to stop the exercise test is moderately severe angina (level 3 on a scale of 1 to 4; see Display 19-3), which should correspond with pain that would normally cause the patient to stop daily activities or take a sublingual nitroglycerin pill.[27,67]

Dyspnea may be the predominant symptom in some patients with CAD, but it is more often associated with reduced left ventricular function or chronic obstructive pulmonary disease. In both conditions, it may be the predominant factor causing poor exercise capacity. Dyspnea is also commonly quantified using a scale of 1 to 4 (see Display 19-3). Claudication is indicative of peripheral vascular disease. If peripheral vascular disease is known or suspected, pretest determination of the presence and strength of peripheral pulses should be made so that posttest comparisons are possible. Leg fatigue not related to claudication is often experienced at maximum exercise; a careful distinction should be made between these two symptoms.

Dizziness and lightheadedness may reflect cerebral hypoxia and may coincide with a feeling of exhaustion at maximum exercise. Lightheadedness can also be a sign of left ventricular dysfunction or hypotension. Dizziness may be accompanied by signs of gray or ashen pallor, diaphoresis, ataxic gait, dyspnea, and strained appearance as blood is maximally shunted to the exercising muscles. Trained observers should be able to recognize these responses and make a determination as to when the test should be stopped.

DISPLAY 19-3 Angina and Dyspnea Scales

Angina Scale

1+	Onset of discomfort
2+	Moderate, bothersome
3+	Moderately severe
4+	Severe; most pain ever experienced

Dyspnea Scale

1+	Mild, noticeable to patient but not observer
2+	Mild, some difficulty, noticeable to observer
3+	Moderate difficulty, but can continue
4+	Severe difficulty, patient cannot continue

TEST TERMINATION

The usual goal of the exercise test in patients with known or suspected disease is to achieve a maximal level of exertion. This permits the greatest information yield from the test. However, achieving a maximal effort should be superseded by any of the clinical indications to stop the test (Display 19-4), by clinical judgment, or

DISPLAY 19-4 Indications for Stopping an Exercise Test

Absolute

- Drop in systolic blood pressure of >10 mm Hg from baseline despite an increase in workload, when accompanied by other evidence of ischemia
- Moderate to severe angina
- Increasing nervous system symptoms (e.g., ataxia, dizziness, or syncope)
- Signs of poor perfusion (cyanosis or pallor)
- Technical difficulties in monitoring electrocardiogram or systolic blood pressure
- Subject's desire to stop
- Sustained ventricular tachycardia
- ST elevation (≥1.0 mm) in leads without diagnostic Q waves (other than V_1 or aVR)

Relative

- Drop in systolic blood pressure of ≥10 mm Hg from baseline blood pressure despite an increase in workload, in the absence of other evidence of ischemia
- ST or QRS changes such as excessive ST depression (>2 mm of horizontal or downsloping ST-segment depression) or marked axis shift
- Arrhythmias other than sustained ventricular tachycardia, including multifocal PVCs, triplets of PVCs, supraventricular tachycardia, heart block, or bradyarrhythmias
- Fatigue, shortness of breath, wheezing, leg cramps, or claudication
- Development of bundle-branch block or intraventricular conduction delay that cannot be distinguished from ventricular tachycardia
- Increasing chest pain
- Hypertensive response*

*In the absence of definitive evidence, the Committee suggests systolic blood pressure of >250 mm Hg or a diastolic blood pressure of 115 mm Hg.

From Gibbons, R. J., Balady, G. J., Bricker, J. T., et al. (2002). ACC/AHA 2002 guideline update for exercise testing. A report of the ACC/AHA Task Force on Practice Guidelines (Committee on Exercise Testing). *Journal of the American College of Cardiology, 40*, 1531–1540.

by the patient's request to stop. The reason for stopping the test should be carefully recorded because the symptoms or signs manifested by exercise often relate to the mechanism of impairment. Determining the endpoint of an exercise test can be problematic. It requires integration of objective physiologic data and termination criteria with subjective judgment based on clinical experience. Some patients may be unable or unwilling to exercise to an adequate level. In patients with suspected coronary disease, a symptom-limited, maximal test is usually more diagnostic. Thus, patients should be instructed to exercise to the point at which they can no longer continue because of fatigue, dyspnea, or other symptoms. They should be informed that the test will be terminated if abnormal responses are observed by the operators. Although patients should be encouraged to exercise as long as possible, they should not be pushed beyond their capacity and any request to stop the test should be honored. Inability to fully monitor the patient's responses because of technical difficulties should result in immediate termination of the test. Most problems can be avoided by having an experienced physician, nurse, or exercise physiologist standing next to the patient, measuring blood pressure and assessing patient appearance during the test. The exercise technician should operate the recorder and treadmill, take appropriate tracings, enter data on a form, and alert the physician to any abnormalities that may appear on the monitor.

Although many efforts have been made to objectify maximal effort, such as age-predicted maximal heart rate, a plateau in oxygen uptake, exceeding the ventilatory threshold, or a respiratory exchange ratio greater than unity, all have considerable measurement error and intersubject variability.[50,68–71] This variability occurs regardless of the population tested. The 95% confidence limits for maximal heart rate based on age, for example, range considerably (see Fig. 19-3); therefore, this endpoint is maximal for some and submaximal for others.[17] The classic index of a person's cardiopulmonary limits, a plateau in oxygen uptake, is not observed in many patients, is poorly reproducible, and has been confused by the many different criteria applied.[68–71] Although subjective, the Borg Perceived Exertion Scale is helpful for assessing exercise effort[72] (Display 19-5). Good judgment on the part of the physician remains the most effective criterion for terminating exercise.

DISPLAY 19-5 Borg Rating of Perceived Exertion Scale

6	
7	Very, very light
8	
9	Very light
10	
11	Fairly light
12	
13	Somewhat hard
14	
15	Hard
16	
17	Very hard
18	
19	Very, very hard
20	

From Borg, G. A. V. (1985). *An introduction to Borg's RPE scale.* Ithaca, NY: Movement Publications.

RECOVERY PERIOD

Some debate exists as to whether the postexercise recovery period should be an active or passive process. This decision should be made on the basis of the purpose of the exercise test. If the test is performed for diagnostic purposes, then it appears to be of value to place the patient in the supine position immediately after stopping exercise. The increase in venous return to the heart observed in the supine position results in increases in ventricular volume, wall stress, and, consequently, myocardial oxygen demand. Several studies have shown that ST-segment abnormalities are enhanced in the supine position and that an active recovery may attenuate the magnitude of these changes.[4,73] Once thought to be false-positive responses, ST-segment changes 2 to 4 minutes into recovery are now known to be particularly important for the detection of ischemia. Patients with symptom-limiting angina or dyspnea may become more uncomfortable in the supine position and should recover in a seated upright or semirecumbent position. If the test is performed for nondiagnostic purposes such as for a fitness evaluation in a healthy or athletic person, then an active recovery may be safer and more comfortable.

Typically, an active recovery period consists of walking on the treadmill at a speed of 1.5 to 2.0 mph or continuing to pedal the cycle ergometer slowly at a work rate ranging from 0 to 25 W. An active recovery decreases the risk of hypotension and may minimize the risk of dysrhythmias secondary to elevated catecholamines in the postexercise period. Standing recovery should be avoided because of potential complications associated with venous pooling. Regardless of the method of recovery, patients should be monitored for at least 6 to 8 minutes into the postexercise period. Blood pressure, the electrocardiogram, and symptoms should be monitored and recorded at 2-minute intervals for the duration of the recovery period. The recovery period should be extended as long as necessary to resolve symptoms or abnormal hemodynamic or electrocardiographic responses. After completion of the recovery portion of the test, patients should be given posttest instructions that include avoidance of long, hot showers or baths. In addition, patients should be told they may experience fatigue and muscle soreness and to avoid any heavy exertion that day. Any pain or discomfort during the day after the test should be reported to their physician immediately.

ASSESSING TEST ACCURACY

All diagnostic tests misclassify patients a certain percentage of the time. In the context of the exercise test, this is not a trivial issue, because people who are inaccurately identified as having disease may be subjected unnecessarily to additional, more invasive, and costly procedures. When the test is performed properly, it commonly serves the very important purpose of screening those who should or should not undergo these additional procedures. However, a patient with significant CAD who is incorrectly classified as normal may not receive appropriate medical therapy. How accurately the exercise test distinguishes people with disease from those without disease depends on the population tested, the definition of disease, and the criteria used for an abnormal test.

The most common terms used to describe test accuracy are sensitivity and specificity. Sensitivity is the percentage of times a

DISPLAY 19-6 Terms Used to Demonstrate the Diagnostic Value of A Test

Sensitivity	$\frac{TP}{TP + FN} \times 100$
Specificity	$\frac{TN}{TN + FP} \times 100$
Positive predictive value	$\frac{TP}{TP + FP} \times 100$
Negative predictive value	$\frac{TN}{TN + FN} \times 100$

TP, true-positives, or those with abnormal test results and with disease; FN, false-negatives, or those with normal test results with disease; FP, false-positives, or those with abnormal test results and no disease; TN, true-negatives, or those with normal test results and no disease.

test correctly identifies those with CAD. Specificity is the percentage of times a test correctly identifies those without cardiovascular disease. Sensitivity and specificity are inversely related and are affected by the choice of discriminant value for abnormal, the definition of disease, and, most importantly, by the prevalence of disease in the population tested. For example, if the population has a greater prevalence or severity of disease (such as coronary disease in multiple vessels) the test will have a higher sensitivity. Alternatively, the test will have a higher specificity (and low sensitivity) when performed in a group of younger, healthier subjects.

Meta-analysis of the exercise testing literature indicates that the exercise test has, on the average, a sensitivity of approximately 68% and a specificity of approximately 77%.[74] However, these values range widely in the various studies; sensitivity can be as low as 40% among patients with single-vessel disease, but greater than 90% among those with triple-vessel disease. Conversely, the specificity of the test is usually quite low (i.e., 50% to 60%) in patients who have more severe CAD but is quite high in populations that are relatively healthy. These values reported in the literature and the inverse relationship between sensitivity and specificity underscore the importance of considering the patient's pretest characteristics (chest pain and CAD risk factors) before beginning the test. No test result can be interpreted accurately without considering the patient in the context of his or her pretest characteristics.

Another important term that helps define the diagnostic value of a test is the predictive value. The predictive value of an abnormal test (positive predictive value) is the percentage of people with an abnormal test result who have disease. Conversely, the predictive value of a normal test (negative predictive value) is the percentage of people with a normal test result who do not have disease. The predictive value of a test cannot be determined directly from the sensitivity and specificity but is strongly associated with the prevalence of disease in the population tested. The calculations used to determine sensitivity, specificity, and predictive value are presented in Display 19-6.

False-Positive and False-Negative Responses

The factors associated with false-positive or false-negative responses should also be considered before the test. A false-positive response is defined as an abnormal exercise test response in a person *without* significant heart disease and causes the specificity to be decreased. A false-negative response occurs when the test is normal in a person *with* disease and causes the sensitivity of the test to be reduced. Factors associated with false-positive and false-negative responses are listed in Display 19-7. In people in whom the probability of a false-positive or false-negative test is high, an alternative procedure (exercise or pharmacologic echocardiogram or radionuclide test) may be appropriate.

DISPLAY 19-7 Causes of False-Negative and False-Positive Test Results

False-Positive

1. Resting repolarization abnormalities (e.g., left bundle-branch block)
2. Cardiac hypertrophy
3. Accelerated conduction defects (e.g., Wolff–Parkinson–White syndrome)
4. Digitalis
5. Nonischemic cardiomyopathy
6. Hypokalemia
7. Vasoregulatory abnormalities
8. Mitral valve prolapse
9. Pericardial disease
10. Coronary spasm in absence of CAD
11. Anemia
12. Female gender

False-Negative

1. Failure to reach ischemic threshold secondary to medications (e.g., β-blockers)
2. Monitoring an insufficient number of leads to detect electrocardiographic changes
3. Angiographically significant disease compensated by collateral circulation
4. Musculoskeletal limitations preceding cardiac abnormalities

ANCILLARY METHODS FOR THE DETECTION OF CAD

Several ancillary imaging techniques have been shown to provide a valuable complement to exercise electrocardiography for the evaluation of patients with known or suspected CAD. These techniques are particularly helpful among patients with equivocal exercise electrocardiograms or those likely to exhibit false-positive or false-negative responses. They are frequently used to clarify abnormal ST-segment responses in asymptomatic people or those in whom the cause of chest discomfort remains uncertain. When exercise electrocardiography and an imaging technique are combined, the diagnostic and prognostic accuracy is enhanced.[75] For example, patients exhibiting both a positive exercise electrocardiogram and a positive radionuclide scan have been shown to have a 2.6-fold increased risk for subsequent coronary events.[76]

The major imaging procedures are myocardial perfusion and ventricular function studies using radionuclide techniques, exercise echocardiography, and pharmacologic stress testing. Because these techniques are often used in conjunction with or as a surrogate for standard exercise testing, they are briefly discussed here. Detailed reviews of these topics are available elsewhere.[77,78]

Myocardial Perfusion Imaging

The most commonly used technique to evaluate myocardial perfusion is the application of the radionuclide thallium-201. When thallium-201 is injected intravenously at maximal exercise, it is rapidly extracted from the blood by living cells in the myocardium. Uptake of thallium-201 is similar to that of potassium in living cells. Radiologic images are then taken, which reveal areas of absent, poor, or moderately poor uptake of thallium-201. When exercise images are compared with resting images, the differences in uptake of thallium-201 indicate areas of decreased blood flow. At the same time, if areas absent of thallium-201 uptake occur at rest, it can be assumed that this represents areas of myocardial scarring and not ischemia with exercise. This information, along with the exercise test, can be more definitive in the evaluation of the extent and localization of ischemia.

Perfusion imaging with technetium-99m sestamibi has become common. This imaging agent permits higher dosing with less radiation exposure than thallium, resulting in improved images that are sharper and have less artifact and attenuation. Sestamibi is the preferred imaging agent for obtaining tomographic images of the heart using single photon emission computed tomography. Single photon emission computed tomography images are obtained with a gamma camera, which rotates 180 degrees around the patient, stopping at preset angles to record the image. Cardiac images are then displayed in slices from three different axes to allow visualization of the heart in three dimensions. Thus, multiple myocardial segments can be viewed individually, without the overlap of segments that occurs with planar imaging.[77,79] As with thallium-201 imaging, perfusion defects that are present during exercise but not seen at rest suggest ischemia. Perfusion defects that are present during exercise and persist at rest suggest previous MI or scar. In this manner, the extent and distribution of ischemic myocardium can be identified.

Perfusion imaging of the coronary anatomy has been shown to be somewhat more sensitive and specific than the exercise electrocardiogram for detecting CAD. An extensive review of the literature suggested that the sensitivity and specificity of exercise thallium scintigraphy for detecting coronary disease were in the order of 84% and 87%, respectively.[76] This modality also permits the localization of ischemia, which is not possible with ST-segment depression on the electrocardiogram. This technique is especially helpful in patients with equivocal exercise electrocardiograms, those using digoxin, or those with left bundle-branch block, in whom the interpretation of electrocardiographic changes is more problematic.[4,17]

Ventricular Function Studies

Ventricular function is commonly evaluated with the use of the radioisotope technetium-99m. This radioisotope is administered as an intravenous bolus, and its transit through the ventricles is measured by special cameras. Technetium-99m is also used to label red blood cells for equilibrium blood pool studies. Both of these methods have been used extensively in the evaluation of left and right ventricular function after acute MI and other cardiac events. This technique can be performed at rest as well as at maximal exercise. When performed at maximal exercise, it has the capability of determining decreased ventricular function compared with rest measures. This can help in the diagnosis of ischemic abnormalities as well as exercise-induced ventricular dysfunction. In addition to measures of ejection fraction, measures of specific regional wall motion can also be taken.[75,77,79]

The limitations of thallium, sestamibi single photon emission computed tomography, and technetium imaging include their higher cost and exposure of the patient to ionizing radiation. Additional equipment and personnel are also required for image acquisition and interpretation, including a nuclear technician to administer the radioactive isotope and acquire the images and a physician trained in nuclear medicine to reconstruct and interpret the images.

Exercise Echocardiographic Imaging

Echocardiographic imaging of the heart is being increasingly used during exercise and pharmacologic stress testing. This technique is frequently combined with an exercise electrocardiogram to increase the sensitivity and specificity of exercise testing. Typically, a two-dimensional image is taken at rest, and repeat images are obtained at peak exercise or immediately afterward. If images are taken after exercise, they must be obtained within 1 to 2 minutes because abnormal wall motion begins to normalize after this point. Rest and stress images are compared side-by-side in a cine-loop display that is gated during systole from the QRS complex. Myocardial contractility normally increases with exercise, whereas ischemia causes hypokinesis, akinesis, and dyskinesis of the affected segments. Therefore, a test is considered positive if wall motion abnormalities develop in previously normal territories with exercise or worsen in an already abnormal segment.[80]

Some advantages of exercise echocardiography over nuclear imaging include the absence of exposure to ionizing radiation and a shorter amount of time required for testing. Like standard exercise testing and radionuclide techniques, the diagnostic accuracy of echocardiography depends primarily on the specific methodology used and the pretest probability of CAD in the subjects tested. The accuracy of echocardiographic testing also depends on observer experience. Reviews of studies published since the advent of exercise echocardiography in the early 1980s suggest that the average sensitivity and specificity of this technique for detecting coronary disease are both approximately 85%.[81] The limitations of exercise echocardiography include dependence on the operator for obtaining adequate, timely images, and some variation exists in image interpretation. In addition, as many as 20% of patients have inadequate echocardiographic windows secondary to body habitus or lung interference.[82]

Pharmacologic Stress Techniques

It is advantageous to use pharmacologic stress techniques for patients who are unable to exercise on a treadmill or cycle ergometer to an adequate level. These include patients who have orthopedic limitations, peripheral vascular disease, and chronic obstructive pulmonary disease or other limiting pulmonary diseases; elderly patients with low functional capacity; diabetic patients with severe neuropathy; and patients with neuromuscular conditions. For these patients, pharmacologic methods can be extremely useful for evaluating coronary blood flow and myocardial function. Pharmacologic stress is a relatively new area with important applications for echocardiographic and nuclear techniques, but only limited data are available directly comparing pharmacologic stress testing with standard exercise testing.

Two types of pharmacologic stress agents have been used: those that increase coronary blood flow through coronary vasodilation and those that increase myocardial oxygen demand by increasing heart rate. The commonly used coronary vasodilators are adenosine and dipyridamole (Persantine), whereas dobutamine is used to increase myocardial oxygen demand. The vasodilators cause greatly increased endocardial and epicardial blood flow in normal coronary arteries but not in stenotic segments, whereas dobutamine can create an imbalance between myocardial oxygen supply and demand by increasing heart rate and contractility. These drugs are administered intravenously and, when associated with an imaging technique such as thallium-201 scintigraphy, sestamibi, or echocardiography, can provide important information about coronary artery stenosis. Comparisons between dipyridamole and standard exercise testing have demonstrated dipyridamole to have a diagnostic accuracy similar to or slightly better than that of standard exercise testing.[83,84] The disadvantages of dipyridamole and adenosine stress testing include side effects (40% to 50% of patients have minor side effects) and lack of cardiovascular response (approximately 10% of patients).[85,86]

GAS EXCHANGE TECHNIQUES

Because of the inaccuracies associated with estimating oxygen uptake and METs from work rate (i.e., treadmill speed and grade), many laboratories directly measure expired gases. The measurement of gas exchange and ventilatory responses provides an added dimension to the exercise test by increasing the information obtained concerning a patient's cardiopulmonary function. The direct measurement of $\dot{V}o_2$ has been shown to be more reliable and reproducible than estimated values from treadmill or cycle ergometer work rate.[29] Peak $\dot{V}o_2$ is the most accurate measurement of functional capacity and is a useful reflection of overall cardiopulmonary health. Measurement of expired gases is not considered necessary for all clinical exercise testing, but the additional information provides important physiologic data. Heart and lung diseases frequently manifest themselves through gas exchange abnormalities during exercise, and the information obtained is increasingly used in clinical trials to objectively assess the response to interventions. Moreover, a growing body of literature suggests that exercise capacity measured directly by gas exchange techniques provides superior prognostic information relative to exercise time or estimated METs.[7,29,87] Recent studies have demonstrated that indices of ventilatory inefficiency (e.g., the VE/$\dot{V}co_2$ slope, oscillatory breathing patterns, oxygen kinetics) are very powerful predictors of risk for adverse outcomes in patients with heart failure.[7,87] Situations in which gas exchange measurements are appropriate include the following[4,8]:

1. When a precise response to a specific therapeutic intervention is needed for a particular patient
2. When a research question is being addressed
3. When the cause of exercise limitation or dyspnea is uncertain
4. To evaluate exercise capacity in patients with heart failure to assist in the estimation of prognosis and assess the need for transplantation
5. To assist in the development of an appropriate exercise prescription for cardiac rehabilitation

The use of these techniques, however, requires added attention to detail and a working knowledge of the equipment and basic physiology. This is particularly important given advances in automation for the collection and calculation of expired gases.

PROGNOSIS

The exercise test has been shown to be of value for estimating prognosis in patients with a wide range of severity of cardiovascular diseases.[4,7,17,33–35,87–89] One of the most important clinical applications of the exercise test is the identification of low-risk patients in whom catheterization (and revascularization) can be safely deferred. There are several reasons why accurately establishing prognosis is important. An estimate of prognosis provides answers to patients' questions regarding the probable outcome of their illness, which may be useful to the patient in planning return to work or making decisions regarding disability, recreational activities, and finances. A second reason to estimate prognosis is to identify patients for whom interventions might improve outcome. Combining clinical and exercise test information into scores has been shown to improve the estimation risk among men and women undergoing exercise testing.[33,44,90,91]

Although there are many exercise test variables known to be of value for estimating prognosis, including exercise capacity, maximal heart rate, a hypotensive response, ST depression, and symptoms, the most powerful predictor of risk appears to be exercise capacity. Recent studies from Duke University, the Mayo Clinic, the Cleveland Clinic, Boston University and the Veterans Administration have confirmed the value of including exercise capacity in the risk paradigm among patients referred for exercise testing.[33,88,89,92,93] It has also been recently demonstrated that the rate in which heart rate recovers from exercise, long empirically associated with better cardiovascular health, is an important risk marker among patients undergoing exercise testing.[94–96] For example, patients who fail to decrease heart rate more than 12 beats/min, 1 minute after completing the exercise test have four times the risk of mortality over the subsequent 6 years.[94]

EXERCISE TESTING IN SPECIAL POPULATIONS

Women

The interpretation of exercise testing results in women is more challenging than that in men.[4,97,98] Exercise-induced ST-segment depression is less sensitive among women as compared to men.[99,100] Test specificity is also thought to be lower among women, although there is a wide variation in the reported studies.[4] Some of these differences may be explained by differences in the meaning of chest pain presentation between men and women, although typical angina is as meaningful in women older than 60 years as it is in men. Nearly half the women with anginal symptoms in the CASS (who were younger than 65 years) had normal coronary arteries.[101] Other possible explanations for the lower test accuracy in women include lower disease prevalence, higher incidence of mitral valve prolapse and syndrome X (chest pain without coronary disease), differences in microvascular function, and possibly hormonal differences.[4,102]

The accuracy for diagnosing CAD in women has been shown to be improved by the use of multivariate methods[103] and by the addition of nuclear or echocardiographic imaging techniques.[102,104,105] Thus, when exercise testing is performed in women, factors that may affect test accuracy should be carefully considered; if the exercise test results are uncertain or when otherwise appropriate, a radionuclide imaging procedure should be considered. The optimal strategy for circumventing false-positive test results in women remains to be defined. Nevertheless, the current AHA/ACC guidelines suggest that there are insufficient data to justify routine radionuclide imaging procedures as the initial test for CAD in women.[4]

The Elderly

The prevalence of CAD increases with increasing age, and the exercise test can be an extremely useful tool for diagnosing CAD in the elderly. However, exercise testing in the elderly can be problematic given their frequently compromised ability to exercise in the context of an increased prevalence of CAD. The occurrence of fatigue and lightheadedness caused by muscle weakness and deconditioning, vasoregulatory abnormalities, and difficulties with gait are important concerns in these patients. Thus, a test modality and protocol should be chosen that provides the highest degree of safety. For instance, cycle ergometry may be more appropriate for elderly patients who have a residual deficit from a cerebral vascular accident. In addition, the testing protocol should be modified considering the expected levels of exercise tolerance. More gradually incremented protocols, such as the Balke, ramp, or Naughton, are usually more suitable in the elderly population. The elderly are more likely to present with more complex medication regimens, more comorbidities, and increased prevalence of aortic stenosis and other valvular diseases, in addition to more severe CAD. For these reasons, the elderly require particularly close evaluation before clearance for exercise testing, a modified testing protocol, and particular attention to appropriate endpoints.[4,97]

Interpretation of the exercise test in the elderly can also differ significantly from that in younger people. Resting electrocardiographic abnormalities, including previous MI, left ventricular hypertrophy, and intraventricular conduction delays, may compromise the diagnostic accuracy of the exercise test. Nevertheless, the application of standard ST-segment criteria among elderly subjects has been shown to have similar diagnostic characteristics as in younger subjects.[99] No doubt because of the higher prevalence of CAD in the elderly, test sensitivity has even been shown to be comparatively higher among the elderly (84%), although specificity is somewhat lower when compared with younger populations (70%).[106] Thus, despite several problems posed by elderly subjects that require additional attention, exercise testing is not contraindicated in this group.[4]

Patients After Cardiac Transplantation

Over the past two decades, transplantation has become a widely used and successful treatment option for patients with end-stage heart failure. The 1-year survival rate for patients who have undergone this procedure is now approximately 85%, compared with only 50% to 60% in patients with severe heart failure who receive medical treatment.[107] The hemodynamic response to exercise in patients who have undergone cardiac transplantation has been characterized since the early 1970s.[108–110] Because the heart is denervated, some intriguing hemodynamic responses are observed. Orthotopic transplantation removes the nervous system connections to the heart. Thus, the heart is not responsive to the normal actions of the parasympathetic and sympathetic systems. The absence of vagal tone explains the high resting heart rates in these patients (100 to 110 beats/min) and the relatively slow adaptation of the heart to a given amount of submaximal work.[110] This slows the delivery of oxygen to the working tissue, contributing to an earlier than normal metabolic acidosis and hyperventilation during exercise.[108,109,111–113] Although transplantation significantly improves the hemodynamic and ventilatory response to exercise, the transplanted patient still exhibits many of the responses typical of the patient with chronic heart failure.[113] These include heightened ventilatory responses attributable to uneven matching of ventilation to perfusion and an increase in physiologic dead space. Maximal heart rate is lower in transplant recipients compared with normal subjects, which contributes to a reduction in cardiac output and peak $\dot{V}o_2$; the arteriovenous oxygen difference widens as a compensatory mechanism.

The exercise test in patients who have undergone cardiac transplantation is less a diagnostic and more a functional tool. In the latter role, it is useful for assessing and modifying therapy in these patients, in addition to evaluating the appropriateness of daily activities and return to work. Although rare cases of chest pain associated with accelerated graft atherosclerosis have been reported in transplant recipients, decentralization of the myocardium usually eliminates anginal symptoms. Exercise electrocardiography is also inadequate in terms of assessing ischemia, as evidenced by its low sensitivity (21% or less).[114] Thus, radionuclide testing may be more useful for assessing ischemia in these patients.

SUMMARY

Although there have been advances in technologies related to the diagnosis of CAD, the numerous applications and widespread availability of the exercise test continue to make it one of the more important tools in cardiovascular medicine. The test is increasingly being supervised by nonphysicians,[16] and the cardiovascular nurse's role has expanded in many centers to include exercise test supervision. Thus, an understanding of proper methodology, conduct, indications, and the physiology related to exercise testing are increasingly recognized skills. A good understanding of these principles can also assist the nurse in applying the information gained from the exercise test to patients with various cardiovascular diseases. In addition to diagnostic and prognostic information, these applications include the assessment of therapy, exercise prescription, and helping to guide medical/surgical management decisions for the patient.

REFERENCES

1. Ashley, E. A., Myers, J., & Froelcher, V. (2000). Exercise testing in clinical medicine. *The Lancet, 356*, 1592–1597.
2. Marcus, R., Lowe, R., Froelicher, V. F., et al. (1995). The exercise test as gatekeeper: Limiting access or appropriately directing resources? *Chest, 107*, 1442–1446.
3. American Thoracic Society/American College of Chest Physicians. (2003). Statement on cardiopulmonary exercise testing. *American Journal of Respiratory and Critical Care Medicine, 167*, 211–277.
4. Gibbons, R. J., Balady, G. J., Bricker, J. T., et al. (2002). ACC/AHA 2002 guideline update for exercise testing. A report of the ACC/AHA Task Force on Practice Guidelines (Committee on Exercise Testing). *Journal of American College of Cardiology, 40*, 1531–1540.
5. Mehra, M. R., Kobashigawa, J., Starling, R., et al. (2006). Listing criteria for heart transplantation: International Society for Heart and Lung Transplantation guidelines for the care of cardiac transplant candidates—2006. *The Journal of Heart and Lung Tansplantation, 25*, 1024–1042 .

6. Arena, R., Myers, J., & Guazzi, M. (2008). The clinical and research applications of aerobic capacity and ventilatory efficiency in heart failure: An evidence-based review. *Heart Failure Reviews, 13*(2), 245–269.
7. Myers, J. (2005). Applications of cardiopulmonary exercise testing in the management of cardiovascular and pulmonary disease. *International Journal of Sports Medicine, 26*, S49–S55.
8. American College of Sports Medicine. (2006). *Guidelines for exercise testing and prescription* (7th ed.). Baltimore: Lippincott Williams & Wilkins.
9. Working Group on Cardiac Rehabilitation and Exercise Physiology and the Working Group on Heart Failure of the European Society of Cardiology. (2001). Recommendations for exercise testing in chronic heart failure patients. *European Heart Journal, 22*, 37–45.
10. American College of Sports Medicine. (2006). *Resource manual for guidelines for exercise testing and prescription*. Baltimore: Lippincott Williams & Wilkins.
11. Rogers, G. P., Ayanian, J. Z., Balady, G. J., et al. (2000). American College of Cardiology/American Heart Association Clinical Competence Statement on Stress Testing. A report of the ACC/AHA and American Society of Internal Medicine Task Force on Clinical Competence. *Circulation, 102*, 1726–1738.
12. Herbert, D. L., & Herbert, W. G. (2002). *Legal aspects of preventive, rehabilitative, and recreational exercise programs* (4th ed.). Canton, OH: PRC.
13. Miranda, C. P., Lehmann, K. G., & Froelicher, V. F. (1989). Indications, criteria for interpretation, and utilization of exercise testing in patients with coronary disease: Results of a survey. *Journal of Cardiopulmonary Rehabilitation, 9*, 479–484.
14. Myers, J., Voodi, L., Umann, T., et al. (2000). A survey of exercise testing: Methods, utilization, interpretation, and safety in the VAHCS. *Journal of Cardiopulmonary Rehabilitation, 20*, 251–258.
15. Gibbons, L., Blair, S. N., Kohl, H. W., et al. (1989). The safety of maximal exercise testing. *Circulation, 80*, 846–852.
16. Franklin, B. A., Gordon, S., Timmis, G. C., et al. (1997). Is direct physician supervision of exercise stress testing routinely necessary? *Chest, 111*, 262–264.
17. Froelicher, V. F., & Myers, J. (2006). *Exercise and the heart* (5th ed.). Philadelphia: W.B. Saunders.
18. Mason, R. E., & Likar, I. (1966). A new system of multiple-lead exercise electrocardiography. *American Heart Journal, 71*, 196–205.
19. Gamble, P., McManus, H., Jensen, D., et al. (1984). A comparison of the standard 12-lead electrocardiogram to exercise electrode placement. *Chest, 85*, 616–622.
20. Kleiner, J. P., Nelson, W. P., & Boland, M. J. (1978). The 12-lead electrocardiogram in exercise testing. *Archives of Internal Medicine, 138*, 1572–1573.
21. Rautaharju, P. M., Prineas, R. J., Crow, R. S., et al. (1980). The effect of modified limb positions on electrocardiographic wave amplitudes. *Journal of Electrocardiology, 13*, 109–114.
22. Buchfuhrer, M. J., Hansen, J. E., Robinson, T. E., et al. (1983). Optimizing the exercise protocol for cardiopulmonary assessment. *Journal of Applied Physiology, 55*, 1558–1564.
23. Hambrecht, R., Schuler, G. C., Muth, T., et al. (1992). Greater diagnostic sensitivity of treadmill versus cycle exercise testing of asymptomatic men with coronary artery disease. *American Journal of Cardiology, 70*, 141–146.
24. Hermansen, L., & Saltin, B. (1969). Oxygen uptake during maximal treadmill and bicycle exercise. *Journal of Applied Physiology, 26*, 31–37.
25. Myers, J., Buchanan, N., Walsh, D., et al. (1991). Comparison of the ramp versus standard exercise protocols. *Journal of the American College of Cardiology, 17*, 1334–1342.
26. Wicks, J. R., Sutton, J. R., Oldridge, N. B., et al. (1978). Comparison of the electrocardiographic changes induced by maximum exercise testing with treadmill and cycle ergometer. *Circulation, 57*, 1066–1069.
27. Myers, J., & Froelicher, V. F. (1994). Optimizing the exercise test for pharmacologic studies in patients with angina pectoris. In D. Ardissino, S. Savonitto, & L. H. Opie (Eds.), *Drug evaluation in angina pectoris* (pp. 41–52). Pavia, Italy: Kluwer Academic.
28. Webster, M. W. I., & Sharpe, D. N. (1989). Exercise testing in angina pectoris: The importance of protocol design in clinical trials. *American Heart Journal, 117*, 505–508.
29. Myers, J. (1996). *Essentials of cardiopulmonary exercise testing*. Champaign, IL: Human Kinetics.
30. Arena, R., Myers, J., Williams, M. A., et al. (2007). Assessment of functional capacity in clinical and research settings: A scientific statement from the American Heart Association Committee on Exercise, Rehabilitation, and Prevention of the Council on Clinical Cardiology and the Council on Cardiovascular Nursing. *Circulation, 116*, 329–343.
31. Stuart, R. J., & Ellestad, M. H. (1980). National survey of exercise stress testing facilities. *Chest, 77*, 94–97.
32. Weiner, D. A., Ryan, T. J., McCabe, C. H., et al. (1987). Value of exercise testing in determining the risk classification and the response to coronary artery bypass grafting in three-vessel coronary artery disease: A report from the Coronary Artery Surgery Study (CASS) registry. *American Journal of Cardiology, 60*, 262–266.
33. Mark, D. B., Hlatky, M. A., Harell, F. E., et al. (1987). Exercise treadmill score for predicting prognosis in coronary artery disease. *Annals of Internal Medicine, 106*, 793–800.
34. Myers, J., & Gullestad, L. (1998). The role of exercise testing and gas exchange measurement in the prognostic assessment of patients with heart failure. *Current Opinion in Cardiology, 13*, 145–155.
35. Mark, D. B., & Lauer M. S. (2003). Exercise capacity: The prognostic variable that doesn't get enough respect. *Circulation, 108*, 1534–1536.
36. Panza, J., Quyyumi, A. A., Diodati, J. G., et al. (1991). Prediction of the frequency and duration of ambulatory myocardial ischemia in patients with stable coronary artery disease by determination of the ischemia threshold from exercise testing: Importance of the exercise protocol. *Journal of the American College of Cardiology, 17*, 657–663.
37. Redwood, D. R., Rosing, D. R., Goldstein, R. E., et al. (1971). Importance of the design of an exercise protocol in the evaluation of patients with angina pectoris. *Circulation, 43*, 618–628.
38. Wolthius, R. A., Froelicher, V. F., Fischer, J., et al. (1997). New practical treadmill protocol for clinical use. *American Journal of Cardiology, 39*, 697–700.
39. Naughton, J. P., & Haiden, R. (1973). Methods of exercise testing. In J. P. Naughton, H. K. Hellerstien, & L. C. Mohler (Eds.), *Exercise testing and exercise training in coronary heart disease* (pp. 79–91). New York: Academic Press.
40. Astrand, P. O., & Rodahl, K. (1986) *Textbook of work physiology* (3rd ed.). New York: McGraw-Hill.
41. Whipp, B. J., Davis, J. A., Torres, F., et al. (1981). A test to determine parameters of aerobic function during exercise. *Journal of Applied Physiology, 50*, 217–221.
42. Myers, J., Buchanan, N., Smith, D., et al. (1992). Individualized ramp treadmill: Observations on a new protocol. *Chest, 101*, 2305–2415.
43. Porszasz, J., Casaburi, R., Somfay, A., et al. (2003). A treadmill ramp protocol using simultaneous changes in speed and grade. *Medicine Science Sports Exercise, 35*, 1596–1603.
44. Chang, J. A., & Froelicher, V. F. (1994). Clinical and exercise test markers of prognosis in patients with stable coronary artery disease. *Current Problems in Cardiology, 19*, 533–538.
45. Froelicher, E. S. (1994). Usefulness of exercise testing shortly after acute myocardial infarction for predicting 10-year mortality. *American Journal of Cardiology, 74*, 318–323.
46. Olona, M., Candell-Riera, J., Permanyer-Miralda, G., et al. (1995). Strategies for prognostic assessment of uncomplicated first myocardial infarction: 5-year follow-up study. *Journal of the American College of Cardiology, 25*, 815–822.
47. Naughton, J., Balke, B., & Nagle, F. (1964). Refinements in methods of evaluation and physical conditioning before and after myocardial infarction. *American Journal of Cardiology, 14*, 837–843.
48. Froelicher, V. F. (1996). *Exercise test reporting aid (EXTRA) software*. St. Louis: Mosby-Year Book.
49. Myers, M., Tan, S. Y., Abella, J., et al. (2007). Comparison of the chronotropic response to exercise and heart rate recovery in predicting cardiovascular mortality. *European Journal of Cardiovascular Prevention and Rehabilitation, 14*, 215–221.
50. Hammond, K., & Froelicher, V. F. (1985). Normal and abnormal heart rate responses to exercise. *Progress in Cardiovascular Disease, 27*, 271–296.
51. Lauer, M. S., Okin, P. M., Larson, M. G., et al. (1996). Impaired heart rate response to graded exercise: Prognostic implications of chronotropic incompetence in the Framingham Heart Study. *Circulation, 93*, 1520–1526.
52. Graettinger, W., Smith, D., Neutel, J., et al. (1995). Relationship of left ventricular structure to maximal heart rate during exercise. *Chest, 107*, 341–345.
53. Bailey, R. H., & Bauer, J. H. (1993). A review of common errors in the indirect measurement of blood pressure. *Archives of Internal Medicine, 153*, 2741–2748.

54. Iyriboz, Y., & Hearon, C. M. (1992). Blood pressure measurement at rest and during exercise: Controversies, guidelines, and procedures. *Journal of Cardiopulmonary Rehabilitation, 12*, 277–287.
55. Mazzotta, G., Scopinaro, G., Falcidieno, M., et al. (1987). Significance of abnormal blood pressure response during exercise-induced myocardial dysfunction after recent acute myocardial infarction. *American Journal of Cardiology, 59*, 1256–1260.
56. Irving, J. B., & Bruce, R. A. (1977). Exertional hypotension and posexertional ventricular fibrillation in stress testing. *American Journal of Cardiology, 39*, 849–851.
57. Dubach, P., Froelicher, V. F., Klein, J., et al. (1988). Exercise induced hypotension in a male population: Criteria, causes, and prognosis. *Circulation, 78*, 1380–1387.
58. San Marco, M., Pontius, S., & Selvester, R. (1980). Abnormal blood pressure response and marked ischemia by ST segment depression as predictors of severe coronary artery disease. *Circulation, 61*, 572–578.
59. Weiner, D. A., McCabe, C. H., Cutler, S. S., et al. (1982). Decrease in systolic blood pressure during exercise testing: Reproducibility, response to coronary artery bypass surgery and prognostic significance. *American Journal of Cardiology, 49*, 1627–1632.
60. Foster, C., Crowe, A. J., Danies, E., et al. (1996). Predicting functional capacity during treadmill testing independent of exercise protocol. *Medicine and Science in Sports Exercise, 28*, 752–756.
61. Philbrick, J. T., Horowitz, S. W., & Feinstein, A. R. (1989). Methodological problems of exercise testing for coronary artery disease: Groups, analysis and bias. *American Journal of Cardiology, 64*, 1117–1122.
62. Miranda, C. P., Liu, J., Kadar, A., et al. (1992). Usefulness of exercise induced ST segment depression in the inferior leads during exercise testing as a marker for coronary artery disease. *American Journal of Cardiology, 69*, 303–307.
63. Yang, J. C., Wesley, R. C., & Froelicher, V. F. (1991). Ventricular tachycardia during routine treadmill testing: Risk and prognosis. *Archives of Internal Medicine, 151*, 349–353.
64. Beckerman, J., Wu, T., Jones, S., et al. (2005). Exercise test-induced arrhythmias. *Progress in Cardiovascular Disease, 47*, 285–305.
65. Partington, S., Myers, J., Cho, S., et al. (2003). Prevalence and prognostic value of exercise-induced ventricular arrhythmias. *American Heart Journal, 145*, 139–146.
66. Frolkis, J. P., Pothier, C. E., Blackstone, E. H., et al. (2003). Frequent ventricular ectopy after exercise as a predictor of death. *New England Journal of Medicine, 348*, 781–790.
67. Myers, J. N. (1994). Perception of chest pain during exercise testing in patients with coronary artery disease. *Medicine and Science in Sports Exercise, 26*, 1082–1086.
68. Myers, J., Walsh, D., Buchanan, N., et al. (1989). Can maximal cardiopulmonary capacity be recognized by a plateau in oxygen uptake? *Chest, 96*, 1312–1316.
69. Myers, J., Walsh, D., Sullivan, M., et al. (1990). Effect of sampling on variability and plateau in oxygen uptake. *Journal of Applied Physiology, 68*, 404–410.
70. Noakes, T. (1988). Implications of exercise testing for prediction of athletic performance: A contemporary perspective. *Medicine and Science in Sports Exercise, 20*, 319–330.
71. Midgley, A. W., McNaughton, L. R., Polman, R., et al. (2007). Criteria for determination of maximal oxygen uptake: A brief critique and directions for future research. *Sports Medicine, 37*, 1019–1028.
72. Borg, G. A. V. (1998). *Borg's Perceived Exertion and Pain Scale*. Champaign, IL: Human Kinetics.
73. Lachterman, B., Lehmann, K. G., Abrahamson, D., et al. (1990). "Recovery only" ST segment depression and the predictive accuracy of the exercise test. *Annals of Internal Medicine, 112*, 11–16.
74. Gianrossi, R., Detrano, R., Mulvihill, D., et al. (1989). Exercise-induced ST depression in the diagnosis of coronary artery disease: A meta-analysis. *Circulation, 80*, 87–98.
75. Borges-Neto, S. (1997). Perfusion and function assessment by nuclear cardiology techniques. *Current Opinion in Cardiology, 12*, 581–586.
76. Kotler, T. S., & Diamond, G. A. (1990). Exercise thallium-201 scintigraphy in the diagnosis and prognosis of coronary artery disease. *Annals of Internal Medicine, 113*, 684–702.
77. McGie, A. I., & Gould, K. L. (2007). Nuclear cardiology. In J. T. Willerson, J. N. Cohn, H. J. Wallens, et al. (Eds.), *Cardiovascular medicine* (3rd ed., pp. 137–160). London: Springer-Verlag.
78. Klocke, F. J., Baird, M. G., Lorell, B. H., et al. (2003). ACC/AHA/ASNC guidelines for the clinical use of cardiac radionuclide imaging—Executive summary: A report of the American College of Cardiology/American Heart Association Task Force on Practice Guidelines. *Journal of the American College of Cardiology, 42*, 1318–1333.
79. Gibbons, R. J. (1991). Nuclear cardiology. In E. R. Guiliani, V. Fyster, B. J. Gersh, et al. (Eds.), *Cardiology: Fundamentals and practice* (2nd ed., pp. 161–180). St. Louis, MO: CV Mosby.
80. Armstrong, W., & Marcovitz, P. A. (1993). In E. Braunwald (Ed.), *Stress echocardiography: Heart disease updates* (pp. 1–10). Philadelphia: W.B. Saunders.
81. Armstrong, W. F., & Zoghbi, W. A. (2005). Stress echocardiography. Current methodology and clinical applications. *Journal of the American College of Cardiology, 45*, 1739–1747.
82. Schmidt, D. H., Port, S. C., & Gal, R. A. (1995). Nuclear cardiology and echocardiography: Non-invasive tests for diagnosing patients with coronary artery disease. In M. Pollack & D. H. Schmidt (Eds.), *Heart disease and rehabilitation* (3rd ed., pp. 81–94). Champaign, IL: Human Kinetics.
83. Bolognese, L., Sarasso, G., Aralda, D., et al. (1989). High dose dipyridamole echocardiography early after uncomplicated acute myocardial infarction: Correlation with exercise testing and coronary angiography. *Journal of the American College of Cardiology, 14*, 357–363.
84. Severi, S., Picano, E., Michelassi, C., et al. (1994). Diagnostic and prognostic value of dipyridamole echocardiography in patients with suspected coronary artery disease: Comparison with exercise electrocardiography. *Circulation, 89*, 1160–1173.
85. Iskandrian, A. S. (1991). Single-photon emission computed tomographic thallium imaging with adenosine, dipyridamole, and exercise. *American Heart Journal, 122*, 279–284.
86. Ranhosky, A., Kempthorne-Rawson, J., & the Intravenous Dipyridamole Thallium Imaging Study Group. (1990). The safety of intravenous dipyridamole thallium myocardial perfusion imaging. *Circulation, 81*, 1205–1209.
87. Arena, R., Guazzi, M., & Myers, J. (2007). Ventilatory abnormalities during exercise in heart failure: A mini review. *Current Respiratory Medicine Reviews, 3*, 179–187.
88. Myers, J., Prakash, M., Froelicher, V. F., et al. (2002). Exercise capacity and mortality in men referred for exercise testing. *New England Journal of Medicine, 346*, 793–801.
89. Roger, V. L., Jacobsen, S. J., Pellikka, P. A., et al. (1998). Prognostic value of treadmill exercise testing. A population-based study in Olmstead County, Minnesota. *Circulation, 98*, 2836–2841.
90. Ashley, E., Myers, J., & Froelicher, V. (2002). Exercise testing scores as an example of better decisions through science. *Medicine and Science in Sports Exercise, 34*, 1391–1398.
91. Ashley, E., & Myers, J. (2003). New insights into the clinical exercise test. *ACSM's Certified News, 13*, 1–5.
92. Lauer, M. S., Pothier, C. E., Magid, D. J., et al. (2007). An externally validated model for predicting long-term survival after exercise treadmill testing in patients with suspected coronary artery disease and a normal electrocardiogram. *Annals of Internal Medicine, 147*, 821–828.
93. Balady, G. J., Larson, M. G., Vasan, R. S., et al. (2004). Usefulness of exercise testing in the prediction of coronary disease risk among asymptomatic persons as a function of the Framingham risk score. *Circulation, 14*, 1920–1925.
94. Cole, C. R., Blackstone, E. H., Pashkow, F. J., et al. (1999). Heart rate recovery immediately after exercise as a predictor of mortality. *New England Journal of Medicine, 341*, 1351–1357.
95. Cole, C. R., Foody, J. M., Blackstone, E. H., et al. (2000). Heart rate recovery after submaximal exercise testing as a predictor of mortality in a cardiovascular healthy cohort. *Annals of Internal Medicine, 132*, 552–555.
96. Shetler, K., Marcus, R., Froelcher, V. F., et al. (2001). Heart rate recovery: Validation and methodologic issues. *Journal of the American College of Cardiology, 38*, 1980–1987.
97. Bryant, B. A., & Limacher, M. C. (2001). Exercise testing in special populations: Athletes, women, and the elderly. *Primary Care, 28*, 55–72.
98. Giardina, A., De Castro, S., Fedele, F., et al. (2006). Non-invasive testing for coronary artery disease in women. *Minerva Cardioangiologica, 54*, 323–330.
99. Hlatky, M. A., Pryor, D. B., Harrell, F. E., Jr., et al. (1984). Factors affecting sensitivity and specificity of exercise electrocardiography: Multivariable analysis. *American Journal of Medicine, 77*, 64–71.
100. Morise, A. P., & Diamond, G. A. (1995). Comparison of the sensitivity and specificity of exercise electrocardiography in biased and

unbiased populations of men and women. *American Heart Journal, 130*, 741–747.
101. Kennedy, H., Killip, T., Fischer, L., et al. (1977). The clinical spectrum of coronary artery disease and its surgical and medical management: 1974–1979, the Coronary Artery Surgery Study. *Circulation, 56*, 756–761.
102. Cerqueira, M. D. (1995). Diagnostic testing strategies for coronary artery disease: Special issues related to gender. *American Journal of Cardiology, 75*, 52D–60D.
103. Robert, A. R., Melin, J. A., & Detry, J. M. (1991). Logistic discriminant analysis improves diagnostic accuracy of exercise testing for coronary artery disease in women. *Circulation, 83*, 1202–1209.
104. Marwick, T. H., Anderson, T., Williams, M. J., et al. (1995). Exercise echocardiography is an accurate and cost-efficient technique for detection of coronary artery disease in women. *Journal of the American College of Cardiology, 26*, 335–341.
105. Morise, A. P., Diamond, G. A., Detrano, R., et al. (1995). Incremental value of exercise electrocardiography and thallium-201 testing in men and women for the presence and extent of coronary artery disease. *American Heart Journal, 130*, 267–276.
106. Kasser, I. S., & Bruce, R. A. (1969). Comparative effects of aging and coronary heart disease on submaximal and maximal exercise. *Circulation, 39*, 759–774.
107. Hoffman, F. M. (2005). Outcomes and complications after heart transplantation: A review. *Journal Cardiovascular Nursing, 20*, S31–S42.
108. Savin, W., Haskell, W. L., Schroeder, J. S., et al. (1980). Cardiorespiratory responses of cardiac transplant patients to graded, symptom limited exercise. *Circulation, 62*, 55–60.
109. Schroeder, J. S. (1979). Hemodynamic performance of the human transplanted heart. *Transplant Proceedings, 11*, 304–308.
110. Stinson, E. B., Griepp, R. L., Schroeder, J. S., et al. (1972). Hemodynamic observations one and two years after cardiac transplantation in man. *Circulation, 14*, 1181–1193.
111. Brubaker, P. H., Berry, M. J., Brozena, S. C., et al. (1993). Relationship of lactate and ventilatory thresholds in cardiac transplant patients. *Medicine and Science in Sports Exercise, 25*, 191–196.
112. Degre, S. G. L., Niset, G. L., DeSmet, J. M., et al. (1987). Cardiorespiratory response to early exercise testing after orthotopic cardiac transplantation. *American Journal of Cardiology, 60*, 926–928.
113. Marzo, K. P., Wilson, J. R., & Mancini, D. M. (1992). Effects of cardiac transplantation on ventilatory response to exercise. *American Journal of Cardiology, 69*, 547–553.
114. Ehrman, J. K., Keteyian, S. J., Levine, A. B., et al. (1993). Exercise stress tests after cardiac transplantation. *American Journal of Cardiology, 71*, 1372–1373.

CHAPTER 20

Cardiac Catheterization

Michaelene Hargrove Deelstra / Carol Jacobson

Cardiac catheterization is widely used for diagnostic evaluation and therapeutic intervention in the management of patients with cardiac disease. Nurses have an important role in precatheterization teaching, intracatheterization, and postcatheterization care. The many nursing responsibilities related to cardiac catheterization are outlined in the American College of Cardiology/Society for Cardiac Angiography and Interventions (ACC/SCA&I) Clinical Expert Consensus Document on Cardiac Catheterization Laboratory Standards.[1]

Cardiac catheterization developed as a result of 50 years of clinical effort. Werner Forssman performed the first documented cardiac catheterization in 1929. Guided by fluoroscopy, Forssman passed a catheter into his own right heart through an antecubital vein. He then walked upstairs to the radiology department and confirmed the catheter position by radiograph. The techniques of right and left heart catheterization were developed during the 1940s and 1950s.[2–4] In 1953, the percutaneous techniques of arterial catheterization were introduced by Seldinger,[5] and, in 1959, selective coronary arteriography was introduced by Sones et al.[6] Important advances related to cardiac catheterization included the development of the Swan–Ganz catheter in 1970 for measuring right heart pressures and the thermodilution method for determination of cardiac output (CO); percutaneous coronary interventions (PCIs), including percutaneous transluminal coronary angioplasty, atherectomy, laser therapy, and stent placement; electrophysiologic mapping and catheter ablation for the management of arrhythmias; valvuloplasty; and noncoronary devices for patent foramen ovale atrial septal defect closure, and ventricular septal defect closure[1] (Chapter 23).

Although noninvasive diagnostic techniques have an important role, cardiac catheterization remains the most definitive procedure for the diagnosis and evaluation of coronary disease. Coronary angiography together with adjunctive technologies during angiography, including intravascular ultrasound (IVUS), fractional flow reserve (FFR), and coronary flow reserve (CFR), provide direct quantitative measurements to evaluate significance of coronary lesions. This chapter describes cardiac catheterization procedures and their possible complications. It also describes the nursing care given before and after catheterization and the interpretation of data as they relate to coronary artery disease (CAD).

INDICATIONS FOR CARDIAC CATHETERIZATION

Cardiac catheterization is indicated in a wide variety of circumstances. The most frequent use of cardiac catheterization is to confirm or define the extent of suspected CAD. Anatomical and physiologic severity of the disease is determined, the presence or absence of related conditions is explored, and the need for PCI can be determined. Cardiac catheterization also is used for the evaluation of patients with acquired (Chapter 29) or congenital (Chapter 31) heart disease. The ACC and the American Heart Association (AHA) have published guidelines for coronary angiography and indications for cardiac catheterization.[7–9] Indications for coronary angiography are classified for specific clinical presentations, including risk stratification for patients with chronic stable angina and asymptomatic patients with ischemia on noninvasive stress testing, and patients with acute coronary syndrome: non-ST elevation myocardial infarction (NSTEMI) and ST elevation myocardial infarction (STEMI).[8–10]

Recommendations for Coronary Angiography for Risk Stratification in Patients With Chronic Stable Angina: ACC/AHA Practice Guidelines[8]

Class I indications:

1. Patients with disabling (Canadian Cardiovascular Society [CCS] class III and IV) chronic stable angina despite medical therapy. (Level of evidence: B)
2. High-risk criteria on noninvasive testing regardless of anginal severity. (Level of evidence: B) (Display 20-1).
3. Patients with angina who have survived sudden cardiac death or serious ventricular arrhythmia. (Level of evidence: B)
4. Patients with angina and symptoms and signs of heart failure (HF). (Level of evidence: C)
5. Patients with clinical characteristics that indicate a high likelihood of severe CAD. (Level of evidence: C)

Recommendations for Coronary Angiography for Risk Stratification in Asymptomatic Patients: ACC/AHA Practice Guidelines[8]

Class IIa indications:

1. Patients with high-risk criteria suggesting ischemia on noninvasive testing. (Level of evidence: C)

Class IIb indications:

1. Patients with inadequate prognostic information after noninvasive testing. (Level of evidence: C)
2. Patients with clinical characteristics that indicate a high likelihood of severe CAD. (Level of evidence: C)

DISPLAY 20-1 Noninvasive Tests Results Predicting High Risk for Adverse Outcome

1. Severe resting left ventricular dysfunction (LVEF <0.35)
2. High-risk treadmill score
3. Severe exercise left ventricular dysfunction (exercise LVEF <0.35)
4. Stress-induced large perfusion defect (particularly if anterior)
5. Stress-induced multiple perfusion defects of moderate size
6. Large, fixed perfusion defect with left ventricular dilatation or increased lung uptake (thallium-201)
7. Stress-induced moderate-size perfusion defect with left-ventricular dilatation or increased lung uptake (thallium-201)
8. Echocardiographic wall motion abnormality (involving more than two segments) developing at low-dose dobutamine or at low heart rate
9. Stress echocardiographic evidence of extensive ischemia

LVEF, left ventricular ejection fraction.
Adapted from Gibbons, R. J., Abrams, J., Chatterjee, K., et al. (2003) ACC/AHA 2002 guideline update for the management of patients with chronic stable angina. *Journal of American College of Cardiology, 41*, 159–168.

Recommendations for Coronary Angiography in Patients With Unstable Angina (UA/NSTEMI: ACC/AHA Practice Guidelines)[9]

Class I indications:

1. An early invasive strategy (i.e., diagnostic angiography with intent to perform revascularization) is indicated in UA/NSTEMI patients who have refractory angina or hemodynamic or electrical instability (without serious comorbidities or contraindications to such procedures). (Level of evidence: C) (See Table 20-1).
2. An early invasive strategy (i.e., diagnostic angiography with intent to perform revascularization) is indicated in initially stabilized UA/NSTEMI patients (without serious comorbidities or contraindications to such procedures) who have an elevated risk for clinical events. (Level of evidence: A)

Patients with UA/NSTEMI who have had prior PCI or coronary artery bypass graft surgery should be considered for early coronary angiography, unless data from previous coronary angiography indicate that further revascularization is unlikely to be possible.[9]

Recommendations for Coronary Angiography in Patients With Variant (Prinzmetal's) Angina: ACC/AHA Practice Guidelines[9]

Class I indications:

1. Diagnostic investigation is indicated in patients with a clinical picture suggestive of coronary spasm, with investigation for the presence of transient myocardial ischemia and ST-segment elevation during chest pain. (Level of evidence: A)
2. Patients with episodic chest pain accompanied by transient ST-segment elevation. (Level of evidence: B)

Recommendations for Coronary Angiography in Patients With Postrevascularization Ischemia: ACC/AHA Practice Guidelines[7]

Class I indications:

1. Suspected abrupt closure or subacute stent thrombosis after percutaneous revascularization. (Level of evidence: B) (Chapter 23).
2. Recurrent angina or high-risk criteria on noninvasive evaluation within 9 months of percutaneous revascularization. (Level of evidence: C) (Display 20-1).

Recommendations for Coronary Angiography in Patients During the Initial Management of Acute Myocardial Infarction: ACC/AHA/Society for Cardiovascular Angiography and Interventions (SCAI) Practice Guidelines[11]

Class I indications:

1. Coronary angiography and primary PCI should be performed in patients with STEMI or myocardial infarction (MI) with new or presumably new left bundle-branch block who can undergo PCI of the infarct artery within 12 hours of symptom onset. (Level of evidence: A)
2. Patients younger than 75 years with ST elevation or presumably new left bundle-branch block who develop shock within 36 hours of MI and are suitable for revascularization that can be performed within 18 hours of shock. (Level of evidence: A)
3. Patients with severe congestive heart failure and/or pulmonary edema and onset of symptoms within 12 hours. (Level of evidence: B)

Recommendations for Patients After Fibrinolytic Therapy: ACC/AHA Practice Guidelines[12]

Class I indications:

1. A strategy of coronary angiography with intent to perform PCI (or emergency coronary artery bypass graft surgery) is recommended for patients who have received fibrinolytic therapy and have any of the following:
   a. Cardiogenic shock in patients younger than 75 years who are suitable candidates for revascularization. (Level of evidence: B)
   b. Severe congestive HF and/or pulmonary edema. (Level of evidence: B)
   c. Hemodynamically compromising ventricular arrhythmias. (Level of evidence: C)

Care of patients with STEMI is presented in Chapter 22.

Table 20-1 ■ SHORT-TERM RISK OF DEATH OR NONFATAL MI IN PATIENTS WITH UNSTABLE ANGINA/NSTEMI*

Feature	High Risk	Intermediate Risk	Low Risk
	At least one of the following features must be present:	*No high-risk feature, but must have one of the following:*	*No high- or intermediate-risk feature but may have any of the following features:*
History	Accelerating tempo of ischemic symptoms in preceding 48 hours	Prior MI, peripheral or cerebrovascular disease, or CABG; prior aspirin use	
Character of pain	Prolonged ongoing (more than 20 minutes) rest pain	Prolonged (more than 20 minutes) rest angina, now resolved, with moderate or high likelihood of CAD Rest angina (more than 20 minutes) or relieved with rest or sublingual NTG Nocturnal angina New-onset or progressive CCS class III or IV angina in the past 2 weeks without prolonged (more than 20 minutes) rest pain but with intermediate or high likelihood of CAD	Increased angina frequency, severity, or duration Angina provoked at a lower threshold New onset angina with onset 2 weeks to 2 months prior to presentation
Clinical findings	Pulmonary edema, most likely due to ischemia New or worsening MR murmur S_3 or new/worsening crackles Hypotension, bradycardia, tachycardia Age greater than 75 years	Age greater than 70 years	
ECG	Angina at rest with transient ST-segment changes greater than 0.5 mm Bundle-branch block, new or presumed new Sustained ventricular tachycardia	T-wave changes Pathological Q waves or resting ST-depression less than 1 mm in multiple lead groups (anterior, inferior, lateral)	Normal or unchanged ECG
Cardiac markers	Elevated cardiac TnT, TnI, or CK-MB (e.g., TnT or TnI >0.1 ng/mL)	Slightly elevated cardiac TnT, TnI, or CK-MB (e.g., TnT >0.01 but <0.1 ng/mL)	Normal

*Estimation of the short-term risks of death and nonfatal cardiac ischemic events in UA (or NSTEMI) is a complex multivariable problem that cannot be fully specified in a table such as this; therefore, this table is meant to offer general guidance and illustration rather than rigid algorithms.

CABG, coronary artery bypass graft surgery; CCS, Canadian Cardiovascular Society; CK-MB, creatine kinase MB fraction; MR, mitral regurgitation; NTG, nitroglycerin; TnI, troponin I; TnT, troponin T.

Anderson, J. L., Adams, C. D., Antman, E. M., et al. (2007). ACC/AHA 2007 guidelines for the management of patients with unstable angina/NSTEMI. *Journal of American College of Cardiology, 50,* 1–157.

Adapted from AHCPR Clinical Practice Guidelines No. 10, Unstable Angina: Diagnosis and Management, May 1994 (124).

CONTRAINDICATIONS FOR CARDIAC CATHETERIZATION

Cardiac catheterization has relatively few contraindications. Any correctable illness or condition that, if corrected, would improve the safety of the procedure should be managed before catheterization. These conditions include uncontrolled ventricular irritability, uncorrected hypokalemia or digitalis toxicity, decompensated HF, and severe renal insufficiency or anuria unless dialysis is planned after the procedure. Preexisting renal insufficiency, particularly in patients with diabetes, and patients with prior anaphylactic reaction to contrast medium require special treatment before the procedure. Other relative contraindications are recent stroke (within 1 month); active gastrointestinal bleeding; active infection; severe, uncontrolled hypertension; and the patient's refusal of the therapeutic procedures to be directed by the catheterization results.[13]

Anticoagulation is a relative contraindication. Routinely, oral anticoagulants should be withheld for 48 to 72 hours before catheterization to achieve an international normalized ratio below 2.0. In patients who must remain on anticoagulants, such as patients with prosthetic heart valves or hypercoagulable states, bridging therapy with heparin is used while prothrombin time is reversed or allowed to return to normal. Immediate reversal of prothrombin time can be facilitated by fresh frozen plasma and vitamin K administration.[14]

PATIENT PREPARATION

Patients suspected of having an acute coronary syndrome would have a cardiac catheterization performed during their hospitalization. Elective cases are usually admitted for cardiac catheterization the day of the procedure. The physician performing the catheterization explains the procedure and obtains informed consent before procedure admission.

Precatheterization orders usually include the following:

1. Standard 12-lead electrocardiogram (ECG).
2. Laboratory tests: complete blood count including platelets and differential, electrolytes, blood urea nitrogen (BUN), and creatinine.

3. Nothing by mouth after midnight (or after a light breakfast if catheterization is to be in the afternoon).
4. Premedication with a mild sedative may be given. During the procedure, a procedural sedation protocol should be followed.
5. Patients with renal insufficiency should be adequately hydrated before and after the procedure and a minimum amount of radiographic low-osmolar contrast medium should be used. The combination of *N*-acetylcysteine and sodium bicarbonate infusion before and after contrast infusion has shown to reduce the risk of contrast induced nephropathy in patients with renal insufficiency.[15]
6. Patients with a history of allergy to previous contrast administration, asthma, or drug or food allergies with iodine-containing substances should receive low-osmolar contrast medium and pretreatment with steroids, antihistamine (diphenhydramine), and an H_2 blocker (cimetidine or ranitidine) are also sometimes used.[16]
7. Patients who are fasting should take a reduced dose of insulin or hold dose as directed by physician. Oral diabetic agents are usually held the morning of the procedure. Metformin is held the day of the procedure and 48 hours after the catheterization.
8. Anticoagulation issues are directed by the physician. Acetylsalicylic acid (ASA) and antiplatelet medications are usually given before catheterization. Warfarin is generally discontinued 3 to 4 days before the procedure until the international normalized ratio is <2.0. Warfarin can be reversed with vitamin K or fresh frozen plasma. If the patient is receiving heparin therapy, heparin can be continued during the catheterization and discontinued for sheath removal.
9. Patient to void before going to catheterization laboratory.
10. There is no evidence-based data to support the prophylactic use of antibiotics.
11. Patients who wear dentures, glasses, or hearing aids should be sent to the laboratory wearing them. The patient is better able to communicate when dentures and hearing aids are in place. Glasses allow the patient to view the angiogram on the monitor and help keep the patient oriented to the surroundings.

Nursing Assessment and Patient Teaching

Nursing assessment and teaching are important parts of patient preparation. The nursing assessment includes the patient's heart rate and rhythm, blood pressure, evaluation of the peripheral pulses of the arms and legs, and assessment of heart and lung sounds. The sites for best palpation of the patient's dorsalis pedis and posterior tibial pulses are marked on the skin. This information will be used for comparison in evaluating peripheral pulses after the catheterization procedure. A procedural sedation assessment is performed, including assessment of the patient's cardiovascular, respiratory, and renal systems. Care is taken to identify characteristics or conditions that may cause the patient to be at greater risk for complications associated with procedural sedation, such as a history of difficult intubation; history of difficulty with sedation; morbid obesity; sleep apnea; extremes of age; severe cardiac, respiratory, renal, hepatic, or central nervous system disease; and history of substance abuse.[17] The nursing assessment also includes an evaluation of the patient's emotional status and attitude toward catheterization.

1. Is this the patient's first cardiac catheterization?
2. What are the patient's apprehensions about the procedure?
3. What has the patient heard about cardiac catheterization? (Patients have sometimes heard "horror stories" from friends or acquaintances about catheterization experiences and may, therefore, need reassurance about the safety of the procedure.)
4. What decisions are being faced? (Patients may be facing good or bad news about the absence or presence and extent of disease. Thus, the period before catheterization most likely is a time of anxiety and fear for a variety of reasons. Discussion and reassurance may help to relieve some of these feelings.)

The catheterization laboratory confronts the patient with new sights, sounds, and experiences that may be intimidating and frightening. Teaching is aimed at preparing the patient for this experience and should begin in the physician's office. In some institutions, patients are given a video to view before the procedure. A printed booklet to which the patient can refer is also helpful. The following points should be covered in patient teaching:

1. The patient is given nothing by mouth for 6 to 8 hours before the catheterization and is asked to void before arriving at the catheterization laboratory.
2. Medication is given before or during the procedure, if prescribed, but the patient is awake during the procedure.
3. The patient should be instructed in deep breathing, how to stop a breath without bearing down, and in coughing on request. With deep inspiration, the diaphragm descends, preventing it from obstructing the view of the coronary arteries in some radiographic projections. Bearing down (Valsalva maneuver) increases intra-abdominal pressure and may raise the diaphragm, obstructing the view. After the injection of contrast medium, coughing is requested to help clear the material from the coronary arteries. The rapid movement of the diaphragm also acts as a mechanical stimulant to the heart and helps prevent the bradycardia that may accompany the injection of contrast medium.[18,19]
4. The appearance of the laboratory should be explained to the patient, including the general function of the equipment.
5. The patient wears a gown to the laboratory.
6. The patient lies on a table that is hard and narrow.
7. The catheter insertion site is washed with an antibacterial scrub and hair is removed using a shaver. Usually, both groins are prepped to provide easy access to the other side for patients with peripheral vascular disease and obstructive disease preventing catheter advancement or sudden instability during the procedure requiring an intra-aortic balloon pump (IABP). The right groin is generally used because the operator standing on that side of the table has easier access.
8. The expected length of the procedure should be explained to the patient (approximately 1 hour for coronary angiogram and 2 hours with PCI). Complex procedures will be longer.
9. The patient is given a local anesthetic at the catheter entry site.
10. The patient may have warm sensation or experience nausea during injection of the coronary arteries with contrast medium, most commonly occurring with the injection of the ventricle during ventriculogram.

11. The patient should report angina, shortness of breath (SOB), and other symptoms to the staff.
12. The patient should be told the expected length of bed rest after the catheterization.

Outpatient Cardiac Catheterization

Improvements in cardiac procedures and decline in risk associated with diagnostic cardiac catheterizations have increased the number of outpatient procedures. Advantages include decreased costs and avoidance of an unnecessary overnight hospital stay. Patients considered for outpatient cardiac catheterization are those with stable coronary symptoms. Patients in whom the outpatient procedure is contraindicated include those with ACS (UA, NSTEMI, or STEMI); uncompensated HF; severe aortic stenosis; suspected left main coronary disease; known bleeding disorders; and metabolically unstable patients.

Patients needing preadmission to the hospital for cardiac catheterization include those who require continuous anticoagulation or who have significant renal insufficiency or brittle diabetes mellitus. Noninvasive testing may identify patients with high-risk coronary or valvular disease before catheterization. Additional considerations include the distance the patient lives from the hospital and the availability of someone to drive the patient home.[1] Freestanding cardiac catheterization laboratories that are not physically attached to a hospital facility are available and are used for diagnostic studies. It is the responsibility of each freestanding laboratory to have a formal relationship with a referral hospital for emergency services. Patients studied at freestanding laboratories require thorough screening. High-risk patients must be excluded to avoid complications that require emergency services.[1]

Preprocedure teaching is best done before hospital admission. The content is similar to that for patients undergoing an inpatient procedure. Patients who have significant CAD or left main coronary disease or complications during the procedure are usually admitted to the hospital for overnight observation (Display 20-2).

After a diagnostic procedure, the patient spends 2 to 6 hours in a short-stay unit, ambulatory recovery, or similar setting. Postprocedure orders are the same for inpatient and outpatient cardiac catheterization. After the required period of bed rest, postural blood pressure and heart rate are obtained and the patient is observed for 30 to 60 minutes while sitting, standing, and walking. During this time, discharge instructions are reviewed. The patient is then allowed to leave. Results of the catheterization are reviewed with the patient and/or family after the procedure by the cardiologist or before discharge. Patients who have had PCI routinely stay overnight for observation and monitoring and are discharged the following morning.

DISPLAY 20-2 General Exclusion Criteria for Early (<2–6 Hour) Discharge After Invasive Cardiac Procedure in Adults

- High risk due to identification of left main disease
- New York Heart Association class III or IV HF
- Unstable ischemic symptoms at any time after the procedure
- Recent MI with postinfarction ischemia
- Pulmonary edema thought to be caused by ischemia
- Severe aortic stenosis with LV dysfunction
- Severe aortic insufficiency with a pulse pressure >80 mm Hg
- Poorly controlled systemic hypertension
- Inadequate or unreliable follow-up over the next 24 hours
- Generalized debility or dementia
- Renal insufficiency (creatinine >1.8 mg/dL)
- Need for continuous anticoagulation therapy or treatment of a bleeding diathesis
- Large hematoma or vascular complication

Adapted from Bashore, T. M., Bates, E. R., Berger, P. B., et al. (2001). American College of Cardiology/Society for Cardiac Angiography and Interventions Clinical Expert Consensus Document on cardiac catheterization laboratory standards: A report of the American College of Cardiology Task Force on Clinical Expert Consensus Documents (ACC/SCA&I Committee to Develop an Expert Consensus Document on Cardiac Catheterization Laboratory Standards). *Journal of the American College of Cardiology, 37,* 2170–2214.

PROCEDURE

Cardiac Catheterization Laboratory

The cardiac catheterization laboratory is a specially equipped radiologic laboratory for the study of children and adults with known or suspected heart disease. The primary technical focus is the generation, recording, and display of high-quality x-ray images during diagnostic and interventional procedures. The ongoing trend toward more complex interventional procedures results in greater exposure to radiation for the patient and laboratory staff. This radiation exposure is monitored for safety.[1]

The technique of imaging has moved away from cineangiographic to digital images in most laboratories. The laboratory usually has the following equipment:

1. A patient support table, adjustable height, flat top whose locks can be released to allow the table top to move horizontally head-to-toe and side-to-side for "panning."
2. Equipment for monitoring intracardiac pressures, CO determination, and physiologic recordings.
3. A suspended C-arm that rotates around the patient and allows variable angulations of the x-ray beam.
4. The image chain consists of a generator and cine pulse system, an x-ray tube, an image intensifier, an optical distributor, a 35-mm cine camera, and a television camera and monitor. The image chain produces fluoroscopy, which is the continuous presentation of an x-ray image on a fluorescent screen, allowing the viewing of structures in motion. The image intensifier receives the fluoroscopic image and increases its brightness, permitting filming (cinefluoroscopy) or digital acquisition of motion pictures and viewing of the image with a television camera, television screen, and videotape recorder. Although 35-mm film was originally used for recording, since 1998 all new images are permanently recorded digitally.
5. Single or biplane imaging system can be used. Biplane imaging provides simultaneous viewing of cardiac structures from two angles, which is helpful for congenital heart disease, transseptal punctures, and electrophysiology ablations.
6. Advanced cardiac life support drugs and equipment with a cardioverter–defibrillator available for emergency treatment.
7. Monitoring electrocardiographic activity with continuous ECG monitor display.

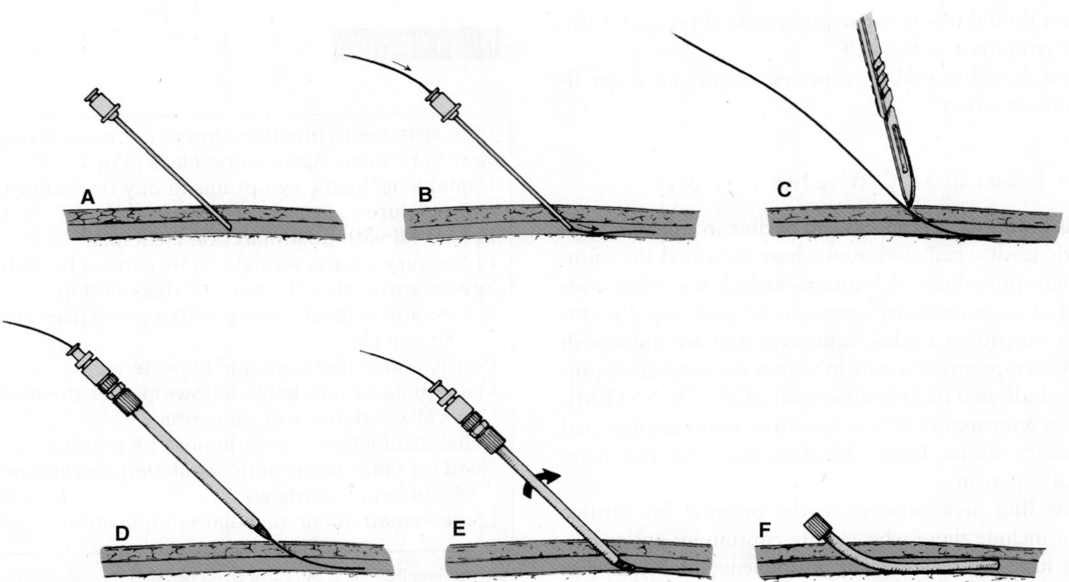

■ **Figure 20-1** Modified Seldinger technique for percutaneous catheter sheath introduction. (A) Vessel is punctured by needle. (B) Flexible guidewire placed in vessel through needle. (C) Needle removed, guidewire left in place, and hole in skin around wire enlarged with scalpel. (D) Sheath and dilator placed over guidewire. (E) Sheath and dilator advanced over guidewire and into vessel. (F) Dilator and guidewire removed while sheath remains in vessel. (From Hill, J. A., Lambert, C. R., Vuestra, R. E., et al. [1998]. Review of techniques. In J. C. Pepine, J. A. Hill, & C. R. Lambert [Eds.], *Diagnostic and therapeutic cardiac catheterization* [3rd ed., p. 107]. Baltimore: Williams & Wilkins.)

8. A standby pacemaker, either a temporary transvenous electrode and pulse generator system or an external transthoracic pacemaker.
9. IABP.

Catheterization Approach

Percutaneous Catheterization

Percutaneous catheterization is accomplished using the modified technique initially described by Seldinger (Fig. 20-1).[5] The same technique is used for both arterial and venous entry. Using the modified Seldinger technique, the vessel is located and a local anesthetic is used to numb the puncture area. The percutaneous needle, with fluid-filled syringe attached, is inserted through the skin nearly parallel to the vessel and enters the front wall of the vessel. Entry of the needle into the vessel is verified by blood return into the syringe with aspiration. The syringe is removed, and a guidewire is passed through the needle into the vessel. The needle is then removed, and a nick is made in the skin with a no. 11 blade to create a hole large enough for a hemostatic introducer sheath to be advanced over the guidewire and placed within the vessel. Catheters are exchanged by inserting a guidewire into the catheter and inserting the catheter with the guidewire through the introducer sheath, into the vessel. A guidewire of length 4 to 6 cm is advanced past the distal end of the catheter so the wire leads as the catheter and wire are advanced to the aortic arch. The guidewire is removed from the catheter completely before catheter placement.

The femoral approach is the preferred site for catheterization. Location of the femoral stick is important to avoid vascular complications. The ideal puncture site should be in the common femoral artery (Fig. 20-2B). Puncture of the artery at or above the inguinal ligament makes catheter advancement difficult and predisposes to inadequate compression, hematoma formation, and retroperitoneal bleeding. Puncture of the artery more than 3 cm below the inguinal ligament increases the chance that the femoral artery will divide into its profunda and superficial branches. Puncture into these branches can cause development of a pseudoaneurysm or thrombotic occlusion of a small vessel.[20]

Alternative arterial puncture sites include the brachial and radial arteries (Fig. 20-2A). The brachial artery may be used in cases of known vascular disease of the abdominal aorta or iliac or femoral arteries. Before using the radial artery, an Allen test is performed to verify patency of the ulnar artery to ensure circulation to the hand. The small caliber of the radial artery mandates the use of small catheters. Injection of lidocaine, nitroglycerin, or calcium channel blocker through the sheath arm is usually necessary to control local spasm in the radial artery. Use of the radial or brachial approach allows for easier control of bleeding at the access site, eliminates the need for bed rest after the procedure, and facilitates earlier discharge of outpatients. Radial artery thrombosis is a potential complication of this approach.

Direct Brachial Approach

The direct brachial approach is rarely used. It requires a cutdown in the antecubital fossa to isolate the brachial artery and vein. A cardiologist trained in brachial cutdown and vascular repair of the artery and vein is required for this procedure. An incision is made over the medial vein for right heart catheterization or over both the vein and the brachial artery if right and left heart catheterization is planned. The vein and artery are approached by blunt dissection and are brought to the surface and tagged with surgical tape. Venotomy and arteriotomy are performed using scissors or a scalpel. The distal segment of the artery is flushed with heparinized saline to prevent clotting from distal arterial stasis. The catheterization is performed. After catheterization, the distal brachial artery is aspirated until a forceful backflow is achieved,

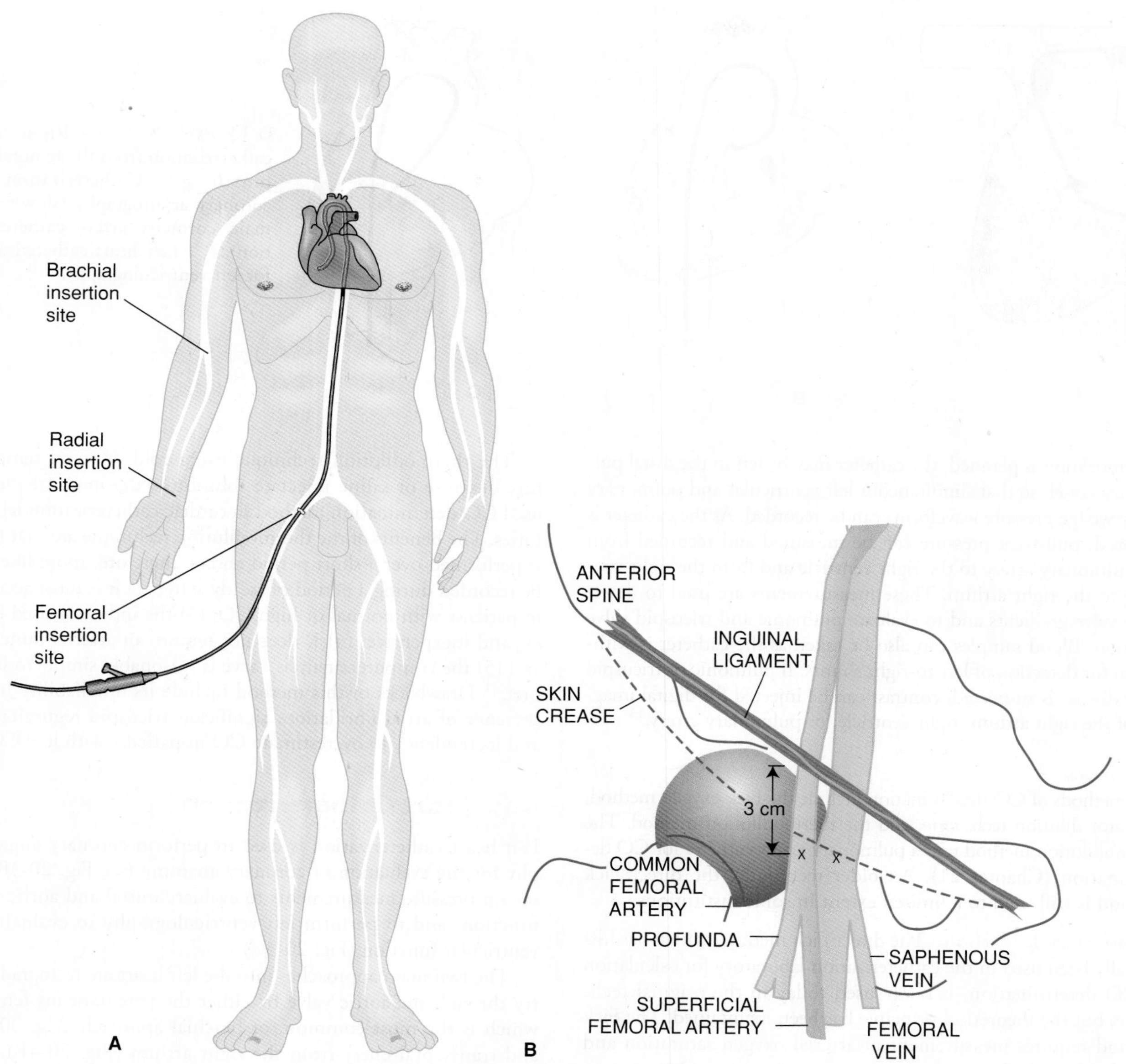

■ **Figure 20-2** (A) Commonly used catheterization sites. The femoral approach is preferred, and the catheter is advanced in a retrograde direction up the aorta, around the aortic arch, and then into the ostia of the coronary arteries or across the aortic valve into the left ventricle. (B) Schematic diagram showing the right femoral artery and vein coursing underneath the inguinal ligament. The arterial skin nick (indicated by X) should be placed approximately 3 cm below the ligament and directly over the femoral arterial pulsation. The venous skin nick should be placed at the same level but approximately one fingerbreadth more medial. (*B* from Baim, D. S., & Simon, D. I. [2006]. Percutaneous approach, including transseptal and apical puncture. In D. S. Baim & W. Grossman [Eds.], *Grossman's cardiac catheterization, angiography, and intervention* [7th ed., p. 81]. Philadelphia: Lippincott Williams & Wilkins.)

and heparinized saline is injected. The arterial incision is then sutured. The patient may sit up in chair or bed after the procedure with arm held straight on an arm board. Distal pulses, sensation, and motor function are checked every 15 minutes for 2 hours.

Right Heart Catheterization

Right heart catheterization (Fig. 20-3A) is used to obtain right heart pressures, to evaluate the pulmonic and tricuspid valves, to sample blood oxygen content of right heart chambers for detection of left-to-right shunt, to determine CO, and to evaluate mitral valve stenosis or mitral valve insufficiency by the transseptal approach.

The right heart can be approached through the femoral, internal jugular or subclavian veins. Once the inferior vena cava or superior vena cava is reached, the catheter is advanced through the right atrium, right ventricle, and pulmonary artery to a distal pulmonary vessel. Right ventricular irritability may be noted when the catheter tip passes through the right ventricle. The course of the catheter is followed with pressure monitoring through the catheter and with fluoroscopy. When indicated, blood samples are taken, and pressures are recorded as the catheter is advanced. If left heart

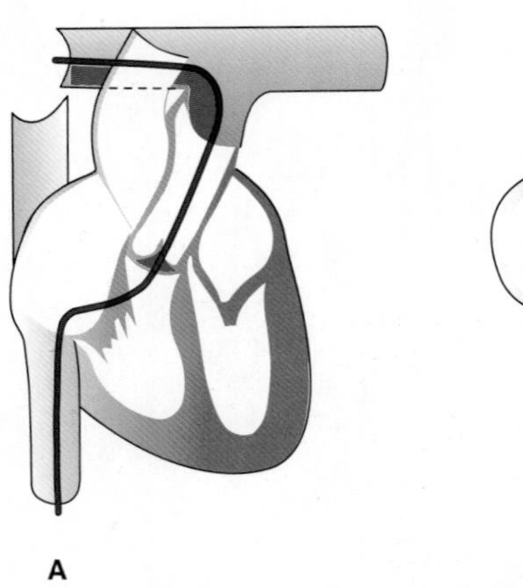

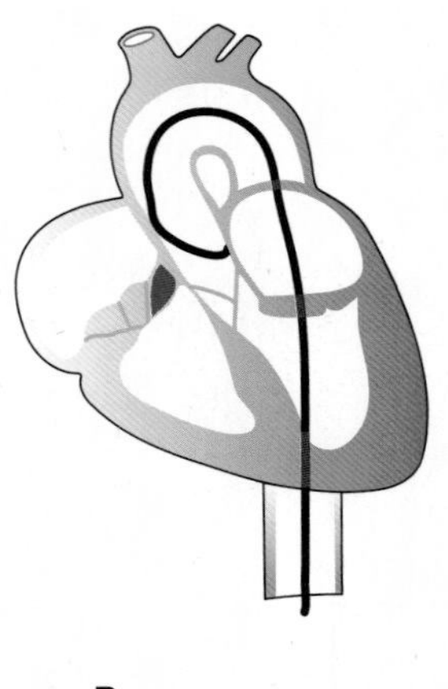

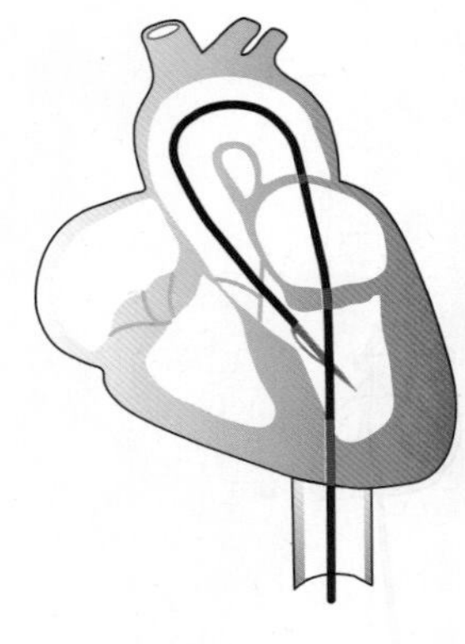

■ **Figure 20-3** (A) Right heart catheterization from the femoral approach. (B) Catheterization for coronary arteriography (shown: left main coronary artery catheterization). (C) Left heart catheterization for left ventriculography.

catheterization is planned, the catheter may be left in the distal pulmonary vessel, so that simultaneous left ventricular and pulmonary artery wedge pressure waveforms can be recorded. As the catheter is removed, pull-back pressure can be measured and recorded from the pulmonary artery to the right ventricle and from the right ventricle to the right atrium. These measurements are used to determine valve gradients and to evaluate pulmonic and tricuspid valve function. Blood samples can also be taken as the catheter is withdrawn for detection of left-to-right shunts. If pulmonic or tricuspid valve disease is suspected, contrast can be injected for digital imaging of the right atrium, right ventricle, or pulmonary artery.[13]

CO Studies

The methods of CO determination include the Fick oxygen method, indicator dilution technique, and the thermodilution method. The thermodilution method uses a pulmonary artery catheter for CO determination (Chapter 21). An older technique, the direct Fick method is still used to a limited extent in some institutions.

Direct Fick Method. The direct Fick method, which has historically been used in the catheterization laboratory for calculation of CO determination, is rarely used today in the original technique, but the theoretical principle has been maintained. The Fick method requires measurement of arterial oxygen saturation and mixed venous (pulmonary artery) oxygen saturation. Oxygen consumption ideally is a measured value obtained during catheterization. The methods of measuring oxygen consumption are extremely cumbersome and time consuming and, in general, not routinely employed in modern catheterization laboratories. Alternatively, oxygen consumption can be assumed on the basis of the patient's body surface area. This is not as accurate a measurement, but it is acceptable. The Fick method of CO determination is helpful in cases where the patient is in atrial fibrillation, has significant tricuspid regurgitation, or a low CO state. It has largely been replaced by the thermodilution method for CO determination.

Thermodilution and Indicator Dilution Methods. Thermodilution and indicator dilution methods are based on the principle that if a known amount of an indicator is added to an unknown quantity of flowing liquid and the concentration of the indicator is then measured downstream, the time course of its concentration gives a quantitative index of the flow. Applied to the circulatory system, the amount of indicator, its dilution within the circulation, and the time during which the first circulation of the substance occurs can be used to compute CO.[21]

The thermodilution technique using cold or room temperature dextrose or saline injectate solution is the most frequently used CO determination method in cardiac catheterization laboratories. The benefits of the thermodilution technique are that (1) it is performed over a short period and is, therefore, more likely to be recorded during a period of steady state; (2) it is most accurate in patients with normal or high CO; (3) the indicator used is inert and inexpensive; (4) it does not require an arterial puncture; and (5) the computer analysis curve is reasonably simple to interpret.[21] Drawbacks of this method include its unreliability in the presence of atrial fibrillation, significant tricuspid regurgitation, and its tendency to overestimate CO in patients with low CO.

Left Heart Catheterization

Left heart catheterization is used to perform coronary angiography for the evaluation of coronary anatomy (see Fig. 20-3B), to obtain pressure measurements to evaluate mitral and aortic valve function, and to perform left ventriculography to evaluate left ventricular function (Fig. 20-3C).

The two main approaches into the left heart are retrograde entry through the aortic valve by either the percutaneous femoral, which is the most common, or brachial approach (Fig. 20-3C) and transseptal entry from the right atrium (Fig. 20-4B). The progress of the catheter in both approaches is followed by fluoroscopy and pressure measurement. In the retrograde approach, the catheter is threaded along the aorta and across the aortic valve to the left ventricle. For mitral valve studies, simultaneous pulmonary artery wedge and left ventricular pressures or simultaneous left atrial and left ventricular pressures are recorded to evaluate pressure differences across the valve. To evaluate aortic valve function, pull-back pressure is recorded as the catheter is withdrawn from the left ventricle to the aorta. Digital imaging may be performed during contrast injection of the left atrium, left ventricle, or aortic root to evaluate valve function further.

Transseptal Left Heart Catheterization

The transseptal approach to left heart catheterization involves crossing from the right atrium to the left atrium through the fossa ovalis (Fig. 20-4B). This technique is infrequently done for diagnostic catheterizations but can be used in the rare situation when retrograde left heart catheterization is not possible due to severe aortic stenosis or a prosthetic valve that cannot be adequately evaluated by echocardiogram or transesophageal echocardiography.

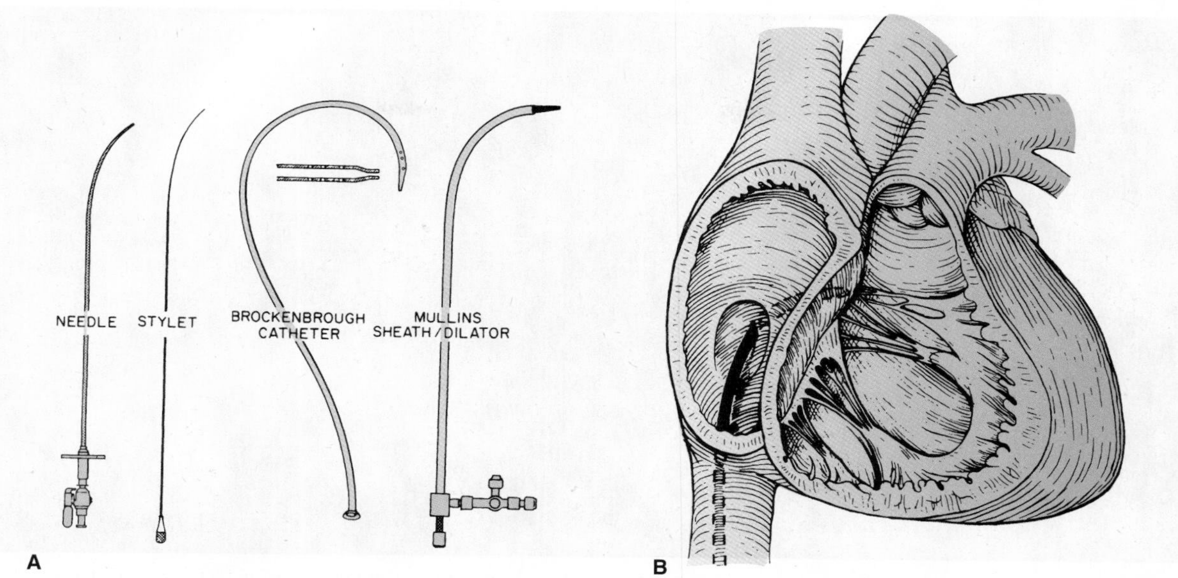

Figure 20-4 Transseptal catheterization. (A) Equipment for transseptal puncture. From left to right: the Brockenbrough needle, Bing stylet, Brockenbrough catheter, Mullins sheath/dilator system. (B) Front of right atrium and ventricle cut away to show the catheter entering the right atrium via the inferior vena cava and crossing the septum into the left atrium. (*A* from Baim, D. S., & Simon, D. I. [2006]. Percutaneous approach, including transseptal and apical puncture. In D. S. Baim & W. Grossman [Eds.], *Grossman's cardiac catheterization, angiography, and intervention* [7th ed., p. 102]. Philadelphia: Lippincott Williams & Wilkins. *B* from Hill, J. A., Lambert, C. R., Vuestra, R. E., et al. [1998]. Review of techniques. In J. C. Pepine, J. A. Hill, & C. R. Lambert [Eds.], *Diagnostic and therapeutic cardiac catheterization* [3rd ed., p. 116]. Baltimore: Williams & Wilkins.)

More common uses of the transseptal approach include mitral valvuloplasty, electrophysiology studies requiring access to the left atrium or left ventricle, and transcatheter closure of patent foramen ovale or atrial septal defects.

Transseptal catheterization is done only through the right femoral vein and inferior vena cava, using percutaneous techniques and the needle and catheter described by Brockenbrough and Braunwald.[22] The transseptal catheter is threaded into the right atrium over a guidewire, which is then removed. The transseptal needle, with a blunt stylet extending beyond its tip to prevent the needle from puncturing the catheter (Fig. 20-4A), is threaded up the catheter, the stylet is withdrawn, and the needle is connected to a pressure transducer. The catheter and needle are guided together to the fossa ovalis, where the needle is advanced to perforate the atrial septum. After perforation of the septum, left atrial pressure is recorded and a blood sample is drawn to confirm the catheter location. The catheter and needle are advanced well into the left atrium, the needle is withdrawn, and the desired studies are performed. The catheter may also be advanced to enter the left ventricle.

Transseptal puncture of the fossa ovalis is safe, but the danger in this approach is that the needle or catheter will inadvertently puncture an adjacent structure such as the posterior free wall of the right atrium, the coronary sinus, or the aortic root causing myocardial hemorrhage, tamponade, or death. The risk is higher in patients who are taking anticoagulants. If the patient is not taking anticoagulants and the perforation is limited to the needle puncture, it is usually benign. However, if the catheter is advanced into the pericardium or aortic root, potentially fatal complications can occur. To minimize risk, the operator must have a detailed familiarity of the regional anatomy of the atrial septum, which can be distorted in aortic and mitral valve disease. When location of the necessary anatomic landmarks is impossible, as in patients who have severe chest deformities, abnormal heart position, a huge right atrium, or in those who cannot lie flat, the transseptal approach is not recommended.[23]

Ventriculography

Ventriculography is performed to evaluate valve structure or function, to define ventricular anatomy, and to evaluate ventricular function. Ventriculography is accomplished by opacifying the ventricular cavity with contrast medium and filming ventricular motion (Fig. 20-5). Digital image acquisition by biplane or single-plane left ventriculography provides information on the location and severity of segmental wall motion abnormalities. The ventriculogram may be performed before the coronary arteriogram because intracoronary contrast medium may have a depressant effect on ventricular function. In very sick patients, coronary angiography may be performed first because it is usually better tolerated than ventriculogram.

The catheter used for contrast injection during ventriculography delivers a large amount of contrast medium (30 to 36 mL) in a short period (10 to 12 mL/s). Many types of catheters are available for ventricular injections (Fig. 20-6). Catheters with side holes, with or without an end hole, are preferred to end-hole catheters because they have less tendency to recoil. Catheter stability is also important to minimize the risk of ventricular arrhythmias during injection. Arrhythmias change the quality of contraction and, thus, make it impossible to use ventriculography for studies of ventricular function.[24]

Contrast injection is accomplished by power injection. Before the power injection is performed, it is important to verify that the

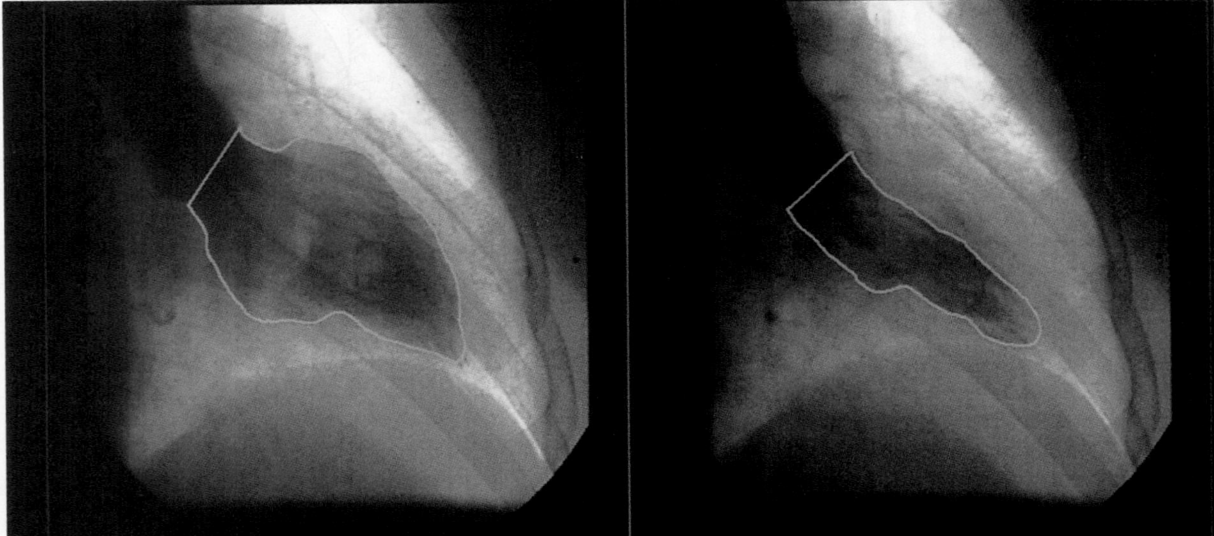

■ **Figure 20-5** Left ventriculogram. Two frames in right anterior oblique (RAO) projection showing the left ventricle in diastole *(left)* and in systole *(right)*. (Courtesy of Swedish Medical Center, Seattle, Washington.)

injection syringe is free of air to prevent air embolism. A low-pressure injection is done to ensure proper catheter placement, then the power injection is done. Patients often feel a hot flash for 30 seconds after injection, resulting from the vasodilatation caused by the contrast agent throughout the arterial system. Occasionally, the patient may experience nausea with the injection, or may vomit. The principal complications of injection are arrhythmias, intramyocardial or endocardial injection of contrast medium, transient left anterior fascicular block, and embolism from injection of air or thrombi.[24]

Coronary Arteriography

Coronary arteriography is performed most commonly by the percutaneous femoral approach. Preformed polyurethane catheters (most commonly Judkins or Amplatz catheters) are used for

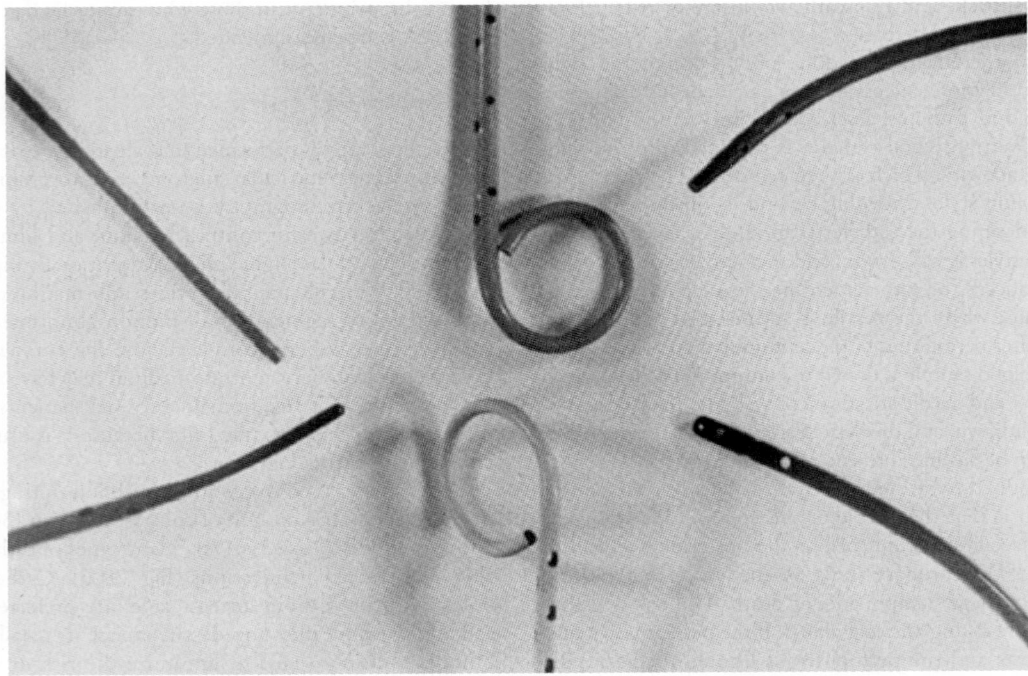

■ **Figure 20-6** Examples of ventriculographic catheters in current use (clockwise from the top): pigtail 8 French (F) (Cook); Gensini 7F; NIH 8F; pigtail 8F (Cordis); Lehman ventriculographic 8F; Sones 7.5F tapering to a 5.5F tip. (From Baim, D. S., & Hill, L. D. [2006]. Cardiac ventriculography. In D. S. Baim & W. Grossman [Eds.], *Grossman's cardiac catheterization, angiography, and intervention* [7th ed., p. 223]. Philadelphia: Lippincott Williams & Wilkins.)

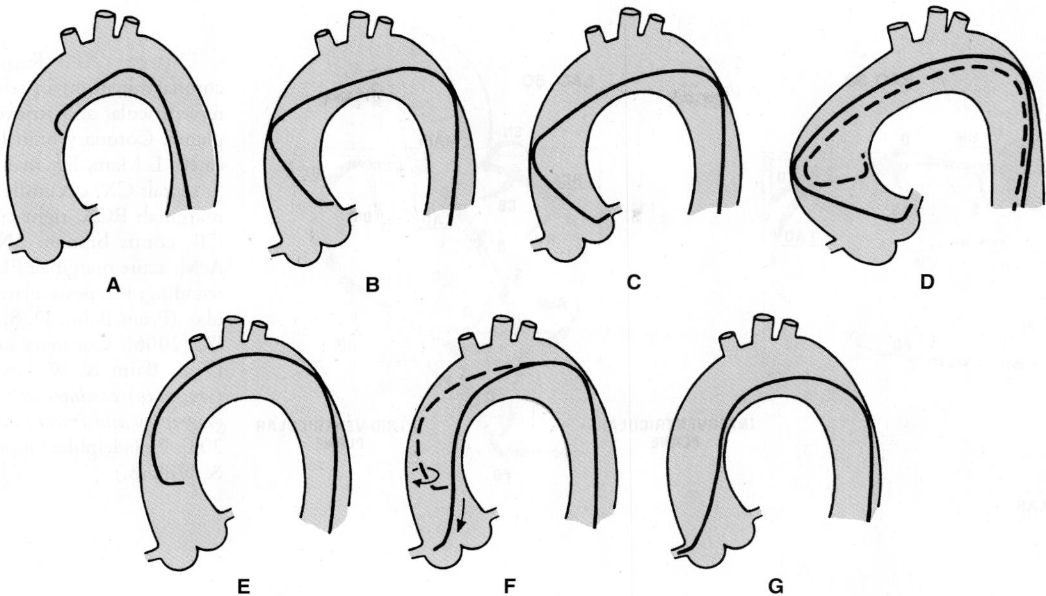

■ **Figure 20-7** Judkins technique for catheterization of the left and right coronary arteries as viewed in the left anterior oblique (LAO) projection. In a patient with a normal size aortic arch, advancement of a JL4 catheter leads to intubation of the left coronary ostium **(A, B,** *and* **C)**. In a patient with an enlarged aortic root **(D)** the arm of the JL4 may be too short, causing the catheter tip to point upward or even flip back into its packaged shape (*dotted line*). A catheter with an appropriately longer arm (a JL5 or JL6) is required. To catheterize the right coronary ostium, the Judkins catheter is advanced around the aortic arch with its tip directed leftward, as viewed in the LAO projection, until it reaches a position 2–3 cm above the level of the left coronary ostium **(E)**. Clockwise rotation causes the catheter tip to drop into the aortic root and point anteriorly **(F)**. Slight further rotation causes the catheter tip to enter the right coronary ostium **(G)**. (From Baim, D. S., & Grossman, W. [2006]. Coronary angiography. In D. S. Baim & W. Grossman [Eds.], *Grossman's cardiac catheterization, angiography, and intervention* [7th ed., p. 192]. Philadelphia: Lippincott Williams & Wilkins.)

catheterization of the right and left coronary arteries (Figs. 20-7 and 20-8).[25] The catheters are guided over a guidewire through the distal aortic arch to the coronary ostium, the guide is withdrawn, and the catheter is filled with contrast medium. Figure 20-9 shows the coronary anatomy as viewed from the right anterior oblique (RAO) and left anterior oblique (LAO) projections.

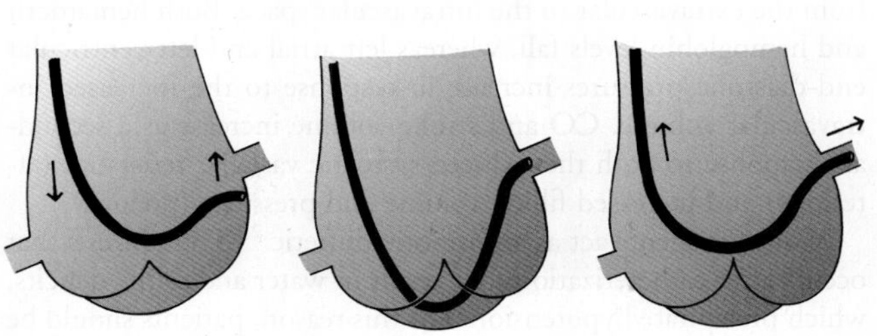

■ **Figure 20-8** Catheterization of the left coronary artery with an Amplatz catheter. The catheter is advanced into the ascending aorta with its tip pointing downward. As the catheter is advanced into the left sinus of Valsalva, its tip initially lies below the left coronary ostium *(left)*. Further advancement causes the tip to ride up the aortic wall and enter the ostium *(center)*. Subsequently, slight withdrawal of the catheter causes the tip to seat more deeply in the ostium *(right)*. (From Baim, D. S., & Grossman, W. [2006]. Coronary angiography. In D. S. Baim & W. Grossman [Eds.], *Grossman's cardiac catheterization, angiography, and intervention* [7th ed., p. 193]. Philadelphia: Lippincott Williams & Wilkins.)

Images of both the right and left coronary arteries are recorded in the LAO and RAO views to ensure that all coronary segments are seen. The image intensifier can also be angulated toward the head (cranial) or the foot (caudal) to better visualize specific lesions (Figs. 20-10 and 20-11). A common sequence of angiographic views for the left coronary artery includes:

1. RAO-caudal: to visualize the left main, proximal left anterior descending (LAD) and proximal circumflex coronary arteries
2. RAO-cranial: to visualize the middle and distal LAD without overlap of septal or diagonal branches
3. LAO-cranial: to visualize the middle and distal LAD in an orthogonal projection
4. LAO-caudal: to visualize the left main and proximal circumflex
5. Left lateral: to visualize the LAD

A common sequence of angiographic views for the right coronary includes:

1. LAO: to visualize the proximal right coronary artery
2. RAO-cranial: to visualize the posterior descending and posterolateral branches
3. Right lateral: to visualize the middle right coronary artery

The patient is asked to take a deep breath and hold it without bearing down, just before the injection, to clear the diaphragm from the field. After the injection, the patient is told to breathe and cough, which helps clear the contrast medium from the coronary arteries. Imaging of the coronary arteries may also be

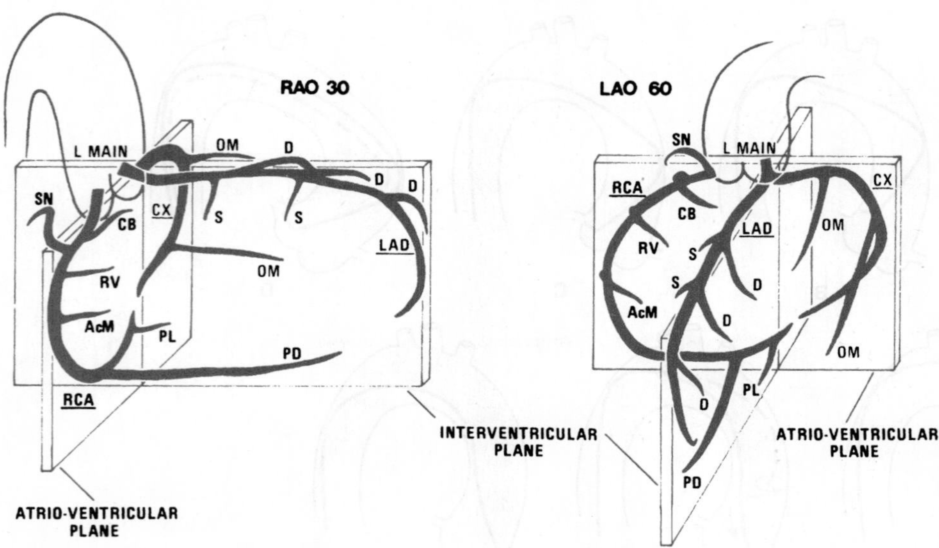

■ **Figure 20-9** Representation of coronary anatomy in relation to the interventricular and atrioventricular valve planes. Coronary branches are as indicated: L Main, left main; D, diagonal; S, septal; CX, circumflex; OM, obtuse marginal; RCA, right coronary artery; CB, conus branch; SN, sinus node; AcM, acute marginal; PD, posterior descending; PL, posterolateral left ventricular. (From Baim, D. S., & Grossman, W. [2006]. Coronary angiography. In D. S. Baim & W. Grossman [Eds.], *Grossman's cardiac catheterization, angiography, and intervention* [7th ed., p. 203]. Philadelphia: Lippincott Williams & Wilkins.)

performed after the administration of nitroglycerin or other vasodilators to evaluate possible vasospasm effects on the coronary circulation, including the collateral vessels.

Angiographic Contrast Agents

Iodinated radiocontrast agents are either ionic or nonionic and have variable osmolality. First-generation contrast agents are the high-osmolar ionic agents and have osmolalities as high as six times that of blood; second-generation agents are lower-osmolar nonionic agents that have an osmolality approximately two to three times that of blood. The newest nonionic agents are iso-osmolal and have an osmolality similar to that of blood.[26] Contrast agents contain iodine, which absorbs x-rays and, thus, provides their imaging properties. The hemodynamic and other side effects of contrast agents are related to their osmolality and their chemical and pharmacologic differences. Low-osmolal and iso-osmolal nonionic agents are associated with fewer side effects and less dramatic hemodynamic reactions than high-osmolar ionic agents, particularly in high-risk patients. Nonionic agents are more costly than ionic agents.[16,26,27]

Most catheterization laboratories use nonionic low-osmolar or iso-osmolar agents. Specific indications for use of low-osmolar agents include unstable ischemic syndromes including acute MI, HF with hemodynamic instability, diabetes mellitus, ejection fraction less than 0.30, acute or chronic renal insufficiency, severe bradycardia, and history of contrast allergy. Nonionic low-osmolar agents are also used for internal mammary artery injection to avoid central nervous system toxicity by reflux of hyperosmolar ionic contrast up the vertebral arteries, and for PCI, which requires larger amounts of contrast.[28] The newest iso-osmolal nonionic agent, iodixanol, appears to reduce the risk of contrast-induced nephropathy in high-risk patients (i.e., diabetics with renal insufficiency).[26] The hemodynamic effects of contrast agents are well documented. These effects vary with the site and volume of the injection as well as with the osmolality, sodium content, and calcium concentration of the agent used. Immediate effects (10 to 120 seconds) are seen with both ventriculography and coronary angiography, whereas long-term effects are seen primarily with ventriculography or other injections that require large amounts of contrast medium.[29]

After left ventricular injection, there is depression of left ventricular contractility, an increase in intravascular volume, and a rise in left ventricular end-diastolic pressure. As contrast reaches the systemic arterial system, there is arteriolar vasodilation; this response increases with the osmolality of the agent used. There is a corresponding decrease in arterial pressure. These effects peak within 2 to 3 minutes, and values return to normal within 5 minutes.[29]

With coronary arteriography, immediate effects of contrast may include sinus bradycardia, systemic arterial hypotension, an increase in left ventricular end-diastolic pressure, arrhythmias, myocardial ischemia, and T-wave changes on the ECG. Usually, these changes revert quickly to normal when the catheter is withdrawn from the coronary ostia and the patient coughs, clearing the contrast medium from the coronary arteries.

The high osmolarity of contrast medium raises serum osmolality. In response, plasma volume increases when water moves from the extravascular to the intravascular space. Both hematocrit and hemoglobin levels fall, whereas left atrial and left ventricular end-diastolic pressures increase in response to the increased intravascular volume. CO and stroke volume increase as a secondary response to both the reduced systemic vascular resistance (afterload) and increased filling volume and pressures (preload).

Contrast agents act as an osmotic diuretic.[29] The diuresis that occurs after catheterization may result in water and saline deficits, which precipitate hypotension. For this reason, patients should be given intravenous (IV) replacement or be encouraged to drink liquids on returning from the laboratory. Hydration is also important for patients with preexisting renal insufficiency.

QUANTITATIVE ANGIOGRAPHY

Quantitative angiography involves adjunctive imaging with IVUS and measurement of coronary physiology in the catheterization laboratory, enhancing clinical decision making. Determination of

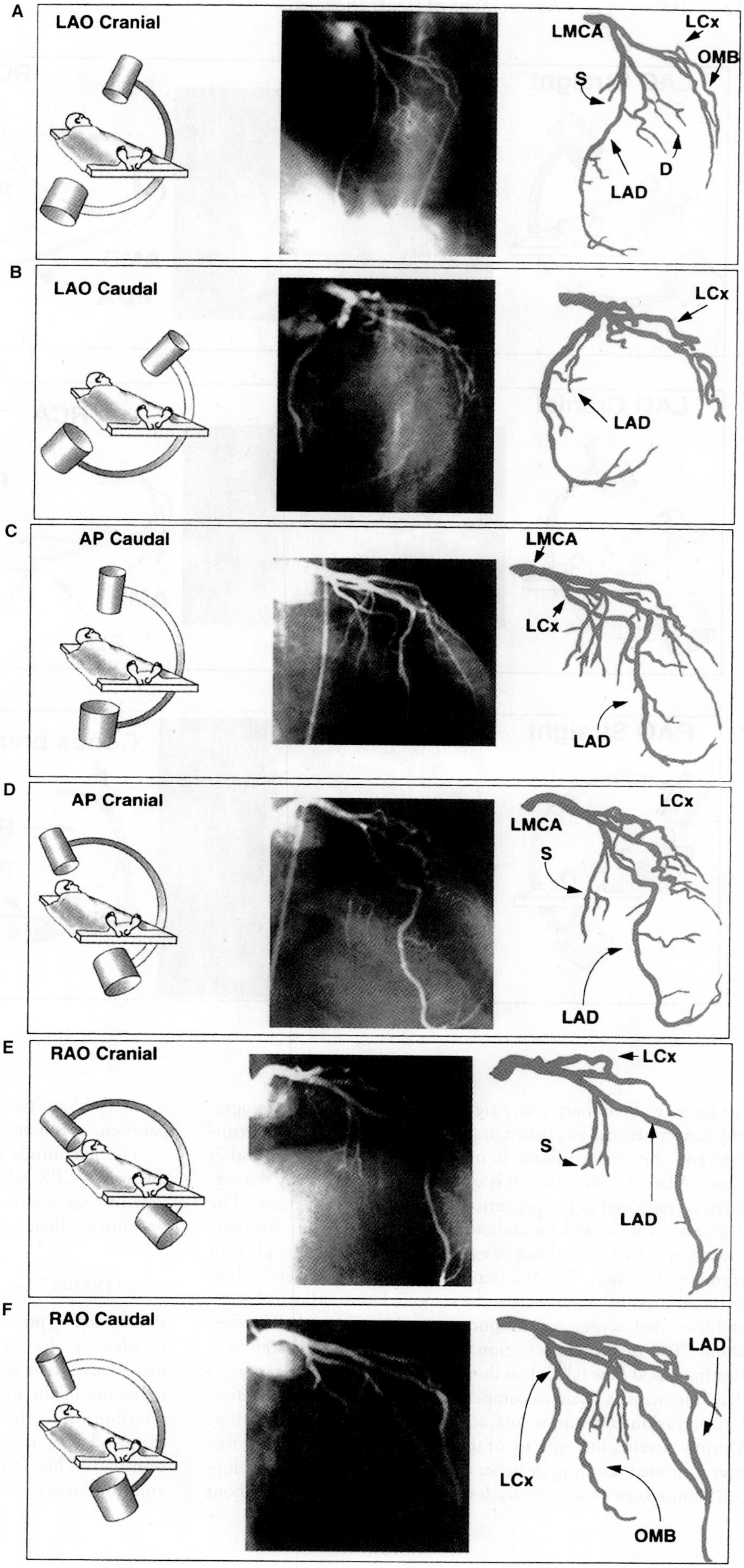

Figure 20-10 Angiographic views of the left coronary artery. The approximate position of the x-ray tube and image intensifier are shown for each of the commonly used angiographic views. (A) 60-degree LAO view with 20 degrees of cranial angulation (LAO cranial) shows the ostium and distal portion of the left main coronary artery (LMCA), the middle and distal portions of the LAD artery, septal perforators (S), diagonal branches (D), and the proximal left circumflex (LCx) and superior obtuse marginal branch (OMB). (B) 60-degree LAO with 25 degrees of caudal angulation (LAO caudal) shows the proximal LMCA and the proximal segments of the LAD and LCx. (C) Anteroposterior projection with 20 degrees of caudal angulation (AP caudal) shows the distal LMCA and proximal segments of the LAD and LCx. (D) Anteroposterior projection with 20 degrees cranial angulation (AP cranial) also shows the midportion of the LAD and its septal (S) branches. (E) 30-degree RAO with 20 degrees of cranial angulation (RAO cranial) shows the course of the LAD and its septal (S) and diagonal branches. (F) 30-degree RAO with 25 degrees of caudal angulation (RAO caudal) shows the LCx and obtuse marginal branches (OMB). (From Popma, J. J., & Bittl, J. [2001]. Coronary angiography and intravascular ultrasonography. In E. Braunwald, D. P. Zipes, & P. Libby [Eds.], *Heart disease: A textbook of cardiovascular medicine* [6th ed., p. 395]. Philadelphia: W.B. Saunders.)

A
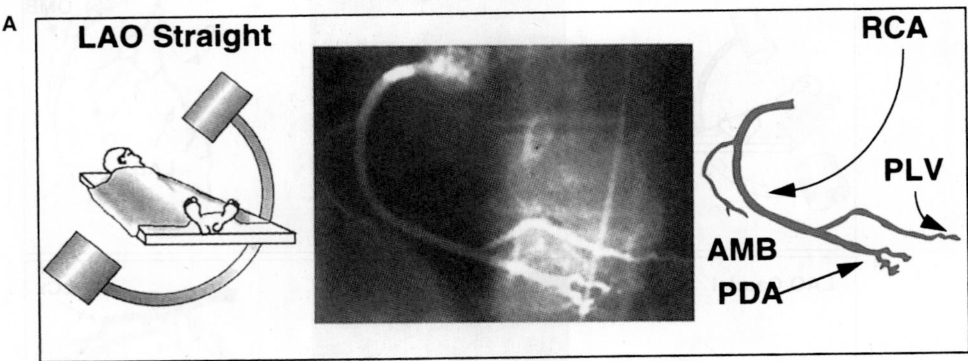

B
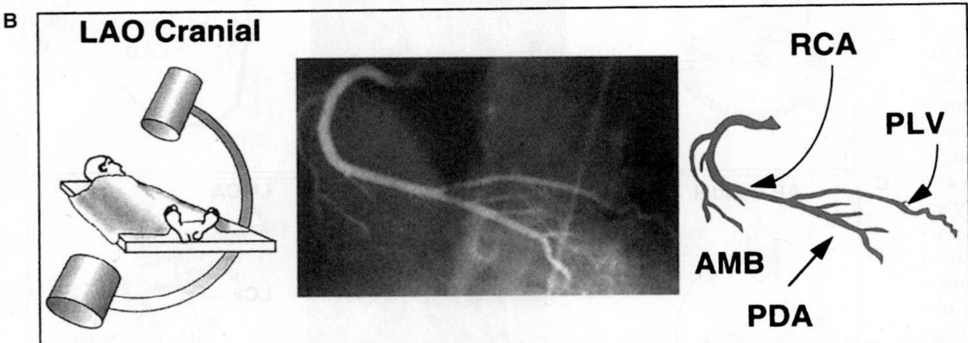

C
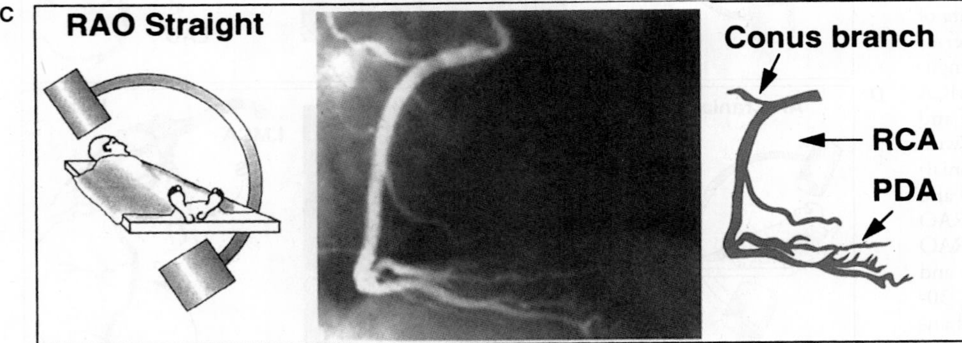

■ **Figure 20-11** Angiographic views of the right coronary artery (RCA). The approximate position of the x-ray tube and image intensifier are shown for each of the commonly used angiographic views. (A) 60-degrees LAO view shows the proximal and midportions of the RCA as well as the acute marginal branches (AMB) and termination of the RCA in the posterior left ventricular branches (PLV). (B) 60-degree LAO view with 25 degrees of cranial angulation (LAO cranial) shows the midportion of the RCA and the origin and course of the posterior descending artery (PDA). (C) 30-degree RAO view shows the midportion of the RCA, the conus branch, and the course of the PDA. (From Popma, J. J., & Bittl, J. [2001]. Coronary angiography and intravascular ultrasonography. In E. Braunwald, D. P. Zipes, & P. Libby [Eds.], *Heart disease: A textbook of cardiovascular medicine* [6th ed., p. 396]. Philadelphia: W.B. Saunders.)

the severity of coronary artery stenoses during coronary angiography can sometimes be challenging when the stenosis is indeterminate and appears significant in one planar view but not in other views. When a stenotic lesion is evaluated by angiography the segment is compared to the presumed-normal adjacent segment. The degree of stenosis can be underestimated when there is diffuse narrowing in the artery and can be exaggerated when there is adjacent coronary dilatation.[30,31] As a stenosis develops in an artery, a drop in blood pressure occurs across the stenotic lesion. Maximal stress and increased oxygen consumption cause blood flow to fall when about 70% of the cross-sectional area of an artery is stenosed. Resting blood flow falls when the stenosis reaches 85% or more.[30] The microvessels dilate to compensate for the reduced distal arterial perfusion pressure to maintain normal resting blood flow. During exercise, the capacity of the microcirculation to dilate further is limited resulting in ischemia. Determination of physiological significance of a coronary lesion provides information about coronary blood flow and the extent of myocardial perfusion impairment at rest and during stress.

The magnitude of the obstruction can be measured as a reduction in CFR, which is the ability of an artery to increase blood flow in response to a physiologic stimulus or as FFR, which is a pressure gradient across the stenotic lesion.

Intravascular Ultrasound Imaging

IVUS imaging provides a transluminal 360-degree scan of the vessel to identify the blood/intima (vessel lumen) border and the media/adventitia interface. IVUS enables cross-sectional measurements of the diameter of the vessel and identification of the distribution of the plaque, either concentric or eccentric, and plaque characteristics such as soft plaque, thrombus, or calcification. IVUS has facilitated improvement in PCI device selection and outcomes. IVUS involves placement of an ultrasound catheter into the coronary artery during left heart catheterization. The catheter is placed distal to the segment of interest and gradually pulled back to visualize the vessel wall. The two-dimensional images are displayed on a monitor that allows evaluation of lesion stenosis, extent of disease and assessment of post intracoronary stent placement.

IVUS Imaging During PCI: ACC/AHA/SCAI Practice Guidelines[11]

Class IIa indications:

1. Assessment of the adequacy of deployment of coronary stents, including the extent of stent apposition and determination of the minimum luminal diameter within the stent. (Level of evidence: B)
2. Determination of the mechanism of stent restenosis and to enable selection of appropriate therapy. (Level of evidence: B)
3. Evaluation of coronary obstruction at a location difficult to image by angiography in a patient with suspected flow-limiting stenosis. (Level of evidence: C)
4. Assessment of a suboptimal angiographic result after PCI. (Level of evidence: C)
5. Establishment of the presence and distribution of coronary calcium in patients for whom adjunctive rotational atherectomy is contemplated. (Level of evidence: C)

Coronary Flow Reserve (CFR)

The normal physiologic response to increased myocardial demand is enhanced blood flow by vasodilatation of epicardial and resistance vessels. The ability to increase coronary blood flow by reducing vasomotor tone to meet myocardial demand in response to a physiologic stimulus is called CFR. In the presence of a significant lesion, the epicardial artery and microvascular coronary bed compensate by vasodilation. In response to a physiological or pharmacological stress, the flow resistance in the coronary vasculature is unable to increase myocardial demand further by vasodilating, causing a state of impaired CFR. Measurement of CFR in the catheterization laboratory is performed by placement of an intracoronary Doppler wire into the coronary artery and administration of an adenosine infusion as a stress agent to evaluate the microcirculation.[32]

Fractional Flow Reserve (FFR)

The FFR is the fraction of maximal coronary blood flow that goes through the stenotic vessel. The FFR calculates a ratio of distal coronary pressure to aortic pressure measured during maximal hyperemia or vasodilatation (when minimal resistance is present across both the epicardial and microvascular beds), reflecting myocardial perfusion. A pressure wire is placed across the suspected lesion and an adenosine infusion is administered. Normal FFR is 1.0; a value less than 0.75 is abnormal and associated with abnormal stress tests and inducible myocardial ischemia. Revascularization is recommended for coronary lesions with an FFR less than 0.75.[31]

Adjunctive in-laboratory coronary physiological measurements facilitate clinical decisions to treat or defer PCI or coronary artery bypass graft surgery in patients who have intermediate stenoses. Decisions based on quantitative angiography have shown equivalent clinical outcomes in patients deferred for revascularization without the cost of PCI and the risk of restenosis.

FFR and Coronary Vasodilatory Reserve During PCI: ACC/AHA/SCAI Practice Guidelines[11]

Class IIa indications:

1 It is reasonable to use intracoronary physiologic measurements in the assessment of the effects of intermediate coronary stenoses (30% to 70% luminal narrowing) in patients with angina symptoms. Coronary pressure or Doppler velocimetry may also be useful as an alternative to performing noninvasive functional testing to determine whether an intervention is warranted. (Level of evidence: B)

NURSING CARE OF PATIENTS UNDERGOING CARDIAC CATHETERIZATION

Nurses working in cardiac catheterization laboratories fill many roles. The basic roles needed in a catheterization laboratory during a procedure are scrubber, recorder, and circulator. In some laboratories, the nurses scrub and assist in the procedure; in others, they are responsible for monitoring pressure and cardiac rhythm, assisting with hemodynamic studies such as CO determination, and administering IV procedural sedation. The nurse may visit the patient before the procedure to teach and help in preparing the patient or after the procedure to evaluate puncture site stability. Ideally, the nurse has a background in intensive or coronary care and a thorough knowledge of cardiovascular drugs, arrhythmias, the principles of IV procedural sedation, sterile technique, cardiac anatomy and physiology, pacemakers, and the concepts of catheter management for coronary angiography and intervention. Changes in the patient's emotional status, alertness, vocal responses, and facial expressions are important indices of the patient's tolerance of the procedure. The nurse's alertness to these clues and early intervention with reassurance or appropriate medication may help to prevent more serious events. Training in advanced cardiac life support is a requirement for catheterization laboratory nurses and those nurses caring for patients after the procedure.

Complications and Nursing Care During Cardiac Catheterization

The nursing care of patients both during and after cardiac catheterization is directed toward the prevention and detection of complications. The risk of a major complication (myocardial infarction, death, or major embolization) during diagnostic cardiac catheterizations is below 1%.

The risk of an adverse event is dependent on individual comorbidities, cardiovascular anatomy, and type of procedure. Severe peripheral vascular disease is a risk factor for major complication with all procedures. The SCAI registry reported the incidence of complications during cardiac catheterization and coronary angiography: vascular complications, 0.43%; contrast reactions, 0.37%; MI, 0.05%; cerebrovascular accident, 0.07%; and mortality, 0.11%.[33]

Lower complication rates were noted with experienced operators and the use of a smaller catheter size (6 Fr or less). Higher complication rates were noted in patients having right and left heart catheterizations, use of catheters greater than 6 Fr, and increased vascular complications in patients with higher body weight.[34] Although complications are rare, they do occur and may be life threatening. Early detection and intervention are essential in prevention.

Local vascular problems at the catheter entry site are the most commonly seen complications after cardiac catheterization procedures. These problems include minor or major oozing, ecchymosis, hematoma, or poorly controlled bleeding at the puncture site. Other vascular complications that are less common are vessel thrombosis, distal embolization, or dissection, pseudoaneurysm and arteriovenous fistula. A complete list of complications is discussed in Chapter 23.

Ventricular arrhythmias occur in response to catheter manipulation or contrast medium injection and tend not to recur after the predisposing stimulus is removed. Atrial and junctional arrhythmias and varying degrees of blocks also occur in response to these stimuli. Bradycardia is common in response to injection of the coronary arteries with contrast or during sheath insertion or removal.

Allergic reactions to the contrast medium may occur. Sneezing, itching of the eyes or skin, urticaria, bronchospasm, or other beginning signs of allergy are treated with antihistamines and corticosteroids. Anaphylactic reactions are treated with intramuscular or subcutaneous (SQ) epinephrine (1:10,000 concentration), aminophylline, steroids, an antihistamine (diphenhydramine), vasopressors, and wide-open normal saline IV to support blood pressure. For patients with increased risk of an adverse reaction to contrast medium, low-osmolar, nonionic contrast agent and a premedication strategy including corticosteroids have shown a reduction in adverse reactions. Contrast reactions can occur despite premedication strategies and the staff must be prepared to treat an anaphylactic reaction. Patients with known or suspected allergies to iodine-containing substances, such as seafood or with a prior allergic reaction to radiographic contrast, should be pretreated with prednisone from 24 to 48 hours before contrast injection. Premedication consists of an H_1 antihistamine (diphenhydramine) or occasionally an H_2 blocker (cimetidine or ranitidine).[16,35]

The catheterization laboratory nurse must be familiar with IABP set-up and management, because the IABP is often used when patients become hemodynamically unstable during a catheterization procedure (Chapter 26). The nurse must also be familiar with other equipment used in the laboratory—IVUS, Doppler and pressure wires, balloon catheters and stents, thrombectomy devices, and atherectomy equipment. Additional skills include access site management, including sheath removal, manual pressure for hemostasis, and use of closure devices or FemoStop for hemostasis, and a thorough knowledge of drugs commonly used during a procedure, such as heparin, bivalirudin, low-molecular-weight heparins, glycoprotein IIb/IIIa receptor inhibitors, antiarrhythmics, vasoactive drugs, and drugs used for procedural sedation.

Postprocedure Care

After the procedure, the patient may be transferred to an observation unit, telemetry unit, interventional cardiology unit, or intensive care unit depending on the type of procedure done and the patient's condition. In most facilities, patients undergoing diagnostic catheterization are cared for in an observational unit, such as an ambulatory care unit or same day surgery unit, for up to 6 hours and then discharged if stable. Patients who have undergone interventional procedures often stay overnight and are cared for in a telemetry unit or interventional cardiology unit where nurses are specially trained and experienced in postprocedure care and have more in-depth knowledge of cardiovascular drugs, arrhythmia interpretation, advanced cardiac life support skills, and management of access sites. If the patient is hemodynamically unstable or has a complication of the procedure, such as MI, severe respiratory distress, acute or threatened vessel closure post-PCI, tamponade, unstable arrhythmias, or requires close observation or intensive nursing care, he or she is transferred to an intensive care unit.

After a diagnostic procedure, the femoral arterial or venous introducer sheaths are removed and manual or mechanical pressure is applied to the access site until hemostasis is achieved. Compression devices or vascular closure devices may be used to achieve hemostasis after a diagnostic or interventional procedure (Chapter 23). For interventional procedures in which extensive anticoagulation was used or IV antiplatelet therapy (i.e., glycoprotein IIb/IIIa receptor inhibitors) is to be continued for several hours, the sheath is often left in place until the activated clotting time is below a critical level and then removed by either catheterization laboratory staff or nurses in the postprocedure unit. Nurses caring for patients after cardiac catheterization must be prepared to perform sheath removal according to institutional policies and guidelines, and must be able to recognize complications associated with this procedure.[36–38]

After returning from the laboratory, the patient must be thoroughly assessed. Information about the approach used, the procedures performed, and any complications experienced during the catheterization should be obtained from the physician, nurse, or technician. Display 20-3 lists typical postcatheterization protocols. The elements of the nursing assessment and intervention and potential findings are listed and explained in the following sections.

Psychological Assessment and Patient Teaching

Patients are often tired, hungry, and uncomfortable when they return from the laboratory. They are usually relieved that the procedure is over and may already know the preliminary findings of their study. This news may be good or bad, and it is important to find out what the patient has been told and what this means to the patient. The patient may have questions about surgery or about what to expect next. Some patients are anxious or depressed. Giving patients the opportunity to express their feelings about the procedure helps to calm and relax them. Reassure the patient by describing the sensations that can be expected, such as thirst and the frequent need to urinate although the patient has had nothing to eat or drink for several hours. Reemphasize the need for bed rest and the need to keep the catheterized limb immobile. Let the patient know that frequent checking of vital signs is routine and not a cause for alarm. Before hospital discharge, the patient should be instructed regarding symptoms for which to call the physician and procedures for site care (Display 20-4).

DISPLAY 20-3 Postcatheterization Protocols

General Guidelines

1. Assess vital signs every 15 minutes for 1 hour, every 30 minutes for 1 hour, and hourly for 4 hours or until discharge.
2. Assess catheterization site for bleeding, hematoma formation, and swelling. Assess peripheral pulses and neurovascular status every 15 minutes for 1 hour, every 30 minutes for 1 hour, and hourly for 4 hours or until discharge.
3. Resume precatheterization diet and medications.
4. Administer analgesic agents as needed.
5. Notify physician if any of the following occur:
   a. Decrease in peripheral pulses
   b. New hematoma or increase in size of existing hematoma
   c. Unusually severe catheter insertion site pain or affected extremity pain
   d. Onset of chest discomfort or shortness of breath

Femoral Approach

6. Order bed rest for 4–6 hours depending on sheath size. The head of the bed may be raised to 30 degrees.
7. Instruct patient not to flex or hyperextend the hip joint of the affected leg for 4–6 hours, and to use the bed controls to elevate the head of the bed or lower the foot of the bed.
8. Compression device may be applied. Monitor peripheral pulses as per protocol.

Brachial or Radial Approach

9. Order bed rest for 2–3 hours. The patient may sit up in bed. Pressure dressing or Ace bandage may be applied to the affected arm.
10. Monitor distal pulses every 15 minutes for 1 hour, every 30 minutes for 1 hour, and hourly for 4 hours until discharge or stable.
11. Instruct patient not to keep the arm in a flexed position for an extended period of time, hyperextend or lie on the affected arm for 24 hours.
12. Instruct patient to observe for bleeding or hematoma. If sutures were used, instruct patient regarding suture removal.

Circulatory Integrity of Access Site

Careful assessment of the access site and limb is an important element of postcatheterization nursing care. The site should be checked for visible bleeding, swelling, or tenderness. The arterial pulse at the site and at points distal to it should be compared with pulses on the opposite limb and those recorded before the procedure. Capillary filling and the warmth of the limb should also be evaluated. Blanching, cramping, coolness, pain, numbness, or

DISPLAY 20-4 Patient Discharge Instructions for Inpatient and Outpatient Catheterization

1. Report the following symptoms to your physician if they occur:
   a. New bleeding or swelling at the catheterization site. (If marked bleeding occurs, press hand firmly over the area of bleeding and call 911.)
   b. Increased tenderness, redness, drainage, or pain at the catheterization site
   c. Fever
   d. Change in color (pallor), temperature (coolness), or sensation (numbness) in the leg or arm used for catheterization
2. Acetaminophen or other non-aspirin-containing analgesic may be taken every 4 hours as needed for pain unless contraindicated
3. If stitches are present, wear an adhesive bandage and remove as directed by physician. Otherwise, cover site with an adhesive bandage for 24 hours
   a. Patient may shower the day after the procedure
   b. Tub bath should be avoided for 3 days after the procedure
4. Patient to see physician for follow-up appointment ____
5. Continue prescribed medications as before unless otherwise indicated by your physician
6. Avoid strenuous activity for 48 hours. Do not lift anything heavier than 5 lb for the next 48 hours
7. Limit excessive stair climbing
8. Patient must be driven home and be accompanied by a responsible adult until the next morning
9. If pain or pressure occurs in chest, arms, shoulders, neck, or jaw:
   a. Take nitroglycerin if it is prescribed for the patient
   b. Notify cardiologist of chest pain if it is relieved with nitroglycerin
   c. If chest pain is not relieved, call 911
10. Follow diet as prescribed by cardiologist, usually a low-salt, low-fat diet.

tingling may indicate reduced perfusion and must be carefully evaluated. A diminished or absent pulse is a sign of serious arterial occlusion, which often constitutes a surgical emergency. The first step, if any of these signs occur, is to check the compression device (if used) and release pressure. If symptoms do not resolve, the physician should be notified immediately and steps should be taken to preserve the limb.

Manual pressure or pressure with a compression device such as a FemoStop is used for hemostasis at the time of sheath removal and when bleeding continues or recurs after initial hemostasis. When pressure is applied at an arterial site, the pulse distal to the site may be safely occluded for 2 to 5 minutes, and then pressure is released until the pulse returns. Distal pulses should remain palpable during the remainder of pressure application, which continues for 15 to 20 minutes. If oozing from the sheath insertion tract continues after initial hemostasis, infiltration of the tract with a solution of lidocaine and epinephrine (1:100,000 strength) followed by 2 to 5 minutes of light manual pressure is usually effective to control bleeding.

Blood Pressure

Evaluation of the blood pressure after cardiac catheterization should include comparison of preprocedure and postprocedure pressures, checking for orthostatic hypotension once the bed rest period is over, and monitoring for paradoxical pulse. Mild systolic hypotension frequently occurs after cardiac catheterization and is usually not of concern. Angiographic contrast medium acts as an osmotic diuretic, and patients frequently return with signs of volume depletion, including orthostatic hypotension. Therefore, patients are kept on bed rest until fluid balance is restored with oral liquids or by IV replacement. *Hypotension* may also be a response to the drugs given during the procedure. If the blood pressure is consistently low, other causes need to be investigated, such as possible blood loss or arrhythmias. Patient assessment needs to be performed and the physician notified. *Paradoxical pulse* suggests pericardial tamponade, which is very rare but may occur as a result of perforation of a coronary artery or the myocardium. In patients with known perforation, this sign should be specifically assessed with each blood pressure measurement, and, if it occurs, the physician should be notified. *Hypertension* can also occur and may contribute to access site bleeding if not controlled.

Heart Rate and Rhythm

Patients who have had an interventional procedure should be on a cardiac monitor for rhythm and ST-segment monitoring. A mild sinus tachycardia (100 to 120 beats per minute) is not unusual after catheterization and may be a sign of anxiety, an indication of saline and water loss due to diuresis, or a reaction to medication such as atropine. Fluids, time, and reassurance often bring the heart rate down to more normal levels. Heart rates above 120 beats per minute should be evaluated for other causes such as hemorrhage, more severe fluid imbalance, fever, or arrhythmias. Bradycardia may indicate vasovagal responses, arrhythmias, or infarction and should be assessed by 12-lead ECG and correlated with other clinical signs, such as pain and blood pressure. Vasovagal reactions are fairly common and can occur immediately or hours after sheath removal. Cardiac monitoring for ST-segment displacement is useful to detect acute reocclusion of the artery or MI after an interventional procedure.[39,40]

Temperature

Early increases in temperature may occur because of the fluid loss that occurs with catheterization. More persistent elevations may indicate infection or pyrogenic reactions.

Urinary Output

Because angiographic contrast medium acts as an osmotic diuretic, patients have an increase in urine output for a short time after catheterization. IV fluids are often continued for a variable time after the procedure, and oral fluids should be encouraged unless the patient has been ordered nothing by mouth for some reason.

Table 20-2 ■ NORMAL ADULT VALUES FOR DATA COLLECTED DURING CARDIAC CATHETERIZATION

Pressures	mm Hg
Systemic arterial	
Peak-systolic	100–140
End-diastolic	60–90
Mean	70–105
Left ventricular	
Peak-systolic	100–140
End-diastolic	3–12
Left atrial	
Left atrial mean (or PAWP)	1–10
a wave	3–15
v wave	3–12
Pulmonary artery	
Peak-systolic	15–30
End-diastolic	3–12
Systolic Mean	9–16
Right ventricular	
Peak-systolic	15–30
End-diastolic	0–8
Right atrial	
Mean	8–10
a wave	2–10
v wave	2–10
Left Ventricular Volumes	
End-systolic volume (mL/m^2)	20–30
End-diastolic volume (mL/m^2)	70–79
Ejection fraction	.58–.72
Resistance (dynes/s/cm^{-5})	
Total systemic resistance	900–1,440
Pulmonary arteriolar (vascular) resistance	37–97
Flow	
CO (L/min)	4.0–8.0
Cardiac index (L/min/m^2)	2.5–4.0
Stroke index (mL/beat/m^2)	35–70
Stroke volume (mL/beat)	60–130
Oxygen consumption (mL/min/m^2)	125
Oxygen Saturation (%)	
Right atrium	60–75
Right ventricle	60–75
Pulmonary artery	60–75
Left atrium	95–99
Left ventricle	95–99
Aorta	95–99

PAWP, pulmonary artery wedge pressure.

From Kucher, N., & Goldhaber, S. Z. (2006). Pulmonary angiography. In Baim, D. S. (Ed.), *Grossman's cardiac catheterization, angiography, and intervention* (7th ed., p. 236). Philadelphia: Lippincott Williams & Wilkins.

Other Possible Problems

MI, stroke, and HF are very rare complications after cardiac catheterization. However, the nurse caring for patients after cardiac catheterization should be aware of the signs and symptoms of these complications.

INTERPRETATION OF DATA

Table 20-2 lists normal ranges for some of the data gathered during cardiac catheterization. The assessment of CAD involves evaluation of the coronary vasculature and left ventricular function.

The first step in evaluating the coronary arteriogram is to determine whether the coronaries are unobstructed and free of lesions. Each major artery is traced along its entire length, and branches and collaterals are noted and evaluated for irregularities or narrowing. When occlusion is present, the degree of disease and the suitability of the artery for revascularization are of primary concern.

In addition to grading the occlusion, the condition of the distal artery must be evaluated. The distal artery may be identified by antegrade or collateral flow, and its caliber and suitability as a recipient for bypass grafting are evaluated. Arteries with diffuse atherosclerotic plaquing and small distal targets are less suitable for bypass grafting. The proximity of the occlusion determines the amount of myocardium in jeopardy. A subjective evaluation of the degree of arterial flow is made by observing the time required for perfused arteries to fill and clear. Contrast medium clears faster with higher flow rates. Intermittent luminal obstruction due to systolic constriction from encircling muscle bands or to coronary artery spasm is also observed, and its degree, distribution, and pattern are evaluated. If bypass grafts have been injected, they are evaluated in the same manner for patency, flow indices, and the condition of the perfused artery. Figures 20-12 and 20-13 show normal angiograms of the right and left coronary arteries.

Evaluation of myocardial function is an important part of the evaluation of CAD. Patterns of ventricular contraction are evaluated by ventriculography and estimated ejection fraction. The anteriolateral, apical, inferior, and posterobasal segments of the left ventricle can be examined in the RAO projection. In the LAO projection, the basal septal, apical septal, apical lateral, and basal lateral segments can be evaluated. Regional contraction may be classified as follows:

1. Normal
2. Mild hypokinesis—mild reduction in myocardial contraction
3. Severe hypokinesis—more severe reduction in myocardial contraction
4. Akinesis—total absence of wall motion in a discrete area
5. Dyskinesis—disturbance causing abnormal movement of left ventricular wall contraction
6. Aneurysm—paradoxical systolic expansion of a portion of the left ventricular wall

The reversibility of myocardial contraction abnormalities is an important consideration in the decision for surgery and long-term prognosis. Improved function is more common with hypokinesis than with akinesis or dyskinesis. The presence of collateral vessels and the lack of Q waves favor the reversibility of hypokinesis.[41]

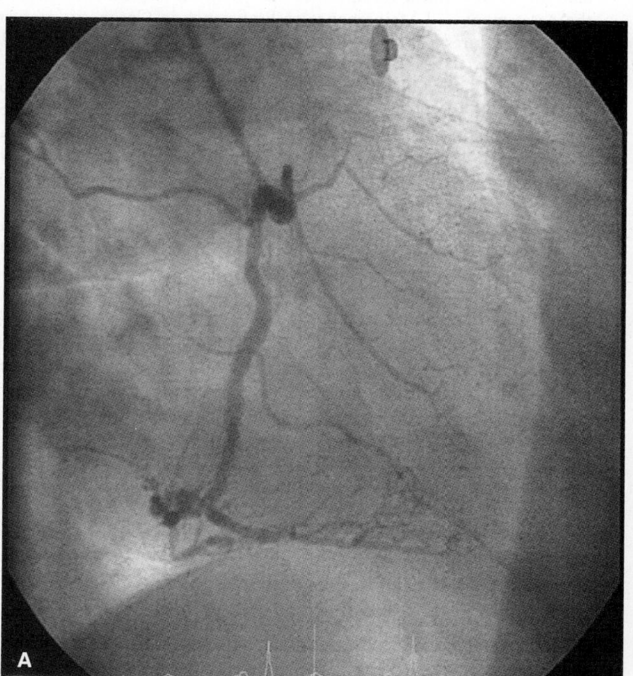

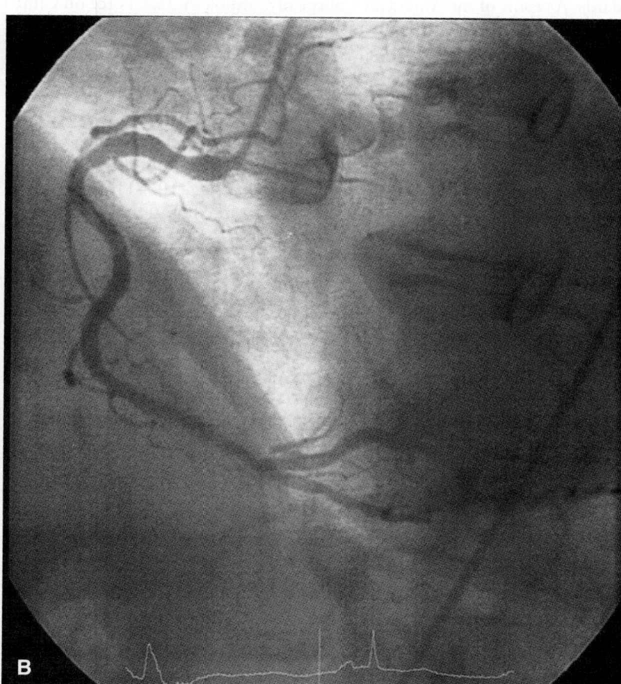

■ **Figure 20-12** Normal RCA shown in (A) RAO projection and (B) LAO projection. (Courtesy of Swedish Medical Center, Seattle, Washington.)

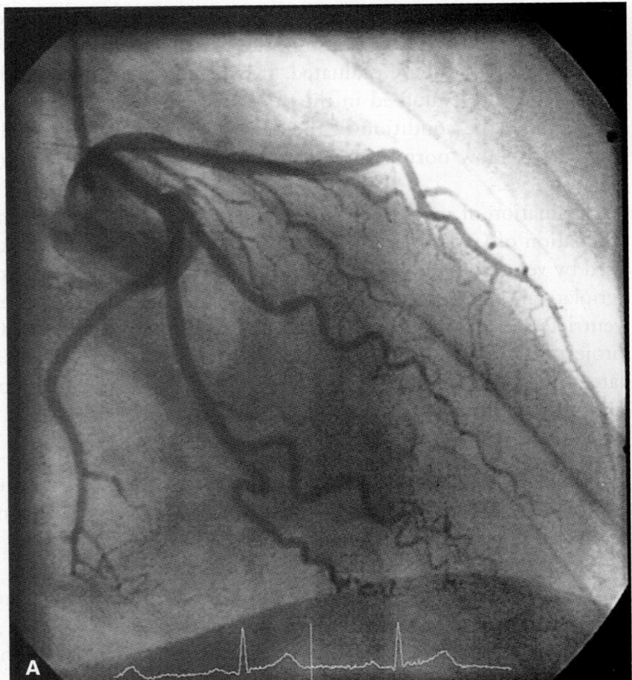

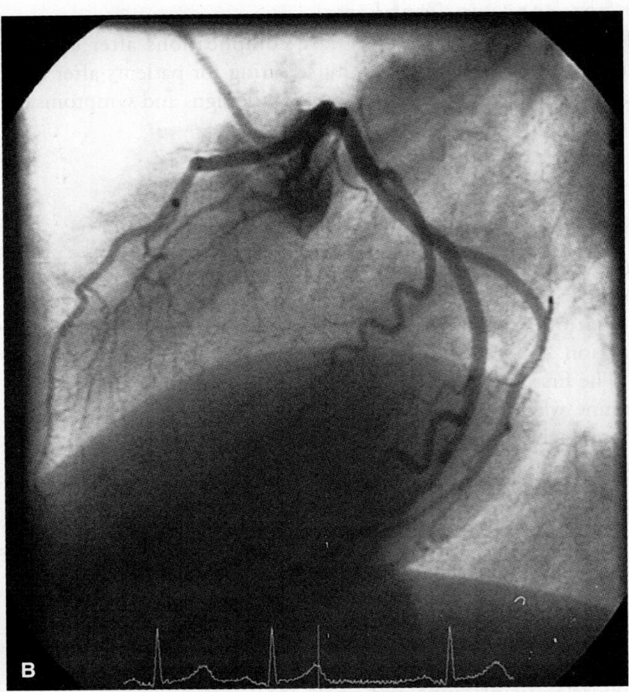

■ **Figure 20-13** Normal left coronary arteries shown in **(A)** RAO projection and **(B)** LAO projection. (Courtesy of Swedish Medical Center, Seattle, Washington.)

REFERENCES

1. Bashore, T. M., Bates, E. R., Berger, P. B., et al. (2001). American College of Cardiology/Society for Cardiac Angiography and Interventions Clinical Expert Consensus Document on cardiac catheterization laboratory standards: A report of the American College of Cardiology Task Force on Clinical Expert Consensus Documents. *Journal of the American College of Cardiology, 37*(8), 2170–2214.
2. Cournand, A. F., & Ranges, C. S. (1941). Catheterization of the right auricle in man. *Proceedings of the Society for Experimental Biology and Medicine, 46*, 462–470.
3. Cournand, A. F., Riley, R. L., & Breed, E. S. (1945). Measurement of cardiac output in man using the technique of catheterization of the right auricle or ventricle. *Journal of Clinical Investigation, 24*, 106–116.
4. Richards, D. W. (1945). Cardiac output by catheterization technique in various clinical conditions. *Federal Proceedings, 4*, 215–220.
5. Seldinger, S. I. (1953). Catheter replacement of the needle in percutaneous arteriography. *Acta Radiologica, 29*, 368–376.
6. Sones, F. M., Shirey, E. K., & Prondfit, W. L. (1959). Cine-coronary arteriography. *Circulation, 20*, 773.
7. Scanlom, P. J., Faxon, D. P., Audet, A.-M., et al. (1999). ACC/AHA guidelines for coronary angiography: Executive summary and recommendations: A report of the American College of Cardiology/American Heart Association Task Force on Practice Guidelines (Committee on Coronary Angiography). Developed in collaboration with the Society for Cardiac Angiography and Interventions. *Circulation, 99*, 2345–2357.
8. Gibbons, R. J., Abrams, J., Chatterjee, K., et al. (2003). ACC/AHA 2002 guideline update for the management of patients with chronic stable angina—Summary article. *Journal of the American College of Cardiology, 41*(1), 159–168.
9. Anderson, J. L., Adams, C. D., Antman, E. M., et al. (2007). ACC/AHA 2007 guidelines for the management of patients with unstable angina/non-ST-elevation myocardial infarction: Executive summary: A repot of the American College of Cardiology/American Heart Association Task Force on Practice Guidelines (Writing Committee to Revise the 2002 Guidelines for the Management of Patients With Unstable Angina/Non-ST-Elevation Myocardial Infarction). *Journal of the American College of Cardiology, 50*, e1–e157.
10. King, S. B., Aversano, T., Ballard, W. L., et al. (2007). ACCF/AHA/SCAI 2007 update of the clinical competence statement on cardiac interventional procedures: A report of the American College of Cardiology Foundation/American Heart Association/American College of Physicians Task Force on Clinical Competence and Training (Writing Committee to Update the 1998 Clinical Competence Statement on Recommendations for the Assessment and Maintenance of Proficiency in Coronary Interventional Procedures). *Journal of the American College of Cardiology, 50*(1), 2–27.
11. Smith, S. C., Feldman, T. F., Hirshfeld, J. W., et al. (2006). ACC/AHA/SCAI 2005 guideline update for percutaneous coronary intervention: A report of the American College of Cardiology/American Heart Association Task Force on Practice Guidelines (ACC/AHA/SCAI Writing Committee to update the 2001 Guidelines for Percutaneous Coronary Intervention). *Journal of the American College of Cardiology, 47*, 216–235.
12. Antman, E. M., Hand, M., Armstrong, P. W., et al. (2008). 2007 Focused Update of the ACC/AHA 2004 Guidelines for the Management of Patients With ST-Elevation Myocardial Infarction. *Circulation, 117*, 296–329.
13. Baim, D. S. (Ed.). (2006). *Grossman's cardiac catheterization, angiography, and interventions* (7th ed.). Philadelphia: Lippincott Williams & Wilkins.
14. Salem, D. N., Stein, P. D., Al-Ahmad, A., et al. (2004). Antithrombotic therapy in valvular heart disease–native and prosthetic: The Seventh ACCP Conference on Antithrombotic and Thrombolytic Therapy. *Chest, 126*, 457–498.
15. Briguori, C., Airoldi, F., D'Andrea, D., et al. (2007). Renal Insufficiency Following Contrast Media Administration Trial (REMEDIAL): A randomized comparison of 3 preventive strategies. *Circulation, 115*, 1211–1217.
16. Cohan, R. H., Ellis, J. H., & Dunnick, N. R. (1995). Use of low-osmolar agents and premedication to reduce the frequency of adverse reactions to radiographic contrast media: A survey of the Society of Uroradiology. *Radiology, 194*, 357–364.
17. Kixmiller, J. M., & Schick, L. (1997). Procedural sedation in cardiovascular procedures. *Critical Care Nursing Clinics of North America, 9*, 301–312.
18. Owens, P., & Bashore, T. M. (1990). The preparation and care of the patient and the laboratory. In T. M. Bashore (Ed.), *Invasive cardiology principles and techniques* (pp. 19–39). Toronto, Ontario, Canada: B. C. Decker.

19. Schultz, D. D., & Olivas, G. S. (1986). The use of cough cardiopulmonary resuscitation in clinical practice. *Heart & Lung, 5*, 273–280.
20. Spector, K. S., & Lawson, W. E. (2001). Optimizing safe femoral access during cardiac catheterization. *Catheterization and Cardiovascular Interventions, 53*, 209–212.
21. Grossman, W. (2006). Blood flow measurement: Cardiac output and vascular resistance. In D. S. Baim (Ed.), *Grossman's cardiac catheterization, angiography, and intervention* (7th ed., pp. 148–162). Philadelphia: Lippincott Williams & Wilkins.
22. Brockenbrough, E. C., & Braunwald, E. (1960). A new technique for left ventricular angiography and transseptal left heart catheterization. *American Journal of Cardiology, 6*, 1062–1064.
23. Baim, D. S., & Simon, D. I. (2006). Percutaneous approach, including transseptal and apical puncture. In D. S. Baim & W. Grossman (Eds.), *Grossman's cardiac catheterization, angiography, and intervention* (7th ed., pp. 79–106). Philadelphia: Lippincott Williams & Wilkins.
24. Baim, D. S., & Hillis, D. (2006). Cardiac ventriculography. In D. S. Baim (Ed.), *Grossman's cardiac catheterization, angiography, and intervention* (7th ed., pp. 222–233). Philadelphia: Lippincott Williams & Wilkins.
25. Judkins, M. P. (1968). Percutaneous transfemoral selective coronary arteriography. *Radiology Clinics of North America, 6*, 467–492.
26. Rudnick, M. R., & Tumlin, J. A. (2008). Prevention of radiocontrast media-induced acute renal failure. *UptoDate*. Retrieved April, 2008, from www.uptodate.com/online
27. Rudnick, M. R., & Tumlin, J. A. (2006, September 15). Radiocontrast media-induced acute renal failure. *UptoDate*. Retrieved December 5, 2006, from www.uptodate.com
28. Baim, D. S. (2006). Coronary angiography. In D. S. Baim (Ed.), *Grossman's cardiac catheterization, angiography, and intervention* (7th ed., pp. 187–221). Philadelphia: Lippincott Williams & Wilkins.
29. Hirshfeld, J. W. (1990). Cardiovascular effects of iodinated contrast agents. *American Journal of Cardiology, 66*, 9F–17F.
30. Wilson, R. F. (1996). Assessing the severity of coronary artery stenoses. *New England Journal of Medicine, 334*, 1735–1737.
31. Pijls, N. H. J., Bruyne, B., Peels, K., et al. (1996). Measurement of fractional flow reserve to assess the functional severity of coronary artery stenoses. *New England Journal of Medicine, 334*, 1703–1708.
32. Kern, M. J., & Lim, M. J. (2006). Evaluation of myocardial blood flow and metabolism. In D. S. Baim (Ed.), *Grossman's cardiac catheterization, angiography, and intervention* (7th ed., pp. 335–370). Philadelphia: Lippincott Williams & Wilkins.
33. Noto, T. J., Johnson, L. W., Krone, R., et al. (1991). Cardiac catheterization 1990: A report of the Registry of the Society for Cardiac Angiography and Interventions (SCA&I). *Catheterization and Cardiovascular Diagnosis, 24*, 75.
34. Ammann, P., Brunner-La Rocca, H., Angehrn, W., et al. (2003). Procedural complications following diagnostic coronary angiography are related to the operator's experience and the catheter size. *Catheterization and Cardiovascular Diagnosis, 59*, 13–18.
35. Hong, S. J., & Cochran, S. T. (2008). Immediate hypersensitivity reactions to radiocontrast media. *UptoDate*. Retrieved April 2008, from www.uptodate.com/online
36. Juran, M. P., Rouse, C. L., Smith, D. D., et al. (1999). Nursing interventions to decrease bleeding at the femoral access site after percutaneous coronary intervention. *American Journal of Critical Care, 8*(5), 303–313.
37. Smith, T. T., & Labriola, R. (2001). Developing best practice in arterial sheath removal for registered nurses. *Journal of Nursing Quality Assurance, 16*(1), 61–67.
38. Dressler, D. K., & Dressler, K. K. (2006). Caring for patients with femoral sheaths: After percutaneous coronary intervention, sheath removal and site monitoring are the nurse's responsibility. *American Journal of Nursing, 106*(5), 64A–64H.
39. Drew, B. J., & Tisdale, L. A. (1993). ST-segment monitoring for coronary artery reocclusion following thrombolytic therapy and coronary angioplasty: Identification of optimal bedside monitoring leads. *American Journal of Critical Care, 2*, 280–292.
40. Jacobson, C. (2006). Bedside cardiac monitoring. In S. Burns (Ed.), *AACN protocols for practice: Noninvasive monitoring* (2nd ed., pp. 3–30). Boston: Jones and Bartlett Publishers.
41. Fifer, M. A., & Douglas, J. S. (2006). Measurement of ventricular volumes, ejection fraction, mass, wall stress, and regional wall motion. In D. S. Baim (Ed.), *Grossman's cardiac catheterization, angiography, and intervention* (7th ed., pp. 304–314). Philadelphia: Lippincott Williams & Wilkins.

CHAPTER 21

Hemodynamic Monitoring

Elizabeth J. Bridges

Cardiovascular support of critically ill patients requires noninvasive and invasive monitoring of physiological indicators of cardiovascular function, including factors that affect cardiac performance (preload, afterload, contractility, and heart rate [HR]) and the balance between O_2 supply and demand. This chapter reviews technologies for hemodynamic monitoring (arterial blood pressure (BP) monitoring, central venous pressure (CVP)/ pulmonary artery (PA) catheterization, and cardiac output (CO) and $S\bar{v}O_2$ monitoring) and discusses the current recommendations for the effective use of hemodynamic monitoring in optimizing patient outcomes. Newer techniques such as central venous oxygenation saturation ($ScvO_2$) and functional hemodynamic monitoring and new technologies such as transpulmonary indicator dilution (TPID) CO, pulse contour analysis, transesophageal Doppler, partial CO_2 rebreathing, and microcirculation and tissue oxygenation monitoring techniques are introduced.

TECHNICAL ASPECTS OF INVASIVE PRESSURE MONITORING

Referencing

Pressure in blood vessels has three components: dynamic BP (i.e., the BP generated by the heart), hydrostatic pressure (related to fluid density, gravitational acceleration, and height of the column of blood between the heart and the vessels), and static pressure (related to the volume of blood in the vascular system at zero flow).[1] The BP is the same at all points along a horizontal level. However, pressure at different vertical levels reflects not only the dynamic pressure but also the hydrostatic pressure.

Referencing, which is performed to correct for the change in hydrostatic pressure in vessels above and below the heart, is accomplished by placing the air–fluid interface (stopcock) of the catheter system at the level of the heart to negate the weight effect of the catheter tubing. All invasive cardiovascular pressure-monitoring systems (PA, CVP, and arterial) are referenced to the heart, not to the catheter tip or the site of insertion.[1–3]

The phlebostatic axis and phlebostatic level are the most commonly used reference points for the mid-right atrium (RA) and left atrium (LA) (Fig. 21-1).[4,5] As the patient moves from the flat to the backrest elevated position, the phlebostatic level rotates on the axis and remains horizontal (Fig. 21-2). In patients with normal chest wall configuration, the midaxillary line (MAL) is a valid reference level for the RA and the LA; however, use of the MAL in patients with varied chest configuration may result in a pressure difference of up to 6 mm Hg.[6]

Although the phlebostatic axis is the most commonly cited reference level, other reference levels have been suggested. For CVP measurements Magder suggests using a reference point 5 cm below the angle of the sternum, as this point reflects mid-RA, which remains the same up to a backrest elevation of 60 degrees. Use of this reference, which is also the same reference recommended for the evaluation of jugular venous distention, gives a CVP measurement that is 3 mm Hg lower than a measurement from a system referenced to the phlebostatic axis.[7,8] There is no general consensus on which reference is most accurate; however, these studies highlight the importance of using a standardized reference and also interpreting the absolute pressure measurements relative to the different reference levels.

Previous research on the effect of position on hemodynamic pressure measurements has been limited by the use of incorrect reference points. In many of these studies, attainment of accurate PA pressures was not possible because the use of a reference point above or below the LA resulted in the inclusion of hydrostatic pressure component; thus, the measured pressures were underestimated or overestimated.[9] For every 1 cm the reference point is above the LA; the measured pressure decreases by 0.73 mm Hg. Conversely, for every 1 cm the reference point is below the LA, the measured pressure increases by 0.73 mm Hg. The position-specific reference points are summarized in Display 21-1. In the lateral position, reference points have been validated for the 30- and 90-degree lateral positions with a 0-degree backrest elevation. Further study of the lateral position with varying degrees of backrest elevation is needed. In studies performed to evaluate the effects of prone position on hemodynamic indices, the MAL or the midanteroposterior diameter of the chest have been used as the reference point.[15–21]

Zeroing Versus Referencing

Zeroing is performed by opening the system to air to establish atmospheric pressure as zero, although changes in barometric pressure have minimal effect on measured pressure.[22] In addition, zeroing is performed to compensate for offset caused by hydrostatic pressure or offset in the pressure transducer, amplifier, oscilloscope, recorder, or digital delays. The act of simultaneously zeroing and referencing ensures that intracardiac pressures are being measured (Display 21-2).

Infection Control

Catheter-related infection remains the leading cause of nosocomial infections, particularly in critical care and are associated with increased length of hospital stay and resource use.[24] In a study of 1,140 central venous and 1,038 arterial catheters, both *in situ* for an average of 9.5 days, the catheter-related blood stream infection (CR-BSI) incidence was 4.6% and 3.7%, respectively.[25] A systematic review of 200 studies found a CR-BSI incidence for nonmedicated central catheters of 2.9/1,000 catheter days (95% cardiac index [CI] = 2.6 to 3.2) and 1.4/1,000 catheter days (95% CI = 0.8 to 2.0) for peripheral arterial lines.[26]

Evidence-based guidelines exist for the prevention of CR-BSI (Table 21-1).[42,43] In 2006, the results of the effect of an

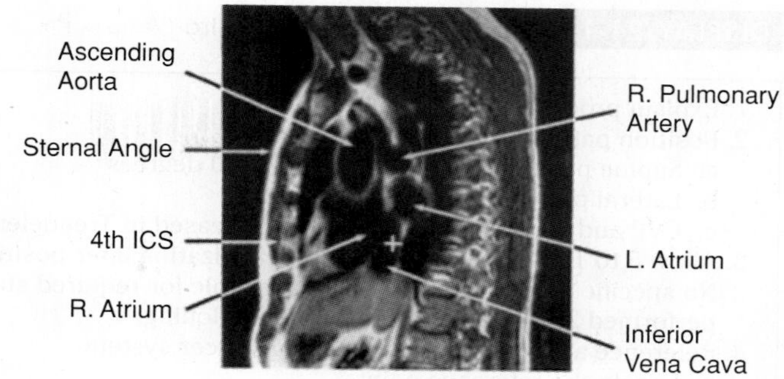

■ **Figure 21-1** Magnetic resonance image of a 43-year-old man. White cross marks the phlebostatic axis. (Reproduced from McGee, S. R. [1998]. Physical examination of venous pressure. *American Heart Journal, 136*[1], 10–18.)

Fourth intercostal space
Lateral margin of sternum
A
Outermost point of posterior chest
Outermost point of sternum
45°
20°
0°
B
AIR-FLUID INTERFACE
PHLEBOSTATIC LEVEL
C

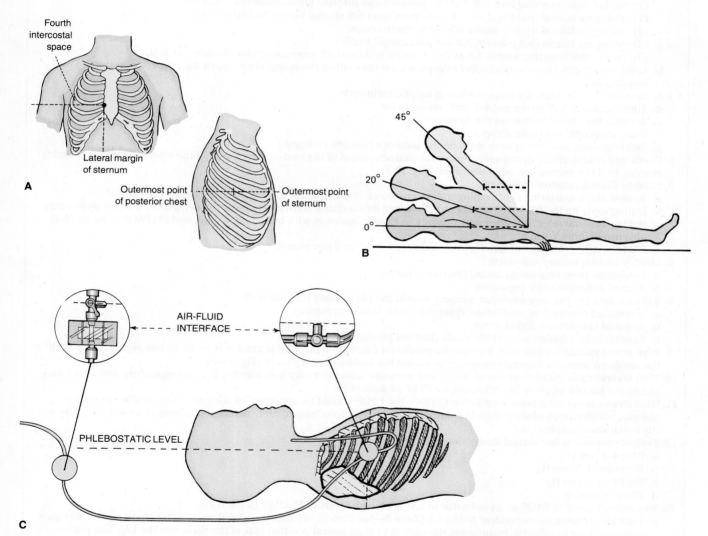

■ **Figure 21-2** The phlebostatic axis and the phlebostatic level. **(A)** The *phlebostatic axis* is the intersection of two reference lines: first, an imaginary line from the fourth ICS at the point where it joins the sternum, drawn out to the side of the body; second, a line drawn *midway* between the anterior and posterior surfaces of the chest. **(B)** The phlebostatic level is a horizontal line through the phlebostatic axis. The air–fluid interface of the stopcock of the transducer must be level with this axis for accurate measurements. Moving from the flat to erect positions, the patient moves the chest and therefore the reference level; the phlebostatic level stays horizontal through the same reference point. (Adapted from Shinn, J. A., Woods, S. L., Huseby, J. S. [1979]. Effect of intermittent positive pressure ventilation upon pulmonary capillary wedge pressures in acutely ill patients. *Heart & Lung, 8*, 324.) **(C)** Two methods for referencing the pressure system to the phlebostatic axis. The system can be referenced by placing the air–fluid interface of either the in-line stopcock or the stopcock on top of the transducer at the phlebostatic level. (From Bridges, E. J., & Woods, S. L. [1993]. Pulmonary artery pressure measurement: State of the art. *Heart & Lung, 22*, 101.)

DISPLAY 21-1 Protocol for Obtaining Central Venous Pressure, PA Pressure, and PAOP

1. Explain procedure to patient
2. Position patient in
   a. Supine position with backrest up to 60 degrees
   b. Lateral position at 30 or 90 degrees
   c. CVP and PA pressures are falsely increased in Trendelenburg and should not be used[10]
3. Allow 5 to 15 minutes for pressure stabilization after position change depending on the patients underlying LV function. No specific recommendations are available for required stabilization after prone positioning; measurements have been performed 20 to 60 minutes after repositioning.
4. Reference and zero the pressure-transducer system
   a. Locate the reference point
      (1) Supine: line bisecting fourth ICS at the sternum and one-half anteroposterior diameter
      (2) 30-degree lateral (right and left): 1/2 distance from left sternal border to surface of bed
      (3) 90-degree lateral (right): fourth ICS at the midsternum
      (4) 90-degree lateral (left): fourth ICS left parasternal border
      (5) Prone: line bisecting fourth ICS at the sternum and one-half anteroposterior diameter or MAL
   b. Level the air–fluid interface with the reference level (use either the in-line stopcock or the stopcock on the top of the transducer)
   c. Remove the cap from the stopcock using aseptic technique
   d. Turn stopcock "off" to the patient and "open" to air
   e. Activate the "Zero" button on the monitor
   f. Close stopcock and replace cap
   g. Reference and zero the system anytime the patient's position changes
5. Check and troubleshoot the dynamic response characteristics of the system every shift, if the waveform characteristics change, or if the system has been disturbed (Fig. 21-3)
6. Confirm Zone 3 catheter placement[11]
   a. Review anteroposterior chest radiograph to ensure catheter is below LA (LA is ~3 cm below the carina.
   b. During wedging the PA waveform should (1) flatten into a characteristic atrial waveform (distinct a and v waves may not be discernible), (2) immediately return to a PA configuration with balloon deflation, and (3) PAOP $<$ mean PA in absence of large V wave.
   c. PAEDP–PAOP gradient $>$ 4 mm Hg (may indicate Zone 1 or 2 placement).
7. Identify end-expiratory waveform
   a. Determine pressures using analog (graphic) tracing
   b. Record end-expiratory pressures
8. If digital data are the only available method, record the PAOP using the following:
   a. Controlled mechanical ventilation: diastolic mode (lowest pressure)
   b. Assisted ventilation: digital mean
   c. Spontaneous ventilation: systolic mode (highest pressure)
9. With active exhalation (suspect if respiratory-induced fluctuation in PAOP is greater than 10–15 mm Hg) read the PAOP at the midpoint between the end-expiratory peak and the end-inspiratory nadir (Fig. 21-5)
10. With inverse-ratio ventilation use of the airway pressure waveform may help identify the end-expiratory phase and consideration should be given to correcting for PEEP or auto-PEEP.
11. With airway pressure release ventilation (APRV), the PAOP should be measured at the end of the positive pressure plateau, which can be observed on the ventilator and is the point immediately before the release of airway pressure and the initiation of inspiration.[12]
12. Evaluate pressures for normal fluctuation and trends
    a. PAS: 4–7 mm Hg
    b. PA mean: 4–5 mm Hg
    c. PAEDP: 4–7 mm Hg
    d. PAOP: 4 mm Hg
13. Improve accuracy of PAOP as an indicator of LAP with high levels of PEEP ($>$10 cm H_2O)
    a. Position catheter tip dependent to the LA (Zone 3—See step 6) or position patient so catheter tip is below LA (e.g., if catheter tip is in right PA, positioning the patient in right lateral position places the tip below the LA). Use angle-specific reference.
    b. Analyze the pulmonary capillary occlusion blood. This confirms correct wedging but does not confirm that PAOP is an accurate indicator of LAP.
    c. Estimate effect of increased transmural pressure on PAOP. Subtract ½ applied PEEP (1 cm H_2O = 0.73 mm Hg) from measured PAOP.[13] Example: 15 cm H_2O PEEP; measured PAOP = 18 mm Hg:

$$15 \text{ cm } H_2O \times 0.73 = 11.1 \text{ mm Hg}$$
$$18 \text{ mm Hg} - \tfrac{1}{2}(11.1 \text{ mm Hg})$$
$$\text{Estimated PAOP} = 12.4 \text{ mm Hg}$$

    This is the largest pressure correction possible. Decreased compliance may lessen the effect; for example, with ARDS only 1/3 of the PEEP may be transmitted to the pleural space.[14]
    d. Suspect non-zone 3 placement if with an increase in PEEP, the PAOP increases greater than ½ the applied PEEP increment (i.e., PEEP increased by 5 cm H_2O (3.7 mm Hg), and PAOP increases greater than 1.8 mm Hg (3.7 mm Hg/2 = 1.8 mm Hg).

DISPLAY 21-2 Preparation of Invasive Pressure Monitoring System[22]

1. Wash hands
2. Gather supplies: bag of intravenous normal saline, pressure monitoring kit, 10 cc luer-lock syringe, and pressure bag with self-venting gauge
3. Prime pressure monitoring system to remove all air
   a. Remove pressure monitoring kit from package, open blood salvage reservoir, tighten connections, close roller clamp, turn stopcock OFF to patient (off toward distal end), and remove vented (white) stopcock cap
   b. Remove IV port cover and pressure monitoring line spike cover
   c. Invert IV bag to orient bag upside down and using sterile technique, insert spike into IV bag
   d. Leave the spiked bag upside down, open roller clamp, and simultaneously pull (activate) fast-flush device (pigtail) continuously while *gently squeezing* to apply pressure to IV bag to slowly clear air from IV bag and drip chamber. Completely fill the drip chamber with IV fluid.
   e. Turn IV bag upright once fluid is advanced sufficiently past the drip chamber
   f. Apply gentle pressure to the IV bag (or hang the bag ~30 in. above distal end of tubing) and pull fast-flush device, advance fluid, priming the stopcock
   g. Orient fluid so that air will be completely removed by the advancing fluid (tilt distal end of reservoir upright at 45° angle)
   h. Pull (activate) fast-flush device while holding blood reservoir at angle, continuing to flush until the entire line is primed
   i. Close blood reservoir, advancing all reservoir fluid through line
   j. Perform Rocket Flush (*Do not perform rocket flush if pressure line is attached to patient.*)
      (1) Turn stopcock off to distal end of catheter ("off to patient")
      (2) Attach a 10-mL syringe to the stopcock near the transducer using sterile technique and slowly withdraw IV fluid to fill syringe
      (3) Turn stopcock off to transducer ("off to monitor")
      (4) Flush line quickly with 10 mL NS from syringe to remove any remaining air bubbles; avoid instilling any air into the line
      (5) Turn stopcock off to port and remove syringe
      (6) Cap stopcock using sterile technique with solid blue cap
4. Place IV bag into self-venting pressure bag and inflate to reach 250 to 300 mm Hg and recheck for air in line
5. Inspect line, remove any remaining air by flushing line using Rocket Flush as indicated by the dynamic response of the system (goal—adequate or optimal system)[23]

Reproduced with permission from Bridges, E. J., Schmelz, J., & Kelley, P. W. (2008). Military nursing research: Translation to disaster response and day-to-day critical care nursing. *Critical Care Nursing Clinics of North America, 20*(1), 121–131.

evidence-based bundle of the procedures aimed at decreasing CR-BSI was published.[44] Use of this bundle, which includes hand washing, using full-barrier precautions during the insertion of central venous catheters, cleaning the skin with chlorhexidine, avoiding the femoral site if possible, and removing unnecessary catheters along with staff education and empowerment and the use of champions, significantly decreased the incidence of CR-BSI from 2.7/1,000 catheter days to 1.4/1,000 catheter days 18 months after the intervention.[44,45] Other studies that emphasize the effect of staff education, multifaceted interventions, and performance feedback have also led to a significant decrease in CR-BSI.[31,46,47] Despite the risk for CR-BSI from arterial lines there are only limited recommendations for arterial line insertion and care, and consideration should be given to using the Centers for Disease Control and Prevention (CDC) recommendations and procedure bundle for central lines for arterial line maintenance.[28,48–50]

Dynamic Response Characteristics

The dynamic response characteristics of the catheter–transducer system reflect the system's ability to faithfully reproduce a pressure waveform. The dynamic response can be determined by evaluating the system's damping coefficient and natural (resonant) frequency (Fig. 21-3). The damping coefficient is a measure of how quickly the system dampens and eventually arrests the oscillations. A certain degree of damping is desirable for optimal fidelity and suppression of unwanted high-frequency vibration or noise. The natural frequency (F_n) refers to the frequency at which the system oscillates when shock excited.[51] As seen in Figure 21-4, the higher the F_n, the greater the range of acceptable damping. The F_n can be quickly assessed by measuring the horizontal distance between the points of two oscillations (each small box equals 1 mm) and dividing the paper speed (25 mm/s) by this value. For example, if there are two small boxes between oscillations, then the $F_n = 25/2 = 12.5$ Hz, which is marginally acceptable. Optimizing the F_n has the greatest effect on the reproduction of a waveform. The F_n of the catheter–transducer system decreases over time,[52] indicating the need to routinely evaluate the dynamic response characteristics of the system.

An underdamped system results in falsely high systolic (15 to 30 mm Hg) and low diastolic pressures. An overdamped system loses its characteristic landmarks, and the waveform appears unnaturally smooth with a diminished or absent dicrotic notch. An overdamped system causes falsely low systolic and high diastolic pressure readings. PA catheters have a decreased F_n compared with arterial pressure lines[52]; thus, taking steps to optimize the system is imperative. The simpler the system (e.g., shorter tubing and fewer stopcocks) the better its ability to reproduce faithfully the pressure waveforms.[23,51,53] Use of in-line blood conservation devices decrease the F_n of the system, resulting in an underdamped system.[54]

Table 21-1 ■ CR-BSI CONTROL

Steps	Comments
Skin antisepsis	• Skin antisepsis with a 2% chlorhexidene preparation is superior to 10% povidone–iodine or 70% alcohol in preventing catheter colonization[27]
Insertion technique	• Central venous catheter: maximum sterile technique for insertion (cap, mask, sterile gloves, sterile gown, large sterile drapes) • Arterial line (not specifically addressed): technique similar to short-term central venous catheter
Hand hygiene	• Perform hand hygiene before and after manipulating catheters/catheter site • Use of gloves does not obviate the need for good hand washing
Location of insertion site	• Higher BSI rates associated with internal jugular or femoral vain insertion site compared to subclavian vein insertion site; avoid lower extremity if possible • Higher contamination and BSI incidence with femoral artery insertion site compared with radial artery insertion site[28–30] • Increased BSI with reinsertion over a guidewire at old insertion site
Antimicrobial catheters	• Antibiotic-impregnated catheters (minocyclin/rifampicin) decrease the risk of CR-BSIs compared with standard catheters and chlorhexidene/silver sulfadiazine catheters[31–34] • Catheters coated with chlorhexidene/silver sulfadiazine and heparin bonding may decrease the risk of CR-BSI[31,40–42] • Consider use of antimicrobial catheters if catheter is to remain in place >5 days and current hospital BSI rate exceeds 2%[35] or NNIS standards
Catheter sleeve (PA catheter)	• Use sterile sleeve during PA catheter insertion
Frequency of catheter change	• Routine catheter replacement is not recommended[36] • Change PA catheters no more frequently than every 7 days[37] • Arterial line (manage similar to short-term central venous catheters)—no specific CDC recommendations for catheters that need to be in place >5 days. • Risk for colonization increases wither greater than 4 days *in situ*;[28,29] however, there are no studies suggesting a need for routine catheter replacement for infection control prevention • Evaluate daily the patients need for central and arterial catheters
Dressing	• Use sterile gauze or sterile, transparent semipermeable membrane dressing • Change gauze dressing every 2 days and transparent dressing at least every 7 days, when the dressing becomes, damp, loose, or soiled or for site inspection
Flush solution	• Do not administer dextrose-containing solutions through the pressure monitoring system
Administration set	• Continuous-flush device • Replace pressure transducers and all tubing and flush solution every 96 hours
Obtaining cultures from central venous and arterial catheters	• Drawing cultures from only one lumen of a multilumen catheter has a 60% chance of detecting significant colonization. If only one lumen is sampled a negative culture does not necessarily rule out the CVC as a source of infection.[38] Colonization of the medial lumen is an independent risk factor for CR-BSI[39] • Cultures obtained through a central venous or arterial catheter have a lower positive predictive value and similar or better negative predictive values compared with peripheral cultures, which indicates that additional cases of bacteremia may be identified from the catheter culture in addition to peripheral cultures[40,41]

CDC, Centers for Disease Control and Prevention; NNIS, National Nosocomial Infections Surveillance System

Blood Drawing From Arterial and Central Venous Catheters

Arterial blood gases, serum electrolytes, and coagulation studies can be drawn from an arterial line. To avoid contamination of the specimen with saline and/or heparin, two times the deadspace volume (volume from the catheter tip to the aspiration site) or two times the deadspace plus 2 mL (approximately equivalent to six times the deadspace) should be withdrawn for arterial blood gases and electrolytes.[56] For coagulation studies (e.g., PT/aPTT), the discard volume should be four to six times the deadspace volume.[57,58] If an in-line blood conservation set is used, caution must be exercised to ensure that an adequate discard volume is obtained.[59] If heparin is used in the flush solution and the coagulation results are abnormal, consideration should be given to using a venipuncture specimen to confirm the results.

Serum sodium and glucose can be obtained from the infusion port of the PA catheter if the dwell volume plus 2 mL of additional blood is discarded.[60] No published research was found regarding measurement of potassium or other electrolytes from PA catheters; however, in a study of central venous lines it was found that a discard volume of 3 mL (corresponding to six times the catheter deadspace) was sufficient after initially flushing the line with 5 mL of saline.[61] Coagulation studies (Activated clotting time [ACT]) drawn from heparin-bonded PA catheters,[62] and the introducer side-port when the PA catheter is present[63] are significantly increased compared with specimens obtained from an arterial catheter although baseline specimens can be obtained from the introducer before placement of the PA catheter.[64]

DIRECT ARTERIAL PRESSURE MONITORING

Indications

Intra-arterial monitoring is indicated when precise and continuous monitoring is required. Examples of clinical conditions warranting direct arterial pressure monitoring include acute hypertensive crises, hypotension, any shock state, frequent drawing of arterial blood samples, monitoring of vasoactive pharmacologic support, and during aggressive respiratory support (e.g., high positive end-expiratory pressures [PEEP]).

Arterial Catheter Placement

Important considerations in site selection for arterial catheters include patient comfort, avoidance of insertion sites at increased risk

Decision Making Algorithm

How to Assess Dynamic Response Characteristics

1. Determine Natural Frequency of System (Fn)
   a. Fast Flush System and Record Strip
   b. Measure period (t) of once cycle
   c. Fn=Paper speed (mm/sec)/one cycle (mm)
2. Determine Amplitude Ratio
   Compare the amplitude of two successive peaks (A2/A1)
3. Plot Amplitude Ratio Against Natural Frequency
   -Apply algorithm if system other than OPTIMAL or ADEQUATE

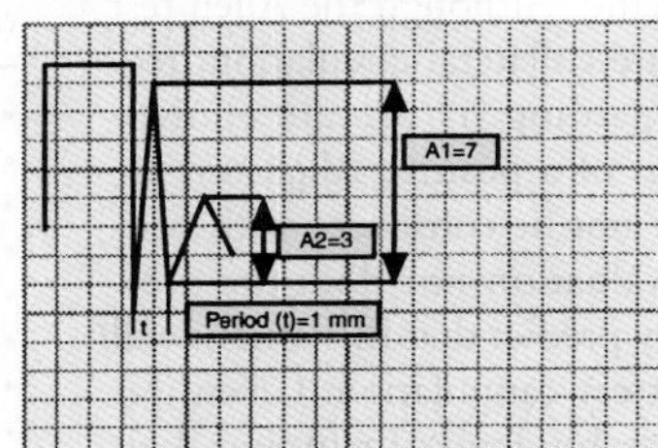

Example:
1) Determine Fn
Paper Speed=25 mm/sec
t=1 mm
Fn=25/1=25 cycles/sec
2) Determine Amplitude
A2/A1=3/7=0.43
3) Plot on graph=ADEQUATE

Frequency versus Amplitude Ratio Plot

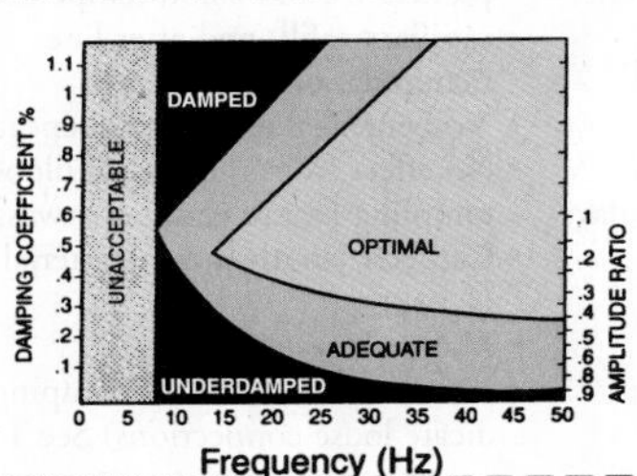

Frequency versus damping coefficient plot that illustrates the five areas into which the catheter, tubing, and transducer systems fall. Systems in the optimal area reproduce even the most demanding (fast heart rate and rapid systolic upstroke) waveforms without distortion. Systems in the adequate area reproduce the most typical waveforms with little or no distortion. All other areas cause serious wave distortion. (Gardner, RM Hollingsworth, KW: Optimizing the electrocardiogram and pressure monitoring. Crit Care Med 14: 651-658m 1986. With permission).

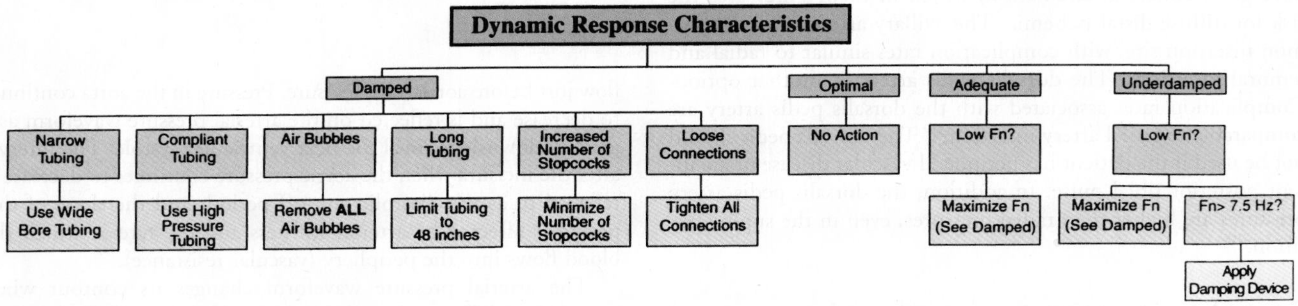

■ **Figure 21-3** Dynamic response characteristics. (Adapted with permission from Bridges, E. J., & Middleton, R. [1997]. Direct arterial vs. oscillometric monitoring of blood pressure: Stop comparing and pick one [a decision-making algorithm]. *Critical Care Nurse, 17*[3], 58–72.)

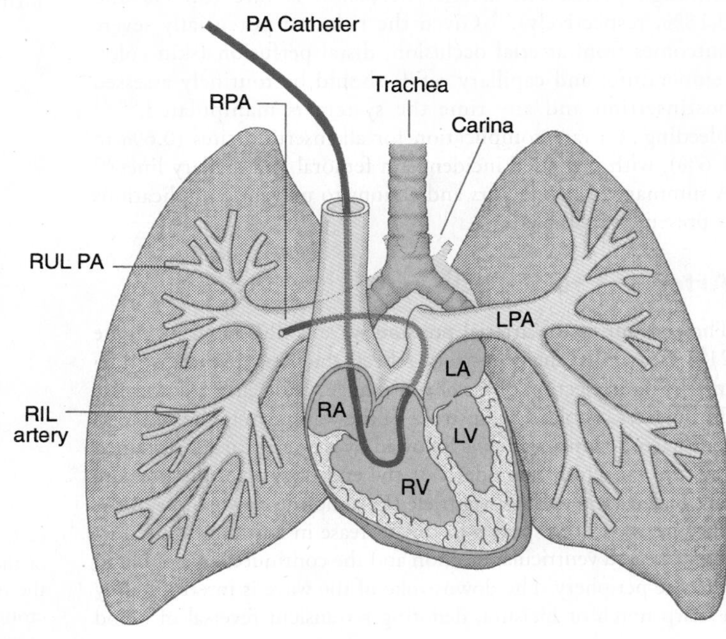

■ **Figure 21-4** Schema of the cardiopulmonary structures demonstrating the relationship between the LA, PA, and pulmonary vasculature, with a correctly positioned PA catheter. RUL PA, right upper lobe PA; RIL, right interlobar PA; RPA, right PA; LPA, left PA; RV, right ventricle; .

for infection, and adequate collateral circulation.[65] The most common insertion site is the radial artery due to the presence of collateral circulation, which decreases the risk of vascular complications. The radial and ulnar artery/superficial palmar arteries provide a dual blood supply to the hand. Although the Allen test has traditionally been used to evaluate collateral circulation, recommendations in the literature regarding its use are equivocal.[66,67] In addition, the implications of a positive Allen test are equivocal. The positive findings may not be consistent with concurrent Doppler ultrasonography evaluation nor does the presence of an abnormal Allen test reliably predict that the patient will develop hand ischemia after radial artery cannulation. Given this limited diagnostic accuracy, newer technologies including digit pressure measurement and plethysmography and Doppler ultrasonography should be considered, particularly for patients who are at increased risk for complications from the catheterization (e.g., peripheral vascular disease or diabetes, previous extremity surgery or trauma, current anticoagulation or vasopressor therapy, and hypotension).[68]

The femoral artery is often an alternative to the radial artery. However, there is an increased risk of infection with the femoral site. The brachial artery is used less frequently because it does not have good collateral circulation, which in theory increases the risk for diffuse distal ischemia. The axillary artery is a less common insertion site, with complication rates similar to radial and femoral insertions. The dorsalis pedis artery is another option. Complication rates associated with the dorsalis pedis artery are comparable to radial artery insertion.[69] The dorsalis pedis should not be used if the patient has peripheral vascular disease or an absent posterior tibial pulse. In addition, the dorsalis pedis artery pressures are higher than radial pressures, even in the supine position.[70]

Complications Related to Arterial Catheterization

The most common complication from arterial cannulation is temporary occlusion of the artery (radial 19.7%; femoral 1.5%), although permanent arterial occlusion is rare (0.09% and 0.18%, respectively).[65] Given the risk and potentially severe outcomes from arterial occlusion, distal perfusion (skin color, temperature, and capillary refill) should be routinely assessed postinsertion and any time the system is manipulated.[68,71] Bleeding is a rare complication for all insertion sites (0.6% to 1.6%), with increased incidence in femoral and axillary lines.[65] A summary of risk factors and actions to prevent complications is presented in Table 21-2.

Arterial Pressure Wave

The contour of the arterial pressure wave is illustrated in Figure 21-5. The initial sharp upstroke reflects the pressure increase during the rapid ejection phase of ventricular systole and a slower rise during later systole. The upstroke of the waveform is referred to as the anacrotic limb, which is followed by a brief, peaked, sustained pressure (anacrotic shoulder). At the end of systole, the pressure falls in the aorta and left ventricle (LV) and the downstroke of the pressure wave corresponds to the decrease in aortic pressure during decreased ventricular ejection and the continued flow of blood into the periphery. The downstroke of the wave is interrupted by a sharp notch or incisura, denoting a transient reversal of blood flow just before aortic valve closure. Pressure in the aorta continues to decrease and is reflected on the arterial pressure waveform as a gradual downslope until the next ventricular systole. The interval after the incisura when the aortic pressure continues to decrease is referred to as the diastolic run-off period, and the slope of this period is affected by arterial stiffness and the rate at which the blood flows into the periphery (vascular resistance).[79]

The arterial pressure waveform changes its contour when recorded at different sites along the arterial circuit[80] (Fig. 21-6). The pulse pressure and the systolic pressure increase, and the ascending limb of the waveform becomes steeper. In addition, the incisura is gradually replaced by a later diastolic wave (dicrotic notch). The change in amplitude and contour of the arterial waveform is primarily caused by peripheral pulse wave reflection.[81]

Table 21-2 ■ RISK FACTORS AND ACTIONS TO PREVENT COMPLICATIONS ASSOCIATED WITH ARTERIAL CATHETERIZATION

Risk Factors	Preventive Actions
• Catheter >20 gauge • Catheter in place >3 days • Female • Low CO/hypotension • Peripheral vascular disease • Vasopressor agents	• Use of heparinized flush solution to maintain patency is equivocal. Consideration should also be given to risk of heparin-induced thrombocytopenia.[72–77]
• Anticoagulation (↓ risk) • Femoral (↓ risk) • Systemic antithrombotics or anticoagulants (↓ risk) • Insertion site (femoral or axillary)	• Aspirate clot or discontinue line if thrombosis is suspected • Perform routine monitoring of distal perfusion (skin color, temperature and capillary refill) and after line manipulation
• Insertion site preparation • Catheter in place >5–7 days • Insertion site	• No beneficial effect from repeated flushes • No effect from method of blood sampling (waste versus nonwaste)[78] • Catheter length sheaths/arterial lines (↓ risk) • Maintain system integrity • Monitor waveform for damping (may indicate loose connections) See Table 21-1

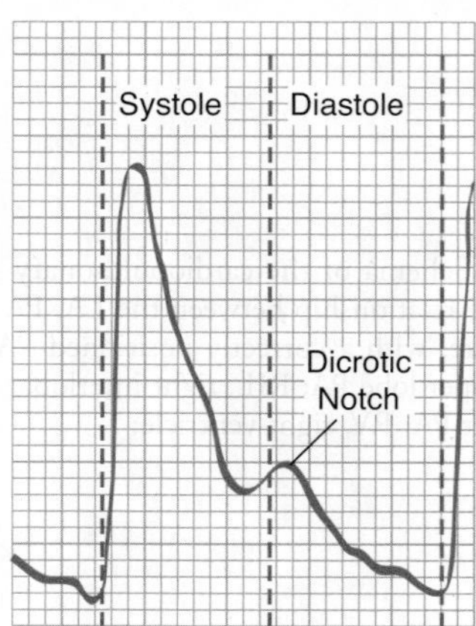

■ **Figure 21-5** Components of the arterial waveform. The upstroke of the arterial waveform, which begins approximately 0.2 second after the onset of the QRS complex indicates the onset of systole. The dicrotic notch reflects closure of the aortic valve and the onset of diastole.

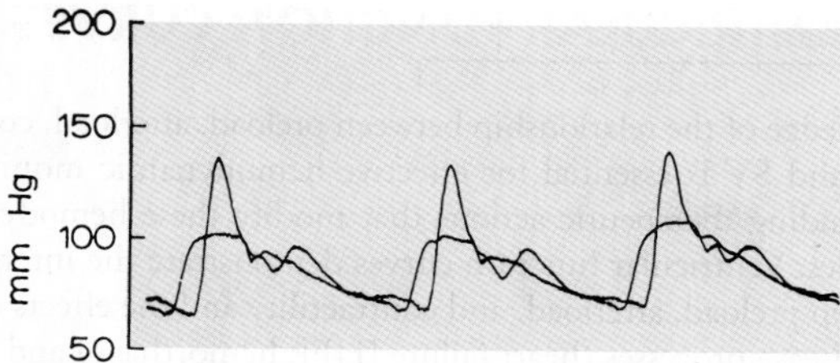

■ **Figure 21-6** Simultaneous recordings of aortic and radial arterial pressure waves. (From Rowell, L. D., Brengelmann, G. L., Blackmon, R. J. et al. [1968]. Disparities between aortic and peripheral pulse pressures induced by upright exercise and vasomotor changes in man. *Circulation, 37*, 954–964.)

Reflection occurs when flow is impeded (i.e., when low-resistance arteries terminate in high-resistance vessels) and the pressure wave is reflected in a retrograde (backward) fashion. This retrograde pressure wave combines with the antegrade (forward) pressure pulse, and the arterial pressure is augmented.

The timing of the return of the reflected pressure wave from the periphery is important because if the reflected wave arrives during systole it increases LV workload.[82,83] In young individuals, the reflected waves arrive at the heart after closure of the aortic valves, which beneficially augments the diastolic blood pressure (DBP) and thus coronary perfusion. However, with aging or increased stiffness of the arteries (i.e., hypertension), the retrograde pulse wave arrives back at the heart during systole, which increases the systolic blood pressure (SBP).[82,83]

Recognition of central aortic systolic pressure augmentation is important in evaluating the effects of various vasodilator agents. Nitroglycerin and nitroprusside substantially decrease aortic pressure without a clinically measurable change in brachial pressure.[84,85] This effect, which is the result of the reduction in pulse–wave reflection (Fig. 21-7), may explain why a patient may "look better" after the initiation of vasodilator therapy even though there has been no marked decrease in peripheral BP or preload. Conversely, vasoconstrictive agents (e.g., norepinephrine) increase peripheral pulse pressure and central aortic pressure, with femoral pressure higher than radial pressure.[86,87]

Interpretation of Arterial Pressure Data

The mean arterial pressure (MAP), which represents the average pressure through a cardiac cycle, is affected by the CO and systemic vascular resistance (SVR) as described by the following equation:

$$\text{MAP} = \text{CO} \times \text{SVR}$$

Recall of the factors that affect SBP, DBP, and MAPs is important when assessing changes in BP. The SBP is affected by left ventricular stroke volume (SV), peak rate of ejection, and distensibility of the vessel walls. The DBP is primarily affected by arterial peripheral resistance. The pulse pressure, which is the difference between systolic and diastolic pressures, is determined by SV, peak rate of ventricular ejection, and the distensibility of the arterial walls.

On average, more central SBP (aortic, femoral, or brachial) is lower than radial SBP by 7 to 14 mm Hg and central DBP similar to or higher than radial DBP by 1 to 9 mm Hg, while the MAP is unchanged and may be a more consistent value to evaluate and guide therapy.[88–90] The SBP differences change with aging (radial SBP $\approx$ aortic SBP),[91,92] vasoconstriction (radial $<$ brachial and femoral),[86,87] vasodilation (femoral $\approx$ radial; aortic $\leq$ radial),[93,94] and exercise (peripheral SBP may be as much as 80 mm Hg higher than central aortic pressure).[80] Both peripheral wave reflection and the end-pressure product, which is the result of the conversion of kinetic energy from flowing blood into pressure as the blood strikes the upstream-looking arterial catheter, cause augmentation of the peripheral SBP.[95] Regardless of the source or site of BP measurement, a key point is that BP and perfusion are not synonymous, and a higher BP does not necessarily translate to higher perfusion.[96]

Direct Arterial Versus Cuff Pressure

There is no basis for the practice of comparing the intra-arterial BP with the auscultatory or oscillometric BP to determine if one system should be followed to guide therapy. The direct method is based on pressure, whereas the oscillometric method depends on flow-induced oscillations in the arterial wall. An erroneous assumption is that pressure equals flow. As described by

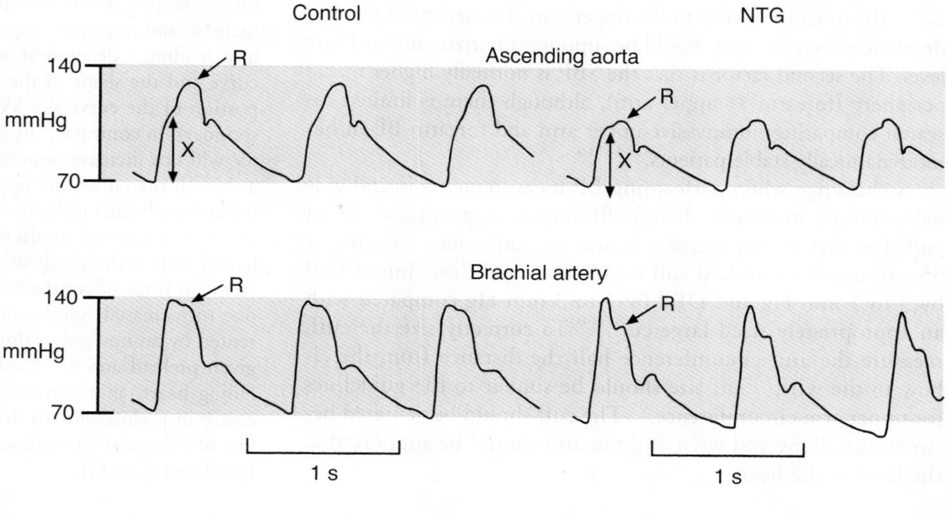

■ **Figure 21-7** Pressure wave recorded directly in a central and peripheral artery. Nitroglycerine 0.3 mg (SL) on average caused a fall of 11 mm Hg in aortic systolic pressure more than the decrease in the brachial systolic pressure. Note the effect on the reflected (R) wave. (From Kelly, R. P., Gibbs, H. H., O'Rourke, M. F., et al. [1990]. Nitroglycerine has more favourable effects on left ventricular afterload than apparent from measurement of pressure in a peripheral artery. *European Heart Journal, 11*, 138–144.)

a derivation of Ohm's law (pressure = flow × resistance), if resistance remains constant, there is a direct relationship between pressure and flow. However, clinically, resistance is seldom constant. Thus, BP may appear adequate while flow is decreased, or conversely BP may be low although perfusion remains adequate. Algorithms and evidence-based guidelines are available to guide assessment of the physiological and technical factors that affect direct and indirect BP measurements and outline the correct performance and interpretation of these BP measurements.[22,23,97,98]

In addition to the physical factors that cause the differences in arterial pressure measured in various locations in the body, there are also technical factors that affect measurement accuracy (see Fig. 21-3).[23,99,100] In addition, the oscillometric system directly measures the mean pressure and extrapolates the systolic and diastolic pressure based on an algorithm, which may affect the accuracy of the systolic and diastolic pressure measurements.

For direct and oscillometric BP monitoring the correct reference is the heart. If the transducer or the arm is positioned above the heart, there will be a decrease in the measured pressure. Conversely, if the transducer/arm is positioned below the heart, there will be an increase in the measured pressure.[101–103] When the patient is in the sitting position, for oscillometric or auscultated BP measurements, the arm should be supported at the level of the heart (level of the midsternum). If the arm is parallel to the patient or supported on the armrest the SBP and DBP may be 10 mm Hg higher than if the arm is supported horizontally at heart level (level of the midsternum)[104–109] and in patients with hypertension the difference in arm position may cause a 20 mm Hg overestimation of SBP.[108] If the patient is in a lateral recumbent position, the noninvasive BP measurements taken from the "up arm" may be 13 to 17 mm Hg lower than those if the patient is in supine position, and BP measurements from the "down arm" are similar to those taken at supine position or inconsistent.[110–112] If the "up arm" is used, the measured pressure can be corrected by measuring the distance from the angle-specific phlebostatic axis (see Display 21-1) and correcting the pressure (1 cm = 0.73 mm Hg or 1 in. = 1.8 mm Hg).

Forearm BP measurements may be necessary in cases in which access to the upper arm is not possible or an appropriate cuff is not available (i.e., the existence of morbid obesity or a conical-shaped arm).[113] Two factors need to be considered when comparing the BP from the upper arm and the forearm. First, if the arm is in a dependent position, the hydrostatic pressure increases the BP in the forearm relative to the upper arm. To correct for this hydrostatic effect, the arm should be supported horizontally at heart level. The second factor is that the SBP is normally higher in the periphery (forearm > upper arm), although there is limited research comparing noninvasive upper arm and forearm BP in hemodynamically stable patients.[114–116]

A challenge when performing BP measurements in individuals who are morbidly obese is finding an appropriately sized cuff. For every 5 cm increase in arm circumference (starting at 35 cm) use of a standard cuff leads to an overestimation of SBP by 3 to 5 mm Hg and DBP by 1 to 3 mm Hg compared with an appropriately sized large cuff.[100] To correctly size the cuff, measure the arm circumference half the distance from the elbow to the wrist. Cuff size should be similar to the guidelines for upper arm circumference.[97] The cuff should be centered between the elbow and wrist and the arm should be supported at the level of the heart.

VENTRICULAR FUNCTION CURVES

Knowledge of the relationship between preload, afterload, contractility, and SV is essential for effective hemodynamic monitoring and guiding therapeutic actions that modify these hemodynamic variables. Ventricular function curves demonstrate the interaction between preload, afterload, and contractility and the effects of various disease processes (heart failure [HF], hemorrhage) and therapeutic actions (vasodilator or inotropic drug therapy) on SV and CO (Fig. 21-8). The family of curves varies for each patient but is useful in predicting and evaluating the effects of various therapeutic interventions. The curves are constructed by plotting the PA occlusion pressure (PAOP) (or some measure of end-diastolic volume or preload) on the horizontal axis and the CO, CI, or SV on the vertical axis. A key point is that an increase in SV in response to a fluid bolus (change in preload) cannot be reliably predicted on the basis of the standard preload indices (CVP, PAOP) or volumetric indices (right ventricular [RV] end-diastolic volume, global end-diastolic volume), because the response depends on ventricular function, as indicated by the slope of the ventricular function curve.[117] The traditional preload indices remain useful in the differential diagnosis and determining a patient's risk for pulmonary edema.

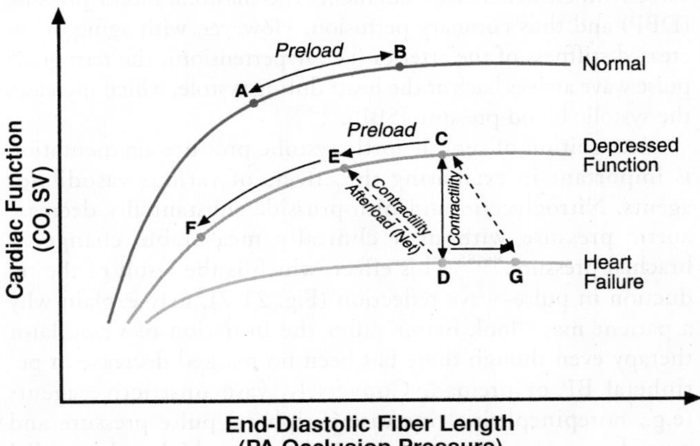

■ **Figure 21-8** Family of ventricular function curves representing normal, depressed, and severely depressed function. A change in preload is represented by a move up or down a single curve (Frank–Starling principle). Point A to point B and point B to point A reflect an increase and decrease, respectively, in preload. The response to volume loading is dependent on the position on the ventricular function curve and the shape of the curve. If both ventricles are on the steep portion of the curve the SV will increase in response to volume (responder). In contrast if the heart is on the flat portion of the curve the SV will not increase (nonresponder). A change in afterload results in a shift in the curve that appears similar to that caused by contractility, although the mechanism is different. Point D to E reflects the net effect of a decrease in afterload on a failing heart. This upward and lateral shift is the result of two actions. Point D to C reflects an increase in force of contraction and point C to E a decrease in preload due to increased systolic ejection. A change in contractility is represented by an upward or downward shift of the curve, that is, for any given preload and afterload, the CO is increased or decreased. In a failing heart, an additional effect of decreased contractility is an increase in preload due to decreased systolic ejection; thus, the net effect of a decrease in contractility is to shift the curve down and to the left (Point C to G).

CVP MONITORING

The CVP directly reflects right atrial pressure (RAP) and indirectly reflects the preload of the right ventricle or RV end-diastolic pressure. The CVP is determined by vascular tone, the volume of blood returning to the heart, the pumping ability of the heart, and patient position (supine, standing).

The CVP is measured in the superior vena cava and the RAP is measured from the proximal port of the PA catheter. The CVP and RAP are generally similar as long as there is no vena caval obstruction. Normally, the CVP ranges from 3 to 8 cm H_2O or 2 to 6 mm Hg (1 mm Hg = 1.36 cm H_2O). In the supine/flat position, a CVP of less than 2 mm Hg may indicate hypovolemia, vasodilation, or increased myocardial contractility. An increased CVP may indicate increased circulatory blood volume, vasoconstriction, or decreased myocardial contractility. An increased CVP is also observed in RV failure, tricuspid insufficiency, positive-pressure breathing, pericardial tamponade, pulmonary embolus, and obstructive pulmonary disease.

Indications

The placement of a central venous or RA catheter is indicated to secure venous access, to administer vasoactive drugs and parenteral nutrition, and to monitor right heart preload. Hemodynamic monitoring using a CVP is most often performed when cardiopulmonary function is relatively normal. Monitoring the CVP has regained importance with the recognition of the effect of right heart function on left heart function.[7]

Effect of Catheter Type and Location on CVP

The CVP may be monitored via a central venous catheter or the distal port of a multilumen catheter.[118] One study also suggests that measurements obtained via tunneled catheters are comparable to direct RA pressure measurements.[119]

In cases where placement of a central venous catheter is not possible, recent studies suggest that the CVP can be indirectly measured from a peripheral venous catheter inserted in the forearm or dorsal hand veins[120,121] or from a lower extremity insertion site.[122] A key to the use of peripheral venous pressure (PVP) measurements is ensuring that there is continuity between the central and venous systems, which can be assessed by observing for an increase in the PVP with a sustained inspiratory effort (Valsalva) or the occlusion of the arm or leg above the catheter insertion site (Fig. 21-9).[122,123] The PVP–CVP difference decreases with increasing CVP,[124] which may reflect vascular continuity. No significant pressure differences were found on the basis of catheter size (14 to 20 gauge) and patient position (as long as the system was referenced to the phlebostatic axis)[120,122] in patients who were hemodynamically unstable,[125] had a decreased ejection fraction (EF), or were receiving vasoactive medications.[121] In general, changes in CVP were mirrored by changes in PVP, which suggests that trends in PVP may be useful. However, clinically significant PVP–CVP differences (>2 to 3 mm Hg) may occur; thus, caution must be exercised when interpreting the absolute PVP values.[120,121,123–128]

There is limited evidence that suggests that CVP measurements can be obtained through an open-ended peripherally inserted central venous catheter (PICC).[129–131] Measurements from the PICC, overestimate measurements from a central catheter by approximately 1 mm Hg and changes in the PICC CVP are closely related to central line CVP measurements.[129,131] Accurate PICC CVP measurements require correct positioning of the PICC tip (at the junction of the vena cava and RA). Passive hydrostatic pressure equilibration across the PICC line takes approximately 60 minutes, but this pressure gradient can be overcome immediately with a pressure line infusing fluid at 3 mL/h.[129] The CVP cannot be measured if the system has a valve (e.g., Groshong, PASV, or PowerPICC SOLO). A limitation of the use of peripheral versus central line during resuscitation is that the peripheral catheter cannot be used to obtain central venous oxygen saturation, which is an end-point of resuscitation.[132]

Limitations

The CVP is not an accurate indicator of LV function or left heart preload.[133] In the presence of normal right heart function, severe deterioration of LV function may not be reflected by a change in

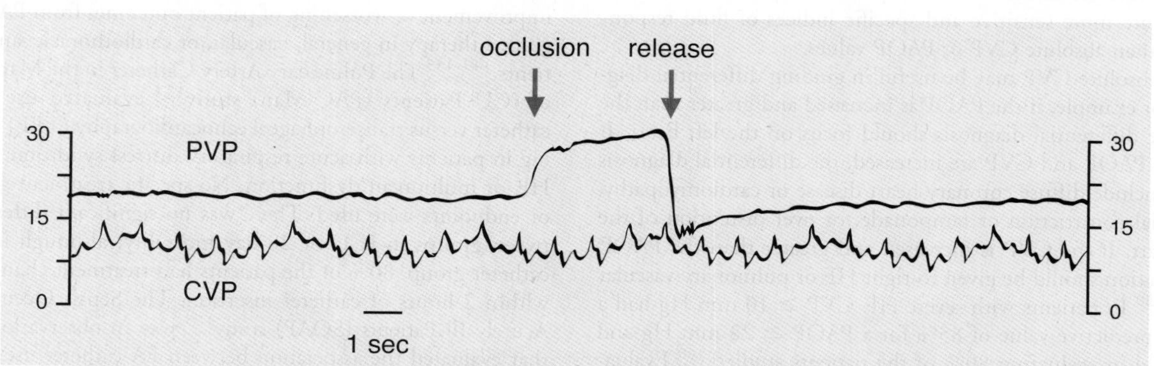

Figure 21-9 Pressure waveforms from simultaneous PVP and CVP measurements demonstrating the effect of manual, circumferential, proximal arm occlusion followed by release. This increase indicates there is continuity between the central and peripheral venous systems. The PVP should not be used if this response is absent. (From Munis, J. R., Bhatia, S., Lozada, L. J. [2001]. Peripheral venous pressure as a hemodynamic variable in neurosurgical patients. *Anesthesia & Analgesia, 92,* 174[.)

CVP. An increased CVP is usually an indication of later stages of LV failure, although the CVP may remain normal even in the presence of high PA pressures and pulmonary edema.

Complications

Complications associated with CVP monitoring include localized infection, arrhythmias, vessel laceration, RV perforation, thrombophlebitis, hematoma formation at the insertion site, and pneumothorax or a malpositioned catheter.[134] The most common predictor of complications, particularly pneumothorax, is the number of needle insertions required to access the vein. There is an increased risk of arterial puncture, but fewer malpositioned catheters, with the jugular approach.[134] Conversely, there may be a decreased risk of infection with a subclavian versus jugular or femoral insertion.[35,135]

Measurement Technique

The CVP system is referenced by placing the air–fluid interface of the stopcock at the level of the phlebostatic axis (see + in Fig. 21-1) or at a point 5 cm below the sternal angle. With correct referencing, the hemodynamically stable patient can be positioned up to 45 degrees for CVP measurements.[136]

An area of confusion when measuring the CVP from a triple lumen catheter is the question of which port to transduce. There are no research-based recommendations regarding port selection. The differences in pressures measured from the various ports are small (<1.5 mm Hg).[118] When the distal port is used there is limited effect from fluids administered via the more proximal ports.[137] Because of the potential for a clinically significant change in pressure depending on the port transduced, it seems prudent to transduce consistently one port, and if a change in the site of monitoring is necessary, to annotate the change on the flowsheet.

Interpretation of CVP Data

There has been increased use of CVP to guide therapy due to the decreased use of PA catheters and results of a study in patients with acute lung injury, which suggests that outcomes from therapy guided by central venous catheter measurements are similar to those guided by PA pressure measurements.[138] Assessment of the dynamic changes in the CVP in response to a fluid bolus or respiration are more sensitive and specific indices of fluid responsiveness than absolute CVP or PAOP values.

The absolute CVP may be useful in guiding differential diagnosis. For example, if the PAOP is increased and greater than the CVP, the differential diagnosis should focus on the left heart. If both the PAOP and CVP are increased, the differential diagnosis should include diffuse coronary heart disease or cardiomyopathy, pericardial constriction or tamponade, or over distention of the right heart. If the CVP is increased and greater than the PAOP, consideration should be given to right HF or pulmonary vascular disease.[139] In patients with severe HF, CVP $\geq$ 10 mm Hg had a positive predictive value of 85% for a PAOP $\geq$ 22 mm Hg and was useful in evaluating 80% of the patients studied.[140] Evaluation of left heart function should always include consideration of right heart function. Correct interpretation of the CVP requires knowledge of the patient's CO. For example, the treatment would be different for a patient with a low CVP and normal CO versus low CO.[141]

CVP is measured at end-diastole, although consideration must also be given to the effect of the maximal pressure. Useful clinical information can also be obtained by examining the CVP/RAP waveforms. There are five mechanical components (a, c, v waves and *x* and *y* descent) of the CVP waveform. A dual-channel strip chart recorder should be used to identify the corresponding venous pressure waves with the electrical events on the ECG (Display 21-3). The mean CVP is determined by bisecting the a, c, and v waves so that there are equal areas above and below the bisection or measured at the leading edge of the c wave (also known as the "z" point). The z point reflects the final pressure in the RA just before the onset of RV systole and the closure of the AV valves; thus, this point represents the RV end-diastolic pressure (preload). Alternatively, if the a and c waves cannot be visualized, draw a straight line through the Q wave or the upstroke of the arterial pressure waveform to identify end-diastole.[7] If there are large A and V waves, the CVP measurement should be made at the z point or the base of the a wave if the z point cannot be identified.[142] If there is a large A or V wave, the peak A or V wave pressure indicates increased upstream hydrostatic pressures (e.g., hepatic, renal). The CVP tracing may be useful in the diagnosis of wide-complex tachyarrhythmias of unknown origin, tricuspid regurgitation (large V wave that begins with the onset of systole), restriction of RV filling due to ventricular stiffness or volume overload (*y* descent > 4 mm Hg—these patients are not likely to respond with increased CO if given a fluid bolus),[143] pericardial tamponade (loss of x and *y* descent) (Fig. 21-10), and constrictive pericarditis.

PA PRESSURE MONITORING

Indications

Between 1993 and 2004, the use of PA catheters has decreased 65%,[144] with the greatest decrease occurring after the publication of a study of 5,735 patients in 1996, which suggested that PA catheter use may increase morbidity and mortality.[145] Since this study, several consensus conferences[146–148] identified patient populations for which PA pressure monitoring may be beneficial or additional outcome studies are needed and that there is a need for standardized education of critical care providers.

In response to the consensus conference recommendations a number studies have been completed. Several studies found no improvement or worsening of patient outcomes from PA catheter guided therapy in general, vascular, or cardiothoracic surgical patients.[149–153] The Pulmonary Artery Catheter in the Management of ICU Patients (PAC-Man) study[154] evaluated use of a PA catheter versus transesophageal echocardiography (TEE) monitoring in patients with acute respiratory distress syndrome (ARDS), HF, or multiorgan dysfunction. No specific treatment guidelines or endpoints were used. There was no significant difference between groups in ICU or 28-day mortality; although in the PA catheter group, 80% of the patients had treatment changes made within 2 hours of catheter insertion. The Sepsis Occurrence in Acutely Ill Patients (SOAP) study[155] was an observational study that evaluated the association between PA catheter use and outcome. Although the patients with PA catheters had a higher mortality rate, when confounding factors such as acuity, age, organ dysfunction, and comorbidities were controlled for, the use of a PA catheter was not associated with increased 60-day mortality. An interesting aspect of the secondary analysis of the SOAP study

DISPLAY 21-3 Relation of Central Venous/Right Atrial and PA Pressures to ECG

Pressures/Waveforms	Mechanical Event	ECG Findings	Example
RA Pressure (2–6 mm Hg)			
a wave	RA systole	80–100 milliseconds after P wave	
x descent	RA relaxation	(Downslope of the a wave)	
c wave	Tricuspid valve closure	After the QRS (follows the a wave by a time interval = PR)	**Interpretation:** RAP tracing from patient on mechanical ventilation. The RAP is a mean pressure (bisect an end-expiratory waveform so that the areas above and below are equal or measure at the onset of the c wave). RAP = 15 mm Hg
v wave	RA filling against closed tricuspid valve	Peak of the T wave	
y descent	RA emptying with opening of tricuspid valve (onset of RV diastole)	(Downslope of the v wave)	
PA Pressures			
Systolic (15–25 mm Hg) Diastolic (8–12 mm Hg) Mean (9–18 mm Hg)	RV ejection of blood into pulmonary vasculature Indirect indicator of LVEDP	T wave (read at peak of waveform 0.08 second after onset of QRS (Determine by bisecting the wave)	**Interpretation:** PA pressure waveform from spontaneously breathing patient
PAOP (6–12 mm Hg)			
a wave	Left atrial systole	~200–240 milliseconds after P wave	**Interpretation:** PAOP tracing from spontaneously breathing patient. The PAOP is a mean pressure (bisect an end-expiratory waveform so that the areas above and below are equal). PAOP = 6 mm Hg
x descent	Left atrial relaxation		
c wave		(Downslope of the a wave)	
v wave	Left atrial filling against closed mitral valve	TP interval	
y descent	Left atrial emptying associated with opening of mitral valve (onset of LV diastole)	(Downslope of the v wave)	

Bridges, E. J. (2000). Monitoring pulmonary artery pressures: Just the facts. *Critical Care Nurse, 20*(6), 59–80.
See Appendix A for a full version of Display 21-3 with the pertinent strips at the end of Book on page 938–939.

is that there was no significant difference in outcomes between patients managed with a PA catheter or other flow measuring device and those who did not have a flow measuring device, nor was there a difference in outcomes between patients managed with a PA catheter versus another flow measuring device.[156] In another study of patients with shock or ARDS there was no difference in 14- or 28-day mortality in patients with a PA catheter compared to those who received standard care without a PA catheter.[157] The Evaluation Study of Congestive Heart Failure and Pulmonary Artery Catheter Effectiveness (ESCAPE) evaluated the effect in therapy guided by clinical presentation only versus therapy guided by PAC indices in 433 patients with severe, acute, or chronic HF.[158] The targets were a resolution of pulmonary congestion and for the PA catheter group a PAOP $<$ 15 mm Hg and an RAP $<$ 8 mm Hg. Results indicated that there was no significant difference between groups in days alive out of the hospital within the first 6 months, 6-month mortality, or the number of days hospitalized. Patients in the PA catheter group did have a significantly higher time-trade-off than those in the control group. One possible explanation for this latter finding is the continued presence of increased PAOP and RAP (hemodynamic congestion) in the absence of clinical congestion.[159] There is clinical sequelae associated with hemodynamic congestion, which may have been relieved in the PA catheter group. A limitation of this study was the exclusion of patients with the most advanced HF (e.g., patients with severe renal dysfunction, prior use of inotropes, and the use of mechanical circulatory support devices or mechanical ventilation).[160,161]

A criticism of these studies is that they did not use a standardized, evidence-based protocol; rather they simply compared the outcomes related to the presence or absence of a PA catheter. In 2006, the ARDSNet Fluids and Catheters Treatment Trial (FACTT) used a standardized protocol to guide fluid therapy (liberal versus conservative),[162] and also compared standardized fluid therapy guided by either a PA catheter or CVP.[138] Compared with therapy guided by a CVP, there was no increased benefit (or harm) from the PA catheter in terms of 60-day mortality, days in the ICU, or ventilator-free days. However, there were improved outcomes in patients in the conservative fluid therapy versus liberal fluid group, regardless of monitoring method (PA catheter vs. CVP). A retrospective study of 53,312 patients in a trauma database (1,933 with PA catheter), found that after controlling for injury severity, there was a survival benefit associated with the use of a PA catheter for patients who presented with more severe injuries in shock or increased age (61 to 90 years).[163]

Results of these studies, meta-analyses,[164,165] and a consensus conference on the use of hemodynamic monitoring in shock[166] indicate that the *routine* use of a PA catheter is not warranted. However, the PA catheter in a patient with a complex presentation (Table 21-3) and there may be subsets of patients

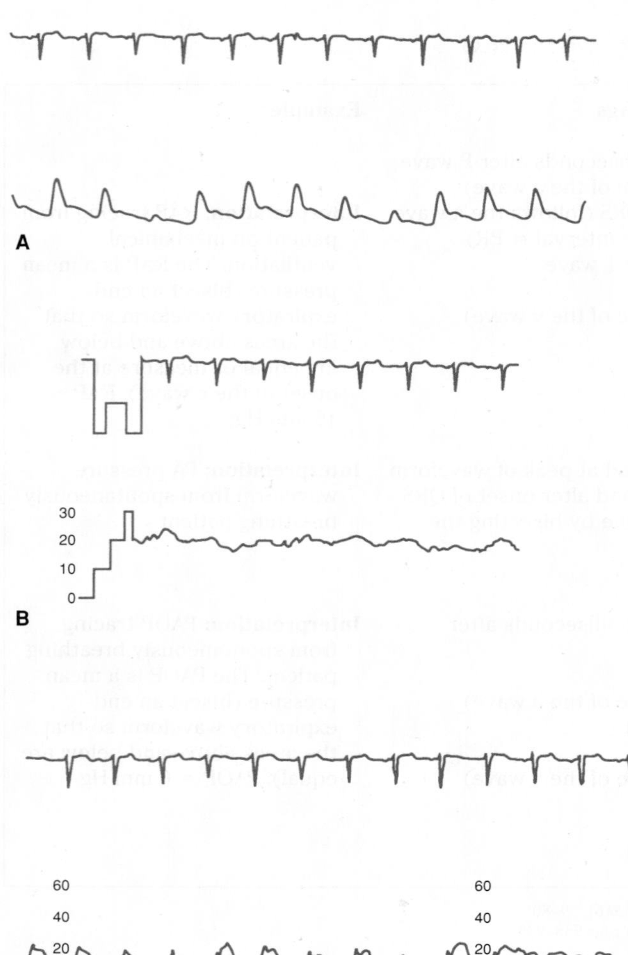

■ **Figure 21-10** Pericardial tamponade in a spontaneously breathing patient. (A) Arterial waveform. Note the electrical alternans, alternating height or duration of the QRS complex, and *pulsus paradoxus* on the arterial waveform. (B) RAP = 20 mm Hg. (C) PA to PAOP. PAS pressure = 26 mm Hg; PAEDP = 17 mm Hg; PA mean pressure = 19 mm Hg; PAOP = 20 mm Hg. Equalization of the diastolic pressures is the result of circumferential compression of all cardiac chambers.

who may benefit from the use of a PA catheter to guide and evaluate therapy (Display 21-4).

With the decreased use of PA catheters, one of the challenges for clinicians will be to maintain clinical proficiency in the use of PA catheters and the hemodynamic data obtained (e.g., CO, $S\bar{v}O_2$). The Pulmonary Artery Catheter Education Program (www.PACEP.org) and the American Thoracic Society Pulmonary Artery Catheter Primer are excellent resources for standardized education.[170,171] Consideration should also be given to the creation of a team of nurses who provide care to patients requiring PA catheterization.

Description of the PA Catheter

The PA catheter is a multilumen, polyvinylchloride catheter with a variable external diameter. Many models of PA catheters are available (Fig. 21-11). The thermodilution catheter is 7.5 Fr in diameter and 110 cm long and is marked in 10-cm increments. The balloon is inflated with a maximum of 1.5 mL of air.

Insertion of the PA Catheter

The catheter is inserted percutaneously. Once the RA is reached, the balloon, located on the distal end of the catheter, is inflated and the catheter is "floated" through the RA and RV and out into the PA, where it occludes a branch of the PA. After the characteristic PAOP tracing has been obtained, the balloon is deflated, allowing the catheter to recoil slightly into the PA. The catheter is left in the balloon-down position to prevent pulmonary infarction. The nursing responsibilities during insertion of the PA catheter are summarized in Display 21-5.

PA Waveform Characteristics

As the catheter passes through the heart, three pressure waveforms can be visualized using a PA catheter: RA, PA, and PAOP (Fig. 21-12*A*).

PA Pressure

PA pressures provide an index of the pressure within the pulmonary vasculature and are affected by compliance of the LV, pulmonary vascular pressure, CO, and the state of the lung tissue. In individuals without preexisting cardiopulmonary disease, PA pressure increases slightly with age (older than 60 years, PA mean ≅ 16 ± 3 mm Hg; younger than 60 years, PA mean ≅ 12 ± 2 mm Hg).[172] Similarly, in individuals with hypertension without other cardiac disease there is also an age-related increase in PA pressures (aged less than 45 years, PA mean ≅ 17 ± 5 mm Hg; aged 45 to 64 years, PA mean ≅ 18 ± 6 mm Hg, and aged greater than or equal to 65 years, PA mean ≅ 21 ± 8 mm Hg).[173]

Three PA pressures are measured: systolic, diastolic, and mean. The PA systolic (PAS) pressure reflects the flow of blood into the PA from the RV. In the absence of elevated pulmonary vascular pressure or RV outflow obstruction, PAS pressure is equal to RV systolic pressure. The PAS is affected by PA compliance and RV ejection. During diastole, the mitral valve is open, and a continuous column of blood from the PA to the LA and LV exists; therefore, the pressure just before contraction (end-diastole) is approximately equal in the PA, LA, and LV. As a result of the diastolic equalization, the PA end-diastolic pressure (PAEDP) is often used as an indirect indicator of PAOP and LV end-diastolic pressure (LVEDP). The difference between the RV end-diastolic pressure and PAEDP (an increase in the diastolic pressure as the catheter passes across the pulmonic valve) is an important characteristic in determining whether the catheter tip is correctly positioned in the PA or has flipped back into the right ventricle (Fig. 21-12*A*).

Pulmonary Artery Occlusion Pressure

The PAOP is obtained by inflation of the balloon on the distal end of the PA catheter, which allows the catheter to float forward to occlude a segment of the PA. The occluded catheter creates a static column of blood through the pulmonary vasculature (Fig. 21-12*B*). This static column acts as an extension of the fluid within the catheter system and allows retrograde transmission of left heart pressures to the distal port of the catheter.

There is, in general, a good relationship between the mean PAOP and mean LAP. At end-diastole, pressure equalizes between

Table 21-3 ■ HEMODYNAMIC CHARACTERISTICS OF VARIOUS PATHOLOGICAL CONDITIONS

	Hemodynamic Findings					
Pathophysiology	**RAP**	**PA**	**PAOP**	**SV**	**CO**	**Additional Findings**
Pericardial tamponade	↑	↑	↑	↓	↓	Equalization (within 5 mm Hg) of RAP = PAEDP = PAOP; RAP waveform: prominent *x* descent with attenuated or absent *y* descent (d/t decreased ventricular filling); *pulsus paradoxus* (↓SBP > 10 mm Hg and ↓pulse pressure during inspiration; DBP unchanged); *pulsus alternans* (Fig. 21-10); absent S_3 heart sound; cardiacpressures may be normal if the patient is hypovolemic
Pericardial constriction	↑	↑	↑	↓	N/↓	RAP waveform: steep *x* and *y* descent resulting in an "M"- or "W"-shaped waveform; RAP ≅ PAEDP ≅ PAOP (if no tricuspid or mitral regurgitation); decreased respiratory variation in RAP; Kussmaul's sign (inspiratory increase in RAP in severe pericardial constriction); *pulsus paradoxus* (approximately 33% of cases). CO maintained by tachycardia
Massive pulmonary embolism	↑	↑	↑/N/↓	↓	↓	Increased RA v wave with steep *y* descent due to tricuspid regurgitation, increased alveolar–arterial oxygen gradient (normal value does not rule out pulmonary embolism), tachypnea, dyspnea, increased pulmonic component of S_2, pleuritic chest pain
Mitral regurgitation			↑			If amplitude of V wave 10 mm Hg or more than *a* wave amplitude, read PAOP at nadir (base) of the *x* descent (Fig. 21-13*C*); PAOP > PAEDP (regurgitant v wave)
Left ventricular failure	N/↑	↑	↑	↓	↓	Pulmonary congestion or edema, S_3 or S_4, increased *a* wave height (due to decreased ventricular compliance); increased v wave height due to mitral regurgitation, pulsus alternans. Approximately 50% of patients with HF have mild or no impairment in systolic function
RV infarction	↑	↑/↓	↑/↓	N/↓	N/↓	RAP > PAOP or RAP 1 to 5 mm Hg > PAOP, or RAP > 10 mm Hg, RA tracing with prominent x and *y* descent (M configuration), increased jugular venous pressure, systemic venous congestion, RV gallop, split S_2, positive hepatojugular reflux, increased RA *a* wave, positive Kussmaul's sign (increased RAP with inspiration), RV S_3 or S_4
Acute ventral septal defect	↑	↑	↑	↓	↓	Acute hypotension and pulmonary congestion, systolic thrill, holosystolic murmur, acute right HF with increased jugular venous pressure, late PAOP v wave, oxygen step up of >10% RA and PA
Hypovolemia	↓	↓	↓	↓	↓/N	Increased SVR (compensatory), decreased $S\bar{v}o_2$
Septic shock (hyperdynamic)	↓	↓	↓/N/↑	N/↑	N/↑	Systemic hypotension, SBP < 90 mm Hg, metabolic acidosis with compensatory hyperventilation (respiratory alkalosis), decreased vascular resistance (↓ SVR) and ↑$S\bar{v}o_2$. This profile may be accompanied by distributive shock.
Septic shock (hypodynamic)		↑↓	↑↓	↓	↓	Systemic hypotension, SBP < 90 mm Hg, systemic vasoconstriction (increased SVR), decreased $S\bar{v}o_2$. During the early phase of septic shock, this profile may reflect inadequate fluid resuscitation. This profile also reflects cardiogenic shock.

N, normal; ↓, decreased; ↑, increased.

DISPLAY 21-4 Indications for PA Catheterization[158,160,161,163,164,166–169]

- Evaluation/guiding therapy in patients who remain hypotensive/hypoperfused after adequate volume resuscitation or standard therapy
- Preoperative evaluation of patients who are candidates for cardiac transplantation
- Evaluation/management of patients with pulmonary hypertension
- Trauma victims: severely injured and older patients
- Evaluation/management of patients with HF for the following conditions: failure of initial therapy, uncertain hemodynamic status (e.g., concomitant pulmonary disease or acute coronary syndrome and HF or uncertain volume or vascular resistance status), clinically significant hypotension or worsening renal/hepatic function, to optimize dosing of diuretics, inotropes, or vasoactive medications. Routine use for ADHF is not recommended.

the LA and ventricle; thus, the PAOP is used as an indirect measure of LV pressure. The assumption in using pressure as surrogate indicator of volume (preload) is that an increase in pressure indicates an increase in volume, and as described by Starling's law of the heart, an increase in CO. However, there are several factors that limit the use of pressure as an indicator of volume. First, the relationship between pressure and volume is curvilinear, not linear; thus, an absolute change in pressure (e.g., PAOP) is not associated with an absolute change in volume. Second, any alteration in myocardial compliance may affect the pressure–volume relation and limit the usefulness of the PAOP as an indicator of left heart preload. Absolute PAOP values should be used with caution in any situation that alters myocardial compliance, such as LV dysfunction or myocardial infarction (MI) (particularly involving the posteroinferior surface of the heart).[174] Third, the PAOP is affected by changes in pericardial pressure; thus, the PAOP may not accurately reflect transmural pressure. Finally, although the PAOP is useful for differential diagnosis and assessing the risk for pulmonary edema, it does not predict if a patient will respond to a

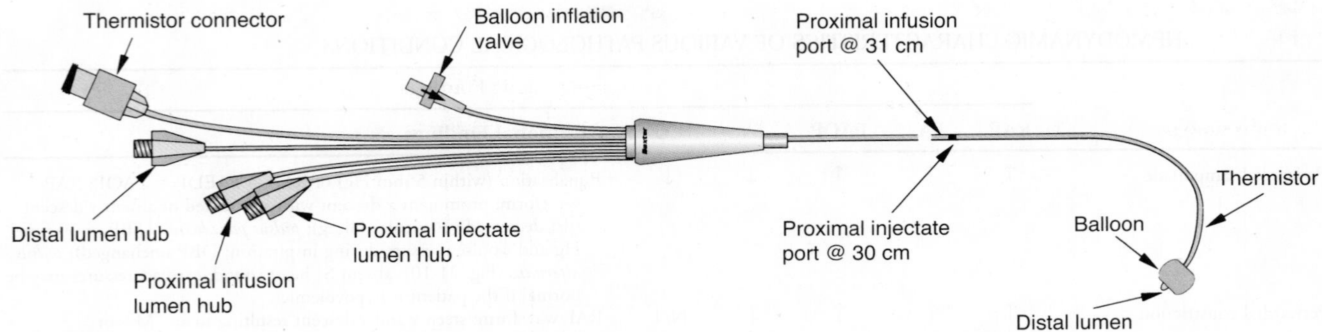

■ **Figure 21-11** Venous infusion port PA catheter. (Courtesy of Baxter Healthcare Corporation, Edwards Critical Care Division, Santa Ana, California.)

fluid bolus with an increase in SV.[175] Functional hemodynamic indices address this limitation.

In addition to being an indirect indicator of LVEDP, the PAOP is also an *estimate* of the capillary pressure (P_{cap}), which is the most important factor in the development of hydrostatic pulmonary edema. If the alveolar epithelium is intact, an increase in P_{cap} greater than 18 to 20 mm Hg causes increased fluid flux across the alveolar-capillary membrane and alveolar flooding. For example, in patients with an acute MI, an increase in PAOP to a value greater than 18 mm Hg is associated with the onset of pulmonary congestion, as exemplified in the Forrester subsets.[176] In contrast, some patients with chronic HF tolerate a substantially higher PAOP without the development of pulmonary edema.[177]

Hydrostatic pulmonary edema can be present with a PAOP less than 18 mm Hg under conditions of transient LV dysfunction that have resolved, massive sympathetic discharge that increases P_{cap} (heroin overdose, intracerebral hemorrhage), and increased pulmonary venous vascular resistance (ARDS).[174,178] Other factors that may increase the PAOP to greater than 18 mm Hg without the onset of pulmonary edema include increased pleural pressure, hyperinflation, and active expiration.[174]

DISPLAY 21-5 Nursing Responsibilities During PA Catheter Insertion

1. Prepare equipment (see Display 21-2 for line preparation)
2. Assist during insertion
   a. Attach pressure tubing to proximal and distal ports and flush system.
   b. Determine integrity of balloon (the provider inserting PA catheter will inflate the balloon); the balloon should be symmetric and not cover the catheter tip.
   c. Transduce the distal lumen on monitor
   d. Inflate balloon at provider's direction (generally after catheter reaches RA).
   e. Monitor oscilloscope for characteristic waveform changes (see Fig. 21-12*A*) and ectopy.
   f. Record waveforms and pressures as catheter passes from RA to PAOP position.
   g. Deflate balloon once PAOP has been obtained, and note return of characteristic PA waveform.
   h. Secure catheter and note insertion distance.
   i. Apply sterile occlusive dressing (see infection control guidelines—Table 21-1).
   j. Obtain chest radiograph to confirm catheter placement.

PA Waveform Interpretation

PA waveform interpretation can be simplified by remembering that electrical activity, as indicated by the ECG, precedes mechanical activity (see Display 21-3).[179] PA pressure waveforms are useful in the diagnosis of various cardiac abnormalities.

Pulmonary Artery Occlusion Pressure

The PAOP waveform is similar to the LAP waveform but is slightly damped and phase delayed (50 to 70 milliseconds) because of pulmonary vascular transmission (Fig. 21-13*A*). The PAOP is a mean pressure and is determined by bisecting the a and v waves, so there is an equal area above and below the bisection.

1. Elevated a wave: conditions that increase resistance to LV filling
   a. Mitral stenosis
   b. LV failure (Fig. 21-13*B*)
   c. Acutely ischemic LV
2. Elevated v wave: conditions that cause increased LA filling during ventricular systole
   a. Acute mitral insufficiency (Fig. 21-13*C*)
   b. Ventricular septal defect
   c. Aortic regurgitation

The giant V wave in acute mitral regurgitation and ventricular septal defect is caused by augmented LA filling. The height of the v wave is determined by LA loading volume and compliance and LV afterload and the presence or absence of a v wave may vary depending on whether there is acute or chronic mitral regurgitation.[180] The height and the presence or absence of a V wave are not indicators of the severity or mitral regurgitation.[181] In the presence of a large V wave (V wave 10 mm Hg greater than a wave or the mean PAOP), LVEDP is best correlated ($r = 0.89$) with the trough or nadir of the *x* descent[182] (Fig. 21-13*C*). The mean PAOP and peak of the a wave overestimate the LVEDP. The clinical importance of the giant V wave, regardless of cause, is the marked increase in P_{cap}, with the potential development of pulmonary edema. The ECG is useful in differentiating a bifid PA waveform (V wave apparent in the PA tracing) from a PAOP with a large V wave (Fig. 21-14).

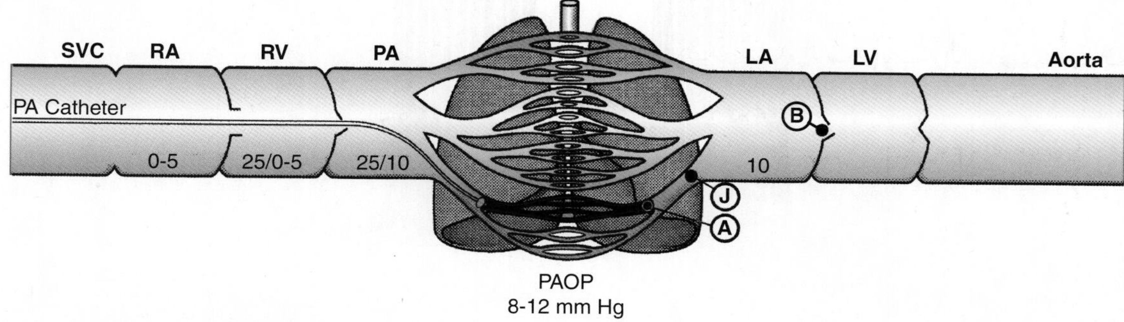

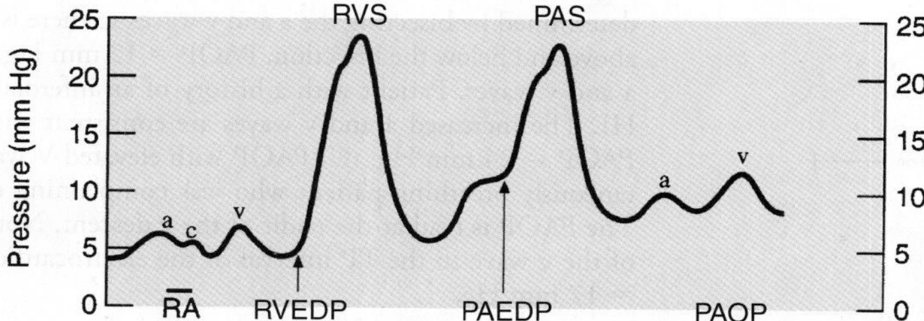

■ **Figure 21-12** (A) Schema of the principle underlying the use of the PAOP as an indicator of LV preload. When the inflated balloon on the catheter obstructs arterial flow, the catheter records the pressure at the junction of the static column of fluid and flowing venous channels (J-point). The J-point occurs in the venous system, approximately 1.5 cm from the LA. The PAOP underestimates P_{cap} when there is increased resistance in the postcapillary vessels proximal to the J-point (point A). The PAOP overestimates LVEDP if there is obstruction distal to the J-point (point B; e.g., mitral stenosis, left atrial myxoma), whereas the PAOP underestimates the LVEDP in the presence of premature closure of the mitral valve as a result of aortic insufficiency. (B) Characteristic waveforms observed as the PA catheter is "floated" from the RA through the right ventricle and into the PA, where it wedges. Note that the mean RAP is similar to the RVEDP, the RV systolic and PAS pressures are similar, and there is a step-up in pressure as the catheter crosses the pulmonic valve and enters the PA. In a correctly positioned catheter, the PAOP is lower than the mean PA pressure and has a waveform that is relatively similar to the RAP (although slightly delayed relative to the ECG).

3. Elevated a and v waves
   a. Cardiac tamponade (Fig. 21-10)
   b. Hypervolemia
   c. Constrictive pericarditis
   d. LV failure (Fig. 21-13*B*)
   e. Mitral stenosis

In mitral stenosis the PAOP is generally similar to LAP (except if PAOP is >25 mm Hg when it may vary as much as 10 mm Hg compared with the LAP[180]) and the height of the v wave is strongly associated with PA pressure.[183] However, because a pressure gradient develops between the LA and LV the PAEDP and PAOP are not accurate indices of LV pressure.[180]

PA Pressure

The PAS pressure is represented by a steep rise during RV ejection and usually occurs after the QRS complex or near the T wave of the ECG (Display 21-3). The PAEDP is measured 0.08 second after the onset of the QRS,[184] and the PA mean pressure is determined by bisecting the end-expiratory waveform, so there is an equal area above and below the bisection. In the presence of LV dysfunction, the presystolic a wave may provide a more consistent index of LVEDP than PAEDP or PAOP; however, the presence of this wave is variable.

Elevated PA pressures occur with:

1. Increased PVR (Fig. 21-15*A*)
   a. Pulmonary hypertension
   b. Chronic obstructive pulmonary disease
   c. ARDS
   d. Hypoxia
   e. Pulmonary embolus
2. Increased pulmonary venous pressure
   a. LV failure
   b. Mitral stenosis
3. Increased pulmonary blood flow
   a. Hypervolemia
   b. Atrial and ventricular septal defects
4. Mitral insufficiency (Fig. 21-15*B*)

Use of PA Catheter for HF and Pulmonary Hypertension

Two areas where PA catheter use is recommended are the management of acute decompensated heart failure (ADHF) after initial therapy has failed and the diagnosis and management of pulmonary hypertension. In patients with ADHF, interpreting the hemodynamic data and undertaking appropriate therapy requires

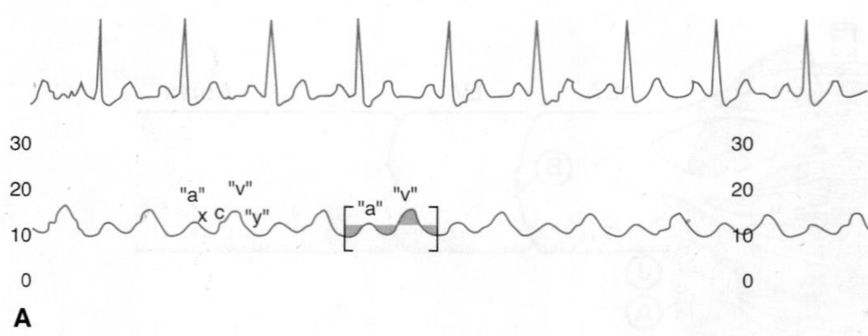

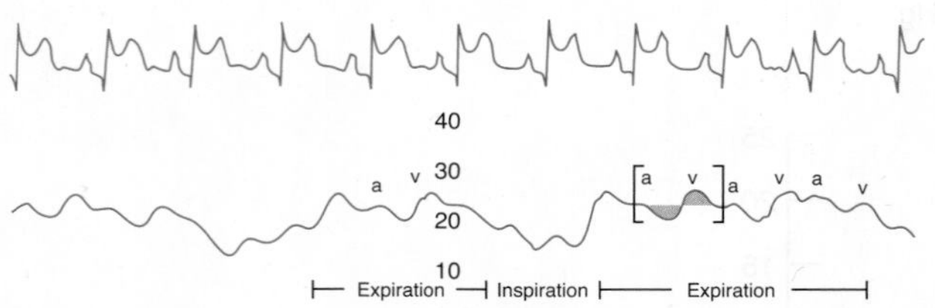

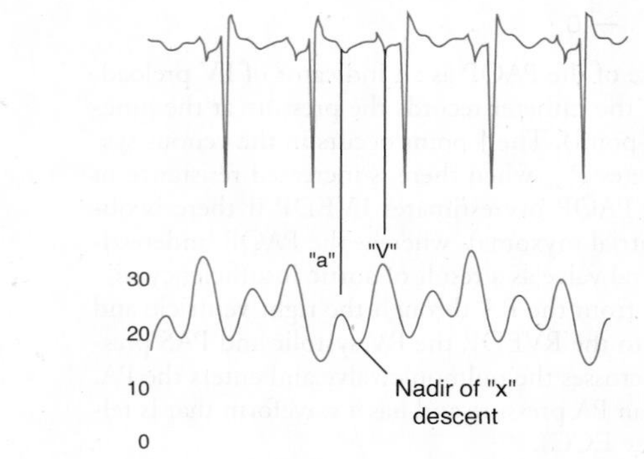

■ **Figure 21-13** PAOP determination. (A) Normal PAOP tracing. The mean PAOP is read at end-expiration waveform and is determined by bisecting the a and v waves so there is an equal area above and below the bisection. PAOP = 12 mm Hg. (B) Elevated a and v waves. Patient with a history of an inferolateral MI with HF. The increased a and v waves are consistent with LV failure. PAOP = 24 mm Hg. (C) PAOP with elevated V wave in a spontaneously breathing patient who was complaining of chest pain. The PAOP is read at the nadir of the *x* descent. Note the relation of the v wave to the TP interval of the electrocardiogram. PAOP = 17 mm Hg.

an understanding of the different causes of the HF. For example, in patients with diastolic dysfunction with a normal EF the increased PAOP reflects the primary disease. In contrast, in patients with systolic dysfunction with a decreased EF, the increased PAOP is secondary to a decrease in CO and the subsequent neurohormonal activation.[185] Further discussion of the management of HF is presented in Chapter 24.

PA catheterization (along with Doppler echocardiography) is part of the diagnosis and management of patients with pulmonary hypertension.[186,187] Idiopathic (formerly referred to as primary) pulmonary arterial hypertension is defined as a mean pulmonary artery pressure (PAM) $\geq$ 25 mm Hg in a setting of a PAOP $\leq$ 15 mm Hg and a normal or decreased or CO or by a PVR > 3 Wood units (>240 dynes/s/cm^{-5}).[188] Secondary pulmonary hypertension is often associated with pulmonary venous hypertension caused by left-sided cardiac disease (e.g., HF, mitral or aortic valvular disease). Pulmonary hypertension is a progressive disorder that may lead to severe RV dysfunction.

PA catheterization is used for the confirmation and differential diagnosis of pulmonary hypertension (idiopathic versus secondary), measurement of cardiac pressures, PVR and vasoreactivity testing. Vasoreactivity testing is performed to determine if a patient will respond favorably to vasodilator therapy (e.g., calcium channel blocker, epoprostenol, inhaled nitric oxide) as indicated by a decrease in PAM greater than 10 mm Hg to a PAM < 40 mm Hg, with an unchanged or increased CO.[186] Table 21-4 presents typical hemodynamic profiles for patients with compensated pulmonary hypertension (maintain normal RAP and CO), decompensated pulmonary hypertension (increased RAP and decreased CO) and pulmonary venous hypertension (increased PAOP associated with left heart disease).[189] Other conditions associated with pulmonary hypertension include pulmonary stenosis and the three hemodynamic profiles associated with advanced liver disease or portal hypertension.

PA perforation or rupture is often cited as a risk of PA catheterization in patients with pulmonary hypertension. However, the pathophysiological thickening of the vasculature may provide some protection and research indicates that at experienced medical facilities the performance of PA catheterization in these patients is a safe procedure (serious adverse events 1.1%), with the most frequent complications related to central line placement (e.g., hemothorax, pneumothorax).[190] One factor that limits the utility of PA catheterization and CO measurement in patients with pulmonary hypertension is severe tricuspid regurgitation, which generally causes an underestimation of the actual CO.[191,192] In the case of tricuspid regurgitation or a very low CO, the Fick method can be used to estimate CO.[193]

Technical Aspects of PA Pressure Monitoring

Numerous research studies have evaluated the technical aspects of PA pressure measurement.[14,194] Incorrect techniques may

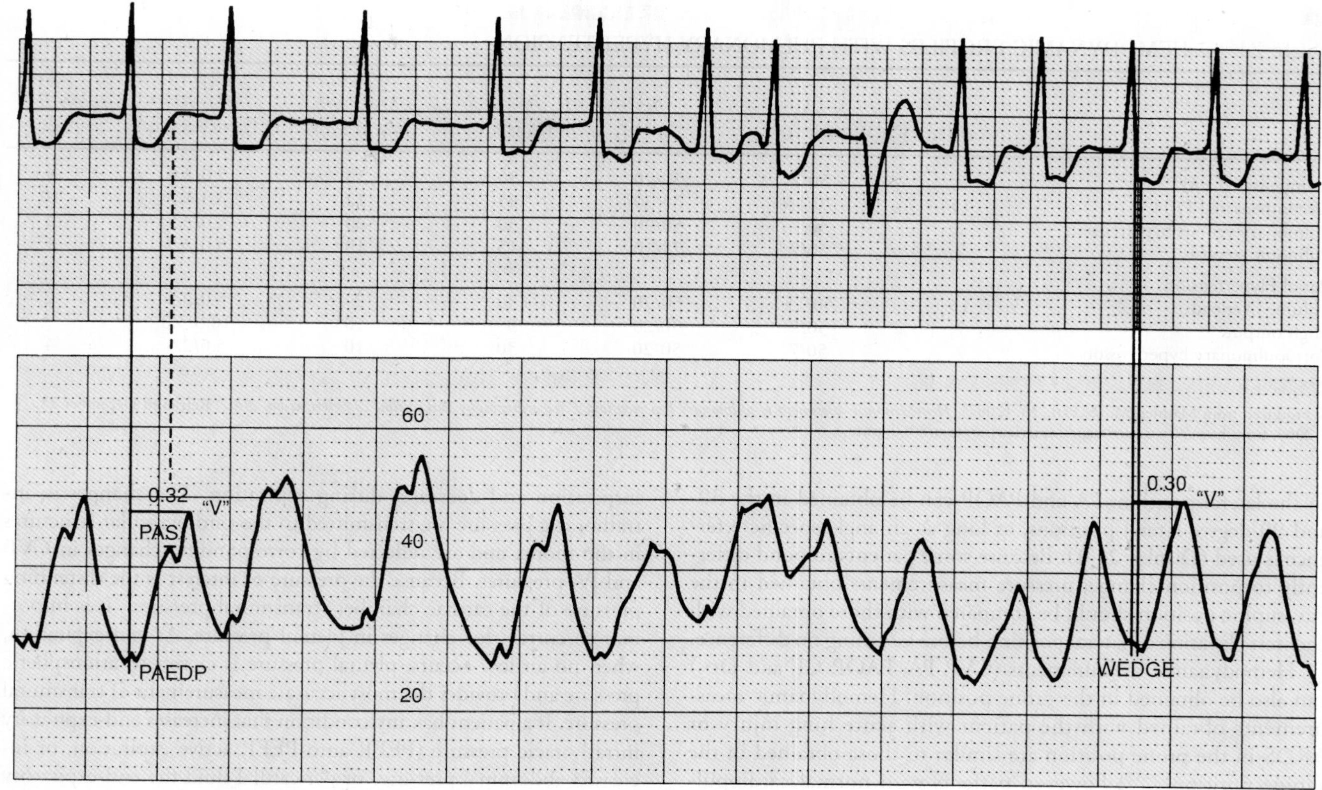

■ **Figure 21-14** PA pressure or PAOP? In the presence of a large V wave, the PAOP tracing may mimic a PA tracing. Comparison of the PA and PAOP relative to the ECG reveals the following: (1) the v wave of the PAOP occurs during the TP interval, whereas the initial systolic upstroke of PA waveform is closely related to the end of the QRS complex; and (2) the PA v wave is a sharp upward deflection on the descending limb of the PA pressure curve, having the same temporal relation as the v wave in the PAOP tracing. PAOP = 30 mm Hg.

introduce error into pressure measurements and potentiate therapeutic mismanagement of critically ill patients.

Positioning

Traditionally, PA and PAOP measurements have been obtained with the patient in the flat, supine position; however, this position may be poorly tolerated in patients with increased intracranial pressure or cardiopulmonary dysfunction. Research has shown that in a wide variety of critically ill patients, accurate PA pressures can be obtained in the supine position with legs extended and a backrest elevation up to 60 degrees.[195] Measurement of PA pressures in the sitting position (legs dependent) is not recommended.

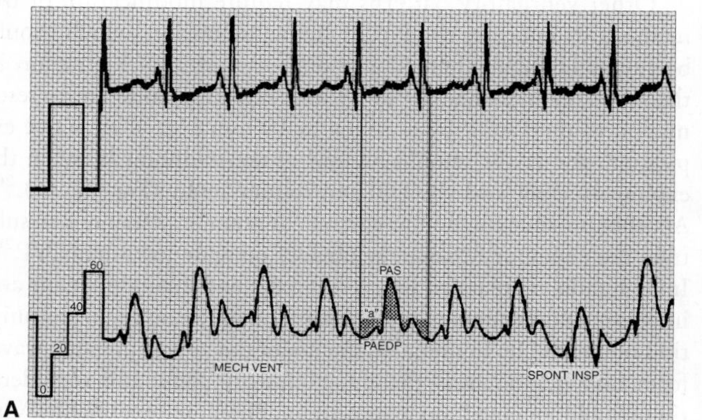

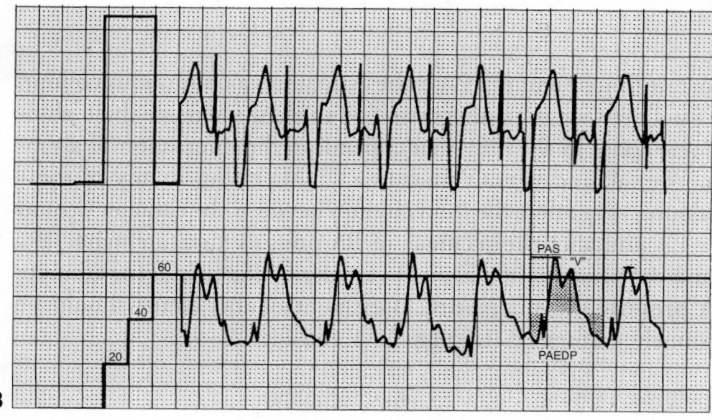

■ **Figure 21-15** PA pressure determination. (A) Elevated PA pressure related to LV failure and ARDS. Patient is on intermittent mandatory ventilation. PAS = 58 mm Hg; PAEDP = 30 mm Hg; PA mean = 38 mm Hg. (B) Patient with vegetation on mitral valve resulting in acute mitral insufficiency. Note the v wave on the downstroke of the PA waveform (bifid waveform). PAS = 68 mm Hg; PAEDP = 32 mm Hg; PAM = 48 mm Hg.

Table 21-4 ■ HEMODYNAMIC PROFILES WITH PULMONARY HYPERTENSION

	CVP (mm Hg)	RV (mm Hg)	PA (mm Hg)	PAM (mm Hg)	PAOP (mm Hg)	CO; CI (L/min; L/min/m^2)	PVR (Wood units)
Compensated PAH	7	50/7	50/20	30	10	5.0/2.5	4
Decompensated PAH	15	70/15	70/30	45	12	3.3/1.7	10
Pulmonary venous hypertension	7	50/7	50/20	30	20	5.0/2.5	2
Pulmonic stenosis	7	50/7	22/10	15	10	5.0/2.5	1
Portal Hypertension							
Volume overload	15	50/15	50/20	30	20	5.0/2.5	2
High output	7	50/7	50/20	30	10	10.0/5.0	2
Portopulmonary hypertension	7	50/7	50/20	30	10	5.0/2.5	4

Reproduced from Mathier, M., & Park, M. (2007). *Hemodynamic assessment of pulmonary hypertension: Echocardiography and cardiac catheterization, 2007.* Retrieved December 28, 2007, from http://www.medscape.com/viewprogram/8360_pnt.

In the lateral position, PA and PAOP can be obtained in the 30- and 90-degree lateral positions, as long as an angle-specific reference is used (Display 21-1). Because some patients respond differently to position change, pressure measurements obtained in the flat, supine position should be compared with those obtained with backrest elevation or lateral position before assuming no difference.

Hemodynamic measurements (CVP, PA, PAOP, CI, and Do_2) can also be obtained in the prone position. Hemodynamic measurements obtained with the patient with acute lung injury or ARDS in the prone position are similar to those obtained in the supine position[15–19]; however, patients with normal cardiopulmonary function[196,197] may demonstrate a decrease in end-diastolic volume and CI without a change in CVP. The amount of time after proning before the measurements can be obtained has not been defined. Most studies evaluated the changes 60 to 90 minutes after the prone positioning. The shortest stabilization period was 15 minutes in healthy patients undergoing lumbar spine surgery,[197] after 20 to 30 minutes in patients with acute lung injury,[15,19] and 20 minutes after stabilization of Spo_2 (60 to 90 minutes after proning) in patients with ARDS.[17] Although abdominal pressure increases slightly in the prone position, there is no effect on the measured cardiac indices.[16,20] Areas for future research include evaluation of the measurements in automated proning beds, description of the time to stabilization of hemodynamic indices after proning, and evaluation of the effect of proning on abdominal and cardiac pressures in patients with intraabdominal hypertension or abdominal compartment syndrome.

Pulmonary Effects

Correct function of the PA catheter requires a continuous column of fluid between the catheter tip and the LA. There are three physiologic zones in the lung that depend on the interaction of alveolar, arterial, and venous pressures.[198] Alteration in any of these pressures may affect the fluid column between the catheter tip and the LA and alter the accuracy of PA pressure measurements. Because the presence of a Zone-3 vascular bed is crucial for accurate PA pressure measurements, assessment of this factor should be routinely performed (Display 21-1 and Fig. 21-4).

Spontaneous Versus Mechanical Ventilation

During spontaneous ventilation, the alveolar pressure decreases during inspiration and increases during expiration. Conversely, during positive-pressure ventilation, intrathoracic pressure increases during inspiration and decreases during expiration. The changes in intrathoracic pressure are transmitted to the cardiovascular structures in the thorax and are reflected by corresponding changes in CVP and PA pressures. Because the pressure of interest is the distending pressure of the cardiac chamber (transmural pressure), it is important to correct for changes in pleural pressure. At end-expiration, when no airflow occurs, pleural pressure is closest to atmospheric pressure and provides the most accurate measurement of transmural pressure. If a patient has any condition that increases end-expiratory intrathoracic pressure (PEEP, auto-PEEP, active expiration, or increased abdominal pressure) or pericardial fluid the end-expiratory intracardiac pressure measurements will overestimate true transmural pressure.

In patients with respiratory variation in the PA waveform tracing, the digital readings are unreliable because of the unselective nature of electrical averaging.[199,200] In addition, the "stop cursor" method (freezing the monitor screen) is less reliable than the graphic method.[200] The analysis of graphic recordings to identify the end-expiratory phase remains the recommended method for interpreting PA waveforms.[201] The validation of accurate pressure measurements in the medical record is imperative as electronic records may "pull" data from the digital readings, and these data may be less accurate than those obtained using the stop cursor or analog approach. The addition of an airway pressure tracing may further improve the accuracy of the measurements.[202] Display 21-1 reviews guidelines for recording PA pressure measurements.

Other ventilatory patterns may require modification of the methods to interpret the PAOP. Active expiration, which should be suspected when there is a respiratory-induced fluctuation in the PAOP greater than 10 to 15 mm Hg, may cause an overestimation of the PAOP by as much as 10 mm Hg. With active expiration, the PAOP should be read at the midpoint between the expiratory peak and the end-inspiratory nadir (Fig. 21-16).[203] Another possible method to correct for active expiration is to subtract the expiratory change in bladder pressure from the CVP.[204] Inverse ratio ventilation, which decreases end-expiratory time and increases end-expiratory lung volume, may cause an overestimation of the PAOP. In this case, the use of the airway pressure waveform may help identify the end-expiratory phase and consideration should be given to correcting for PEEP or auto-PEEP. With airway pressure release ventilation, the PAOP should be measured at the end of the positive pressure plateau, which can be observed on the ventilator and is the point immediately before the release of airway pressure and the initiation of inspiration.[205]

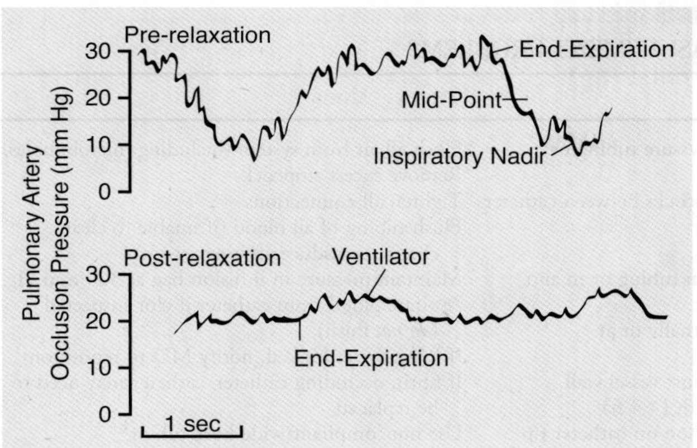

Figure 21-16 *(Top)* PAOP tracings showing the end expiratory, end inspiratory (nadir) and the midpoint values in a patient with marked respiratory variation. *(Bottom)* PAOP in same patient post muscle relaxation with paralytic. (Reprinted with permission from Hoyt, J. D., Leatherman, J. W. [1997]. Interpretation of the pulmonary artery occlusion pressure in mechanically ventilated patients with large respiratory excursion in intrathoracic pressure. *Intensive Care Medicine, 23*[11], 1126.)

Manipulation/Removal of PA Catheter

To safely manipulate or discontinue the catheter, critical care nurses must have knowledge of the correct technique for catheter insertion, be able to interpret waveforms (normal and abnormal) to confirm catheter position, to have knowledge of the appropriate action required should an abnormal waveform occur, and be able to troubleshoot the catheter system[206] (Table 21-5). Potential complications during repositioning include PA rupture, cardiac perforation or tamponade, thrombus formation, sepsis or catheter-related infection, and cardiac arrhythmias.

Factors that contribute to PA rupture include balloon hyperinflation, peripheral location of the catheter tip, and hypothermia. Steps to avoid these risks are to slowly inflate the balloon to volume (1.25 to 1.5 mL of air, never fluids), at which time the pressure tracing should change from a PA to a PAOP waveform, and to limit inflation time to less than 15 seconds. If an overwedge is observed, stop immediately. To avoid distal migration of the catheter, the PA tracing should be continuously monitored and the chest radiograph should be assessed to determine if the tip of the catheter is correctly positioned within 5 cm of the mediastinum.

During PA catheter removal (Display 21-6), additional risks include air embolism, arrhythmias, and myocardial or valvular damage. Risk factors for air embolization include a decreased intravascular pressure (hypovolemia, tachycardia), negative intrathoracic pressure (tachypnea, upright position, catheter removal during deep inspiration), an incompetent diaphragm on the introducer, and right to left intracardiac shunt. To minimize the risk of an air embolism, the patient should be placed in a supine/flat position and the catheter removed during breath holding at the end of a deep inspiration or positive pressure ventilation (to increase CVP). After removal of the catheter, the introducer should be sealed with a sterile obturator or a male cap. The incidence of cardiac arrhythmias during catheter removal ranges from 5% to 19%, with a small percentage of arrhythmias considered life threatening.[207] Patients at increased risk for arrhythmias are those with electrolyte imbalances myocardial ischemia or infarction, CI < 2.5 L/min/m^2 or prolonged manipulation time. The use of a steady, continuous withdrawal of the catheter may decrease the incidence of arrhythmias. Myocardial or valvular damage can occur because of kinking or knotting of the catheter around cardiac structures or failure to deflate the balloon before withdrawal of the catheter. Caution should be taken if the patient has another cardiac catheter (i.e., transvenous pacemaker) or excessive catheter length (dilated heart).

DISPLAY 21-6 Removal of PA Catheter

1. Verify the order to remove the catheter
2. Assemble necessary equipment
3. Document on the flow sheet the ECG rhythm and vital signs before initiating the procedure
4. Explain the procedure to the patient
5. Transfer IV infusions from PA catheter ports to side port of introducer or discontinue IV solutions if appropriate
6. Ensure that the patient remains in hemodynamically stable condition after transfer of infusions to side port
7. Turn off any remaining infusions to distal and proximal ports
8. Ensure that the balloon is deflated by lining up the red lines on the balloon port, drawing back on the syringe, and then discontinuing the syringe
9. Place the patients supine and turn the patient's head away from the insertion site
10. Open the sterile obturator/introducer cap, ensuring that sterility of the cap is maintained
11. Put on examination gloves
12. If the catheter dressing is nonocclusive or covers the introducer, after putting on a mask, remove the dressing
13. Instruct the patients to inspire deeply and hold their breath (or apply positive pressure breath on ventilator) during withdrawal of the catheter
14. Unlock the catheter shield from the introducer
15. While securing the introducer with nondominant hand, withdraw the catheter with dominant hand, using a constant steady continuous motion
16. Observe the ECG continuously during withdrawal of the catheter
17. If any resistance is met, do not continue to remove the catheter, and notify the physician immediately
18. Once the PA catheter has been removed, don sterile gloves and insert a sterile adaptor cap into the diaphragm site of the introducer
19. If necessary, reapply a sterile dressing to the catheter site according to policy
20. Elevate head of bed and return patient to position of comfort
21. Examine balloon and catheter to ensure that they are intact. If they are not intact, notify the physician immediately
22. Document on flow sheet the patient's response to procedure, including vital signs and ECG rhythm

Zevola, D. R., & Maier, B. (1999). Improving the care of cardiothoracic surgery patients through advanced nursing skills. *Critical Care Nurse, 19*(1), 34–44.

Table 21-5 ■ TROUBLESHOOTING THE PA CATHETER AND MEASUREMENT PROBLEMS

Clinical Problem	Implications	Possible Causes	Interventions
Overdamped pressure tracing	Falsely low systolic readings Falsely increased diastolic readings	Air bubbles in the pressure tubing or transducer More than three stopcocks between catheter and transducer Loose connections Collection of blood in tubing or in and around transducer Catheter kinked internally or at insertion site Catheter wedged against vessel wall Excessive tubing length (>4 ft) Clot or fibrin deposition on catheter tip	Flush all air from system (including microbubbles). Remove excess stopcocks Tighten all connections Flush tubing of all blood (if unable to clear, change transducer-tubing set-up) Maintain pressure in infusion bag at 300 mm Hg Aspirate blood from catheter if clot suspected (*do not* flush) If PA catheter kinked, notify MD to reposition If fibrin occluding catheter, catheter may need to be replaced Use noncompliant/wide-bore tubing
Underdamped pressure tracing	Overestimation of systolic pressure Underestimation of diastolic pressure	Air bubbles in tubing, stopcocks, or transducer Excessive tubing length (>4 ft) Excess number of stopcocks	Remove all air bubbles from system Limit tubing to 4 ft maximum Remove unnecessary stopcocks If all attempts to resolve unsuccessful, consider the addition of an in-line damping device
Catheter whip (fling) or artifact	Overestimation of systolic pressure Underestimation of diastolic pressure Difficult interpretation of waveform	Location of distal tip of PA catheter near pulmonic valve Hyperdynamic heart Looping of PA catheter in RV External disruption of PA catheter system	Assess dynamic response characteristics (troubleshoot system) Notify MD or qualified RN to reposition PA catheter If fling fails to resolve, use mean pressure
Absence of PA occlusion tracing	Potential for air embolism or blood leaking from balloon port	Balloon rupture Improper positioning of PA catheter	If balloon is inflated without return of air into syringe on passive deflation, assess for signs of air embolism (if present, place in Trendelenburg in left lateral decubitus position, treat symptoms, notify MD) If stable, label balloon port "DO NOT WEDGE." Notify MD of need to replace catheter If balloon is inflated to 1.5 mL, without change in waveform from PA to PA wedge pattern, notify MD or qualified RN of need to reposition catheter Once catheter is repositioned, assess the amount of air required for wedge (ideal volume 1.25–1.5 mL)
Migration of the PA catheter into the RV	Presence of RV arrhythmias Decreased diastolic pressure (equal to RAP)	Accidental or spontaneous withdrawal of catheter into the RV	Inflate the balloon fully to engulf the tip of the catheter and reduce ectopy Notify MD or, if approved for RN, reposition catheter into PA If compromised by arrhythmias, ensure balloon is deflated and withdraw catheter into RA (15–20 cm marking on PA catheter and RAP waveform observed from distal port)
Overwedging	Overwedging (eccentric balloon inflation or inflation in a small vessel) is potential risk for PA perforation and rupture	Catheter migration Balloon position in small pulmonary vessel	Slowly inflate balloon while constantly observing the waveform If overwedge pattern observed, immediately stop inflation and allow balloon to deflate passively Notify MD or, if approved for RN, reposition catheter
Spontaneous wedge	Potential for loss of blood supply to branch of pulmonary vessel and risk of PA infarction	Catheter migration (patient movement, warming up of catheter after placement)	Turn patient to side opposite catheter placement. Have patient straighten arm or turn head to dislodge catheter Have patient gently cough Notify MD or RN, reposition catheter

Modified from Gardner, P. E. (1993). Pulmonary artery pressure monitoring. *AACN Clinical Issues in Critical Care Nursing, 4*, 98–119.

Despite the potential complications associated with manipulating and removing the PA catheter, properly educated and qualified nurses can safely and successfully manipulate and remove PA catheters.[208] For example, in 125 patients with PA catheters, 39 (31%) of the catheters were incorrectly positioned (35 required advancement, 4 required withdrawal), of which 36 were repositioned by a critical care nurse (without complication).[206] In a recent study,[209] which evaluated the performance of the correct steps for removal of PA catheters in 60 patients (30 removed by RN/30 removed by MD), there was no significant difference in the incidence of complications associated with PA catheter removal. Of note, the nurses performed correct patient positioning and provided instructions to the patient on breathe holding during the procedure 100% of the time in contrast to the physicians

Table 21-6 ■ RIGHT HEART FUNCTION VARIABLES

Variable	Normal
SV	60–100 mL/beat
Stroke volume index	33–46 mL/beat/m^2
RVEF	40%–60%
RV end-systolic index	30–60 mL/m^2
RVEDVI	60–100 mL/m^2

who performed these steps 33% and 70% of the time, respectively. These studies support that nurses who are educated in the correct procedure for PA catheter removal can do so safely.

Volumetric Measures

Although the focus of hemodynamic monitoring has been predominantly on left heart function, awareness of RV function on global cardiac function is equally important[210] as RV function affects fluid responsiveness.[211,212] RV function is altered in sepsis, ARDS, traumatic myocardial contusion, with the application of PEEP, and during liver transplantation.

A new technology allows for continuous RV end-diastolic volume (CEDV) and continuous cardiac output (CCO).[213] The system uses small pulses of heat from a coil on the PA catheter and creates a curve that resembles a thermodilution washout curve.[214] Simultaneous recording of the CCO and the ECG allows for the measurement of the RV ejection fraction (RVEF) and CEDV = (CCO/HR)/RVEF. The CEDV equation suggests that caution must be taken when interpreting the absolute CEDV as it will change with variations in the RVEF (Table 21-6).

Although earlier studies[215,216] suggested that right ventricular end-diastolic volume index (RVEDVI) may be useful endpoint for resuscitation, RV indices were not mentioned as endpoints of resuscitation at the 2006 International Consensus Conference on hemodynamics in shock.[166] The CEDV catheter may be useful in monitoring changes in RVEF and RVEDVI during liver transplantation,[217–219] but this utility was not found in cardiac surgery patients.[220]

While the RVEDVI and CEDV are more closely correlated with SV than CVP or PAOP,[217,221–223] there is marked heterogeneity in these indices. Of note, similar results have been observed for global end-diastolic volume and intrathoracic blood volume, which are measured using the TPID technique (discussed below).[224,225] No specific thresholds have been identified for any of these volumetric indices to predict fluid responsiveness.[214,224,226,227]

FUNCTIONAL HEMODYNAMIC INDICES

The administration of fluids to augment preload and thus increase CO is a mainstay of the treatment of shock. However, the administration of fluids is not free of risk. After appropriate initial resuscitation of shock, excess fluids may increase morbidity and mortality.[162,228,229] Therefore, a key clinical question is whether a patient will respond to volume loading with increased SV or whether volume administration will cause or worsen cardiopulmonary compromise?

Table 21-7 ■ DIFFERENCES IN CVP AND PAOP BETWEEN FLUID RESPONDERS (R) AND NONRESPONDERS (N)

Patients	R (mm Hg)	N (mm Hg)	p
CVP			
Critically ill/cardiac[232]	5 ± 1	5 ± 2	NS
Sepsis/septic shock[233]	9 ± 3	9 ± 4	NS
Sepsis[175]	8 ± 4	9 ± 4	NS
PAOP			
Critically ill/cardiac[232]	8 ± 1	7 ± 2	NS
Trauma[221]	16 ± 6	15 ± 5	NS
Septic shock[234]	10 ± 4	12 ± 3	NS
Postcardiac surgery[235]	12 ± 2	16 ± 3	<.01
Sepsis/septic shock[233]	10 ± 3	11 ± 2	NS
Sepsis[175]	10 ± 4	11 ± 4	NS

Static preload indices (e.g., CVP or PAOP) are not good predictors of fluid responsiveness.[175,230,231] As demonstrated in Table 21-7, the CVP and PAOP do not differentiate between patients who will or will not respond to fluids.

The limitations of CVP and PAOP highlight an important concept that preload is not preload (or fluid) responsiveness.[117,236] Fluid responsiveness depends not only on the baseline preload, but also on the ventricular contractility and the slope of the ventricular function curve. For example, if the preload is low or if the heart is on the steep portion of the curve, a fluid bolus should increase the SV (preload dependent). However, if the preload is in an intermediate range or the slope of the curve is flattened (indicative of failure), there may only be a small change in the SV (preload independent); thus, the interpretation of an absolute preload value as predictive of fluid responsiveness will be difficult.[117] Patients will be "responders" to volume expansion only if both ventricles operate on the ascending portion of the curve. In contrast, if one or both of the ventricles is operating on the flat portion of the curve, the patient will be a "nonresponder."[211] While the assessment of fluid responsiveness provides insight into ventricular function; the finding that a patient is fluid responsive does not necessarily mean that the patient requires fluids. The decision to administer fluids should be based on indications of altered cardiovascular function that would benefit from increased preload versus the risk for the development of pulmonary edema. Functional hemodynamic indices, which are used to predict if a patient will respond to volume loading, reflect spontaneous and mechanical ventilation-induced changes in intrathoracic pressure, with subsequent changes in CVP, BP, and SV.

Spontaneous Ventilation

During spontaneous inspiration, pleural and intrathoracic pressure decreases with a resultant decrease in CVP. With a decrease in CVP, which is the backpressure to venous filling, venous return increases transiently. This increase in venous return results in an inspiratory increase in RV preload and output (assuming that the right ventricle is on the steep portion of the ventricular function curve). However, if the right ventricle cannot dilate further (i.e., RV failure), the CVP will not decrease during inspiration, which indicates that the RA/ventricle is on the flat portion of the cardiac function curve, and the administration of additional volume will not increase RV output.[237–239]

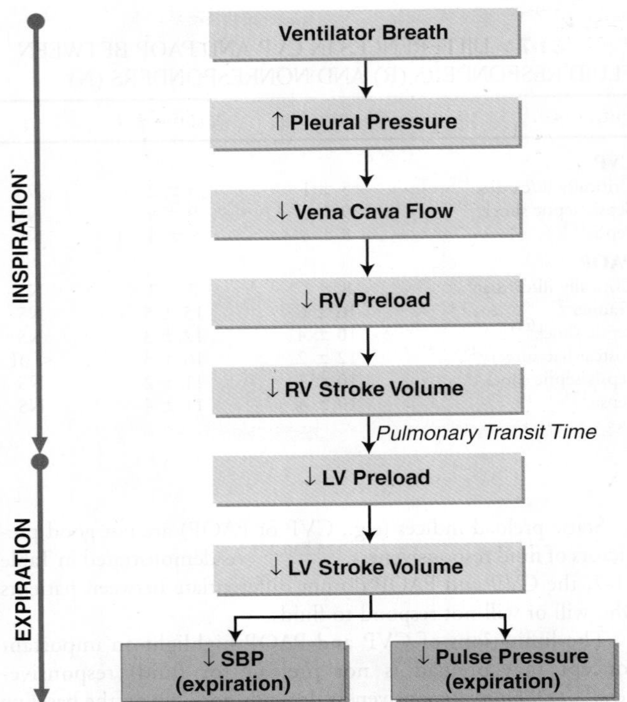

Figure 21-17 Primary mechanism for ventilator-induced variation in SV, SBP, and pulse pressure. The cyclic changes in LV stroke volume are mainly related to the expiratory decrease in LV preload due to the inspiratory decrease in RV filling and output.

Mechanical Ventilation

During positive pressure mechanical ventilation, the inspiratory increase in intrathoracic pressure decreases venous return to the heart and increases RV afterload. These changes lead to a decrease in RV SV during inspiration. The decreased RV output causes a decrease in LV preload, which subsequently decreases LV SV during expiration. Thus, the LV SV increases during inspiration because of compression of the pulmonary bed and decreases during expiration, primarily because of the decreased RV output (Fig. 21-17).[211,239]

Observation of the ventilator-induced changes in SV can be exploited on the basis of the finding that RV preload and SV changes are greater when the ventricle is on the steep versus the flat portion of ventricular function curve. The increased RV output is transmitted to the left heart, and if both ventricles are preload dependent, the increased LV preload will be observed as a cyclic change in LV SV. The cyclic changes in LV SV are important, because the SV is a primary contributor to the SBP and pulse pressure. The assumption underlying the interpretation of the cyclic SV changes is that a greater cyclic change is indicative of fluid responsiveness (i.e., a patient who will respond to volume loading with an increase in SV), whereas a smaller SV change indicates preload independence (fluid nonresponder). Patients who are preload independent will not increase their SV in response to volume loading and may be compromised by the excess fluid. Variations in these hemodynamic indices may help predict fluid responsiveness. A number of functional hemodynamic indices have been evaluated.

Respiratory Variation in CVP

Although, the patient is more likely to respond to a fluid bolus if they have a lower CVP, in general the absolute CVP is not predictive of a patient's fluid responsiveness and over time a patient may respond differently to fluids despite a similar CVP.[141,175,231] For example, in cardiac surgery patients, 25% of patients with a CVP between 0 and 5 mm Hg did not respond to a fluid bolus; although, if their CVP was greater than 13 mm Hg, the likelihood of increasing the CI > 300 mL/min/m^2 in response to a fluid bolus was low.[141] Consideration of the limitations of the absolute CVP is important as sepsis guidelines direct that in the presence of continued hypoperfusion, volume resuscitation should be undertaken to achieve a CVP > 8 mm Hg.[132,240] It is possible that despite a low CVP some of these patients may not respond to fluids, which may exacerbate their condition. An alternate way to evaluate the CVP is not whether the patient requires fluids but rather if the patient will respond to fluids. The inspiratory change in RAP (ΔRAP) may be a useful predictor of fluid responsiveness,[237,241] and unlike other functional indices, the ΔRAP can be evaluated in spontaneously breathing patients.[242] For example, in medical and cardiac surgery patients with an adequate spontaneous inspiratory effort (i.e., an inspiratory decrease of >2 mm Hg in PAOP), a spontaneous inspiratory decrease of ≥ 1 mm Hg in RAP predicted a positive response (responder), whereas a decrease of <1 mm Hg was a negative response (nonresponder)[241] (Fig. 21-18). The value of the ΔRAP is the identification of patients who will not respond to fluids. In addition, if a patient has a ΔRAP greater than 1 mm Hg, they may also be at risk for decreased CO if their PEEP is increased.[243]

Respiratory Variation in SBP

In patients who are mechanically ventilated, the SBP decreases during expiration and increases during inspiration. The difference between inspiratory increase and expiratory decrease for a given ventilatory cycle is the systolic pressure variation (SPV) (Fig. 21-19). The SPV is calculated using the following equation:

$$SPV = SPV_{max} - SPV_{min}$$

The second method (SPV%) may be more sensitive and specific during periods of hemodynamic instability,[244] although recent

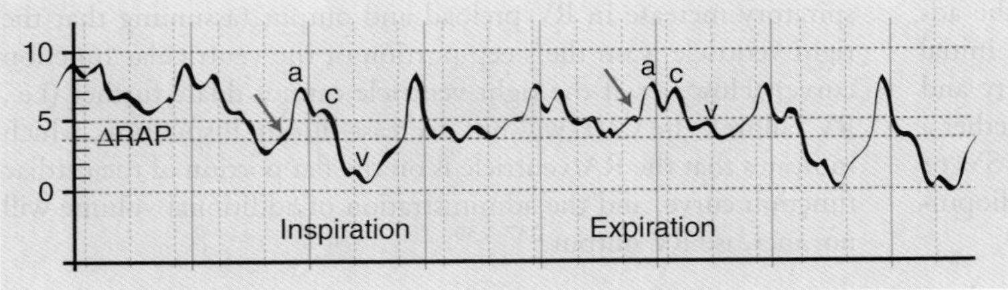

Figure 21-18 Example of the evaluation of ΔRAP in a spontaneously breathing patient. The CVP (RAP) is read at the base of the "a" wave or the base of the "c" wave. The ΔRAP is 1.5 mm Hg, indicating that the patient is likely to respond to a fluid bolus.

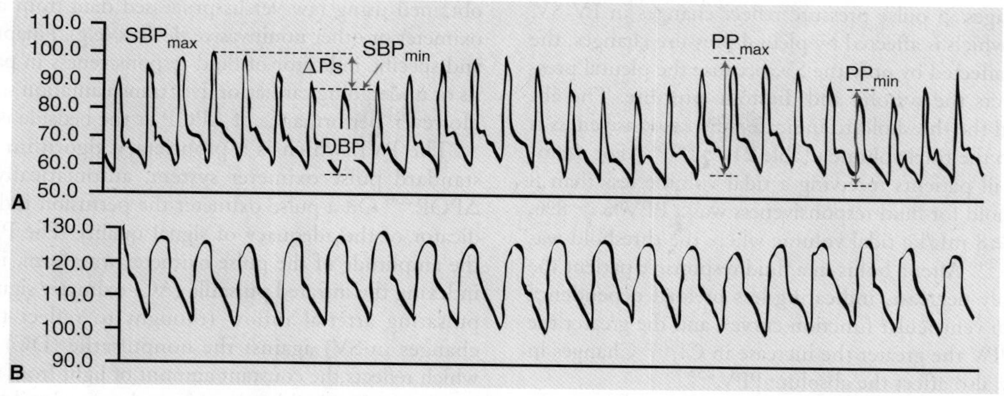

■ **Figure 21-19** Example of SPV and PPV. **(A)** This analog tracing was obtained from the bedside monitor with the paper speed decreased to 6.25 mm/s. In this case, the patient is demonstrating marked variation in their SPV (e.g., SPV = 9 mm Hg) indicating fluid responsiveness. **(B)** In this case, there is minimal variation in the functional indices (e.g., SPV = 4 mm Hg) indicating that the patient would not be fluid responsive and other methods, such as a vasopressor, should be considered to treat the patient's hypoperfusion.

studies suggest that it may be artificially increased during hypotension,[245] uses the following equation:

$$SPV\% = \frac{(SBP_{max} - SBP_{min})}{[(SBP_{max} + SBP_{min})/2]} \times 100$$

The absolute SPV and SPV% are directly related to the tidal volume (Table 21-8). In patients with acute circulatory failure caused by sepsis who were receiving an 8 to 11 mL/kg VT, SPV greater than 10 mm Hg was predictive of fluid responsiveness.[234] Additional research is needed to identify a threshold for these indices with smaller tidal volumes (<8 mL/kg).

Pulse Pressure Variation

Arterial pulse pressure is the difference between the arterial systolic and diastolic pressure (Fig. 21-19). Pulse pressure variation (PPV) is measured using the following equation[254]:

$$PPV\% = \frac{(PP_{max} - PP_{min})}{[(PP_{max} + PP_{min})/2]} \times 100$$

Three factors affect the pulse pressure: LV SV, arterial resistance, and arterial compliance. Of note, the latter two factors do not change significantly during a single breath[255]; therefore, the

Table 21-8 ■ FUNCTIONAL HEMODYNAMIC INDICATOR THRESHOLDS

Population	Response Threshold	VT (mL/kg)	Threshold	Sensitivity	Specificity
Septic shock[234]	↑SV ≥ 15%	8–11	SPV ≥ 10 mm Hg	NR	NR
			PAOP > 11 mm Hg	NR	NR
ARDS or septic shock[233]	↑CI ≥ 15%	8–12	PPV > 13%	94%	96%
			PAOP (no threshold)		
			CVP (no threshold)	—	—
Critically ill[246]	↑CI ≥ 15%	<8	PPV ≥ 12%	39%	65%
		<8	PPV ≥ 8%	66%	65%
		≥8	PPV > 12%	88%	89%
		All VT	PPV > 12%	60%	74%
Acute circulatory failure[247]	↑SV ≥ 15%	~8	PPV ≥ 10%	89%	83%
Postcardiac surgery[248]	↑CO ≥ 12%	8–10	PPV% ≥ 11%	100%	93%
			SPV%	NR	NR
			PAOP (no threshold)	—	—
			CVP (no threshold)	—	—
Postcardiac surgery LVEF < 35%[249]	↑SVI ≥ 5%	10	SVV ≥ 9.5%	71%	80%
			PAOP ≥ 7 mm Hg	79%	70%
			CVP ≥ 6 mm Hg	50%	90%
LVEF > 50%			SVV > 9.5%	79%	85%
			PAOP > 8 mm Hg	59%	75%
			CVP > 10 mm Hg	71%	62%
Septic shock[250]	↑CI ≥ 10%	PS	SVV—no threshold	—	—
Postcardiac surgery[251]	↑CI ≥ 15%	8–10	PPV > 11.8%	95%	92%
			SVV—no threshold		
ARDS[252]	↑CI ≥ 15%	5–8	PPV > 11.8%	68%	100%
Postcardiac surgery[253]	↑CI ≥ 15%	8	PPV > 12%	97%	95%

NR = not reported; PS = pressure support; LVEF, left ventricular ejection fraction.

beat-to-beat changes in pulse pressure reflect changes in LV SV. Unlike the SBP, which is affected by pleural pressure changes, the pulse pressure is affected by only the SV, because the pleural pressure equally affects the systolic and diastolic pressure. The absolute PPV% and the threshold to indicate fluid responsiveness is directly related to the tidal volume (Table 21-8).[246,256] For example, in critically ill patients receiving a tidal volume less than 8 mL/kg the threshold for fluid responsiveness was a PPV% > 8%, in contrast to a ≥8 mL/kg tidal volume where the threshold was a PPV% > 12%.[246] After a bolus in a fluid responsive patient the PPV will generally decrease, indicating less preload dependence (a shift up a given ventricular function curve), and the greater the decrease in the PPV the greater the increase in CI.[233] Changes in contractility may also affect the absolute PPV.[256]

Detection of Occult Hemorrhage

The changes in SPV or PPV may also be useful indicators of hemorrhage or occult blood loss.[257] In experimental hemorrhage in cardiac surgery patients, a change in SPV greater than 4 mm Hg was indicative of a significant blood loss.[258] Conversely, in patients undergoing therapeutic phlebotomy, SPV less than 5 mm Hg was considered to indicate an absence of hypovolemia.[259] In a recent animal study, the PPV% increased significantly (12.6% ± 1.4% to 15.8% ± 2.0%, $p < .05$) with 18% blood loss, whereas the HR, MAP, CVP, PAOP, and SPV did not change significantly until there was a 36% blood loss.[260] Caution must be exercised when interpreting these values as the VT varied between studies. In addition, hypotension may artificially increase the SPV% and PPV% because of the inclusion of absolute SBP or PP (pulse pressure) in the denominator of the equation.[245]

Stroke Volume Variation

Stroke volume variation (SVV), which is a derived volumetric indicator, can be continuously measured using pulse contour analysis or esophageal Doppler. The SVV is defined as the change in SV over a 30-second period.

$$SVV\% = \frac{(SV_{max} - SV_{min})}{[(SV_{max} + SV_{min})/2]} \times 100$$

The assumption underlying SVV is that the observed SV changes are respiratory-induced variations. The absolute SVV is also directly related to VT (Table 21-8), and as with other volumetric measurements, the SVV is more closely associated with changes in SV than are changes in PAOP and CVP.[249,261]

Concern has been voiced regarding the method used to measure the SVV (direct SV measurement versus pulse contour analysis)[262] as reflected in the contradictory results of the ability of SVV to predict fluid responsiveness.[263,264] The contradictory results may reflect differences in the tidal volume, which affects the absolute SVV,[265] or the hemodynamic status of the patients studied (stable versus hypovolemic). Finally, to achieve a stable tidal volume, SVV analysis can be performed only in patients who are on controlled mechanical ventilation and are heavily sedated/paralyzed.

Pleth Variability Index

A new noninvasive functional indicator that is under investigation is the pleth variability index (PVI).[266] The respiratory variation in pulse oximeter plethysmographic amplitude (ΔPOP), which is obtained using raw versus processed data from a standard pulse oximeter or other noninvasive devices (e.g., Finapres) is a sensitive and specific indicator of fluid responsiveness in patients with sepsis or undergoing cardiac or liver transplantation surgery.[251,267–270] However, performance of ΔPOP at the bedside is not feasible.

The PVI, which is a proprietary algorithm embedded in a standard pulse oximeter system, automatically calculates the ΔPOP.[266] On a pulse oximeter the perfusion index (PI) is an indicator of the adequacy of signal quality. The PI, which reflects the amplitude of the pulse oximeter waveform, is determined by indexing the infrared pulsatile (AC) oximeter signal caused by the pulsating arterial inflow (thought to reflect the beat-to-beat changes in SV) against the nonpulsatile (DC) infrared signal, which reflects the constant amount of light from the pulse oximeter that is absorbed by the skin and nonpulsatile blood flow. The PVI reflects the change in the PI amplitude over a single respiratory cycle (PVI = [(PImax − PImin)/PImax] × 100). In 25 cardiac surgery patients with a tidal volume of 8 to 10 mL/kg, a PVI > 14% discriminated between responders (↑CI ≥ 15%) and nonresponders with a sensitivity of 81% and 100% specificity, area under the curve (AUC = 0.92), and the PVI was comparable to PPV% (AUC = 0.94) and ΔPOP (AUC = 0.94).[271] In spontaneously breathing patients, the ΔPOP detects changes in intravascular volume[272] and ΔPOP[273] and PVI (threshold > 19%, sensitivity = 82%, specificity = 57%) also predict fluid responsiveness in conjunction with passive leg raising (PLR).[274]

Factors that may affect the PVI measurement include location of the oximeter probe (finger versus ear or forehead),[275,276] arm position as it affects venous congestion (DC portion of the PI measurement), and the loss of the signal with severe vasoconstriction. PVI measurements cannot be obtained in patients with cardiac arrhythmias, and variations in tidal volume will affect the absolute PVI values and threshold interpretation. Further research is needed in unstable patients, particularly those with changes in vascular tone, in different patient populations and using different proprietary systems as the algorithms and thus the PVI values may vary between systems.

Limitations of Functional Measures

There are limitations to the use of functional measurements. The SPV, PPV, and SVV cannot be monitored in a spontaneously breathing patient due to variation in pleural pressure change,[277] although PLR (described below) and evaluation of the ΔRAP can be performed in these patients.[278] Patients with cardiac arrhythmias have been excluded from all studies; thus, the use of these measures cannot be recommended in this population. There is also limited research in patients with decreased ventricular function.[249]

Changes in tidal volume,[246,279] PEEP,[280] and pulmonary compliance will alter the magnitude of the ventilator-induced change in these indices. The absolute values of these indices are directly related to VT (see Table 21-8). The VT also affects the sensitivity and specificity of the threshold values. In addition, at a low VT (6 mL/kg) the patient may be fluid responsive, yet not reach the threshold because of insufficient ventilator-induced variation.[281] Conversely, at a high VT the patient may exceed the threshold because of increased swings in pleural pressure and not fluid responsiveness.

A change in vascular tone may also affect the absolute values and the thresholds indicating fluid responsiveness. For example, in an animal model of hemorrhage, the SPV% and PPV% increased with hemorrhage (PPV% baseline 12% ± 9%, posthemorrhage 28% ± 11%, $p < .001$; SPV% baseline 12.5% ± 6.5%, posthemorrhage 21% ± 8, $p < .05$). The increase in values reflects increased fluid responsiveness, but may also reflect the effect of decreased SBP and pulse pressure on the absolute values. In the same animals, the subsequent addition of norepinephrine caused a decrease in PPV (14.5% ± 6.2%) and SPV (15.5% ± 4.5%). In this case, the decrease in SPV and PPV does not reflect resolution of the intravascular volume deficit, but rather an increase in vascular tone. In contrast, nitroprusside will increase variation.[282] Treatment would be a decrease in the vasodilator, not a fluid bolus. As described below, the integration of standard and functional indices may aid in tailoring therapy for a patient.

The mode of ventilation may affect the absolute values of the functional indices. In an animal model, under conditions of normovolemia and moderate hypovolemia the mode of ventilation (pressure versus volume controlled) does not affect the absolute values of the functional indices. With severe hypovolemia (hemorrhage = 30% estimated blood volume), functional indices are higher with volume-controlled versus pressure-controlled ventilation, which reflects the variable effects of the ventilator modes on intrathoracic pressure.[283] In addition, ventilation with variable VT (e.g., pressure support ventilation) also affects the accuracy of these measurements.[250]

Intra-abdominal hypertension (intra-abdominal pressure [IAP] > 12 mm Hg), may occur in up to 50% of ICU patients.[284] Absolute functional hemodynamic indicator values are affected by intra-abdominal hypertension. In an animal model, independent of intravascular volume, as the IAP increased the SPV, PPV, and SVV also increased.[285] Caution should be exercised when interpreting functional indices if the IAP is greater than RAP.[285,286] In patients with intra-abdominal hypertension or perhaps during laparoscopic surgery where a pneumoperitoneum is created, the use of PPV or SVV are recommended over the SPV or static indices (CVP or PAOP), as the PPV and SVV are less affected by the initial ventilator-induced increase in venous return that occurs with moderate increases in IAP.[286,287] If the IAP and pleural pressure are not changing, then changes in the functional indices may reflect fluid responsiveness, but absolute thresholds indicative of fluid responsiveness remain to be defined.

Passive Leg Raising

Evaluation of the reversible change in flow-related indices (e.g., aortic blood flow or SV by transthoracic echocardiography or TEE, transpulmonary thermodilution (TPTD) CO, arterial pulse pressure, or PVI) in response to PLR is another method to assess fluid responsiveness.[274,278,288–293] The PLR maneuver, which is performed by either elevating the legs to 30 to 45 degrees with the thorax horizontal or moving the patient from a head of bed elevated position to a horizontal position and concurrently elevating the legs to 30 to 45 degrees, causes a reversible translocation (autotransfusion) of approximately 300 mL of blood from the legs to the central circulation and increases RV preload.[294] If the patient is fluid responsive, the increased RV preload causes an increase in left ventricular preload and if the LV is also fluid responsive, the SV and CO increase. The increase in SV and CO occurs immediately and reaches a maximum approximately 1 minute after starting the PLR maneuver,[278] with evaluation of SV or pulse pressure 30 to 90 seconds after the PLR maneuver. For example, in patients with septic shock, a PLR-induced increase of ≥10% in aortic blood flow (as measured by TEE) predicted a fluid bolus-induced increase of ≥15% in aortic blood flow (sensitivity = 97%, specificity = 94%).[278] On the basis of the random and systematic variability in CO measurements, De Backer[291] recommends that at a minimum a 15% PLR-induced change in CO or SV be the threshold to predict fluid responsiveness. In contrast to earlier research that demonstrated a strong correlation ($r = 0.89$, $p < .001$) between PLR-induced change in pulse pressure and the response to a 300-mL fluid bolus,[288] a PLR-induced increase of ≥12% in pulse pressure was not as useful a marker of fluid responsiveness (sensitivity = 60%, specificity = 85%).[278]

Interpretation of the PLR-induced change is based on the assumption that there is adequate volume translocation from the legs to the central circulation and a change in ventricular preload, which can be assessed with a change in CVP or an echocardiographic preload indicator (e.g., FTc) or end-diastolic volume.[293] Of note, the change in preload is greater with a position transfer from the semirecumbent to the flat, supine position with legs raised versus the flat, supine position with the legs raised and provides a more sensitive and specific indicator of fluid responsiveness.[295] In contrast to other functional indices, evaluation of fluid responsiveness with PLR can be performed in patients who are spontaneously breathing or have arrhythmias.[278,292,296,297] PLR can cause RV compromise and should be performed cautiously in patients with decreased RVEF (<40%)[298] and care should be taken to avoid any noxious stimuli during the maneuver as this may cause changes in vascular tone and affect the response.

CO MEASUREMENT

Measurement of CO by the thermodilution method (thermodilution CO [TDCO]) is based on the injection of a known volume of cold or room temperature sterile D5W through the proximal port of the PA catheter into the RA. The blood is temporarily cooled by the injectate, and the change in temperature is sensed by a thermistor on the distal end of the PA catheter. A computer connected to the PA catheter calculates the CO on the basis of the area under the curve (AUC) using the Stewart–Hamilton equation. The temperature of the blood is assumed to be stable; thus, theoretically any change in blood temperature is caused by the injectate. This assumption may be incorrect, particularly if a patient is on mechanical ventilation, which causes a ventilator-induced variability in blood temperature or during rapid core temperature changes (induced hypothermia or rewarming). Most CO computers display the CO time–temperature curve, which allows for confirmation of a correct waveform.

Factors Influencing Thermodilution CO Measurement

Technical factors that affect the accuracy of thermodilution CO measures include the catheter position, site of injection, use of the correct calibration constant, injection technique, and volume and temperature of the injectate (Display 21-7). Pathophysiological conditions, such as tricuspid insufficiency and ventricular septal defect, inhibit adequate mixing of the thermal indicator and blood before it is sensed by the thermistor, and may cause underestimation of the TDCO.[191]

DISPLAY 21-7 PA Thermodilution CO

Factor	Notes	
Catheter position	• Distal port (catheter tip) must be in the PA (confirm by observing PA waveform) • Proximal port should be positioned in RA (verify by observing RA waveform) • Ensure catheter not wedged	
Injection port	• Inject into the proximal port (RA), venous infusion port, or RV port • Injections through side-port less accurate than injections through infusion port • Ensure exit of proximal port is outside of introducer sheath	
Calibration constant (CC) (see manufacturer's insert for catheter-specific CC)	• A factor that corrects for the gain of heat from the tubing and thermistor • Specific to (1) catheter type, (2) volume (5 vs. 10 mL), (3) temperature (iced vs. room temperature), (4) solution type (D5W vs. NS)	
Injection technique		
• Injection rate of 4 seconds	• Injection rate demonstrated to produce accurate results 5 to 10 mL injectate	
• Avoid handling syringe barrel	• Heat transfer from hands will alter accuracy of measurements	
• Inject at end-expiration or throughout respiratory cycle	• Respiratory-induced changes in CO, with up to 30% variability between inspiration/expiration • Measurements obtained at end-expiration decrease variability in measures (may overestimate CO by 1–1.5 times) • Measurements obtained with random injection throughout respiration increases validity of measures	
• Allow ~60 seconds between measures (monitor will indicate "READY")		
• Perform four TDCO measurements (may require more with room temperature injectate or 5 mL vs. 10 mL)	• To determine the CO, average three measurements that are within 10% of median value (e.g., if median value = 5 L/min, include all measures 4.5–5.5 L/min) or average the four measurements to provide 95% confidence that the CO is within 5% of "true" CO[299]	
Injectate temperature/volume • Temperature between injectate and blood should be ≥10°C • There is increased variability in CO measurements between cold and room temperature injectate particularly in patients with a low EF (<30%)[300]	Iced injectate (0–5°C) • 5 mL ≅ 10 mL • Low and high CO • Hyperdynamic patients • 10 mL iced is considered the standard*	Room temperature (19–25°C) • 10 mL RT ≅ 10 mL IT • CO within normal limits (5 mL IT ≅ 10 mL RT) • Normothermia (5 mL if fluid restricted) • Hyperdynamic patients • Hypothermia

Concomitant infusion	• Increased variability with concomitant infusion
	  • Consider discontinuation of infusion if there is not risk to the patient
	  • Avoid performance of TDCO during bolus infusion[301]
	• Remove all vasoactive medications from proximal port to avoid inadvertent bolus	

Patient position	• Reproducible TDCO measures with backrest up to 20 degrees (Note: CCO reproducible up to 40 degrees backrest elevation)[302] • 250 to 500 mL/min position-related change CO in 20-degree sidelying position • Compare sidelying CO to supine CO	
Concurrent use of sequential compression devices (SCDs)	• Note the effect of SCDs on CO measurements—decrease CO an average of 24% during inflation cycle[303]	

*It is not necessary to prime the catheter with cold solution before CO measurements

CO Measurement During Therapeutic Hypothermia

There is limited research on the effect of therapeutic hypothermia on CO measurement. During rapid changes in core body temperature there may be thermal instability or thermal noise in PA blood temperature, which increases the error in CO measurements most likely due to baseline drift in temperature immediately preceding the CO measurement. In cardiac surgery patients, TDCO and CCO were similar pre- and postoperatively, but during the early phase of bypass when there was a decrease in core temperature the TDCO and CCO were significantly different; however, determining which method was most accurate was not possible.[304] A newer technology (TPTD—PiCCO), which uses a cold injectate to calibrate the system, was found in two case studies to have clinically significant increase in variability at colder core temperature, which resolved with normothermia.[305,306] Rewarming may also increase thermal noise. Further research is needed to determine the most accurate method for CO measurement during therapeutic hypothermia.

Clinically Important Changes in CO

In general, a change of greater than 10% to 15% in CO is considered to be physiologically important. This criterion is based on studies that demonstrate that on average normal physiological variability ranges from approximately 4.8% to 9.9%,[307,308] although individual variation may be larger.[309] In atrial fibrillation, where there is increased CO variability, two sets of measurements must vary more than 15% before one can be 95% confident that a real change has occurred.[310] In assessing changes in CO, it is important to evaluate technical (Display 21-7), physiological, and pathophysiological factors related to the CO. The characterization of a CO change as clinically important should not be based on the absolute change in CO, but rather the patient's tolerance to the

Table 21-9 ■ HEMODYNAMIC INDICES

Indices/Equations	Normal Values	Interpretation
Preload		
RAP or CVP	2–6 mm Hg	RV filling pressure—does not predict fluid responsiveness
PAEDP	8–12 mm Hg	Indirect indicator of LV filling pressure and capillary filling pressure (P_{cap})
PAOP	6–12 mm Hg	Indirect indicator of LV filling pressure and capillary filling pressure (P_{cap})—does not predict fluid responsiveness
Afterload		
SBP	120 mm Hg	Clinical indicator of pressure that must be overcome during ejection phase of cardiac cycle.
SVR	800–1200 dynes/s/cm^{-5}	Measure of systemic vascular tone (one factor that affects cardiac afterload, but it is not synonymous with afterload;[311] increased SVR manifested by increased MAP)
SVRI	1900–2400 dynes/s/cm^{-5}/m^2	SVR indexed to BSA
Pulmonary vascular resistance	70–80 dynes/s/cm^{-5} or 1 Wood unit	Measure of resistance to RV ejection
Force of Contraction		
SV	60–180 mL/beat	Amount of blood ejected during each ventricular contraction
Stroke Volume Index	33–47 mL/beat/m^2	SVR indexed to BSA
RV stroke work index (RVSWI) RVSWI = SVI(MAP − CVP) × 0.0136	5–10 g-m/m^2/beat	Work performed by the right ventricle to eject blood into the pulmonary vasculature. Stroke work determines the energy expenditure (oxygen consumption) of the heart.
Left ventricular stroke work index (LVSWI)	45–65 g · m/m^2/beat	Work performed by the LV to eject blood into the aorta. The factor 0.0136 is used to convert pressure and volume to units of work.
LVSWI = SVI(MAP − PAOP) × 0.0136		With high filling pressures or hypotension, this equation may underestimate the amount of work performed.
RAP variation (ΔRAP)	ΔRAP > 1	Spontaneous inspiratory decrease in RAP > 1 mm Hg (on or off the ventilator) predictive of volume response
SPV	≥7–10 mm Hg depending on VT	With VT > 8 mL/kg an SPV > 10 mm Hg indicates fluid responsiveness. Unpublished animal research (VT = 8 mL/kg) identified an SPV ≥ 7 mm Hg as predictive of fluid responsiveness (sensitivity = 0.74/specificity 0.71, AUC = 0.75) (Bridges, 2008). Increased ΔSPV associated with in ΔCI for any given volume infused Patient must be on mechanical ventilation with minimal spontaneous ventilation and stable VT
SPV%	> 10% predictive in one study	Unpublished animal research (VT = 8 mL/kg) identified an SPV% > 7% as predictive of fluid responsiveness (sensitivity = 0.75, specificity = 0.69, AUC = 0.8). May be artificially increased with severe hypotension Patient must be on mechanical ventilation with minimal spontaneous ventilation and stable VT
PPV%	PPV > 12% (VT >8 mL/kg) PPV > 10% (VT = 8 mL/kg) PPV ≥ 8% (VT < 8 mL/kg	Affected only by change in SV (assuming arterial resistance and compliance do not acutely change during a single breath) May be a more reliable indicator than SPV or SPV% May be artificially increased with severe hypotension Patient must be on mechanical ventilation with minimal spontaneous ventilation and stable VT
SVV%	> 10% (VT = 10 mL/kg)	Requires proprietary technology Patient must be on mechanical ventilation with minimal spontaneous ventilation and stable VT No studies at lower VT
PVI	> 14% (VT 8–10 mL/kg)	Only one study describing thresholds. Further research required in unstable patients and patients with changing vascular tone

BSA, body surface area.

change based on indications of adequacy of oxygenation and perfusion. The direct and derived indices used in a comprehensive hemodynamic assessment are outlined in Table 21-9.

CONTINUOUS CARDIAC OUTPUT

CCO is performed using a PA catheter with a heating filament located in the RA or RV (14 to 25 cm from the catheter tip) that produces pseudorandom heat pulses in an on/off pattern. The heat pulses (0.02°C to 0.07°C) are detected by a thermistor on the distal end of the catheter. The heat pulses replace the cold bolus injection that is normally used for TDCO measurements. The CCO measurements are comparable with TDCO over a wide range of COs and temperatures, although increased variability exists between the two methods of measurements.[312–316]

The CCO measurements can be obtained with blood temperatures between 31°C and 41°C, although there is decreased accuracy above 38.5°C[312,317] and during induced hypothermia.[304] Of note, no studies have been done regarding the accuracy of CCO during induced hypothermia and rewarming postcardiac arrest. The CCO is accurate at low flow rates (0.5 to 3 L/min),[318] and during tachycardia or atrial fibrillation.[319] However, at higher flow rates, there is an increased difference between the absolute CCO and TDCO, although the percent difference remains similar.[312,320] The CCO on average overestimates the CO from a left ventricular assist device by approximately 0.5 L/min.[321]

A limitation of the CCO system is the delay between a change in CO and display of the change.[322,323] The displayed CO is updated every 30 seconds and represents the average CO over the previous 3 to 6 minutes. Although newer technology has decreased the response time, when the two systems most commonly used in practice were exposed to a 4-L/min CO change, they detected 20% of the change in 5.3 to 6.5 minutes, 50% change in 7.6 to 8.8 minutes, and 80% change in 10.8 to 11.1 minutes. When flow was changed by 1 L every 2 minutes, neither system detected the change.[324] The observed changes in CO also lag behind changes in MAP, HR, and $S\bar{v}o_2$ and TDCO.[315,325] The use of the STAT mode may be an option. In contrast to the concern that more frequent measurements may result in increased "noise," the bias (−0.04 to 0.18 L/min) and precision (0.61 to 0.84 L/min) of STAT mode versus TDCO were comparable to values comparing the TDCO with normal CCO.[326]

Several other factors may affect the accuracy and repeatability of CCO measurements. The infusion of a cold solution may cause overestimation of CCO measurements, although CCO measurements are minimally affected by fluctuations in PA temperatures.[304,327] In addition, fluid boluses cause an underestimation of CO in low flow states (CO < 4 L/min). Intracardiac shunt, tricuspid regurgitation, and incorrect catheter placement (thermal filament in the vena cava or in contact with the heart) decrease the accuracy of CCO measures.

LESS INVASIVE METHODS FOR CO MONITORING

Over the past decade, there has been increased emphasis on developing less invasive methods for CO monitoring. Intermittent CO measurements using the TPID technique involve injection of an indicator into the venous circulation with a sensor in the systemic arterial circulation. There are currently two TPID CO techniques that have been validated against other CO measurement methods.[328] The Transpulmonary Thermodilution (TPID) method uses a 10 to 15 mL injection of iced D5W or saline via a central catheter (subclavian or jugular) as the indicator with a 4-Fr thermistor-tipped arterial catheter placed in the femoral, brachial, or axillary artery (PiCCO; Pulsion Medical Systems, Munich, Germany). Recently, a study suggests that the thermistor-tipped catheter may also be placed in the radial artery.[329] Injection of the cold solution through the femoral vein also produces reliable estimates, but absolute CO values are higher than those obtained using the jugular vein due to increased transit time. The LiDCO system (LiDCO; London, UK) uses a subtherapeutic bolus of lithium injected via a peripheral or central catheter as the indicator. The lithium bolus is detected and a time curve, which is used to derive the CO, is created by a lithium-sensitive electrode attached to an arterial pressure monitoring line.[330] The dose of lithium is too small to create a pharmacological effect;[331] however, LiDCO measurements cannot be performed in patients receiving lithium and neuromuscular blocking agents may also interfere with calibration.

The TPID methods are now used primarily to calibrate the pulse contour. For thermodilution pulse contour analysis, calibration is based on the analysis of the area under the systolic portion of the thermodilution curve and a coefficient characterizing vascular compliance. Once calibrated, the system (PiCCO) provides a beat-to-beat analysis of SV. The lithium-based system uses pulse power analysis, which uses a series of approximations regarding the relationship between radial artery pressure, aortic pressure, aortic flow, and CO.[332] The LiDCO is then used to calibrate the system and convert the derived CO into a patient-specific CO. There have been concerns raised regarding the ability of these systems to accurately reflect the absolute or relative change in SV during periods of marked hemodynamic instability, although the data remain equivocal.[333,334]

The FloTrac/Vigileo System (Edwards Lifesciences, Irvine, California) also provides continuous SV monitoring. The system uses a proprietary sensor that can be attached to any arterial line. This system does not require external calibration, rather the SV is derived using the following equation ($SV = K \times$ pulsatility), where the calibration constant (K) characterizes the patient's vascular resistance and arterial compliance based on their sex, height, weight, and age and the pulse pressure waveform characteristics, and pulsatility is derived from continuous analysis of the arterial pressure waveform.[328,335] The early evaluation of this device found only moderate agreement with other CO methods;[316,336–343] however, derived CO measurements using a new algorithm (version 1.10), which updates the calibration every minute, is generally comparable to other CO measurement devices.[344,345] However, in hemodynamically unstable patients there was an unacceptable difference (56%) in FloTrac CO compared with thermodilution CO.[346,347]

A concern regarding these noninvasive indices is that changes in vascular resistance may necessitate recalibration of the system. The manufacturers recommend recalibration of the LiDCO and PiCCO systems every 8 hours or with marked changes in hemodynamic status.[348,349] Unfortunately, there is no standard definition of what a "marked change" in hemodynamics is. One study found that while small changes in SVR (<20%) do not affect the pulse contour measurements, a greater than 50% increase in SVR increases the bias between PiCCO and TDCO measurements.[350] In a recent study using the PiCCO system, while the TPTD and the derived CO correlated over an 8-hour period ($r^2 = 0.68$) the difference between the value was less than 30% for only the first hour after calibration and when the SVR changed more than 15% the error was 36%.[351] In another study, the LiDCO CO was within acceptable levels of agreement for only 4 hours after recalibration[352] and in an animal model of acute hemorrhage the LiDCO overestimated CO, suggesting the need to recalibrate with acute changes in preload, afterload, or contractility.[353] An algorithm for the PiCCO system that accounts for vascular compliance and resistance was studied in postoperative cardiac surgery patients with CO changes greater than 20% (ΔCO 40% ± 27%) and a wide range of SVRs (450 to 2,360 dynes/s/cm^{-5}). The PiCCO CO was closely correlated ($r = 0.88$) and similar to TDCO measures (bias = −0.2 ±1.2 L/min), although there was increased variability in the CO in contrast to hemodynamically stable patients.[349] These data suggest that the systems need to be recalibrated when there is a greater than 15% to 20% change in SVR or CO.

Another concern about using these less invasive methods is the lack of information about the risk for pulmonary edema. Transpulmonary indicator thermodilution methods allow for the measurement of both intrathoracic blood volume and extravascular lung water (EVLW).[225] The EVLW is normally between 3 and

7 mL/kg and is generally greater than 10 mL/kg with cardiogenic and permeability pulmonary edema.[354] The EVLW may have prognostic implications;[355] however, results are equivocal on whether it aids in the differential diagnosis of cardiogenic versus permeability pulmonary edema. There is no current research regarding the use of EVLW to guide fluid therapy and EVLW cannot be measured using TPTD in patients who have a large pulmonary vascular obstruction, focal lung injury, or a lung resection.

Limitations of TPID Method

A decrease in the accuracy of TPID measurements may occur with any condition that alters the transfer of the indicator across the heart and lungs (e.g., intracardiac shunts, aortic aneurysm/stenosis, pneumonectomy, and pulmonary embolism), arrhythmias, rapidly changing temperature, and during extracorporeal circulation or intra-aortic balloon pump. A relative contraindication to pulse contour analysis is the presence an extremely damped arterial waveform.[350] Of interest, in a study of LiDCO, 68% of the catheters were underdamped; however, this did not affect the relationship between the continuous LiDCO and intermittent CO measurements.[356] Similar research is needed on PiCCO and the FloTrac systems.

Doppler Ultrasound

Doppler ultrasound is performed using an internal probe (esophagus or endotracheal tube) or via a transcutaneous approach via the suprasternal notch. This section focuses on the esophageal Doppler monitor (EDM). Blood flow measurements using ultrasound are based on the Doppler principle. The system emits an ultrasound beam that is directed toward flowing blood. The ultrasound wave is reflected by the blood moving toward the signal, causing the signal to shift in frequency. The magnitude of the frequency shift is proportional to blood flow velocity. Blood flow is equal to the cross-sectional area of the column (i.e., the aorta) times the flow velocity. Stroke volume is derived by multiplying the cross-sectional area times the area under the flow curve. Inaccurate cross-sectional area measurement and altered distribution of blood flow between the aorta and brachiocephalic vessels leads to inaccurate estimation of the CO.

The EDM probe, which is embedded in a 6- to 7-mm diameter tube, is positioned at the midthoracic level (approximately 30 to 40 cm from the teeth) and measures blood flow in the descending aorta (Fig. 21-20*A*). Correct positioning of the probe is determined by the observation of an optimal cardiac signal. EDM should not be used if the patient has esophageal disease.

Clinical Applications of EDM

In addition to measuring the CO, the indices obtained from the Doppler flow wave also provide information regarding preload, contractility, and afterload (Table 21-10 and Fig. 21-20*B* and *C*). The intraoperative use of the EDM to guide optimization of

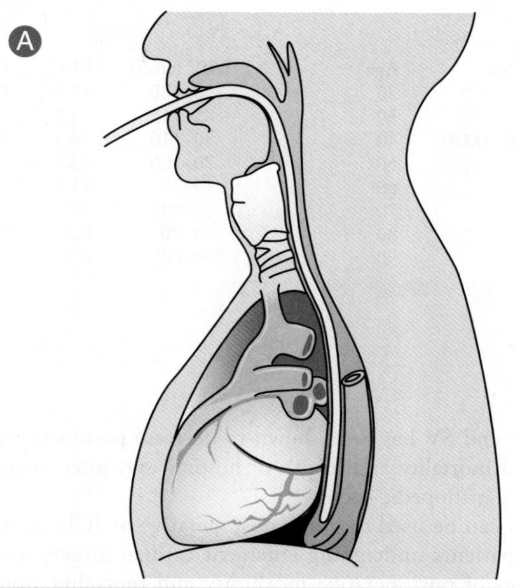

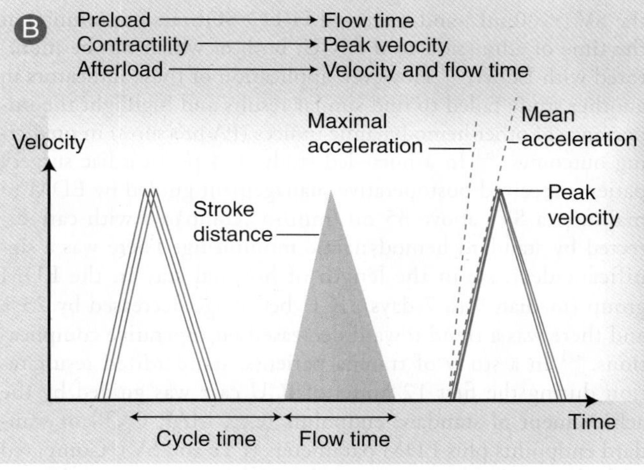

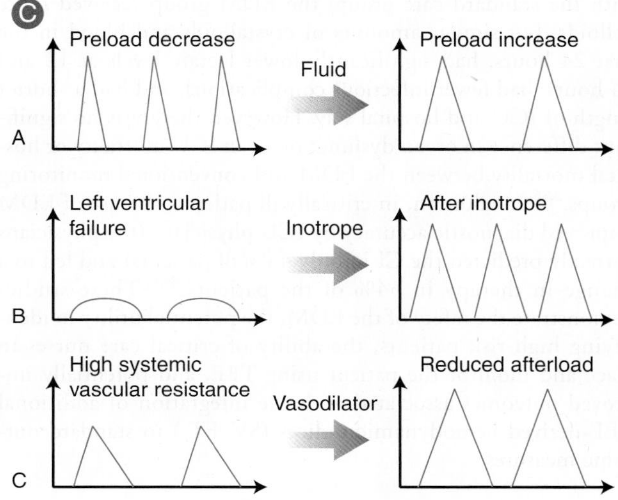

■ **Figure 21-20** (A) Correct positioning of the esophageal Doppler probe. (Reproduced courtesy of Deltex Medical.) (B) Doppler flow velocity waveform. (C) EDM waveforms. The first graph shows the components of the normal Doppler waveform and the effect of increasing preload, which corresponds to an increased FT_c. The second graph displays poor contractility (decreased PV), which responds to inotropes by increasing PV. The last graph displays increased afterload (decreased FT_c and decreased PV) and the effects of afterload reduction (increased FT_c and increased PV) (Gan, T. [2000]. The esophageal Doppler as an alternative to the pulmonary artery catheter. *Current Opinion in Critical Care, 6*, 214–221.)

Table 21-10 ■ DOPPLER INDICES

Indices	Normal Value			Interpretation
Flow time corrected (FT_c)	330–360 milliseconds			Correction in flow time for HR. The FT_c is an indicator of preload.[311] The FTc may also be affected by factors that affect vascular resistance.[357] Example: ↓ FT_c (narrow base of waveform)—hypovolemia/decreased preload (may reflect changes in preload or preload-CO-induced changes in vascular resistance). ↑ FT_c—increased preload—decreasing vascular resistance.
Peak velocity (PV)	Age	PV (cm/s)	MA	Peak velocity of blood (apex of waveform) during the systolic ejection phase. Provides an index of contractility. ↑ PV—increased contractility
	20	90–120	15.6	
	30	85–115	14.9	
Mean acceleration (MA)	40	80–110	14.1	MA: Maximum slope of the velocity curve as a function of time (derivative of the velocity). Indicator of contractility.
	50	70–100	12.7	
	60	60–90	11.2	
	70	50–80	9.7	
	80	40–70	8.2	*↑ afterload: ↓ PV (decreased contractile force) and ↓ FTc (decreased ejection time)
	90	30–60	6.7	

volume status and SV has been shown to decrease postoperative morbidity and mortality and length of hospital stay after major abdominal and orthopedic surgery.[358–361]

EDM also can be used to guide postoperative or ICU management. In patients undergoing emergent cardiac surgery, the best indicators of postoperative morbidity and mortality were the SV (<60 mL) and increased HR (>90 beats per minute) at the time of admission to the ICU, both of which can be monitored with EDM.[362] However, application of these indicators in another study failed to find similar results and highlight the importance of other hemodynamic indices (PA pressures) in predicting outcomes.[363] In a nurse-led study, 174 post-cardiac surgery patients received postoperative management guided by EDM to maintain a SVI above 35 mL/min/m^2 compared with care directed by standard hemodynamic monitoring. There was a significant decrease in the length of hospital stay in the EDM group (median 9 to 7 days), ICU bed usage decreased by 23% and there was a trend toward decreased postoperative complications.[364] In a study of trauma patients, standardized resuscitation during the first 12 hours of ICU care was guided by the achievement of standard endpoints (e.g., MAP, CVP) or standard endpoints plus EDM parameters (FTc and SV). Compared with the standard care group, the EDM group received more colloids, but similar amounts of crystalloids and blood in the first 24 hours, had significantly lower lactate levels at 12 and 24 hours, had fewer infectious complications, and had a shorter length of ICU and hospital stay. However, there was no significant difference in organ dysfunction or in ICU mortality or hospital mortality between the EDM and conventional monitoring groups.[365] In addition, in critically ill patients, the use of EDM improved diagnostic accuracy by ICU physicians (the physicians correctly predicted the CI in only 44% of patients) and led to a change in therapy in 54% of the patients.[366] These studies demonstrate the safety of the EDM, the potential utility in identifying high-risk patients, the ability of critical care nurses to place and monitor the patient using TEE, and potentially improved outcomes associated with the integration of additional TEE-derived hemodynamic indices (SV, FT_c) to standard outcome measures.

Echocardiography

Doppler echocardiography provides information on CO and estimates of intracardiac pressures, global and regional LV and RV systolic and diastolic function, end-diastolic area (preload), and regional wall motion abnormalities.[367] Echocardiography is also useful in the diagnosis of traumatic aortic injury after blunt chest trauma, cardiac tamponade, mechanical complications after an acute MI (e.g., mitral valve dysfunction, free wall rupture, septal defect), sepsis-induced myocardial dysfunction, and the cause of a pulseless electrical activity cardiac arrest.[368–370] Echocardiography or the measurement of CO should be considered in patients with clinical evidence of ventricular failure and persistent shock despite adequate fluid resuscitation.[166]

TEE in the ICU

In the ICU, TEE rather than transthoracic echocardiography may be necessary when there is interference with imaging caused by subcutaneous air, chest wall edema, the presence of mediastinal or pleural tubes, mechanical ventilation, or surgical dressings. TEE is typically used for a single monitoring event in sedated/anesthetized patients. The use of TEE improves diagnostic accuracy in critically ill patients compared with PA catheter-derived diagnosis, particularly in cases of unexplained hypotension, abnormal ventricular function, cardiac tamponade, and the determination of preload status.[371–374] However, results are variable from studies comparing the agreement and correlation of TEE–CO with TDCO and Fick–CO measurements;[375–377] thus, CO–TEE can be used to follow trends, but caution must be taken when interpreting absolute values.

TEE also can be used to evaluate respiratory-induced changes in peak aortic flow velocity and vena caval diameter as indicators of preload responsiveness.[378,379] However, ventricular volume measurement (left ventricular end-diastolic area) does not predict fluid responsiveness,[235] which highlights the difference between preload and preload responsiveness.

Although TEE is a relatively safe procedure, complications can occur (major complications <0.02%).[380] The patient should be monitored for hypotension, arrhythmias, and vomiting and aspiration during placement of the probe. Additional complications include pharyngeal, laryngeal, or esophageal trauma and dental damage.

Impedance Cardiography

Impedance cardiography (ICG) or thoracic electrical bioimpedance (TEB) measures the electrical resistance of the thorax to a high-frequency, low-amplitude current. Bioreactance technology, which is a modification of the TEB technology, may improve the signal-to-noise ratio seen with TEB and decrease the variability in the measurement.[381,382] With TEB, the current is passed through the thorax and the voltage change with each systole is measured. This change in voltage is the result of a change in TEB, which corresponds with systole.[383] The TEB is inversely proportional to the content of thoracic fluids (i.e., when thoracic fluids increase the TEB decreases). Three factors affect TEB: (1) change in tissue fluid volume; (2) respiratory-induced changes in pulmonary and venous volume; and (3) changes in aortic blood flow. The change in aortic blood flow can be measured by the change in TEB, assuming that the other factors remain stable or are filtered.[384] The system consists of specialized electrodes placed laterally on the neck and at the lateral aspect of the lower thorax (at the level of the xiphisternal junction). The electrical voltage (2 to 4 mA), which is safe and not felt by the patient, is passed longitudinally through the thorax between electrodes.[383] Whole body ICG uses electrodes placed on the wrists and ankles and a different algorithm to estimate CO.[385]

Factors that affect the accuracy of ICG measures include the positioning of the electrodes (i.e., the electrodes must be in exactly the same position for each measurement), any factor that interferes with electrode contact (e.g., perspiration), an irregular heart rhythm, altered tissue water content (chest wall edema, pulmonary edema, or pleural effusions), aortic valve disease, abnormalities of the aorta (coarctation or aortic aneurysm), and cardiac shunts. Obesity does not appear to affect the accuracy of ICG measurements.[386]

A meta-analysis published in 1997 suggested that ICG-CO might be useful for trend analysis, but absolute ICG-CO measurements may not be accurate.[387] Since then, there have been changes to the algorithm and technology. In a study of cardiothoracic patients using the BioZ (CardioDynamics, San Diego, CA) and the most current algorithms there was good agreement between ICG-CO and TDCO (bias = −0.17 L/min, precision = 1.09 L/min).[388] Similar results were found in post-operative cardiac surgery patients using the Aesculon (Osypka Medical, Berlin, Germany)[389] and in cardiac surgery and medical-surgical cardiac patients using whole body impedance.[385,390] However, in a recent study of 15 medical and surgical ICU patients, the bias and precision between Fick and TDCO was 1.7 ± 3.8 L/min, Fick and ICG-CO (BioZ, CardioDynamics) 2.4 ± 4.7 L/min, and TDCO and ICG-CO 0.7 ± 2.9 L/min; although there was less internal agreement for TDCO (±8%), which was measured throughout the respiratory cycle, than for ICG-CO (±4%).[391] In perioperative cardiac surgery the ICG SV measured with the HL-4 (Hemologic, Amersfoort, the Netherlands) and three different algorithms was not comparable to TDCO. However, the ICG-CO was less variable than TDCO, which was measured throughout the respiratory cycle.[392] These studies demonstrate the need to identify which monitor and the algorithm are used in a given study, the limitations of using TDCO as the standard for comparison, and the potentially large bias in the ICG-CO measurements compared with other CO measurement methods. These results support the recommendation to follow the ICG-CO for trends and to cautiously interpret absolute CO values.

Clinical Applications of ICG

Despite the concerns regarding the comparability of ICG-CO with other CO measures, ICG has been used for intraoperative monitoring and in outpatient and emergency department settings for the diagnosis and management of patients. For example, in hemodynamically unstable ICU patients, the physicians were only accurate in their assessment of CO and thoracic fluid content in 57% and 48% of the patients, respectively, compared with ICG-derived values.[393] A unique variable provided by ICG is a measure of thoracic fluid status (Zo), which is a composite measure of interstitial, alveolar, and intracellular fluid and is the inverse of thoracic fluid content.[394] A normal Zo is 20 to 30 Ω for men and 25 to 30 Ω for women, although there is individual variability and the Zo values can be affected by other thoracic conditions (e.g., emphysema, pneumonia).[395] In patients with HF, there was an inverse relationship between Zo and chest radiograph findings of pulmonary edema, and a Zo less than 19 Ω was highly sensitive and specific for identifying radiographic findings of pulmonary edema. Interstitial edema was present at Zo = 18.5 ± 7.1 Ω and alveolar edema was present at 14.8 ± 5 Ω.[396] Use of ICG may aid in the differential diagnosis of shortness of breath. In patients with suspected HF and shortness of breath, the Zo was significantly different in those with radiographic evidence of cardiomegaly (17.5 ± 5 Ω) and pulmonary edema (17.2 ± 4.2 Ω) than those with normal radiographs (23.4 ± 5.4 Ω).[397]

In patients with HF or acute coronary syndrome, ICG has been used to measure CO and cardiac power (the product of simultaneously measured CO, MAP, and SVR). Measurement of CO, SVR, and cardiac power has been found to be useful in the differential diagnosis of different acute HF syndromes (e.g., cardiogenic shock, hypertensive crisis, ADHF, and pulmonary edema)[398] and in the titration of vasodilator agents for patients with acute HF.[385] However, for the detection of a CI $\leq$ 2.2 L/min/m^2 as determined by TDCO, the ICG had a sensitivity of 62%, specificity of 79%, and a positive predictive value of 68%, again highlighting the limitations in using absolute ICG values rather than following trends.[399] In patients with chronic HF, ICG measures of cardiac reserve (i.e., increased CO with exercise or a stress test) were inversely related to exercise intolerance.[400] In addition, bioimpedance measures of CO reserve during exercise and cardiac power during dobutamine stress echocardiography identified patients with multivessel coronary artery disease or stress-induced ischemia.[398,401]

ICG monitoring also has been used for the management of patients with HF.[394,402–404] Intrathoracic impedance monitoring described below may also be beneficial for these patients.[395] In patients with resistant hypertension, therapy guided by ICG monitoring resulted in a greater improvement in control rates compared with management by an experienced clinician (56% vs. 34%, $p < .05$)[405] and ambulatory impedance monitoring, which uses ambulatory ICG and BP monitoring may provide further insight into the patient's hemodynamic status (LV function, SVR, BP) during daily activity and allow for further tailoring of therapy.[406,407] The ICG has also been used to optimize pacemaker therapy.[408,409] However, ICG monitoring is *absolutely contraindicated* in patients who have pacemakers that use "minute ventilation" to guide the firing rate. In this case, the ICG signal interferes with the pacemaker signal and potentially cause a rapid increase in firing rate.[410]

ICG monitoring also has been performed in the emergency department to describe cardiopulmonary and tissue perfusion patterns in survivors and nonsurvivors of trauma or septic shock, which may aid in the earlier identification and treatment of patients with occult hypoperfusion or cardiovascular impairment.[411–413] For example, in acute trauma patients, CI by ICG and thermodilution agreed (-0.07 ± 0.47 L/min/m^2) and noninvasive CI (along with other MAP and other oxygenation and perfusion indices) was higher in survivors versus nonsurvivors.[414] In addition, indices obtained with noninvasive monitoring of cardiac, pulmonary, and perfusion indices (CI, SpO_2, and transcutaneous O_2/FiO_2) were predictors of morbidity and mortality.[414,415]

Implantable Hemodynamic Monitors

Although the hemodynamic profile of ADHF is often thought to reflect low CO, preliminary analysis of data from 107,362 patients in the Acute Decompensate Heart Failure Registry (ADHERE) suggest that a typical hemodynamic profile is increased PAOP and vascular resistance with a CO within normal range. Forty-six percent of the patients had mild or no impairment in systolic function and 50% presented with an SBP > 140 mm Hg. In these patients the primary cause of admission was volume overload.[416] In the Organized Program to Initiate Lifesaving Treatment in Hospitalized Patients with Heart Failure (OPTIMIZE-HF) study, which had more than 34,000 patients in the registry, 47% of the patients had preserved LV function and 48% had an SBP > 140 mm Hg, and in a study of 3,580 patients in the EuroHeart Failure Survey II (EHFS II), 34% of the patients had preserved systolic function (EF > 45%).[417] In all these studies, less than 2% of patients presented with an SBP < 90 mm Hg or cardiogenic shock.

Two subtypes of acute HF have been suggested: (1) acute decompensated cardiac failure, characterized by deterioration of cardiac performance over days to weeks leading to decompensation; and (2) acute vascular failure, characterized by acute hypertension and increased vascular stiffness.[418] Dividing acute HF into these subtypes suggests the need for different types of monitoring and therapies. Although use of a PA catheter in patients with HF was not found to improve outcomes in patients who presented with severe HF (average left ventricular ejection fraction = 19%),[158] implantable hemodynamic monitors (IHMs) may allow for earlier detection of hemodynamic deterioration (ADHF) before the onset of symptoms and the initiation of preventative measures.[419,420] These early preventive measures may be important as there are negative effects from hemodynamic congestion (e.g., increased LV wall stress with increased myocardial remodeling and hypertrophy, increased angiotensin II release, subendocardial ischemia) that occur before the onset of signs and symptoms (clinical congestion—dyspnea, jugular vein distention, peripheral edema, pulmonary crackles/rales).[159]

Intrathoracic Impedance Monitoring

Intrathoracic impedance monitoring is based on a software that is integrated into a cardiovascular resynchronization therapy pacemaker and/or implantable cardioverter–defibrillators. Intrathoracic impedance is measured between the RV lead and the device casing. There is an inverse relationship between intrathoracic impedance and PAOP, LVEDP, and the degree of pulmonary fluid and congestion. In the Medtronic Impedance Diagnostics in Heart Failure Patients trial (MidHeFT), which evaluated intrathoracic impedance using the OptiVol device (Medtronic, Minneapolis, Minnesota) in patients with NYHA Class III/IV HF, intrathoracic impedance decreased on average 15 days before the onset of symptoms,[419] and results from the Fluid Accumulation Status Trial (FAST) suggest that decreasing impedance can predict health care use (e.g., hospitalization for HF, modification of diuretic therapy).[421] A threshold trigger of 60 Ω is also a sensitive but not specific indicator of clinical deterioration independent of clinical signs and symptoms.[422] However, the important clinical question that has not yet been answered is whether use of these devices improves the tailoring of therapy, decreases hospitalizations, and improves quality of life for these individuals.

Other factors that may decrease intrathoracic impedance include pneumonia, pleural effusions, and revision of the pocket for implantation of the device (must wait 34 days before beginning to use the device). An increase in intrathoracic impedance may also occur with dehydration or decreased intravascular volume, pneumothorax, and increased air trapping (e.g., chronic obstructive pulmonary disease or positive pressure ventilation).

Implantable Continuous Pressure Monitoring

Research is ongoing using an IHM that provides a continuous estimation of the PAEDP from a lead placed permanently in the RV outflow track.[423] The Chronicle Offers Management to Patients with Advanced Signs and Symptoms of Heart Failure (COMPASS-HF) study, which compared the effect of HF management using standard therapy versus standard therapy plus IHM data, failed to find any difference in HF-related events, although the IHM group had a significantly longer time to the first HF-related hospitalization.[424] The HeartPod, which is a device that is implanted into the left atrial septum and provides continuous monitoring of left atrial pressures, is also under investigation.[425,426] Similar to continuous intrathoracic impedance monitoring, it remains to be demonstrated if use of IHM technology improves outcomes for individuals with HF.[427]

OXYGEN SUPPLY AND DEMAND

In critically ill patients, the monitoring and evaluation of specific indicators of tissue hypoxia are warranted, because the standard indices of hemodynamic stability (i.e., BP, HR, and urine output [UOP]) may be normal in the presence of continued tissue hypoxia (e.g., occult hypoperfusion or cryptic shock). For example, 36 critically ill patients who despite being resuscitated to a HR of 50 to 120 bpm and a MAP of 70 to 110 mm Hg continued to have signs of tissue hypoxia (lactate >2 mmol/L and a central venous oxygen saturation [$ScvO_2$] < 65%). Although interventions were undertaken to improve tissue oxygenation for these patients (as indicated by a decrease in lactate and an increase in $ScvO_2$), there were no changes in the BP or HR.[428] Similar results were observed in patients with cardiogenic shock[429] and trauma victims.[430] Use of standard endpoints (e.g., MAP > 60 mm Hg) may also be insufficient in ensuring adequate tissue perfusion. For example, in patients with septic shock whose MAP was increased with norepinephrine from 65 to 85 mm

Hg, while the CI increased there was no improvement in indicators of tissue perfusion.[96] Therefore, standard hemodynamic indices may not be sensitive to changes in tissue oxygenation, and the use of global ($\dot{D}o_2$, $\dot{V}o_2$, serum lactate, and $S\bar{v}o_2$ or $Scvo_2$) and regional indices (transcutaneous O_2 and CO_2 saturation, near-infrared spectroscopy (NIRS) and sublingual microcirculation assessment) may offer additional targeted information.

Global Indicators of Oxygen Supply and Demand

Oxygen delivery depends on the amount of O_2 in the blood and how much blood is delivered to the tissues (CO). The O_2 delivery ($\dot{D}o_2$) and O_2 consumption ($\dot{V}o_2$) equations are outlined in Table 21-11. An understanding of the factors that affect $\dot{D}o_2$ and $\dot{V}o_2$ is important to guide therapeutic decision, although the use of absolute $\dot{D}o_2$ and $\dot{V}o_2$ values as endpoints for resuscitation has not been found to improve outcomes.

Mixed Venous Oxygen Saturation

Although CO provides important information about the capacity of the cardiopulmonary system to deliver O_2 to the tissues, it does not necessarily depict the adequacy of O_2 supply at the tissue level. The $S\bar{v}o_2$, which is a global measure of the balance between total body O_2 delivery and consumption,[431] is affected by factors that affect O_2 delivery (CO, Hb, Sa_{o2}) and consumption ($\dot{V}o_2$) as described by the following equation:

$$S\bar{v}o_2 = Sa_{O2} - \left(\frac{\dot{V}o_2}{CO} \times 1.36 \times Hgb\right)$$

The assumption is that if the Hgb and Sa_{o2} are not changing; the change in $S\bar{v}o_2$ reflects a change in CO. However, a decreased $S\bar{v}o_2$ may also be caused by arterial hypoxemia, increased $\dot{V}o_2$, or a decreased Hgb; and in patients with severe HF (EF $<$ 30%) the $S\bar{v}o_2$ is not an adequate indicator of changes in CO.[432] Conversely, in septic shock an increased $S\bar{v}o_2$ may indicate inadequate O_2 utilization.[431]

Technical Aspects of Monitoring

Components of a continuous $S\bar{v}o_2$ monitoring system include the fiberoptic PA catheter, the optical module, and the microprocessor. The fiberoptic catheter is a quadruple-lumen PA catheter with fiberoptic channels running the length of the catheter. The optical module contains diodes that emit light pulses through one of the fiberoptic channels in the tip of the catheter. The second fiberoptic channel returns reflected light to a photodetector in the optical module (reflected spectrometry). The amount of light reflected depends on the amount of saturated Hgb, because oxygenated and deoxygenated Hgb have different reflections. The light is relayed electronically to the microprocessor, which interprets the light signal and determines the ratio between oxygenated and deoxygenated blood. The $S\bar{v}o_2$ is based on this ratio.

Indications

Continuous $S\bar{v}o_2$ monitoring has been recommended for monitoring and as an outcome measure in patients with sepsis/septic shock, cardiac surgery, complicated MI (i.e., cardiogenic shock), or patients with respiratory failure requiring PEEP. $S\bar{v}o_2$ monitoring is also recommended in the absence of hypotension when shock is suspected by history and physical examination.[166]

Clinical Application

The $S\bar{v}o_2$ normally ranges from 70% to 75%, which is associated with a Pvo_2 of 40 mm Hg. An $S\bar{v}o_2$ of less than 40% is usually accompanied by anaerobic metabolism, and an $S\bar{v}o_2$ between 40% and 60% indicates inadequate $\dot{D}o_2$ or excessive O_2 demand. In response to increased O_2 demand, the body either increases CO to deliver more O_2 or increases the extraction of O_2 from the blood. Although the $S\bar{v}o_2$ reflects the O_2 balance for the entire body, it does not provide information on the adequacy of oxygenation for individual organs.

When the Sa_{o2} is maintained near 100%, there is a strong relationship between the $S\bar{v}o_2$ and the O_2 extraction ratio (O_2ER), as defined by the equation:

$$S\bar{v}o_2 = 1 - O_2ER.$$

Increased O_2 extraction decreases Hgb saturation, which is reflected as a decrease in $S\bar{v}o_2$. In general, as long as O_2 delivery is

Table 21-11 ■ OXYGEN TRANSPORT EQUATIONS

Variables	Equation/Example	Normal
Arterial oxygen content (Ca_{o2})	$(Hgb \times 1.36 \times Sa_{o2}) + (0.003 \times Pa_{o2})$ $(15 \times 1.36 \times 0.99) + (0.003 \times 100)$	20 mL/dL
Venous oxygen content (Cv_{o2})	$(Hgb \times 1.36 \times S\bar{v}o_2) + (0.003 \times PvO_2)$ $(15 \times 1.36 \times 0.75) + (0.003 \times 40)$	15 mL/dL
Oxygen Delivery ($\dot{D}O_2$)	$CO \times Ca_{o2} \times 10$ $5 \times (15 \times 1.36 \times 0.99) \times 10$	1000 mL/min
Oxygen Delivery Index ($\dot{D}o_2I$)	$CI \times Ca_{o2} \times 10$ $3.5 \times (15 \times 1.36 \times 0.99) \times 10$	600 mL/min/m^2
Oxygen Consumption ($\dot{V}o_2$)	$CO \times 1.36 \times Hgb\ (Sa_{o2} - S\bar{v}o_2)$ $5 \times 1.36 \times 15\ (1.0 - 0.75)$	250 mL/min
Oxygen Consumption Index ($\dot{V}o_2I$)	$CI \times 1.36 \times Hgb\ (Sa_{o2} - S\bar{v}o_2)$ $3.5 \times 1.36 \times 15\ (1.0 - 0.75)$	125 mL/min/m^2
Oxygen Extraction Ratio (O_2ER)	$\dot{D}o_2/\dot{V}o_2$ $(Ca_{o2} - Cv_{o2})/\ Ca_{o2}$ $[(Hgb \times 1.36 \times Sa_{o2}) - (Hgb \times 1.36 \times S\bar{v}o_2)]/(Hgb \times 1.36 \times Sa_{o2})$ $(Sa_{o2} - S\bar{v}O_2)/\ Sa_{o2}$	25%
Cardiac Index/Oxygen Extraction Ratio	$CI/O_2ER\ (3.0 \div 0.25)$	10–12

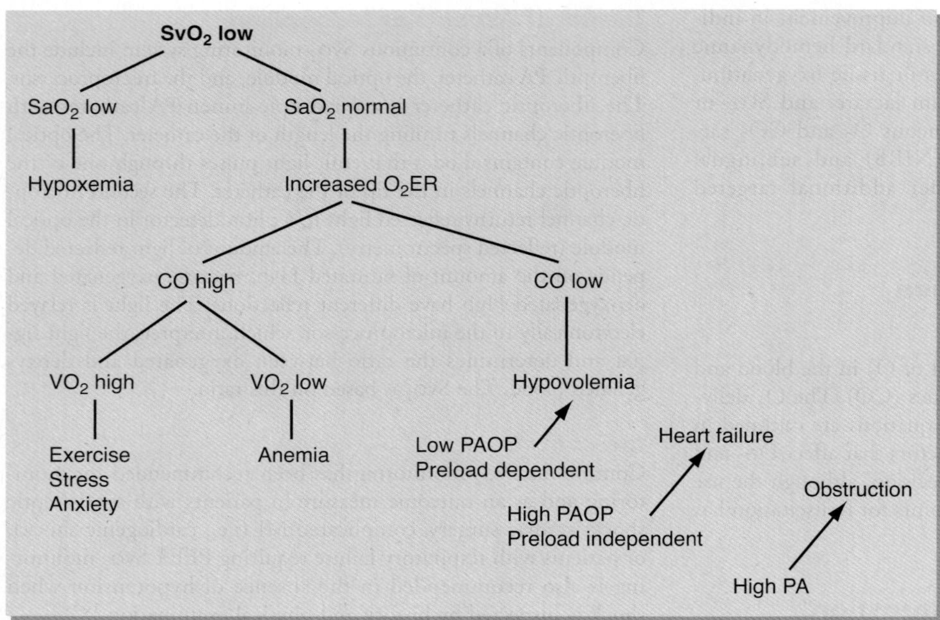

■ **Figure 21-21** Interpretation of hemodynamic data starting with mixed venous O_2 saturation (Svo_2), O_2ER, O_2 extraction ratio; $\dot{V}o_2$, O_2 uptake. (Vincent, J. L., De Backer, D. [2002]. Cardiac output measurement: Is least invasive always the best? *Critical Care Medicine, 30*[10], 2381).

adequate to meet tissue O_2 demands, the $S\bar{v}o_2$ remains within 60% to 80%. Decreases in $S\bar{v}o_2$ occur with an increase in O_2 demand (e.g., fever, shivering, and recovery from anesthesia, pain, agitation, or seizures) or decreased O_2 delivery (e.g., cardiac failure, obstructive shock, hemorrhage, hypoxia, hypovolemia, and arrhythmias). Conversely, increased $S\bar{v}o_2$ (>80%) may be the result of decreased O_2 demand (e.g., hypothermia, sedation, neuromuscular blockade) or is an indicator of maldistribution or impaired cellular use of O_2 in sepsis. Technical causes of a high $S\bar{v}o_2$ include a wedged PA catheter or deposits of fibrin on the tip of the catheter, or during manual sampling when the rapid withdrawal of blood from the catheter results in a specimen contaminated with capillary blood.

The interpretation of CO should not be in terms of "normal," but rather in terms of adequacy of perfusion. The interpretation of CO relative to $S\bar{v}o_2$ and the O_2ER may provide an indication of adequacy of perfusion (Fig. 21-21). Vincent et al. suggest that $S\bar{v}o_2$ is the most important factor in the determination of adequate hemodynamic status, particularly if it is low.[433] In the presence of anemia, when the $S\bar{v}o_2$ is low, the creation of CI/O_2ER diagram may also be helpful.[433,434]

Continuous $S\bar{v}o_2$ is useful in evaluating the effect of O_2-sensitive nursing and interdisciplinary interventions. Interventions such as a bed bath, positioning, or chest physiotherapy increase O_2 consumption.[435–437] For example, in patients with an EF $\leq$ 30%, the $S\bar{v}o_2$ decreased immediately after turning,[432] and in patients with anemia (Hgb <10 g/dL) and low $\dot{D}o_2I$ (<500 mL/min/m^2), the $S\bar{v}o_2$ decreased acutely with turning and remained lower for 10 minutes than in patients with Hgb more than 10 g/dL.[438] These results are important given the current practice to liberalize the trigger for blood transfusions to 8 g/dL for patients without cardiac disease and 10 g/dL for patients with cardiac disease.[439] Modification of the plan of care may be particularly important in patients with increased baseline $\dot{V}o_2$ (sepsis, trauma, pain) who also have limited capacity to increase O_2 delivery (HF). An interdisciplinary plan of care aimed at balancing O_2 supply and demand may include actions to decrease $\dot{V}o_2$ (antipyretics, pain medications, sedation) and limit or reorganize nursing activities (i.e., avoiding clustering of activities) in high-risk patients.

Central Venous Oxygen Saturation

Central venous O_2 saturation ($Scvo_2$) has been used as an alternative to the $S\bar{v}o_2$. The $Scvo_2$ can be measured continuously using an oximetric catheter[440,441] or intermittently from a central line (including a PICC) positioned in the superior vena cava.[130] The $Scvo_2$ primarily reflects the O_2 supply and demand relationship in the head, neck, and upper arms in contrast to the $S\bar{v}o_2$, which reflects the entire body. In general, changes in the $Scvo_2$ match changes in $S\bar{v}o_2$.[442,443] The $Scvo_2$ tends to overestimate the $S\bar{v}o_2$ by approximately 5%. However, wide variability of differences between $Scvo_2$ and $S\bar{v}o_2$ can occur; thus, the absolute values are not interchangeable.[443–448] For example, in post-cardiac surgery patients, while the bias between $S\bar{v}o_2$ and $Scvo_2$ was small, there was a lack of precision (bias = 0.6% ± 9.4%; 95% CI = −19.2% to 18%).[448] Similarly, in another group of cardiac surgery patients, the $Scvo_2$ significantly overestimated the $S\bar{v}o_2$, particularly when the $S\bar{v}o_2$ was less than 70%.[449]

Clinically, the $Scvo_2$ may be useful in tracking changes in $S\bar{v}o_2$,[442] as a low $Scvo_2$ (60%), which indicates an even lower $S\bar{v}o_2$, may be an indicator of impaired O_2 delivery.[450] The $Scvo_2$ may also be a marker of unresolved tissue hypoxia, despite normalization of vital signs. For example, in critically ill patients who were resuscitated to normal vital signs, 50% continued to have increased lactate levels and decreased $Scvo_2$ levels,[451] and in patients with acutely decompensated HF, clinical presentation and vital signs did not differentiate between those with and without severe hypoperfusion, while lactate and $Scvo_2$ clearly differentiated the patients.[429] The $Scvo_2$ may also be an indicator of risk for increased morbidity and mortality. For example, a low $Scvo_2$ (<60%) on admission to the ICU,[452] perioperative (<73%)[453] and postsurgery (<64%)[454] were associated with increased morbidity and mortality. The $Scvo_2$ is a goal for resuscitation ($Scvo_2$

> 70%) for adult patients with severe sepsis and septic shock,[132,240] and use of $Scvo_2$ as an endpoint has been found to improve outcomes in pediatric and adolescent patients with septic shock.[455]

Caution must be exercised when using $Scvo_2$ as an endpoint of resuscitation as the exact threshold to optimize outcomes has not been identified[456] and interventions to increase $Scvo_2$ may vary between different patient populations. The benefits of $Scvo_2$ monitoring have been described only with continuous monitoring. Recent research found that intermittent measurements missed between 29% and 62% of clinically significant changes in $Scvo_2$, which supports the need for continuous monitoring (Pambianco, unpublished data, 2008). Other factors to consider when deciding on whether to use continuous versus intermittent monitoring include the risk of intermittent blood draws (infection and iatrogenic anemia) and the cost of intermittent laboratory testing versus purchasing catheters for continuous monitoring.

Lactate

Lactate is an end product of anaerobic metabolism, and an increased level (>2 mmol/L) is a surrogate indicator of tissue hypoxia. Although hyperlactatemia is indicative of tissue hypoxia, because the liver has a large capacity to oxidize lactate, a normal serum lactate level does not rule out tissue hypoperfusion and anaerobic metabolism. In addition, localized hypoperfusion may be insufficient to increase systemic levels. Therefore, lactate is a late, and often insensitive, indicator of hypoperfusion. Conversely, increased lactate occurs with factors other than hypoxia, including increased glycolysis (e.g., increased Na^+, K^+-ATPase activity, hypermetabolic state, catecholamine administration, diabetes mellitus, trauma, burns, sepsis) and impaired lactate clearance (hepatic dysfunction, pyruvate dehydrogenase dysfunction). Despite these limitations tissue hypoxia should be ruled out before assuming that other factors are causing increased lactate.[457]

Increased lactate is associated with increased morbidity and mortality. In patients with a suspected infection, a lactate >4 mmol/L was associated with mortality, independent of BP and other covariates.[458] In patients who underwent emergent repair of a ruptured aortic aneurysm, an immediate postoperative lactate ≥4 mmol/L or a base deficit <−7 were associated with a 95% probability of death[459] and in cardiac surgery patients a lactate >3 mmol/L during surgery or on admission to the ICU was associated with increased morbidity and mortality.[460,461]

Although increased levels of lactate (>4 mmol/L) is a trigger for the initiation of goal-directed therapy in patients with sepsis,[132] the use of lactate levels as an indicator of tissue hypoxia in these patients is complicated.[462] In septic shock, increased lactate levels may occur when there is adequate O_2 delivery and, conversely, when the O_2 delivery increases lactate levels may not decrease. Factors that may be associated with this discordant response include an increase in glycolysis caused by an inflammatory increase in pyruvate or increased levels of endogenous or exogenous epinephrine and decreased lactate clearance.[462,463]

General recommendations for the use of lactate are to follow trends rather than a single measurement. Hyperlactatemia (lactate >2 mmol/L) persisting for more than 6 hours after admission is predictive of increased mortality in ICU and trauma patients.[464] A decrease in lactate of 10% per hour is usually indicative of adequate response to treatment, whereas no change or an increase in lactate is an ominous sign.[465] Research is ongoing to determine if early lactate-directed therapy has an effect on outcomes in patients with sepsis and septic shock.

Optimizing Resuscitation

The current endpoints for resuscitation are based on optimizing the patient's physiological status.[166] A major criticism of research related to optimization is that in many cases resuscitation is not initiated until after organ failure had occurred. Evidence suggests that although achieving normal O_2 delivery is important, the timing of the initiation of goal-directed therapy may be the more critical factor in decreasing morbidity and mortality.[240,466,467] Two meta-analyses found no decrease in mortality if attempts to improve tissue perfusion were taken after the onset of organ failure. In contrast, beneficial effects were observed when attempts to improve oxygenation were taken preoperatively or before the onset of organ failure.[466,467]

In 2001, a study was conducted to determine the effect of early goal-directed therapy with patients who presented to the emergency department with severe sepsis or septic shock.[240] The patients in the experimental group received 6 hours of early goal-directed therapy, including volume resuscitation, blood transfusions, and vasopressor therapy, aimed at optimizing tissue oxygenation (CVP 8 to 12 mm Hg, MAP ≥ 65 mm Hg, UOP ≥ 0.5 mL/kg/h, and $Scvo_2$ > 70%) in contrast to the patients in control group whose therapy was guided only by standard hemodynamic indices. An interesting finding in this study was that on admission, despite relatively normal vital signs in both the control and experimental groups, both groups had indications of tissue hypoxia. Early goal-directed therapy was associated with a 16% absolute reduction in mortality compared with standard care. Although there was no difference between the routine care and experimental group in length of ICU stay, the experimental group was also less acutely ill during the first 3 days in the ICU and had a shorter length of hospitalization. Subsequent studies have also demonstrated morbidity and mortality benefits from the initiation of early goal-directed therapy for patients presenting with severe sepsis,[468–470] and a recent systematic analysis of 39 goal-directed therapy studies found that all studies had a relative risk reduction of 25% or greater and an absolute risk reduction greater than 9%.[470] In addition, in community hospitals the benefits of the early recognition of hypoperfusion or shock from any cause and the early initiation of therapy have also been shown. Research is ongoing to determine if the benefits in these studies are related to the Early Goal-Directed Therapy (EGDT) Protocol or simply the provision of focused care (in a manner similar to the response to trauma, cardiac arrest, or stroke).[471–474] This research will also aid in further description of the triggers for the administration of blood products and to determine if $Scvo_2$ monitoring is necessary during EGDT.

There is less literature on goal-directed therapy in cardiac surgery.[475] Goal-directed therapy to optimize oxygenation and perfusion ($S\bar{v}o_2$ > 70% and lactate < 2 mmol/L) in addition to standard hemodynamic endpoints (CI, BP, PAOP, Hgb) during the first 8 hours after cardiac surgery was associated with decreased morbidity and shorter hospitalization compared with patients whose care was aimed at optimizing standard endpoints.[476] Based on a review of the literature[475] the following primary endpoints for resuscitation have been suggested for high-risk cardiac surgery patients: normal perfusion pressure (MAP 70–90 mm Hg), SVI > 35 mL/beat/m^2, and $S\bar{v}o_2$ > 70%. Secondary endpoints include CVP < 15 mm Hg, PAEDP < 20 mm Hg, lactate < 2 mmol/L

DISPLAY 21-8 Integrated Approach to Fluid Resuscitation

1. Is there an indication of end-organ hypoperfusion?
2. Measure MAP/functional indicators
3. If functional indicator > threshold—give 500 mL bolus over 15 minutes and reassess
4. Repeat boluses every 15 minutes until functional indicator < threshold, then stop
5. If MAP remains < 60 mm Hg after initial fluid bolus—start norepinephrine
6. If functional indicator < threshold and vasopressor therapy is still required—evaluate cardiac contractility (echo)
7. If contractility is impaired -consider dobutamine

Adapted from Pinsky, M. (2002). Functional hemodynamic monitoring: Applied physiology at the bedside. In J. L. Vincent (Ed.), *Intensive care medicine. Annual update 2002* (pp. 537–552). Berlin, Germany: Springer-Verlag.

and UOP > 0.5 mL/kg/h. Further research to evaluate protocols to achieve these endpoints and the effect of this goal-directed approach needs to be conducted.

Integration of Functional Hemodynamic Indices Into the Plan of Care

Similar to other studies there was no significant difference in outcomes between patients monitored with a PA catheter versus PiCCO.[477] However, the use of functional indices may provide insight into the adequacy of resuscitation. For example, in organ donors a PPV > 13% (indicating under-resuscitation) was associated with higher interleukin-6 and a decreased number of organs taken for transplant.[478] A limitation of these studies is that the functional indices were not used as part of an integrated plan of care.[479]

Research is now being conducted to evaluate the use of functional indices or less invasive CO monitoring as part of an integrated plan of care. For example, high-risk surgical patients were randomized to receive postoperative fluid resuscitation guided by CVP (fluid boluses administered to achieve a sustained increased in CVP of 2 mm Hg lasting for at least 20 minutes) compared with patients receiving fluids to increase their SV by >10% for at least 20 minutes and dopexamine if their $\dot{D}O_2I$ did not exceed 600 mL/min/m^2. Patients in the goal-directed group had few complications and a shorter length of stay. Although this study used an LiDCO monitor, which provides functional indices, because many of the patients were extubated early, the functional indices were not used as part of the protocol to determine if fluid therapy was the appropriate intervention. It would be interesting to determine the effect of additional tailoring of fluid administration using prospective functional indices, rather than retrospectively depending on the SV response.

Pinsky[255] proposed an algorithm that integrates functional and standard hemodynamic indices to guide resuscitation (Display 21-8). Functional and standard hemodynamic indices can also be used to guide titration of vasopressors (Fig. 21-22).[480]

Recent studies addressed whether the use of an integrated goal-directed approach that includes functional indices improves patient outcomes. In a study, which used the functional indices as the endpoint for resuscitation, high-risk surgery patients received either standard intraoperative monitoring or care or they were resuscitated to maintain a PPV% < 10%.[481] The PPV group received more fluids during surgery but had a significantly shorter postoperative length of stay (7 days versus 17 days, $p < .001$) and fewer postoperative complications (1.4 ± 2.1 versus 3.9 ± 2.8,

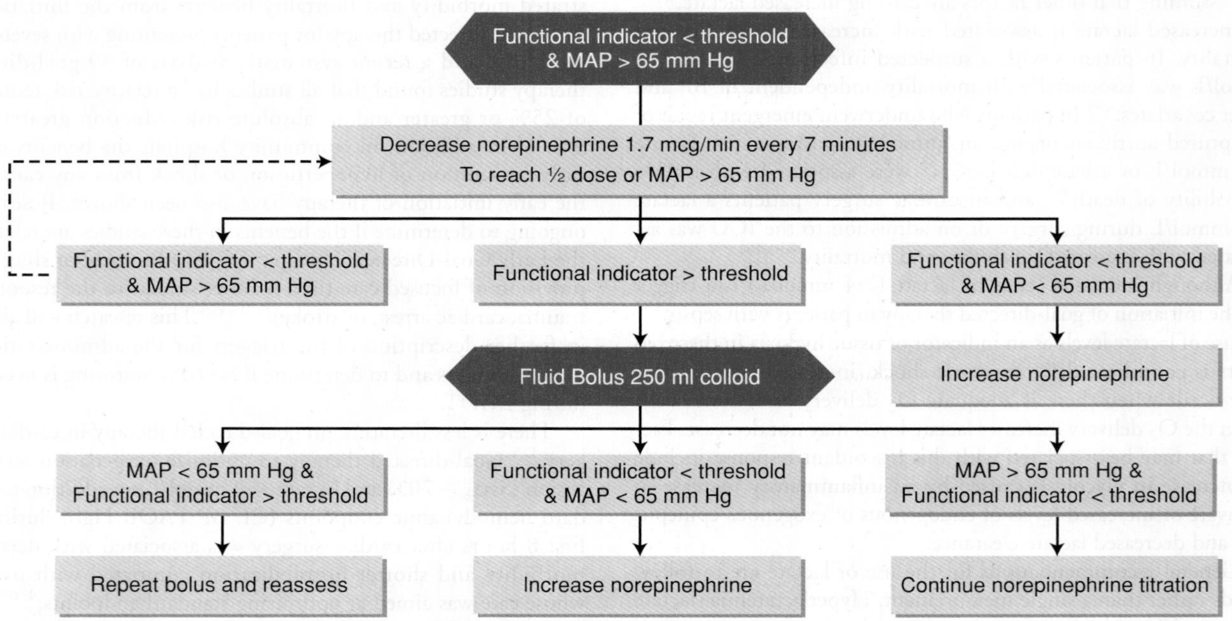

■ **Figure 21-22** Use of standard and functional hemodynamic indices to guide titration of vasoactive medications. (Modified from Vallet, B., Tygat, H., Lebuffe, G. [2007]. How to titrate vasopressor against fluid loading in sepsis. *Advances in Sepsis, 6*[2], 38.)

$p < .05$). In a study of moderate to high-risk cardiac surgery patients, postoperative goal-directed therapy integrated standard hemodynamic indices, oxygenation indices ($\dot{D}O_2I$, $ScvO_2$) and FloTrac indices (CI, SV, SVV) were compared with a standard care group (HR, MAP, Sp_{O2}, CVP).[482] In the goal-directed group if the CI was <2.5 L/min/m^2, the CVP was less than 6 mm Hg or the SVV was >10% fluid boluses were administered to optimize these parameters. Vasoactive medications and red blood cells were subsequently added to increase the SVI > 30 mL/min/m^2 and to achieve an $ScvO_2$ > 70%. The goal-directed group had fewer hours of mechanical ventilation and shorter period of ICU and hospital stay. Further research is needed to determine if this integrated goal-directed approach works in different patient populations.

Regional Indicators

Monitoring of regional indices of oxygenation (gut mucosa, subcutaneous tissue, and muscle tissue) is based on the assumption that these areas serve as early markers of systemic hypoperfusion. The next section summarizes the current use of regional indicators to detect and guide therapy to treat hypoperfusion.

Tissue Perfusion Monitoring

Tissue or peripheral perfusion monitoring may augment global hemodynamic and oxygenation monitoring. In hypoperfusion and shock, blood is shunted away from less vital areas including the skin and muscle to vital organs and these areas regain normal perfusion after restoration of circulation in other vital areas; thus, monitoring of these areas may be useful in the early detection of hypoperfusion and evaluating the adequacy of resuscitation. The two most common technologies used for tissue perfusion monitoring are NIRS and transcutaneous tissue monitoring.

Near-Infrared Spectroscopy

NIRS uses a probe placed on the thenar eminence or deltoid that emits near-infrared light. NIRS monitoring is based on the finding that hemoglobin, myoglobin, and cytochrome oxidase alter their absorption of near-infrared light with changes in oxygenation, with hemoglobin providing the major contribution. The NIRS signal is a measure of tissue hemoglobin O_2 saturation (StO_2).

In trauma patients and patients undergoing cardiac surgery changes in StO_2 were found to mirror changes in global oxygenation indices.[483,484] In contrast, in patients with left ventricular failure or sepsis the StO_2 and $S\bar{v}O_2$ were not correlated;[485] thus, specific recommendations for the use of StO_2 as a surrogate for $S\bar{v}O_2$ under different shock conditions remain to be resolved.[486] StO_2 or skeletal muscle oxygenation monitoring may be useful in identifying occult hypoperfusion. For example, during cardiac surgery the lowest StO_2 value preceded the highest lactate value by 90 minutes,[484] and in critically ill trauma victims who were considered adequately resuscitated the average StO_2 was 63% ± 27%, which suggests incomplete resuscitation.[487]

The utility of NIRS to identify the severity of shock in trauma patients is equivocal. In trauma patients the StO_2 differentiated between normals (83% ± 6%) and trauma patients without shock (83% ± 10%) and those with severe shock (45% ± 26%). However, NIRS StO_2 did not differentiate patients with mild (83% ± 10%) or moderate shock (80% ± 12%),[488] which may limit its utility as an early indicator of blood loss[489] or to guide resuscitation. Another limitation is interpreting absolute StO_2 values and using StO_2 as an endpoint for resuscitation.[486] An StO_2 threshold of 75% within the first hour of traumatic shock resuscitation has been identified as a critical predictor of organ dysfunction and mortality[490] and the severity of outcomes increases with a lower StO_2.[491] However, there is wide individual variability in StO_2. For example, in the study by Ikossi et al.[487] the StO_2 in patients deemed to be adequately resuscitated was 63% ± 27%, and the average StO_2 in patients who required massive transfusions was 58% ± 22% in contrast to patients who did not required a massive transfusion (67% ± 19%).[491]

Recently, changes in StO_2 that are created using an arterial or venous occlusion test (forearm compression with a cuff to create transient venous obstruction or ischemia) have been used to describe microcirculatory reactivity and local O_2 consumption.[492,493] When the cuff is released reactive hyperemia occurs, which reflects the local response to hypoxia and microcirculatory function. In patients with sepsis, microvascular reactivity was impaired compared with other critically ill patients or normal control subjects.[494–496] In addition, microvascular reactivity was higher in survivors versus nonsurvivors[496] and the impairment was worse in patients who developed more severe organ failure.[497] In patients who are septic, muscle O_2 consumption is also decreased, which may reflect cytopathic hypoxia or impaired blood flow.[493,497]

Transcutaneous Tissue Monitoring

Transcutaneous tissue O_2 ($P_{tc}O_2$) reflects tissue oxygenation from the cell mitochondria to the venous capillary in contrast to pulse oximetry, which reflects arterial oxygenation. In normal subjects, the $P_{tc}O_2$ is estimated to be approximately 80% of the Pa_{O2} and in a recent study the $P_{tc}O_2$ was 61% ± 15% in normal subjects and 48% ± 13% in individuals who were morbidly obese.[498] In nonshock states the $P_{tc}O_2$ varies with Pa_{O2}, but in shock states the $P_{tc}O_2$ mirrors changes in CO and $\dot{D}O_2$ with minimal response to an increase in Fi_{O2} or Pa_{O2}. This lack of increase is thought to reflect increased O_2 consumption by ischemic cells; thus, the $P_{tc}O_2$ provides insight into cellular oxygenation that may not be apparent from global hemodynamic indices.

The $P_{tc}O_2$ and transcutaneous CO_2 ($P_{tc}CO_2$) values may be early indicators of hypoperfusion and have prognostic implications. In trauma patients the $P_{tc}O_2/Fi_{O2}$ was significantly higher in survivors (220 ± 132) than nonsurvivors (117 ± 100) and the $P_{tc}CO_2$ was significantly lower (46 ± 16 mm Hg versus 52 ± 13 mm Hg).[413,414] However, these results were not found in patients with severe sepsis and septic shock.[499,500]

In contrast to absolute values, in patients with sepsis and septic shock the response to an oxygen challenge test (OCT), which evaluates a change in $P_{tc}O_2$ after 5 minutes of Fi_{O2} of 1.0, is associated with morbidity and mortality. A positive OCT, which is defined as a baseline $P_{tc}O_2$ of 30 mm Hg or more and the ability to achieve an increase in $P_{tc}O_2$ of 25 to 40 mm Hg or more after 5 minutes of Fi_{O2} of 1.0, is associated with decreased morbidity and mortality.[499,500] The OCT has also been used as an endpoint for resuscitation. Using a standardized protocol, patients with severe sepsis and septic shock were resuscitated to $\dot{D}O_2$ and $S\bar{v}O_2$ goals or an OCT response of 40 mm Hg or more. Mortality was significantly lower in the OCT group (13%) versus the $\dot{D}O_2$–$S\bar{v}O_2$ group (40%). Similar to earlier research related to achieving supranormal oxygenation goals, patients who were unable to achieve the OCT goal had increased mortality.

Transcutaneous tissue monitoring uses an electrode placed on the anterior chest below the clavicle that heats the skin (44°C) and changes the structures of the stratum corneum from the gel to the sol state, which allows rapid diffusion of O_2 and CO_2 from the

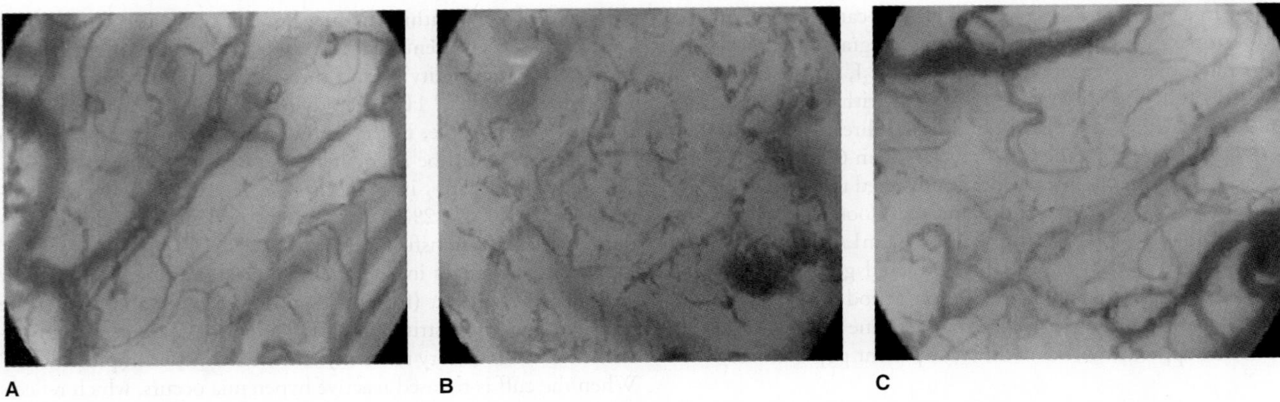

■ **Figure 21-23** Representative examples of the sublingual microcirculation in (A) control patient (B) cardiogenic shock,[512] and (C) septic shock.[513] Note the decrease in the density of small vessels in the patient with severe cardiac failure and the decreased vascular density and increased heterogeneity of perfusion in the patient with septic shock. (Reproduced from De Backer, D., Creteur, J., Dubois, M. J., et al. [2004]. Microvascular alterations in patients with acute severe HF and cardiogenic shock. *American Heart Journal, 147,* 95 and De Backer, D., Creteur, J., Preiser, J.-C., et al. [2002]. Microvascular flow is altered in patients in sepsis. *American Journal of Respiratory and Critical Care Medicine, 166,* 99.)

subcutaneous tissue to the electrode. To avoid electrode-induced burns the probe must be moved every 4 hours. Of note in several studies there were no thermal burns if these safety guidelines were followed.[413,499,500] With each application of the electrode the system requires a 10- to 15-minute recalibration.

Sublingual Capnography

Perfusion to the gut is often considered the "canary of the body,"[501] providing an indicator of circulatory redistribution during hemodynamic compromise. Gastric tonometry was used to study alterations in gut perfusion. However, this procedure was difficult to perform at the bedside and affected by factors such as the concurrent administration of H_2-blockers, proton-pump inhibitors or antacids and the need to stop enteral feedings before obtaining the measurements. The sublingual mucosa was considered an alternative site for assessment and monitoring as the sublingual and mesenteric vascular structures share a common embryonic origin and changes in sublingual PCO_2 and mirror those in splanchnic vessels.[502] Assessment of the microcirculation is important as persistent microvascular alterations (despite normalization of global hemodynamics) are associated with increased morbidity and mortality.[503,504]

Sublingual capnography, which is performed with a disposable sensor that detects sublingual CO_2, is used to measure $PslCO_2$.[505,506] As described by the Fick equation, the two determinants of tissue PCO_2 are CO_2 production and tissue blood flow and there is an inverse relationship between perfusion and $PslCO_2$.[507,508] With acute perfusion failure there is an increase in O_2 extraction, hydrogen ion concentration, and tissue CO_2, with a subsequent increase in venous PCO_2 and the venoarterial PCO_2 gradient.[503,505] In a recent study in patients with sepsis the difference between arterial PCO_2 and $PslCO_2$ ($PslCO_2gap$) decreased as the proportion of well-perfused capillaries increased, and changes in $PslCO_2$ mirrored changes in gastric CO_2 demonstrating the relationship between sublingual perfusion and gut perfusion[502]. Sublingual capnometry may provide a rapid, noninvasive method to monitor microcirculatory status and provide an early indication of tissue hypoperfusion and to assess the patient's response to therapy. However, use of the sublingual probe requires a specialized holder to maintain the probe in the correct position, which may limits its utility for continuous bedside monitoring. Recent research using a buccal PCO_2 ($PbuCO_2$) probe in animal models of hemorrhagic shock have demonstrated similar results[509,510] and the buccal probe may be easier to use at the bedside.

Microcirculatory Monitoring

Currently, two technologies (orthogonal polarization spectral imaging and sidestream dark-field imaging) are being used to visualize and assess sublingual microcirculatory flow.[511] These techniques use specialized light probes, with the sublingual mucosa as the primary site of analysis. The probes emit light and the scattered light, which is absorbed by hemoglobin of red blood cells in superficial vessels, and allows for the direct visualization of the microcirculation and the qualitative evaluation of vascular density, capillary perfusion, and perfusion heterogeneity, which reflects the distribution of perfused and nonperfused capillaries (Fig. 21-23*A* and *B*). Sidestream dark-field imaging and orthogonal polarization spectral imaging, which have been used primarily under experimental conditions, are limited by motion artifact (requires the patient be heavily sedated) and differences in data interpretation. Further research is needed before this technology will be available for routine bedside clinical use.

Microcirculatory derangements vary depending on the cause of shock (e.g., distributive, hemorrhagic, cardiogenic).[514] For example, in patients with severe sepsis and septic shock microcirculatory derangements are more severe in nonsurvivors and those with more severe global cardiovascular dysfunction.[515] In addition, during early goal-directed therapy, survivors demonstrate improvement in microcirculatory function in contrast to nonsurvivors and improvement in microcirculatory flow was greater in patients who did not develop organ failure.[511] In an animal model, microcirculatory derangements were more severe in septic animals compared with animals with hemorrhagic shock, independent of BP and CI, and with fluid resuscitation there was normalization of microcirculation in the hemorrhagic shock group but not the septic group.[516] Patients with severe HF and cardiogenic shock had a lower proportion of perfused small vessels than cardiac patients without HF independent of

CO and BP, and survivors had better preserved perfusion than nonsurvivors.[512,513]

These varying microcirculatory derangements occur even though the global hemodynamic indicators are similar and alterations in microcirculatory perfusion are often independent of changes in MAP and CO.[96,504,513,515,517] These results suggest a potential role for microcirculatory analysis as an early indicator of hypoperfusion, as a method to evaluate a patient's response to therapy and as a target for resuscitation. For example, studies evaluating the effects of dobutamine and activated protein C in patients with sepsis, both demonstrated increased capillary perfusion independent of systemic hemodynamics.[517,518] These studies also demonstrate the need to target both global (or macro) hemodynamics (e.g., CO, $S\bar{v}O_2$) and microhemodynamics ($PslCO_2$ or microcirculation with orthogonal polarization spectral imaging or sidestream dark-field imaging) and reiterate the limitations of solely using endpoints such as MAP and CO to guide resuscitation.

REFERENCES

1. Bridges, E., Bond, E., Ahrens, T., et al. (1997). Ask the experts: Direct arterial vs oscillometric monitoring of blood pressure: Stop comparing and pick one. *Critical Care Nurse, 17,* 96–97, 101–102.
2. Courtois, M., Fattal, P., Kovacs, S., et al. (1995). Anatomically and physiologically based reference level for measurement of intracardiac pressures. *Circulation, 92,* 1994–2000.
3. McCann, U., Schiller, H., Carney, D., et al. (2001). Invasive arterial BP monitoring in trauma and critical care. *Chest, 120,* 1322–1326.
4. Kee, L. L., Simonson, J. S., Stotts, N. A., et al. (1993). Echocardiographic determination of valid zero reference levels in supine and lateral positions. *American Journal of Critical Care, 2,* 72–80.
5. Paolella, L., Dortman, G., Cronan, J., et al. (1988). Topographic location of the left atrium by computed tomography: Reducing pulmonary artery catheter calibration errors. *Critical Care Medicine, 16,* 1154–1156.
6. Bartz, B., Maroun, C., & Underhill, S. (1988). Differences in midanteroposterior level and midaxillary level of patients with a range of chest configurations. *Heart & Lung, 17,* 309.
7. Magder, S. (2006). Central venous pressure monitoring. *Current Opinion in Critical Care, 12,* 219–227.
8. Bafaqeeh, F., & Magder, S. (2004). CVP and volume responsiveness of cardiac output. *American Journal of Respiratory and Critical Care Medicine, 169,* A344.
9. Bridges, E. J., Woods, S. L., Brengelmann, G. L., et al. (2000). Effect of the 30 degree lateral recumbent position on pulmonary artery and pulmonary artery wedge pressures in critically ill adult cardiac surgery patients. *American Journal Critical Care, 9,* 262–275.
10. Reuter, D. A., Felbinger, T. W., Schmidt, C., et al. (2003). Trendelenburg positioning after cardiac surgery: Effects on intrathoracic blood volume index and cardiac performance. *European Journal of Anaesthesiology, 20,* 17–20.
11. Teboul, J., Besbes, M., Axler, D., et al. (1988). A bedside index for determination of zone III condition of pulmonary artery (PA) catheters tips during mechanical ventilation. *American Review of Respiratory Disease, 137,* A137.
12. Kaplan, L., & Bailey, H. (200). A comparison of pulmonary artery occlusion pressure (PaOP) measurements using pressure controlled ventilation (PCV) versus airway pressure release ventilation. *Critical Care, 4,* P7.
13. Marini, J., O'Quin, R., Culver, B., et al. (1982). Estimation of transmural cardiac pressure during ventilation with PEEP. *Journal of Applied Physiology, 53,* 384–391.
14. Bridges, E. J. (2006). Pulmonary artery pressure monitoring: When, how, and what else to use. *AACN Advanced Critical Care, 17,* 286–303.
15. Vollman, K., & Bander, J. (1996). Improved oxygenation using a prone positioner in patients with acute respiratory distress syndrome. *Intensive Care Medicine, 22,* 1105–1111.
16. Hering, R., Vorwerk, R., Wrigge, H., et al. (2002). Prone positioning, systemic hemodynamics, hepatic indocyanine green kinetics, and gastric intramucosal energy balance in patients with acute lung injury. *Intensive Care Medicine, 28,* 53–58.
17. Hering, R., Wrigge, H., Vorwerk, R., et al. (2001). The effects of prone positioning on intraabdominal pressure and cardiovascular and renal function in patients with acute lung injury. *Anesthesia & Analgesia, 92,* 1226–1231.
18. Blanch, I., Mancebo, J., Perez, M., et al. (1997). Short-term effects of prone position in critically ill patients with acute respiratory distress syndrome. *Intensive Care Medicine, 23,* 1033–1039.
19. Jolliet, P., Bulpa, P., & Chevrolet, J. C. (1998). Effects of the prone position on gas exchange and hemodynamics in severe acute respiratory distress syndrome. *Critical Care Medicine, 26,* 1977–1985.
20. Matejovic, M., Rokyta, R., Jr., Radermacher, P., et al. (2002). Effect of prone position on hepato-splanchnic hemodynamics in acute lung injury. *Intensive Care Medicine, 28,* 1750–1755.
21. Borelli, M., Lampati, L., Vascotto, E., et al. (2000). Hemodynamic and gas exchange response to inhaled nitric oxide and prone positioning in acute respiratory distress syndrome patients. *Critical Care Medicine, 28,* 2707–2712.
22. Bridges, E., Evers, K. G., Schmelz, J., et al. (2005). Invasive pressure monitoring at altitude. *Critical Care Medicine, 33,* A13.
23. Bridges, E., & Middleton, R. (1997). Direct arterial vs oscillometric monitoring of blood pressure: Stop comparing and pick one (A decision-making algorithm). *Critical Care Nurse, 17,* 58–72.
24. Ramritu, P., Halton, K., Cook, D., et al. (2008). Catheter-related bloodstream infections in intensive care units: A systematic review with meta-analysis. *Journal of Advanced Nursing, 62,* 3–21.
25. Esteve, F., Pujol, M., Limon, E., et al. (2007). Bloodstream infection related to catheter connections: A prospective trial of two connection systems. *Journal of Hospital Infections, 67,* 30–34.
26. Maki, D. G., Kluger, D. M., & Crnich, C. J. (2006). The risk of bloodstream infection in adults with different intravascular devices: A systematic review of 200 published prospective studies. *Mayo Clinic Proceedings, 81,* 1159–1171.
27. Mimoz, O., Villeminey, S., Ragot, S., et al. (2007). Chlorhexidine-based antiseptic solution vs alcohol-based povidone-iodine for central venous catheter care. *Archives of Internal Medicine, 167,* 2066–2072.
28. Koh, D. B., Gowardman, J. R., Rickard, C. M., et al. (2008). Prospective study of peripheral arterial catheter infection and comparison with concurrently sited central venous catheters. *Critical Care Medicine, 36,* 397–402.
29. Khalifa, R., Dahyot-Fizelier, C., Laksiri, L., et al. (2008). Indwelling time and risk of colonization of peripheral arterial catheters in critically ill patients. *Intensive Care Medicine, 34,* 1820–1826.
30. Lorente, L., Santacreu, R., Martin, M. M., et al. (2006). Arterial catheter-related infection of 2,949 catheters. *Critical Care, 10,* R83.
31. Ramritu, P., Halton, K., Collignon, P., et al. (2008). A systematic review comparing the relative effectiveness of antimicrobial-coated catheters in intensive care units. *American Journal of Infection Control, 36,* 104–117.
32. Niel-Weise, B. S., Stijnen, T., & van den Broek, P. J. (2007). Anti-infective-treated central venous catheters: A systematic review of randomized controlled trials. *Intensive Care Medicine, 33,* 2058–2068.
33. Gilbert, R. E., & Harden, M. (2008). Effectiveness of impregnated central venous catheters for catheter related blood stream infection: A systematic review. *Current Opinion in Infectious Disease, 21,* 235–245.
34. Hockenhull, J. C., Dwan, K., Boland, A., et al. (2008). The clinical effectiveness and cost-effectiveness of central venous catheters treated with anti-infective agents in preventing bloodstream infections: A systematic review and economic evaluation. *Health Technology Assessment, 12,* 1–154.
35. Taylor, R. W., & Palagiri, A. V. (2007). Central venous catheterization. *Critical Care Medicine, 35,* 1390–1396.
36. Timsit, J. F. (2000). Scheduled replacement of central venous catheters is not necessary. *Infection Control and Hospital Epidemiology, 21,* 371–374.
37. Chen, Y. Y., Yen, D. H., Yang, Y. G., et al. (2003). Comparison between replacement at 4 days and 7 days of the infection rate for pulmonary artery catheters in an intensive care unit. *Critical Care Medicine, 31,* 1353–1358.
38. Dobbins, B. M., Catton, J. A., Kite, P., et al. (2003). Each lumen is a potential source of central venous catheter-related bloodstream infection. *Critical Care Medicine, 31,* 1688–1690.
39. Sirvent, J. M., Vidaur, L., Garcia, M., et al. (2006). Colonization of the medial lumen is a risk factor for catheter-related bloodstream infection. *Intensive Care Medicine, 32,* 1404–1408.
40. Beutz, M., Sherman, G., Mayfield, J., et al. (2003). Clinical utility of blood cultures drawn from central vein catheters and peripheral venipuncture in critically ill medical patients. *Chest, 123,* 854–861.
41. Falagas, M. E., Kazantzi, M. S., & Bliziotis, I. A. (2008). Comparison of utility of blood cultures from intravascular catheters and peripheral veins: A systematic review and decision analysis. *Journal of Medical Microbiology, 57,* 1–8.

42. O'Grady, N. P., Alexander, M., Dellinger, E. P., et al. (2002). Guidelines for the prevention of intravascular catheter-related infections. Centers for Disease Control and Prevention. *Morbidity and Mortality Weekly Report. Recommendations and Reports, 51*, 1–29.
43. Pratt, R. J., Pellowe, C. M., Wilson, J. A., et al. (2007). epic2: National evidence-based guidelines for preventing healthcare-associated infections in NHS hospitals in England. *Journal of Hospital Infections, 65*(Suppl. 1), S1–S64.
44. Pronovost, P., Needham, D., Berenholtz, S., et al. (2006). An intervention to decrease catheter-related bloodstream infections in the ICU. *New England Journal of Medicine, 355*, 2725–2732.
45. Berenholtz, S. M., Pronovost, P. J., Lipsett, P. A., et al. (2004). Eliminating catheter-related bloodstream infections in the intensive care unit. *Critical Care Medicine, 32*, 2014–2020.
46. Warren, D. K., Zack, J. E., Mayfield, J. L., et al. (2004). The effect of an education program on the incidence of central venous catheter-associated bloodstream infection in a medical ICU. *Chest, 126*, 1612–1618.
47. Safdar, N., & Abad, C. (2008). Educational interventions for prevention of healthcare-associated infection: A systematic review. *Critical Care Medicine, 36*, 933–940.
48. Mermel, L. A. (2008). Arterial catheters are not risk-free spigots. *Critical Care Medicine, 36*, 620–622.
49. Traore, O., Liotier, J., & Souweine, B. (2005). Prospective study of arterial and central venous catheter colonization and of arterial- and central venous catheter-related bacteremia in intensive care units. *Critical Care Medicine, 33*, 1276–1280.
50. Rijnders, B. J. (2005). Catheter-related infection can be prevented ... if we take the arterial line seriously too! *Critical Care Medicine, 33*, 1437–1439.
51. Gardner, R. (1981). Direct blood pressure measurement. Dynamic response requirements. *Anesthesiology, 54*, 227–236.
52. Promonet C., Anglade D., Menaouar A., et al. (2000). Time-dependent pressure distortion in a catheter-transducer system: Correction by fast flush. *Anesthesiology, 92*, 208–218.
53. Gore, S., Middleton, R., & Bridges, E. (1995). Analysis of an algorithm to guide decision making regarding direct and oscillometric blood pressure measurement. *American Journal of Respiratory and Critical Care Medicine, 151*, A331.
54. Woda, R. P., Dzwonczyk, R., Buyama, C., et al. (1999). On the dynamic performance of the Abbott Safeset™ blood-conserving arterial line system. *Journal of Clinical Monitoring and Computing, 15*, 215–221.
55. Bridges, E. J., Schmelz, J., & Kelley, P. W. (2008). Military nursing research: Translation to disaster response and day-to-day critical care nursing. *Critical Care Nursing Clinics of North America, 20*, 121–131.
56. Rickard, C. M., Couchman, B. A., Schmidt, S. J., et al. (2003). A discard volume of twice the deadspace ensures clinically accurate arterial blood gases and electrolytes and prevents unnecessary blood loss. *Critical Care Medicine, 31*, 1654–1658.
57. Laxson, C. J., & Titler, M. G. (1994). Drawing coagulation studies from arterial lines: An integrative literature review. *American Journal of Critical Care, 3*, 16–22.
58. Heap, M. J., Ridley, S. A., Hodson, K., et al. (1997). Are coagulation studies on blood sampled from arterial lines valid? *Anaesthesia, 52*, 640–645.
59. Hoste, E. A., Roels, N. R., Decruyenaere, J. M., et al. (2002). Significant increase of activated partial thromboplastin time by heparinization of the radial artery catheter flush solution with a closed arterial catheter system. *Critical Care Medicine, 30*, 1030–1034.
60. Carlson, K., Snyder, M., LeClair, H., et al. (1990). Obtaining reliable sodium and glucose determinations from pulmonary artery catheters. *Heart & Lung, 19*, 613–619.
61. Odum, L., & Drenck, N. (2002). Blood sampling for biochemical analysis from central venous catheters: Minimizing the volume of discarded blood. *Clinical Chemistry and Laboratory Medicine, 40*, 152–155.
62. McNulty, S., Maguire, D., & Thomas, R. (1998). Effect of heparin-bonded pulmonary artery catheters on activated coagulation time. *Journal of Cardiothoracic and Vascular Anesthesia, 12*, 533–535.
63. Leyvi, G., Zhuravlev, I., Inyang, A., et al. (2004). Arterial versus venous sampling for activated coagulation time measurements during cardiac surgery: A comparative study. *Journal of Cardiothoracic Vascular Anesthesia, 18*, 573–580.
64. Haering, J., Maslow, A., Parker, R., et al. (2000). The effect of heparin-coated pulmonary artery catheters on activated coagulation time in cardiac surgical patients. *Journal of Cardiothoracic and Vascular Anesthesia, 14*, 260–263.
65. Scheer, B., Perel, A., & Pfeiffer, U. J. (2002). Clinical review: Complications and risk factors of peripheral arterial catheters used for haemodynamic monitoring in anaesthesia and intensive care medicine. *Critical Care, 6*, 199–204.
66. Barone, J. E., & Madlinger, R. V. (2006). Should an Allen test be performed before radial artery cannulation? *Journal of Trauma, 61*, 468–470.
67. Jarvis, M. A., Jarvis, C. L., Jones, P. R., et al. (2000). Reliability of Allen's test in selection of patients for radial artery harvest. *Annals of Thoracic Surgery, 70*, 1362–1365.
68. Wallach, S. G. (2004). Cannulation injury of the radial artery: Diagnosis and treatment algorithm. *American Journal of Critical Care, 13*, 315–319.
69. Martin, C., Saux, P., Papazian, L., et al. (2001). Long-term arterial cannulation in ICU patients using the radial artery or dorsalis pedis artery. *Chest, 119*, 901–906.
70. Parry, T., Hirsch, N., & Fauvel, N. (1995). Comparison of direct pressure measurement at the radial and dorsalis pedis arteries during surgery in the horizontal and reverse Trendelenburg positions. *Anaesthesia, 50*, 553–555.
71. Lipsitz, E. C. (2004). Cannulation injuries of the radial artery. *American Journal of Critical Care, 13*, 314, 319.
72. AACN. (1993). Evaluation of the effects of heparinized and nonheparinized flush solutions on the patency of arterial pressure monitoring lines: The AACN Thunder Project. *American Journal of Critical Care, 2*, 3–15.
73. Randolph, A. G., Cook, D. J., Gonzales, C. A., et al. (1998). Benefit of heparin in peripheral venous and arterial catheters: Systematic review and meta-analysis of randomised controlled trials. *BMJ, 316*, 969–975.
74. Zevola, D. R., Dioso, J., & Moggio, R. (1997). Comparison of heparinized and nonheparinized solutions for maintaining patency of arterial and pulmonary artery catheters. *American Journal of Critical Care, 6*, 52–55.
75. Hall, K. F., Bennetts, T. M., Whitta, R. K., et al. (2006). Effect of heparin in arterial line flushing solutions on platelet count: A randomised double-blind study. *Critical Care and Resuscitation, 8*, 294–296.
76. Whitta, R. K., Hall, K. F., Bennetts, T. M., et al. (2006). Comparison of normal or heparinised saline flushing on function of arterial lines. *Critical Care Resuscitation, 8*, 205–208.
77. Bradley, C., & Munro, P. (2000). The effect of using a heparin-free flush system for central venous and pulmonary artery catheters on a general medical and surgical intensive care unit. *Critical Care, 4*, P35.
78. Kaye, J., Heald, G. R., Morton, J., et al. (2001). Patency of radial arterial catheters. *American Journal of Critical Care, 10*, 104–111.
79. O'Rourke, M. F., & Mancia, G. (1999). Arterial stiffness. *Journal of Hypertension, 17*, 1–4.
80. Rowell, L., Brengelmann, G., Blackmon, J., et al. (1968). Disparities between aortic and peripheral pulse pressures induced by upright exercise and vasomotor changes in man. *Circulation, 37*, 954–964.
81. O'Rourke, M. (1993). Wave travel and reflection in the arterial system. In M. O'Rourke, M. Safar, & V. Dzau (Eds.), *Arterial vasodilation* (pp. 10–22). Philadelphia: Lea & Febiger.
82. O'Rourke, M. F., & Hashimoto, J. (2007). Mechanical factors in arterial aging: A clinical perspective. *Journal of the American College of Cardiology, 50*, 1–13.
83. Nichols, W. W., Denardo, S. J., Wilkinson, I. B., et al. (2008). Effects of arterial stiffness, pulse wave velocity, and wave reflections on the central aortic pressure waveform. *Journal of Clinical Hypertension (Greenwich), 10*, 295–303.
84. Kelly, R., Gibbs, H., O'Rourke, M., et al. (1990). Nitroglycerin has more favourable effects on left ventricular afterload than apparent from measurement of pressure in a peripheral artery. *European Heart Journal, 11*, 138–144.
85. Westerbacka, J., Tamminen, M., Cockcroft, J., et al. (2004). Comparison of in vivo effects of nitroglycerin and insulin on the aortic pressure waveform. *European Journal of Clinical Investigations, 34*, 1–8.
86. Mignini, M. A., Piacentini, E., & Dubin, A. (2006). Peripheral arterial blood pressure monitoring adequately tracks central arterial blood pressure in critically ill patients: An observational study. *Critical Care, 10*, R43.
87. Pytte, M., Dybwik, K., Sexton, J., et al. (2006). Oscillometric brachial mean artery pressures are higher than intra-radial mean artery pressures in intensive care unit patients receiving norepinephrine. *Acta Anaesthesiologica Scandinavica, 50*, 718–721.
88. Umana, E., Ahmed, W., Fraley, M. A., et al. (2006). Comparison of oscillometric and intraarterial systolic and diastolic blood pressures in lean, overweight, and obese patients. *Angiology, 57*, 41–45.
89. Manios, E., Vemmos, K., Tsivgoulis, G., et al. (2007). Comparison of noninvasive oscillometric and intra-arterial blood pressure measurements in hyperacute stroke. *Blood Pressure Monitoring, 12*, 149–156.
90. Smulyan, H., Sheehe, P. R., & Safar, M. E. (2008). A preliminary evaluation of the mean arterial pressure as measured by cuff oscillometry. *American Journal of Hypertension, 21*, 166–171.

91. Fournier, A., & Safar, M. (2003). Accurate measurement of blood pressure. *JAMA, 289,* 2793; author reply 2793–2794.
92. Pauca, A. L., Kon, N. D., & O'Rourke, M. F. (2004). The second peak of the radial artery pressure wave represents aortic systolic pressure in hypertensive and elderly patients. *British Journal of Anaesthesia, 92,* 651–657.
93. Yazigi, A. (2002). Blood pressure measurements in the radial and femoral artery [Letter to the editor]. *Acta Anaesthesiologica Scandinavica, 46,* 1176–1178.
94. Soderstrom, S., Sellgren, J., & Ponten, J. (1999). Aortic and radial pulse contour: Different effects of nitroglycerin and prostacyclin. *Anesthesia & Analgesia, 89,* 566–572.
95. Grossman, W. (2005). Pressure measurement. In D. Baim (Ed.), *Grossman's cardiac catheterization, angiography, and intervention* (pp. 133–147). Philadelphia: Lippincott Williams & Wilkins.
96. LeDoux, D., Astiz, M. E., Carpati, C. M., et al. (2000). Effects of perfusion pressure on tissue perfusion in septic shock. *Critical Care Medicine, 28,* 2729–2732.
97. Pickering, T. G., Hall, J. E., Appel, L. J., et al. (2005). Recommendations for blood pressure measurement in humans: An AHA scientific statement from the Council on High Blood Pressure Research Professional and Public Education Subcommittee. *Journal of Clinical Hypertension (Greenwich), 7,* 102–109.
98. Rauen, C. A., Chulay, M., Bridges, E., et al. (2008). Seven evidence-based practice habits: Putting some sacred cows out to pasture. *Critical Care Nurse, 28,* 98–124.
99. Bur, A., Herkner, H., Vlcek, M., et al. (2003). Factors influencing the accuracy of oscillometric blood pressure measurement in critically ill patients. *Critical Care Medicine, 31,* 793–799.
100. Fonseca-Reyes, S., De Alba-Garcia, J. G., Parra-Carrillo, J. Z., et al. (2003). Effect of standard cuff on blood pressure readings in patients with obese arms. How frequent are arms of a 'large circumference'? *Blood Pressure Monitoring, 8,* 101–106.
101. Kirchoff, K., Rebenson-Piano, M., & Patel, M. (1984). Mean arterial pressure readings: Variations with positions and transducer level. *Nursing Research, 33,* 343–345.
102. McCann, U., Schiller, H., Carney, D., et al. (1999). Proper transducer level for arterial blood pressure measurement. *Chest, 116,* 281S.
103. Netea, R. T., Lenders, J. W., Smits, P., et al. (2003). Both body and arm position significantly influence blood pressure measurement. *Journal of Human Hypertension, 17,* 459–462.
104. Pickering, T. G. (1993). Blood pressure variability and ambulatory monitoring. *Current Opinion in Nephrology and Hypertension, 2,* 380–385.
105. Netea, R. T., Lenders, J. W., Smits, P., et al. (1999). Arm position is important for blood pressure measurement. *Journal of Human Hypertension, 13,* 105–109.
106. Netea, R. T., Elving, L. D., Lutterman, J. A., et al. (2002). Body position and blood pressure measurement in patients with diabetes mellitus. *Journal of Internal Medicine, 251,* 393–399.
107. Adiyaman, A., Verhoeff, R., Lenders, J. W., et al. (2006). The position of the arm during blood pressure measurement in sitting position. *Blood Pressure Monitoring, 11,* 309–313.
108. Mourad, A., Carney, S., Gillies, A., et al. (2003). Arm position and blood pressure: A risk factor for hypertension? *Journal of Human Hypertension, 17,* 389–395.
109. Familoni, O. B., & Olunuga, T. O. (2005). Comparison of the effects of arm position and support on blood pressure in hypertensive and normotensive subjects. *Cardiovascular Journal of South Africa, 16,* 85–88.
110. Newton, K. M. (1981). Comparison of aortic and brachial cuff pressures in flat supine and lateral recumbent positions. *Heart & Lung, 10,* 821–826.
111. van der Steen, M. S., Pleijers, A. M., Lenders, J. W., et al. (2000). Influence of different supine body positions on blood pressure: Consequences for night blood pressure/dipper-status. *Journal of Hypertension, 18,* 1731–1736.
112. Cavelaars, M., Tulen, J. H., Man in 't Veld, A. J., et al. (2000). Assessment of body position to quantify its effect on nocturnal blood pressure under ambulatory conditions. *Journal of Hypertension, 18,* 1737–1743.
113. Pickering, T. G., Hall, J. E., Appel, L. J., et al. (2005). Recommendations for blood pressure measurement in humans and experimental animals. Part 1: Blood pressure measurement in humans: A statement for professionals from the Subcommittee of Professional and Public Education of the American Heart Association Council on High Blood Pressure Research. *Circulation, 111,* 697–716.
114. Schell, K., Bradley, E., Bucher, L., et al. (2005). Clinical comparison of automatic, noninvasive measurements of blood pressure in the forearm and upper arm. *American Journal of Critical Care, 14,* 232–241.
115. Singer, A. J., Kahn, S. R., Thode, H. C., Jr., et al. (1999). Comparison of forearm and upper arm blood pressures. *Prehospital Emergency Care, 3,* 123–126.
116. Schell, K., Lyons, D., Bradley, E., et al. (2006). Clinical comparison of automatic, noninvasive measurements of blood pressure in the forearm and upper arm with the patient supine or with the head of the bed raised 45 degrees: A follow-up study. *American Journal of Critical Care, 15,* 196–205.
117. Michard, F., & Reuter, D. A. (2003). Assessing cardiac preload or fluid responsiveness? It depends on the question we want to answer. *Intensive Care Medicine, 29,* 1396.
118. Scott, S., Guiliano, K., Pysznik, E., et al. (1998). Influence of port site on central venous pressure measurements from triple-lumen catheters in critically ill adults. *American Journal of Critical Care, 7,* 60–63.
119. Blot, F., Laplanche, A., Raynard, B., et al. (2000). Accuracy of totally implanted ports, tunnelled, single- and multiple-lumen central venous catheters for measurement of central venous pressure. *Intensive Care Medicine, 26,* 1837–1842.
120. Tugrul, M., Camci, E., Pembeci, K., et al. (2004). Relationship between peripheral and central venous pressures in different patient positions, catheter sizes, and insertion sites. *Journal of Cardiothoracic and Vascular Anesthesia, 18,* 446–450.
121. Desjardins, R., Denault, A. Y., Belisle, S., et al. (2004). Can peripheral venous pressure be interchangeable with central venous pressure in patients undergoing cardiac surgery? *Intensive Care Medicine, 30,* 627–632.
122. Cox, P., Johnson, J. O., & Tobias, J. D. (2005). Measurement of central venous pressure from a peripheral intravenous catheter in the lower extremity. *Southern Medical Journal, 98,* 698–702.
123. Munis, J. R., Bhatia, S., & Lozada, L. J. (2001). Peripheral venous pressure as a hemodynamic variable in neurosurgical patients. *Anesthesia & Analgesia, 92,* 172–179.
124. Cave, G., & Harvey, M. (2008). The difference between peripheral venous pressure and central venous pressure (CVP) decreases with increasing CVP. *European Journal of Anaesthesiology, 25,* 1037–1040.
125. Hoftman, N., Braunfeld, M., Hoftman, G., et al. (2006). Peripheral venous pressure as a predictor of central venous pressure during orthotopic liver transplantation. *Journal of Clinical Anesthesia, 18,* 251–255.
126. Amar, D., Melendez, J. A., Zhang, H., et al. (2001). Correlation of peripheral venous pressure and central venous pressure in surgical patients. *Journal of Cardiothoracic and Vascular Anesthesia, 15,* 40–43.
127. Charalambous, C., Barker, T. A., Zipitis, C. S., et al. (2003). Comparison of peripheral and central venous pressures in critically ill patients. *Anaesthesia and Intensive Care, 31,* 34–39.
128. Choi, S. J., Gwak, M. S., Ko, J. S., et al. (2007). Can peripheral venous pressure be an alternative to central venous pressure during right hepatectomy in living donors? *Liver Transplantation, 13,* 1414–1421.
129. Black, I. H., Blosser, S. A., & Murray, W. B. (2000). Central venous pressure measurements: Peripherally inserted catheters versus centrally inserted catheters. *Critical Care Medicine, 28,* 3833–3836.
130. Lopez, A., Thompson, D., Dauenhauer, C., et al. (2003). *Accuracy of peripherally inserted central catheters (PICCs) for hemodynamic monitoring and central venous oximetry 2003.* Seattle: American Thoracic Society.
131. McLemore, E. C., Tessier, D. J., Rady, M. Y., et al. (2006). Intraoperative peripherally inserted central venous catheter central venous pressure monitoring in abdominal aortic aneurysm reconstruction. *Annals of Vascular Surgery, 20,* 577–581.
132. Dellinger, R. P., Levy, M. M., Carlet, J. M., et al. (2008). Surviving Sepsis Campaign: International guidelines for management of severe sepsis and septic shock: 2008. *Critical Care Medicine, 36,* 296–327.
133. Forrester, J., Diamond, G., Mchugh, T., et al. (1971). Filling pressures in the right and left sides of the heart in acute myocardial infarction. A reappraisal of central-venous pressure monitoring. *New England Journal of Medicine, 285,* 190–192.
134. Schummer, W., Schummer, C., Rose, N., et al. (2007). Mechanical complications and malpositions of central venous cannulations by experienced operators. A prospective study of 1794 catheterizations in critically ill patients. *Intensive Care Medicine, 33,* 1055–1059.
135. Ruesch, S., Walder, B., & Tramer, M. R. (2002). Complications of central venous catheters: internal jugular versus subclavian access—A systematic review. *Critical Care Medicine, 30,* 454–460.
136. Wilson, A. E., Bermingham-Mitchell, K., Wells, N., et al. (1996). Effect of backrest position on hemodynamic and right ventricular measurements in critically ill adults. *American Journal of Critical Care, 5,* 264–270.
137. Lakhal, K., Ferrandiere, M., Lagarrigue, F., et al. (2006). Influence of infusion flow rates on central venous pressure measurements through

multi-lumen central venous catheters in intensive care. *Intensive Care Medicine, 32*, 460–463.

138. Wheeler, A. P., Bernard, G. R., Thompson, B. T., et al. (2006). Pulmonary-artery versus central venous catheter to guide treatment of acute lung injury. *New England Journal of Medicine, 354*, 2213–2224.
139. Magder, S. (1998). More respect for the CVP. *Intensive Care Medicine, 24*, 651–653.
140. Drazner, M. H., Hamilton, M. A., Fonarow, G., et al. (1999). Relationship between right and left-sided filling pressures in 1000 patients with advanced heart failure. *Journal of Heart and Lung Transplantation, 18*, 1126–1132.
141. Magder, S., & Bafaqeeh, F. (2007). The clinical role of central venous pressure measurements. *Journal of Intensive Care Medicine, 22*, 44–51.
142. Magder, S. (2005). How to use central venous pressure measurements. *Current Opinion in Critical Care, 11*, 264–270.
143. Magder, S., Erice, F., & Lagonidis, D. (2000). Determinants of the 'y' descent and its usefulness as a predictor of ventricular filling. *Journal of Intensive Care Medicine, 15*, 262–269.
144. Wiener, R. S., & Welch, H. G. (2007). Trends in the use of the pulmonary artery catheter in the United States, 1993–2004. *JAMA, 298*, 423–429.
145. Connors, A., Speroff, T., Dawson, N., et al. (1996). The effectiveness of right heart catheterization in the initial care of critically ill patients. *JAMA, 276*, 889–897.
146. Pulmonary Artery Catheter Consensus Conference: Consensus statement. (1997). *New Horizons, 5*, 175–194.
147. Bernard, G. R., Sopko, G., Cerra, F., et al. (2000). Pulmonary artery catheterization and clinical outcomes: National Heart, Lung, and Blood Institute and Food and Drug Administration Workshop Report. Consensus Statement. *JAMA, 283*, 2568–2572.
148. Practice guidelines for pulmonary artery catheterization: An updated report by the American Society of Anesthesiologists Task Force on Pulmonary Artery Catheterization. (2003). *Anesthesiology, 99*, 988–1014.
149. Afessa, B., Spencer, S., Khan, W., et al. (2001). Association of pulmonary artery catheter use with in-hospital mortality. *Critical Care Medicine, 29*, 1145–1148.
150. Barone, J. E., Tucker, J. B., Rassias, D., et al. (2001). Routine perioperative pulmonary artery catheterization has no effect on rate of complications in vascular surgery: A meta-analysis. *American Surgery, 67*, 674–679.
151. Polanczyk, C. A., Rohde, L. E., Goldman, L., et al. (2001). Right heart catheterization and cardiac complications in patients undergoing noncardiac surgery: An observational study. *JAMA, 286*, 309–314.
152. Rhodes, A., Cusack, R. J., Newman, P. J., et al. (2002). A randomised, controlled trial of the pulmonary artery catheter in critically ill patients. *Intensive Care Medicine, 28*, 256–264.
153. Sandham, J. D., Hull, R. D., Brant, R. F., et al. (2003). A randomized, controlled trial of the use of pulmonary-artery catheters in high-risk surgical patients. *New England Journal of Medicine, 348*, 5–14.
154. Harvey, S., Harrison, D. A., Singer, M., et al. (2005). Assessment of the clinical effectiveness of pulmonary artery catheters in management of patients in intensive care (PAC-Man): A randomised controlled trial. *Lancet, 366*, 472–477.
155. Sakr, Y., Vincent, J. L., Reinhart, K., et al. (2005). Use of the pulmonary artery catheter is not associated with worse outcome in the ICU. *Chest, 128*, 2722–2731.
156. Harvey, S. E., Welch, C. A., Harrison, D. A., et al. (2008). Post hoc insights from PAC-Man—The U.K. pulmonary artery catheter trial. *Critical Care Medicine, 36*, 1714–1721.
157. Richard, C., Warszawski, J., Anguel, N., et al. (2003). Early use of the pulmonary artery catheter and outcomes in patients with shock and acute respiratory distress syndrome: A randomized controlled trial. *JAMA, 290*, 2713–2720.
158. Binanay, C., Califf, R. M., Hasselblad, V., et al. (2005). Evaluation study of congestive heart failure and pulmonary artery catheterization effectiveness: The ESCAPE trial. *JAMA, 294*, 1625–1633.
159. Gheorghiade, M., Filippatos, G., De Luca, L., et al. (2006). Congestion in acute heart failure syndromes: An essential target of evaluation and treatment. *American Journal of Medicine, 119*, S3–S10.
160. Shah, M. R., & Miller, L. (2007). Use of pulmonary artery catheters in advanced heart failure. *Current Opinion in Cardiology, 22*, 220–224.
161. Cotter, G., Cotter, O. M., & Kaluski, E. (2008). Hemodynamic monitoring in acute heart failure. *Critical Care Medicine, 36*, S40–S43.
162. Wiedemann, H. P., Wheeler, A. P., Bernard, G. R., et al. (2006). Comparison of two fluid-management strategies in acute lung injury. *New England Journal of Medicine, 354*, 2564–2575.
163. Friese, R. S., Shafi, S., & Gentilello, L. M. (2006). Pulmonary artery catheter use is associated with reduced mortality in severely injured patients: A National Trauma Data Bank analysis of 53,312 patients. *Critical Care Medicine, 34*, 1597–1601.
164. Shah, M. R., Hasselblad, V., Stevenson, L. W., et al. (2005). Impact of the pulmonary artery catheter in critically ill patients: Meta-analysis of randomized clinical trials. *JAMA, 294*, 1664–1670.
165. Harvey, S., Young, D., Brampton, W., et al. (2006). Pulmonary artery catheters for adult patients in intensive care. *Cochrane Database Systematic Reviews, 3*, CD003408.
166. Antonelli, M., Levy, M., Andrews, P. J., et al. (2007). Hemodynamic monitoring in shock and implications for management: International Consensus Conference, Paris, France, 27–28 April 2006. *Intensive Care Medicine, 33*, 575–590.
167. Pinsky, M. R., & Vincent, J. L. (2005). Let us use the pulmonary artery catheter correctly and only when we need it. *Critical Care Medicine, 33*, 1119–1122.
168. Leier, C. V. (2007). Invasive hemodynamic monitoring the aftermath of the ESCAPE trial. *Cardiology Clinics, 25*, 565–571; vi.
169. Stevenson, L. W. (2006). Are hemodynamic goals viable in tailoring heart failure therapy? Hemodynamic goals are relevant. *Circulation, 113*, 1020–1027; discussion 1033.
170. PACEP Collaborative. (2006). *Pulmonary Artery Catheter Education Project (PACEP): PACEP Collaborative, 2006*. Retrieved September 15, 2008, from http://www.pacep.org
171. American Thoracic Society. (2006). *Pulmonary artery catheter primer*. Retrieved September 15, 2008, from http://www.thoracic.org/sections/clinical-information/critical-care/hemodynamic-monitoring/pulmonary-artery-catheter-primer
172. Davidson, W., & Fee, E. (1990). Influence of aging on pulmonary hemodynamics in a population free of coronary artery disease. *American Journal of Cardiology, 65*, 1454–1458.
173. Ghali, J. K., Liao, Y., Cooper, R. S., et al. (1992). Changes in pulmonary hemodynamics with aging in a predominantly hypertensive population. *American Journal of Cardiology, 70*, 367–370.
174. Pinsky, M. R. (2003). Clinical significance of pulmonary artery occlusion pressure. *Intensive Care Medicine, 29*, 175–178.
175. Osman, D., Ridel, C., Ray, P., et al. (2007). Cardiac filling pressures are not appropriate to predict hemodynamic response to volume challenge. *Critical Care Medicine, 35*, 64–68.
176. Forrester, J. S., Diamond, G. A., & Swan, H. J. (1977). Correlative classification of clinical and hemodynamic function after acute myocardial infarction. *American Journal of Cardiology, 39*, 137–145.
177. Chakko, S., Woska, D., Martinez, H., et al. (1991). Clinical, radiographic, and hemodynamic correlations in chronic congestive heart failure: Conflicting results may lead to inappropriate care. *American Journal of Medicine, 90*, 353–359.
178. Pinsky, M. R. (2003). Pulmonary artery occlusion pressure. *Intensive Care Medicine, 29*, 19–22.
179. Bridges, E. (2000). Monitoring pulmonary artery pressures: Just the facts. *Critical Care Nurse, 20*, 59–78.
180. Ragosta, M. (2008). Mitral valve disorders. In M. Ragosta (Ed.), *Textbook of clinical hemodynamics* (pp. 50–67). Philadelphia: Saunders.
181. Freihage, J. H., Joyal, D., Arab, D., et al. (2007). Invasive assessment of mitral regurgitation: Comparison of hemodynamic parameters. *Catheterization and Cardiovascular Interventions, 69*, 303–312.
182. Haskell, R., & French, W. (1988). Accuracy of left atrial and pulmonary artery wedge pressure in pure mitral regurgitation in predicting left ventricular end-diastolic filling pressure. *American Journal of Cardiology, 61*, 136–141.
183. Ha, J. W., Chung, N., Jang, Y., et al. (2000). Is the left atrial v. wave the determinant of peak pulmonary artery pressure in patients with pure mitral stenosis? *American Journal of Cardiology, 85*, 986–991.
184. Lipp-Ziff, E. L., & Kawanishi, D. T. (1991). A technique for improving accuracy of the pulmonary artery diastolic pressure as an estimate of left ventricular end-diastolic pressure. *Heart & Lung, 20*, 107–115.
185. Le Jemtel, T. H., & Alt, E. U. (2006). Are hemodynamic goals viable in tailoring heart failure therapy? Hemodynamic goals are outdated. *Circulation, 113*, 1027–1032.
186. Badesch, D. B., Abman, S. H., Simonneau, G., et al. (2007). Medical therapy for pulmonary arterial hypertension: Updated ACCP evidence-based clinical practice guidelines. *Chest, 131*, 1917–1928.
187. Celermajer, D. S., & Marwick, T. (2008). Echocardiographic and right heart catheterization techniques in patients with pulmonary arterial hypertension. *International Journal of Cardiology, 125*, 294–303.
188. McLaughlin, V. V., & McGoon, M. D. (2006). Pulmonary arterial hypertension. *Circulation, 114*, 1417–1431.

189. Mathier, M., & Park, M. (2007). *Hemodynamic assessment of pulmonary hypertension: Echocardiography and cardiac catheterization, 2007*. Retrieved December 28, 2007, from http://www.medscape.com/viewprogram/8360_pnt.
190. Hoeper, M. M., Lee, S. H., Voswinckel, R., et al. (2006). Complications of right heart catheterization procedures in patients with pulmonary hypertension in experienced centers. *Journal of the American College of Cardiology, 48*, 2546–2552.
191. Balik, M., Pachl, J., Hendl, J., et al. (2002). Effect of the degree of tricuspid regurgitation on cardiac output measurements by thermodilution. *Intensive Care Medicine, 28*, 1117–1121.
192. Hoeper, M. M., Tongers, J., Leppert, A., et al. (2001). Evaluation of right ventricular performance with a right ventricular ejection fraction thermodilution catheter and MRI in patients with pulmonary hypertension. *Chest, 120*, 502–507.
193. Guillinta, P., Peterson, K. L., & Ben-Yehuda, O. (2004). Cardiac catheterization techniques in pulmonary hypertension. *Cardiology Clinics, 22*, 401–415.
194. American Association of Critical Care Nurses. (2004). *Practice alert: Pulmonary artery pressure monitoring*. Retrieved October 10, 2008, from http://www.aacn.org/WD/Practice/Docs/PAP_Measurement_05-2004.pdf.
195. Bridges, E. (2000). Hemodynamic monitoring. In S. Woods, E. Sivarajan Froelicher, & S. Underhill Motzer (Eds.), *Cardiac nursing* (pp. 427–478). Philadelphia: Lippincott.
196. Schaefer, W. M., Lipke, C. S., Kuhl, H. P., et al. (2004). Prone versus supine patient positioning during gated 99mTc-sestamibi SPECT: Effect on left ventricular volumes, ejection fraction, and heart rate. *Journal of Nuclear Medicine, 45*, 2016–2020.
197. Toyota, S., & Amaki, Y. (1998). Hemodynamic evaluation of the prone position by transesophageal echocardiography. *Journal of Clinical Anesthesia, 10*, 32–35.
198. West, J., Dollery, C., & Naimark, A. (1964). Distribution of blood flow in isolated lung; relation to vascular and alveolar pressures. *Journal of Applied Physiology, 19*, 713–724.
199. Johnson, M., & Schumann, L. (1995). Comparison of three methods of measurement of pulmonary artery catheter readings in critically ill patients. *American Journal of Critical Care, 4*, 300–307.
200. Lundstedt, J. (1997). Comparison of methods measuring pulmonary artery pressure. *American Journal of Critical Care, 6*, 324–332.
201. Ahrens, T. S., & Schallom, L. (2001). Comparison of pulmonary artery and central venous pressure waveform measurements via digital and graphic measurement methods. *Heart & Lung, 30*, 26–38.
202. Rizvi, K., Deboisblanc, B. P., Truwit, J. D., et al. (2005). Effect of airway pressure display on interobserver agreement in the assessment of vascular pressures in patients with acute lung injury and acute respiratory distress syndrome. *Critical Care Medicine, 33*, 98–103.
203. Hoyt, J. D., & Leatherman, J. W. (1997). Interpretation of the pulmonary artery occlusion pressure in mechanically ventilated patients with large respiratory excursions in intrathoracic pressure. *Intensive Care Medicine, 23*, 1125–1131.
204. Qureshi, A. S., Shapiro, R. S., & Leatherman, J. W. (2007). Use of bladder pressure to correct for the effect of expiratory muscle activity on central venous pressure. *Intensive Care Medicine, 33*, 1907–1912.
205. Vender, J. S., & Franklin, M. (2004). Hemodynamic assessment of the critically ill patient. *International Anesthesiology Clinics, 42*, 31–58.
206. Antle, D. E. (2000). Ensuring competency in nurse repositioning of the pulmonary artery catheter. *Dimensions in Critical Care Nursing, 19*, 44–51.
207. Baldwin, I. C., & Heland, M. (2000). Incidence of cardiac dysrhythmias in patients during pulmonary artery catheter removal after cardiac surgery. *Heart & Lung, 29*, 155–160.
208. Zevola, D. R., & Maier, B. (1999). Improving the care of cardiothoracic surgery patients through advanced nursing skills. *Critical Care Nurse, 19*, 34–44.
209. Oztekin, D. S., Akyolcu, N., Oztekin, I., et al. (2008). Comparison of complications and procedural activities of pulmonary artery catheter removal by critical care nurses versus medical doctors. *Nursing in Critical Care, 13*, 105–115.
210. Leeper, B. (2003). Monitoring right ventricular volumes: A paradigm shift. *AACN Clinical Issues, 14*, 208–219.
211. Michard, F., & Teboul, J. L. (2000). Using heart–lung interactions to assess fluid responsiveness during mechanical ventilation. *Critical Care, 4*, 282–289.
212. Magder, S. (2007). The left heart can only be as good as the right heart: Determinants of function and dysfunction of the right ventricle. *Critical Care and Resuscitation, 9*, 344–351.
213. Zink, W., Noll, J., Rauch, H., et al. (2004). Continuous assessment of right ventricular ejection fraction: New pulmonary artery catheter versus transoesophageal echocardiography. *Anaesthesia, 59*, 1126–1132.
214. Wiesenack, C., Fiegl, C., Keyser, A., et al. (2005). Continuously assessed right ventricular end-diastolic volume as a marker of cardiac preload and fluid responsiveness in mechanically ventilated cardiac surgical patients. *Critical Care, 9*, R226–R233.
215. Chang, M. C., & Meredith, J. W. (1997). Cardiac preload, splanchnic perfusion, and their relationship during resuscitation in trauma patients. *Journal of Trauma, 42*, 577–582.
216. Miller, P., Meredith, J., & Chang, M. (1998). Randomized, prospective comparison of increased preload versus inotropes in the resuscitation of trauma patients: Effects on cardiopulmonary function and visceral perfusion. *Journal of Trauma, 44*, 107–113.
217. Della Rocca, G. D., Costa, M. G., Feltracco, P., et al. (2008). Continuous right ventricular end diastolic volume and right ventricular ejection fraction during liver transplantation: A multicenter study. *Liver Transplantation, 14*, 327–332.
218. De Wolf, A. M., & Aggarwal, S. (2008). Monitoring preload during liver transplantation. *Liver Transplantation, 14*, 268–269.
219. Gouvea, G., Diaz, R., Auler, L., et al. (2008). Evaluation of the right ventricular ejection fraction during orthotopic liver transplantation under propofol anaesthesia. *British Journal of Anaesthesia, 101*, 161–165.
220. Hofer, C. K., Furrer, L., Matter-Ensner, S., et al. (2005). Volumetric preload measurement by thermodilution: A comparison with transoesophageal echocardiography. *British Journal of Anaesthesia, 94*, 748–755.
221. Diebel, L., Wilson, R. F., Heins, J., et al. (1994). End-diastolic volume versus pulmonary artery wedge pressure in evaluating cardiac preload in trauma patients. *Journal of Trauma, 37*, 950–955.
222. Diebel, L. N., Wilson, R. F., Tagett, M. G., et al. (1992). End-diastolic volume. A better indicator of preload in the critically ill. *Archives of Surgery, 127*, 817–821.
223. Siniscalchi, A., Pavesi, M., Piraccini, E., et al. (2005). Right ventricular end-diastolic volume index as a predictor of preload status in patients with low right ventricular ejection fraction during orthotopic liver transplantation. *Transplantation Proceedings, 37*, 2541–2543.
224. Michard, F., Alaya, S., Zarka, V., et al. (2003). Global end-diastolic volume as an indicator of cardiac preload in patients with septic shock. *Chest, 124*, 1900–1908.
225. Della Rocca, G., Costa, M. G., & Pietropaoli, P. (2007). How to measure and interpret volumetric measures of preload. *Current Opinion in Critical Care, 13*, 297–302.
226. Wagner, J. G., & Leatherman, J. W. (1998). Right ventricular end-diastolic volume as a predictor of the hemodynamic response to a fluid challenge. *Chest, 113*, 1048–1054.
227. Tokuda, Y., Song, M. H., Mabuchi, N., et al. (2007). Right ventricular end-diastolic volume in the postoperative care of cardiac surgery patients: A marker of the hemodynamic response to a fluid challenge. *Circulation Journal, 71*, 1408–1411.
228. Bagshaw, S. M., & Bellomo, R. (2007). The influence of volume management on outcome. *Current Opinion in Critical Care, 13*, 541–548.
229. Pepe, P. E., Dutton, R. P., & Fowler, R. L. (2008). Preoperative resuscitation of the trauma patient. *Current Opinion in Anaesthesiology, 21*, 216–221.
230. Michard, F., & Teboul, J. L. (2002). Predicting fluid responsiveness in ICU patients: A critical analysis of the evidence. *Chest, 121*, 2000–2008.
231. Kumar, A., Anel, R., Bunnell, E., et al. (2004). Pulmonary artery occlusion pressure and central venous pressure fail to predict ventricular filling volume, cardiac performance, or the response to volume infusion in normal subjects. *Critical Care Medicine, 32*, 691–699.
232. Calvin, J., Driedger, A., & Sibbald, W. (1981). Does pulmonary capillary wedge pressure predict left ventricular preload in critically ill patients? *Critical Care Medicine, 9*, 437–443.
233. Michard, F., Boussat, S., Chemla, D., et al. (2000). Relation between respiratory changes in arterial pulse pressure and fluid responsiveness in septic patients with acute circulatory failure. *American Journal of Respiratory Critical Care Medicine, 162*, 134–138.
234. Tavernier, B., Makhotine, O., Lebuffe, G., et al. (1998). Systolic pressure variation as a guide to fluid therapy in patients with sepsis-induced hypotension. *Anesthesiology, 89*, 1313–1321.
235. Tousignant, C. P., Walsh, F., & Mazer, C. D. (2000). The use of transesophageal echocardiography for preload assessment in critically ill patients. *Anesthesia & Analgesia, 90*, 351–355.
236. Pinsky, M. R., & Teboul, J. L. (2005). Assessment of indices of preload and volume responsiveness. *Current Opinion in Critical Care, 11*, 235–239.

237. Magder, S., Georgiadis, G., & Cheong, T. (1992). Respiratory variation in right atrial pressure predict the response to fluid challenge. *Journal of Critical Care, 7,* 76–85.
238. Magder, S. (2006). Central venous pressure: A useful but not so simple measurement. *Critical Care Medicine, 34,* 2224–2227.
239. Pinsky, M. R. (2007). Heart-lung interactions. *Current Opinion in Critical Care, 13,* 528–531.
240. Rivers, E., Nguyen, B., Havstad, S., et al. (2001). Early goal-directed therapy in the treatment of severe sepsis and septic shock. *New England Journal of Medicine, 345,* 1368–1377.
241. Magder, S., & Lagonidis, D. (1999). Effectiveness of albumin versus normal saline as a test of volume responsiveness in post-cardiac surgery patients. *Journal of Critical Care, 14,* 164–171.
242. Magder, S. (2006). Predicting volume responsiveness in spontaneously breathing patients: Still a challenging problem. *Critical Care, 10,* 165.
243. Magder, S., Lagonidis, D., & Erice, F. (2001). The use of respiratory variations in right atrial pressure to predict the cardiac output response to PEEP. *Journal of Critical Care, 16,* 108–114.
244. Pizov, R., Ya'ari, Y., & Perel, A. (1988). Systolic pressure variation is greater during hemorrhage than during sodium nitroprusside-induced hypotension in ventilated dogs. *Anesthesia & Analgesia, 67,* 170–174.
245. Berkenstadt, H., Friedman, Z., Preisman, S., et al. (2005). Pulse pressure and stroke volume variations during severe haemorrhage in ventilated dogs. *British Journal of Anaesthesia, 94,* 721–726.
246. De Backer, D., Heenen, S., Piagnerelli, M., et al. (2005). Pulse pressure variations to predict fluid responsiveness: Influence of tidal volume. *Intensive Care Medicine, 31,* 517–523.
247. Charron, C., Fessenmeyer, C., Cosson, C., et al. (2006). The influence of tidal volume on the dynamic variables of fluid responsiveness in critically ill patients. *Anesthesia & Analgesia, 102,* 1511–1517.
248. Kramer, A., Zygun, D., Hawes, H., et al. (2004). Pulse pressure variation predicts fluid responsiveness following coronary artery bypass surgery. *Chest, 126,* 1563–1568.
249. Reuter, D. A., Kirchner, A., Felbinger, T. W., et al. (2003). Usefulness of left ventricular stroke volume variation to assess fluid responsiveness in patients with reduced cardiac function. *Critical Care Medicine, 31,* 1399–1404.
250. Perner, A., & Faber, T. (2006). Stroke volume variation does not predict fluid responsiveness in patients with septic shock on pressure support ventilation. *Acta Anaesthesiologica Scandinavica, 50,* 1068–1073.
251. Wyffels, P. A., Durnez, P. J., Helderweirt, J., et al. (2007). Ventilation-induced plethysmographic variations predict fluid responsiveness in ventilated postoperative cardiac surgery patients. *Anesthesia & Analgesia, 105,* 448–452.
252. Huang, C. C., Fu, J. Y., Hu, H. C., et al. (2008). Prediction of fluid responsiveness in acute respiratory distress syndrome patients ventilated with low tidal volume and high positive end-expiratory pressure. *Critical Care Medicine, 36,* 2810–2816.
253. Auler, J. O., Jr., Galas, F. R., Sundin, M. R., et al. (2008). Arterial pulse pressure variation predicting fluid responsiveness in critically ill patients. *Shock, 30*(Suppl. 1), 18–22.
254. Michard, F., Chemla, D., Richard, C., et al. (1999). Clinical use of respiratory changes in arterial pulse pressure to monitor the hemodynamic effects of PEEP. *American Journal of Respiratory and Critical Care Medicine, 159,* 935–939.
255. Pinsky, M. (2002). Functional hemodynamic monitoring: Applied physiology at the bedside. In J. L. Vincent (Ed.), *Intensive care medicine. Annual update 2002* (pp. 537–552). Berlin, Germany: Springer-Verlag.
256. Kim, H. K., & Pinsky, M. R. (2008). Effect of tidal volume, sampling duration, and cardiac contractility on pulse pressure and stroke volume variation during positive-pressure ventilation. *Critical Care Medicine, 36,* 2858–2862.
257. Preisman, S., DiSegni, E., Vered, Z., et al. (2002). Left ventricular preload and function during graded haemorrhage and retransfusion in pigs: Analysis of arterial pressure waveform and correlation with echocardiography. *British Journal of Anaesthesia, 88,* 716–718.
258. Ornstein, E., Eidelman, L. A., Drenger, B., et al. (1998). Systolic pressure variation predicts the response to acute blood loss. *Journal of Clinical Anesthesia, 10,* 137–140.
259. Rooke, G. A., Schwid, H. A., & Shapira, Y. (1995). The effect of graded hemorrhage and intravascular volume replacement on systolic pressure variation in humans during mechanical and spontaneous ventilation. *Anesthesia & Analgesia, 80,* 925–932.
260. Westphal, G., Garrido Adel, P., de Almeida, D. P., et al. (2007). Pulse pressure respiratory variation as an early marker of cardiac output fall in experimental hemorrhagic shock. *Artificial Organs, 31,* 284–289.
261. Cope, T., Marx, G., McCrossan, L., et al. (2002). Stroke volume variation for assessment of cardiac responsiveness to volume loading in severe sepsis. *Intensive Care Medicine, 28,* S81.
262. Pinsky, M. R. (2003). Probing the limits of arterial pulse contour analysis to predict preload responsiveness. *Anesthesia & Analgesia, 96,* 1245–1247.
263. Reuter, D. A., Felbinger, T. W., Schmidt, C., et al. (2002). Stroke volume variations for assessment of cardiac responsiveness to volume loading in mechanically ventilated patients after cardiac surgery. *Intensive Care Medicine, 28,* 392–398.
264. Wiesenack, C., Prasser, C., Rodig, G., et al. (2003). Stroke volume variation as an indicator of fluid responsiveness using pulse contour analysis in mechanically ventilated patients. *Anesthesia & Analgesia, 96,* 1254–1257.
265. Reuter, D. A., Bayerlein, J., Goepfert, M., et al. (2003). Functional preload monitoring by arterial pulse contour analysis: Influence of tidal volume on left ventricular stroke volume variations (abstract). *Critical Care Medicine, 30,* A19.
266. Cannesson, M., Delannoy, B., Morand, A., et al. (2008). Does the Pleth variability index indicate the respiratory-induced variation in the plethysmogram and arterial pressure waveforms? *Anesthesia & Analgesia, 106,* 1189–1194.
267. Natalini, G., Rosano, A., Franceschetti, M. E., et al. (2006). Variations in arterial blood pressure and photoplethysmography during mechanical ventilation. *Anesthesia & Analgesia, 103,* 1182–1188.
268. Cannesson, M., Attof, Y., Rosamel, P., et al. (2007). Respiratory variations in pulse oximetry plethysmographic waveform amplitude to predict fluid responsiveness in the operating room. *Anesthesiology, 106,* 1105–1111.
269. Feissel, M., Teboul, J. L., Merlani, P., et al. (2007). Plethysmographic dynamic indices predict fluid responsiveness in septic ventilated patients. *Intensive Care Medicine, 33,* 993–999.
270. Solus-Biguenet, H., Fleyfel, M., Tavernier, B., et al. (2006). Non-invasive prediction of fluid responsiveness during major hepatic surgery. *British Journal of Anaesthesia, 97,* 808–816.
271. Cannesson, M., Desebbe, O., Rosamel, P., et al. (2008). Pleth variability index to monitor the respiratory variations in the pulse oximeter plethysmographic waveform amplitude and predict fluid responsiveness in the operating theatre. *British Journal of Anaesthesiology, 101,* 200–206.
272. Gesquiere, M. J., Awad, A. A., Silverman, D. G., et al. (2007). Impact of withdrawal of 450 ml of blood on respiration-induced oscillations of the ear plethysmographic waveform. *Journal of Clinical Monitoring and Computing, 21,* 277–282.
273. Delerme, S., Renault, R., Le Manach, Y., et al. (2007). Variations in pulse oximetry plethysmographic waveform amplitude induced by passive leg raising in spontaneously breathing volunteers. *American Journal of Emergency Medicine, 25,* 637–642.
274. Keller, G., Cassar, E., Desebbe, O., et al. (2008). Ability of pleth variability index to detect hemodynamic changes induced by passive leg raising in spontaneously breathing volunteers. *Critical Care, 12,* R37.
275. Shelley, K. H., Jablonka, D. H., Awad, A. A., et al. (2006). What is the best site for measuring the effect of ventilation on the pulse oximeter waveform? *Anesthesia & Analgesia, 103,* 372–377.
276. Michard, F. (2007). Using pulse oximetry waveform analysis to guide fluid therapy: Are we there yet? *Anesthesia & Analgesia, 104,* 1606–1607.
277. Heenen, S., De Backer, D., & Vincent, J. L. (2006). How can the response to volume expansion in patients with spontaneous respiratory movements be predicted? *Critical Care, 10,* R102–R108.
278. Monnet, X., Rienzo, M., Osman, D., et al. (2006). Passive leg raising predicts fluid responsiveness in the critically ill. *Critical Care Medicine, 34,* 1402–1407.
279. Renner, J., Cavus, E., Meybohm, P., et al. (2007). Stroke volume variation during hemorrhage and after fluid loading: Impact of different tidal volumes. *Acta Anaesthesiologica Scandinavica, 51,* 538–544.
280. Kubitz, J. C., Annecke, T., Kemming, G. I., et al. (2006). The influence of positive end-expiratory pressure on stroke volume variation and central blood volume during open and closed chest conditions. *European Journal of Cardiothoracic Surgery, 30,* 90–95.
281. Michard, F. (2005). Volume management using dynamic parameters: The good, the bad, and the ugly. *Chest, 128,* 1902–1903.
282. Pizov, R., Segal, E., Kaplan, L., et al. (1990). The use of systolic pressure variation in hemodynamic monitoring during deliberate hypotension in spine surgery. *Journal of Clinical Anesthesia, 2,* 96–100.
283. Fonseca, E. B., Otsuki, D. A., Fantoni, D. T., et al. (2008). Comparative study of pressure- and volume-controlled ventilation on pulse pressure variation in a model of hypovolaemia in rabbits. *European Journal of Anaesthesiology, 25,* 388–394.

284. Malbrain, M. L., Chiumello, D., Pelosi, P., et al. (2004). Prevalence of intra-abdominal hypertension in critically ill patients: A multicentre epidemiological study. *Intensive Care Medicine, 30*, 822–829.
285. Duperret, S., Lhuillier, F., Piriou, V., et al. (2007). Increased intra-abdominal pressure affects respiratory variations in arterial pressure in normovolaemic and hypovolaemic mechanically ventilated healthy pigs. *Intensive Care Medicine, 33*, 163–171.
286. Malbrain, M. L., & De Laet, I. (2008). Functional haemodynamics during intra-abdominal hypertension: What to use and what not use. *Acta Anaesthesiologica Scandinavica, 52*, 576–577.
287. Bliacheriene, F., Machado, S. B., Fonseca, E. B., et al. (2007). Pulse pressure variation as a tool to detect hypovolaemia during pneumoperitoneum. *Acta Anaesthesiologica Scandinavica, 51*, 1268–1272.
288. Boulain, T., Achard, J. M., Teboul, J. L., et al. (2002). Changes in BP induced by passive leg raising predict response to fluid loading in critically ill patients. *Chest, 121*, 1245–1252.
289. Lafanechere, A., Pene, F., Goulenok, C., et al. (2006). Changes in aortic blood flow induced by passive leg raising predict fluid responsiveness in critically ill patients. *Critical Care, 10*, R132–R139.
290. Ridel, C., Lamia, B., Monnet, X., et al. (2006). Passive leg raising and fluid responsiveness during spontaneous breathing: Pulse contour evaluation. *Intensive Care Medicine, 32*, S81.
291. De Backer, D. (2006). Can passive leg raising be used to guide fluid administration? *Critical Care, 10*, 170–171.
292. Lamia, B., Ochagavia, A., Monnet, X., et al. (2007). Echocardiographic prediction of volume responsiveness in critically ill patients with spontaneously breathing activity. *Intensive Care Medicine, 33*, 1125–1132.
293. Monnet, X., & Teboul, J. L. (2008). Passive leg raising. *Intensive Care Medicine, 34*, 659–663.
294. Caille, V., Jabot, J., Belliard, G., et al. (2008). Hemodynamic effects of passive leg raising: An echocardiographic study in patients with shock. *Intensive Care Medicine, 34*, 1239–1245.
295. Jabot, J., Teboul, J. L., Richard, C., et al. (2008). Passive leg raising for predicting fluid responsiveness: Importance of the postural change. *Intensive Care Medicine, 34*, S187.
296. Maizel, J., Airapetian, N., Lorne, E., et al. (2007). Diagnosis of central hypovolemia by using passive leg raising. *Intensive Care Medicine, 33*, 1133–1138.
297. Teboul, J. L., & Monnet, X. (2008). Prediction of volume responsiveness in critically ill patients with spontaneous breathing activity. *Current Opinion in Critical Care, 14*, 334–339.
298. Bertolissi, M., Broi, U. D., Soldano, F., et al. (2003). Influence of passive leg elevation on the right ventricular function in anaesthetized coronary patients. *Critical Care, 7*, 164–170.
299. Nilsson, L. B., Nilsson, J. C., Skovgaard, L. T., et al. (2004). Thermodilution cardiac output—are three injections enough? *Acta Anaesthesiologica Scandinavica, 48*, 1322–1327.
300. McCloy, K., Leung, S., Belden, J., et al. (1999). Effects of injectate volume on thermodilution measurements of cardiac output in patients with low ventricular ejection fraction. *American Journal of Critical Care, 8*, 86–92.
301. Griffin, K., Benjamin, E., DelGiudice, R., et al. (1997). Thermodilution cardiac output measurement during simultaneous volume infusion through the venous infusion port of the pulmonary artery catheter. *Journal of Cardiothoracic and Vascular Anesthesia, 11*, 437–439.
302. Giuliano, K. K., Scott, S. S., Brown, V., et al. (2003). Backrest angle and cardiac output measurement in critically ill patients. *Nursing Research, 52*, 242–248.
303. Killu, K., Oropello, J. M., Manasia, A. R., et al. (2007). Effect of lower limb compression devices on thermodilution cardiac output measurement. *Critical Care Medicine, 35*, 1307–1311.
304. Bottiger, B. W., Rauch, H., Bohrer, H., et al. (1995). Continuous versus intermittent cardiac output measurement in cardiac surgical patients undergoing hypothermic cardiopulmonary bypass. *Journal of Cardiothoracic and Vascular Anesthesia, 9*, 405–411.
305. Ong, T., Gillies, M. A., & Bellomo, R. (2004). Failure of continuous cardiac output measurement using the PiCCO Device during induced hypothermia: A case report. *Critical Care Resuscitation, 6*, 99–101.
306. Sami, A., Rochdil, N., Hatem, K., et al. (2007). PiCCO monitoring accuracy in low body temperature. *American Journal of Emergency Medicine, 25*, 845–846.
307. Sasse, S., Chen, P., Berry, R., et al. (1994). Variability of cardiac output over time in medical intensive care unit patients. *Critical Care Medicine, 22*, 225–232.
308. Huang, C. C., Tsai, Y. H., Chen, N. H., et al. (2000). Spontaneous variability of cardiac output in ventilated critically ill patients. *Critical Care Medicine, 28*, 941–946.
309. Nguyen, T. V., & Hillman, K. M. (2001). On the analysis and interpretation of spontaneous variability of cardiac output. *Critical Care Medicine, 29*, 220–221.
310. Østergaard, M., Nilsson, L. B., Nilsson, J. C., et al. (2005). Precision of bolus thermodilution cardiac output measurements in patients with atrial fibrillation. *Acta Anaesthesiologica Scandinavica, 49*, 366–372.
311. Chemla, D., & Nitenberg, A. (2006). Systolic duration, preload, and afterload: Is a new paradigm needed? *Intensive Care Medicine, 32*, 1454–1455.
312. Sun, Q., Rogiers, P., Pauwels, D., et al. (2002). Comparison of continuous thermodilution and bolus cardiac output measurements in septic shock. *Intensive Care Medicine, 28*, 1276–1280.
313. Bendjelid, K., Schutz, N., Suter, P. M., et al. (2006). Continuous cardiac output monitoring after cardiopulmonary bypass: A comparison with bolus thermodilution measurement. *Intensive Care Medicine, 32*, 919–922.
314. Zollner, C., Goetz, A. E., Weis, M., et al. (2001). Continuous cardiac output measurements do not agree with conventional bolus thermodilution cardiac output determination. *Canadian Journal of Anaesthesia, 48*, 1143–1147.
315. Bao, F. P., & Wu, J. (2008). Continuous versus bolus cardiac output monitoring during orthotopic liver transplantation. *Hepatobiliary & Pancreatic Disease International, 7*, 138–144.
316. Button, D., Weibel, L., Reuthebuch, O., et al. (2007). Clinical evaluation of the FloTrac/Vigileo™ system and two established continuous cardiac output monitoring devices in patients undergoing cardiac surgery. *British Journal of Anaesthesia, 99*, 329–336.
317. Luchette, F., Johannigman, J., Branson, R., et al. (1995). Effect of body temperature on accuracy of continuous cardiac output measurements. *Critical Care Medicine, 23*, A137.
318. O'Malley, P., Smith, B., Hamlin, R., et al. (2000). A comparison of bolus versus continuous cardiac output in an experimental model of heart failure. *Critical Care Medicine, 28*, 1985–1990.
319. Boyle, M., Jacobs, S., Torda, T. A., et al. (1997). Assessment of the agreement between cardiac output measured by bolus thermodilution and continuous methods, with particular reference to the effect of heart rhythm. *Australian Critical Care, 10*, 5–8, 10–11.
320. Medin, D., Brown, D., Onibene, F., et al. (1997). Comparison of cardiac output measurements by bolus thermodilution technique and continuous automated thermal technique in critically ill patients. *Critical Care Medicine, 25*, A81.
321. Mets, B., Frumento, R. J., Bennett-Guerrero, E., et al. (2002). Validation of continuous thermodilution cardiac output in patients implanted with a left ventricular assist device. *Journal of Cardiothoracic and Vascular Anesthesia, 16*, 727–730.
322. Lazor, M. A., Pierce, E. T., Stanley, G. D., et al. (1997). Evaluation of the accuracy and response time of STAT-mode continuous cardiac output. *Journal of Cardiothoracic and Vascular Anesthesia, 11*, 432–436.
323. Boyle, M., Murgo, M., Lawrence, J., et al. (2007). Assessment of the accuracy of continuous cardiac output and pulse contour cardiac output in tracking cardiac index changes induced by volume load. *Australian Critical Care, 20*, 106–112.
324. Aranda, M., Mihm, F. G., Garrett, S., et al. (1998). Continuous cardiac output catheters: Delay in vitro response time after controlled flow changes. *Anesthesiology, 89*, 1592–1595.
325. Poli de Figueiredo, L. F., Malbouisson, L. M., Varicoda, E. Y., et al. (1999). Thermal filament continuous thermodilution cardiac output delayed response limits its value during acute hemodynamic instability. *The Journal of Trauma, 47*, 288–293.
326. Singh, A., Juneja, R., Mehta, Y., et al. (2002). Comparison of continuous, stat, and intermittent cardiac output measurements in patients undergoing minimally invasive direct coronary artery bypass surgery. *Journal of Cardiothoracic and Vascular Anesthesia, 16*, 186–190.
327. Haller, M., Zollner, C., Briegel, J., et al. (1995). Evaluation of a new continuous thermodilution cardiac output monitor in critically ill patients: A prospective criterion standard study. *Critical Care Medicine, 23*, 860–866.
328. Bridges, E. J. (2008). Arterial pressure-based stroke volume and functional hemodynamic monitoring. *Journal of Cardiovascular Nursing, 23*, 105–112.
329. de Wilde, R. B., Breukers, R. B., van den Berg, P. C., et al. (2006). Monitoring cardiac output using the femoral and radial arterial pressure waveform. *Anaesthesia, 61*, 743–746.
330. Pearse, R. M., Ikram, K., Barry, J. (2004). Equipment review: An appraisal of the LiDCO plus method of measuring cardiac output. *Critical Care, 8*, 190–195.

331. Linton, R. A., Band, D. M., & Haire, K. M. (1993). A new method of measuring cardiac output in man using lithium dilution. *British Journal of Anaesthesiology, 71*, 262–266.
332. Jonas, M. M., & Tanser, S. J. (2002). Lithium dilution measurement of cardiac output and arterial pulse waveform analysis: An indicator dilution calibrated beat-by-beat system for continuous estimation of cardiac output. *Current Opinion in Critical Care, 8*, 257–261.
333. Felbinger, T. W., Reuter, D. A., Eltzschig, H. K., et al. (2005). Cardiac index measurements during rapid preload changes: A comparison of pulmonary artery thermodilution with arterial pulse contour analysis. *Journal of Clinical Anesthesia, 17*, 241–248.
334. Gunn, S. R., Kim, H. K., Harrigan, P. W., et al. (2006). Ability of pulse contour and esophageal Doppler to estimate rapid changes in stroke volume. *Intensive Care Medicine, 32*, 1537–1546.
335. Manecke, G. R. (2005). Edwards FloTrac sensor and Vigileo monitor: Easy, accurate, reliable cardiac output assessment using the arterial pulse wave. *Expert Review of Medical Devices, 2*, 523–527.
336. Sander, M., Spies, C. D., Grubitzsch, H., et al. (2006). Comparison of uncalibrated arterial waveform analysis in cardiac surgery patients with thermodilution cardiac output measurements. *Critical Care, 10*, R164–R173.
337. Cannesson, M., Attof, Y., Rosamel, P., et al. (2007). Comparison of FloTrac cardiac output monitoring system in patients undergoing coronary artery bypass grafting with pulmonary artery cardiac output measurements. *European Journal of Anaesthesiology, 24*, 832–839.
338. de Waal, E. E., Kalkman, C. J., Rex, S., et al. (2007). Validation of a new arterial pulse contour-based cardiac output device. *Critical Care Medicine, 35*, 1904–1909.
339. Lorsomradee, S., Lorsomradee, S. R., Cromheecke, S., et al. (2007). Continuous cardiac output measurement: Arterial pressure analysis versus thermodilution technique during cardiac surgery with cardiopulmonary bypass. *Anaesthesia, 62*, 979–983.
340. Manecke, G. R., Jr., & Auger, W. R. (2007). Cardiac output determination from the arterial pressure wave: Clinical testing of a novel algorithm that does not require calibration. *Journal of Cardiothoracic and Vascular Anesthesia, 21*, 3–7.
341. Mayer, J., Boldt, J., Schollhorn, T., et al. (2007). Semi-invasive monitoring of cardiac output by a new device using arterial pressure waveform analysis: A comparison with intermittent pulmonary artery thermodilution in patients undergoing cardiac surgery. *British Journal of Anaesthesiology, 98*, 176–182.
342. Opdam, H. I., Wan, L., & Bellomo, R. (2007). A pilot assessment of the FloTrac cardiac output monitoring system. *Intensive Care Medicine, 33*, 344–349.
343. Sakka, S. G., Kozieras, J., Thuemer, O., et al. (2007). Measurement of cardiac output: A comparison between transpulmonary thermodilution and uncalibrated pulse contour analysis. *British Journal of Anaesthesiology, 99*, 337–342.
344. Prasser, C., Trabold, B., Schwab, A., et al. (2007). Evaluation of an improved algorithm for arterial pressure-based cardiac output assessment without external calibration. *Intensive Care Medicine, 33*, 2223–2225.
345. Mayer, J., Boldt, J., Wolf, M. W., et al. (2008). Cardiac output derived from arterial pressure waveform analysis in patients undergoing cardiac surgery: Validity of a second generation device. *Anesthesia & Analgesia, 106*, 867–872.
346. Compton, F. D., Zukunft, B., Hoffman, A. H., et al. (2008). Performance of a minimally invasive cardiac output monitoring system (Flotrac/Vigileo). *British Journal of Anaesthesiology, 101*, 279–280.
347. Compton, F. D., Zukunft, B., Hoffmann, C., et al. (2008). Performance of a minimally invasive uncalibrated cardiac output monitoring system (Flotrac/Vigileo) in haemodynamically unstable patients. *British Journal of Anaesthesiology, 100*, 451–456.
348. Linton, N. W., & Linton, R. A. (2001). Estimation of changes in cardiac output from the arterial blood pressure waveform in the upper limb. *British Journal of Anaesthesiology, 86*, 486–496.
349. Godje, O., Hoke, K., Goetz, A. E., et al. (2002). Reliability of a new algorithm for continuous cardiac output determination by pulse-contour analysis during hemodynamic instability. *Critical Care Medicine, 30*, 52–58.
350. Rodig, G., Prasser, C., Keyl, C., et al. (1999). Continuous cardiac output measurement: Pulse contour analysis vs thermodilution technique in cardiac surgical patients. *British Journal of Anesthesiology, 82*, 525–530.
351. Hamzaoui, O., Monnet, X., Richard, C., et al. (2008). Effects of changes in vascular tone on the agreement between pulse contour and transpulmonary thermodilution cardiac output measurements within an up to 6-hour calibration-free period. *Critical Care Medicine, 36*, 434–440.
352. Cecconi, M., Fawcett, J., Grounds, R. M., et al. (2008). A prospective study to evaluate the accuracy of pulse power analysis to monitor cardiac output in critically ill patients. *BMC Anesthesiology, 8*, 3.
353. Cooper, E. S., & Muir, W. W. (2007). Continuous cardiac output monitoring via arterial pressure waveform analysis following severe hemorrhagic shock in dogs. *Critical Care Medicine, 35*, 1724–1729.
354. Michard, F. (2007). Bedside assessment of extravascular lung water by dilution methods: Temptations and pitfalls. *Critical Care Medicine, 35*, 1186–1192.
355. Sakka, S. G., Klein, M., Reinhart, K., et al. (2002). Prognostic value of extravascular lung water in critically ill patients. *Chest, 122*, 2080–2086.
356. Pittman, J., Bar-Yosef, S., SumPing, J., et al. (2005). Continuous cardiac output monitoring with pulse contour analysis: A comparison with lithium indicator dilution cardiac output measurement. *Critical Care Medicine, 33*, 2015–2021.
357. Singer, M. (2006). The FTc is not an accurate marker of left ventricular preload. *Intensive Care Medicine, 32*, 1089; author reply 1091.
358. Gan, T. J., Soppitt, A., Maroof, M., et al. (2002). Goal-directed intraoperative fluid administration reduces length of hospital stay after major surgery. *Anesthesiology, 97*, 820–826.
359. Sinclair, S., James, S., & Singer, M. (1997). Intraoperative intravascular volume optimisation and length of hospital stay after repair of proximal femoral fracture: Randomised controlled trial. *BMJ, 315*, 909–912.
360. Wakeling, H. G., McFall, M. R., Jenkins, C. S., et al. (2005). Intraoperative oesophageal Doppler guided fluid management shortens postoperative hospital stay after major bowel surgery. *British Journal of Anaesthesiology, 95*, 634–642.
361. Abbas, S. M., & Hill, A. G. (2008). Systematic review of the literature for the use of oesophageal Doppler monitor for fluid replacement in major abdominal surgery. *Anaesthesia, 63*, 44–51.
362. Poeze, M., Ramsay, G., Greve, J. W., et al. (1999). Prediction of postoperative cardiac surgical morbidity and organ failure within 4 hours of intensive care unit admission using esophageal Doppler ultrasonography. *Critical Care Medicine, 27*, 1288–1294.
363. Rady, M. Y. (2000). Prediction of postoperative cardiac surgical morbidity and organ failure at admission to the intensive care unit using esophageal Doppler ultrasonography. *Critical Care Medicine, 28*, 3368–3369.
364. McKendry, M., McGloin, H., Saberi, D., et al. (2004). Randomised controlled trial assessing the impact of a nurse delivered, flow monitored protocol for optimisation of circulatory status after cardiac surgery. *BMJ, 329*, 258.
365. Chytra, I., Pradl, R., Bosman, R., et al. (2007). Esophageal Doppler-guided fluid management decreases blood lactate levels in multiple-trauma patients: A randomized controlled trial. *Critical Care, 11*, R24.
366. Iregui, M. G., Prentice, D., Sherman, G., et al. (2003). Physicians' estimates of cardiac index and intravascular volume based on clinical assessment versus transesophageal Doppler measurements obtained by critical care nurses. *American Journal of Critical Care, 12*, 336–342.
367. Ahmed, S., Syed, F., & Porembka, D. (2007). Echocardiographic evaluation of hemodynamic parameters. *Critical Care Medicine, 35*, S323–S329.
368. Beaulieu, Y., & Marik, P. (2005). Bedside echocardiography in the ICU: Part 2. *Chest, 128*, 1766–1781.
369. Beaulieu, Y. (2007). Bedside echocardiography in the assessment of the critically ill. *Critical Care Medicine, 35*, S235–S249.
370. Douglas, P. S., Khandheria, B., Stainback, R. F., et al. (2007). ACCF/ASE/ACEP/ASNC/SCAI/SCCT/SCMR 2007 appropriateness criteria for transthoracic and transesophageal echocardiography: A report of the American College of Cardiology Foundation Quality Strategic Directions Committee Appropriateness Criteria Working Group, American Society of Echocardiography, American College of Emergency Physicians, American Society of Nuclear Cardiology, Society for Cardiovascular Angiography and Interventions, Society of Cardiovascular Computed Tomography, and the Society for Cardiovascular Magnetic Resonance endorsed by the American College of Chest Physicians and the Society of Critical Care Medicine. *Journal of the American College of Cardiology, 50*, 187–204.
371. Bruch, C., Comber, M., Schmermund, A., et al. (2003). Diagnostic usefulness and impact on management of transesophageal echocardiography in surgical intensive care units. *American Journal of Cardiology, 91*, 510–513.
372. Bouchard, M. J., Denault, A., Couture, P., et al. (2004). Poor correlation between hemodynamic and echocardiographic indexes of left ventricular performance in the operating room and intensive care unit. *Critical Care Medicine, 32*, 644–648.
373. Colreavy, F. B., Donovan, K., Lee, K. Y., et al. (2002). Transesophageal echocardiography in critically ill patients. *Critical Care Medicine, 30*, 989–996.

374. Fontes, M. L., Bellows, W., Ngo, L., et al. (1999). Assessment of ventricular function in critically ill patients: Limitations of pulmonary artery catheterization. *Journal of Cardiothoracic and Vascular Anesthesia, 13,* 521–527.
375. Jaeggi, P., Hofer, C. K., Klaghofer, R., et al. (2003). Measurement of cardiac output after cardiac surgery by a new transesophageal Doppler device. *Journal of Cardiothoracic and Vascular Anesthesia, 17,* 217–220.
376. Dark, P. M., & Singer, M. (2004). The validity of trans-esophageal Doppler ultrasonography as a measure of cardiac output in critically ill adults. *Intensive Care Medicine, 30,* 2060–2066.
377. Sharma, J., Bhise, M., Singh, A., et al. (2005). Hemodynamic measurements after cardiac surgery: Transesophageal Doppler versus pulmonary artery catheter. *Journal of Cardiothoracic and Vascular Anesthesia, 19,* 746–750.
378. Feissel, M., Michard, F., Faller, J. P., et al. (2004). The respiratory variation in inferior vena cava diameter as a guide to fluid therapy. *Intensive Care Medicine, 30,* 1834–1837.
379. Feissel, M., Michard, F., Mangin, I., et al. (2001). Respiratory changes in aortic blood velocity as an indicator of fluid responsiveness in ventilated patients with septic shock. *Chest, 119,* 867–873.
380. Peterson, G. E., Brickner, M. E., & Reimold, S. C. (2003). Transesophageal echocardiography: Clinical indications and applications. *Circulation, 107,* 2398–2402.
381. Squara, P., Denjean, D., Estagnasie, P., et al. (2007). Noninvasive cardiac output monitoring (NICOM): A clinical validation. *Intensive Care Medicine, 33,* 1191–1194.
382. Raval, N. Y., Squara, P., Cleman, M., et al. (2008). Multicenter evaluation of noninvasive cardiac output measurement by bioreactance technique. *Journal of Clinical Monitoring and Computing, 22,* 113–119.
383. Moshkovitz, Y., Kaluski, E., Milo, O., et al. (2004). Recent developments in cardiac output determination by bioimpedance: Comparison with invasive cardiac output and potential cardiovascular applications. *Current Opinion in Cardiology, 19,* 229–237.
384. Albert, N. M. (2006). Bioimpedance cardiography measurements of cardiac output and other cardiovascular parameters. *Critical Care Nursing Clinics of North America, 18,* 195–202.
385. Cotter, G., Moshkovitz, Y., Kaluski, E., et al. (2004). Accurate, noninvasive continuous monitoring of cardiac output by whole-body electrical bioimpedance. *Chest, 125,* 1431–1440.
386. Brown, C. V., Martin, M. J., Shoemaker, W. C., et al. (2005). The effect of obesity on bioimpedance cardiac index. *American Journal of Surgery, 189,* 547–550.
387. Raaijmakers, E., Faes, T. J., Scholten, R. J., et al. (1999). A meta-analysis of three decades of validating thoracic impedance cardiography. *Critical Care Medicine, 27,* 1203–1213.
388. Van De Water, J. M., Miller, T. W., Vogel, R. L., et al. (2003). Impedance cardiography: The next vital sign technology? *Chest, 123,* 2028–2033.
389. Suttner, S., Schollhorn, T., Boldt, J., et al. (2006). Noninvasive assessment of cardiac output using thoracic electrical bioimpedance in hemodynamically stable and unstable patients after cardiac surgery: A comparison with pulmonary artery thermodilution. *Intensive Care Medicine, 32,* 2053–2058.
390. Kaukinen, S., Koobi, T., Bi, Y., et al. (2003). Cardiac output measurement after coronary artery bypass grafting using bolus thermodilution, continuous thermodilution, and whole-body impedance cardiography. *Journal of Cardiothoracic and Vascular Anesthesia, 17,* 199–203.
391. Engoren, M., & Barbee, D. (2005). Comparison of cardiac output determined by bioimpedance, thermodilution, and the Fick method. *American Journal of Critical Care, 14,* 40–45.
392. de Waal, E. E., Konings, M. K., Kalkman, C. J., et al. (2008). Assessment of stroke volume index with three different bioimpedance algorithms: Lack of agreement compared to thermodilution. *Intensive Care Medicine, 34,* 735–739.
393. Stout, C. L., Van de Water, J. M., Thompson, W. M., et al. (2006). Impedance cardiography: Can it replace thermodilution and the pulmonary artery catheter? *American Surgery, 72,* 728–732.
394. Lasater, M., & Von Rueden, K. T. (2003). Outpatient cardiovascular management utilizing impedance cardiography. *AACN Clinical Issues, 14,* 240–250.
395. Albert, N. M. (2006). Bioimpedance to prevent heart failure hospitalization. *Current Heart Failure Report, 3,* 136–142.
396. Milzman, D. P., Hogan, C., Han, C., et al. (1997). Continuous, noninvasive cardiac output monitoring quantified acute congestive heart failure in the ED. *Critical Care Medicine, 25,* 17.
397. Peacock, W. I., Albert, N. M., Kies, P., et al. (2000). Bioimpedance monitoring: Better than chest x-ray for predicting abnormal pulmonary fluid? *Congestive Heart Failure, 6,* 86–89.
398. Cotter, G., Moshkovitz, Y., Kaluski, E., et al. (2003). The role of cardiac power and systemic vascular resistance in the pathophysiology and diagnosis of patients with acute congestive heart failure. *European Journal of Heart Failure, 5,* 443–451.
399. Drazner, M. H., Thompson, B., Rosenberg, P. B., et al. (2002). Comparison of impedance cardiography with invasive hemodynamic measurements in patients with heart failure secondary to ischemic or nonischemic cardiomyopathy. *American Journal of Cardiology, 89,* 993–995.
400. Samejima, H., Omiya, K., Uno, M., et al. (2003). Relationship between impaired chronotropic response, cardiac output during exercise, and exercise tolerance in patients with chronic heart failure. *Japanese Heart Journal, 44,* 515–525.
401. Weiss, S. J., Ernst, A. A., Godorov, G., et al. (2003). Bioimpedance-derived differences in cardiac physiology during exercise stress testing in low-risk chest pain patients. *Southern Medical Journal, 96,* 1121–1127.
402. Folan, L., & Funk, M. (2008). Measurement of thoracic fluid content in heart failure: The role of impedance cardiography. *AACN Advanced Critical Care, 19,* 47–55.
403. Summers, H. R., Woodward, L. H., Thompson, J. R., et al. (2008). Impedance cardiographic waveform changes in response to treatment of acute heart failure: A case study. *Congestive Heart Failure, 14,* 157–160.
404. Summers, R. L., Parrott, C. W., Quale, C., et al. (2004). Use of noninvasive hemodynamics to aid decision making in the initiation and titration of neurohormonal agents. *Congestive Heart Failure, 10,* 28–31.
405. Taler, S. J., Textor, S. C., & Augustine, J. E. (2002). Resistant hypertension: Comparing hemodynamic management to specialist care. *Hypertension, 39,* 982–988.
406. Parry, M. J., & McFetridge-Durdle, J. (2006). Ambulatory impedance cardiography: A systematic review. *Nursing Research, 55,* 283–291.
407. McFetridge-Durdle, J., Routledge, F., Parry, M., et al. (2008). Ambulatory impedance cardiography in hypertension: A validation study. *European Journal of Cardiovascular Nursing, 7,* 204–213.
408. Braun, M. U., Schnabel, A., Rauwolf, T., et al. (2005). Impedance cardiography as a noninvasive technique for atrioventricular interval optimization in cardiac resynchronization therapy. *Journal of Interventional Cardiac Electrophysiology, 13,* 223–229.
409. Heinroth, K. M., Elster, M., Nuding, S., et al. (2007). Impedance cardiography: A useful and reliable tool in optimization of cardiac resynchronization devices. *Europace, 9,* 744–750.
410. Belott, P. (1999). Bioimpedance in the pacemaker clinic. *AACN Clinical Issues, 10,* 414–418.
411. Shoemaker, W. C., Wo, C. C., Yu, S., et al. (2000). Invasive and noninvasive haemodynamic monitoring of acutely ill sepsis and septic shock patients in the emergency department. *European Journal of Emergency Medicine, 7,* 169–175.
412. Shoemaker, W. C., Wo, C. C., Chan, L., et al. (2001). Outcome prediction of emergency patients by noninvasive hemodynamic monitoring. *Chest, 120,* 528–537.
413. Shoemaker, W. C., Wo, C. C., Chien, L. C., et al. (2006). Evaluation of invasive and noninvasive hemodynamic monitoring in trauma patients. *Journal of Trauma, 61,* 844–853.
414. Shoemaker, W. C., Wo, C. C., Lu, K., et al. (2006). Noninvasive hemodynamic monitoring for combat casualties. *Military Medicine, 171,* 813–820.
415. Shoemaker, W. C., Wo, C. C., Lu, K., et al. (2006). Outcome prediction by a mathematical model based on noninvasive hemodynamic monitoring. *Journal of Trauma, 60,* 82–90.
416. Adams, K. F., Jr., Fonarow, G. C., Emerman, C. L., et al. (2005). Characteristics and outcomes of patients hospitalized for heart failure in the United States: Rationale, design, and preliminary observations from the first 100,000 cases in the Acute Decompensated Heart Failure National Registry (ADHERE). *American Heart Journal, 149,* 209–216.
417. Nieminen, M. S., Brutsaert, D., Dickstein, K., et al. (2006). EuroHeart Failure Survey II (EHFS II): A survey on hospitalized acute heart failure patients: Description of population. *European Heart Journal, 27,* 2725–2736.
418. Cotter, G., Felker, G. M., Adams, K. F., et al. (2008). The pathophysiology of acute heart failure—Is it all about fluid accumulation? *American Heart Journal, 155,* 9–18.
419. Yu, C. M., Wang, L., Chau, E., et al. (2005). Intrathoracic impedance monitoring in patients with heart failure: Correlation with fluid status and feasibility of early warning preceding hospitalization. *Circulation, 112,* 841–848.

420. Piccini, J. P., & Hranitzky, P. (2007). Diagnostic monitoring strategies in heart failure management. *American Heart Journal, 153*, 12–17.
421. Abraham, W. T., Foreman, B., Fishel, R., et al. (2005). Fluid Accumulation Status Trial (FAST). *Heart Rhythm, 2*, S65–S66.
422. Ypenburg, C., Bax, J. J., van der Wall, E. E., et al. (2007). Intrathoracic impedance monitoring to predict decompensated heart failure. *American Journal of Cardiology, 99*, 554–557.
423. Wadas, T. M. (2005). The implantable hemodynamic monitoring system. *Critical Care Nurse, 25*, 14–16, 18–20, 22–24.
424. Bourge, R. C., Abraham, W. T., Adamson, P. B., et al. (2008). Randomized controlled trial of an implantable continuous hemodynamic monitor in patients with advanced heart failure: The COMPASS-HF study. *Journal of the American College of Cardiology, 51*, 1073–1079.
425. Ritzema, J., Melton I. C., Richards, A. M., et al. (2007). Direct left atrial pressure monitoring in ambulatory heart failure patients: Initial experience with a new permanent implantable device. *Circulation, 116*, 2952–2959.
426. Walton, A. S., & Krum, H. (2005). The Heartpod implantable heart failure therapy system. *Heart, Lung & Circulation, 14*(Suppl. 2), S31–S33.
427. Teerlink, J. R. (2008). Learning the points of COMPASS-HF: Assessing implantable hemodynamic monitoring in heart failure patients. *Journal of the American College of Cardiology, 51*, 1080–1082.
428. Rady, M. Y., Rivers, E. P., & Nowak, R. M. (1996). Resuscitation of the critically ill in the ED: Responses of blood pressure, heart rate, shock index, central venous oxygen saturation, and lactate. *American Journal of Emergency Medicine, 14*, 218–225.
429. Ander, D. S., Jaggi, M., Rivers, E., et al. (1998). Undetected cardiogenic shock in patients with congestive heart failure presenting to the emergency department. *American Journal of Cardiology, 82*, 888–891.
430. Wo, C. C., Shoemaker, W. C., Appel, P. L., et al. (1993). Unreliability of blood pressure and heart rate to evaluate cardiac output in emergency resuscitation and critical illness. *Critical Care Medicine, 21*, 218–223.
431. Bauer, P., Reinhart, K., & Bauer, M. (2008). Significance of venous oximetry in the critically ill. *Medicina Intensiva / Sociedad Española de Medicina Intensiva y Unidades Coronarias, 32*, 134–142.
432. Gawlinski, A. (1998). Can measurement of mixed venous oxygen saturation replace measurement of cardiac output in patients with advanced heart failure? *American Journal of Critical Care, 7*, 374–380.
433. Vincent, J. L., & De Backer, D. (2004). Oxygen transport–the oxygen delivery controversy. *Intensive Care Medicine, 30*, 1990–1996.
434. Yalavatti, G. S., De Backer, D., & Vincent, J. L. (2000). Assessment of cardiac index in anemic patients. *Chest, 118*, 782–787.
435. Atkins, P., Hapshe, E., & Riegel, B. (1994). Effects of bedbath on mixed venous oxygen saturation and heart rate in coronary artery bypass graft patients. *American Journal of Critical Care, 3*, 107–115.
436. Horiuchi, K., Jordan, D., Cohen, D., et al. (1997). Insights into the increased oxygen demand during chest physiotherapy. *Critical Care Medicine, 25*, 1347–1351.
437. Banasik, J. L., & Emerson, R. J. (2001). Effect of lateral positions on tissue oxygenation in the critically ill. *Heart & Lung, 30*, 269–276.
438. Reed, S., Jesurum-Urbaitis, J., Kumpula, J., et al. (2003). The effect of lateral positioning on tissue oxygenation in cardiovascular surgical patients with anemia. *American Journal of Critical Care, 12*, 279–280.
439. Hébert, P. C. (1998). Transfusion requirements in critical care (TRICC): A multicentre, randomized, controlled clinical study. Transfusion Requirements in Critical Care Investigators and the Canadian Critical Care Trials Group. *British Journal of Anaesthesiology, 81*(Suppl. 1), 25–33.
440. Rivers, E. P., Ander, D. S., & Powell, D. (2001). Central venous oxygen saturation monitoring in the critically ill patient. *Current Opinion in Critical Care, 7*, 204–211.
441. Molnar, Z., Umgelter, A., Toth, I., et al. (2007). Continuous monitoring of ScvO(2) by a new fibre-optic technology compared with blood gas oximetry in critically ill patients: A multicentre study. *Intensive Care Medicine, 33*, 1767–1770.
442. Dueck, M. H., Klimek, M., Appenrodt, S., et al. (2005). Trends but not individual values of central venous oxygen saturation agree with mixed venous oxygen saturation during varying hemodynamic conditions. *Anesthesiology, 103*, 249–257.
443. Reinhart, K., Kuhn, H. J., Hartog, C., et al. (2004). Continuous central venous and pulmonary artery oxygen saturation monitoring in the critically ill. *Intensive Care Medicine, 30*, 1572–1578.
444. Edwards, J. D., & Mayall, R. M. (1998). Importance of the sampling site for measurement of mixed venous oxygen saturation in shock. *Critical Care Medicine, 26*, 1356–1360.
445. Turnaoglu, S., Tugrul, M., Camci, E., et al. (2001). Clinical applicability of the substitution of mixed venous oxygen saturation with central venous oxygen saturation. *Journal of Cardiothoracic and Vascular Anesthesia, 15*, 574–579.
446. Chawla, L. S., Zia, H., Gutierrez, G., et al. (2004). Lack of equivalence between central and mixed venous oxygen saturation. *Chest, 126*, 1891–1896.
447. Varpula, M., Karlsson, S., Ruokonen, E., et al. (2006). Mixed venous oxygen saturation cannot be estimated by central venous oxygen saturation in septic shock. *Intensive Care Medicine, 32*, 1336–1343.
448. Yazigi, A., El Khoury, C., Jebara, S., et al. (2008). Comparison of central venous to mixed venous oxygen saturation in patients with low cardiac index and filling pressures after coronary artery surgery. *Journal of Cardiothoracic and Vascular Anesthesia, 22*, 77–83.
449. Sander, M., Spies, C. D., Foer, A., et al. (2007). Agreement of central venous saturation and mixed venous saturation in cardiac surgery patients. *Intensive Care Medicine, 33*, 1719–1725.
450. Rivers, E. (2006). Mixed vs central venous oxygen saturation may be not numerically equal, but both are still clinically useful. *Chest, 129*, 507–508.
451. Rady, M. Y. (1992). The role of central venous oximetry, lactic acid concentration and shock index in the evaluation of clinical shock: A review. *Resuscitation, 24*, 55–60.
452. Bracht, H., Hanggi, M., Jeker, B., et al. (2007). Incidence of low central venous oxygen saturation during unplanned admissions in a multidisciplinary intensive care unit: An observational study. *Critical Care, 11*, R2–R9.
453. Collaborative Study Group on Perioperative $ScvO_2$ Monitoring. (2006). Multicentre study on peri- and postoperative central venous oxygen saturation in high-risk surgical patients. *Critical Care, 10*, R158–R165.
454. Pearse, R., Dawson, D., Fawcett, J., et al. (2005). Changes in central venous saturation after major surgery, and association with outcome. *Critical Care, 9*, R694–R699.
455. de Oliveira, C. F., de Oliveira, D. S., Gottschald, A. F., et al. (2008). ACCM/PALS haemodynamic support guidelines for paediatric septic shock: An outcomes comparison with and without monitoring central venous oxygen saturation. *Intensive Care Medicine, 34*, 1065–1075.
456. Varpula, M., Karlsson, S., Ruokonen, E., et al. (2007). Mixed venous oxygen saturation cannot be estimated by central venous oxygen saturation in septic shock. *Intensive Care Medicine, 33*, 545; author reply 546.
457. Bakker, J., & Jansen, T. C. (2007). Don't take vitals, take a lactate. *Intensive Care Medicine, 33*, 1863–1865.
458. Howell, M. D., Donnino, M., Clardy, P., et al. (2007). Occult hypoperfusion and mortality in patients with suspected infection. *Intensive Care Medicine, 33*, 1892–1899.
459. Singhal, R., Coghill, J. E., Guy, A., et al. (2005). Serum lactate and base deficit as predictors of mortality after ruptured abdominal aortic aneurysm repair. *European Journal of Vascular and Endovascular Surgery, 30*, 263–266.
460. Maillet, J. M., Le Besnerais, P., Cantoni, M., et al. (2003). Frequency, risk factors, and outcome of hyperlactatemia after cardiac surgery. *Chest, 123*, 1361–1366.
461. Ranucci, M., De Toffol, B., Isgro, G., et al. (2006). Hyperlactatemia during cardiopulmonary bypass: Determinants and impact on postoperative outcome. *Critical Care, 10*, R167–R175.
462. Levy, B. (2006). Lactate and shock state: The metabolic view. *Current Opinion in Critical Care, 12*, 315–321.
463. Levy, B., Gibot, S., Franck, P., et al. (2005). Relation between muscle Na^+K^+ ATPase activity and raised lactate concentrations in septic shock: A prospective study. *Lancet, 365*, 871–875.
464. Suistomaa, M., Ruokonen, E., Kari, A., et al. (2000). Time-pattern of lactate and lactate to pyruvate ratio in the first 24 hours of intensive care emergency admissions. *Shock, 14*, 8–12.
465. Nguyen, H. B., Rivers, E. P., Knoblich, B. P., et al. (2004). Early lactate clearance is associated with improved outcome in severe sepsis and septic shock. *Critical Care Medicine, 32*, 1637–1642.
466. Kern, J. W., & Shoemaker, W. C. (2002). Meta-analysis of hemodynamic optimization in high-risk patients. *Critical Care Medicine, 30*, 1686–1692.
467. Poeze, M., Greve, J. W., & Ramsay, G. (2005). Meta-analysis of hemodynamic optimization: Relationship to methodological quality. *Critical Care, 9*, R771–R779.
468. Shapiro, N. I., Howell, M. D., Talmor, D., et al. (2006). Implementation and outcomes of the Multiple Urgent Sepsis Therapies (MUST) protocol. *Critical Care Medicine, 34*, 1025–1032.
469. Nguyen, H. B., Corbett, S. W., Steele, R., et al. (2007). Implementation of a bundle of quality indicators for the early management of severe sepsis and septic shock is associated with decreased mortality. *Critical Care Medicine, 35*, 1105–1112.
470. Rivers, E. P., Coba, V., & Whitmill, M. (2008). Early goal–directed therapy in severe sepsis and septic shock: A contemporary review of the literature. *Current Opinion in Anaesthesiology, 21*, 128–140.

471. Sebat, F., Johnson, D., Musthafa, A. A., et al. (2005). A multidisciplinary community hospital program for early and rapid resuscitation of shock in nontrauma patients. *Chest, 127*, 1729–1743.
472. Sebat, F., Musthafa, A. A., Johnson, D., et al. (2007). Effect of a rapid response system for patients in shock on time to treatment and mortality during 5 years. *Critical Care Medicine, 35*, 2568–2575.
473. Kortgen, A., Niederprum, P., & Bauer, M. (2006). Implementation of an evidence-based "standard operating procedure" and outcome in septic shock. *Critical Care Medicine, 34*, 943–949.
474. Otero, R. M., Nguyen, H. B., Huang, D. T., et al. (2006). Early goal-directed therapy in severe sepsis and septic shock revisited: Concepts, controversies, and contemporary findings. *Chest, 130*, 1579–1595.
475. Heringlake, M., Heinze, H., Misfeld, M., et al. (2008). Goal-directed hemodynamic optimization in high-risk cardiac surgery patients: A tale from the past or a future obligation? *Minerva Anestesiologica, 74*, 251–258.
476. Polonen, P., Ruokonen, E., Hippelainen, M., et al. (2000). A prospective, randomized study of goal-oriented hemodynamic therapy in cardiac surgical patients. *Anesthesia & Analgesia, 90*, 1052–1059.
477. Uchino, S., Bellomo, R., Morimatsu, H., et al. (2006). Pulmonary artery catheter versus pulse contour analysis: A prospective epidemiological study. *Critical Care, 10*, R174–R183.
478. Murugan, R., Venkataraman, R., Madden, N., et al. (2008). *Preload responsiveness is associated with increased IL-6 and lower organ yield from cadaveric donors, 2008*. Retrieved October 10, 2008, from http://www.lidco.com/archives/abstract-IL-6.pdf.
479. Pinsky, M. R., & Payen, D. (2005). Functional hemodynamic monitoring. *Critical Care, 9*, 566–572.
480. Vallet, B., Tygat, H., & Lebuffe, G. (2007). How to titrate vasopressors against fluid loading in sepsis. *Advances in Sepsis, 6*, 34–40.
481. Lopes, M. R., Oliveira, M. A., Pereira, V. O., et al. (2007). Goal-directed fluid management based on pulse pressure variation monitoring during high-risk surgery: A pilot randomized controlled trial. *Critical Care, 11*, R100–R108.
482. Malhotra, K., Kakani, M., Chowdhury, U., et al. (2008). Early goal-directed therapy in moderate to high-risk cardiac surgery patients. *Annals of Cardiac Anaesthesia, 11*, 27–34.
483. McKinley, B. A., Marvin, R. G., Cocanour, C. S., et al. (2000). Tissue hemoglobin O_2 saturation during resuscitation of traumatic shock monitored using near infrared spectrometry. *Journal of Trauma, 48*, 637–642.
484. Putnam, B., Bricker, S., Fedorka, P., et al. (2007). The correlation of near-infrared spectroscopy with changes in oxygen delivery in a controlled model of altered perfusion. *American Surgery, 73*, 1017–1022.
485. Podbregar, M., & Mozina, H. (2007). Skeletal muscle oxygen saturation does not estimate mixed venous oxygen saturation in patients with severe left heart failure and additional severe sepsis or septic shock. *Critical Care, 11*, R6–R13.
486. Puyana, J. C., & Pinsky, M. R. (2007). Searching for non-invasive markers of tissue hypoxia. *Critical Care, 11*, 116–117.
487. Ikossi, D. G., Knudson, M. M., Morabito, D. J., et al. (2006). Continuous muscle tissue oxygenation in critically injured patients: A prospective observational study. *Journal of Trauma, 61*, 780–788.
488. Crookes, B. A., Cohn, S. M., Bloch, S., et al. (2005). Can near-infrared spectroscopy identify the severity of shock in trauma patients? *Journal of Trauma, 58*, 806–813.
489. Soller, B. R., Ryan, K. L., Rickards, C. A., et al. (2008). Oxygen saturation determined from deep muscle, not thenar tissue, is an early indicator of central hypovolemia in humans. *Critical Care Medicine, 36*, 176–182.
490. Cohn, S. M., Nathens, A. B., Moore, F. A., et al. (2007). Tissue oxygen saturation predicts the development of organ dysfunction during traumatic shock resuscitation. *Journal of Trauma, 62*, 44–54.
491. Moore, F. A., Nelson, T., McKinley, B. A., et al. (2008). Massive transfusion in trauma patients: Tissue hemoglobin oxygen saturation predicts poor outcome. *Journal of Trauma, 64*, 1010–1023.
492. Creteur, J. (2008). Muscle StO_2 in critically ill patients. *Current Opinion in Critical Care, 14*, 361–366.
493. Skarda, D. E., Mulier, K. E., Myers, D. E., et al. (2007). Dynamic near-infrared spectroscopy measurements in patients with severe sepsis. *Shock, 27*, 348–353.
494. De Blasi, R. A., Palmisani, S., Alampi, D., et al. (2005). Microvascular dysfunction and skeletal muscle oxygenation assessed by phase-modulation near-infrared spectroscopy in patients with septic shock. *Intensive Care Medicine, 31*, 1661–1668.
495. Pareznik, R., Knezevic, R., Voga, G., et al. (2006). Changes in muscle tissue oxygenation during stagnant ischemia in septic patients. *Intensive Care Medicine, 32*, 87–92.
496. Creteur, J., Carollo, T., Soldati, G., et al. (2007). The prognostic value of muscle StO_2 in septic patients. *Intensive Care Medicine, 33*, 1549–1556.
497. Doerschug, K. C., Delsing, A. S., Schmidt, G. A., et al. (2007). Impairments in microvascular reactivity are related to organ failure in human sepsis. *American Journal of Physiology. Heart and Circulatory Physiology, 293*, H1065–H1071.
498. Nishiguchi, B. K., Yu, M., Suetsugu, A., et al. (2008). Determination of reference ranges for transcutaneous oxygen and carbon dioxide tension and the oxygen challenge test in healthy and morbidly obese subjects. *Journal of Surgical Research, 150*, 204–211.
499. Yu, M., Chapital, A., Ho, H. C., et al. (2007). A prospective randomized trial comparing oxygen delivery versus transcutaneous pressure of oxygen values as resuscitative goals. *Shock, 27*, 615–622.
500. Yu, M., Morita, S. Y., Daniel, S. R., et al. (2006). Transcutaneous pressure of oxygen: A noninvasive and early detector of peripheral shock and outcome. *Shock, 26*, 450–456.
501. Dantzker, D. R. (1993). The gastrointestinal tract. The canary of the body? *JAMA, 270*, 1247–1248.
502. Creteur, J., De Backer, D., Sakr, Y., et al. (2006). Sublingual capnometry tracks microcirculatory changes in septic patients. *Intensive Care Medicine, 32*, 516–523
503. Marik, P. E., & Bankov, A. (2003). Sublingual capnometry versus traditional markers of tissue oxygenation in critically ill patients. *Critical Care Medicine, 31*, 818–822.
504. Sakr, Y., Dubois, M. J., De Backer, D., et al. (2004). Persistent microcirculatory alterations are associated with organ failure and death in patients with septic shock. *Critical Care Medicine, 32*, 1825–1831.
505. Marik, P. E. (2006). Sublingual capnometry: A non-invasive measure of microcirculatory dysfunction and tissue hypoxia. *Physiological Measurement, 27*, R37–R47.
506. Creteur, J. (2006). Gastric and sublingual capnometry. *Current Opinion in Critical Care, 12*, 272–277.
507. Weil, M. H., Nakagawa, Y., Tang, W., et al. (1999). Sublingual capnometry: A new noninvasive measurement for diagnosis and quantitation of severity of circulatory shock. *Critical Care Medicine, 27*, 1225–1229.
508. Povoas, H. P., Weil, M. H., Tang, W., et al. (2001). Decreases in mesenteric blood flow associated with increases in sublingual PCO2 during hemorrhagic shock. *Shock, 15*, 398–402.
509. Pellis, T., Weil, M. H., Tang, W., et al. (2005). Increases in both buccal and sublingual partial pressure of carbon dioxide reflect decreases of tissue blood flows in a porcine model during hemorrhagic shock. *Journal of Trauma, 58*, 817–824.
510. Cammarata, G. A., Weil, M. H., Castillo, C. J., et al. (2009). Buccal capnometry for quantitating the severity of hemorrhagic shock. *Shock, 31*, 207–211.
511. Trzeciak, S., McCoy, J. V., Dellinger, R. P., et al. (2008). Early increases in microcirculatory perfusion during protocol-directed resuscitation are associated with reduced multi-organ failure at 24 h in patients with sepsis. *Intensive Care Medicine, 34*, 2210–2217.
512. De Backer, D., Creteur, J., Dubois, M. J., et al. (2004). Microvascular alterations in patients with acute severe heart failure and cardiogenic shock. *American Heart Journal, 147*, 91–99.
513. De Backer, D., Creteur, J., Preiser, J. C., et al. (2002). Microvascular blood flow is altered in patients with sepsis. *American Journal of Respiratory Critical Care Medicine, 166*, 98–104.
514. Elbers, P. W., & Ince, C. (2006). Mechanisms of critical illness–classifying microcirculatory flow abnormalities in distributive shock. *Critical Care, 10*, 221–228.
515. Trzeciak, S., Dellinger, R. P., Parrillo, J. E., et al. (2007). Early microcirculatory perfusion derangements in patients with severe sepsis and septic shock: Relationship to hemodynamics, oxygen transport, and survival. *Annals of Emergency Medicine, 49* , 88–98.e2.
516. Fang, X., Tang, W., Sun, S., et al. (2006). Comparison of buccal microcirculation between septic and hemorrhagic shock. *Critical Care Medicine, 34*, S447–S453.
517. De Backer, D., Creteur, J., Dubois, M. J., et al. (2006). The effects of dobutamine on microcirculatory alterations in patients with septic shock are independent of its systemic effects. *Critical Care Medicine, 34*, 403–408.
518. De Backer, D., Verdant, C., Chierego, M., et al. (2006). Effects of drotrecogin alfa activated on microcirculatory alterations in patients with severe sepsis. *Critical Care Medicine, 34*, 1918–1924.

PART

IV Pathophysiology and Management of Heart Disease

CHAPTER

22 Acute Coronary Syndromes

Jean Marie Blue Verrier / Michaelene Hargrove Deelstra

In 2005, there were an estimated 16 million people in the United States with coronary heart disease (CHD), translating to approximately 1 in every 15 Americans. Of these cases, 1.2 million were new or recurrent CHD. There were 451,300 CHD-related deaths in 2004.[1]

Acute coronary syndromes (ACS) have evolved over the last 10 years into an operational term referring to a constellation of clinical symptoms that equate to myocardial ischemia. Ischemic heart disease is one type of CHD. ACS encompasses ST-elevation myocardial infarction (STEMI), non-ST-elevation myocardial infarction (NSTEMI), and unstable angina (UA). Identification of ACS at the earliest point in the health care continuum allows paramedics to initiate immediate cardiac medications and route patients to the most appropriate facilities for care. The shortest time to reperfusion is the most desirable goal of treatment and management of the patient population with ACS.[2,3]

UA/NSTEMI constitutes a clinical syndrome that is a subset of ACS. UA/NSTEMI is usually, but not always, caused by atherosclerotic coronary artery disease (CAD, a type of CHD) and is associated with an increased risk of cardiac mortality.[4] CAD is also associated with an increased incidence of myocardial infarction (MI). As a subset of ACS, UA/NSTEMI is defined by electrocardiographic ST-segment depression or prominent T-wave inversion. Biomarkers of myocardial necrosis, such as troponin, may or may not be present. No ST-segment elevation is present on electrocardiogram (ECG). The patient typically has chest discomfort or an anginal equivalent.[4]

Variant (Prinzmetal's) angina is an unusual form of UA that occurs spontaneously and frequently is not related to exertion. The chest discomfort tends to be prolonged and severe. It is caused by spasm of the epicardial coronary artery/arteries and classically is characterized by transient ST-segment elevation that resolves with nitroglycerin (NTG) use.

Patients presenting with STEMI have a high likelihood of coronary thrombus causing a complete occlusion of the artery. Angiographic evidence of coronary thrombus formation is seen in more than 90% of patients with STEMI but in only 35% to 75% of patients presenting with UA/NSTEMI. There is ST-segment elevation evident on ECG. Biomarkers of myocardial necrosis such as troponin are typically elevated. The patient generally has chest discomfort or an anginal equivalent.[2]

In the last several years, there has been an unprecedented focus on quantifying and improving health care delivery. The American College of Cardiology (ACC) and the American Heart Association (AHA) jointly have developed a long-term strategy to improve clinical care. The initial phase created practice guidelines that synthesized available evidence to guide care. The second phase developed performance measures to assess and improve the quality of cardiovascular care. Table 22-1 presents the ACC/AHA STEMI/NSTEMI performance measurement set developed in January 2006.[5] The measures include aspirin therapy at arrival and at discharge; β-blocker therapy at arrival and at discharge; low-density lipoprotein cholesterol (LDL-C) assessment; lipid-lowering therapy at discharge; angiotensin-converting enzyme inhibitor (ACEI) and/or angiotensin II receptor blocker (ARB) therapy for left ventricular (LV) systolic dysfunction; time-to-fibrinolytic therapy; time-to-percutaneous coronary intervention (PCI); reperfusion therapy; and adult smoking cessation advice/counseling.[5] Pathogenesis of ACS is presented in Chapter 5. PCI is presented in Chapter 23. ACS risk factors are presented in Chapter 32. For a complete presentation of the care of patients with STEMI and UA/NSTEMI, refer to the original sources for the ACC/AHA STEMI[2,3] and NSTEMI Guidelines,[4] which simply are abstracted here for purposes of this chapter.

PRESENTATION OF ACS

Morbidity and mortality from ACS can be reduced significantly if symptoms are recognized early. The symptoms of UA/NSTEMI and STEMI include midsternal or substernal compression or crushing chest discomfort. The patient may describe it as a cramping, burning, or an aching sensation in the midsternal area. The discomfort may also be described as pressure, tightness, or heaviness in the chest. Unexplained indigestion or belching with or without epigastric pain is also a common subjective complaint. The pain may radiate to the neck, jaw, shoulders, back, or one or both arms. Commonly there is associated dyspnea, nausea and/or vomiting, and diaphoresis. Women more often than men present with atypical chest pain. Patients with diabetes also may present atypically due to diabetes-associated autonomic dysfunction.

Table 22-1 ■ ACC/AHA STEMI/NSTEMI PERFORMANCE MEASUREMENT SET: DIMENSIONS OF CARE INPATIENT MEASURES MATRIX

Performance Measure	Diagnostics	Patient Education	Treatment	Self-Management	Monitoring of Disease Status*
1. Aspirin at arrival			✔		
2. Aspirin prescribed at discharge			✔		
3. β-Blocker at arrival			✔		
4. β-Blocker prescribed at discharge			✔		
5. LDL-C assessment	✔				
6. Lipid-lowering therapy at discharge			✔		
7. ACEI or ARB for LVSD			✔		
8. Time to fibrinolytic therapy			✔		
9. Time to PCI			✔		
10. Reperfusion therapy			✔		
11. Adult smoking cessation advice/counseling		✔			

*Although no current measures exist for these dimensions of care for the inpatient setting, future measure development efforts will examine how to address this gap in the measurement set.

LVSD, left ventricular systolic dysfunction.

Anderson, J.L., Bennett, S.J., Brooks, N.H., et al. (2006). ACC/AHA clinical performance measures for adults with ST-elevation and non-ST-elevation myocardial infarction: A report of the American College of Cardiology/American Heart Association task force on performance measures. *JACC, 47,* 236–65.

Older adults can present with stroke, syncope, a change in mental status, and/or generalized weakness.

There are three common principal presentations of UA.[4] Resting angina pectoris, as the name implies, occurs during a period of nonexertion. Exertion in this setting can be physical exertion with routine activities, exercise, emotional exertion, and/or stress. The emotional exertion or stress can be related to any strong emotional reaction, such as excitation over a ball game or an event that provokes excitation, anxiety, or anger. The second principal presentation of UA is classified as new-onset angina that has its onset in less than 2 months. The third presentation is crescendo or increasing angina.[6] The increase can reflect intensity, duration, and/or frequency of anginal symptoms. Compared with UA, NSTEMI generally presents as prolonged, more intense resting angina or an anginal equivalent, such as shortness of breath, or jaw or arm pain.

Variant angina usually does not progress to MI. Uncommonly, prolonged vasospasm can result in MI, atrioventricular block, ventricular tachycardia, or sudden death.[4] Attacks can be precipitated by emotional stress, hyperventilation, exercise, or exposure to cold. The anginal attacks tend to occur more in the morning. Patients with variant angina tend to be younger with fewer coronary risk factors. This type of angina is usually responsive to NTG, long-acting nitrates, and calcium antagonists, all of which are first-line therapies.[4] Smokers should stop smoking. Prognosis with medical therapy is usually good, particularly in the presence of a normal coronary angiogram. If CAD is present on angiogram, then the prognosis is not as good.

Refer to Chapter 10 for a complete discussion of the cardiovascular history and physical examination, and to Chapters 11 and 15 for details of cardiac biomarker and 12-lead ECG interpretation, respectively.

INITIAL EVALUATION AND MANAGEMENT OF PATIENTS WITH ACS

The ACC/AHA 2007 recommendations for initial evaluation and management follow.[4] Table 22-2 illustrates the classification and certainty of treatment effect for these recommendations.

1. Patients with symptoms suggestive of ACS should be instructed to call 911 and should be transported to the emergency department by ambulance rather than by private transport. (Class I, level of evidence: B)
2. The prehospital emergency medical providers should administer at this time aspirin 162 to 325 mg to the patient suspected of ACS unless contraindicated or if already taken by the patient. More rapid buccal absorption occurs with nonenteric-coated formulations and is recommended. (Class I, level of evidence: C)
3. Health care providers performing initial assessment of a patient suspected of ACS that has had NTG prescribed should instruct the patient not to take more than one dose of NTG sublingually in response to chest discomfort. If chest discomfort is unimproved or is worsening 5 minutes after dosing, it is recommended that the patient or family member call 911 immediately to access emergency medical services (EMS). In patients with chronic stable angina whose symptoms have improved after one NTG, it is appropriate to instruct the patient to repeat NTG every 5 minutes for a maximum of three doses. If symptoms do not resolve completely after three doses, 911 should be called for evaluation and treatment of symptoms. (Class I, level of evidence: C)
4. Patients with suspected ACS who have chest discomfort or other ischemic symptoms at rest for greater than 20 minutes, hemodynamic instability, or recent presyncope/syncope should be referred immediately to an emergency department for further evaluation. Patients experiencing less severe symptoms and who have none of the high-risk features described in the next section can be seen initially in an outpatient facility able to provide an acute evaluation. This recommendation would include patients who responded to an NTG dose. (Class I, level of evidence: C)
5. If the EMS providers have the capability, a 12-lead ECG should be performed in the field and transmitted to an emergency physician. The ECG assists in triage decisions, allowing transport to the most appropriate emergency department. ECGs with validated computer-generated interpretation are recommended in this setting. (Class IIa, level of evidence: B)

Table 22-2 ■ APPLYING CLASSIFICATION OF RECOMMENDATIONS AND LEVEL OF EVIDENCE

Size of Treatment Effect →

ESTIMATE OF CERTAINTY (PRECISION) OF TREATMENT EFFECT

	Class I *Benefit >>> Risk*	**Class IIa** *Benefit >> Risk* *Additional studies with focused objectives needed*	**Class IIb** *Benefit ≥ Risk* *Additional studies with broad objectives needed; Additional registry data would be helpful*	**Class III** *Risk ≥ Benefit* *No additional studies needed*
	Procedure/Treatment SHOULD be performed/ administered	IT IS REASONABLE to perform procedure/ administer treatment	Procedure/Treatment MAY BE CONSIDERED	Procedure/Treatment should NOT be performed/ administered SINCE IT IS NOT HELPFUL, AND IT MAY BE HARMFUL
Level A *Multiple (3–5) population risk strata evaluated** *General consistency of direction and magnitude of effect*	• Recommendation that procedure or treatment is useful/effective • Sufficient evidence from multiple randomized trials or meta-analyses	• Recommendation in favor of treatment or procedure being useful/effective • Some conflicting evidence from multiple randomized trials or meta-analyses	• Recommendation's usefulness/efficacy less well established • Greater conflicting evidence from multiple randomized trials or meta-analyses	• Recommendation that procedure or treatment is not useful/effective and may be harmful • Sufficient evidence from multiple randomized trials or meta-analyses
Level B *Limited (2–3) population risk strata evaluated**	• Recommendation that procedure or treatment is useful/effective • Limited evidence from single randomized trials or non-randomized studies	• Recommendation in favor of treatment or procedure being useful/effective • Some conflicting evidence from single randomized trial or non-randomized studies	• Recommendation's usefulness/efficacy less well established • Greater conflicting evidence from single randomized trial or non-randomized studies	• Recommendation that procedure or treatment is not useful/effective and may be harmful • Limited evidence from single randomized trial or non-randomized studies
Level C *Very limited (1–2) population risk strata evaluated**	• Recommendation that procedure or treatment is useful/effective • Only expert opinion, case studies, or standard-of-care	• Recommendation in favor of treatment or procedure being useful/effective • Only diverging expert opinion, case studies, or standard-of-care	• Recommendation's usefulness/efficacy less well established • Only diverging expert opinion, case studies, or standard-of-care	• Recommendation that procedure or treatment is not useful/effective and may be harmful • Only expert opinion, case studies, or standard-of-care
Suggested phrases for writing recommendations†	Should Is recommended Is indicated Is useful/effective/beneficial	Is reasonable Can be useful/effective/ beneficial Is probably recommended or indicated	May/might be considered May/might be reasonable Usefulness/effectiveness is unknown/unclear/uncertain or not well established	Is not recommended Is not indicated Should not Is not useful/effective/ beneficial May be harmful

†In 2003, the ACC/AHA Task Force on Practice Guidelines developed a list of suggested phrases to use when writing recommendations. All guideline recommendations have been written in full sentences that express a complete thought, such that a recommendation, even if separated and presented apart from the rest of the document (including headings above sets of recommendations), would still convey the full intent of the recommendation. It is hoped that this will increase readers' comprehension of the guidelines and will allow queries at the individual recommendation level.

*Data available from clinical trials or registries about the usefulness/efficacy in different subpopulations, such as gender, age, history of diabetes, history of prior myocardial infarction, history of heart failure, and prior aspirin use. A recommendation with Level of Evidence B or C does not imply that the recommendation is weak. Many important clinical questions addressed in the guidelines do not lend themselves to clinical trials. Even though randomized trials are not available, there may be very clear clinical consensus that a particular test or therapy is useful or effective.

Anderson, L. J, Bennett, S. J., Brooks, N. H., et al. (2006). ACC/AHA clinical performance measures for adults with ST-elevation and non-ST-elevation myocardial infarction: A report of the American College of Cardiology/American Heart Association task force on performance measures. *JACC, 47,* 236–65.

Early Risk Stratification

An estimation of risk is useful in selection of the initial medical and interventional therapies. Generally, risk is highest at the time of presentation and declines subsequently but remains elevated even beyond the acute phase. In patients with symptoms suggestive of ACS, the initial medical history, physical examination, ECG, and assessment of renal function and cardiac biomarker can be integrated into an estimation of the risk of mortality or a nonfatal cardiac event.

The five most important factors on the initial history are the nature of the anginal symptoms, a prior history of CAD, sex, age, and the number of risk factors present. In patients without preexisting clinical CHD, older age is the most important factor.[4]

A history of MI increases the risk of obstructive and multivessel CAD. Traditional risk factors are only weakly predictive of the likelihood of acute ischemia, and they are less important than symptoms, ECG findings, and cardiac biomarkers.[7] Diabetes mellitus and extracardiac disease are major risk factors for poor outcomes in patients with ACS.[4] The ECG is central to the diagnostic and triage pathway for ACS. Figure 22-1 illustrates practice guidelines recommended for ACS and demonstrates the pivotal role the 12-lead ECG plays in treatment course selection. Transient ST-segment changes greater than or equal to 0.05 mV or 0.5 mm that develop during the time the patient is symptomatic at rest is strongly suggestive of myocardial ischemia due to severe CAD.

Patients who present with ST-segment depression could have either UA or NSTEMI. The distinction is made by the later detection of biomarkers of myocardial necrosis. Inverted T waves, particularly if greater than or equal to 2 mm, can also be indicative of UA/NSTEMI. Q waves are suggestive of prior MI and indicate high likelihood of CAD. A normal ECG does not completely exclude ACS; 1% to 6% of patients with documented NSTEMI and 4% of patients with documented UA will have a normal ECG. Serial ECGs increase diagnostic sensitivity and are recommended because ST-segment elevation on the 12-lead ECG

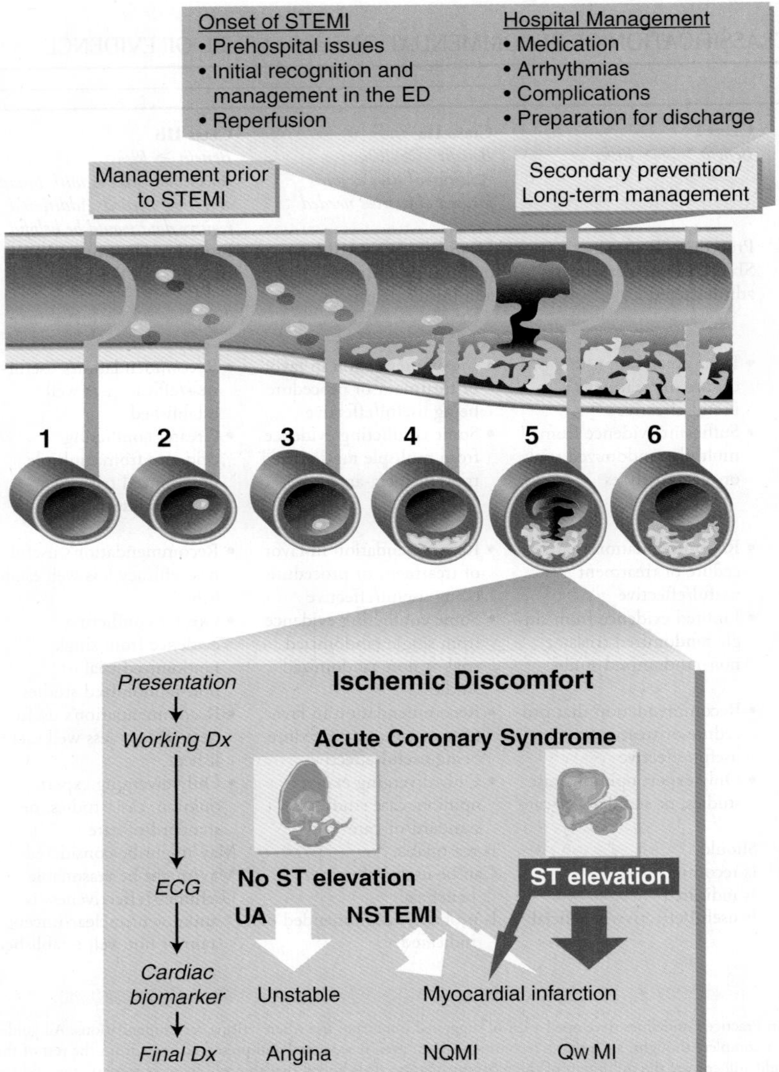

■ **Figure 22-1** Acute Coronary Syndromes. The top half of the figure illustrates the chronology of the interface between the patient and the clinician through the progression of plaque formation, onset, and complications of UA/NSTEMI, along with relevant management considerations at each stage. The longitudinal section of an artery depicts the "timeline" of atherogenesis from (1) a normal artery to (2) lesion initiation and accumulation of extracellular lipid in the intima, to (3) the evolution to the fibrofatty stage, to (4) lesion progression with procoagulant expression and weakening of the fibrous cap. An ACS develops when the vulnerable or high-risk plaque undergoes disruption of the fibrous cap (5); disruption of the plaque is the stimulus for thrombogenesis. Thrombus resorption may be followed by collagen accumulation and smooth muscle cell growth (6). After disruption of a vulnerable or high-risk plaque, patients experience ischemic discomfort that results from a reduction of flow through the affected epicardial coronary artery. The flow reduction may be caused by a completely occlusive thrombus (bottom half, right side) or subtotally occlusive thrombus (bottom half, left side). Patients with ischemic discomfort may present with or without ST-segment elevation on the ECG. Among patients with ST-segment elevation, most (thick red arrow in bottom panel) ultimately develop a Q-wave MI (QwMI), although a few (thin red arrow) develop a non-Q-wave MI (NQMI). Patients who present without ST-segment elevation are suffering from either UA or a non-ST-segment elevation MI (NSTEMI) (thick white arrows), a distinction that is ultimately made on the basis of the presence or absence of a serum cardiac marker such as CK-MB or a cardiac troponin detected in the blood. Most patients presenting with NSTEMI ultimately develop an NQMI on the ECG; a few may develop a QwMI. The spectrum of clinical presentations ranging from UA through NSTEMI and STEMI is referred to as the ACSs. This UA/NSTEMI guideline, as diagrammed in the upper panel, includes sections on initial management before UA/NSTEMI, at the onset of UA/NSTEMI, and during the hospital phase. Secondary prevention and plans for long-term management begin early during the hospital phase of treatment. Dx, diagnosis; NQMI, non-Q-wave MI; QwMI, Q-wave MI. (From Anderson, J. L., Adams, C. D., Antman, E. M., et al. (2007). ACC/AHA 2007 guidelines for the management of patients with unstable angina/non-ST-elevation myocardial infarction: A report of the American College of Cardiology/American Heart Association Task Force on Practice Guidelines. *Journal of American College of Cardiology, 50*(7), e1–e157.)

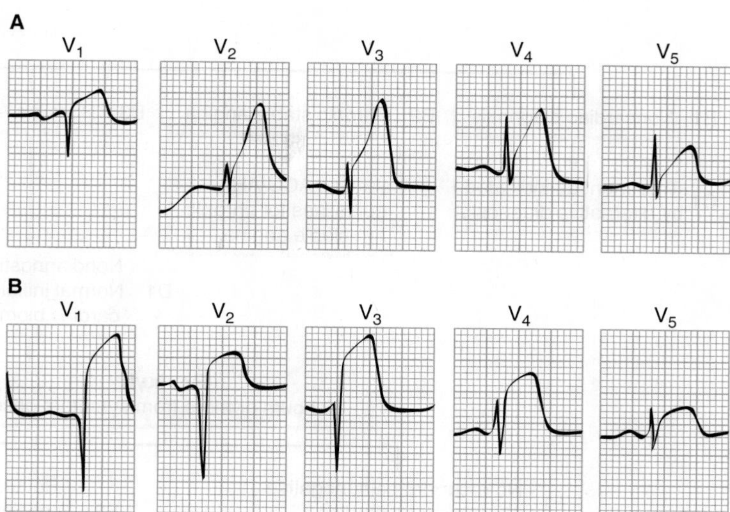

Figure 22-2 Chest leads from a patient with acute anterior wall infarction. (A) In the earliest phase of the infarction, tall, positive (hyperacute) T waves are seen in leads V_2 to V_5. (B) Several hours later, marked ST depression is seen in the same leads and abnormal Q waves are seen in leads V_1 and V_2. (From Goldberger, A. L. [1999]. *Clinical electrocardiography: A simplified approach* [6th ed.]. St. Louis, MO: C.V. Mosby.)

is the principal criterion for reperfusion therapy. Figure 22-2 shows anterior ST-segment elevation indicative of acute anterior STEMI.

Potential precipitating factors of myocardial ischemia, such as uncontrolled hypertension, thyrotoxicosis, or gastrointestinal bleeding, are identified on physical examination. Identification of any comorbid conditions, such as pulmonary disease or malignancy, is critical because both therapeutic risk and clinical decision making could be altered. Immediate evaluation is important to rule out alternative diagnoses of noncardiac chest pain, including aortic dissection (suggestive with findings of unequal pulses or a loud new aortic murmur), acute pericarditis (presents with pleuritic chest pain and/or the presence of a friction rub), pulmonary embolism, tension pneumothorax, myocarditis, perforating peptic ulcer, and esophageal rupture.[2] The physical examination will also give indications as to the hemodynamic effect of the myocardial ischemia, such as hypotension and organ hypoperfusion seen in cardiogenic shock—a medical emergency. Practice guidelines for patient management in the early risk stratification phase follow[4]:

1. A rapid clinical determination of risk for obstructive CAD that focuses on history, physical findings, ECG findings, and cardiac biomarker integration should be made in all patients experiencing chest discomfort suggestive of ACS. (Class I, level of evidence: C)
2. A 12-lead ECG should be performed and evaluated by an emergency department physician of any patient with chest discomfort or anginal equivalent within 10 minutes of arrival to the facility. (Class I, level of evidence: C)
3. If the initial ECG demonstrates no evidence of ischemia but the patient remains symptomatic, serial ECGs at 15- to 30-minute intervals should be performed to detect the development of ST-segment elevation or depression. (Class I, level of evidence: B)
4. Cardiac biomarkers should be measured in all patients who present with chest discomfort indicative of ACS. Cardiac-specific troponin is the preferred biomarker and should be measured in all patients presenting with chest discomfort suggestive of ACS. Patients with negative cardiac biomarkers within 6 hours from the onset of symptoms should have biomarkers re-measured in 8 to 12 hours after the onset of symptoms. (Class I, level of evidence: B)
5. For patients with suspected ACS, troponin-I is the laboratory marker of choice as it is found exclusively in the myocardium. Because of its specificity and sensitivity for detecting myocardial ischemia, troponin-I has become the preferred method of measurement. Other markers of pathophysiologic mechanisms implicated in ACS are under investigation, including markers of coagulation, platelet activation, inflammation, and heart failure. B-type natriuretic peptide, used to indicate the presence of heart failure, has been shown to provide incremental prognostic value in patient cohorts with STEMI and UA/NSTEMI.[8–10]
6. Various forms of imaging are often used to evaluate patients with symptoms that are suggestive of ACS. Bedside echocardiography is useful for diagnosis and risk stratification of patients with ACS in the emergency department.[2] A portable chest radiograph is a Class I recommendation by the ACC guidelines in STEMI. It should not however delay reperfusion strategies.

Immediate Patient Management

Following are the ACC/AHA guidelines for immediate patient management of patients with ACS.[2,4] An in-depth discussion of the medications used in ACS is presented later in this chapter. Figure 22-3 illustrates the ACC/AHA algorithm for the management of ACS. Figure 22-4 illustrates AHA's Advanced Cardiac Life Support algorithm for chest discomfort suggestive of ischemia.

1. The history, physical examination, 12-lead ECG, and initial cardiac biomarkers should be utilized to categorize the chest discomfort into one of four groups: noncardiac diagnosis, chronic stable angina, possible ACS, and definite ACS. (Class I, level of evidence: C)
2. Patients with possible ACS but whose initial 12-lead ECG and cardiac biomarker levels are normal should be observed with ongoing cardiac monitoring, serial ECGs, and repeat biomarker measurement. (Class I, level of evidence: B)
3. In patients with symptoms suggestive of ACS in whom ischemic heart disease is present or suspected, but the follow-up 12-lead ECG and cardiac biomarkers measurements are normal, a stress test (exercise or pharmacologic) to provoke ischemia should be performed in the emergency department within 72 hours of discharge. (Class I, level of evidence: C)
4. In the patient population recommended for outpatient stress testing, precautionary appropriate pharmacotherapy should be prescribed including aspirin, β-blockers, and/or sublingual NTG. If the patient is discharged from the emergency

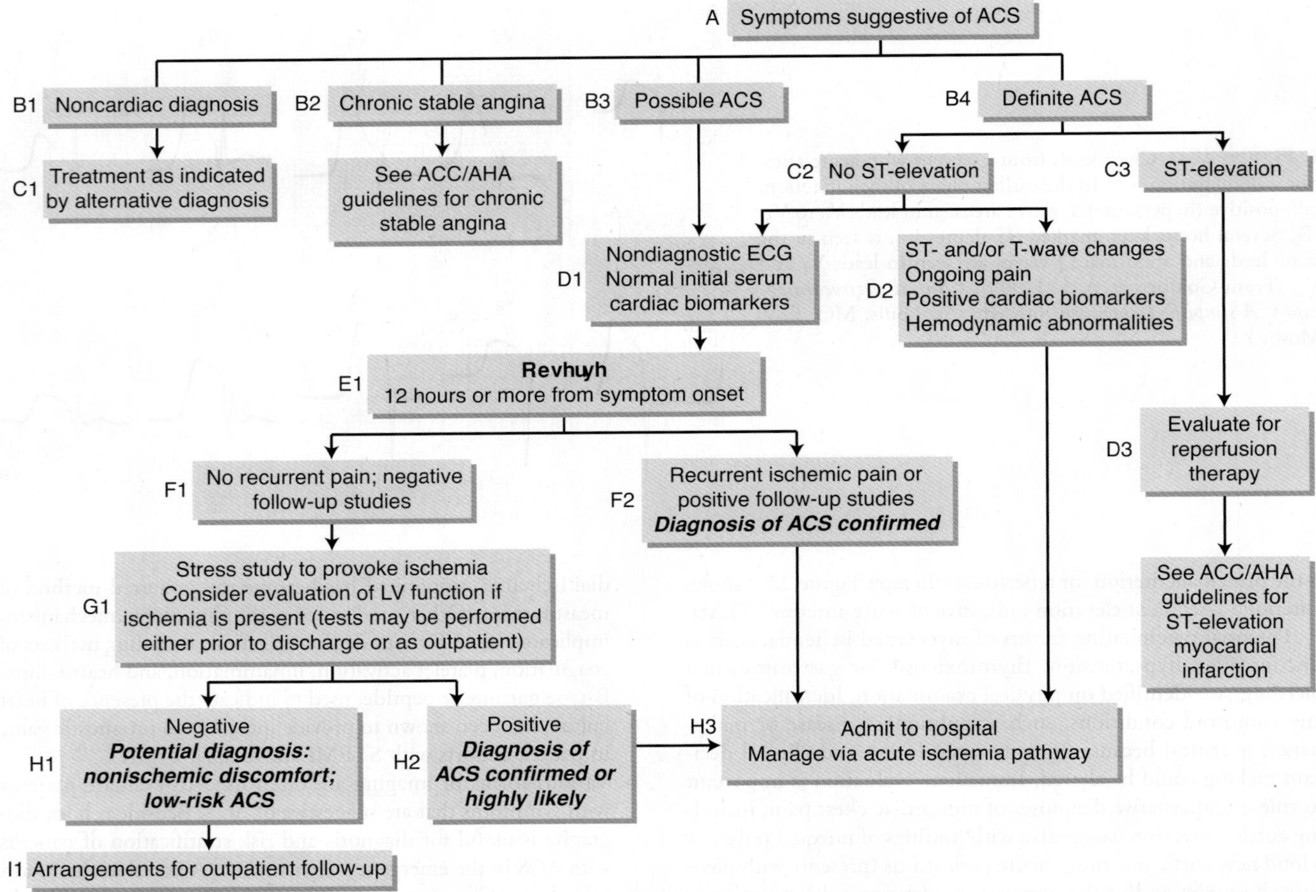

■ **Figure 22-3** Algorithm for the evaluation and management of patients suspected of having ACS. (Reproduced with permission of the American Heart Association, 2006.)

department for outpatient stress testing he/she should receive instruction on activity, medication, and follow-up care with an appropriate health care provider. Patients with definite ACS and ongoing ischemia, positive cardiac biomarkers, new ST-segment deviations, new deep T-wave inversions, hemodynamic abnormalities, or a positive stress test in the emergency department should be admitted to the hospital for further treatment and possible invasive management. Admission to the critical care unit is advised for those patients with active, ongoing ischemia and hemodynamic or electrical instability. (Class I, level of evidence: C)

5. Any patient presenting with STEMI, new or presumed new left bundle-branch block (LBBB) should be evaluated for immediate reperfusion therapy (Class I, level of evidence: A)
6. At this point, bed rest should be maintained to decrease activity and myocardial oxygen consumption. Supplemental oxygen should be administered to patients with ACS particularly if any degree of respiratory insufficiency or hypoxia is present. Oral or intravenous (IV) β-blocker therapy should be administered to those patients with STEMI without a contraindication, irrespective of concomitant fibrinolytic therapy or performance of primary PCI (Class I, level of evidence: A)
7. In the absence of contraindications, morphine sulfate is the analgesic of choice for the management of pain associated with STEMI (Class I, level of evidence: C). Analysis of retrospective data has raised a question as to the potentially adverse effects of morphine in patients with UA/NSTEMI.[1] As a result morphine use in that patient population has been reduced to a Class IIa recommendation.
8. IV NTG is recommended for ongoing chest discomfort unrelieved by sublingual NTG dosing, control of hypertension, or management of pulmonary congestion (Class I, level of evidence: C)

CORONARY REVASCULARIZATION STRATEGIES AND REPERFUSION THERAPIES

Coronary revascularization strategies include PCI, pharmacologic reperfusion, and coronary artery bypass graft (CABG) surgery. Coronary revascularization is performed to improve prognosis, relieve symptoms, prevent ischemic complications, and improve functional capacity. CABG is primarily indicated for patients with left main CAD, three-vessel disease with LV dysfunction, or for those patients for whom PCI is not optimal. Table 22-3 presents the ACC/AHA guidelines for selecting a reperfusion strategy. A full discussion of indications for PCI and CABG can be found in Chapters 23 and 25, respectively.

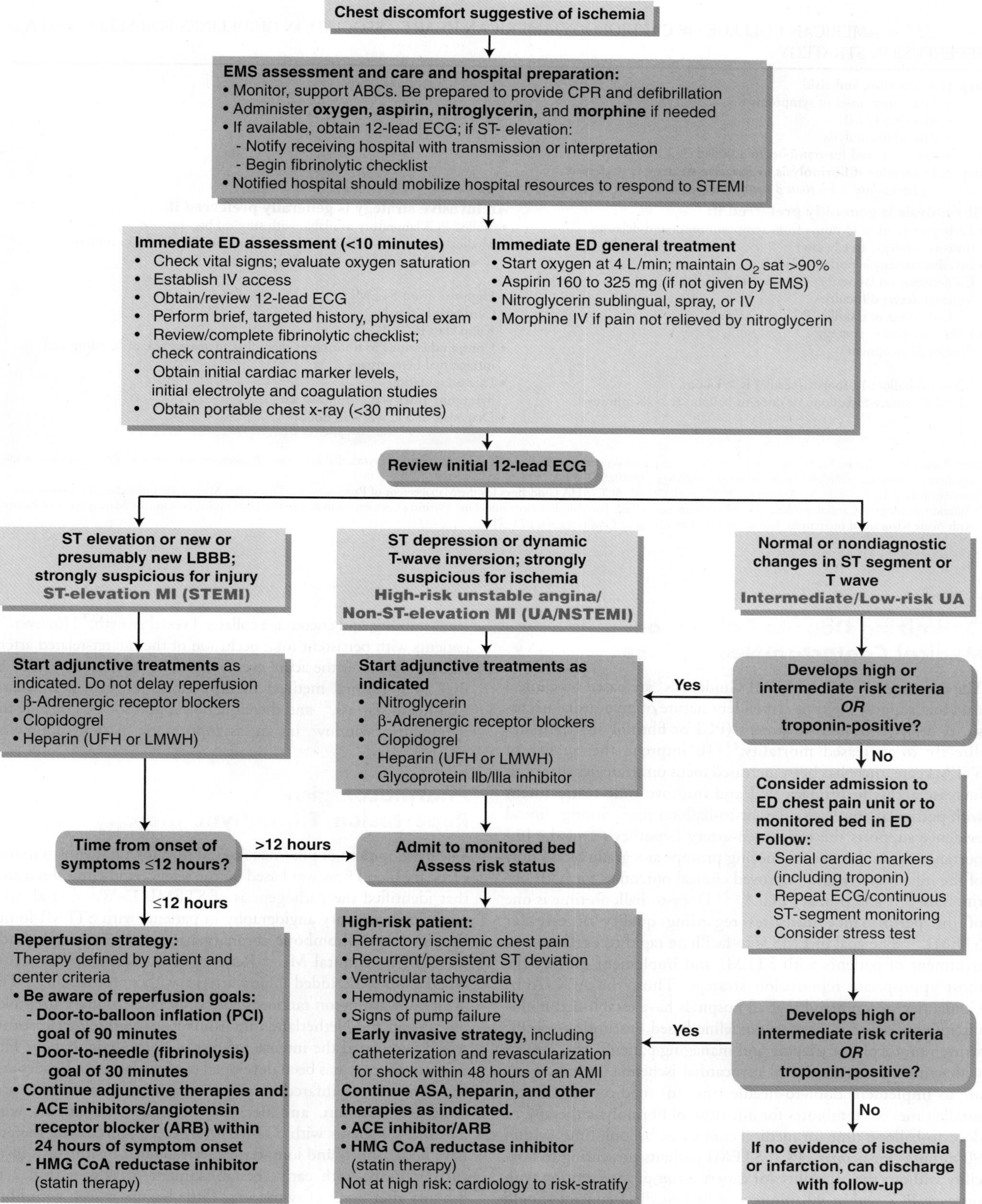

■ **Figure 22-4** ACSs algorithm for chest discomfort suggestive of ischemia. (Reproduced with permission of the American Heart Association, 2006.)

Table 22-3 ■ AMERICAN COLLEGE OF CARDIOLOGY/AMERICAN HEART ASSOCIATION GUIDELINES FOR SELECTING A REPERFUSION STRATEGY

Step 1: Assess time and risk

- Time since onset of symptoms
- Risk of STEMI
- Risk of fibrinolysis
- Time required for transport to a skilled PCI laboratory

Step 2: Determine if fibrinolysis or invasive strategy is preferred

If presentation is less than 3 hours and there is no delay to an invasive strategy, there is no preference for either strategy

Fibrinolysis is generally preferred if:	An invasive strategy is generally preferred if:
• Early presentation (3 hours from symptom onset and delay to invasive strategy) (see below)	• Skilled PCI laboratory available with surgical backup Medical contact-to-balloon or door-to-balloon time is <90 minutes (Door-to-balloon)-(door-to-needle) time is <1 hour
• Invasive strategy is not an option Catheterization laboratory occupied/not available Vascular access difficulties Lack of access to a skilled PCI laboratory	• High risk from STEMI Cardiogenic shock Killip class is ≥ 3
• Delay to invasive strategy Prolonged treatment (Door-to-balloon)-(door-to-needle) is >1 hour Medical contact-to-balloon or door-to-balloon is >90 minutes	• Contraindications to fibrinolysis including increased risk of bleeding and intracranial hemorrhage • Late presentation Symptom onset was >3 hours ago • Diagnosis of STEMI is in doubt

From Boden, W. E., Eagle, K., & Granger, C. B. (2007). Reperfusion strategies in acute ST-segment elevation myocardial infarction: A comprehensive review of contemporary management options. *Journal of American College of Cardiology, 50*(10), 917–929.

From Antman, J. L., Anbe, D. T., Armstrong, P. W., et al. (2004). ACC/AHA Guidelines for the Management of Patients with ST-elevation Myocardial Infarction: A report of the American College of Cardiology/American Heart Association Task Force on Practice Guidelines (Writing Committee to Revise the 1999 Guidelines for the Management of Patients with Acute Myocardial Infarction). *Journal of American College of Cardiology, 44*, 671–719.

Optimizing Door-to-Balloon or Medical Contact-to-Needle Time

The current ACC/AHA STEMI Guidelines[2] are based on clinical data that support the time-dependent nature of myocardial necrosis. A delay in time-to-treatment (PCI or fibrinolysis) translates directly to increased mortality.[11] To improve the quality of STEMI care, there has been increased focus on strategies that both increase access to primary PCI and improve time-to-treatment with particular emphasis on door-to-balloon time. Strong clinical evidence supports the early-open-artery hypothesis[12] of the important relation between achieving prompt antegrade blood flow of the infarct artery and improved clinical outcomes for both fibrinolysis[13–15] and primary PCI.[16–20] Door-to-balloon time is one of the performance measures regarding quality of care for STEMI.[2,3] The goal of EMS is to facilitate rapid recognition and treatment of patients with STEMI and implement quickly the most appropriate reperfusion strategy. Thus, the ACC/AHA Guidelines[2] recommend that all hospitals have established multidisciplinary teams to develop guideline-based, institution-specific written protocols for triaging and managing patients who present with symptoms suggestive of myocardial ischemia. Specific goals are to implement door-to-needle time (or medical contact-to-needle time) of 30 minutes for initiation of fibrinolytic therapy, or door-to-balloon time (or medical contact-to-balloon time) within 90 minutes for primary PCI. STEMI patients presenting to a facility without the capability for expert, prompt intervention with primary PCI within 90 minutes of first medical contact should undergo fibrinolysis within 30 minutes unless contraindicated. (Class I, level of evidence: B)[3]

The late-open-artery hypothesis proposed that late reestablishment of antegrade flow would improve LV function, enhance electrical stability, and encourage collateral vessel growth.[3] However, in patients with persistent total occlusion of the infarct-related artery 3 to 28 days after the acute event, there was no delayed benefit of PCI over optimal medical therapy alone (aspirin, β-blockers, ACEI, and statins),[21] and therefore no support for PCI outside the therapeutic window in an asymptomatic patient following STEMI.[3,12]

Pharmacological Reperfusion/Fibrinolytic Therapy

The development of pharmacological fibrinolytic agents to restore coronary blood flow was based on the science and clinical research that identified the pathogenesis of STEMI. DeWood et al. who performed coronary angiography in patients with STEMI found that 85% had thrombotic coronary artery occlusion in the early hours of transmural MI.[22] Rentrop et al. demonstrated acute reperfusion of occluded infarct arteries with streptokinase.[23] The Western Washington randomized trial of intracoronary streptokinase[24] and the Netherlands Interuniversity Cardiology Institute trial[25] stimulated the intense interest in fibrinolytic therapy. Fibrinolytic therapy has been developed over the last two decades and shown to restore infarct artery patency, reduce infarct size, preserve LV function, and decrease mortality in patients with STEMI.[26] Patients with STEMI who receive fibrinolytic therapy have better short- and long-term survival when treatment is instituted rapidly, with early reestablishment of flow within 2 to 3 hours after onset of symptoms. Little benefit is seen with fibrinolytic therapy after 12 hours, which is theorized to be related to thrombus organization within the coronary artery over time and loss of an opportunity for restoration of blood flow and myocardial salvage.[27]

Table 22-4 ■ COMPARISON OF FIBRINOLYTIC AGENTS

	Streptokinase	Alteplase	Reteplase	Tenecteplase-tPA
Dose	1.5 million units over 30 to 60 minutes	Up to 100 mg in 90 minutes (based on weight)*	10 U × 2 each over 2 minutes	30 to 50 mg based on weight†
Bolus administration	No	No	Yes	Yes
Antigenic	Yes	No	No	No
Allergic reactions (hypotension most common)	Yes	No	No	No
Systemic fibrinogen depletion	Marked	Mild	Moderate	Minimal
90-minute patency rates, approximate %	50	75	7	75
TIMI grade 3 flow, %	32	54	60	63
Cost per dose (US$) in 2004	$613	$2,974	$2,750	$2,833 for 50 mg

*Bolus 15 mg, infusion 0.75 mg/kg times 30 minutes (maximum 50 mg), then 0.5 mg/kg not to exceed 35 mg over the next 60 minutes to an overall maximum of 100 mg.
†Thirty milligrams for weight less than 60 kg; 35 mg for 60 to 69 kg; 40 mg for 70 to 79 kg; 45 mg for 80 to 89 kg; 50 mg for 90 kg or more.
Antman, J.L., Anbe D.T., Armstrong P.W., et al. (2004). ACC/AHA Guidelines for the Management of Patients with ST-elevation Myocardial Infarction: A report of the American College of Cardiology/American Heart Association task force on Practice Guidelines (writing Committee to Revise the 1999 Guidelines for the Management of Patients with Acute Myocardial Infarction). *JACC,* e3–e170.

Indications for Fibrinolysis

In the absence of contraindications, fibrinolytic therapy should be administered to STEMI patients who have onset of symptoms within the previous 12 hours and (1) ST-segment elevation greater than 0.1 mV in at least two contiguous precordial leads or at least two adjacent limb leads or (2) new or presumably new LBBB (Class I, level of evidence: A).[2] The failure of IV fibrinolytic therapy to improve clinical outcomes in the absence of STEMI or LBBB was demonstrated in the Thrombolysis in Myocardial Ischemia 111B (TIMI 111B),[28] International Study of Infarct Survival 2 (ISIS-2),[29] and Gruppo Italiano per lo Studio della Streptochinasi nell'Infarto Miocardico 1 (GISSI 1) trials.[30] Fibrinolytic therapy has no significant benefit for management of patients with UA/NSTEMI without STEMI, true posterior MI, or a presumed new LBBB, and therefore is not recommended.[28–30] Table 22-4 compares characteristics of the fibrinolytic agents. Contraindications and cautions of fibrinolytic agents are presented in Table 22-5.

Prehospital Fibrinolytics

Multiple trials[31–34] have demonstrated that prehospital fibrinolytic administration can significantly decrease time from symptom onset to treatment.[12] Compared with historical control patients, patients who received prehospital fibrinolysis achieved more rapid resolution of ST-segment elevation.[32] A meta-analysis[31] of six randomized trials[33–38] demonstrated improved outcomes and lower mortality with prehospital fibrinolysis.

Prehospital fibrinolysis protocols are reasonable if physicians are present in the ambulance or if well-organized EMS systems are in place and meet the following criteria: (1) paramedics are full time employees, can transmit 12-lead ECGs, and have initial and ongoing training in ECG interpretation and STEMI treatment; (2) an online medical command and a medical director with training/experience in STEMI management are available; and (3) an ongoing continuous quality-improvement program has been implemented (Class IIa, level of evidence: B).[2] If the EMS are capable of providing fibrinolysis, and if the patient qualifies for fibrinolytic therapy, fibrinolysis should begin within 30 minutes of EMS arrival on scene.[3]

Fibrinolytic Agents

There are two major categories of fibrinolytic agents: fibrin nonselective and fibrin selective. A summary of the most commonly used fibrinolytic agents is presented below. Also see Tables 22-4 and 22-5.

Streptokinase. First-generation nonselective fibrinolytics include streptokinase and urokinase, which activate plasminogen systemically and are not fibrin specific. IV urokinase is not approved for STEMI. Tillet and Garner[39] discovered in 1933 that several strains of *Streptococcus hemolyticus* could dissolve human

Table 22-5 ■ CONTRAINDICATIONS AND CAUTIONS FOR FIBRINOLYSIS USE IN STEMI

Absolute Contraindications

- Any prior intracranial hemorrhage
- Known structural cerebral vascular lesion (e.g., AVM)
- Known malignant intracranial neoplasm (primary or metastatic)
- Ischemic stroke within 3 months EXCEPT acute ischemic stroke within 3 hours
- Suspected aortic dissection
- Active bleeding or bleeding diathesis (excluding menses)
- Significant closed head or facial trauma within 3 months

Relative Contraindications

- History of chronic severe, poorly controlled hypertension
- Severe uncontrolled hypertension on presentation (SBP >180 mm Hg or DBP >110 mm Hg)†
- History of prior ischemic stroke greater than 3 months, dementia, or known intracranial pathology not covered in contraindications
- Traumatic or prolonged (greater than 10 minutes) CPR or major surgery (less than 3 weeks)
- Recent (within 2 to 4 weeks) internal bleeding
- Noncompressible vascular punctures
- For streptokinase/anistreplase: prior exposure (more than 5 days ago) or prior allergic reaction to these agents
- Pregnancy
- Active peptic ulcer
- Current use of anticoagulants: the higher the INR, the higher the risk of bleeding

*Viewed as advisory for clinical decision making and may not be all-inclusive or definitive.
†Could be an absolute contraindication in low-risk patients with STEMI.
AVM, arteriovenous malformation; SBP, systolic BP; DBP, diastolic BP; CPR, cardiopulmonary resuscitation; INR, international normalized ratio.
Antman, JL., Anbe, DT., Armstrong, PW., et al. (2004). ACC/AHA Guidelines for the Management of Patients with ST-elevation Myocardial Infarction: A report of the American College of Cardiology/American Heart Association task force on Practice Guidelines (writing Committee to Revise the 1999 Guidelines for the Management of Patients with Acute Myocardial Infarction). JACC, e3–e170.

thrombus. Streptokinase is a single chain polypeptide protein derived from β-hemolytic streptococcus. It binds to plasminogen to form the streptokinase–plasminogen activator complex and then converts plasminogen to plasmin, which initiates fibrinolysis. As described by Bates,[40] early studies of IV streptokinase showed inconsistent improvement in LV function and mortality, likely because doses were inconsistent and administered too late. With improvements in both time-to-administration and consistent dosing protocol (1.5 million units of streptokinase infused over 60 minutes), patency rates at 60 to 90 minutes and at 2 to 3 hours of approximately 50% and 70%, respectively, were attained.

Streptokinase is antigenic and can cause immunologic sensitization with repeat administration. Major reactions of anaphylaxis are rare and occur in <0.5% of cases. Less severe symptoms with administration include shivering, pyrexia, rash, or hypotension that may occur in 10% of patients.[41] Bleeding is the most common complication, with minor bleeding at puncture sites occurring in 3% to 4% of patients; major bleeding and stroke occurs in <1% and 1.6%, respectively, in patients older than 70 years.[42]

Tissue Plasminogen Activator (t-PA) and Recombinant t-PA (rt-PA; Alteplase). The second-generation fibrinolytics are fibrin selective and have demonstrated improved patency rates for reperfusion in STEMI. The fibrinolytic t-PA occurs as a serine protease that is secreted naturally by vascular endothelium. rt-PA is known as alteplase. Both native t-PA and rt-PA (alteplase) preferentially activate plasminogen at the fibrin clot and cause lysis of thrombus, although systemic plasminogen activation occurs at clinical doses.[41]

Accelerated or front-loaded alteplase, weight adjusted and administered with heparin for 24 to 48 hours, has proven to be the best fibrinolytic strategy of the second-generation agents with 90-minute patency rates of approximately 82%.[41] Alteplase has a short half-life (3 to 4 minutes), requiring heparin infusion for at least 24 hours after administration. Alteplase has not been associated with allergic reactions or hypotensive reactions.

Reteplase (r-PA), Tenecteplase (TNK-t-PA), and Lanoteplase (n-PA). The third-generation fibrinolytics include reteplase, tenecteplase, and lanoteplase. STEMI treatment advancement with these third-generation agents has been in the fine-tuning of protocols and administration of adjunctive treatments rather than in the synthesis of new compounds.[43] Reteplase, a nonglycosylated deletion mutant of wild-type t-PA,[43,44] has preferential activation of fibrin-bound plasminogen, a longer half-life, enhanced fibrinolytic potency, and lower affinity for endothelial cells than does t-PA.[43] Tenecteplase is a genetically engineered, multiple point mutant of t-PA that has a longer plasma half-life, allowing single IV bolus injection and more fibrin specificity than standard t-PA. Clinical trials involving reteplase and tenecteplase have found similar efficacy and safety results as with alteplase, but these agents are easier and more convenient to use because of bolus administration rather than infusion.[44,45]

Ancillary Anticoagulation to Support Reperfusion Therapy

To prevent reocclusion of the infarct vessel, the ACC/AHA STEMI fibrinolysis guidelines recommend ancillary anticoagulant therapy for a minimum of 48 hours (level of evidence: C) but optimally for the duration of hospitalization. Unfractionated heparin (UFH) is recommended only for the first 48 hours because of the risk of heparin-induced thrombocytopenia with prolonged UFH exposure (level of evidence: A)[3] unless there are ongoing indications for anticoagulation.[2,46,47] The 2004 ACC/AHA STEMI ancillary anticoagulation recommendations are[2]:

1. Patients undergoing percutaneous or surgical revascularization should receive UFH. (Class I, level of evidence: C)
2. UFH should be given intravenously to patients undergoing reperfusion therapy with alteplase, retaplase, or tenecteplase. (Class I, level of evidence: C)
3. UFH should be given intravenously to patients treated with nonselective fibrinolytic agents (streptokinase, anistreplase, urokinase) who are at high risk for systemic emboli (large anterior MI, atrial fibrillation, previous embolus, or known LV thrombus). (Class I, level of evidence: B)
4. Platelet counts should be monitored daily in patients taking UFH. (Class I, level of evidence: C)

A number of studies[48–52] have compared alternative anticoagulant protocols with UFH or placebo. According to the 2007 ACC/AHA STEMI focused update[3] there are three currently recommended ancillary anticoagulant regimens that have established efficacy:

1. UFH as initial bolus (60 U/kg, with maximum of 4,000 U) followed by 12 U/kg/h (maximum 1000 U/h), adjusted to maintain activated partial thromboplastin time (aPTT) at 1.5 to 2 times (approximately 50 to 70 seconds) (level of evidence: C).
2. Enoxaparin (if serum creatinine level <2.5 mg/dL in men or <2.0 mg/dL in women): for patients younger than 75 years, as initial 30 mg IV bolus followed 15 minutes later by subcutaneous (SC) injection of 1.0 mg/kg every 12 hours. For patients at least 75 years old, initial IV bolus is eliminated and SC injection is reduced to 0.75 mg/kg every 12 hours. Regardless of patient age, if creatinine clearance is <30 mL/min, SC protocol is 1.0 mg/kg every 24 hours. Continue enoxaparin for duration of index hospitalization (up to 8 days). (level of evidence: A)
3. Fondaparinux (if serum creatinine level <3.0 mg/dL): initial dose 2.5 IV, followed by 2.5 mg SC daily. Continue fondaparinux for duration of index hospitalization (up to 8 days). (level of evidence: B)

Cautions, Complications, and Contraindications for Fibrinolytic Agents

The ACC/AHA STEMI Guidelines recommend the following actions to prevent complications[2]:

1. Health care providers should ascertain whether the patient has neurological contraindications to fibrinolytic therapy, including any history of intracranial hemorrhage (ICH) or significant closed head or facial trauma within the past 3 months, uncontrolled hypertension, or ischemic stroke within the past 3 months. (Class I, level of evidence: A)
2. Patients with STEMI at substantial (>4%) risk of ICH should be treated with PCI rather than fibrinolytic therapy. (Class I, level of evidence: A)

Complications of Fibrinolytic Therapy. Most complications associated with second- and third-generation fibrinolytic agents are minor bleeding. Major bleeding occurs in approximately 5% to 6% of patients treated with fibrinolytics. Although the fibrin-specific agents were expected to result in fewer bleeding complications, the larger comparative studies showed no difference in bleeding or transfusion rates compared with streptokinase. Severe bleeding complications such as ICH occur in 1% to 2% of patients and more commonly in the elderly.[12]

1. The occurrence of a change in neurological status during or after reperfusion therapy, particularly within the first 24 hours after initiation of treatment, is considered to be due to ICH until proven otherwise. Fibrinolytic, antiplatelet, and anticoagulant therapies should be discontinued until brain imaging scan shows no evidence of ICH. (Class I, level of evidence: A)
2. Neurology and/or neurosurgery or hematology consultations should be obtained for patients with STEMI who have ICH, as dictated by clinical circumstances. (Class I, level of evidence: C)
3. In patients with ICH, infusions of cryoprecipitate, fresh frozen plasma, protamine, and platelets should be given, as dictated by clinical circumstances. (Class I, level of evidence: C)2

Contraindications of Fibrinolytic Therapy. There are both absolute and relative contraindications to fibrinolytic therapy. Contraindications are listed in Table 22-5.

Combination Therapy: Fibrinolytic Agents and Glycoprotein (GP) IIb/IIIa Inhibitors

Pharmacological reperfusion with fibrinolytic agents does not produce complete restoration of coronary blood flow and TIMI flow 3 in all patients.[53] (See Display 22-1.) Further clinical studies to improve reperfusion with STEMI involved the use of GP IIb/IIIa inhibitors. Intracoronary thrombus formation occurs when fibrinogen and other adhesive proteins bind to adjacent platelets by means of the GP IIb/IIIa receptor sites. Blocking the GP IIb/IIIa receptors can decrease thrombus formation. There are three GP IIb/IIIa receptor inhibitors currently available for clinical use: abciximab, tirofiban, and eptifibatide. Abciximab, a monoclonal antibody, is directed against the receptor, while tirofiban and eptifibatide are high affinity nonantibody receptor inhibitors.[54]

The use of GP IIb/IIIa inhibitors alone was examined in patients with STEMI and the ability to restore TIMI flow 3. These agents in isolation do not adequately restore reperfusion to make GP IIb/IIIa inhibitors alone a viable pharmacological strategy for STEMI.[55–57]

Combination therapy has been proposed as a method to increase reperfusion rates. Two randomized studies (Global Utilization of Strategies to open Occluded Coronary Arteries-V [GUSTO V] and Assessment of the Safety and Efficacy of a New Thrombolytic-III [ASSENT III]) evaluated the effect on mortality and cardiovascular clinical events in STEMI.[58] The GUSTO V trial compared half-dose reteplase and abciximab with full-dose reteplase. No improvement in mortality was demonstrated with combination therapy but there was a modest reduction in clinical events, such as reinfarction, ventricular fibrillation, and ventricular septal defect.[58,59] However, there was an increase in bleeding complications and transfusion rates with combination therapy. Patients older than 75 years had a higher incidence of ICH.[59]

The ASSENT III trial compared full-dose tenecteplase (TNK-t-PA) plus standard dose UFH, full-dose tenecteplase (TNK-t-PA) plus enoxaparin, and half-dose tenecteplase (TNK-t-PA) plus abciximab. The combination therapy had no survival advantage after 30 days and had increased bleeding complications.[60] Combination therapy has no mortality advantage in STEMI but is associated with slight reductions in cardiovascular clinical events.[58]

The ACC/AHA guidelines for STEMI state that combination pharmacological reperfusion with half-dose reteplase or tenecteplase may be considered for the prevention of reinfarction and other complications of STEMI in selected patients meeting the following criteria: anterior MI, younger than 75 years, and no risk factors for bleeding in whom an early referral for angiography and PCI is planned.[2]

DISPLAY 22-1 Timi Flow Grade[98]

The TIMI (Thrombolysis in Myocardial Infarction) trial flow grade classification characterizes coronary blood flow in the infarct-related artery, which is usually measured at 60 to 90 minutes after the administration of fibrinolytic therapy

TIMI 0 refers to the absence of any antegrade flow beyond a coronary occlusion.

TIMI 1 flow is faint antegrade coronary flow beyond the occlusion, although filling of the distal coronary bed is incomplete.

TIMI 2 flow is delayed or sluggish antegrade flow with complete filling of the distal territory.

TIMI 3 flow is normal flow, which fills the distal coronary bed completely.

From Chesebro, J. H., Knatterud, G., Roberts, R., et al. (1987). Thrombolysis in Myocardial Infarction (TIMI) Trial, Phase I: A comparison between intravenous tissue plasminogen activator and intravenous streptokinase. Clinical findings through hospital discharge. *Circulation, 76*(1), 142–154.

REPERFUSION STRATEGIES FOR STEMI AND UA/NSTEMI

Prompt and complete restoration of blood flow in the infarct artery is necessary to prevent myocardial necrosis and improve short- and long-term outcomes. Immediate reperfusion therapy can be achieved by pharmacological therapy (fibrinolysis), PCI (balloon angioplasty with or without deployment of an intracoronary stent) with pharmacological measures to prevent thrombosis. Surgical reperfusion in a timely manner is not usually possible in STEMI; candidates for reperfusion routinely receive either fibrinolysis or a catheter-based treatment.[2]

ACC/AHA Guidelines for Management of Patients with STEMI[2] recommend that all STEMI patients should undergo rapid evaluation for reperfusion therapy and have a reperfusion strategy implemented promptly after contact with the medical system (Class I, level of evidence: A). In STEMI, rapid primary PCI results in superior clinical outcomes compared to fibrinolysis.[61–66] However, the preferred reperfusion therapy for STEMI must take into account the location of the patient, the response time and the expertise of the paramedical/ambulance personnel, their relationship to the regional health care facility, and the availability, capability, and expertise of the medical personnel at the facility[12] (Table 22-3).

Primary PCI for STEMI

Guidelines from the ACC/AHA/European Society of Cardiology recommend a treatment goal of 90 minutes or less for door-to-balloon time (or time from initial medical contact to treatment). This measure is incorporated into national, publicly reported quality measures for hospital performance. The Health Quality Alliance program, which is a combined effort of the Centers for Medicare and Medicaid Services and the Joint Commission, includes door-to-balloon time among its core measures of quality of care for acute MI. When both reperfusion strategies can be rapidly performed current evidence supports the use of primary PCI based on its superiority in establishing coronary blood flow and lower risk of reinfarction and intracerebral hemorrhage.[11]

PCI is the best option for patients with cardiogenic shock and the only option for patients with contraindications to fibrinolytic therapy. However, fibrinolytic therapy remains a practical option for patients with no immediate access to a catheter-based procedure or a catheterization laboratory.

Coronary Angiography for STEMI

According to the ACC/AHA STEMI guidelines,[2] diagnostic coronary angiography should be performed:

1. In candidates for primary or rescue PCI. (Class I, level of evidence: A)
2. In patients with cardiogenic shock who are candidates for revascularization. (Class I, level of evidence: A)
3. In candidates for surgical repair of ventricular septal rupture or severe mitral regurgitation. (Class I, level of evidence: B)
4. In patients with persistent hemodynamic and/or electrical instability. (Class I, level of evidence: C)

Primary PCIs for STEMI

The ACC/AHA STEMI guidelines[2] recommend that, if immediately available, primary PCI should be performed in patients with STEMI (including true posterior MI) or MI with new or presumably new LBBB who can undergo PCI of the infarct artery within 12 hours of symptom onset, if performed in a timely fashion (balloon inflation within 90 minutes of presentation) by persons skilled in the procedure. The procedure should be supported by experienced personnel in an appropriate laboratory environment. (Class I, level of evidence: A)

Specific considerations for primary PCI are[2]:

1. Primary PCI should be performed as quickly as possible with the goal of a medical contact-to-balloon or door-to-balloon interval of within 90 minutes. (Class I, level of evidence: B)
2. If symptom duration is within 3 hours and the expected door-to-balloon time minus the expected time is within 1 hour, primary PCI is generally preferred. (Class I, level of evidence: B). However, if symptom onset is greater than 1 hour, fibrinolytic therapy (fibrin-specific agents) is generally preferred. (Class I, level of evidence: B)
3. If symptom duration is greater than 3 hours, primary PCI is generally preferred and should be performed with a medical contact-to-balloon or door-to-balloon interval as short as possible and a goal within 90 minutes. (Class I, level of evidence: B)
4. Primary PCI should be performed for patients younger than 75 years with ST elevation or LBBB who develop shock within 36 hours of MI and are suitable for revascularization that can be performed within 18 hours of shock unless further support is futile because of patient's wishes or contraindications/unsuitability for further invasive care. (Class I, level of evidence: A)
5. Primary PCI should be performed in patients with severe congestive heart failure (CHF) and/or pulmonary edema (Killip class 3) and onset of symptoms within 12 hours. The medical contact-to-balloon or door-to-balloon time should be as short as possible. (Class I, level of evidence: B)

Reperfusion Strategies for UA/NSTEMI

In the patient with UA/NSTEMI, the decision for initial conservative versus initial invasive strategies is evaluated. An early invasive strategy with diagnostic angiography and intent to perform revascularization is indicated in patients with UA/NSTEMI if the anginal symptoms are refractory and/or hemodynamic or electrical instability are present unless there are known contraindications to PCI (Class I, level of evidence: B).[4] If the patient presenting with UA/NSTEMI has a subsequent troponin that is positive for MI, the patient should be considered for an invasive strategy of revascularization (Class I, level of evidence: A). If an invasive strategy is undertaken in the patient presenting with UA/NSTEMI, PCI is recommended for one to two vessel CAD with or without significant proximal left anterior descending disease but with a large area of viable myocardium (Class I, level of evidence: B). PCI is recommended in this patient population with multivessel CAD if suitable coronary anatomy is present with normal LV function and the absence of diabetes mellitus. (Class I, level of evidence: A).[4]

Early, Late, and Long-Term Care of Patients With ACS

Early Hospital Care

Patients with definite or probable UA/NSTEMI who are hemodynamically stable should be admitted to the inpatient unit for bed rest with ongoing monitoring of cardiac rhythm and careful observation for recurrent ischemic symptoms. Supplemental oxygen should be administered to all patients (UA/NSTEMI and STEMI) with arterial oxygen desaturation less than 90% (Class IIa, level of evidence: C).[2,4] High-risk UA/NSTEMI patients with ongoing chest discomfort, those with hemodynamic instability, and STEMI patients who are unstable after initial reperfusion should be admitted to a cardiac care unit (CCU) for 24 hours of observation.[4]

After admission, optimal management for the UA/NSTEMI patient has dual goals: relieve ischemia and prevent serious adverse outcomes. These goals are accomplished through antiischemic drug therapy, anticoagulation, and ongoing risk stratification to determine the appropriate use of invasive reperfusion strategies. Assessment of LV function by echocardiogram is recommended for immediate and ongoing patient management. If a patient with UA/NSTEMI has recurrent symptoms or there is ongoing evidence of ischemia after initiation of medical therapy, coronary angiography is indicated.[4]

Late Hospital Care

In preparation for discharge from the hospital, it is important to use two patient-centered goals to guide management: (1) Prepare the patient and his/her family as much as possible to resume their normal activities of daily living; and (2) utilize this acute event as an opportunity to reevaluate the patient and family lifestyle, and if warranted, institute aggressive risk factor modification. There is little time to educate patients as to lifestyle changes necessary for risk factor modification during acute hospitalization. Patients who have undergone successful PCI are typically discharged the following day. Uncomplicated CABG length of stay is typically 4 to 7 days. Patients who have undergone noninvasive testing usually are discharged in 1 to 2 days.[4]

A further barrier to education is that frequently patients are under emotional stress due to the crisis, which hinders their absorption of information necessary for change. However, it is important to use this time when the event is fresh in the patient's and family's minds to introduce the concept of risk factor modification. Written materials given to the patient during the acute phase are helpful and can be reviewed on an outpatient basis during subsequent clinic visits.[4]

At discharge, detailed written and verbal instruction for the post-ACS patient should include education on medications, diet, exercise, and smoking cessation if appropriate.[4] Pharmacotherapies started in the inpatient setting, such as oral antiischemic, antiplatelet, and antihypertensive medications are continued after discharge. Referral to cardiac rehabilitation (if ordered by the provider) and scheduling of a timely outpatient appointment should be done prior to discharge from the hospital. Scheduling of a timely outpatient appointment should occur before discharge as well. Minimizing the risk of recurrent cardiovascular events requires ongoing patient compliance with prescribed therapies and recommended lifestyle modification. Patient-specific risk for postdischarge mortality after ACS can be predicted on the basis of clinical information and the ECG. The Platelet Glycoprotein IIb/IIIa in Unstable Angina: Receptor Suppression Using Integrilin Therapy (PURSUIT), TIMI, and Global Registry of Acute Coronary Events (GRACE) risk models are helpful in completing this risk assessment and have been validated for patients experiencing UA/NSTEMI.[4,67–71]

Long-Term Medical Therapy

A team of health care providers in the outpatient setting should work with patients and their families to aggressively manage CAD risk factors. Section V, Health Promotion and Disease Prevention, details CAD risk factor modification strategies. Cardiac rehabilitation personnel are particularly instrumental in patient education due to frequent patient contact. This recommendation is inclusive of patients who have undergone primary revascularization.[72] Patient education should be focused on detailed information regarding specific targets for LDL-C and high density lipoprotein cholesterol (HDL-C),[4,5] blood pressure (BP),[73] diabetes mellitus, diet and weight management,[5] physical activity,[5] and tobacco cessation.[5] Once informed, patients are in a better position to take responsibility for the management of their coronary risk factors.

All patients with elevated systolic or diastolic BPs should be educated and attempt to achieve BPs less than 140 mm Hg systolic and 80 mm Hg diastolic.[4] Patients with diabetes, chronic renal failure, and/or LV dysfunction should achieve a lower range.[3,73]

Every means available should be utilized in assisting patients to be successful at smoking cessation. Tobacco cessation programs, health provider counseling, and the use of pharmacologic agents are recommended to maximize the potential for success.[74,75]

In patients with diabetes and ACS, normoglycemia (a blood glucose level in the range of 80 to 110 mg/dL) is the glycemic goal.[4] For diabetics with ACS, lipid-lowering agents are important to achieve target LDL-C levels of 70 mg/dL or less.[76] Patients who are overweight should be instructed in diets for weight loss and the important role exercise plays in maintaining ideal body mass index. Exercise also plays a pivotal role in decreasing insulin resistance and improving overall well-being.[77,78]

Daily walking can be encouraged immediately for all patients. Patients with residual ischemia should be cautioned to rest should any symptoms occur and to notify their health care provider of symptom recurrence. Cardiac rehabilitation programs have demonstrated effectiveness in improving exercise tolerance without increasing cardiovascular complications. The exercise program and the support to adhere to prescribed management regimes improves both blood lipid and blood glucose levels.[79] Comprehensive cardiac rehabilitation involves individualized risk factor assessment, education, and modification, in addition to prescribed monitored exercise. Cardiac rehabilitation programs can contribute to return to work.[80]

In patients who are stable at discharge from the hospital without complications, sexual activity with the usual partner can be resumed within 7 to 10 days. If otherwise in compliance with state laws, the patient can begin driving a car one week after discharge from the hospital. In patients with complicated MI or evidence of life-threatening arrhythmias, driving should not resume for 2 to 3 weeks after discharge from the hospital or after an outpatient visit with a cardiologist or cardiology nurse practitioner.

PHARMACOLOGICAL MANAGEMENT OF ACS

Optimal medical management includes a regimen that provides resolution of ischemia, relief from discomfort, and prevention of adverse outcomes. Medical management for ACS includes antiischemic agents, analgesia, ACEI, antiplatelet, and anticoagulants therapies.[4]

Antiischemic Therapies

Nitrates

Actions/Indications. NTG promotes vasodilatation of vascular smooth muscle in the peripheral and coronary arteries. Reduction in ischemia and angina results from decrease in systemic vascular resistance (afterload) and decrease in myocardial oxygen demand. NTG promotes dilatation of coronary arteries and collateral blood flow to improve coronary blood flow into ischemic regions of the myocardium. NTG also causes dilatation to a lesser extent of veins and capillaries which decreases venous return and reduces preload.[4,81] NTG is indicated for ischemic discomfort of acute and chronic stable angina.

Contraindications/Adverse Reactions. NTG is contraindicated in patients who take phosphodiestererase inhibitors for erectile dysfunction (sildenafil citrate within previous 24 hours or tadalafil within 48 hours) because of increased and prolonged NTG-mediated vasodilatation with these medications.[4]

Nitrates can cause a sudden decrease in BP and should be avoided in patients with an initial BP less than 90 mm Hg, or 30 mm Hg or more below their baseline, and/or with marked bradycardia or tachycardia.[4] Headache is a common side effect of nitrate therapy.

Administration. Sublingual NTG 0.4 mg tablets should be used every 5 minutes until symptoms are relieved or three doses are taken. Patients who continue to have angina not relieved by sublingual NTG while in the hospital can be started on an IV infusion. IV NTG is indicated for ongoing ischemic discomfort, control of hypertension, or management of pulmonary edema.[2] Topical or oral nitrates can be used as an alternative for patients with stable angina symptoms and used to transition from an NTG infusion.

Nursing Implications. Use of all forms of NTG in ACS requires monitoring of hemodynamic status and response to therapy. Tolerance to the therapeutic effects of nitrates is dose- and duration dependent. After 24 hours of continuous therapy with all NTG medications, titration should be attempted with a regimen that includes a nitrate-free interval. Abrupt cessation of IV NTG has caused recurrent ischemia. Therefore, a decreasing titration of dose is recommended.[4]

β-Adrenergic Blockers

Action/Indications. β-Blockers act by competitively blocking the effects of catecholamines on cell membrane β-receptors. β_1-Adrenergic receptors located in the myocardium inhibit catecholamine activity at receptor sites and reduce myocardial contractility, sinus node rate, and AV node conduction velocity.[4] β_2-Adrenergic receptors present in vascular and bronchial tissue mediate arteriolar dilation and bronchial smooth muscle relaxation. β_1-Selective blockers (i.e., atenolol, metoprolol, and esmolol) are considered cardioselective. They are recommended in patients who have a history of chronic obstructive pulmonary disease because they are less likely to cause bronchospasm.

β-Blockers are indicated for the treatment of angina pectoris, compensated CHF with a combination medical regimen, arrhythmias, and hypertension. The primary benefits of β-blockers are due to a decreased cardiac output and myocardial oxygen demand, slower heart rate that increases the diastolic duration and filling time, which increases both coronary and collateral blood flow.[4] Oral β-blockers are recommended to be initiated promptly in patients with UA/NSTEMI in the absence of contraindication within the first 24 hours. Oral β-blockers are recommended for secondary prevention before hospital discharge.[4]

Contraindications/Adverse Reactions. The benefits of routine early IV use of β-blockers in patients with acute MI have been challenged by the randomized Clopidogrel and Metoprolol in Myocardial Infarction Trial/Second Chinese Cardiac Study (COMMIT/CCS/2). A total of 45,852 patients were randomized within 24 hours of onset of suspected MI to receive IV metoprolol followed by oral metoprolol or placebo for a mean of 15 days. There was no difference in mortality. The use of early β-blocker therapy in acute MI reduced the risk of reinfarction and ventricular fibrillation, but increased the risk of cardiogenic shock, hypotension, and bradycardia seen in the first day after hospitalization primarily in those patients who were hemodynamically compromised.[4,82] Early aggressive IV β-blocker use is suggested with greater caution in patients with STEMI; it should only be used in specific patients and should be avoided in patients with heart failure, hypotension, and/or hemodynamic instability.[4]

Nursing Implications. Monitoring during IV β-blocker therapy should include frequent checks of heart rate and BP and continuous ECG monitoring because of the risk of significant bradycardia and hypotension. Nursing assessment should include auscultation for crackles or wheezes during initiation of β-blocker therapy because there is a possibility of vasoconstriction and bronchoconstriction, resulting in pulmonary edema or bronchospasm.

Calcium Channel Blockers

Actions/Indications. Calcium channel blockers are potent vasodilators that block the inflow of calcium in smooth muscle cells. Calcium channel blocker activity results in peripheral arterial vasodilatation and relaxation of smooth muscle and coronary artery dilatation. Commonly used calcium channel blockers include amlodipine, nifedipine, diltiazem and verapamil. Amlodipine and nifedipine have the most potent peripheral arterial dilatory effect. Diltiazem and verapamil, in addition to vasodilatation effects, also decrease sinus node and atrial–ventricular node conduction causing decreased heart rates. Negative inotropic effects have been reported in varying degrees with calcium channel blockers.[81]

Calcium channel blockers are indicated for patients with chronic stable angina, variant (Prinzmetal's) angina, and in patients with CAD without CHF and an ejection fraction 0.30 or greater. Calcium channel blockers may be used in patients who are unresponsive or intolerant to nitrates or β-blockers. A calcium channel blocker may be added to the medical regimen of a patient who is adequately treated with nitrates and a β-blocker but still has angina.[4] Beneficial effects of calcium channel blockers in chronic stable angina are reduction in peripheral vascular resistance, decreased afterload, decreased myocardial oxygen demand, and increased exercise tolerance.[81]

Contraindications/Adverse Reactions. Patients can have severe hypotension, postural hypotension, or heart block associated with calcium channel blockers. Caution should be used with patients who have a systolic BP less than 90 mm Hg and/or on diuretic therapy. Peripheral edema is a common side effect.[81]

Rapid-release nifedipine must not be used in the absence of β-blockers. Diltiazem and verapamil should be avoided in patients with pulmonary edema, severe LV dysfunction, or heart block.[4] Patients who are already on a β-blocker should use calcium channel blockers cautiously because of synergistic depression of LV function and sinus and AV node conduction.[4] Calcium channel blockers are not indicated for STEMI.

Nursing Implications. When calcium channel blockers are initiated, patients should be monitored for hypotension and arrhythmias (i.e., bradycardia or heart block). Calcium channel blockers can be safely used in patients with chronic obstructive pulmonary disease.

Analgesia

IV Morphine Sulfate

Actions/Indications. Morphine sulfate is a potent narcotic that produces analgesia and sedation. Morphine sulfate is used for pain associated with ischemia and is the analgesia of choice for STEMI.[2] IV doses of morphine starting at 1 to 2 mg are used for patients whose chest pain/discomfort is not relieved with NTG or is recurrent despite antiischemic therapies.[4] Morphine reduces myocardial oxygen demand because of its venodilation properties, modest reductions in heart rate (through increased vagal tone) and systolic BP, and stress reduction via pain relief.

Contraindications/Adverse Reactions. Based on retrospective data concerning the safety of morphine for patients with UA/NSTEMI, the ACC/AHA guidelines recommend using caution when administering morphine to those patients.[4] The major adverse reaction to morphine is an exaggeration of its therapeutic effect, causing hypotension especially in the presence of volume depletion and/or vasodilator therapy. Nausea and vomiting occurs in 20% of patients. Respiratory depression is the most serious complication with severe hypoventilation requiring intubation.

Nursing Implications. Patients who develop hypotension should be placed supine or in the Trendelenburg position, given IV saline boluses or infusions, and IV atropine if the hypotension is accompanied by bradycardia. Antiemetics are used to control nausea and vomiting. Naloxone (0.4 to 2.0 mg IV) may be administered for morphine overdose with respiratory or circulatory depressions. Other narcotics may be used for pain relief in patients allergic to morphine.

Oral Analgesia

There is an increased risk of cardiovascular events among patients taking cyclooxygenase-2 inhibitors and other nonsteroidal antiinflammatory drugs. These events include increased mortality, reinfarction, hypertension, heart failure, and myocardial rupture with STEMI.[3] Patients who present with STEMI or UA/NSTEMI should stop these drugs immediately. An alternative pain treatment plan for chronic pain should be instituted as soon as possible and would begin with acetaminophen or aspirin, small doses of narcotics, or nonacetylated salicylates. If pain relief is inadequate, a nonselective, nonsteroidal anti-inflammatory drug, such as naproxen, is a possible alternative.[3]

Angiotensin Converting Enzyme Inhibitors

Actions/Indications. ACEIs block the conversion of angiotensin I to angiotensin II, a potent vasoconstrictor. The use of this class of drugs has been shown to reduce mortality rates in patients with STEMI, NSTEMI with LV systolic dysfunction, diabetes mellitus with LV dysfunction, and severe CAD.[4] Angiotensin receptor blockers (ARBs) may be used in patients intolerant to ACEI.

Contraindications/Adverse Reactions. ACEI should be used cautiously in patients who are hemodynamically unstable, particularly in the presence of extracellular fluid deficit, because the vasodilatation caused with ACEI therapy can produce marked hypotension. ACEI are used cautiously in patient with renal insufficiency, necessitating close surveillance of renal function. ACEIs are contraindicated in patients with bilateral renal artery stenosis.

Nursing Implications. Before initiation of ACEI therapy, baseline BP measurement and serum creatinine level should be obtained. Monitor the patient for hypotension after initiation of therapy, and know the parameters for holding or stopping medication. Serum creatinine levels are monitored closely; a significant elevation or trend in elevation is reported promptly so that discontinuation of therapy can be considered by the provider.

Antiplatelet Agents

A combination of aspirin (acetylsalicylic acid or ASA), an anticoagulant, and antiplatelet therapy represent the most effective therapy for ACS.

Aspirin

Actions/Indications. ASA inhibits COX-1 within platelets, which prevents the formation of thromboxane A2, diminishing the platelet aggregation promoted by this pathway. Patients who have not taken aspirin before presentation with STEMI should chew soluble aspirin 162 to 325 mg. Although some trials have used enteric-coated aspirin for initial dosing, more rapid buccal absorption occurs with non-enteric-coated aspirin formulations.[2] Aspirin is continued indefinitely in patients with CAD unless contraindicated.

Contraindications/Adverse Reactions. Aspirin is contraindicated for patients with a known sensitivity to the drug. Patients with a history of gastrointestinal bleeding should use ASA with caution, take enteric-coated aspirin, and have supplemental therapy to prevent recurrence of bleeding.

Nursing Implications. Aspirin should be taken with meals to avoid gastric irritation. Teach patients to monitor for possible bleeding or allergic reaction. Periodic hemoglobin and hematocrit levels should be monitored.

Adenosine Diphosphate Receptor Antagonists

Actions/Indications. The adenosine diphosphate (ADP) receptor antagonists are agents that selectively inhibiting ADP binding to its receptor and prevent activation of the GP IIb/IIIa complex needed for platelet aggregation.[81] Two oral ADP receptor antagonists currently used for ACS and PCI include clopidogrel and ticlopidine. Clopidogrel and ticlopidine irreversibly modify the platelet ADP receptor for the life of the platelet. Dose-dependent inhibition of the platelet is seen after 2 hours of a single dose. Clopidogrel is the primary chosen ADP receptor antagonist and preferred to ticlopidine because of more rapid inhibition of platelets, once-a-day dosing, and a favorable safety profile that is comparable to aspirin.[83] A loading dose for clopidogrel is 300 to 600 mg and recommended in ACS and PCI with stenting for rapid platelet inhibition.[53] Inhibition reaches a steady state after 3 to 7 days. Platelet aggregation and bleeding time gradually returns to normal after 5 days of drug cessation.[81]

Contraindications/Adverse Reactions. Contraindications include known hypersensitivity to the drug or any drug components, or any active bleeding. Serious adverse effects include neutropenia, thrombotic thrombocytopenic purpura, and gastrointestinal or cerebral hemorrhage.[84] Other adverse effects include gastrointestinal problems (diarrhea, abdominal pain, nausea, vomiting) and rash.

Nursing Implications. Patients who have received a stent with primary PCI must understand the importance and necessity of continued daily use of clopidogrel (or ticlopidine if allergic to clopidogrel) for a specified duration as prescribed. Acute stent closure and the potential for MI or death have been reported with premature cessation of clopidogrel or ticlopidine.

Patients taking ticlopidine must be aware of the need to monitor complete blood cell count with differential every 2 weeks for the first 3 months of therapy to screen for neutropenia. Patients should be told that it might take them longer than usual to stop bleeding when they are taking clopidogrel or ticlopidine, and that they should report unusual bleeding. Patients should advise their physicians and dentists that they are taking clopidogrel or ticlopidine before a surgery is scheduled; patients should not stop taking the medication unless advised by their cardiologist.

IV Antiplatelet Agents

ACC/AHA Guidelines for Antiplatelet Therapy Recommendations.[4] These guidelines are followed by sections on antiplatelet actions/indications, contraindications/adverse reactions, and nursing implications.

1. Aspirin should be administered to UA/NSTEMI patients as soon as possible after hospital presentation and continued indefinitely in patients not known to be intolerant of that medication. (Class I, level of evidence: A)
2. Clopidogrel (loading dose followed by a maintenance dose) should be administered to UA/NSTEMI patients who are unable to take ASA because of hypersensitivity or major gastrointestinal intolerance. (Class I, level of evidence: A) In UA/NSTEMI patients with a history of gastrointestinal bleeding, when ASA and clopidogrel are administered alone or in combination, drugs to minimize the risk of recurrent gastrointestinal bleeding (proton-pump inhibitors) should be prescribed concomitantly. (Class I, level of evidence: B)
3. For UA/NSTEMI patients in whom an initial invasive strategy is selected, antiplatelet therapy in addition to ASA should be initiated before diagnostic angiography and either clopidogrel or an IV GP IIb/IIIa inhibitor. (Class I, level of evidence: A)

4. For UA/NSTEMI patients in whom an initial conservative strategy is selected, clopidogrel should be added to ASA and anticoagulant therapy as soon as possible after admission and administered for at least 1 month (Class I, level of evidence: A) and ideally up to 1 year. (Class I, level of evidence: B)
5. For UA/NSTEMI patients in whom an initial conservative strategy is selected, if recurrent symptoms/ischemia, heart failure, or serious arrhythmias subsequently appear, then diagnostic angiography should be performed. (Class I, level of evidence: A) Either an IV GP IIb/IIIa inhibitor or clopidogrel should be added to ASA and anticoagulant therapy before diagnostic angiography. (Class I, level of evidence: C)

Actions/Indications. There are three IV antiplatelet agents, abciximab, eptifibatide, and tirofiban, which are classified as GP IIb/IIIa receptor antagonists. The smaller molecules, tirofiban and eptifibatide, are less expensive to manufacture than abciximab, a monoclonal antibody.[85] Abciximab has a short half-life but a strong affinity for the GP IIb/IIIa receptor. Platelet aggregation gradually returns to normal in 48 hours after discontinuation of abciximab, although the drug remains in the circulation for 10 to 15 days in a platelet-bound state, resulting in sustained antiplatelet activity.[4] Abciximab is indicated for patients with ACS who undergo PCI and for patients treated with conventional medical therapy with planned PCI within 24 hours. Abciximab has been studied primarily in PCI trials with clinical reduction in rates of MI and need for urgent revascularization.[4]

Eptifibatide and tirofiban are synthetic receptor antagonists that bind to the GP IIb/IIIa receptor. Receptor occupancy with these two agents is reversible. Platelet aggregation returns to normal 4 to 8 hours following cessation of the infusion. Eptifibatide and tirofiban are indicated for patients with ACS who are managed medically and with PCI.[4]

Contraindications/Adverse Reactions. GP IIb/IIIa inhibitors should not be used in patients with a known hypersensitivity; history of bleeding tendency or evidence of active bleeding within previous 30 days; severe hypertension (systolic BP > 180 mm Hg or diastolic BP > 110 mm Hg); major surgery within previous 4 to 6 weeks; history of stroke within 30 days or hemorrhagic stroke; international normalized ratio greater than 1.2; prior administration of a GP IIb/IIIa inhibitor within the previous 24 to 48 hours; acute pericarditis; presumed or documented vasculitis; platelet count less than 100,000/mm^3; and creatinine level greater than 4.0 mg/dL (eptifibatide).[85]

Administration of abciximab may result in antibody formation that could potentially cause allergic or hypersensitivity reactions including anaphylaxis. The most common adverse reactions of GP IIb/IIIa antagonists include minor bleeding from access sites and rarely major bleeding including ICH. There is a potential increase in bleeding risk with combination use of anticoagulants or fibrinolytics. Severe thrombocytopenia (platelets <50,000/mm^3) has been reported in 0.5% patients receiving GP IIb/IIIa antagonists. Although thrombocytopenia is reversible, it is associated with increased risk of bleeding.[86,87]

Nursing Implications. Monitor the complete blood cell count and differential and platelet count prior to treatment, 2 to 4 hours following the bolus dose, and at 24 hours or prior to discharge. If a patient experiences an acute decrease in platelets, the drug should be discontinued and additional platelet counts should be monitored until the platelet count returns to normal. Platelet infusions may be needed for an acute drop in platelets and/or with bleeding associated with thrombocytopenia. Monitor for potential bleeding at arterial and venous puncture sites and gastrointestinal, genitourinary, and retroperitoneal sites. Postural BPs should be measured prior to ambulation to rule out potential extracellular fluid volume deficit secondary to bleeding. If an allergic reaction occurs, stop the drug immediately and initiate resuscitative measures if indicated.

Anticoagulant Agents

For patients with STEMI and UA/NSTEMI, anticoagulant therapy should be initiated at the time of presentation to prevent thrombus-related events.[2,4]

UFH and Low-Molecular-Weight Heparin

Actions/Indications. UFH accelerates the action of circulating antithrombin, which inactivates factor IIa (thrombin), factor IXa, and factor Xa. UFH prevents thrombus propagation but does not cause lysis of existing thrombi. UFH binds to a number of plasma proteins, blood cells, and endothelial cells leading to poor bioavailability and marked variability in anticoagulant response. The anticoagulant effect of heparin requires monitoring with aPTT. A weight-adjusted dosing regimen is needed to provide more predictable anticoagulation.[4]

Enoxaparin has been studied more frequently than other low-molecular-weight heparin (LMWH) preparations. It has antithrombotic properties with inhibition of factor Xa and antithrombin (factor IIa) occurring 3 to 5 hours after SC injection. Enoxaparin has a longer half-life than does UFH, resulting in a more predictable and sustained anticoagulant effect. Enoxaparin is weight-based, administered once or twice a day subcutaneously, and does not require laboratory monitoring. Enoxaparin does not prolong routine coagulation tests (i.e., prothrombin time, aPTT, or activated clotting time) in a predictable manner, thus monitoring is not suitable to evaluate level of anticoagulation.[4] Consequently, UFH is frequently preferred during PCI to allow close monitoring of anticoagulation and reversibility if the patient is going to undergo CABG.

Patients with ACS/NSTEMI who are treated with conservative medical management can be treated with either UFH or LMWH. Several trials have found a benefit with enoxaparin over UFH with conservative management in ACS, demonstrating reductions in death and nonfatal MI.[88,89] The ACC/AHA recommends an anticoagulant preference of fondaparinux, enoxaparin, and UFH for patients with a noninvasive strategy.[4] Patients with ACS/NSTEMI who are treated with an early aggressive approach were evaluated in the SYNERGY (Superior Yield of the New strategy of Enoxaparin, Revascularization and GlYcoprotein IIb/IIIa inhibitors) trial.[90] Enoxaparin was found to be safe and an effective alternative to UFH but without significant advantage. There was a modest increase in major bleeding with enoxaparin compared with UFH. The advantage of LMWH is the ease of SC administration and the absence of monitoring. Compared with UFH, LMWH stimulates platelets less and is less frequently associated with heparin-induced thrombocytopenia. However, compared with UFH, the anticoagulant effect of LMWH is less effectively reversed with protamine. When LMWH is administered during PCI, the activated clotting time cannot be monitored so that the degree of anticoagulation cannot be monitored.[2]

Contraindications/Adverse Reactions. Heparin is contraindicated in patients with a history or current diagnosis of heparin-induced thrombocytopenia, allergy, or acute cerebrovascular accident or a history of life-threatening gastrointestinal bleeding.

Nursing Implications. Obtain a baseline aPTT before starting therapy with UFH, and again every 6 hours after any dosage change or significant change in clinical status. The dosage of UFH is adjusted so that the aPTT is within the therapeutic range. Daily complete blood cell count with differential should be evaluated for bleeding or thrombocytopenia. Although aPTT and prothrombin times are not monitored with LMWH, a complete blood cell count with differential should be evaluated for bleeding or thrombocytopenia.

Direct Thrombin Inhibitors

Actions/Indications. The naturally occurring anticoagulant hirudin (the active principal component in the salivary secretion of leeches) and bivalirudin, its synthetic analog, are direct thrombin inhibitors. Thus, they are able to inactivate thrombin in blood clots, which is in contrast to the action of UFH, which targets only soluble thrombin.[91]

The ACC/AHA UA/NSTEMI guidelines for the use of direct thrombin inhibitors are the following[4,91]:

1. For patients in whom an invasive strategy is selected, bivalirudin is recommended as the anticoagulant of choice, with enoxaparin, UFH, and fondaparinux (see the following section) as acceptable alternatives. When bivalirudin is selected, a GP IIb/IIIa inhibitor may be omitted before diagnostic angiography and PCI as long as clopidogrel (at least 300 mg) was administered within 6 hours.
2. For patients in whom CABG is selected following coronary angiography, discontinue bivalirudin 3 hours before CABG and switch to UFH per institutional protocol.
3. For patients in whom medical therapy is selected following coronary angiography and bivalirudin was administered prior to angiography, either discontinue bivalirudin or continue administration for up to 72 hours at the discretion of the physician.

Contraindications/Adverse Reactions. The major contraindications are hypersensitivity to hirudins and active major bleeding, which can occur at any site. In the ISAR-REACT 3 (Intracoronary Stenting and Antithrombotic Regimen: Rapid Early Action for Coronary Treatment 3) clinical trial, the incidence of major bleeding was 33% lower with bivalirudin (3.1%) compared with UFH (4.6%). The incidence of minor bleeding was also significantly less with bivalirudin. However, transfusion and thrombocytopenia incidence were similar.[92] Back pain, headache, and hypotension are the most common adverse reactions.[93]

Nursing Implications. Bivalirudin is administered intravenously and has a short (25 minutes) half-life.[93] Monitor for major and minor bleeding, including evaluation of hemoglobin and hematocrit and assessment of vascular access sites.

Factor Xa Inhibitor: Fondaparinux

Actions/Indications. Fondaparinux is a synthetic heparin pentasaccharide that selectively binds to antithrombin III, consequently inhibiting factor Xa,[81] interrupting the blood coagulation cascade, and thus inhibiting thrombin formation and thrombus development. Compared with UFH, fondaparinux has decreased plasma-protein and endothelial-cell binding; dose-independent clearance; and longer half-life, allowing a more predictable and sustained anticoagulant effect for once-a-day, fixed-dose SC administration.[4] Fondaparinux does not affect thrombin that is already present, a possible reason for the increased rate of catheter-associated thrombosis with fondaparinux.[53]

The ACC/AHA UA/NSTEMI guidelines for fondaparinux use are the following[4,94]:

1. For patients undergoing early invasive strategies, fondaparinux (along with enoxaparin, UFH, and bivalirudin) has established efficacy for patients undergoing an early invasive strategy. However, if fondaparinux is selected, supplemental UFH should be administered during PCI,[4] leading others not to recommend its use in patients undergoing an invasive strategy.[94]
2. For patients selected for a conservative strategy, fondaparinux and LMWH are considered preferable to UFH.
3. For patients in whom CABG is planned within 24 hours, UFH is preferred to fondaparinux or LMWH, because its anticoagulant effect can be more rapidly reversed.
4. For patients at increased risk of bleeding, fondaparinux is recommended as the anticoagulant of choice.

Contraindications/Adverse Reactions. Contraindications include hypersensitivity to fondaparinux or any of its components, severe renal impairment (creatinine clearance <30 mL/min), low body weight (<50 kg), active major bleeding, bacterial endocarditis, and thrombocytopenia associated with a positive *in vitro* test for antiplatelet antibody in the presence of fondaparinux. The major adverse event is bleeding at any site. Risk for adverse reactions may be increased in patients with renal dysfunction, whose age is greater than 75 years, and whose weight is less than 50 kg.[95]

Nursing Implications. Following sheath removal, do not resume fondaparinux for at least 2 hours in patients with UA/NSTEMI and 3 hours in patients with STEMI.[95] Periodically monitor complete blood cell count and serum creatinine, but as with LMWH, fondaparinux does not require laboratory coagulation monitoring. Monitor all puncture sites for potential bleeding and test for occult blood in the stool.

COMPLICATIONS OF MI

Ventricular Free Wall Rupture

Ventricular free wall rupture may account for up to 10% of acute MI-associated mortality. It occurs in near equal frequency in both anterior and inferior MI, typically within the first week after infarction. Clinical presentations are pulseless electrical activity and sudden death. Attempts at resuscitation are futile. Accurately identifying patient populations at high risk for ventricular free wall rupture is difficult. Large Q-wave infarcts are more likely to demonstrate rupture than others. The risk of this devastating complication increases with the age of the patient.[2]

Ventricular Septal Rupture

Ventricular septal rupture occurs in 1% to 3% of acute MIs.[4] It tends to occur from 3 to 7 days post-MI, and clinically presents with abrupt, severe LV failure, a new loud holosystolic murmur, and systemic hypoperfusion due to left-to-right shunting. Diagnosis is made with echocardiography to visualize the ventricular septum.

The treatment is emergency surgical repair preceded by intra-aortic balloon counterpulsation and nitroprusside infusion. The mortality rate is greater than 20% in 24 hours and 40% in 1 week.

Mitral Regurgitation

Mitral regurgitation may occur early in the course of acute MI due to ischemia of the valve or papillary muscles. It occurs most frequently with inferior MI or non-Q-wave MI.[2] The onset of regurgitant flow is usually within the first week following MI. Diagnosis is made with echocardiography. Pulmonary congestion as a result of mitral valve dysfunction may be intermittent or persistent. Mitral valve dysfunction may require urgent revascularization if the papillary muscle dysfunction is due to ischemia. However, if the ischemic event causes papillary muscle rupture, ejection fraction declines rapidly, requiring intra-aortic balloon counterpulsation and the infusion of NTG or sodium nitroprusside before emergency surgical repair[96] (see Chapter 29).

Arrhythmias

Arrhythmias can occur in the course of infarction due to electrophysiological alterations in ischemic myocardium, pharmacotherapeutic interventions, electrolyte imbalances, or endogenous catecholamine release.[4] Arrhythmias that occur late may be due to poor systolic function or ventricular aneurysm. Ventricular tachyarrhythmias are not uncommon following MI. Approximately 7% of patients with acute MI have ventricular fibrillation and cardiac arrest. A similar number of patients experience recurrent ventricular tachycardia.[4] Low levels of potassium and magnesium can precipitate ventricular fibrillation in this patient population and should be monitored closely. Bradyarrhythmias are more common in inferior wall MI. Sinus bradycardia, sinus arrest, and second- and third-degree atrioventricular block occur more commonly in right ventricular (RV) infarction. Complete heart block occurs up to 20% of all patients with acute RV infarction.[4] Bradyarrhythmias are treated with atropine or transvenous pacing. Sinus bradycardia is treated only if the patient is symptomatic. β-Blockers are contraindicated in this setting despite their clear benefit in MI and angina pectoris. Anterior wall MI is much more likely to cause infranodal conduction abnormalities, characterized by wide complex idioventricular rhythms[4] (see Chapter 16).

Pericarditis

Pericarditis most commonly occurs as a complication of MI several weeks following the event as a result of a localized inflammatory response. Post-MI, pericarditis is also referred to as Dressler's syndrome. Pericarditis can occur acutely following MI, and in that case, typically is isolated to the pericardium adjacent to the infarcted area. The diagnosis is made by history, physical examination, and evaluation of the ECG. Typically the patient describes sharp, substernal, severe chest pain that can radiate to the neck, shoulders, or back. The pain is worsened with deep inspiration or when reclining. A pericardial friction rub may be auscultated on physical examination. The classic multilead ST-segment elevation is present with diffuse pericarditis but not present if the pericarditis is localized to the infarct region (Chapter 30). Thrombolytic therapy has decreased the incidence of this complication significantly.[2]

Heart Failure and Cardiogenic Shock

Cardiogenic shock, characterized by systemic hypoperfusion due to low cardiac output despite high filling pressures, complicates approximately 7% of all cases of acute MI, with the majority resulting from LV pump failure.[45,97] The remaining patients with MI who develop shock do so from mechanical complications, such as ventricular septal rupture, mitral regurgitation, or tamponade. Modern therapy, including aggressive revascularization and intra-aortic balloon support, has contributed to an improvement in survival. However, the overall 30-day mortality associated with this catastrophic complication of acute MI remains more than 50% (Chapter 24).

NURSING MANAGEMENT OF ACS*

Nursing management of the patient with ACS involves caring for the patient during varying stages of the disease process: During acute onset of chest discomfort, as the diagnosis is confirmed, at hospital discharge, during convalescence, or on an ongoing basis with the goal to prevent recurrence of angina or MI. The focus of this section is on the nursing management of angina pectoris or during the acute phase of MI.

Chest Discomfort

Diagnosis

Chest discomfort, related to an imbalance in myocardial oxygen supply and demand, manifested by patient complaints of chest discomfort, with or without radiation to arms, neck, back, or jaw, by nonverbal expressions of discomfort (facial grimacing, Levine sign), and increases in heart rate, BP, respiratory rate, and by cool, clammy skin.

Goals

1. To detect chest discomfort and associated ECG and hemodynamic changes early.
2. To reduce or eliminate chest discomfort.
3. To prevent the occurrence of the discomfort.

Interventions

Nursing interventions are directed toward assessment and improvement of the myocardial ischemia. Ischemia can be improved by interventions that decrease myocardial oxygen consumption or increase coronary perfusion. Examples of nursing interventions for the hospitalized patient with angina or acute MI follow

For Goal 1

Teach the patient to report chest discomfort immediately on a scale of 1 to 10 (with 10 being the worst) at the onset of the discomfort and proceed as follows:

1. Assess and document the patient's description of the discomfort including location, radiation, duration, intensity, and any factors that exacerbate or improve the discomfort.
2. Assess BP, heart rate and rhythm, and respiratory rate and rhythm.
3. Assess the skin for temperature and moistness.
4. Obtain a 12-lead ECG during chest discomfort.

*Contributed by Sherri Del Bene and Anne Vaughan.

5. Consider ST-segment monitoring to detect silent ischemia or to evaluate the relation between patient care activities and ischemia.
6. Report the findings of the above assessment to the physician.

For Goal 2

1. Immediately reduce the patient's physical activity to the level before occurrence of the discomfort.
2. Administer oxygen, morphine sulfate if ordered, and NTG or other medications as ordered, and continuously evaluate the patient's response to therapy.
3. Provide a restful environment and maximize; and promote the patient's physical comfort by elevating the head of the bed to 20 to 30 degrees or higher and by individualizing basic patient care.

For Goal 3

1. Provide care in a calm, competent manner.
2. Provide a restful, quiet environment.
3. Provide small portions of easily digestible food.
4. Assist the patient with activities of daily living.
5. Teach patient to exhale with physical movement (to avoid Valsalva maneuver), and as necessary, offer stool softeners and laxatives to prevent straining.
6. Teach patient to recognize precipitating factors and alter behavior accordingly.
7. Teach patient to practice relaxation techniques.

Outcome Criteria

Goal 1: Chest discomfort, 12-lead ECG changes indicative of ischemia, and changes in vital signs and hemodynamic responses are detected at the onset.

Goal 2: Within 5 minutes of the intervention, patient states that chest discomfort is relieved or reduced; patient appears comfortable, heart and respiratory rates and BP are returning or have returned to the baseline level before the onset of chest discomfort, ST segments and T waves revert to pattern seen before the onset of chest discomfort, and skin is warm and dry.

Goal 3: Patient denies chest discomfort, patient appears comfortable, heart and respiratory rates and BP are within patient's normal range, and skin is warm and dry (Display 22-2).

DISPLAY 22-2 Selected Therapies to Reduce Ischemia

Decrease Myocardial O_2 Consumption

- Narcotic analgesics
- β-Blocking agents
- Maintain BP within normal limits
- Maintain normal sinus rhythm with medications, pacing, or cardioversion
- Selected diet (initially clear liquids followed by small, frequent, easily digested meals)
- Stress reduction techniques
- Anxiolytics as indicated
- Maintain quiet environment
- Stool softeners and laxatives
- Rest with backrest elevation 20 to 30 degrees
- Gradually increase physical activity

Increase Myocardial O_2 Supply

- Oxygen
- NTG
- Aspirin
- Anticoagulants
- Reperfusion
  - Thrombolytics
  - PCI
  - CABG

Decreased Myocardial Tissue Perfusion

Diagnosis

Decreased myocardial tissue perfusion related to an imbalance between myocardial oxygen supply and demand and manifested by chest discomfort, arrhythmias, conduction disturbances, and/or heart failure. Refer to previous diagnosis of chest discomfort for goals, interventions, and outcome criteria for chest discomfort.

Goals

1. To detect early manifestations (specify) and etiologies of decreased myocardial tissue perfusion.
2. To reduce or eliminate manifestations (specify) of decreased myocardial tissue perfusion.
3. To prevent, when possible, manifestations (specify) of decreased myocardial tissue perfusion and extension of MI or progression to infarction in patients with angina.

Interventions

Interventions are designed to detect the manifestations of the imbalance between myocardial oxygen supply and demand and to improve this imbalance. Interventions to meet each goal include:

For Goal 1

1. The patient's heart rate and rhythm should be monitored frequently during the acute phase of MI. Assess and document cardiac rhythm every 1 to 4 hours depending on patient condition, before and after each dose of antiarrhythmic or vasoactive drug (or any drug with cardiovascular effects), and when patient status indicates. Assess BP and obtain 12-lead ECG with changes in cardiac rhythm or if patient complains of palpitations.
2. If the patient experiences arrhythmias, perform a cardiovascular examination; obtain venous blood for electrolytes, hemoglobin, and, if appropriate, drug levels; obtain arterial blood for blood gas analysis; and obtain a chest radiograph as ordered by the physician.
3. Initially, every 4 to 8 hours, and during chest discomfort, assess, document, and report to the physician the following: new S_3 or S_4 gallops or a new murmur of mitral regurgitation, new or increasing crackles, and reduced activity tolerance.

For Goal 2

1. Immediately reduce patient's physical activity to the level of activity before occurrence of manifestations of decreased myocardial tissue perfusion.
2. Administer oxygen and antiarrhythmic and other medications (positive inotropic, afterload-reducing, and preload-reducing agents) as ordered and continuously evaluate the patient's response to therapy.
3. Provide a restful environment; and promote the patient's physical comfort by elevating head of bed to 20 to 30 degrees or higher and providing individualized basic nursing care.

For Goal 3

1. Provide small portions of easily digested, low-sodium, low saturated fat foods.
2. Provide a restful environment; as needed, assist the patient in a supportive, calm, competent manner with activities of daily living.
3. Teach patient to exhale with physical movement; as necessary.
4. Offer stool softeners and laxatives to prevent straining with bowel movements, and teach patient relaxation techniques.

Outcome Criteria

Goal 1: Arrhythmias and conduction disturbances and signs and symptoms of heart failure are detected at onset.

Goal 2: Immediately after intervention, the patient's cardiac rate and rhythm return to patient's normal range. Patient states that palpitations are relieved or reduced; patient appears comfortable; and BP is returning or has returned to baseline level. S_3 or S_4 gallops or the murmurs of mitral regurgitation disappear or do not increase in intensity; crackles are eliminated or reduced; and activity tolerance is maintained or improved.

Goal 3. The patient denies chest discomfort. The patient appears comfortable. Heart and respiratory rates and BP are within the patient's normal range. The skin is warm and dry. There are no S_3 or S_4 gallops, no murmur of mitral regurgitation, and no crackles. The patient's activity tolerance is maintained.

Decreased Systemic Perfusion

Diagnosis

Decreased systemic tissue perfusion related to a decrease in cardiac output from arrhythmias and conduction disturbances and from heart failure, manifested by abnormal pulse rate and rhythm; abnormal respiratory rate and rhythm; deterioration of other hemodynamic parameters; decreased mentation; decreased urine output; individually defined undue or excess fatigue; and moist, cool, cyanotic skin.

Goals

1. Detect early manifestations and etiologies of decreased systemic tissue perfusion.
2. Reduce or eliminate manifestations of decreased systemic tissue perfusion.
3. Prevent manifestations of decreased systemic tissue perfusion.

Interventions

Interventions are designed to detect the manifestations of the imbalance between systemic oxygen supply and demand and to improve this imbalance by restoring the balance between myocardial oxygen supply and demand. Interventions to meet each goal include:

For Goal 1

On admission, every 4 hours, and during chest discomfort, assess, document, and report to the physician the following: abnormal heart rate and rhythm; hypotension; narrowing pulse pressure; abnormal respiratory rate and rhythm; decreased mentation; decreased urine output; increasing fatigue; and moist, cool, cyanotic skin.

For Goal 2

1. Immediately reduce patient's physical activity to the level of activity before occurrence of manifestations of decreased systemic tissue perfusion.
2. Administer oxygen and antiarrhythmic and other medications (positive inotropic, afterload-reducing, and preload-reducing agents) as ordered, and continuously evaluate the patient's response to therapy.
3. Provide a restful environment; promote the patient's physical comfort by elevating head of bed to 20 to 30 degrees or higher, or by providing a cardiac chair (depending on BP response), and by giving individualized basic nursing care.

For Goal 3

1. Provide small portions of easily digestible, low-sodium, low saturated fat foods. Provide a restful environment; as needed, assist the patient in a supportive, calm, competent manner with activities of daily living.
2. Teach patient to exhale with physical movement.
3. Offer stool softeners and laxatives to prevent straining with bowel movements. Teach patient to recognize precipitating factors of decreased systemic tissue perfusion and to alter behavior accordingly.

Outcome Criteria

Goal 1

Signs and symptoms of decreased systemic tissue perfusion are detected early.

Goal 2

BP and pulse pressure are returning or have returned to baseline level. Respiratory rate and rhythm are returning or have returned to patient's baseline. Patient remains fully alert and oriented, without personality change. Urine output remains greater than 250 cc per 8 hours. Patient's complaints of fatigue are reduced. Patient is able to carry out activities of daily living within prescribed activity limits. Extremities remain warm, dry, and of normal color.

Goal 3

Normal sinus rhythm without arrhythmia or conduction disturbance is maintained. BP and pulse pressure are maintained at patient's baseline level. Respiratory rate and rhythm are maintained at patient's baseline. Patient remains fully alert and oriented, without mental status change. Urine output remains greater than 250 cc per 8 hours. Patient does not complain of worsening fatigue. Patient is able to carry out activities of daily living within prescribed activity limits. Extremities remain warm, dry, and of normal color.

Fear or Anxiety

Diagnosis

Decreased systemic tissue perfusion related to a decrease in cardiac output from arrhythmias and conduction disturbances and from heart failure, manifested by abnormal pulse rate and rhythm; abnormal respiratory rate and rhythm; deterioration of other hemodynamic parameters; decreased mentation; decreased urine output; individually defined undue or excess fatigue; and moist, cool, cyanotic skin.

Goals

1. Detect early manifestations and etiologies of decreased systemic tissue perfusion.
2. Reduce or eliminate manifestations of decreased systemic tissue perfusion.
3. Prevent manifestations of decreased systemic tissue perfusion.

Interventions

Interventions are designed to detect the manifestations of the imbalance between systemic oxygen supply and demand and to improve this imbalance by restoring the balance between myocardial oxygen supply and demand. Interventions to meet each goal include:

For Goal 1

1. On admission, every 4 hours, and during chest discomfort, assess, document, and report to the physician the following: abnormal heart rate and rhythm; hypotension; narrowing pulse pressure; abnormal respiratory rate and rhythm; decreased mentation; decreased urine output; increasing fatigue; and moist, cool, cyanotic skin.

For Goal 2

1. Immediately reduce patient's physical activity to the level of activity before occurrence of manifestations of decreased systemic tissue perfusion.
2. Administer oxygen and antiarrhythmic and other medications (positive inotropic, afterload-reducing, and preload-reducing agents) as ordered, and continuously evaluate the patient's response to therapy.
3. Provide a restful environment; and promote the patient's physical comfort by elevating head of bed to 20 to 30 degrees or higher, or by providing a cardiac chair (depending on BP response), and by giving individualized basic nursing care.

For Goal 3

1. Provide small portions of easily digested, low-sodium, low saturated fat foods. Provide a restful environment; as needed, assist the patient in a supportive, calm, competent manner with activities of daily living.
2. Teach patient to exhale with physical movement.
3. Offer stool softeners and laxatives to prevent straining with bowel movements. Teach patient to recognize precipitating factors of decreased systemic tissue perfusion and to alter behavior accordingly.

Outcome Criteria

Goal 1

Signs and symptoms of decreased systemic tissue perfusion are detected early.

Goal 2

BP and pulse pressure are returning or have returned to baseline level. Respiratory rate and rhythm are returning or have returned to patient's baseline. Patient remains fully alert and oriented, without personality change. Urine output remains greater than 250 cc per 8 hours. Patient's complaints of fatigue are reduced. Patient is able to carry out activities of daily living within prescribed activity limits. Extremities remain warm, dry, and of normal color.

Goal 3

Normal sinus rhythm without arrhythmia or conduction disturbance is maintained. BP and pulse pressure are maintained at patient's baseline level. Respiratory rate and rhythm are maintained at patient's baseline. Patient remains fully alert and oriented, without mental status change. Urine output remains greater than 250 cc per 8 hours. Patient does not complain of worsening fatigue. Patient is able to carry out activities of daily living within prescribed activity limits. Extremities remain warm, dry, and of normal color.

Knowledge Deficit

Diagnosis

Knowledge deficit about acute MI and CHD, the medical or surgical management plan, risk factor modifications, or the return to usual activities of daily living are related to fear and anxiety, lack of recall, non-use of information, misinterpretation, cognitive limitations, disinterest, lack of familiarity with available resources, or denial of angina or acute MI; knowledge deficit is manifested by the patient being unable to describe the disease process, unable to explain the rationale behind the diagnosis, treatment, and prognosis of acute MI and CHD, unaware of activity limitations and prescribed medications, unaware of cardiac risk factors in general, or unaware of specific risk factors and how to modify them.

Goals

1. Early detection, reduction or elimination, and prevention of the specific knowledge deficit and maintenance of heart-healthy behaviors in the patient and family.
2. Specific goals should be based on each identified knowledge deficit.

Interventions

Development of a teaching plan to enables all nurses to provide standardized content to each patient.

1. Teach patient to decrease activity and take NTG as prescribed during periods of angina.
2. Teach patient to seek medical attention immediately if relief of chest discomfort has not occurred within 30 minutes; call the physician if there is a change in the pattern of angina.
3. Diagnostic procedures and interventions may be a source of anxiety and fear. Provide concrete information about procedures and describe sensory experiences that they may have. For example, "the dye (during cardiac catheterization) will make you feel hot and flushed for about 15 seconds" or "the room (cardiac catheterization laboratory) will be dimly lit and cool."
4. Teach the patient and family the content necessary for them to modify their lifestyles. Provide information about modification of risk factors such as elevated cholesterol levels, smoking, hypertension, and physical activity. Advise the patient to adhere to the prescribed therapeutic plan (diet, medication, and activity level).
5. Encourage active participation in cardiac rehabilitation programs.
6. To prevent myocardial ischemia from progressing to infarction or reinfarction, teach the patient to be aware of physiologic (such as activity during cold weather, after a heavy meal, or with sexual intercourse) and psychological (such as anger or grief) precipitating factors.
7. Teach the patient to reduce precipitating factors by taking prophylactic NTG, reducing specific physical activity and psychological stress that often result in chest discomfort, and countering emotional stress by regular physical exercise.

Outcome Criteria

The patient and family are able to describe the disease process and explain the rationale behind the diagnosis, treatment, and prognosis of acute MI and CHD. The patient and family describe activity limitations and prescribed medications. The patient and family list general and specific cardiac risk factors and describe strategies they will use to modify risk factors.

NURSING MANAGEMENT OF PATIENTS WITH RV INFARCTION

An important initial nursing consideration is to suspect RV infarction in any person admitted to an intensive care unit with an

Nursing Care Plan 22-1 ■ The Patient with RV Infarction.

Nursing Diagnosis ➧ Decreased cardiac output, related to dilated and noncompliant right ventricle, manifested by decreased BP, decreased pulmonary artery wedge pressure (PAWP), decreased urine output, cool moist skin, cyanosis, and mental confusion

Nursing Goal 1 ➧ To detect early the signs of RV dysfunction secondary to RV infarction

Outcome Criteria ➧ During hospitalization, the following signs are detected, documented, and immediately reported to the physician:

1. Physical assessment features: jugular venous distention, RV S_3 or S_4 gallop, systolic murmur of tricuspid regurgitation, hepatomegaly, peripheral edema, hypotension, urine output less than 0.5 mL/kg/h or 4 mL/k/8 h, cool, moist skin, cyanosis, mentation change
2. Right precordial electrocardiographic (ECG) features:
   ST elevation of ≥0.5–1 mm in lead V_4R
   ST elevation of ≥1 mm in lead V_4R–V_6R or V_6R only
   QS pattern in lead V_4R or V_3R–V_4R
   ST elevation in lead V_4R that is greater than the ST elevation in V_1–V_3
   ST depression in lead V_2 that is 50% or less than the magnitude of ST elevation in aVF
3. Hemodynamic profile characteristics:
   RA pressure >10 mm Hg and RA: PAWP ration ≥0.8
   RA waveform: prominent *y* descent that is at least as great as the *x* descent
   RV waveform: diastolic dip-plateau pattern ("square-root sign")
   Cardiac index <2.2 L/min/m^2

NURSING INTERVENTIONS	RATIONALE
1. On admission, every 4 hours, and with chest pain, assess, document, and report to the physician the following: a. Jugular venous distention b. RV S_3 or S_4 gallop c. Systolic murmur of tricuspid regurgitation d. Hepatomegaly e. Peripheral edema f. Clear lungs g. Hypotension h. Urine output less than 0.5 mL/kg/h or 4 mL/k/8 h i. Cool, moist, cyanotic extremities j. Mentation change	1. Required to detect changes.
2. On admission, every 8 hours the first 25 hours, and every 24 hours for at least 3 days obtain standard 12-lead ECG and right precordial ECG.	2. ST segment elevation suggestive of RV infraction may disappear in less than 10 hours from onset of chest pain, necessitating frequent serial recordings to allow documentation.
3. Continually monitor the V_4R lead in addition to conventional leads, and record a rhythm strip every 4 hours and during chest discomfort.	3. ST segment and QRS morphologic changes thought to be indicative or RV infarction frequently involve lead V_4R. Continual monitoring of this lead may provide early ECG clues to the occurrence of RV infarction and subsequently expedite appropriate treatment.
4. Assess serial (as stated in number 2) right precordial ECG for the following changes: a. ST elevation of ≥0.5–1 mm is lead V_4R b. ST elevation of ≥1 mm is lead V_4R–V_6R or V_6R only c. QS pattern in lead V_4R or V_3–V_4R d. ST elevation in V_4R greater than the ST elevation in V_1–V_3 e. ST depression in V_2 that is 50% or less than the magnitude of ST elevation in aVF	4. Clinical studies suggest that these ECG features may suggest an evolving RV infarction.
5. Record and document pressures and obtain pressure tracings as the pulmonary artery catheter is inserted into the RA, RV, pulmonary artery, and wedge position.	5. These measurements and tracings serve as a baseline for comparison of later data. Also, the hemodynamic diagnosis of RV infarction may be missed with exclusion of this step, precluding prompt treatment.
6. Measure RA pressure, PAWP, and cardiac index, and derive pulmonary and systemic vascular resistance every hour.	6. Early frequent recordings of hemodynamic parameters may aid in the recognition of low cardiac output secondary to RV infarction.

Nursing Care Plan 22-1 ■ *(continued)*

NURSING INTERVENTIONS	RATIONALE
7. Observe, document, and report the following hemodynamic patterns: **a.** RA pressure >10 mm Hg and RA:PAWP ratio of ≥ 0.8 **b.** RA waveform: prominent *y* descent that is at least as great as the *x* descent **c.** RV waveform: diastolic dip-plateau pattern ("square-root sign") **d.** Cardiac index <2.2 L/min/m^2	**7.** Investigative reports suggest that these hemodynamic criteria may be indicative of RV infarction.

Nursing Goal 2 ➧ To eliminate the signs of RV dysfunction secondary to RV infarction.

Outcome Criteria ➧ During hospitalization, the following signs are observed and documented: SBP >90 mm Hg
PAWP of 15–20 mm Hg
Urine output = at least 0.5 mL/kg/h or 4 mL/kg/8h
Cardiac index >2.2 L/min/m^2
Skin pink, warm, dry
Mentation unchanged

NURSING INTERVENTIONS	RATIONALE
1. Infuse IV fluid bolus per physician protocol to attain a PAWP of 15–20 mm Hg.	**1.** Initial rapid volume expansion increases RV end-diastolic volume, which may optimize contractility of a diastolic noncompliant RV.
2. Administer positive inotropic agents such as dobutamine or dopamine per physician protocol. Monitor heart rate and rhythm for development of tachycardia or tachyarrhythmias.	**2.** Dobutamine (2–20 μg/kg/min) and dopamine (2–10 μg/kg/min) directly stimulate β-adrenergic myocardial receptors, resulting in increased contractility and cardiac output. Although dobutamine is less arrhythmogenic than dopamine, both agents may precipitate tachycardia and tachyarrhythmias, resulting in decreased diastolic filling and reduced cardiac output.
3. Administer peripheral vasodilators such as nitroprusside or hydralazine per physician protocol. Monitor pulmonary and systemic vascular resistance at least every hour.	**3.** These agents decrease RV and LV afterload, thereby enhancing RV and LV stroke volume. Hydralazine may be preferable because it selectively vasodilates arterioles and should not decrease preload. Pulmonary and systemic vascular resistance parameters are necessary to optimize preload and afterload.
4. When pacing therapy is indicated, institute atrial or atrioventricular sequential method per physician protocol.	**4.** Preservation of atrioventricular synchronous contraction maximizes contractility and cardiac output.
5. Avoid administration of drugs and performance of maneuvers that decrease preload: **a.** Diuretics **b.** Venodilators (NTG, morphine) **c.** Sitting up in bed **d.** Valsalva maneuver	**5.** Filling of the left ventricle is dependent on distention of the right ventricle. These actions decrease preload, thereby reducing stretch of the RV myocardial fibers and further compromising the ability of the noncompliant chamber to propel blood forward. Reduced cardiac output results.

*Contributed by Sherri Del Bene and Anne Vaughan.

acute inferior or posterior LV infarction. A right precordial ECG should be obtained for any patient with evidence of an inferior MI. Initial clues to the development of RV dysfunction may be subtle. In addition, the low cardiac output syndrome may be thought secondary to primary LV dysfunction. The major differences between the low cardiac output state of predominant RV and LV infarction are listed in Table 22-6. Critical care nurses can facilitate the diagnosis and appropriate management of patients with RV infarction through awareness of the usual clinical features and electrocardiographic changes associated with RV infarction and the systematic and continual assessment of these features as well as the evaluation of the patient's response to therapy.

Patients with RV infarction experience similar alterations in functional health status as those with LV infarction. Nursing Care Plan 22-1 encompasses altered health patterns of patients with MI. In the setting of RV infarction, however, decreased cardiac output is a potential nursing problem that requires a different approach in terms of detection, assessment, and treatment.

Table 22-6 ■ MAJOR DIFFERENCES IN THE LOW CARDIAC OUTPUT SYNDROMES OF PREDOMINANT RIGHT VENTRICULAR VERSUS LEFT VENTRICULAR INFARCTION

	Right Ventricle	Left Ventricle
Physical examination	Clear lungs Systemic venous congestion Jugular venous distention S_3 or S_4 may be present Tricuspid regurgitation	Crackles, pulmonary edema No systemic venous congestion Normal jugular veins S_3 or S_4 may be present Mitral regurgitation
Hemodynamic profile	CI <2.2 L/min/m^2	CI <2.2 L/min/m^2 PAWP >18 mm Hg Decreased preload
Treatment	Increase preload Volume dependent Avoid diuretics and nitrates Give inotropes Reduce RV afterload by decreasing PA pressure (milrinone) Reperfuse	Decrease preload Limit volume administration Give diuretics and nitrates Give inotropes Reduce LV afterload and increase myocardial perfusion with IABP Reperfuse

CI, cardiac index; PAWP, pulmonary artery wedge pressure; IABP, intra-aortic balloon pump.

REFERENCES

1. American Heart Association. (2008). *Heart disease and stroke statistics—2008 update.* Dallas, TX: Author.
2. Antman, E. M., Anbe, D. T., Armstrong, P. W., et al. (2004). ACC/AHA guidelines for the management of patients with ST-elevation myocardial infarction—Executive summary. A report of the American College of Cardiology/American Heart Association Task Force on Practice Guidelines (Writing Committee to Revise the 1999 Guidelines for the Management of Patients With Acute Myocardial Infarction). *Journal of American College of Cardiology, 44*(3), 671–719.
3. Antman, E. M., Hand, M., Armstrong, P. W., et al. (2008). 2007 Focused update of the ACC/AHA 2004 guidelines for the management of patients with ST-elevation myocardial infarction: A report of the American College of Cardiology/American Heart Association Task Force on Practice Guidelines: Developed in collaboration with the Canadian Cardiovascular Society endorsed by the American Academy of Family Physicians: 2007 Writing Group to Review New Evidence and Update the ACC/AHA 2004 Guidelines for the Management of Patients With ST-Elevation Myocardial Infarction, Writing on Behalf of the 2004 Writing Committee. *Circulation, 117*(2), 296–329.
4. Anderson, J. L., Adams, C. D., Antman, E. M., et al. (2007). ACC/AHA 2007 guidelines for the management of patients with unstable angina/non-ST-elevation myocardial infarction: A report of the American College of Cardiology/American Heart Association Task Force on Practice Guidelines (Writing Committee to Revise the 2002 Guidelines for the Management of Patients With Unstable Angina/Non-ST-Elevation Myocardial Infarction) developed in collaboration with the American College of Emergency Physicians, the Society for Cardiovascular Angiography and Interventions, and the Society of Thoracic Surgeons endorsed by the American Association of Cardiovascular and Pulmonary Rehabilitation and the Society for Academic Emergency Medicine. *Journal of American College of Cardiology, 50*(7), e1–e157.
5. Krumholz, H. M., Anderson, J. L., Brooks, N. H., et al. (2006). ACC/AHA clinical performance measures for adults with ST-elevation and non-ST-elevation myocardial infarction: A report of the American College of Cardiology/American Heart Association Task Force on Performance Measures (Writing Committee to Develop Performance Measures on ST-Elevation and Non-ST-Elevation Myocardial Infarction). *Journal of American College of Cardiology, 47*(1), 236–265.
6. Moliterno, D. J., & Saw, J. (2005). Differences between unstable angina and acute myocardial infarction: Pathophysiological and clinical spectrum. In E. Topol (Ed.), *Acute coronary syndromes* (3rd ed., (pp. 637–687). New York: Marcel Dekker.
7. Jayes, R. L., Jr., Beshansky, J. R., D'Agostino, R. B., et al. (1992). Do patients' coronary risk factor reports predict acute cardiac ischemia in the emergency department? A multicenter study. *Journal of Clinical Epidemiology, 45*(6), 621–626.
8. Galvani, M., Ottani, F., Oltrona, L., et al. (2004). N-terminal pro-brain natriuretic peptide on admission has prognostic value across the whole spectrum of acute coronary syndromes. *Circulation, 110*(2), 128–134.
9. Morrow, D. A., de Lemos, J. A., Sabatine, M. S., et al. (2003). Evaluation of B-type natriuretic peptide for risk assessment in unstable angina/non-ST-elevation myocardial infarction: B-type natriuretic peptide and prognosis in TACTICS-TIMI 18. *Journal of American College of Cardiology, 41*(8), 1264–1272.
10. Palazzuoli, A., Deckers, J., Calabro, A., et al. (2006). Brain natriuretic peptide and other risk markers for outcome assessment in patients with non-ST-elevation coronary syndromes and preserved systolic function. *American Journal of Cardiology, 98*(10), 1322–1328.
11. Newell, M., Browning, J., Larson, D., et al. (2008). Optimizing door-to-ballon times: A useful measure of STEMI for hospitals of all levels. *Cardiac Interventions Today, 2*, 32–35.
12. Boden, W. E., Eagle, K., & Granger, C. B. (2007). Reperfusion strategies in acute ST-segment elevation myocardial infarction: A comprehensive review of contemporary management options. *Journal of American College of Cardiology, 50*(10), 917–929.
13. Boersma, E., Maas, A. C., Deckers, J. W., et al. (1996). Early thrombolytic treatment in acute myocardial infarction: Reappraisal of the golden hour. *Lancet, 348*(9030), 771–775.
14. Fibrinolytic Therapy Trialists' (FTT) Collaborative Group. (1994). Indications for fibrinolytic therapy in suspected acute myocardial infarction: Collaborative overview of early mortality and major morbidity results from all randomised trials of more than 1000 patients. *Lancet, 343*(8893), 311–322.
15. The GUSTO investigators. (1993). An international randomized trial comparing four thrombolytic strategies for acute myocardial infarction. *New England Journal of Medicine, 329*(10), 673–682.
16. Berger, P. B., Ellis, S. G., Holmes, D. R., Jr., et al. (1999). Relationship between delay in performing direct coronary angioplasty and early clinical outcome in patients with acute myocardial infarction: Results from the global use of strategies to open occluded arteries in Acute Coronary Syndromes (GUSTO-IIb) trial. *Circulation, 100*(1), 14–20.
17. Brodie, B. R., Hansen, C., Stuckey, T. D., et al. (2006). Door-to-balloon time with primary percutaneous coronary intervention for acute myocardial infarction impacts late cardiac mortality in high-risk patients and patients presenting early after the onset of symptoms. *Journal of American College of Cardiology, 47*(2), 289–295.

18. Cannon, C. P., Gibson, C. M., Lambrew, C. T., et al. (2000). Relationship of symptom-onset-to-balloon time and door-to-balloon time with mortality in patients undergoing angioplasty for acute myocardial infarction. *JAMA, 283*(22), 2941–2947.
19. De Luca, G., van't Hof, A. W. J., de Boer, M. J., et al. (2004). Time-to-treatment significantly affects the extent of ST-segment resolution and myocardial blush in patients with acute myocardial infarction treated by primary angioplasty. *European Heart Journal, 25*(12), 1009–1013.
20. Shavelle, D. M., Rasouli, M. L., Frederick, P., et al. (2005). Outcome in patients transferred for percutaneous coronary intervention (a national registry of myocardial infarction 2/3/4 analysis). *American Journal of Cardiology, 96*(9), 1227–1232.
21. Hochman, J. S., Lamas, G. A., Buller, C. E., et al. (2006). Coronary intervention for persistent occlusion after myocardial infarction. *New England Journal of Medicine, 355*(23), 2395–2407.
22. DeWood, M. A., Spores, J., Notske, R., et al. (1980). Prevalence of total coronary occlusion during the early hours of transmural myocardial infarction. *New England Journal of Medicine, 303*(16), 897–902.
23. Rentrop, K. P., Blanke, H., Karsch, K. R., et al. (1979). Acute myocardial infarction: Intracoronary application of nitroglycerin and streptokinase. *Clinical Cardiology, 2*(5), 354–363.
24. Kennedy, J. W., Ritchie, J. L., Davis, K. B., et al. (1983). Western Washington randomized trial of intracoronary streptokinase in acute myocardial infarction. *New England Journal of Medicine, 309*(24), 1477–1482.
25. Simoons, M. L., Serruys, P. W., vd Brand, M., et al. (1985). Improved survival after early thrombolysis in acute myocardial infarction. A randomised trial by the Interuniversity Cardiology Institute in The Netherlands. *Lancet, 2*(8455), 578–582.
26. Gruppo Italiano per lo Studio della Streptochinasi nell'Infarto Miocardico (GISSI). (1986). Effectiveness of intravenous thrombolytic treatment in acute myocardial infarction. *Lancet, 1*(8478), 397–402.
27. Nallamothu, B. K., Bradley, E. H., & Krumholz, H. M. (2007). Time to treatment in primary percutaneous coronary intervention. *New England Journal of Medicine, 357*(16), 1631–1638.
28. Thrombolysis in Myocardial Ischemia (TIMI) Investigators. (1994). Effects of tissue plasminogen activator and a comparison of early invasive and conservative strategies in unstable angina and non-Q-wave myocardial infarction. Results of the TIMI IIIB Trial. *Circulation, 89*(4), 1545–1556.
29. Baigent, C., Collins, R., Appleby, P., et al. (1998). ISIS-2: 10 year survival among patients with suspected acute myocardial infarction in randomised comparison of intravenous streptokinase, oral aspirin, both, or neither. The ISIS-2 (Second International Study of Infarct Survival) Collaborative Group. *BMJ, 316*(7141), 1337–1343.
30. Franzosi, M. G., Santoro, E., De Vita, C., et al. (1998). Ten-year follow-up of the first megatrial testing thrombolytic therapy in patients with acute myocardial infarction: Results of the Gruppo Italiano per lo Studio della Sopravvivenza nell'Infarto-1 study. The GISSI Investigators. *Circulation, 98*(24), 2659–2665.
31. Morrison, L. J., Verbeek, P. R., McDonald, A. C., et al. (2000). Mortality and prehospital thrombolysis for acute myocardial infarction: A meta-analysis. *JAMA, 283*(20), 2686–2692.
32. Morrow, D. A., Antman, E. M., Sayah, A., et al. (2002). Evaluation of the time saved by prehospital initiation of reteplase for ST-elevation myocardial infarction: Results of The Early Retavase-Thrombolysis in Myocardial Infarction (ER-TIMI) 19 trial. *Journal of American College of Cardiology, 40*(1), 71–77.
33. The European Myocardial Infarction Project Group. (1993). Prehospital thrombolytic therapy in patients with suspected acute myocardial infarction. *New England Journal of Medicine, 329*(6), 383–389.
34. Weaver, W. D., Cerqueira, M., Hallstrom, A. P., et al. (1993). Prehospital-initiated vs hospital-initiated thrombolytic therapy. The Myocardial Infarction Triage and Intervention Trial. *JAMA, 270*(10), 1211–1216.
35. Castaigne, A. D., Herve, C., Duval-Moulin, A. M., et al. (1989). Prehospital use of APSAC: Results of a placebo-controlled study. *American Journal of Cardiology, 64*(2), 30A–33A; discussion 41A–42A.
36. GREAT Group. (1992). Feasibility, safety, and efficacy of domiciliary thrombolysis by general practitioners: Grampian region early anistreplase trial. *BMJ, 305*(6853), 548–553.
37. Roth, A., Barbash, G. I., Hod, H., et al. (1990). Should thrombolytic therapy be administered in the mobile intensive care unit in patients with evolving myocardial infarction? A pilot study. *Journal of American College of Cardiology, 15*(5), 932–936.
38. Schofer, J., Buttner, J., Geng, G., et al. (1990). Prehospital thrombolysis in acute myocardial infarction. *American Journal of Cardiology, 66*(20), 1429–1433.
39. Tillett, W. S., & Garner, R. L. (1933). The fibrinolytic activity of hemolytic streptococci. *Journal of Experimental Medicine, 58*, 485–502.
40. Bates, E. R. (2008). Infusion fibrinolytic therapy. In E. R. Bates (Ed.), *Reperfusion therapy for acute myocardial infarction* (pp. 43–58). New York: Informa Heath Care.
41. Bates, E. R. (2005). Fibrinolysis for ST-elevation myocardial infarction: First and second generation agents. In E. J. Topol (Ed.), *Acute coronary syndromes* (3rd ed., pp. 199–216). New York: Informa Health Care.
42. The Global Use of Strategies to Open Occluded Coronary Arteries (GUSTO III) Investigators. (1997). A comparison of reteplase with alteplase for acute myocardial infarction. *New England Journal of Medicine, 337*(16), 1118–1123.
43. Brener, S. J. (2005). Third-generation fibrinolytic agents and combined fibrinoplatelet lysis for acute myocardial infarction. In E. J. Topol (Ed.), *Acute coronary syndromes* (3rd ed., pp. 217–232). New York: Informa Health Care.
44. Bode, C., Smalling, R. W., Berg, G., et al. (1996). Randomized comparison of coronary thrombolysis achieved with double-bolus reteplase (recombinant plasminogen activator) and front-loaded, accelerated alteplase (recombinant tissue plasminogen activator) in patients with acute myocardial infarction. The RAPID II Investigators. *Circulation, 94*(5), 891–898.
45. Van De Werf, F., Adgey, J., Ardissino, D., et al. (1999). Single-bolus tenecteplase compared with front-loaded alteplase in acute myocardial infarction: The ASSENT-2 double-blind randomised trial. *Lancet, 354*(9180), 716–722.
46. Thompson, P. L., Aylward, P. E., Federman, J., et al. (1991). A randomized comparison of intravenous heparin with oral aspirin and dipyridamole 24 hours after recombinant tissue-type plasminogen activator for acute myocardial infarction. National Heart Foundation of Australia Coronary Thrombolysis Group. *Circulation, 83*(5), 1534–1542.
47. Warkentin, T. E., Levine, M. N., Hirsh, J., et al. (1995). Heparin-induced thrombocytopenia in patients treated with low-molecular-weight heparin or unfractionated heparin. *New England Journal of Medicine, 332*(20), 1330–1335.
48. Antman, E. M., Morrow, D. A., McCabe, C. H., et al. (2006). Enoxaparin versus unfractionated heparin with fibrinolysis for ST-elevation myocardial infarction. *New England Journal of Medicine, 354*(14), 1477–1488.
49. Gibson, C. M., Murphy, S. A., Montalescot, G., et al. (2007). Percutaneous coronary intervention in patients receiving enoxaparin or unfractionated heparin after fibrinolytic therapy for ST-segment elevation myocardial infarction in the ExTRACT-TIMI 25 trial. *Journal of American College of Cardiology, 49*(23), 2238–2246.
50. Giraldez, R. R., Nicolau, J. C., Corbalan, R., et al. (2007). Enoxaparin is superior to unfractionated heparin in patients with ST elevation myocardial infarction undergoing fibrinolysis regardless of the choice of lytic: An ExTRACT-TIMI 25 analysis. *European Heart Journal, 28*(13), 1566–1573.
51. White, H. D., Braunwald, E., Murphy, S. A., et al. (2007). Enoxaparin vs. unfractionated heparin with fibrinolysis for ST-elevation myocardial infarction in elderly and younger patients: Results from ExTRACT-TIMI 25. *European Heart Journal, 28*(9), 1066–1071.
52. Yusuf, S., Mehta, S. R., Chrolavicius, S., et al. (2006). Effects of fondaparinux on mortality and reinfarction in patients with acute ST-segment elevation myocardial infarction: The OASIS-6 randomized trial. *JAMA, 295*(13), 1519–1530.
53. King, S. B., III, Smith, S. C., Jr., Hirshfeld, J. W., Jr., et al. (2008). 2007 focused update of the ACC/AHA/SCAI 2005 guideline update for percutaneous coronary intervention: A report of the American College of Cardiology/American Heart Association Task Force on Practice guidelines. *Journal of American College of Cardiology, 51*(2), 172–209.
54. Becker, R. C. (2008). Clinical trials of platelet glycoprotein IIb/IIIa receptor inhibitors in coronary heart disease: Intravenous agents. *UpToDate*. Retrieved August, 2008, http://www.uptodateonline.com/online/content/topic.do?topicKey=chd/31791&selectedTitle=6~150&source=search_result.
55. Brener, S. J., Zeymer, U., Adgey, A. A., et al. (2002). Eptifibatide and low-dose tissue plasminogen activator in acute myocardial infarction: The integrilin and low-dose thrombolysis in acute myocardial infarction (INTRO AMI) trial. *Journal of American College of Cardiology, 39*(3), 377–386.
56. Gold, H. K., Garabedian, H. D., Dinsmore, R. E., et al. (1997). Restoration of coronary flow in myocardial infarction by intravenous chimeric 7E3 antibody without exogenous plasminogen activators. Observations in animals and humans. *Circulation, 95*(7), 1755–1759.
57. SPEED Investigators. (2000). Trial of abciximab with and without low-dose reteplase for acute myocardial infarction. Strategies for Patency Enhancement in the Emergency Department (SPEED) Group. *Circulation, 101*(24), 2788–2794.

58. Eisenberg, M. J., & Jamal, S. (2003). Glycoprotein IIb/IIIa inhibition in the setting of acute ST-segment elevation myocardial infarction. *Journal of American College of Cardiology, 42*(1), 1–6.
59. Topol, E. J. (2001). Reperfusion therapy for acute myocardial infarction with fibrinolytic therapy or combination reduced fibrinolytic therapy and platelet glycoprotein IIb/IIIa inhibition: The GUSTO V randomised trial. *Lancet, 357*(9272), 1905–1914.
60. ASSENT-3 Investigators. (2001). Efficacy and safety of tenecteplase in combination with enoxaparin, abciximab, or unfractionated heparin: The ASSENT-3 randomised trial in acute myocardial infarction. *Lancet, 358*(9282), 605–613.
61. Aversano, T., Aversano, L. T., Passamani, E., et al. (2002). Thrombolytic therapy vs primary percutaneous coronary intervention for myocardial infarction in patients presenting to hospitals without on-site cardiac surgery: A randomized controlled trial. *JAMA, 287*(15), 1943–1951.
62. Garcia, E., Elizaga, J., Perez-Castellano, N., et al. (1999). Primary angioplasty versus systemic thrombolysis in anterior myocardial infarction. *Journal of American College of Cardiology, 33*(3), 605–611.
63. Grines, C. L., Browne, K. F., Marco, J., et al. (1993). A comparison of immediate angioplasty with thrombolytic therapy for acute myocardial infarction. The Primary Angioplasty in Myocardial Infarction Study Group. *New England Journal of Medicine, 328*(10), 673–679.
64. Ribichini, F., Steffenino, G., Dellavalle, A., et al. (1998). Comparison of thrombolytic therapy and primary coronary angioplasty with liberal stenting for inferior myocardial infarction with precordial ST-segment depression: Immediate and long-term results of a randomized study. *Journal of American College of Cardiology, 32*(6), 1687–1694.
65. The Global Use of Strategies to Open Occluded Coronary Arteries in Acute Coronary Syndromes (GUSTO IIb) Angioplasty Substudy Investigators. (1997). A clinical trial comparing primary coronary angioplasty with tissue plasminogen activator for acute myocardial infarction. *New England Journal of Medicine, 336*(23), 1621–1628.
66. Zijlstra, F., de Boer, M. J., Hoorntje, J. C., et al. (1993). A comparison of immediate coronary angioplasty with intravenous streptokinase in acute myocardial infarction. *New England Journal of Medicine, 328*(10), 680–684.
67. Antman, E. M., Cohen, M., Bernink, P. J., et al. (2000). The TIMI risk score for unstable angina/non-ST elevation MI: A method for prognostication and therapeutic decision making. *JAMA, 284*(7), 835–842.
68. Boersma, E., Pieper, K. S., Steyerberg, E. W., et al. (2000). Predictors of outcome in patients with acute coronary syndromes without persistent ST-segment elevation. Results from an international trial of 9461 patients. The PURSUIT Investigators. *Circulation, 101*(22), 2557–2567.
69. Eagle, K. A., Lim, M. J., Dabbous, O. H., et al. (2004). A validated prediction model for all forms of acute coronary syndrome: Estimating the risk of 6-month postdischarge death in an international registry. *JAMA, 291*(22), 2727–2733.
70. Granger, C. B., Goldberg, R. J., Dabbous, O., et al. (2003). Predictors of hospital mortality in the global registry of acute coronary events. *Achieves of Internal Medicine, 163*(19), 2345–2353.
71. Pollack, C. V., Jr., Sites, F. D., Shofer, F. S., et al. (2006). Application of the TIMI risk score for unstable angina and non-ST elevation acute coronary syndrome to an unselected emergency department chest pain population. *Academic Emergency Medicine, 13*(1), 13–18.
72. Flaker, G. C., Warnica, J. W., Sacks, F. M., et al. (1999). Pravastatin prevents clinical events in revascularized patients with average cholesterol concentrations. Cholesterol and Recurrent Events CARE Investigators. *Journal of American College of Cardiology, 34*(1), 106–112.
73. Chobanian, A. V., Bakris, G. L., Black, H. R., et al. (2003). The Seventh Report of the Joint National Committee on Prevention, Detection, Evaluation, and Treatment of High Blood Pressure: the JNC 7 report. *JAMA, 289*(19), 2560–2572.
74. Agency for Health Care Policy & Research. (1996). *Clinical practice guidelines: Number 18: Smoking cessation* (AHCPR Publication No. 96-0692). Retrieved from.
75. Tonstad, S., Tønnesen, P., Hajek, P., et al. (2006). Effect of maintenance therapy with varenicline on smoking cessation: A randomized controlled trial. *JAMA, 296*(1), 64–71.
76. Ahmed, S., Cannon, C. P., Murphy, S. A., et al. (2006). Acute coronary syndromes and diabetes: Is intensive lipid lowering beneficial? Results of the PROVE IT-TIMI 22 trial. *European Heart Journal, 27*(19), 2323–2329.
77. Thompson, P. D. (2005). Exercise prescription and proscription for patients with coronary artery disease. *Circulation, 112*(15), 2354–2363.
78. Thompson, P. D., Buchner, D., Pina, I. L., et al. (2003). Exercise and physical activity in the prevention and treatment of atherosclerotic cardiovascular disease: A statement from the Council on Clinical Cardiology (Subcommittee on Exercise, Rehabilitation, and Prevention) and the Council on Nutrition, Physical Activity, and Metabolism (Subcommittee on Physical Activity). *Circulation, 107*(24), 3109–3116.
79. Balady, G. J., Ades, P. A., Comoss, P., et al. (2000). Core components of cardiac rehabilitation/secondary prevention programs: A statement for healthcare professionals from the American Heart Association and the American Association of Cardiovascular and Pulmonary Rehabilitation Writing Group. *Circulation, 102*(9), 1069–1073.
80. Smith, S. C., Jr., Allen, J., Blair, S. N., et al. (2006). AHA/ACC guidelines for secondary prevention for patients with coronary and other atherosclerotic vascular disease: 2006 update endorsed by the National Heart, Lung, and Blood Institute. *Journal of American College of Cardiology, 47*(10), 2130–2139.
81. Cullen, B. (2007). *Physicians' desk reference* (Vol. 61). New York: Thompson PDR, Simon & Schuster.
82. Chen, Z. M., Pan, H. C., Chen, Y. P., et al. (2005). Early intravenous then oral metoprolol in 45,852 patients with acute myocardial infarction: Randomised placebo-controlled trial. *Lancet, 366*(9497), 1622–1632.
83. CAPRIE Steering Committee. (1996). A randomised, blinded, trial of clopidogrel versus aspirin in patients at risk of ischaemic events (CAPRIE). *Lancet, 348*(9038), 1329–1339.
84. Kulkarni, R. A. (2000). Clopidogrel in cardiovascular disorders. *Journal of Postgraduate Medicine, 46*(4), 312–313.
85. Hofmann, L. V., Razavi, M., Arepally, A., et al. (2001). GPIIb-IIIa receptor inhibitors: What the interventional radiologist needs to know. *Cardiovascular and Interventional Radiology, 24*(6), 361–367.
86. Berkowitz, S. D., Sane, D. C., Sigmon, K. N., et al. (1998). Occurrence and clinical significance of thrombocytopenia in a population undergoing high-risk percutaneous coronary revascularization. Evaluation of c7E3 for the Prevention of Ischemic Complications (EPIC) Study Group. *Journal of American College of Cardiology, 32*(2), 311–319.
87. McClure, M. W., Berkowitz, S. D., Sparapani, R., et al. (1999). Clinical significance of thrombocytopenia during a non-ST-elevation acute coronary syndrome. The platelet glycoprotein IIb/IIIa in unstable angina: Receptor suppression using integrilin therapy (PURSUIT) trial experience. *Circulation, 99*(22), 2892–2900.
88. Antman, E. M., McCabe, C. H., Gurfinkel, E. P., et al. (1999). Enoxaparin prevents death and cardiac ischemic events in unstable angina/non-Q-wave myocardial infarction. Results of the thrombolysis in myocardial infarction (TIMI) 11B trial. *Circulation, 100*(15), 1593–1601.
89. Cohen, M., Demers, C., Gurfinkel, E. P., et al. (1997). A comparison of low-molecular-weight heparin with unfractionated heparin for unstable coronary artery disease. Efficacy and Safety of Subcutaneous Enoxaparin in Non-Q-Wave Coronary Events Study Group. *New England Journal of Medicine, 337*(7), 447–452.
90. Ferguson, J. J., Califf, R. M., Antman, E. M., et al. (2004). Enoxaparin vs unfractionated heparin in high-risk patients with non-ST-segment elevation acute coronary syndromes managed with an intended early invasive strategy: Primary results of the SYNERGY randomized trial. *JAMA, 292*(1), 45–54.
91. Simons, M. (2008). Direct thrombin inhibitors. Anticoagulant therapy in unstable angina and acute non-ST elevation myocardial infarction. UpToDate Online, version 16.3, accessed August, 2008
92. Kastrati, A., Neumann, F. J., Mehilli, J., et al. (2008). Bivalirudin versus unfractionated heparin during percutaneous coronary intervention. *New England Journal of Medicine, 359*(7), 688–696.
93. Aschenbrenner, D. S. (2009). Drugs affecting coagulation. In D. S. Aschenbrenner & S. J. Venable (Eds.), *Drug therapy in nursing* (3rd ed., pp. 594–626). Philadelphia: Lippincott Williams & Wilkins.
94. Simons, M. (2008). Fondaparinux. Anticoagulant therapy in unstable angina and acute non-ST elevation myocardial infarction UpToDate Online, version 16.3, retrieved date August, 2008
95. Fondaparinux Drug Information. (2008). UpToDate Online, version 16.3, Accessed January 2009.
96. Antman, E. M., & Braunwald, E. (2001). Acute myocardial infarction. In E. Braunwald (Ed.), *Heart disease: A textbook of cardiovascular medicine* (6th ed., Vol. 2, pp. 1114–1231). St. Louis, MO: W.B. Saunders.
97. Dzavik, V., & Hochman, J. S. (2005). Cardiogenic shock and heart failure complicating acute myocardial infarction. In E. Topol (Ed.), *Acute coronary syndromes* (3rd ed., pp. 657–687). New York: Marcel Dekker.
98. Chesebro, J. H., Knatterud, G., Roberts, R., et al. (1987). Thrombolysis in Myocardial Infarction (TIMI) Trial, Phase I: A comparison between intravenous tissue plasminogen activator and intravenous streptokinase. Clinical findings through hospital discharge. *Circulation, 76*(1), 142–154.

CHAPTER 23

Interventional Cardiology Techniques: Percutaneous Coronary Intervention

Michaelene Hargrove Deelstra

More than 30 years has passed since the introduction of coronary angioplasty by Andreas Gruentzig in 1977.[1] Interventional cardiology has continued to evolve and improve techniques and procedures for percutaneous treatment of coronary heart disease (CHD). Interventional coronary devices used to restore or enhance myocardial blood flow include angioplasty balloons, atherectomy devices, and intracoronary stents. Pharmacological therapies have been an important partner in the development of device technology. This interventional cardiology chapter provides a review and understanding of the evolution of device technology, patient management, the current trends and devices used in the catheterization laboratory today to treat CHD, and a look at percutaneous devices used for the treatment of cardiac structural abnormalities.

The term *percutaneous coronary intervention* (*PCI*) refers to the collective group of interventional procedures performed through a percutaneous approach in the coronary arteries. PCI was initially limited to balloon angioplasty but now encompasses other procedures using atherectomy devices, thrombectomy devices, and bare metal and drug-eluting stents (DES). Factors that have improved the overall success and complication rates include operator experience, modifications in procedural instruments, newer interventional devices, and advances in adjunctive pharmacologic therapy. These improvements have led to the expansion of interventional cardiology treatment to higher risk patients with more complex coronary lesions and comorbidities. These improvements have influenced the short- and long-term success of PCI.[2]

PATIENT SELECTION FOR PCI

The American College of Cardiology/American Heart Association/ Society for Cardiovascular Angiography and Interventions (ACC/AHA/SCAI) task force provides broad guidelines and recommendations for appropriate application of PCI technology based on scientific evidence for revascularization. Recommendations for revascularization with PCI include patients presenting with significant ischemia on noninvasive testing, unstable angina, and acute coronary syndrome (ACS). When the patient is considered for revascularization with PCI, the potential risks and benefits should be discussed in detail with the patient and family and be weighed against alternative therapies such as medical therapy or coronary artery bypass graft (CABG) surgery. Patients should understand the possible complications associated with the procedure, the possibility of restenosis, stent thrombosis (see complications) postprocedure, and the potential for incomplete revascularization in patients with diffuse coronary artery disease (CAD). The clinical and angiographic variables associated with increased mortality include advanced age, female sex, diabetes mellitus, prior myocardial infarction (MI), multivessel disease, left main disease or equivalent (severe stenosis of the left anterior descending artery and circumflex arteries proximal to any major branch), a large area of myocardium at risk, pre-existing impairment of left ventricular (LV) function or renal function, and collateral vessels supplying significant areas of myocardium that originate distal to the segment to be treated.[3]

ACC/AHA/SCAI[4] recommends an early invasive strategy with PCI in patients with unstable angina/non-ST-elevation MI (NSTEMI) who exhibit the following:

- Recurrent angina, ischemia at rest or with low-level activities despite intensive medical therapy
- Elevated cardiac biomarkers, new or presumed new ST-segment depression
- Signs or symptoms of heart failure or new worsening mitral regurgitation
- High-risk findings on noninvasive testing or hemodynamic instability
- Sustained ventricular tachycardia and prior CABG or reduced LV ejection fraction <.40.
- PCI is not indicated for a persistently occluded infarct-related artery after NSTEMI or ST-elevation MI (STEMI) older than 24 hours in a stable, asymptomatic patient.

In patients with stable CAD optimal medical therapy alone can be considered versus PCI with optimal medical therapy. PCI when added to optimal medical therapy in stable angina has been shown to reduce the prevalence of angina symptoms but not to reduce long-term rates of death, MI, or hospitalization for ACS.[5]

Special Subgroups of Patients Receiving PCI

Patients Receiving Fibrinolytic Therapy

Facilitated PCI refers to a strategy of planned immediate PCI after the administration of an initial pharmacological regimen intended to improve coronary patency before the procedure. Clinical trials of facilitated PCI have not demonstrated benefit in reducing infarct size or improving outcomes. In patients with STEMI, a planned reperfusion strategy using full-dose fibrinolytic therapy (Chapter 22) followed by immediate PCI may be harmful and is not advocated.

Coronary angiography and intent to perform revascularization are recommended for patients who have received fibrinolytic therapy, are in cardiogenic shock, are candidates for PCI, and have severe heart failure or pulmonary edema or hemodynamically significant ventricular arrhythmias. Rescue PCI should be considered in patients with STEMI who have received fibrinolytic agents and have evidence of failed reperfusion (ST-segment resolution <50%) 90 minutes after initiation of fibrinolytic therapy, and have a moderate-to-large area of myocardium at risk.[4]

Women

Women presenting with CHD frequently have increased severity of disease at time of presentation. Women are generally older when they present with their first coronary event, and often have have diffuse atherosclerotic disease and a higher incidence of co-morbidities, including hypertension, diabetes mellitus, hypercholesterolemia, peripheral vascular disease, and unstable angina. Women have an excellent long-term prognosis after a successful procedure even though coronary vessel lumen may be smaller. Although newer revascularization procedures with stents and concomitant use of glycoprotein (GP) IIb/IIIa receptor inhibitors have shown similar benefit in women as men, these interventions have not eliminated the gender difference in mortality that has persistently shown higher rates with device treatment in the setting of ACS and elective procedures in women.[3,6]

Patients With Diabetes Mellitus

Patients with diabetes mellitus account for about 20% of revascularization procedures. PCI in patients with diabetes is associated with less favorable long-term outcomes, need for repeat intervention because of restenosis, multivessel disease, and possible progression of underlying disease. Current guidelines have favored CABG surgery for patients with diabetes who have two-or-three vessel disease because of more complete revascularization and decreased need for repeat intervention.[7–9] Use of DES has improved the long-term outcomes in patients with diabetes who have single-vessel disease.[10] An intravenous GP IIb/IIIa receptor inhibitor should be administered for diabetic patients with unstable angina or NSTEMI; GP IIb/IIIa receptor inhibitors appear to improve the outcome of PCI with reduced death, MI and repeat revascularization.[11]

Patients With Multivessel CAD

The two primary interventions for multivessel CAD are PCI and CABG. Several randomized and observation studies have compared the long-term outcomes of these two interventions before the introduction of DES. These trials demonstrated that in appropriately selected patients with multivessel coronary disease, an initial strategy of standard PCI with bare metal stent (BMS) yields similar overall outcomes to initial revascularization with CABG. An important exception is in the subgroup of patients with diabetes mellitus who had reduced cardiac mortality with CABG compared to PCI. Patient preference, patient compliance with dual antiplatelet therapy, surgical risk, angiographic characteristics, LV function, and co-morbid issues need to be considered before a treatment strategy is selected.[12]

An observational study from the New York State Registry identified patients with multivessel disease who received DES or underwent CABG. Conclusions from the registry indicated lower mortality rates and repeat revascularization with CABG compared to DES.[13] Currently, ongoing multicenter, randomized, controlled trials such as SYNTAX (Synergy between PCI with Taxus and Cardiac Surgery) and FREEDOM (Future Revascularization Evaluation in Patients With Diabetes Mellitus—Optimal Management of Multivessel Disease), are evaluating multivessel DES versus bypass surgery in different subsets of patients and will provide guidance for selection of treatment that will benefit specific groups of patients.[12]

Older Adults

Patients aged 75 years and older should be considered for PCI in a similar manner as younger patients. Decisions should not be based solely on chronologic age but should be patient centered with consideration of the patient's general health, functional and cognitive status, comorbidities, life expectancy, and preference and goals. Clinical trials have shown benefits from early invasive procedures with similar success rates as younger patients but with higher risks of bleeding and vascular complications. Older adults often have altered pharmacokinetics, risk of drug interactions, and polypharmacy contributing to complications.[14] Increased risk of neurological events secondary to diffuse atherosclerotic disease has also been seen in older adults.

PERCUTANEOUS TRANSLUMINAL CORONARY ANGIOPLASTY

Dotter and Judkins first proposed the concept of transluminal angioplasty in 1964.[15] Gruentzig initially applied the technique of percutaneous transluminal coronary angioplasty (PTCA) to human coronary arteries in 1977.[1] Since the first PTCA, advances in catheter and balloon techniques have improved immediate and long-term success. Although conventional balloon angioplasty is a core procedure in the catheterization laboratory, it is usually not a stand-alone procedure but is now augmented by adjunctive stenting, which greatly improves procedural success and reduces complication rates.

The desired therapeutic effect of balloon angioplasty is the enlargement of the internal luminal diameter of the diseased artery. Application of balloon pressure to an atherosclerotic lesion results in plaque rupture, disruption of the endothelium, and stretching of the vessel segment, which enlarges the vessel lumen size (Fig. 23-1).

Guiding catheters are used to cannulate the coronary artery and to provide support for delivery of guidewires and interventional devices. In the catheterization laboratory, after the guide catheter is placed and the wire crosses the lesion, a balloon catheter is selected that most closely approximates the diameter of the nondiseased reference segment adjacent to the site to be treated. The prepared and flushed balloon is loaded onto the free end of the guidewire. The balloon is passed into the guide catheter, down the proximal vessel, and across the lesion. Once the balloon catheter is positioned across the lesion, the balloon is inflated using a handheld inflation device equipped with a pressure dial. Multiple balloon inflations of variable pressure and duration are used depending on the type of lesion and the physician preference. The response of the lesion to dilatation is assessed by contrast injection and repeat angiography through the guiding catheter with the guidewire in place. When the lesion in successfully dilated, the balloon apparatus is removed and multiple angiographic projections are reviewed. The guidewire and guiding catheter are removed after an adequate result is obtained.

Cutting Balloon Angioplasty

Cutting balloon angioplasty uses a balloon designed with three-to-four microscopic blades or atherotomes mounted on the balloon surface that protrude slightly above the balloon surface when inflated (Fig. 23-2). The mechanism of action referred to as atherotomy utilizes the balloon device to make three-to-four controlled incisions that score the plaque in an atherosclerotic coronary artery. The noncompliant balloon then dilates the incised areas resulting

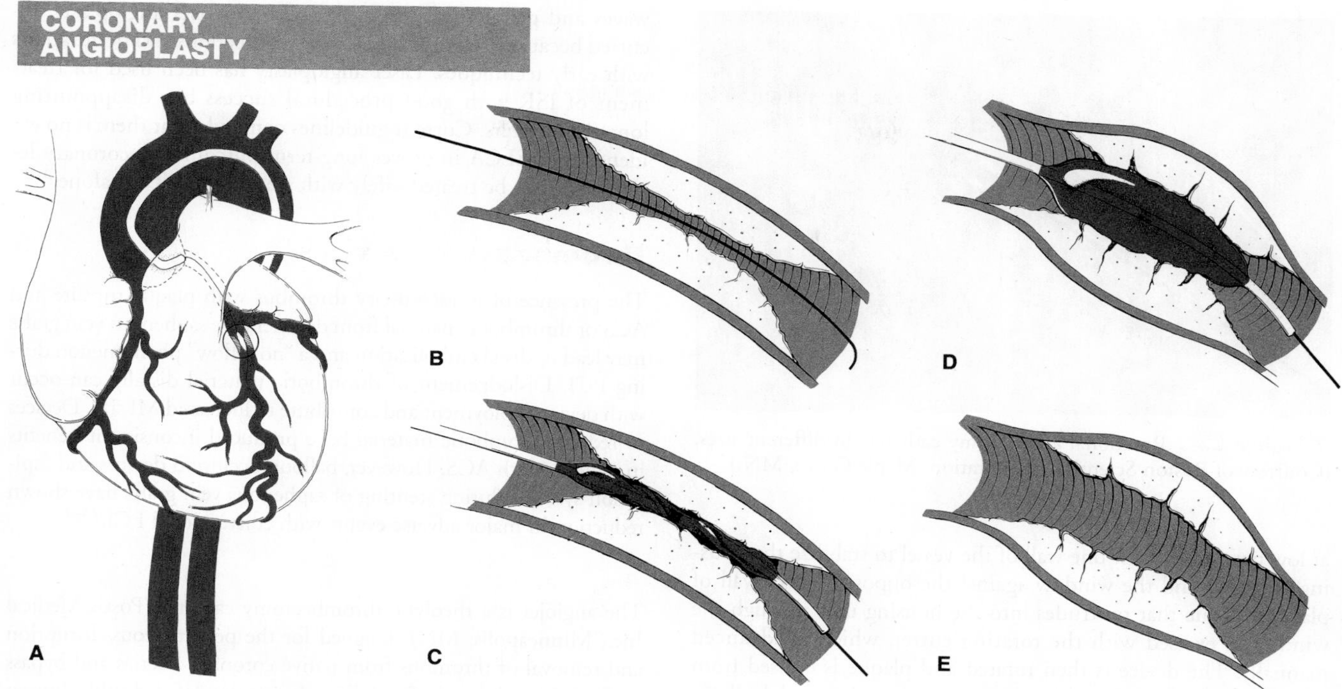

■ **Figure 23-1** Mechanism of intracoronary balloon angioplasty. (A) A balloon catheter is introduced into the coronary artery through a guide catheter in the aorta. (B) A guidewire is advanced across the area of narrowing. (C) The balloon catheter is advanced over the wire across the lesion. (D) The balloon is inflated. (E) Coronary artery after PTCA. (Courtesy of Boston Scientific Corporation, Maple Grove, MN.)

in plague compression and less vessel wall expansion. This type of dilatation may reduce the force needed to dilate an obstructed lesion. The cutting balloon has specific, limited indications: lesions that are resistant to dilatation by traditional angioplasty balloons, such as calcific, elastic, and fibrotic lesions; and in-stent restenosis (ISR) to avoid slipping-induced vessel trauma during PCI.[16,17] The cutting balloon may be used alone or in combination with stents.

CORONARY ATHERECTOMY, ATHEROABLATIVE, AND THROMBECTOMY DEVICES

Coronary atherectomy (directional and rotational) and excimer laser coronary angioplasty (ELCA) were developed and approved by the FDA for coronary artery use in the late 1980 to 1990s, with hopes of resolving the limitations of PTCA. Atherectomy device technique involves reduction of the severity of coronary blockage by removal of atheromatous plaque rather than compressing and/or fracturing the plaque, or stretching the arterial wall. In theory, this approach was developed to permit a more controlled vascular injury, minimize the degree of arterial mural stretch, create a smoother surface by debulking the vessel, and removal of atherosclerotic plaque that is frequently resistant to balloon dilatation.

Atherectomy devices have been used successfully to remove atherosclerotic plaque but were associated with increased complication rates and restenosis rates similar to PTCA from neointimal hyperplasia. Atherectomy devices now account for less than 3% of current PCI and are being used in very specific subsets of patients. Clinical trials have shown no improvement in long-term results with these devices; many atherectomy devices no longer are used.[18,19]

Atherectomy

Directional Coronary Atherectomy

The directional coronary atherectomy (DCA) catheter (Guidant Corporation, Santa Clara, CA) consists of a catheter-mounted, cylindrical metallic housing unit (collection chamber, window, and cup-shaped cutter) and a small balloon attached to the housing. When the catheter is placed at the lesion, a balloon is inflated

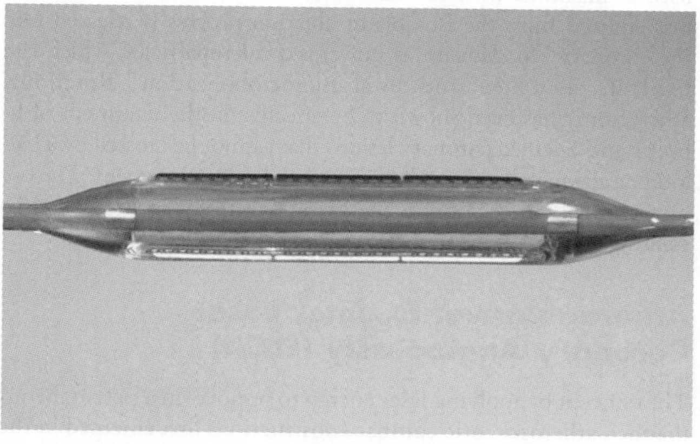

■ **Figure 23-2** The cutting balloon. (Courtesy of Boston Scientific Corporation, Maple Grove, MN.)

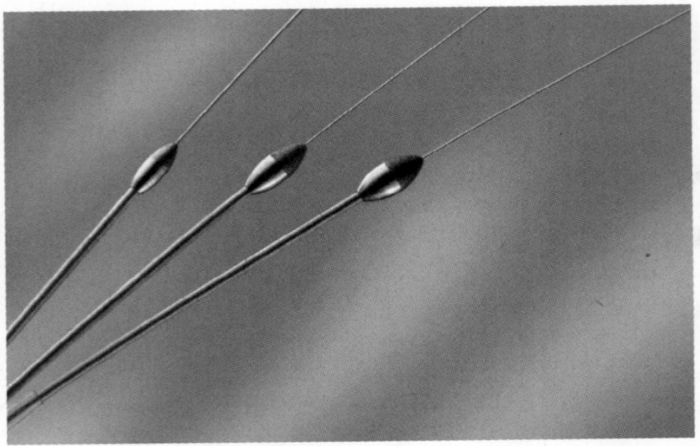

■ **Figure 23-3** Rotational atherectomy catheters in different sizes. (Courtesy of Boston Scientific Corporation, Maple Grove, MN.)

at low pressure against one wall of the vessel to stabilize the housing chamber and the window against the opposite vessel wall of plaque. Plaque that protrudes into the housing unit through the window is excised with the rotating cutter, which is advanced manually. The device is then rotated and plaque is excised from around the lumen. Combination aggressive plaque debulking with DCA and stenting did not improve short- or long-term clinical outcomes over stenting alone; there is no well-established evidence for efficacy of DCA use in coronary arteries.[3,19,20] A modified device is currently used in peripheral vascular interventions.

Rotational Atherectomy

The rotational atherectomy device (Rotablator/Boston Scientific, Maple Grove, MN) uses a high-speed, rotating, elliptical burr coated with diamond chips 20 to 30 microns in diameter that form an abrasive surface (Fig. 23-3). When the burr is spun at a high speed (140,000 to 180,000 rpm, depending on burr size), it preferentially removes atheroma because of its selective differential cutting of inelastic plaque rather than elastic normal tissue. The process involves a stepwise incremental increase in burr size to provide a "sanding effect." Gradual advancement and withdrawal of the burr in 2- to 5-second intervals for up to 20 to 30 seconds in the lesion allows for heat dissipation, improved distal perfusion, and washout of particulate debris. The postablation vessel diameter is equal to the largest burr size used. Adjunctive PTCA and stenting is used to maximize final coronary artery luminal diameter. The debris emitted from the Rotablator ablation process is released into the coronary bloodstream as pulverized microparticles, which can result in "slow flow" and distal microembolization. Rotational atherectomy has been shown to be effective in the treatment of fibrotic and calcified coronary lesions that cannot be crossed by a balloon or adequately dilated before planned stent placement. The use of rotational atherectomy is used very selectively as an adjunct to stenting and was not supported in clinical trials for ISR.[17,21]

Atheroablative: Excimer Laser Coronary Angioplasty (ELCA)

The concept of applying laser energy to remove, in a percutaneous manner, atherosclerotic coronary obstructions first emerged in the late 1980s. The ELCA produces monochromatic light energy to cause ablation of plaque via the generation of heat and shock waves and plaque disruption. A decline in laser angioplasty occurred because of significant coronary dissections and perforations with early techniques. Laser angioplasty has been used for treatment of ISR with good procedural success but disappointing long-term results. Current guidelines conclude that there is no evidence that ELCA improves long-term outcomes in coronary lesions that can be treated safely with stenting or PTCA alone.[3,22]

Thrombectomy Devices

The presence of intracoronary thrombus with plaque rupture and ACS or thrombotic material from degenerative saphenous vein grafts may lead to distal embolization and a "no reflow" phenomenon during PCI. Dislodgement of thrombotic material distally can occur with device deployment and contribute to increased MI size. Devices to reduce thrombotic material have produced inconsistent benefits in patients with ACS. However, balloon occlusion devices and aspiration systems during stenting of saphenous vein grafts have shown reduction in major adverse events with conventional PCI.[23–25]

Angiojet

The angiojet is a rheolytic thrombectomy catheter (Possis Medical Inc., Minneapolis, MN) designed for the percutaneous disruption and removal of thrombus from native coronary arteries and bypass grafts using high-velocity saline. It consists of a double lumen catheter. The smaller lumen of the catheter is used to supply the catheter tip with saline jets that are generated by an external drive unit. These jets aid in the formation of a recirculation pattern that fragments the thrombotic material and creates a "Venturi effect" that aids in evacuation of the macerated thrombotic material.[23,26]

Aspiration Thrombectomy

Aspiration thrombectomy catheters are used to manually extract thrombus. These catheters are advanced into the coronary artery and, while suction is applied, pulled back through the thrombus. After aspiration of the thrombus material, PCI with PTCA or stent is performed.

Distal Protection Devices

These devices are designed to provide protection of the distal microcirculation during PCI. One device type is a balloon occlusive system that temporarily occludes the distal vessel during the intervention followed by the aspiration of liberated atheromatous and thrombotic material before it reaches that arteriolar and capillary bed. The other device type is a nonocclusive, filter-based system that preserves coronary blood flow through tiny pores, as low as 100 microns. Atheromatous and thrombotic material is trapped in the filter-based systems and then removed with the retrieval of the device through a retrieval catheter. These techniques can reduce the incidence of cardiac enzyme elevation post-PCI.

CORONARY STENTS

The majority of current PCI involve coronary stenting as a primary procedure or as an adjunct to balloon angioplasty. When PTCA was first introduced, it was plagued by two major limitations: acute or subacute closure, and restenosis. Subsequently, improved intracoronary stent design, techniques, and pharmacological management have contributed to the success of catheter-based revascularization with stents, reducing the incidence of these two major complications

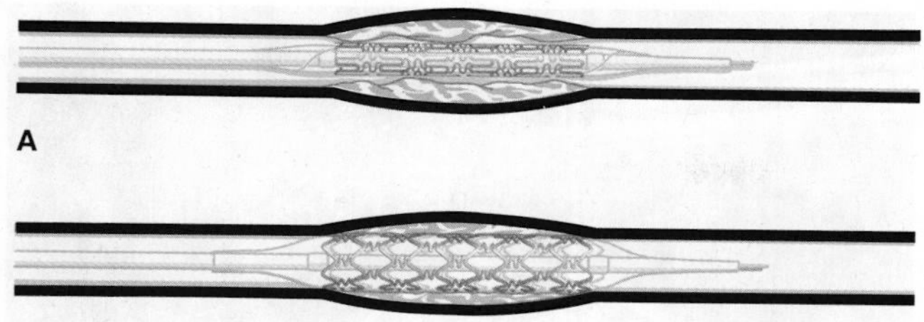

■ **Figure 23-4** Stent deployment. **(A)** Stent in the closed position across lesion on the balloon delivery system. **(B)** Stent in open position in coronary artery after balloon inflation. (Courtesy of Cordis, A Johnson & Johnson Company, Miami Lakes, FL.)

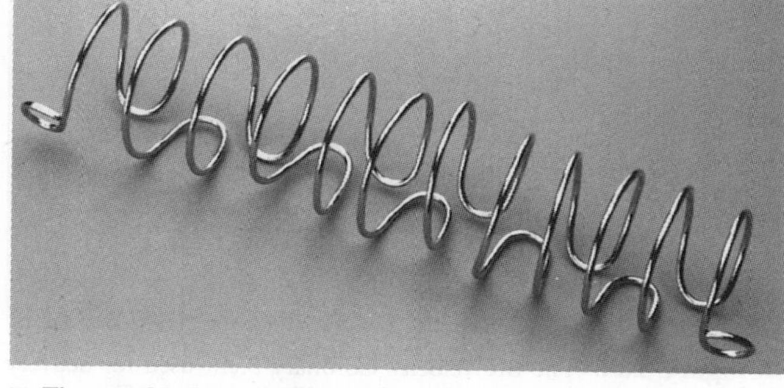

■ **Figure 23-5** The Gianturco-Roubin Flex-Stent. (Courtesy of Cook, Inc., Bloomington, IN.)

of PCI. The optimal stent should be easily and safely deliverable to various locations in coronary arteries and have the following properties: are flexible, low profile, radiopaque, smooth contour, sufficient radial strength, and tissue and blood compatible.[27]

Dotter first demonstrated the concept of stenting an injured vessel in 1960s. In 1986, Sigwart et al.[28] reported use of a percutaneous, self-expanding metallic stent in coronary vessels in humans. The development of intracoronary stents was initiated to provide structural support to an artery opposing elastic recoil preventing vasoconstriction, and preventing or treating dissections of the arterial wall seen with other coronary devices. The stent procedure is similar in preparation to PTCA with a guide catheter in the ostium of the coronary artery and a guidewire passed across the lesion. The lesion can be predilated with an angioplasty balloon or the stent placed without predilatation (primary stenting).

There are a variety of different types of intracoronary stents, categorized by mechanism of deployment, structure, metals, sizes, and stent coating (including bare-metal, drug-eluting, and covered). Stents are deployed using balloon-expandable or self-expandable mechanisms. The most commonly used stents are balloon-expandable and delivered over a guidewire into the coronary artery in a collapsed state and mounted on a balloon delivery system. Self-mounted stents are available in Europe. Once the balloon is positioned correctly across the lesion, the balloon is inflated, expanding the stent. The balloon delivery system is removed and a high-pressure balloon is frequently used to postdilate the stent to assure its full expansion (Fig. 23-4). Adequate apposition of the stent to the arterial wall has been found to be very important for long-term success and reduction of major cardiac events secondary to thrombotic complications. The self-expanding stents are used less frequently in the coronary arteries and more frequently in the peripheral vasculature. They are placed on the delivery system in a collapsed state with a retaining outer membrane. Retraction of the membrane after the delivery system is across the lesion allows the stent to expand. A high-pressure balloon can be used after deployment to completely expand the stent.

Bare Metal Stent (BMS)

Two of the first FDA-approved stents were the Gianturco-Roubin Flex-Stent (Fig. 23-5), which reduced the incidence of emergency CABG surgery associated with PTCA,[29] and the Palmaz-Schatz coronary stent. Two landmark clinical stent trials that empowered the stent revolution were randomized trials comparing the Palmaz-Schatz Stent with PTCA. The Stent Restenosis Trial (STRESS) and the Belgium Netherlands Stent Trial (Benestent) found that patients with an intracoronary stent in a de novo lesion had a higher procedural success rate and a less frequent need for revascularization than patients with balloon angioplasty.[30,31] However, this benefit was achieved at the cost of a significantly higher risk of vascular bleeding complications and a longer hospital stay. An aggressive regimen of adjunctive pharmacologic agents was used during these trials and during the initial experience of stenting, including ASA (acetylsalicylic acid or aspirin), dipyridamole, warfarin, heparin, and dextran. The initial stent trials were hindered by a high rate of subacute stent thrombosis, embolization of stents, difficulty in stent placement, and groin complications. Improvement in stent deployment techniques, operator experience, elimination of aggressive anticoagulation regimens, and the introduction of antiplatelet therapy facilitated wide spread acceptance of coronary stenting with less complications.

These first-generation BMS designs have provided the initial stent model but have been replaced by newer designs with better flexibility, and a wide variety of sizes and lengths. BMSs currently have an excellent procedure success rate of 20% but restenosis rates of approximately 25%.[32,33]

Drug-Eluting Stent (DES)

Bare metal stents dramatically decreased acute and threatened closure with PTCA but did not eliminate the significant problem of restenosis. The development of the next generation of stents with drug-eluting properties provides successful treatment of coronary lesions with low complications rates and mechanisms to limit the development of neointimal hyperplasia, leading to restenosis seen with PTCA, atherectomy devices, and BMS. Since 2002, randomized trials have shown that DESs, as compared to BMSs, reduce the need for subsequent revascularization procedures and as a result, the use of DES has increased rapidly with current rates in excess of 80% of all stenting procedures.

The concept behind DES is to prevent neointimal hyperplasia and allow normal development of endothelial lining on the stent struts. Endothelialization is important for preventing direct contact between bare metal and circulating blood, a circumstance that can lead to clot formation and stent thrombosis. The stent platform is coated with a polymer that allows the intended antiproliferative drug to adhere to the stent struts and allow local delivery. The stent design, balloon delivery system, drug mechanisms, type of polymer, and release pattern of the drug all are important for effective dilatation and compression of the coronary plaque, ability to safely dispense the drug, and prevention of cell death and necrosis of the

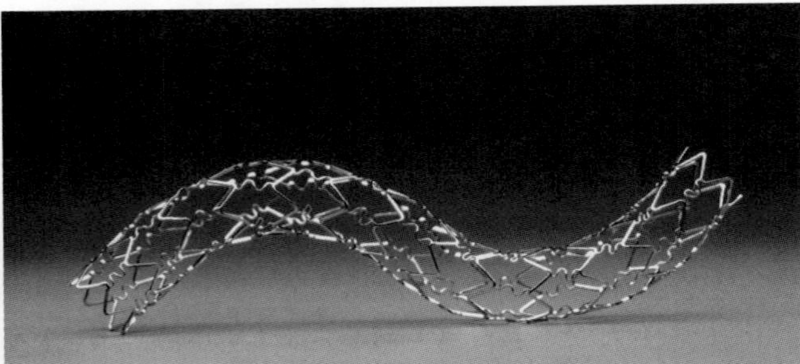

■ **Figure 23-6** The BX Velocity Coronary Stent used for delivery of Sirolimus: The CYPHER™ Sirolimus-Eluding Stent. (Courtesy of Cordis, A Johnson & Johnson Company, Miami Lakes, FL.)

coronary vessel leading to vascular complications. The clinical success of this technology depends on the complex interaction between the stent, coating matrix, drug, and vessel wall.[34]

Sirolimus-Eluting Stent (SES)

The first DES approved for use in PCI by the FDA in 2003 was the CYPHER™ sirolimus-eluting stent (Fig. 23-6). The CYPHER stent has a stainless steel stent platform, the BX Velocity, covered with a thin polymer coating containing the drug sirolimus. The slow-release formulation inhibits cell proliferation by targeting smooth muscle cells, while simultaneously reducing inflammatory cytokine production and resultant vessel wall inflammation.[35]

Paclitaxel-Eluting Stent (PES)

The second DES approved by the FDA in 2004 was the TAXUS™ paclitaxel-eluting stent (Fig. 23-7). The Express-2 stent is used as

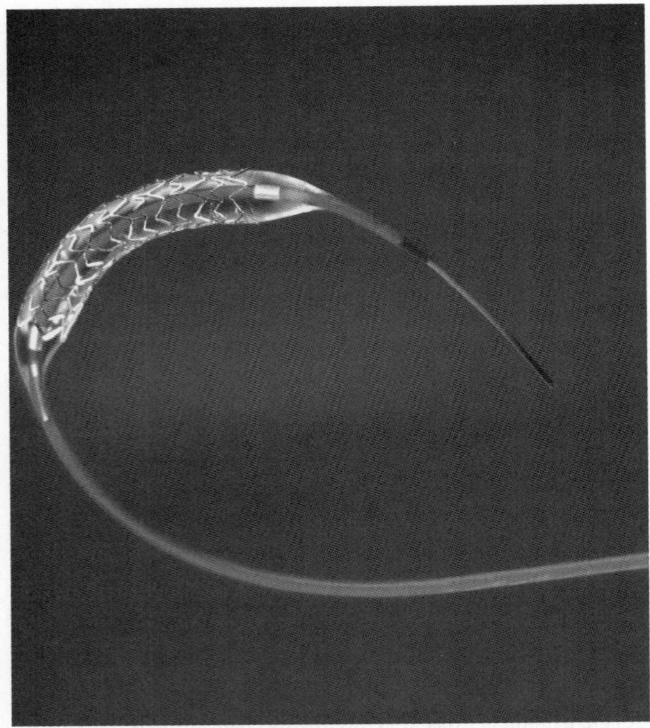

■ **Figure 23-7** The TAXUS™ Stent on the Balloon Delivery System. (Courtesy of Boston Scientific Corporation, Maple Grove, MN.)

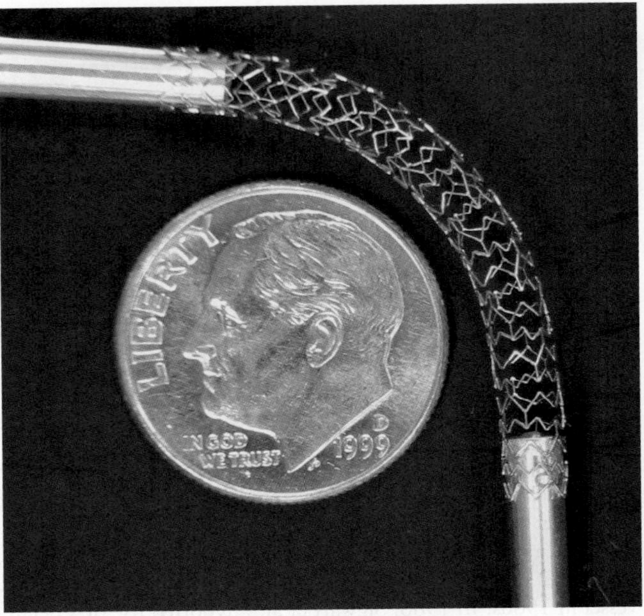

■ **Figure 23-8** The TAXUS™ Stent. The Express 2 Stent is used as the platform for the Paclitaxel-Eluting Stent. A dime is placed next to the device to represent size. (Courtesy of Boston Scientific Corporation, Maple Grove, MN.)

the stent platform and the drug paclitaxel is placed on the stent with a copolymer coating. Paclitaxel is a potent antiproliferative agent released in a biphasic manner, with an initial burst in the first 2 days, followed by lower-level sustained release for 10 days (Fig. 23-8).[36] Safety and efficacy have been shown with repeat intervention rates at 30 months to be approximately 10% for SES and 13% for PES.[37]

MANAGEMENT OF THE PATIENT DURING PCI

Preprocedure Management

Preparation for elective or acute PCI requires informed consent after physician discussion of risks and benefits, provisional consent for emergency CABG surgery, and patient education. Patient education includes expectations during the procedure and postprocedural care using visual, written, and verbal information. The nursing history (including all current medications and herbal supplements) and physical examination are documented, with abnormalities reported to the physician and catheterization laboratory staff prior to the PCI.

Patients with Diabetes Mellitus

Oral hypoglycemic agents are usually held prior to the PCI. The combination of contrast medium and metformin should be completely avoided in patients with renal dysfunction, hepatic dysfunction, alcohol abuse, or severe congestive heart failure because all these conditions limit metformin excretion and can increase lactate production, possibly leading to fatal lactic acidosis.[38] Insulin dosage adjustments are ordered by the physician. In general, one-half the usual dose of insulin is given with continued surveillance of blood glucose before and after the procedure. Insulin drips are used for patients with Type I diabetes mellitus, difficult glycemic control, ACS, or who are otherwise unstable.

Patients With Renal Insufficiency

Patients with pre-existing renal insufficiency and/or diabetes mellitus have an increased risk of contrast-induced nephropathy with contrast medium used during PCI. Renal dysfunction is present when creatinine clearance is less than 60 mL/min or serum creatinine is >1.5 mg/dL. Creatinine clearance should be estimated and medication dosage adjusted in patients with altered renal function. Isosmolar contrast agents should be used during PCI. The major preventive strategy includes adequate hydration before and after the procedure. The combination of N-acetylcysteine and sodium bicarbonate infusion before and after contrast administration has been reported to reduce the risk of contrast-induced nephropathy in patients with renal insufficiency.[39]

Intraprocedure Management

Patient preparation is similar to the patient having a diagnostic cardiac catheterization (Chapter 20). Conscious sedation is given at the discretion of the cardiologist and the patient monitored by the catheterization laboratory staff as per protocol. A sheath is placed in the femoral artery, which is the most common arterial access site. Alternatively, the brachial or radial artery can be used for arterial access.

A bolus of heparin is given to maintain an activated clotting time (ACT) of 250 to 300 seconds. ACT below 250 seconds has been associated with thrombotic complications during PCI with multiple catheters, wires, or devices being placed in the aorta and coronary arteries. Use of low-molecular-weight heparin (LMWH) or direct thrombin inhibitors can be used as an alternative to heparin (see anticoagulation options for PCI).[40,41] For patients who undergo PCI with LMWH, specific dosage regimens are available. When fondaparinux (an LMWH) is used prior to intervention, additional intravenous treatment with an anticoagulant possessing anti-IIa activity (such as unfractionated heparin, or UFH) should be used because of the risk of catheter thrombosis.[4] Baseline angiographic views are obtained of the coronary artery to be treated using the standard diagnostic catheter or the guiding catheter. Coronary injections may be repeated after administration of intracoronary nitroglycerin to exclude spasm as a significant component of the target stenosis and to minimize the occurrence of coronary spasm during the PCI. The appropriate guiding catheter is positioned in the coronary ostium and a guidewire is directed across the stenotic lesion. After the wire tip is confirmed to be in the distal portion of the coronary artery to be treated, the angioplasty balloon or other device is selected. The patient is monitored for hemodynamic stability and electrocardiographic changes during the procedure.

During the procedure additional heparin or a direct thrombin inhibitor is given by the cardiologist to maintain an adequate ACT and anticoagulation status. A GP IIb/IIIa receptor inhibitor infusion may be selected for patients with ACS or angiographic thrombus. After the procedure is complete, the patient is prepared for transfer to the postinterventional ward. Vital signs are monitored and patient placed on a portable monitor for transfer. The arterial access site is assessed for bleeding or hematoma prior to transfer. Report is called to the receiving staff, including type of procedure performed, specific artery treated, vital signs, status of the arterial sheath, and other pertinent information. (See vascular sheath removal under postprocedure management.)

Postprocedure Management

The interventional patient is monitored for manifestations of myocardial ischemia, such as chest pain, electrocardiogram (ECG) changes, arrhythmias, or hemodynamic instability. A 12-lead ECG is obtained postprocedure to establish a baseline for comparison. Laboratory tests are drawn and should minimally include hematocrit, platelet count, blood urea nitrogen, and creatinine. All patients who have unstable angina, MI, or a complicated procedure should have CK-MB and troponin measured. Patients may be relatively extracellular fluid (ECF) depleted after PCI because of nothing-by-mouth status and radiographic contrast-induced diuresis. Hydration is maintained by normal or half-normal saline until oral intake is sufficient to meet patient requirements. Anticoagulants, antithrombin agents, or GP IIb/IIIa receptor inhibitors infusions are continued as per institutional protocol or physician orders.

Vascular Sheath Removal

Vascular sheath removal, mobilization, and ambulation protocols vary according to the device protocol and hospital policies. In general, the sheaths are removed 4 to 6 hours after the procedure, when the ACT falls below 180 seconds, by either the patient care unit nursing staff or catheterization technician. Vascular sheaths are removed by manual pressure and either an adjunctive compression device or a vascular closure device. Manual pressure is applied for at least 20 minutes or longer, as warranted, to provide homeostasis with strict attention to the arterial site and distal circulation. Recognition and treatment of complications are essential to prevent peripheral vascular injuries. The vascular site is monitored for bleeding, hematoma formation, distal circulation, and sensation, initially every 15 minutes and advancing to every hour until stable. Manual compression remains the standard method for femoral sheath removal worldwide. Passive closure techniques enhance manual pressure utilizing (a) external patches with prothrombotic coatings (Syvek Patch, Marine Polymer Technologies, Danvers, MA); (b) wire-stimulated tract thrombosis (Boomerang Wire, Cardiva Medical, Mountainview, CA); or (c) assisted compression devices (Femostop, RADI Medical system Inc., Wilmington MA; or Safeguard, Datascope Corp. Montvale, NJ). Pressure dressings and sand bags to groin sites have been found to be ineffective in controlling recurrent or persistent bleeding and cause discomfort.[42] Minor or tract oozing after a compression or a vascular closure device can be managed with light manual pressure, injection of xylocaine with epinephrine, or light pressure dressing.

Vasovagal reactions can occur at the time of sheath insertion or removal. Common symptoms associated with a vasovagal reaction include hypotension, nausea, vomiting, yawning, and diaphoresis. This syndrome is triggered by pain and anxiety, particularly in the setting of ECF deficit.[43] Treatment includes cessation of painful stimuli, rapid volume administration with normal saline, and atropine intravenously. If hypotension persists, additional hemodynamic support with intravenous vasopressor agents may be needed.

Use of Vascular Closure Devices

Vascular closure devices (VCDs) for rapid hemostasis after femoral sheath removal became available in the early 1990s. The use of the VCD evolved to allow early sheath removal and hemostasis of femoral access sites, increased patient comfort, decreased compression time by hospital staff, and early ambulation. Despite advances in VCD technique, improved patient comfort, and earlier ambulation, VCDs have not been routinely adapted. Their limited use reflects concerns about complications, device cost, and lack of evidence-based superiority over manual compression.[44] The most commonly used closure devices with active hemostasis components include collagen plugs (Angio-Seal, St. Jude Medical, St. Paul, MN), suture devices (Perclose, Abbott Vascular, Redwood City, CA), and surgical staples/clips (StarClose, Abbott Vascular, Redwood City, CA). The use of arterial closure devices requires specific training by the cardiologist and the catheterization staff.

ANTICOAGULATION OPTIONS FOR PCI

Arterial injury at the PCI site and indwelling angioplasty equipment serve as potent stimuli for thrombus formation during PCI. Anticoagulation and antiplatelet agents are administered routinely to reduce the risk of an acute thrombotic complication. See Table 22-2, Applying Classification of Recommendations and Level of Evidence, in the previous chapter.

Oral Antiplatelet Therapy[3]

Class I recommendations:

1. Patients already on ASA should take 75 to 325 mg before the PCI. (Level of evidence: A)
2. Patients not already on chronic ASA should be pretreated with ASA 75 to 325 mg at least 2 hours before and preferably 24 hours before PCI is performed. (Level of evidence: C)
3. After the PCI, in patients with neither ASA resistance, allergy, or risk of increased bleeding, ASA 75 to 325 mg daily should be given for at least 1 month for BMS, 3 months for SES, and 6 months for PES. Then all patients should take daily chronic ASA 75 to 162 mg indefinitely. (Level of evidence: B)
4. A loading dose of clopidogrel should be administered before PCI. (Level of evidence: A) The recommended dose of clopidogrel dose of 300 mg at least 6 hours before PCI has the best evidence of efficacy. (Level of evidence: B)
5. After PCI, patients should be given clopidogrel 75 mg daily for at least 1 month after BMS, 3 months after SES, 6 months after PES, and ideally up to 12 months. (Level of evidence: C)

Recent clinical studies evaluated a 600 mg loading dose of clopidogrel given 2 hours before PCI. This dose was found to be safe, and provide faster and greater platelet inhibition than the lower dose.[45,46] Risk of thrombocytopenia with clopidogrel requires surveillance of platelet counts before and after PCI. Patients who are allergic to clopidogrel should be given ticlopidine. When using ticlopidine, there is a risk of neutropenia requiring monitoring a complete blood count with differential before and then again 7 to 10 days after PCI.

Antithrombotic Therapy[3]

Class I recommendations:

1. UFH should be administered to patients undergoing PCI. (Level of evidence: C)
2. For patients with heparin-induced thrombocytopenia, it is recommended that bivalirudin or argatroban (direct thrombin inhibitors) be used to replace heparin. (Level of evidence: B)

Class IIa recommendations:

1. Bivalirudin may be used as an alternative to UFH and GP IIb/IIIa inhibitors in low-risk patients undergoing elective PCI.
2. LMWH is an alternative to UFH in patients with unstable angina/NSTEMI undergoing PCI. Enoxaparin can be used without crossover to another agent. Fondaparinux should not be used as the sole anticoagulant during PCI but should be coupled with UFH or bivalirudin.[4]

Patients undergoing PCI who are treated with LMWH (enoxaparin) require no additional dosing if the last dose of enoxaparin was given less than 8 hours before PCI. If the last dose was administered more than 8 hours previously, an IV bolus is given per protocol.[47,48] LMWH is less frequently used in the catheterization laboratory with PCI and sheath management because of the longer half-life and the inability to monitor ACT or PTT to establish anticoagulation status. The direct thrombin inhibitor, bivalirudin, prolongs the ACT allowing monitoring of the dose during PCI similar to UFH.

GP IIb/IIIa Receptor Inhibitors[3]

The GP IIb/IIIa receptor inhibitors are a class of drugs used intravenously before and during interventional cardiology procedures and ACS. The final common pathway to platelet aggregation and coronary thrombus involves the activation of the platelet GP IIb/IIIa receptor. The GP IIb/IIIa receptor inhibitors act by occupying the receptors, preventing fibrinogen from binding and thereby preventing platelet aggregation. There are three GP IIb/IIIa receptor antagonists available for intravenous use to block platelet aggregation: abciximab, tirofiban, and eptifibatide. GP IIb/IIIa receptor antagonists diminish ischemic complications associated with PCI (Chapter 20).[3,46–52]

Class I recommendations:

1. In patients with unstable angina or NSTEMI undergoing PCI without clopidogrel administration, a GP IIb/IIIa receptor inhibitor (abciximab, tirofiban, and eptifibatide) should be given. (Level of evidence: A)

COMPLICATIONS ASSOCIATED WITH PCI

Chest Pain or Discomfort Post-PCI

Persistent or recurrent chest pain/discomfort after PCI requires immediate evaluation. It may be caused by acute or threatened closure, MI, loss of coronary artery side branch, distal embolization, vessel perforation, vascular spasm, or may be residual chest pain associated with vessel dilatation and stretch. Obtaining full details of the PCI and patient information including presenting symptoms, procedure type, results, and procedural complications is valuable in evaluating the chest pain symptoms.

Anatomic improvement after a PCI correlates with elimination of angina symptoms. Persistent chest pain or recurrent chest pain should be monitored and reported to the cardiologist if there is a change in intensity. Residual chest discomfort should be transient and dissipate in severity over several hours of PCI. If ongoing angina persists, an ECG should be obtained for comparison and if new or suspicious ECG changes are present, the patient must return to the catheterization laboratory for repeat coronary angiography and possible intervention.

Abrupt Vessel Closure

Coronary artery plaque disruption or dissection is caused by a controlled injury resulting from balloon dilatation with PTCA or atherectomy device. However, large progressive dissections may interfere with blood flow; cause compression of the true lumen by the dissection flap; cause superimposed thrombus formation, platelet adhesion, or vessel spasm; and lead to a total occlusion of the treated artery—a phenomenon known as abrupt closure. Vessel wall damage activates the GP IIb/IIIa receptor on the platelet surface causing platelet aggregation and thrombosis formation. Abrupt or acute vessel closure causes acute myocardial ischemia with chest pain and ECG changes. If the coronary artery is not successfully reopened percutaneously, the event may progress to MI, require emergency CABG surgery, and/or lead to death. With the use of stents and GP IIb/IIIa receptor inhibitors, the incidence of abrupt closure and the need for emergency bypass surgery has been reduced to less than 0.5% of patients.[53]

Acute Stent Thrombosis

Acute stent thrombosis is a potential catastrophic complication resulting in acute closure of the coronary vessel. The metallic surface of the stent contributes to the thrombogenic potential seen with BMS and DES. Risks associated with acute stent thrombosis include stenting in ACS, inadequate deployment of the stent, or propagation of thrombus from inadequate anticoagulation or antiplatelet therapies. Use of the current antiplatelet regimen before and after the procedure has reduced the incidence of acute stent thrombosis. Intravascular ultrasound (IVUS) has provided an evaluation tool to assess stent expansion and full apposition of the stent struts to the vessel wall preventing inflow and outflow obstruction in the coronary artery leading to thrombus formation. Acute stent thrombosis rates have decreased to less than 0.5% with current treatment regimens.[53]

Non-ST-Elevation MI

Elevation of cardiac enzymes occurs after uncomplicated PCI in up to 38% of patients, with isolated serum troponin elevation in 20% of patients. The most common causes are distal microembolization or loss of small coronary artery side branches. Distal embolization of friable plaque or thrombus can be released into the microcirculation during PCI and atherectomy procedures. Release of a large burden of embolic debris into the coronary circulation with rotational atherectomy, an ACS, or during treatment of a saphenous vein graft creates a "no-flow" phenomenon with transient occlusion of the distal coronary vessel, causing myocardial necrosis and elevation of CK-MB and/or troponin. Patients with CK-MB elevations have shown increased incidence of adverse long-term events, while isolated troponin elevation has conflicting prognostic significance. Treatment with GP IIb/IIIa receptor inhibitors, distal protection devices, and statin therapy are recommended to prevent microembolization in high-risk patients.[54]

Loss of a side branch of a major coronary artery occurs when a stent is placed across the side branch and poststent dilatation occludes the branch. The occlusion can be transient or result in stent-induced occlusion of the branch ("stent jail") and result in myocardial ischemia. Treatment options for side-branch occlusions include placing a guidewire into the "jailed" side branch and dilating the lesion through the stent struts with an angioplasty balloon.

ST-Elevation MI

STEMI, as documented by ECG changes (including new Q waves, new LBBB pattern) or cardiac enzyme elevation greater than three times upper level of normal occurs in less than 1% of patients after PCI. STEMI is usually due to an ACS, abrupt vessel closure, acute stent thrombosis, or loss of a major side branch originating within or in close proximity to the lesion being treated. Patients are treated as per protocol for MI (Chapter 22).

Coronary Vessel Perforation

Perforation or frank rupture of a coronary artery may lead to rapid hemodynamic collapse and cardiac tamponade. Perforation is an infrequent event with PTCA, occurring in less than 0.6% of PCIs but up to 2.0% with directional and rotational atherectomy.[55] Mechanisms of perforation with a guidewire include forceful advancement, crossing of a chronic total occlusion, passage of a device over a wire that is extra luminal or into a septal branch. Anticoagulation during PCI complicates the management of wire perforation. Vessel perforation may also occur with an oversized balloon or stent, atherectomy devices, or high postdilatation pressures.

Management of coronary perforation includes pain management, close hemodynamic monitoring, and early echocardiography. The administration of intravenous fluids and vasopressor agents may be required. Cessation of GP IIb/IIIa receptor inhibitors and reversal of anticoagulation with protamine is recommended only with frank rupture and hemopericardium. Balloon inflation at the perforation site can occlude the perforation and prevent further extravasation of blood. The polytetrafluoroethylene membrane-covered stent graft is the most effective device for urgent management of perforation to tack up the perforation and prevent further extravasation into the pericardium. Patients with limited pericardial blood can be managed conservatively and followed with echocardiogram surveillance. If there is a significant leak into the pericardial space resulting in hemopericardium and potential cardiac tamponade, pericardiocentesis is required. If unable to manage the bleeding in the catheterization laboratory, emergency cardiac surgery may be necessary.[56]

Vascular Spasm

Vascular spasm at the site or distal to the treated site is a potential cause of acute chest pain or ischemia during or after PCI. Vascular spasm is most common with atherectomy devices, particularly the high-speed rotational atherectomy device. It may occur at the treated site, in the proximal vessel secondary to guide catheter-related injury, or in the distal vessels. Vascular spasm is usually transient, can cause chest pain and hypotension, and is most commonly seen in the catheterization laboratory. Treatment includes nitroglycerin or a low-pressure balloon. If spasm is significant, the patient may be maintained on nitroglycerin and intravenous fluids overnight.

Arrhythmias and Conduction Disturbances

Ischemia during treatment can cause ECG changes, including transient heart block, atrial arrhythmias, or ventricular arrhythmias. Significant arrhythmias occur in approximately 1% of PCI, usually as a result of prolonged ischemia during balloon inflation or luminal occlusion with devices.[57]

Contrast Medium-Related Complications

Hypersensitivity reactions to radiocontrast medium are independent of amount or rate of infusion. This reaction can occur immediately (within 1 hour) or delayed (from 1 hour to 1 week). Signs and symptoms include pruritus, urticaria, angioedema, laryngospasm, bronchospasm, hypotension with loss of consciousness, and rarely hypovolemic shock and death. Risks of hypersensitivity reactions are previous anaphylactoid reaction to contrast, asthma, a history of allergic rhinitis, or drug or food allergies. Strategies to prevent recurrent reactions include use of low osmolar contrast and a prednisone regimen (premedicate with prednisone 13 hours before the procedure, administer a second dose at 7 hours before the procedure, and administer a third dose 1 hour before the procedure), an H1 antihistamine (diphenhydramine) 1 hour before the procedure, and possibly an H2 blocker (cimetidine or ranitidine), which has shown conflicting benefit prior to the procedure. For emergency procedures, an intravenous steroid (hydrocortisone) should be given immediately and every 4 hours until completion of procedure and diphenhydramine 1 hour before the procedure.[38]

Contrast-induced nephropathy can cause temporary or permanent renal dysfunction. Patients with diabetes or preexisting renal insufficiency, and older adults are at highest risk. Limiting volume of contrast and hydration prior to PCI remains the best preventive strategy.

Volume overload (ECF, water, or both; Chapter 7) can be due to hypertonic contrast agents, myocardial depression secondary to ischemia, poor baseline ventricular function, routine diuretics and other medication held prior to PCI, and excessive volume preloading. Prevention involves continued monitoring of ECF and water status before and after the procedure, particularly in patients with LV dysfunction, and reinstituting routine medications. Additional diuretics may be needed.

Cerebrovascular Complications

Transient ischemic attacks or cerebral vascular accidents secondary to plaque disruption may occur from manipulation of catheters and devices during intervention in patients with diffuse atherosclerotic disease.[58] A rare complication is spontaneous intracerebral hemorrhage with aggressive anticoagulation and antiplatelet agents.

Groin Complications

Bleeding post-PCI is an independent predictor for short- and long-term clinical events with increased mortality and morbidity.[59,60] The incidence of vascular complications among patients undergoing PCI is 0.8% to 5.5%, and has decreased significantly from earlier experiences. Decreased incidence of complications has been seen with the decrease in sheath size and the current standard drug regimen for stent management.

Hematoma formation or ecchymosis is frequent and self-limiting. It usually requires no intervention other than comfort measures.

Retroperitoneal bleeding caused by large hematomas dissecting into the retroperitoneum are life threatening and need prompt attention by the nursing and medical staff. Inadvertent puncture of the artery proximal to the inguinal ligament (i.e., the external iliac artery) while placing the arterial sheath is frequently the cause. There is less supporting tissue in this area, and it is more difficult to compress the puncture site. Retroperitoneal bleeding is characterized by lumbar or groin pain, a significant drop in hematocrit, hypotension, and possible bradycardia or tachycardia. Diagnosis is confirmed by a computed tomography scan. Treatment involves transfusion and fluid resuscitation to maintain adequate blood pressure, reversal of anticoagulation and occasionally surgical repair of the artery.

Arterial thrombosis at the puncture site may lead to occlusion of the artery or distal thrombosis into the extremity. Preexisting peripheral vascular disease increases the risk of a thromboembolic event. Surveillance of distal circulation and sensory checks should be continued after sheath removal. Signs of loss of pulse, color changes, decreased sensation, decreased temperature, or decreased motor function are potential indicators of thrombosis.

Pseudoaneurysm is an extra-luminal cavity in communication with an adjacent artery, usually the femoral artery. Inadvertent puncture of the superficial femoral or profunda femoris artery increases the incidence of arterial complications. Contributing factors include inadequate compression of the puncture site, heparin use, intramural arterial calcifications, and hypertension. On physical examination, the patient may have a pulsatile mass, systolic bruit, normal distal arterial pulses, and pain in the groin. Doppler ultrasound and color flow imaging are used to confirm the diagnosis and delineate the location and size of the pseudoaneurysm. Although most small pseudoaneurysms spontaneously close in 4 to 8 weeks without sequelae, they may enlarge or hemorrhage, especially in patients with prolonged anticoagulation. Treatment includes ultrasound-guided compression, thrombin injection with ultrasound guidance, or surgical closure.[61]

Arteriovenous (AV) fistula is a communication between an artery and vein. The mechanism of injury involves a puncture through both the femoral artery and vein, which results in a false communication. On physical examination, the patient may have a pulsatile mass in the groin and a continuous systolic–diastolic bruit; over time, temperature of the extremity decreases due to high flow through the fistula and ischemia of the extremity; a thrill may be present at the site; and heart failure may result if the fistula is persistent. Doppler ultrasound and color flow imaging confirm diagnosis. Surgical treatment may be necessary for closure and repair of the peripheral vasculature.

Septic endarteritis is rare and has been implicated in chronic intimal damage and stasis due to flow turbulence in the region of a pseudoaneurysm or AV fistula, multiple procedures through the same access site, obesity, or sheaths left in place for over 24 hours. In high-risk patients, antibiotics are given postprocedure and may be continued postdischarge if warranted.[62]

VCD complications include infection, femoral artery compromise, arterial laceration, uncontrolled bleeding, pseudoaneurysm, AV fistula, as well as device embolism and limb ischemia. These events include all types of VCD utilization. The use of VCD has not shown superiority over manual compression or reduction in groin complications. The severity of bleeding complications may be worse after a failed VCD compared to manual compression because the VCD is deployed at maximal anticoagulation while manual compression is delayed until the ACT is below 180 seconds. Device embolism and limb ischemia require emergency vascular surgery for device removal.[44]

Stent Thrombosis

Stent thrombosis can occur at different time intervals after implantation. Stent thrombosis events have been identified as early-acute (within 24 hours), subacute (within 30 days), late (>30 days to 1 year), and very late (>1 year after stent implantation).[63] Stent thrombosis that results in closure of the stent or threatened closure is a potentially life-threatening complication. It can occur with all stents regardless of design or composition. The patient usually presents with severe ischemia or acute MI. Stent thrombosis was more commonly seen in early stenting experiences with BMS, but has decreased with improved pharmacological therapy and IVUS-facilitated, stent deployment. Thrombotic events with BMS are uncommon after 30 days with dual antiplatelet treatment. Complete endothelialization of the BMS has been confirmed angioscopically within 3 to 6 months.

Since 2003 there has been a rapid increase in the use of DES. There is an increased risk of late (between 7 and 18 months) stent thrombotic events with DES compared to BMS, resulting in cardiac death and nonfatal MI in patients after discontinuation of clopidogrel at 6 months. The presumed mechanism is delayed or incomplete endothelialization or localized hypersensitivity to the polymer on the DES.[64] Resistance to the antiplatelet effects of aspirin and clopidogrel has been associated with platelet hyperreactivity. A strong independent predictor of stent thrombosis is nonresponsiveness to clopidogrel. Further assessment tools to identify nonresponders and alternative pharmacological strategies may be indicated for this group of patients.[65,66] The incidence of very late thrombosis with DES is about 0.2% events per year after 1 year and up to 0.6% at 3 to 4 years compared to BMS.[67] There was no significant increase of death or MI reported at 4 years with DES compared to BMS. Similar mortality and morbidity results may reflect a counter balance of an increase in late stent thrombosis with DES but a higher incidence of restenosis with BMS and the need for repeat target vessel revascularization. Treatment for stent thrombosis is emergency PCI or, less commonly, fibrinolysis to restore vessel patency.

Stent thrombosis is associated with a suboptimal angiographic result and incomplete stent apposition (defined as the stent strut not having full contact with the vessel at implantation or late after vessel remodeling leading to thrombosis). Other risk factors for thrombosis include specific high-risk lesion characteristics (such as small vessels and bifurcation lesions), "off-label" use of stents, and high-risk patients, such as those with diabetes, renal failure, ACS, and localized hypersensitivity to the stent polymer. Early cessation of dual antiplatelet therapy is a major cause of stent thrombosis. Obtaining a good angiographic result and administering aspirin and a thienopyridine (clopidogrel or ticlopidine) are the cornerstones of stent thrombosis prevention.

Concerns about the prolonged risk of stent thrombosis have resulted in the empirical practice of extending dual antiplatelet therapy for 12 months or longer. The medical decision-making process and risks and benefits of therapy should be thoroughly discussed with the patient and documented in the medical record. Patients should be reassured that the implantation of a DES after careful consideration with the physician remains a very effective treatment for CAD.[3]

With Noncardiac Surgery and Invasive Procedures

When noncardiac surgery or invasive procedures are performed early after stent placement before complete stent endothelialization has occurred, the risk of stent thrombosis is increased. Antiplatelet therapy is discontinued in the perioperative period; surgery itself creates a prothrombotic state increasing the risk of stent thrombosis. Antiplatelet bridging strategies with DES have not been well studied. The ACC/AHA[68] has proposed several important points to consider and recommendations for perioperative patient management with PCI.

Perioperative management of patients with recent coronary stents and PTCA[68] is important to reduce the risk of stent thrombosis.

- Patients undergoing noncardiac surgery within 1 to 2 weeks after a BMS are at high risk of stent thrombosis and death if antiplatelet therapy is discontinued in the perioperative period.
- Surgery should be avoided for at least 4 weeks after BMS implantation.
- Perioperative stent thrombosis is associated with high mortality and morbidity.
- Revascularization does not improve perioperative outcomes in patients with stable CAD; stenting prior to noncardiac surgery should be avoided.
- If PCI is necessary in a patient undergoing surgery, PTCA only may be a useful option. In such a case, surgery should be delayed by a week to permit vascular healing.
- A patient requiring stent who may also need surgery in the foreseeable future should receive a BMS.

Perioperative management of patients with recent DES[68] also is important in prevention of DES thrombosis. The optimal delay of noncardiac surgery after a DES is unknown, but a delay of 1 year is recommended. Perioperative thrombosis of DES has been reported as late as 21 months after stent implantation. Primary PCI is the preferred treatment strategy for patients who develop perioperative stent thrombosis. Consultation with cardiology prior to surgery and disposition to the telemetry floor or surgical floor after surgery are at the discretion of the cardiologist. When clopidogrel is continued throughout surgery, the anesthesiologist will be unable to perform spinal or epidural therapies.

Proposed recommendations for patients with DES who need surgery early after stent implantations[68]:

- Continue dual antiplatelet therapy in the perioperative period for patients at low risk of bleeding.
- Discontinue dual antiplatelet therapy; bridge with heparin and GP IIb/IIIa receptor inhibitors for the perioperative period, with early resumption of oral antiplatelet therapy postoperatively.
- Stop dual antiplatelet agents preoperatively and restart as early as feasible with clopidogrel loading.

RESTENOSIS

Restenosis is defined as a coronary luminal re-narrowing after PCI that is documented by repeat coronary angiography or other intracoronary imaging modalities. Clinical restenosis or ischemia noted on noninvasive testing frequently requires additional revascularization procedures, exposing patients to additional cardiovascular risks and causing substantial health care expenditures. Mechanical devices developed to limit restenosis, such as rotational atherectomy, DCA, and laser angioplasty, failed to reduce the restenosis rate. Coronary stents were the first devices with documented reduction in restenosis compared to PTCA and atherectomy. Restenosis rates are variable from reports of clinical trials, but are reported to be 30% to 40% with PTCA, 35% to 50% with atherectomy, and 20% to 30% with BMS.[19,20,69–71] Diffuse CHD, long lesions, small vessel size, bifurcation lesions, multiple stents, and diabetes have shown a higher incidence of restenosis.

Restenosis after PTCA and atherectomy involves a series of mechanisms with vessel lumen loss due to the elastic recoil; a wound-healing process including thrombotic, inflammatory, and cell growth proliferation that form neointimal hyperplasia; and remodeling of the treated vessel causing shrinkage. Restenosis usually occurs within 3 to 6 months and rarely 12 months after PTCA and atherectomy. Stents limit two of the three major mechanisms of restenosis: acute elastic recoil after dilatation and vessel shrinkage due to remodeling. However, stents enhance neointimal proliferation.[37]

Stents provide a larger arterial lumen diameter (acute gain) but the reparative response of neointimal hyperplasia (late loss) is still present. ISR occurs when neointimal hyperplasia after stenting causes significant narrowing and results in a positive stress test or return of symptoms. The time interval for restenosis with BMS is usually seen within the first 6 to 12 months and rarely after 1 year, similar to PTCA and atherectomy. The antiproliferative activity with DESs has significantly decreased the neointimal hyperplasia at the treatment site compared to PTCA, atherectomy, and BMS, but has a small increased risk of very late stent thrombosis.[72]

Treatment Options for In-Stent Restenosis

Treatment options for ISR initially included repeat PTCA, cutting balloon, atherectomy (DCA, rotational, and laser), and repeat BMS. These procedures provide an immediate technical success and a low rate of ischemic events, but 30% to 60% required repeat target vessel revascularization secondary to recurrent neointimal hyperplasia and no significant improvement in long-term results.[3,73,74]

Vascular Brachytherapy

Brachytherapy is a Class IIa recommendation for the treatment of ISR (Evidence level: A). Brachytherapy is similar to PTCA but involves placement of a catheter containing a radioactive source (γ or β radiation) across the dilated lesion. An initial PTCA is performed, the coronary lesion is dilated within the stent, and then a catheter containing a radioactive source is placed across the dilated restenotic portion. Both γ and β radiation reduce neointimal proliferation associated with ISR. Although brachytherapy can be an effective treatment for ISR, the benefits of radiation therapy have been mitigated by safety concerns and late complications. The following potential limitations have been observed with the use of brachytherapy to treat ISR: edge stenoses or geographic miss, acute thrombosis, late thrombosis and occlusion (up to 14%), increased plague burden outside the stent, IVUS echolucent areas, and very late catch-up phenomenon or delayed restenosis.[3,72,74]

Drug-Eluting Stents

It is reasonable to perform PCI for ISR within a DES and place a new DES for patients who develop ISR if anatomic factors are appropriate. (Class IIb recommendation; level of evidence: B).[3] Recent randomized trials comparing DES to β-emitting brachytherapy and PTCA for ISR have indicated superiority for long-term results with DES. The better results were related to the greater acute gain and late loss similar to or lower than brachytherapy.[75,76] Therefore, DESs are currently the treatment of choice for ISR.[74]

ADJUNCTIVE MODALITIES: QUANTITATIVE ANGIOGRAPHY

Coronary angiography alone sometimes may not provide sufficient information to distinguish ischemia-producing coronary lesions from non-ischemia-producing, intermediate coronary lesions. Nuclear perfusion imaging and stress echocardiography are noninvasive tests that can be used to guide treatment (Chapter 14). Invasive modalities used for diagnostic purposes are IVUS, coronary flow reserve, and fractional flow reserve. Coronary flow reserve and fractional flow reserve are described in Chapter 20.

Intravascular Ultrasound

IVUS has become an important procedure used during PCI to enhance procedure results, providing a detailed cross-sectional image of the vessel wall. This method of direct visualization of the arterial wall and lesion at the site of a planned intervention has improved clinical and angiographic outcomes. A miniaturized ultrasound transducer is placed on the distal end of a flexible catheter and advanced down the coronary artery. IVUS can be used during cardiac catheterization to evaluate plaque and tissue characteristics and during interventional procedures to verify adequate results and stent deployment. Colombo et al.[73] recognized with the use of IVUS that stent deployment techniques were inadequate and that the stents frequently were not completely expanded in the vessel, contributing to subacute closure. As a result of these findings, the use of high-pressure balloon dilatation after stent deployment to ensure full stent expansion was instituted, significantly affecting stenting practices and decreasing thrombotic complications.[77] (Fig. 23-9).

NONCORONARY DEVICES FOR TREATMENT OF CONGENITAL HEART DEFECTS

Percutaneous treatment of congenital heart defects (Chapter 31) requires special training by an interventional cardiologist with extensive knowledge of structural cardiac anatomy. The diagnosis of congenital abnormalities is confirmed by trans-thoracic or trans-esophageal echocardiography (Chapter 13). Use of noncoronary devices for treatment of atrial septal defect (ASD) and patent foramen ovale (PFO) are described below.

Atrial Septal Defect

Secundum ASD is the most common congenital heart defect to present into adulthood. Untreated, ASD produces right heart volume overload, atrial arrhythmias, CHF, and pulmonary hypertension. Initial techniques of percutaneous ASD closure were impractical for younger patients because of the size of the delivery

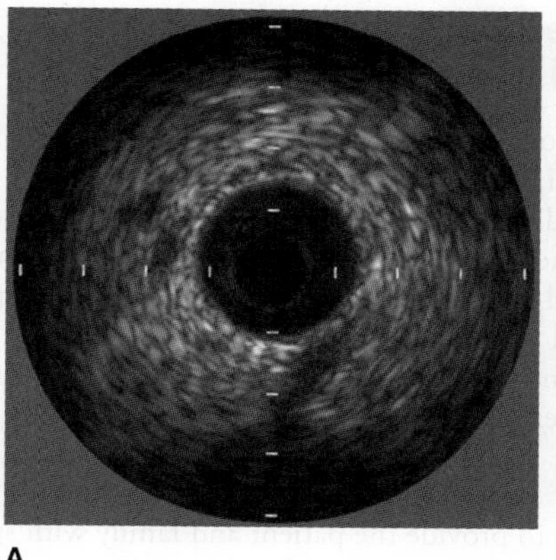

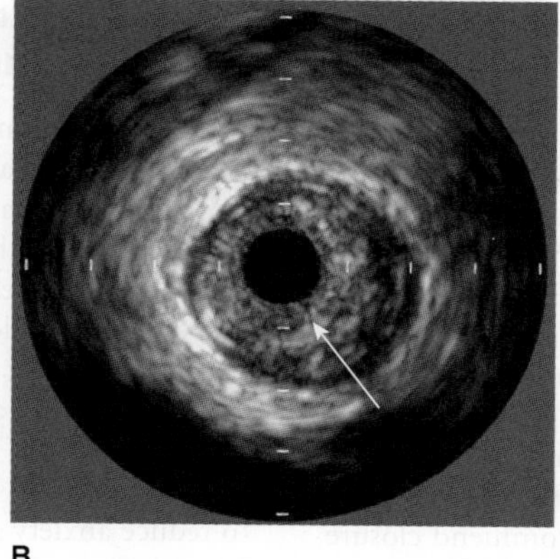

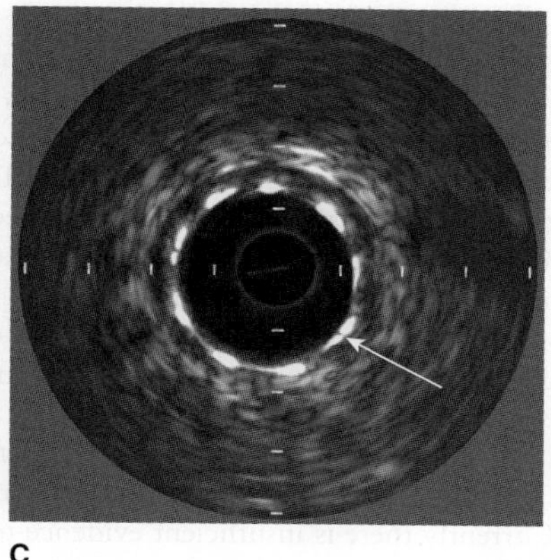

■ **Figure 23-9** Intravascular ultrasound. (A) Normal coronary artery. (B) Atherosclerotic plaque inside coronary artery; arrow points to plaque. (C) Coronary artery after stent placement; arrow points to stent struts. (Courtesy Volcano Corporation Rancho Cordova, CA.)

system. Improvements in device design and techniques have led to transcatheter closure systems.[78]

ASD closure devices include Amplatzer Atrial Septal Occluder (AGA Medical, Golden Valley, MN), CardioSeal and Star Flex (NMT Medical, Inc., Boston, MA), and HELEX Septal Occluder (W.L. Gore & Associates, Flagstaff, AZ).[79,80] The CardioSeal device has a clamshell design with four nitinol struts on each half of the shell that are draped with biocompatible knitted polyester fabric (Fig. 23-10). The Amplatzer Occluder is a self-expandable, double-disc device composed of flexible nitinol wire mesh lined with thin polyester fabric sewn into each disc (Fig. 23-11). The device implantation is performed with a single femoral venous puncture under fluoroscopy. Appropriate placement of the device is evaluated by use of trans-thoracic or trans-esophageal echocardiography, intracardiac echocardiography, or injection of contrast into the right atrium through the introducer. In the USA, the CardioSeal and the Amplatzer Septal Occluder are used also for VSD closure.

Patent Foramen Ovale

There is an association between PFO and ischemic stroke of undetermined cause (cryptogenic stroke) in young adults. The pathogenic mechanism is theorized to be a right-to-left shunt with thromboembolic material that crosses the septum through the PFO and then enters the cerebral circulation, termed a "paradoxical embolism." PFO is common and the prevalence varies from 34% in patients under the age of 35 years to 20% in those over the age of 80 years. There is conflicting evidence about the atrial abnormalities (i.e., an atrial septal aneurysm) with the PFO possibly mediating an increased incidence of stroke.[81]

No prospective trial of percutaneous closure of PFO among patients who have experienced cryptogenic stroke has been completed, and no device has been approved by the FDA for PFO closure after cryptogenic stroke. Therefore, the safety and effectiveness of devices for this indication are unknown. In 2007, the FDA Circulatory System Devices panel convened a meeting to discuss the necessity of randomized trials to answer the clinical utility of PFO closure devices. Devices approved for ASD and

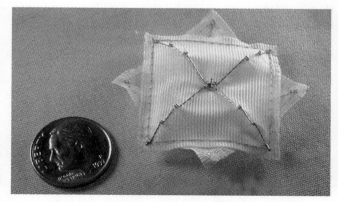

■ **Figure 23-10** The CardioSeal septal occlusion system. A dime is placed next to the device to represent size. (Courtesy of NMT Medical, Inc., Boston, MA.)

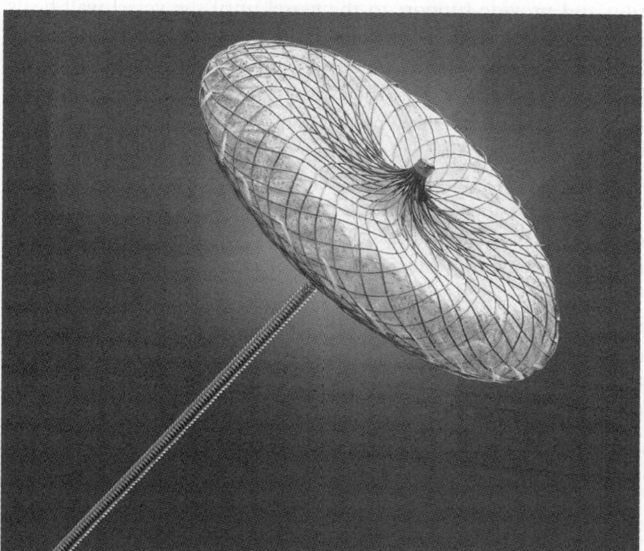

■ **Figure 23-11** The Amplatzer Septal Occluder for atrial septal defect closure. (Courtesy of AGA Medical Corporation, Golden Valley, MN; Courtesy of Boston Scientific Corporation, Maple Grove, MN.)

VSD (ventricular septal defect) closure have been used for a brief time as humanitarian device exemptions in high-risk patients with presumed paradoxical embolism.[82] Patients are currently treated with PFO devices through enrollment into clinical trials.

Paradoxical embolism is often invoked as a cause of stroke when no other cause can be easily identified. Between 30% and 40% of strokes in young patients (less than 55 years) have no identifiable cause. The association between a PFO and stroke is stronger in younger patients. A review of observational studies suggested a rate of recurrent events in patients undergoing percutaneous closure of a PFO to be 0% to 4.9% compared with 3.8% to 12% in medically treated patients. Major complications occur in 1.5% of patients undergoing percutaneous PFO closure.[82]

Currently there is insufficient evidence to recommend closure of PFO in patients with a first stroke and PFO.[82,83] A transcatheter PFO closure may be considered in patients with recurrent cryptogenic stroke despite optimal medical therapy (Class IIb recommendation:).[83]

An incidental finding in some patients with migraine with aura was the presence of a PFO. A recent trial confirmed the high prevalence of right-to-left shunt in patients with migraine with aura, and supports further need for investigation. Larger trials are currently underway in the USA and Europe.[84]

FUTURE DIRECTIONS FOR PCI

Interventional cardiology has expanded to provide an array of treatment options for CAD. DESs have significantly decreased restenosis and repeat revascularization but with the small but devastating risk of very late stent thrombosis. New antiproliferative drug coatings (zotarolimus and everolimus) for stents are coming to market with promising results.[85,86]

Bioabsorbable stents and nonpolymer technology (polymers in some patients cause a hypersensitivity reaction) with potential to reduce stent thrombosis are currently in clinical trials. The bioabsorbable stent is designed to mechanically reduce the coronary lesion and provide support to the vessel until the vessel wall heals and endothelialization is complete. Unlike the metallic stents, a bioabsorbable stent is designed to be slowly metabolized by the body and completely absorbed over time. A preliminary clinical trial with bioabsorbable stents has shown clinical safety in patients with CAD. This platform of stents, if successful, has potential for reducing stent thrombosis.[87]

Longitudinal databases need to be created to follow patient outcomes more consistently and identify the risks and benefits of the interventional procedures. A comprehensive database combined with continued research with interventional devices will help determine future recommendations. The percutaneous treatment of congenital abnormalities with noninvasive techniques will continue to evolve as outcome data become available. The cost for new technology and research will continue to be a challenge.

NURSING MANAGEMENT OF PATIENTS UNDERGOING PCI

Nursing management focuses on identification and preparation of eligible patients before treatment and on prevention, detection, and treatment of potential complications after interventional cardiology measures.

Anxiety Related to Uncertainty About PCI and Its Outcomes

At the time of admission, anxiety may occur related to unfamiliar environment, unfamiliar treatment modality, and uncertainty of outcome. Chest pain/discomfort related to myocardial ischemia if the patient is in the acute phase of MI or unstable angina may contribute to increased anxiety causing increased pulse rate, respiratory rate, and blood pressure. Patients may exhibit inability to focus attention or signs of anxiety such as facial grimaces, hand clutched to chest, anger, and moaning.

Goals

To reduce anxiety and to provide the patient and family with sufficient information to allow appropriate decision making.

Interventions

Provide concise explanations of all procedures and a calm, organized delivery of care to alleviate anxiety. Perform history and physical assessment of the patient under consideration for PCI. Obtain baseline ECG and laboratory data. Implement conventional measures to relieve ischemic chest pain. Utilize skilled assessment to distinguish pain from anxiety (many indices of anxiety are also cues to pain; anxiety also increases myocardial oxygen demand and may contribute to ischemic pain). Assess patient/family level of understanding about PCI and postprocedure care. (Risks, potential complications, and alternative therapies are part of informed consent and should be addressed by the cardiologist.) Provide patients with alternative means of coping with stress and anxiety, such as music therapy, meditation, and relaxation techniques.

Outcome Criteria

Outcomes include reduction of inappropriately elevated heart rate, respiratory rate, and blood pressure; reduction in magnitude and numbers of verbal and nonverbal indices of anxiousness; patient/family self-reports of questions answered; patient/family engages in decision making.

Risk of Altered Myocardial Tissue Perfusion Causing Chest Pain/Discomfort Related to Myocardial Ischemia

The risk of recurrent chest pain/discomfort is related to ongoing ischemia and decreased myocardial tissue perfusion secondary to abrupt closure, vascular spasm, loss of coronary artery side branch, distal microembolization, or slow flow secondary to thrombus burden in ACS. The patient may return to the floor with complaints of continuing or recurring chest pain/discomfort, and may still have residual chest pain related to MI, or procedural event.

Goals

To prevent, detect, and treat chest pain/discomfort and inadequate myocardial tissue perfusion.

Interventions

Obtain baseline vital signs, ECG, and place patient on telemetry monitor with lead that reflects the lesion treated. Compare current ECG and ECG taken prior to procedure. Administer nitroglycerin as ordered. If patient had an MI or vascular spasm, or has a potential for distal microembolization, continue nitroglycerin drip until pain free or as directed. Notify cardiologist of significant changes in vital signs, ECG, or escalation of chest pain pattern. Maintain anticoagulant infusions to prevent myocardial ischemia as prescribed and monitor ordered coagulation tests. Re-occlusion of the stenotic coronary artery or intracoronary stent is signaled by sudden onset of chest pain and return of ST-segment elevation on the ECG. Lead selection for continuous ECG monitoring should be based on knowledge of the involved vessels to allow early detection of ST-segment changes that may occur in the absence of chest pain. Treatment is the same as described for the patient with myocardial ischemia.

Outcome Criteria

Outcome criteria include patient remains free of chest pain and ECG manifestations of acute injury, and coagulation tests remain within therapeutic range. Chest pain, and ECG and hemodynamic changes are noted and reported within 15 minutes of onset.

Risk of Decreased Cardiac Output Related to Arrhythmias

Cardiac ischemia, reperfusion, injection of contrast, and fluctuating fluid and electrolyte status place patients receiving interventional cardiac therapies at risk for cardiac arrhythmias. The severity of the drop in cardiac output determines the patient's response to arrhythmias. Some arrhythmias are well tolerated and require only identification, assessment of hemodynamic response, and documentation.

Goals

To detect early, identify, and treat arrhythmias, and assess and treat hemodynamic responses to arrhythmias.

Interventions

Continuously monitor cardiac rhythm to detect arrhythmias after PCI. Identify and document the arrhythmia and associated hemodynamic responses. The most common reperfusion arrhythmia is accelerated idioventricular rhythm; it usually requires no additional intervention. Ventricular tachycardia, atrial arrhythmias, bradycardia, and atrioventricular block may occur after reperfusion and intervention. Specific therapies are determined by the type of arrhythmia and severity of alteration in cardiac output.

Outcome Criteria

Outcome criteria include detection at onset of arrhythmias and accompanying hemodynamic responses, and immediate institution of appropriate interventions to stop the arrhythmia or stabilize hemodynamic parameters.

ECF DEFICIT RELATED TO CONTRAST-INDUCED DIURESIS, RESTRICTED ORAL INTAKE, HEMORRHAGE FROM DELAYED COAGULATION

An ECF deficit may further compound myocardial ischemia, and hemodynamic and rhythm instability. There is a risk of bleeding or hemorrhage related to delayed clot formation secondary to anticoagulant and antiplatelet agents, or groin complications. Aggressive anticoagulation, antiplatelet agents, or direct thrombin inhibitors, vessel trauma from the intravascular sheaths for mechanical interventions place the patient at risk for arterial access bleeding. Bleeding at puncture sites occurs from delayed or inadequate hemostasis after diagnostic angiography or interventions. This type of access bleeding is a risk for all patients receiving some type of interventional cardiac therapy because aggressive intraoperative and postprocedure anticoagulation and antiplatelet therapies result in delayed clot formation. Access-site bleeding ranges from oozing at the site of puncture to hematoma formation or retroperitoneal bleeding if the femoral approach is used.

Goals

To prevent, detect early, and treat ECF deficit. To prevent, detect early, and treat bleeding at puncture sites.

Interventions

Evaluate serum electrolytes, blood pressure, heart rate and rhythm, urine output, central pressures (central venous pressure, pulmonary artery wedge pressure if possible) or jugular venous distension, or reports of dizziness/lightheadedness when standing. Infuse intravenous fluids (normal saline, lactated Ringer's) as ordered and provide oral rehydration with electrolyte-containing fluids unless contraindicated. Evaluate patient complaints of thirst. Check postural blood pressures before ambulating postprocedure (Chapters 7 and 10). Prevent access site bleeding by leaving arterial and venous sheaths in place until heparin or a direct thrombin inhibitor can be interrupted or discontinued and ACT returns to normal. Systematic monitoring and assessment of access sites for bleeding and serial laboratory evaluation of patient platelet count, hemoglobin, and hematocrit aid in detection of bleeding. Care is also guided by institutional protocols and standing orders specific to each type of intervention.

Outcome Criteria

Outcome criteria are absence of changes in heart rate and rhythm, blood pressure, central pressures, urine output, dizziness, or lightheadedness. There are no reliable laboratory indicators of ECF deficit. Signs of ECF deficit and bleeding are detected early and reported.

REFERENCES

1. Gruentzig, A. R., & Meier, B. (1983). Percutaneous transluminal coronary angioplasty. The first five years and the future. *International Journal of Cardiology, 2*(3–4), 319–323.
2. King, S. B., III, Aversano, T., Ballard, W. L., et al. (2007). ACCF/AHA/SCAI 2007 update of the clinical competence statement on cardiac interventional procedures: A report of the American College of Cardiology Foundation/American Heart Association/American College of Physicians Task Force on Clinical Competence and Training (writing Committee to Update the 1998 Clinical Competence Statement on Recommendations for the Assessment and Maintenance of Proficiency in Coronary Interventional Procedures). *Journal of the American College of Cardiology, 50*(1), 82–108.
3. Smith, S. C., Jr., Feldman, T. E., Hirshfeld, J. W., Jr., et al. (2006). ACC/AHA/SCAI 2005 guideline update for percutaneous coronary intervention-summary article: A report of the American College of Cardiology/American Heart Association Task Force on Practice Guidelines (ACC/AHA/SCAI Writing Committee to Update the 2001 Guidelines for Percutaneous Coronary Intervention). *Journal of the American College of Cardiology, 47*(1), 216–235.
4. King, S. B., III, Smith, S. C., Jr., Hirshfeld, J. W., Jr., et al. (2008). 2007 focused update of the ACC/AHA/SCAI 2005 guideline update for percutaneous coronary intervention: A report of the American College of Cardiology/American Heart Association Task Force on Practice guidelines. *Journal of the American College of Cardiology, 51*(2), 172–209.

5. Boden, W. E., O'Rourke, R. A., Teo, K. K., et al. (2007). Optimal medical therapy with or without PCI for stable coronary disease. *New England Journal of Medicine, 356*(15), 1503–1516.
6. Jacobs, A. K. (2003). Coronary revascularization in women in 2003: Sex revisited. *Circulation, 107*(3), 375–377.
7. Sedlis, S. P., Morrison, D. A., Lorin, J. D., et al. (2002). Percutaneous coronary intervention versus coronary bypass graft surgery for diabetic patients with unstable angina and risk factors for adverse outcomes with bypass: Outcome of diabetic patients in the AWESOME randomized trial and registry. *Journal of the American College of Cardiology, 40*(9), 1555–1566.
8. The Bypass Angioplasty Revascularization Investigation (BARI) Investigators. (1996). Comparison of coronary bypass surgery with angioplasty in patients with multivessel disease. The Bypass Angioplasty Revascularization Investigation (BARI) Investigators. *New England Journal of Medicine, 335*(4), 217–225.
9. The Bypass Angioplasty Revascularization Investigation (BARI) Investigators. (2000). Seven-year outcome in the Bypass Angioplasty Revascularization Investigation (BARI) by treatment and diabetic status. *Journal of the American College of Cardiology, 35*(5), 1122–1129.
10. Baumgart, D., Klauss, V., Baer, F., et al. (2007). One-year results of the SCORPIUS study: A German multicenter investigation on the effectiveness of sirolimus-eluting stents in diabetic patients. *Journal of the American College of Cardiology, 50*(17), 1627–1634.
11. Anderson, J. L., Adams, C. D., Antman, E. M., et al. (2007). ACC/AHA 2007 guidelines for the management of patients with unstable angina/non-ST-Elevation myocardial infarction: A report of the American College of Cardiology/American Heart Association Task Force on Practice Guidelines (Writing Committee to Revise the 2002 Guidelines for the Management of Patients With Unstable Angina/Non-ST-Elevation Myocardial Infarction) developed in collaboration with the American College of Emergency Physicians, the Society for Cardiovascular Angiography and Interventions, and the Society of Thoracic Surgeons endorsed by the American Association of Cardiovascular and Pulmonary Rehabilitation and the Society for Academic Emergency Medicine. *Journal of the American College of Cardiology, 50*(7), e1–e157.
12. Wali, A. (2007). Multivessel stenting in the current DES era. *Cardiac Interventions Today, 1*(1), 39–42.
13. Hannan, E. L., Wu, C., Walford, G., et al. (2008). Drug-eluting stents vs. coronary-artery bypass grafting in multivessel coronary disease. *New England Journal of Medicine, 358*(4), 331–341.
14. Wiemer, M., Langer, C., Kottmann, T., et al. (2007). Outcome in the elderly undergoing percutaneous coronary intervention with sirolimus-eluting stents: Results from the prospective multicenter German Cypher Stent Registry. *American Heart Journal, 154*(4), 682–687.
15. Dotter, C. T., & Judkins, M. P. (1989). Transluminal treatment of arteriosclerotic obstruction. Description of a new technic and a preliminary report of its application. 1964. *Radiology, 172*(3, Pt. 2), 904–920.
16. Kondo, T., Kawaguchi, K., Awaji, Y., et al. (1997). Immediate and chronic results of cutting balloon angioplasty: A matched comparison with conventional angioplasty. *Clinical Cardiology, 20*(5), 459–463.
17. Silber, S., Albertsson, P., Aviles, F. F., et al. (2005). Guidelines for percutaneous coronary interventions. The Task Force for Percutaneous Coronary Interventions of the European Society of Cardiology. *European Heart Journal, 26*(8), 804–847.
18. Bittl, J. A., Chew, D. P., Topol, E. J., et al. (2004). Meta-analysis of randomized trials of percutaneous transluminal coronary angioplasty versus atherectomy, cutting balloon atherotomy, or laser angioplasty. *Journal of the American College of Cardiology, 43*(6), 936–942.
19. Topol, E. J., Leya, F., Pinkerton, C. A., et al. (1993). A comparison of directional atherectomy with coronary angioplasty in patients with coronary artery disease. The CAVEAT Study Group. *New England Journal of Medicine, 329*(4), 221–227.
20. Holmes, D. R., Jr., Topol, E. J., Califf, R. M., et al. (1995). A multicenter, randomized trial of coronary angioplasty versus directional atherectomy for patients with saphenous vein bypass graft lesions. CAVEAT-II Investigators. *Circulation, 91*(7), 1966–1974.
21. Teirstein, P. S., Warth, D. C., Haq, N., et al. (1991). High speed rotational coronary atherectomy for patients with diffuse coronary artery disease. *Journal of the American College of Cardiology, 18*(7), 1694–1701.
22. Dahm, J. B., Kuon, E., Vogelgesang, D., et al. (2002). Relation of degree of laser debulking of in-stent restenosis as a predictor of restenosis rate. *American Journal of Cardiology, 90*(1), 68–70.
23. Ali, A., Cox, D., Dib, N., et al. (2006). Rheolytic thrombectomy with percutaneous coronary intervention for infarct size reduction in acute myocardial infarction: 30-day results from a multicenter randomized study. *Journal of the American College of Cardiology, 48*(2), 244–252.
24. Kaltoft, A., Bottcher, M., Nielsen, S. S., et al. (2006). Routine thrombectomy in percutaneous coronary intervention for acute ST-segment-elevation myocardial infarction: A randomized, controlled trial. *Circulation, 114*(1), 40–47.
25. V. Korn, H., Ohlow, M., Donev, S., et al. (2007). Export aspiration system in patients with acute coronary syndrome and visible thrombus provides no substantial benefit. *Catheterization and Cardiovascular Interventions, 70*(1), 35–42.
26. Silva, J. A., Ramee, S. R., Cohen, D. J., et al. (2001). Rheolytic thrombectomy during percutaneous revascularization for acute myocardial infarction: Experience with the AngioJet catheter. *American Heart Journal, 141*(3), 353–359.
27. Colombo, A., Stankovic, G., & Moses, J. W. (2002). Selection of coronary stents. *Journal of the American College of Cardiology, 40*(6), 1021–1033.
28. Sigwart, U., Puel, J., Mirkovitch, V., et al. (1987). Intravascular stents to prevent occlusion and restenosis after transluminal angioplasty. *New England Journal of Medicine, 316*(12), 701–706.
29. Roubin, G. S., Cannon, A. D., Agrawal, S. K., et al. (1992). Intracoronary stenting for acute and threatened closure complicating percutaneous transluminal coronary angioplasty. *Circulation, 85*(3), 916–927.
30. Fischman, D. L., Leon, M. B., Baim, D. S., et al. (1994). A randomized comparison of coronary-stent placement and balloon angioplasty in the treatment of coronary artery disease. Stent Restenosis Study Investigators. *New England Journal of Medicine, 331*(8), 496–501.
31. Serruys, P. W., de Jaegere, P., Kiemeneij, F., et al. (1994). A comparison of balloon-expandable–stent implantation with balloon angioplasty in patients with coronary artery disease. Benestent Study Group. *New England Journal of Medicine, 331*(8), 489–495.
32. Klein, L. W. (2006). Are drug-eluting stents the preferred treatment for multivessel coronary artery disease? *Journal of the American College of Cardiology, 47*(1), 22–26.
33. Weisz, G., Leon, M. B., Holmes, D. R., Jr., et al. (2006). Two-year outcomes after sirolimus-eluting stent implantation: Results from the Sirolimus-Eluting Stent in de Novo Native Coronary Lesions (SIRIUS) trial. *Journal of the American College of Cardiology, 47*(7), 1350–1355.
34. Serruys, P. W., Kutryk, M. J., & Ong, A. T. (2006). Coronary-artery stents. *New England Journal of Medicine, 354*(5), 483–495.
35. Moses, J. W., Leon, M. B., Popma, J. J., et al. (2003). Sirolimus-eluting stents versus standard stents in patients with stenosis in a native coronary artery. *New England Journal of Medicine, 349*(14), 1315–1323.
36. Grube, E., Silber, S., Hauptmann, K. E., et al. (2003). TAXUS I: Six- and twelve-month results from a randomized, double-blind trial on a slow-release paclitaxel-eluting stent for de novo coronary lesions. *Circulation, 107*(1), 38–42.
37. Schomig, A., Dibra, A., Windecker, S., et al. (2007). A meta-analysis of 16 randomized trials of sirolimus-eluting stents versus paclitaxel-eluting stents in patients with coronary artery disease. *Journal of the American College of Cardiology, 50*(14), 1373–1380.
38. Cohan, R. H., Ellis, J. H., & Dunnick, N. R. (1995). Use of low-osmolar agents and premedication to reduce the frequency of adverse reactions to radiographic contrast media: A survey of the Society of Uroradiology. *Radiology, 194*(2), 357–364.
39. Briguori, C., Airoldi, F., D'Andrea, D., et al. (2007). Renal Insufficiency Following Contrast Media Administration Trial (REMEDIAL): A randomized comparison of 3 preventive strategies. *Circulation, 115*(10), 1211–1217.
40. Antman, E. M. (2003). Should bivalirudin replace heparin during percutaneous coronary interventions? *JAMA, 289*(7), 903–905.
41. Lincoff, A. M., Bittl, J. A., Harrington, R. A., et al. (2003). Bivalirudin and provisional GP IIb/IIIa blockade compared with heparin and planned GP IIb/IIIa blockade during percutaneous coronary intervention: REPLACE-2 randomized trial. *JAMA, 289*(7), 853–863.
42. Juran, N. B., Rouse, C. L., Smith, D. D., et al. (1999). Nursing interventions to decrease bleeding at the femoral access site after percutaneous coronary intervention. SANDBAG Nursing Coordinators. Standards of Angioplasty Nursing Techniques to Diminish Bleeding Around the Groin. *American Journal of Critical Care, 8*(5), 303–313.
43. Landau, C., Lange, R. A., Glamann, D. B., et al. (1994). Vasovagal reactions in the cardiac catheterization laboratory. *American Journal of Cardiology, 73,* 95–97.
44. Dauerman, H. L., Applegate, R. J., & Cohen, D. J. (2007). Vascular closure devices: The second decade. *Journal of the American College of Cardiology, 50*(17), 1617–1626.

45. Cuisset, T., Frere, C., Quilici, J., et al. (2006). Benefit of a 600-mg loading dose of clopidogrel on platelet reactivity and clinical outcomes in patients with non-ST-segment elevation acute coronary syndrome undergoing coronary stenting. *Journal of the American College of Cardiology, 48*(7), 1339–1345.
46. Kastrati, A., Mehilli, J., Neumann, F. J., et al. (2006). Abciximab in patients with acute coronary syndromes undergoing percutaneous coronary intervention after clopidogrel pretreatment: The ISAR-REACT 2 randomized trial. *JAMA, 295*(13), 1531–1538.
47. Antman, E. M., Morrow, D. A., McCabe, C. H., et al. (2006). Enoxaparin versus unfractionated heparin with fibrinolysis for ST-elevation myocardial infarction. *New England Journal of Medicine, 354*(14), 1477–1488.
48. Collet, J. P., Montalescot, G., Lison, L., et al. (2001). Percutaneous coronary intervention after subcutaneous enoxaparin pretreatment in patients with unstable angina pectoris. *Circulation, 103*(5), 658–663.
49. EPIC Investigators. (1994). Use of a monoclonal antibody directed against the platelet glycoprotein IIb/IIIa receptor in high-risk coronary angioplasty. The EPIC Investigation. *New England Journal of Medicine, 330*(14), 956–961.
50. EPILOG Investigators. (1997). Platelet glycoprotein IIb/IIIa receptor blockade and low-dose heparin during percutaneous coronary revascularization. The EPILOG Investigators. *New England Journal of Medicine, 336*(24), 1689–1696.
51. EPISTENT Investigators. (1998). Randomised placebo-controlled and balloon-angioplasty-controlled trial to assess safety of coronary stenting with use of platelet glycoprotein-IIb/IIIa blockade. *Lancet, 352*(9122), 87–92.
52. PRISM-PLUS Investigators. (1998). Inhibition of the platelet glycoprotein IIb/IIIa receptor with tirofiban in unstable angina and non-Q-wave myocardial infarction. Platelet Receptor Inhibition in Ischemic Syndrome Management in Patients Limited by Unstable Signs and Symptoms (PRISM-PLUS) Study Investigators. *New England Journal of Medicine, 338*(21), 1488–1497.
53. Moreno, R., Fernandez, C., Hernandez, R., et al. (2005). Drug-eluting stent thrombosis: Results from a pooled analysis including 10 randomized studies. *Journal of the American College of Cardiology, 45*(6), 954–959.
54. Cavallini, C., Savonitto, S., Violini, R., et al. (2005). Impact of the elevation of biochemical markers of myocardial damage on long-term mortality after percutaneous coronary intervention: Results of the CK-MB and PCI study. *European Heart Journal, 26*(15), 1494–1498.
55. Ramana, R. K., Arab, D., Joyal, D., et al. (2005). Coronary artery perforation during percutaneous coronary intervention: Incidence and outcomes in the new interventional era. *Journal of Invasive Cardiology, 17*(11), 603–605.
56. Klein, L. W. (2006). Coronary artery perforation during interventional procedures. *Catheterization and Cardiovascular Interventions, 68*(5), 713–717.
57. Baim, D. S., & Simon, D. I. (2006). Complications and optimal use of adjunctive pharmacology. In D. S. Baim (Ed.), *Grossman's cardiac catheterization, angiography, and intervention* (7th ed., pp. 36–76). Philadelphia: Lippincott Williams & Wilkins.
58. Laskey, W., Boyle, J., & Johnson, L. W. (1993). Multivariable model for prediction of risk of significant complication during diagnostic cardiac catheterization. The Registry Committee of the Society for Cardiac Angiography & Interventions. *Catheterization and Cardiovascular Diagnosis, 30*(3), 185–190.
59. Bogart, D. B., Bogart, M. A., Miller, J. T., et al. (1995). Femoral artery catheterization complications: A study of 503 consecutive patients. *Catheterization and Cardiovascular Diagnosis, 34*(1), 8–13.
60. Kinnaird, T. D., Stabile, E., Mintz, G. S., et al. (2003). Incidence, predictors, and prognostic implications of bleeding and blood transfusion following percutaneous coronary interventions. *American Journal of Cardiology, 92*(8), 930–935.
61. Agrawal, S. K., Pinheiro, L., Roubin, G. S., et al. (1992). Nonsurgical closure of femoral pseudoaneurysms complicating cardiac catheterization and percutaneous transluminal coronary angioplasty. *Journal of the American College of Cardiology, 20*(3), 610–615.
62. Frazee, B. W., & Flaherty, J. P. (1991). Septic endarteritis of the femoral artery following angioplasty. *Reviews Infectious Diseases, 13*(4), 620–623.
63. Laskey, W. K., Yancy, C. W., & Maisel, W. H. (2007). Thrombosis in coronary drug-eluting stents: Report from the meeting of the Circulatory System Medical Devices Advisory Panel of the Food and Drug Administration Center for Devices and Radiologic Health, 7–8 December 2006. *Circulation, 115*(17), 2352–2357.
64. Pfisterer, M., Brunner-La Rocca, H. P., Buser, P. T., et al. (2006). Late clinical events after clopidogrel discontinuation may limit the benefit of drug-eluting stents: An observational study of drug-eluting versus bare-metal stents. *Journal of the American College of Cardiology, 48*(12), 2584–2591.
65. Buonamici, P., Marcucci, R., Migliorini, A., et al. (2007). Impact of platelet reactivity after clopidogrel administration on drug-eluting stent thrombosis. *Journal of the American College of Cardiology, 49*(24), 2312–2317.
66. Lev, E. I., Patel, R. T., Maresh, K. J., et al. (2006). Aspirin and clopidogrel drug response in patients undergoing percutaneous coronary intervention: The role of dual drug resistance. *Journal of the American College of Cardiology, 47*(1), 27–33.
67. Bavry, A. A., Kumbhani, D. J., Helton, T. J., et al. (2006). Late thrombosis of drug-eluting stents: A meta-analysis of randomized clinical trials. *American Journal of Medicine, 119*(12), 1056–1061.
68. Brilakis, E. S., Banerjee, S., & Berger, P. B. (2007). Perioperative management of patients with coronary stents. *Journal of the American College of Cardiology, 49*(22), 2145–2150.
69. Deelstra, M. H. (1993). Coronary rotational ablation: An overview with related nursing interventions. *American Journal of Critical Care, 2*(1), 16–25; quiz 26–17.
70. Ellis, S. G., Savage, M., Fischman, D., et al. (1992). Restenosis after placement of Palmaz-Schatz stents in native coronary arteries. Initial results of a multicenter experience. *Circulation, 86*(6), 1836–1844.
71. Haude, M., Baumgart, D., & Ge, J. (2000). The restenotic lesion. In S. G. Ellis & D. R. Holmes (Eds.), *Strategic approaches in coronary intervention* (2nd ed., pp. 296–324). Philadelphia: Lippincott Williams & Wilkins.
72. Teirstein, P. S., & Kuntz, R. E. (2001). New frontiers in interventional cardiology: Intravascular radiation to prevent restenosis. *Circulation, 104*(21), 2620–2626.
73. Colombo, A., Hall, P., Nakamura, S., et al. (1995). Intracoronary stenting without anticoagulation accomplished with intravascular ultrasound guidance. *Circulation, 91*(6), 1676–1688.
74. Mukherjee, D., & Moliterno, D. J. (2006). Brachytherapy for in-stent restenosis: A distant second choice to drug-eluting stent placement. *JAMA, 295*(11), 1307–1309.
75. Holmes, D. R., Jr., Teirstein, P., Satler, L., et al. (2006). Sirolimus-eluting stents vs vascular brachytherapy for in-stent restenosis within bare-metal stents: The SISR randomized trial. *JAMA, 295*(11), 1264–1273.
76. Stone, G. W., Ellis, S. G., O'Shaughnessy, C. D., et al. (2006). Paclitaxel-eluting stents vs vascular brachytherapy for in-stent restenosis within bare-metal stents: The TAXUS V ISR randomized trial. *JAMA, 295*(11), 1253–1263.
77. Hasdai, D., Holmes, D. R., & Lerman, A. (2000). Evaluating stenosis severity: Quantitative angiography, coronary flow reserve, and intravascular ultrasound. In S. G. Ellis & D. R. Holmes (Eds.), *Strategic approaches in coronary intervention* (2nd ed., pp. 175–184). Philadelphia: Lippincott Williams & Wilkins.
78. King, T. D., Thompson, S. L., Steiner, C., et al. (1976). Secundum atrial septal defect. Nonoperative closure during cardiac catheterization. *JAMA, 235*(23), 2506–2509.
79. Amin, Z., Hijazi, Z. M., Bass, J. L., et al. (2004). Erosion of Amplatzer septal occluder device after closure of secundum atrial septal defects: Review of registry of complications and recommendations to minimize future risk. *Catheterization and Cardiovascular Interventions, 63*(4), 496–502.
80. Jones, T. K., Latson, L. A., Zahn, E., et al. (2007). Results of the U.S. multicenter pivotal study of the HELEX septal occluder for percutaneous closure of secundum atrial septal defects. *Journal of the American College of Cardiology, 49*(22), 2215–2221.
81. Di Tullio, M. R., Sacco, R. L., Sciacca, R. R., et al. (2007). Patent foramen ovale and the risk of ischemic stroke in a multiethnic population. *Journal of the American College of Cardiology, 49*(7), 797–802.
82. Slottow, T. L., Steinberg, D. H., & Waksman, R. (2007). Overview of the 2007 Food and Drug Administration Circulatory System Devices Panel meeting on patent foramen ovale closure devices. *Circulation, 116*(6), 677–682.
83. Sacco, R. L., Adams, R., Albers, G., et al. (2006). Guidelines for prevention of stroke in patients with ischemic stroke or transient ischemic attack: A statement for healthcare professionals from the American Heart Association/American Stroke Association Council on Stroke: Co-sponsored by the Council on Cardiovascular Radiology and Intervention: The American

Academy of Neurology affirms the value of this guideline. *Circulation, 113*(10), e409–e449.

84. Dowson, A., Mullen, M. J., Peatfield, R., et al. (2008). Migraine Intervention With STARFlex Technology (MIST) trial: A prospective, multicenter, double-blind, sham-controlled trial to evaluate the effectiveness of patent foramen ovale closure with STARFlex septal repair implant to resolve refractory migraine headache. *Circulation, 117*(11), 1397–1404.
85. Kandzari, D. E., Leon, M. B., Popma, J. J., et al. (2006). Comparison of zotarolimus-eluting and sirolimus-eluting stents in patients with native coronary artery disease: A randomized controlled trial. *Journal of the American College of Cardiology, 48*(12), 2440–2447.
86. Serruys, P. W., & Ruygrok, P. (2006). A randomized comparison of an everolimus-eluting coronary stent with a paclitaxel-eluting coronary stent: The SPIRIT II trial. *Eurointervention, 2*, 286–294.
87. Ormiston, J. A., Serruys, P. W., Regar, E., et al. (2008). A bioabsorbable everolimus-eluting coronary stent system for patients with single de-novo coronary artery lesions (ABSORB): A prospective open-label trial. *Lancet, 371*(9616), 899–907.

CHAPTER 24

Heart Failure and Cardiogenic Shock

Laurie A. Soine

HEART FAILURE

Heart failure (HF) is a pathophysiologic state in which an abnormality of cardiac function is responsible for inadequate systemic perfusion. HF is not an event or disease but rather a constellation of signs and symptoms that represent the final pathway of a heterogeneous group of diseases, the end result of most cardiovascular disease states.[1] The extent and severity by which cardiac function is impaired varies greatly. It is the primary reason people over the age of 65 are hospitalized in the United States.[2,3] Three-month rehospitalization rates for recurrent failure are as high as 79%.[3]

The prevalence of the syndrome of HF has increased dramatically throughout the world over the last decade, attributable to both the general aging of the worlds' population and advances in the treatment of acute cardiac disease. Over 5 million people carry the diagnosis, with approximately 550,000 new cases diagnosed annually.[4] While the syndrome of HF has been extensively researched and intensively studied, it remains a significant and growing health problem in the United States and worldwide. There is an increasing incidence of HF in the aging population, with a prevalence of approximately 10% by age 70 years. For HF occurring in the absence of myocardial infarction (MI), the lifetime risk is 1 in 9 for men and 1 in 6 for women; the increase in HF is largely attributable to hypertension.[5] The American Heart Association estimates that greater than $33 billion is spent on the syndrome of HF annually.[4]

As many as 20 million people in the United States who have asymptomatic impairment of cardiac function are likely to develop symptoms of HF within 5 years.[4] In the past decade, experimental and clinical studies have demonstrated altered neurohormonal activity as a major pathophysiologic component of HF. The quality of life, exercise capacity, and perhaps the life expectancy of patients with HF can be altered by the introduction of appropriate medical and nursing interventions.

This chapter reviews major physiologic and pathophysiologic concepts of chronic HF as a basis for understanding its underlying causes as well as its clinical and physical findings. Emphasis also is placed on the various diagnostic tests, the vast array of pharmacologic agents, and medical and nursing interventions in the adult patient with ventricular dysfunction. With this knowledge, the nurse is able to develop and implement a plan of care, to identify patients at risk for developing the syndrome, and to optimize the functional capacity and outcome of patients living with the syndrome of HF. Although pharmacologic agents are reviewed in this chapter, refer to current sources of information for specifics of use and dose.

Historic Perspective

The understanding of the syndrome of HF has evolved dramatically in the last 100 years. Advances in our understanding of the syndrome have evolved secondary to the tools available to detect and mark the disease progression. During the nineteenth century the altered architecture of the failing heart was implicated as the cause of patient's symptoms. In 1832, James Hope first described *backward failure* as the failure that results as the ventricle fails to pump its volume, causing blood accumulation and subsequent increase in ventricular, atrial, and venous pressures. A primary cause of backward failure was mechanical cardiac obstruction. The term *forward failure*, proposed by MacKenzie in 1913, was applied to a situation in which the primary pathologic process was decreased cardiac output, which ultimately leads to a decrease in vital organ perfusion, and to water and sodium retention.[6] MacKenzie was the first to propose that intrinsic myocardial abnormalities lead to the death of patients with this syndrome.[7] By the mid-1920s Starling and colleagues revolutionized the understanding of the syndrome with their animal studies describing the effect of alterations in pressure and flow on myocardial performance. This work formed the basis upon which the syndrome was understood until almost the end of the twentieth century. The hemodynamic derangement secondary to pressure and flow abnormalities became the accepted paradigm, explaining the therapeutic interventions of the time. If pressure and volume where the two components of myocardial contractility—causing reduced cardiac output, therapeutic interventions were aimed at accurately assessing and altering hemodynamics. While we now know that cardiac hemodynamics play a role in the syndrome of HF, therapeutic intervention targeted at normalization of hemodynamic derangement did not translate to improved outcomes in patients.

Advances in cellular biochemistry and biophysics in the 1970s to 1980s lead to a widening of the lens through which the complexity and progression of the HF syndrome emerged. Patients with HF were noted to have markedly elevated levels of stress hormones such as norepinephirine. These discoveries led some to hypothesize that while myocardial dysfunction begins the syndrome, progression and subsequent death of the patients may be attributable to dramatic neurohormonal abnormalities. By the early 1990s studies of medications aimed at altering the neurohormonal milieu within the body solidly supported the neurohormonal/neuroendocrine hypothesis that remains the target of many of our current interventions.[8] However, by the turn of the twentieth century advances in the ability to measure molecular changes in myocytes has lead to an ever complex understanding of the collection of complex genetic and molecular disorders that lead to and perpetuate the syndrome.

Etiologies and Definitions

HF is a complex clinical syndrome manifested by shortness of breath, fatigue, and characterized by abnormalities of left ventricular

Table 24-1 ■ CONDITIONS ASSOCIATED WITH HEART FAILURE

Abnormal Volume Load	Abnormal Pressure Load	Myocardial Abnormalities	Filling Disorders	Increased Metabolic Demand
Aortic valve incompetence	Aortic stenosis	Cardiomyopathy	Mitral stenosis	Anemias
Mitral valve incompetence	Hypertrophic cardiomyopathy	Myocarditis	Tricuspid stenosis	Thyrotoxicosis
Tricuspid valve incompetence	Coarctation of the aorta	Coronary heart disease	Cardiac tamponade	Fever
Left-to-right shunts	Hypertension	Ischemia	Restrictive pericarditis	Beriberi
Secondary hypervolemia	Primary	Infarction	Restrictive cardiomyopathy	Paget's disease
	Secondary	Arrhythmias		Arteriovenous fistulas
		Toxic disorders		Pulmonary emboli
		Alcohol		Systemic emboli
		Cocaine		
		Administration of cardiac depressants agents or salt-retaining drugs		

(LV) function and neurohormonal regulation.[1] Any disorder that places the heart under an increased volume or pressure load or that produces primary damage or an increased metabolic demand on the myocardium may result in HF (Table 24-1). Over the last decade there has been a primary shift in the etiology of HF with coronary artery disease (CAD) surpassing hypertension or valvular heart disease.[5] As treatment modalities for both the acute and chronic treatment of CAD improve, the number of patients living with CAD grows.

Ventricular dysfunction begins with injury. It is vital for the clinician to identify the underlying and the precipitating causes of HF. CAD is the underlying cause of HF in two thirds of patients with systolic dysfunction. Hypertension is implicated in both systolic and diastolic dysfunctions. Arrhythmias are common in patients with underlying structural heart disease; and they commonly precipitate an acute decompensation in patients with stable HF. These arrhythmias may take the form of tachyarrhythmias (most commonly atrial fibrillation), marked bradycardia, degrees of heart block, and abnormal intraventricular conduction, such as left bundle-branch block or ventricular arrhythmias. Other precipitating factors include systemic infections, anemias, and pulmonary emboli that all place increased metabolic and hemodynamic demand on the heart. Administration of cardiac depressants or salt-retaining drugs may precipitate HF; examples may include corticosteroids, nondihydropyridine calcium-channel antagonists, and nonsteroidal anti-inflammatory drugs (NSAIDs). Alcohol is a potent myocardial depressant and may be responsible for the development of cardiomyopathy. Inappropriate reduction in therapy is perhaps the most common cause of decompensation in a previously compensated patient, with reduction in pharmacological therapy or dietary excess of sodium.

Stages of HF

The writing committee of the American College of Cardiology and the American Heart Association (ACC/AHA) Task Force decided to emphasize the evolution and progression of HF in their most recent revision of the guidelines.[1] This classification recognizes that HF, like CAD, has established risk factors, that the progression of HF has asymptomatic and symptomatic phases, and that treatments prescribed at each stage can reduce morbidity and mortality. Four stages of HF were identified. Stage A identifies the patient who is at high risk but has no structural heart disease; stage B refers to a patient with structural heart disease but no symptoms of HF; stage C denotes the patient with structural heart disease and current or previous symptoms of HF; and stage D describes the patient with end-stage disease that requires special interventions (Fig. 24-1). The importance of this staging system arises from the fact that, while treatment options for HF have advanced in the last decade, once myocyte, myocardial, and systemic changes have begun, the only treatment option is altering the trajectory of the syndrome as cure is seldom an option.

As the understanding of the mechanisms underlying both the development and progression of the syndrome have evolved, much attention of late has been placed on identifying the factors that put patients at risk for developing the syndrome (Table 24-2). While it is not surprising that advancing age, history of CAD, MI, or hypertension are associated with developing HF, a robust association has been seen in patients with both Type II diabetes mellitus (DM)[9,10] and obesity, and the subsequent syndrome of HF. The worldwide epidemic of Type II DM and obesity make them potentially modifiable targets to reduce incidence of HF.

The clinical manifestations of acute and chronic failure depend on how rapidly the syndrome of HF develops. Acute HF may be the initial manifestation of heart disease but is more commonly an acute exacerbation of a chronic cardiac condition. The marked decrease in LV function may be caused by acute MI or acute valvular dysfunction. The events occur so rapidly that the sympathetic nervous system compensation is ineffective, resulting in the rapid development of pulmonary edema and circulatory collapse (cardiogenic shock). Chronic HF develops over time and is usually the end result of an increasing inability of physiologic mechanisms to compensate.

Low and High Cardiac Output Syndromes

In response to high blood pressure and hypovolemia, low cardiac output syndrome can appear. The word *syndrome* implies that the failure represents a reaction rather than a primary pathologic process. Low cardiac output syndrome is evidenced by impaired peripheral circulation and peripheral vasoconstriction.

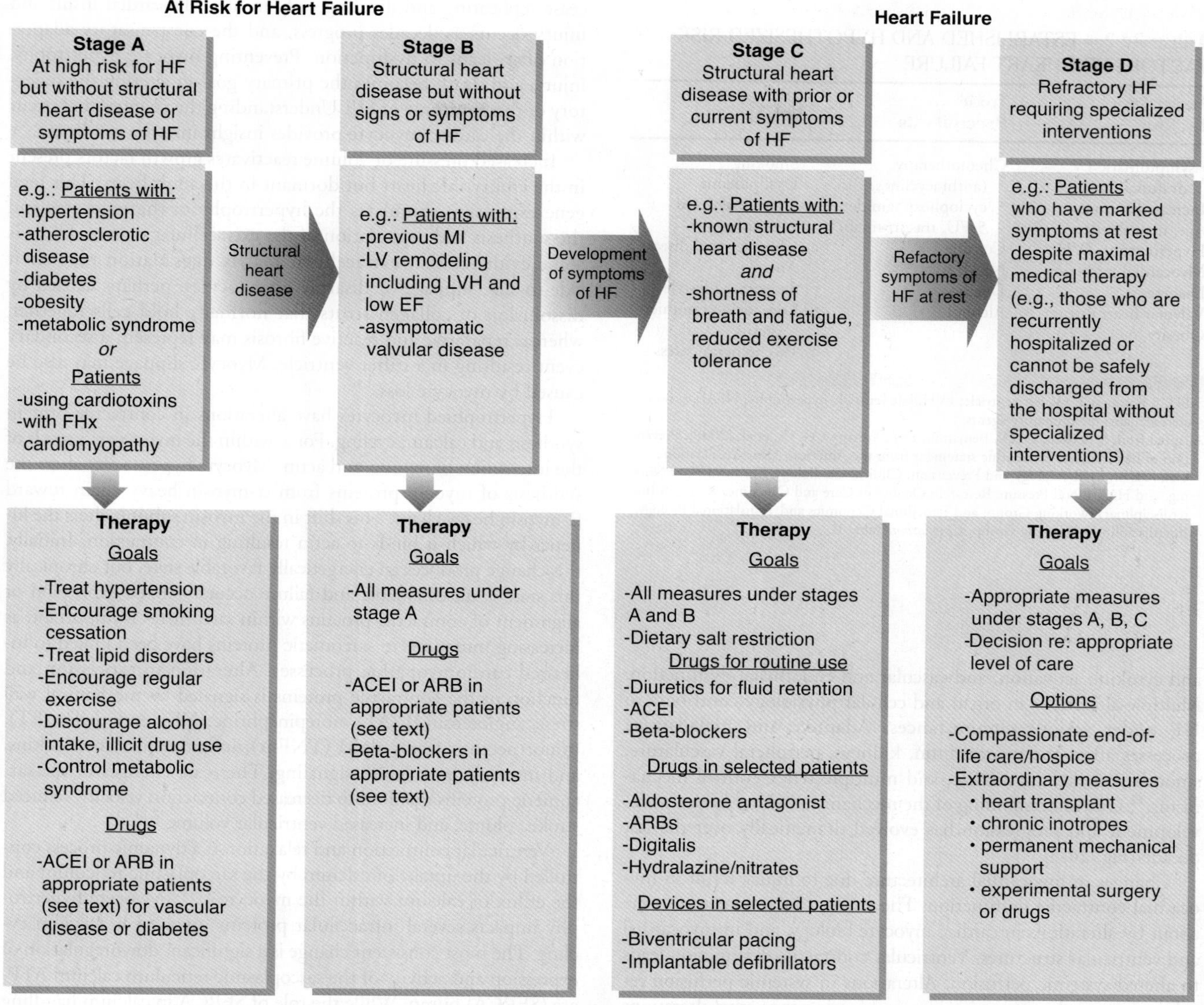

At Risk for Heart Failure
Heart Failure
Stage A
At high risk for HF but without structural heart disease or symptoms of HF
e.g.: Patients with:
-hypertension
-atherosclerotic disease
-diabetes
-obesity
-metabolic syndrome
or
Patients
-using cardiotoxins
-with FHx cardiomyopathy
Structural heart disease
Stage B
Structural heart disease but without signs or symptoms of HF
e.g.: Patients with:
-previous MI
-LV remodeling including LVH and low EF
-asymptomatic valvular disease
Development of symptoms of HF
Stage C
Structural heart disease with prior or current symptoms of HF
e.g.: Patients with:
-known structural heart disease
and
-shortness of breath and fatigue, reduced exercise tolerance
Refactory symptoms of HF at rest
Stage D
Refractory HF requiring specialized interventions
e.g.: Patients who have marked symptoms at rest despite maximal medical therapy (e.g., those who are recurrently hospitalized or cannot be safely discharged from the hospital without specialized interventions)
Therapy
Goals
-Treat hypertension
-Encourage smoking cessation
-Treat lipid disorders
-Encourage regular exercise
-Discourage alcohol intake, illicit drug use
-Control metabolic syndrome
Drugs
-ACEI or ARB in appropriate patients (see text) for vascular disease or diabetes
Therapy
Goals
-All measures under stage A
Drugs
-ACEI or ARB in appropriate patients (see text)
-Beta-blockers in appropriate patients (see text)
Therapy
Goals
-All measures under stages A and B
-Dietary salt restriction
Drugs for routine use
-Diuretics for fluid retention
-ACEI
-Beta-blockers
Drugs in selected patients
-Aldosterone antagonist
-ARBs
-Digitalis
-Hydralazine/nitrates
Devices in selected patients
-Biventricular pacing
-Implantable defibrillators
Therapy
Goals
-Appropriate measures under stages A, B, C
-Decision re: appropriate level of care
Options
-Compassionate end-of-life care/hospice
-Extraordinary measures
• heart transplant
• chronic inotropes
• permanent mechanical support
• experimental surgery or drugs

■ **Figure 24-1** Stages in the development of heart failure/recommended therapy by stage. (From Hunt, S. A., Abraham, W. T., Chin, M. H., et al. [2005]. ACC/AHA 2005 Guideline Update for the Diagnosis and Management of Chronic Heart Failure in the Adult: A Report of the American College of Cardiology/American Heart Association Task Force on Practice Guidelines [Writing Committee to Update the 2001 Guidelines for the Evaluation and Management of Heart Failure]: Developed in Collaboration With the American College of Chest Physicians and the International Society for Heart and Lung Transplantation: Endorsed by the Heart Rhythm Society. *Circulation, 112*[12], e154–e235.) CM, cardiomyopathy; ACEI, angiotensin converting enzyme inhibitor; ARB, angiotensin II receptor blocker; LVH, left ventricular hypertrophy

Any condition that causes the heart to work harder to supply blood may be categorized as high cardiac output syndrome. High cardiac output states require an increased oxygen supply to the peripheral tissues, which can occur only with an increased cardiac output. Reduced systemic vascular resistance (SVR) is characteristic of this condition; it augments peripheral circulation and venous return, which in turn increases stroke volume and cardiac output. High cardiac output states may be caused by increased metabolic requirements, as seen in hyperthyroidism, fever, and pregnancy, or may be triggered by hyperkinetic conditions such as arteriovenous fistulas, anemia, and beriberi. While the terms *low-output* and *high-output syndromes* are not commonly used in practice, recognizing that processes occur is important.

Pathogenesis and Pathophysiology

While the root of HF is altered myocardial function, a host of compensatory systemic responses lead to the subsequent progressive clinical syndrome (Fig. 24-2). Altered myocardial function, ventricular remodeling, altered hemodynamics, neurohormonal

Table 24-2 ■ ESTABLISHED AND HYPOTHESIZED RISK FACTORS FOR HEART FAILURE

Major Risk Factors	Toxic Precipitants	Minor Risk Factors
Asymptomatic LV dysfunction	Chemotherapy (anthracyclines, cyclophosphamide, 5-FU, trastuzumab)	Smoking
Increased LV mass		Dyslipidemia
Age, male gender		Sleep-disordered breathing
Hypertension, LVH	Cocaine	Chronic renal disease
Myocardial infarction	NSAIDs	Anemia
Diabetes	Doxazosin	Sedentary lifestyle
Valvular heart disease	Alcohol	Low socioeconomic status
Obesity		Psychological stress

5-FU, 5-florouracil; LV, left ventricle; LVH, left ventricle hypertrophy; NSAIDs, nonsteroidal anti-inflammatory agents.

Adapted from Schocken, D. D., Benjamin, E. J., Fonarow, G. C., et al. [2008]. Prevention of heart failure. A scientific statement from the American Heart Association Councils on Epidemiology and Prevention, Clinical Cardiology, Cardiovascular Nursing, and High Blood Pressure Research; Quality of Care and Outcomes Research Interdisciplinary Working Group; and Functional Genomics and Translational Biology Interdisciplinary Working Group. *Circulation*, Table 1.

and cytokine activation, and vascular and endothelial dysfunction. Multiple alterations in organ and cellular physiology contribute to HF under various circumstances. Adaptive and maladaptive processes affect the myocardium, kidneys, peripheral vasculature, smooth and skeletal muscle, and multiple reflex control mechanisms.[11] Our understanding of the mechanism behind both the development and progression has evolved dramatically over the last decade (Fig. 24-3).

Changes in myocardial architecture due to injury result in myocardial contractile dysfunction. The changes in architecture come about by alterations in cardiac myocyte biology, and in myocardial and ventricular structures. Ventricular contractile dysfunction leads to altered systemic perfusion. Alterations in systemic perfusion result in neuroendocrine activation resulting in progressive alterations in myocardial architecture and contractile function. In short, myocardial injury leads to altered systemic perfusion causing neuroendorine changes that result in further ventricular dysfunction. The remainder of this section examines more closely each of the steps in this process. It is important to recognize that understanding the interplay between each of these steps is a dynamic and rapidly expanding venture.

Histologically there are four prominent features of the failing heart: (1) hypertrophy of the myocytes, (2) fibrosis, (3) myocyte disarray (or unordered appearance), and (4) apoptosis. These histological processes occur secondary to myocardial ischemia, infarction, or hemodynamic overload.[12] Ventricular hypertrophy is defined by an increase in ventricular mass attributable to increase in the volume of cardiac cells. The increase in ventricular mass is due to an increase in the size of the myocytes, increased number of fibroblasts, and an increase in the extracellular matrix proteins (collagen and fibronectin).

Myocyte Pathophysiology

The primary goal in preventing and ultimately managing HF is protection and preservation of the myocyte. Cardiac myocytes cease replicating and dividing early in life. Myocardial insult and injury occurs as decades progress, and the compensatory adaptation often leads to dysfunction. Preventing myocyte hypertrophy, injury, and death becomes the primary goal in altering the trajectory of the syndrome of HF. Understanding the changes that occur within the cardiac myocyte provides insight into the syndrome.

Increased pressure or volume reactivates growth factors present in the embryonic heart but dormant in the adult heart. This fetal gene expression stimulates the hypertrophy of the myocytes and the synthesis and degradation of the extracellular matrix. There is some evidence that extracellular matrix degradation may elicit side-to-side slippage or disarray of myocytes, perhaps caused by dissolution of collagen struts that normally hold cells together, whereas reparative and reactive fibrosis may represent a secondary event resulting in a stiffer ventricle. Myocyte slippage may also be caused by myocyte loss.[13]

Hypertrophied myocytes have alterations in contractile protein synthesis and calcium cycling. Force within the myocyte is a result of the interaction of myosin and actin. Myocyte hypertrophy alters the synthesis of myocin proteins from α-myosin heavy chain toward β-myosin heavy chain. This shift in the myosin subunit alters the kinetics by which it binds to actin resulting in contraction. Initially, this change produces an energetically favorable state, but chronically this state is unsustainable and failure occurs. Altered expression or alignment of contractile proteins within sarcomeres is important, as increasing mutations in sarcomeric proteins have been linked to inherited cardiomyopathic processes. Alteration in expression and function of the contractile proteins is signaled by mechanical wall stress, angiotensin II (AT), norepinephrine (NE), endothelin (ET), tumor necrosis factor-alpha (TNF-α), inflammatory interleukins, and intracellular calcium signaling. There are changes in the sarcomeric proteins that lead to decreased contraction velocity, reduced stroke volume, and increased ventricular volume.[7,11]

Ventricular contraction and relaxation is a dynamic process controlled by the uptake of calcium by the sarcoplasmic reticulum and the efflux of calcium within the myocyte.[11–13] Myocyte hypertrophy impacts several intracellular proteins involved in calcium cycling. The most consistent change is a significant downregulation of expression and activity of the sarcoplasmic reticulum calcium ATPase (SERCA) pump. While the role of SERCA in calcium handling within the myoctye is complex and remains the topic of study, the net result is a reduction in the availability of peak systolic calcium, and an elevation and prolongation in diastolic calcium, resulting in reduced systolic contraction and delayed diastolic relaxation.

The paracrine function of the heart is markedly altered in HF. Paracrine action is the release of a locally acting endocrine substance, a system in which the target cells are close to the signaling cells. The signal transduction system in the failing myocardium is profoundly altered. The failing myocardium is induced to secrete both atrial and b-type natriuretic peptides (ANP and BNP, respectively).

Actual myocyte loss may also occur by one of two mechanisms: apoptosis or necrosis. Apoptosis is a programmed cell death that is energy-dependent, producing cell dropout. Apoptosis is a highly regulated process that causes the cell to shrink, yielding cell fragments that are surrounded by plasma membrane. This process does not invoke an inflammatory or fibrotic response. Apoptosis is stimulated by hypoxia, AT II, TNF-α, myocyte calcium overload, and mitochondrial or cell injury.[14] Two forms of apoptosis appear to affect the course of postinfarction remodeling: ischemic-driven apoptosis at the site of the infarction and load-dependent

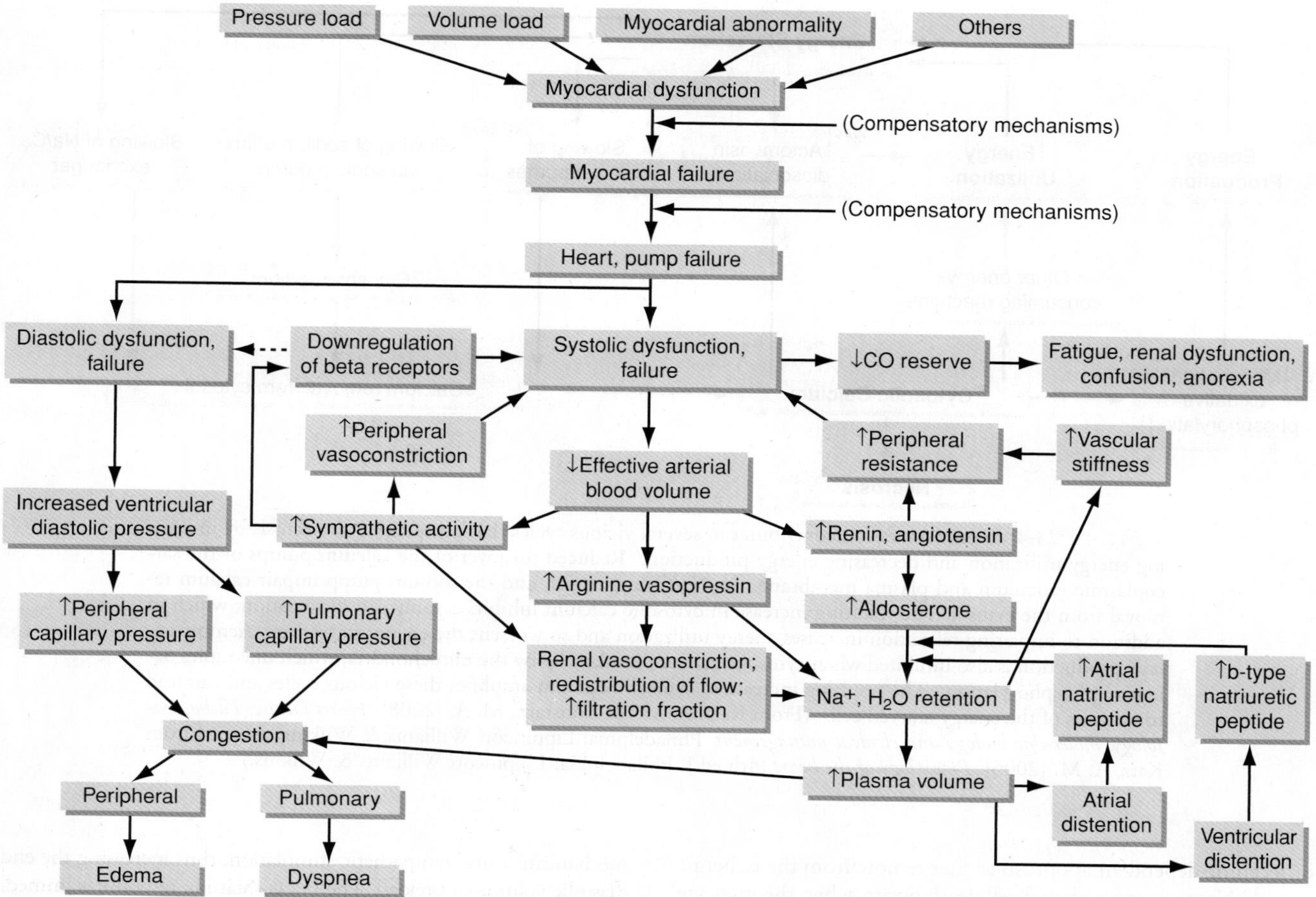

■ **Figure 24-2** Sequence of events in heart failure. An increased load or myocardial abnormality leads to myocardial failure and eventually heart failure, resulting in increased sympathetic activity, increased activity of the renin–angiotensin–aldosterone system, pulmonary and peripheral congestion and edema, and decreased cardiac output reserve. Both the atrial natriuretic and b-type natriuretic plural–peptides are also released in response to increased plasma volume. (From Francis, G. S., Gassler, J. P., & Sonneblick, E. H. [2001]. Pathophysiology and diagnosis of heart failure. In J. W. Hurst [Ed.], *The heart* [10th ed.]. New York: McGraw-Hill.)

Evolution of Heart Failure

Risk Factors		Cellular Pathophysiology		Venticular Remodeling		Venticular Dysfunction
Aging Hypertension Smoking Dyslipidemia Diabetes Obesity Toxins Genes	→	Hypertrophy Infarction Accelerated apoptosis Fibrosis	→	LVH Dilatation Both	→	Systolic Diastolic Both
		Structural Heart Disease without Symptoms				Symptomatic Heart Failure
Stage A		**Stage B** **AHA/ACC Stages of Heart Failure**				**Stages C and D**

■ **Figure 24-3** The evolution of HF along AHA/ACC guidelines for the diagnosis and management of HF clinical stages. (From Schocken, D. D., Benjamin, E. J., Fonarow, G. C. , et al. [2008]. Prevention of heart failure. A scientific statement from the American Heart Association Councils on Epidemiology and Prevention, Clinical Cardiology, Cardiovascular Nursing, and High Blood Pressure Research; Quality of Care and Outcomes Research Interdisciplinary Working Group; and Functional Genomics and Translational Biology Interdisciplinary Working Group. *Circulation*, CIRCULATIONAHA. 107.188965.)

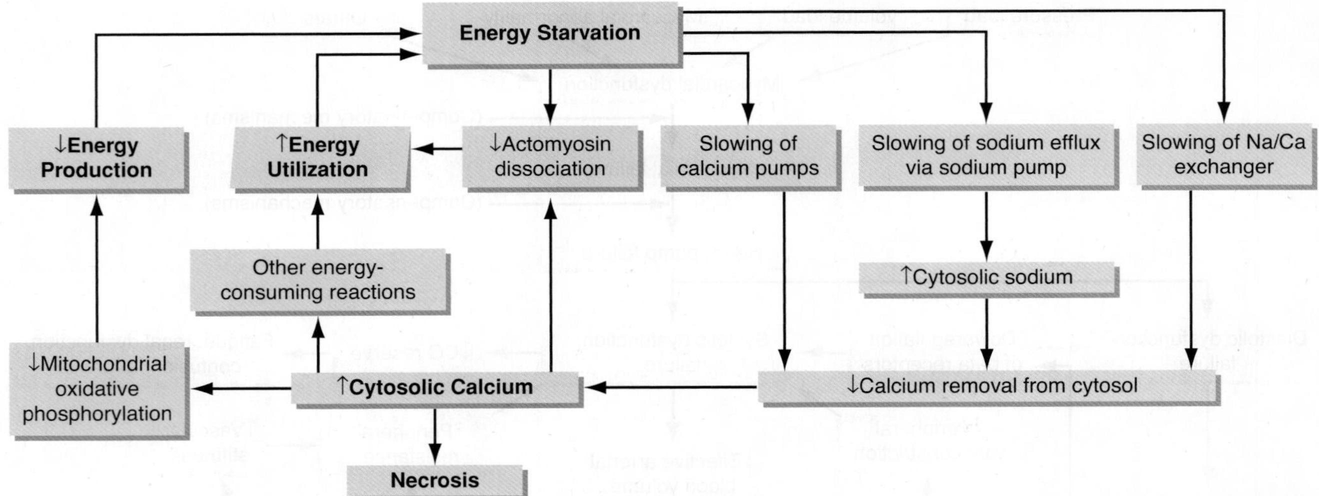

■ **Figure 24-4** Energy starvation contributes to several vicious cycles that cause myocyte necrosis by increasing energy utilization and decreasing energy production. Reduced turnover of the calcium pumps of the sarcoplasmic reticulum and plasma membrane, the Na/Ca exchanger, and the sodium pump impair calcium removal from the cytosol. The resulting increase in cytosolic calcium inhibits actomyosin dissociation, which in addition to impairing relaxation increases energy utilization and so worsens the energy starvation. Aerobic energy production is also inhibited when cytosolic calcium is taken up by the mitochondria, which uncouples oxidative phosphorylation. The resulting increase in cytosolic calcium amplifies these vicious cycles and can lead to necrosis of the energy-starved cells. (From Katz, A. M., & Konstam, M. A. [2008]. *Heart failure: Pathophysiology, molecular biology and clinical management.* Philadelphia: Lippincott Williams & Wilkins; adapted from Katz, A. M. [2006]. *Physiology of the heart* [4th ed.]. Philadelphia: Lippincott Williams & Wilkins.)

or receptor-dependent apoptosis at sites remote from the ischemic areas.[15] Necrosis or accidental cell death occurs when the myocyte is deprived of oxygen or energy. Energy starvation of the myocyte results from an increase in energy demand and a reduced capacity for energy production.[11] The inflammatory response that is induced by overload elevates circulating levels of cytokines that in turn release reactive oxygen species and free radicals. Calcium overload increases energy expenditure and slows energy production. All these processes lead to the loss of cellular membrane integrity, causing the cell to swell and eventually burst. This loss of cellular membrane integrity releases proteolytic enzymes that cause cellular disruption. The release of cell contents initiates an inflammatory reaction that leads to scarring and fibrosis. Myocyte necrosis may be localized, as in an MI, or diffuse, as from myocarditis or idiopathic cardiomyopathy.[6,7] The vicious cycle of the overloaded heart is depicted in Figure 24-4.

Ventricular Remodeling

Myocardial remodeling in the failing myocardium involves complex events at the molecular and cellular levels.[16] When the heart is presented with an increased workload by either pressure or volume overload, or by myocardial abnormality, a number of physiologic alterations are evoked in an attempt to maintain normal cardiac pumping function. Myocardial contractility (inotropy) and relaxation (lusitropy) are impaired in patients with HF. In addition, systemic hemodynamics, which include both preload and afterload, and ventricular architecture (shape, cavity size, and wall thickness) determine ejection and filling of a failing heart (Fig. 24-5).[7] As diastolic filling increases, ventricular dilatation occurs in response to maladaptive growth response and remodeling of the damaged or chronically overloaded heart. Renal compensatory mechanisms cause sympathetic stimulation, thus increasing the end-diastolic volume or preload. The Frank–Starling response is immediately activated as a consequence of increased diastolic volume. According to the Frank–Starling law, length-dependent changes in contractile performance during diastole increases the force of contraction during systole. The increased preload augmenting contractility is the major mechanism by which the ventricles

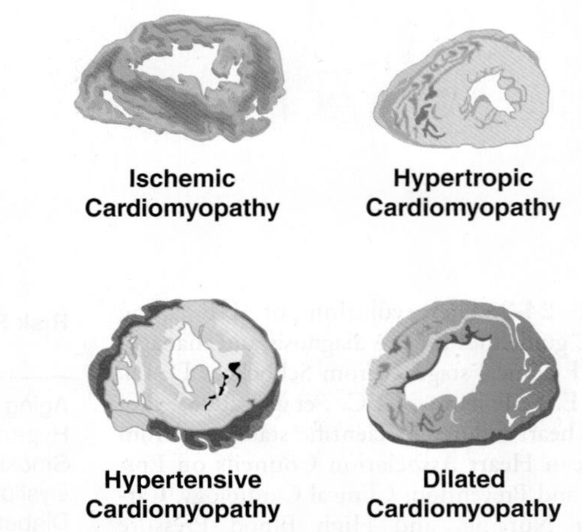

■ **Figure 24-5** Patterns of ventricular hypertrophy and remodeling in various forms of cardiomyopathy. (From Katz, A. M., & Konstam, M. A. [2008]. *Heart failure: Pathophysiology, molecular biology and clinical management.* Philadelphia: Lippincott Williams & Wilkins; adapted from Konstam, M. A. [2003]. Systolic and diastolic dysfunction in heart failure? Time for a new paradigm. *Journal of Cardiac Failure, 9*[1], 1–3.)

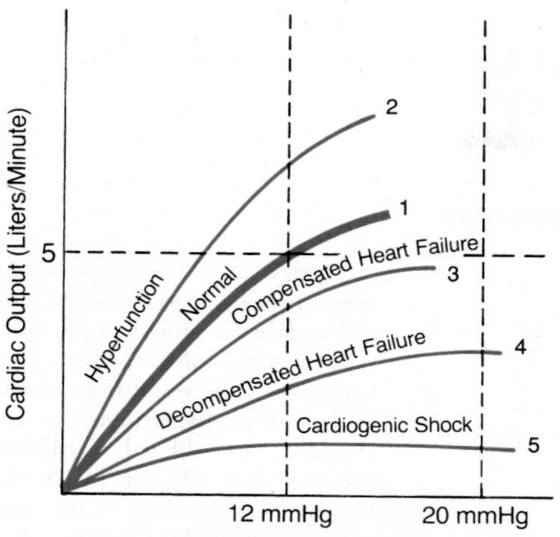

■ **Figure 24-6** Left ventricular function curves. Curve 1: Normal function curve, with a normal cardiac output at optimal filling pressures. Curve 2: Cardiac hyperfunction, with an increased cardiac output at optimal filling pressures. Curve 3: Compensated heart failure, with normal cardiac outputs at higher filling pressures. Curve 4: Decompensated heart failure, with a decrease in cardiac output and elevated filling pressures. Curve 5: Cardiogenic shock, with extremely depressed cardiac output and marked increase in filling pressures. (Adapted from Michaelson, C. R. [1983]. *Congestive heart failure* [p. 61]. St. Louis: CV Mosby.)

maintain an equal output as their stroke volumes vary.[7,11] It may be useful to consider normal and impaired myocardial function within the framework of the Frank–Starling mechanism, as illustrated by analysis of LV function curves (Fig. 24-6). Cardiac output or cardiac index (CI) is used as a measure of ventricular work; LV end-diastolic pressure or pulmonary artery wedge pressure (PAWP) is used as a reflection of preload. The normal relation between ventricular end-diastolic volume and ventricular work is shown in Figure 24-6 by curve 1. Optimal contractility occurs at a diastolic volume of 12 to 18 mm Hg. If the heart is physiologically stressed, as occurs in acute MI, the initial drop in cardiac output stimulates the sympathetic nervous system. An increase in sympathetic tone elevates heart rate and contractility, illustrated in Figure 24-6 by curve 2. As the cardiac workload increases and myocardial dysfunction persists, HF progresses. HF progression is reflected by further elevation of end-diastolic volume (preload) and ventricular dilatation. This increased preload, in turn, may further contribute to depressed ventricular contractility and the development of congestive symptoms (Fig. 24-6, curve 3).[17]

The normal left ventricle is able to adjust to large changes in aortic impedance (afterload) with small changes in output, in part by calling on the Frank–Starling response and, perhaps, by augmenting the contractile force as an intrinsic property of the normal myocardium. In contrast, the damaged left ventricle loses this compensatory ability and becomes sensitive to even small changes in impedance.[18] Because increased activity of the sympathetic nervous system or the renin–angiotensin–aldosterone system (RAAS) results in vasoconstriction of the small arteries and arterioles, increased impedance of LV filling is imposed, decreasing the stroke volume and cardiac output. Because HF is characterized by heightened activity of these neurohormonal vasoconstrictor systems, a positive-feedback loop can be generated in which impaired pump performance increases impedance to LV ejection, further impairing pump performance.

Changes in the composition of the myocardium occur in response to injury or overload and result in structural remodeling, divided into both cellular and noncellular changes. Several of the cellular changes have be discussed in the prior section and include changes within the cardiomyocytes (hypertrophy, apoptosis, and necrosis) but several alterations in other cell types, such as fibroblasts, vascular smooth muscle cells, monocytes and macrophages, also contribute to ventricular remodeling. Noncellular components of the myocardium likewise contribute to remodeling. There is an increase in interstitial deposition of collagen fibers and an increase in perivascular deposition of collagen, leading to thickening of the walls of the small intramyocardial arteries and arterioles.

Throughout the body there is a fine balance of synthesis and degradation. Fibroblasts within the myocardium produce collagen. Excesses in ventricular collagen are thought to be caused by both an increase in collagen synthesis by the myofibroblasts and an associated reduction in collagenase activity.[19] The balance of synthesis and degradation of myocardial fibrosis is complex. But it is intriguing that many of the substances known to be elevated in patients with HF are highly profibrotic and include angiotensin II, ET, NE, aldosterone, and interleukin-6. In contrast many substances that facilitate degradation seem to be lacking in patients with HF, including bradykinin, prostaglandins, and TNF-α.[11] Thus, myocardial fibrosis, which accounts for a large part of the structural changes seen in patients with HF, may be the consequence of the loss of regulation that exists between synthesis and degradation.

Neurotransmitters such as NE, secreted at sympathetic nerve junctions within the myocardium, attempt to help the myocardium meet the increasing demands of the body. β-Receptors located within the myocardium serve as the portal to activation. Stimulation of β_1-receptors leads to increased heart rate, contractility, and speed of relaxation. Myocardial injury leads to neurohormonal activation that prompts a dramatic reduction of both the number and function of β-receptors within the myocardium, resulting in impaired signal transduction and disturbances in myocellular calcium metabolism.

The metabolism of the failing myocardium likewise is altered adversely. In fact, the hyperadrenergic state of HF initiates a metabolic vicious cycle. The principal energy source in a normal myocardium is free fatty acids, but in hypertrophic states, switches to glucose utilization. Myocardial energy generation and utilization may have a profound effect on cellular energy levels. Altered myocardial carbohydrate metabolism and related insulin resistance are currently variables of interest in abnormal myocardial energetics.

Ventricular volume overload and increased diastolic wall stress lead to replication of sarcomeres, elongation of myocytes, and ventricular dilatation or eccentric hypertrophy. Maladaptive growth and changing myocyte phenotype leads to myocyte thickening (seen in diastolic dysfunction and concentric hypertrophy) and myocyte elongation (seen in systolic dysfunction and eccentric hypertrophy).[20] These large, genetically abnormal cells cannot contract as efficiently as normal cells (Fig. 24-7).

Concentric and eccentric hypertrophy impair ventricular filling. Decreased cavity size, as seen in concentric hypertrophy, decreases compliance and thus impedes venous return. Eccentric hypertrophy, which increases end-diastolic volume and pressure,

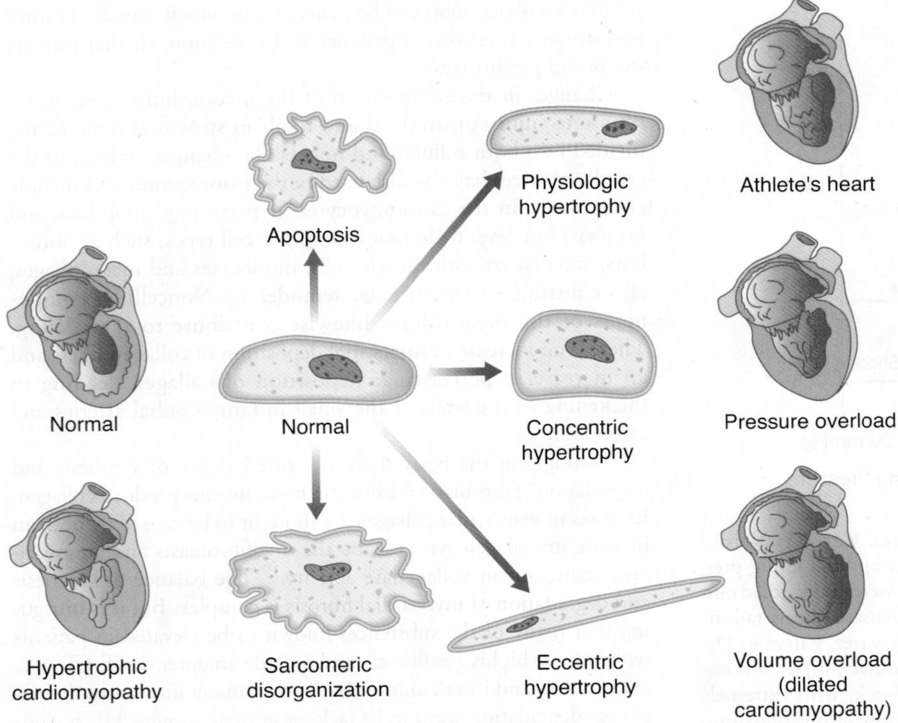

■ **Figure 24-7** Phenotype change of the heart at the cellular and organ levels. Normal muscle can grow in a physiologic way, as seen in the athlete's heart. Concentric hypertrophy can result from pressure overload; eccentric hypertrophy due to volume overload, or dilated cardiomyopathy. (Adapted from Drexler, H., & Hasenfuss, G. [2001]. Physiology of the normal and failing heart. In M. Crawford, & J. P. DiMarco [Eds.], *Cardiology.* London: Mosby.)

is also accompanied by a decrease in compliance.[12] Mechanisms responsible for diastolic dysfunction include hypertrophy, as described, which causes an increase in passive chamber stiffness (decreased compliance) and decreased active relaxation. Decreased levels of activity of SERCA (sarco/endoplasmic reticulum calcium ATPase) to remove calcium from the cytosol and increased levels of phospholamban (a SERCA inhibitory protein) lead to a net effect of impaired relaxation. This same net effect is seen in myocardial ischemia, abnormal ventricular loading (e.g., in hypertrophic or dilated cardiomyopathy), asynchrony, abnormal flux of calcium ions, and hypothyroidism. Of interest, SERCA decreases with age, coincident with impaired diastolic dysfunction.[6,21] Wall stiffness and associated decreased compliance is increased with age and is caused, in part, by diffuse fibrosis. Decreased compliance is also noted in patients with focal scar or aneurysm after MI. Infiltrative cardiomyopathies (e.g., amyloidosis) can also increase wall stiffness. Pericardial constriction or tamponade causes mechanical increased resistance to filling of part or all of the heart.[20] Interactions with LV hypertrophy (LVH), ischemia, and diastolic dysfunction create a vicious cycle in which LVH predisposes to ischemia, the ischemia causes impairment of relaxation in the heart with LVH, and the severity of subendocardial ischemia worsens. Several mechanisms appear to lower subendocardial perfusion pressure. Coronary vascular remodeling occurs with increased medial thickness and perivascular fibrosis. The increased LV mass and inadequate vascular growth results in a loss of coronary vasodilator reserve so that there is a limited ability to increase myocardial perfusion in response to an increased oxygen demand. In addition, increased diastolic pressure exerts a compressive force against the subendocardium and restricts subendocardial perfusion.[20]

Altered Systemic Perfusion Results in Neuroendocrine Activation

The major elements of the neuroendocrine response may be described as activation of the sympathetic nervous system, RAAS, and inflammatory systems. While each of these homeostatic mechanisms represents a beneficial short-term response to impaired cardiac function, they also are associated with detrimental maladaptive long-term consequences (Table 24-3).[7]

The systemic response to a decrease in cardiac output accelerates heart rate, vasoconstricts arteries and veins, increases the ejection fraction and, by promoting salt and water retention by the kidneys, increases blood volume. Salt and water retention, vasoconstriction, and cardiac stimulation are mediated by signaling molecules that play a regulatory and counter-regulatory role in HF (Table 24-4). The various mediators evoke similar and often overlapping responses. When a regulatory signal turns on a process, counter-regulatory signals are released to turn off the process.[7,22]

Activation of the Sympathetic Nervous System. The most important stimulus for vasoconstriction in HF is sympathetic activation that releases catecholamines. Plasma levels of NE become elevated. NE binds to α_1-adrenergic receptors increasing vascular tone to raise SVR (afterload) and mean systemic filling pressure, thereby augmenting venous return or preload (Fig. 24-8).[23]

In HF, stimulation of the sympathetic nervous system represents the most immediately responsive mechanism of compensation. Stimulation of the β-adrenergic receptors in the heart causes an elevation in heart rate and contractility to raise stroke volume and cardiac output. Sympathetic over-activity in HF may exert adverse effects on the structure and function of the myocardium

Table 24-3 ■ NEUROHORMONAL RESPONSE: SHORT- AND LONG-TERM RESPONSES

Mechanism	Short-Term Adaptive	Long-Term Maladaptive
Functional	**Adaptive Response**	**Maladaptive Consequences**
Salt and water retension	↑Preload, maintain cardiac output	Edema, anasarca, pulmonary congestion
Vasoconstriction	↑Afterload, maintain blood pressure	↓ Cardiac output, ↑energy expenditure, cardiac necrosis
Cardiac β-adrenergic drive	↑Contractility, ↑Relaxation ↑Heart rate	↑ Cytosolic calcium (arrhythmias, sudden death ↑ Cardiac energy demand (cardiac necrosis)
Proinflammatory	**"Anti-Other"** Antimicrobial, antihelminthic Adaptive hypertophy	**"Anti-Self"** Cachexia (skeletal catabolism) Skeletal muscle myopathy
Proliferative	**Adaptive Hypertrophy**	**Maladaptive Hypertrophy**
Transcriptional activation More sarcomeres	Cell thickening (normalize wall stress, maintain cardiac output) ↑ Sarcomere number	Cell elongation (dilation, remodeling, increased wall stress) Apoptosis ↑ Cardiac energy demand (cardiac myocyte necrosis)

Adapted from Katz, A. M., & Konstam, M. A. (2008). *Heart failure: Pathophysiology, molecular biology and clinical management.* Philadelphia: Lippincott Williams & Wilkins.

by the process of remodeling. Myocardial remodeling involves hypertrophy and apoptosis of myocytes, regression to a cellular phenotype, and changes in the nature of the extracellular matrix.[11,23]

Attenuating the myocardial response to NE is an important counter-regulatory change in patients with HF. Chronic sympathetic stimulation inhibits β-receptor synthesis and reduces the ability of the β-receptor to respond to the stimulus of NE. β-Receptor downregulation reduces the amount of receptors available to bind to NE. Mechanisms responsible for β_1-receptor downregulation help protect the failing heart from the adverse effects of sustained sympathetic stimulation.

Table 24-4 ■ REGULATORY AND COUNTER REGULATORY SIGNALING MOLECULES

I. Signaling Molecules Whose Major Role is Regulatory

Mediators
Catecholamines (peripheral effect)
Renin–angiotensin–aldosterone system (angiotensin II)
Arginine vasopressin or ADH
Endothelin

Responses
Retention of fluid by kidneys
Vasoconstriction
Stimulation of cell growth and proliferation
Increased contractility, relaxation, heart rate

II. Signaling Molecules Whose Major Role is Counter Regulatory

Mediators
Catecholamines (peripheral effect)
Dopamine
Atrial natriuretic peptide
Nitric oxide
Bradykinin

Effects
Reduced fluid retention by the kidneys
Vasodilatation
Decreased cardiac contractility, relaxation, heart rate
Inhibition of cell growth and proliferation

Adapted from Katz, A. M., & Konstam, M. A. (2008). *Heart failure: Pathophysiology, molecular biology and clinical management.* Philadelphia: Lippincott Williams & Wilkins.

Activation of the RAAS. The RAAS plays an important role in HF; AT has a vast range of biologic activities (Fig. 24-9). In addition to stimulating aldosterone, AT is a potent vasoconstrictor.[11] There are four recognized AT receptor sites, but the AT1 receptors, which predominate in adult hearts, exert their regulatory effects in myocytes: vasoconstriction, increased myocardial contractility,

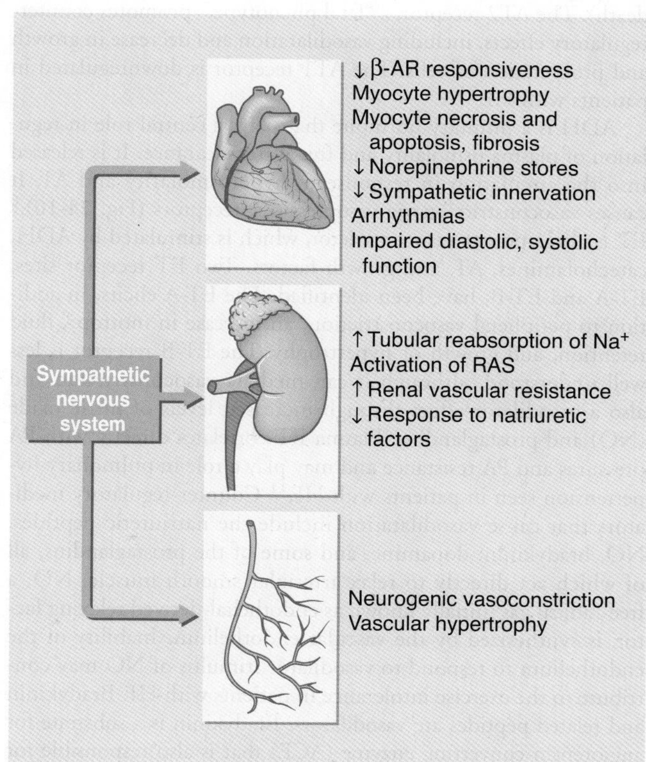

■ **Figure 24-8** Increased sympathetic activity may contribute to the pathophysiology of HF by multiple mechanisms. (B-AR, postsynaptic β-adrenergic receptor; RAS, renin–angiotensin system. (Adapted from Floras, J. S. [1993]. Clinical aspects of sympathetic activation and parasympathetic withdrawal in heart failure. *Journal of American College of Cardiology, 22*[4, Suppl. A], 72A–84A.)

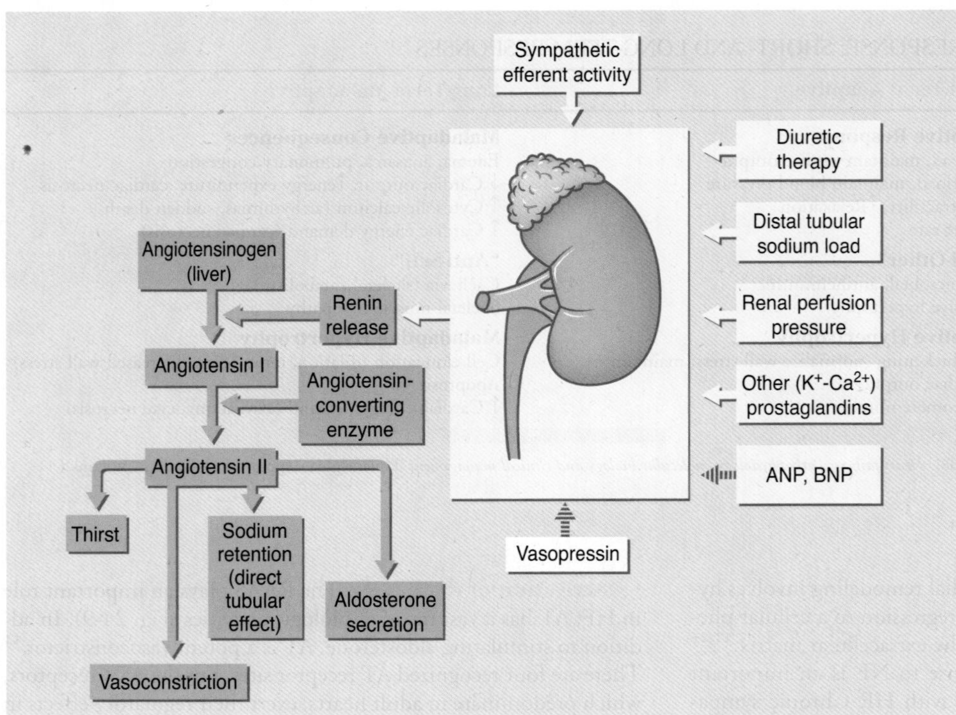

■ **Figure 24-9** The renin–angiotensin–aldosterone system is activated in patients with heart failure. Multiple stimuli may contribute to renal release of renin into the systemic circulation, including increased sympathetic efferent activity, decreased tubular sodium delivery, reduced renal perfusion, and diuretic therapy. Natriuretic peptides (ANP, BNP), and vasopressin (ADH) (*striped arrows*) may inhibit release of renin. Angiotensin I is converted to angiotensin II, which is a potent vasoconstrictor; it promotes sodium reabsorption by increasing aldosterone secretion, and by a direct effect on the tubules, stimulates water intake by acting on the thirst center. (Adapted from Paganelli, W. C., Craeger, M. A., & Dzau, V. J. [1986]. Cardiac regulation of renal function. In T. O. Cheung [Ed.], *International textbook of cardiology.* New York: Bergamman Press.)

cell growth (hypertrophy), and apoptosis (programmed cell death). The AT2 receptor, a "fetal phenotype," promotes counter-regulatory effects, including vasodilatation and decrease in growth and proliferation of cells. The AT1 receptor is downregulated in patients with HF.[24]

ADH is a pituitary hormone that plays a central role in regulation of plasma osmolality and free water clearance. It is released into the circulation in response to hyperosmolarity and AT. It causes vasoconstriction via vasopressin 1 receptors (Fig. 24-10).[6] ET is also a potent vasoconstrictor, which is stimulated by ADH, catecholamines, AT, and growth factors. Two ET receptor sites, ET-A and ET-B, have been identified. The ET-A elicits, in addition to peripheral vasoconstriction, an increase in inotropy, fluid retention, and growth or hypertrophy. The ET-B receptor is less well understood, although it can mediate vasoconstriction and also a vasodilator effect through increased levels of nitric oxide (NO) and prostaglandins. Plasma ET correlates directly with PA pressures and PA resistance and may play a role in pulmonary hypertension seen in patients with HF.[11] Counter-regulatory mediators that cause vasodilatation include the natriuretic peptides, NO, bradykinin, dopamine, and some of the prostaglandins, all of which act directly to relax arteriolar smooth muscle. NO, a free-radical gas initially known as endothelial-derived relaxing factor, is synthesized by the vascular endothelium. Inability of the endothelium to respond to vasodilator stimulus of NO may contribute to the exercise intolerance in patients with HF. Bradykinin and related peptides are vasodilators. Bradykinin is a substrate for angiotensin-converting enzyme (ACE) that is also responsible for the production of AT. In addition, bradykinin also inhibits maladaptive growth.[6,7] Adrenomedullin is a peptide with vasodilating and natriuretic properties. It also has positive inotropic effects. The clinical importance of these effects on HF is not fully established.[25] Dopamine, which is a precursor to NE, is a catecholamine that has central and peripheral effects. At low concentrations, dopamine relaxes smooth muscle; this vasodilatation lowers peripheral resistance and dilates renal blood vessels. Prostaglandin synthesis is stimulated by NE, AT, and ADH. The vasodilators are prostacyclin (PGI_2) and prostaglandin E_2. Because they are short-lived, they act locally to exert their effects, either released from one cell to work on another (paracrine effect) or binding to the same cell that released the prostaglandin (autocrine effect). In patients with HF, these counter-regulatory effects are often overwhelmed by the vasoconstrictor response.[11]

Renal compensation is triggered initially by a decrease in kidney perfusion, which decreases glomerular filtration rate (GFR) and activates the RAAS, resulting in an increased SVR and increased sodium and water absorption.[22] Under normal physiologic conditions these pathways act in concert to maintain volume status, vascular tone, and optimize cardiac output. However, chronic activation of these systems leads to worsening of the syndrome.[26] Mediators of the selective vasoconstrictor response include NE, ADH, AT, and ET.[27] Aldosterone, a steroid hormone, increases tubular sodium reabsorption along with AT and NE. ADH acts on the collecting ducts to promote water reabsorption. In early HF, catecholamine, ADH, and ET play the major role in stimulating aldosterone secretion.[23] In patients with advanced HF, the most important stimulus for aldosterone release is AT, whose levels are increased with diuretic therapy.[22]

Natriuretic peptides are counter-regulatory mediators produced in the body. This family of peptides includes ANP, BNP, and clearance natriuretic peptide (CNP). The heart itself produces ANP and BNP. ANP is stored mainly in the right atria, and an increase in atrial distending pressure, however produced, leads to the release of ANP. BNP, identified initially in the brain, is synthesized in the ventricles and is released in response to increased ventricular pressure.[27] CNP is produced in blood vessels and in the brain. CNP appears to act primarily as a clearance receptor that regulates levels of the peptides and reduces vascular resistance

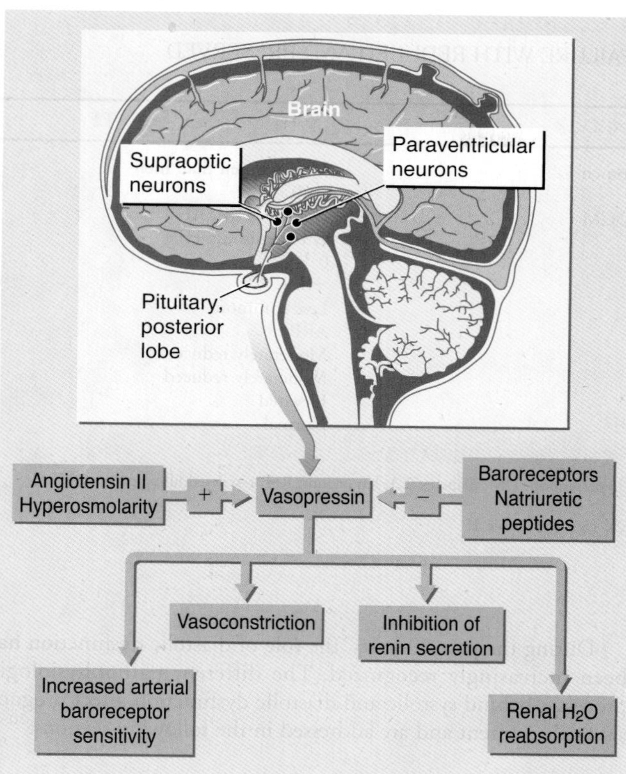

Figure 24-10 Arginine vasopressin (ADH) is a peptide released from the posterior pituitary gland. Angiotensin II and osmoreceptors stimulate vasopressin release; the natriuretic peptides (ANP, BNP) inhibit vasopressin secretion. Vasopressin causes vasoconstriction, renal reabsorption of water, and renal secretion of renin. (Cusco, J. A. & Creager, M. A. [1999]. Neurohumoral, renal, and vascular adjustments in heart failure. In W. S. Colucci & E. Braunwald (Eds.), *Atlas of heart failure. Cardiac function and dysfunction* [2nd ed.]. Philadelphia: Blackwell Science.)

but has no natriuretic property. Both ANP and BNP promote vasodilatation and sodium excretion.[28] They may also attenuate sympathetic tone, RAAS activity (see Fig. 24-9), ADH, and the growth or hypertrophy of the ventricle.[6,11] All three peptides are elevated in HF[29] (see Fig. 24-10).

The syndrome of HF is more accurately a syndrome of concomitant cardiac and renal dysfunction, each accelerating the progression of the other. Renal dysfunction in patients with HF is common and is an independent risk factor for morbidity and mortality.[30,31] Studies have demonstrated that for every 0.5 mg/dL increase in serum creatinine there is an associated 7% risk of death.[26] Interestingly, renal dysfunction is equally prevalent in patients with HF with either preserved or reduced ejection fractions.[32] What is not known is whether worsening renal function itself leads to increased morbidity and mortality or if it is a marker of more severe cardiac and renal diseases.

Inflammation. Local and systemic inflammation plays an important role in HF, particularly in regard to disease progression.[33] Cytokines are signaling peptides whose actions include cell growth and cell death through direct toxic effects on the heart and peripheral circulation. The proinflammatory or "stress-activated" cytokines include TNF-α and some interleukins (e.g., IL-1α, IL-6, IL-8, IL-12). The cardiac myocytes themselves are capable of synthesizing these proinflammatory cytokines in response to various forms of cardiac injury.[34] The local inflammatory response can appear within minutes of an abnormal stress. Local inflammation of the cytokines and other mediators includes deleterious effects of LV remodeling, which include myocyte hypertrophy, alteration in fetal gene expression, contractile defects, and progressive myocyte loss through apoptosis. In addition, there may be promotion of LV remodeling through alterations of the extracellular matrix. A number of studies have shown that the local proinflammatory molecules are activated as early as New York Heart Association (NYHA) class I, which is before some of the classic neurohormonal responses, that tend to be activated in the latter stages (NYHA II thru IV). There are important signaling interactions between the RAAS and the sympathetic nervous system, along with the proinflammatory cytokines.[35]

Activation of the systemic inflammatory response is found in advanced HF. Cardiac cachexia and skeletal muscle myopathy, which contributes to the fatigue and muscle weakness seen in HF, is a part of the systemic inflammatory response; the elevation of the proinflammatory cytokines correlates with the severity of the syndrome. The knowledge of the role of inflammation remains incomplete. As with the hemodynamic defence reaction, the inflammatory response may be initially beneficial, but when sustained becomes deleterious.

Systolic and Diastolic Dysfunction

HF is commonly subdivided into two entities. Patients with symptoms of HF and a reduction in left ventricular ejection fraction (LVEF) (<0.50) are classified as having systolic dysfunction. Patients with symptoms and preserved LVEF are classified as having diastolic dysfunction. While these labels are somewhat useful in describing the pattern of LV dysfunction, they grossly oversimplify the underlying pathophysiology. In fact, there is little pathophysiologic evidence to support this subdivision. Instead HF might best be thought of as a continuous spectrum of closely related clinical entities. As our understanding grows of the dynamic and complex processes that result in effective myocardial contractility, this distinction may no longer be appropriate.[36]

Table 24-5 describes the clinical features of HF in patients with reduced and preserved LVEFs. Interestingly, survival of patients with clinical HF symptoms is similar regardless of whether LVEF is reduced or preserved.[37]

HF With Reduced LVEF. Systolic dysfunction is determined by an impaired pump function with LVEF less than 0.50 and an enlarged end-diastolic chamber volume. The ventricle is dilated, often thin-walled, and may be eccentrically hypertrophied. Systolic dysfunction can be regional, as in MI, or global, as in dilated cardiomyopathy.[16] The principal clinical manifestations of LV systolic dysfunction result from inadequate cardiac output and fluid retention. Systolic dysfunction is thought to account for approximately 50% of patients with symptoms of HF.[38] The etiology is most commonly secondary to long-standing chronic ischemic heart disease attributable to CAD.

HF With Preserved LVEF. Diastolic HF implies normal systolic function in the presence of clinical HF, and is characterized by an increased resistance to filling, with one or both ventricles becoming stiff or noncompliant. Diastolic dysfunction is related to reduction in early LV relaxation compromising the transfer of blood from the atrium into the ventricle. It is typically characterized by

Table 24-5 ■ COMPARISON OF CLINICAL FEATURES OF HEART FAILURE WITH REDUCED AND PRESERVED EJECTION FRACTIONS

	HF with Reduced LVEF	HF with Preserved LVEF
Sex	More men than women	More women than men
Age (years)	50–60	>60
Etiology	MI or idiopathic DCM	HTN + DM, AF
Clinical progress	Persistent HF	Often episodic HF
↑ LV volumes	+++	0
LV hypertrophy	+ / −	+++
Desynchronize	Common	Less common
Mitral inflow pattern	RFP or ARP	ARP
Peak mitral annular systolic velocity	Greatly reduced	Moderately reduced
Peak mitral annular early diastolic velocity	Greatly reduced	Moderately reduced
LA pressure	Elevated	Elevated
LA volume	Elevated	Normal

AF, atrial fibrillation; ARP, abnormal relaxation pattern; DCM, dilated cardiomyopathy; HTN, hypertension; DM, diabetes; LA, left atrium; RFP, restricted filling pattern; MI, myocardial infarction.
Adapted from Sanderson, J. E. (2007). Heart failure with a normal ejection fraction. *Heart, 93*(2), 155–158. Table 1.

delayed ventricular relaxation most commonly due to distortion of the ventricular chamber and prolongation of the ventricular ejection. Advances in imaging of the myocardium both with echocardiograms and functional MRI have led to increased understanding of the factors that lead to diastolic dysfunction. Qualitatively, ventricle walls are thick, there is an increase in left atrial (LA) size and reduction in mitral annulus motion.[36] LA volume is often viewed as a morphologic expression of LV diastolic dysfunction. When the mitral valve is open during diastole, the LA is exposed to the loading pressures of the LV. As the LA is chronically exposed to the increased filling pressure of LV, remodeling occurs and results in increased LA size and volume.[39]

The LV has passive compliance or elastic property that characterizes wall stiffness. Diastolic function can be impaired by four types of lusitropic abnormalities: slowed relaxation with decreased rate of pressure fall ($-dP/dt$) during isovolumetric relaxation, delayed filling during early diastole, incomplete relaxation with reduced filling throughout diastole, and decreased compliance or increased stiffness in late diastole. These changes cause abnormal pressure–volume relationships and produce a higher pressure for any given volume. The pressure is transmitted backwards to the atria, and the pulmonary, and systemic circulation, as noted by elevated pulmonary pressures and decreased cardiac output, leading to dyspnea and fatigue during exercise.[7]

LV failure is caused by diastolic dysfunction in up to 40% of cases. The etiology is most commonly secondary to long-standing systemic hypertension, but CAD; diabetes; obesity; sleep disorders; hypertrophic, infiltrative, and restrictive cardiomyopathies; and primary valve disorders also can lead to diastolic HF.[20] Pure diastolic dysfunction has also been observed immediately after cardiac surgery.[20] Changes that occur in the cardiovascular system as a result of aging have a greater impact on diastolic function than on systolic function. Consistency of the association of female sex with HF and preserved LV function across numerous subgroups of patients implies that sex itself is an important determinant of LV adaptation, regardless of the underlying pathophysiologic process.[40,41] The major consequence of diastolic failure relates to elevation of ventricular filling pressures, causing pulmonary and/or systemic congestion.

During the past 20 years, the role of diastolic dysfunction has been increasingly recognized. The different pathophysiologic processes behind systolic and diastolic dysfunction affect prognosis and treatment and are addressed in the following sections.[20]

Left-Sided HF

Left-sided HF, associated with elevated pulmonary venous pressure and decreased cardiac output, appears clinically as breathlessness, weakness, fatigue, dizziness, confusion, pulmonary congestion, hypotension, and death.

Weakness or fatigue is precipitated by decreased perfusion to the muscles. Abnormalities of skeletal muscle histology and biochemistry also play a role, along with deficient endothelial function. Patients describe a feeling of heaviness in their arms and legs, and there is a reduction in exercise capacity. Cardiac cachexia is a severe complication of HF and is considered a terminal manifestation. Circulating cytokines are known to be important in tissue catabolism.

Decreased cerebral perfusion caused by low cardiac output leads to changes in mental status, such as restlessness, insomnia, nightmares, or memory loss. Anxiety, agitation, paranoia, and feelings of impending doom may develop as the syndrome progresses.

During the course of HF, pulmonary congestion progresses through three stages: stage 1, early pulmonary congestion; stage 2, interstitial edema; and stage 3, alveolar edema.[27] During the early phase, little measurable increase in interstitial lung fluid is noted. There are few clinical manifestations during this phase.

Interstitial edema usually occurs when the PAWP exceeds 18 mm Hg, leading to a net filtration of fluid into the interstitial space. Clinical manifestations of interstitial edema are varied. Engorged pulmonary vessels, elevated PA pressure, and reduced lung compliance cause increased exertional dyspnea.[22] If LV function is severely impaired, orthopnea or a nonproductive cough may be present. Paroxysmal nocturnal dyspnea may also occur because of postural redistribution of blood flow that increases venous return and pulmonary vascular pressure when the patient is in a recumbent position. Congestion of the bronchial mucosa that increases airway resistance and the work of breathing may also contribute to paroxysmal nocturnal dyspnea.

Pulmonary crackles are first noted over the lung bases, and as the PAWP increases, they progress toward the apices.

Stage 3 occurs when the PAWP rises to 25 to 28 mm Hg, causing rapid movement of fluid out of the intravascular and interstitial spaces into the alveoli. As the edema progresses, the alveoli no longer remain open because of the large fluid accumulation. At this point, the alveolar–capillary membrane is disrupted, fluid invades the large airways, and the patient describes or exhibits frothy, pink-tinged sputum. Acute pulmonary edema is a catastrophic indicator of HF. These pulmonary congestion stages are broad categories. The correlation between a patient's PCWP and clinical symptoms is highly variable and most likely dependent upon the duration of illness and individual compensatory mechanisms.

Right-Sided HF

Right-sided HF, associated with increased systemic venous pressure, gives rise to the clinical signs of jugular venous distension, hepatomegaly, dependent peripheral edema, and ascites.[22] Dependent ascending peripheral edema is a manifestation in which edema begins in the lower legs and ascends to the thighs, genitalia, and abdominal wall. Patients may notice their shoes fitting tightly or marks left on the feet from their shoes or socks. Weight gain is what most patients recognize; consistent self-weighing in the morning helps to detect subtle changes in fluid status. An adult may retain 10 to 15 lb (4 to 7 L) of fluid before edema occurs.

Congestive hepatomegaly characterized by a large, tender, pulsating liver, and ascites also occurs. Liver engorgement is caused by venous engorgement, whereas ascites results from transudation of fluid from the capillaries into the abdominal cavity. Gastrointestinal symptoms such as nausea and anorexia may be a direct consequence of the increased intra-abdominal pressure.

Another finding related to fluid retention is diuresis at rest. When at rest, the body's metabolic requirements are decreased, and cardiac function improves. This decreases systemic venous pressure, allowing edema fluid to be mobilized and excreted. Recumbency also increases renal blood flow and GFR, also increasing diuresis. Table 24-6 lists the various subjective and objective indicators for LV and right ventricular (RV) failure.

Table 24-6 ■ CLINICAL INDICATORS AND PHYSICAL FINDINGS OF LEFT AND RIGHT VENTRICULAR FAILURE

Left Ventricular Failure	Right Ventricular Failure
Subjective Findings	
Breathlessness	Lower extremity heaviness
Cough	Abdominal distention
Fatigue and weakness	Gastric distress
Memory loss and confusion	Anorexia, nausea
Diaphoresis	
Palpitations	
Anorexia	
Insomnia	
Objective Findings	
Weight gain	Weight gain
Tachycardia	Neck vein pulsations and distention
Decreased S_1	Increased jugular venous pressure (increased central venous pressure)
S_3 and S_4 gallops	Edema
Crackles (rales)	Hepatomegaly
Pleural effusion	Positive hepatojugular reflux
Diaphoresis	Ascites
Pulsus alternans	
Increased pulmonary artery wedge pressure	
Decreased cardiac index	
Increased systemic vascular resistance	

Diagnosis and Clinical Manifestations

The predominant symptoms of HF are breathlessness or dyspnea and fatigue. Orthopnea and paroxysmal nocturnal dyspnea occur in the more advanced stages of HF. For more detail, refer to "Part III/Assessment of Heart Disease."

History

A careful history is important to ascertain possible causes of HF and identify patients at increased risk for HF. The history should include past medical history and a thorough review of systems. Table 24-7 lists the vital elements in a thorough history, including a history of CAD, hypertension, valvular heart disease, congenital heart defects, or diabetes. Other endocrine abnormalities include a history of thyroid disease or a family history of cardiomyopathy or CAD should be explored. Ascertain if the patient is using possible toxic agents, such as alcohol or cocaine, or has been exposed to radiation or chemotherapy. Patients with a history of central sleep apnea may also have impaired autonomic control and increased cardiac arrhythmias.[42] Precipitating factors for HF should be assessed, such as anemia, infection, or pulmonary embolism. Obtaining a description of a patient's exercise capacity and ability to perform activities of daily living may be useful in assessing their degree of limitation. Patients who describe symptoms of presyncope or syncope should be evaluated for arrhythmias, because atrial fibrillation and ventricular arrhythmias are commonly found in this patient population. Sudden death is responsible for up to 40% to 50% of fatal events in HF.[43] In patients with decompensation of existing HF, dietary or medication noncompliance, or exacerbating mediations (like NSAIDs) should be investigated.

Physical Examination

A major goal in assessing the patient with HF is to determine the type and severity of the underlying disease causing HF and the extent of the HF syndrome. Physical examination of the patient with HF focuses on the cardiovascular and pulmonary systems, as well as relevant aspects of the integumentary and gastrointestinal systems (See Chapter 10.)

Cardiovascular Assessment. Determination of the rate, rhythm, and character of the pulse is important in patients with HF. The pulse rate is usually elevated in response to a low cardiac output. Pulsus alternans (alternating pulse) is characterized by an altering strong and weak pulse with a normal rate and interval. Pulsus alternans is associated with altered functioning of the LV causing variance in LV preload. An irregular pulse is usually indicative of an arrhythmia. Increased heart size is common in patients with HF. This cardiac enlargement is detected by precordial palpation, with the apical impulse displaced laterally to the left and downward. In patients with HF, there maybe a third heart sound (S_3) that is associated with a reduced EF and impaired diastolic function as determined by the peak filling rate.[44] A fourth heart sound (S_4) may occur, although it is not in itself a sign of failure but rather a reflection of decreased ventricular compliance associated with ischemic heart disease, high blood pressure, or hypertrophy. When the heart rate is rapid, these two diastolic sounds may merge

Table 24-7 ■ EVALUATION OF THE CAUSE OF HEART FAILURE

Patient History to Include	Family History to Include
Hypertension	Predisposition to atherosclerotic disease
Diabetes	Sudden cardiac death
Dyslipidemia	Myopathy
Valvular heart disease	Conduction system disease
Coronary or peripheral vascular disease	Tachyarrhythmias
Myopathy	Cardiomyopathy (unexplained HF)
Rheumatic fever	Skeletal myopathies
Mediastinal irradiation	
History or symptoms of sleep disorders	
Exposure to cardiotoxic agents	
Current or past heavy alcohol consumption	
Smoking	
Collagen vascular disease	
Thyroid disease	
Pheochromocytoma	
Obesity	

Adapted from Hunt, S. A., Abraham, W. T., Chin, M. H., et al. (2005). ACC/AHA 2005 Guideline Update for the Diagnosis and Management of Chronic Heart Failure in the Adult: A Report of the American College of Cardiology/American Heart Association Task Force on Practice Guidelines (Writing Committee to Update the 2001 Guidelines for the Evaluation and Management of Heart Failure): Developed in Collaboration With the American College of Chest Physicians and the International Society for Heart and Lung Transplantation: Endorsed by the Heart Rhythm Society. *Circulation, 112*(12), e154–e235. Table 2.

into a single loud sound or summation gallop. Patients with HF frequently have a murmur of mitral regurgitation, which radiates to the axilla. Jugular venous pulses are a means of estimating venous pressure. The a and v waves rise as the mean right atrial (RA) pressure rises. The hepatojugular reflux is also associated with HF.

Pulmonary Assessment. Persistently elevated PA pressures result in the transudation of fluid from the capillaries into the interstitial spaces and, eventually, into the alveolar spaces. The accumulated fluid may result in pulmonary crackles. Initially, the crackles are heard at the most dependent portions of the lungs; but later, as pulmonary congestion increases, crackles become diffuse and are heard over the entire chest.[44] Respiratory rate and pattern reflect the severity of the pulmonary compromise, with rapid breathing (tachypnea) or periodic respiratory (Cheyne–Stokes) being noted.[42]

Integumentary Assessment. Patients with HF often present with dependent edema. It is most often detected in the feet, ankles, or sacral area. Color and temperature of the skin are also assessed, with major findings being pallor, decreased temperature, cyanosis, and diaphoresis. Cardiac cachexia, with a decrease in tissue mass, may be evident in patients with long-standing HF. Cachexia is defined as a documented, unintentional, nonedematous weight loss of 5 kg or more with a body mass index of less than 24 kg/m^2.

Gastrointestinal Assessment. Characteristically, HF results in hepatomegaly. The liver span is increased and the liver is usually palpable well below the right costal margin. An enlarged spleen may also be palpated in advanced HF.

Imaging and Laboratory Studies

Transthoracic Doppler two-dimensional echocardiography coupled with Doppler flow studies is the single most valuable tool and is of particular benefit for specifically assessing ventricular mass, chamber size, valvular changes, pericardial effusion, and systolic and diastolic dysfunctions.[1] (See Chapter 13.) Systolic dysfunction is defined as an EF less than 0.35 to 0.40. Diastolic dysfunction appears with concentric LV hypertrophy, LA enlargement, an EF of 0.45 to 0.55, a reduced rate of LV filling, and a prolonged time to peak filling.[45,46] Studies have shown LV mass/volume were increased in diastolic dysfunction but not in systolic dysfunction.[18,40,47] Radionuclide studies are a precise and reliable measurement of EF and have also become important in providing clues to the presence and cause of HF.[1] Myocardial perfusion studies are also a valuable tool in assessing myocardial ischemia, myocardial infarction and myocardial viability to help determine patients who might benefit from revascularization.[1,47] (See Chapter 14.)

Cardiac catheterization/coronary arteriography is used in patients with angina or large areas of ischemic or hibernating myocardium, and is also the best quantitative evaluation of diastolic dysfunction and shows an increase in PAWP or LV end-diastolic pressure.[1,48] (See Chapter 20.)

A number of routine laboratory tests useful in the evaluation of HF, including a chest radiograph, should also be included to assess the size of the heart and the pulmonary vascular markings (Chapter 12). The electrocardiogram (ECG) is not helpful in assessing the presence or degree of HF, but it demonstrates patterns of ventricular hypertrophy, arrhythmias, and any degree of myocardial ischemia, injury, or infarction (Chapter 15).

Laboratory tests include blood chemistries, complete blood count, and urinalysis (Chapter 11). Measurement of hemoglobin and hematocrit is useful to exclude anemia in patients with HF.[1] Anemia was found to be a common factor in patients with HF and an independent prognostic factor for mortality.[31,49] Electrolyte imbalances in HF reflect complications of failure as well as the use of diuretics and other drug therapy. Disturbances in sodium, potassium, and magnesium are particularly significant. In patients with severe HF, an increase in total-body water dilutes body fluid and is reflected by a decrease in the serum sodium. Diuretics may also contribute to low serum sodium. Hypokalemia, or low serum potassium level, and low serum magnesium may occur as the result of the use of diuretics such as thiazides and furosemides, because these diuretics may lead to excessive excretion of potassium and magnesium. Hyperkalemia, or elevated potassium level, may occur secondary to depressed effective renal blood flow and low GFR.

Any impairment of kidney function may be reflected by elevated blood urea nitrogen, creatinine, and uric acid.[31] Elevated levels of bilirubin, aspartate aminotransferase and lactate dehydrogenase result from hepatic congestion. Urinalysis may reveal proteinuria, red blood cells, and high specific gravity. Thyroid-stimulating hormone in patients with unexplained HF may also be helpful. Elevated serum glucose (diabetes) and lipid abnormalities are risk factors, and these should also be measured.[9]

In patients with decompensation of HF, arterial blood gases usually show a decrease in Pa_{O_2} (partial pressure of oxygen in arterial blood; hypoxemia) and a low Pa_{CO_2} (partial pressure of carbon dioxide in arterial blood). In the clinical situation of HF, the alveoli become filled with fluid, causing a decrease in Pa_{O_2}, whereas the compensatory attempt to increase the Pa_{O_2} by hyperventilating causes a decrease in the Pa_{CO_2}, resulting in a mild respiratory alkalosis. Later changes caused by decreased peripheral perfusion result in a build-up of lactic acid, causing metabolic acidosis (Chapter 7).

Measurement of BNP has become a recent laboratory value that is measured as a means to identify patients with elevated LV filling

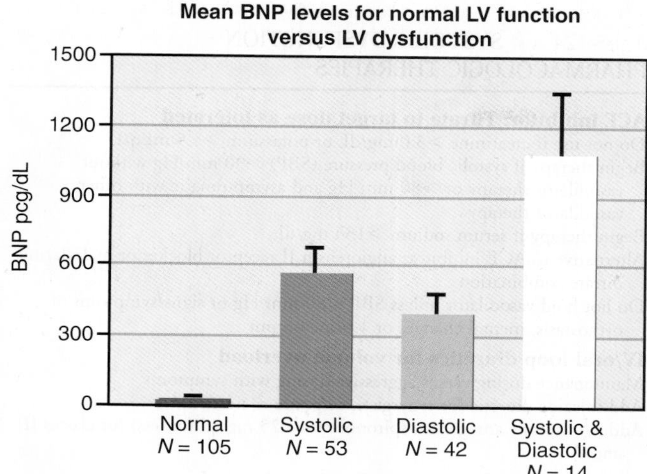

■ **Figure 24-11** BNP values for the different subclasses of LV dysfunction. Normal BNP levels are less than 100 pg/mL. (From Maisel, A. S., Koon, J., Krishnaswamy, P., et al. [2001]. Utility of B-natriuretic peptide as a rapid, point-of-care test for screening patients undergoing echocardiography to determine left ventricular dysfunction. *American Heart Journal, 141*[3], 369.)

pressures. It is increased in patients with systolic and diastolic dysfunction, and although it cannot distinguish between the two dysfunctions, it is being widely investigated as a biochemical marker for morbidity and mortality.[50–52] It is very helpful in differentiating dyspnea caused by HF from other causes. The normal level of BNP is less than 100 pg/mL (Fig. 24-11).

Although not a general test for HF, plasma homocysteine has been recently associated with an increased risk of vascular disease. There is some evidence that increased plasma homocysteine level independently predicts risk of the development of HF in adults without previous MI.[53]

Prognosis

Despite many advances in the treatment of HF in the last decade it remains a highly lethal syndrome, with more than 50,000 deaths reported annually in the United States.[54] Most patients with HF will die from the syndrome. The mode of death is typically either secondary to progressive LV dysfunction with systemic malperfusion or via a sudden arrhythmic event. Two-year mortality rates of approximately 20% and 6-year rates of 50% have been reported in population-based studies.[55] A large community-based cohort study revealed that the number of new cases of HF has not declined over the past 20 years but survival has. The incidence of HF was highest among men and survival after onset was worse in men. However, the largest survival gains over the last 20 years were seen in the men and younger patients, with less improvement in women and patients over the age of 75.[56]

While complex algorithms and computer tools have been created and tested in the last few years to aid in estimating prognosis,[57] it is important to remember that likelihood of survival can only be determined in populations not in individuals. A large, population-based study examined the association between application of the AHA/ACC HF staging system and survival. The following 5-year survival rates in patients were determined: stage 0, 99%; stage A, 97%; stage B, 96%; stage C, 75%; and stage D, 20%.[58] Historically, mortality has been linked to NYHA functional class (i.e., patient's symptoms); newer algorithms include laboratory measures and quantitative data regarding LV status. Clinical factors associated with a lower survival rates include older age; hyponatremia, decreased hematocrit; widened QRS; and worsening LVEF, NYHA functional class, peak exercise oxygen uptake (V_{O_2} max), and renal function.[43] While studies have demonstrated an association between elevated circulating neurohormones (BNP, ET, and NE) and outcome, neurohormonal levels are not used commonly in the clinical area to predict survival. Sudden cardiac death (SCD; Chapter 27) remains an ever-present risk. It is estimated that approximately 50% of patients with systolic dysfunction will die of a sudden tachycardic or bradycardiac rhythm. Predicting SCD in this population has proven difficult; thus, primary prevention measures, such as implantation of implantable cardioverter defibrillators (ICDs) is indicated in patients with LVEF less than 0.35.[59]

As imperfect as the ability to predict the outcome for individual patients, candid discussions regarding prognosis must occur between providers, families, and patients such that expectations can be aligned and plans made. As the tools to detect, quantify, diagnose, and treat the syndrome of HF improve, the life trajectory of patients has improved.[43]

Approach to Treatment

Patients with LV dysfunction often present with exercise intolerance, shortness of breath, and/or fluid retention. Incidental findings of dysfunction also may be found in asymptomatic patients. All patients presenting with HF should undergo a detailed evaluation to: (1) determine the type of cardiac dysfunction, (2) uncover correctable causative factors, (3) determine prognosis, and (4) guide treatment. Recognition of signs and symptoms resulting from an inadequate cardiac output and from systemic and pulmonary congestion is accomplished through a careful history, physical examination, routine laboratory analyses, and diagnostic studies.[1]

There are various principles that guide management of HF. The first and most important step begins with early identification of patients who we know to be at risk for developing the syndrome. The first step is identification and correction of the underlying pathogenic processes, as appropriate, such as aggressive medical management of hypertension, coronary revascularization procedures for CAD or surgical correction of structural abnormalities.[1] The second step is the removal of the compounding or precipitating causes, such as infection, arrhythmia, and pulmonary emboli. The third step is the treatment and control of HF. Therapy for HF is directed at reducing the workload of the heart and manipulating the various factors that determine cardiac performance, such as contractility, heart rate, preload, and afterload. The greatest advance has been in agents that inhibit harmful neurohormonal systems that are activated in support of the failing heart, specifically the RAAS and sympathetic nervous system.[60] Treatment of HF is based on the manner in which the patient clinically presents, which may encompass the extremes from asymptomatic LV failure to acute cardiogenic shock.

HF ranges clinically from acute cardiogenic shock, acute decompensation of chronic HF, to compensated chronic HF. The goal of therapy is support of pump function, which may include positive inotropic agents, vasodilator therapy, and/or, if extremely severe, mechanical devices. In the case of ischemia caused by CAD, treatment of the underlying process is the management goal. The combination of ischemia and LV dysfunction carries a poor prognosis, and it is this patient group that may benefit from revascularization by percutaneous coronary intervention techniques (Chapter 23) or urgent cardiac surgery (Chapter 25).

Systolic Dysfunction

Coronary heart disease, hypertension, and dilated cardiomyopathy are the most commonly identified causes of LV systolic dysfunction. The writing committee of the ACC/AHA[1] based the therapy guidelines on the four stages of evolution of HF (Fig. 24-1). *Stage A* includes patients who are at high risk for HF but do not have LV dysfunction. Treatment is aimed at risk factor modification, including management of hypertension, diabetes and lipids, cessation of smoking, and counseling to avoid alcohol and illicit drugs. Patients are encouraged to exercise on a regular basis. Obesity increases the risk of diabetes and hypertension, and steps should be taken to promote strategies to maintain optimal weight. An angiotensin-converting enzyme inhibitor (ACE-I) is indicated in patients with a history of atherosclerotic vascular disease, hypertension, or diabetes.

Stage B includes patients who are asymptomatic but who have LV systolic dysfunction and are at significant risk for HF. All of stage A therapies are needed, with the addition of an ACE-I and β-adrenergic blockers unless contraindicated. Valve replacement or repair should be undertaken in patients with hemodynamically significant valvular stenosis or regurgitation.

Stage C includes patients with LV dysfunction with current or previous symptoms and who need to be treated with all measures used for stages A and B. They should be managed routinely with four types of drugs: a diuretic, an ACE-I, a β-adrenergic blocker agent, and digitalis. For those patients with an intolerance to ACE inhibitors, an angiotensin receptor blocker (ARB) can be used. For those patients with renal insufficiency or angioedema, a hydralazine/nitrate combination can be substituted. The use of an aldosterone antagonist (i.e., spironolactone) for NYHA Classes III and IV symptoms should be considered. Avoid the use of antiarrhythmics, NSAIDs, and most calcium-channel blockers. Calcium-channel blockers are not of proven benefit for patients with systolic dysfunction and may be harmful. Such risks may not extend to the use of longer-acting calcium-channel blockers (e.g., amlodipine), which currently are undergoing further evaluation. Nonpharmacologic therapies include a 2 to 3 g sodium diet, encouragement of physical activity with possible referral for cardiac rehabilitation and exercise training, and administration of influenza and pneumococcal vaccines.

Stage D includes patients with refractory end-stage HF. They should be treated with all measures used for stages A, B, and C. An overview of the specific pharmacologic therapy for systolic dysfunction is described in Table 24-8. It is critical in this group of patients to have meticulous control of fluid retention. Patients who are at the end stage of their disease are at particular risk for hypotension and may be able to tolerate only a small dose of ACE inhibitors or β-blockers, or they may not be able to tolerate them at all. Despite optimal treatment, some patients do not improve. For these patients, specialized treatment strategies include mechanical circulatory support, continuous inotropic therapy, referral for cardiac transplantation, or hospice care.

Circulatory support may include LV assistance devices (LVADs) or extracorporeal devices.[1] For patients who cannot be sustained on medical therapy, LVAD has been a successful bridge to transplantation. Portable devices have been approved by the FDA (Chapter 26). Low-dose dopamine, dobutamine, or milrinone on an outpatient basis may benefit patients with refractory HF. However, the intermittent or chronic use of these positive inotropic agents remains an area of controversy. All of these agents have been associated with an increase in mortality as a result of markedly higher occurrences of sudden death. Cardiac transplantation plays a role in end-stage patients without contraindications to this procedure and offers excellent long-term outcomes. The goal of therapy for those patients not desiring or eligible for cardiac transplantation is symptom relief. End-of-life considerations deserve attention for this patient population as well, with the focus of hospice care extending to the relief of symptoms.

Table 24-8 ■ SYSTOLIC DYSFUNCTION PHARMACOLOGIC THERAPIES

ACE inhibitor: Titrate to target dose as tolerated
Do not use if creatinine >3.0 mg/dL or potassium >5.5 mEq/L
Begin therapy if systolic blood pressure (SBP) >90 mm Hg without vasodilator therapy or >80 mm Hg and asymptomatic with other vasodilator therapy
Begin therapy if serum sodium >134 mg/dL
Alternative to ACE inhibitor: angiotensin II receptor blocker or hydralazine/nitrate combination
Do not hold vasodilator unless SBP <80 mm Hg or signs/symptoms of orthostasis, mental changes or ↓ urine output

IV/oral loop diuretics for volume overload
Maintenance dosing versus aggressive dosing with symptoms
Add thiazide diuretic for synergistic response as needed
Add aldosterone antagonist, spironolactone 25 mg qd (or less) for classes III and IV

β-blocker: Titrate to target dose as tolerated
Use in NYHA Classes II and III patients.* May use in NYHA Class I patients with history of myocardial infarction or hypertension.†
May use in NYHA Class IV patients* who are euvolemic without significant signs/symptoms of volume overload
Do not initiate therapy if history of bronchospasm, heart block, or sick sinus syndrome without permanent pacemaker, hepatic failure, overt congestion, symptomatic hypotension

Digoxin: Dose is based on weight, age, sex, creatinine clearance, and concomitant medication
Given at a low dose of 0.125 mg qd. Maintain serum digoxin level of 0.8 to 2.0 ng/dL

*Carvedilol (Coreg) is the only β-blocker indicated in mild, moderate, and severe HF and essential hypertension.
†Carvedilol (Coreg) is not indicated in NYHA Class I.

Diastolic Dysfunction

Several myocardial disorders are associated with diastolic dysfunction, including restrictive, infiltrative, and hypertrophic cardiomyopathy. The affects of aging that occur in the cardiovascular system have a greater impact on diastolic function than on systolic performance. HF associated with preserved systolic function is predominantly a disease of older women, most with hypertension and LV hypertrophy. In contrast to systolic dysfunction, there are few studies on therapy for diastolic dysfunction.[45] The difference in pharmacologic therapy is that the goal of drug therapy in diastolic dysfunction is to reduce symptoms by lowering the elevated filling pressures without significantly reducing cardiac output (Table 24-9). The treatment of HF caused by

Table 24-9 ■ DIASTOLIC DYSFUNCTION GENERAL TREATMENT

Goal	Treatment
Reduce venous pressure	Decrease central blood volume Salt restriction Diuretics Venodilation ACE inhibitors Angiotensin II receptor blockers Nitrates Morphine
Maintain atrial contraction, synchrony	Electrical or pharmacologic cardioversion Sequential AV pacing Biventricular pacing
Prevent tachycardia	Digitalis in atrial fibrillation β-adrenergic blockers Calcium-channel blockers (verapamil, diltiazem)
Treat and prevent ischemia	Nitrates, β-adrenergic blockers, calcium-channel blockers Coronary revascularization (percutaneous coronary intervention or bypass surgery)
Control hypertension and promote regression of hypertrophy	ACE inhibitors, other antihypertensive agents Surgical intervention (e.g., aortic valve repair)
Attenuate neurohormonal activation	ACE inhibitors, β-adrenergic blockers
Prevent fibrosis and promote regression of fibrosis	ACE inhibitor or angiotensin II receptor blockers Spironolactone Anti-anginal agents
Improve ventricular relaxation	β-adrenergic blocker Calcium-channel blockers (in hypertropic cardiomyopathy) Systolic unloading agents

Adapted from Gaasch, W. H., & Shick, E. C. (2000). Heart failure with normal left ventricular ejection fraction: A manifestation of diastolic dysfunction. In M. H. Crawford & J. P. DiMarco (Eds.), *Cardiology* (Section 5, pp 6.1–6.8). London: Mosby.

diastolic dysfunction has similarities and dissimilarities to the treatment of HF caused by systolic dysfunction.[1] The first step is the treatment of the underlying cause. Ischemia is relieved through standard medical management and revascularization for CAD. Medical management extends to the use of nitrates, β-adrenergic blockers, and calcium-channel blockers. Volume reduction with diuretics is used to control pulmonary congestion and peripheral edema; diuretics should be titrated carefully. Control of systemic hypertension is important, with ACE-I assisting in normalizing blood pressure and reducing LV mass in patients with hypertension-induced LVH. Other antihypertensive agents also may be needed.

Tachycardia is poorly tolerated, and atrial tachyarrhythmias and even sinus tachycardia have a negative impact on diastolic function. Allowing maximum time for diastolic filling and lowering diastolic filling pressure can be accomplished by rate-slowing agents. Benefits of a slower rate include increased coronary perfusion time, decreased myocardial oxygen requirements, and increased myocardial efficiency. β-Adrenergic blockers and calcium-channel blockers (amlodipine or diltiazem) have been used to prevent excessive tachycardia and also have been shown to improve some exercise parameters. Calcium-channel blockers have important lusitropic effects that enhance ventricular relaxation, with verapamil usually the drug of choice, particularly in hypertrophic cardiomyopathy. β-Adrenergic blockers also improve LV relaxation by decreasing myocardial oxygen consumption and ischemia.

Atrial fibrillation with rapid ventricular response is poorly tolerated, and electrical or chemical cardioversion should be performed to restore normal sinus rhythm. β-Blockers and/or amiodarone may be required to control and prevent atrial fibrillation. Radiofrequency ablation and atrioventricular pacing may also be used. Agents with positive inotropic actions are not indicated if systolic function is normal; these agents appear to provide little benefit and have the potential to worsen pathophysiologic processes, such as myocardial ischemia.

Specific Strategies

Anticoagulation. Patients with increased LV volumes and reduced function are at increased risk for LV thrombus formation. Embolization of these thrombi into the systemic circulation can result in transient ischemic attacks and cerebrovascular accidents.[61] Several studies have attempted to determine whether chronic anticoagulation reduces this transient ischemic attack/cerebrovascular accident risk, but their results are mixed.[62,63] Therefore, routine anticoagulation with warfarin is recommended only for patients with atrial fibrillation, a previous history of systemic pulmonary embolism, or mobile ventricular thrombi.[1] Use of warfarin for patients with LVEF of 0.35 or less may be considered, but careful assessment of the risks and benefits should be undertaken.

Device Therapy. Device therapy extends to biventricular pacing and ICDs. Cardiac resynchronization therapy by simultaneous pacing of the LV and RV through biventricular pacing may be an advantageous therapy that, in patients with severe HF and intraventricular conduction delay, improves ventricular coordination and hemodynamics.[64] By synchronizing LV contraction, there is improvement of LV dP/dT, EF, and cardiac output, as well as reduction of wall stress and LV filling pressures.[65]

ICDs are the treatment of choice in patients with LV dysfunction who have documented ventricular tachycardia or ventricular fibrillation.[1,66] Because HF patients are at high risk for SCD, these patients should be evaluated for ICD indication criteria: LVEF less than 0.35, previous MI, and/or nonsustained ventricular tachycardia.[66] Combined device therapy includes ICD with pacemaker capabilities (Chapter 28).

Surgical Therapy. Cardiac transplantation is an established long-term surgical treatment for HF.[1] However, the scarcity of available organs and strict eligibility criteria make this an option for only approximately 2000 people in the United States each year.[67] Mitral regurgitation occurs to some extent in the remodeled, dilated ventricle, and mitral valve reconstruction has been undertaken. LVADs are emerging as destination therapy in some patients with end-stage HF. Mechanical support of the failing myocardium is currently an area of widening investigation and application (Chapter 26).

Inhibitors of the RAAS

Angiotensin-Converting Enzyme Inhibitors. The use of ACE-I has been conclusively shown to improve long-term prognosis in HF.[68–70] ACE-I block the formation of AT, which reverses vasoconstriction (reducing afterload), and inhibit endocrine, paracrine, and cellular growth effect of AT.[71] ACE-I also diminish release of aldosterone (inhibiting sodium retention) and produce venodilation (reducing preload). In addition to blocking AT formation, this drug class increases levels of bradykinin, promotes vasodilatation, and inhibits maladaptive growth, including ventricular remodeling, hypertrophy, fibrosis, and improves endothelial and vascular function. The unique characteristics of this class of neurohormonal inhibitors support the use of ACE-I as first-line drugs in all patients with HF or asymptomatic LV systolic dysfunction.[1,72] Clinical benefits also extend to patients with evidence of atherosclerotic disease. The doses used should be titrated to target levels. NSAIDs should be avoided in patients in HF, and particularly in those patients using ACE-I therapy.

AT Receptor Blockers. AT receptor blockers differ in their mechanism of action compared to ACE-I. Rather than inhibiting the production of angiotensin by blockade of the ACE, ARBs block the cell surface receptor for AT_1.[70] Hemodynamic effects are similar to those of ACE-I with respect to reducing preload and afterload and increasing cardiac output. The potential concern of this class of drug is that the blockade of AT_1 elevates serum AT, which, because the AT_2 receptors are not blocked, can increase counter regulatory actions of AT_2 activation.[73]

There is ongoing interest in and investigation of combination therapy with ACE-I and ARBs,[74] but at the present time this combination cannot be recommended as routine therapy. ACE-I rather than ARBs continue to be the agent of choice for blockade of the RAAS in HF, and the use of ARBs are usually reserved for patients truly intolerant to ACE inhibitor because of cough.[73,75]

Aldosterone Antagonists. ACE-I do completely block the effect of the RAAS. After several months of ACE-I treatment, there can be an increase in aldosterone levels. Aldosterone promotes sodium retention (edema) and release of cytokines and growth factors, and causes myocardial and vascular fibrosis (autocrine or paracrine effects), baroreceptor dysfunction, and progressive remodeling.[76–78] The addition of low-dose spironolactone to standard therapy for patients with ACC/AHA stage C and/or D (NYHA Classes III and IV) promotes a therapeutic effect and reduces morbidity and mortality.[79] The benefit of this class of drug is not primarily a diuretic effect; spironolactone lessens myocardial fibrosis, significantly reduces plasma BNP levels, and improves LV remodeling and cardiac sympathetic nerve activity (which may reduce ventricular arrhythmias and SCD).[79]

β-Adrenergic Blockers. Cardiac myocytes have three adrenergic receptors (β_1, β_2, and α_1) that are coupled with positive inotropic and chronotropic response, cardiac myocyte growth, toxicity, and apoptosis.[80] Although β_1 and β_2 receptors are present in the normal human myocardium, because β_1 receptors are down-regulated, β_2 receptors predominate in the failing myocardium. Neurohormonal activity in HF can be blunted by β-adrenergic blockers.[81] Second- and third-generation β-adrenergic blockers have been used in HF.[82] Metoprolol and bisoprolol are second-generation selective β_1-adrenergic blockers.[83] Carvedilol is a nonselective β-adrenergic (blocking β_1 and β_2 receptors), as well as an α-blocking agent. At low doses, carvedilol exhibits β_1 selectivity; at higher target doses, it blocks all three adrenergic receptors, allowing for renal and systemic vasodilatation. β-Adrenergic blockers protect the failing myocardium from the deleterious effects of the neurohormonal activity associated with the syndrome of HF. β-Adrenergic blockers should be administered routinely to clinically stable patients who are on standard therapy (usually ACE-I and diuretic). ACC/AHA stages B, C, and D therapy should be initiated at low doses and up-titrated slowly, generally no sooner than at 2-week intervals (Table 24-10).[1] Table 24-11 describes strategies for management of side effects during titration of β-adrenergic blockers. β-Adrenergic blockers have been shown in multiple studies to reduce mortality, morbidity, and improve symptoms.[84–89] The safety of beta-blockers in asymptomatic LV dysfunction has not been tested.

Diuretics. The kidney is the target organ of many of the neurohormonal and hemodynamic changes that occur in HF.[90] Diuretics and dietary salt restriction exert their primary benefit by decreasing extracellular fluid and intravascular blood volume. The elimination of dependent edema helps reduce tissue pressure, oppose venous pooling, and therefore improve the capacitance of the venous system. Similarly, the decrease in intravascular volume also reduces ventricular preload directly, thereby helping to diminish the filling pressures in the pulmonary and systemic circulations. Thiazide diuretics may be helpful in patients with mild fluid overload and normal renal function, but most patients require loop diuretics. Administration of the aldosterone antagonist spironolactone should be considered (see previous section). With advanced HF and compromised renal function, multiple diuretics with different sites of renal action are usually needed.[1]

Digitalis Glycosides. The cardiac glycosides have important effects in HF, including augmenting contractility (positive inotropy),

Table 24-10 ■ PHARMACOLOGIC THERAPIES

Medication	Start (mg)	Target (mg)	Maximum (mg)
Angiotensin Converting Enzyme Inhibitors and Vasodilators			
Captopril	6.25–12.5 tid	50 tid	100 tid
Enalapril	2.5–5 bid	10 bid	20 bid
Lisinopril	2.5–5 qd	20 qd	40 bid
Ramipril	1.25–2.5 bid	5 bid	10 bid
Quinipril	5 bid	20 bid	20 bid
Fosinorpil	2.5–5 bid	20 bid	20 bid
Hydralazine	25 qid	50–75 bid to tid	100 qid
Isosorbide dinitrate	10–20 tid	20–80 tid	80 tid
Isosorbide mononitrate	30 qd	60–120 qd	240 qd
Diuretics			
Furosemide*	20–40 qd	As required	480 qd
Torsemide*	10–20 qd	As required	200 qd
Hydochlorothiazide†	25 qd	As required	200 qd
Metolazone*†	2.5 qd	As required	5 qd
Spironolactone‡	25 qd	As required	50 bid
β-Blockers			
Carvedilol	3.125 bid	6.35–25 bid	50 bid
Metoprolol succinate	6.25–25 qd	50–200 qd	200 qd
Bisoprolol	1.25 qd	10 qd	10 qd
Angiotensin II Receptor Blockers			
Ibersartan	150 qd	300 qd	300 qd
Candesartan	16 qd	32 qd	32 qd
Losartan	12.5–25	50 qd	50–100 qd
Valsartan	80 qd	160 qd	320 qd

*Watch potassium carefully; may cause hypokalemia
†Give 30 minutes before loop diuretic
‡May increase serum potassium; do not give if serum potassium >4.7 mEq/L

Table 24-11 ■ MANAGING SIDE EFFECTS DURING TITRATION OF β-BLOCKERS

Vasodilator Effects (Dizziness or Light Headedness)
Give drug with food
Give drug 2 hours before vasodilator agents or stagger doses of vasodilator medications or other medications affecting blood pressure
Reduce diuretic or vasodilator therapy temporarily
Reduce β-blocker dose if symptoms persist after diuretic and vasodilator decreased two times

Significant Bradycardia (<60–65 bpm with Symptoms)
Reduce β-blocker dose
Clarify digoxin dosage
  Temporarily stop digoxin or reduce digoxin dose
  Monitor digoxin levels
Clarify concomitant drug use
  Amiodarone
  Calcium-channel blockers (verapamil or diltiazem)

Worsening Heart Failure (Dyspnea, Weight gain, Edema)
Increase diuretic dose (if qd increase to bid; if bid, consider increasing the dose)
Intensify salt restriction
Reduce β-blocker dose (if symptoms persist after diuretic increased)

slowing of the sinus pacemaker and atrioventricular conduction (negative chronotropy and dromotrophy), and neurohormonal modulating effects including a sympathoinhibitory effect.[91] Little controversy exists as to the benefit of digoxin in patients with symptomatic systolic dysfunction and concomitant atrial fibrillation, but the debate still continues over its current role in patients in normal sinus rhythm. Digoxin should be considered as a fourth-line medication in patients who have LV systolic dysfunction while receiving standard therapy.[1,92] In the majority of patients with HF and normal sinus rhythm, the starting dosage of digoxin should be 0.125 or 0.25 mg once daily (no loading dose) based on ideal body weight, age, and renal function. In patients with HF and rapid ventricular response, higher doses are not recommended. If amiodarone is added, the dose of digoxin should be reduced. Studies support a lower-serum digoxin concentration target in the range of 0.5 to 0.8 ng/dL, because higher concentrations were associated with increased mortality.[93,94]

Vasodilator Therapy. The venous and arterial beds are often inappropriately constricted. Venoconstriction tends to displace blood in the thorax causing pulmonary congestion, whereas arteriolar constriction increases the impedance to LV emptying. Arteriolar dilatation results in a reduction of afterload and may augment cardiac output, whereas venodilatation tends to produce a reduction in preload, lowers ventricular filling pressure, and reduces symptoms of pulmonary congestion. Vasodilators may be separated into three categories: venous dilators (preload reducers), arterial dilators (afterload reducers), and mixed venous and arterial dilators (preload and afterload reducers).

Venous Dilators. Nitroglycerin and the closely related isosorbide dinitrate are primarily reducers of preload because they dilate the systemic veins and reduce venous return, ultimately to reduce LV filling pressure. Nitrates are indicated for the treatment of angina in patients with HF.[1] A combination of hydralazine with isosorbide dinitrate combines the effect of improved preload and afterload (see next section on hydralazine) and may be administered to patients on standard therapy who cannot be administered an ACE inhibitor because of renal insufficiency or true intolerance.

Arterial Dilators. As a direct arteriolar vasodilator with direct inotropic effects, hydralazine can improve LV function by reducing afterload and myocardial oxygen consumption, augmenting stroke volume, and improving cardiac output. It is used in combination as described in the previous section.

Calcium-Channel Blockers. The net benefits of calcium-channel blocker use rest in their ability to decrease afterload and to exert anti-ischemic effects. Calcium-channel blockers are a diverse group of agents with complex actions. They do not seem to have a place in systolic dysfunction and may be harmful, although risks may not accompany the use of the longer-acting agents (e.g., amlodipine) in patients with concomitant hypertension or angina. Calcium-channel blockers may be of benefit in diastolic dysfunction because of improvement of diastolic relaxation, control of blood pressure, and prevention of myocardial ischemia, and they may reverse LVH.

Natriuretic Peptides. Natriuretic peptides such as nesiritide are intravenously delivered compounds that promote diuresis and have vasodilator properties that suppress neurohormonal activation and indirectly improve myocardial performance.[95,96] Nesiritide in the acute setting has been shown to rapidly reduce symptoms of congestion, but the effects on morbidity and mortality remain unclear.[97] There are recent data linking nesiritide use to worsening renal function and increased mortality and thus it should be used cautiously.[54,98]

Antiarrhythmics. HF is the most arrhythmogenic disorder in cardiovascular disease. Management of arrhythmias in this group of patients is difficult and remains far from satisfactory. Many patients with HF experience frequent and complex ventricular tachyarrhythmias, and the imminent risk of sudden death appears to be present for all patients with HF. Experimental and clinical evidence indicates that circulatory neurohormonal and electrolyte deficits (potassium and magnesium) interact to provoke malignant ventricular ectopic rhythms. In general, antiarrhythmic therapy in patients with HF is reserved for symptomatic arrhythmias or for control of ventricular responses to atrial fibrillation.[1] Class 1 antiarrhythmics demonstrated an increase in mortality in patients with ventricular arrhythmias in HF.[99] β-Blockers can prevent up to 40% to 50% of SCD, which adds to their benefit in managing patients with HF.[86] Amiodarone has undergone the most extensive evaluation for efficacy and safety in LV dysfunction, but has had equivocal effect on SCD. Survival of patients with life-threatening arrhythmias is improved with ICD placement as compared with antiarrhythmic therapy.[100,101] Amiodarone is the preferred drug in patients with HF with supraventricular tachycardia not controlled by β-blocker or digoxin, or for those patients who are not candidates for ICD placement.[1,102]

Other Important Considerations

Diabetes Mellitus. An association between Type II DM and HF has been clearly seen now for over a decade, the question remains *does insulin resistance (IR) cause a cardiomyopathic process that leads to HF and/or does HF lead to IR?* Diabetes affects 20 million Americans; it is highly associated with factors known to cause HF, such as hypertension and CAD. In addition, diabetes has long been known to be an independent risk factor for the development of HF.[10] Therefore, anomalies in glucose metabolism may synergistically act to increase the prevalence of HF. There are several genetic disorders (Alström syndrome and Bardet–Biedl syndrome) associated with both severe IR and fatal hyperglycemia. Such association gives pause to examine the mechanistic impact of IR on the myocardium. A more common thought is that HF predisposes a person to developing IR or Type II DM. There are data to suggest that 43% of patient with HF exhibit abnormal glucose metabolism.[103] A recent prospective study suggested a one standard deviation decrease in insulin sensitivity increased the risk of HF by one third.[104] Previous studies have shown that even a 1% increase in hemoglobin A1c increases the risk of HF by 15%.[105] One must recognize that while systemic IR (Type II DM) is associated with increased mortality in patients with HF,[106] systemic and myocardial IR may be different. Interestingly, cardiac positron emission tomography studies suggest that a failing myocardium has reduced glucose uptake in favor of free fatty acid uptake; in patients with Type II DM, myocardial glucose uptake is even lower.[107]

Smoking Cessation. Cessation of smoking has a dramatic effect on improvement in health status. Smoking contributes to 32% of all deaths due to cardiovascular disease in the United States.[108] Patients with HF who continue to smoke have an approximately 30% to 50% higher risk hospitalization for HF, MI, and death than patients who do not smoke.[109,110] While many patients with HF who have smoked long periods of time may question the benefit of quitting seemingly late in the course of their lives, there is strong evidence to support that within 2 years of quitting, the increased relative risk of both hospitalization for HF and MI drop similar to those levels in persons who have never smoked.[110] In fact mortality benefits associated with smoking cessation exceed those of many of the standard pharmacologic treatment regimes, such as ACE-I and β-blocker therapy in patients with HF. The benefits of smoking cessation accrue rapidly (within one year) in patients with HF. Despite this clear benefit, many nurses and health care providers are hesitant to address this issue with this patient population.[111] Data suggest that only 9% of smokers hospitalized with HF are counseled to quit smoking.[112] However, there is mounting evidence that smokers who received assistance from a nurse have a 28% greater probability of quitting.[113] Documentation of assessment of tobacco use and subsequent smoking cessation counseling is now an indicator of quality under new Joint Commission on the Accreditation of Healthcare Organizations standards of practice for all patients hospitalized for HF (Chapter 34).[114]

Anemia. Anemia is a common problem in patients with HF and reduced LVEFs. Some estimates suggest that the incidence is as high as 60%.[115] While the precise prevalence is unknown, anemia does appear more common in HF patient groups with other comorbidities, such as renal dysfunction and advanced age. Anemia occurs secondary to a deficiency in new erythrocyte production relative to the rate of removal of aged erythrocytes. Erythropoetin, primarily produced by the kidneys, is the key component in red blood cell mass. Abnormalities that impact renal perfusion impact the body's response to erythropoetin. In addition, iron deficiency is present in about 30% of anemic patients with HF.[116] Age, female sex, decreased GFR, decreased body mass index, use of ACE-I, increased jugular venous pressure, and lower extremity edema have all been associated with anemia.[117,118]

Chronic anemia is associated with sodium and water retention, reduction of renal blood flow, and neurohormonal activation—all defining characteristics of the syndrome of HF. While reduction in hemoglobin in patients with HF has been shown to be an independent predictor of mortality and rehospitalization in many studies,[49,57,119] it is difficult to determine if the HF outcome is worsened by the anemia or the anemia is secondary to worsening HF. There are currently no recommendations to treat anemia in patients with HF. Diagnosis and evaluation of potential reversible causes, such as nutritional deficiencies, should be undertaken, but given the absence of long-term clinical trials, aggressive treatment with transfusions or exdogenous erythropoetin is not recommended.[120]

Interestingly, perhaps an alternative hypothesis may be that the anemia associated with HF is an adaptive mechanism. Hemoglobin is high in oxidative stress and as such reduction in trafficking of such an agent may be in fact a compensatory mechanism. Further work in this area is ongoing and highlights an important point that observations made in the patient with HF cannot automatically be converted to treatment options without prospective, well-done randomized clinical trials.[118]

Depression. Patients living with HF have a significant burden of symptoms. Optimizing their health status is an important goal of therapy, yet specific factors influencing health status are just now being studied. Significant depressive symptoms is reported by approximately 30% to 50% of patients with HF.[121,122] These depressed patients report a significantly higher symptom burden, lower physical and social function, and lower quality of life compared to nondepressed patients with HF. In fact, depressive symptoms are some of the strongest predictors of decline in health status in patients with HF.[121] Symptoms of depression have been associated with a 56% increase likelihood of death or hospitalization for HF even after controlling for other markers of disease severity.[123] What remains unclear and is the focus of ongoing study are the effect of interventions aimed at treatment of depression in this population.[124,125]

Sleep Disturbances. The link between sleep disordered breathing and HF has recently been made. Patients with obstructive sleep apnea have a 2.4 times higher risk of developing HF independent of other risk factors.[42] Interestingly, the risk of HF associated with obstructive sleep apnea exceeds that of hypertension, CAD, and stroke. Respiratory events during sleep have long been known to cause hypoxemia, systemic and pulmonary hypertension, sympathetic activation and reduced stroke volume.[126] Patients with sleep apnea have dynamic ST-segment and T-wave changes on ambulatory ECG monitoring consistent with myocardial ischemia.[127,128] While the many mechanisms that might link the broad spectrum of sleep disturbances to clinical HF remain uncertain, several hypotheses are plausible. Obstructive sleep apnea is associated with sympathetic hyperactivity,[129] which can cause hypoxia—a putative atherogenic factor[130]—and pulmonary hypertension;[131] sympathetic hyperactivity and pulmonary hypertension both lead to and exacerbate the syndrome of HF. While there is no current evidence that treating sleep disorders will prevent HF, data are beginning to suggest that treatment of HF with continuous positive airway pressure improves outcomes in patients with documented sleep apnea.[132]

Cognitive Dysfunction. Cognitive dysfunction, including impairments in memory, attention, learning, psychomotor ability, perceptual skills, and language are common in patients with HF.[133] Difficulties with memory and concentration are very common in patients with HF.[134] It has been reported recently that 30% to 50% of patients with HF will have diminished cognition.[134,135]

Baseline intelligence and NYHA functional class have been shown to predict the degree of impairment.[136] Increased age, presence of comorbidities, and abnormalities of serum sodium, potassium, albumin, and glucose all increased the relative risk of cognitive impairment.[137] While the precise mechanisms of impairment remain unclear, included in the list of hypotheses are chronic cerebral hypoperfusion and/or hypoxia, and repeated cerebral microembolic events. Small observational studies of patients with HF have shown an association between diminished cerebral blood flow as measured by single photon emission computed tomography brain imaging and abnormalities noted on neuropsychological testing.[138]

Cognition changes are often barriers to a patient's ability to engage in self-care behaviors. A conceptual framework of cognitive defects in patients with HF has recently been proposed[139] (Fig. 24-12). While this model continues to evolve, and perhaps should include an expanded list of contributing factors, it forms an initial platform to develop interventions aimed at improving cognition.

Disease Management Programs

Whether in a hospital, clinic, nursing home, or patient's home, the nurse cares for patients in all stages and phases of the syndrome of HF. The nurse may be the first person to identify the risk factors for or presence of HF. The best means for reducing the number of patients with HF is by prevention, early identification of HF risk, and implementation of targeted interventions. The importance of early diagnosis is highlighted by evidence that treatment of asymptomatic patients can slow progression and improve clinical outcomes.[69,140] Screening for high blood pressure, diabetes, dyslipidemia, metabolic syndrome, smoking, atherosclerosis, and breathing and valvular disorders may ensure aggressive treatment and may prevent the subsequent syndrome of HF.

Once a diagnosis of HF has been established, a major goal is determining the type and severity of the underlying disease and the extent of the syndrome. HF remains the number one reason

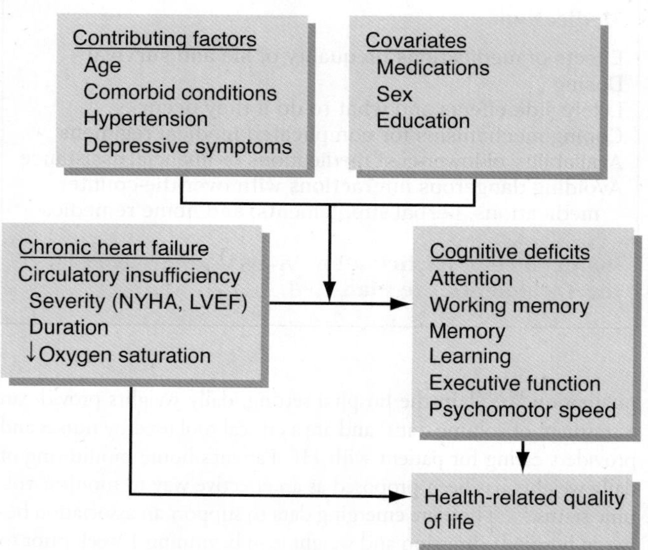

■ **Figure 24-12** Conceptual model of cognitive deficits in heart failure. (From Bennett, S. J., Sauve, M. J., & Shaw, R. M. [2005]. A conceptual model of cognitive deficits in chronic heart failure. *Journal of Nursing Scholarship, 37*[3], 222–228.)

why patients over the age of 65 years require hospitalization.[4] Three-month rehospitalization rates exceed 50%.[141] The primary reason for rehospitalization is volume overload followed by angina and arrhythmias.[142] Common precipitants of readmission include medication nonadherence, dietary indiscretion, inappropriate medications, and delay in seeking care.[143] Identification of the early onset of HF symptoms may prompt therapeutic interventions instituted on an ambulatory basis and prevent rehospitalization. Coordination of care by a nurse-directed multidisciplinary team (including nurses, cardiologists, primary care providers, case managers, dieticians, pharmacists, and cardiac rehabilitation specialists) can provide HF initiatives to guide evidence-based practice, enable self-care at home, and coordinate clinical care across the continuum.[144] A growing trend has been to have advanced practice nurses coordinate these programs.[145]

The goal of HF disease management programs is to reduce symptom burden, improve functional capacity, reduce hospital visits, and reduce rehospitalization. Components of disease management programs include discharge planning, education and counseling, medication optimization, early attention to deterioration and vigilant follow-up. HF disease management programs have been shown to improve quality of life[141] and patient satisfaction with care.[146] Application of these strategies by nurses has been shown to reduce the likelihood of 90-day readmission by 56%[141,147] and to improve significantly 1-year survival without readmission.[148,149] There is mounting evidence to suggest that HF disease management programs reduce not only readmission but also mortality.[150]

Patient and Family Education. The health care community is increasingly faced with a growing division between what is known to improve patient outcome and our ability to encourage, apply, and teach these behaviors to the patients and populations we serve. An early study demonstrated that education successfully alters adherence in patients living with chronic diseases.[151] Education and support have been shown to improve self-care behaviors in patients with chronic HF.[152,153] Multidisciplinary education and support interventions have been shown to reduce rehospitalization rates in this patient population.[148,154] Comprehensive discharge planning and postdischarge follow-up of elderly patients with HF has been shown to not only reduce the need for rehospitalization but may even reduce 1-year mortality.[155] However, education alone certainly does not predict patient behavior in the home setting.[156]

Several investigators have described a relationship between social support and health outcomes in this patient population.[148,153] Patient-related decompensation of chronic HF can be attributed to knowledge deficit of the disease, diet and medications; nonadherence to medication and diet; inability to recognize signs and symptoms of HF; inadequate social support; and inability to access health care providers. Several clinical studies have demonstrated a decline in hospital readmissions by as much as 50% with aggressive telephone follow-up care. Telemanagement of HF undertaken by advanced practice nurses,[157] has been shown to promote consistency of care across health care sites. Even short one-on-one teaching sessions can significantly reduce need for rehospitalization and death.[158]

Specialized HF centers are being established to oversee therapeutic options, including complex polypharmacy, device therapy, and investigational agents.[159] Nursing plays a key role in these centers and clinics, coordinating care that impacts the physical, psychological, and social challenges that these patients face. In addition to morbidity and mortality, quality of life is an equally important outcome in patients with HF.[160] Risk factor modification, management of nutrition, biobehavioral therapy, drug management, and exercise training are just some of the interventions shown to benefit patients with HF.[160] Home management of HF may relate to stabilizing the patient's condition after hospital discharge, providing care before cardiac transplantation, or hospice care for those patients with end-stage HF.[161]

When the patient is admitted to the hospital, the problems associated with HF may have become more advanced and may require supervised administration of medications as well as other measures to reduce edema and improve myocardial performance. The overall plan of care for patients with HF is to reduce cardiac workload, improve cardiac output, prevent complications, and educate the patient regarding follow-up care. Display 24-1 presents topics for patient, family, and caregiver education.

Self-Care Expectations. Self-care is the process by which persons function on their own behalf to promote health and to prevent and treat disease.[162] Important components of self-care in patients living with HF include recognizing symptoms, weighing daily, and adhering to activity recommendations and medications.[162] Self-care behaviors have been shown to improve in patients involved in HF disease management programs.[144,149,153] Self-care in patients with HF has been divided into "maintenance" and "management" processes. Reigel et al.[163] classified the concrete "rule following" activities of patients with HF as "maintenance" behaviors. However, a patient's independent decision or choice to engage in these activities (restricting dietary sodium intake, home daily weights, and daily exercise) remains complex. Sneed and Paul[164] found that while most patients report consistently adhering to recommended "maintenance" behaviors, only 39% reported engaging in regular exercise while 94% reported consumption of a high-sodium food product within the preceding 24 hours.[163,164] "Management" behaviors, as Reigel et al. have labeled the behaviors that required integration of multifaceted data, include the perception and/or recognition of symptoms, decisions involved in articulating and reporting changes in status, independent or guided alternatives in treatment plans and complex evaluation of responses.[163,165] Each of these vital steps is linked to the aforementioned complexity of the phenomena we term behavior.

Complexity of Patient Behavior. Patient behavior is a complex phenomenon. Knowledge, motivation,[166] hope,[149] self-efficacy, health beliefs, social support,[167] cognitive capacity,[134] and perceived support[168] are just a few of the variables that have been shown to impact behavior of patients with HF. Each of these variables serves as a filter through which patients perceive and integrate information, and establish resultant behavior. While patients' perceptions of the severity of symptoms of HF have been shown to correlate with the assessments of their health care providers,[169] the studies in this area are few. In a small, prospective qualitative study, Reigel and Carlson[165] explored the impact of HF on patients' lives and identified symptoms and misconceptions as major barriers to performing self-care behaviors. Patient education and symptom severity predicted behavior, such as recognizing, reporting, and evaluating symptoms.[170] Reflective listing, negotiating a plan, and bridging the transition to home also lead to a patient's successful adherence to self-care regimens.[162]

Daily Weight. Lack of adherence to a prescribed outpatient regimen, resulting in volume overload and leading to shortness of breath, has been cited as the primary reason patients require rehospitalization.[143,171] In the hospital setting, daily weights provide an assessment of volume status and are a critical tool used by nurses and providers caring for patient with HF. Patient's home monitoring of daily weights has been proposed as an effective way to monitor volume status.[154] There are emerging data to support an association between hospital admission and weight gain beginning 1 week prior to admission.[172] However, little is known about the home self-weighing behavior experience of patients with chronic HF.

Patient-directed home monitoring of daily weights can be an effective tool to detect subtle (2 to 5 lb) changes in volume status,

DISPLAY 24-1 Topics for Patient, Family, and Caregiver Education and Counseling

General Counseling, with Explanations of

- Heart failure and the reason for symptoms
- Cause or probable cause of heart failure
- Expected symptoms
- Symptoms of worsening heart failure
- What to do if symptoms worsen
- Self-monitoring with daily weights
- Treatment/care plan
- Patient responsibilities
- Importance of cessation of tobacco use
- Role of family members or other caregivers in the treatment/care plan
- Availability and value of qualified local support group
- Importance of obtaining vaccinations against influenza and pneumococcal disease

Prognosis

- Life expectancy
- Advance directives
- Advice for family members in the event of sudden death

Activity Recommendations

- Recreation, leisure, and work activity
- Exercise
- Sexual activity, sexual difficulties, and coping strategies

Dietary Recommendations

- Consistent and restricted sodium intake (2 to 5 mg/day)
- Relationship of excess sodium intake to subsequent symptoms or weight gain
- Fluid moderation, no restriction
- Small, frequent meals
- Calorie-appropriate diet
- Alcohol moderation or restriction if heart failure secondary to alcohol use

Medications

- Effects of medications on quality of life and survival
- Dosing
- Likely side effects and what to do if they occur
- Coping mechanisms for complicated medical regimens
- Availability of lower-cost medications or financial assistance
- Avoiding dangerous interactions with over-the-counter medications, herbal supplements, and home remedies

Importance of Participation in and Adherence to the Treatment/Care Plan

often prior to the development of overt symptoms. Two small studies have shown that while most patients with HF recall being asked to monitor their weights at home, and describe this behavior as "important," only approximately 30% reported engaging in the behavior.[154, 173] Daily weights were among the five least frequently performed self-care behaviors.[152]

Most patients with HF are instructed to weigh themselves one time per day. Although the ideal time of this weight has not been studied, it is most likely not as important as the fact that it is performed at a consistent time each day. Patients are typically asked to weigh upon rising in the morning, after urinating and prior to dressing or eating. The accuracy or precision of the home device (scale) used for weighing has likewise not been studied. However, the accuracy of the measurement probably is not as important as its reproducibility. Recognizing mild volume overload early on increases the efficacy of treatment interventions, such as augmentation of diuretic dose and heightened sodium restriction. These interventions can interrupt the cycle of progressive myocardial that results in reduced renal perfusion and consequent sodium and water retention, manifested clinically as shortness of breath, paroxysmal nocturnal dyspnea, and lower extremity edema.

Activity and Exercise. A classic symptom associated with HF is exercise intolerance, characterized by fatigue or shortness of breath. Exploring the pathophysiologic mechanisms underlying these symptoms has been the focus of much study over the last decade.[174] Figure 24-13 depicts the mechanisms for augmenting cardiac output in the patient with and without HF. The mechanisms involve both myocardial and peripheral abnormalities, including altered cardiac output in response to exercise, abnormal redistribution of blood flow, reduced mitochondrial volume density, impaired vasodilatory capacity, heightened sympathetic vascular resistance, and impaired sympathetic tone.[175–177]

Until recently, patients with HF have been instructed to avoid exercise. In the late 1990s there was mounting evidence from small controlled studies that neurohormonal activation, symptoms, resting cardiac function, and quality of life appeared to improve with exercise.[174] Larger well-controlled trials now demonstrate a clear morbidity, mortality, and the quality of life benefit of low- and moderate-level exercise training.[178–181] While stable patients benefit from exercise training, Table 24-12 highlights a subset of patients for whom exercise prescriptions should be altered.

Table 24-12 ■ RELATIVE AND ABSOLUTE CONTRAINDICATIONS TO EXERCISE TRAINING AMONG PATIENTS WITH STABLE CHRONIC HEART FAILURE

Relative Contraindications	Absolute Contraindications
>4 lb wt gain over previous 1 to 3 days	Progressive dyspnea at rest over previous 5 days
Continuous or intermittent dobutamine	Ischemia at low levels of exercise
↓ In systolic BP with exercise	Uncontrolled diabetes
NYHA IV	Acute systemic illness or fever
Complex ventricular arrhythmia at rest	Recent embolism
Complex ventricular arrhythmia with exercise	Thrombophlebitis
Supine resting HR >100 beats/min	Active pericarditis or myocarditis
	Severe aortic stenosis
	Myocardial infarction within previous 3 weeks
	New onset atrial fibrillation with rapid ventricular response

Wt, weight; BP, blood pressure; NYHA, New York Heart Association functional class; HR, heart rate.

Adapted from Working Group on Cardiac Rehabilitation & Exercise Physiology and Working Group on Health Failure of the European Society of Cardiology. (2001). *European Heart Journal, 22*, 125–135.

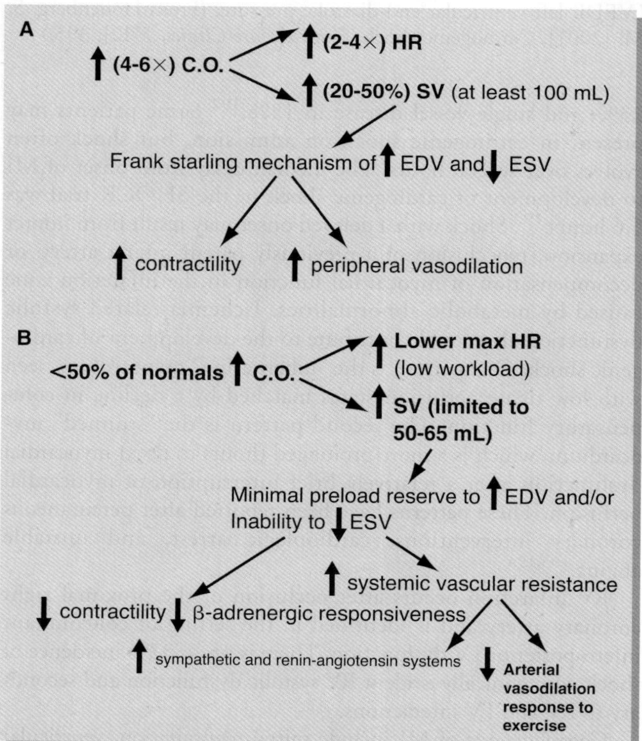

■ **Figure 24-13** Mechanisms to augment cardiac output (from Pina, I. L., Apstein, C. S., Balady, G. J., et al. [2003]. Exercise and heart failure: A statement from the American Heart Association Committee on exercise, rehabilitation, and prevention. *Circulation, 107*[8], 1210–1225.) A series indicates cardiac output augmentation in a normal heart. B series indicates cardiac output augmentation in HF.

Diet. Patients with HF frequently lack a clear understanding of the dietary recommendations. While there is a lack of clinical trials evaluating the effect of many of the dietary recommendations made to patients with HF, the general consensus is that limiting sodium intake lessens the risk of volume overload. While most clinicians agree that limiting sodium intake is important, incorporation of this strategy into the lives of patients is more complex. Lack of knowledge, reduced food selection, cost, and interference with socialization have been identified as factors associated with patient nonadherence to a low-sodium diet.[182] However, the findings of a recent study suggests that if patients perceive the positive link between low or consistent sodium intake (i.e., avoiding episodic high sodium items) and reduced risk of hospitalization for volume overload (i.e., HF), they are more likely to adhere to a reduced sodium diet.[183] Thus, Bennett et al. validated the common sense association that if patients understand the rationale behind the treatment recommendations, adherence is more likely improved. Fluid restriction has not been shown to be effective in either short- or long-term volume management[184] in this population.

Medications. Important advances have been made in the pharmacologic treatment of patients with HF. But, there are clearly many barriers to medication adherence in patients with HF. Common sense tells us that if patients are unable to obtain medications or to take their medications correctly, the favorable outcomes observed in clinical trails will not be seen clinically. Medication nonadherence is highly prevalent in patients with HF.[143,185,186] However, a positive association between patients' perception of the effects of a medication and subsequent adherence has been demonstrated.[187] Education and support have likewise been shown to significantly increase adherence resulting in improvements in functional outcome and reduced emergency room visits and hospitalization.[188,189]

Social Support and Quality of Life. There is evidence that a relationship between social support and health outcomes in patients with HF exists. Feldman et al.[144] evaluated the impact of sending e-mail reminders regarding HF-specific clinical recommendations to home health nurses. Patients cared for by nurses receiving the prompts were significantly more likely to recognize their medications, less likely to report salting their food, and more likely to weigh themselves. The Kansas City Cardiomyopathy Questionnaire score and health-related quality of life were significantly higher in the patients receiving care from a nurse receiving the prompts. This study is of interest, as it attempts to demonstrate and measure the link between self-care practice and functional outcomes. Was the improvement in outcome related to improved knowledge and adherence or augmented provider patient interaction? These are questions for future studies.

CARDIOGENIC SHOCK

Acute HF is a true medical emergency that warrants an expedient diagnosis. If appropriate treatment is not instituted within a short time course, then irreversible decompensation may ensue, leading to a progressive syndrome of shock.[190] As the endpoint on the clinical continuum of LV failure, cardiogenic shock includes shock caused by ineffective cardiac contractility and myocardial failure. The complexity of acute HF has diverse potential etiologies making a precise definition difficult.

Shock is a complex clinical syndrome characterized by impaired cellular metabolism caused by decreased tissue perfusion. The inadequacy of tissue perfusion results in cellular hypoxia, the accumulation of cellular metabolic wastes, cellular destruction, and ultimately, organ and system failure. The syndrome begins as an adaptive response to some insult or injury and progresses to multiple organ system failure. The pathophysiologic mechanisms of shock include decreased circulating blood volume, decreased cardiac contractility, and increased venous capacitance.[191]

Atherosclerotic heart disease and the complications of ischemia and infarction are the most common causes of acute HF.[191] Acute coronary occlusion first impairs diastolic function, with later diminished systolic function, stroke volume, and blood pressure. This downward spiral leads to progressive myocardial dysfunction and possibly death (Fig. 24-14).[190] Shock occurs in approximately 8% of patients with acute LV MI, most often of the anterior wall. Angiographic findings of the SHOCK (Should We Emergently Revascularize Occluded Coronaries for Cardiogenic Shock) trial showed left main coronary artery occlusion in 20% of patients, three-vessel disease in 64%, two-vessel disease in 23%, and single-vessel disease in 13%.[192] Some patients may present in cardiogenic shock on admission, but shock often evolves over several hours. The median delay from onset of MI to development of cardiogenic shock in the SHOCK trial was 5.6 hours.[192] Shock with a delayed onset may result from infarct expansion, reocclusion of a previously patent infarct artery, or decompensation of myocardial function in the infarction zone caused by metabolic abnormalities. Ischemia-related systolic dysfunction also could contribute to the development of cardiogenic shock. One pattern is the "hibernating" myocardium, seen with low tissue perfusion states matched by a decline in compensatory function. The second pattern is the "stunned" myocardium, which is a more prolonged (hours to days) myocardial dysfunction after a relatively brief interruption of myocardial perfusion. These patterns have been reported after percutaneous coronary interventions, cardioplegic arrest, and unstable angina.[193,194]

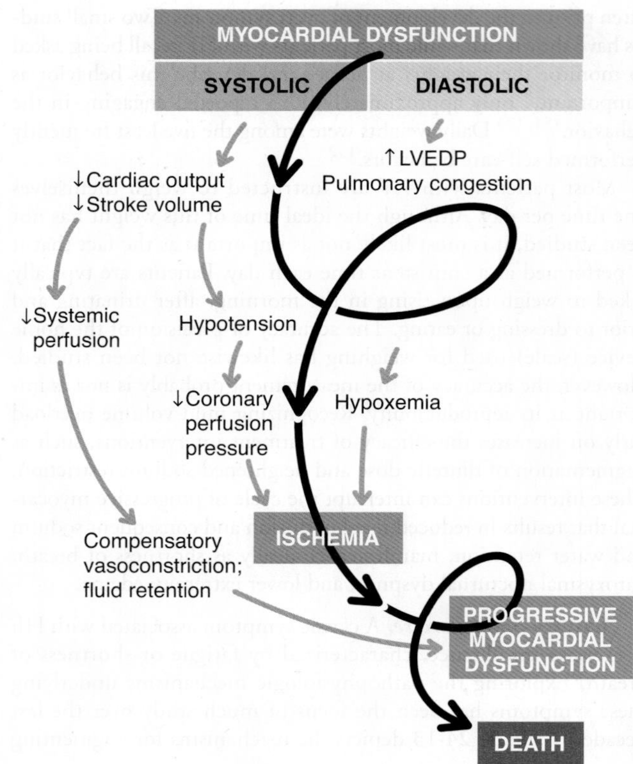

■ **Figure 24-14** The downward spiral in cardiogenic shock. LVEDP, left ventricular end-diastolic pressure. (From Hollenberg, S. M. [2001]. Cardiogenic shock. *Critical Care Clinics, 17*[2], 395.)

RV infarction occurs after occlusion of the proximal right coronary artery and is identified in the setting of concomitant infero-posterior LV dysfunction. There is up to 32% incidence of shock with clinically evident RV systolic dysfunction and secondary to RV and LV interactions.

Complications of MI include mitral regurgitation, ventricular septal defect (VSD), and free-wall rupture. Significant mitral regurgitation patterns are seen clinically: papillary muscle (usually the posterior papillary muscle) or chordal rupture caused by MI, and mitral regurgitation associated with LV dilatation. Acute VSD abruptly increases pulmonary blood flow and leads to symptoms of biventricular failure within hours to days if not corrected. LV free-wall rupture occurs in less than 1% of acute MIs but carries a high mortality rate.[195]

Non-MI-related acute valvular problems involve the mitral and aortic valve. Acute mitral regurgitation can be caused by spontaneous chordal rupture, infective endocarditis, inflammatory disorders (e.g., rheumatic fever), or trauma. Acute aortic insufficiency may be caused by infective endocarditis with leaflet destruction (most common), acute aortic dissection, or traumatic injury. Shock may be caused by aortic stenosis with increasing metabolic demands or with concomitant LV failure. Mitral stenosis rarely causes shock without rapid atrial fibrillation.[195] Prosthetic valve dysfunction, especially left-sided, most often causes shock because of valvular insufficiency. Acute prosthetic valvular insufficiency occurs because of dehiscence of the sewing ring, infective endocarditis, or catastrophic mechanical failure.

Infiltrative disease, such as amyloidosis, sarcoidosis, and hemochromatosis, are examples of infiltrative diseases in their later stages that may be associated with shock. Shock caused by trauma is usually seen secondary to myocardial or aortic rupture, or caused by acute volume loss secondary to hemorrhage.

Acute decompensation of chronic HF represents a somewhat different pathophysiologic state, because these patients have a marked reduction in LV systolic function at baseline as compared to those patients with acute HF without prior LV dysfunction.[190] Patients with chronic HF are likely to be using combination therapy, usually an ACE-I, diuretic, β-blocker, and/or digoxin. There is already activation of the neurohormonal compensatory mechanisms, including increased sympathetic stimulation of the heart, activation of the RAAS, increased vasoconstriction, fluid retention by the kidneys, increased ventricular preload, and LV hypertrophy and remodeling. When a precipitating event occurs, there is further derangement of these compensatory mechanisms. Factors leading to acute decompensation in chronic HF may include the following: acute myocardial ischemia, poorly treated or untreated hypertension, new-onset atrial fibrillation, concurrent infections (e.g., pneumonia, influenza), medication noncompliance, excess dietary sodium, cardiac depressant drugs, NSAIDs, and endocrine abnormalities (e.g., poorly controlled diabetes, hyperthyroidism).[190] Table 24-13 compares clinical and pathophysiologic features of acute and chronic HF.

Extracardiac Obstructive Shock

Pericardial Tamponade

The accumulation of fluid within the pericardial sac increases pressure, causing extracardiac obstruction to filling that results in a decrease in ventricular preload and cardiac output. What determines whether pericardial effusion will cause shock is how rapidly the fluid accumulates. Patients at risk for shock caused by tamponade are those with malignancy (especially lung and breast cancer, lymphoma, leukemia, or melanoma), infection, aortic dissection, or severe pericarditis.

Pulmonary Embolism

When embolic material, such as thrombus, fat, tumor, or air, obstructs 30% or more or the pulmonary vasculature, the RV cannot provide adequate pressure to compensate for the increased resistance to blood flow. RV failure ensues, with increased RV end-diastolic and RA pressures, and finally a decrease in cardiac output and shock.

Compensatory Mechanisms

The following equations illustrate the physiologic relation of the hemodynamic variables. Here CO, cardiac output; SV, stroke volume; HR, heart rate; MAP, mean arterial pressure; and SVR, systemic vascular resistance compose the equations:

$$CO = SV \times HR$$
$$MAP = CO \times SVR$$

In the pathophysiologic state of cardiogenic shock, the decrease in MAP is brought about by an alteration in one of the variables. The reduction in cardiac output results from a decrease in stroke volume:

$$\downarrow CO = \downarrow SV \times HR$$

The deduction in MAP results from the decrease in cardiac output:

$$\downarrow MAP = \downarrow CO \times SVR$$

Compensatory mechanisms consist of reflex reactions to an initial fall in blood pressure. They are activated immediately and

Table 24-13 ■ COMPARISON OF ACUTE AND CHRONIC HEART FAILURE

Clinical Feature	Acute Heart Failure	Decompensated Chronic Heart Failure	Stable Chronic Heart Failure
Symptom severity (shortness of breath and fatigue)	Marked and sudden	Moderate to severe	None to Mild or moderate
Pulmonary edema	Common	Frequent	Rare
Peripheral edema	Rare	Frequent	Occasional
Weight gain	None to mild	Very frequent	Occassional
Total body volume	No change to mild increase	Marked increase	Mild increase
Cardiomegaly	Uncommon	Common	Common
LV systolic function	Hypo-, normo- or hypercontractile	Normal to reduced	Normal to reduced
LV wall stress	Marked increase	Marked increase	Elevated
Activation of sympathetic nervous system	Marked increase	Marked increase	Mild to marked increase
Activation of RAAS	Marked increase	Marked increase	Mild to marked increase
Myocardial ischemia*	Common	Occasional	Rare
Hypertensive crisis	Common	Occasional	Rare

*For example, acute coronary syndrome, acute mitral regurgitation, aortic stenosis, or ventricular septal defect.
LV, left ventricle; RAAS, renin–angiotensin–aldosterone system.

increase in intensity in an attempt to restore adequate tissue perfusion.[190] The compensatory mechanisms are directed at the restoration and maintenance of adequate blood volume, cardiac output, and vascular tone. The initial compensatory mechanisms vary with the primary pathophysiologic derangement, but the intermediate and final stages are similar. The initial compensatory mechanisms in cardiogenic shock are an increased heart rate and increased SVR.

Initial Stage

In cardiogenic shock, the decreased coronary blood flow results in profound local compensatory events. Figure 24-15 graphically displays the compensatory mechanisms activated in the initial states of an acute reduction in cardiac output. There is an increase in myocardial oxygen extraction and dilatation of the coronary arteries. The myocardial cells shift to anaerobic metabolism and use glycolysis in the production of adenosine triphosphate (ATP).[196,197] These events occur immediately in response to myocardial ischemia. If compensatory mechanisms are inadequate, myocardial contractility decreases, leading to a decrease in cardiac output and systemic hypoperfusion.

A reduction in arterial blood pressure secondary to decreased blood volume, decreased cardiac output, or increased venous capacitance initiates the body's compensatory mechanisms to maintain adequate tissue perfusion. These mechanisms serve to increase cardiac output and arterial blood pressure through increasing heart rate, enhancing myocardial contractility, providing selective vasoconstriction, conserving sodium and water, and shifting fluid from the interstitial to the intravascular space.

Specialized nerve endings (mechanoreceptors) in the carotid sinus, aortic arch, heart, and lungs sense the decrease in blood pressure and transmit their impulses to the vasomotor center. The vasomotor center stimulates the sympathetic nervous system, inhibits the parasympathetic nervous system, and initiates the secretion of catecholamines from the adrenal gland. Sympathetic nervous system stimulation unopposed by parasympathetic effects results in increased heart rate, increased myocardial contractility, and selective vasoconstriction. Reflexes of the sympathetic nervous system are active within 30 seconds of an acute decrease in circulating blood volume and are able to compensate for a 20% loss in blood volume by increasing cardiac output by 20% to 25%.[196] In response to ischemia and sympathetic

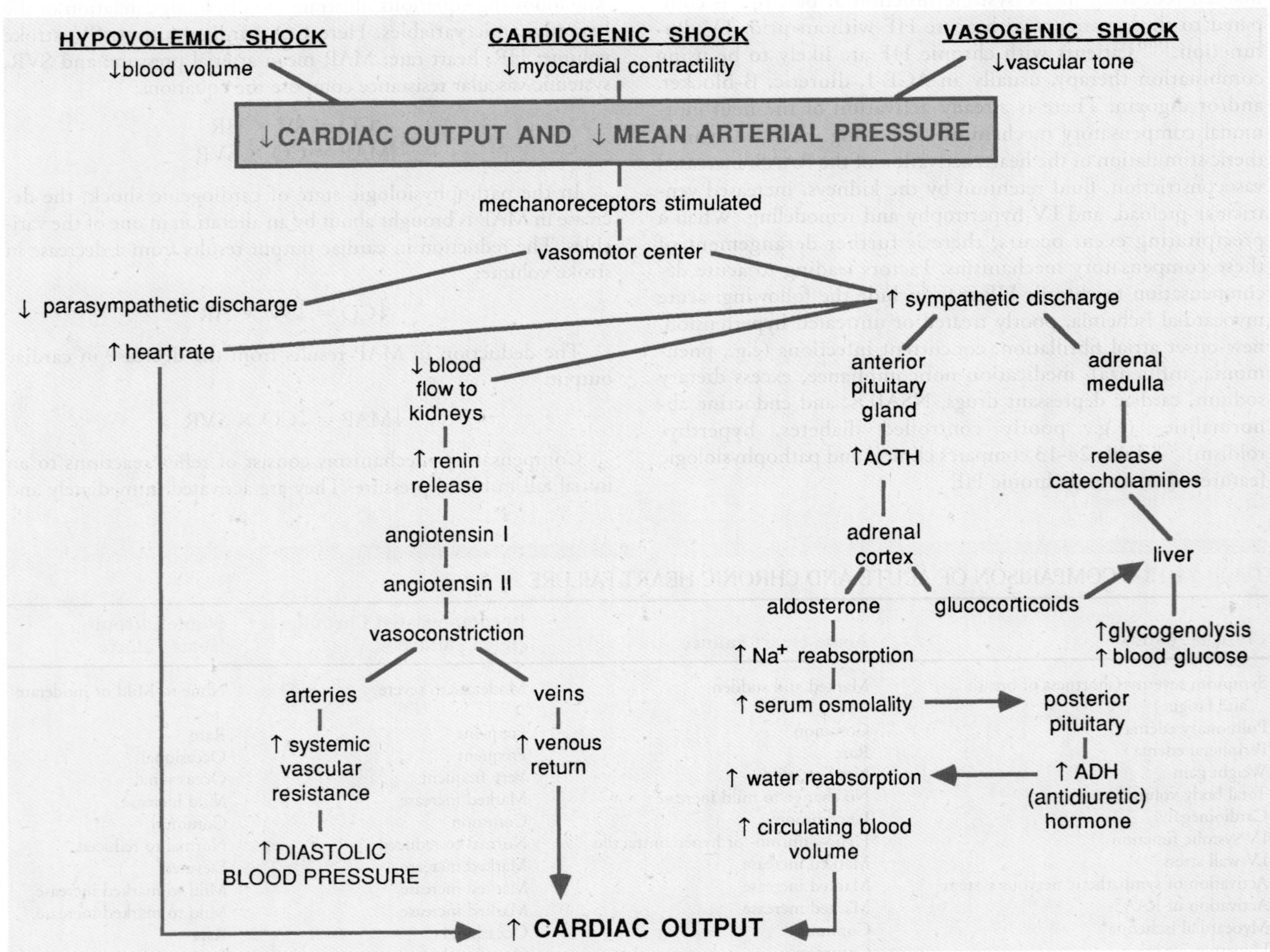

■ **Figure 24-15** In the initial stage of shock, all three types of shock lead to a decrease in mean arterial pressure. Compensatory mechanisms attempt to reduce the effects of this decreased mean arterial pressure and, if successful, lead to an increase in cardiac output and mean arterial pressure.

stimulation, hormones are released from the adrenal medulla, adrenal cortex, anterior and posterior pituitary gland, and kidneys, which further compensate for decreased circulating blood volume. The adrenal medulla releases epinephrine and NE, which enhance vasoconstriction and myocardial contractility, and increase heart rate.[13] Epinephrine and NE also stimulate glycogenolysis, thus increasing serum glucose. The adrenal cortex releases glucocorticoids, which also increase serum glucose. Decreased renal blood flow results in the release of renin, which initiates a series of reactions in the liver and elsewhere, resulting in the production of angiotensin. Angiotensin promotes the release of aldosterone by the adrenal cortex and, in situations of hypovolemia, promotes profound vasoconstriction. Aldosterone enhances renal sodium reabsorption accompanied by increased water reabsorption. Antidiuretic hormone is released from the posterior pituitary and further enhances renal water reabsorption. Thirst is stimulated and also causes increased fluid intake.[11] As a result of decreased capillary pressure, Starling capillary forces are altered, and fluid is transferred from the interstitial space to the capillary.

Intermediate Stage

If shock is not recognized and reversed in the initial compensatory stage, it progresses (Fig. 24-16). Compensatory mechanisms are no longer able to maintain homeostasis and may become counterproductive. For example, continued profound vasoconstriction in the presence of decreased MAP promotes inadequate tissue perfusion and cellular hypoxia.

Decreased delivery of oxygen and nutrients causes cells to shift to anaerobic metabolic pathways.[7] Increasing amounts of lactic acid are produced and accumulate in the cells because of decreased perfusion. Because anaerobic metabolism is less efficient in meeting the energy requirements of the cells, ATP is depleted. Reduction in the available ATP results in failure of the membrane transport mechanisms, intracellular edema, and rupture of the cell membrane. Progressive tissue ischemia results in increased anaerobic metabolism and the further production of metabolic acidosis.[190]

Impairment of cellular function disrupts all body organs and organ systems. Splanchnic ischemia results in the release of endotoxin from the intestine. The reticuloendothelial (tissue macrophage) system is suppressed by splenic and hepatic ischemia. The continued renal response to ischemia leads to further vasoconstriction, stimulating the release of aldosterone from the adrenal gland and promoting the reabsorption of sodium in the kidney. This response is no longer useful because the increased volume cannot be pumped by the failing heart and

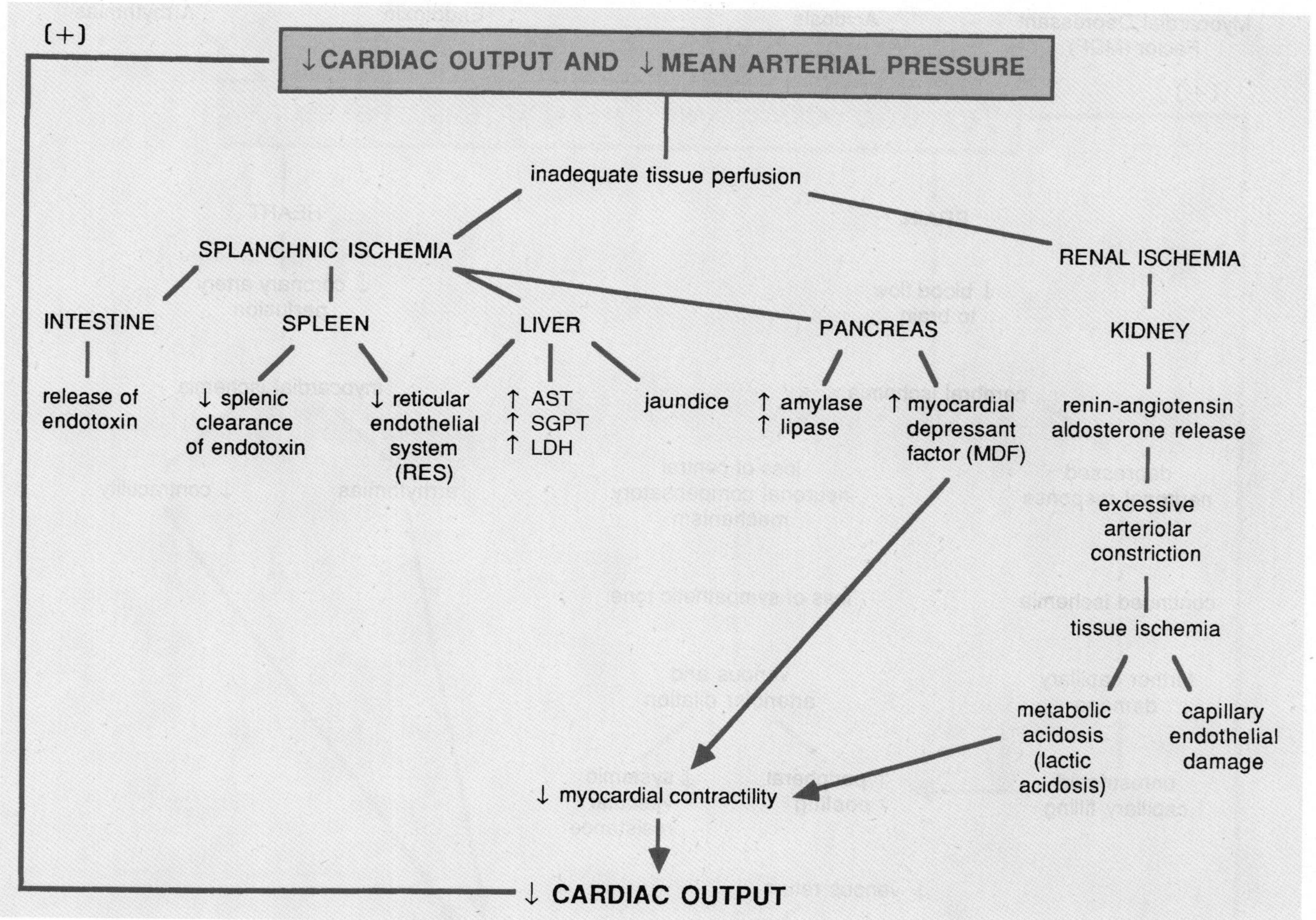

■ **Figure 24-16** In the intermediate stage of shock, compensatory mechanisms fail, resulting in decreased tissue perfusion and organ function. Decreased myocardial contractility leading to a decrease in cardiac output sets up a positive feedback mechanism (+) to decrease further cardiac output and mean arterial pressure. AST, aspartate aminotransferase; SGPT, serum glutamic pyruvic transaminase; LDH, lactate dehydrogenase.

results in ventilatory failure. The increased volume begins to pool in tissues secondary to profound venoconstriction and increased capillary permeability.

If the myocardial ischemia is severe and prolonged enough, myocardial cellular injury becomes irreversible.[190] Cytokines are signaling peptides whose actions include cell growth and cell death through direct toxic effects on the heart and peripheral circulation. The proinflammatory or "stress-activated" cytokines include TNF-α and some interleukins (i.e., IL-1β, IL-6, IL-8, IL-12). The cardiac myocytes themselves are capable of synthesizing these proinflammatory cytokines in response to various forms of cardiac injury. The local inflammatory response can appear within minutes of an abnormal stress. Local inflammation of the cytokines and other mediators includes deleterious effects of LV remodeling, which include myocyte hypertrophy, alteration in fetal gene expression, contractile defects, and progressive myocyte loss through apoptosis.[198] In addition to the direct detrimental effects of myocardial ischemia, there is some evidence that a peptide secreted by the pancreas, the myocardial depressant factor, may further depress myocardial function.[11] Myocardial depressant factor has been identified in the serum of patients in the early stages of septic shock. Its presence in other forms of shock remains controversial.

Irreversible Stage

In this stage, the compensatory mechanisms are nonfunctioning or no longer effective, and hypotension has reached the critical level of adversely affecting the heart and brain (Fig. 24-17). Myocardial hypoperfusion, resulting from hypotension and tachycardia, produces acidosis, which leads to further depression of myocardial function. Decreased cerebral blood flow leads to depressed neuronal function and activity and loss of the central neuronal compensatory mechanisms.[197]

The progressive general hypoxia and reduction in cardiac output further deprive body cells of oxygen and nutrients needed for cell growth and result in microcirculatory insufficiency. The microcirculation responds by vasodilatation to secure the necessary nutrients and oxygen for the deprived cells. Microcirculatory vasodilatation, in association with systemic vasoconstriction, results in the sequestration of blood in the capillary beds, further limiting

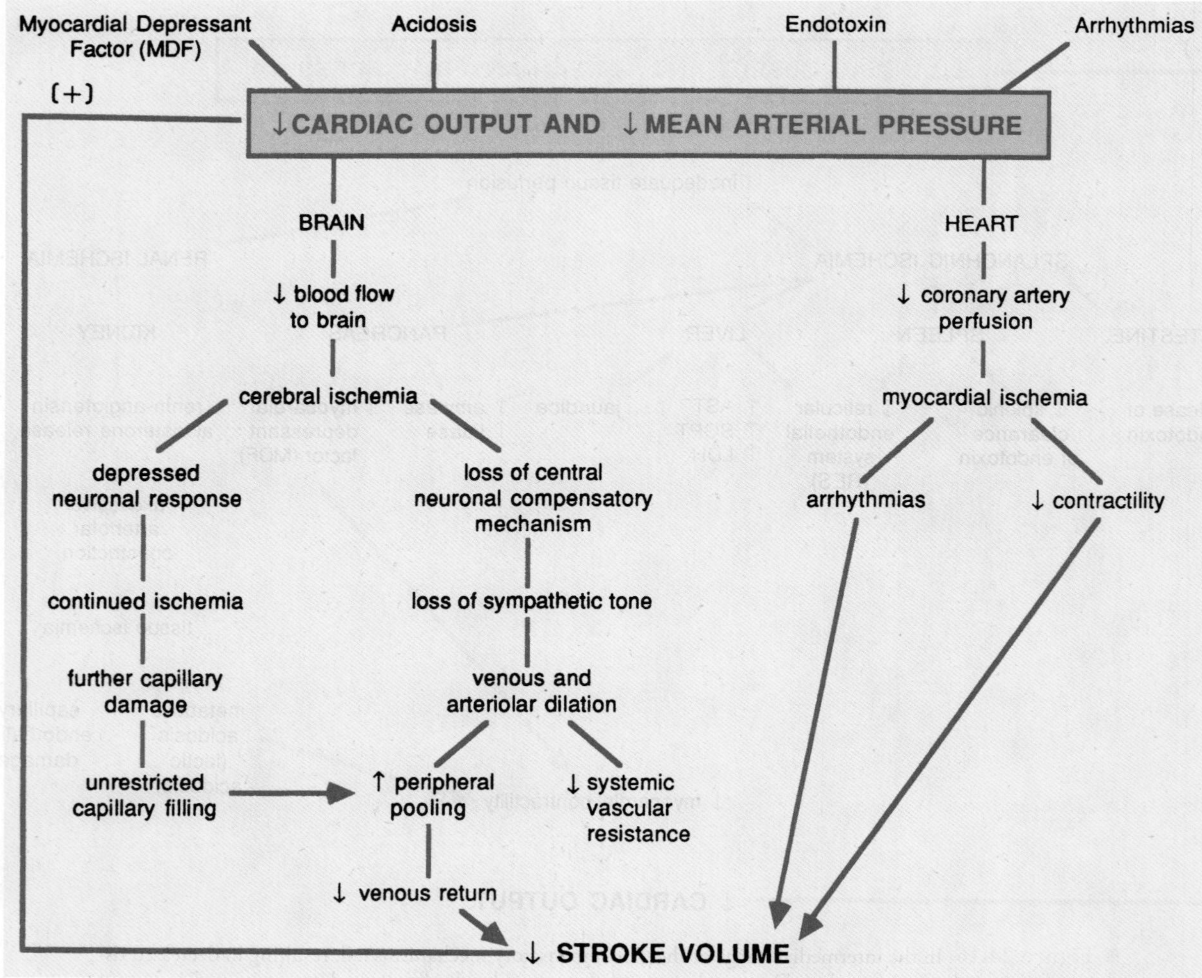

■ **Figure 24-17** In the irreversible stage of shock, a prolonged decrease in cardiac output and mean arterial pressure leads to cellular necrosis and multiple organ failure.

the volume of blood returning to the systemic circulation. This loss of circulating blood volume and impaired capillary flow results in reduced venous return, further reducing cardiac output and arterial pressure. This situation creates a positive feedback mechanism in which the low-flow state produces a further reduction in flow.[197]

Diagnosis and Clinical Manifestations

The diagnosis of shock is made by the history, physical examination, and collection of data from adjunctive diagnostic tests.

History

Most patients who present with cardiogenic shock have either a history of cardiovascular disease or risk factors for cardiovascular disease. Obtaining a thorough medical and surgical history is vital to plan life-saving interventions. Much like chronic HF, a history may provide possible causes of the acute decompensation.

Physical Examination

Ongoing assessment of the patient at risk for or in shock, with early detection of subtle changes in the patient's condition, is essential. Subjective and objective data must be correlated with adjunctive clinical measurements, such as the measurement of cardiac output and oxygen consumption. The clinical assessment of the patient provides the basis for medical and nursing interventions.

Cardiovascular Assessment. Low blood pressure is one of the defining characteristics of shock. A MAP of 65 mm Hg is required to maintain adequate myocardial and renal perfusion. Shock is defined clinically as the pathophysiologic state that results from a MAP of less than 65 mm Hg over time. Narrowing of the pulse pressure indicates arteriolar vasoconstriction and a decreasing cardiac output.[1,197] Heart rate usually increases in response to sympathetic stimulation to compensate for decreased stroke volume and to maintain cardiac output. In cardiogenic shock the pulse is weak and thready.

Distended neck veins may be seen with cardiogenic shock.[44] The presence of an RV heave, jugular venous V waves, and right-sided S_3 or S_4 gallops may suggest pulmonary emboli. Distant heart sounds and an exaggerated pulsus paradoxus ($>$10 mm Hg) suggest cardiac tamponade. A laterally displaced and sustained LV apical impulse with left-sided S_3 and/or S_4 suggests LV dysfunction.[44]

Pulmonary Assessment. The lungs are fairly resistant to short-term ischemia. Thus, it is unlikely that low blood flow is the sole cause of pulmonary insufficiency associated with shock. Other contributory factors have been implicated, including thromboemboli or fat emboli in the pulmonary tree, and the toxic effects of fibrin degradation products that result from intravascular coagulation and serum complement depletion with sequestration of granulocytes in the lung. These factors lead to increased pulmonary capillary permeability. As the ensuing alveolar edema impairs surfactant production, massive atelectasis develops, clinically termed shock lung, systemic inflammatory response syndrome, adult respiratory distress syndrome, or primary pulmonary edema. These conditions are characterized by severe hypoxemia, dyspnea, a marked reduction in lung compliance, and the presence of extensive lung infiltrates.[196]

In cardiogenic shock, failure of the left ventricle leads to acute cardiogenic pulmonary edema. Because of the increase in LV end-diastolic pressure, there is an increase in LA pressure and dilation. Pressure is increased within the pulmonary capillary bed, forcing plasma or whole blood into the pulmonary interstitial compartment and, finally, into the pulmonary alveoli.

Respiratory rate and depth are initially increased in all forms of shock, and patients may experience dyspnea or air hunger. This increased ventilation represents the body's attempt to eliminate lactic acid resulting from decreased tissue perfusion. Increased respiratory depth also enhances blood return to the right heart. Arterial blood gases initially reveal respiratory alkalosis. As shock progresses, a combined metabolic and respiratory acidosis follows.

Neuroregulatory Assessment. Decreased cerebral blood flow and coagulopathy can lead to a cerebral infarction or cerebral thrombus formation. Alterations in cellular metabolism throughout the body, metabolic acidosis, and the accumulation of toxins further depress cerebral function. Lethargy, stupor, and coma develop as shock progresses. Finally, in the irreversible stage of shock, the vasomotor center in the brain is disrupted, causing failure of the circulatory mechanisms.[196]

Level of consciousness is an indicator of the adequacy of cerebral blood flow. With cerebral ischemia, the patient initially exhibits hypervigilance, restlessness, agitation, and mild confusion. Persistent cerebral hypoxia results in progressive unresponsiveness to verbal stimuli with eventual coma.

Gastrointestinal Assessment. Compensatory vasoconstriction in shock may result in mucosal ischemia, an ileus, and full-thickness gangrene of the bowel. If the bowel wall becomes disrupted, the normal bacterial flora of the intestines enters the abdomen and can then enter the circulation. Gastrointestinal bleeding may also occur. Factors that cause damage to the liver include decreased blood flow, splanchnic vasoconstriction, pooling of blood in the microcirculation, right HF, and bacterial invasion. The subsequent changes include loss of reticuloendothelial (tissue macrophage) system function, increasing the risk of infection; a decreased lactic acid conversion, contributing to metabolic acidosis; altered protein, fat, and carbohydrate metabolism; and altered bilirubin function.[197] Jaundice, increased serum bilirubin levels, and increased serum enzymes are early indicators of liver damage associated with shock. Serum globulin is increased, and serum albumin is decreased.[196]

Renal Assessment. Adequate renal perfusion produces a minimum of 400 mL urine/24 hours, or 20 mL/h. Impaired renal perfusion in shock results in hourly urine outputs of less than 20 mL/h.[198] The excretion of high volumes of low solute urine may also represent renal hypoperfusion. Prolonged hypoperfusion may lead to acute tubular necrosis and acute renal failure. Urine output is an indicator of the adequacy of renal perfusion and may decrease early in cardiogenic shock. Oliguria is defined by a urine output of less than 20 mL/h. Urine osmolarity and specific gravity increase, and urine sodium decreases with decreased urine output. An elevated serum creatinine is an early, nonspecific indicator of impaired renal perfusion.

Integumentary Assessment. Skin appearance and temperature provide a clinical measure of peripheral circulation. Progressive peripheral vasoconstriction results in a change from the initial normal skin appearance to cool, moist, pale skin with mottling. In cardiogenic shock, cool, moist skin with barely perceptible peripheral pulses is commonly observed. Capillary refill and peripheral pulses are other indicators of the relative adequacy of cardiac output. Normal capillary refill is almost instantaneous; in cardiogenic shock, capillary refill is often prolonged.

Diagnostic Tools

The primary measurements that document the relative adequacy of blood flow include continuous monitoring of arterial blood pressure and monitoring of the ECG with rhythm analysis. The ECG can be diagnostic in the setting of MI. Most patients in shock are tachycardic and may show evidence of supraventricular or ventricular arrhythmias. Low QRS voltage and/or electrical alternans can be seen in cardiac tamponade.[199]

Transthoracic echocardiography is an excellent tool to obtain noninvasive information regarding the overall and regional systolic and diastolic function, intravascular volume, cardiac hemodynamics, myocardial abnormalities.[46] Echocardiography can rapidly assess for mechanical causes, such as severe mitral regurgitation and papillary muscle rupture, acute VSD, free-wall rupture, and tamponade. Predictors of short- and long-term mortality from cardiogenic shock relate to the LVEF and mitral regurgitation on presentation, supporting early use of echocardiography in the course of cardiogenic shock.[46]

Chest radiography may suggest a specific diagnosis. Continuous measurement of urine output and mental status are good indicators of adequate organ perfusion. A complete blood count and serial cardiac enzymes should be obtained. Serial measurements of arterial blood gases reflect the overall metabolic state of the patient, the adequacy of ventilation, and the adequacy of the circulation in providing for oxygen and metabolic needs. Measurement of mixed venous oxygen content ($S\bar{v}O_2$) by direct blood sampling or by continuous invasive monitoring reflects peripheral oxygen extraction and use. Serial arterial lactate levels can also be measured because the presence of lactic acidosis helps identify critical hypoperfusion as marked by anaerobic metabolism.[46]

Measurement of serum BNP has become a recent laboratory value that is measured as a means to identify those patients with LV dysfunction[28] (see Figure 24-11). Elevation of other substances in the blood that reflect the function of specific organs, such as blood urea nitrogen, creatinine, bilirubin, aspartate aminotransferase, and lactate dehydrogenase, may be useful in the diagnosis of shock.

In seriously ill patients, direct determination of intra-arterial pressure with an arterial line is necessary because systemic arterial pressure determines the perfusion pressure of various organ systems and is predominantly the product of cardiac output and SVR. In HF, a drop in cardiac output is compensated for by an increased SVR in an attempt to maintain the arterial blood pressure in normal range.

Right-sided heart catheterization with a PA quadruple lumen thermodilution catheter can aid in the diagnosis and assessment of the severity of HF (Chapter 21). This invasive hemodynamic monitoring can be useful in excluding volume depletion, RV infarction, and mechanical problems (e.g., acute mitral regurgitation). It is also useful for monitoring the response to treatment (including volume, diuretics, inotropic support, vasoactive agents, natriuretic peptide) and manipulation of the variables of cardiac output, preload, and afterload.[190] The hemodynamic variables measured by this catheter are cardiac output by thermodilution; RA pressure; and PA systolic, diastolic, and wedge pressures. The cardiac output is decreased in HF, whereas the RA pressure or central venous pressure is elevated. The PAWP indirectly measures the LV end-diastolic pressure, which is a measure of end-diastolic volume or preload and is elevated in HF.

Derived parameters that may be obtained by the use of the PA catheter include CI and SVR. Body surface area (BSA), measured in square meters, is correlated with the volume of cardiac output (CO) to establish the CI:

$$CI = \frac{CO}{BSA}$$

SVR, measured in dynes/s/cm^5, reflects the pressure difference of the systemic arteries to the veins.

$$SVR = \frac{MAP - RAP}{CO} \times 80$$

Besides offering diagnostic information, hemodynamic variables show a strong prognostic value for short-term survival. Forrester et al.[201] classified patients with acute MI into four subsets with different mortality rates (see Fig. 24-18). They showed that clinical signs of hypoperfusion occur with a CI of less than 2.2 L/min per m^2 and clinical signs of pulmonary congestion occur with a PAWP greater than 18 mm Hg. Subset I shows a patient with normal CI and normal PAWP with no evidence of pulmonary congestion or peripheral hypoperfusion (warm and dry). Subset III shows a patient with a low CI and PAWP, reflecting peripheral hypoperfusion without pulmonary conges-

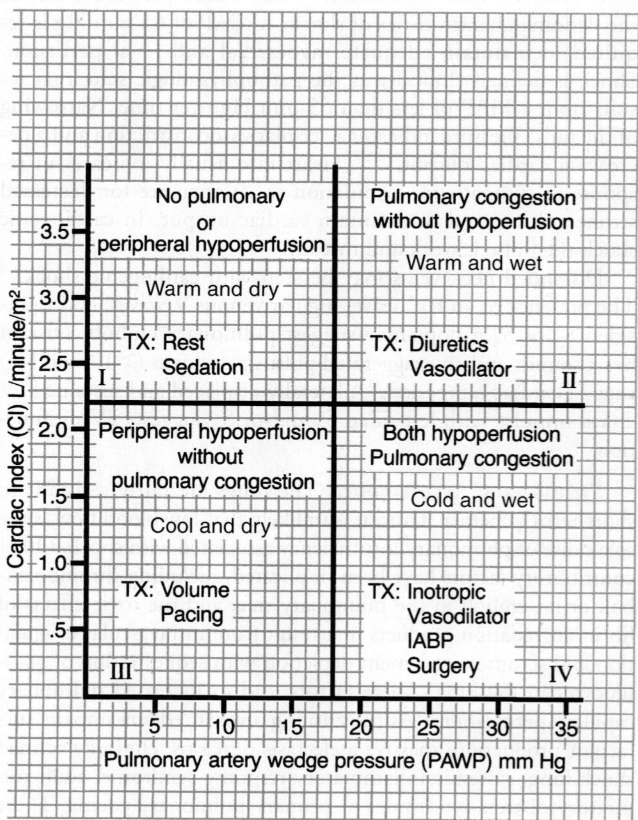

■ **Figure 24-18** Forrester subsets: clinical states and therapy. IABP, intra-aortic balloon pumping.

tion (cool and dry) as seen in patients with hypovolemia. Subset II describes the patient with pulmonary edema with an elevated PAWP but without peripheral hypoperfusion (warm and wet), which may be seen in acute HF or decompensated chronic HF. Subset IV describes the patient with pulmonary edema with hypoperfusion (cold and wet), as seen in cardiogenic shock.[201]

Assessment of tissue metabolism, which is determined by mixed venous oxygen saturation, conventionally required sending a PA blood sample to the laboratory for interpretation. Some PA catheters are designed with a fiberoptic photometric lumen, allowing for continuous monitoring of mixed venous oxygen saturation. Although PA catheters have been widely used for almost 40 years, there has been controversy because there are data to suggest increased mortality in critically ill patient who had PA lines.[202] Current consensus is that PA catheters are useful in settings MI and cardiogenic shock.[1]

Prognosis

The stages of shock depict a series of pathophysiologic changes that occur if medical and nursing interventions are delayed or inappropriate. The stages do not progress at the same speed in all patients. The length of time tissues are hypoxic is a major factor in determining the occurrence of complications. The initial and intermediate stages of shock are reversible with aggressive management. The irreversible stage is caused by cellular necrosis and multiple organ failure. Thus, the chance of recovery in the irreversible stage without permanent injury is low. In cardiogenic shock, patients with a CI less than 1.81 L/min per m^2 have a 70% mortality rate.[200] Patients with $S\bar{v}O_2$ less than 55% also have a high mortality rate.[190]

Approach to Treatment

The main goal of treatment of the metabolic defects produced by shock is the restoration of adequate tissue perfusion.[197]

Initial general management for patients is placement of large-bore venous catheters, and continuous monitoring of blood pressure, pulse oximetry, and ECG. If respiratory failure is imminent with patients with severe hypoxemia, hypercarbia, or metabolic acidosis, then endotracheal intubation may be required with mechanical ventilation. A PA catheter may be placed. Volume expansion may be needed to restore adequate circulation to maintain a PAWP of 14 to 16 mm Hg. Vasopressor support should be used only after preload is adequate to restore the blood pressure. The choice of a particular vasopressor/inotropic agent depends on the clinical circumstance (Table 24-14).

Acute manifestations of HF can be either in the setting of a new onset or in patients with established chronic HF. It is critical to establish the diagnosis and determine the hemodynamic status: pulmonary congestion without peripheral hypoperfusion versus shock/hypoperfusion (Fig. 24-19). The three major goals of treatment of acute HF, acute decompensated chronic HF, and cardiogenic shock are (1) to increase the oxygen supply to the myocardium; (2) to maximize the cardiac output; and (3) to decrease the workload of the left ventricle.

Goal 1: Increase Oxygen Supply to the Myocardium

Increased inspired oxygen concentrations, including the institution of mechanical ventilation with positive end-expiratory pressure, may be required to maintain arterial blood gases within normal limits. Narcotic analgesics are used to control the patient's pain and aid in reducing myocardial oxygen demands.

Aggressive reperfusion of the coronary arteries can be undertaken by invasive and noninvasive approaches, including percutaneous transluminal coronary angioplasty, atherectomy or stent placement, use of adjunctive antiplatelet therapy, thrombolytic therapy, and coronary artery bypass grafting, which were all associated with lower in-hospital mortality rates than treatment with standard medical therapy.[195] Studies suggest that immediate revascularization with percutaneous coronary intervention, which may include angioplasty, stent placement, and atherectomy, along with adjunctive antiplatelet therapy, improves outcomes in patients with cardiogenic shock.[203] Improvement is seen in wall motion in the infarct territory, with increased perfusion of the infarct zone augmenting contraction of remote myocardium, possibly because of recruitment of collateral blood

Table 24-14 ■ VASOPRESSORS AND INOTROPES USED IN CARDIOGENIC SHOCK

Feature	Dopamine		Dobutamine	Norepinephrine	Epinephrine	Phenylephrine	Milrinone
Dosage (mcg/kg/min)	1–4	4–20	2.5–20	0.05–1	0.05–2	0.5–5	0.375–0.750
Receptor							
α	+	+++	+	++++	++++	++++	0
β_1	+	++	+++	+	++++	0	0
β_2	0	0	++	0	++	0	0
Dopaminergic	+++	++	0	0	0	0	0
Chronotropic (HR)	+	++	++	+	+++	0	+
Inotropic (stroke volume/cardiac output)	+	++/+++	+++	+	+++	0	+++
SVR (afterload)	↓	↑↑	↓↓	↑↑↑↑	↓↓↑↑	↑↑↑↑	↓↓↓
Filling pressure (preload)	↓	↔↑↑	↓↓	↔↑↑	↔	↔	↓↓
Comments	Improves renal flow in low dose; first-line drug to restore BP		First-line agent to improve CO, but may be arrhythmogenic	Pure vasoconstrictor compared to dopamine	Increases MVO_2, supports BP	Purest vasoconstrictor	Inotrope of choice in pulmonary hypertension

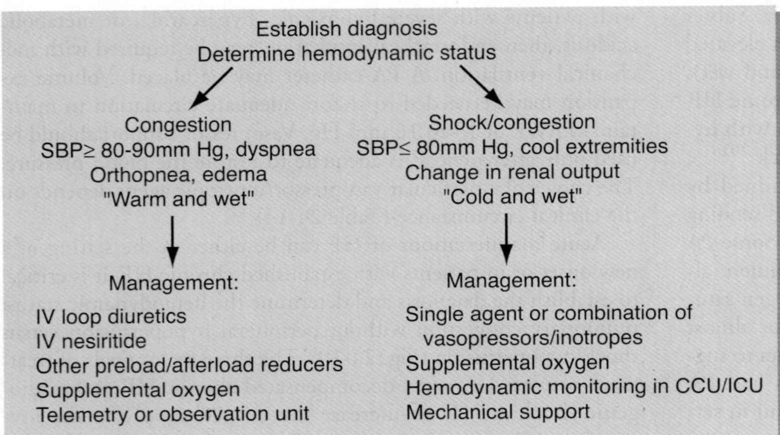

■ **Figure 24-19** Algorithm for establishing the diagnosis of acute heart failure/acute decompensation of chronic heart failure with pulmonary congestion versus cardiogenic shock with hypoperfusion and pulmonary congestion. General management principles for each diagnosis are listed. SBP, systolic blood pressure; IV, intravenous, IABP, intra-aortic balloon pump. (Adapted from Lyengar, S., Hass, G., & Young, J. [2006]. Acute heart failure. In E. J. Topol [3rd ed.], Textbook of cardiovascular medicine [pp. 1845–1898]. Philadelphia: Lippincott Williams & Wilkins.)

flow. Reperfusion therapy with thrombolytic agents has decreased the occurrence of cardiogenic shock in patients with persistent ST-segment elevation MI, but thrombolytic therapy for patients in whom shock has already developed is disappointing and may be attributed to low perfusion pressure.[195] For hospitals without revascularization capability, early thrombolytic therapy along with intra-aortic balloon pumping followed by immediate transfer for percutaneous coronary intervention or coronary artery bypass grafting may be appropriate.[204] There are data to support favorable outcomes for patients undergoing emergent coronary artery bypass grafting.[192]

Goal 2: Maximize Cardiac Output

Because the cardiac output is already compromised, arrhythmias, which occur as a result of ischemia, acid–base alterations, or MI, can cause a further decline in cardiac output. Electrolyte abnormalities should be corrected, because hypokalemia and hypomagnesemia predispose to ventricular arrhythmias. Antiarrhythmic agents, pacing, or cardioversion may be used to maintain a stable heart rhythm. Volume loading is undertaken with caution and in the presence of adequate hemodynamic monitoring. Optimal preload (LV end-diastolic pressure or PAWP) ranges between 14 and 18 mm Hg. However, fluid loading must be abandoned when the increase in filling pressure occurs without increase in cardiac output.

Unlike patients with acute HF, patients with chronic HF are usually using chronic pharmacologic therapy (i.e., diuretic, ACE-I, β-blocker, and digitalis). Treatment of acute episodes in these two scenarios are similar, with the exception of the higher incidence of reparable lesions in acute HF (e.g., acute occlusion of major coronary artery, ruptured chordae tendineae).[205] The Forrester subsets (see Fig. 6-18) can be used as guidelines for these patients in pulmonary edema (warm and wet).[201] In subset II, the goal of therapy is to reduce the PAWP below a level that causes pulmonary congestion but above a level that causes a deleterious reduction in cardiac output by the Starling mechanism. There are several options because diuretics, peripheral vasodilators, and inotropic agents all reduce PAWP (Tables 24-14 and 24-15). The management strategy for the patient in acute cardiogenic pulmonary edema is outlined in Display 24-2.

An intravenous diuretic such as furosemide is administered when symptoms of pulmonary edema occur. Nesiritide (BNP) represents a recent drug class for acute decompensated HF. Nesiritide affords a unique combination of hemodynamic effects as a

Table 24-15 ■ PRELOAD- AND AFTERLOAD-REDUCING AGENTS FOR ACUTE/DECOMPENSATED HEART FAILURE

Drug	Dosing	Advantages	Disadvantages
Nitroglycerin	Sublingual: 0.4 mg (or 1 to 2 sprays) at 5-minute intervals intravenous: 0.4 μg/kg/min initially; increase as needed	+ Effect on coronary vasculature and in myocardial ischemia infarction	Hypotension; drug tolerance; inadequate afterload reduction in catastrophic disorders (e.g., acute valve insufficiency)
Nitroprusside	Intravenous: 0.1 μg/kg/min initially; increase as needed	Powerful afterload reducer	Hypotension; infusion needs to be watched closely; less favorable effects on coronary vasculature and myocardial ischemia; thiocyanate or cyanide toxicity during high-dose or prolonged infusion; particularly in renal failure
Nesiritide	Intravenous: bolus of 2 μg/kg, followed by 0.01 μg/kg/min infusion; may rebolus 1 μg/kg 1, and increase infusion up to maximum, which is 0.03 μg/kg/min	Useful afterload reducer and diuretic; use in acute decompensated heart failure	Hypotension; has been linked to progressive renal dysfunction; not to be used in patients in cardiogenic shock, moderate renal dysfunction or systolic BP <90 mm Hg

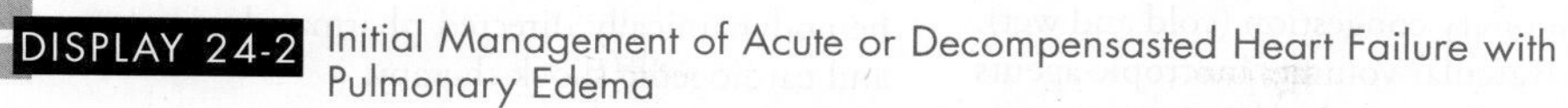

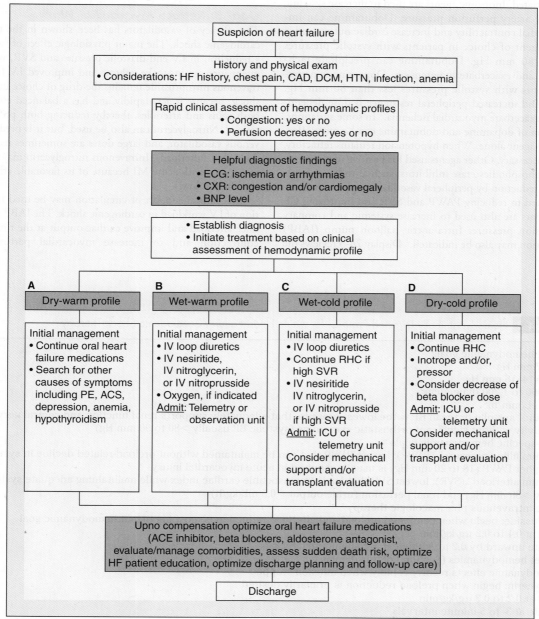

DISPLAY 24-2 Initial Management of Acute or Decompensasted Heart Failure with Pulmonary Edema

Suspicion of heart failure

History and physical exam
- Considerations: HF history, chest pain, CAD, DCM, HTN, infection, anemia

Rapid clinical assessment of hemodynamic profiles
- Congestion: yes or no
- Perfusion decreased: yes or no

Helpful diagnostic findings
- ECG: ischemia or arrhythmias
- CXR: congestion and/or cardiomegaly
- BNP level

- Establish diagnosis
- Initiate treatment based on clinical assessment of hemodynamic profile

A — Dry-warm profile

Initial management
- Continue oral heart failure medications
- Search for other causes of symptoms including PE, ACS, depression, anemia, hypothyroidism

B — Wet-warm profile

Initial management
- IV loop diuretics
- IV nesiritide, IV nitroglycerin, or IV nitroprusside
- Oxygen, if indicated

Admit: Telemetry or observation unit

C — Wet-cold profile

Initial management
- IV loop diuretics
- Continue RHC if high SVR
- IV nesiritide IV nitroglycerin, or IV nitroprusside if high SVR

Admit: ICU or telemetry unit

Consider mechanical support and/or transplant evaluation

D — Dry-cold profile

Initial management
- Continue RHC
- Inotrope and/or, pressor
- Consider decrease of beta blocker dose

Admit: ICU or telemetry unit

Consider mechanical support and/or transplant evaluation

Upno compensation optimize oral heart failure medications (ACE inhibitor, beta blockers, aldosterone antagonist, evaluate/manage comorbidities, assess sudden death risk, optimize HF patient education, optimize discharge planning and follow-up care)

Discharge

Adapted from Lyengar, S., Hass, G., & Young, J. (2006). Acute heart failure. In E. J. Topol (3rd ed.), *Textbook of cardiovascular medicine* (pp. 1845–1898). Philadelphia: Lippincott Williams & Wilkins.

venous and arterial vasodilator, reducing preload and afterload while increasing cardiac output (indirectly) without increasing heart rate. It also has neurohormonal (inhibition of the RAAS and NE) and renal (diuresis and natreiuresis) effects.[190] Nesiritide is best used early in conjunction with intravenous diuretics. ACE-I and/or β-blocker therapy may be continued for those patients with decompensated chronic HF. Many patients are also receiving digoxin. Digoxin levels should be measured because they may be abnormally increased during acute decompensation and adjustments of the daily dose may be necessary. Once the patient is compensated and free from congestion, nesiritide can be discontinued, and oral medications for HF should be optimally maximized. Nesiritide should not be used in renal failure, cardiogenic or distributive shock, severe valvular stenosis, restrictive or obstructive cardiomyopathy, or constrictive pericarditis and pericardial tamponade.[98,206]

Because patients in cardiogenic shock are in the high-risk Forrester subset IV (see Fig. 24-18), simultaneous improvement of both CI and PAWP is the goal of therapy.[197] These patients are hypoperfused and have pulmonary congestion (cold and wet). For patients with adequate intravascular volume, inotropic agents should be initiated. Inotropic agents are used to increase systemic and coronary artery perfusion pressure. Dobutamine can improve myocardial contractility and increase cardiac output and is usually the agent of choice in patients with systolic pressures greater than 80 mm Hg. Dobutamine can precipitate tachyarrhythmias and exacerbate hypotension. Dopamine is preferable in patients with systolic pressures less than 80 mm Hg. Tachycardia and increased peripheral resistance is dose dependent, and can exacerbate myocardial ischemia.[1] In some situations, a combination of dopamine and dobutamine can be more effective than one agent alone. When hypotension remains refractory, NE may be necessary. Other agents used for positive inotropic effect include phosphodiesterase inhibitors, such as milrinone.

Afterload reduction by peripheral vasodilators appears particularly well suited to reducing PAWP and SVR and improving CI. Inotropic agents are also used to increase systemic and coronary artery perfusion pressure. Intra-aortic balloon pump (IABP) counterpulsation may also be indicated.[1] Display 24-3 reviews the hemodynamically directed pharmacologic protocol for acute HF and cardiogenic shock therapy.

Goal 3: Reduce Myocardial Work

The efficacy of vasodilators has been shown in the treatment of cardiogenic shock. The major physiologic effect of vasodilators is a reduction in LV end-diastolic pressure and SVR, with a subsequent increase in stroke volume and improved LV function. Intravenous nitroprusside remains the drug of choice in cardiogenic shock, because it acts rapidly and has a balanced effect, dilating both veins and arterioles, thereby reducing both preload and afterload. Nitroglycerin can also be used, but it is predominantly a venous vasodilator, and large doses are sometimes required to reduce SVR (afterload). Intravenous nitroglycerin may be preferred in patients with acute MI because of its favorable effect on coronary blood flow.[1]

Mechanical support of circulation may be used in the reduction of LV workload in cardiogenic shock. The IABP is used to reduce afterload and improve cardiac output at the time of systolic contraction and to increase myocardial perfusion during

DISPLAY 24-3 Hemodynamically Directed Protocol for Acute Heart Failure/Cardiogenic Shock Therapy

I. General hemodynamic goals
   RAP ≤7 mm Hg
   PAWP =14–16 mm Hg
   SVR 1,000 to 1,200 dyne/s/cm^5
   CI > 2.5 L/min/m^2
   "Optimum" systolic or mean BP is the lowest pressure that adequately supports renal function and central nervous system activity without significant orthostatic symptoms (systolic BP usually >80 to 90 mm Hg)
II. Patient-specific hemodynamic goals
   "Optimum filling pressure" (PAWP): lowest PAWP that can be maintained without preload-related decline in systolic BP or CI. A higher PAWP (18 to 20 mm Hg) is usually required in acute myocardial injury
   "Optimum afterload" (SVR): lowest SVR that leads to reasonable cardiac index while maintaining adequate systolic BP (usually >80 mm Hg) and renal perfusion (urine output >0.5 mL/kg/h)
III. Specific intravenous pharmacologic therapy
   Nitroprusside: begin when combined preload and afterload reduction is most important hemodynamic goal
      Start at 0.1 to 0.2 μg/kg/min
      Titrate upward by 0.2 μg/kg/min at 3- to 5-minute intervals
      Target hemodynamics (Section I of this display)
      Hemodynamic effects resolve rapidly when infusion stopped
   Nitroglycerin: begin when preload reduction is primarily desired
      Start at 0.2 to 0.3 μg/kg/min
      Titrate at 3- to 5-minute intervals
      Be aware of tolerance
      Target hemodynamics (Section I of this display)
      Effects resolve rapidly when infusion stopped
   Dobutamine: begin when both inotropic and vasodilating effects desired but inotropic effects most important
      Start at 2.5 μg/kg/min
      Attempt to keep dose <15 μg/kg/min; avoid significant tachycardia
      Consider adding low-dose dopamine to assist with augmenting renal perfusion or milrinon to achieve hemodynamic endpoints
      Hemodynamic effects resolve over minutes to hours when infusion stopped
   Milrinone: begin when both vasodilating and inotropic effects desired
      Dose range is 0.375 to 0.75 μg/kg/min (usual is 0.5 μg/kg/min)
      Target hemodynamics (Section I of this display)
      Prolonged hemodynamic effects after drug is stopped

BP, blood pressure; CI, cardiac index; PAWP, pulmonary artery wedge pressure; RAP, right atrial pressure; SVR, systemic vascular resistance.
Adapted from text Lyengar, S., Hass, G., & Young, J. (2006). Acute heart failure. In E. J. Topol (3rd ed.), *Textbook of cardiovascular medicine* (pp. 1845–1898). Philadelphia: Lippincott-Williams & Wilkins.

diastole.[197] Other mechanical assist devices may be used. Chapter 26 provides an in-depth discussion of circulatory assist devices.

Other Considerations

Right Ventricular Infarction. Interventions include correction of hypovolemia with fluid administration and maintaining RV preload to a mean RA pressure of 15 mm Hg. Inotropic therapy with dobutamine can be used to support cardiac output. Atrioventricular (AV) synchrony is also important, and AV sequential pacing can improve blood pressure and cardiac output. Reperfusion of the occluded coronary artery is also crucial.[205]

Acute Mitral Regurgitation. Management includes afterload reduction, usually with nitroprusside, and IABP as temporizing measures. Inotropic or vasopressor support may also be needed to support blood pressure and cardiac output. Surgical valve repair or replacement is the definitive treatment.[205]

Ventricular Septal Wall Rupture. IABP and supportive pharmacologic agents are necessary. Operative repair is the only option. The timing of the repair remains controversial, although most feel repair should be undertaken within 48 hours of the rupture.[207,208]

Cardiac Free-Wall Rupture. This condition usually occurs during the first week after MI. This is a catastrophic event. Possible salvage is possible with rapid recognition, pericardiocentesis to relieve acute tamponade, and thoracotomy with repair.[208–210]

Valvular Heart Disease. Emergency surgery is indicated for aortic dissection that results in acute aortic regurgitation. In cases of severe mitral stenosis, decreasing the heart rate to improve diastolic filling time improves cardiac output. Mitral valvuloplasty or surgical intervention is indicated.

Extracardiac Obstructive Shock. Pulmonary embolism is best treated with thrombolytic therapy.[210] Cardiac tamponade initially needs volume support, but definitive therapy is pericardiocentesis and possible pericardial window.[208]

REFERENCES

1. Hunt, S. A., Abraham, W. T., Chin, M. H., et al. (2005). ACC/AHA 2005 Guideline Update for the Diagnosis and Management of Chronic Heart Failure in the Adult: A Report of the American College of Cardiology/American Heart Association Task Force on Practice Guidelines (Writing Committee to Update the 2001 Guidelines for the Evaluation and Management of Heart Failure): Developed in Collaboration With the American College of Chest Physicians and the International Society for Heart and Lung Transplantation: Endorsed by the Heart Rhythm Society. *Circulation, 112*(12), e154–e235.
2. Fonarow, G. C. (2008). Epidemiology and risk stratification in acute heart failure. *American Heart Journal, 155*(2), 200–207.
3. Gwadry-Sridhar, F. H., Flintoft, V., Lee, D. S., et al. (2004). A systematic review and meta-analysis of studies comparing readmission rates and mortality rates in patients with heart failure. *Archives of Internal Medicine, 164*(21), 2315–2320.
4. Rosamond, W., Flegal, K., Furie, K., et al. (2008). Heart disease and stroke statistics—2008 update: A report from the American Heart Association Statistics Committee and Stroke Statistics Subcommittee. *Circulation, 117*(4), e25–e146.
5. Lloyd-Jones, D. M., Larson, M. G., Leip, E. P., et al. (2002). Lifetime risk for developing congestive heart failure: The Framingham Heart Study. *Circulation, 106*(24), 3068–3072.
6. Colluci, W., & Braunwald, E. (2001). *Heart disease: A textbook of cardiovascular medicine.*
7. Katz, A. M. (2000). *Heart failure: Pathophysiology, molecular biology and clinical management.* Philadelphia: Lippincott Williams & Williams.
8. Packer, M. (1992). The neurohormonal hypothesis: A theory to explain the mechanism of disease progression in heart failure. *Journal of the American College of Cardiology, 20*(1), 248–254.
9. Bell, D. S. (2003). Heart failure: The frequent, forgotten, and often fatal complication of diabetes. *Diabetes Care, 26*(8), 2433–2441.
10. Kannel, W. B., & McGee, D. L. (1979). Diabetes and cardiovascular disease. The Framingham study. *JAMA, 241*(19), 2035–2038.
11. Bock, G., & Goode, J. (2006). *Heart failure: Molecules, mechanisms and therapeutic targets.* Chichester, UK: John Wiley & Sons Ltd.
12. Katz, A. M. (1998). Evolving concepts of heart failure: Cooling furnace, malfunctioning pump, enlarging muscle. Part II: Hypertrophy and dilatation of the failing heart. *Journal of Cardiac Failure, 4*(1), 67–81.
13. Dorn, G. W., II, & Molkentin, J. D. (2004). Manipulating cardiac contractility in heart failure: Data from mice and men. *Circulation, 109*(2), 150–158.
14. Mani, K., & Kitsis, R. N. (2003). Myocyte apoptosis: Programming ventricular remodeling. *Journal of the American College of Cardiology, 41*(5), 761–764.
15. Abbate, A., Biondi-Zoccai, G. G., Bussani, R., et al. (2003). Increased myocardial apoptosis in patients with unfavorable left ventricular remodeling and early symptomatic post-infarction heart failure. *Journal of the American College of Cardiology, 41*(5), 753–760.
16. Sanderson, J. E. (2007). Heart failure with a normal ejection fraction. *Heart, 93*(2), 155–158.
17. Weil, J., Eschenhagen, T., Hirt, S., et al. (1998). Preserved Frank-Starling mechanism in human end stage heart failure. *Cardiovascular Research, 37*(2), 541–548.
18. Sokolovsky, R. E., Zlochiver, S., & Abboud, S. (2008). Stroke volume estimation in heart failure patients using bioimpedance: A realistic simulation of the forward problem. *Physiological Measurement, 29*(6), S139–S149.
19. Lopez, B., Gonzalez, A., & Diez, J. (2004). Role of matrix metalloproteinases in hypertension-associated cardiac fibrosis. *Current Opinion in Nephrology and Hypertension, 13*(2), 197–204.
20. Lester, S. J., Tajik, A. J., Nishimura, R. A., et al. (2008). Unlocking the mysteries of diastolic function: Deciphering the Rosetta Stone 10 years later. *Journal of the American College of Cardiology, 51*(7), 679–689.
21. Tang, W. H., & Francis, G. S. (2007). The year in heart failure. *Journal of the American College of Cardiology, 50*(24), 2344–2351.
22. Cotter, G., Felker, G. M., Adams, K. F., et al. (2008). The pathophysiology of acute heart failure—Is it all about fluid accumulation? *American Heart Journal, 155*(1), 9–18.
23. Felker, G. M., & Cotter, G. (2006). Unraveling the pathophysiology of acute heart failure: An inflammatory proposal. *American Heart Journal, 151*(4), 765–767.
24. Mazhari, R., & Hare, J. M. (2007). Advances in cell-based therapy for structural heart disease. *Progress in Cardiovascular Disease, 49*(6), 387–395.
25. Szokodi, I., Kinnunen, P., Tavi, P., et al. (1998). Evidence for cAMP-independent mechanisms mediating the effects of adrenomedullin, a new inotropic peptide. *Circulation, 97*(11), 1062–1070.
26. Smith, G. L., Lichtman, J. H., Bracken, M. B., et al. (2006). Renal impairment and outcomes in heart failure: Systematic review and meta-analysis. *Journal of the American College of Cardiology, 47*(10), 1987–1996.
27. Liang, K. V., Williams, A. W., Greene, E. L., et al. (2008). Acute decompensated heart failure and the cardiorenal syndrome. *Critical Care Medicine, 36*(1, Suppl.), S75–S88.
28. Anand, I. S., Fisher, L. D., Chiang, Y. T., et al. (2003). Changes in brain natriuretic peptide and norepinephrine over time and mortality and morbidity in the Valsartan Heart Failure Trial (Val-HeFT). *Circulation, 107*(9), 1278–1283.
29. Aronson, D., & Burger, A. J. (2003). Neurohumoral activation and ventricular arrhythmias in patients with decompensated congestive heart failure: Role of endothelin. *Pacing and Clinical Electrophysiology, 26*(3), 703–710.
30. Bibbins-Domingo, K., Lin, F., Vittinghoff, E., et al. (2004). Renal insufficiency as an independent predictor of mortality among women with heart failure. *Journal of the American College of Cardiology, 44*(8), 1593–1600.

31. Ezekowitz, J., McAlister, F. A., Humphries, K. H., et al. (2004). The association among renal insufficiency, pharmacotherapy, and outcomes in 6,427 patients with heart failure and coronary artery disease. *Journal of the American College of Cardiology, 44*(8), 1587–1592.
32. Owan, T. E., Hodge, D. O., Herges, R. M., et al. (2006). Secular trends in renal dysfunction and outcomes in hospitalized heart failure patients. *Journal of Cardiac Failure, 12*(4), 257–262.
33. Mann, J. F., Sheridan, P., McQueen, M. J., et al. (2008). Homocysteine lowering with folic acid and B vitamins in people with chronic kidney disease—Results of the renal Hope-2 study. *Nephrology Dialysis Transplantation, 23*(2), 645–653.
34. Mann, D. L. (2006). Heart failure: Beyond practice guidelines. *Texus Dialiasis Heart Institute Journal, 33*(2), 201–203.
35. Mann, D. L. (2004). Basic mechanisms of left ventricular remodeling: The contribution of wall stress. *Journal of Cardiac Failure, 10*(6, Suppl.), S202–S206.
36. De Keulenaer, G. W., & Brutsaert, D. L. (2007). Diastolic heart failure: A separate disease or selection bias? *Progress in Cardiovascular Disease, 49*(4), 275–283.
37. Bhatia, R. S., Tu, J. V., Lee, D. S., et al. (2006). Outcome of heart failure with preserved ejection fraction in a population-based study. *New England Journal of Medicine, 355*(3), 260–269.
38. Sanderson, J. E., & Tse, T. F. (2003). Heart failure: A global disease requiring a global response. *Heart, 89*(6), 585–586.
39. Lang, R. M., Bierig, M., Devereux, R. B., et al. (2005). Recommendations for chamber quantification: A report from the American Society of Echocardiography's Guidelines and Standards Committee and the Chamber Quantification Writing Group, developed in conjunction with the European Association of Echocardiography, a branch of the European Society of Cardiology. *Journal of the American Society of Echocardiography, 18*(12), 1440–1463.
40. Kitzman, D. W., Little, W. C., Brubaker, P. H., et al. (2002). Pathophysiological characterization of isolated diastolic heart failure in comparison to systolic heart failure. *JAMA, 288*(17), 2144–2150.
41. Brucks, S., Little, W. C., Chao, T., et al. (2005). Contribution of left ventricular diastolic dysfunction to heart failure regardless of ejection fraction. *American Journal of Cardiology, 95*(5), 603–606.
42. Shahar, E., Whitney, C. W., Redline, S., et al. (2001). Sleep-disordered breathing and cardiovascular disease: Cross-sectional results of the Sleep Heart Health Study. *American Journal of Respiratory and Critical Care Medicine, 163*(1), 19–25.
43. Patel, J., & Heywood, J. T. (2007). Mode of death in patients with systolic heart failure. *Journal of Cardiovascular Pharmacology and Therapeutics, 12*(2), 127–136.
44. Bates, B. (1991). *A guide to physical examination and history taking* (5th ed.). Philadelphia: J.B. Lippincott Company.
45. Angeja, B. G., & Grossman, W. (2003). Evaluation and management of diastolic heart failure. *Circulation, 107*(5), 659–663.
46. Glassberg, H., Kirkpatrick, J., & Ferrari, V. A. (2008). Imaging studies in patients with heart failure: Current and evolving technologies. *Critical Care Medicine, 36*(1, Suppl.), S28–S39.
47. Velazquez-Cecena, J. L., Sharma, S., Nagajothi, N., et al. (2008). Left ventricular end diastolic pressure and serum brain natriuretic peptide levels in patients with abnormal impedance cardiography parameters. *Archives of Medical Research, 39*(4), 408–411.
48. Van Mieghem, C. A. G., McFadden, E. P., de Feyter, P. J., et al. (2006). Noninvasive detection of subclinical coronary atherosclerosis coupled with assessment of changes in plaque characteristics using novel invasive imaging modalities: The integrated biomarker and imaging study (IBIS). *Journal of the American College of Cardiology, 47*(6), 1134–1142.
49. Anand, I. S., Kuskowski, M. A., Rector, T. S., et al. (2005). Anemia and change in hemoglobin over time related to mortality and morbidity in patients with chronic heart failure: Results from Val-HeFT. *Circulation, 112*(8), 1121–1127.
50. Maisel, A. S., Koon, J., Krishnaswamy, P., et al. (2001). Utility of B-natriuretic peptide as a rapid, point-of-care test for screening patients undergoing echocardiography to determine left ventricular dysfunction. *American Heart Journal, 141*(3), 367–374.
51. Lubien, E., DeMaria, A., Krishnaswamy, P., et al. (2002). Utility of B-natriuretic peptide in detecting diastolic dysfunction: Comparison with Doppler velocity recordings. *Circulation, 105*(5), 595–601.
52. Nielsen, O. W., McDonagh, T. A., Robb, S. D., et al. (2003). Retrospective analysis of the cost-effectiveness of using plasma brain natriuretic peptide in screening for left ventricular systolic dysfunction in the general population. *Journal of American College of Cardiology, 41*(1), 113–120.
53. Vasan, R. S., Beiser, A., D'Agostino, R. B., et al. (2003). Plasma homocysteine and risk for congestive heart failure in adults without prior myocardial infarction. *JAMA, 289*(10), 1251–1257.
54. Aaronson, K. D., & Sackner-Bernstein, J. (2006). Risk of death associated with nesiritide in patients with acutely decompensated heart failure. *JAMA, 296*(12), 1465–1466.
55. Mosterd, A., Cost, B., Hoes, A. W., et al. (2001). The prognosis of heart failure in the general population: The Rotterdam Study. *European Heart Journal, 22*(15), 1318–1327.
56. Roger, V. L., Weston, S. A., Redfield, M. M., et al. (2004). Trends in heart failure incidence and survival in a community-based population. *JAMA, 292*(3), 344–350.
57. Mozaffarian, D., Anker, S. D., Anand, I., et al. (2007). Prediction of mode of death in heart failure: The Seattle Heart Failure Model. *Circulation, 116*(4), 392–398.
58. Ammar, K. A., Jacobsen, S. J., Mahoney, D. W., et al. (2007). Prevalence and prognostic significance of heart failure stages: Application of the American College of Cardiology/American Heart Association heart failure staging criteria in the community. *Circulation, 115*(12), 1563–1570.
59. Parkash, R., Stevenson, W. G., Epstein, L. M., et al. (2006). Predicting early mortality after implantable defibrillator implantation: A clinical risk score for optimal patient selection. *American Heart Journal, 151*(2), 397–403.
60. Linseman, J. V., & Bristow, M. R. (2003). Drug therapy and heart failure prevention. *Circulation, 107*(9), 1234–1236.
61. Fuster, V., Gersh, B. J., Giuliani, E. R., et al. (1981). The natural history of idiopathic dilated cardiomyopathy. *American Journal of Cardiology, 47*(3), 525–531.
62. Al-Khadra, A. S., Salem, D. N., Rand, W. M., et al. (1998). Warfarin anticoagulation and survival: A cohort analysis from the studies of left ventricular dysfunction. *Journal of the American College of Cardiology, 31*(4), 749–753.
63. Dries, D. L., Domanski, M. J., Waclawiw, M. A., et al. (1997). Effect of antithrombotic therapy on risk of sudden coronary death in patients with congestive heart failure. *American Journal of Cardiology, 79*(7), 909–913.
64. Lindenfeld, J., Feldman, A. M., Saxon, L., et al. (2007). Effects of cardiac resynchronization therapy with or without a defibrillator on survival and hospitalizations in patients with New York Heart Association class IV heart failure. *Circulation, 115*(2), 204–212.
65. Auricchio, A., Metra, M., Gasparini, M., et al. (2007). Long-term survival of patients with heart failure and ventricular conduction delay treated with cardiac resynchronization therapy. *The American Journal of Cardiology, 99*(2), 232–238.
66. Mehta, P. A., Dubrey, S. W., McIntyre, H. F., et al. (2008). Mode of death in patients with newly diagnosed heart failure in the general population. *European Journal of Heart Failure, 10*(11), 1108–1116.
67. Miller, L. W. (1998). Listing criteria for cardiac transplantation: Results of an American Society of Transplant Physicians—National Institutes of Health conference. *Transplantation, 66*(7), 947–951.
68. Effects of enalapril on mortality in severe congestive heart failure. Results of the Cooperative North Scandinavian Enalapril Survival Study (CONSENSUS). The CONSENSUS Trial Study Group. (1987). *New England Journal of Medicine, 316*(23), 1429–1435.
69. Effect of enalapril on survival in patients with reduced left ventricular ejection fractions and congestive heart failure. The SOLVD Investigators. (1991). *New England Journal of Medicine, 325*(5), 293–302.
70. Howard, P. A., Cheng, J. W. M., Crouch, M. A., et al. (2006). Drug therapy recommendations from the 2005 ACC/AHA guidelines for treatment of chronic heart failure. *The Annals of Pharmacotherapy, 40*(9), 1607–1616.
71. Shibata, M. C., Tsuyuki, R. T., & Wiebe, N. (2008). The effects of angiotensin-receptor blockers on mortality and morbidity in heart failure: A systematic review. *International Journal of Clinical Practice, 62*(9), 1397–1402.
72. Aronow, W. S. (2003). Epidemiology, pathophysiology, prognosis, and treatment of systolic and diastolic heart failure in elderly patients. *Heart Disease, 5*(4), 279–294.

73. Cohn, J. N., & Tognoni, G. (2001). A randomized trial of the angiotensin-receptor blocker valsartan in chronic heart failure. *New England Journal of Medicine, 345*(23), 1667–1675.
74. McMurray, J. J., Ostergren, J., Swedberg, K., et al. (2003). Effects of candesartan in patients with chronic heart failure and reduced left-ventricular systolic function taking angiotensin-converting-enzyme inhibitors: The CHARM-added trial. *Lancet, 362*(9386), 767–771.
75. Granger, C. B., McMurray, J. J., Yusuf, S., et al. (2003). Effects of candesartan in patients with chronic heart failure and reduced left-ventricular systolic function intolerant to angiotensin-converting-enzyme inhibitors: The CHARM-alternative trial. *Lancet, 362*(9386), 772–776.
76. Struthers, A. D. (2004). Aldosterone blockade in cardiovascular disease. *Heart, 90*(10), 1229–1234.
77. Chai, W., Garrelds, I. M., de Vries, R., et al. (2005). Nongenomic effects of aldosterone in the human heart: Interaction with angiotensin II. *Hypertension, 46*(4), 701–706.
78. Khan, N. U., & Movahed, A. (2004). The role of aldosterone and aldosterone-receptor antagonists in heart failure. *Reviews in Cardiovascular Medicine, 5*(2), 71–81.
79. Pitt, B., Zannad, F., Remme, W. J., et al. (1999). The effect of spironolactone on morbidity and mortality in patients with severe heart failure. Randomized Aldactone Evaluation Study Investigators. *New England Journal of Medicine, 341*(10), 709–717.
80. Azuma, J., & Nonen, S. (2008). Chronic heart failure: Beta-blockers and pharmacogenetics. *European Journal of Clinical Pharmacology*.
81. Fonarow, G. C. (2008). A review of evidence-based beta-blockers in special populations with heart failure. *Reviews in Cardiovascular Medicine, 9*(2), 84–95.
82. Bristow, M. R., Krause-Steinrauf, H., Nuzzo, R., et al. (2004). Effect of baseline or changes in adrenergic activity on clinical outcomes in the beta-blocker evaluation of survival trial. *Circulation, 110*(11), 1437–1442.
83. Gilbert, E. M., O'Connell, J. B., & Bristow, M. R. (1991). Therapy of idiopathic dilated cardiomyopathy with chronic beta-adrenergic blockade. *Heart and Vessels Supplement, 6*, 29–39.
84. Tate, C. W., III, Robertson, A. D., Zolty, R., et al. (2007). Quality of life and prognosis in heart failure: Results of the Beta-Blocker Evaluation of Survival Trial (BEST). *Journal of Cardiac Failure, 13*(9), 732–737.
85. Varadarajan, P., Joshi, N., Appel, D., et al. (2008). Effect of beta-blocker therapy on survival in patients with severe mitral regurgitation and normal left ventricular ejection fraction. *American Journal of Cardiology, 102*(5), 611–615.
86. Hjalmarson, A., Goldstein, S., Fagerberg, B., et al. (2000). Effects of controlled-release metoprolol on total mortality, hospitalizations, and well-being in patients with heart failure: The Metoprolol CR/XL Randomized Intervention Trial in Congestive Heart Failure (MERIT-HF). *JAMA, 283*(10), 1295–1302.
87. O'Connor, C. M., Gattis, W. A., Zannad, F., et al. (1999). Beta-blocker therapy in advanced heart failure: Clinical characteristics and long-term outcomes. *European Journal of Heart Failure, 1*(1), 81–88.
88. Houghton, T., Freemantle, N., & Cleland, J. G. (2000). Are beta-blockers effective in patients who develop heart failure soon after myocardial infarction? A meta-regression analysis of randomised trials. *European Journal of Heart Failure, 2*(3), 333–340.
89. Tatli, E., & Kurum, T. (2005). A controlled study of the effects of carvedilol on clinical events, left ventricular function and proinflammatory cytokines levels in patients with dilated cardiomyopathy. *Canadian Journal of Cardiology, 21*(4), 344–348.
90. Cohn, J. N. (2001). Optimal diuretic therapy for heart failure. *American Journal of Medicine, 111*(7), 577.
91. Harjola, V. P., Oikarinen, L., Toivonen, L., et al. (2008). The hemodynamic and pharmacokinetic interactions between chronic use of oral levosimendan and digoxin in patients with NYHA Classes II–III heart failure. *International Journal of Clinical Pharmacology and Therapeutics, 46*(8), 389–399.
92. Dulin, B. R., & Krum, H. (2006). Drug therapy of chronic heart failure in the elderly: The current state of clinical-trial evidence. *Current Opinion in Cardiology, 21*(4), 393–399.
93. Ahmed, A., Pitt, B., Rahimtoola, S. H., et al. (2008). Effects of digoxin at low serum concentrations on mortality and hospitalization in heart failure: A propensity-matched study of the DIG trial. *International Journal of Cardiology, 123*(2), 138–146.
94. Leibundgut, G., Pfisterer, M., & Brunner-La Rocca, H. P. (2007). Drug treatment of chronic heart failure in the elderly. *Drugs and Aging, 24*(12), 991–1006.
95. Rutten, J. H. W., Steyerberg, E. W., Boomsma, F., et al. (2008). N-terminal pro-brain natriuretic peptide testing in the emergency department: Beneficial effects on hospitalization, costs, and outcome. *American Heart Journal, 156*(1), 71–77.
96. Owan, T. E., Chen, H. H., Frantz, R. P., et al. (2008). The effects of nesiritide on renal function and diuretic responsiveness in acutely decompensated heart failure patients with renal dysfunction. *Journal of Cardiac Failure, 14*(4), 267–275.
97. Elkayam, U., Bitar, F., Akhter, M. W., et al. (2004). Intravenous nitroglycerin in the treatment of decompensated heart failure: Potential benefits and limitations. *Journal of Cardiovascular Pharmacology and Therapeutics, 9*(4), 227–241.
98. Sackner-Bernstein, J. D., Skopicki, H. A., & Aaronson, K. D. (2005). Risk of worsening renal function with nesiritide in patients with acutely decompensated heart failure. *Circulation, 111*(12), 1487–1491.
99. Echt, D. S., Liebson, P. R., Mitchell, L. B., et al. (1991). Mortality and morbidity in patients receiving encainide, flecainide, or placebo. The Cardiac Arrhythmia Suppression Trial. *New England Journal of Medicine, 324*(12), 781–788.
100. Chapa, D. W., Lee, H. J., Kao, C. W., et al. (2008). Reducing mortality with device therapy in heart failure patients without ventricular arrhythmias. *American Journal of Critical Care, 17*(5), 443–452; quiz 453.
101. Russo, A. M., Poole, J. E., Mark, D. B., et al. (2008). Primary prevention with defibrillator therapy in women: Results from the Sudden Cardiac Death in Heart Failure Trial. *Journal of Cardiovascular Electrophysiology, 19*(7), 720–724.
102. Bardy, G. H., Lee, K. L., Mark, D. B., et al. (2005). Amiodarone or an implantable cardioverter-defibrillator for congestive heart failure. *New England Journal of Medicine, 352*(3), 225–237.
103. Suskin, N., McKelvie, R. S., Burns, R. J., et al. (2000). Glucose and insulin abnormalities relate to functional capacity in patients with congestive heart failure. *European Heart Journal, 21*(16), 1368–1375.
104. Ingelsson, E., Sundstrom, J., Arnlov, J., et al. (2005). Insulin resistance and risk of congestive heart failure. *JAMA, 294*(3), 334–341.
105. Stratton, I. M., Adler, A. I., Neil, H. A., et al. (2000). Association of glycaemia with macrovascular and microvascular complications of type 2 diabetes (UKPDS 35): Prospective observational study. *BMJ, 321* (7258), 405–412.
106. Kostis, J. B., & Sanders, M. (2005). The association of heart failure with insulin resistance and the development of type 2 diabetes. *American Journal of Hypertension, 18*(5, Pt. 1), 731–737.
107. Dutka, D. P., Pitt, M., Pagano, D., et al. (2006). Myocardial glucose transport and utilization in patients with type 2 diabetes mellitus, left ventricular dysfunction, and coronary artery disease. *Journal of the American College of Cardiology, 48*(11), 2225–2231.
108. *Annual U.S. Deaths Attributable to Smoking 1997–2001*. (2005). Center for Disease Control and Prevention.
109. Bibbins-Domingo, K., Lin, F., Vittinghoff, E., et al. (2004). Predictors of heart failure among women with coronary disease. *Circulation, 110*(11), 1424–1430.
110. Suskin, N., Sheth, T., Negassa, A., et al. (2001). Relationship of current and past smoking to mortality and morbidity in patients with left ventricular dysfunction. *Journal of the American College of Cardiology, 37*(6), 1677–1682.
111. Goldstein, M. G., Niaura, R., Willey-Lessne, C., et al. (1997). Physicians counseling smokers. A population-based survey of patients' perceptions of health care provider-delivered smoking cessation interventions. *Archives of Internal Medicine, 157*(12), 1313–1319.
112. Nohria, A., Chen, Y. T., Morton, D. J., et al. (1999). Quality of care for patients hospitalized with heart failure at academic medical centers. *American Heart Journal, 137*(6), 1028–1034.
113. Rice, V. H., & Stead, L. F. (2008). *Cochrane Database System Review*, 1: CD00118.
114. Fonarow, G. C., Yancy, C. W., Heywood, J. T., et al. (2005). Adherence to heart failure quality-of-care indicators in US hospitals: Analysis of the ADHERE registry. *Archives of Internal Medicine, 165*(13), 1469–1477.
115. Androne, A. S., Katz, S. D., Lund, L., et al. (2003). Hemodilution is common in patients with advanced heart failure. *Circulation, 107*(2), 226–229.

116. Handelman, G. J., & Levin, N. W. (2008). Iron and anemia in human biology: A review of mechanisms. *Heart Failure Reviews, 13*(4), 393–404.
117. Dzudie, A., Kengne, A. P., Mbahe, S., et al. (2008). Chronic heart failure, selected risk factors and co-morbidities among adults treated for hypertension in a cardiac referral hospital in Cameroon. *European Journal of Heart Failure, 10*(4), 367–372.
118. Westenbrink, B. D., de Boer, R. A., Voors, A. A., et al. (2008). Anemia in chronic heart failure: Etiology and treatment options. *Current Opinion in Cardiology, 23*(2), 141–147.
119. Maggioni, A. P., Opasich, C., Anand, I., et al. (2005). Anemia in patients with heart failure: Prevalence and prognostic role in a controlled trial and in clinical practice. *Journal of Cardiac Failure, 11*(2), 91–98.
120. Pfeffer, M. A., Solomon, S. D., Singh, A. K., et al. (2005). Uncertainty in the treatment of anemia in chronic kidney disease. *Reviews Cardiovascular Medicine, 6*(Suppl. 3), S35–S41.
121. Rumsfeld, J. S., Havranek, E., Masoudi, F. A., et al. (2003). Depressive symptoms are the strongest predictors of short-term declines in health status in patients with heart failure. *Journal of the American College of Cardiology, 42*(10), 1811–1817.
122. Vaccarino, V., Kasl, S. V., Abramson, J., et al. (2001). Depressive symptoms and risk of functional decline and death in patients with heart failure. *Journal of the American College of Cardiology, 38*(1), 199–205.
123. Sherwood, A., Blumenthal, J. A., Trivedi, R., et al. (2007). Relationship of depression to death or hospitalization in patients with heart failure. *Archives of Internal Medicine, 167*(4), 367–373.
124. Sullivan, M., Simon, G., Spertus, J., et al. (2002). Depression-related costs in heart failure care. *Archives of Internal Medicine, 162*(16), 1860–1866.
125. Sullivan, M. D., Levy, W. C., Crane, B. A., et al. (2004). Usefulness of depression to predict time to combined end point of transplant or death for outpatients with advanced heart failure. *American Journal of Cardiology, 94*(12), 1577–1580.
126. Parish, J. M., & Shepard, J. W., Jr. (1990). Cardiovascular effects of sleep disorders. *Chest, 97*(5), 1220–1226.
127. Hanly, P., Sasson, Z., Zuberi, N., et al. (1993). ST-segment depression during sleep in obstructive sleep apnea. *American Journal of Cardiology, 71*(15), 1341–1345.
128. Guilleminault, C., Connolly, S. J., & Winkle, R. A. (1983). Cardiac arrhythmia and conduction disturbances during sleep in 400 patients with sleep apnea syndrome. *American Journal of Cardiology, 52*(5), 490–494.
129. Fletcher, E. C., Miller, J., Schaaf, J. W., et al. (1987). Urinary catecholamines before and after tracheostomy in patients with obstructive sleep apnea and hypertension. *Sleep, 10*(1), 35–44.
130. Gainer, J. L. (1987). Hypoxia and atherosclerosis: Re-evaluation of an old hypothesis. *Atherosclerosis, 68*(3), 263–266.
131. Bradley, T. D. (1992). Right and left ventricular functional impairment and sleep apnea. *Clinics in Chest Medicine, 13*(3), 459–479.
132. Mansfield, D. R., Gollogly, N. C., Kaye, D. M., et al. (2004). Controlled trial of continuous positive airway pressure in obstructive sleep apnea and heart failure. *American Journal of Respiratory and Critical Care Medicine, 169*(3), 361–366.
133. Dickson, V. V., Tkacs, N., & Riegel, B. (2007). Cognitive influences on self-care decision making in persons with heart failure. *American Heart Journal, 154*(3), 424–431.
134. Bennett, S. J., & Sauve, M. J. (2003). Cognitive deficits in patients with heart failure: A review of the literature. *Journal of Cardiovascular Nursing, 18*(3), 219–242.
135. Zuccala, G., Onder, G., Pedone, C., et al. (2001). Hypotension and cognitive impairment: Selective association in patients with heart failure. *Neurology, 57*(11), 1986–1992.
136. Vogel, R. (2007). Profile of cognitive impairment in chronic heart failure. *Journal of the American Geriatric Society, 55*(11), 1764–1770.
137. Zuccola, T. (2006). Correlates of cognitive impairment among patients with heart failure: Results of a multicenter survey. *American Journal of Medicine, 118*(5), 496–502.
138. Alves, T. C., Rays, J., Fraguas, R., Jr., et al. (2005). Localized cerebral blood flow reductions in patients with heart failure: A study using 99mTc-HMPAO SPECT. *Journal of Neuroimaging, 15*(2), 150–156.
139. Bennett, S. J., Sauve, M. J., & Shaw, R. M. (2005). A conceptual model of cognitive deficits in chronic heart failure. *Journal of Nursing Scholarship, 37*(3), 222–228.
140. Hernandez, A. F., & O'Connor, C. M. (2003). Sparing a little may save a lot: Lessons from the Studies of Left Ventricular Dysfunction (SOLVD). *Journal of the American College Cardiology, 42*(4), 709–711.
141. Rich, M. W., Beckham, V., Wittenberg, C., et al. (1995). A multidisciplinary intervention to prevent the readmission of elderly patients with congestive heart failure. *New England Journal of Medicine, 333*(18), 1190–1195.
142. Bennett, S. J., Huster, G. A., Baker, S. L., et al. (1998). Characterization of the precipitants of hospitalization for heart failure decompensation. *American Journal of Critical Care, 7*(3), 168–174.
143. Vinson, J. M., Rich, M. W., Sperry, J. C., et al. (1990). Early readmission of elderly patients with congestive heart failure. *Journal of the American Geriatric Society, 38*(12), 1290–1295.
144. Feldman, P. H., Murtaugh, C. M., Pezzin, L. E., et al. (2005). Just-in-time evidence-based e-mail "reminders" in home health care: Impact on patient outcomes. *Health Services Research, 40*(3), 865–885.
145. Ansari, M., Shlipak, M. G., Heidenreich, P. A., et al. (2003). Improving guideline adherence: A randomized trial evaluating strategies to increase [beta]-blocker use in heart failure. *Circulation, 107*(22), 2799–2804.
146. Riegel, B., Carlson, B., Kopp, Z., et al. (2002). Effect of a standardized nurse case-management telephone intervention on resource use in patients with chronic heart failure. *Archives of Internal Medicine, 162*(6), 705–712.
147. Kimmelstiel, C., Levine, D., Perry, K., et al. (2004). Randomized, controlled evaluation of short- and long-term benefits of heart failure disease management within a diverse provider network: The SPAN-CHF Trial. *Circulation, 110*(11), 1450–1455.
148. Krumholz, H. M., Amatruda, J., Smith, G. L., et al. (2002). Randomized trial of an education and support intervention to prevent readmission of patients with heart failure. *Journal of the American College of Cardiology, 39*(1), 83–89.
149. Stromberg, A., Martensson, J., Fridlund, B., et al. (2003). Nurse-led heart failure clinics improve survival and self-care behaviour in patients with heart failure: Results from a prospective, randomised trial. *European Heart Journal, 24*(11), 1014–1023.
150. Inglis, S. C., Pearson, S., Treen, S., et al. (2006). Extending the horizon in chronic heart failure: Effects of multidisciplinary, home-based intervention relative to usual care. *Circulation, 114*(23), 2466–2473.
151. Mazzuca, S. A. (1982). Does patient education in chronic disease have therapeutic value? *Journal of Chronic Disease, 35*(7), 521–529.
152. Artinian, N. T., Magnan, M., Sloan, M., et al. (2002). Self-care behaviors among patients with heart failure. *Heart & Lung, 31*(3), 161–172.
153. Jaarsma, T., Halfens, R., Huijer Abu-Saad, H., et al. (1999). Effects of education and support on self-care and resource utilization in patients with heart failure. *European Heart Journal, 20*(9), 673–682.
154. Sulzbach-Hoke, L. M., Kagan, S. H., & Craig, K. (1997). Weighing behavior and symptom distress of clinic patients with CHF. *Medical Surgical Nursing, 6*(5), 288–293, 314.
155. Baker, D. W., Asch, S. M., Keesey, J. W., et al. (2005). Differences in education, knowledge, self-management activities, and health outcomes for patients with heart failure cared for under the chronic disease model: The improving chronic illness care evaluation. *Journal of Cardiac Failure, 11*(6), 405–413.
156. Lee, N. C., Wasson, D. R., Anderson, M. A., et al. (1998). A survey of patient education postdischarge. *Journal of Nursing Care Quality, 13*(1), 63–70.
157. Mueller, T. M., Vuckovic, K. M., Knox, D. A., et al. (2002). Telemanagement of heart failure: A diuretic treatment algorithm for advanced practice nurses. *Heart & Lung, 31*(5), 340–347.
158. Koelling, T. M., Johnson, M. L., Cody, R. J., et al. (2005). Discharge education improves clinical outcomes in patients with chronic heart failure. *Circulation, 111*(2), 179–185.
159. Fonarow, G. C. (2001). Quality indicators for the management of heart failure in vulnerable elders. *Annals of Internal Medicine, 135*(8, Pt. 2), 694–702.
160. Grady, K. L., Dracup, K., Kennedy, G., et al. (2000). Team management of patients with heart failure: A statement for healthcare professionals from The Cardiovascular Nursing Council of the American Heart Association. *Circulation, 102*(19), 2443–2456.
161. Bither, C. J., & Apple, S. (2001). Home management of the failing heart. Inotropic therapy in the outpatient setting. *American Journal of Nursing, 101*(12), 41–45.

162. Riegel, B., Dickson, V. V., Hoke, L., et al. (2006). A motivational counseling approach to improving heart failure self-care: Mechanisms of effectiveness. *Journal of Cardiovascular Nursing, 21*(3), 232–241.
163. Riegel, B., Carlson, B., & Glaser, D. (2000). Development and testing of a clinical tool measuring self-management of heart failure. *Heart & Lung, 29*(1), 4–15.
164. Sneed, N. V., & Paul, S. C. (2003). Readiness for behavioral changes in patients with heart failure. *American Journal of Critical Care, 12*(5), 444–453.
165. Riegel, B., & Carlson, B. (2002). Facilitators and barriers to heart failure self-care. *Patient Education and Counseling, 46*(4), 287–295.
166. Happ, M. B., Naylor, M. D., & Roe-Prior, P. (1997). Factors contributing to rehospitalization of elderly patients with heart failure. *Journal of Cardiovascular Nursing, 11*(4), 75–84.
167. Koenig, H. G. (1998). Depression in hospitalized older patients with congestive heart failure. *General Hospital Psychiatry, 20*(1), 29–43.
168. Yu, D. S., Lee, D. T., & Woo, J. (2004). Health-related quality of life in elderly Chinese patients with heart failure. *Research in Nursing & Health, 27*(5), 332–344.
169. Subramanian, U., Fihn, S. D., Weinberger, M., et al. (2004). A controlled trial of including symptom data in computer-based care suggestions for managing patients with chronic heart failure. *The American Journal of Medicine, 116*(6), 375–384.
170. Chriss, P. M., Sheposh, J., Carlson, B., et al. (2004). Predictors of successful heart failure self-care maintenance in the first three months after hospitalization. *Heart & Lung, 33*(6), 345–353.
171. Welsh, J. D., Heiser, R. M., Schooler, M. P., et al. (2002). Characteristics and treatment of patients with heart failure in the emergency department. *Journal of Emergency Nursing, 28*(2), 126–131.
172. Chaudhry, S. I., Wang, Y., Concato, J., et al. (2007). Patterns of weight change preceding hospitalization for heart failure. *Circulation, 116*(14), 1549–1554.
173. Ni, H., Nauman, D. J., & Hershberger, R. E. (1999). Analysis of trends in hospitalizations for heart failure. *Journal of Cardiac Failure, 5*(2), 79–84.
174. Pina, I. L., Apstein, C. S., Balady, G. J., et al. (2003). Exercise and heart failure: A statement from the American Heart Association Committee on exercise, rehabilitation, and prevention. *Circulation, 107*(8), 1210–1225.
175. Drexler, H., & Coats, A. J. (1996). Explaining fatigue in congestive heart failure. *Annual Review of Medicine, 47*, 241–256.
176. Kitzman, D. W. (2005). Exercise intolerance. *Progress in Cardiovascular Disease, 47*(6), 367–379.
177. Myers, J., & Froelicher, V. F. (1991). Hemodynamic determinants of exercise capacity in chronic heart failure. *Annals of Internal Medicine, 115*(5), 377–386.
178. Larsen, A. I., & Dickstein, K. (2005). Exercise training in congestive heart failure. A review of the current status. *Minerva Cardioangiologica, 53*(4), 275–286.
179. Belardinelli, R. (2007). Exercise training in chronic heart failure: How to harmonize oxidative stress, sympathetic outflow, and angiotensin II. *Circulation, 115*(24), 3042–3044.
180. Belardinelli, R., Capestro, F., Misiani, A., et al. (2006). Moderate exercise training improves functional capacity, quality of life, and endothelium-dependent vasodilation in chronic heart failure patients with implantable cardioverter defibrillators and cardiac resynchronization therapy. *European Journal of Cardiovascular Prevention and Rehabilitation, 13*(5), 818–825.
181. Giada, F., Carlon, R., Delise, P., et al. (2007). [Consensus Statement of Multisocietary Task Force—prescription of physical exercise in the cardiological environment (third part)]. *Monaldi Archives of Chest Disease, 68*(3), 134–148.
182. Bentley, B., De Jong, M. J., Moser, D. K., et al. (2005). Factors related to nonadherence to low sodium diet recommendations in heart failure patients. *European Journal of Cardiovascular Nursing, 4*(4), 331–336.
183. Bennett, S. J., Lane, K. A., Welch, J., et al. (2005). Medication and dietary compliance beliefs in heart failure. *Western Journal of Nursing Research, 27*(8), 977–993; discussion 994–979.
184. Travers, B., O'Loughlin, C., Murphy, N. F., et al. (2007). Fluid restriction in the management of decompensated heart failure: No impact on time to clinical stability. *Journal of Cardiac Failure, 13*(2), 128–132.
185. Monane, M., Bohn, R. L., Gurwitz, J. H., et al. (1994). Noncompliance with congestive heart failure therapy in the elderly. *Archives of Internal Medicine, 154*(4), 433–437.
186. Bagchi, A. D., Esposito, D., Kim, M., et al. (2007). Utilization of, and adherence to, drug therapy among Medicaid beneficiaries with congestive heart failure. *Clinical Therapeutics, 29*(8), 1771–1783.
187. Ekman, I., Fagerberg, B., & Lundman, B. (2002). Health-related quality of life and sense of coherence among elderly patients with severe chronic heart failure in comparison with healthy controls. *Heart & Lung: The Journal of Acute and Critical Care, 31*(2), 94–101.
188. Goodyer, L. I., Miskelly, F., & Milligan, P. (1995). Does encouraging good compliance improve patients' clinical condition in heart failure? *British Journal of Clinical Practice, 49*(4), 173–176.
189. Murray, M. D., Young, J., Hoke, S., et al. (2007). Pharmacist intervention to improve medication adherence in heart failure: A randomized trial. *Annals of Internal Medicine, 146*(10), 714–725.
190. Reynolds, H. R., & Hochman, J. S. (2008). Cardiogenic shock: Current concepts and improving outcomes. *Circulation, 117*(5), 686–697.
191. Gheorghiade, M., Sopko, G., De Luca, L., et al. (2006). Navigating the crossroads of coronary artery disease and heart failure. *Circulation, 114*(11), 1202–1213.
192. Hochman, J. S., Sleeper, L. A., Webb, J. G., et al. (1999). Early revascularization in acute myocardial infarction complicated by cardiogenic shock. SHOCK investigators: Should we emergently revascularize occluded coronaries for cardiogenic shock. *New England Journal of Medicine, 341*(9), 625–634.
193. Bonow, R. O. (1995). The hibernating myocardium: Implications for management of congestive heart failure. *American Journal of Cardiology, 75*(3), 17A–25A.
194. Bolli, R. (1998). Basic and clinical aspects of myocardial stunning. *Progress in Cardiovascular Disease, 40*(6), 477–516.
195. Babaev, A., Frederick, P. D., Pasta, D. J., et al. (2005). Trends in management and outcomes of patients with acute myocardial infarction complicated by cardiogenic shock. *JAMA, 294*(4), 448–454.
196. Topalian, S., Ginsberg, F., & Parrillo, J. E. (2008). Cardiogenic shock. *Critical Care Medicine, 36*(1, Suppl.), S66–S74.
197. Hollenberg, S. M. (2001). Cardiogenic shock. *Critical Care Clinics, 17*(2), 391–410.
198. Mann, D. L. (2005). Cardiac remodeling as therapeutic target: Treating heart failure with cardiac support devices. *Heart Failure Review, 10*(2), 93–94.
199. Oliver, C., Marin, F., Pineda, J., et al. (2002). Low QRS voltage in cardiac tamponade: A study of 70 cases. *International Journal of Cardiology, 83*(1), 91–92.
200. Forrester, J. S., Diamond, G., Chatterjee, K., et al. (1976). Medical therapy of acute myocardial infarction by application of hemodynamic subsets (second of two parts). *New England Journal Medicine, 295*(25), 1404–1413.
201. Forrester, J. S., & Waters, D. D. (1978). Hospital treatment of congestive heart failure. Management according to hemodynamic profile. *American Journal of Medicine, 65*(1), 173–180.
202. Connors, A. F., Jr., Speroff, T., Dawson, N. V., et al. (1996). The effectiveness of right heart catheterization in the initial care of critically ill patients. SUPPORT investigators. *JAMA, 276*(11), 889–897.
203. Lindholm, M. G., Kober, L., Boesgaard, S., et al. (2003). Cardiogenic shock complicating acute myocardial infarction; prognostic impact of early and late shock development. *European Heart Journal, 24*(3), 258–265.
204. Sanborn, T. A., Sleeper, L. A., Bates, E. R., et al. (2000). Impact of thrombolysis, intra-aortic balloon pump counterpulsation, and their combination in cardiogenic shock complicating acute myocardial infarction: A report from the SHOCK Trial Registry. Should we emergently revascularize occluded coronaries for cardiogenic shock? *Journal of the American College of Cardiology, 36*(3, Suppl. A), 1123–1129.
205. Jeger, R. V., Harkness, S. M., Ramanathan, K., et al. (2006). Emergency revascularization in patients with cardiogenic shock on admission: A report from the SHOCK trial and registry. *European Heart Journal, 27*(6), 664–670.
206. Hollenberg, S. M. (2007). Vasodilators in acute heart failure. *Heart Failure Review, 12*(2), 143–147.

207. Killen, D. A., Piehler, J. M., Borkon, A. M., et al. (1997). Early repair of postinfarction ventricular septal rupture. *Annals of Thoracic Surgery, 63*(1), 138–142.
208. Slater, J., Brown, R. J., Antonelli, T. A., et al. (2000). Cardiogenic shock due to cardiac free-wall rupture or tamponade after acute myocardial infarction: A report from the SHOCK Trial Registry. Should we emergently revascularize occluded coronaries for cardiogenic shock? *Journal of the American College of Cardiology, 36*(3, Suppl. A), 1117–1122.
209. Reardon, M. J., Carr, C. L., Diamond, A., et al. (1997). Ischemic left ventricular free wall rupture: Prediction, diagnosis, and treatment. *Annals of Thoracic Surgery, 64*(5), 1509–1513.
210. Meneveau, N., Schiele, F., Metz, D., et al. (1998). Comparative efficacy of a two-hour regimen of streptokinase versus alteplase in acute massive pulmonary embolism: Immediate clinical and hemodynamic outcome and one-year follow-up. *Journal of the American College of Cardiology, 31*(5), 1057–1063.

CHAPTER 25

Cardiac Surgery

Denise Ledoux* / Helen Luikart†

Surgical intervention continues to be a mainstay of treatment for acquired heart disease even though catheter-based interventional cardiology techniques have continued to expand and medical management has improved. This chapter focuses on surgical interventions for acquired heart disease, including coronary artery bypass grafting (CABG), minimally invasive cardiac surgery, transmyocardial revascularization, cardiomyoplasty, aortic surgery, and cardiac transplantation. Surgical intervention for valvular heart disease is briefly discussed in this chapter and is more extensively covered in Chapter 29.

EVOLVING TRENDS IN CARDIAC SURGERY

Cardiac surgical operative techniques continue to evolve. Arterial bypass conduits such as the internal mammary artery (IMA) are the preferred graft because of excellent long-term patency. Additional arterial conduits have expanded to include radial artery grafts and the gastroepiploic artery (GEA). Spawned by laparoscopic approaches in other surgical subspecialties, minimally invasive cardiac surgery (with and without cardiopulmonary bypass [CPB]) has rapidly developed. Computer-assisted, robotic CABG, and mitral valve surgical procedures have been preformed world wide on highly selected patients.[1] Shorter intubation times and "rapid recovery" programs have led to shorter intensive care unit stays with overall reduced length of stay and decreased cost associated with cardiac surgery.

As cardiac surgery techniques evolve, the population changes as well. Interventional cardiology approaches such as coronary angioplasty, atherectomy, and stenting have delayed or replaced surgical revascularization in patients with coronary lesions amenable to catheter-based interventions.

PREOPERATIVE ASSESSMENT AND PREPARATION

Before referral for cardiac surgery, patients complete their cardiac work-up, which includes cardiac catheterization to define coronary artery anatomy and target vessels for revascularization; stress testing to verify areas of ischemia; nuclear scans to identify areas of myocardial viability and ventricular function; and echocardiography to delineate valvular lesions, ventricular function, and focal wall-motion abnormalities. Usually, most of the preoperative medical evaluation is completed before the patient enters the hospital. Prior to cardiac surgery, the patient should have a complete physical examination with special attention given to the cardiovascular examination. A new history and physical examination, chest radiograph, electrocardiogram (ECG), complete blood count, serum electrolytes, coagulation screen, and typing and crossmatching of blood are performed. Preoperative anemia increases the risk of postoperative adverse events.[2] These data provide information about other disease conditions and cardiac problems. Patients are admitted to the hospital early on the morning of their surgery. Patients with symptomatic carotid bruits should undergo carotid duplex to assess for carotid stenosis. Patients with pre-existing cerebrovascular disease are at increased risk for neurological complications postoperative.[3] Patients with chronic lung disease should undergo pulmonary function testing and arterial blood gas testing because they may have difficulty weaning from the ventilator. Patients undergoing valve surgery should complete a dental evaluation and work before valve repair or replacement to reduce the chance of dental disease being a source of bacteremia and possible prosthetic valve endocarditis. Patients are maintained on antianginal, antihypertensives, and heart failure medications until surgery. Antiplatelet medications are usually discontinued before surgery: aspirin, clopidogrel, and nonsteroidal anti-inflammatory agents should be stopped before surgery to prevent perioperative bleeding. The Society of Thoracic Surgeon's workforce recommends that for elective patients and for high-risk aspirin-sensitive patients that aspirin should be stopped 3 to 5 days before surgery.[4] Patients on warfarin usually have their dose withheld 3 to 5 days preoperatively. Patients on warfarin for previous mechanical valve replacements may be admitted 1 to 2 days before surgery for intravenous heparin. Heparin is withheld 1 to 2 hours before surgery, whereas enoxaparin is usually stopped 12 hours beforehand. In a study by Jones et al.,[5] patients on preoperative enoxaparin demonstrated a higher rate of bleeding requiring re-exploration for bleeding (7.9% versus 3.7% in the unfractionated heparin group, $P = 0.03$).

The preoperative nursing assessment should be thorough and well documented because it provides baseline data for postoperative comparison. The history should include a social assessment of family roles and support systems, and a description of the patient's usual functional level and typical activities. Elderly patients or those with limited social and emotional support may need additional assistance from social service for effective discharge and rehabilitation planning. The patient with acute coronary heart disease (CHD) may be hospitalized for only hours or days before surgery. A myocardial infarction may have occurred, or the patient may be experiencing unstable angina. In either case, if CABG surgery is being considered, then a cardiac catheterization must be performed to determine if surgery is indicated and to define coronary anatomy.

*Author of the section on cardiac surgery.
†Author of the section on cardiac transplantation.

SURGICAL TECHNIQUES

Minimally Invasive Techniques

In standard cardiac surgery, the heart is arrested and circulation is maintained by placing the patient on CPB. Although this procedure has been used successfully for more than three decades, it has drawbacks such as physiologic derangements associated with CPB and long hospital stays. Minimally invasive cardiac surgery has evolved out of laparoscopic techniques originally used in general and gynecologic surgery. The term *minimally invasive* covers a variety of techniques rather than referring only to one surgical procedure. Minimally invasive techniques include CABG surgery performed by standard sternotomy but without the use of CPB (off-pump or OPCAB), CABG surgery performed off-pump through a small left anterior thoracotomy (minimally invasive direct coronary artery bypass [MIDCAB]), valve surgery performed on-pump but through "mini-sternotomy," and computer-enhanced robotic system techniques that allow CABG and valve surgery to be performed on-pump through a small incision with videoscopic assistance and femoral bypass.[6] Techniques are rapidly evolving that are geared toward multivessel revascularization through port access on a beating heart. Rather than just one approach for all patients, cardiac surgeons have a variety of surgical techniques available depending on the patient's anatomy, medical history, and comorbid conditions. Further discussion of these surgical methodologies is found in the coronary bypass and valve surgery sections of this chapter.

Cardiopulmonary Bypass

CPB comprises an extracorporeal circuit that circulates systemic throughout the body during periods of time the heart and lungs are not functioning during cardiac surgical procedures. CPB has been the standard method used during cardiac surgery for diverting blood from the heart and lungs to provide a stationary, bloodless surgical field and to promote preservation of optimal organ function. Blood is removed from the right atrium or vena cava by one or two cannula, routed through the CPB machine, and returned to the patient by a cannula in the ascending aorta or the femoral artery.

The CPB system has several components, including venous and arterial cannula; a membrane or bubble oxygenator that oxygenates the blood, removal of carbon dioxide, and delivery of anesthetic gases; a heat exchanger that allows the blood to be either heated or cooled by conduction; a pump, which keeps the blood moving at a constant speed; filters, which remove particulate or gas emboli and plasma protein or platelet aggregates; a left ventricular vent to prevent distention of the left ventricle during aortic cross-clamp; cardiotomy suction to aspirate blood from the operative field; and sensors, which detect air bubbles, low levels of oxygen saturation, and low levels of blood in collection chambers.[7,8] Heparin is used for anticoagulation during CPB to prevent clotting in the CPB circuit. Before initiation of CPB, a heparin dose of 3 mg/kg is administered through a central line. Activated clotting time is monitored a minimum of every 30 minutes during CPB. Once CPB is completed, heparin is reversed using protamine sulfate.[7] Care is taken to administer protamine slowly and watch for a possible protamine reaction, which may vary from mild hypotension to full-blown anaphylaxis. Patients at greater risk for protamine reaction include those with insulin-dependent diabetes and those with an allergy to fish. While the patient is connected to the CPB machine, the surgeon, anesthetist, and CPB perfusionists control many physiologic variables. Hemodilution with crystalloid solutions is used to reduce hematocrit and the blood's viscosity. CPB flow rates are controlled to maintain a cardiac index of 2.2 L/min/m^2 and a mean arterial pressure around 60 mm Hg. Blood may be cooled to reduce metabolic demands or warmed to normothermia toward the end of the procedure.

CPB produces a systemic inflammatory response that releases biologically active substances that impair coagulation and the immune response. Proinflammatory cytokines contribute to neutrophil adhesion.[9] In response to the vascular permeability changes that occur with CPB and to the decrease in plasma oncotic pressure that occurs with hemodilution, large amounts of fluid move from intravascular to interstitial spaces. Movement of fluid into interstitial spaces causes postoperative edema. This generalized edema that occurs after CPB resolves after the first few days postoperative or fluid mobilization may be facilitated with the use of diuretics. The longer the CPB time, the more severe the physiologic derangements during the postoperative recovery.

Systemic warming is started approximately 30 minutes before the anticipated time of discontinuing CPB. If the left atrium, left ventricle, or aorta has been entered, air must be evacuated before aortic cross-clamp removal to prevent air embolism. The heart is warmed and resumes spontaneous rhythm or is paced with epicardial wires. Ventricular fibrillation may occur and is converted with internal defibrillation. Under the direction of the surgeon and anesthesiologist, CPB weaning begins by ventilation of the lungs. CPB is gradually weaned by decreasing the amount of blood diverted through the CPB circuit. When the heart is functioning normally with adequate blood pressure and adequate cardiac index, CPB is discontinued, heparin is reversed, and cannulae are removed. If the heart cannot support an adequate cardiac index and mean arterial pressure after weaning from CPB, the patient may have to be placed back on CPB to rest the heart, and other measures for heart failure may need to be instituted, such as inotropic treatment or intra-aortic balloon pump. In patients who continue to have severe hemodynamic compromise, ventricular assist devices may be used.

Myocardial Protection

Myocardial protection is the intraoperative techniques intended to protect the myocardium from damage resultant from the ischemic state that occurs with CPB. In cardiac surgical procedure requiring CPB, cross clamping of the aorta without the use of myocardial protection would result in anaerobic metabolism and depletion of myocardial energy stores. Cross-clamping the aorta without protection for more than 15 to 20 minutes would result in profound myocardial dysfunction.[8] Cardioplegia is infused to arrest the heart and provide a bloodless, motionless operative field as well as protect the heart during cardiac surgery. Cardioplegic solution is infused into the aorta or coronary sinus or into the coronary arteries themselves to cause cardiac arrest. Debate continues over the best type of cardioplegia, what is the best temperature (hypothermic vs. normothermic), whether cardioplegia should be infused antegrade or retrograde, and timing of infusion (intermittent or continuous). Most cardiac surgery programs use a combination of the myocardial protection techniques discussed here.

Cardioplegia solutions are made of crystalloid, oxygenated crystalloid, or crystalloid–blood mixtures. Although cardioplegic solutions vary widely, typical components include potassium, magnesium, or procaine to provide immediate diastolic arrest; oxygen, glucose, glutamate, or aspartate as energy substrate; bicarbonate or phosphate to buffer acidosis; and calcium, steroids, or procaine to stabilize membranes. The solution should be hyperosmolar to edema. Cardioplegia is infused continuously or intermittently.

Cardioplegia can be normothermic or hypothermic. Hypothermic techniques were originally used as a means to reduce metabolic demands during arrest. A cooled nonbeating heart uses less oxygen than a warm-beating or fibrillating heart. Cold cardioplegic solutions are commonly cooled to 15°C to 20°C to reduce oxygen demand. Normothermic cardioplegia has been used at both the induction of cardioplegic arrest and at the termination of arrest. Warm, oxygenated, hyperkalemic blood cardioplegia maintains arrest while supplying oxygenated blood to myocardial cells. "Hot shots" are warm cardioplegic infusions administered at the end of the surgical procedure, before removal of the aortic cross-clamp.

Cardioplegia solution can be delivered antegrade into the ascending aorta, after which it flows through the coronary circulation and returns to the heart through the coronary sinus. Although antegrade cardioplegia has been the standard in cardiac surgery for many years, its delivery may be inadequate. Antegrade cardioplegia infusion through coronary arteries that are severely stenosed or occluded is uneven. Hearts with left ventricular hypertrophy may receive incomplete delivery to the subendocardium. In patients with aortic insufficiency, the left ventricle may become distended because of the retrograde flow of cardioplegia across the valve. Although cardioplegia can be delivered through saphenous vein grafts, it cannot be delivered through IMA grafts. Insufficient delivery of cardioplegia results in poor myocardial protection, which results in postoperative myocardial damage and dysfunction. Because of inadequate delivery using antegrade techniques, retrograde delivery systems were developed. Retrograde cardioplegia is infused under low pressure through catheters inserted directly into the coronary sinus. Cardioplegia flows retrograde through the coronary veins to capillaries to the coronary arterial bed, and exits at the coronary ostia, where effluent is removed by vent and suction. Retrograde and combined retrograde–antegrade techniques allow for optimal delivery and myocardial protection.

Deep Hypothermic Circulatory Arrest

Circulatory arrest (interruption of circulation through the ascending aorta for an extended period of time) may be necessary in procedures involving the ascending aorta and aortic arch. Profound hypothermia is used to protect the brain and other vital organs. The patient's body temperature is lowered to 18°C and CPB is stopped. Operative procedures are performed expediently because of the interruption of circulation to vital organs. In general, deep hyperthermic arrest can be used up to 60 minutes.[8] After repair, the patient is placed back on CPB and is gradually rewarmed.

CARDIAC SURGERY PROCEDURES FOR CORONARY ARTERY REVASCULARIZATION

Coronary Artery Bypass Surgery

Indications for Surgical Revascularization

CABG surgery is done primarily to alleviate anginal symptoms as well as improve survival. CABG surgery is among the most common surgical procedures preformed worldwide. The American College of Cardiology and the American Heart Association Task Force on Practice Guidelines was formed to recommend appropriate use of diagnostic tests and therapies. Based on both literature review and expert opinion, the ACC/AHA updated the guidelines for CABG in 2004. Class I guideline indications for CABG are described as conditions for which there is evidence and/or general agreement that a given procedure or treatment is useful and effective. Class I recommendations for CABG surgery include: significant left main coronary artery stenosis or equivalent; three-vessel coronary disease; two-vessel coronary disease and an ejection fraction less than 50%; one- or two-vessel disease with a large amount of viable myocardium at risk; and one- or two-vessel disease with severe angina despite maximal medical therapy.[10] Other class I indications for CABG include failed angioplasty with persistent pain or hemodynamic instability, postinfraction ventricular septal defect (VSD) or postinfarction mitral insufficiency, cardiogenic shock in patients less than age 75.[10] In comparison with drug-eluting stents for patients with multivessel coronary disease, CABG is associated with lower mortality rates and lower rates of repeat revascularization.[11]

Relative Contraindications

Conditions that greatly increase the mortality risk during surgery and anatomic limitations are relative contraindications to CABG surgery. Lack of adequate conduit, coronary arteries distal to the stenosis smaller than 1 to 1.5 mm, and severe aortic atherosclerosis are anatomic abnormalities that may limit the success of the revascularization for technical reasons. Severe left ventricular failure and coexisting pulmonary, renal, carotid, and peripheral vascular disease may significantly increase the risk of surgery by predisposing to complications during the perioperative period. Patients with low ejection fraction are sicker at baseline and more than four times the mortality than patients with high ejection fraction.[12]

Bypass Conduits

Coronary artery revascularization is accomplished most commonly with the IMA in combination with saphenous vein grafts. Because of the excellent patency associated with IMA grafts, other arterial conduits are now accepted for bypass surgery. Use of the right GEA as a pedicle graft to the right coronary or as a free graft to the left coronary system requires a more extensive surgery because the abdomen must be entered. Radial artery grafts were initially used in the early 1970s but were abandoned because of their tendency to spasm and their poor short-term patency. With the advent of calcium-channel blockers, radial artery grafts have enjoyed renewed interest. Greater saphenous vein from the legs is the most commonly used venous conduit. Because of patient anatomy, history of vein stripping, or previous revascularizations, alternative conduits may be necessary. Veins harvested from the

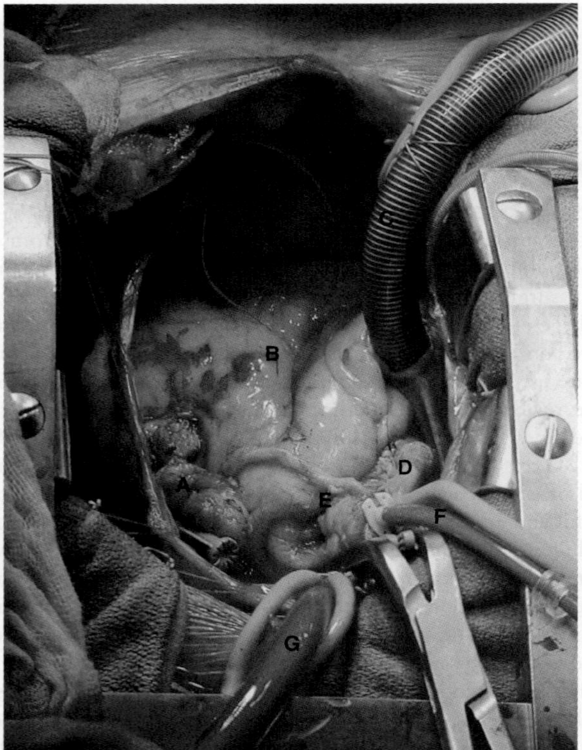

■ **Figure 25-1** View of completed internal mammary and saphenous vein grafts. View from the head of the operating table shows: (A) internal mammary graft to left anterior descending coronary artery; (B) temporary epicardial pacing wires inserted into the right ventricle; (C) venous cannula into right atrium; (D) ascending aorta; (E) saphenous vein graft; (F) cardioplegia delivery catheter; (G) aortic cannula. (Photo by D. LeDoux, 2003.)

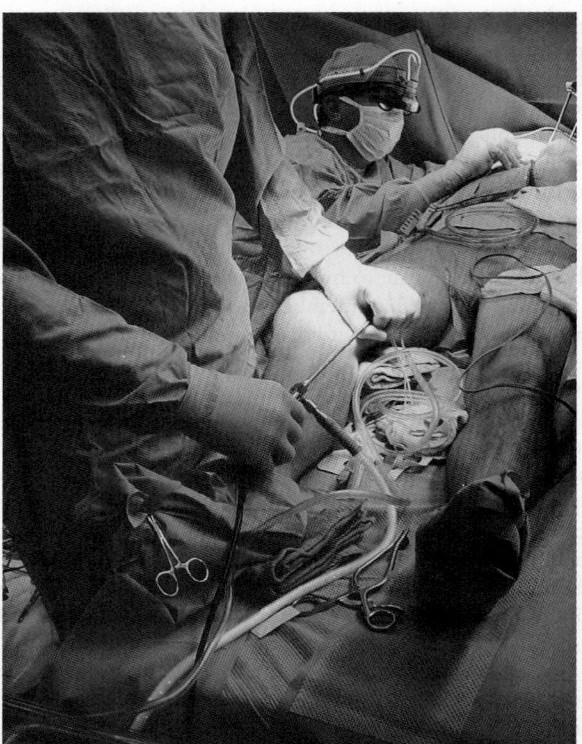

■ **Figure 25-2** Saphenous vein is dissected out by video-assisted endoscopic approach while the internal mammary is dissected down from the retrosternal bed. (Photo by D. LeDoux, 2003.)

arms, such as the cephalic or basilic, make poor bypass conduits because of their calibre and high incidence of aneurysm formation. Lesser saphenous vein located on the posterior aspect of the lower leg may be used, but may be small calibre and difficult to harvest. Cadaveric and synthetic bypass grafts have also been attempted but are not commonly used due to poor patency rates. Because of long-term patency, the left IMA is most commonly used to bypass the left anterior descending (LAD) artery. The right IMA may also be used to bypass the LAD, artery as well as the right coronary artery. When multiple grafts are required, single or bilateral IMA grafts in combination with other arterial conduit and saphenous vein grafts can be used to accomplish complete revascularization (Fig. 25-1). Many authors recommended complete arterial revascularization in young patients in hopes of avoiding additional revascularizations later in life.

Saphenous Vein Bypass Grafts. While the sternal incision is made and the patient is readied for CPB, the saphenous vein is prepared. Traditionally, saphenous vein is harvested using standard incisions. With the advent of minimally invasive surgery, saphenous vein can be harvested using endoscopic techniques and small incisions at the same time that the IMA graft is taken down from the retrosternal bed (Fig. 25-2). A long segment of vein is carefully exposed, the branches are ligated and divided, and the vein is removed. The vein is flushed with a cold heparinized solution and checked for leaks. One side of the untwisted vein is marked with a surgical pencil, and the vein is filled with and stored in a cold solution. CPB is instituted, a clamp is placed across the distal aorta, and cold cardioplegia is injected into the aortic root. Portions of saphenous vein are sutured to coronary arteries beyond the arterial stenoses. Distal anastomoses to the LAD artery are usually made first, followed by distal anastomoses to the coronary arteries located on the back of the heart. After all distal anastomoses are completed, the aortic cross-clamp is removed and patient warming is begun. Small openings in the ascending aorta are made with a punch, and the proximal end of the saphenous vein is anastomosed to the aorta. After the proximal anastomoses are completed, CPB is discontinued and the chest is closed.

IMA Bypass Grafts. Harvesting the IMA is technically more difficult than harvesting the saphenous vein graft. After the sternum is cut open, the IMA is dissected away from the chest wall. A special retractor is used to expose the IMA in the retrosternal bed.[13] A 2-cm-wide pedicle strip is removed from the chest-wall muscle, fat, and pleura that surround the IMA. The pedicle strip, with the IMA lying in the center, is exposed from the IMA origin at the subclavian artery down to the level of the fourth to sixth intercostal space. The branches of the IMA are exposed, divided, and ligated. An incision is made into the coronary artery to be bypassed (usually the LAD) and the distal end of the IMA is sutured into place. The IMA can be used as a free graft rather than a pedicle graft if it is not long enough to reach the target.

Radial Artery Bypass Grafts. The radial artery graft is used for bypass conduit only after collateral circulation of the ulnar artery has been assessed by vascular ultrasound or Allen's test. Although both radial arteries can be used, the radial artery from the patient's nondominant hand is the usual choice and can be harvested before the chest is opened. Because the radial artery is very thick-walled and prone to spasm, after harvesting, papaverine may be used to flush and dilate the artery before grafting. During and after surgery, nitrates and calcium-channel blockers are used to prevent spasm, although duration of administration of these agents has not been standardized.[14] The radial graft is a desirable conduit because of its length and ability to reach most distal targets. Postoperative nursing care includes evaluation of ulnar pulse and distal circulation.

Gastroepiploic Graft. The right GEA is a branch of the gastroduodenal artery that supplies blood to the greater curvature of the stomach. The GEA can be used as an in situ graft on the posterior surfaces of the heart or as a free graft to other vessels. Harvesting of the GEA graft requires laparotomy in addition to the sternotomy or thoracotomy incisions required for CABG. Longer operative times and abdominal surgery increase the complexity of the surgery.

Operative Results

Coronary bypass surgery is done to improve quality of life by relieving anginal symptoms, or to prolong life. Although angina pectoris is relieved in more than 90% of patients who undergo CABG surgery, Canadian Cardiovascular Society class III angina reoccurs in 5% to 10% of patients at 3 years and gradually increases because of graft stenosis or progression of native disease.[15] The overall rate is thought to have increased because of the changing population referred for cardiac surgery. In a retrospective cohort study by Guru et al.,[16] women had a higher early mortality rate than men although long-term mortality appeared to be equivalent as early as 1 year after surgery.[16] The advent of interventional cardiology and improved medical management, patients now referred for CABG surgery are older, sicker, and have more complex disease.

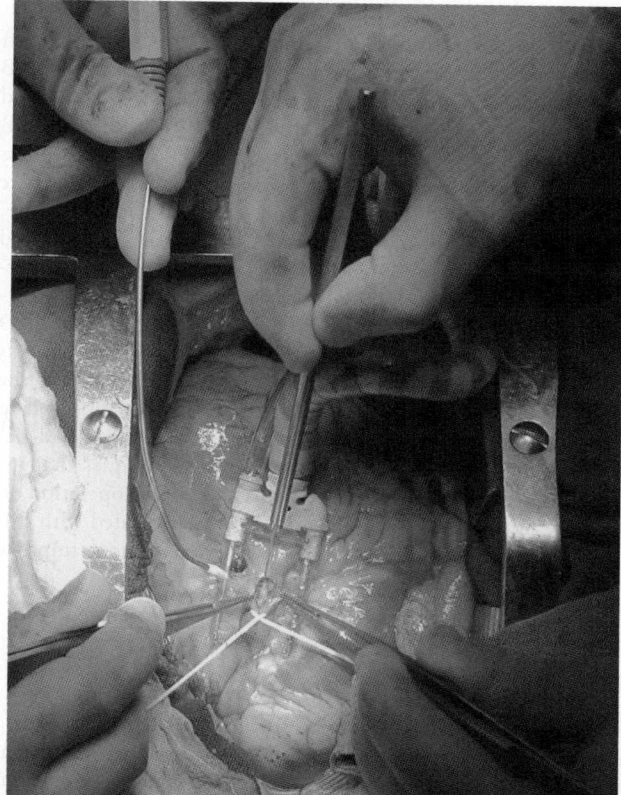

■ **Figure 25-3** A two-pronged stabilizer immobilizes the surrounding myocardium and coronary artery in off-pump bypass surgery done on a beating heart. A snare is used proximal to the incision on the left anterior descending coronary artery. Forceps hold open the incision on the LAD open, and the internal mammary pedicle will be sewn into place. (Photo by D. LeDoux, 2003.)

Minimally Invasive Coronary Artery Bypass Surgery

MIDCAB is CABG surgery performed through a left anterior small thoracotomy, a short parasternal incision, or small incisions using port access and video-assisted technology. Because the small incisions limit the surgical approach, MIDCAB is usually confined to proximal disease of the LAD or right coronary artery with IMA as conduits to these sites. Radial artery, GEA, and saphenous vein grafts have also been used if the IMA graft could not be used or if more distal targets required grafting. Surgery is performed on the beating heart. To allow suturing of the graft anastomosis to the beating heart, pharmacologic measures such as adenosine and β-blockers are used to slow or temporarily stop the heart, in conjunction with mechanical stabilizers that immobilize the portion of the coronary artery where the graft anastomosis is sutured (Fig. 25-3). Transesophageal echocardiography is used to assess for wall-motion abnormalities that would signal ischemia. CPB is on standby during each MIDCAB procedure if emergent conversion to standard sternotomy and CPB is required. The advantages of MIDCAB surgery are coronary revascularization without the physiologic derangements of CPB and avoidance of the traditional sternotomy incision. As a result, patients have less pain, need fewer blood transfusions, and have reduced overall length of hospital stay. Robotic totally endoscopic coronary artery bypass surgery as a totally endoscopic, closed-chest procedure but is limited primarily to the LAD and diagonal branches on the anterior surface of the heart. For patients with multivessel disease, integrated or hybrid revascularization may combine totally endoscopic coronary artery bypass with percutaneous techniques to provide for complete revascularization.[17]

Coronary artery bypass surgery performed by median sternotomy but without the use of CPB is known as OPCAB. Like MIDCAB, grafts are performed on the beating heart. Avoidance of CPB and aortic cross clamping may be desirable in patients with poor ventricular function or severe atherosclerosis of the aorta who may not tolerate aortic cross clamping. Median sternotomy allows for better exposure than in MIDCAB techniques. While it has been suggested that OPCAB offers neurologic protection, a randomized controlled trial comparing neurologic outcome of OPCAB to CABG with CPB demonstrated improved neurologic outcomes at 3 months but this difference became negligible at 12 months.[18] In a follow-up multicenter randomized controlled trial, avoiding CPB had no effect on 5-year cognitive outcomes.[19]

Operative Results for MIDCAB and OPCAB

Midterm results in patients undergoing MIDCAB through left anterior small thoracotomy and using the left IMA and OPCAB have been encouraging. In a multicenter, randomized controlled trial comparing OPCAB and CABG with CPB,[20] the OPCAB group had less use of blood products ($p < 0.01$) and 41% less release of creatinine kinase (CK; $p < 0.01$), but otherwise there were no significant differences in complications, quality of life, length of stay, or recurrent angina. A prospective randomized trial was conducted by Drenth et al.[21] comparing coronary artery percutaneous transluminal coronary angioplasty with stenting (PCI) to OPCAB in patients for high-grade proximal LAD lesions. In a mean follow-up time of 3 years, angina pectoris class was lower in the OPCAB group ($p = 0.02$) as well as the need for antianginal medication ($p = 0.01$) when compared to the PCI group. OPCAB is technically more difficult and demanding for surgeons.[22] Because operative techniques that involve minimally invasive incisions, port access, and operation on a beating heart have a learning curve, results associated with this newer operative technology are expected to continue to improve over time.

Transmyocardial Laser Revascularization

Transmyocardial laser revascularization (TMLR or TMR) is a technique under investigation in patients with refractory angina. In TMLR, carbon dioxide, holmium-YAG (yttrium–aluminum garnet), or excimer lasers[23] are used to produce multiple channels from the endocardial surface of the ventricular wall in an effort directly to improve blood flow to areas of myocardium that cannot be revascularized using traditional techniques. It has also been postulated that myocardial blood flow is enhanced by angiogenesis that occurs with TMLR, although this is still unproven. Left anterolateral thoracotomy is most often used to provide exposure, although TMLR can also be done by standard median sternotomy if it is performed at the same time as standard CABG to other vessels. TMLR is done on a beating heart. The laser is synchronized with the patient's R-wave. Transesophageal echocardiography is used to detect steam or bubbles that verify channel creation. Epicardial surface seals off with gentle pressure, leaving an endocardial channel in which blood flows. TMLR is recognized by the Society of Thoracic Surgery as acceptable as either sole therapy or as an adjunct to a selected subset of patients with refractory angina be cannot be revascularized by the more traditional methods of bypass surgery or percutaneous intervention.[24]

CARDIAC SURGERY PROCEDURES FOR ACQUIRED STRUCTURAL HEART DISEASE

Acquired Valvular Heart Disease

Valvular Repair

Surgical repair of a stenotic or incompetent mitral valve is performed frequently. The reparative surgeries, mitral commissurotomy (in which the fused valve cusps are split open) and annuloplasty (in which the large orifice of an incompetent valve is made smaller) are discussed in Chapter 29. Care of the patient after surgical repair of valves is similar to that of the patient after CABG surgery.

Valvular Replacement

If a dysfunctional mitral or aortic valve is not suitable for repair, valve replacement is undertaken. Valvular heart surgery can be accomplished through a standard median sternotomy incision, through a small parasternal incision, or through port access using small incisions and endoscopic techniques. Because valve surgery requires an arrested, open heart, CPB must be used and can be done by the standard method or by femorofemoral cannulation. Surgical techniques for mitral valve replacement (MVR) and aortic valve replacement (AVR), types of prosthetic heart valves, and indications for valvular replacement are discussed in Chapter 29.

Mitral Valve Repair or Replacement. The routine medical care after MVR surgery is similar to that after CABG surgery. Early after MVR surgery, a patient is more likely to have important cardiovascular or pulmonary dysfunction than a patient who has undergone CABG surgery. Late after surgery, problems related to the prosthetic device may occur. Prognosis and outcome after MVR are related to severity of the left ventricular and right ventricular dysfunction before surgery.

Aortic Valve Replacement. The routine medical care after AVR surgery is similar to that after CABG surgery. Early after AVR surgery, a patient is more likely to have arrhythmia, decreased cardiac output, or neurologic dysfunction than a patient who has undergone CABG surgery. Late after surgery, arrhythmia, heart failure, or problems related to the prosthetic device may occur. Prognosis and outcome after AVR are related to severity of left ventricular dysfunction before surgery.

Surgical Techniques for the Failing Heart

As an alternative to cardiac transplant, number surgical techniques are evolving. In the Dor procedure, the left ventricular cavity is opened and monofilament sutures placed circumferentially above the boarder of the diseased muscle, restoring the normal contour of the ventricle.[25] The reduction ventriculoplasty was pioneered by Batitista as a surgical option for patients with cardiomyopathy who cannot undergo cardiac transplantation. To decrease wall tension and ventricular size in the dilated left ventricular, an oval-shaped portion of myocardium is removed from apex to base. Although Batitista reported encouraging results in his own series, this procedure after being introduced in the United States has had mixed results.[25] While the Cleveland Clinic series reported midterm results with a 30-day mortality rate of 3.2%,[26] other series have reported high mortality rates.[25]

Dynamic cardiomyoplasty is an alternative to heart transplantation for patients with end-stage heart failure. Surgery is accomplished through a left thoracotomy incision, and CPB is not required. The latissimus dorsi muscle is placed into the thoracic cavity through a space where the second rib has been resected. Intramuscular pacing electrodes are inserted in the proximal portion of the muscle. The patient is then repositioned, and a sternal incision is made to complete the muscle wrap around the heart. A cardiomyostimulator (a pacemaker especially designed for cardiomyoplasty) is implanted beneath the rectus muscle and activated 2 weeks after surgery, allowing the muscle to rest and develop collateral circulation before pacing is started. Stimulation is gradually introduced by a stimulated pulse synchronized to every other cardiac cycle. Long-term survival after cardiomyoplasty has been reported as high as 50% at 8 years.[27] Although cardiomyoplasty is not a replacement for cardiac transplantation, it may have a limited role in patients who would not be candidates for transplantation.

Acquired VSD Repair

Rupture of the intraventricular septum after MI is a rare complication that can occur with acute MI. The infarct that accompanies VSD is usually extensive and transmural. Thinning and dilatation of the infarcted portion of septum, which evolves to rupture 1 to 7 days after MI, causes biventricular failure as the left ventricle shunts blood into the right ventricle, causing right-sided heart failure and pulmonary edema. Clinical signs of acquired VSD include rapid-onset biventricular failure or cardiogenic shock, pansystolic murmur, and a sequential increase in venous oxygen saturation from the right atrium to the pulmonary artery. Bedside cardiac output measures done with the pulmonary artery catheter by thermodilution are falsely elevated because of the left-to-right ventricular shunt. The anatomy and size of the septal rupture is diagnosed by echocardiography and cardiac catheterization.

Stabilization of the patient with septal rupture is aimed at afterload reduction. Using pharmacologic vasodilators and intra-aortic balloon pumping, forward flow is improved and the left-to-right shunt fraction is reduced. The VSD is repaired by patching the defect with a Dacron-covered patch, which is then lined, if possible, with pericardium to make it leak proof. In patients with significant coronary artery stenosis, CABG surgery may also be added to the operative procedure. Even with surgical repair, the hospital mortality rate after VSD repair remains 10% to 40%.[28] The important risk factors associated with early death are poor preoperative hemodynamic state and acute right ventricular dysfunction.

Repair of Ascending Aortic Aneurysm or Dissection

Aortic aneurysm is used to describe localized dilatation of the aorta. Causes of ascending aortic aneurysm include hypertension, Marfan's syndrome, and cystic medial necrosis. The likelihood of aortic aneurysm rupture is related to size. The more the aorta is stretched, the greater the tension and wall stress forces. If the ascending aorta is aneurysmal, the cusps of the aorta may be distorted, resulting in aortic insufficiency and acute or chronic heart failure.

Aortic dissection occurs secondary to disruption of the intimal layer of the aorta and is a true medical emergency. Blood enters the intimal tear and dissects a false lumen in the abnormal medial layer, with blood flowing retrograde and antegrade, separating layers of the intimal and adventitial layers. The dissection is propagated by hypertension and elevated force of contraction. In the Stanford classification, type A describes dissection of the ascending aorta and transverse arch, whereas type B is used to describe dissections of the descending thoracic aorta. Aortic dissection has a grave prognosis and requires prompt surgical intervention.

Ascending aortic dissection and aneurysm are treated with surgical resection of the involved portion of aorta and replacement with prosthetic tubular graft. In ascending aortic aneurysm or type A dissection, if the aortic valve is regurgitant, it is replaced. In the case of aneurysm alone, it may be possible to spare the aortic valve by resuspending it within the prosthetic graft of the ascending aorta (David procedure). If surgery involves the aortic arch, deep hypothermic circulatory arrest is used (see the "Surgical Techniques" section).

Routine Postoperative Care

Immediate postoperative care is similar for patients undergoing any cardiac surgical procedure, including CABG, MIDCAB, valve repair or replacement, and cardiac transplantation. After cardiac surgery, the patient is admitted to an intensive care unit for close monitoring for 6 to 24 hours after surgery. On arrival in the intensive care unit, the critical care nurse performs a number of rapid assessments to ensure patient stability. Routine care includes continuous ECG monitoring, measurement of blood pressure by arterial line, pulse oximetry, pulmonary artery pressures, and body temperature measurement. Intermittent parameters may include cardiac output measurement as well as calculation of derived hemodynamic parameters, such as afterload, cardiac index, and contractility indices. Specialty pulmonary artery catheters, such as the continuous cardiac output pulmonary artery catheter, may be used to evaluate minute-to-minute changes in cardiac output. Oximetry pulmonary artery catheters may be used continuously to monitor mixed venous oxygen concentration, and values can be used to calculate oxygen consumption and delivery parameters during periods of critical illness.

Sinus bradycardia or other hemodynamically significant bradycardic dysrhythmias such as accelerated junctional rhythm can occur postoperatively and may be treated with an atrial or atrioventricular pacemaker set at a rate of 70 or 100 beats/min. Heart block may occur after valve repair or replacement because of edema and trauma at the suture lines close to the conduction system. Hypertension may be treated with either intravenous nitrates or sodium nitroprusside. Hypotension occurs often during the first 12 hours after surgery as the patient warms and as systemic vascular resistance decreases to normal levels. Hypovolemia (right or left atrial or pulmonary artery wedge pressure of less than 8 to 10 mm Hg) may be present because of the fluid volume alterations that occur with CPB or if diuretic was administration at the end of CPB. Hypovolemia may be treated with crystalloid or colloid volume expanders such as 5% albumin or hetastarch, or with crystalloid. If the patient's hemoglobin is less than 8 g/dL, packed red blood cells or whole blood may be administered. Blood may be recovered through the chest tubes for autotransfusion during the first 4 to 12 hours after surgery. If patients are normovolemic, they are usually placed on a salt and free-water restriction. Potassium replacement is often necessary. Patients are usually maintained on a respirator for the first 1 or 2 hours after surgery, until the effects of anesthesia have reversed. Patients are on prophylactic antibiotics, usually a second-generation cephalosporin, to prevent wound infection for 48 hours or less. Antibiotic prophylaxis beyond 48 hours is not associated with decreased infections.[29]

Because of improved anesthesia and surgical techniques and a shift from acute care resulting from changes in reimbursement, cardiac surgery has evolved to include same day admission and shortened length of stay. Stable, uncomplicated patients are earmarked to "fast track" by extubating early and minimizing their intensive care unit and hospital stay. Patient care is directed by an established care map or "roadmap." In the operating room, patients receive lower doses of opioids with the aim of extubation within 1 or 2 hours after arrival in the intensive care unit. The patient is kept sedated with short-acting agents such as propofol or midazolam intravenous infusions. When the patient is hemodynamically stable and bleeding is under control, the patient can be extubated. As a result, cardiac surgery patients may stay in the intensive care unit as little as 8 to 12 hours, thus freeing up critical care beds and reducing costs to the patient. Patients who are "fast tracked" in rapid recovery programs are discharged 3 to 5 days after surgery. Nurse practitioners or physician assistants in collaboration may manage cardiac surgery patients with the physician. Atrial arrhythmias and pulmonary complications are the most common variances that keep patients in hospital longer than planned by the care map.

Early Complications After Cardiac Surgery

Cardiovascular

Cardiovascular dysfunction or low cardiac output syndrome can occur after cardiac surgery. Low cardiac output syndrome may be related to reduced preload, increased afterload, arrhythmias, cardiac tamponade, or myocardial depression with or without myocardial necrosis. Excessive bleeding can occur secondary to coagulopathy, uncontrolled hypertension, or inadequate hemostasis. Perioperative MI and pericarditis can occur as a result of cardiac surgery.

Postoperative Bleeding. Pleural and mediastinal tubes are attached to water-seal and 20-cm suction to drain mediastinal shed blood. Although blood may clot in these chest tubes, they should not be stripped because stripping may cause excessive suction, which may increase bleeding or cause damage to grafts.[30] Excessive postoperative bleeding (mediastinal drainage of more than >500 mL for the first hour after surgery or drainage, totaling >200 mL/h thereafter) usually is mechanical in nature and caused by bleeding from suture lines, but it may be caused by the presence of pericardial adhesions from an earlier surgery or to a coagulopathy. Postoperative bleeding is usually venous rather than arterial. Coagulopathies may occur in patients with prolonged CPB times or excessive intraoperative bleeding. If patients are bleeding excessively, coagulation panels should be obtained immediately to evaluate for coagulopathy. Coagulopathies caused by depletion of factors should be treated with administration of depleted factors, such as fresh-frozen plasma, platelets, and cryoprecipitate. Autotransfusion may be used to replace red blood cells, but filtered blood lacks adequate clotting factors. In an observational study of 8004 coronary artery bypass patients,[31] having a lower nadir hematocrit is associated with increased risk of developing low output heart failure and that risk was increased further with transfusion of packed red blood cells as a significant independent predictor of low output heart failure (adjusted odds ratio, 1.27; 95% CI, 1.00 to 1.61; $p = 0.047$).

Pharmacologic means of controlling postoperative hemorrhage include a variety of nonhematogenous therapies. Aminocaproic acid is an antifibrinolytic medication that inhibits conversion of plasminogen to plasmin. Desmopressin (DDAVP) may be infused intravenously in patients with severe platelet dysfunction after prolonged CPB or uremia. DDAVP shortens bleeding time and improves platelet function by increasing circulating levels of von Willebrand factor. DDAVP also increases factor VIII C levels, which shorten the partial prothrombin time. In the past, aprotinin had been used extensively to limit bleeding especially in redo operations, the safety of aprotinin came under scrutiny. An observational study by Mangano et al.[32] of 4,374 patient undergoing revascularization found a doubling of the risk of renal failure (95% CI), 55% increased risk of MI or heart failure ($p < 0.001$), and 181% increase in risk of stroke or encephalopathy ($p = 0.001$). In a retrospective analysis by Shaw et al.,[33] patients who received aprotinin had higher mortality rate and larger increase in serum creatinine than those who received Aminocaproic or no antifibrinolytic agent.

Protamine also may be administered intravenously in patients who had inadequate reversal of heparin or in those with heparin rebound. Protamine must be administered as a slow intravenous infusion to prevent hypotension. Patients with insulin-dependent diabetes or allergy to fish are more likely to have allergic reactions to protamine. If postoperative bleeding continues and coagulation tests are normal, bleeding may be mechanical or may result from suture line or venous bleeding. Adequate control of hypertension with sodium nitroprusside may also help control bleeding. If coagulopathies were corrected and bleeding continues, mediastinal re-exploration is advised to decrease the risk of cardiac tamponade.

Cardiac Tamponade. Cardiac tamponade is a life-threatening emergency that may occur immediately postoperative. Compression of the right heart with blood and/or clot decreases left ventricular preload and consequently, cardiac output that results in causes hemodynamic deterioration.[34] Cardiac tamponade is suspected as a cause of low cardiac output if right and left heart pressures increase and equalize. Physical exam findings, hemodynamic parameters, and diagnostic tests for tamponade include: decreased cardiac index, mediastinal drainage that may increase as well as decrease or stop, radiography shows widening of the cardiac silhouette, neck vein distention, a pulsus paradoxus is noted by arterial line or by auscultation, or narrow pulse pressure is present. Although tachycardia is a sign of classic tamponade, the cardiac surgical patient may be unable to generate a compensatory tachycardia because of heart block or previously administered β-blockers or calcium-channel blockers. Echocardiography provides rapid confirmation of pericardial fluid and tamponade physiology, facilitating intervention with echo-guided pericardiocentesis, or open pericardial drainage in the operating room.

Myocardial Depression. Myocardial depression (impaired myocardial contractility) may be reversible or irreversible after cardiac surgery. If a patient is not acidotic or hypoxemic and has evidence of decreased cardiac contractility, myocardial cell dysfunction or necrosis is suspected. Treatment of low cardiac output secondary to myocardial dysfunction first involves treatment of hypoxemia, acidosis, heart rate and rhythm abnormalities, decreased preload, and increased afterload. If a patient continues to have a low cardiac output after these maneuvers, inotropes or intra-aortic balloon pump therapy is instituted. A variety of inotropes and vasoactive medications may be employed postoperatively (Table 25-1). Dobutamine, dopamine, epinephrine, norepinephrine, and milrinone intravenous infusions are frequently used for inotropic support of myocardial depression after cardiac surgery. If the patient's cardiac index is normal to high and hypotension is related to vasodilation, pressers such as vasopressin

Table 25-1 ■ INOTROPES AND VASODILATOR INTRAVENOUS INFUSIONS COMMONLY USED AFTER CARDIAC SURGERY

Medication	Dose Range	Mechanism of Action	Indications	Heart Rate	Blood Pressure	Cardiac Output
Dobutamine	2–15 mcg/kg/min	Primarily β1-adrenergic receptor stimulation	Low cardiac output after cardiac surgery	+	+/0/−	++
Dopamine	1–2 mcg/kg/min for renal effect 5–20 mcg/kg/min for inotropy and increased vascular resistance	Stimulation of dopaminergic and a drenergic receptors	Treatment of shock and hypotension after cardiac surgery in patient who has been volume resuscitated	+	++	++
Epinephrine	0.01–0.1 mcg/kg/min to high dose 0.3–0.3 mcg/kg/min	Stimulation of α- and β1- and β2-adrenergic receptors	Treatment of low cardiac output and shock after cardiac surgery	++	++	++
Isoproterenol	0.01–0.1 mcg/kg/min	Stimulation of β1- and β2-adrenergic receptors	Used after heart transplantation and in patients with severe bradycardia to stimulate heart rate	+++	+	++
Milrinone	0.25–0.75 mcg/kg/min	Phosphodiesterase inhibition resulting in increase inotropy and vasodilation	Low cardiac output after cardiac surgery; may require use of adrenergic agent to maintain blood pressure	0/+	−	+
Nitroglycerin	5–200 mcg/min	Dilates coronary arteries and reduces myocardial oxygen demand, reduce ventricular pressures	Used to prevent spasm in arterial grafts after cardiac surgery as well as may be used to reduce preload and afterload	−/+	−	−
Nitroprusside	0.3–5 mcg/kg/min (high doses may result in thiocyanate toxicity)	Cause peripheral vasodilation by acting directly on smooth muscle in the venous and arterial circulation	Used to decreased blood pressure and afterload	−	−	0/+
Norepinephrine	0.01–0.1 mcg/min	Stimulation of α- and β-adrenergic receptors (α effects are predominate)	Used for shock and low systemic vascular resistance after cardiac surgery	+/−	++	+
Phenylephrine	0.1–0.3 mcg/kg/min	Potent α-adrenergic stimulator	Used to increase systemic vascular resistance and blood pressure cardiac output is maintained but blood pressure is low	0/−	++	−
Vasopressin	0.01–0.1 units/min	Potent vasoconstrictor	Used to treat shock and increase systemic vascular resistance and blood pressure cardiac output is maintained but blood pressure is low	−	++	−

+, increase; 0, no change; −, decrease.

and phenylephrine may be used A variety of vasodilating agents such as sodium nitroprusside, nitroglycerin, and angiotensin-converting enzyme inhibitors may be used to reduce afterload in low cardiac output syndrome as well as hypertension. Intra-aortic balloon pump therapy is frequently used in patients with severe cardiac dysfunction that is not adequately supported with medications alone.

Perioperative Myocardial Infarction. Despite improved methods of myocardial protection, perioperative MI continues to be a serious complication. Diagnosis of perioperative MI is made from a variety of diagnostic tests including ECG, echocardiography, and cardiac enzymes. MI related to cardiac surgery may be secondary to spasm of grafts, emboli of air or debris, or insufficient myocardial protection. CK is routinely elevated immediately after cardiac surgery and usually drops after 12 to 16 hours. CK peaks associated with perioperative MI occur 16 to 24 hours after surgery. More recently, troponin I has been used for the diagnosis of perioperative MI. Postoperative troponin I levels in patients without perioperative MI peak at 8 to 10 hours, whereas in patients with perioperative MI, troponin I levels peak in 20 hours and at higher concentrations.[35] A study by Lasocki et al.[36] found that elevated troponin I levels more than 13 ng/mL was an independent predictor of in-hospital mortality. The interpretation of troponin release is complex due to a variety of potential underlying reasons.[37] New wall-motion abnormalities noted on echocardiography are another way to verify perioperative MI. Postoperative pericarditis may mimic myocardial ischemia with chest pain and widespread ST-segment elevation. ECG changes associated with pericarditis are J-point changes, concave rather than convex, and do not result in pathologic Q waves.

Arrhythmias. Arrhythmias are common after cardiac surgery and are a prevalent cause of increased length of stay after cardiac surgery. Bradyarrhythmias are common after CABG and valve surgeries and may require temporary pacing via epicardial pacing wires placed at the time of surgery. Bradycardia or heart block following cardiac surgery is often hemodynamically significant may require placement of permanent transvenous pacers before discharge. Atrial arrhythmias are the most common after cardiac surgery. Contributing factors of atrial fibrillation (AF) may include electrolyte or metabolic disturbances, increased circulating catecholamines, volume overload, hypoxia, and myocardial ischemia or MI. Although atrial tachyarrhythmias may occur any time during the first few days to weeks after cardiac surgery, they frequently peak around the second or third day postoperative. Atrial fibrillation after cardiac surgery may be associated with important complications including stroke, renal dysfunction, and prolonged hospitalization.[38] Risk factors for postoperative AF include advanced age, history of congestive heart failure or AF, chronic obstructive lung disease, male sex, history of rheumatic heart disease, prolonged aortic cross-clamp time, and bicaval cannulation.[39] The onset of tachyarrhythmias is often preceded by frequent premature atrial contractions. Medications commonly used to control the ventricular response in AF and flutter include diltiazem (either intravenous drip or orally), digoxin, and β-blockers (orally or by intravenous drip, such as esmolol). Medications used to promote conversion of AF include procainamide, amiodarone, and sotalol. While multiple medications have been studied, β-blockers have been the only medication consistently shown across clinical studies that reduce the frequency of postoperative AF.[40] β-Blockers should be considered early during the postoperative course, especially if the patient was on β-blockers preoperatively. Although β-blockers, atrial pacing, antiarrhythmic medications, or a combination of these therapies may reduce the incidence or duration of AF, optimal strategies are still being defined.[41]

Postoperative arrhythmia diagnosis and treatment is facilitated by the presence of atrial epicardial pacemaker wires. Atrial activity is more pronounced when recorded in atrial ECGs than when recorded in a normal surface ECG (Fig. 25-4). When atrial activity is accentuated, differentiation between supraventricular and ventricular arrhythmias, and AF and flutter is made easier. If the ventricular response to AF exceeds 110 beats/min, then the patient's rate should be controlled.

If pharmacologic modalities fail to convert the patient to a sinus rhythm, electrical therapies may be used. Atrial flutter may be converted using rapid atrial pacing. To perform rapid atrial pacing, both atrial epicardial wires are connected to the rapid atrial pacemaker. The pacemaker output is set between 10 and 20, and the pacemaker rate is set approximately 20% faster than the existing atrial rate (atrial rate can be determined on the atrial ECG). Rapid atrial pacing continues for 30 seconds or until the atrial ECG complex changes from a negative to a positive deflection in lead II. Rapid atrial pacing is then abruptly discontinued, which allows the atria to resume a normal sinus rhythm (Fig. 25-5). Patients with chronic AF may be refractory to either pharmacologic or electrical conversion. If the AF is new in onset (<1 year), the patient may be successfully cardioverted by synchronized cardioversion. If the patient has been in AF or flutter longer than 48 hours or the AF remains paroxysmal, it is desirable to anticoagulate for 3 to 4 weeks to prevent thromboembolism, and then have the patient return for elective cardioversion if they remain in AF or flutter.

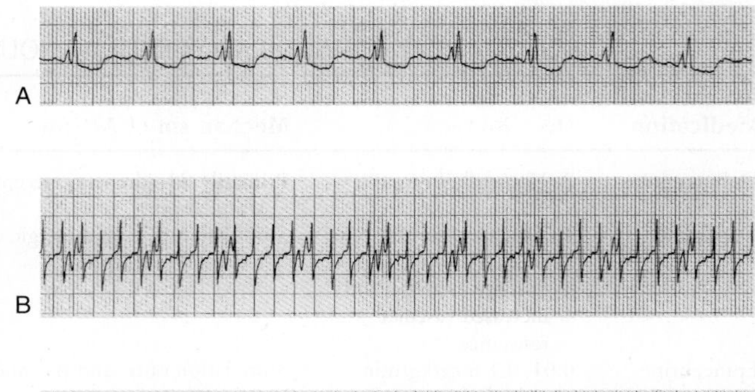

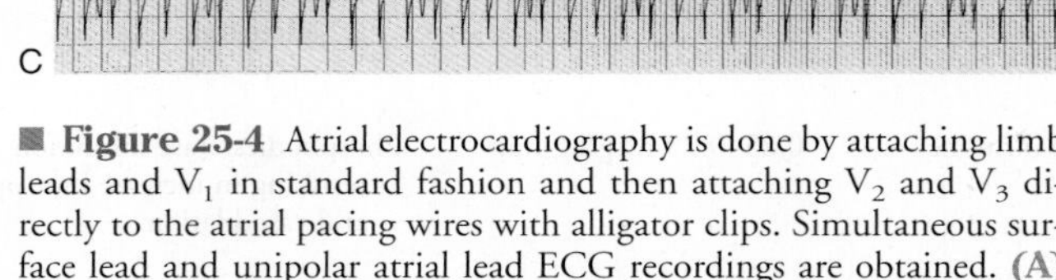

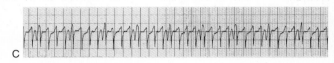

■ **Figure 25-4** Atrial electrocardiography is done by attaching limb leads and V_1 in standard fashion and then attaching V_2 and V_3 directly to the atrial pacing wires with alligator clips. Simultaneous surface lead and unipolar atrial lead ECG recordings are obtained. **(A)** Lead V_1 is the surface or reference lead. There is no atrial enhancement. **(B, C)** Leads V_2 and V_3 are unipolar atrial leads that accentuate the atrial activity and demonstrate an atrial rate of approximately 300 beats/min that was not apparent on the surface lead or standard 12-lead ECG.

While premature ventricular contractions and nonsustained runs of ventricular tachycardia may occur commonly after cardiac surgery, sustained ventricular tachycardia and ventricular fibrillation are rare but associated with a poor prognosis.[42] Premature ventricular contractions and nonsustained runs of ventricular tachycardia should be treated with correction of electrolytes, reduction or elimination of arrhythmogenic drugs such as catecholamines, and ruled out for ischemia. Sustained ventricular tachycardia should be cardioverted and antiarrhythmic agents such as amiodarone or lidocaine should be instituted.[42] Electrophysiology studies and implantable defibrillators may be used in selected cases.

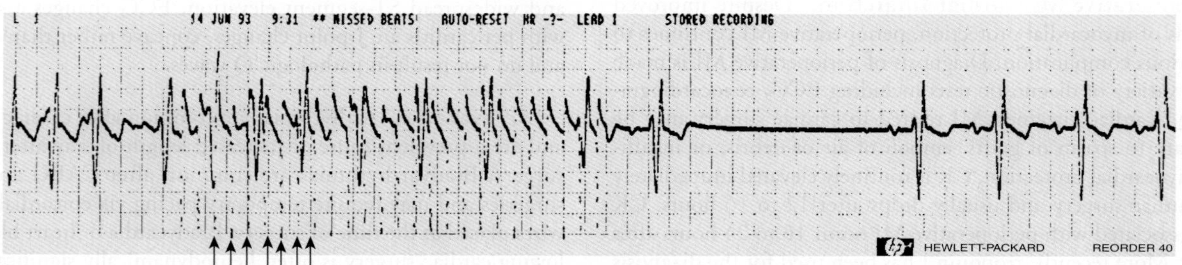

■ **Figure 25-5** Recording of a burst of rapid atrial pacing used to overdrive and convert this atrial flutter to sinus rhythm. *Arrows* denote atrial pacing spikes.

Pulmonary

Routinely, patients are intubated and ventilated for 2 to 4 hours after cardiac surgery. Pulmonary function is monitored with continuous pulse oximetry as well as intermittent arterial blood gases and chest radiographs. Mild pulmonary dysfunction is common after cardiac surgery. Pathophysiologic changes that occur after CPB include increased capillary permeability, increased pulmonary vascular resistance, and intrapulmonary aggregation of leukocytes and platelets. A noncardiac pulmonary edema may occur immediately after CPB or during the first several days after surgery. Comparative studies between OPCAB and CABG with CPB suggest that CPB alone may not be the major cause of the development of postoperative pulmonary dysfunction.[9] In a prospective, controlled trial by Roosens et al.,[43] both patients with and without CPB had dramatic impairment of respiratory system mechanic postoperatively. Severe pulmonary dysfunction is uncommon and may be related to preexisting lung disease. Although severe lung injury after cardiac surgery is rare, it continues to be a major impact on morbidity and mortality as well as related cost of hospitalization.[9] In a case controlled study by Milot et al.[44] in 3,278 patients, adult respiratory distress syndrome after cardiac surgery was rare (0.4%) but carried a 15% mortality rate. Independent predicators of adult respiratory distress syndrome in cardiac surgery patients include number of blood products transfused, shock, and previous cardiac surgery.[44] Chest radiographs should be performed as part of the fever work-up to rule out atelectasis and pneumonia. Atelectasis may occur secondary to hypoventilation related to sternal incision discomfort. Pain from chest tubes and sternotomy incision interferes with normal respiration and pulmonary toilet, making adequate pain control a high priority. Diminished breath sounds and lung fields at the bases that are dull to percussion indicate significant pleural effusions. Pneumothorax may occur any time during the postoperative period or at the time of pleural chest tube removal. Phrenic nerve damage may result in diaphragmatic paralysis or dysfunction but is uncommon with today's surgical techniques.

Pulmonary embolism is uncommon after cardiac surgery. Factors associated with a higher incidence of pulmonary emboli include AF, heart failure, obesity, hypercoagulable states, and immobilization. Diagnostic work-up for pulmonary emboli includes arterial blood gas, ventilation perfusion scan, CT scan, or pulmonary angiogram. Treatment with continuous intravenous heparin is begun once the diagnosis of pulmonary emboli is established, and warfarin is started for long-term anticoagulation. In patients in whom anticoagulation is contraindicated, an inferior vena caval filter may be placed. Surgical pulmonary embolectomy may be used in patients with large pulmonary emboli and associated clinical presentation of right-side heart failure.

Renal

While the pathogenesis of renal failure after cardiac surgery is multifactorial, CPB represents a specific risk.[45] Radiocontrast used during coronary angiography before cardiac surgery can further reduce renal function. Nonoliguric renal failure after cardiac surgery occurs most commonly after cardiac surgery. If renal dysfunction progresses to oliguric renal failure, serum potassium levels may increase rapidly and maintenance of normovolemia may be difficult without hemofiltration or dialysis. Nephrotoxic medications such as aminoglycoside antibiotics, radiographic contrast, and nonsteroidal anti-inflammatory drugs must be avoided in postoperative renal failure, and many other medications, such as antibiotics and digoxin, must be adjusted for decreased renal clearance. When renal failure after cardiac surgery is severe enough to require renal replacement therapy, the mortality rate is close to 60%.[46]

Gastrointestinal

Serious gastrointestinal complications can occur after cardiac surgery. Abdominal distention can occur during the first days after surgery secondary to decreased motility related to anesthesia, narcotics, and diabetic gastroparesis. If ileus and abdominal distention do not resolve with fasting and suppository or enema treatments, the etiology of the distention should be explored further. Gastroduodenal bleeding can result from erosive gastritis or esophagitis, or frank ulceration, especially in patients with a previous history of peptic ulcer disease. Patients after cardiac surgery usually are placed on prophylactic gastrointestinal agents such as antacids, sucralfate, histamine blockers such as famotidine or ranitidine, or proton-pump inhibitors such as pantoprazole. Cholecystitis presents with right upper quadrant pain and can be evaluated with abdominal ultrasound. After cardiac surgery or critical illness, cholecystitis commonly occurs in its acalculous (no stones) form. Mild elevations of hepatic transaminases also occur commonly after CPB. Severe hepatic dysfunction or "shock liver syndrome" with massive increases in liver enzymes most often occurs as a result of global hypoperfusion and end-organ damage. Acute hemorrhagic pancreatitis is uncommon after CABG surgery, but it has high rates of mortality and morbidity. If the patient continues to remain acidotic and the diagnostic work-up fails to identify another cause, abdominal exploration is done in the hope of finding a correctable source such as necrotic bowel. Diarrhea may occur with enteral feedings and medications such as quinidine or procainamide, or may be the result of *Clostridium difficile* infection. Patients with diarrhea should have stool samples sent to test for *C. difficile* toxin and are treated with oral administration of metronidazole or vancomycin.

Neuropsychological

Neuropsychological dysfunction after cardiac surgery can be either central or peripheral. Cognitive decline after CPB has been estimated from 3% to 50%, depending on definitions and time of assessment and stroke in approximately 3% of patients undergoing CABG surgery.[18] Embolization is the most common etiology of stroke during cardiac surgery but hypoperfusion may also play a role.[47]

Two types of peripheral neurologic deficits, brachial plexus injury and ulnar nerve injury, are described after cardiac surgery. The brachial plexus is susceptible to stretch injury and can occur with sternal retraction is a key factor responsible for injury.[48] In addition to a history of upper extremity pain and paresthesia, examination for brachial plexus injury includes evaluation of motor function of muscle groups innervated by the brachial plexus and sensation to pin prick.[48] Ulnar nerve injury, a result of nerve compression, is frequently described by patients after cardiac surgery as paresthesias in the affected arm below the elbow in the ulnar distribution involving the third, fourth, and fifth digits.

Postcardiotomy delirium occurs 2 to 5 days after cardiac surgery and is manifested as mild confusion, somnolence, agitation, or hallucinations. Memory and alertness are frequently preserved but psychosis may occur.[47] While postcardiotomy delirium is usually self-limiting, it may put the patient at increased risk for self-injury and prolonged hospitalization. Haloperidol is often used for sedation.

Late Postoperative Complications

After the fourth postoperative day, most cardiac surgery patients have short, uncomplicated hospital stays and are discharged to home. However, postpericardiotomy syndrome, cardiac tamponade, or incisional wound infection may occur during the last postoperative period.

Postpericardiotomy syndrome occurs when traumatized tissue in the pericardial cavity triggers an autoimmune response. Postpericardiotomy syndrome usually occurs weeks to months after surgery and results from inflammation of the pleura and pericardium causes aching pericardial pain and severe pleuritic pain. Pleural and pericardial effusions may accompany the inflammation. Treatment is with ibuprofen, indomethacin, or a brief course of prednisone. Large or symptomatic pleural effusions should be drained by thoracentesis (Fig. 25-6).

Late cardiac tamponade may occur several days to weeks after surgery and is seen more frequently in patients on warfarin or other anticoagulants. The incidence ranges from 0.5% to 2.0% of cardiac surgeries and late tamponade may be related or unrelated to postpericardiotomy syndrome.[34] While the clinical findings of tachycardia, decreased cardiac output, and enlarged cardiac silhouette may be present, late tamponade may present with patient symptoms of increasing shortness of breath, decreased exercise tolerance, and near syncope. Late tamponade is most often treated with pericardiocentesis.

Wound infection after CABG surgery occurs despite perioperative antibiotics and aseptic technique. Sternal wound infections typically present 4 to 14 days after surgery with fever, leukocytosis, and inflammatory wound with purulent drainage. Sternal wounds are often associated with a sternal click and sternal instability. Staphylococci, both *Staphylococcus aureus* and coagulase-negative staphylococcus, are the most common causative organism.[49] Superficial chest wounds are treated with antibiotics and local drainage. Deep sternal wounds and mediastinitis are treated with surgical débridement and closure or plastic surgical closure with muscle flap. The incidence of deep sternal infections range from 0.25% to 4% and the superficial sternal wound infections are seen in 2% to 6% after cardiac surgery, both of which prolong care and increase cost.[29] Infections at the venectomy donor sites may also occur and are usually treatable with oral antibiotics, but severe infections may require open drainage and intravenous antibiotics.

CARDIAC TRANSPLANTATION

Cardiac transplantation is an accepted therapy for end-stage heart disease. Impressive improvements in survival, refinement of immunosuppressive therapy, and improvements in monitoring techniques have prompted many new centers to initiate cardiac transplantation programs. Worldwide, 76,538 heart transplantations have been performed, with 3,040 performed in June of 2005 to June of 2006.[50] The 1-year actuarial survival rate for patients

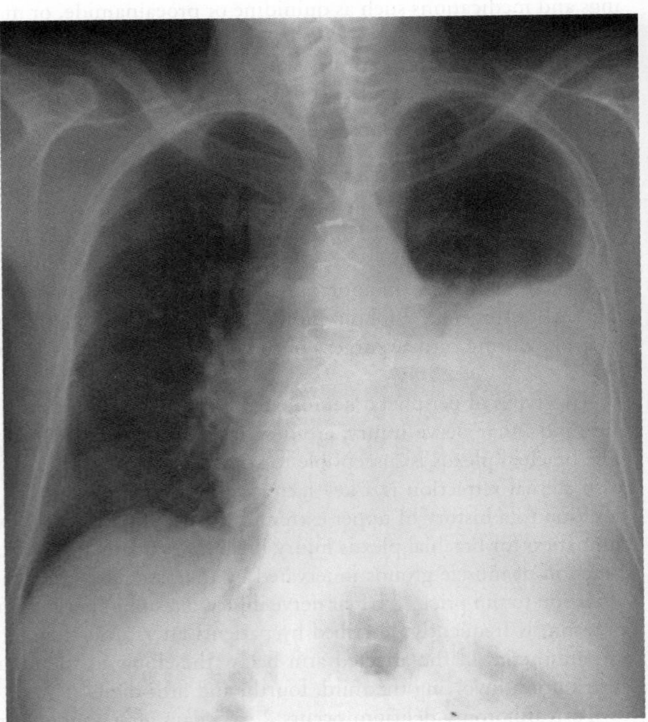
A

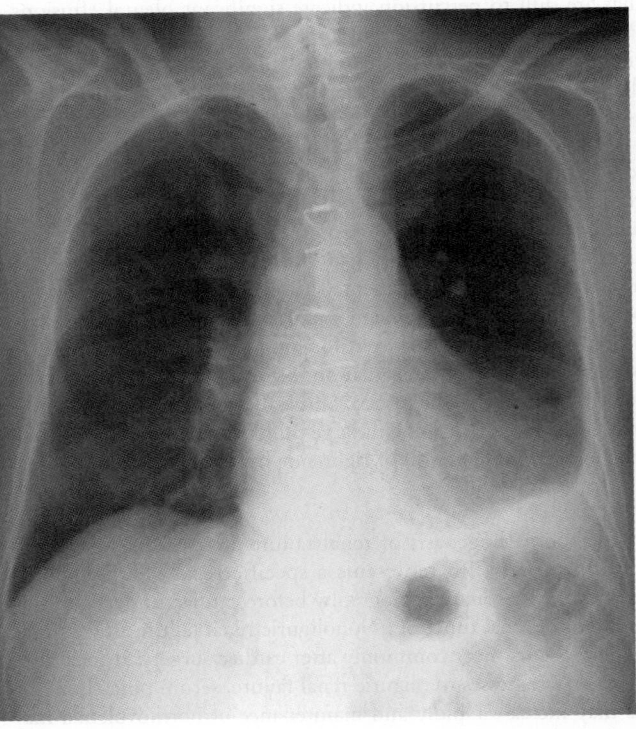
B

Figure 25-6 Left pleural effusion after coronary bypass surgery. (A) Chest radiograph shows large pleural effusion obscuring the left heart border. (B) Chest radiograph film shows decrease in effusion after 1,500 mL of serosanguineous fluid was aspirated by thoracentesis.

after heart transplantation is 87%, the 5-year survival rate is 71%, and the 10-year survival rate is 52%.[50] These figures represent patients who underwent transplantation from 1987 to 2006. This section outlines expectations, therapeutic treatment regimes, and a plan of nursing care.

Progress in Cardiac Transplantation

One-year survival rates after cardiac transplantation have improved from 22% in 1968 to more than 87% in 2006.[50] In 1974, major changes in survival were attributed to the introduction of the endomyocardial biopsy technique for monitoring rejection, to the treatment of rejection, and to the introduction of polyclonal antibodies. Survival results took another upward leap after the introduction of cyclosporine therapy in 1980. We are now benefiting from better prevention, diagnosis, and management of rejection and the complications of immunosuppressive therapy.

The calcinurin inhibitors, cyclosporine and tacrolimus, are the most effective immunosuppressant drugs available and are capable of specific immunosuppressant activity to control rejection without totally suppressing the body's ability to fight infection.[51,52] Cyclosporine contributed to an approximate 20% increase in 1-year patient survival in the early 1980s. This increase is caused in large part by cyclosporine's superior ability selectively to inhibit T-cell proliferation and reduce the incidence of rejection.

Improved survival has led to alterations in patient selection criteria with respect to age. Other selection criteria have changed little since the earlier years of cardiac transplantation. Before the introduction of cyclosporine therapy, an upper age limit of 50 years and a lower age limit of adult-sized adolescence were followed. Earlier data indicated that patients older than age 50 years did not tolerate immunosuppression and had poorer survival.[53] Because calcinurin inhibitors do not totally suppress the entire immune system, older patients are considered for transplantation. The general trend is to define the upper age limit as 60 to 65 years. The current age range is from newborn to 75.3 years, with a mean age of 45 years.[50] Before 1980, children younger than 10 years of age were not considered to be transplantation candidates. This criterion was reevaluated. Before 1980, each year, fewer than five children (18 years of age or younger) underwent heart transplantation. In 2006 to 2007, 102 transplantations were performed in children from newborn to 1 year of age, and 242 transplantations were performed in children between 1 and 18 years of age.[54] Actuarial 1-year survival for pediatric patients less than 1 year is 80% and around 90% for children 1 to 17 years. The primary causes of death for patients surviving greater than 1 year are coronary vasculopathy, acute rejection, and malignancy (including lymphoma).[54]

Distant organ procurement enables transplantation centers to increase the number of transplantations performed. A surgical team can be dispatched from the transplantation center and can travel up to 500 miles to retrieve the needed heart. An ischemic time of up to 4 hours is considered acceptable. This allowable ischemic time permits an approximate travel time of 2.5 hours, with the remaining time required to implant the heart into the patient. Greater public awareness and media attention focused on the need for donors have also contributed to an increase in the available donor pool and transplantation activity. Legislation in some states requires that a family of a potentially eligible donor be asked if that person wished organ donation. However, the limiting factor in solid organ transplantation continues to be organ donation. The success of heart transplantation has created an ever-increasing gap between the number of transplantation candidates and usable heart donors. In March 2008, there were 2,656 patients waiting for a heart donor and 2,210 transplantations in the United States from January 1, 2007 to January 1, 2008.[55] Transplant centers and organ procurement organizations work together to promote organ donation by providing public and health care professional education.[56]

With a greater number of centers involved in transplantation and listing potential recipients in organ registries, the average wait for a donor heart has increased dramatically. As a result, the patients often become sicker while waiting. Because of the increasingly sophisticated management of the patient with heart failure, the use of β-blockers to produce hemodynamic and symptomatic improvement, and the pressure for transplant physicians to manage patients on an outpatient basis, patients are put on an acuity scale (status) of need that includes strict definitions of illness. Medical review boards are used to monitor transplant centers listing criteria.

Evaluation of Recipients

Candidates for cardiac transplantation should have severe functional limitation and poor life expectancy from their heart disease. The candidates should be without the established contraindications or usual exclusions. The most frequent medical diagnoses of these patients are cardiomyopathy of various origins (idiopathic, viral, or valvular) and ischemic heart disease.[57] Candidate criteria have been established for use in the evaluation process to identify patients most likely to benefit from the operation. Table 25-2 outlines contraindications to cardiac transplantation.

Pediatric patients who may benefit from cardiac transplantation include those with cardiomyopathy and those with structural heart disease without severe pulmonary vascular disease.[58] These patients might have been treated surgically initially, but progressive, severe ventricular dysfunction or progressive pulmonary vascular disease limits further therapeutic options. A child with severe pulmonary vascular disease is not a cardiac transplant candidate because of the likelihood of irreversible right ventricular failure after transplantation. Pediatric transplantation has been at a plateau since the early nineties. Neonatal transplantation is performed on a smaller scale. In 2007, 102 children younger than age 1 year underwent transplantation; less than 1% of this donor population cause of death was from sudden infant death syndrome.[55] Once a child reaches late adolescence, it becomes feasible to use adult donor hearts, and organ procurement is no more difficult than it is with adults. However, there has been a trend over the past 10 years to transplant pediatric donor hearts into children because the allocation policy gives preference for the pediatric recipient to receive the pediatric donor organ.[59]

As previously indicated, the potential transplant recipient must not have fixed irreversible pulmonary hypertension, which is defined as a pulmonary vascular resistance greater than 6 to 8 Wood units. The presence of severe pulmonary hypertension would result in certain right ventricular failure in a newly transplanted heart. The transplanted heart is developed normally and not accustomed to pumping against such elevated pressures. Irreversible hepatic and renal failure also may preclude transplantation. Some dysfunction may exist, but this should be because of the patient's low cardiac output and is expected to reverse with replacement with a healthy heart. Cyclosporine, tacrolimus, and mycophenolate

Table 25-2 ■ CONTRAINDICATIONS TO CARDIAC TRANSPLANTATION

Condition	Rationale
Age older than 70 years	Older patients do not tolerate immunosuppression well, and poor survival is likely.
Severe pulmonary vascular hypertension: PVR >5 wood units PA systolic pressure >50 to 60 mm Hg	Normal transplanted right ventricle fails when faced with acute, severe increase in workload.
Irreversible end-organ failure	Organs are damaged further by immunosuppressive therapy; poor survival is likely.
Active or recent malignancy, severe peripheral, or cerebrovascular disease	These conditions limit long-term survival.
Diabetes Mellitus with: End-organ damage (neuropathy, nephropathy, retinopathy) Poor glycemic control (HbA1c >7.5)	Conditions are exacerbated by steroid therapy. Diabetic patients are prone to poor wound healing and may be more prone to infection.
Active infection	Infection is exacerbated by immunosuppression; poor risk for survival.
Potential sites of infection (recent pulmonary infarction, embolus, open wounds)	High risk of infection.
History of substance abuse that resulted in previous noncompliance with a medical regime or interfered with work performance or family relationships. Careful individual evaluation indicated.	A history of poor compliance and disruption of work and family relationships may indicate the patient is at high risk for future noncompliance. This may not be a contraindication if patient has successfully recovered from previous substance abuse problem.

mofetil may have untoward side effects on renal and hepatic functions. Irreversible failure in either organ limits the possibility of survival.

Other systemic conditions that contraindicate transplantation include malignancy, severe peripheral disease, or severe cerebrovascular disease. Insulin-dependent diabetes does not appear to effect outcome and does not contraindicate transplantation unless associated with severe end-organ disease.[60] Patients with mild diabetes may be candidates. Most centers also view cured (no evidence of disease for more than 5 years), nonmetastatic malignancies as a relative contraindication.[61] All these conditions may limit long-term survival, and the required steroid therapy would exacerbate insulin-dependent diabetes. Any active infection would progress rapidly after immunosuppression; patients with active infection are excluded for that reason, until proven free of infection. Any patient with a condition that places him or her at high risk for infection is also excluded. Because the lungs are the most frequent site of infections, patients who had a recent pulmonary infarction or embolus are excluded until these conditions resolve.

Donor Characteristics

It is widely recognized that pronouncement of death can be based on neurologic criteria.[62] People who have sustained complete and irreversible destruction of the brain, and have met the criteria for brain death may become heart donors. The most common causes of brain death among heart donors are blunt head trauma, gunshot wounds, intracerebral hemorrhage, and cerebral anoxia. Donors are typically men younger than 34 years of age. Donor age ranges from newborn to 70 years of age, with the average being 26.7 years. Seventy percent of donors are men.[55] Male heart donors may be considered up to the age of 40 to 45 years, however older donors are considered based on need, negative cardiac history, negative echocardiogram, and/or negative preprocurement coronary angiography.[63]

Nurses play an important role in managing the care of heart donors. Once brain death has occurred, hemodynamic instability potentially can develop in donors because of several factors. Hypotension in a donor may be caused by multiple contributing clinical conditions. Pre-existing fluid deficits may be present in donors who were treated with diuretics to decrease cerebral edema and may precipitate hypotension. In addition, with the death of the brainstem and loss of the vasomotor center, vascular tone is lost, resulting in vascular dilatation and subsequent hypotension. It is crucial to restore intravascular volume to avoid serious hypotension. With loss of pituitary function, antidiuretic hormone secretion ceases. This change contributes to the development of diabetes insipidus and subsequent decreased intravascular volume. After correcting intravascular volume deficits with fluid administration, vasomotor tone may be supported with a vasopressor agent. Dopamine hydrochloride is used most often because of its property of renovascular dilatation and its beneficial effects on renal perfusion. Diabetes insipidus is treated with aqueous vasopressin, which increases reabsorption of water by the renal tubules.

Donor heart allocation oversight is done by the United National Organ Sharing (UNOS), a contracted organization that manages the sharing arrangement and agreement of solid organ allocation under the Department of Health and Human Services. Thoracic organs are allocated locally first, then within zones in a sequence of delineated circles with the donor hospital at the center. Allocation is done by blood type, weight and size, time on list, and acuity.

Surgical Procedure

Once accepted into a transplantation program, the recipient must wait for the donor heart. A residence close to the hospital is required. Recipients often carry telepagers or beepers, and are "on call" for a donor heart. When a donor is available, the recipient is admitted rapidly to the hospital and prepared for surgery. Because little time is available for preoperative teaching and preparation for the recovery process, the major portion of that is performed during the initial candidacy evaluation and during the process of informed consent.

Donor and recipient are matched by ABO blood group, weight, and body size. Lymphocyte crossmatch is necessary for those recipients whose lymphocytes react to crossmatch testing (performed when recipients are accepted as transplantation candidates) against standard pools of lymphocytes from multiple serum donors. This result is reported in a percentage of panel reactive antibody (% PRA). Patients with a known positive reaction, a positive PRA for example of 50%, will have additional HLA testing to identify those specific circulating antibodies. These candidates are identified as "sensitized" such that the candidates antibodies could react to certain donor cell antigens and result in antibody-mediated rejection. Therapies are available to reduce these antibodies.

The original surgical technique for orthotopic heart transplantation described by Shumway et al.[64] has remained the standard procedure. After a median sternotomy and the initiation of CPB, the recipient's heart is removed, leaving the posterior walls of the atria intact (Fig. 25-7). The inflows of the two venae cavae and the pulmonary veins are left in place and unaltered. Both the aorta and pulmonary artery are transected. Then the atrial walls of the donor heart are anastomosed to the recipient atria, with care taken to avoid injury to the donor heart's sinus node. After atrial anastomosis, the donor pulmonary artery and aorta are anastomosed to the recipient vessels. On completion of the procedure, temporary epicardial atrial and frequently ventricular pacing wires are placed. Before closing the chest, mediastinal drainage tubes are secured as with any cardiac surgical procedure.

An alternative technique is referred to as total orthotopic heart transplantation or the bicaval and pulmonary venous anastomosis. The basic features of the bicaval method are complete excision of the recipient atria and donor heart implantation with bicaval end-to-end anastomosis. Proponents of this technique cite the potential for more synchronous atrial contraction, and reduction of pacemaker implantation and atrioventricular valve regurgitation.[65]

Medical Management

In the immediate postoperative period, postoperative care is similar to that of any cardiac surgical patient. Transplant recipients are intubated and mechanically ventilated for 12 to 24 hours and require hemodynamic stabilization. Differences in care revolve around the patient's likely debilitated preoperative status, potential manifestations of ischemia in the donor heart, potential cardiac rejection, and immunosuppression.

Impact of Preoperative Status

Cardiac transplant recipients were in chronic low cardiac output states before transplantation surgery. They likely had poor nutritional status and were relatively immobile. Many were hospitalized

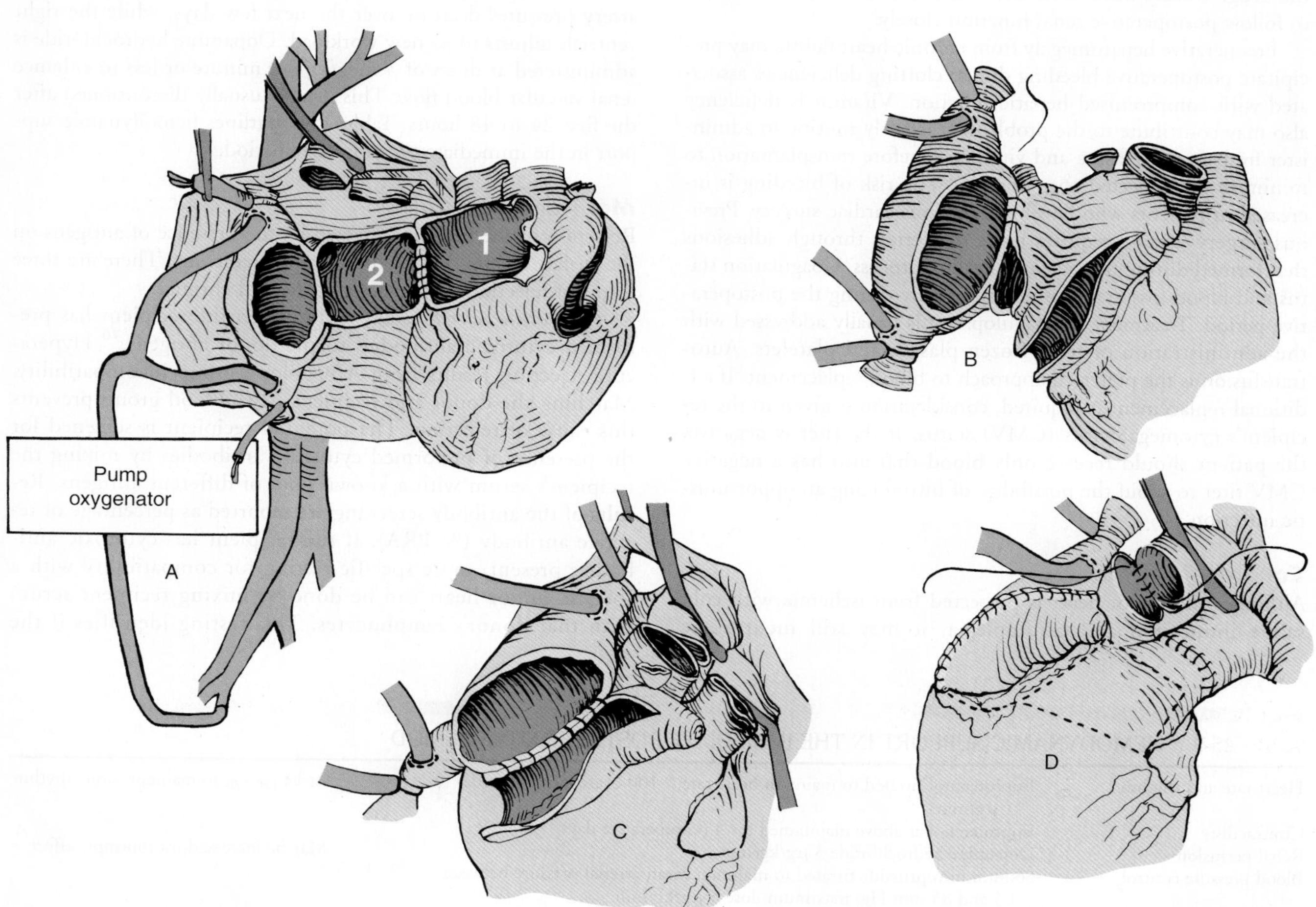

■ **Figure 25-7** (A) Cardiac transplantation begins by suturing the donor left atrium (1) to the posterior wall of the recipient left atrium (2). (B) The intra-atrial septa are anastomosed, followed by (C) anastomosis of the right atrial wall. (D) The final step is the anastomosis of the donor and recipient great vessels. (Adapted from Cooley, D. A., & Norman, J. L. [1975]. *Techniques in cardiac surgery* [p. 220]. Houston: Texas Medical Press.)

with an acute exacerbation of heart failure and, in some cases, cardiogenic shock. Maintenance of adequate nutrition during the preoperative phase is difficult because of the anorexia, nausea, and impaired digestion and absorption associated with serious cardiac failure.

After transplantation, interventions to improve nutritional status are important because the patient is immunosuppressed. Postoperative basal metabolic requirements are increased at the same time corticosteroid therapy is accelerating protein catabolism. Maintaining adequate nutrition is important to minimize postoperative complications and to facilitate recovery and rehabilitation.[66] Diet becomes an important factor in minimizing some of the side effects of corticosteroid therapy.[67] Diet can be supplemented with hyperalimentation and intravenous lipid preparations in sicker patients.

Preoperative cardiac failure potentially contributes to postoperative renal and hepatic dysfunctions as a result of the chronic low cardiac output state. Elevated serum creatinine levels are evidence of renal dysfunction. Because cyclosporine and tacrolimus may induce nephrotoxicity, careful attention must be given to monitoring renal status. An elevated preoperative serum creatinine may be an indication to reduce cyclosporine/tacrolimus dosage or even delay by a few days postoperative administration of the drug. Weekly urine creatinine clearance tests may be ordered to follow postoperative renal function closely.

Preoperative hepatomegaly from chronic heart failure may precipitate postoperative bleeding due to clotting deficiencies associated with compromised hepatic function. Vitamin K deficiency also may contribute to the problem. It is fairly routine to administer fresh-frozen plasma and vitamin K before transplantation to minimize the expected coagulopathy. The risk of bleeding is increased in patients who have had previous cardiac surgery. Previous surgery usually requires more dissection through adhesions that formed during the previous healing process. Coagulation status and blood loss are monitored carefully during the postoperative period. Treatment of coagulopathy is usually addressed with the administration of fresh-frozen plasma and platelets. Autotransfusion is the preferred approach to blood replacement. If additional replacement is required, consideration is given to the recipient's cytomegalovirus (CMV) status. If the titer is negative, the patient should receive only blood that also has a negative CMV titer to avoid the possibility of introducing an opportunistic infection.

Cardiac Function

Although the donor heart is protected from ischemia with cold saline immersion and cardioplegia, it may still incur some ischemia that is evident during the immediate postoperative period. The transplanted heart benefits from pharmacologic β-receptor stimulation in the early postoperative period. Isoproterenol is used routinely for up to 4 days to augment contractility, atrioventricular conduction, and heart rate. The denervated heart cannot respond to the autonomic nervous system and depends on circulating catecholamines. Atrial pacing is now commonly used to support heart rate and dopamine is used to support contractility. Underlying bradycardia and junctional rhythms are not uncommon during this time. Because node dysfunction can occur as a result of injury during procurement, surgery, or distortion of the atria with transplantation, or it may be acquired as the result of cardiac rejection.[68] Temporary atrial pacing may also be used for arrhythmia issues during the immediate postoperative period. Once the heart has recovered from the trauma of surgery, a normal intrinsic donor heart rate of approximately 95 to 110 beats/min becomes evident. Sinus node dysfunction is common, and 6% to 10% of patients may require permanent pacemaker implantation.[69]

Blood pressure control with sodium nitroprusside therapy is usually required for the first 24 to 48 hours after surgery. In patients with high preoperative pulmonary artery pressures, inhaled nitric oxide therapy may be used to dilate the pulmonary vascular bed and reduce afterload in the graft right ventricle. Pulmonary artery pressures decrease over the next few days, while the right ventricle adjusts to its new workload. Dopamine hydrochloride is administered at doses of 3 mcg/kg per minute or less to enhance renal vascular blood flow. This drug is usually discontinued after the first 24 to 48 hours. Table 25-3 outlines hemodynamic support in the immediate postoperative period.

Monitoring Rejection

Rejection of the heart is triggered by the presence of antigens on the surface of the cells of the transplanted heart. There are three forms of rejection: hyperacute, acute, and chronic.

Hyperacute rejection may occur when the recipient has preformed cytotoxic antibodies to the donor antigens.[70] Hyperacute rejection results from ABO blood group incompatibility. Matching the donor and recipient ABO blood group prevents this cause of rejection. The potential recipient is screened for the presence of preformed cytotoxic antibodies by mixing the recipient's serum with a known pool of different antigens. Results of the antibody screening are reported as percentage of reactive antibody (% PRA). If the recipient has cytotoxic antibodies present, more specific testing for compatibility with a specific donor heart can be done by mixing recipient serum with that donor's lymphocytes. This testing identifies if the

Table 25-3 ■ HEMODYNAMIC SUPPORT IN THE IMMEDIATE POSTOPERATIVE PERIOD

Heart rate and rhythm	Isoproterenol titrated to maintain heart rate >100 beats/min; range 0.5 to 1 μg/min	Atrial pacing to maintain sinus rhythm
Contractility	Isoproterenol as above maintained for 4 postoperative days	
Renal perfusion	Dopamine hydrochloride 3 μg/kg/min	May be increased for inotropic effect
Blood pressure control	Sodium nitroprusside titrated to maintain mean arterial pressure between 65 and 85 mm Hg; maximum dose 5 μg/kg/min	
Volume therapy	Normal saline, plasma expanders, or blood products to maintain central venous pressure 8 to 12 mm Hg	
Pulmonary vasodilation	Prostaglandin E_1 used for elevated pulmonary vascular resistance or long donor ischemic times associated with right ventricular dysfunction	

potential recipient has cytotoxic antibodies that will react to that specific donor heart.

Acute rejection is the most frequently occurring form of rejection and is a major cause of death within the first year after transplantation.[54] Preoperative immunosuppressive therapy is begun for prevention of acute cardiac rejection. Routine monitoring for acute rejection is centered around endomyocardial biopsy. With cyclosporine/tacrolimus therapy, there are few clinically evident signs and symptoms of acute rejection. The objective is to detect acute rejection in its early stages at a time when the process can be reversed, thus preventing serious, permanent damage to the new heart. Therefore, biopsy remains the gold standard for monitoring and early detection of acute rejection. Because acute rejection is expected to occur during the first 3 months after surgery, biopsy is performed within the first 14 days after transplantation, and then up to once per week during this crucial time interval. Any time that rejection is detected, biopsies are performed frequently to monitor the progress of antirejection treatment. By 1 month, the biopsy schedule is tapered to every other week, then once per month after the third month. Patients are then monitored indefinitely by biopsy every 4 months to annually, depending on the transplant center. Many centers stop biopsy surveillance 5 years posttransplant, unless clinically indicated.

The biopsy procedure is routinely performed in the catheterization laboratory but may be performed in the operating room or echocardiography laboratory. It can be performed in 15 to 30 minutes and requires only local anesthesia. Figure 25-8 illustrates the technique of endocardial specimen retrieval from the right ventricle. A standardized cardiac biopsy grading scale was revised in 2004. Mild rejection may resolve spontaneously and is often not treated. It is characterized by endocardial and interstitial infiltrate, International Society of Heart and Lung Transplantation (ISHLT) grade 1R (old scales 1A, 1B, and 2). Moderate rejection is characterized by the presence of myocyte necrosis and perivascular, endocardial, and interstitial infiltration of immunoblasts ISHLT grade 2R (old scale 3A). Severe rejection results in myocyte and vascular necrosis with hemorrhage and a mixed infiltrate of immunoblasts and neutrophils ISHLT grade 3R (old scales 3B and 4).[71] Resolving rejection is evidenced by active fibrosis, which represents reparative changes. Table 25-4 outlines the heart biopsy grading system adopted by the ISHLT in 1990,[72] and revised in 2005. Treatment of rejection depends on the grade of rejection, length of time from transplantation, clinical findings, symptoms, and the presence or absence of hemodynamic compromise.

Table 25-4 ■ INTERNATIONAL SOCIETY OF HEART AND LUNG TRANSPLANTATION STANDARD GRADING OF CARDIAC REJECTION

Revised Grade (2004)	Old Grade	Nomenclature
0R	0	No rejection
1R	1	A, Focal, mild
		B, Diffuse, mild
	2	One aggressive infiltrate, focal moderate
2R	3	A, Multifocal aggressive, moderate
3R		B, Diffuse inflammatory process
	4	Diffuse, aggressive, with necrosis, severe acute rejection

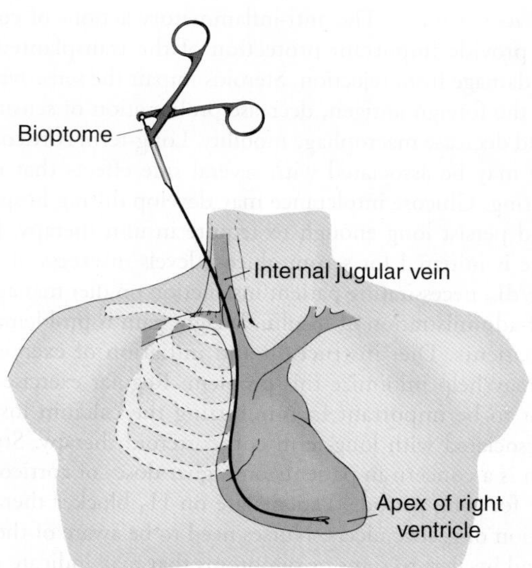

■ **Figure 25-8** To perform a biopsy, a bioptome is introduced by way of the internal jugular vein and advanced to the right ventricular apex, where several pieces of tissue are retrieved for analysis.

An alternative strategy in detecting rejection is gene expression profiling. Gene expression profiling uses a quantitative polymerase chain reaction test that measures the expression of genes associated with cardiac allograft rejection in peripheral mononuclear cells. It has a high-negative predictive value and may be useful to identify low-risk patients who can be safely managed without routine invasive endomyocardial biopsy.[73] The blood test is used in conjuction with echocardiograpy and physical exam for rejection assessment. Treatment of moderate to high acute cellular rejection is usually treated with high dose methylprednisolone (500 to 1000 mg) for 3 days with or without cytolitic therapy depending on the degree of cardiac dysfunction.

Humoral rejection or antibody-mediated rejection is an uncommon form of rejection that is caused by antibody and complement accumulation in the tissue and blood. It is confimed by evidence of graft dysfunction, features in the heart biopsy, which include myocardial capillary swelling with or without a positive immunofluorescence staining (+C4d). Antibody-mediated rejection can occur days to years after transplant, although it is more frequently seen in the first 6 months. It is associated with a high mortality rate and is a strong risk factor for the development of accelerated transplant vasculopathy.[74,75]

Cardiac allograft vasculopathy (CAV) also referred to as accelerated graft CHD, graft atherosclerosis, or chronic rejection, may be present in up to 50% of patients 5 years after transplantation.[76] (See "complications" section.)

Monitoring for Infection

Infection is an ever-present threat to the immunosuppressed cardiac transplant recipient and is almost inevitable at some point during the postoperative course. It is a major cause of morbidity and mortality.[61,77] Patients on multiple immunosuppressants at high doses are at greater risk. Bacterial infections are the most common form of infection. Fungal, viral, and protozoan infections are the most difficult to treat. Prophylactic regimes have been shown to be effective in transplant recipients to prevent or attenuate opportunistic infections. Trimethoprim–sulfamethoxazole is used against *Pneumocystis carinii*. CMV prophylaxisis includes intravenous ganciclovir postoperatively for several days then oral ganciclovir for 6 weeks up to a year to atenuate activation or reactivation. In addition, hyperimmune globulin (CMVIG) may be used in high risk patients who are CMV sero-negative recipients of a seropositive donor.[61,78] In addition, antifungal mouth losengers are used to prevent oral candidiasis, some centers have patients take oral antifungals to help prevent aspirgillious infections.

Hand washing and universal precautions are used as the mainstays of protection in the hospitalized patient. Infection is monitored for closely. Because the lungs are the primary site of infection, daily chest radiographs are performed immediately after surgery as well as chest auscultation are performed every 4 hours. Good pulmonary assessment is extremely important. Incentive spirometry, early mobility, and coughing and deep breathing are used to minimize atelectasis and possible infection. A temperature rise over 37°C, changes on the chest radiograph, or development of a cough are indications for obtaining sputum cultures. A temperature increase more than 38°C is an indication for blood cultures. Otherwise, routine laboratory screening for infection is performed on a weekly basis, except white blood cell counts, which are performed daily.

Monitoring for Immunosuppressive Drug Side Effects

Specific adverse effects and clinical manifestations of common immunosuppressive drugs are outlined in Table 25-5. Several side effects have implications for patient teaching and coaching and warrant further discussion. Nurses play a key role in providing patients with knowledge of drug side effects and methods of self-monitoring. It is important that patients are able to detect problems that can be injurious to their health and know when to seek medical attention. A knowledgeable patient also can take steps to minimize some of these problems. Some of the drug side effects may be particularly emotionally troublesome for patients. Nurses can do much to prepare them for this and assist them with strategies for coping with these side effects.

Calcineurin Inhibitors

Cyclosporine. Cyclosporine (Sandimmune, Neoral, Gengraf, Eon) is a natural metabolite found in a fungus. It is a lymphokine-synthesis inhibitor that profoundly inhibits cell-mediated immunity. It also impairs interleukin secretion by macrophages. Cyclosporine selectively interferes in the immune system, specifically targeting T cells; this specificity allows the body to retain some ability to protect itself from infection.[51,52] The drug must be used cautiously and monitored closely. Cyclosporine is nephrotoxic, leading to a decrease in glomerular filtration rate, renal plasma, and blood flow.[79,80] Calcineurin inhibitor-induced arterial hypertension has been reported to be as high as 100% and is a difficult problem to control in the long-term survivor.[81] It is important to maintain a consistent administration time for cyclosporine. Equally important is timely acquisition of blood specimens for cyclosporine levels after the last dose of the drug. Cyclosporine and tacrolimus has numerous drug interactions with common medications. Cyclosporine and tacrolimus are metabolized by the cytochrome P-450 system, so drugs that affect the P-450 system alter the metabolism of these drugs.[82] It is extremely important for nurses to know most of these interactions to avoid adverse side effects, in addition to understanding the pharmacology of calcineurin inhibitors. Patients are taught to take this drug after meals to decrease the possibility of gastrointestinal intolerance and to promote absorption.

Hypertension is a serious side effect that often is difficult to control. Patients need to monitor their hypertension and should be taught how to take an accurate blood pressure. They are also sent home with an understanding of what symptoms, such as headaches, may indicate their hypertension has become uncontrolled.

Cyclosporine therapy does result in changed bodily appearance, particularly diffuse increased hair growth. Changed bodily appearance was reported in 34% of 44 patients on cyclosporine and corticosteroid protocols.[83] Excessive hair growth was reported in 45% of the patients. Nurses can coach patients to prepare for this side effect and provide ideas for managing this problem. Cyclosporine can also cause neurotoxicity, and patients may exhibit tremors and report headache.

Tacrolimus. Tacrolimus (Prograf), formally referred to as FK506, is a potent immunosuppressive macrolide antibiotic. Tacrolimus acts by inhibition of the earliest steps of T-cell activation in a manner similar to that of cyclosporine. It was initially used in liver and kidney transplantation with successful results, and it is now used as a frequent alternative to cyclosporine. It is used as an effective agent for rescue therapy in refractory cardiac rejection and as a primary immunosuppressant in many centers.[84]

Tacrolimus has demonstrated that it is well tolerated in general. It is nephrotoxic, as is cyclosporine, and has a slightly higher diabetogenic effect. Tacrolimus does not cause hirsutism, gingival hyperplasia, or facial dysmorphism as cyclosporine can. Its primary side effects are headache, nausea, and tremors. It is important to monitor patient blood levels, kidney function, and blood glucose. Tacrolimus is also similar to cyclosporine in that it is metabolized through the P-450 system; therefore, similar drug interactions are present.[82]

Corticosteroids. The anti-inflammatory actions of corticosteroids provide important protection of the transplanted heart against damage from rejection. Steroids impair the sensitivity of T cells to the foreign antigen, decrease proliferation of sensitized T cells, and decrease macrophage mobility. Long-term corticosteroid therapy may be associated with several side effects that require monitoring. Glucose intolerance may develop during hospitalization and persist long enough to require insulin therapy. Insulin coverage is initiated for serum glucose levels in excess of 200 to 250 mg/dL, necessitating patient instruction on diet management and self-administration of insulin. Weight gain is problematic for many patients. Diet instruction and initiation of exercise programs may help minimize this problem. Regular exercise is also thought to be important in minimizing the calcium loss from bone associated with long-term corticosteroid therapy. Stress ulceration is a concern in patients on higher doses of corticosteroid therapy for long periods. Patients are on H_2 blocker therapy for prevention of gastric ulcers. Nurses need to be aware of the possibility and be alert to signs or symptoms that may indicate a problem. It is also necessary to teach the importance of good skin care. Fragile skin that heals poorly may become a problem with the long-term patient. Patients should be taught to monitor the

Table 25-5 ■ MAJOR ADVERSE SIDE EFFECTS OF IMMUNOSUPPRESSIVE AGENTS AND CLINICAL MANIFESTATIONS

Drug	Adverse Effects	Clinical Manifestations
Cyclosporine	Nephrotoxicity	Elevated BUN and creatinine.
		Decreased urine output
		Weight gain, edema
	Hypertension	Elevated blood pressure
	Hepatotoxicity	Elevated bilirubin
		Elevated alkaline phosphatase, AST, and ALT levels
		Jaundice
	Hypertrichosis	Excessive hair growth all over body
	Tremors, seizures	Fine motor tremors, especially hands
		Associated paresthesias
		Seizure activity
	Increased risk of malignancy when associated with high doses of multiple agents	Dependent on type and location of malignancy
	Gingival hyperplasia	Growth of gums over teeth
		Bleeding of gums
Tacrolimus	Nephrotoxicity associated with high doses	Elevated BUN and creatinine
		Decreased urine output
	Hyperkalemia	Elevated potassium levels
	Insomnia	Sleep disturbances
	Malaise	Headaches, nausea, and vomiting associated with IV administration
	Hyperglycemia	Elevated serum glucose
	Hypertension	Elevated blood pressure
Corticosteroids	Aseptic necrosis of bone, osteoporosis	Pain in weight-bearing joints
		Pathologic fractures
	Hyperglycemia, steroid-induced diabetes mellitus	Elevated serum glucose
		Polydipsia, polyuria
	Salt and water retention	Weight gain or fluctuations associated with edema
	Hypertension	Elevated blood pressure
	Skin alterations	
	Acne	Rash or pimples on face and trunk
	Sun sensitivity	Susceptibility to sunburn
		Skin malignancies
	Hirsutism	Excessive hair growth on face, trunk, and extremities
	Growth retardation in children	Failure to reach normal height for age
	Gastritis/gastrointestinal ulcerations	Abdominal pain, dysphagia
		Hematemesis, guaiac-positive stools
	Cataracts	Visual acuity problems
Azathioprine	Bone marrow depression	Leukopenia, thrombocytopenia, anemia
	Hepatotoxicity	Elevated bilirubin
		Elevated alkaline phosphatase, AST, and ALT levels
		Jaundice
	Increased risk of malignancy when associated with high doses of multiple agents	Dependent on type and location of malignancy
	Sun sensitivity of skin	Susceptibility to sunburn
		Skin malignancies
Orthocione OKT3	Pyrexia, malaise	Fever, chills, influenza-like symptoms
		Headache, diarrhea
	Respiratory distress associated with initial doses and fluid overload	Chest tightness, dyspnea, wheezing
	Increased risk of malignancy when associated with high doses of multiple agents	Dependent on type and location of malignancy
Antithymocyte preparations	Anaphylactic reactions	Hypotension, dyspnea, wheezing, fever, chills
	Serum sickness associated with antibody formation to foreign protein	Fever, joint pain
		Elevation of BUN and creatinine
	Bone marrow depression associated with prolonged use in conjunction with azathioprine	Leukopenia
		Thrombocytopenia
		Anemia
	Local inflammatory reactions associated with intramuscular administration	Pain, redness, extreme muscle soreness, swelling
	Increased risk of malignancy when associated with high doses of multiple agents	Dependent on type and location of malignancy
Mycophenolate mofetil	Bone marrow suppression	Neutropenia
	Gastrointestinal disturbance	Nausea, vomiting, diarrhea, constipation
	Malaise	Headache, nausea

(table continues on page 614)

Table 25-5 ■ MAJOR ADVERSE SIDE EFFECTS OF IMMUNOSUPPRESSIVE AGENTS AND CLINICAL MANIFESTATIONS (continued)

Drug	Adverse Effects	Clinical Manifestations
Rapammune	Bone marrow suppression	Anemia, thrombocytopenia
	Hypercholesteremia	Elevated serum cholesterol, elevated triglycerides
	Hyperlipidemia	Elevated serum lipid levels
	Hypertension	Elevated blood pressure
	Lower extremity edema	Swelling of lower extremites
	Interstitial pneumonitis	Crackles over lung fields, shortness of breath
	Oral ulcerations	Pain in and around mouth and lips

ALT, alanine aminotransferase; AST, aspartate aminotransferase; BUN, blood urea nitrogen.
From Urden, L. D., Stacy, K. M., & Lough, M. E. (Eds.). (2002). *Critical care nursing: Diagnosis and management* (4th ed., pp. 998–1001). St. Louis: Mosby; Micromedex Healthcare Series: Micromedex, Inc. Breenwood Village, CO (edition expires 9/03). Available: http://hcs.mdx.com (accessed April 2003); Luikart, H. (2001). Pediatric transplantation: Management issues. *Journal of Pediatric Nursing, 16*, 320–331.)

condition of their skin and be alert for lesions that do not heal well or that become infected.

Fragile skin and bruising were reported to occur often or always in up to 60% of patients on corticosteroid and azathioprine protocols. Changed facial and bodily appearance was reported by 43%. Poor vision, a problem associated with corticosteroid therapy, was "quite a bit" or "extremely" upsetting to 30% of patients.[83,85]

Mycophenolate Mofetil. Mycophenolate mofetil (CellCept) is an immunosuppressive agent that inhibits the de novo pathway of purine synthesis in activated lymphocytes. Mycophenolate mofetil works at a late stage in T-cell activation, in contrast to cyclosporine and tacrolimus, which inhibit the earliest events. Mycophenolate mofetil has been shown to have activity against B cells; therefore, it may have a role in preventing graft atherosclerosis.[82]

Multicenter trials have shown that mycophenolate mofetil is an effective immunosuppressant, safe and well tolerated in kidney and heart transplant recipients. It is less myelosuppressive than azathioprine, thereby avoiding the neutropenia and anemia, and less hepatotoxic as well. Its major side effects are gastrointestinal disturbances. Nausea, vomiting, and diarrhea are the most frequently reported symptoms. These symptoms are usually self-limiting and dose dependent.[53]

Sirolimus and Everolimus

Sirolimus. Sirolimus (Rapamune) and its derivative everolimus (Certican, Rad) is an antibiotic and in a class of drugs called mTOR (mammalian targets of rapamycin) inhibitors. Sirolimus prevents cell cycle activation and T-cell proliferation. Sirolimus and its derivatives may be synergistic with the calcineuron inhibitors. These drugs are dosed orally once or twice daily. Blood trough levels are measured for dose monitoring. Research studies suggest that rapamycin treatment may prevent or even reverse allograft vascular disease.[52] The common side effects of sirolimus are increased levels of triglycerides, decrease in hemoglobin and platelet counts, tremors, peripheral edema, arthralgias, and the potential for slow wound healing.[51]

Azathioprine. Azathioprine (Imuran) can be used as a maintenance drug to prevent activation and proliferation of T cells in response to the foreign antigen or the transplanted heart. It is an antimetabolite that interferes with purine synthesis. Purine synthesis is necessary for antibody production and for synthesis of nucleic acids in rapidly proliferating cells, such as the cells of the immune system.[86] Prevention of this cell proliferation can also impair other rapidly proliferating cells in the body and cause conditions such as leukopenia, thrombocytopenia, and anemia. It is important to monitor the patient's white blood cell count closely and to titrate the dose of the drug accordingly.

Antilymphocyte Antibodies

Orthoclone OKT3. Orthoclone OKT3 is a monoclonal antibody that is targeted to remove T cells from circulation through the formation of antigen–antibody complexes.[86] It can be used initially after transplantation as an induction agent to eliminate the T-cell response in the first 14 postoperative days, or can be used to treat a later rejection episode. Patients can acquire sensitivity to the drug and form antibodies against the foreign protein. For that reason, usually only one 5-day course of the drug is given. Adverse effects are caused by the massive lysis of T cells, resulting in general malaise, fever, and chills.

Antithymocyte Preparations. Thymoglobulin is rabbit γ immune globulin and is an antithymocyte preparation that uses antibodies produced by animals in response to foreign human T cells. They are polyclonal preparations pooled from multiple animals. These preparations are used as an induction therapy and to treat severe rejection after standard antirejection therapy has failed. Its possible mechanisms of action include T-cell clearance from the circulation and modulation of T-cell activation. The course of therapy is typically 2 to 5 days. As with orthoclone OKT3, adverse effects are associated with the massive lysis of T cells, causing fever and chills.[86] Although rare, patients can have anaphylactic reactions to the foreign animal protein.

Daclizumab and Basiliximab. Daclizumab and basiliximab are monoclonal antibodies used as induction agents. They are hybrid, humanized interleukin-2 receptor antibodies. The advantage of these agents is the minimal administration side effects that other monoclonal have exhibited, and the apparent usefulness in preventing early rejection.[51,52]

Complications

Hypertension

Hypertension is a long-term, ever-present complication that requires considerable attention. Hypertension is caused in large part

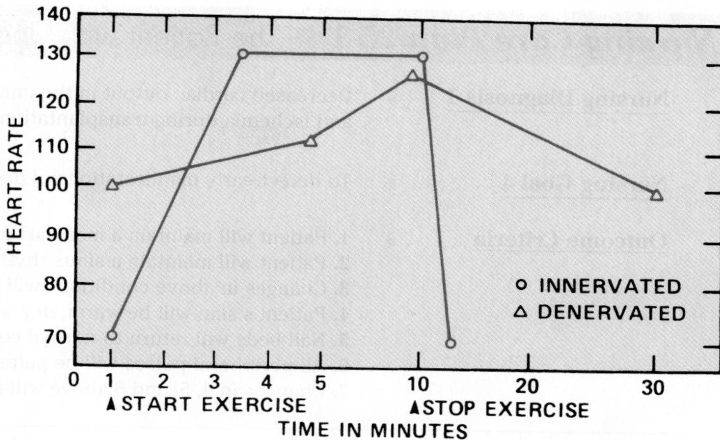

■ **Figure 25-9** Sample differences in response to exercise between an innervated and denervated heart. (From McKelvey, S. A. [1985]. Effects of denervation in the cardiac transplant recipient. In M. K. Douglas & J. A. Shinn [Eds.], *Advances in cardiovascular nursing* [p. 201]. Rockville, MD: Aspen Systems.)

by the calcineurin inhibitors that are known to cause chronic nephropathy; in addition, cyclosporine is implicated in the activation of the sympathetic nervous system, resulting in hypertension.[87] Patients are managed on one, two, or three agents because of the tenacity of the hypertension.

Transplant Vasculopathy

CAV is an accelerated and diffuse form of CHD unique to the transplanted heart. It is the major cause of death in the long-term heart transplant patient.[61] CAV is a peculiar kind of vasculopathy characterized by diffuse and concentric vascular inflammation and smooth muscle proliferation. It results in coronary lumen loss, ischemia, silent MI, and graft loss, which can present as a sudden death.[88] Treatment of CAV is limited because of the diffuse nature of the disease, and it is not typically amenable to usual palliative interventions such as angioplasty, atherectomy, or coronary artery bypass. Retransplantation is the only definitive treatment, and it is fraught with high morbidity and mortality rates, and brings fourth the debate regarding the use of limited donor supply.

Sexual Dysfunction

Sexual dysfunction is a prevalent problem in cardiac transplantation recipients. Impotence is not uncommon, and much of it can be attributed to the requirement for antihypertensive therapy. Patients would benefit from knowing that these occurrences are not uncommon. They need to feel comfortable voicing concerns and reporting future problems so that appropriate counseling or other assistance can be provided.

Conditioning and Exercise Training

Physical rehabilitation is a necessary part of the posttransplantation patient recovery program. Physical therapy is needed to ameliorate the deconditioning of the pretransplantation, heart failure state and to decrease the sequelae of the immunosuppressants and surgical procedure.[89] Low-level exercise is begun with extremity and shoulder flexion, extension, and abduction exercises. The intensity and duration are progressed to the patient's tolerance.[90] These low-level exercises serve as warm-up for more intensive exercises once the patient can complete the low-level program without undue fatigue or balance loss. Bicycle ergometry is usually introduced within 3 days. Intensity and duration are gradually progressed according to patient response. By discharge, most patients are able to cycle for 20 minutes without resistance and for 5 minutes with resistance. With cardiac denervation, heart rate response to exercise is abnormal.

The ability to perform any exercise beyond mild in intensity depends on circulating catecholamines to increase heart rate, contractility, and cardiac output. The normal, immediate increase in heart rate induced by exercise is absent in the denervated heart, and several minutes are required before heart rate can increase. Warm-up exercise is necessary before vigorous activity, and its duration should be approximately 5 minutes. Deceleration of heart rate after exercise is prolonged. The patient's heart rate may not return to resting levels for up to 20 minutes after cessation of the activity. Prolonged cool-down periods are also necessary. Figure 25-9 illustrates a typical response to exercise.

Patients need to understand how their response to exercise is different after transplantation. Self-monitoring techniques are taught before discharge, and continued regular exercise is encouraged. Patients are taught to use dyspnea as a guide for activity intensity rather than heart rate. The dyspnea index is presented in Table 25-6. Patients are coached not to exceed a dyspnea index greater than level 2. The rating of perceived exertion is a widely used self-monitoring tool for transplant recipient. The Borg scale is a rating of perceived exertion that is scaled from 6 (very, very

Table 25-6 ■ CARDIAC TRANSPLANT RECIPIENTS' DYSPNEA INDEX FOR EXERCISE TRAINING

Level 0	No shortness of breath Can count to 15 without taking a breath
Level 1	Mild shortness of breath Counts to 15 and requires one breath in the sequence: continue at this intensity
Level 2	Moderate shortness of breath counts to 15 and requires two breaths in the same sequence; this is the desired level of intensity
Level 3	Definite shortness of breath Must take three breaths in the sequence of counting to 15; reduce the intensity of exercise
Level 4	Severe shortness of breath Unable to count or speak; cease activity

Adapted with permission from Sadowsky, H. S., Rohrkemper, K. F., & Quon, S. (1986). *Rehabilitation of cardiac and cardiopulmonary recipients,* appendix 1. Stanford, CA: Stanford University Hospital.

Nursing Care Plan 25-1 ■ The Patient with Uncomplicated Cardiac Transplantation

Nursing Diagnosis 1 ➧ Decreased cardiac output in the immediate postoperative period related to cardiac denervation and ischemia during transplantation, manifested by bradycardia and hypotension.

Nursing Goal 1 ➧ To detect early manifestations of decreased cardiac output.

Outcome Criteria ➧

1. Patient will maintain a mean arterial blood pressure (MAP) between 70 and 90 mm Hg.
2. Patient will maintain a sinus rhythm with a heart rate (HR) of 100 to 110 beats/min.
3. Changes in above conditions will be detected within 20 minutes of occurrence.
4. Patient's skin will be warm, dry, and normal in color.
5. Nail beds will return to normal color after blanching from pressure over the capillary bed.
6. All peripheral pulses will be palpable. Urine output will be >30 mL/h.
7. Changes in 4, 5, and 6 above will be detected within an hour of occurrence.

NURSING INTERVENTIONS	RATIONALE
1. Assess and document MAP, HR, and rhythm continuously.	1. Required to detect changes.
2. Report any HR <100, loss of sinus rhythm, or MAP <70 mm Hg to physician.	2. An HR <100 may be considered bradycardic for the immediate postoperative transplantation period and may indicate the need for more isoproterenol support. Myocardial edema and manipulation of the heart during surgery increase the risk of bradycardia. Junctional rhythms occur at lesser degrees of bradycardia in the transplant recipient and loss of sinus rhythm may indicate the need for atrial pacing. Loss of blood pressure may be a result of bradycardia or loss of sinus rhythm.
3. Evaluate volume status; a central venous pressure (CVP) <8 mm Hg may indicate need for fluid. If MAP <60 mm Hg with an adequate CVP, hypotension may be a result of decreased contractility. Notify physician if these findings occur.	3. Hypotension also may be an indication of hypovolemia or a depressed inotropic state related to ischemia incurred during surgery and organ donation. Further evaluation is required.
4. Assess and document skin temperature, color, moisture, capillary filling, quality of peripheral pulses, and urine output hourly as needed. Report abnormal findings to physician.	4. Low cardiac output will be manifested by decreased peripheral perfusion and decreased renal vascular blood flow, resulting in decreased glomerular filtration and subsequent urine output.

Nursing Goal 2 ➧ To reduce or eliminate manifestations of decreased cardiac output specifically bradycardia or hypotension

Outcome Criteria ➧

1. Within 15 minutes of intervention, HR returns to >100 beats/min.
2. Within 15 minutes of intervention, MAP returns to >70 mm Hg.
3. Within 30 minutes of intervention, good peripheral pulses are present, skin is warm, dry, and of normal color.

NURSING INTERVENTIONS	RATIONALE
1. Connect pacing wires to a temporary pacemaker. Obtain an order for pacing support and appropriate settings. HR is usually maintained at 100 beats/min minimum.	1. Temporary pacing may be indicated to maintain an HR in the prescribed parameters.
2. Notify physician if a junctional rhythm develops and results in bradycardia or hypotension.	2. Sinus node function may be impaired due to myocardial edema in the area of the sinus node. Atrial pacing may be indicated.
3. Verify that CVP is between 8 and 12 mm Hg and administer ordered replacement fluid if CVP is below ordered minimum (usually <8 mm Hg).	3. Hypotension may be the result of hypovolemia: a denervated heart depends on a large stroke volume to stretch myocardial fibers (Starling mechanism) and produce a strong contraction.
4. Notify physician if hypotension does not respond to volume therapy or is present with an adequate CVP.	4. Hypotension may be the result of decreased contractility, and further inotropic support is needed.

Nursing Care Plan 25-1 (continued)

Nursing Diagnosis 2 ➧ Potential for infection related to immunosuppression manifested by a temperature >37.5°C, a rising white blood cell count, or a change in pulmonary secretions.

Nursing Goal 1 ➧ To prevent conditions and situations that predispose the patient to increased risk of infection.

Outcome Criteria ➧
1. Patient will maintain a temperature, 37°C.
2. Patient will maintain a white blood cell count between 5,000 and 10,000.
3. Patient will have normal breath sounds without cough and a clear chest radiograph.

NURSING INTERVENTIONS	RATIONALE
1. Maintain protective protocols and monitor protective technique of all visitors and staff entering the patient's room.	1. Poor technique may put the patient at risk for infection by organisms carried in the room from the outside environment.
2. Restrict plants, flowers, and unpeeled fruit from the room.	2. Plants, flowers, and unpeeled fruit, such as oranges, may harbor fungus and put the patient at risk for fungal infection.
3. Teach each patient technique for wearing mask when leaving the room. Explain rationale. (May not be required in all institutions.).	3. It is important for the patient to begin to assume responsibility for health maintenance. The hospital environment is contaminated with multiple organisms and potentially resistant strains that may jeopardize the patient not knowledgeable in precautionary techniques.
4. Monitor visitors and personnel for signs of infection and decline entry into room.	4. Some visitors and personnel may be unaware of the potential threat of a seemingly benign infection. Viral infections such as herpes simplex or colds, or infected cuts and other skin lesions, are of particular concern.
5. Change all wound, CVP insertion site, and pacemaker wire exit site dressings daily. Use absolute sterile technique.	5. Conscientious attention to potential ports of entry reduces the potential for wound, systemic, or pacemaker wire-borne infection.
6. Change all intravenous solutions, tubings, stopcocks, and any heparin-locked lines daily. (Individual program guidelines may vary from 24 to 48 hours.)	6. Intravenous lines that are frequently accessed for specimens and medications increase risk of introducing organisms into the bloodstream.
7. Monitor patient technique of self-administration of antibiotic and antifungal mouthwashes. Ensure that mouthwashes are swished throughout the mouth, are allowed to linger, and are taken after meals. Teach patient not to perform toothbrushing or eat immediately after the administration of mouthwashes.	7. The patient is at risk for opportunistic oral infection, and care must be taken to ensure that medications are used appropriately. Mouthwashes should be allowed to linger and not be followed by eating, drinking, or other rinsing, which reduce mouthwash effectiveness.
8. Notify physician if white blood cell count falls below 5,000.	8. Patient is at greatest risk for infection during augmented immunosuppression and any time the white blood cell count falls below target suppression level. A fall in this count indicates a need for adjustment of dosage.
9. Provide aggressive pulmonary care, including inspirometers, deep breathing, coughing, and early mobility to prevent atelectasis.	9. Atelectasis is a risk after surgery, and its development increases the risk of pulmonary infection.

Nursing Goal 2 ➧ To detect early manifestations of infection to ensure prompt medical attention and intervention

Outcome Criteria ➧
1. Patient will have negative cultures 7 days after course of antimicrobial therapy.
2. Patient will have a white blood cell count between 5,000 and 10,000 after antimicrobial therapy.
3. Patient's temperature will return to less than 37°C after antimicrobial therapy.

NURSING INTERVENTIONS	RATIONALE
1. Obtain weekly urine, sputum, and viral cultures as ordered. Ensure that daily white blood cell counts and chest radiographs are obtained.	1. Absolute vigilance in monitoring for infection and identifying organisms is crucial to successful, early treatment of infection.
2. Auscultate breath sounds every 4 hours. Document and immediately report changes in secretions or aeration. 3. Monitor for and report any productive or nonproductive cough.	2–4. Nurses are often the first to identify changes in pulmonary status. The lungs are a likely site of infection, and prompt medical evaluation is important. Cultures are necessary to identify appropriate antimicrobial therapy.

(care plan continues on page 618)

Nursing Care Plan 25-1 (continued)

NURSING INTERVENTIONS	RATIONALE
4. Obtain sputum cultures if quantity, composition, color, or odor changes dramatically.	
5. Observe all wound, intravenous, and pacemaker wire sites daily for signs of suspect drainage, redness, swelling, or heat, and report any of these findings to the physician. 6. Obtain cultures of any suspicious drainage.	5–6. Wound and insertion site infections can be well established by the time overt signs are present in the immunosuppressed patient. Prompt treatment and insertion site changes are indicated.
7. Obtain temperature every 4 hours. Immediately document and report any temperature greater than 37°C. 8. Obtain aerobic and anaerobic blood cultures if temperature is greater than 37°C.	7–8. Corticosteroid therapy reduces normal basal and maximal body temperature. A temperature rise greater than 37°C may indicate the presence of systemic infection. It is important to obtain cultures when the temperature elevation occurs to identify possible organisms and appropriate antimicrobial therapy.

Nursing Diagnosis 3 ➧ Activity intolerance related to preoperative deconditioned state manifested by easy fatigue, decreased muscle strength, and inability to ambulate outside of room without assistance.

Nursing Goal 1 ➧ To increase activity intolerance and muscle strength to level compatible with requirements for activities of daily living and recreational exercise

Outcome Criteria ➧

1. Patient will be able to ambulate independently by third postoperative day (POD).
2. Patient will be able to cycle on stationary bicycle for 20 minutes at dyspnea level 2 by discharge.
3. Patient will self-monitor exercise tolerance by discharge.

NURSING INTERVENTIONS	RATIONALE
1. Obtain physical therapy consult and evaluation 2 days after transplantation.	1. Reconditioning exercises can begin as soon as the patient is alert, extubated, and hemodynamically stable. Further inactivity may contribute to existing deconditioned state.
2. Begin supine in-bed exercises on first postoperative day after extubation (one session per day).	2. Patients are mobile enough to perform ankle pumps and flexion and abduction of hips and shoulders.
3. Progress patient activity to include shoulder circles, trunk rotation, and knee flexion and extension when stable in a sitting position (one session per day). 4. When patient is able to stand with sufficient balance, include toe raises, trunk lateral flexion, backward and forward bends, and arm circles in the exercise program (one session per day). 5. When able to complete previous activities without undue fatigue or balance loss, initiate light weight resistance exercises, and stationary cycling (two sessions per day). 6. Monitor and document blood pressure, dyspnea, and heart rate response to exercise. Monitor and document symptom occurrence with exercise. Stop exercise: a. Systolic blood pressure increases greater than 40 mm Hg or decreases more than 15 mm Hg from baseline. b. HR increases greater than 30 beats/min over baseline. c. Dyspnea index is greater than level 2. d. Patient has vertigo, excessive fatigue, or ST segment increase or decrease greater than 1 mm. Report any findings to physician, and reevaluate exercise progression with physical therapist.	3–6. Slow progression of conditioning can coincide with increasing patient strength and endurance. Progression can be guided by patient tolerance and is only decreased during rejection episodes. Once rejection resolves, activity progression resumes.
7. Revert to l low-level activity if moderate or severe rejection occurs, and consult physician for guidelines.	7. It is important to limit the amount of stress on the rejecting heart. Exercise capacity is decreased during this time.
8. Teach patient the dyspnea index and how to obtain a pulse. Assess and document patient learning.	8. Patient must acquire self-monitoring skills for continuation of safe exercise after discharge.

Nursing Care Plan 25-1 ■ (continued)

Nursing Diagnosis 4 ➧ Potential disturbance in self-concept related to changes in facial appearance secondary to immunosuppressive drug therapy, manifested by subjective complaints.

Nursing Goal 1 ➧ To assist patient with identifying strategies to enhance appearance and self-esteem

Outcome Criteria ➧
1. Patient will identify methods to minimize hirsutism and increased body hair.
2. Patient will identify methods to de-emphasize cushingoid facial features.
3. Patient will remain socially involved.
4. Patient will take initiative to seek resources for enhancing appearance if desired.

NURSING INTERVENTIONS	RATIONALE
1. Introduce patient to a transplantation support group or to other patients who have had a cardiac transplantation.	1. Transplant recipients achieve a better understanding of positive adaptive measures used by other patients who have experienced transplantation.
2. Offer female patients possible solutions to increased body hair growth and hirsutism if perceived as disturbing. Shaving, bleaching, and cream hair removers may be suggested. Caution patient not to apply to inflamed, broken, or chapped skin.	2. Cyclosporine stimulates hair follicles, causing a diffuse increase in hair growth (hypertrichosis). Corticosteroid steroid therapy contributes to the development of hirsutism. Male patients may not view this as problematic, but female patients may find this side effect to be troublesome.

Nursing Diagnosis 5 ➧ Potential knowledge deficit about medications related to lack of familiarity, manifested by inability to self-administer medications correctly.

Nursing Goal 1 ➧ To provide patient with knowledge and skills that will allow patient to self-administer medications correctly by discharge.

Outcome Criteria ➧
1. Patient will identify each medication by name, proper dose, dose schedule, and potential side effects by discharge.
2. Patients will self-administer medications at correct time on a consistent basis by discharge.

NURSING INTERVENTIONS	RATIONALE
1. Set realistic goals for self-administration. Consider patient's previous experience with self-medication, present state of recovery, ability to concentrate and read printed material. Include patient in planning realistic time frames.	1. It is unrealistic to expect patients to learn multiple medications in a short time. They also may not be feeling well and may not be able to concentrate on instruction while still experiencing discomforts from surgery. Rushing learning may only increase anxiety about their capabilities.
2. Medication lists are available with color pictures of exact medication, use, side effects and precautions. 3. Provide patient with a variety of materials to assist with learning, such as flashcards, posters, and written material.	2–3. An actual picture allows the patient visual and written information about medications. Its format allows for independent review at the patient's directed pace. Learning is more successful when a variety of materials are used.
4. Allow patient to assume gradually total responsibility for self-administration of medication. Patient's significant other will be a active participant in all education. Acknowledge accomplishments.	
5. Monitor patient's progress in ability to self-administer medications and document.	

Note: There are many other areas of potential knowledge deficit. These include the following:
- Prevention of infection
- Signs and symptoms of infection
- Monitoring activity progression at home
- Diet
- Treatment of rejection
- Seeking medical attention for illness or unusual symptoms
- Follow-up care
- Management of health care insurance and other financial issues
- Return to work

easy) to 12 to 14 (somewhat hard), to 15 to 20 (very, very difficult). Patients are instructed to continue their exertion until they perceive their exercise has become somewhat hard.[89] Patients are also counseled to decrease their duration of exercise if they experience excessive fatigue during or after exercise.

Corticosteroid therapy, cyclosporine, and tacrolimus are detrimental to bone density and structure. Potential corticosteroid-induced osteoporosis puts the patient in greater jeopardy of bone fractures. Several types of medications are available to treat transplantation osteoporosis such as bisphosphonates, calcitonin, estrogen, and vitamin D. Bisphosphonates, such as alendronate, inhibit bone resorption and can prevent bone loss. Calcitonin is another antiresorptive drug. Estrogen therapy effectively prevents bone loss related to estrogen deficiency.[91,92]

Regular exercise programs help patients to control weight and to minimize calcium loss from bone. Approximately 86% of transplant recipients are considered to have class I New York Heart Association functional status. More than 90% of the recipients report having no activity limitations up to 5 years posttransplant.[77] They are capable of performing most recreational activities and are advised against contact sports or other sports with high risk of injury, such as alpine skiing, unless the recipient was previously accomplished in the sport. Physician approval is recommended if patients wish to pursue vigorous running or jogging. The additional benefit of improved collateral circulation is important if chronic rejection develops at a later time.

Preparation for Discharge

Patient preparation for discharge begins in the intensive care unit and continues until discharge, which can be as early as 7 days. It is important that patients fully understand their condition and the implications of cardiac denervation. They need to adapt to a new medical regime and must understand its importance in maintaining their state of health. Patients are discharged with multiple medications and must understand their purpose, actions, and side effects. This understanding is facilitated by a patient medication self-administration list that is easily interpreted, followed, and changeable. Many variations are available online and can be translated to several languages. By discharge, it is important that they assume total responsibility for self-care. Bedside flow sheets can be used by the nursing staff to indicate the progress of the patient's learning. Patients are taught how to detect signs of infection and to monitor their temperature. Cardiac risk factors should be evaluated with the patient so that strategies can be outlined to decrease risk. In addition to the primary nurse, dietitians, social workers, physical therapists, and the nurse transplantation coordinators can all contribute to patient instruction. It is important for a nurse to have good teaching skills, sensitivity to the patient's psychological needs, and an ability to communicate. These skills can greatly enhance the patient's success in learning.

Nursing Management Plan

Nursing care of the transplant recipient is, for the most part, interdependent with medical management. The exception to this is the provision of patient teaching. Nonetheless, several nursing diagnoses can be identified for the patient after cardiac transplantation. This management plan focuses on diagnoses, goals, and interventions unique to the transplant recipient. Because this patient has undergone cardiac surgery, many diagnoses used for the cardiac surgical patient can be used with the transplant recipient. Nursing Care Plan 25-1 is an outline of a nursing management plan for an uncomplicated cardiac transplantation recipient. Sample nursing diagnoses are presented. Not all possibilities have been discussed. Other diagnoses that the nurse may assess for include the following:

- Potential fluid volume excess related to sodium and water retention from corticosteroid therapy
- Potential altered nutrition: more than body requirement related to appetite increase from corticosteroid therapy
- Potential fear or anxiety related to the possibility of rejection and death from complications
- Altered family processes related to disruption of family life from prolonged hospitalization and need to reside in the local area for 2 to 3 months after discharge
- Potential for noncompliance related to the complexity of the prescribed medical regime

REFERENCES

1. Diodato Jr., M. D., Maniar, H. S., Prasad, S. M., et al. (2003). Robotics in cardiac surgery. In K. L. Franco & E. D. Verrier (Eds.), *Advanced therapy in cardiac surgery* (pp. 102–114). Hamilton, Ontario: BC Decker.
2. Kulier, A., Levin, J. Moser, R., et al. (2007). Impact of preoperative anemia on outcome in patients undergoing coronary artery bypass graft surgery. *Circulation, 116*, 471–479.
3. McKhann, G. M., Grega, M. A., Borowicz, L. M. et al. (2006). Stroke and encephalopathy after cardiac surgery an update. *Stroke, 37*, 562–571.
4. Ferraris, V. A., Ferraris, S. E., Moliterno, D. J., et al. (2005). The society of thoracic surgeons practice guideline series: Aspirin and other antiplatelet agents during operative coronary revascularization (executive summary). *Annals of Thoracic Surgery, 79*, 1454–1461.
5. Jones, H. U., Muhlestein, J. B., Jones, K. W., Bair, T. L., et al. (2002). Preoperative use of enoxaparin compared with unfractionated heparin increases the incidence of re-exploration for postoperative bleeding after open-heart surgery in patients who present with an acute coronary syndrome. *Circulation, 106*(Suppl. I), I-19–I-22.
6. Falk, V., Jacobs, S., Walther, T., et al. (2003). Total endoscopic bypass grafting. In K. L. Franco & E. D. Verrier (Eds.), *Advanced therapy in cardiac surgery* (pp. 119–123). Hamilton, Ontario: BC Decker.
7. Seifert, P. C. (2002a). Basic cardiac surgical procedures. In P. C. Seifert, *Cardiac surgery: Perioperative patient care* (pp. 213–257). St Louis: Mosby.
8. Bojar, R. M. (1999). Intraoperative considerations in cardiac surgery. In R. M. Bojar & K. G. Warner, *Manual of perioperative care in cardiac surgery* (3rd ed., pp. 93–106). Malden: Blackwell Science.
9. Ng, C. S. H., Wan, S., Yim, A. P. C., et al. (2002). Pulmonary dysfunction after cardiac surgery. *Chest, 121*(4), 1269–1277.
10. Eagle, K. A., Guyton, R. A., Davidoff, R., et al. (2004). ACC/AHA guideline update for coronary artery bypass graft surgery: Summary article: A report of the American College of Cardiology/American Heart Association Task Force on Practice Guidelines (Committee to update the 1999 guidelines for coronary bypass surgery). *Circulation, 110*, 1168–1176.
11. Hannan, E. L., Wu, C., Walford, G., et al. (2008). Drug-eluting stents vs. coronary artery bypass grafting in multivessel coronary disease. *New England Journal of Medicine, 358*, 331–341.
12. Topkara, V. K., Cheema, F. H., Kesavaramanujam, S., et al. (2005) *Circulation, 114*(Suppl. I), I-344–I-350.
13. Seifert, P. C. (2002b). Surgery for coronary artery disease. In P. C. Seifert, *Cardiac surgery: Perioperative patient care* (pp. 258–306). St Louis: Mosby.
14. Acorda, R., Kraus, T., & Casey, P. E. (2000). Advances in surgical treatment of coronary artery disease. *Nursing Clinics of North America, 35*, 913–932.
15. Chatterjee, K. (1998). Recognition and management of patients with stable angina pectoris. In L. Goldman & E. Brauwnwald (Eds.), *Primary cardiology* (pp. 234–256). Philadelphia: WB Saunders.
16. Guru, V., Fremes, S. E., and Tu, J. V. (2004). Time-related mortality for women after coronary artery bypass graft surgery: A population-based study. *Journal Thoracic and Cardiovascular Surgery, 127*, 1158–1165.

17. Katz, M. R., Van Praet, F., de Canniere, D., et al. (2006). Integrated coronary revascularization percutaneous coronary intervention plus robotic totally endoscopic coronary artery bypass. *Circulation, 114*(Suppl. I), I-473–I-476.
18. Van Dijk, D., Jansen, E. W., Hijman, R., et al. (2002). Cognitive outcomes after off-pump and on-pump coronary artery bypass surgery. *JAMA, 287,* 1405–1412.
19. Van Dijk, D., Spoor, M., Hijman, R., et al. (2007). Cognitive and cardiac outcomes 5 years after off-pump vs. on-pump coronary artery bypass surgery. *JAMA, 297,* 701–708.
20. Van Dijk, D., Nierch, A. P., & Jansen, E. W. L. (2001). Early outcomes after off-pump coronary bypass surgery. *Circulation, 104,* 1761–1766.
21. Drenth, D. J., Veeger, N. J., & Winter, J. B. (2002). A prospective randomized trail comparing stenting with off-pump coronary surgery for high-grade stenosis of the left anterior descending coronary artery: Three-year follow-up. *Journal of the American College of Cardiology, 40,* 1955–1960.
22. Mangino-Blanchard, L. (2002). Off-pump coronary revascularization: Is it all that it's cracked up to be? *Dimensions of Critical Care Nursing, 21*(5), 190–194.
23. Frazier, O. H., Kadipasaoglu, K. A., & Cooley, D. A. (1998). Transmyocardial laser revascularization: Does it have a role in treatment of ischemic heart disease? *Texas Heart Institute Journal, 25,* 24–29.
24. Bridges, C. R., Horvath, K. A., Nugent, W. C., et al. (2004). The society of thoracic surgeons practice guidelines series: Transmyocardial laser revascularization. *Annals Thoracic Surgery, 77,* 1494–1502.
25. Calafiore, A. M., Di Mauro, M., & Contini, M. (2003). Left ventricular volume reduction for dilated cardiomyopathy. In K. L. Franco & E. D. Verrier (Eds.), *Advanced therapy in cardiac surgery* (pp. 415–430). Hamilton, Ontario: BC Deck.
26. Franco-Cereceda, A., McCarthy, P. M., & Blackstone, E. H. (2001). Partial left ventriculectomy for dilated cardiomyopathy: Is this an alternative to transplantation? *Journal of Thoracic Cardiovascular Surgery, 121,* 879–893.
27. Chachques, J. C., Cattadori, B., & Carpentier, A. (2003). Dynamic to cellular cardiomyoplasty. In K. L. Franco & E. D. Verrier (Eds.), *Advanced therapy in cardiac surgery* (pp. 431–438). Hamilton, Ontario: BC Decker.
28. King, R. C., & Verrier, E. V. (2003). Postinfarction ventricular septal defect repair. In K. L. Franco & E.D. Verrier (Eds.), *Advanced therapy in cardiac surgery* (pp. 83–88). Hamilton, Ontario: BC Decker.
29. Edwards, F. H., Engelman, R. M., Houck, P., et al. (2006). The society of thoracic surgeons practice guideline series: Antibiotic prophylaxis in cardiac surgery, part I: Duration. *Annals Thoracic Surgery, 81,* 397–404.
30. Duncan, C., & Erickson, R. (1982). Pressures associated with chest tube stripping. *Heart and Lung, 11*(2), 166–171.
31. Surgenor, S. D., DeFoe, G. R., Fillinger, M. P., et al. (2006). Intraoperative red blood cell transfusion during coronary artery bypass graft surgery increases the risk of postoperative low-output heart failure. *Circulation, 114*(Suppl. I), I-43–I-48.
32. Mangano, D. T., Tudor, I. C, & Dietzel, C. (2006). The risk associated with aprotinin in cardiac surgery. *New England Journal of Medicine, 354,* 353–365.
33. Shaw, A. D., Stafford-Smith, M., White, W.D., et al. (2008). The effect of aprotinin on outcome after coronary artery bypass grafting. *New England Journal of Medicine, 358,* 784–793.
34. Braile, D., & Petrucci, O. (2000). Cardiac tamponade. In P. P. Soltoski, H. L. Karamanoukian, & T. A. Salerno, *Cardiac surgery secrets* (pp. 228–229). Philadelphia: Hanley & Belfus.
35. Dehoux, M., Provenchere, S., Benessiano, J., et al. (2001). Utility of cardiac troponin measurement after cardiac surgery. *Clinica Chimica Acta, 311,* 41–44.
36. Lasocki, S., Provenchere, S., Benessiano, J., et al. (2002). Cardiac troponin I is an independent predictor of in-hospital death after cardiac surgery. *Anesthesiology, 97,* 405–411.
37. Croal, B. L., Hillis, G. S., Gibson, P. H., et al. (2006). Relationship between postoperative cardiac troponin I levels and outcome of cardiac surgery. *Circulation, 114,* 1468–1475.
38. Mathew, J. P., Fontes, M. L., Tudor, I. C., et al. (2004). A multicenter risk index for atrial fibrillation after cardiac surgery. *JAMA, 291,* 1720–1729.
39. Cleveland Jr., J. C., & Grover, F. L. (2003). Prophylaxis against atrial fibrillation following open heart surgery. In K. L. Franco & E. D. Verrier (Eds.), *Advanced therapy in cardiac surgery* (pp. 22–26). Hamilton, Ontario: BC Decker.
40. Hill, L. L., DeWat, C., & Hogue Jr, C. W. (2002). Management of atrial fibrillation after cardiac surgery, part II: Prevention and treatment. *Journal of Cardiothoracic and Cardiovascular Anesthesia, 16,* 626–637.
41. Maisel, W. H., Rawn, J. D., & Stevenson, W. G. (2001). Atrial fibrillation after cardiac surgery. *Annals of Internal Medicine, 135,* 1061–1073.
42. Rho, R. W., Bridges, C. R., & Kocovic, D. (2000). Management of postoperative arrhythmias. *Seminars in Thoracic and Cardiovascular Surgery, 12,* 349–361.
43. Roosens, C., Heerman, J., DeSomer, F., et al. (2002). Effects of off-pump coronary surgery on the mechanics of the respiratory system, lung, and chest wall: Comparison with extracorporeal circulation. *Critical Care Medicine, 30,* 2430–2437.
44. Milot, J., Perron, J., Lacasse, Y., et al. (2001). Incidence and predictors of ARDS after cardiac surgery. *Chest, 119,* 884–888.
45. Loef, B. G., Epema, A. H., Navi, G., et al. (2002). Off-pump coronary revascularization attenuates transient renal damage compared to on-pump revascularization. *Chest, 121,* 1190–1194.
46. Bove, T., Landoni, G., Grazia Calabro`, M., et al. (2005). Renoprotective action of fenoldopam in high-risk patients undergoing cardiac surgery. A prospective, double-blind, randomized clinical trial. *Circulation, 111,* 3230–3235.
47. Lopes, D. K. (2000). Neurologic complications of cardiac surgery. In P. P. Soltoski, H. L. Karamanoukian, & T. A. Salerno, *Cardiac surgery secrets* (pp. 253–257). Philadelphia: Hanley & Belfus.
48. Sharma, A. D., Parmley, C. L., & Sreeram, G. (2000). Peripheral nerve injuries during cardiac surgery: Risk factors, diagnosis, prognosis, and prevention. *Anesthesia and Analgesia, 91,* 1358–1369.
49. Gardlund, B., Bitkover, C. Y., & Vaage, J. (2002). Postoperative mediastinitis in cardiac surgery-microbiology and pathogenesis. *European Journal of Cardio-thoracic Surgery, 21,* 825–830.
50. Trulock, E. P., Edwards, L. B., Taylor, D. O., et al. (2007). Registry of the International Society for Heart and Lung Transplantation: Twenty-fourth official adult lung and heart–lung transplantation report-2006. *International Society for Heart and Lung Transplantation: The Journal of Heart and Lung Transplantation, 26,* 763–807.
51. Baran, D. A., Galin, I. D., & Gass, A. L. (2002). Current practices: Immunosuppression induction, maintenance, and rejection regimens in contemporary post-heart transplant patient treatment. *Current Opinion in Cardiology, 17,* 165–170.
52. Taylor, D. O. (2000). Immunosuppressive therapies after heart transplantation: Best, better, and beyond. *Current Opinion Cardiology, 15,* 108–114.
53. Kirklin, J. K., Bourge, R. C., & Naftel, D. C. (1994). Treatment of recurrent heart rejection with mycophenolate mofetil (RS-61443): Initial clinical experience. *Journal of Heart and Lung Transplantation, 13,* 444–450.
54. International Society of Heart and Lung Transplant (ISHLT) Registry Quarterly Report in North America. Available from http://www.ishlt.org/registries/quartleydatareports.asp. (2 March 2008).
55. The Organ Procurement and Transplantation Network (OPTN). Current U.S. waiting list. Available from www.optn.org/latestdata/RPT (13 March 2008).
56. Brown, M. (1995). Thoracic transplantation: Procurement and organization. In N. E. Shumway & S. J. Shumway (Eds.), *Thoracic Transplantation* (pp. 79–83). Cambridge: Blackwell Science.
57. Mehra, M. R., Kobashigawa, J., Starling R. (2006). Listing criteria for heart transplantation: ISHLT guidelines for the care of cardiac transplant candidates-2006. *Journal of Heart and Lung Transplantation, 25,* 1024–1042.
58. Boucek, M. M., Edwards, L. B., Keck, B. M., et al. (2003). The Registry of the International Society for Heart and Lung Transplantation: Sixth Official Pediatric Report-2003. *Journal of Heart and Lung Transplantation, 22,* 636–652.
59. *2006 Annual Report of the U.S. Organ Procurement and Transplantation Network and the Scientific Registry of Transplant Recipients: Transplant data 1996–2005.* Department of Health and Human Services, Health Resources and Services Administration. Office of Special Programs, Division of Transplantation, Rockville, MD; United Network for Organ Sharing, Richmond, VA; University Renal Research and Education Association, Ann Arbor, MI.
60. Frazier, O. H. (1996). Patient selection for heart transplantation. In O. H. Frazier, M. P. Macris, & B. Radovancevic (Eds.), *Support and replacement of the failing heart* (pp. 59–68). Philadelphia: JB Lippincott.
61. Deng, M. C. (2002). Cardiac transplantation. *Heart, 87,* 177–184.
62. Veith, F. J., Fein, J. M., Tendler, M. D., et al. (1978). Brain death: I. A status report of medical and ethical considerations. *JAMA, 238,* 1651–1655.
63. Zaroff, J. G., Rosengard, B. R., Armstrong, W. F., et al. (2002). Consensus Conference Report. Maximizing use of organs recovered from the cadaver donor: Cardiac recommendations. *Circulation, 106,* 836–841.

64. Shumway, N. E., Lower, R. R., & Stofer, C. (1966). Transplantation of the heart. *Advances in Surgery, 2*, 265–284.
65. Trento, A., Takkenberg, J. M., Czer, L. S. C., et al. (1996). Clinical experience with one hundred consecutive patients undergoing orthotopic heart transplantation with bicaval and pulmonary venous anastomosis. *Journal of Thoracic Cardiovascular Surgery, 112*, 1496–1503.
66. Frazier, D. H., VanBuren, C. T., & Poindexter, S. M. (1985). Nutritional management of the heart transplant recipient. *Heart Transplantation, 4*, 450–452.
67. Shinn, J. A. (1985). New issues in cardiac transplantation. In M. K. Douglas & J. A. Shinn (Eds.), *Advances in cardiovascular nursing* (pp. 185–195). Rockville: Aspen Systems.
68. Bexton, R. S., Nathan, A. W., Hellestrand, K. J., et al. (1984). Sinoatrial function after cardiac transplantation. *Journal of the American College of Cardiology, 13*, 712–723.
69. DiBiase, A., Tse, T. M., Schnittger, I., et al. (1991). Frequency and mechanism of bradycardia in cardiac transplant recipients and need for pacemakers. *American Journal of Cardiology, 67*, 1385–1389.
70. Rose, A. G. (1986). Endomyocardial biopsy diagnosis of cardiac rejection. *Heart Failure, 2*(2), 64–72.
71. Stewart, S., Winters, G. L, & Fishbein, M. C. (2005). Revision of the 1990 working formulation for the standardization of nomenclature in the diagnosis of heart rejection. *Journal of Heart and Lung Transplantation, 24*, 1710–1720.
72. Billingham, M. E., Cary, N. R. B., Hammond, M. E., et al. (1990). A working formulation for the standardization of nomenclature in the diagnosis of heart and lung rejection: Heart rejection study group. *Journal of Heart Transplantation, 9*, 587–591.
73. Starling, R. C., Pham, M., Valantine, H., et al. (2006). Working group on molecular testing in cardiac transplantation. Molecular testing in the management of cardiac transplant recipients: Initial clinical experience. *Journal of Heart and Lung Transplantation, 25*(12), 1389–1395.
74. Uber, W. E., Self, S. E., Bakel, A. B., Van Bakel, A. B., & Pereira, N. C. (2007). Acute antibody-mediated rejection following heart transplantation. *American Journal of Transplantation, 7*, 2064–2074.
75. Almuti, K., Haythe, J., Dwyer, E., Silviu, I., et al. (2007). The changing pattern of humoral rejection in cardiac transplant recipients. *Transplantation, 84*, 498–503.
76. Ramzy, D., Rao, V., Brahm, J., et al. (2005). Cardiac allograft vasculopathy: A review. *Canadian Journal of Surgery, 48*, 319–327.
77. Hertz, M. I, Taylor, D. O., Trulock, E. P., et al. (2002). The Registry of the International Society for Heart and Lung Transplantation: Nineteenth official report-2002. *Journal of Heart and Lung Transplantation, 21*, 950–970.
78. Valantine, H. A. (1995). Prevention and treatment of cytomegalovirus disease in thoracic organ transplant patients: Evidence for a beneficial effect of hyperimmune globulin. *Transplant Proceedings, 27*, 49–57.
79. Moran, M., Tomlanovich, S., & Myers, B. D. (1985). Cyclosporin-induced nephropathy in human recipients of cardiac allografts. *Transplant Proceedings, 17*(Suppl. 1), 185–190.
80. Myers, B. D., Ross, J., Newton, L., et al. (1984). Cyclosporin associated chronic nephrotoxicity. *New England Journal of Medicine, 311*, 699–705.
81. Thompson, M. E., Shapiro, M. E., Johnsen, A. M., et al. (1983). New onset of hypertension following cardiac transplantation. *Transplant Proceedings, 25*(Suppl. 1), 2573–2577.
82. Wagoner, L. W. (1997). Management of the cardiac transplant recipient: Roles of the transplant cardiologist and primary care physician. *American Journal of Medical Science, 324*, 173–184.
83. Lough, M. E., Lindsey, A. M., Shinn, J. A. (1987). Impact of symptom frequency and symptom distress on self-reported quality of life in heart transplant recipients. *Heart and Lung, 16*, 193–200.
84. Przepiorka, D. (1992). Tacrolimus: Preclinical and clinical experience. In D. Przepioka & H. Sollinger (Eds.), *Recent developments in transplantation medicine: New immunosuppressive drugs* (pp. 29–50). Glenview, IL: Physicians and Scientist Publishing.
85. Lough, M. E., Lindsey, A. M., & Shinn, J. A. (1985). Life satisfaction following heart transplantation. *Heart Transplantation, 4*, 446–449.
86. Crandell, B. (1990). Immunosuppression. In K. M. Sigardson-Poor & L. M. Haggerty (Eds.), *Nursing care of the transplant recipient* (pp. 53–85). Philadelphia: WB Saunders.
87. Eisen, H. J. (2003). Hypertension in heart transplant recipients: More than just cyclosporine. *Journal of the American College of Cardiology, 41*(3), 433–434.
88. Aranda, J. M., & Hill, J. (2000). Cardiac transplant vasculopathy. *Chest, 118*, 1792–1800.
89. Sadowsky, H. S. (1996). Cardiac transplantation: A review. *Physical Therapy, 76*, 498–515.
90. Sadowsky, H. S., & Fries, K. (1986). *Introduction to the treatment of cardiac and cardiopulmonary transplant patients.* Stanford, CA: Department of Physical and Occupational Therapy, Stanford University Hospital.
91. Shane, E., Addesso, V., Namerow, P. B., et al. (2004). Alendronate versus calcitrol for the prevention of bone loss after cardiac transplantation. *New England Journal of Medicine, 350*, 767–769.
92. Rodino, M. A., & Shane, E. (1998). Osteoporosis after organ transplantation. *American Journal of Medicine, 104*(5), 459–469.

CHAPTER 26

Mechanical Circulatory Assist Devices

Michael A. Chen*

Mechanical circulatory assist devices have been used since the 1960s. Intra-aortic balloon pump (IABP) catheters are the most commonly used devices. Other circulatory support devices, once restricted to a few large centers, are now becoming more widely available for temporary use in the cardiac catheterization laboratory, as an adjunct to cardiac surgery, as well as being implanted for short-, intermediate-, and even long-term ventricular assistance (i.e., "destination therapy"). Such devices are used to support circulation temporarily when the injured (left or right) ventricular myocardium cannot generate adequate cardiac output. One such device has been used successfully to support a patient for nearly seven and a half years.[1] With the aging of the population and the improved treatment of coronary artery disease and myocardial infarction (MI), the incidence of heart failure is increasing; in the coming years the numbers of patients who have acute severe and end-stage heart failure will increase. Typically, less than 2,500 patients per year receive cardiac transplants in the United States due to a limited donor pool, making mechanical assist devices an important long-term therapy as well.[2] In November 2002, the Food and Drug Administration approved the use of the HeartMate (Thoratec Laboratories, Inc., Pleasanton, CA) left ventricular assist device (LVAD) for permanent or destination therapy in patients who are not appropriate candidates for heart transplantation.[3]

With early recognition, the often rapid hemodynamic deterioration of patients with acute left ventricular (LV) failure can be arrested with circulatory assist devices. The type of device used depends on the degree of myocardial injury, the degree of LV functional impairment, the anticipated length of therapy as well as other factors (including what is available locally). The purpose of therapy is to stabilize the patient until: (1) the left ventricle recovers from acute injury; (2) mechanical problems causing acute failure (e.g., ruptured ventricular septum) can be surgically corrected; (3) heart transplantation can be performed; or (4) a decision is made to place a device as "destination therapy," for patients who are not candidates for transplant. The goal of a circulatory assist device is to stabilize or improve hemodynamics and secondary organ function. The major principles governing all devices are that they: (1) decrease or take over LV workload; (2) enhance oxygen supply to the myocardium; and (3) partially or totally support the systemic circulation and thus, other organ perfusion. The extent to which each principle can be achieved depends on the type of device used. An IABP offers only partial support, whereas implantable right ventricular assist devices (RVADs), LVADs, and BiVADs can assume the total workload of the right, left, or both ventricles, respectively. In addition, there are devices that provide intermediate levels of support. Most cardiovascular critical care nurses encounter patients requiring IABP support. In addition, this chapter will describe other types of circulatory assist devices.

INTRA-AORTIC BALLOON PUMP COUNTERPULSATION

The IABP was introduced in the late 1960s as a therapy for cardiogenic shock after MI.[4] Since then, its application has expanded to include patients with other etiologies of acute LV failure, including before or after cardiac surgery, from acute myocarditis, and in patients with chronic heart failure who experience acute hemodynamic deterioration. Other indications include support during high-risk percutaneous coronary intervention (PCI), reducing major adverse coronary events and procedural complications.[5,6] They can be used for patients with unstable angina, refractory ventricular arrhythmias (particularly when ischemia driven), and for patients with mechanical complications of acute MI, such as papillary muscle rupture or ventricular septal rupture, as a bridge to surgical repair. It is estimated that over 70,000 IABP are placed each year in the United States alone.[4] Display 26-1 lists the most common indications for IABP placement from a review of nearly 17,000 patients who received the therapy from 1996 to 2000.[7]

Description

The intra-aortic balloon is constructed of a biocompatible, nonthrombogenic material and mounted on a catheter constructed of the same material. An opening at the catheter–balloon connection allows pressurized gas (usually helium) to move in and out of the balloon, causing inflation and deflation to occur. Most catheters have two lumens: an inner lumen for central pressure monitoring at the catheter tip and a second lumen for the gas. Properly positioned, the distal tip of the balloon catheter rests just distal to the origin of the left subclavian artery and the proximal end of the balloon is positioned proximal to the renal arteries. Figure 26-1 illustrates proper anatomic position of the IABP catheter. (See Figure 12-3 in Chapter 12.) The tip of the catheter is radio-opaque so that its position can be verified with a chest x-ray. The catheter is inserted via a direct femoral or iliac arteriotomy or by percutaneous insertion using the Seldinger technique with or without a sheath. Although a direct arteriotomy approach is rarely used today, prior designs made it mandatory, and it may still be the optimal choice for a patient with severe peripheral vascular disease (when direct visualization is desired) or for pediatric patients. The approach requires an incision in the groin for access to the femoral or iliac artery. This technique is more invasive and time consuming, and requires surgical removal. The percutaneous technique is faster, less

*Debra Laurent and Julie A. Shinn are authors of Nursing Care Plan 26-1

DISPLAY 26-1 Major Indications for Intra-aortic Balloon Pump Therapy in 16,909 Patient (1996 to 2000)

Hemodynamic support during or after cardiac catheterization (21%)
Cardiogenic shock (19%)
Weaning from cardiopulmonary bypass (13%)
Refractory unstable angina (12%)
Refractory heart failure (6.5%)
Mechanical complications of acute myocardial infarction (5.5%)
Intractable ventricular arrhythmias (1.7%)

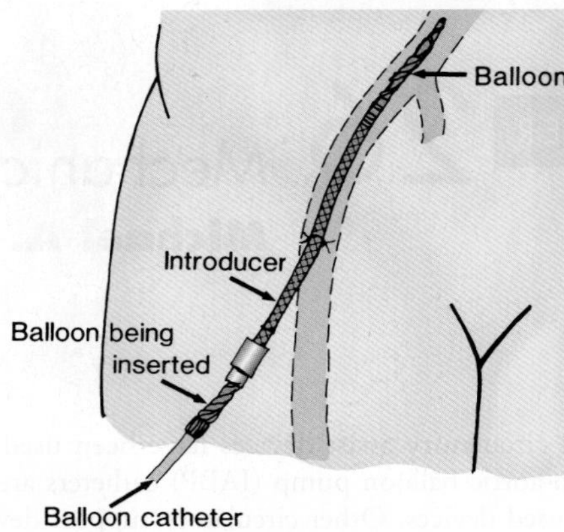

■ **Figure 26-2** Percutaneous insertion of the balloon catheter through an introducer or sheath. Note the right wrap of the balloon. (From Bull, S. O. [1983]. Principles and techniques of intra-aortic balloon counterpulsation. In S. L. Woods [Ed.], *Cardiovascular critical care nursing* [p. 171]. New York: Churchill Livingstone.)

invasive and allows for easy bedside removal. In all catheters, the balloon is wrapped tightly around its own guide wire so that it slides easily through a sheath or directly into the artery. Once in proper position, the balloon is inflated, resulting in unwrapping of the balloon, allowing inflation and deflation to commence. This catheter is secured to the skin by sutures. Figure 26-2 illustrates the percutaneous insertion technique utilizing an introducer sheath.

A newer design (SupraCor) has recently been introduced. This device can be placed in the ascending aorta for use after cardiac surgery. In an animal model, the device was shown to increase blood flow in saphenous vein and internal mammary bypass grafts, when a standardly placed IABP did not.[8]

Physiologic Principles

The two goals of IABP therapy are to increase coronary artery perfusion pressure and thus coronary artery blood flow, and to decrease LV workload by lowering LV afterload. These goals are achieved by displacement of volume in the aorta during systole and diastole with alternating inflation and deflation of the balloon. A typical adult-sized balloon contains 40 mL of gas or volume. For smaller adult patients, a 35-mL balloon is available; for larger patients, a 50-mL balloon is available. Placing a smaller-sized balloon (shorter) in smaller patients is important because a larger (longer) balloon could extend into the abdominal aorta, potentially compromising blood flow to the renal vasculature or even the lower extremities and exposes the balloon to abrasion (and even rupture) from calcified abdominal aortic atherosclerotic plaques.

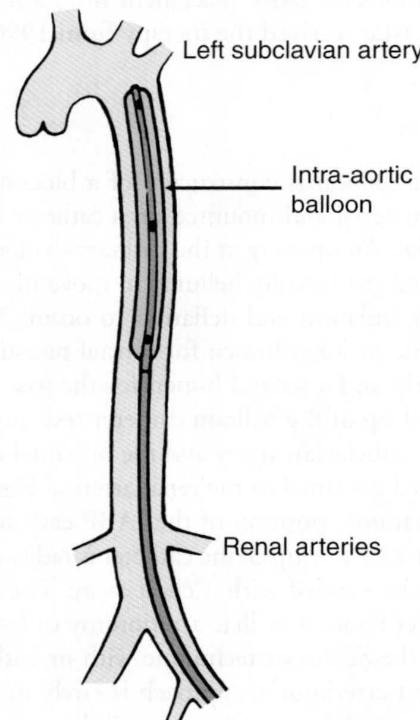

■ **Figure 26-1** Proper placement of the intra-aortic balloon catheter is just distal to the left subclavian artery and proximal to the renal arteries. (From Shinn, J. A. [1986]. Intra-aortic balloon pump counterpulsation. In C. M. Hudak, B. M. Gallo, & T. S. Lohr [Eds.], *Critical care nursing: A holistic approach* [4th ed., p. 190]. Philadelphia: J.B. Lippincott).

The size of the catheters range from 7 to 9.5 French. When the balloon is rapidly inflated at the onset of diastole, an additional 35 to 50 mL (depending on the balloon size) of volume is suddenly added to the aorta. This acute increase in volume creates an early diastolic pressure rise in the aortic root (where the coronary ostia lie), increasing coronary artery perfusion pressure. Figure 26-3 illustrates this effect. Because ischemic coronary beds are maximally vasodilated, no further autoregulatory increases in flow are possible, and flow is pressure dependent.[9–11] IABP inflation provides this enhanced pressure. The early diastolic pressure increase is referred to as the *diastolic augmentation*. Diastolic augmentation increases coronary perfusion pressure and in addition, by increasing overall mean arterial pressure, also contributes to enhanced flow to other organs.

This augmented diastolic pressure gradually falls, as diastolic pressure normally does when diastolic run-off occurs. Rapid evacuation of gas out of the balloon during deflation removes 35 to 50 mL of volume (the same amount used in inflation) out of the aorta. This sudden drop in aortic volume rapidly decreases pressure. Deflation is timed to occur at the end of diastole, just before the patient's next systole. Effective deflation, which decreases end-diastolic pressure, decreases the impedance or afterload that the ventricle must contract against to open the aortic valve and sustain ejection during systole. The lower the impedance, the lower the wall stress, and, therefore, the lower the LV workload. In cardiogenic shock, high systemic vascular resistance contributes to greater impedance, resulting in a greater workload for the failing

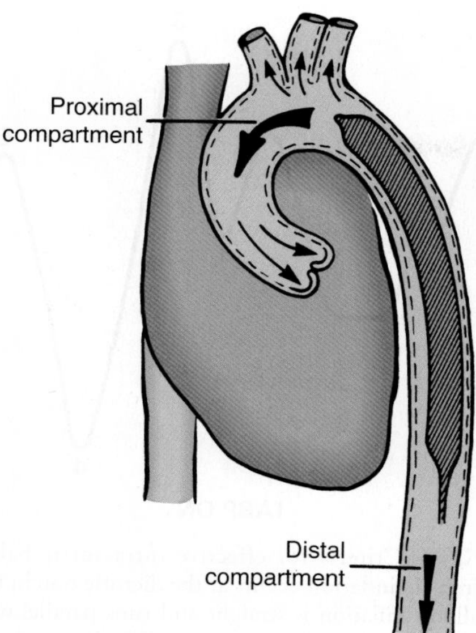

■ **Figure 26-3** Balloon inflation during diastole displaces volume retrograde toward the aortic root. The result is increased coronary artery perfusion pressure. Enhanced distal flow may also occur. (From Quaal, S. J. [1984]. *Comprehensive intra-aortic balloon pumping* [p. 82]. St. Louis: C.V. Mosby.)

left ventricle. With properly timed deflation, which lowers end-diastolic pressure and impedance to ejection, the LV workload is reduced. Figure 26-4 illustrates this effect. Systolic pressure is decreased when deflation of the balloon is timed properly. As a result of decreased afterload, there is more effective forward flow during systole. Improved forward flow contributes to decreased end-

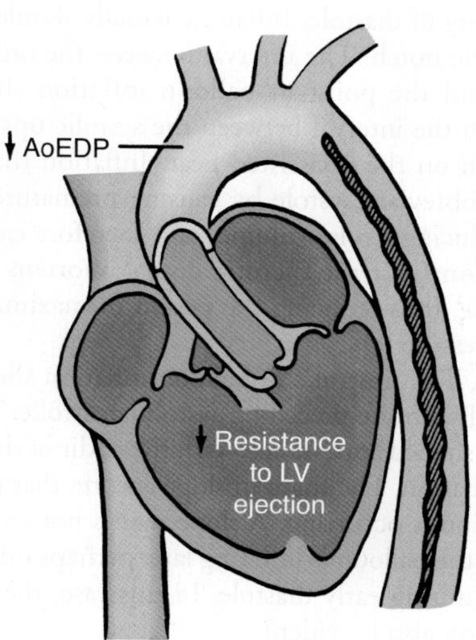

■ **Figure 26-4** Impedance or resistance to left ventricular (LV) ejection is decreased by abrupt balloon deflation before systole. Properly timed deflation decreases aortic end-diastolic pressure (A_0EDP), which decreases the workload of the left ventricle. (From Quaal, S. J. [1984]. *Comprehensive intra-aortic balloon pumping* [p. 83]. St. Louis: C.V. Mosby.)

DISPLAY 26-2 Physiologic Effects and Expected Clinical Outcomes of Balloon Inflation

Physiologic effects

Increased early diastolic pressure (by about 30%)
Diastolic augmentation
Increased aortic root pressure
Enhanced coronary artery perfusion pressure
Improved oxygen delivery
Decreased ischemia

Clinical outcomes

Early diastolic pressure ≥ systolic pressure
Decreased angina
Decreased signs of ischemia on the electrocardiogram
Decreased ventricular ectopy of ischemic origin

systolic volume in the ventricle. Improved emptying leads to decreased subsequent preload, which also contributes to decreasing LV workload. Cardiac output is increased and so is the mean arterial pressure. The need for compensatory tachycardia is reduced and heart rate is expected to fall, further decreasing myocardial oxygen demand. Better systemic perfusion helps to reverse the acidosis often seen in shock and improves secondary organ dysfunction related to the previous hypoperfused state. Although there is significant patient-to-patient variability, the expected beneficial outcomes of IABP therapy are listed in Displays 26-2 and 26-3.[10,12]

DISPLAY 26-3 Physiologic Effects and Expected Clinical Outcomes of Balloon Deflation

Physiologic effects

End-diastolic drop in aortic pressure
Decreased afterload
Lower systolic pressure (by about 20%)
Decreased calculated peak LV wall stress (by about 14%)
Improved contractility
Increased forward flow during systole
Improved secondary organ perfusion
Increased efficiency of left ventricular work (decreased oxygen demand)

Clinical outcomes

Improved forward flow
Decreased preload
Decreased pulmonary capillary wedge pressure (by about 20%)
Decreased crackles in the lung fields
Increased cardiac output (by about 20%)
Increased mean blood pressure
Improved urine output
Improved peripheral pulses and warm skin temperature
Clearer sensorium
Decreased heart rate (by less than 20%)

Contraindications

Because inflation of the balloon during diastole increases pressure in the aortic root, significant aortic regurgitation is a contraindication to IABP therapy. Inflation would otherwise increase regurgitation and thus LV workload. The presence of an aortic aneurysm is also a contraindication to IABP therapy. Trauma or rupture of the aneurysm can occur during IABP insertion. Dislodgement of adjacent thrombus can occur during insertion or from balloon inflation resulting in embolization. These risks are all unacceptable. Severe peripheral vascular occlusive disease in the femorial or iliac artery contraindicates IABP therapy. Catheter insertion may be difficult or impossible, and occlusion of the affected vessel, dissection, and dislodgement of plaque from the vessel wall are all possibilities as well. These potential problems can be avoided by selecting an alternate method of insertion. In the cardiac surgery patient, the catheter may be inserted directly into the thoracic aorta, although this method requires reopening the sternotomy incision to remove the catheter. The catheter can also be placed antegrade in the aorta via the right subclavian/axillary artery.[13] This approach requires a subperiosteal clavicular resection to access the artery, but is less invasive than a sternotomy incision. Newer catheters of smaller diameter minimize the risk of occluding distal blood flow. In addition, the ascending aorta device described above (SupraCor) could be considered. Uncontrolled sepsis and coagulopathy are other contraindications. Lastly, if invasive therapies are contrary to the goals of care (e.g., comfort care in a patient who is very unlikely to survive despite even heroic measures), IABP therapy should not be utilized.

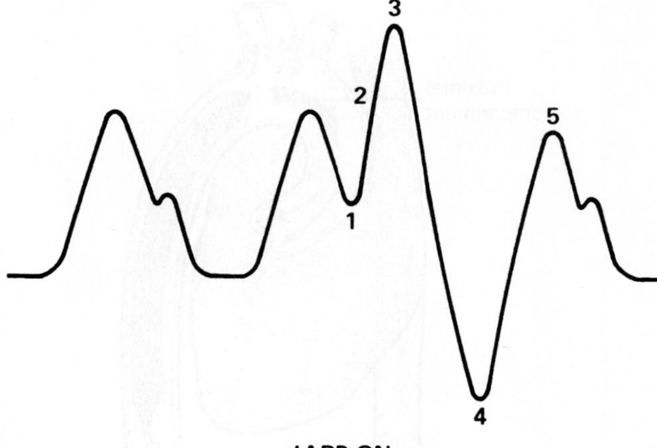

■ **Figure 26-5** Criteria for effective intra-aortic balloon pump (IABP) timing: (1) inflation occurs at the dicrotic notch; (2) the slope of rise of balloon inflation is straight and runs parallel with the preceding systolic upstroke; (3) augmented diastolic pressure is at least equal to the preceding systolic pressure; (4) end-diastolic pressure at balloon deflation is lower than the preceding unassisted end-diastolic pressure; (5) the next systolic pressure is assisted systole and is lower than the preceding systole, which was not affected by balloon deflation. (From Shinn, J. A. Intra-aortic balloon pump counterpulsation. In C. M. Hudak, B. M. Gallo, & T. S. Lohr [Eds.], *Critical care nursing: A holistic approach* [5th ed., p. 213]. Philadelphia: J.B. Lippincott, 1990.)

Proper Timing and Expected Clinical Outcomes

Proper timing of IABP therapy is crucial to achieving the beneficial hemodynamic changes described above. Proper timing requires coordination of inflation and deflation of the balloon with the patient's cardiac cycle. To evaluate balloon timing properly, the assist ratio is set at 1:2, meaning the balloon is assisting every other cardiac cycle. In this way, the observer can compare the effect of balloon inflation and deflation with unassisted beats. Most patients tolerate this ratio well, at least for a brief period. The R wave from the ECG, pacemaker spikes on the ECG, or the arterial systolic pressure can be used to identify individual cardiac cycles. Each can act as signals for the IABP console to discriminate systole from diastole. The R wave signals the onset of electrical depolarization, which immediately precedes mechanical systole. A ventricular pacemaker spike essentially represents the same event. Arterial systolic pressure signals the onset of mechanical systole. Any of these reference points can be used to determine when deflation of the balloon should optimally occur. An arterial waveform is necessary to determine the onset of mechanical diastole and systole and to verify timing. Diastole has begun when the dicrotic notch (which results from aortic valve closure) appears on the arterial waveform. Balloon inflation is timed to occur at this point in the cardiac cycle. The deflation point can be optimally adjusted by observing the end-diastolic drop in pressure created by balloon deflation. The goal is to create the greatest pressure drop possible. Ideally, there would be at least a 10 mm Hg difference between end-diastolic pressure without the balloon effect and the end-diastolic pressure created by balloon deflation. Evidence that afterload reduction has occurred is seen in the following systolic pressure. With afterload reduction, the next systolic pressure after balloon deflation is lower than the systolic pressure with no balloon effect, which is evidence that LV workload has been decreased. Five criteria can be used to determine the effectiveness of IABP timing, as illustrated on the arterial pressure tracing (Fig. 26-5) and detailed below.

- *Criterion 1.* Inflation must occur at the dicrotic notch, which is the beginning of diastole. Inflation actually should be timed to obliterate the notch. The interval between the onset of systolic upstroke and the point of balloon inflation should not be shorter than the interval between the systolic upstroke and dicrotic notch on the unassisted beat. Inflation that occurs too early can abbreviate systole by causing premature aortic valve closure, reducing stroke volume, and therefore cardiac output. Late inflation (past the dicrotic notch) shortens the duration of assistance, thus reducing the period of maximal augmented diastolic pressure.
- *Criterion 2.* The upstroke of balloon inflation should be sharp and parallel with the preceding systolic upstroke. This inflation creates a V-shaped appearance, with the nadir of the V being the point of inflation. The sharp upslope ensures that maximal early augmentation is occurring. A slope that is not straight may indicate that the balloon is inflating late, perhaps mistiming off of an artifact during early diastole. In this case, the loss of the V configuration also is evident.
- *Criterion 3.* The augmented diastolic pressure peak should be at least equal to the preceding systolic pressure peak. A decrease in this pressure peak may indicate gas loss from the balloon. This loss can occur by natural diffusion. A balloon normally requires refilling every 1 to 2 hours because of natural diffusion of gas through the membrane. Most consoles automatically purge and

refill the balloon and catheter at least every 2 hours. An abrupt loss of the pressure peak may indicate the development of a balloon or catheter leak. Occasionally, augmentation greater than the systolic pressure is not achievable because the balloon is too small relative to the aorta. Ideally, the balloon should occlude 85% to 90% of the aorta when fully inflated. If there is a size mismatch, diastolic augmentation pressure may be reduced, and may even be less than the patient's systole.

- *Criterion 4.* The balloon deflation should occur at the end of diastole. Proper deflation results in a drop in pressure at the end of diastole. This drop in pressure creates an end-diastolic pressure much lower than diastolic pressure without the balloon effect. Timing is adjusted so that the lowest pressure possible is achieved. It is important to make sure that the systolic upstroke that follows is straight and that a sharp, V-shaped configuration is present. The V shape indicates that systole began immediately after deflation. Any plateau indicates that deflation occurred too early, diminishing (or obliterating) the intended reduction in afterload. Late deflation, on the other hand, results in higher impedance because the balloon remains inflated at the onset of systolic ejection, creating more work for the LV. An end-diastolic pressure that is the same or greater than the end-diastolic pressure without balloon assistance is evidence of late deflation. The systolic pressure in the following beat may be the same or lower than the unassisted systole because of the inability of the failing ventricle to work against the higher impedance to ejection.
- *Criterion 5.* Finally, the observer should note what effect balloon deflation has on the next systolic pressure, for the reasons just described. The goal is to ensure that the lower systolic pressure that follows balloon deflation is caused by afterload reduction and not by improper timing, which resulted in late deflation. Proper balloon fit has an impact on the ability to achieve afterload reduction. If the balloon size is small, then volume displacement may have less of an effect on lowering end-diastolic pressure. Figure 26-6 illustrates the four possible errors that can occur with timing.

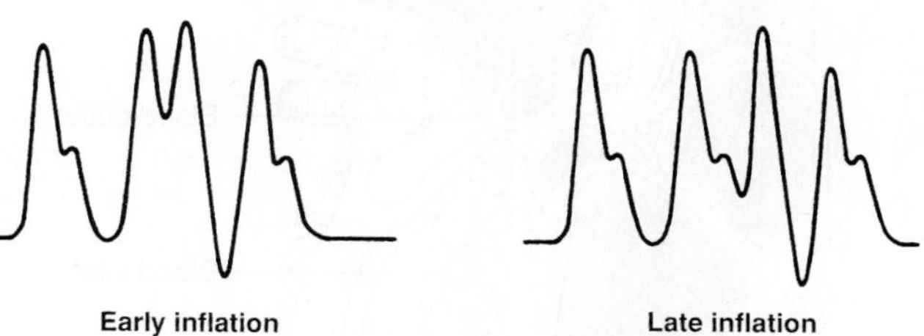

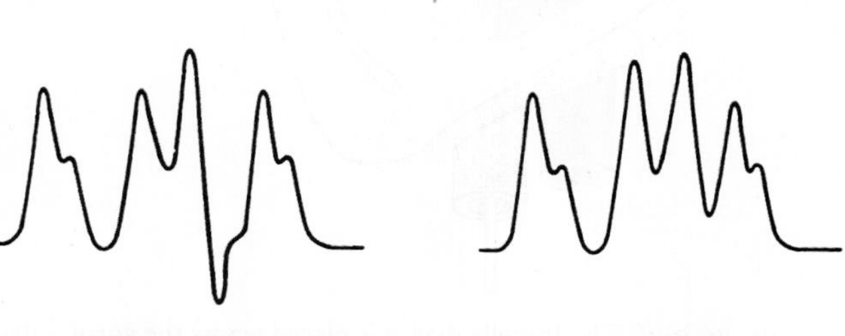

Figure 26-6 Possible errors in balloon timing. (From Shinn, J. A. [1986]. Intra-aortic balloon pump counterpulsation. In C. M. Hudak, B. M. Gallo, & T. S. Lohr [Eds.], *Critical care nursing: A holistic approach* [4th ed., p. 198]. Philadelphia: J.B. Lippincott.)

Complications

IABP therapy carries a relatively low risk of additional morbidity in a generally sick population. In the series of nearly 17,000 patients with IABPs placed (from 1996 to 2000) mentioned above, the incidence of any complication was 7% and major complications (i.e., severe bleeding, major acute limb ischemia, death from IABP insertion, or failure) was 2.6%.[7] Vascular complications have been reported to range from 6% to 25% of cases depending on the report.[14–16] Vascular injuries include plaque dislodgement, dissection, laceration, and compromise of the circulation to the distal extremity. Peripheral nerve injury is another possible complication of insertion (particularly if a cut down approach is used). Compromised circulation can occur any time during IABP therapy as a result of the presence of the indwelling catheter, compartment syndrome, or embolus from thrombus formation along the catheter or on the balloon.[17] The incidence of limb ischemia ranges from 5% to 35%.[17,18] Although intravenous heparin is generally used with IABP, there is little evidence that heparin reduces limb ischemia, and one randomized trial of 153 patients did not find a difference in such events.[19]

Complications are more common in patients with peripheral vascular occlusive disease, in women, those who are smaller (body surface area [BSA] <1.8 m^2), and in patients with a history of stroke, transient ischemic attacks, and diabetes.[7,17,20–23] Risk is decreased with sheathless insertion and with smaller balloon sizes.[22,24,25] In addition, operator's and hospital-staff's experience likely play a part.[26] Nurses monitor for and prevent compromised circulation by carefully assessing peripheral perfusion; preventing the patient from flexing the hip of the affected extremity, which may compromise blood flow; and maintaining coagulation times within prescribed parameters by careful titration of any prescribed anticoagulants. The nurse should be aware that multiple or prolonged attempts at insertion increase the risk of vascular injury and thrombus formation. Infection at the insertion site is reported to occur in less than 5% of patients, with an increase risk after 7 days of therapy. Insertion site infections may dictate the removal of the IABP catheter. Careful efforts must be made to maintain the sterility of insertion site dressings. Other problems that may be encountered include thrombocytopenia; compromised circulation to the left subclavian, renal, or mesenteric arteries because of balloon malposition; and bleeding from the insertion site or other line insertion sites. Mechanical problems related to the balloon include improper timing or a leak or perforation in the balloon, necessitating its removal. A leak in the balloon becomes evident as augmentation becomes less effective. Eventually, blood backs up in the catheter and can be detected. When a leak has occurred, the balloon must be removed immediately to avoid the possibility of gas embolus or balloon entrapment. Entrapment occurs when blood enters the balloon and becomes a large, hardened mass. The size makes it difficult to remove without a surgical intervention.

Nursing Management Plan

Meticulous cardiovascular assessment of the patient provides indicators that IABP therapy is effectively assisting LV function. Assessment includes vital signs, cardiac output, heart rhythm, signs of myocardial ischemia, urine output, color, peripheral perfusion, and mentation. If IABP treatment is effective, these parameters improve. The patient using IABP therapy is relatively immobile because of the need to avoid hip flexion and the presence of multiple invasive monitoring and infusion lines. Often, due to their critical condition, patients will be intubated and on ventilator support. Care must be taken to prevent or minimize atelectasis. These patients also are at greater risk for respiratory tract infection. Careful suctioning technique and prevention of aspiration reduce this risk.

Prolonged hypotension from the shock state may jeopardize renal function. Monitoring urine output and quality closely may contribute to early recognition and treatment of renal dysfunction, thus avoiding acute renal failure. Psychosocial support of the patient and family is also important. The patient requires interventions that minimize stress, disorientation, and sleep deprivation. Families benefit from honest communication and help with the interpretation of the patient's condition. Nursing Care Plan 26-1 outlines a plan of care for the patient on IABP therapy. Because this patient is experiencing acute LV failure or cardiogenic shock, many nursing diagnoses used for those conditions apply. The plan of care that is outlined focuses on issues unique to IABP therapy. The Nursing Care Plan, originally written by Laurent and Shinn for the 5th edition of *Cardiac Nursing,* has been placed at the end of this chapter.

OTHER MECHANICAL CIRCULATORY ASSIST DEVICES

An IABP is only able to augment cardiac output marginally (500 to 800 mL/min). Thus, with profound ventricular failure, IABP therapy may provide insufficient assistance, and more aggressive therapy may need to be considered. In recent years, a number of other mechanical circulatory assist devices have been developed for short-, intermediate-, and long-term use.

Indications and Contraindications

Indications for mechanical assistance include support/off-loading of the heart during high-risk PCI, weaning from cardiopulmonary bypass, as a bridge to recovery (from acute MI or acute myocarditis), as a bridge to transplant, or as a bridge to another device (e.g., a more permanent device) or for so-called "destination therapy" in patients who are not transplant candidates. Device selection depends on patient factors such as anticipated duration of need, patient size, as well as local experience and patient preference.

Contraindications to most of these devices include severe aortic or peripheral vascular disease (i.e., dissection, atherosclerosis, or aneurysm), LV or atrial thrombi, coagulopathy, uncontrolled sepsis, significant aortic valve stenosis or regurgitation, recent stroke or neurologic injury, or when invasive or heroic therapy would clearly be futile or inappropriate.

Mechanism of Support

Most (but not all) circulatory assist devices are designed to replace the pumping function of the left (or sometimes right or both) ventricles by diverting blood outside the normal blood flow circuit. Some derive their inflow from the left atrium or ventricle and return it to the aorta (LVAD) or receive blood from the right atrium or ventricle and return it to the pulmonary artery (RVAD). Blood may be returned to the aorta with continuous flow from the pump or in a pulsatile fashion with pump ejection occurring during the patient's diastole or asynchronous with their cardiac cycle. Although it was previously thought that pulsatile flow patterns were more desirable, studies have shown equivalent flow generation and clinical outcomes.[27,28] Continuous flow pumps are generally smaller, because they do not require a reservoir chamber. The remainder of this section will describe several assistive devices in order of increasing durations of use.

Short-Term Ventricular Assist Devices

Percutaneous Axial Flow Pump

Axial flow pumps work on the principle of the Archimedes screw. They are composed of a single cannula which is placed retrograde across the aortic valve into the left ventricle. Although they may be placed surgically, a femoral artery approach can be used.[29,30] The screw turns and draws blood out of the LV and ejects it into the ascending aorta beyond the aortic valve. Figure 26-7 depicts the device. Currently available devices include the Impella 2.5 and 5.0 microaxial flow devices (Abiomed, Inc., Danvers, MA). Because the position of the outflow area must be confirmed to be on the aortic side of the aortic valve, either fluoroscopic or echocardiographic guidance must be utilized. These devices can generate (nonpulsatile) flows of up to 2.5 or 5.0 L/min (depending on the model). Anticoagulation is required. Risks include hemolysis and thrombocytopenia, which are often transient; significant aortic valve disease (stenosis or regurgitation) can contraindicate its use.[31]

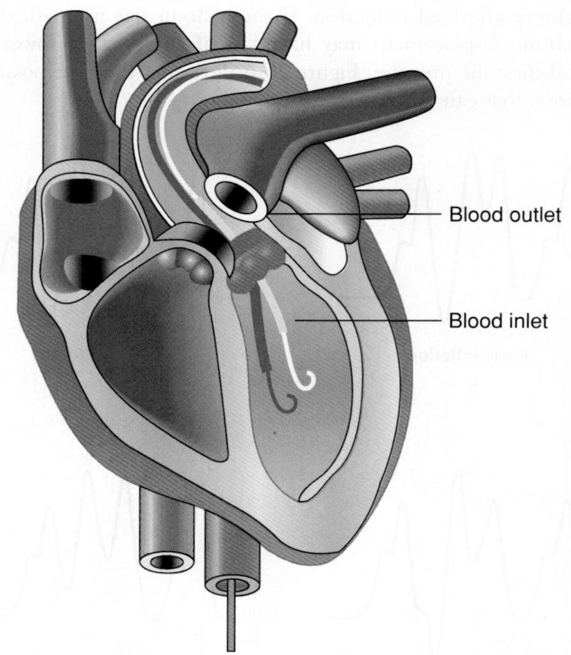

Figure 26-7 The Impella device is placed across the aortic valve, which allows the pump to aspirate blood from the left ventricle and expel it into the ascending aorta. (Courtesy of Abiomed, Danvers, MA; also from Figure 17, Lee, M. S., & Makkar, R. R. [2006]. Percutaneous left ventricular support devices. *Cardiology Clinics, 24*(2), 265–275, vii.)

Percutaneous Centrifugal Pumps

Another percutaneously placed VAD is the left atrial to femoral artery VAD (e.g., Tandem Heart™). A venous catheter is placed in the left atrium via transseptal puncture from the right atrium. An arterial cannula is inserted in the iliac artery. The pump is a centrifugal model providing continuous flow. The device is used for short-term stabilization, for hemodynamic support during PCIs, or as a bridge to recovery or surgical treatment. It requires anticoagulation (ideal activated clotting time of 250 to 350 seconds). Studies have shown improvement in cardiac output (the pump can move 4 to 5 L/min of blood), cardiac index, and other metabolic parameters. Mortality rates were comparable between IABP and VAD, but there were more complications (e.g., bleeding, acute limb ischemia) with VAD than with IABP.[32]

Another centrifugal percutaneous VAD is the Biomedicus (Medtronic, Inc., Minneapolis, MN) system. It is a centrifugal-kinetic energy pump that provides continuous flow via rotating cones that pull blood into the resulting vortex. It can be placed at the bedside with cannulae inserted in the femoral vessels, thus not requiring that the patient be brought to the catheterization laboratory; it can also be placed surgically. Compared to cardiopulmonary bypass or roller pumps, trauma to blood cells is decreased and heparinization is not required if flow rates are sufficiently maintained.[33]

Extracorporeal membrane oxygenation devices are designed to remove carbon dioxide from and to add oxygen to venous blood. Blood passes through an artificial membrane lung, bypassing the pulmonary circulation and returning to either the venous or arterial bloodstream. In severe respiratory failure the veno-venous route is used. In severe heart failure, veno-arterial bypass is utilized. When used in cardiogenic shock, extracorporeal membrane oxygenation is usually paired with either IABP or another mechanical assist device to augment cardiac output. Hemolysis and thromboembolism are significant barriers to extended use.[34]

Cardiopulmonary Assist Devices

Some assistive devices (e.g., the Abiomed AB5000, which is the follow-up to the Abiomed BVS 5000 VAD; Abiomed, Inc., Danvers, MA) must be placed surgically. It is a paracorporeal system, FDA approved for use in any potentially reversible acute cardiogenic shock. It is a versatile device that can be used as an LVAD, RVAD, or BiVAD for up to several weeks. Via a cannula in the right or left atrium, blood fills the atrial chamber of the pump by gravity and then flows across polyurethane valves into a ventricular chamber. Then it is pumped back via a coated graft into the pulmonary artery or the aorta. Flow is driven by the amount of drainage received by the atrial chamber, so volume depletion needs to be avoided. Heparanization is needed as clots can form in the cannulae or on the valve surface. The maximum output is about 5 L/min. Hemolysis and bleeding have been observed complications.[35]

Long-Term Ventricular Assist Devices

These devices can be used as bridges to recovery or transplant, or for destination therapy. Thoratec (Thoratec Laboratories Inc., Pleasanton, CA) produces both a paracorporeal (TLC-II) and an implanted (intra-abdominal, IVAD) assist device. They are pneumatic pump systems in which pulsatile flow is created by air compression of a polyurethane sac that contains 65 mL of blood. Positive air pressure compresses the sac, causing ejection from the LVAD to the aorta (or into the pulmonary artery if it is in RVAD configuration). Negative pressure is applied after ejection, causing the blood sac to fill. Backward flow is prevented by placement of inflow and outflow disk valves in the pump. The blood sac is filled by means of a cannula placed in either the left atrium or the LV. It can be controlled in one of three modes: (1) a fixed rate that is asynchronous with the patient's heart and delivers variable stroke volumes, (2) triggering of the pump by the R wave of the ECG (not practical for long-term support or in ambulatory patients), or (3) triggering of pump ejection by reaching full-fill (also called *fill-to-empty mode*).[36] Infectious risk is increased in the paracorporeal device (where the pump is external). Conduits from the atrium or ventricle and the return conduits to the aorta are tunneled through the chest and connected to the external pump (Fig. 26-8). For longer-term support, the preference is to cannulate the ventricle as larger flows can be obtained. Epithelial cells grow into the Dacron-covered conduits and protect the patient from infection. Tissue growth acts as a seal from the surface of the body.

The Novacor pump (World Heart Corp, Oakland, CA) is electrically driven and is fully implanted in a preperitoneal pocket just anterior to the posterior rectus sheath. Chronic support is possible because electrical energy can be stored in battery cells that are small enough to implant, although the electric power unit currently used is an exchangeable 5-hour battery. Filling of the pump occurs from a cannula that is placed in the LV apex. The cannula is tunneled through to the preperitoneal pocket, where the pump

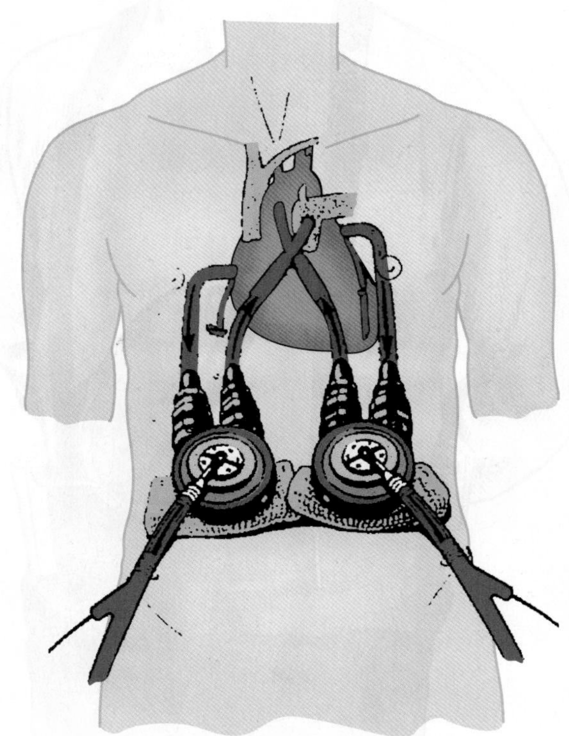

■ **Figure 26-8** Cannula placement of two Thoratec pumps during support of both right and left ventricles. Arrows indicate direction of blood flow. (From Ruzevich, S. A., Swartz, M. I., & Pennington, D. G. [1988]. Nursing care of the patient with a pneumatic ventricular assist device. *Heart & Lung, 17*, 399–405.)

is implanted. Blood is returned to the ascending aorta through another cannula. The device also uses inflow and outflow tissue valves. Ejection is triggered by a fixed rate, changes in the velocity of filling, or in a fill-to-empty mode. When the blood sac is filled, or when the trigger is recognized, two electrically powered pusher plates compress the blood sac, which is located between the two plates. Ejection occurs when the sac is compressed.[37] The major advantages are the implantability, which reduces infectious risk, and the ability of the patient to be ambulatory and possibly discharged from the hospital. Figure 26-9 illustrates the appearance of the device. Patients wear a controller on either on a belt or in a vest, and carry two batteries with them. One battery serves as a reserve supply when the patient switches from AC power to battery operation, and vice versa. The other primary battery pack can supply power for up to 5 hours, allowing the patient freedom from a tethered set-up. Figure 26-10 shows the first patient in the United States to receive the wearable system.

The HeartMate vented electric system (Thoratec, Pleasanton, CA) is also designed for long-term use. The HeartMate pump is electrically driven, with a controller and battery pack system similar to those of the Novacor pump. Ejection occurs as a result of compression of the blood sac by a single, motor-driven pusher plate.[38] Both the Novacor and HeartMate systems can support patients for extended periods with a relatively low risk of thromboembolism or mechanical problems. They can be used to support patients awaiting heart transplantation, and because they are portable, allow patients to be ambulatory and live in the community. This device was evaluated in the REMATCH trial, which randomized end-stage, NYHA class IV patients who were not eligible for transplantation to LVAD or optimal medical therapy. It revealed a higher survival (23% vs. 8%) and improved quality of life for patients randomized to LVAD. However there were adverse events, such as infection, bleeding, and device malfunction (which was 35% at 2 years).[39]

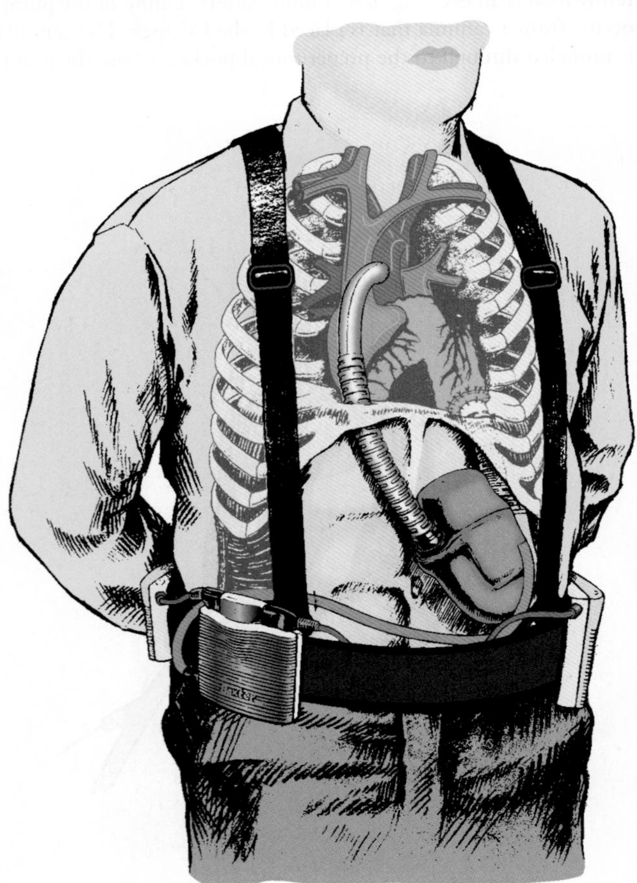

■ **Figure 26-9** Illustration of the Novacor left ventricular assist device shows the design of the implanted system. Power is transmitted through a percutaneous lead to the implanted pump. The patient either wears portable batteries or can be connected to an AC power source when at rest. (Courtesy of World Heart Inc. Oakland, CA.)

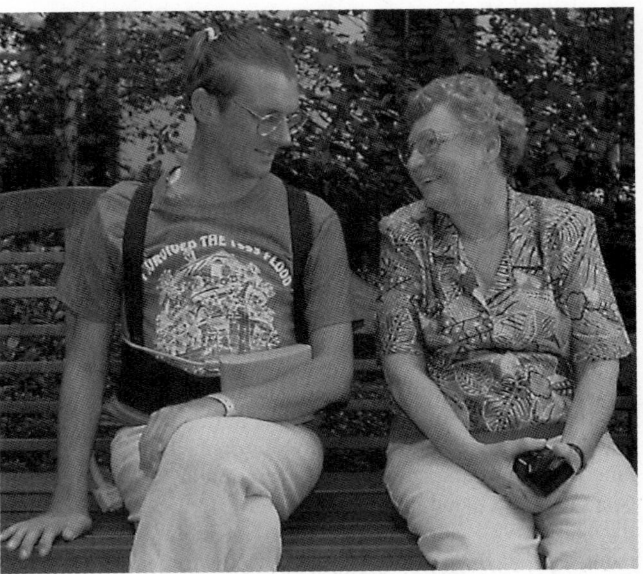

■ **Figure 26-10** A patient with the wearable Novacor left ventricular assist system. The patient carries a 5-hour battery pack on a specially designed belt, allowing him to be totally untethered to a heavy operating console, as with many other types of devices. This patient is shown at approximately 3 weeks after implantation and is waiting for a donor heart.

The HeartMate II (Thoratec, Pleasanton, CA) device is a continuous axial flow device. Unlike the pulsatile devices, which need a compliance chamber, the HeartMate II is much smaller but also requires somewhat higher levels of anticoagulation. Figure 26-11 depicts the device. The inflow cannula is placed in the LV apex and the outflow cannula is anastamosed to the ascending aorta. The VAD pump is placed in the abdominal or peritoneal cavity, with a percutaneous lead carrying the electrical cable to an electronic controller and battery packs, which are worn on a belt and shoulder holster. This device was recently evaluated in 133 patients as a bridge to transplant. Survival was 75% at 6 months and 68% at 1 year. Functional status and quality of life were improved when measured at 3 months. Bleeding, stroke, right heart failure, and percutaneous lead infection were seen, but rates compared favorably with those reported for pulsatile flow pumps. However, two patients sustained HeartMate II pump thrombosis.[40]

Other Continuous Flow Devices

Several promising devices are under active investigation but not yet FDA approved: the MicroMed-DeBakey VAD (MicroMed

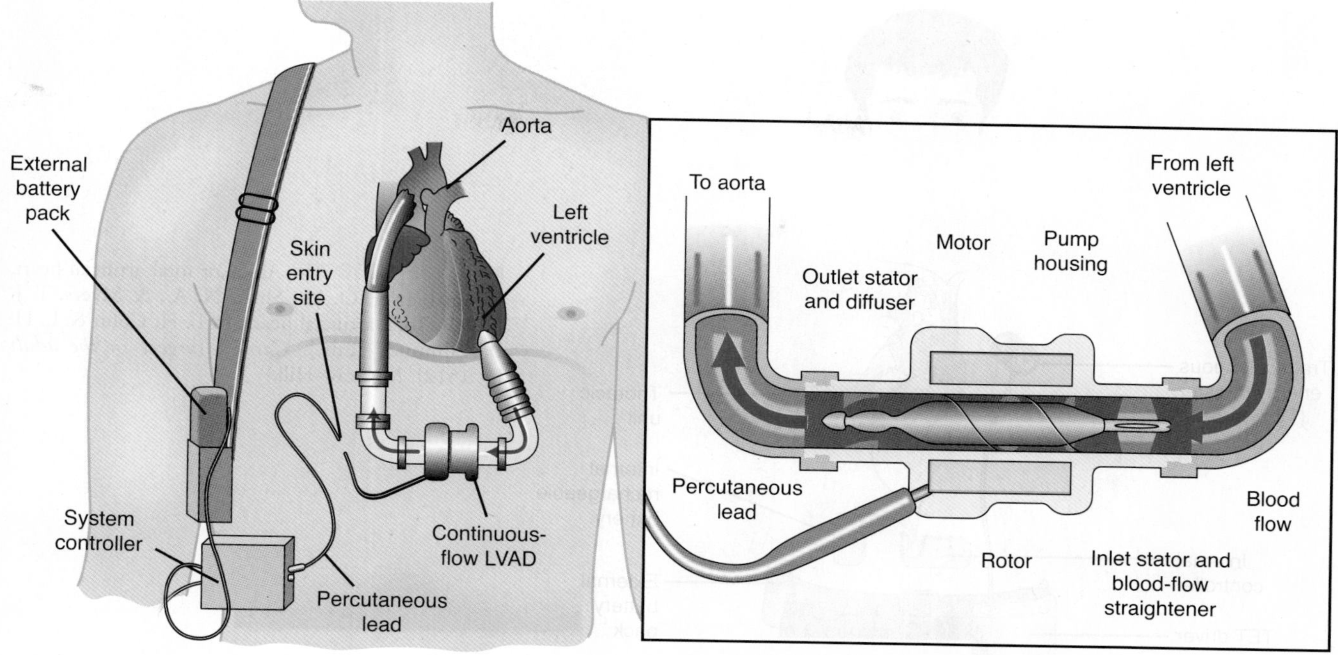

■ **Figure 26-11** The HeartMate II LVAD is composed of an inflow cannula inserted into the apex of the left ventricle, an outflow cannula that is anastomosed to the ascending aorta and a pump that is placed within the abdominal wall or peritoneal cavity. A percutaneous lead carries the electrical cable to an electronic controller and battery packs, which are worn on a belt and shoulder holster, respectively. (From Figure 1, Miller, L., Pagani, F., Russell, S., et al. [2007]. Use of a continuous-flow device in patients awaiting heart transplantation. *The New England Journal of Medicine, 357*, 885–896.)

Cardiovascular, Inc., Houston, TX) and the Jarvik 2000 (Jarvik Heart Inc., New York, NY). In Europe, the InCorBerlinHeart (Berlin Heart, Inc., Berlin, FR, German), and in Australia the VentrAssist are available. These axial flow pumps are capable of generating upward of 10 L/min of continuous flow, which more effectively rests the left ventricle.[41,42]

Total Artificial Heart

Total artificial hearts are devices that are placed in the chest after the patient's native heart has been removed. Complications such as thromboembolism, infection, and bleeding have limited their development. The CardioWest total artificial heart (SynCardia Systems, Tucson, AZ) is a pneumatic total artificial heart that has been studied as a bridge to transplant. In a nonrandomized prospective, multicenter trial using historical controls, 81 patients who received the device were followed after implantation. The rate of survival to transplantation was 79% (95% confidence interval, 68 to 87%). Of the 35 control patients who met the same entry criteria but did not receive the artificial heart, 46% survived to transplantation. Overall, the 1-year survival rate among the patients who received the artificial heart was 70%, as compared with 31% percent among the controls. One- and 5-year survival rates after transplantation among patients who had received a total artificial heart as a bridge to transplantation were 86% and 64%, respectively.[43] This device is depicted in Figure 26-12.

The AbioCor total artificial heart (Abiomed, Inc., Danvers, MA) is uniquely designed to use low-viscosity oil that is shunted

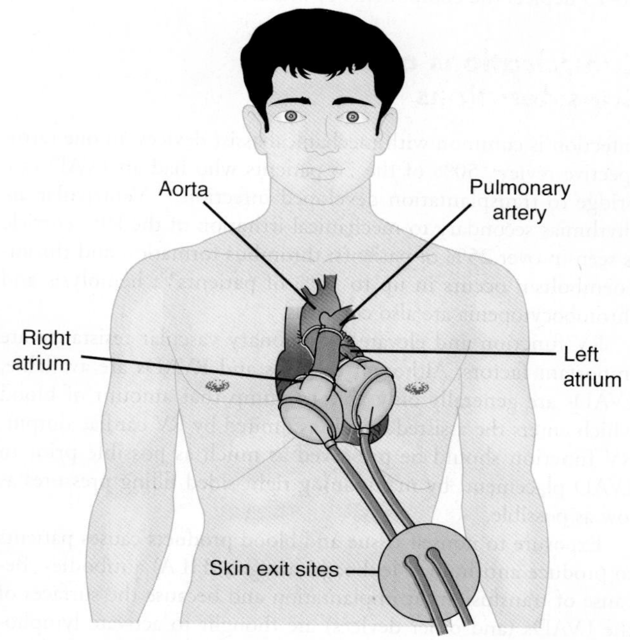

■ **Figure 26-12** The CardioWest total artificial heart (From Figure 1, Copeland, J. G., Smith, R. G., Arabia, F. A., et al. [2004]. Cardiac replacement with a total artificial heart as a bridge to transplantation. *The New England Journal of Medicine, 351*, 859–867.)

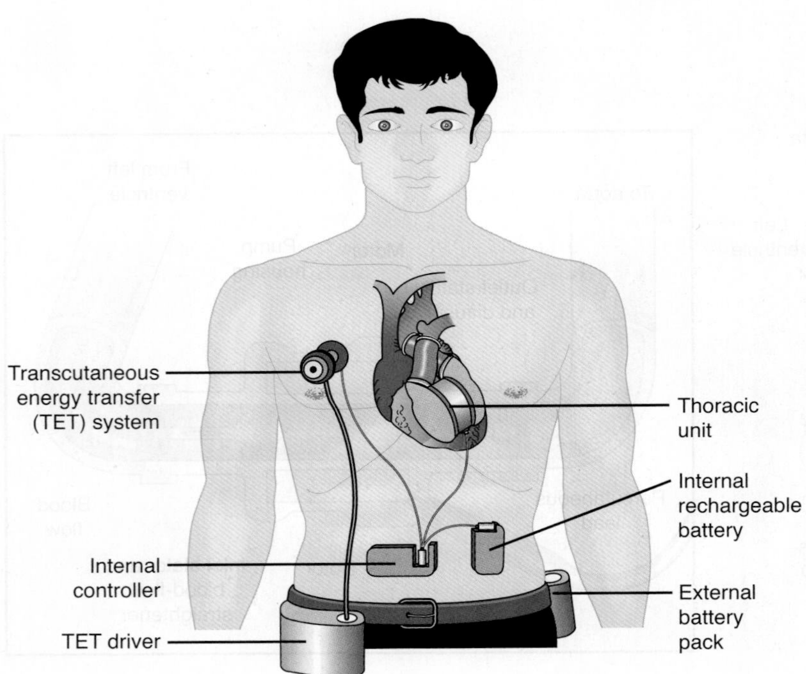

■ **Figure 26-13** The AbioCor total artificial heart. (From Frazier, O. H., Shah, N. A., & Myers, T. J. [2003]. Total artificial heart. In L. H. Cohn & L. H. Jr. Edmunds [Eds.]. *Cardiac surgery in the adult* [p. 1512]. McGraw-Hill.)

via a rotary pump between the right and left ventricles. This decompression shunt obviates the need for a compliance chamber reducing the size of the device. An electrical wire implanted around the abdomen acts as a conduction cable through which the battery energy can be provided percutaneously. No wires protrude out of the skin, however. The device is available via the FDA's humanitarian device exception at several US centers. Figure 26-13 depicts the components of the device.

Complications and Other Considerations

Infection is common with mechanical assist devices; in one retrospective review, 50% of the 76 patients who had an LVAD as a bridge to transplantation developed infection.[44] Ventricular arrhythmias secondary to mechanical irritation of the left ventricle is seen in over 25% of patients; thrombus formation and thromboembolism occurs in up to 16% of patients[45]; hemolysis and thrombocytopenia are also concerns.

RV function and elevated pulmonary vascular resistance are important factors. Although BiVADs and RVADs are available, LVADs are generally only able to pump that amount of blood which enters the assisted circuit as limited by RV cardiac output. RV function should be preserved as much as possible prior to LVAD placement, by maintaining right-sided filling pressures as low as possible.

Exposure to nonself tissue and blood products causes patients to produce anti-human leukocyte antigen (HLA) antibodies. Because of transfusions at implantation and because the surfaces of the LVADs (and other devices) are thought to activate lymphocytes, patients with LVADs have increased anti-HLA antibody production. These antibodies are associated with transplant rejection and decreased allograft survival,[46] and is an area of active research.

Ventricular Recovery and Device Removal

Intriguing research has demonstrated myocardial changes suggestive of "reverse remodeling," that may indicate that support could lead to significant myocardial recovery and explantation without need for transplant. Favorable findings include normalization of LV chamber geometry, regression of myocyte hypertrophy and fibrosis, improvement in myocyte contractile force, restoration of β-adrenergic responsiveness, and altered expression of genes involved in metabolism and apoptosis.[47–52] In one clinical study, 15 patients with nonischemic cardiomyopathies had aggressive medical therapy (which was composed of an angiotensin-converting enzyme inhibitor, two β-blockers, an aldosterone antagonist, and an angiotensin receptor antagonist) plus LVAD. Of these patients, 11 had sufficient recovery of ventricular function (mean ejection fraction of 0.12 before and 0.64 after) to have the devices explanted.[53] Two of the 11 explanted patients died: one of arrhythmias 24 hours after explant and the other of lung cancer. After a mean 4-year follow-up on the surviving nine patients, the ejection fraction remained normal, and recurrent heart failure was experienced by only one patient (after a period of high alcohol intake).

Given the anticipated expansion of the population of patients meeting indications for mechanical circulatory assistive devices, the progress already made and the research and development that are ongoing, there is tremendous hope for better devices, and more importantly, even better outcomes in the future.

Nursing Care Plan 26-1 ■ The Patient with an Intra-Aortic Balloon Pump

Nursing Diagnosis 1 ➧ Potential impaired tissue perfusion in the lower extremities related to catheter obstruction, emboli, or thrombosis, manifested by signs and symptoms of decreased perfusion in legs.

Nursing Goal 1 ➧ To minimize risk of decreased tissue perfusion in lower extremities.

Outcome Criteria ➧
1. Appropriate level of anticoagulation will be maintained as prescribed.
2. Dorsalis pedis and posterior tibial pulses will be palpable and of equivalent strength to baseline assessment.
3. Patient's skin will be warm, dry, and of normal color.
4. Patient will be knowledgeable about proper hip position.

NURSING INTERVENTIONS	RATIONALE
1. Record quality of peripheral pulses before insertion of the intra-aortic balloon pump (IABP) catheter.	**1.** Required to establish a baseline so changes will be detectable.
2. Evaluate quality of peripheral pulses, skin color, capillary refill, and temperature at least hourly.	**2.** Required to detect changes.
3. Maintain anticoagulation level at prescribed range by accurate monitoring or heparin or dextran infusion.	**3.** Thrombus could form along catheter or on balloon if anticoagulation falls below therapeutic range. Any thrombus may potentially break loose with balloon movement, causing emboli. In addition, excessive anticoagulation may lead to bleeding.
4. Assist patient with ankle flexion and extension every 1 to 2 hours.	**4.** Exercise of calf muscles will minimize venous stasis and potential for deep venous thrombosis.
5. Maintain cannulated extremity in a straight position, avoiding hip flexion. Use a brace or soft restraint as needed.	**5–7.** Hip flexion will decrease flow in the cannulated artery, potentially compromising distal circulation.
6. Keep head of bed at a 15-degree backrest position or lower. If it is desirable to elevate the head of the bed for pulmonary care issues, put the patient in reverse Trendelenburg to achieve the desired elevation without hip flexion.	
7. If patient is alert, instruct patient in importance of avoiding hip flexion.	
8. Maintain continuous alternating inflation and deflation of the balloon.	**8.** Continuous motion minimizes the possibility of thrombus formation on the balloon. Thrombus can occur rapidly on a motionless balloon, with subsequent risk of vascular occlusion or embolization.

Nursing Diagnosis 2 ➧ To detect early manifestations of decreased tissue perfusion in lower extremities.

Outcome Criteria ➧
1. Patient will maintain palpable dorsalis pedis and posterior tibial pulses equivalent to baseline.
2. Patient's skin will be warm, dry, and of normal color.
3. These changes will be detected within 1 hour of occurrence.

NURSING INTERVENTIONS	RATIONALE
1. Monitor quality of peripheral pulses, capillary refill, skin temperature, and color hourly.	**1.** Required to detect changes.
2. Notify physician if pulses diminish or become absent in the cannulated extremely.	**2.** Circulatory compromise may progress slowly as thrombus grows larger or rapidly as a result of an embolus.
3. If patient complains of leg pain, promptly evaluate peripheral perfusion. Notify physician of any changes.	**3.** Leg pain may be occurring as a result of ischemia. Ischemia is an indication for removal of the IABP catheter.
4. Monitor for swollen limb that is tense on palpation, if the patient complains of continuous pressure, and/or pain induced with passive stretching of the affected muscle.	**4.** These signs and symptoms may indicate the presence of compartment syndrome.

Nursing Care Plan 26-1 ■ (continued)

Nursing Diagnosis 2 ➧ Decreased cardiac output related to suboptimal IABP therapy, manifested by lowered mean arterial blood pressure with requirement for high-dose inotropic support.

Nursing Goal 1 ➧ To prevent decreases in cardiac output as a result of suboptimal IABP therapy.

Outcome Criteria ➧
1. Mean arterial blood pressure will be 60 to 70 mm Hg or higher.
2. IABP timing will be correct with:
   Inflation occurring at the dicrotic notch
   Optimal diastolic augmentation
   Deflation at end-diastole wit a drop in pressure of at least 8 to 10 mm Hg below unassisted end-diastole.
3. Balloon will be refilled before large gas losses secondary to diffusion.
4. Patient will have decreasing requirements for inotropic support over the course of IABP assistance.

NURSING INTERVENTIONS	RATIONALE
1. Verify correct timing of IABP hourly. Make correction as needed.	1. Timing may be altered if the heart rate changes or systolic function improves.
2. Document settings for inflation, deflation, and systolic, end-diastolic, and mean arterial pressures with IABP assistance.	2. Documentation will illustrate trends, improvement, and necessary interventions to achieve optimal assistance.
3. Document level of diastolic augmentation, evaluate for a decrease in augmentation. 4. Maintain proper volume of balloon to ensure optimal diastolic augmentation.	3–4. A decrease in diastolic augmentation may indicate a need to refill the balloon. A major loss of diastolic augmentation in a short time may indicate a tear or leak in the balloon (Check catheter for evidence of blood backing up from aorta.)
5. Ensure that the balloon is refilling every 1 to 2 hours, depending on the type of machine.	5. An optimally filled balloon is necessary for optimal diastolic augmentation.

Nursing Goal 2 ➧ To reduce or eliminate situations that will interfere with maintenance of proper IABP timing assist ratio (i.e., assistance of every beat).

Outcome Criteria ➧
1. Patient will have a regular heart rhythm.
2. There will be no interference of trigger signal to IABP console.
3. Timing will be corrected with changes in heart rate.
4. Balloon will be free of kinking.

NURSING INTERVENTIONS	RATIONALE
1. Re-evaluate timing anytime there is greater than a 10- to 20-beat change in heart rate on onset of new arrhythmias. Use the automatic timing feature on the IABP console if available.	1. A 10- to 20-beat or greater change in heart rate alters the systole-to-diastole ratio in each cardiac cycle. Previous inflation and deflation settings may be inappropriate for a change in this ratio (i.e., the time spent in diastole is longer at slower heart rates and shorter at rapid heart rates) unless the IABP console has an automatic timing feature.
2. Maintain adequate electrocardiogram (ECG) trigger signals to IABP console. Change any ECG electrodes that become loose, placing new ones on clean, dry skin.	2. Loss of trigger signals impairs IABP ability to assist the heart with each cardiac cycle.
3. Notify physician of any dysrhythmias. Secure cardiac pacing parameters if dysrhythmia is irregular and is impairing IABP tracking. Administer antiarrhythmic agents as ordered.	3. Irregular rhythms may impair IABP ability to assist each cardiac cycle. Pacing can stabilize this situation so that systole-to diastole ratio is the same for each cardiac cycle. The pacemaker spike may be used as the trigger for IABP timing.
4. Maintain patient in proper body position (head of bed 15 degrees and no hip flexion). Use leg brace and soft restraint as necessary. Log roll patient when turning. 5. Instruct x-ray technicians and other personnel not to sit patient upright.	4–5. Sitting the patient upright or elevating head of bed may cause hip flexion and subsequent catheter kinking. Kinking impairs the flow of gas in and out of balloon. An upright position also may cause the catheter to advance up the aorta with potential migration into an aortic arch vessel.

Nursing Care Plan 26-1 ■ (continued)

Nursing Diagnosis 3 ➧ Sensory/perceptual alterations: sensory overload related to intensive care unit environment and the need for frequent monitoring, manifested by disorientation, anxiety, restlessness, and sleeplessness.

Nursing Goal 3 ➧ To reduce or eliminate excessive sensory stimuli that might impair sleep–wake cycles

Outcome Criteria ➧
1. There will be no excessive or unnecessary noise in patient's environment.
2. Patient will have progressive blocks of undisturbed time for sleep.

NURSING INTERVENTIONS	RATIONALE
1. Maintain monitor "bleep" volume at lowest audible level. **2.** Minimize amount of extraneous noise from other equipment in patient's room. **3.** Minimize unnecessary noise caused by staff conversations in patient's room.	**1–3.** Unnecessary noise disturbs patient's sleep and creates higher levels of stress during wakefulness.
4. Turn down lights in patient's room during the night.	**4.** Darkening the room during the night helps patient distinguish day from night and provides a better environment for sleep at night.
5. Organize nursing care so patient has uninterrupted time for sleep during the night, amount to be determined by patient's condition.	**5.** Organized care can provide patients with up to 2-hour periods when it is unnecessary directly to touch the patient. As the patient's condition improves, longer blocks of time are feasible.

Nursing Goal 2 ➧ To assist patient with maintaining orientation and some degree of control of self.

Outcome Criteria ➧
1. Patient will be oriented to date, time, and place.
2. Patient will be able appropriately to interpret his or her environment.

NURSING INTERVENTIONS	RATIONALE
1. Talk with patient while administering care. Explain noises, activity, and procedures to be done.	**1.** Explanations assist the patient to interpret the environment appropriately and minimize stress and anxiety associated with a fear of the unknown.
2. Involve patient in decision making about care if possible (e.g., which direction to turn next). When patient is able, teach patient to do ankle flexion exercises and deep breathing exercises, which can be done independently by patient.	**2.** Involvement in decisions helps the patient maintain some degree of control.
3. Frequently inform patient of the time and date and orient to surroundings.	**3.** Frequently reorienting the patient helps prevent disorientation.
4. Place familiar objects such as pictures within patient view; involve family in the process.	**4.** Familiar objects may help maintain orientation.

Nursing Diagnosis 4 ➧ Ineffective family coping related to inadequate support, knowledge deficit, fear of patient dying, and fear of the intensive care unit environment, manifested by requests for help or inappropriate behavior.

Nursing Goal ➧ To assist family with development of ability to cope.

Outcome Criteria ➧
1. The family members will acknowledge their fears and concerns.
2. The family will verbalize a decrease in their level of fear and will appear calmer.
3. The family will demonstrate an ability to cope effectively.

Nursing Care Plan 26-1 ■ (continued)

NURSING INTERVENTIONS	RATIONALE
1. Encourage family members to express feelings, and convey understanding of their concerns and emotional stress.	**1.** Expression of concerns promotes effective coping.
2. Provide the family with honest information about the patient's condition to reduce fears. Keep the family informed of changes.	**2–3.** Fear is reduced by clarifying misunderstandings. Information decreases fear of the unknown.
3. Set aside time during visiting hours to spend with the family, and encourage family members to ask questions. Offer explanations about the intensive care unit environment.	
4. Encourage realistic hope based on the patient's progress. Point out progress to the family.	**4.** Hope helps the family with coping.
5. Allow family to participate in care as appropriate.	**5.** Participation decreases feelings of helplessness in aiding the recovery of the patient.
6. Determine how the family has coped with previous stressful situations.	**6.** It is important to identify previous effective coping mechanisms and to promote the use of these mechanisms.

REFERENCES

1. Maugh, T. H. (2007, December 7). Peter Houghton, 68. *Los Angeles Times.*
2. Rosamond, W., Flegal, K., Furie, K., et al. (2008). Heart disease and stroke statistics—2008 update: A report from the American Heart Association Statistics Committee and Stroke Statistics Subcommittee. *Circulation, 117*(4), e25–e146.
3. Deng, M. C., Young, J. B., Stevenson, L. W., et al. (2003). Destination mechanical circulatory support: Proposal for clinical standards. *The Journal of Heart and Lung Transplantation, 22*(4), 365–369.
4. Kantrowitz, A. (1990). Origins of intra-aortic balloon pumping. *The Annals of Thoracic Surgery, 50,* 672–674.
5. Mishra, S., Chu, W. W., Torguson, R., et al. (2006). Role of prophylactic intra-aortic balloon pump in high-risk patients undergoing percutaneous coronary intervention. *American Journal of Cardiology, 98,* 608.
6. Brodie, B. R., Stuckey, T. D., Hansen, C., et al. (1999). Intra-aortic balloon counterpulsation before primary percutaneous transluminal coronary angioplasty reduces catheterization laboratory events in high-risk patients with an acute myocardial infarction. *American Journal of Cardiology, 84,* 18.
7. Ferguson, J. J., Cohen, M., Freedman, R. J., et al. (2001). The current practice of intra-aortic balloon counterpulsation: Results from the Benchmark registry. *Journal of the American College of Cardiology, 38,* 1456.
8. Gitter, R., Cate, C. M., Smart, K., et al. (1998). Influence of ascending versus descending balloon counterpulsation on bypass graft blood flow. *The Annals of Thoracic Surgery, 65,* 365.
9. Mueller, H., Ayres, S. M., Conklin, E. F., et al. (1971). The effects of intra-aortic counterpulsation on cardiac performance and metabolism shock associated with acute myocardial infarction. *The Journal of Clinical Investigation, 50,* 1885.
10. Scheidt, S., Wilner, G., Mueller, H., et al. (1973). Intraaortic balloon counterpulsation in cardiogenic shock. *The New England Journal of Medicine, 288,* 979.
11. Kern, M. J., Aguirre, F. V., Tatineni, S., et al. (1993). Enhanced coronary blood flow velocity during intraaortic balloon counterpulsation in critically ill patients. *Journal of the American College of Cardiology, 21,* 359.
12. Urschel, C. W., Eber, L., Forrester, J., et al. (1970). Alteration of mechanical performance of the ventricle by intraaortic balloon counterpulsation. *The American Journal of Cardiology, 25,* 546.
13. McBride, L. R., Miller, L. W., & Nauheim, K. S. (1989). Axilliary artery insertion of an intra-aortic balloon pump. *The Annals of Thoracic Surgery, 48,* 874–875.
14. Funk, M., Ford, C. F., Foell, D. W., et al. (1992). Frequency of long-term lower limb ischemia associated with intraaortic balloon pump use. *The American Journal of Cardiology, 70,* 1195.
15. Barnett, M. G., Swartz, M. T., Peterson, G. J., et al. (1994). Vascular complications from intraaortic balloons: Risk analysis. *Journal of Vascular Surgery, 19,* 81.
16. Patel, J. J., Kopisyansky, C., Boston, B., et al. (1995). Prospective evaluation of complications with percutaneous intraaortic balloon counterpulsation. *The American Journal of Cardiology, 76,* 1205.
17. Cohen, M., Dawson, M. S., Kopistansky, C., et al. (2000). Sex and other predictors of intra-aortic balloon counter pulsation-related complications: Prospective study of 1119 consecutive patients. *American Heart Journal, 139,* 282–287.
18. Arafa, O. E., Pedersen, T. H., Svennevig, J. L., et al. (1999). Vascular complications of the intra-aortic pump in patients undergoing open heart operations: 15 year experience. *The Annals of Thoracic Surgery, 67,* 645–651.
19. Jiang, C. Y., Zhao, L. L., Wang, J. A., et al. (2003). Anticoagulation therapy in intra-aortic balloon counterpulsation: Does IABP really need anti-coagulation? *Journal of Zhejiang University SCIENCE, 4,* 607–611.
20. Gottlieb, S. O., Brinker, J. A., Borkon, A. M., et al. (1984). Identification of patients at high risk for complications of intraaortic balloon counterpulsation: A multivariate risk factor analysis. *The American Journal of Cardiology, 53,* 1135.
21. Eltchaninoff, H., Dimas, A. P., Whitlow, P. L. (1993). Complications associated with percutaneous placement and use of intraaortic balloon counterpulsation. *The American Journal of Cardiology, 71,* 328.
22. Tatar, H., Cicek, S., Demirkilic, U., et al. (1993). Vascular complications of intraaortic balloon pumping: Unsheathed versus sheathed insertion. *The Annals of Thoracic Surgery, 55,* 1518.
23. Scholz, K. H., Ragab, S., von zur Muhlen, F., et al. (1998). Complications of intra-aortic balloon counterpulsation: The role of catheter size and duration of support in a multivariate analysis of risk. *European Heart Journal, 19,* 458.
24. Meharwal, Z. S., & Trehan, N. (2002). Vascular complications of intra-aortic balloon insertion in patients undergoing coronary revascularization: Analysis of 911 cases. *European Journal of Cardiothoracic, 21,* 741.
25. Erdogan, H. B., Goksedef, D., Erentug, V., et al. (2006). In which patients should sheathless IABP be used? An analysis of vascular complications in 1211 cases. *Journal of Cardiac Surgery, 21,* 342.
26. Chen, E. W., Canto, J. G., Parsons, L. S., et al. (2003). Relation between hospital intra-aortic balloon counterpulsation volume and mortality in acute myocardial infarction complicated by cardiogenic shock. *Circulation, 108,* 951.

27. Radovancevic, B., Vrtovec, B., de Kort, E., et al. (2007). End-organ function in patients on long-term circulatory support with continuous- or pulsatile-flow assist devices. *The Journal of Heart and Lung Transplantation*, 26, 815–818.
28. Feller, E. D., Sorensen, E. N., Haddad, M., et al. (2007). Clinical outcomes are similar in pulsatile and nonpulsatile left ventricular assist device recipients. *The Annals of Thoracic Surgery, 83*, 1082–1088.
29. Siegenthaler, M. P., Brehm, K., Strecker, T., et al. (2004). The Impella recover microaxial left ventricular assist device reduces mortality for postcardiotomy failure: A three-center experience. *The Journal of Thoracic and Cardiovascular Surgery, 127*, 812.
30. Jurmann, M. J., Siniawski, H., Erb, M., et al. (2004). Initial experience with miniature axial flow ventricular assist devices for postcardiotomy heart failure. *The Annals of Thoracic Surgery, 77*, 1642.
31. Thiele, H., Smalling, R. W., Schuler, G. C. (2007). Percutaneous left ventricular assist devices in acute myocardial infarction complicated by cardiogenic shock. *European Heart Journal, 28*, 2057–2063.
32. Thiele, H., Sick, P., Boudriot, E., et al. (2005). Randomized comparison of intra-aortic balloon support with a percutaneous left ventricular assist device in patients with revascularized acute myocardial infarction complicated by cardiogenic shock. *European Heart Journal, 26*, 1276.
33. Noon, G. P., Lafuente, J. A., Irwin, S. (1999). Acute and temporary ventricular support with BioMedicus centrifugal pump. *The Annals of Thoracic Surgery, 68*, 650–654.
34. Rastan, A. J., Lachmann, N., Walther, T., et al. (2006). Autopsy findings in patients on postcardiotomy extracorporeal membrane oxygenation (ECMO). *The International Journal of Artificial Organs, 29*, 1121–1131.
35. Samuels, L. E., Holmes, E. C., Garwood, P., et al. (2005). Initial experience with the Abiomed AB5000 ventricular assist device system. *The Annals of Thoracic Surgery, 80*, 309–312.
36. Maroney, D. A., & Reedy, J. E. (1994). Understanding ventricular assist devices: A self-study guide. *Journal of Cardiovascular Nursing, 8*(2), 1–12.
37. Shinn, J. A., & Oyer, P. E. (1993). Novacor ventricular assist system. In S. Quaal (Ed.), *Cardiac mechanical assist beyond balloon pumping* (pp. 99–115). St. Louis: C.V. Mosby.
38. Hunt, S. A., Frazier, O. H., & Myers, T. J. (1998). Mechanical circulatory support and cardiac transplantation. *Circulation, 97*, 2079–2090.
39. Rose, E. A., Gelijns, A. C., Moskowitz, A. J., et al. (2001). Long-term mechanical left ventricular assistance for end-stage heart failure. *The New England Journal of Medicine, 345*(20), 1435–1443.
40. Miller, L., Pagani, F., Russell, S., et al. (2007). Use of a continuous-flow device in patients awaiting heart transplantation. *The New England Journal of Medicine, 357*, 885–896.
41. Frazier, O. H., Myers, T. J., Gregoric, I. D., et al. (2002). Initial clinical experience with the Jarvik 2000 implantable axial-flow left ventricular assist system. *Circulation, 105*, 2855–2860.
42. Koerner, M. M., & Jahanyar, J. (2008). Assist devices for circulatory support in therapy-refractory acute heart failure. *Current Opinion in Cardiology, 23*, 99–406.
43. Copeland, J. G., Smith, R. G., Arabia, F. A., et al. (2004). Cardiac replacement with a total artificial heart as a bridge to transplantation. *The New England Journal of Medicine, 351*, 859–867.
44. Simon, D., Fischer, S., Grossman, A., et al. (2005). Left ventricular assists device-related infection: Treatment and outcome. *Clinical Infectious Disease, 40*, 1108.
45. Reilly, M. P., Wiegers, S. E., Cucchiara, A. J., et al. (2000). Frequency, risk factors, and clinical outcomes of left ventricular assist device-associated ventricular thrombus. *The American Journal of Cardiology, 86*, 1156.
46. Itescu, S., Ankersmit, J. H., Kocher, A. A., et al. (2000). Immunobiology of left ventricular assist devices. *Progress in Cardiovascular Diseases, 43*, 67.
47. Dipla, K., Mattiello, J. A., Jeevanandam, V., et al. (1998). Myocyte recovery after mechanical circulatory support in humans with end-stage heart failure. *Circulation, 97*, 2316.
48. Heerdt, P. M., Holmes, J. W., Cai, B., et al. (2000). Chronic unloading by left ventricular assist device reverses contractile dysfunction and alters gene expression in end-stage heart failure. *Circulation, 102*, 2713.
49. Bruckner, B. A., Stetson, S. J., Perez-Verdia, A., et al. (2001). Regression of fibrosis and hypertrophy in failing myocardium following mechanical circulatory support. *The Journal of Heart and Lung Transplantation, 20*, 457.
50. Madigan, J. D., Barbone, A., Choudhri, A. F., et al. (2001). Time course of reverse remodeling of the left ventricle during support with a left ventricular assist device. *The Journal of Thoracic and Cardiovascular Surgery, 121*, 902.
51. Ogletree-Hughes, M. L., Stull, L. B., Sweet, W. E., et al. (2001). Mechanical unloading restores beta-adrenergic responsiveness and reverses receptor downregulation in the failing human heart. *Circulation 104*, 881.
52. Vatta, M., Stetson, S. J., Perez-Verdia, A., et al. (2002). Molecular remodelling of dystrophin in patients with end-stage cardiomyopathies and reversal in patients on assistance-device therapy. *The Lancet, 359*, 936.
53. Birks, E. J., Tansley, P. D., Hardy, J., et al. (2006). Left ventricular assist device and drug therapy for the reversal of heart failure. *The New England Journal of Medicine, 355*, 1873.

CHAPTER 27

Sudden Cardiac Death and Cardiac Arrest

Donna Gerity

Sudden cardiac death (SCD) is a major clinical and public health problem in the United States. The incidence of SCD is difficult to measure due to inconsistent methodology in classifying deaths. Various estimates of annual SCD events in the United States range from 200,000 to 450,000. The most widely used estimate is in the range of 300,000 to 350,000 deaths annually. Even with significant advances in management of coronary artery disease (CAD), and the treatment of heart failure, the overall incidence has remained unchanged as our population ages.[1] CAD is present in as many as 80% of those individuals who experience SCD. Autopsy studies show that 50% of these sudden death patients have acute changes in coronary status, such as plaque, rupture, or thrombus.[2] Survival rates for out-of-hospital sudden cardiac arrest (SCA) victims are low, with only 2% to 25% surviving to discharge in the United States. Those survivors of SCA have a high risk for future events. Therefore, the aim at decreasing SCD is to better identify and treat potential victims of SCD. Future events will be minimized if the incidence of CAD is reduced and primary and secondary prevention is provided.[3,4]

DEFINITION OF SUDDEN DEATH

SCD is defined as an unexpected death caused by cardiac causes that occurs within 1 hour of symptom onset. The person may or may not have known pre-existing heart disease. Cardiac arrest, usually caused by cardiac arrhythmias, is the term used to describe the sudden collapse, loss of consciousness and loss of effective circulation that precedes biologic death.[5,6] A subclassification of sudden death uses the term *instantaneous death*, a death with immediate collapse without preceding symptoms. Other causes of death may also be instantaneous, such as stroke, massive pulmonary embolism, or rupture of an aortic aneurysm. It is also important to note that not all arrhythmic deaths are sudden. A patient may be successfully resuscitated from a cardiac arrest but may die days later from complications.[7]

PATHOPHYSIOLOGY AND CAUSE OF SCA

The epidemiology of SCD tends to follow that of coronary heart disease (CHD). The incidence of SCD increases with the aging population in both men and women, whites and nonwhites, just as ischemic heart disease increases. SCD occurs 75% more often in men. Hypertension, left ventricular hypertrophy (LVH), intraventricular conduction defect, hypercholesterolemia, vital capacity, smoking, relative weight, and heart rate were all noted as risk factors per the 26-year follow-up of the Framingham Study.[8] SCD does appear to be increasing in women. From 1989 to 1999, SCD increased by 21% among women aged 35 to 44 years in the United States. During this same time frame there was a 2.8% decline among men of the same age group.[1,9] Risk profiling for CAD is useful for identifying populations and individuals at risk, but does not identify an individual patient at risk for SCD. The inability to identify individuals is a major reason why SCD remains an important public health problem.[10]

There are several different arrhythmia mechanisms responsible for SCD. The most common arrhythmia leading to SCD appears to be ventricular tachycardia (VT) accelerating into ventricular fibrillation (VF), often followed by asystole or pulseless electrical activity (PEA). Acquired structural and functional changes that occur in a diseased heart, and genetic factors may contribute to sudden death. However, the mechanism that produces the potentially fatal arrhythmia among patients with CAD is difficult to define.[11,12]

The episode could be caused from pure ischemic injury because of occlusion of a major artery in a patient with a normal ventricle in whom VF develops in the first minutes of an acute infarction. The other type of mechanism is one in which a patient with a previous myocardial infarction (MI) has postinfarction scarring that provides the anatomic substrate for VT that leads to hemodynamic collapse and SCD. Patients could also have complex substrates consisting of dense scar tissue with aneurysms or other areas where disorganized arrhythmias predominate. This complex interaction and multiplicity of influences that occur in a cardiac arrest episode differ for all patients.[2,7]

Structural Abnormalities

Coronary Heart Disease

CHD is the major structural abnormality found in most SCA victims. In 80% of patients who have had an SCA, CAD is present. SCA is often the first manifestation of CHD.[10,13] Pathology studies of SCD patients have shown that coronary atherosclerosis is the major predisposing cause. Plaque rupture and plaque erosion are the underlying pathologies in the majority of cases of SCD. Evidence shows a difference in the mechanism of MI and death between men and woman. Men tend to have coronary plaque rupture, while women tend to have plaque erosion.[14] Data from the Nurses' Health Study of 121,701 women have shown that 94% of women who had SCD had one risk factor for heart disease.[9] The evolution and clinical manifestation of CHD leading to SCA has been identified as four separate stages (Fig. 27-1). The first stage is *atherogenesis*, which is the beginning of plaque formation and occurs over a long period of time. This stage should be thought of as the stage that determines risks for CHD. The

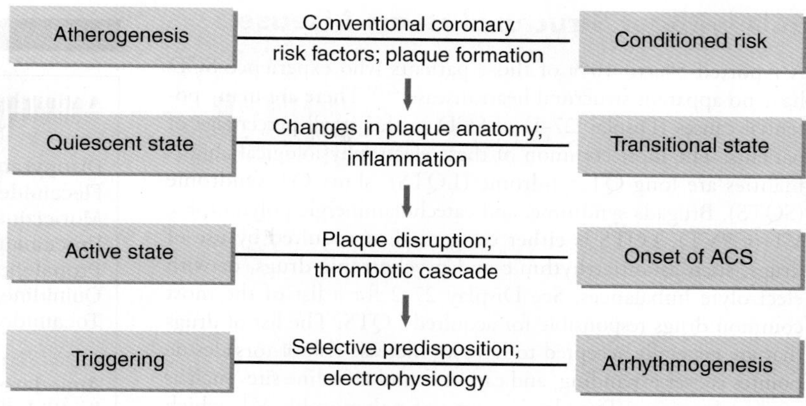

Figure 27-1 Evolution and clinical manifestations of risk for sudden cardiac death due to coronary artery disease. The cascade identifies four levels of progression beginning with plaque formation and development, progressing to an active state, then to acute coronary syndromes (ACS), and ending with life-threatening arrhythmias of SCD. (Used with permission from Myerburg, R. J. [2002]. Scientific gaps in the prediction and prevention of sudden cardiac death. *Journal of Cardiovascular Electrophysiology, 13*, 709–723.)

second stage is the *transitional stage* where changes in plaque anatomy and pathophysiology are taking place. During this stage, the disease has moved from quiet to active. The third level of the process is the *acute coronary syndrome* phase when the acute ischemic event may be triggered by plaque disruption and the onset of the thrombotic process. The time to a fatal arrhythmia is close, leaving less time for preventative actions. The final phase is the *arrhythmogenesis*, when an interaction is occurring between the active ischemic process and the onset of cardiac arrhythmias.[15]

Changes in coronary artery blood flow from other causes such as coronary vasospasms or nonatherosclerotic coronary artery abnormalities can also provoke ischemia and create myocardial electrical disturbances and the development of VF. Structural coronary artery abnormalities without atherosclerosis are rare and include congenital lesions, coronary artery emboli from aortic valve endocarditis, or from thrombotic material released from prosthetic aortic or mitral valve.[16]

Cardiomyopathy

The second largest group of patients who experience SCD includes patients with cardiomyopathy. Severely depressed left ventricular function is an independent predictor of SCD in patients with ischemic and nonischemic cardiomyopathy. An ejection fraction equal to or less than 0.35 is considered the most powerful predictor of SCD. Improved treatment options for patients with heart failure provide them with better long-term survival. However, there is an increasing proportion of patients with heart failure who die suddenly.[16] Three primary prevention studies have shown reduction in total mortality for ischemic and nonischemic cardiomyopathy patients. The Multicenter Automatic Defibrillator Implantation Trial (MADIT II) has shown that the implantable cardioverter defibrillator (ICD) will reduce total mortality in patients with ischemic cardiomyopathy with ejection fractions less that 0.30. The Sudden Cardiac Death in Heart Failure Trial (SCD-HeFT) enrolled patients with either ischemic or nonischemic cardiomyopathy with ejection fractions less than 0.35, and NYHA classes II and III heart failure. The results confirmed reduced mortality in the ischemic patients, but also in the nonischemic cardiomyopathy patients. The Defibrillators in Nonischemic Cardiomyopathy Treatment Evaluation (DEFINITE) trial also showed reduction in death from arrhythmias with ICD therapy.[17–19]

LVH has been established as an independent risk factor for SCD. ECG changes consistent with LVH and echocardiography evidence have both been associated with sudden and unexpected cardiac death.[8,20] The underlying causes for myocardial hypertrophy include hypertensive or valvular heart disease, obstructive and nonobstructive hypertrophic cardiomyopathy (HCM), and right ventricular hypertrophy secondary to pulmonary hypertension or congenital heart disease. All of these conditions are associated with increased risk of SCD, but it has been suggested that people with severely hypertrophic ventricles are especially susceptible to SCD.[16]

HCM is a familial cardiac disease that occurs in 1 out of 500 people. Often the disease goes undiagnosed and is the most common cause of sudden death in people under 30 years of age.[21,22] Sudden death often occurs with vigorous exercise is this group of patients. Various risk factors for SCD with HCM include family history of sudden death, documented nonsustained VT, recurrent and unexplained syncope, and extreme thickness of 30 mm or more of the left ventricle. Polymorphic VT and VF are thought to be the initial rhythm for patients with HCM who experience SCD.[7,16] Genetic studies of HCM have confirmed autosomal dominate inheritance patterns. Typically HCM is caused by mutations in any one of 10 genes that encode proteins of the cardiac sarcomere. DNA testing can identify patients with HCM at an early onset, helping to modify medical therapy and recommendations for placement of an implantable defibrillator, or withdrawing from intense physical activities and competitive sports.[22]

Valvular Heart Disease

The risk of sudden death in patients with valve disease is low but present. After prosthetic or heterograft aortic valve replacements, patients are at risk for SCD caused by arrhythmias, prosthetic valve dysfunction, or existing CHD. The risk of SCD after surgery peaks at 3 weeks and plateaus after 8 weeks. Sudden death can also occur with exertion in young adults with congenital aortic stenosis. The mechanism is uncertain but thought to be from sudden changes in ventricular filling or aortic obstruction with secondary arrhythmias.[7] Mitral valve prolapse is associated with a high incidence of symptomatic atrial and ventricular arrhythmias; however, whether it causes SCD is unresolved.[16]

Rare reports of sudden death have been reported from coronary embolism due to valvular vegetations, which trigger a fatal ischemic arrhythmia. Endocarditis of the aortic or mitral valve may cause deterioration of the valvular apparatus, and abscesses of the valvular rings or septum leading to sudden death.[16]

SCD without Structural Heart Disease

A reported 5% to 10% of those patients who experience SCD have no apparent structural heart disease.[2,20] There are many potential causes (Display 27-1) of SCD in this small percentage of patients. The most common of these electrophysiological abnormalities are long QT syndrome (LQTS), short QT syndrome (SQTS), Brugada syndrome, and catecholaminergic polymorphic VT (CPVT). LQTS is either congenital or acquired by use of drugs, such as antiarrhythmic and psychotropic drugs, or with electrolyte imbalances. See Display 27-2 for a list of the most common drugs responsible for acquired LQTS. The list of drugs that are generally accepted to have an increase risk of torsades de pointes is ever expanding, and can be found at online sites such as www.qtdrugs.org. Torsades is a type of polymorphic VT, which leads to syncope or SCD. SQTS is relatively newly defined syndrome, with short refractory periods both in the atria and the ventricles. Brugada syndrome is a genetic disease characterized by a right ventricular conduction delay. CPVT is characterized by

DISPLAY 27-1 Causes of Sudden Death

Cardiac Causes

- Acute myocarditis
- Aortic or ventricular aneurysm with dissection or rupture
- Aortic stenosis
- Cardiomyopathies
  - Ischemic cardiomyopathy
  - Nonischemic dilated cardiomyopathy
  - Hypertrophic cardiomyopathy
  - Alcoholic cardiomyopathy
- Chagas disease
- Congenital heart disease
- Coronary artery abnormalities
  - Myocardial infarction
  - Coronary artery spasm
  - Coronary artery embolism
- Endocarditis
- Electrophysiologic abnormalities
  - Brugada syndrome
  - Complete AV block
  - Wolff–Parkinson–White
  - Long QT syndrome—congenital and acquired
  - Catecholaminergic polymorphic ventricular tachycardia
- Prolapsed mitral valve syndrome
  - Prosthetic aortic or mitral valves
- Right ventricular dysplasia
- Sarcoidosis

Noncardiac Causes

- Cerebral or subarachnoid hemorrhage
- Choking
- Dissecting aneurysm of the aorta
- Electrolyte abnormalities
- Metabolic disturbances
- Pulmonary hypertension (primary, particularly during pregnancy)
- Pulmonary embolism
- Sudden infant death syndrome (should at least in part be included in cardiac causes)

DISPLAY 27-2 Drugs that Potentially Prolong the QT Interval (Generic Name/Brand Name)

Antiarrhythmic Agents

Class I

Disopyramide/Norpace
Flecainide/Tambocor
Moricizine/Ethmozine
Procainamide/Pronestyl
Propafenonel/Rhythmol
Quinidine/Quinidex
Tocainide/Tonocard

Class III

Amiodarone/Cordarone
Ibutilide/Corvert
Sotalol/Betapace
Dofetilide/Tikosyn

Class IV

Bepridil/Vascor

Antihistamines

Terfenadine/Seldane (Off U.S. Market)
Astemizole/Histamil (Off U.S. Market)

Antimicrobials

Ampicillin/Polycillin
Clarithromycin/Biaxin
Erythromycin/E-mycin
Pentamidine/Pentam
Trimethoprim-sulfamethoxazole/Bactrim

Antidepressants

Amitriptyline/Elavil
Amoxapine/Asendin
Clomipramine/Anafranil
Desipramine/Norpramin
Imipramine/Tofranil
Maprotiline/Ludiomil
Nortriptyline/Pamelor
Protriptyline/Vivactil

Antipsychotics

Chlorpromazine/Thorazine
Perphenazine/Trilafon
Risperidone/Risperdal
Thioridazine/Mellaril
Thiothixene/Navane
Trifluoperazine/Stelazine

Antiemetics

Droperidol/Inapsine
Prochlorperazine/Compazine

Gastrointestinal Agents

Cisapride/Propulsid
Ipecac syrup

Lipid-Lowering Agents

Probucol/Lorelco

Adapted from 2005 American Heart Association Guidelines for CPR and ECG.

ventricular arrhythmias that develop during physical activity in the presence of a normal resting ECG.[20,23]

Congenital Long QT Syndrome

Patients with the classic long QT intervals corrected for heart rate (QTc interval) are at increased risk for torsades.[20,23,24] Congenital long QT is hereditary; mutations in eight genes have been identified. The most common mutations are LQT1 (42%), LQT2 (45%), and LQT3 (8%). Most mutations affect the cardiac potassium-channel genes KCNQ1 and KCNH2 and cause the most frequent forms of long QT. An impaired sodium channel gene, SCN5A, is the cause for LQT3. However, the mutation LQT4 has been identified as a mutation from a membrane adaptor protein, and not an ion channel.[12,23] QT interval duration was identified as the strongest predictor of SCD, even before genetic mutation identification. A QTc greater than 500 ms in a patient identified with an affected gene carries the highest risk of syncope or SCD by the age of 40.[20] Two patterns of long QT have been reported: the Romano Ward syndrome, which is an autosomal dominant syndrome, and the Jervell and Lange-Nielsen syndrome. The latter is autosomal recessive, more severe, and often associated with congenital deafness.[20,25]

In individuals with long QT, ventricular arrhythmias often occur in the setting of stress and activity, but also can occur during rest and sleep. Exercise, particularly swimming, is often a trigger for arrhythmias in the LQT1 patients. LQT2 patients have arrhythmias that are triggered during both rest and emotion, often associated with acoustic stimuli. The LQT3 patients are more prone to having arrhythmias at rest and during sleep.[20,26] Avoidance of competitive sports is recommended for LQT1 and LQT2 patients, but not for LQT3 patients.[22]

Brugada Syndrome

Brugada syndrome is an inherited disease that is associated with a high incidence of sudden death. A mutation of cardiac sodium-channel gene SCN5A, has been identified in about 20% of persons with the syndrome, and occurs more often in men. The Brugada syndrome is confirmed with ST-segment elevation in the precordial leads, right bundle-branch block (RBBB) conduction pattern, and history of SCD. The ECG changes may be present all the time or elicited when antiarrhythmic drugs are given that block sodium channels (Chapter 15).[20,27,28] Fever has been reported to unmask ECG changes of Brugada syndrome and elicit an electrical VT storm.[29] Globally, the syndrome is more prevalent in areas of southeast Asia.[23]

Wolff–Parkinson–White Syndrome

Wolff–Parkinson–White (WPW) is associated with an accessory pathway that allows for conduction between the atria and ventricles. Normally, WPW is associated with nonlethal arrhythmias. However, if atrial fibrillation develops and conduction is rapid over the accessory pathway, the ventricular rate can become so fast that the rhythm degenerates into VF. SCD in the setting of WPW is quite low, and has been reported at 0.39% per year.[23,30]

Catecholaminergic Polymorphic Ventricular Tachycardia

CVPT is a catecholamine-dependent arrhythmia that occurs in the absence of a long QT interval. The arrhythmia often occurs during physical activity or emotional distress; therefore, β-adrenoceptor-blocking agents can be helpful in treating this condition. The first episode often occurs during childhood. The arrhythmia is characterized by bidirectional and polymorphic VT. The condition is rare, and is related to a genetic disorder. CPVT is caused by mutations involving the cardiac ryanodine receptor, and calsequestrin, a calcium-buffering protein.[20,23,31]

MANAGEMENT OF SCA

The outcome of cardiac arrest is determined by how promptly treatment is initiated with advanced cardiac life support (ACLS). To improve outcome from SCA, the following must occur as rapidly as possible: (1) early recognition of warning signs, (2) early activation of the emergency medical system, (3) early basic cardiopulmonary resuscitation (CPR), (4) early defibrillation, and (5) early ACLS. These events have been described as "links in a chain of survival," because they are all connected and indispensable to the overall success of emergency cardiac care.[32,33]

Although this section summarizes ACLS recommendations for the adult patient, it is not a complete reference. For each cardiac nurse, participation in an ACLS provider course by the American Heart Association (AHA) is strongly recommended. In addition, the most current version of *Emergency Cardiac Care, Basic Life Support for Healthcare Providers,* and *The Textbook of Advanced Cardiac Life Support* should be used as definitive references.

Adult Advanced Cardiac Life Support

ACLS teaches the appropriate skills and knowledge, as determined by leaders in emergency cardiovascular care (ECC), to improve survival from SCA and acute life-threatening cardiopulmonary events. ACLS includes early recognition of prearrest, basic life support, the use of airway and circulation adjuncts, cardiac monitoring, and defibrillation and other arrhythmia control techniques. ACLS also includes establishment of intravenous access, drug therapy, and postresuscitation care. This section focuses on defibrillation and ACLS management of pulseless cardiac arrest. Postresuscitation management of SCA survivors is also included. For discussions of basic and complex arrhythmias, conduction disturbances, electrophysiology studies, hemodynamic monitoring, acute coronary syndrome, pacemakers, and implantable defibrillators, respectively, refer to Chapters 15, 16, 18, 21, 22, and 28, respectively.

In 2005, the AHA updated the guidelines for CPR and ECC.[32] The guidelines are based on the 2005 International Consensus Conference on Cardiopulmonary Resuscitation and Emergency Cardiovascular Care Science with Treatment Recommendations. The classes of recommendation for ACLS management are based on evidence evaluation (Display 27-3).

Electrical Therapy of Malignant Arrhythmias

Defibrillation and cardioversion are a delivery of electrical energy that totally depolarizes and stuns the myocardium, which allows the sinus node to resume its function as the pacemaker for the heart. Defibrillation is, by definition, the therapy for VF. Cardioversion, which is a synchronized shock, is the electrical therapy for all other tachyarrhythmias. Transcutaneous and transvenous pacing are additional types of electrical therapy used in ACLS

DISPLAY 27-3 2005 AHA Classification Guidelines Using Level of Evidence Criteria

Class I	Class IIA	Class IIb	Class III	Indeterminate
Benefit >>> risk Procedure, treatment, or test should be performed or administered. Supported by high level prospective studies	Benefit >> risk It is reasonable to perform procedure, treatment/test. The weight of evidence supports action or therapy. It is considered acceptable and useful	Benefit ≥ risk Procedure, treatment or test may be considered. Evidence documents short-term benefit or positive results with lower levels of evidence	Risk ≥ benefit Procedure, treatment or test should not be performed or administered. May be harmful	Risk/benefit unknown Research just starting or ongoing. Further research needed before recomm-endations established

Adapted from 2005 American Heart Association Guidelines for CPR and ECG.

for patients with hemodynamically compromised bradycardias (Chapter 28).

Early Defibrillation

VT and VF are the most common arrhythmias during cardiac arrest, although the incidence of VF seems to be declining as reported by two studies from European cities, and from analysis of cardiac arrest events in Seattle, Washington from 1980 to 2000.[33,34] Defibrillation is the definitive therapy for cardiac arrest caused by VF. Rapid, early defibrillation is a key step and the most important intervention likely to save lives. Survival rates are best when immediate bystander CPR is provided and defibrillation occurs within 3 to 5 minutes.[35,36] A major obstacle to rapid, early defibrillation is that most cardiac arrests occur outside of the hospital, indicating a need for public health initiatives to improve early recognition of heart attack signs and symptoms.[1] The widespread use of automated external defibrillators (AEDs) assists in making early defibrillation a reality by expanding the number of rescuers available to treat SCD. The AHA integrates the use of AEDs with basic life support skills because VF is the most common rhythm found in adults with witnessed, nontraumatic SCA.[32,33]

Defibrillators. Defibrillators are the power source used to deliver the electrical therapy. Defibrillators typically include a capacitor charger, a capacitor to store energy, a charge switch, and discharge switch to complete the circuit from the capacitor to the electrodes. The capacitor charger converts power from a low-voltage source, such as direct current, to a voltage level sufficient for a shock. Portable defibrillators derive their power from a battery, which must be kept charged. Electrical output of defibrillators is quantified in terms of Joules (J), or watt-seconds, of energy.[33]

Defibrillators deliver energy to the electrode in either a biphasic or a monophasic waveform. Biphasic waveforms deliver current in a positive direction for a specific duration, and then reverse the current to a negative direction for the remaining discharge. A monophasic waveform delivers the current in one polarity or direction. Studies show that biphasic waveforms achieve shock success rates at lower energies, 150 J compared to 200 J, and produce less ST-segment change than shocks delivered with monophasic waveforms.[37–39] Lower energy requirements reduce the size and weight of the defibrillator, which in turn increases public access to AEDs because they are easier to handle, less expensive, and more convenient.

Rapid defibrillation can be performed with manual, automatic, or semiautomatic external defibrillators. Well-trained personnel, often ACLS responders, who are able to interpret cardiac rhythms on a rhythm strip or monitor, must operate manual defibrillators. Automatic advisory or semiautomatic external defibrillators have been developed for use by first responders. AEDs are accurate and easy to use and, unlike standard defibrillators, have detection systems that analyze the rhythm and advise the operator to shock when VF/VT characteristics are determined. Thus, successful defibrillation can be achieved without requiring the operator to have rhythm recognition skills. AEDs are attached to the patient with the use of adhesive sternal and apex pads that are connected to a cable, allowing for "hands-free defibrillation." AEDs were shown to help emergency personnel deliver the first shock on an average of 1 minute sooner than personnel using conventional defibrillators.[40] Early defibrillation with an AED has been shown to significantly increase survival in both out-of-hospital and in-hospital cardiopulmonary arrests.[32,41]

Transthoracic Impedance. The ability to defibrillate requires the passage of sufficient electric current through the heart. Current flow is determined by transthoracic impedance (TTI), or resistance to current flow, and the selected energy (Joules). If TTI is high, a low-energy shock may fail to produce sufficient current to defibrillate. The factors that determine TTI include energy setting, electrode size and composition, electrode–skin interface, number of and time between previous electrical discharges, electrode pressure, ventilation phase, and electrode placement.[42,43]

Resistance between the electrode and the chest wall must be minimized. Bare electrodes produce high resistance to electrical flow. Defibrillation electrode gel or paste, made specifically for defibrillation, will help to decrease impedance. Self-adhesive monitor or defibrillator pads are also available and effective. The adhesive defibrillator pads are thought to be more convenient and safer, as they reduce the possibility of electrical arcing. AHA recommends the use of adhesive pads. The pads can be placed as the patients condition deteriorates, allowing for monitoring of the patients heart rhythm and providing the ability to deliver a shock rapidly if necessary.[32,33]

Elevated TTI reduces the chance of successful defibrillation. Common causes of increased TTI include chest hair, which can increase impedance by 35%, and improper paddle position.[43,44] The optimal paddle size for adults in hand-held and self-adhesive pads are 8.5 to 12 cm in diameter, although defibrillation success may be higher with the electrodes that are 12 cm in diameter.[40]

Energy Requirements. Energy recommendations for defibrillation were changed with the 2005 AHA Guidelines.[32] The type of waveform the defibrillator delivers determines the amount of energy required to convert VF or pulseless VT. Defibrillators available today deliver either a monophasic waveform or one of two types of biphasic waveforms. A single immediate defibrillation must be performed followed by CPR, instead of the previously recommended three-stacked shocks. Both low-energy and high-energy biphasic waveform shocks are effective. There is no evidence to support that escalating energy or nonescalating energy is more effective.[32,33] AHA stresses that the most important factor in surviving an adult VF arrest is rapid defibrillation by either a monophasic or biphasic defibrillator.

Biphasic defibrillators use either a biphasic truncated exponential waveform that delivers an effective shock of 150 to 200 J, or a rectilinear biphasic waveform that is effective with a 120 J shock. AHA recommends that subsequent shocks remain the same, but can also be increased if the defibrillator is capable of delivering higher energy shocks. If a manual biphasic defibrillator is in use and the rescuer does not know the effective shock range for that particular defibrillator, the first shock should be 200 J. If an older model monophasic defibrillator is used, the rescuer should always select 360 J for all shocks. All defibrillators should be clearly labeled, so that the rescuer knows the starting effective energy level. All health care providers should be familiar with all models of defibrillators in their facility as there are many different models available. Rescuers who perform defibrillation must announce that they are about to deliver a shock. They must then check that all personnel are clear of the patient and stretcher before defibrillating. If the first shock successfully terminates VF but the patient subsequently goes back into VF, the energy should be kept at the last successful level rather than increasing the energy level.[32,33]

Electrode Position. Electrode placement is critical in ensuring that a critical mass of myocardium is depolarized. Any of three electrode positions may be used. *Standard* or *anterolateral* electrode placement involves one electrode being placed to the right of the upper sternum just below the right clavicle. The other electrode is placed on the left chest, lateral to the left breast in the mid-axillary line (Fig. 27-2). Two other patch positions are listed as class IIa recommendations in the updated AHA Guidelines[32]: patches on the lateral chest wall on the right and left sides (biaxillary); or one patch in the standard left apical position and the other pad on the right or left upper back. In patients with permanent pacemakers, electrode placement should be as far as possible from the pacemaker pulse generator, and when possible an anterior–posterior position should be considered. Refer to Chapter 28 for information on paddle placement for patients with ICDs.

Defibrillation Procedure. Identify the rhythm as VF. If the rhythm appears to be asystole, check the rhythm in another lead to confirm that the rhythm is not fine VF.

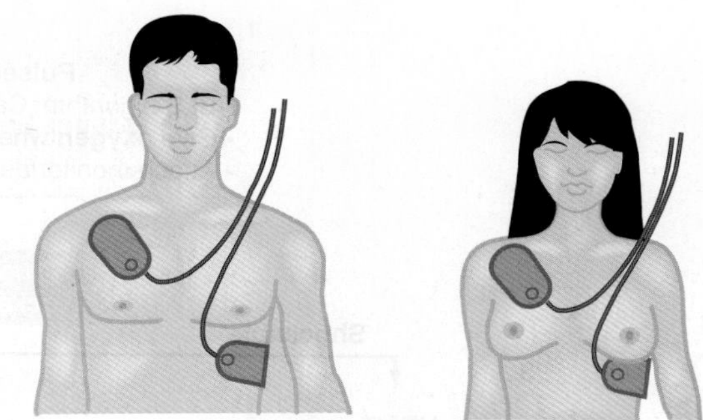

Figure 27-2 Standard positioning of defibrillator paddles.

- Turn on the defibrillator.
- Apply the adhesive pads in proper electrode position. The chest may need to be shaved, as hair will increase impedance. If electrode paddles are used, apply conductive materials.
- Set energy level to 120 to 200 J for biphasic defibrillator (device specific) and 360 J for monophasic defibrillator.
- Charge capacitors. Charging may take several seconds. Many defibrillators emit a sound or light signal, or both, to indicate that the unit has charged.
- Ensure proper electrode placement on chest.
- If using paddles, apply pressure of 25 lb per paddle. Do not lean forward because of the danger of the paddles slipping.
- Scan the area to ensure that no personnel are in contact directly or indirectly with the patient. Make sure there is no flowing oxygen source in electrical field.
- State firmly, "all clear" or other warning chant.
- Check rhythm—if patient remains in VF, deliver shock by depressing both buttons simultaneously on the paddles or discharge button on defibrillator.
- Start CPR immediately, beginning with compressions and resume for five cycles.
- Repeat assessment procedure. Continue with 200 J shock for biphasic defibrillator. (If biphasic defibrillator has ability to increase energy level a higher dose can be selected.) Continue with 360 J for monophasic defibrillator. Scan for personnel in contact with the patient, giving a warning signal prior to delivering shock.
- Resume CPR immediately beginning with compressions. If VF continues, refer to management of pulseless arrest algorithm (Fig. 27-3).

Management of Cardiac Arrest—ACLS Algorithms

A general framework for the use of ACLS algorithms is outlined in Display 27-4. The initial approach to the management of cardiac arrest is outlined in the ACLS pulseless arrest algorithm (Fig. 27-3). ACLS providers must always start with this algorithm by activating the emergency medical system and beginning basic life support (BLS). The basics of airway, breathing, and circulation remain important during the entire resuscitation continuum. Once the patient is attached to a monitor, determine the rhythm

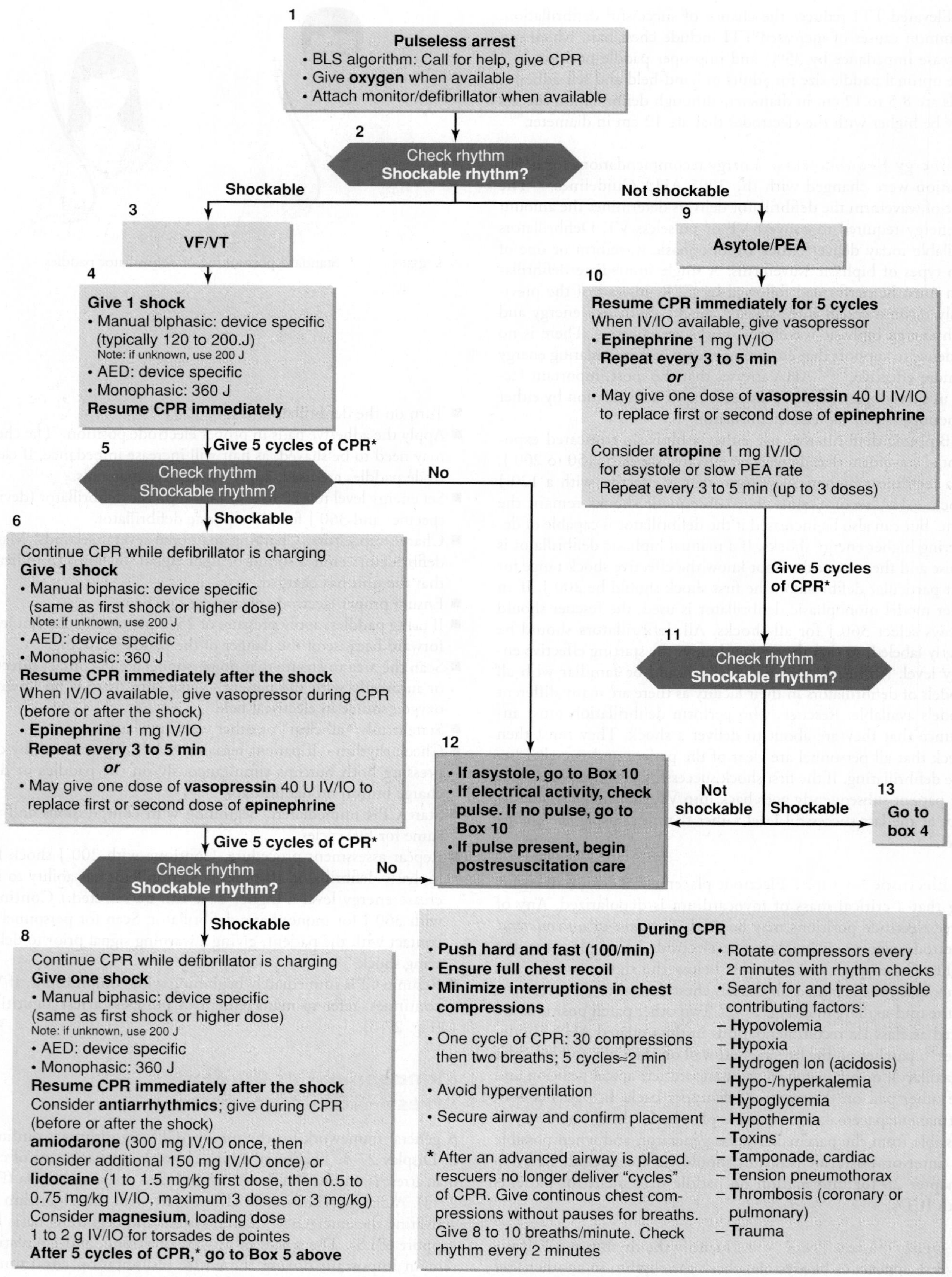

■ **Figure 27-3** Algorithm for pulseless arrest. The left side of the algorithm is for VT/VF; the right side for asystole/PEA. (From American Heart Association [2005]. *ACLS provider manual* [p. 42]. Dallas, TX: AHA.)

DISPLAY 27-4 The Algorithm Approach to Emergency Cardiac Care

The American Heart Association Guidelines use algorithms as an educational tool. They are an illustrative method to summarize information. Providers of emergency care should view algorithms as a summary and a memory aid. They provide ways to treat a broad range of patients. Algorithms by nature oversimplify. The effective teacher and care provider uses them wisely, not blindly. Some patients may require care not specified in the algorithms. When clinically appropriate, flexibility is accepted and encouraged. Many interventions and actions are listed as "considerations" to help providers think. These lists should not be considered endorsements or requirements or "standard of care" in a legal sense. Algorithms do not replace clinical understanding. Although the algorithms provide a good "cookbook," the patient always requires a "thinking cook."

The following clinical recommendations apply to all treatment algorithms:

- First, treat the patient, not the monitor.
- Algorithms for cardiac arrest presume that the condition under discussion continually persists, that the patient remains in cardiac arrest, and that CPR is always performed. The foundation of ACLS is good BLS.
- Apply different interventions whenever appropriate indications exist.
- Priorities during cardiac arrest are CPR with proper ventilation and chest compressions, and defibrillation. Administration of medications and insertion of an advanced airway are considered secondary importance.
- Providers may establish interosseous (IO) cannulation for IV fluids, drug administration and blood sampling if IV access is available (class IIa). If IV and IO access cannot be established some drugs can be given via the endotracheal route (lidocaine, epinephrine, atropine, naloxone, and vasopressin). Drugs given into the trachea have decreased absorption, and should be given in doses 2 to 2.5 times the recommended IV dose.
- With a few exceptions, intravenous medications should always be administered rapidly, by a bolus method.
- After each intravenous medication, give a 20- to 30-mL bolus of intravenous fluid and immediately elevate the extremity. This will enhance delivery of drugs to the central circulation, which may take 1 to 2 minutes.
- Last, treat the patient, not the monitor.

From American Heart Association. (2005). American Heart Association Guidelines for cardiopulmonary resuscitation and emergency cardiovascular care. *Supplement to Circulation, 112* (Suppl. IV), IV-19–IV-34.

and potential cause for the arrest. If VF or pulseless VT is present, the left side of the algorithm should be followed. If electrical activity is present without a pulse, or asystole is present then the right side of the algorithm should be followed.

Cardiac arrest should be managed by an ACLS team composed of a team leader and one or more team members. Priorities for resuscitation are:

- Effective CPR: minimizing interruptions of chest compressions and pushing hard and fast. Always ventilate not hyperventilate.
- Assess—then perform appropriate action.
- Rapid, early defibrillation for VF or pulseless VT.
- Vasopressin single dose or epinephrine given every 3 to 5 minutes to maintain coronary and cerebral perfusion.
- Differential diagnosis: search for and treat any reversible causes.

VF and Pulseless VT

In an *unwitnessed arrest*, the most critical intervention in the first few minutes of VF or pulseless VT is immediate CPR for at least 2 minutes, followed by rapid defibrillation. Providers should give one shock, rather than the three-stacked shocks that were recommended from previous versions of ACLS. Immediate CPR increases survival, and provides blood flow to the brain and heart, which keeps the heart in VF (as opposed to asystole) for a longer period. Defibrillation allows the normal pacemakers of the heart to restart after interrupting fibrillatory electrical activity.[4,45] After the single shock, CPR should be resumed immediately, beginning with compressions.

In a *witnessed arrest*, CPR should be started immediately, and a shock should be delivered as soon as VF/VT has been confirmed and a defibrillator is available. It is not necessary to perform the 2 minutes of CPR prior to the shock for a witnessed arrest. CPR should be initiated immediately after the shock.[32,33] Although studies comparing one shock to three shocks have not been conducted, evidence shows that interruption of chest compression decreases coronary perfusion. With previous algorithms that called for three-stacked shocks, there was noted to be a delay of nearly 40 seconds to the time CPR was resumed.[4,46,47] Delays in resuming CPR longer than 15 to 20 seconds have been shown to be a predictor of low survival, decreased myocardial function, and poor neurological outcome.[48,49]

The VF and pulseless VT algorithm directs rescuers to give either epinephrine or a one-time dose of vasopressin after the second shock and five cycles of CPR if the patient remains in VF/VT. Vasopressors remain an extremely important drug for patients in cardiac arrest. The beneficial effects of both vasopressin (non-adrenergic vasopressor) and epinephrine (adrenergic vasopressor) during cardiac arrest come from vasoconstriction, which increases aortic diastolic pressure, coronary perfusion pressure, and coronary blood flow.[32,33] Studies have not shown improved outcome using high-dose or escalating doses of epinephrine. The epinephrine dose remains 1 mg intravenous/intraosseus every 3 to 5 minutes.[4,32,33]

An antiarrhythmic drug can be considered after the second cycle of CPR, ventilations, and defibrillations. There is no evidence that giving antiarrhythmic drugs during cardiac arrest increases survival to hospital discharge, and the optimal number of cycles before drug administration has not been determined.[32,33] Amiodarone has been shown to increase survival to hospital admission when compared with lidocaine or a placebo (Display 27-5) and is a first-line antiarrhythmic drug for shock-refractory VT or VF (class IIb).[32,50,51] Lidocaine is an alternative antiarrhythmic, but has no proven short- or long-term efficacy in cardiac arrest. Lidocaine is given an indeterminate classification of recommendation.[32] Magnesium has been

DISPLAY 27-5 Arrest and Alive—Scientific Evidence for Use of Amiodarone

ARREST Trial—Amiodarone in Out-of-Hospital **R**esuscitation of **RE**fractory **S**ustained Ventricular **T**achyarrhythmias

Methods: Patients were enrolled if they had three or more unsuccessful shocks for VF or pulseless VT in an out-of-hospital cardiac arrest. In a randomized, double-blind, placebo controlled study patients were either randomly assigned to receive 300 mg of IV amiodarone (246 patients) or placebo (258 patients).

Results: Patients in the amiodarone group were more likely to survive to be admitted to the hospital. Forty-four percent of patients in the amiodarone group survived to hospital admission compared to 34% in the placebo group. There was no statistical difference in survival to hospital discharge between the two groups.

Conclusion: Patients in refractory VT/VF treated with amiodarone in out-of-hospital cardiac arrests have a higher rate of survival to hospital admission. Further investigation is warranted to see if the benefits extend to hospital discharge. (From Kudenchuk, P. J., Cobb, L. A., Copass, M. K., et al. [1999]. Amiodarone for resuscitation after out-of-hospital cardiac arrest due to ventricular fibrillation. *New England Journal of Medicine, 341*, 871–878.)

ALIVE Trial—Amiodarone versus **Li**docaine in Prehospital **V**entricular Fibrillation **E**valuation

Methods: Patients were enrolled if they had an out-of-hospital VF arrest resistant to total of four shocks and one dose of epinephrine; or if they had a recurrence of VF after initial success. Patients were randomized in a double-blind manner to receive either IV amiodarone plus lidocaine placebo (179 patients) or IV lidocaine plus amiodarone placebo (165 patients). The primary endpoint was survival to hospital admission.

Results: Those patients receiving amiodarone had a higher rate of survival to hospital admission than those receiving lidocaine (22.8% in amiodarone group versus 12.0% in lidocaine group). However only 5% of amiodarone group survived to hospital discharge, and 3% of lidocaine group survived to hospital discharge.

Conclusion: Amiodarone shows clinical effectiveness in the early stages of resuscitation. There appears to be no indication for the administration of lidocaine in the out-of-hospital setting for shock-resistant ventricular fibrillation. (From Dorian, P., Cass, D., Schwartz, B., et al. [2002]. Amiodarone as compared with lidocaine for shock-resistant ventricular fibrillation. *New England Journal of Medicine, 346*, 884–890.)

shown to be effective in terminating polymorphic VT associated with long QT (torsades de pointes) (class IIa for torsades). Magnesium has not been shown to be effective with polymorphic VT and normal QT interval.[32] Antiarrhythmic drugs are delivered by a bolus during cardiac arrest; however, after a return of spontaneous circulation (ROSC), they are often converted to infusions.

Asystole

The prognosis for patients in asystole is extremely poor. Asystole usually is the result of end-stage heart disease or prolonged cardiac arrest. The focus for treating asystole is effective CPR with minimal interruptions, providing ventilation with an advanced airway, and treating reversible causes. When asystole is first recognized a second lead configuration should be checked to reconfirm asystole. The defibrillator should also be checked quickly to assure that no leads have been disconnected from the patient or defibrillator/monitor. Vasopressors (epinephrine or vasopressin), and atropine are the treatment options in cardiac arrest with asystole and are used in an attempt to induce spontaneous electrical activity. Asystole should not be defibrillated. There have been no studies that have documented an improvement in survival by shocking asystole. Also, there have been no trials to show benefit from transcutaneous pacing for asystole. Asystole and PEA are both pulseless and nonshockable conditions. The right side of the pulseless arrest algorithm should be utilized to review all the steps to take in treating asystole (Fig. 27-3). CPR and resuscitation efforts should be ceased if it is determined that the patient has a valid do not attempt resuscitation order, has signs of irreversible death, or no physiologic benefit can be expected.[32,33]

Pulseless Electrical Activity

PEA is an organized rhythm without a pulse, and includes electromechanical dissociation, pseudo-electromechanical dissociation, idioventricular rhythms, ventricular escape rhythms, postdefibrillation idioventricular rhythms, and bradysystolic rhythms. Like asystole, the prognosis of patients with PEA is very poor unless the underlying cause can be identified and treated appropriately. Therefore, the highest priority is to find the correctable cause while maintaining the patient's airway, breathing, and circulation. Common correctable causes of electromechanical dissociation include hypovolemia, cardiac tamponade, tension pneumothorax, hypoxemia, and acidosis. Massive damage from MI, prolonged ischemia during resuscitation, and pulmonary embolism are less correctable causes. Patients in profound shock of any cause initially may present with PEA. Hypovolemia is assessed by history and lack of neck vein distension; it is treated by volume replacement. Tension pneumothorax is assessed by history and neck vein distension; it is treated by needle aspiration, chest tube insertion, or both. Cardiac tamponade is assessed by history and neck vein distension; it is treated by pericardiocentesis or thoracotomy. Hypoxemia is assessed by history and arterial blood gases and is treated by improving oxygenation and ventilation. Acidosis is also assessed by history and arterial blood gases, and is treated by improving CPR technique and hyperventilating the patient. If bradycardia is present, then atropine may be administered in an attempt to increase heart rate. ACLS presents the most common cause of PEA as "H's" (hypovolemia, hypoxia, hydrogen ion, hypo-/hyperkalemia, hypoglycemia, hyperthermia) and "T's" (toxins, tamponade, tension pneumothorax, thrombosis, trauma) and can be viewed at the bottom of the pulseless arrest algorithm (Fig. 27-3).[32,33]

Management of Impending Cardiac Arrest

Ventricular and Supraventricular Tachycardia

The tachycardia algorithm (Fig. 27-4) directs rescuers to focus on the patient and determine the hemodynamic stability of the

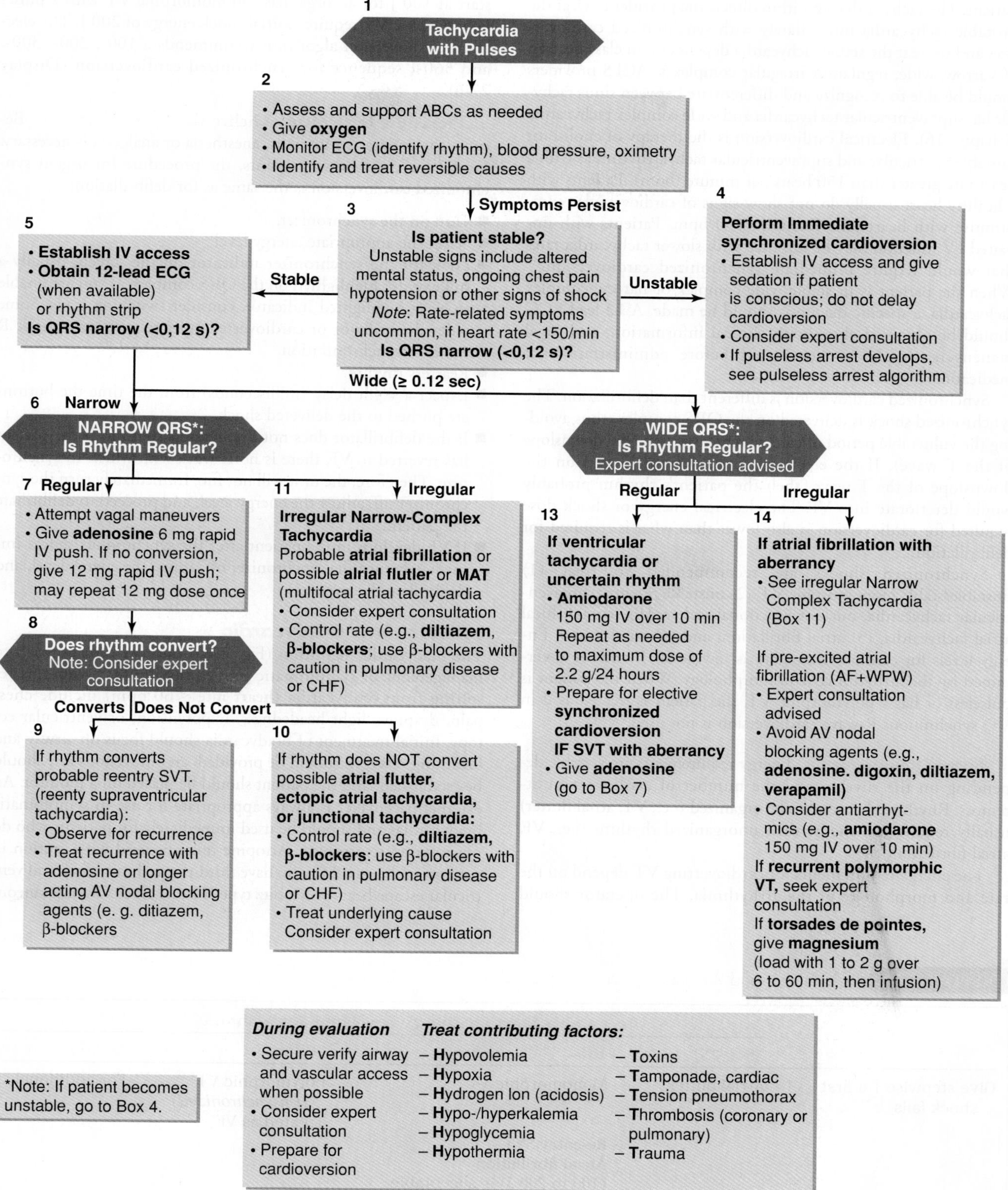

1
Tachycardia with Pulses
2
• Assess and support ABCs as needed
• Give oxygen
• Monitor ECG (identify rhythm), blood pressure, oximetry
• Identify and treat reversible causes
Symptoms Persist
3
Is patient stable?
Unstable signs include altered mental status, ongoing chest pain hypotension or other signs of shock
Note: Rate-related symptoms uncommon, if heart rate <150/min
Is QRS narrow (<0,12 s)?
Stable
Unstable
4
Perform Immediate synchronized cardioversion
• Establish IV access and give sedation if patient is conscious; do not delay cardioversion
• Consider expert consultation
• If pulseless arrest develops, see pulseless arrest algorithm
5
• Establish IV access
• Obtain 12-lead ECG (when available) or rhythm strip
Is QRS narrow (<0,12 s)?
Wide (≥ 0.12 sec)
6 Narrow
NARROW QRS*: Is Rhythm Regular?
WIDE QRS*: Is Rhythm Regular? Expert consultation advised
7 Regular
11 Irregular
Regular
Irregular
• Attempt vagal maneuvers
• Give adenosine 6 mg rapid IV push. If no conversion, give 12 mg rapid IV push; may repeat 12 mg dose once
Irregular Narrow-Complex Tachycardia
Probable atrial fibrillation or possible alrial flutler or MAT (multifocal atrial tachycardia
• Consider expert consultation
• Control rate (e.g., diltiazem, β-blockers; use β-blockers with caution in pulmonary disease or CHF)
13
If ventricular tachycardia or uncertain rhythm
• Amiodarone 150 mg IV over 10 min Repeat as needed to maximum dose of 2.2 g/24 hours
• Prepare for elective synchronized cardioversion
IF SVT with aberrancy
• Give adenosine (go to Box 7)
14
If atrial fibrillation with aberrancy
• See irregular Narrow Complex Tachycardia (Box 11)
If pre-excited atrial fibrillation (AF+WPW)
• Expert consultation advised
• Avoid AV nodal blocking agents (e.g., adenosine. digoxin, diltiazem, verapamil)
• Consider antiarrhytmics (e.g., amiodarone 150 mg IV over 10 min)
If recurrent polymorphic VT, seek expert consultation
If torsades de pointes, give magnesium (load with 1 to 2 g over 6 to 60 min, then infusion)
8
Does rhythm convert? Note: Consider expert consultation
Converts
Does Not Convert
9
If rhythm converts probable reentry SVT. (reenty supraventricular tachycardia):
• Observe for recurrence
• Treat recurrence with adenosine or longer acting AV nodal blocking agents (e. g. ditiazem, β-blockers
10
If rhythm does NOT convert possible atrial flutter, ectopic atrial tachycardia, or junctional tachycardia:
• Control rate (e.g., diltiazem, β-blockers: use β-blockers with caution in pulmonary disease or CHF)
• Treat underlying cause Consider expert consultation
*Note: If patient becomes unstable, go to Box 4.
During evaluation
• Secure verify airway and vascular access when possible
• Consider expert consultation
• Prepare for cardioversion
Treat contributing factors:
– Hypovolemia
– Hypoxia
– Hydrogen Ion (acidosis)
– Hypo-/hyperkalemia
– Hypoglycemia
– Hypothermia
– Toxins
– Tamponade, cardiac
– Tension pneumothorax
– Thrombosis (coronary or pulmonary)
– Trauma

■ **Figure 27-4** Algorithm for tachycardia. Boxes 9, 10, 11, 13, and 14 are designed for in-hospital use with expert consultation available. (From American Heart Association [2005]. *ACLS provider manual* [p. 91]. Dallas, TX: AHA.)

patient. The tachycardia algorithm directs the provider to treat the unstable tachycardia immediately with synchronized cardioversion and to treat the stable tachycardia dependent on classification of narrow, wide, regular, or irregular complexes. ACLS providers should be able to recognize and differentiate between sinus tachycardia, supraventricular tachycardia and wide complex tachycardia (Chapter 16). Electrical cardioversion is the therapy of choice for unstable ventricular and supraventricular tachyarrhythmias with a heart rate greater than 150 beats per minute (bpm). Patients with a healthy heart usually do not show signs of cardiovascular compromise with heart rates less than 150 bpm. Patients with impaired LV function may be unstable with slower tachycardia rates that would require immediate synchronized cardioversion.[32] When the patient is in stable wide-complex or narrow-complex tachycardia, a specific diagnosis should be made. A 12-lead ECG should be obtained along with clinical information, and vagal maneuvers should be considered before administration of medications.

Synchronized cardioversion is different than defibrillation. The synchronized shock is delivered on the QRS complex, thus avoiding the vulnerable period of cardiac repolarization (the downslope of the T wave). If the electrical shock were delivered on the downslope of the T wave, then the patient's rhythm probably would deteriorate into VF. The electrical energy or shock dose required for cardioversion is also lower than what is required for defibrillation.

Synchronized shocks are recommended to treat (1) unstable/stable monomorphic VT, (2) unstable re-entry supraventricular tachycardia, but not junctional tachycardia or multifocal atrial tachycardia, (3) atrial fibrillation, and (4) atrial flutter. Energy levels for cardioversion start as low as 50 J, and are determined by the arrhythmias and morphology. When the patient is pulseless or has a polymorphic VT, the patient is treated as if in VF; synchronous R-wave cardioversion is not used.[32,33]

Energy Requirements. Energy requirements are variable depending on the rhythm and the number of cardioversion attempts. Rhythms that tend to be organized (i.e., VT, atrial flutter) usually require less energy than unorganized rhythms (i.e., VF, atrial fibrillation).

The energy requirements for cardioverting VT depend on the rate and morphology of the arrhythmia. The operator should start at 100 J for an organized, monomorphic VT with a pulse. Polymorphic VT requires initial shock energy of 200 J. The electrical cardioversion algorithm recommends a 100-, 200-, 300-, and 360-J sequence for synchronized cardioversion (Display 27-6).

Procedure for Urgent Synchronized Cardioversion. Because the patient is conscious, anesthesia or analgesia is necessary. Except for the following points, the procedure for urgent synchronized cardioversion is the same as for defibrillation:

- Turn on the synchronizer.
- Select the appropriate energy level.
- Look for the synchronizer indicator on the screen, usually a spike or dot highlighted on the QRS complex. If you are unable to get a highlighted indicator, consider switching leads. Some older defibrillator or cardioverter units require an upright R wave for synchronization.
- Reassess rhythm.
- Expect a slight delay (milliseconds) from the time the buttons are pushed to the delivered shock.
- If the defibrillator does not fire, reassess rhythm. If the patient has reverted to VF, there is no R wave with which to synchronize. Therefore, the unit will not fire. Immediately turn the synchronizer off, adjust the energy level, and proceed to defibrillate the patient.
- If VF develops in the patient after the synchronous shock, immediately turn the synchronizer off, adjust the energy level, and defibrillate the patient.

Symptomatic Bradycardia

The bradycardia algorithm (Fig. 27-5) outlines the approach to management of symptomatic bradyarrhythmias. Symptoms resulting from bradycardia (heart rate <60 bpm) include chest pain, dyspnea, light-headedness, hypotension, or ventricular ectopy. Initial treatment of bradycardia should focus on airway and breathing. Oxygen should be provided, an intravenous line should be established, and the patient should be placed on a monitor. An external pacemaker is always appropriate for use in symptomatic bradycardias and should be used immediately for patients who do not respond to atropine. Atropine must be used with caution in patients with acute MI who have third-degree heart block and ventricular escape beats or Mobitz type II heart block. Transcutaneous

DISPLAY 27-6 Arrhythmias and Recommended Energy Levels for Cardioversion

	Acceptable Starting Energy Levels for Arrhythmias			
	50 J	**100 J**	**200 J**	**≥300 J**
Give stepwise ↑ if first shock fails	Atrial flutter	Monomorphic VT Re-entry SVT Atrial fibrillation (100 to 200 J) is acceptable	Polymorphic VT (*Unsynchronized*) Treated as VF	For additional

Starting energy levels for cardioversion vary with different arrhythmias. Atrial flutter and paroxysmal supraventricular tachycardia (PSVT) can convert to sinus rhythm with energy levels as low as 50 J. If unsuccessful, increase energy level to 100 J for second shock, 200 J for third shock, and 300 J or higher for additional shocks. Start energy level at 100 J for monomorphic VT, SVT, and atrial fibrillation, increasing energy level as needed. Polymorphic VT requires 200 J unsynchronized treated as VF. Energy levels are based on monophasic defibrillators; further data are required before dosing recommendations for cardioversions with biphasic waveforms can be made. (From American Heart Association. [2005]. American Heart Association Guidelines for cardiopulmonary resuscitation and emergency cardiovascular care. *Supplement to Circulation, 112*[Suppl. IV], IV-19–IV-34; American Heart Association. (2006). *ACLS provider manual.* Dallas, TX: AHA)

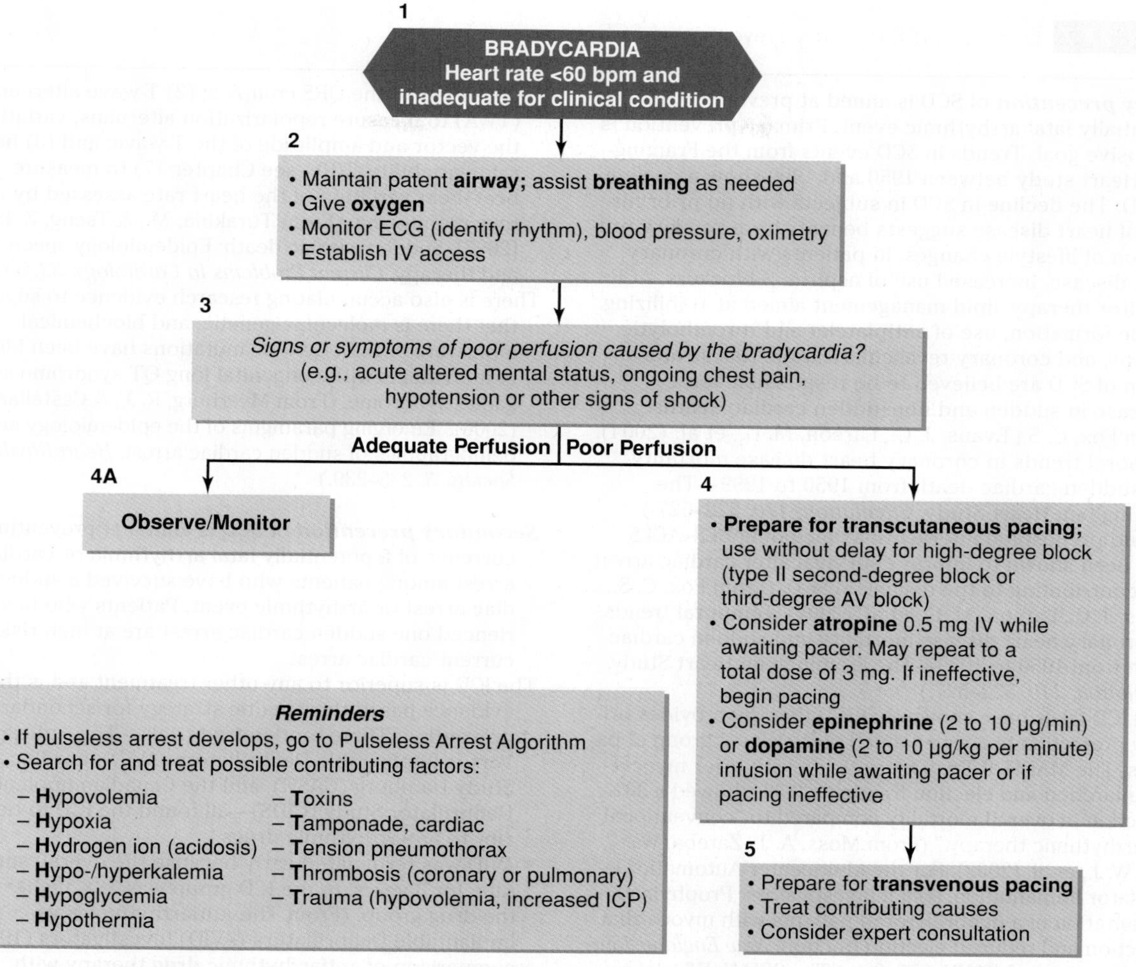

■ **Figure 27-5** Algorithm for bradycardia: atrioventricular blocks, and emergency pacing. (From American Heart Association [2005]. *ACLS provider manual* [p. 81]. Dallas, TX: AHA.)

pacing is first-line therapy for type II second-degree block or third-degree block. Dopamine and epinephrine should be added as the patient's condition worsens. Cardiac arrest from bradyarrhythmias, asystole, and PEA are more common in the secondary forms of cardiac arrest from MI.[32,33]

SURVIVORS OF CARDIAC ARREST

Prognosis

Prognosis of survivors is affected by how promptly definitive therapy is initiated, the rhythm or conduction disturbance initially recognized after cardiac arrest, and whether the patient also has sustained an acute MI. Nearly 80% of patients who experience SCD have an unwitnessed cardiac arrest outside the hospital setting; and only a minority of patients have ROSC. Only about one third of the patients who experience cardiac arrest will receive resuscitation attempts. Patient mortality remains very high after ROSC. Total survival rate with reasonable functional recovery for out-of-hospital cardiac arrests is as low as 2%, and as high as 25% in the United States.[13,32,52] Ongoing changes in CPR Guidelines, with a push for high quality and minimally interrupted CPR, have substantially increased initial survival rates.[53,54] The postresuscitation period is often marked with such complications as renal failure, congestive heart failure, respiratory complications, sepsis, and the potential for multiorgan failure. Protocols for patient management following a cardiac arrest can help to optimize the chance for survival and good neurological outcomes.[52] Postresuscitation care, the so-called "fifth link," has not seen the same standardization and research as BLS and ACLS support. Various interventions, such as percutaneous coronary intervention (PCI) and therapeutic hypothermia, have been associated with increased survival. Ongoing research that helps develop in-hospital guidelines will be beneficial in decreasing mortality postcardiac arrest.[55,56]

SCD survivors have received benefits from AEDs, revascularization procedures, ICDs, antiarrhythmic drugs, radiofrequency ablation of VT, or any combined therapies. Research has focused on providing primary prevention with prophylactic ICD therapy for patients with history of previous MI and LV dysfunction, improving the survival rate of high-risk patients.[17,23] (Display 27-7).

DISPLAY 27-7 Primary and Secondary Prevention of SCD

Primary prevention of SCD is aimed at preventing the first potentially fatal arrhythmic event. Primary prevention is an elusive goal. Trends in SCD events from the Framingham Heart study between 1950 and 1999 show a decline in SCD. The decline in SCD in subjects with no prior history of heart disease suggests benefits from primary prevention of lifestyle changes. In patients with coronary heart disease, increased use of aspirin, β-blockers, ACE inhibitor therapy, lipid management aimed at stabilizing plaque formation, use of antiplatelet and thrombolytic therapy, and coronary revascularization, risk stratification of SCD are believed to be responsible for a decrease in sudden and nonsudden cardiac deaths. (From Fox, C. S., Evans, J. C., Larson, M. G., et al. (2004). Temporal trends in coronary heart disease mortality and sudden cardiac death from 1950 to 1999—The Framingham Heart Study. *Circulation, 110,* 522–527.)

AEDs and prehospital interventions including BLS–ACLS have been shown to improve survival after cardiac arrest also contributing to the decline in SCD. (From Fox, C. S., Evans, J. C., Larson, M. G., et al. (2004). Temporal trends in coronary heart disease mortality and sudden cardiac death from 1950 to 1999—The Framingham Heart Study. *Circulation, 110,* 522–527.)

Several ICD trials have shown that ICD therapy provides primary protection in a well-defined high-risk subgroup of patients. The MADIT II Trial, for patients with prior myocardial infarction and ejection fraction ≤0.30, showed a 30% reduction in overall mortality compared to "conventional antiarrhythmic therapy." (From Moss, A. J., Zareba, W., Hall, W. J., et al. [2002]. For the Multicenter Automatic Defibrillator Implantation Trial II investigators. Prophylactic implantation of a defibrillator in patients with myocardial infarction and reduced ejection fraction. *New England Journal of Medicine, 346*[12], 877–883.) The SCD-HeFT trial results confirmed the benefit of ICD therapy in both ischemic and nonischemic cardiomyopathy patients with an ejection fraction ≤0.35 with a 23% reduction in risk of all-cause mortality. (From Bardy, G. H., Lee, K. L., Mark, D. B., et al. (2005). Amiodarone or an implantable cardioverter defibrillator for congestive heart failure. *New England Journal of Medicine, 352,* 225–327.) The DEFINITE trial showed a trend toward reduced mortality in patients with nonischemic dilated cardiomyopathy who receive an ICD for primary prevention. (From Kadish, A., Dyer, A., Daubert, J. P., et al. (2004). Prophylactic defibrillator implantation in patients with non-ischemic dilated cardiomyopathy. *New England Journal of Medicine, 350,* 2151–2158.)

Other tests available to help determine the risk of SCD include: (1) signal averaged ECG (SAECG) to measure late potentials of the QRS complex; (2) T-wave alternans (TWA) to measure repolarization alternans, variations in the vector and amplitude of the T wave; and (3) heart rate variability (HRV; see Chapter 17) to measure beat–beat variation of the heart rate assessed by ambulatory monitoring. (From Turakhia, M., & Tseng, Z. H. [2007]. Sudden cardiac death: Epidemiology, mechanisms, and therapy. *Current Problems in Cardiology, 32,* 501–546.)

There is also accumulating research evidence to suggest that there is molecular, genetic, and biochemical indicators of SCD. Genetic mutations have been identified in individuals with congenital long QT syndrome and Brugada's syndrome. (From Myerburg, R. J., & Castellanos, A. (2006). Emerging paradigms of the epidemiology and demographics of sudden cardiac arrest. *Heart Rhythm Society, 3,* 235–239.)

Secondary prevention of SCD is aimed at preventing a recurrence of a potentially fatal arrhythmia or cardiac arrest among patients who have survived a sudden cardiac arrest or arrhythmic event. Patients who have experienced one sudden cardiac arrest are at high risk for recurrent cardiac arrest.

The ICD is superior to any other treatment and is the only evidence-based therapeutic strategy for secondary prevention. Three randomized trials—The Antiarrhythmic Versus Implantable Defibrillators (AVID), Cardiac Arrest Study Hamburg (CASH), and the Canadian Implantable Defibrillator Study (CIDS)—all found the ICD to be superior to antiarrhythmic drugs.

- AVID was terminated early because the overall survival rate, for 3 years, in the ICD group was 32% higher than the drug group. (From The Antiarrhythmics vs. Implantable Defibrillators (AVID) Investigators (1997). A comparison of antiarrhythmic drug therapy with implantable defibrillators in patients resuscitated from near fatal ventricular arrhythmias. *New England Journal of Medicine, 337,* 1576–1583.)
- The CASH study showed a 23% lower mortality rate in the ICD group compared to the patients randomized to amiodarone/ metoprolol. (From Kuck, K. H., Cappato, R., Siebels, J., et al. (2000). Randomized comparison of antiarrhythmic drug therapy with implantable defibrillators in patients resuscitated from cardiac arrest: the Cardiac Arrest Study Hamburg (CASH). *Circulation, 102,* 748–754.)
- The CIDS trial showed similar results, with a 19% reduction in mortality in the ICD group compared to patients taking amiodarone. (From Connolly, S. J., Gent, M., Roberts, R. S., et al. (2000). Canadian Implantable Defibrillator Study (CIDS): a randomized trial of the implantable cardioverter defibrillator against amiodarone. *Circulation, 101,* 1297–1302.)

Medical Management of Survivors of Cardiac Arrest

Postresuscitation Goals

- Provide cardiac and respiratory support for optimal tissue perfusion, especially to the brain.
- Transfer the patient to the nearest appropriately equipped emergency department and then to a critical care unit.
- Identify the causes of the arrest.
- Institute medical therapy to prevent arrhythmia recurrence, such as antiarrhythmic drug therapy and correction of underlying abnormalities that may have precipitated the cardiac arrest.
- Institute measures that increase functional neurological outcomes.

Cerebral Resuscitation

The primary goal of cardiopulmonary-cerebral resuscitation is to retain healthy brain function. Unfortunately, neurologic recovery is incomplete after a successful cardiac resuscitation. Cessation of circulation for 10 to 20 seconds results in loss of consciousness caused by lack of oxygen. Within 2 to 4 minutes, glucose and glycogen stores are used up, and after 4 to 5 minutes ATP is exhausted. Hypoxemia and hypercarbia cause loss of cerebral blood flow autoregulation; the brain then becomes dependent on cerebral perfusion pressure.[54,57] Cerebral perfusion pressure is equal to mean arterial pressure minus intracranial pressure (CPP = MAP − ICP). After ROSC, a brief period of hyperemia occurs along with global hypoperfusion resulting in a "no-reflow phenomenon."[32,55] Improvement in cerebral recovery after cardiac arrest results when cardiac arrest and CPR times are short, and ROSC is restored quickly. During the Brain Resuscitation Clinical Trials, a cardiac arrest duration of 6 minutes or longer and an ROSC time of 28 minutes was associated with poor neurologic recovery.[52,58]

Treatment for the unresponsive patient should include optimizing cerebral perfusion pressure by maintaining a normal or slightly elevated mean arterial pressure and reducing intracranial pressure. Hyperthermia and seizures increase the oxygen requirements of the brain; therefore, all attempts at maintaining normothermia should be made. Research has shown induced hypothermia of 32°C to 34°C, improves outcomes in comatose survivors of cardiac arrest; however, optimal duration and temperature range require further investigation. Future studies and clarification of guidelines will help to implement induced hypothermia as a standard of care during postresuscitation support.[54–57,59] AHA recommends therapeutic hypothermia (class IIa) when the initial rhythm for SCD is VF and (class IIb) for non-VF arrest; out-of-hospital or in-hospital arrest.[32]

Electrolyte imbalances are likely to occur. There is an association between hyperglycemia and poor neurologic outcomes. One prospective randomized study has shown that maintaining glucose levels in the normal range reduced hospital mortality rates of critically ill patients, but not necessarily post-SCA patients.[60] The 2005 ECC Guidelines recommend strict glucose control, however acknowledge that additional studies are required to identify the appropriate glucose target range for post-SCA patients.[32]

Seizures are common after cardiac arrest and can delay recovery. They occur in approximately one third of patients. Once seizures are noted they should be treated with anticonvulsive therapy to optimize recovery. The patient's head should be maintained in a midline position and elevated to 30 degrees to increase cerebral venous drainage. Vigilant attention should be made at maintaining oxygenation and perfusion to the brain to maximize the chance for full neurological recovery.[32,52]

Ongoing Medical Care

The medical management for survivors of cardiac arrest depends on the patient's central nervous system function and known preexisting factors. Most survivors of cardiac arrest are comatose, and recovery is far from certain. Prognosis may not be determined for up to 72 hours postarrest.[61] Management of the patient includes providing effective perfusion of organs and tissues while directing diagnostic evaluation and treatment toward ongoing ischemia, LV dysfunction, structural abnormalities, arrhythmias, and other concurrent medical conditions.[32]

Diagnostic Evaluation. The most common substrate of SCD is CAD, seen in 80% of patients. Therefore patients should undergo coronary angiography after successful resuscitation. Decisions regarding timing of angiogram depend on hemodynamic instability, evidence of acute MI, and overall neurological prognosis with an extended cardiac arrest.[52] Studies from Sweden and Norway have shown an increase in survival with early coronary angiography and reperfusion treatment with PCI.[55,56] If the patient sustained cardiac arrest as a result of acute MI, evaluation and treatment are no different from those in any other patient with acute MI. The cardiac arrest produces a period of global ischemia and stunning to the myocardium; potentially, there is a need for either inotropic or intra-aortic counterpulsation to maintain perfusion. Often, ventricular dysfunction improves after the initial injury, and the initial low ejection fraction may not represent a true reading.[7] If the arrest is attributable to proarrhythmic drug effects or electrolyte disturbances, extensive evaluation usually is not indicated. Aggressive evaluation is warranted for most patients whose cardiac arrest was precipitated by coronary atherosclerosis not associated with acute transmural MI, or with other heart disease that can be managed medically or surgically. Diagnostic tests include ECG to rule out ischemia, long QT interval, and WPW. Other diagnostic tests may include cardiac catheterization (Chapter 20), radionuclide stress testing (Chapter 14), echocardiography (Chapter 13), electrophysiologic studies (Chapter 18), and possibly magnetic resonance imaging (Chapter 14) if arrhythmogenic right ventricular dysplasia is suspected. Laboratory tests that focus on possible causes include electrolytes, magnesium, and toxicology screen if drugs suspected (Chapter 11).[7,32,52]

Hemodynamic Support. After resuscitation and transfer to the intensive care unit (ICU), the patient usually will be intubated and will require general support of blood pressure, and heart rate. Patients often require inotropic drugs and fluids to maintain mean arterial pressure >65 to 70 mm Hg to help support coronary and cerebral blood flow.[55] There have been no clinical trials to indicate the optimal mean arterial pressure postcardiac arrest. Restoration of blood pressure and improvement in gas exchange does not necessarily lead to survival. Most postresuscitation deaths have been noted to occur in the first 24 hours.[32] The patient requires ongoing monitoring and treatment of ventricular arrhythmias. Amiodarone has been shown to be superior to placebo for shock-refractory VT and VF.[4,32]

Reduction of Ischemia. Depending on the anatomy and physiology of the disease process, either medical or surgical therapy is indicated. If the patient has had an acute MI, treatment guidelines should be consistent with the ACS algorithm (Chapter 22). Treatment options for secondary prevention of SCD include statins and aspirin to reduce the incidence of coronary plaque rupture or platelet aggregation and thrombosis. β-Blocker therapy stabilizes autonomic balance and helps reduce ischemia; angiotensin converting enzyme (ACE) inhibitors improve survival. β-Blocker therapy in patients with CAD has been shown to decrease total mortality by 20%, and decrease SCD by 30%.[62,63] β-Blockers are also effective in treating ventricular arrhythmias in the setting of increased sympathetic tone.[63] ACE inhibitor use may reduce SCD, as evidenced by the Trandolapril Cardiac Evaluation Trial (TRACE). The benefit is greatest in patients who have had a large MI, reduced ejection fraction, or clinical evidence of CHF.[64]

Myocardial revascularization has been shown to reduce the incidence of SCD in patients with heart disease, both in primary and secondary prevention of SCD. The greatest benefits are seen in those patients with multivessel disease and decreased left ventricular function.[7] Surgery is indicated for those patients with conventional criteria (i.e., uncontrolled angina, or left main or multiple-vessel CHD) or with specific criteria for antiarrhythmic surgery (i.e., discrete ventricular aneurysms or inducible, potentially lethal, arrhythmias not controlled by medication).[7]

Because of the complexity of SCD mechanisms, treatment is geared at delaying further progression of CHD in those patients with known cardiac disease. Long-term treatments include preventing thrombus formation and plaque rupture, preventing arrhythmias, stabilizing autonomic balance, improving pump function, and correcting ischemia.[63]

Antiarrhythmic Therapy. The uses of antiarrhythmic drugs are valuable in the immediate period after resuscitation. Intravenous amiodarone and β-blockers are the most effective antiarrhythmics in the early postarrest phase. However, unlike β-blockers and ACE inhibitors, certain antiarrhythmics, particularly class I drugs, have been associated with increased mortality rates despite suppressing ventricular ectopy.[7] Increased mortality was seen in the Cardiac Arrhythmia Suppression Trial (CAST) study with the use of encainide and flecainide in the patient after acute MI. CAST II showed increased mortality rates in this same group with the use of moricizine.[60] In contrast, several trials have shown a beneficial effect on mortality with the use of amiodarone, a class III drug, in patients after MI. Properties of amiodarone that may help reduce mortality after MI are coronary vasodilatation and heart rate reduction, which serve to reduce ischemia.[32,51]

Implantable Cardioverter Defibrillator. ICD therapy has emerged as the therapy of choice for secondary prevention of SCD in patients with pre-existing heart disease. Three large multicenter trials compared ICD therapy versus antiarrhythmic drug therapy in survivors of SCA and demonstrated ICD therapy was superior to best antiarrhythmic drug therapy (Display 27-7). Recent years have produced dramatic technological improvements in ICDs. Devices are smaller, implantation has been greatly simplified, and therapy options are greater, which help to reduce the number of unnecessary shocks. Treatment of life-threatening ventricular arrhythmias will most likely remain the domain of the ICD in the future. Antiarrhythmic drugs and catheter ablation will continue to complement the ICD, decreasing the frequency of ICD discharges and, hopefully, improving quality of life. (See Chapter 28 for additional ICD information.)

Nursing Management of SCD Survivors

Survivors of cardiac arrest and their families have physiological, psychological, and educational needs that differ from those of the patient with acute myocardial ischemia and infarction. However, if the underlying cause of SCA includes ischemia, management of the patient with ischemia and infarction should be included in nursing care.

Physiological Nursing Management

After cardiac arrest, patients are admitted to the cardiac care unit. A complete evaluation for heart disease is obtained on all patients, and is used as the basis of treatment goals. Occasionally, patients present with an "arrhythmia storm" and are in danger of recurrent VF. The patient will need aggressive correction for acute ischemia, and possibly hemodynamic support.[2] The patient will require continuous ECG monitoring until an ICD is placed. An intravenous line is left in place for immediate venous access. Time of hospital discharge is related to the cause of the cardiac arrest, the type of diagnostic studies required, and the eventual therapies selected by the patient and family. If the patient will be receiving an ICD, the implications of an ICD must be discussed thoroughly, and further educational needs should be evaluated.

Emotional Support

Emotional support given to patients and their families affects their quality of life. Patients and their families experience fear of recurrent cardiac arrest. Fear is exacerbated further at the time of transfer out of the cardiac care unit to a telemetry unit, and further still at the time of discharge from the hospital. Fear of transferring out of the ICU is known as "transfer anxiety," and can lead to physical complaints and symptoms of anxiey.[65] The effect that SCD survival has on quality of life and anxiety is not well defined. Some studies report an increase in stress, anxiety, fear, and memory difficulties associated with cardiac arrest.[66,67] Another study found that emotional distress is similar between cardiac patients, whether patients have had a cardiac arrest or not.[68] Another study has shown a decrease in anxiety after 6 months to 1-year postarrest.[69] However, a consistent theme is that interventions aimed at educating the patient and family about their disease process and ICD decrease anxiety. Cardiac nurses play a major therapeutic role in the management of SCA survivors and their families.

Patient and Family Education

Information regarding the impact of specific education interventions for SCA survivors is limited, and is mostly focused on the patient with an ICD. Cardiac arrest survivors have decreased ability to concentrate when compared to noncardiac arrest patients with heart disease.[68] Hypoxia during cardiac arrest leads to both diffuse brain injury and to injury of focal memory regions of the brain. Studies have documented persistent memory impairment in the VF survivor.[70,71] Knowing that memory is compromised, patient education may be difficult and family members will need to be involved early in the process to help with ongoing patient education and recovery. When Dougherty et al.[72] interviewed partners of SCA survivors who received an ICD during the first year of recovery, the partners conveyed eight major concerns: (1) physical care, (2) emotional care, (3) memory, (4), ICD, (5) money, (6) uncertain future, (7) health care providers, and (8) family. Nurses providing care to SCA survivors and their families should keep these concerns in mind when providing education and support.

All of this information is overwhelming and almost impossible for patients and their families to remember without teaching aids such as booklets, charts, videotapes, and pictures. Family members may also feel particularly overwhelmed by the thought of recurring episodes. Support groups have been shown to provide a means for seeking educational information, and developing camaraderie with others to assist in coping with anxieties.[73,74] Nurses often coordinate ICD support groups, providing an essential role in the education and support of patients and their families as they ask questions and discuss issues.

SUMMARY

Sudden cardiac death remains the primary cause of cardiac death in the United States, despite all the advances in therapy and technology. At present, the pathophysiology of SCD is not clearly understood. Progress has been made on the genotype-phenotype correlations of LQTS patients and other inherited diseases linking genetic substrate as a marker for SCD. Risk factor stratification and an understanding of pathophysiology remain critically deficient. SCD will remain a deadly challenge until these problems are solved. Education and training should continue to focus on initiating the "chain of survival" stressing the importance of CPR, and focusing on post-resuscitation guidelines to increase survival rates for sudden cardiac arrest patients. Stressing prevention is vital because the first symptom is often death.

REFERENCES

1. Zheng, Z. J., Croft, J. B., Giles, W. H., et al. (2001). Sudden cardiac death in the United States, 1989–1998. *Circulation, 104*, 2158–2163.
2. Callans, D. J. (2002). Management of the patient who has been resuscitated from sudden cardiac death. *Circulation, 105*, 2704–2707.
3. Prystowsky, E. N. (2001). Primary and secondary prevention of sudden cardiac death: The role of the implantable cardioverter defibrillator. *Reviews in Cardiovascular Medicine, 2*(4), 197–205.
4. Ali, B., & Zafari, A. M. (2007). Narrative review: Cardiopulmonary resuscitation and emergency cardiovascular care: Review of the current guidelines. *Annals of Internal Medicine, 147*(3), 171–179.
5. Myerburg, R. J., & Castellanos, A. (2004). Cardiac arrest and sudden cardiac death. In D. P. Zipes, R. O. Bonow, & E. Braunwald (Eds.), *E. Braunwald's heart disease: A textbook of cardiovascular medicine* (7th ed., pp. 865–908). Philadelphia: Elsevier Saunders Company.
6. Kusmirek, S. L., & Gold, M. R. (2007). Sudden cardiac death: The role of risk stratification. *American Heart Journal, 153*(4, Suppl. 1), 25–33.
7. Dimarco, J. P. (2003). Sudden cardiac death. In M. H. Crawford (Ed.), *Current diagnosis and treatment in cardiology* (2nd ed., chap. 24). New York: Lange Medical Books/McGraw-Hill.
8. Zipes, D. P., & Wellens, H. J. (1998). Clinical cardiology: New frontiers—Sudden cardiac death. *Circulation, 98*, 2334–2351.
9. Albert, C. M., Chae, C. U., Grostein, F., et al. (2003). Prospective study of sudden cardiac death among women in the United States. *Circulation, 107*, 2096–2101.
10. Myerburg, R. J., & Castellanos, A. (2006). Emerging paradigms of the epidemiology and demographics of sudden cardiac arrest. *Heart Rhythm Society, 3*, 235–239.
11. Lopshire, J. C., & Zipes, D. P. (2006). Sudden cardiac death: Better understanding of risks, mechanism, and treatment. *Circulation, 114*, 1134–1136.
12. Rubart, M., & Zipes, D. P. (2005). Mechanism of sudden cardiac death. *The Journal of Clinical Investigation, 115*, 2305–2315.
13. Eisenberg, M. S., & Mengert, J. T. (2001). Cardiac resuscitation. *New England Journal of Medicine, 344*, 1304–1313.
14. Burke, A. P., Farb, A., Malcom, G. T., et al. (1998). Effect of risk factors on the mechanism of acute thrombosis and sudden coronary death in women. *Circulation, 97*, 2110–2116.
15. Myerburg, R. J. (2002). Scientific gaps in the prediction and prevention of sudden cardiac death. *Journal of Cardiovascular Electrophysiology, 13*, 709–723.
16. Myerburg, R. J., & Castellanos, A. (2007). Cardiac arrest and sudden cardiac death. In P. Libby, R. O. Bonow, D. L. Mann, et al. (Eds.), *Braunwald's heart disease: A textbook of cardiovascular medicine* (8th ed., chap. 36). Philadelphia: Saunders Elsevier.
17. Moss, A. J., Zareba, W., Hall, W. J., et al. (2002). For the Multicenter Automatic Defibrillator Implantation Trial II investigators. Prophylactic implantation of a defibrillator in patients with myocardial infarction and reduced ejection fraction. *New England Journal of Medicine, 346*(12), 877–883.
18. Bardy, G. H., Lee, K. L., Mark D. B., et al. (2005). Amiodarone or an implantable cardioverter defibrillator for congestive heart failure. *New England Journal of Medicine, 352*, 225–237.
19. Kadish, A., Dyer, A., Daubert, J. P., et al. (2004). Prophylactic defibrillator implantation in patients with non-ischemic dilated cardiomyopathy. *New England Journal of Medicine, 350*, 2151–2158.
20. Zipes, D. P., et al. (2006). ACC/AHA/ESC 2006 Guidelines for management of patients with ventricular arrhythmias and the prevention of sudden cardiac death. *Journal of American College of Cardiology, 48*(5), 247–346.
21. Maron, B. J. (2002). Hypertrophic cardiomyopathy—cardiology patient page. *Circulation, 106*, 2419–2421.
22. Maron, B. J., Seidman, J. G., & Seidman, C. E. (2004). Viewpoint—Proposal for contemporary screening strategies in families with hypertrophic cardiomyopathy. *Journal of the American College of Cardiology, 44*(11), 2125–2132.
23. Turakhia, M., & Tseng, Z. H. (2007). Sudden cardiac death: Epidemiology, mechanisms, and therapy. *Current Problems in Cardiology, 32*, 501–546.
24. Imboden, M., Swan, H., Denjoy, I., et al. (2006). Female predominance and transmission distortion in the long-QT syndrome. *New England Journal of Medicine, 355*(26), 2744–2751.
25. Napolitano, C., Priori, S. G., & Schwartz, P. J. (2005). Genetic testing in the long QT syndrome—Development and validation of an efficient approach to genotyping in clinical practice. *JAMA, 294*(23), 2975–2981.
26. Moss, A. J., Robinson, J. L., Gessman, L., et al. (1999). Comparison of clinical and genetic variables of cardiac events associated with loud noise versus swimming among subjects with the long QT syndrome. *American Journal of Cardiology, 84*, 876–879.
27. Priori, S. G., Napolitano, C., Gasparini, M., et al. (2000). Clinical and genetic heterogeneity of right bundle branch block and ST-segment elevation syndrome. A prospective evaluation of 52 families. *Circulation, 102*, 2509–2515.
28. Brugada, P., & Brugada, J. (1992). Right bundle branch block, persistent ST segment elevation and sudden cardiac death: A distinct clinical and electrocardiographic syndrome. *Journal of American College of Cardiology, 20*, 1391–1396.
29. Dinckal, M. H., Davutoglu, V., & Akdemir, I. (2003). Incessant monomorphic ventricular tachycardia during febrile illness in a patient with Brugada syndrome: Fatal electrical storm. *Europace, 5*, 527–261.
30. Pappone, C., Santinelli, V., Rosanio, S., et al. (2003). Usefulness of invasive electrophysiologic testing to stratify the risk of arrhythmic events in asymptomatic patients with Wolff-Parkinson-White syndrome. *Journal of American College of Cardiology, 41*, 239–244.
31. Priori, S. G., & Napolitano, C. (2005). Intracellular calcium handling dysfunction and arrhythmogenesis—A new challenge for the electrophysiologist. *Circulation Research, 97*, 1077–1079.
32. American Heart Association. (2005). American Heart Association Guidelines for cardiopulmonary resuscitation and emergency cardiovascular care. *Supplement to Circulation, 112*(Suppl. IV), IV-19–IV-34.
33. American Heart Association. (2006). *ACLS provider manual.* Dallas, TX: AHA.
34. Cobb, L. A., Fahrenbruch, C. E., Olsufka, M., et al. (2002). Changing incidence of out-of-hospital ventricular fibrillation, 1980–2000. *JAMA, 288*, 3008–3013.
35. Cummins, R. O., Ornato, J. P., Thies, W. H., et al. (1991). Improving survival from sudden cardiac arrest: The "chain of survival" concept. A statement for health professionals from the Advanced Cardiac Life Support Subcommittee and the Emergency Cardiac Care Committee, American Heart Association. *Circulation, 83*, 1832–1847.
36. Wik, L., Hansen, T. B., Fylling, F., et al. (2003). Delaying defibrillation to give basic cardiopulmonary resuscitation to patients with out-of-hospital ventricular fibrillation: A randomized trial. *JAMA, 289*, 1389–1395.
37. Bardy, G. H., Marchlinski, F., Sharma, A., et al. (1996). For the Transthoracic Investigators. Multicenter comparison of truncated biphasic shocks and standard damped sine wave monophasic shocks for transthoracic ventricular fibrillation. *Circulation, 94*, 2507–2514.
38. Morrison, L. J., Dorian, P., Long, J., et al. (2005). Out of hospital cardiac arrest rectilinear biphasic to monophasic damped sine defibrillation waveforms with advanced life support intervention trial (ORBIT). *Resuscitation, 66*, 149–157.
39. Schneider, T., Martens, P. R., Paschen, H., et al. (2000). Multicenter, randomized, controlled trial of 150-J biphasic shocks compared with 200 to 360-J monophasic shocks in the resuscitation of out-of-hospital cardiac arrest victims. Optimized Response to Cardiac Arrest (ORCA) Investigators. *Circulation, 102*, 1780–1787.

40. Stults, K. R., Brown, D. D., Kerber, R. E., et al. (1986). Efficacy of an automated external defibrillator in the management of out-of-hospital cardiac arrest: Validation of the diagnostic algorithm and initial experience in a rural environment. *Circulation, 73*, 701–709.
41. Zafari, A. M., Zarter, S. K., & Wilson, P. (2004). A program encouraging early defibrillation results in improved In-hospital resuscitation efficacy. *Journal of the American College of Cardiology, 44*(4), 846–852.
42. Kerber, R., Kouba, C., Martins, J., et al. (1984). Advance predication of transthoracic impedance in human defibrillation and cardioversion: Importance of impedance in determining success of low energy shocks. *Circulation, 70*, 303–308.
43. Sado, D. M., & Deakin, C. D. (2005). How good is your defibrillation technique? *Journal of the Royal Society of Medicine, 98*, 3–6.
44. Bissing, J., & Kerber, R. (2000). Effect of shaving the chest of hirsute subjects on transthoracic impedance to self-adhesive defibrillation electrode pads. *American Journal of Cardiology, 86*, 587–589.
45. Kern, K. B., Hilwig, R. W., Berg, R. A., et al. (2002). Importance of continuous chest compressions during cardiopulmonary resuscitation: Improved outcome during a simulated single lay rescuer scenario. *Circulation, 105*, 645–649.
46. Van Alem, A. P., Chapman, F. W., Lank, P., et al. (2003). A prospective, randomised and blinded comparison of first shock success of monophasic and biphasic waveforms in out-of-hospital cardiac arrest. *Resuscitation, 58*, 17–24.
47. Berg, M. D., Clark, L. L., & Valenzuela, T. D. (2005). Post-shock chest compression delays with automated external defibrillator use. *Resuscitation, 64*, 287–291.
48. Eftestol, T., Sunde, K., & Steen, P. A. (2002). Effects of interrupting precordial compressions on the calculated probability of defibrillation success during our-of-hospital cardiac arrest. *Circulation, 105*, 2270–2273.
49. Yu, T., Weil, M. H., Tang, W., et al. (2002). Adverse outcomes of interrupted precordial compression during automated defibrillation. *Circulation, 106*, 368–372.
50. Kudenchuk, P. J., Cobb, L. A., Copass, M. K., et al. (1999). Amiodarone for resuscitation after out-of-hospital cardiac arrest due to ventricular fibrillation. *New England Journal of Medicine, 341*, 871–878.
51. Dorian, P., Cass, D., Schwartz, B., et al. (2002). Amiodarone as compared with lidocaine for shock-resistant ventricular fibrillation. *New England Journal of Medicine, 346*, 884–890.
52. Schulman, S. P., Hartmann, T. K., & Geocadin, R. G. (2006). Intensive care after resuscitation from cardiac arrest: A focus on heart and brain injury. *Neurologic Clinics, 24*, 41–59.
53. Rea, T. D., Helbock, M., Perry, S., et al. (2006). Increasing use of cardiopulmonary resuscitation during out-of-hospital ventricular fibrillation arrest: Survival implication of guideline changes. *Circulation, 114*, 2760–2765.
54. Ornato, J. P., & Peberdy, M. A. (2006). Measuring progress in resuscitation—It's time for a better tool. *114*, 2754–2756.
55. Sunde, K., Pytte, M., Jacobsen, D., et al. (2007). Implementation of a standardised treatment protocol for post resuscitation care after out-of-hospital cardiac arrest. *Resuscitation, 73*, 29–39.
56. Werling, M., Thoren, A. B., Axelsson, C., et al. (2007). Treatment and outcome in post-resuscitation care after out-of-hospital cardiac arrest when a modern therapeutic approach was introduced. *Resuscitation, 73*, 40–45.
57. Holzer, M., & The Hypothermia After Cardiac Arrest Study Group. (2002). Mild therapeutic hypothermia to improve the neurologic outcome after cardiac arrest. *New England Journal of Medicine, 346*(8), 549–556.
58. Brain Resuscitation Clinical Trial II Study Group. (1991). A randomized clinical study of a calcium-entry blocker (Lidoflazine) in the treatment of comatose survivors of cardiac arrest. *New England Journal of Medicine, 324*, 1225–1231.
59. Bernard, S. A., Gray, T. W., Buist, M. D., et al. (2002). Treatment of comatose survivors of out-of-hospital cardiac arrest with induced hypothermia. *New England Journal of Medicine, 346*, 549–556.
60. Echt, D. S., Liebson, P. R., Mitchell, L. B., et al. (1991). Mortality and morbidity in patients receiving encainide, flecainide, or placebo. *New England Journal of Medicine, 324*(12), 781–188.
61. Booth, C. M., Boone, R. H., Tominson, G., et al. (2004). Is the patient dead, vegetative, or severely neurologically impaired? Assessing outcome for comatose survivors of cardiac arrest. *JAMA, 291*, 870–879.
62. Singh, B. N. (1990). Advantages of beta-blockers versus antiarrhythmic agents and calcium channel antagonists in secondary prevention after myocardial infarction. *American Journal of Cardiology, 66*(90), 9C–20C.
63. Reynolds, M. R., Pinto, D. S., & Josephson, M. E. (2008). Hurst's the heart, 12th Edition. R. A. Walsh & D. I. Simon (Ed. Online edition), In M. H. Crawford (Ed.), *Sudden Cardiac Death* (chap. 49). McGraw-Hill Company, Inc.
64. Køber, L., Torp-Pederson, C., Carlsen, J. E., et al. (1995). A clinical trial for the angiotensin-converting-enzyme inhibitor trandolapril in patients with left ventricular dysfunction after myocardial infarction. *New England Journal of Medicine, 333*, 1670–1676.
65. Tel, H., & Tel, H. (2006). The effect of individualized education on the transfer anxiety of patients with myocardial infarction and their families. *Heart & Lung, 35*(2), 101–107.
66. Kamphuis, H. C., De Leeuw, R. J., Derksen, R., et al. (2002). A 12-month quality of life assessment of cardiac arrest survivors treated with or without an implantable cardioverter defibrillator. *Europace, 4*, 417–425.
67. Middelkamp, W., Moulaert, V. R., Verbunt, J. A., et al. (2007). Life after survival: Long-term daily life functioning and quality of life of patients with hypoxic brain injury as a result of a cardiac arrest. *Clinical Rehabilitation, 21*, 425–431.
68. Ladwig, K. H., Schoefinius, A., Dammann, G., et al. (1999). Long-acting psychotraumatic properties of a cardiac arrest experience. *American Journal of Psychiatry, 156*, 912–919.
69. Dougherty, C. M. (2001). The natural history of recovery following sudden cardiac arrest and internal cardioverter-defibrillator implantation. *Progress in Cardiovascular Nursing, 16*(4), 163–168.
70. Bunch, T. J., Hammill, S. C., & White, R. D. (2005). Outcomes after ventricular fibrillation out-of-hospital cardiac arrest: Expanding the chain of survival. *Mayo Clinic Proceedings, 80*(6), 774–782.
71. Bunch, T. J., White, R. D., Smith, G. E., et al. (2004). Long-term subjective memory function in ventricular fibrillation out-of-hospital cardiac arrest survivors resuscitated by early defibrillation. *Resuscitation, 60*, 189–195.
72. Dougherty, C. M., Pyper, G. P., & Benoliel, J. Q. (2004). Domains of concern of intimate partners of sudden cardiac arrest survivors after ICD implantation. *Journal of Cardiovascular Nursing, 19*(1), 21–31.
73. Dickerson, S. S., Posluszny, M., & Kennedy, M. C. (2000). Help seeking in a support group for recipients of implantable cardioverter defibrillators and the support persons. *Heart and Lung, 29*(2), 87–96.
74. Shea, J. B. (2004). Quality of life issues in patients with implantable cardioverter defibrillators—Driving occupation, and recreation. *AACN Clinical Issues, 15*(3), 478–489.

CHAPTER 28 Pacemakers and Implantable Defibrillators*

Carol Jacobson / Donna Gerity

PACEMAKERS

Arrhythmia device therapy is becoming more complex with every advance in technology, requiring clinicians to have more knowledge and greater responsibilities than ever before. Early pacemakers were single-chamber devices designed to pace only in the ventricle, and the only programmable parameters were pacing rate and output. With the introduction of dual-chamber pacemakers with the capability of pacing the atria and the ventricles, the number of programmable parameters increased dramatically. Rate-responsive pacemakers came next and are capable of increasing the pacing rate in response to the body's need for increased cardiac output. Antitachycardia devices were developed to terminate supraventricular and ventricular tachyarrhythmias using pacing techniques, cardioversion, or defibrillation. Most recently, the development of biventricular pacing capability allows for pacing to improve hemodynamics and left ventricular (LV) function in patients with heart failure (HF) and cardiomyopathy. There have been tremendous advances in technology of devices for both bradycardia and antitachycardia therapy in recent years, with even more complex devices coming in the future. Given the number of companies in the arrhythmia device market and the increasing complexity of the devices themselves, it has become very difficult for clinicians to stay abreast of device features and function. The goal of this chapter is to present generic concepts of pacemaker and implantable defibrillator functions to provide a basic knowledge background upon which cardiac nurses can build to enhance their understanding of arrhythmia management devices.

Indications for Pacing

Pacemakers were originally designed to treat disorders of impulse initiation or impulse conduction resulting in symptomatic bradycardia. *Symptomatic bradycardia* is a term used to define a bradycardia that is directly responsible for symptoms such as syncope, near syncope, transient dizziness, or light-headedness, and confusion resulting from cerebral hypoperfusion caused by slow heart rate.[1] Other symptoms such as fatigue, exercise intolerance, HF, dyspnea, and hypotension can also result from bradycardia. Symptomatic bradycardia can be caused by sinus node dysfunction or by conduction failure in or below the AV node. Sinus node dysfunction is the most common indication for permanent pacing, followed by AV node dysfunction.[2,3]

In addition to treating symptomatic bradycardia, pacemaker therapy can have beneficial effects on hemodynamics and clinical status by providing rate response for patients whose sinus node is not capable of increasing its rate appropriately in response to the body's need for increased cardiac output (chronotropic incompetence). Dual-chamber pacemaker therapy can improve stroke volume in patients with LV dysfunction, hypertrophic cardiomyopathy, or dilated cardiomyopathy by ensuring AV synchrony and providing optimal AV intervals to enhance ventricular filling.[4,5] Cardiac resynchronization therapy (CRT) with biventricular pacing improves septal wall motion, mitral valve function, and the dynamics of LV contraction in patients with severe HF or dilated cardiomyopathy.[4–11] The use of pacemaker therapy to prevent atrial fibrillation is an area of intense interest and investigation and has proven successful in many patients.[12–18] Other indications for cardiac pacing include hypersensitive carotid sinus syndrome, neurocardiogenic syncope (vasovagal syncope), long QT syndrome, and sleep apnea.[1–4,19]

The American College of Cardiology (ACC), American Heart Association (AHA), and Heart Rhythm Society (HRS) task force on practice guidelines recently updated the guidelines for implantation of pacemakers and antiarrhythmia devices.[1] Display 28-1 lists the indications for permanent pacemaker implantation in selected clinical settings.

Temporary pacing is indicated to treat symptomatic bradycardia after AMI or cardiac surgery, or when associated with hyperkalemia or drug toxicity; bradycardia-dependent ventricular tachycardia (VT); before permanent pacemaker implantation in symptomatic patients; and in reversible conditions that will not likely result in the need for permanent pacing, such as bacterial endocarditis, Lyme disease, or cardiac trauma.[20,21] Temporary pacing in acute myocardial infarction (MI) is still controversial. Inferior MI results in intranodal block that is usually benign and temporary and requires pacing only if it results in symptomatic bradycardia or bradycardia-dependent VT. When atrioventricular (AV) block occurs in anterior MI, it is usually infranodal, involves a large amount of myocardium, and is often symptomatic. Second- or third-degree AV block associated with anterior MI and bundle-branch block usually requires temporary pacing, but the mortality rate is high because of LV dysfunction secondary to the large infarction rather than to the conduction disturbance. Prophylactic temporary pacing is often performed in the presence of new right bundle-branch block (RBBB) with either anterior or posterior hemiblock, in left bundle-branch block (LBBB) with first-degree AV block, and in alternating right and LBBB.

Temporary pacing is often used after cardiac surgery to prevent or treat symptomatic bradycardia and is sometimes used prophylactically in high-risk patients during cardiac catheterization, or with electrical or chemical cardioversion. Overdrive atrial pacing

*Carol Jacobson wrote the section on pacemakers. Donna Gerity wrote the section on implantable defibrillators.

DISPLAY 28-1 Guidelines For Device-Based Therapy of Cardiac Rhythm Abnormalities

This table covers guidelines for pacemaker therapy in selected situations. For the complete guidelines for all situations, refer to the reference at the end of this table. The guidelines for ICD therapy are presented in Display 28-4.

Permanent Pacing in Sinus Node Dysfunction (SND)

Class I
1. SND with documented symptomatic bradycardia, including frequent sinus pauses that produce symptoms. (Level C)
2. Symptomatic chronotropic incompetence. (Level C)

Class IIa
1. SND with heart rate less than 40 bpm when a clear association between significant symptoms consistent with bradycardia and the actual presence of bradycardia has not been documented. (Level C)
2. Syncope of unexplained origin when clinically significant abnormalities of sinus node function are discovered or provoked in EPS. (Level C)

Class IIb
1. Minimally symptomatic patients with chronic heart rate less than 40 bpm while awake. (Level C)

Permanent Pacing in Acquired AV Block in Adults

Class I
1. Third-degree and advanced second-degree AV block at any anatomic level:
   a. Associated with bradycardia with symptoms (including heart failure) or ventricular arrhythmias presumed to be due to AV block. (Level C)
   b. Associated with arrhythmias and other medical conditions that require drug therapy that results in symptomatic bradycardia. (Level C)
   c. In awake, symptom-free patients in sinus rhythm, with documented periods of asystole greater than or equal to 3.0 seconds or any escape rate less than 40 bpm, or with an escape rhythm below the AV node. (Level C)
   d. In awake, symptom-free patients with AF and bradycardia with one or more pauses of at lest 5 seconds or longer. (Level C)
   e. After catheter ablation of the AV junction. (Level C)
   f. Associated with postoperative AV block that is not expected to resolve after cardiac surgery. (Level C)
   g. Associated with neuromuscular diseases with AV block, such as myotonic muscular dystrophy, Kearns–Sayre syndrome, Erb dystrophy, and peroneal muscular atrophy, with or without symptoms. (Level B)
2. Second-degree AV block with associated symptomatic bradycardia regardless of type or site of block. (Level B)
3. Asymptomatic persistent third-degree AV block at any anatomic site with average awake ventricular rates of 40 bpm or faster if cardiomegaly or LV dysfunction is present or if the site of block is below the AV node. (Level B)
4. Second- or third-degree AV block during exercise in the absence of myocardial ischemia. (Level C)

Class IIa
1. Persistent third-degree AV block with an escape rate greater than 40 bpm in asymptomatic patients without cardiomegaly. (Level C)
2. Asymptomatic second-degree AV block at intra- or infra-His levels found at EPS. (Level B)
3. First or second-degree AV block with symptoms similar to those of pacemaker syndrome or hemodynamic compromise. (Level B)
4. Asymptomatic type II second-degree AV block with a narrow QRS. When type II second-degree AV block occurs with a wide QRS, including isolated RBBB, pacing becomes a Class I recommendation. (Level B)

Class IIb
1. Neuromuscular diseases (as listed above) with any degree of AV block (including first degree) with or without symptoms, because there may be unpredictable progression of AV conduction disease. (Level B)
2. AV block in the setting of drug use and/or drug toxicity when the block is expected to recur even after the drug is withdrawn. (Level B)

Permanent Pacing in Chronic Bifascicular Block

Class I
1. Advanced second-degree AV block or intermittent third-degree AV block. (Level B)
2. Type II second-degree AV block. (Level B)
3. Alternating bundle branch block. (Level C)

Class IIa
1. Syncope not demonstrated to be due to AV block when other likely causes have been excluded, specifically ventricular tachycardia. (Level B)
2. Markedly prolonged HV interval (greater than or equal to 100 ms) found at EPS in asymptomatic patients. (Level B)
3. Incidental finding at EPS of pacing induced infra-His block that is not physiological. (Level B)

Class IIb
1. In the setting of neuromuscular disease with any fascicular block, with or without symptoms. (Level C)

Permanent Pacing After the Acute Phase of Myocardial Infarction

Class I
1. Persistent second-degree AV block in the His-Purkinje system with alternating BBB or third-degree AV block within or below the His-Purkinje system after ST segment elevation MI. (Level B)
2. Transient advanced second or third-degree infranodal AV block and associated BBB. (Level B)
3. Persistent and symptomatic second or third-degree AV block. (Level C)

Class IIb
1. Persistent second or third-degree AV block at the AV node level, even in the absence of symptoms. (Level B)

(display continued on page 657)

DISPLAY 28-1 Guidelines For Device-Based Therapy of Cardiac Rhythm Abnormalities (continued)

Permanent Pacing in Hypersensitive Carotid Sinus Syndrome and Neurocardiogenic Syncope

Class I 1. Recurrent syncope caused by spontaneously occurring carotid sinus stimulation and carotid sinus pressure that induces ventricular asystole of more than 3 seconds. (Level C)

Class IIa 1. Syncope without clear, provocative events and with a hypersensitive cardioinhibitory response of 3 seconds or longer. (Level C)

Class IIb 1. Significantly symptomatic neurocardiogenic syncope associated with bradycardia documented spontaneously or at the time of tilt-table testing. (Level B)

Cardiac Resynchronization Therapy in Patients With Severe Systolic Heart Failure

Class I 1. For patients who have LVEF less than or equal to 35%, a QRS duration greater than or equal to 0.12 second, and sinus rhythm, CRT with or without an ICD is indicated for the treatment of NYHA functional Class III or ambulatory Class IV heart failure symptoms with optimal recommended medical therapy.

Class IIa 1. For patients who have LVEF less than or equal to 35%, a QRS Duration greater than or equal to 0.12 second, and AF, CRT with or without an ICD is reasonable for the treatment of NYHA functional class III or ambulatory Class IV heart failure symptoms on optimal recommended medical therapy. (Level B)

2. For patients with LVEF less than or equal to 35% with NYHA functional Class III or ambulatory Class IV symptoms who are receiving optimal recommended medical therapy and who have frequent dependence on ventricular pacing, CRT is reasonable. (Level C)

Class IIb 1. For patients who have LVEF less than or equal to 35% with NYHA functional Class I or II symptoms who are receiving optimal recommended medical therapy and who are undergoing implantation of a permanent pacemaker and/or ICD with anticipated frequent ventricular pacing, CRT may be considered. (Level C)

Permanent Pacing to Prevent Tachycardia

Class I 1. Sustained pause-dependent VT, with or without QT prolongation. (Level C)
Class IIa 1. High-risk patients with congenital long-QT syndrome. (Level C)
Class IIb 1. Prevention of symptomatic, drug-refractory, recurrent AF in patients with coexisting SND. (Level B)

Classification of Recommendations

Class I: Benefit >>> Risk, procedure/treatment SHOULD BE performed/administered.
Class IIa: Benefit >> Risk, IT IS REASONABLE to perform procedure/administer treatment.
Class IIb: Benefit ≥ Risk, procedure/treatment MAY BE CONSIDERED.

Level of Evidence Definitions

Level A: Data derived from multiple randomized clinical trials or meta-analyses.
Level B: Data derived from a single randomized trial or nonrandomized studies.
Level C: Only consensus opinion of experts, case studies, or standard-of-care.

ICD, implantable cardioverter defibrillator; AV, atrioventricular; LV, left ventricular; SND, sinus node dysfunction; EPS, electrophysiology study; AF, atrial fibrillation; RBBB, right bundle branch block; MI, myocardial infarction; LVEF, left ventricular ejection fraction; CRT, cardiac resynchronization therapy; NYHA, New York Heart Association.
Source: Epstein, A. E., DiMarco, J. P., Ellenbogen, K. A., et al. (2008). ACC/AHA/HRS 2008 guidelines for device-based therapy of cardiac rhythm abnormalities. A report of the American College of Cardiology/American Heart Association Task Force on Practice Guidelines (Writing Committee to Revise the ACC/AHA/NASPE 2002 Guideline Update for Implantation of Cardiac Pacemakers and Antiarrhythmia Devices). *Circulation, 117*, e350–e3408.

is sometimes used in an attempt to terminate atrial flutter or fibrillation after cardiac surgery when atrial epicardial leads are in place.

Types of Pacemakers

Refer to Displays 28-2 and 28-3 for definitions of single- and dual-chamber pacemaker terminology. The terms defined there are used throughout the pacemaker section of this chapter and are not defined in the text unless necessary.

Permanent Pacemakers

Permanent pacemakers are usually implanted under local anesthesia in the operating room (OR), electrophysiology laboratory, or cardiac catheterization laboratory. The pulse generator is placed in a subcutaneous pocket in the pectoral area and the pacing lead is inserted either through the cephalic vein or through the subclavian vein and advanced into the right ventricular (RV) apex. If a dual-chamber pacemaker is implanted, then a second lead is placed in the right atrial appendage (Fig. 28-1). Permanent pulse generators are powered by lithium batteries with a lifespan of approximately 10 years, depending on many factors, including how the pacemaker is programmed and the percentage of time that it paces.

Temporary Pacemakers

Temporary pacing can be accomplished with transvenous, epicardial, or transcutaneous methods. Temporary pacing can be per-

(*text continues on page 660*)

DISPLAY 28-2 Single Chamber Pacing Terminology

Asynchronous (fixed rate) pacing: The pacemaker releases a pacing stimulus at the programmed rate regardless of the heart's intrinsic activity. No sensing occurs so the pacemaker fires in competition with the heart's natural rhythm. Examples of asynchronous modes are AOO, VOO, and DOO.

Automatic interval: The time period between two consecutive paced events without an intervening sensed event. Also known as the *basic interval* or *pacing interval.*

Base rate: The rate at which the pacemaker paces when no intrinsic cardiac activity is present. Also known as the *minimum rate* or *lower rate.*

Bipolar: Having two poles. (1) A pacing lead with two electrical poles. The negative pole is the distal tip of the lead and the positive pole is a metal ring located a few millimeters proximal to the distal tip. The stimulating pulse is delivered through the distal tip electrode. (2) A pacing system with both electrical poles in or on the heart.

Capture: Ability of the pacing stimulus to depolarize the chamber being paced. Capture is recognized on the ECG whenever the pacing spike is followed immediately by the appropriate waveform: an atrial spike followed by a P wave or a ventricular spike followed by a wide QRS.

Demand Pacing: The pacemaker only paces when the heart's intrinsic rate is below the pacemakers programmed rate (only when necessary or on demand). This mode means that the pacemaker senses intrinsic cardiac activity and inhibits its output when intrinsic activity is present.

Electrode: The exposed metal tip of a pacing lead that contacts myocardium and directly transmits the pacing stimulus to cardiac tissue.

Electromagnetic interference: Electrical signals from the environment (i.e., radiofrequency waves) which can be sensed by the pacemaker and interfere with pacer function.

Escape interval: The period of time between a sensed cardiac event and the next pacemaker output. The escape interval is usually equal to the basic pacing rate but it can be programmed longer in some pacemakers (hysteresis).

Fusion beat: A cardiac depolarization (either atrial or ventricular) that results from two foci both contributing to depolarization of the chamber. In pacing, a fusion beat results when an intrinsic depolarization and a pacing stimulus occur simultaneously and both contribute to depolarization (usually seen in the ventricle).

Hysteresis: A programmable feature in some pacemakers that allows the escape interval to be programmed longer than the basic pacing interval (the pacing interval following a sensed beat is longer than the basic pacing interval). This allows more time for the heart's intrinsic activity to occur.

Inhibited response: A type of response to sensing that inhibits pacemaker output when an intrinsic beat is sensed. This results in demand pacing, or pacing only when the heart's intrinsic activity is slower than the basic pacing rate.

Lead: The insulated wire and its electrode that transmits the pacing stimulus from the pulse generator to the heart and relays sensed intrinsic activity back to the pulse generator. A single-chamber pacemaker uses one lead and a dual-chamber pacemaker usually uses two leads, one in the atrium and one in the ventricle.

Magnet mode: A term used for the pacemaker's response when a magnet is placed over the pulse generator. A magnet inactivates the sensing circuitry and causes a pacemaker to function asynchronously at a predetermined rate and in a preset manner. The magnet mode differs among manufacturers in pacing rate and number of impulses delivered with the magnet in place. A change is magnet-induced pacing rate is often an indicator of battery depletion and warrants pulse generator replacement.

Myopotential: An electrical signal generated by muscle movement. Myopotentials are sometimes sensed by the pacemaker and cause inhibition of pacemaker output.

Output: The electrical stimulus delivered by the pulse generator, usually defined in terms of pulse amplitude (V = volts) and pulse width (ms = milliseconds).

Oversensing: Detection of inappropriate electrical signals by the pacemaker's sensing circuit, resulting in inappropriate inhibition of pacer output. Sources of oversensing can include electromagnetic interference, myopotentials, T waves, or crosstalk between atrial and ventricular channels in dual-chamber pacemakers.

Pacemaker syndrome: Adverse clinical signs and symptoms due to inadequate timing of atrial and ventricular contraction. The syndrome can be due to loss of AV synchrony in VVI pacing, inappropriate AV interval in dual-chamber pacing, or inappropriate rate modulation. Symptoms include fatigue, confusion, unpleasant pulsations in neck or chest, limited exercise capacity, CHF, hypotension, syncope, or near syncope.

Pacing interval: The time between two consecutive paced events without an intervening sensed event. Measured in milliseconds (ms). AA interval, atrial pacing interval; VV interval, ventricular pacing interval.

Pacer spike: Term used to describe the small vertical "blip" recorded on the ECG with every pacemaker output pulse. The presence of a pacer spike indicates that a stimulus was released by the pacemaker.

Pseudofusion beat: An electrocardiographic phenomenon resulting from delivery of a pacemaker spike into an intrinsic event. In the ventricle, it appears as a pacer spike in an intrinsic QRS complex, but since the ventricle is already depolarized the spike is ineffective but may distort the QRS complex on the ECG.

Pulse generator: The device that contains the power source (battery) and the electronic circuits that control pacemaker function. The term "pacemaker" is commonly used for the pulse generator.

Rate modulation: The ability of a pacemaker to increase the pacing rate in response to physical activity or metabolic demand. The pacemaker uses some type of physiologic sensor to determine the need for increased pacing rate. The most commonly used sensors at the present time are motion sensors and minute ventilation sensors. It is also known as *rate adaptation* or *rate response.*

(display continued on page 659)

DISPLAY 28-2 Single Chamber Pacing Terminology (continued)

Refractory period: (1) In the heart, the period of time during which the myocardium is incapable of responding to a stimulus. (2) In the pacemaker, an interval or timing cycle following a sensed or paced event during which the pacemaker will not respond to incoming signals. A single-chamber pacemaker has one refractory period, a dual-chamber pacemaker has an atrial refractory and a ventricular refractory period.

Sensing: The ability of the pacemaker to recognize and respond to intrinsic cardiac depolarization.

Sensing threshold: The smallest intrinsic atrial or ventricular signal (measured in mV) that can be consistently sensed by the pacemaker.

Stimulation threshold: The minimum amount of voltage necessary to capture the heart consistently. It is also known as *capture threshold* or *pacing threshold.*

Undersensing: Failure of a pacemaker to sense intrinsic cardiac depolarizations. This can result in competition between the pacemaker and the intrinsic rhythm.

Unipolar: Having one pole. (1) A unipolar lead has only one pole, located at the distal tip. (2) A pacing system with one pole in or on the heart and the second pole located remote from the heart to complete the circuit. Permanent unipolar systems utilize the back of the pulse generator as the second pole. Temporary epicardial pacing systems utilize a ground wire in subcutaneous tissue as the second pole.

DISPLAY 28-3 Dual Chamber Pacemaker Terminology

Adaptive AV delay (or rate adaptive AV delay): See AV interval.

Alert period: The portion of the pulse generator's timing cycle during which it can sense and respond to intrinsic cardiac activity. The alert period follows the refractory period.

Atrial escape interval: Period of time form a sensed or paced ventricular event to the next paced atrial event. Also known as the *V–A interval.*

Atrial refractory period: Period of time during which the atrial channel is unable to respond to sensed signals. In dual-chamber pacemakers, the total atrial refractory period is divided into two parts: the AV interval and the postventricular atrial refractory period (PVARP).

Atrial tracking: A state of pacing in which sensed atrial activity triggers a ventricular pacing output at the end of the programmed AV delay. Also known simply as *tracking.*

AV interval (or AV delay): The "electronic PR interval," or the length of time between a sensed or paced atrial event and the delivery of the ventricular pacing output. The AV interval is programmable and is measured in milliseconds (e.g., an AV interval of 120 ms = a PR interval of 0.12 second). Many pacemakers have an *"adaptive AV delay,"* meaning that the AV delay can be programmed to shorten when the intrinsic atrial rate increases, thus mimicking the heart's own physiological increase in AV conduction as heart rate increases. Many devices also have a *"differential AV delay,"* meaning that the AV interval can be programmed to be longer on an atrial paced beat than on an atrial sensed beat (e.g., 200 ms when the atrium is paced and 150 ms when P waves are sensed).

Blanking period: A very short ventricular refractory period that occurs simultaneously with every atrial pacing output to prevent the ventricle from sensing the atrial stimulus. It is intended to prevent inhibition of ventricular output due to crosstalk (see definition below). Many pacemakers allow the blanking period to be programmed longer to prevent crosstalk.

Crosstalk: The sensing of a signal in one chamber by the sensing circuit in the other chamber, usually used in reference to the sensing of the atrial output pulse by the ventricular channel. Crosstalk due to sensing of atrial signals by the ventricular channel causes inhibition of ventricular pacing output because the ventricular channel thinks that the atrial output is a ventricular event.

Differential AV delay: See AV interval.

Endless loop tachycardia: See Pacemaker mediated tachycardia.

Maximum tracking rate (MTR): The programmable upper rate limit of a dual-chamber pacemaker that determines the fastest rate at which 1:1 tracking of atrial-sensed events will occur. The MTR prevents the ventricular channel from pacing faster than the upper rate limit when the intrinsic atrial rate exceeds the programmed MTR. When the intrinsic atrial rate is faster than the upper rate limit, the pacemaker reverts to its "upper rate response" to prevent the ventricular rate from exceeding the MTR. Also known as the *ventricular tracking limit* or *upper rate limit.*

Mode switching: Ability of a dual-chamber pacemaker to switch from an atrial tracking mode (e.g., DDD) to a nontracking mode (e.g., DDI or VVI) when rapid atrial impulses are sensed by the atrial channel. This prevents the pacemaker from pacing the ventricle rapidly and erratically when atrial fibrillation or flutter occur.

Noncompetitive atrial pace (NCAP): A feature in some dual-chamber pacemakers that delays the delivery of the next atrial output when an atrial signal is sensed in the atrial channel's refractory period (e.g., a PAC that occurs in PVARP delays the delivery of the next atrial pacing output). This prevents the delivery of an atrial output during the atrial refractory period in an attempt to prevent induction of atrial fibrillation.

Pacemaker mediated tachycardia: A tachycardia induced by competition between the pacemaker and the intrinsic rhythm and sustained by the continued participation of the pacemaker. Most commonly used to describe the endless loop tachy-

(display continued on page 660)

DISPLAY 28-3 Dual Chamber Pacemaker Terminology (continued)

cardia that results when there is retrograde conduction from the ventricle to the atria, sensing of the retrograde P wave by the atrial channel, and pacing in the ventricle in response to the sensed P wave. This results in a reentry tachycardia in which the pacemaker serves as the antegrade limb of the circuit and the intrinsic conduction system serves as the retrograde limb. Also known as *endless loop tachycardia* or *pacemaker reentry tachycardia.*

Psuedopseudofusion beat: An electrocardiographic phenomenon in which an atrial pacing spike is superimposed on a native QRS complex. The atrial pacing spike cannot contribute to ventricular depolarization, but the presence of the spike can distort the native QRS complex on the ECG.

Postventricular atrial refractory period (PVARP): Part of the total atrial refractory period that begins with a sensed or paced ventricular event. PVARP is a programmable parameter and is intended to prevent the atrial channel from sensing far-field ventricular signals, such as T waves or local myocardial potentials. PVARP can also be programmed to prevent the atrial channel from sensing retrograde P waves, thus preventing PMT.

Rate drop response: Pacing at a rate faster than the programmed pacing rate when the patient's intrinsic heart rate drops suddenly, as in vasovagal syncope or hypersensitive carotid sinus syndrome. Pacing is initiated at a rate up to 110 bpm if bradycardia suddenly occurs.

Rate response: Ability of the pacemaker to increase its pacing rate in response to physical activity or increased metabolic demand. Rate responsive pacemakers have some type of sensor that detects physical activity or a physiological parameter that indicates the need for increased heart rate. Currently, the sensors most commonly used are vibration or motion sensors and minute ventilation sensors. Other sensors being evaluated include blood temperature, blood oxygen content, QT interval, and stroke volume. Also known as *rate modulation* or *rate adaptation.*

Rate smoothing: A programmable function that prevents excessive cycle-to-cycle changes in pacing rate. Atrial tracking and rate response can occur but no sudden acceleration or deceleration in pacing rate can occur.

Safety pacing: The delivery of a ventricular output at a short AV interval whenever a signal is sensed early in the AV delay. The purpose of safety pacing is to prevent crosstalk inhibition of ventricular output. Also known as *nonphysiological AV delay* or *ventricular safety standby.*

Sleep rate: The pacemaker is programmed to gradually decrease the base pacing rate to a lower limit (e.g., a sleep rate of 50 bpm) at bedtime and gradually increase the base pacing rate when the patient awakens.

Total atrial refractory period (TARP): Timing cycle that determines the total length of time that the atrial channel is unresponsive to signals (in effect "has its eyes closed"). TARP is composed of two separately programmable timing cycles during which the atrial channel is refractory: the AV interval and PVARP.

Ventricular refractory period: The amount of time following a ventricular sensed or paced event during which the ventricular channel cannot respond to signals (in effect "has its eyes closed"). The purpose is to prevent the ventricular channel from seeing large repolarization signals (T waves) or other local myocardial signals.

formed in emergency and elective situations, and it is usually performed in a monitored unit such as critical care or telemetry unit. Transcutaneous pacing can also be performed by paramedics or other trained personnel in emergency response vehicles or in the field.

Transvenous Pacing. Transvenous pacing is usually performed by percutaneous puncture of the internal jugular, subclavian, antecubital, or femoral vein and threading a pacing lead into the apex of the right ventricle for ventricular pacing, the right atrium for atrial pacing, or both chambers for dual-chamber pacing (Fig. 28-2). The transvenous pacing lead is attached to an external pulse generator that is kept either on the patient or at the bedside. The procedure is usually performed under fluoroscopy in a cardiac catheterization laboratory but it can be done at the bedside with or without fluoroscopy. Transvenous pacing is usually necessary only for a few days until the rhythm returns to normal or a permanent pacemaker is inserted. Instructions for initiating transvenous pacing are covered later in this chapter.

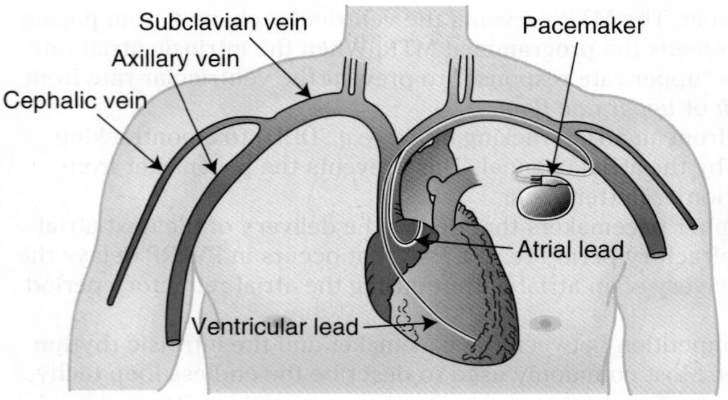

Figure 28-1 Transvenous installation of a permanent dual-chamber pacemaker.

Epicardial Pacing. Epicardial pacing is performed through electrodes placed on the atria or ventricles during cardiac surgery. The pacing electrode end of the lead is attached to the epicardial surface of the atria or ventricles and the other end is pulled through the chest wall, sutured to the skin, and attached to an external pulse generator. A ground wire is often placed subcutaneously in the chest wall and pulled through with the other leads. The number and placement of leads varies with the surgeon; there may be one or two atrial leads, one or two ventricular leads, and one, two, or no ground leads (Fig. 28-3). Instructions for initiating epicardial pacing are covered later in this chapter.

Transcutaneous Pacing. Transcutaneous external pacing is a noninvasive method of pacing used as a temporary measure in emergency situations for treatment of asystole, severe bradycardia, or overdrive pacing for tachyarrhythmias until a transvenous

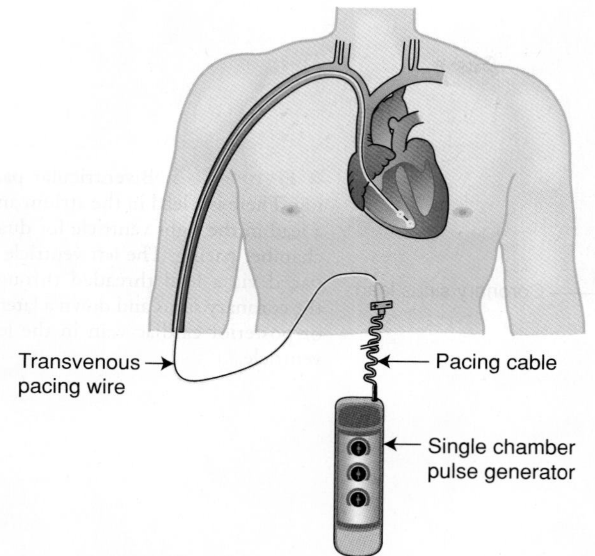

■ **Figure 28-2** Temporary transvenous pacing lead in right ventricle inserted through antecubital vein.

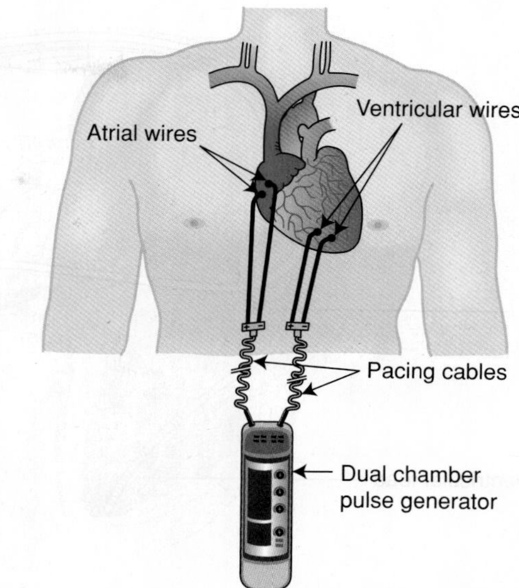

■ **Figure 28-3** Epicardial pacing using atrial and ventricular pacing leads attached to a dual-chamber pacemaker.

pacing lead can be inserted. Large-surface adhesive electrodes are attached to the anterior and posterior chest wall and connected to an external pacing unit (Fig. 28-4). The pacing current passes through skin and chest wall structures to reach the heart; therefore, high energies are required to achieve capture and sedation is usually needed to minimize the discomfort felt during pacing.

Single-Chamber Pacing

Single-chamber pacing means that only the atria or the ventricles, but not both, are paced. This type of pacing requires only one pacing lead inserted into the desired chamber. Single-chamber ventricular pacing is the most frequently used temporary transvenous type of pacing and can also be used for permanent pacing. Single-chamber atrial or ventricular pacing can be performed using epicardial-pacing leads.

Dual-Chamber Pacing

Dual-chamber pacing means that both the atria and the ventricles can be paced. Dual-chamber pacing is a frequently used method of permanent pacing and can also be performed via epicardial-pacing leads. Temporary transvenous dual-chamber pacing can be performed, but it is difficult to place temporary atrial leads and it is not as reliable as ventricular pacing.

Biventricular Pacing

Biventricular pacing means that both ventricles are simultaneously paced via a lead in the RV apex for RV pacing and a lead threaded through the coronary sinus into a lateral or posterior cardiac vein (or less commonly via an epicardial LV lead) for LV pacing. Figure 28-5 illustrates dual-chamber biventricular pacing leads, and this topic is discussed in more detail later in this chapter.

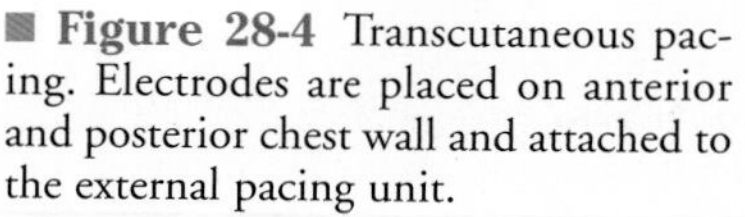

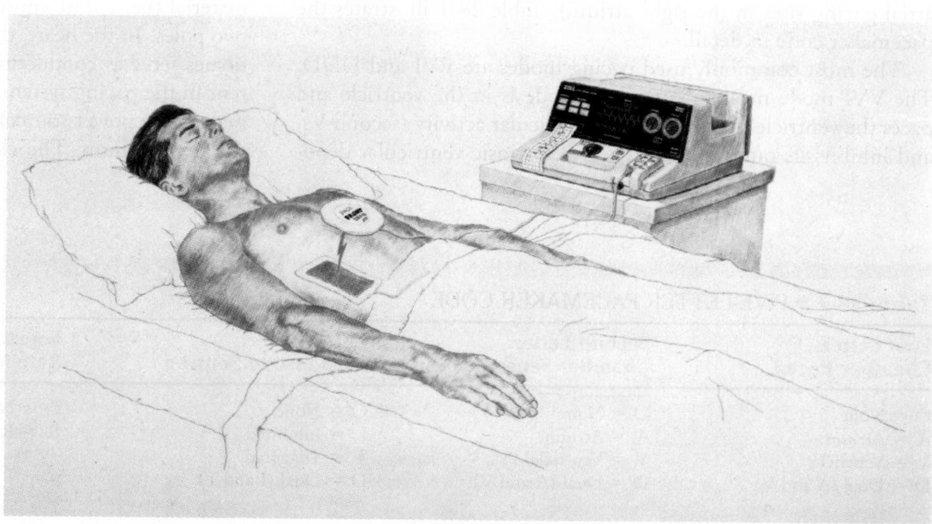

■ **Figure 28-4** Transcutaneous pacing. Electrodes are placed on anterior and posterior chest wall and attached to the external pacing unit.

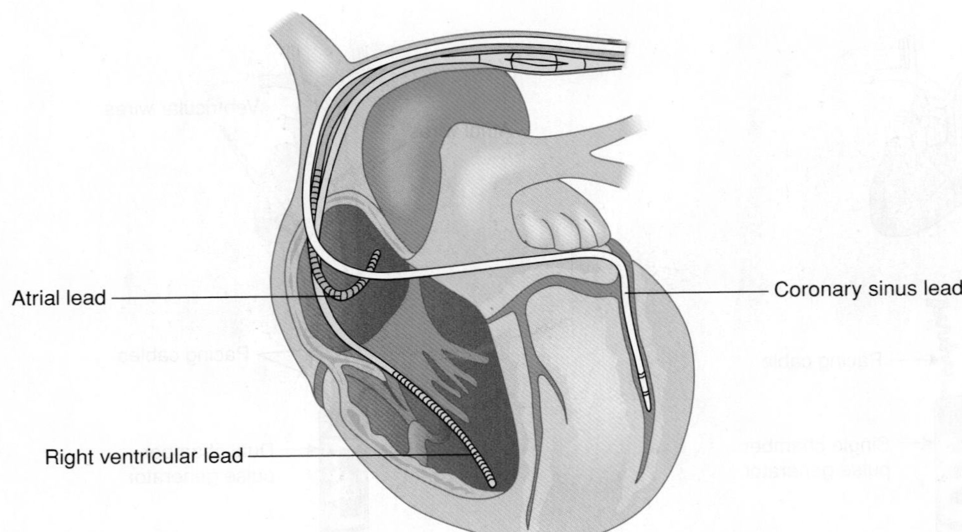

■ **Figure 28-5** Biventricular pacing. There is a lead in the atrium and a lead in the right ventricle for dual-chamber pacing. The left ventricle is paced via a lead threaded through the coronary sinus and down a lateral or posterior cardiac vein in the left ventricle.

Pacing Modes

The current nomenclature used to describe the expected function of a pacemaker was established by members of the North American Society of Pacing and Electrophysiology and the British Pacing and Electrophysiology Group and is designated the NBG code for pacing nomenclature.[22] The code describes the expected function of the device according to the site of the pacing electrodes and the mode of pacing. The first letter describes the chamber that is paced: A, atrium; V, ventricle; D, dual (both atrium and ventricle); O, none. The second letter describes the chamber where intrinsic electrical activity is sensed: A, atrium; V, ventricle; D, dual (both atrium and ventricle); O, none. The third letter describes the pacemaker's response to sensing of intrinsic electrical activity: I, inhibited; T, triggered; D, dual (inhibits or triggers); O, none. The fourth letter denotes the presence or absence of rate modulation (R, rate modulation and O, none). The fifth letter specifies the location or absence of multisite pacing, which includes either biatrial or biventricular pacing, or more than one stimulation site in a single chamber (e.g. two atrial pacing sites in the right atrium). Table 28-1 illustrates the pacemaker code in detail.

The most commonly used pacing modes are VVI and DDD. The VVI mode means that the electrode is in the ventricle and paces the ventricle (first V), senses ventricular activity (second V), and inhibits its output when it senses intrinsic ventricular depolarization (I in third position). VVI is the most commonly used mode of pacing with temporary transvenous leads because it is the quickest and easiest method of pacing in an emergency, and it is difficult to get a temporary atrial lead to stay in place. VVI is also often used with epicardial leads after cardiac surgery, especially if third-degree AV block is present, and is the mode that has to be used for permanent pacing in patients with chronic atrial fibrillation. The DDD mode means that both atrial and ventricular electrodes are present and both chambers are paced (first D), both chambers are sensed (second D), and the device either inhibits or triggers an output in response to sensed intrinsic activity (D in third position means dual-response to sensing). DDD is the most frequently used permanent pacing mode, unless the patient has chronic atrial fibrillation or flutter. Other pacing modes that are sometimes used are AOO, AAI, DVI, DDI, and VDD.

Basics of Pacemaker Operation

Electrical current flows in a closed-loop circuit between two pieces of metal (poles). For current to flow, there must be conductive material (i.e. a lead, muscle, or conductive solution) between the two poles. In the heart, the pacing lead, cardiac muscle, and body tissues serve as conducting material for the flow of electrical current in the pacing system. The pacing circuit consists of the pacemaker (the power source), the conducting lead (pacing lead), and the myocardium. The electrical stimulus travels from the pulse

Table 28-1 ■ FIVE-LETTER PACEMAKER CODE

First Letter: Chamber Paced	Second Letter: Chamber Sensed	Third Letter: Response to Sensing	Fourth Letter: Rate Modulation	Fifth Letter: Multisite Pacing
O = None A = Atrium V = Ventricle D = Dual (A and V)	O = None A = Atrium V = Ventricle D = Dual (A and V)	O = None I = Inhibited T = Triggered D = Dual (I and T)	O = None R = Rate modulation	O = None A = Atrial V = Ventricle D = Dual

generator through the pacing lead to the myocardium, through the myocardium, and back to the pulse generator, thus completing the circuit.[23,24]

Components of a Pacing System

The three basic components of a cardiac pacing system are the pulse generator, the pacing lead, and the myocardium. The *pulse generator* contains the power source (battery) and all of the electronic circuitry that controls pacemaker function. Most pacemakers are powered by a lithium battery. The pulse generator of a permanent pacemaker is small and thin, and is implanted in the pectoral area or sometimes in the abdominal area (see Fig. 28-1). Once a permanent pulse generator is implanted, the only way to alter its pacing parameters is with a programmer that communicates with the pacemaker through a wand placed over the pulse generator. A temporary pulse generator is a box that is kept at the bedside of the patient and is usually powered by a regular 9-volt battery. It has controls on the front that allow the operator to set certain pacing parameters easily (Fig. 28-6).

The *pacing lead* is an insulated wire used to transmit the electrical current from the pulse generator to the myocardium. A unipolar lead contains a single wire and a bipolar lead contains two wires that are insulated from each other. In a unipolar lead, the electrode is an exposed metal tip at the end of the lead that contacts the myocardium and serves as the negative pole of the

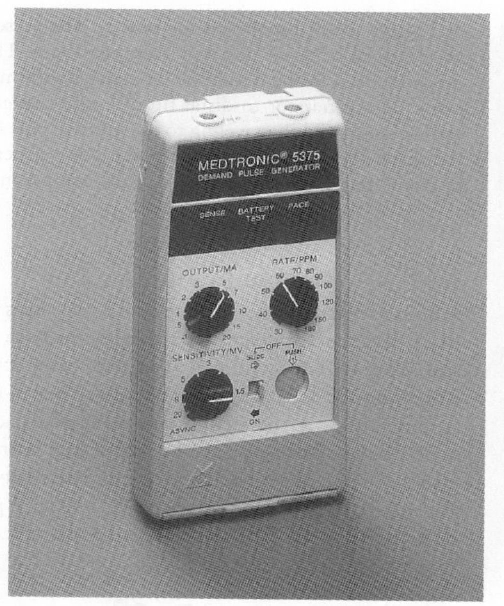

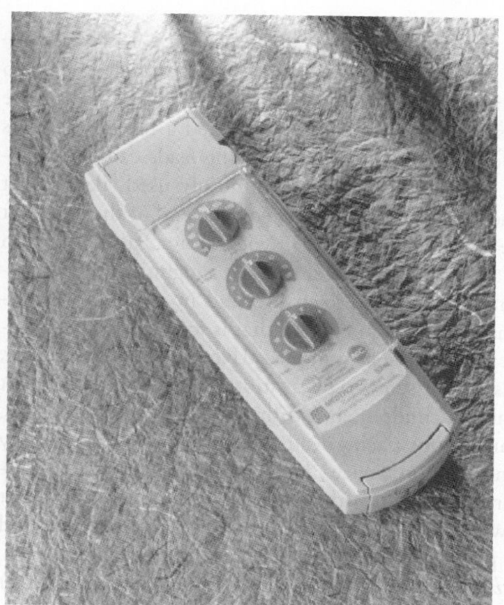

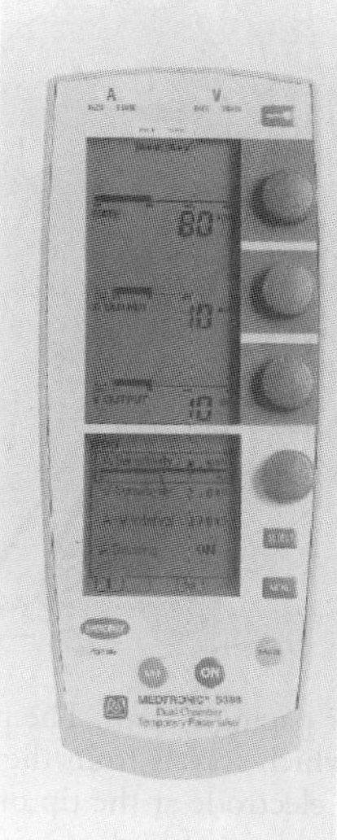

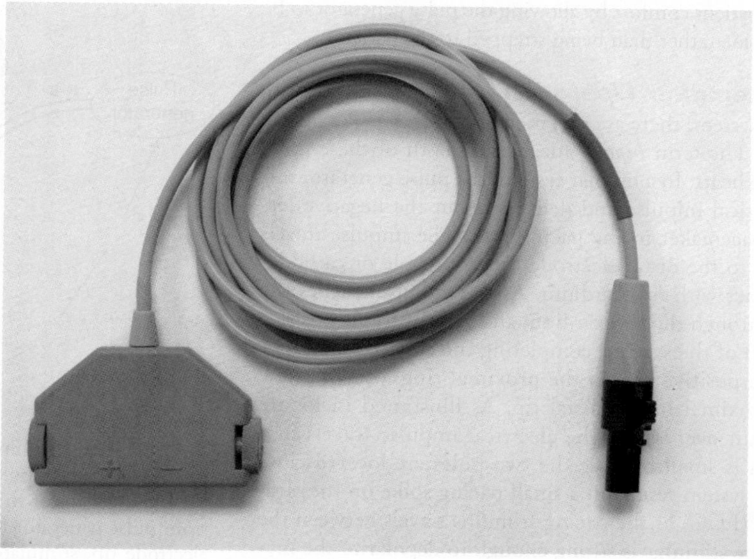

Figure 28-6 Examples of temporary pulse generators and pacing cable. (A) Older model Medtronic single-chamber pacemaker. (B) New model Medtronic single-chamber pacemaker. (C) New model Medtronic dual-chamber pacemaker. (D) Pacing cable used to connect pulse generator to pacing leads.

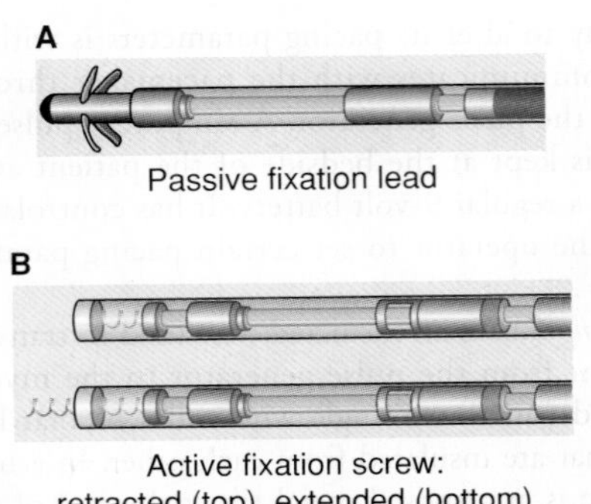

■ **Figure 28-7** Pacing leads. (A) Passive fixation lead with tines on the end to hold lead in position. (B) Active fixation screw lead; top shows screw retracted, bottom shows screw extended.

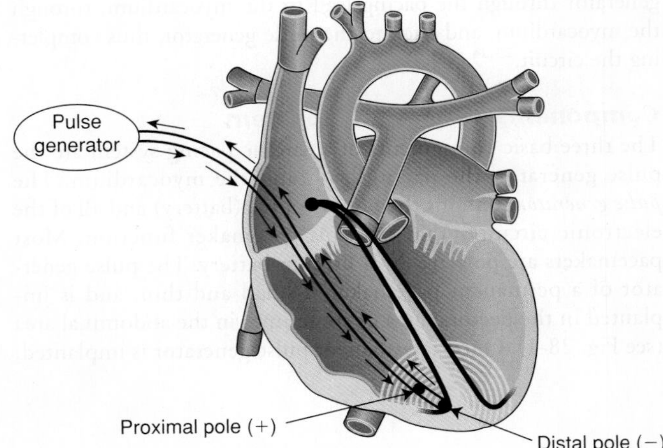

■ **Figure 28-8** Bipolar pacing system. The pulse generator delivers an electrical stimulus at a predetermined rate. The stimulus travels down the lead to the distal pole in contact with myocardium (arrows from pulse generator to distal tip of lead). Current spreads through cardiac muscle while traveling to the positive pole located proximal to the distal tip. Current returns to the pulse generator (arrows from proximal pole back to pulse generator), completing the circuit.

pacing circuit. In a bipolar lead, the end of the lead is a metal tip that contacts myocardium and serves as the negative pole, and the positive pole is an exposed metal ring located a few millimeters proximal to the distal tip. Permanent pacing leads can be unipolar or bipolar, but bipolar is more commonly used. Permanent leads have some type of fixation device on the end of the lead that helps keep the tip in contact with myocardium. Passive-fixation leads usually have tines on the end that get caught in the trabeculae of the right ventricle and keep the lead in position. Active-fixation leads have a screw on the end that is screwed into the ventricular muscle to hold the lead in place (Fig. 28-7). Occasionally, epicardial leads with a screw-type fixation are used in permanent pacing, especially in children, and with implantable defibrillators. Temporary transvenous pacing leads are insulated wires (usually bipolar) with no-fixation device, making them more prone to dislodgment. Temporary epicardial-pacing leads are unipolar or bipolar wires with one end looped through the myocardium and the leads then pulled through the chest wall for easy access.

A *pacing cable* is usually used to connect a temporary pacemaker pulse generator to the pacemaker lead, similar to an extension cord. This enhances patient comfort by allowing the pulse generator to be kept at the bedside rather than being strapped to the patient.

Bipolar Pacemaker Operation

In any pacing system, there are two metal poles that make up the pacing circuit. The term *bipolar* means that both of these poles are in or on the heart. In a bipolar system, the pulse generator initiates the electrical impulse and delivers it out the negative terminal of the pacemaker to the pacing lead. The impulse travels down the lead to the distal electrode (negative pole or cathode) that is in contact with myocardium. As the impulse reaches the tip, it travels through the myocardium and returns to the positive pole (or anode) of the system, completing the circuit. In a bipolar system, the positive pole is the proximal ring located a few millimeters proximal to the distal tip. As illustrated in Figure 28-8, the circuit over which the electrical impulse travels in a bipolar system is small because the two poles are located close together. This system results in a small pacing spike on the electrocardiogram (ECG) as the pacing stimulus travels between the two poles. If the stimulus is strong enough to depolarize the myocardium, then the pacing spike is immediately followed by a P wave if the lead is in the atrium, or a wide QRS complex if the lead is in the ventricle.

Unipolar Pacemaker Operation

A unipolar system has only one of the two poles in or on the heart. In a permanent unipolar pacing system, the back of the pulse generator serves as the second pole. In a temporary epicardial-pacing system, a ground lead placed in the subcutaneous tissue in the mediastinum serves as the second pole. Unipolar pacemakers work the same way as bipolar systems, but the circuit over which the impulse travels is much larger because of the distance between the two poles (Fig. 28-9). This type of system results in a large pacing spike on the ECG as the impulse travels between the two poles.

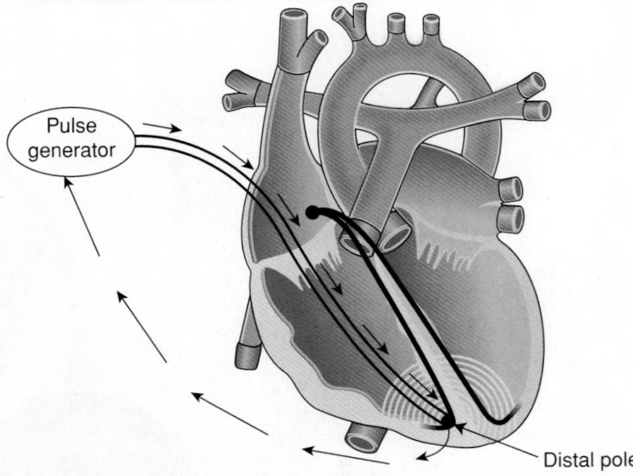

■ **Figure 28-9** Unipolar pacing system. The pulse generator delivers an electrical impulse which travels from the negative terminal of the pulse generator to the electrode at the tip of the catheter (arrows from pulse generator to distal tip of lead). Current exits through the electrode tip, stimulates the myocardium, and completes the circuit by traveling through body tissues to the positive terminal on the back of the pulse generator (arrow from distal tip of pacing lead to pulse generator).

Asynchronous (Fixed-Rate) Pacing

A pacemaker programmed to an asynchronous mode paces at the programmed rate regardless of intrinsic cardiac activity. This mode can result in competition between the pacemaker and the heart's own electrical activity. Asynchronous pacing in the ventricle is unsafe because of the potential for pacing stimuli to fall in the vulnerable period of repolarization and cause ventricular fibrillation (VF). Asynchronous pacing in the atria is less dangerous but can cause atrial fibrillation.

Demand Pacing

The term *demand* means that the pacemaker paces only when the heart fails to depolarize on its own, that is, the pacemaker fires only "on demand." In the demand mode, the pacemaker's sensing circuit is capable of sensing intrinsic cardiac activity and inhibiting pacer output when intrinsic activity is present. Sensing takes place between the two poles of the pacemaker. A bipolar system senses over a small area because the poles are close together, and this can result in "undersensing" of intrinsic signals. A unipolar system senses over a large area because the poles are far apart, and this can result in "oversensing." A unipolar system is more likely to sense myopotentials caused by muscle movement and inappropriately inhibit pacemaker output, potentially resulting in periods of asystole if the patient has no underlying cardiac rhythm. The demand mode should always be used for ventricular pacing to avoid the possibility of VF.

Capture

Capture means that a pacing stimulus results in depolarization of the chamber being paced. Capture is determined by the strength of the stimulus, which is measured in milliamperes (mA), the amount of time the stimulus is applied to the heart (pulse width), and by contact of the pacing electrode with the myocardium. Capture cannot occur unless the distal tip of the pacing lead is in contact with healthy myocardium that is capable of responding to the stimulus. Pacing in infarcted tissue usually prevents capture. Similarly, if the catheter is floating in the cavity of the ventricle and not in direct contact with myocardium, capture will not occur.

In permanent pacing systems, stimulus strength is programmed at implant and can be changed as necessary by using a pacemaker programmer. In temporary pacing, the output dial on the face of the pulse generator controls stimulus strength and can be set and changed easily by the operator. Temporary pulse generators usually are capable of delivering a stimulus of from 0.1 to 20 mA.

Sensing

The sensing circuit controls how sensitive the pacemaker is to intrinsic cardiac depolarizations. Intrinsic activity is measured in millivolts (mV), and the higher the number, the larger the intrinsic signal. For example, a 10-mV QRS complex is larger than a 2-mV QRS. When pacemaker sensitivity needs to be increased to make the pacemaker "see" smaller signals, the sensitivity number must be decreased. For example, a sensitivity of 2 mV is more sensitive than one of 5 mV.

A fence analogy may help explain sensitivity (see Fig. 28-10). Think of sensitivity as a fence standing between the pacemaker and what the pacemaker wants to see—the ventricle, for example. If there is a 10-ft-high fence (or a 10-mV sensitivity) between the two, then the pacemaker may not see what the ventricle is doing. To make the pacemaker able to see, the fence needs to be lowered. Lowering the fence to 2 feet would probably enable the pacemaker to see the ventricle. Changing the sensitivity from 10 to 2 mV is like lowering the fence—the pacemaker becomes more sensitive and is able to "see" intrinsic activity more easily. Thus, to increase the sensitivity of a pacemaker, the millivolt number (fence) must be decreased.

Initiating Temporary Pacing

Transvenous Ventricular Pacing

A transvenous pacing lead is inserted through a peripheral vein, either antecubital or femoral, or through the internal jugular or subclavian vein, and advanced into the apex of the right ventricle. The lead is sutured in place at its insertion site and a dressing is applied. Temporary transvenous pacing leads are bipolar and have two tails, one marked "positive" or "proximal" and the other marked "negative" or "distal." These tails are connected to the pacing cable, which is then connected to the pulse generator. To initiate ventricular pacing using a transvenous lead (Fig. 28-11):

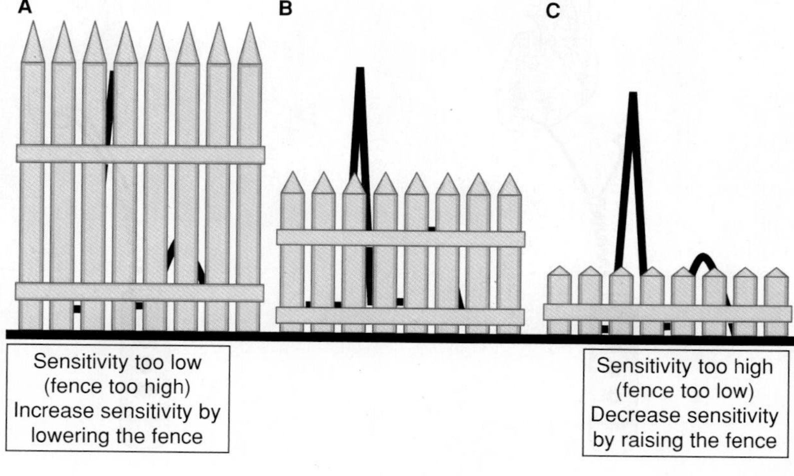

■ **Figure 28-10** The fence analogy for pacemaker sensitivity. The height of the fence is inversely related to the sensitivity of the pacemaker: the taller the fence, the less sensitive the pacemaker is; the shorter the fence the more sensitive the pacemaker is. (A) The fence is too high for the QRS complex behind it to be visible; the pacemaker sensitivity is too low to be able to sense the QRS. (B) The fence is a good height for the pacemaker to be able to see the QRS but not the P wave or T wave or other signals. (C) The fence is too low and now the T wave is visible along with the QRS complex; the pacemaker sensitivity is so high that it senses extraneous signals.

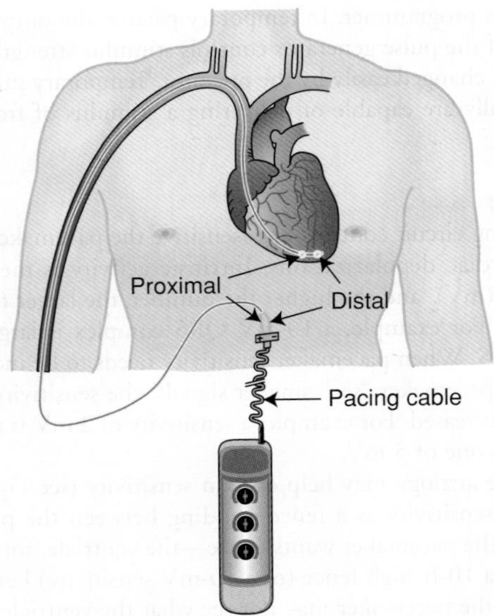

■ **Figure 28-11** Initiating temporary transvenous pacing. The distal tail of the pacing lead is connected to the negative terminal of the pacemaker, and the proximal tail of the pacing lead is connected to the positive terminal of the pacemaker.

1. Connect the pacing cable to the top of the pulse generator (if using an older pacemaker with positive and negative connections on top, make sure cable is connected positive to positive and negative to negative).
2. Connect the other end of the pacing cable to the tails of the pacing wire: proximal tail to positive terminal of pacing cable, and distal tail to the negative terminal of pacing cable.
3. Set the rate at 70 to 80 bpm or as ordered by physician.
4. Set the output at 5 mA and adjust according to stimulation threshold.
5. Set the sensitivity at 2 mV and adjust according to sensitivity threshold.

See the section "Nursing Considerations" for the procedure for performing stimulation and sensitivity threshold tests.

Epicardial Pacing

The number and location of epicardial leads placed in surgery determine connections for epicardial pacing. There may be one or two atrial or ventricular leads with a ground or no ground lead. If only one lead is on a chamber, then unipolar pacing is performed. If there are two leads on a chamber, then bipolar pacing can be performed.

To initiate unipolar atrial or ventricular pacing (Fig. 28-12*A*):

1. Connect the pacing cable to the top of the pulse generator (if using an older pacemaker with positive and negative connections on top, make sure cable is connected positive to positive and negative to negative).
2. Connect the other end of pacing cable to pacing wires: negative terminal of the cable to the atrial or ventricular wire to be paced, positive terminal of the cable to the ground wire.
3. Set the rate at 70 to 80 bpm or as ordered by physician.
4. Set the output at 10 mA for atrial pacing and 5 mA for ventricular pacing, then determine stimulation threshold and set two- to three-times higher.
5. Set the sensitivity at the lowest possible number for atrial pacing and at 2 mV for ventricular pacing.

To initiate bipolar atrial or ventricular pacing (see Fig. 28-12B):

1. Connect the pacing cable to the top of the pulse generator (if using an older pacemaker with positive and negative connections on top, make sure cable is connected positive to positive and negative to negative).
2. Connect the other end of the pacing cable to pacing wires: for atrial pacing, connect one atrial pacing wire to the negative terminal of the pacing cable the other atrial pacing wire to the

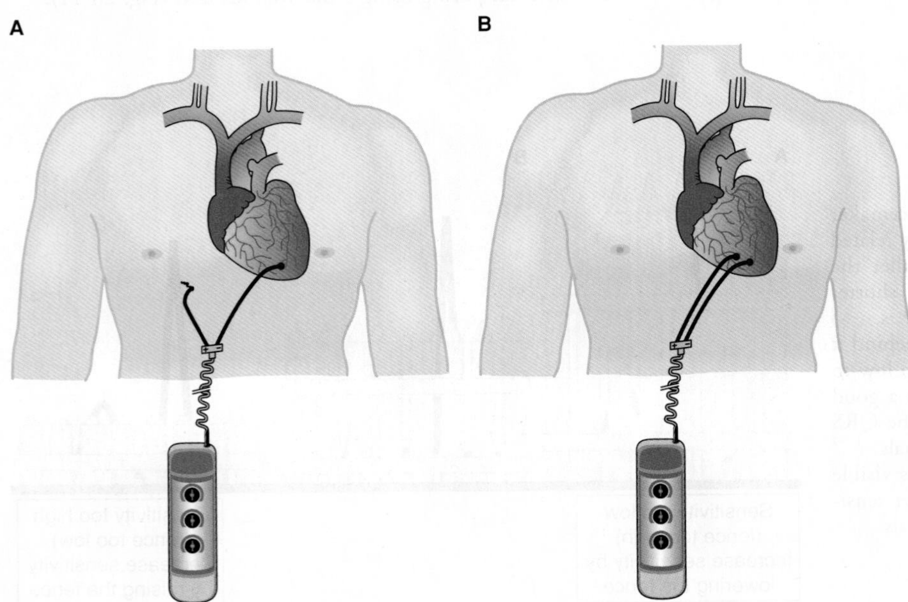

■ **Figure 28-12** Initiating epicardial pacing. (A) Unipolar epicardial pacing. The ventricular lead (or atrial lead for atrial pacing) is connected to the negative terminal of the pacemaker and the ground lead is connected to the positive terminal. (B) Bipolar epicardial pacing. One ventricular lead is connected to the positive terminal and one to the negative terminal of the pacemaker. (For atrial pacing, either atrial lead is connected to the positive terminal and the other atrial lead to the negative terminal of the pacemaker.)

positive terminal of the cable; for ventricular pacing, connect one ventricular pacing wire to the negative terminal of the pacing cable and the other ventricular wire to the positive terminal of the cable.

3. Set the rate at 70 to 80 bpm or as ordered.
4. Set the output at 10 mA for atrial pacing and 5 mA for ventricular pacing, then determine stimulation threshold and set two- to three-times higher.
5. Set the sensitivity at the lowest possible number for atrial pacing and at 2 mV for ventricular pacing.

Dual-Chamber Temporary Pacing

Dual-chamber pacing can be performed through epicardial-pacing leads or with transvenous atrial and ventricular leads. Transvenous dual-chamber pacing is not often performed because of difficulties in placing temporary atrial leads and the unreliable stability of atrial leads. Epicardial dual-chamber pacing is often performed after cardiac surgery, but should be performed only when there are two ventricular leads in place. Two ventricular leads allow for bipolar ventricular pacing and sensing, thus reducing the possibility that the ventricular lead will sense atrial output and inappropriately inhibit ventricular pacing (crosstalk).

Dual-chamber pacing modes available depend on the type of pulse generator used for pacing. Older dual-chamber temporary pulse generators (like that shown in Fig. 28-6A) allow only DVI pacing. The newer dual-chamber units allow for DDD, DVI, DDI, and VDD pacing in addition to the single-chamber options AAI, AOO, and VVI.

To initiate dual-chamber pacing with epicardial leads:

1. Connect two pacing cables to the top of the pulse generator: one to the atrial terminal and one to the ventricular terminal.
2. Connect the atrial pacing cable to the atrial pacing wires: one atrial wire to the positive terminal and one atrial wire to the negative terminal.
3. Connect the ventricular pacing cable to the ventricular wires: one ventricular wire to the positive terminal and one ventricular wire to the negative terminal.
4. Select dual-chamber pacing mode desired (if option is provided): DDD, DDI, DVI, VDD. The DDD mode is almost always used.
5. Set AV delay at 150 milliseconds or as ordered.
6. Set atrial output at 10 mA and ventricular output at 5 mA, then determine stimulation threshold for both chambers and set output two- to three-times higher than threshold.
7. Set atrial or ventricular sensitivity as necessary, depending on pacing mode selected (atrial sensing occurs only in DDD, DDI, and VDD dual-chamber modes).
   a. Set atrial sensitivity at 0.5 mV.
   b. Set ventricular sensitivity at 2 mV.

Nursing Considerations

Nursing care of patients with pacemakers requires an understanding of how pacemakers work and what to expect the pacemaker to do depending on how it is programmed. Clinicians working in pacemaker follow-up clinics or physician offices have the advantage of being able to use the pacemaker programmer and view intracardiac electrograms and marker channels to help evaluate pacemaker function. Bedside nurses in most acute care facilities do not have access to programmers and must be able to evaluate appropriate pacemaker function by looking at the ECG or rhythm strips. The next section of this chapter covers ECG analysis of pacemaker rhythm strips to assist bedside practitioners in evaluating pacemaker function. It is beyond the scope of this chapter to discuss pacemaker follow-up in a clinic or office setting.

An important function for nurses or monitor technicians is to document significant bradycardias that may require pacemaker therapy and to relate these bradycardia events with clinical symptoms whenever possible. The guidelines for pacemaker insertion state, "definite correlation of symptoms with a bradyarrhythmia is required to fulfill the criteria that define symptomatic bradycardia."[1] Many insurance companies will not cover the cost of pacemaker insertion without good clinical documentation of the need. Nurses and monitor technicians are in a prime position to be able to document the bradycardia event by mounting rhythm strips in the patient's chart or getting a 12-lead ECG, and documenting symptoms that occur in conjunction with the bradycardia. Documentation of hypotension, syncope or near syncope, dizziness or light-headedness, confusion, fatigue, exercise intolerance, and development of symptoms of HF associated with bradycardia is an important nursing function.

Permanent Pacemakers

Implantation of a permanent pacemaker is often performed on an outpatient basis, but some patients are kept overnight for observation. The procedure is performed under local anesthesia in the cardiac catheterization laboratory, electrophysiology laboratory, or the OR, and it takes from 1 to 5 hours to complete depending on the number and location of pacing leads being inserted. In addition to routine postoperative care given to any surgical patient, permanent pacemaker insertion usually requires that the patient immobilize the operative arm in a sling for the first 24 hours to prevent lead dislodgment. The nurse must be aware of the potential complications of pacemaker insertion, including the potential for cardiac perforation leading to tamponade, and monitor for those complications. Patient teaching includes information about pacemaker function, how to count the pulse, and importance of follow-up visits to the physician. Because patients are discharged so soon after the procedure, they should be told to take their temperature and monitor the insertion site for signs of infection.

Using a Magnet With a Permanent Pacemaker. Occasionally, the nurse is asked to place a pacemaker magnet over the permanent pulse generator. Use of a magnet usually requires a physician's order or is covered by a written protocol detailing conditions under which a magnet can be used without a direct order.

A magnet inactivates the sensing circuit of a permanent pacemaker and causes it to revert to the asynchronous mode of pacing. This may be performed to verify a pacemaker's ability to pace when it is being inhibited by a patient's own natural rhythm. With a magnet in place, the pacemaker paces at a fixed rate in competition with the patient's rhythm, thus verifying the pacemaker's ability to deliver pacing stimuli. When a paced impulse happens to fall at a time when the ventricle is able to respond, capture should occur, verifying the pacemaker's ability to capture. A magnet may also be used to evaluate battery status if a pacemaker is nearing its end of service. In some older pacemakers the primary indicator of battery depletion is a change in the magnet-induced pacing rate. Some models of pacemakers pace at a faster rate for the first several beats after magnet application and then pace at a slower rate. Some pacemakers remain in the asynchronous pacing mode for the entire duration that the magnet is in place, whereas others only pace asynchronously for a certain number of beats and then revert to normal operation. It is possible to program the magnet operation off in some pacemakers, although this is rarely done. Because of the wide variety of potential responses to magnet application, it is advisable to know what pacemaker is present and what the programmed parameters are whenever possible when using a magnet.

Another indication for magnet use is to terminate a pacemaker-mediated tachycardia (PMT) in a dual-chamber pacemaker (see section "Dual-Chamber Pacing"). When using the magnet, the nurse should have the patient on a cardiac monitor and must be aware of the potential danger of a pacing spike falling in the vulnerable period and causing ventricular arrhythmias. A defibrillator should be immediately available whenever a magnet is used on a permanent pacemaker.

Pacemakers in the OR. The biggest concern regarding pacemakers in the OR is the potential effect of electromagnetic interference (EMI) on pacemaker operation. Cautery used during surgery is a type of EMI that can cause abnormal behavior of the pacemaker. Although modern pacemakers are heavily shielded and protected from many sources of EMI, it is still possible for extraneous signals to enter the pacemaker when detected by the pacing leads. Bipolar pacing systems are less likely to be affected than unipolar systems because the sensing circuit in a bipolar system is much smaller than that in a unipolar system. Possible responses to EMI include: (1) inhibition of pacemaker output; (2) triggering of pacemaker output at rapid rates; (3) asynchronous pacing; (4) mode resetting; (5) damage to the circuitry in the pacemaker; or (6) delivery of inappropriate shocks if the device is an ICD.[25] The most common responses to EMI in the OR are inhibition of pacing or reversion to a "noise mode," usually VOO or DOO pacing (asynchronous pacing). Inhibition of pacing occurs when the pacemaker senses the cautery and interprets those signals as intrinsic ventricular activity. This feature can result in asystole if the patient is pacemaker-dependent with no reliable underlying rhythm and is the most worrisome concern when dealing with pacemakers in the OR. Many pacemakers revert to asynchronous pacing when they sense electrical "noise" from cautery or other sources of EMI. This feature allows pacing to occur in an asynchronous mode, creating the potential problem of pacemaker output occurring during the vulnerable period of ventricular repolarization and resulting in VF.

There are several interventions that can reduce the potential adverse effects of EMI during surgery. If cautery is to be used, then place the grounding pad as far away from the pulse generator as possible (e.g. on a leg rather than on the chest or back), and place it on the opposite side of the body from the pacemaker. Use cautery in short bursts rather than long, continuous applications. Observe the monitor for pacemaker response to cautery, and if cautery appears to cause inhibition of pacing place a magnet over the pacemaker while cautery is being applied. A defibrillator and other emergency equipment should be immediately available during surgery. It is advisable to interrogate a pacemaker both before and after surgical procedures involving cautery or other sources of EMI (i.e. high-intensity radiation, radiofrequency ablation, lithotripsy) to verify programmed parameters before surgery and make sure they have not changed after surgery. If the pacemaker is programmed to a rate-modulated mode (VVIR, DDDR), then it is wise to disable rate modulation by programming to VVI or DDD before surgery, because mechanical ventilators, bone hammers, surgical saws, and other equipment in the surgical environment may trigger the physiological sensors and result in rapid pacing.

Nonmedical Sources of EMI. Pacemakers can be adversely affected by EMI in the environment, and patients should be taught about potential pacemaker interactions with common sources of EMI. Security systems or antitheft devices in department stores can potentially interact with pacemakers and cause intermittent inhibition of pacing output, inappropriate atrial tracking, or asynchronous pacing.[25] Patients should be cautioned not to linger close to a security system but to pass through it and then move away. Metal detectors used in security systems in airports and other places can potentially interact with pacemakers, but this interaction is rare. It is generally safe for people with pacemakers or ICDs to walk through a metal detector gate even though the alarm may be triggered by the device. People with implanted devices can request a manual search rather than a hand-held metal detector search.

Cell phones, personal digital assistants, laptop computers, and other wireless devices are a potential source of EMI that can inhibit pacemaker output, cause asynchronous pacing, or cause inappropriate ventricular tracking in a dual-chamber device.[25] Keeping a cell phone at least 6 inches away from the pacemaker pulse generator prevents interactions. Patients should avoid carrying their cell phone in a pocket near the pulse generator and should use the ear opposite the pacemaker when talking on a cell phone. It is reasonable to consider the hand used to hold a cell phone when selecting the site for pacemaker implantation in individual patients.

Household appliances are safe for use by patients with pacemakers, as are other commonly used electrical or motor-driven appliances like lawn mowers, leaf blowers, and small tools (drills, saws, etc.). Almost all interactions with household appliances (especially washing machines) occur with improper grounding of the appliance.[25]

Cardioversion and Defibrillation. Patients with pacemakers can be safely cardioverted or defibrillated if precautions are taken to protect the pacemaker from high-energy electrical forces. Paddles or defibrillation pads should not be placed directly over the pulse generator. Placing the paddles or pads in the anterior–posterior position is preferred over the standard transthoracic placement (refer to Fig. 28-4, which illustrates anterior–posterior pad placement for external pacing). Use of lower energy shocks is preferable over higher energy shocks whenever possible. The pacemaker should be interrogated after cardioversion or defibrillation to make sure it is still programmed and functioning as intended.

Temporary Pacemakers

In the care of patients with temporary pacemakers, the following additional considerations become important.

Insertion Site Care. A temporary pacing catheter is usually inserted through a venous sheath that is sutured to the skin and treated as any central venous catheter. Maintaining a clean, dry insertion site is important to prevent infection, and hospital policies governing the care of central venous catheters and dressings should be followed. If the pacing catheter is placed via a femoral vein, then the patient needs to be on bed rest with the affected leg straight and head of bed elevated no more than 20 degrees while the femoral sheath is in place.

Care of Epicardial Leads. Epicardial leads exit through the chest and unless they are being used for pacing, they are usually coiled and placed in a gauze dressing until needed. The exit site should be kept clean and dry according to established hospital policies on exit site care. Epicardial leads are easily dislodged, so care must be taken when handling them so as not to pull them out. Use of a pacing cable is recommended to prevent the need to strap the temporary pacemaker directly to the patient's body. The leads and pacing cable must be securely taped to the chest to prevent dislodgement of epicardial leads. Because the exposed metal end of the leads is a direct route for electrical current from the environment to conduct directly to the heart, care must be taken to insulate the leads to prevent cardiac arrhythmias, especially VF (see section "Electrical Safety," for more information).

Electrical Safety. A temporary pacing lead provides a direct pathway for stray electrical current to reach the heart without the protective resistance of the skin. Even a very small electrical current can initiate atrial fibrillation or VF if it is conducted directly to the heart by pacing leads.

Some considerations for electrical safety when caring for patients with temporary pacing leads include:

1. Wear gloves when handling pacing leads.
2. Make sure that all connections between the pulse generator and pacing cable and between pacing cable and pacing leads are tight and inserted completely into their receptacles so no metal is exposed.
3. If using a pacing cable with an alligator clip connector, then wrap a glove around the connections in such a way that they are separated and insulated from each other and from the environment.
4. Cover exposed metal ends of pacing leads that are not in use with some type of insulating material.
   a. Wrap a glove around the ends of transvenous leads and tape loosely.
   b. Place the ends of epicardial leads in a glove (or cut a finger from a glove and place them inside) or place the metal end of each individual lead in a needle cover, small syringe, or some other insulating material.
5. Keep dressings over pacing lead insertion sites dry; wet dressings conduct electricity more easily.
6. Make sure all electrical equipment in the room is grounded and in good working order.
7. Be aware of your own body's static electricity, especially if your unit is carpeted.
   a. Never let the pacing system be the first thing you touch when entering a patient's room.
   b. Be especially careful when using slider boards to transfer patients into and out of bed, because they generate static electricity.

Stimulation Threshold Testing. The stimulation threshold is the minimum pacemaker output necessary to capture the heart consistently. The contact of the pacing lead with the myocardium causes local tissue edema and inflammation that impedes the delivery of current to the myocardium. Peak thresholds occur approximately 3 to 4 weeks after permanent lead placement, and chronic stable thresholds are usually reached at approximately 3 months. Stimulation threshold testing with a temporary pacing system should be performed every shift to ensure an adequate safety margin for capture. The procedure for performing a stimulation threshold test is as follows:

1. Verify that the patient is in a paced rhythm; pacing rate may need to be temporarily increased to override an intrinsic rhythm.
2. Watch the cardiac monitor continuously while gradually decreasing output.
3. Note when loss of capture occurs (pacing spike not followed by appropriate waveform: P wave for atrial pacing, QRS for ventricular pacing).
4. Gradually turn output up until 1:1 capture resumes—this is the stimulation threshold.
5. Set the output two- to three-times higher than threshold to ensure adequate safety margin; for example, if consistent capture is regained at 2 mA, then set the output at 4 to 6 mA.

Sensitivity Threshold Testing. The sensitivity threshold is the minimum voltage of intrinsic cardiac activity that can be sensed by the pacemaker. The pacemaker becomes more sensitive (can sense smaller signals) as the number on the sensitivity control gets smaller (see section "Sensing," for further explanation).

Sensitivity testing can be performed only if the patient has a hemodynamically stable underlying rhythm. If the patient is completely pacemaker-dependent or has a very slow underlying rate, then do not perform sensitivity threshold testing. The procedure for performing a sensitivity threshold test is as follows:

1. Verify that the patient has an intrinsic rhythm (is not being paced); this may require temporarily decreasing the pacing rate to allow the underlying rhythm to emerge.
2. Slowly decrease the pacemaker's sensitivity (by *increasing* the number on the sensitivity control) while watching the sense indicator light on the pulse generator or watching the cardiac monitor.
   a. The sense indicator light flashes with each sensed P wave (for atrial sensing) or QRS (for ventricular sensing).
   b. Pacing remains inhibited and there are no pacing spikes seen on the monitor as long as sensing continues.
3. Note when the sense indicator fails to flash with each P wave or QRS and when pacing spikes begin to appear in competition with the intrinsic rhythm; this is the sensitivity threshold.
4. Set the sensitivity at one-half of the identified threshold to ensure an adequate safety margin; for example, if the threshold is 5 mV, then set the sensitivity at 2.5 mV.

Evaluating Pacemaker Function

This section is directed primarily at temporary pacemakers because nurses can interact more directly with them than with permanent pacemakers. The same concepts apply to permanent pacemakers, but corrective measures require the use of a pacemaker programmer or an actual surgical procedure to reposition pacing leads or replace the pulse generator.

Evaluation of pacemaker function requires knowledge of the mode of pacing expected (e.g. VVI, AAI, DDD); the minimum rate of the pacemaker, or pacing interval; and any other programmed parameters in the pacemaker. The basic functions of a pacemaker include stimulus release, capture, and sensing, and they should be evaluated for both temporary and permanent pacemakers. *Stimulus release* refers to pacemaker output, or the ability of the pacemaker to generate and release a pacing impulse. *Capture* is the ability of the pacing stimulus to cause depolarization of the chamber being paced. *Sensing* is the ability of the pacemaker to recognize and respond to intrinsic electrical activity in the

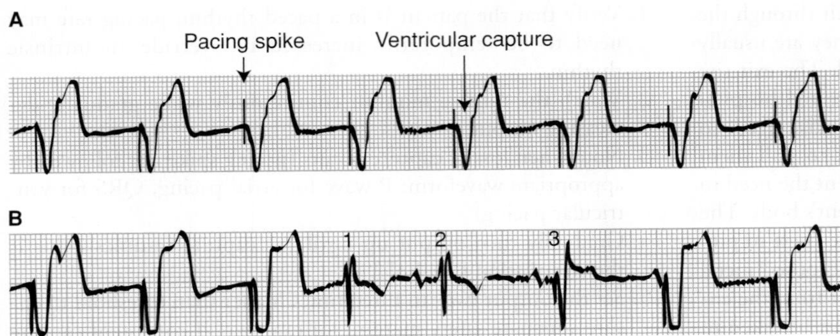

■ **Figure 28-13** Normal VVI pacemaker function. **(A)** Capture is good, but sensing cannot be evaluated because no intrinsic QRS complexes are present. **(B)** Capture and sensing both normal. Beats numbers 1 and 2 are intrinsic QRS complexes that are sensed, inhibit ventricular pacing output, and reset the pacing interval. Beat number 3 is a fusion beat between the intrinsic QRS and the paced beat.

heart. Pacemaker operation is evaluated by assessing these three functions. Single-chamber pacemaker evaluation is much less complicated than dual-chamber evaluation. Because ventricular pacing is the most common type of single-chamber pacing, evaluation of VVI pacemakers is discussed here. The concepts presented for ventricular pacemaker evaluation can also be applied to atrial pacemaker evaluation.

A VVI pacemaker is expected to pace the ventricle at the set rate unless spontaneous ventricular activity occurs to inhibit pacing. The minimum rate of the pacemaker, or pacing interval, is measured from one pacing stimulus to the next consecutive pacing stimulus with no intervening sensed beats between the two. In a normally functioning VVI pacemaker, pacing spikes occur at the preset pacing interval and each spike results in a ventricular depolarization (capture). If spontaneous ventricular activity occurs (either a normally conducted QRS or a PVC), that activity is sensed, the next pacing stimulus is inhibited, and the pacing interval timing cycle is reset. If no intrinsic ventricular activity occurs, a pacing stimulus is released at the end of the timing cycle. Figure 28-13 shows normal VVI pacemaker function.

The pacemaker has a *refractory period*, which is a period of time after either pacing or sensing in the ventricle during which the pacemaker is unable to respond to intrinsic activity. During the refractory period, the pacemaker in effect has its "eyes closed" and is not able to sense spontaneous activity. If an intrinsic QRS should occur during the pacemaker's refractory period, it is not sensed because the pacemaker is "blind" at that time.

Stimulus Release

Stimulus release is verified on the ECG by the presence of a pacing spike. A pacing spike indicates that the pacemaker battery has enough power to initiate a stimulus and that the stimulus was delivered into the body. When evaluating a temporary pacing system, the presence of a pacing spike indicates that the connections between the pulse generator and the pacing cable and between the pacing cable and the pacing leads are intact. If any part of the system becomes disconnected, the stimulus cannot reach the body and a pacing spike is not seen. The presence of a pacing spike alone does not indicate where the stimulus was delivered, only that it entered the body somewhere.

Absence of pacing stimuli when they should be present can indicate a faulty pulse generator or battery, or a break or disconnection in the lead system. Pacing stimuli can also be absent when pacing is inhibited by the sensing of extraneous electrical signals, such as EMI or myopotentials. Figure 28-14 illustrates total loss of stimulus release in a patient whose permanent pacemaker battery was totally depleted.

Capture

Capture is indicated by a wide QRS complex immediately after the pacemaker spike and represents the ability of the pacing stimulus to depolarize the ventricle. Loss of capture is recognized by the presence of pacing spikes that are not followed by paced ventricular complexes (Fig. 28-15). Causes of loss of capture include the following:

1. Inadequate stimulus strength, which can be corrected by increasing the electrical output of the pacemaker (turning up the milliamperage).
2. Pacing lead out of position and not in contact with myocardium, which can sometimes be corrected by repositioning the patient; repositioning the pacing lead is usually not a nursing function and must be performed by a physician or someone trained in intracardiac catheter manipulation.
3. Pacing lead positioned in infarcted tissue, which can be corrected by repositioning the lead to a place where myocardium is healthy and capable of responding to the stimulus.

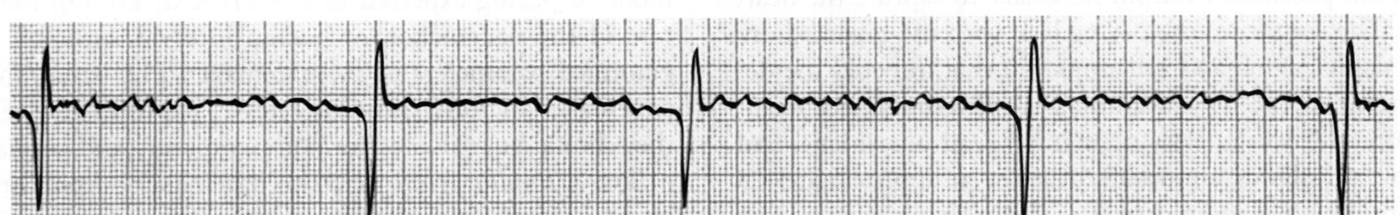

■ **Figure 28-14** Absence of stimulus release in a patient with a permanent pacemaker. Underlying rhythm is atrial fibrillation with complete atrioventricular block and a very slow ventricular rate. The battery in the pacemaker generator was at end of service.

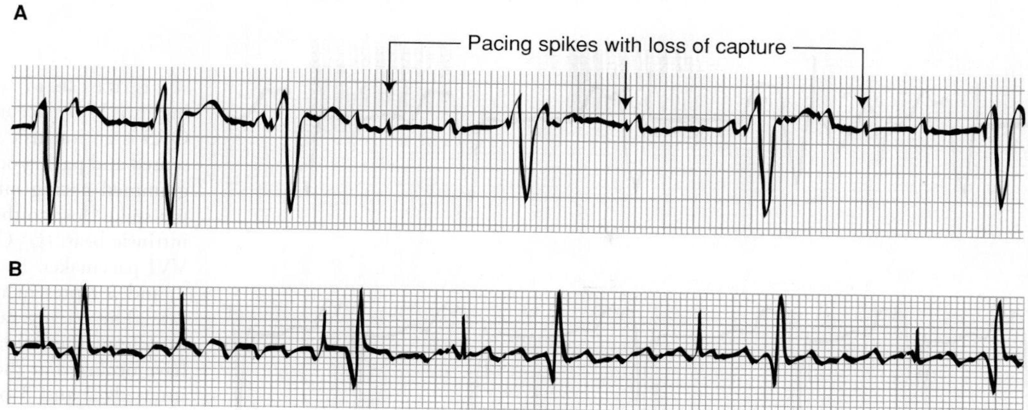

■ **Figure 28-15** (A) VVI pacemaker with intermittent loss of capture. (B) VVI pacemaker with total loss of capture. The underlying rhythm is atrial flutter with a slow ventricular response.

4. Electrolyte imbalances or drugs that alter the ability of the heart to respond to the pacing stimulus.
5. Delivery of a pacing stimulus during the ventricle's refractory period when the heart is physiologically unable to respond to the stimulus; this problem occurs with loss of sensing (undersensing) and can be prevented by correcting the sensing problem (Fig. 28-16A).

Loss of capture in a totally pacemaker-dependent patient is an emergency because without an effective underlying rhythm, the patient may be asystolic or severely symptomatic because of slow, ineffective rate. If the underlying rhythm is ineffective or absent, cardiopulmonary resuscitation must be performed until the capture problem is corrected or until the emergency transcutaneous pacing can be instituted. If loss of capture is intermittent, it may not result in symptoms but should be corrected as soon as possible.

Sensing

Sensing of intrinsic ventricular electrical activity inhibits the next pacing stimulus and resets the pacing interval. Sensing cannot occur unless the pacemaker is given the opportunity to sense. It

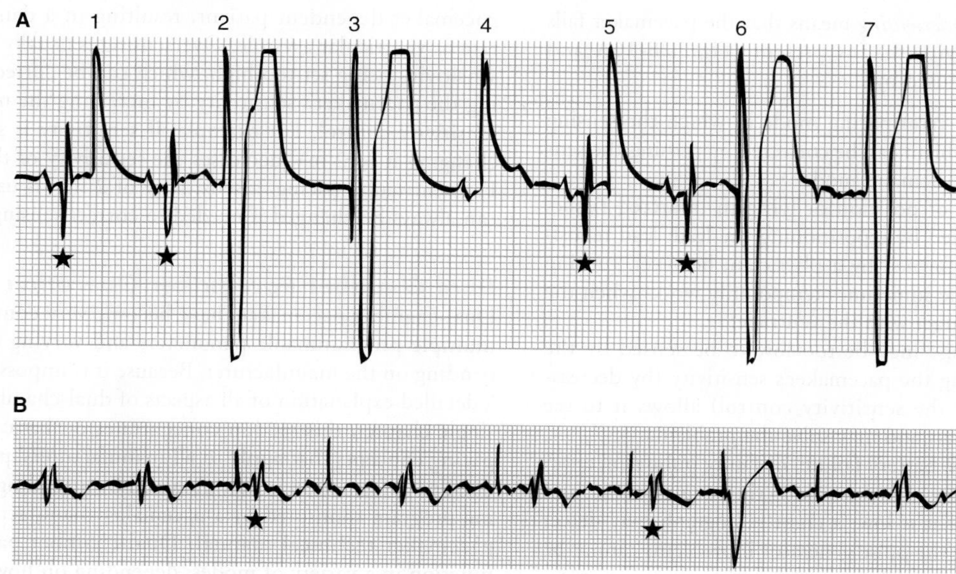

■ **Figure 28-16** (A) Loss of sensing in a VVI pacemaker. Delivery of the pacing stimulus during the heart's refractory period makes it appear that capture is lost as well. Because the heart is physiologically unable to respond to the pacing stimulus when it falls in the refractory period, this is not a problem. The beats marked with stars are beats that were not sensed by the pacemaker. Pacing spikes 1, 2, 5, and 6 should not have occurred; their presence is due to loss of sensing. Pacing spike 4 occurred coincident with the normal QRS complex, resulting in a "pseudofusion" beat, and does not represent loss of sensing. (B) Loss of capture in a VVI pacemaker. Only one pacing spike captures the ventricle. Two QRS complexes marked with stars occur during the pacemaker's refractory period and thus are not sensed. This does not represent loss of sensing because the pacemaker has its "eye closed" during the time intrinsic ventricular activity occurred.

A

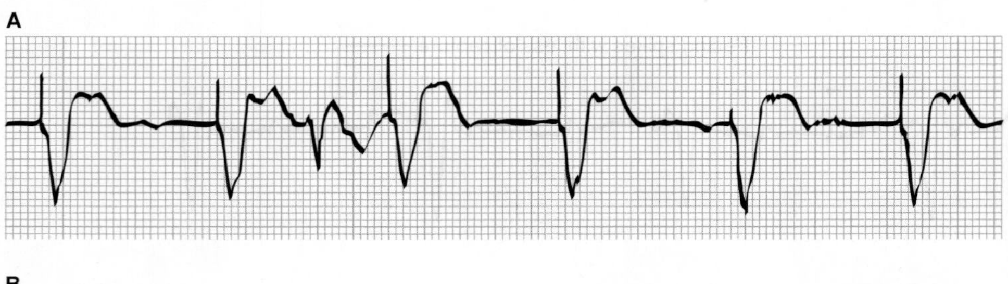

B

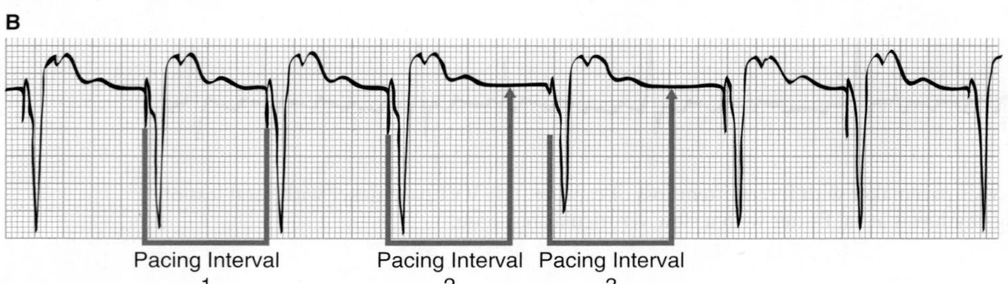

■ **Figure 28-17** (A) Undersensing in a VVI pacemaker. The third QRS is an intrinsic beat that is not sensed and pacing occurs at the programmed pacing interval, resulting is a spike close to the T wave of the intrinsic beat. (B) Oversensing in a VVI pacemaker. Pacing intervals 1, 2, and 3 represent the basic pacing rate. The pacing rate slows in the middle of the strip; pacing should have occurred at the end of pacing intervals 2 and 3 but was delayed because the device sensed something that reset the pacing interval.

must be in the demand mode and there must be intrinsic ventricular activity for the pacemaker to have an opportunity to sense. In Figure 28-13A, sensing cannot be evaluated because there is no intrinsic ventricular activity; therefore, the pacemaker is not given an opportunity to sense. In Figure 28-13B, the occurrence of two spontaneous QRS complexes provides the opportunity to sense. In this example, sensing occurred normally, as indicated by the absence of the next two expected pacing stimuli and resetting of the pacing interval from the intrinsic QRS complex.

Undersensing. *Undersensing* means that the pacemaker fails to sense intrinsic activity that is present (Figs. 28-16A and 28-17A). This can be caused by:

1. Asynchronous (fixed-rate) pacing mode in which the sensing circuit is off; this problem can be corrected by turning the sensitivity control to the demand mode.
2. Pacing catheter out of position or lying in infarcted tissue, which can be corrected by repositioning the lead; lead repositioning must be performed by a physician; however, turning the patient to the side sometimes temporarily works when the pacing lead loses contact with the ventricle.
3. Intrinsic QRS voltage may be too low to be sensed by the pacemaker; increasing the pacemaker's sensitivity (by decreasing the number on the sensitivity control) allows it to see smaller intrinsic signals and may solve the problem.
4. Break in connections, battery failure, or faulty pulse generator; check and tighten all connections along the pacing system, and replace the battery if it is low; a chest radiograph may detect lead fracture; change the pulse generator if problems cannot be corrected any other way.
5. Intrinsic ventricular activity falling in the pacemaker's refractory period; if a spontaneous QRS complex occurs during the time the pacemaker has its "eyes closed," then the pacemaker cannot see it; this may occur when the pacemaker fails to capture, which can allow an intrinsic QRS to occur during the pacemaker's refractory period; this problem is caused by loss of capture and does not reflect a sensing malfunction (see Fig. 28-16B).

Oversensing. *Oversensing* means that the pacemaker is so sensitive that it inappropriately senses internal or external signals as QRS complexes and inhibits its output. Common sources of external signals that can interfere with pacemaker function include electromagnetic or radiofrequency signals or electronic equipment in use near the pacemaker. Internal sources of interference can include large P waves, large T-wave voltage, local myopotentials in the heart, or skeletal muscle potentials. Figure 28-17B illustrates oversensing in a temporary pacemaker. Because a VVI pacemaker is programmed to inhibit its output when it senses, oversensing can be a dangerous situation in a pacemaker-dependent patient, resulting in a dangerously slow rate or ventricular asystole. Oversensing is usually caused by the sensitivity being set too high, which can be corrected by reducing the pacemaker's sensitivity by increasing the number on the sensitivity control. For example, if sensitivity is set at 0.5 mV, changing it to 2 mV decreases the sensitivity of the pacemaker. For ventricular pacing, a sensitivity of 2 mV is usually safe and can always be changed if needed to correct sensing problems.

Dual-Chamber Pacemaker Operation

Dual-chamber pacemakers have become very complicated, with multiple programmable parameters and varying functions, depending on the manufacturer. Because it is impossible to present a detailed explanation of all aspects of dual-chamber pacing in a single chapter, this section concentrates on basic dual-chamber pacing concepts that apply to all manufacturers' products. More detailed information is best obtained by attending a formal pacing program sponsored by a pacemaker manufacturer or from a pacemaker technical manual. Dual-chamber pacemakers can function in a variety of modes, depending on how they are programmed (Table 28-2). Because the DDD mode is most commonly used, basic DDD function is described here. Display 28-3 defines terms commonly used in dual-chamber pacing.

Dual-Chamber Timing Cycles

According to the pacemaker code, DDD means that both chambers (atria and ventricles) are paced, both chambers are sensed, and the mode of response to sensed events is either inhibited or

Table 28-2 ■ DUAL-CHAMBER PACING MODES

Mode	Chamber(s) Paced	Chamber(s) Sensed	Response to Sensing
DVI	Atrium and ventricle	Ventricle	Ventricular sensing inhibits atrial and ventricular pacing
VDD	Ventricle	Atrium and ventricle	Atrial sensing—triggers ventricular pacing Ventricular sensing—inhibits ventricular pacing
DDI	Atrium and ventricle	Atrium and ventricle	Atrial sensing inhibits atrial pacing Ventricular sensing inhibits ventricular pacing
DDD	Atrium and ventricle	Atrium and ventricle	Atrial sensing—inhibits atrial pacing, triggers ventricular pacing Ventricular sensing—inhibits atrial and ventricular pacing

triggered, depending on which chamber is sensed. When atrial activity is sensed, atrial pacing is inhibited and ventricular pacing is triggered at the end of the programmed AV delay. When ventricular activity is sensed, all pacemaker output is inhibited. The following timing cycles determine how a dual-chamber pacemaker functions, and Figure 28-18 illustrates many of these timing cycles[24,26]:

1. Pacing interval (or lower rate limit)—the base rate of the pacemaker, measured between two consecutive atrial pacing stimuli with no intervening sensed events; the pacing interval is a programmable parameter and determines the minimum rate at which the pacemaker paces in the absence of intrinsic cardiac activity.
2. AV delay (or AV interval)—the amount of time between atrial and ventricular pacing, or the "electronic PR interval"; this is measured from the atrial pacing spike to the ventricular pacing spike and is a programmable parameter; the AV delay timer is initiated by a paced or sensed atrial event, and if no intrinsic conduction occurs to the ventricle within that time, a ventricular pacing spike occurs at the end of the programmed AV delay.
3. Atrial escape interval (or ventriculoatrial [VA] interval)—the interval from a sensed or paced ventricular event to the next atrial pacing output; the VA interval represents the amount of time the pacemaker waits after it paces in the ventricle or senses ventricular activity before pacing the atrium; the atrial escape interval is not a programmed parameter, but rather is derived by subtracting the AV delay from the pacing interval; its length can be estimated by measuring from a ventricular spike to the next atrial pacing spike.
4. Total atrial refractory period—the period of time after a sensed P wave or a paced atrial event during which the atrial channel does not respond to sensed events; the total atrial refractory period consists of the AV delay and the postventricular atrial refractory period (PVARP).
5. PVARP—the period of time after an intrinsic QRS or a paced ventricular beat during which the atrial channel is refractory and does not respond to sensed atrial activity; PVARP is a programmable parameter but is not evident on a rhythm strip.
6. Blanking period—the very short ventricular refractory period that occurs with every atrial pacemaker output; the ventricular channel "blinks its eyes" so it will not sense the atrial output and inappropriately inhibit ventricular pacing; the blanking period is a programmable parameter but is not evident on a rhythm strip.
7. Ventricular refractory period—the period of time after a ventricular pacing output or a sensed QRS during which the ventricular channel ignores intrinsic ventricular activity; ventricular refractory period is a programmable parameter but is not evident on a rhythm strip.
8. Maximum tracking interval (or upper rate limit)—the maximum rate at which the ventricular channel tracks atrial activity; the upper rate limit prevents rapid ventricular pacing in response to very rapid atrial activity, such as atrial tachycardia or

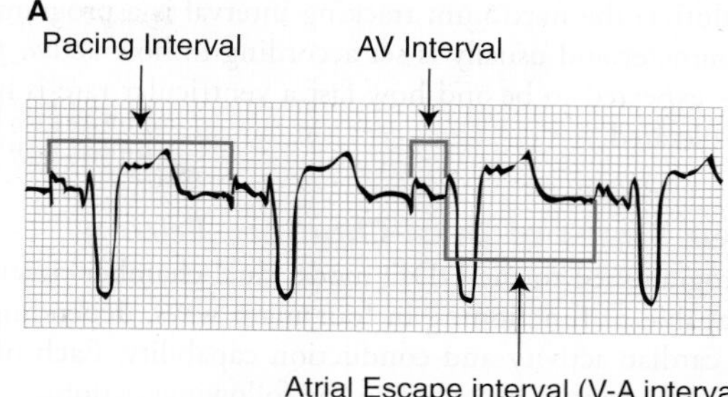

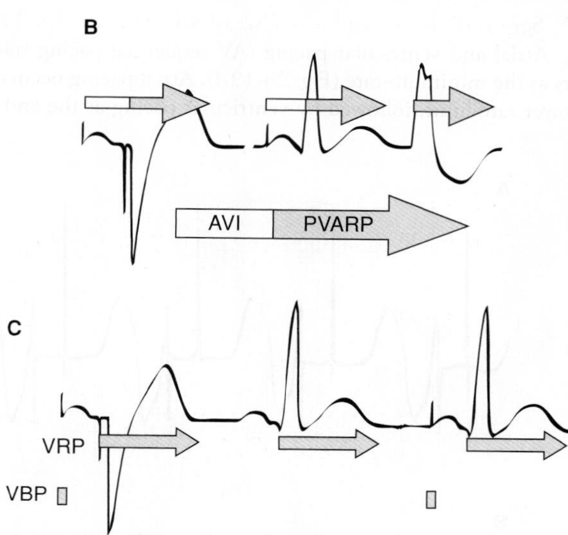

■ **Figure 28-18** Dual-chamber pacemaker timing cycles. (A) The pacing interval represents the minimum pacing rate and is measured from one atrial pacing spike to the next consecutive atrial pacing spike. The atrioventricular interval (AVI) is measured from the atrial pacing spike to the ventricular pacing spike. The atrial escape interval (or V–A interval) is the interval from a sensed or paced ventricular event to the next atrial pacing output and determines when the next atrial output is due. (B) Atrial channel refractory period. The arrows represent the total atrial refractory period, which is composed of the AVI, which begins with an atrial output or sensed P wave, and the postventricular atrial refractory period (PVARP) which begins with a paced or sensed ventricular event. (C) Ventricular channel refractory periods. The ventricular blanking period (VBP) is a brief ventricular refractory period that occurs with every atrial pacer output to prevent sensing of atrial output by the ventricular channel (crosstalk). The ventricular refractory period (VRP) begins with a paced or sensed ventricular event.

atrial flutter; the maximum tracking interval is a programmable parameter and usually is set according to how active a patient is expected to be and how fast a ventricular rate is likely to be tolerated.

The Four States of Dual-Chamber Pacing

When programmed to the DDD mode, dual-chamber pacemakers are capable of functioning in four main ways, depending on intrinsic cardiac activity and conduction capability. Each of the four states of pacing is described in the following sections.

AV Sequential Pacing State (Atrial and Ventricular Pacing). Atrial and ventricular pacing (AV sequential pacing state) occurs at the minimum rate (Fig. 28-19*A*). Atrial pacing occurs at the lower rate limit, followed by ventricular pacing at the end of the programmed AV delay. This type of pacing would occur if the underlying cardiac rhythm were sinus bradycardia with AV block or asystole.

Atrial Pacing State (Atrial Pacing With Ventricular Sensing). Atrial pacing occurs at the minimum rate, but normal conduction to the ventricle occurs before the AV delay times out, resulting in intrinsic QRS complexes after the paced atrial beats (see Fig. 28-19B). This type of pacing would occur if the underlying rhythm were sinus bradycardia with normal conduction through the AV node.

Atrial Tracking State (Atrial Sensing With Ventricular Pacing). Intrinsic P waves are followed by paced ventricular beats (see Fig. 28-19C). Intrinsic atrial activity is sensed by the pacemaker and starts the AV delay. No intrinsic ventricular activ-

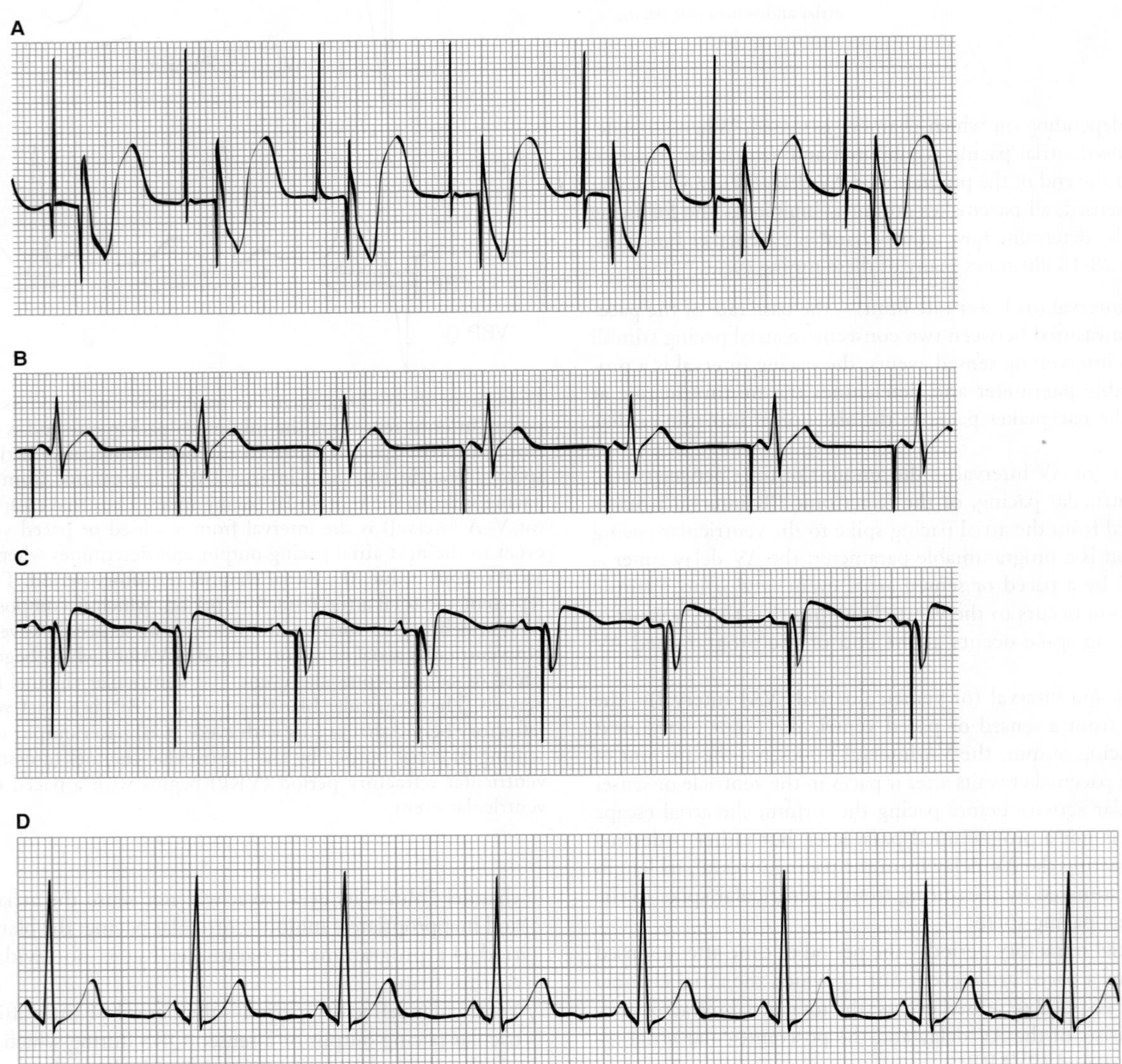

■ **Figure 28-19** The four states of dual-chamber pacing. **(A)** Atrioventricular (AV) sequential pacing state with atrial and ventricular pacing at the minimum pacing rate. **(B)** Atrial pacing, ventricular sensing state: atrial pacing occurs at the minimum rate and there is normal conduction to the ventricles, which inhibits ventricular output and terminates the AV delay. **(C)** Atrial tracking state: the pacemaker senses the patient's intrinsic P waves and paces the ventricle at the end of the AV delay. **(D)** Inhibited state with all pacing inhibited by normal sinus rhythm.

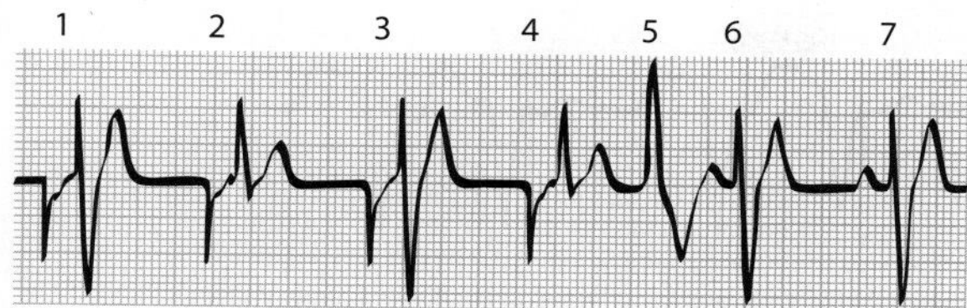

Figure 28-20 DDD pacemaker operating in all four states of pacing (stimulated strip). Beat 1, atrioventricular (AV) sequential pacing; beat 2, atrial pace, ventricular sense; beat 3, AV sequential pacing; beat 4, atrial pace, ventricular sense; beat 5, premature ventricular contraction; beat 6, atrial sense, ventricular pace; and beat 7, atrial sense, ventricular pace. Atrial capture is proven by beats 2 and 4 (atrial spike followed by normal QRS within the programmed AV delay). Atrial sensing is proven by beats 6 and 7 (normal P followed by paced V at end of AV delay). Ventricular capture is verified by beats 1, 3, 6, and 7 (wide-paced QRS following ventricular pacing spike). Ventricular sensing is proven by beats 2 and 4 (atrial spike followed by normal QRS, which inhibited ventricular pacing spike).

ity occurs before the AV delay times out, so a ventricular output is released at the end of the programmed AV delay. This type of pacing would occur if the underlying rhythm were sinus rhythm with complete AV block.

Inhibited State (Atrial and Ventricular Sensing). No pacing occurs in either chamber because intrinsic atrial and ventricular activity is present at a rate faster than the minimum pacing rate (see Fig. 28-19D). This occurs when the underlying rhythm is normal sinus rhythm.

The pacemaker is capable of switching from one state of pacing to another on a beat-to-beat basis depending on intrinsic activity. Figure 28-20 illustrates a DDD pacemaker operating in all four pacing states within a short period of time.

Evaluating Dual-Chamber Pacemaker Function

Because a dual-chamber pacemaker has both atrial and ventricular pacing and sensing functions, evaluation includes assessing atrial capture, atrial sensing, ventricular capture, and ventricular sensing. To evaluate pacemaker function, it is necessary to know the programmed mode (e.g. DDD, DVI), the minimum rate, the upper rate limit, the programmed AV delay, and refractory periods for both channels. In reality, the only time all of this information is available is immediately after an implantation, when the final programmed parameters are in the current patient chart, or in the physician's office records. Therefore, in the real world of bedside nursing, we have to rely on a basic understanding of the issues involved in pacemaker evaluation, often without having all of the necessary information at hand. Some of the needed information can be determined by measuring intervals on a rhythm strip. For example, the AV delay can be measured from atrial spike to ventricular spike if there are any AV sequentially paced beats present. The minimum rate can be determined by measuring the interval between two consecutive atrial pacing spikes, if present. The following sections briefly discuss the issues of assessing atrial and ventricular capture and sensing in a dual-chamber pacing system.

Atrial Capture. Atrial capture can be verified by seeing a P wave in response to every atrial pacing spike, although this is not always easy to see. The atrial response to pacing is often so small that it cannot be seen in many monitoring leads, so we cannot rely on the presence of a P wave after atrial pacing spikes as evidence of atrial capture. In the absence of a clear P wave, atrial capture can be assumed only when an atrial pacing spike is followed by a normally conducted QRS complex within the programmed AV delay. If the atrial spike captures the atrium and there is intact AV conduction, the presence of the normal QRS indicates that the atrium must have been captured for conduction to have occurred into the ventricles before the ventricular pacing stimulus was delivered. Because a DDD pacemaker paces the ventricle at a preset AV delay after atrial pacing, the presence of a ventricular paced beat after an atrial paced beat does not verify atrial capture, because the ventricle paces at the end of the AV delay regardless of whether atrial capture occurs. Therefore, atrial capture can be assumed only when there is an obvious P wave after every atrial pacing spike or when an atrial pacing spike is followed by a normal QRS within the programmed AV delay (see Figs. 28-19B and 28-20).

Atrial Sensing. Atrial sensing is verified by the presence of an intrinsic P wave that is followed by a paced ventricular beat at the end of the programmed AV delay. If a P wave is sensed, it starts the AV delay and ventricular pacing is triggered at the end of the AV delay, unless AV conduction is intact and results in a normal QRS. The presence of a normal P wave followed by a normal QRS proves only that AV conduction is intact, not that the P wave was sensed by the pacemaker. Therefore, atrial sensing is verified by an intrinsic P wave followed by a paced QRS (see Figs. 28-19C and 28-20).

Ventricular Capture. Ventricular capture is recognized by a wide QRS immediately after a ventricular pacing spike. Ventricular capture is much easier to recognize than atrial capture and is the same as with single-chamber ventricular pacing (see Figs. 28-19A and C and 28-20).

Ventricular Sensing. Ventricular sensing can be assessed only if there is intrinsic ventricular activity present for the pacemaker to sense. Ventricular sensing is verified by an atrial pacing spike followed by a normal QRS that inhibits the ventricular pacing spike, which is the same event that proves atrial capture (see Figs. 28-19B and 28-20). If a QRS is sensed before the next atrial pacing spike is due, both the atrial and ventricular pacing stimuli are inhibited and the VA interval (atrial escape interval) is reset.

Other Features of Dual-Chamber Pacemakers

Upper-Rate Behavior. To avoid rapid ventricular pacing in response to atrial arrhythmias, dual-chamber pacemakers have an upper rate limit or maximal tracking rate that limits the rate at which ventricular pacing occurs in response to sensed atrial activity. This upper rate limit applies only to paced tachycardias, not to intrinsic tachycardias. That is, tachycardias that are caused by ventricular pacing in response to rapid atrial rhythms should not exceed the upper rate limit of the pacemaker. However, spontaneous VT or supraventricular tachycardia that conducts to the ventricle through the normal AV node or across an accessory pathway may result in ventricular rates that exceed the upper rate limit of the pacemaker. When an atrial rate being tracked by the ventricular channel of the pacemaker exceeds the upper rate limit, the pacemaker is programmed to limit the ventricular rate. Upper rate responses can be used alone or in combination and include

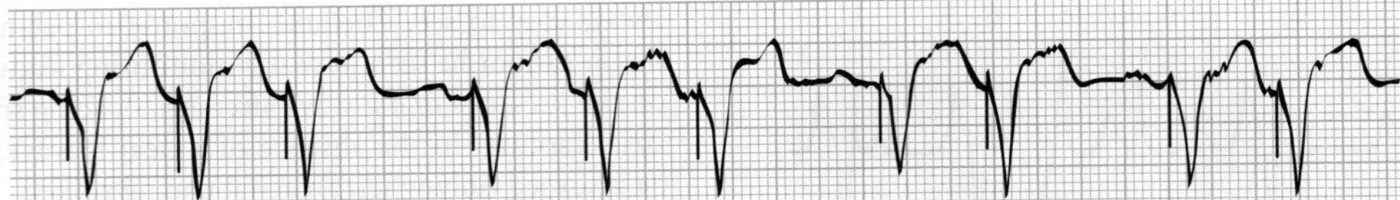

■ **Figure 28-21** Wenckebach upper-rate response. Sinus tachycardia is present at a rate slightly faster than the upper rate limit of about 125 bpm. The pacemaker tracks the intrinsic P waves and ventricular pacing occurs at the upper rate limit with occasional pauses. Note that the atrioventricular delay prolongs on consecutive beats until a P wave falls in the postventricular atrial refractory period, causing a pause in the ventricular paced rhythm.

Wenckebach response, block response, fallback, or rate smoothing. The Wenckebach response and block response are discussed here.

Wenckebach response is the most commonly used upper rate response. As the atrial rate increases above the upper rate limit, P waves fall progressively closer to the preceding ventricular paced beat and the AV interval gets progressively longer. Eventually, a P wave falls in PVARP, where it cannot be sensed. The unsensed P wave does not start an AV delay; therefore, there is no ventricular paced beat after that P wave, and the resulting pause causes the ventricular paced rate to remain at or below the upper rate limit. The ECG shows a gradual lengthening of the AV interval and pauses whenever a P wave falls in PVARP (Fig. 28-21). This pattern presents as group beating just like AV Wenckebach, but the R-R intervals are constant instead of getting shorter. The atrial rate, the upper rate limit, and the PVARP determine the degree of block (e.g., 3:2, 5:4).

In *block response*, 1:1 tracking occurs at a constant AV delay until the atrial rate reaches a critical rate at which a P wave falls in PVARP and sudden block develops. As the atrial rate increases, P waves fall closer to the preceding ventricular paced beat, and eventually a P wave lands in PVARP where it cannot be sensed. The unsensed P wave does not start an AV delay; therefore, there is no ventricular paced beat after that P wave and the resulting pause keeps the ventricular paced rate below the upper rate limit. The ECG shows constant AV intervals with sudden block, often in a 2:1 ratio (Fig. 28-22). This type of response causes an abrupt rate change rather than a more gradual rate change, as occurs with other upper rate responses.

Adaptive AV Delays. Most dual-chamber pacemakers can be programmed with two different AV delays: a shorter AV delay on atrial sensed beats and a longer AV delay on atrial paced beats. Atrial depolarization in response to normal sinus rhythm (atrial sensed event) is quicker than atrial depolarization due to atrial pacing; therefore, a longer AV delay on atrial paced beats helps maintain a more normal atrial–ventricular contraction sequence by delaying ventricular pacing when atrial pacing occurs.

In rate responsive mode (DDDR) the AV delay can be programmed to decrease as the pacing rate increases. This mimics the heart's normal response to an increase in heart rate by decreasing AV conduction time; the pacemaker paces with a shorter AV delay as the pacing rate increases.

Mode Switching. Mode switching is a function that causes a dual-chamber pacemaker to switch to a nontracking mode (i.e., DDI/R or VVI/R) when rapid atrial arrhythmias occur (e.g., atrial flutter or fibrillation). This prevents the ventricular channel from trying to track rapid atrial activity. The nontracking mode continues until the atrial channel senses that atrial rate has returned to normal (i.e., atrial fibrillation converts to sinus rhythm), at which time the device resumes DDD/R operation.

Pacemaker-Mediated Tachycardia. PMT (also called *endless loop tachycardia* or *pacemaker re-entry tachycardia*) is rapid ventricular pacing, usually at the upper rate limit, that can occur in patients with dual-chamber pacemakers when retrograde conduction is present in the normal conduction system or in an accessory pathway. Retrograde conduction means that impulses can conduct backward from ventricle to atrium. Pacemaker units that detect intrinsic atrial activity and stimulate the ventricle after an appropriate AV delay (VDD and DDD modes) can participate in the maintenance of a PMT. The tachycardia circuit consists of the

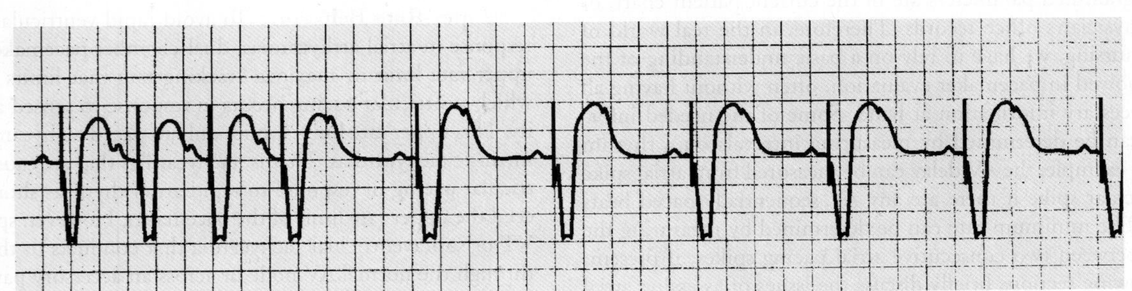

■ **Figure 28-22** Atrioventricular block upper-rate response (simulated strip). Sinus tachycardia is present at a rate of approximately 120 bpm and the upper rate limit is 120 bpm. Atrial tracking occurs at the beginning of the strip. As the sinus rate increases slightly, 2:1 block develops as every other P wave falls in the postventricular atrial refractory period. (From Kenny T. [2005]. *The nuts and bolts of cardiac pacing* [p. 82]. Malden, MA: Blackwell Futura.)

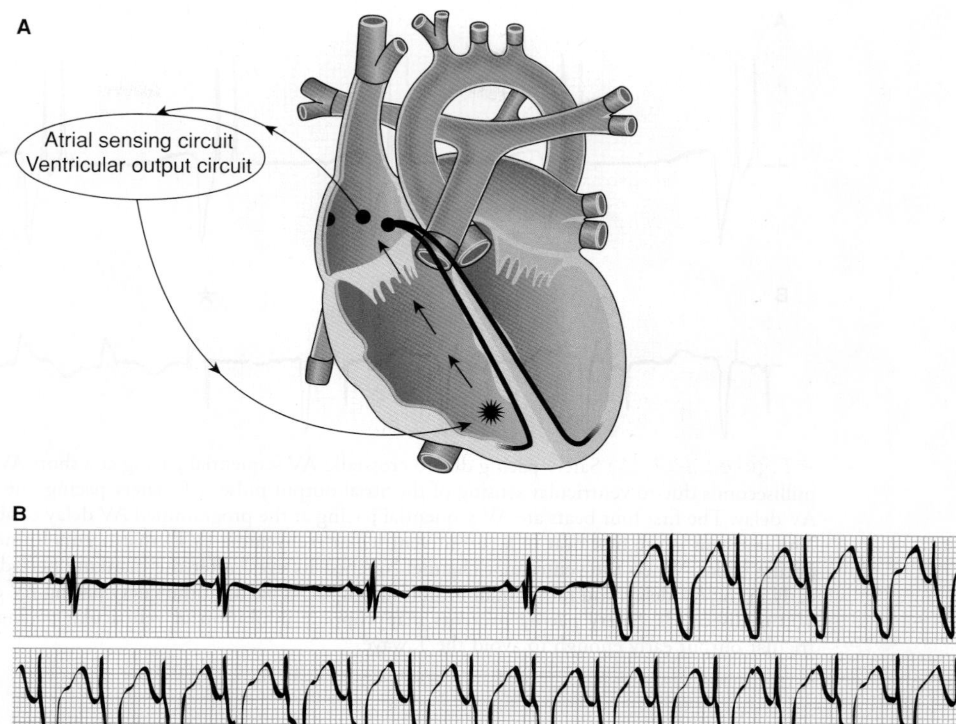

■ **Figure 28-23** (A) Diagram illustrating the mechanism of pacemaker-mediated tachycardia (PMT). A PVC occurs (indicated by *) and conducts retrograde to the atria (represented by the dashed line). The retrograde P wave is sensed by the atrial channel of the pacemaker and a ventricular output is delivered at the end of the programmed AV delay. The reentry circuit consists of the intrinsic conduction system as the retrograde limb and the pacemaker as the antegrade limb. (B) Rhythm strip of PMT. Sinus rhythm is present, and then a ventricular paced beat occurs, probably in response to atrial oversensing of myopotentials or something in the environment. Retrograde conduction occurs to the atria (seen as a P wave after the first ventricular paced beat), which then initiates PMT.

patient's normal AV conduction system (or an accessory pathway) that is capable of retrograde conduction, and the pacemaker's atrial sensing and ventricular output circuits (Fig. 28-23A). Retrograde conduction results in a sensed atrial depolarization, which in turn triggers the ventricular output channel. If this sequence is repeated, a tachycardia is maintained indefinitely until the retrograde pathway fatigues or until the tachycardia is terminated by inactivating the atrial sensing circuit (see Fig. 28-23B). Placing a magnet over the pulse generator inactivates the atrial sensing circuit and terminates PMT.

Conditions necessary for initiation of PMT include loss of AV synchrony, intact retrograde conduction, and VA conduction times longer than PVARP. Any condition that results in the atrium being repolarized and ready to respond to retrograde conduction can initiate PMT. Common initiators include PVCs with retrograde conduction, atrial undersensing, atrial oversensing, and loss of atrial capture.[27] Most newer dual-chamber pacemakers incorporate PMT prevention algorithms, such as extending PVARP after a PVC or temporarily inactivating the atrial sensing circuit after a PVC, in an attempt to prevent the initiation of PMT. Many devices also have PMT termination algorithms that attempt to break the tachycardia if it occurs.

Crosstalk. Crosstalk refers to the sensing of a signal in one chamber by the sensing circuit of the pacemaker in the other chamber. The most common and potentially dangerous type of crosstalk is sensing of the atrial output pulse by the ventricular channel, resulting in inhibition of ventricular output. If the ventricular channel senses the atrial pacing stimulus, it thinks it sees a ventricular event and thus inhibits its next output. This could result in total ventricular asystole in a patient who has no underlying ventricular rhythm. Other manifestations of crosstalk include atrial pacing at a rate faster than the programmed rate and a longer distance from the atrial pacing spike to the conducted QRS than is programmed for the AV delay. The ventricular blanking period and safety pacing are two features of dual-chamber pacemakers whose purpose is to prevent crosstalk.

Blanking Period. The ventricular blanking period is one method of trying to eliminate crosstalk. The blanking period is a very short refractory period that occurs on the ventricular channel during delivery of the atrial output pulse (see Fig. 28-18C). The blanking period "blinds" the ventricular channel for a short time so it cannot see the atrial pacing output. This blinding should prevent crosstalk, but if the blanking period is too short, it may still be possible for the ventricular channel to sense the end of the atrial output pulse. In most pacemakers, the blanking period is programmable and can be made longer if necessary to prevent crosstalk.

Safety Pacing (Nonphysiologic AV Delay). Safety pacing is a mechanism used to prevent the inhibition of ventricular output when crosstalk occurs. Safety pacing results in the delivery of a ventricular pacing spike at a short AV delay (e.g. 100 milliseconds) whenever the ventricular channel senses any signal immediately after the blanking period (Fig. 28-24). Safety pacing prevents inhibition of ventricular pacing and the short AV delay prevents delivery of the ventricular pacing spike on a T wave. Safety pacing presents on the ECG as a shorter than programmed AV interval, and is another way to verify that ventricular sensing is intact, because safety pacing only occurs when the ventricular channel senses something right after the end of the blanking period.

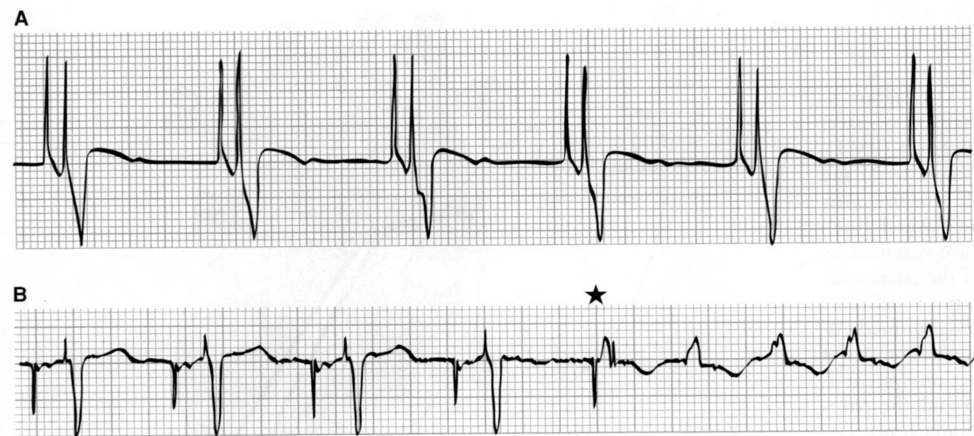

■ **Figure 28-24** (A) Safety pacing due to crosstalk: AV sequential pacing at a short AV interval of about 100 milliseconds due to ventricular sensing of the atrial output pulse. (B) Safety pacing due to sensing early in the AV delay. The first four beats are AV sequential pacing at the programmed AV delay of about 160 milliseconds. The star beat is the first beat in a run of ventricular tachycardia (VT) that occurs immediately after the atrial pacing spike. When the ventricular channel "opened its eyes" after the blanking period, it saw the QRS very early in the AV delay, and rather than inhibit its output, it paced at the safety pacing AV delay of approximately 100 milliseconds. Safety pacing prevents inappropriate inhibition of ventricular pacing but delivers the ventricular output early enough to avoid the T wave.

Rate-Adaptive Pacing. Rate-adaptive pacing is used when the heart is unable to increase its rate appropriately when the body's need for cardiac output increases (chronotropic incompetence). The pacing system contains a physiologic sensor that tells the pacemaker to pace faster in response to the sensed parameter. The most frequently used sensors at this time are motion sensors and minute ventilation sensors. Motion sensors are activated by body movement, such as occurs with exercise, and signal the pacemaker to pace faster. Minute ventilation sensors measure transthoracic impedance and increase the pacing rate when the respiratory rate is increased in response to exercise, emotional states, fever, and so on. Other technologies being investigated include sensors for metabolic parameters like blood temperature and venous oxygen saturation, and sensors of cardiac indices like QT interval, ventricular depolarization gradient, pre-ejection interval, stroke volume, and rate of myocardial wall tension development.[28] It is likely that future pacemakers will combine two or more sensors to get the most physiologic response to the body's needs for increased cardiac output. Figures 28-25 and 28-26 illustrate ECG examples of rate adaptive pacing, which can appear as pacemaker malfunction if the observer is unaware of the rate response feature.

Atrial Overdrive Pacing. Atrial pacing at rapid rates of 200 to 500 impulses/min is used in an attempt to terminate atrial tachyarrhythmias such as atrial tachycardia, atrial flutter, and atrial fibrillation (Fig. 28-27). This type of pacing is most frequently performed using a temporary pulse generator and pacing through epicardial leads in cardiac surgery patients. It can also be performed with a transvenous atrial lead, but this is less effective. Newer dual-chamber temporary pulse generators have overdrive pacing capability. It is extremely important to accurately identify the atrial pacing wires and make sure that rapid pacing is not

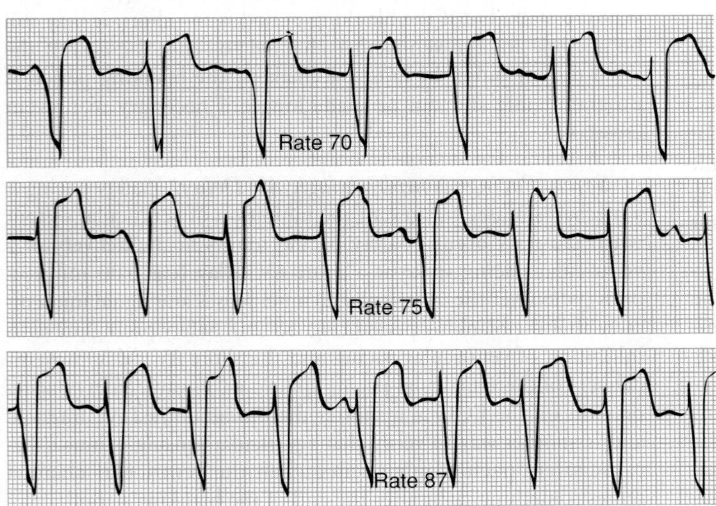

■ **Figure 28-25** VVIR pacing. Note the increase in VVI pacing rate from 70 bpm to 87 bpm with activity.

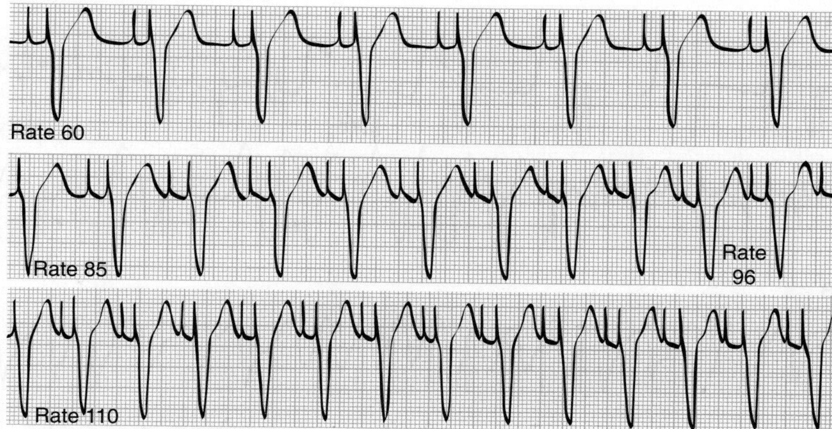

■ **Figure 28-26** DDDR pacing with a gradual increase in AV sequential pacing rate from 60 bpm at rest to 110 bpm with activity. This also illustrates the feature of adaptive AV delay in which the AV interval gradually shortens as the pacing rate increases, mimicking normal AV node physiology.

performed through ventricular leads, because that would most likely result in VF.

Antitachycardia Pacing. Antitachycardia pacing (ATP) involves the delivery of one to several paced impulses to the atria or the ventricles in an attempt to terminate tachycardias. This type of pacing is most often performed in the ventricle to terminate VT, and most ATP is incorporated into implantable defibrillator devices, which are covered later in this chapter. Figure 28-28 shows two examples of ATP during VT in patients with an ICD.

CRT with Biventricular Pacing

Patients with advanced systolic HF have delays in AV conduction, interventricular conduction, and intraventricular conduction that contribute to reduced LV function in several ways.[1,6–9] As many as 30% to 50% of patients with HF have an intraventricular conduction delay, usually due to LBBB, that causes the ventricles to contract asynchronously and contributes to abnormal contraction patterns in the septum and LV.[8,9,11,29]

Ventricular Dysynchrony

The term *ventricular dysynchrony* is used to describe the delayed electrical activation and mechanical contraction abnormalities that contribute to reduced LV performance in patients with advanced HF.

Electrical abnormalities that result from LBBB include the following:

1. RV depolarization occurs before LV depolarization.
2. The septum, which is usually activated in a left-to-right direction from Purkinje fibers that arise from the proximal portion of the left bundle branch, is activated from the right side and depolarizes before the LV free wall.
3. There is slow cell-to-cell depolarization of the LV that causes a wide QRS complex and abnormal spread of electrical activation through the LV.

Mechanical abnormalities that result from abnormal electrical activation include the following:

1. Contraction of the right ventricle before the LV (interventricular dysynchrony).
2. Paradoxical septal wall motion in which the septum contracts before the LV free wall and is finished repolarizing by the time LV contraction begins; this results in the septum moving away from the LV and bulging into the right ventricle during LV systole rather than participating in LV ejection.
3. Mitral regurgitation caused by delayed activation of the LV; the abnormal spread of electrical activation to the lateral wall of the LV causes delayed activation of the papillary muscles that normally contract slightly before the LV free wall and hold the mitral valve closed during LV systole.
4. Abnormally slow depolarization of the LV free wall causes asynchronous contraction patterns within the LV (intraventricular dysynchrony).
5. Delayed contraction of the LV also delays LV relaxation; this causes reduced LV filling because atrial contraction occurs before the LV is relaxed and able to accept the volume of blood being ejected by the contracting left atrium.
6. The combination of abnormal septal motion, mitral regurgitation, abnormal LV contraction patterns, and reduced LV filling contribute to the already reduced stroke volume that occurs in HF.

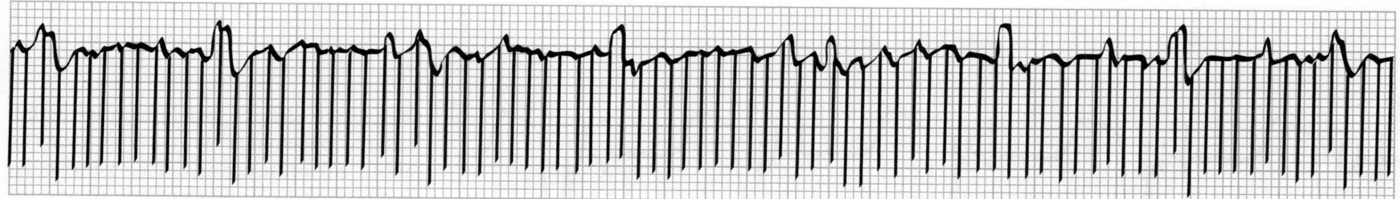

■ **Figure 28-27** Atrial overdrive pacing in attempt to terminate atrial flutter using atrial epicardial wires in a postcardiac surgery patient.

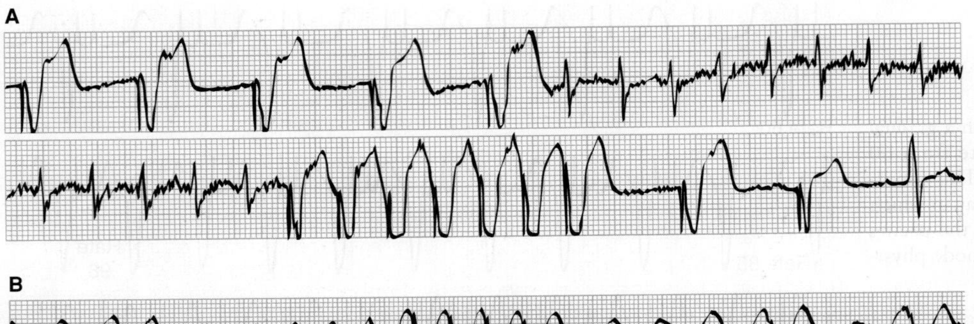

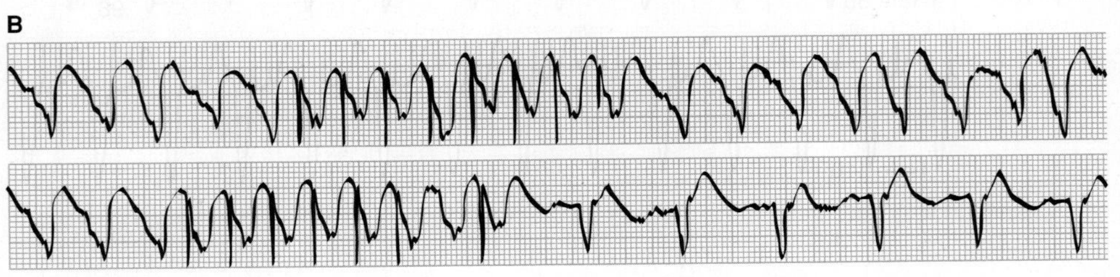

■ **Figure 28-28** Antitachycardia pacing. **(A)** Ventricular pacing is present for five beats and then VT begins. In the second strip, a burst of seven paced beats is delivered into the VT with successful termination. **(B)** Top strip show a burst of eight paced beats into VT, which was unsuccessful in terminating tachycardia. Bottom strip shows a second burst of eight paced beats which terminated the VT.

Ventricular Resynchronization

The use of AV sequential biventricular pacing (also called *atriobiventricular* pacing), in which both ventricles are paced simultaneously, can correct the electrical abnormalities that cause mechanical dysfunction and "resynchronize" ventricular contraction to improve LV function. Simultaneous electrical activation of the ventricles with biventricular pacing forces the septum to contract at the same time as the LV and reduces the adverse effects of paradoxical septal wall motion on stroke volume. Identifying the area of the LV with the most delayed mechanical contraction and then pacing close to that area improves LV intraventricular synchrony and reduces mitral regurgitation by normalizing LV contraction patterns.[29,30] Optimization of the AV interval with dual-chamber pacing improves mitral valve motion and facilitates ventricular filling by optimizing atrial kick. Newer biventricular devices offer a programmable V-V delay which allows the option for simultaneous pacing of both ventricles or for sequential pacing with one ventricle paced a few milliseconds before the other. Some studies suggest that sequential ventricular pacing further improves LV systolic and diastolic function; some patients do better with RV pacing slightly preceding LV pacing and others do better with LV pacing slightly preceding RV pacing (Fig. 28-29).[31,32]

Clinical trials have demonstrated the following beneficial outcomes of CRT, with and without ICD, in patients with advanced HF[6,7,33–36]:

1. Improved exercise capacity (6-minute walk test; peak respiratory O_2 uptake)
2. Improved quality of life (QOL)
3. Improved NYHA functional class (e.g., from NYHA class III to class II)
4. Decreased mitral regurgitation
5. Reduced hospitalizations for HF
6. Reverse ventricular remodeling (reduced end-diastolic pressure and volume)
7. Improved ejection fraction
8. Improvements in morbidity
9. Reduced all-cause mortality

CRT is recommended in patients with severe systolic HF who have LVEF ≤35%, QRS duration ≥0.12 seconds, sinus rhythm, NYHA class III or ambulatory class IV HF symptoms on optimal medical therapy.[1] CRT with biventricular pacing is accomplished by inserting a standard atrial pacing lead in the right atrium, a ventricular lead in the RV apex, and a lead threaded into the coronary sinus and down a posterior or lateral cardiac vein in the LV (see Fig. 28-5).

Evaluating Ventricular Capture in a Biventricular Pacemaker

Evaluating ventricular capture in a biventricular pacemaker is complicated and requires that the clinician be attuned to changes in the shape and width of the QRS complex as well as to changes in the QRS axis.[37] Because both ventricles are paced simultaneously, the paced QRS in biventricular pacing is often narrower than ordinary paced QRS complexes, although in some patients there is not much noticeable difference. The actual shape of the QRS complex during biventricular capture depends on the location of the RV pacing lead (RV apex vs. RV outflow tract) and the LV lead (lateral vs. posterior vein location). As capture is lost in one or the other ventricle, the QRS changes shape and becomes much wider because one ventricle depolarizes before the other.

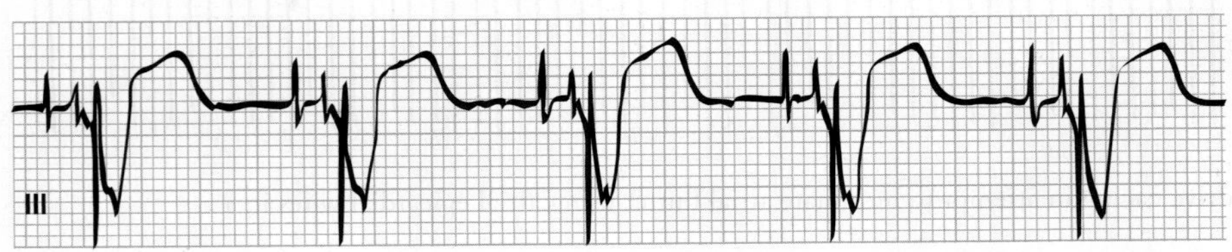

■ **Figure 28-29** Dual-chamber biventricular pacemaker with a V–V delay of about 80 milliseconds. Two ventricular pacing spikes can be seen: one pacing the RV and the other pacing the LV.

When capture is lost in both ventricles, the QRS resumes its prepaced shape and width, usually a pattern of LBBB.

Lead V_1 should logically be a good lead for evaluating ventricular capture in a biventricular pacemaker because of its ability to differentiate RV from LV activation (see discussion of bundle-branch block patterns in Chapter 15). Leads I and III or aVF are often used to evaluate the QRS axis. It is recommended that a total of four 12-lead ECGs should be recorded during implantation of a biventricular device: (1) QRS morphology during intrinsic conduction prior to any pacing, (2) paced QRS complexes during RV pacing alone, (3) paced QRS complexes during LV pacing alone, and (4) paced QRS complexes during biventricular capture.[37] The lead or leads that best show an obvious difference in QRS morphology among these four pacing states should be used as the continuous bedside monitoring lead(s) and during office follow-up visits for pacemaker evaluation.

If monitoring in lead V_1, which is the usual preferred bedside monitoring lead for arrhythmia detection, the following concepts should (but may not always) apply to evaluation of biventricular pacing:

1. Biventricular capture in lead V_1 usually presents with a mostly positive QRS that is often narrower than a paced QRS resulting from RV pacing alone when the RV lead is in the RV apex. Sometimes biventricular capture presents as a mostly negative QRS in V_1, especially if the RV lead is in the outflow tract.[37] The QRS frontal plane axis is usually in a superior direction, resulting in a negative QRS complex in the inferior leads (II, III, aVF). Figure 28-30 shows two examples of biventricular capture in lead V_1.
2. When capture is lost in the RV but is present in the LV, the QRS widens and becomes upright in V_1 (assumes an RBBB morphology) as LV capture causes the LV to depolarize first and the impulse to spread toward the right ventricle, resulting in an upright V_1. This also shifts the QRS axis to the right, resulting in a negative QRS complex in lead I and an upright complex in the inferior leads.
3. When capture is lost in the LV but present in the RV, the QRS widens and becomes negative in V_1 (assumes an LBBB morphology), and looks like an ordinary RV paced beat. The QRS axis shifts to the left; lead I becomes upright and the inferior leads are negative.

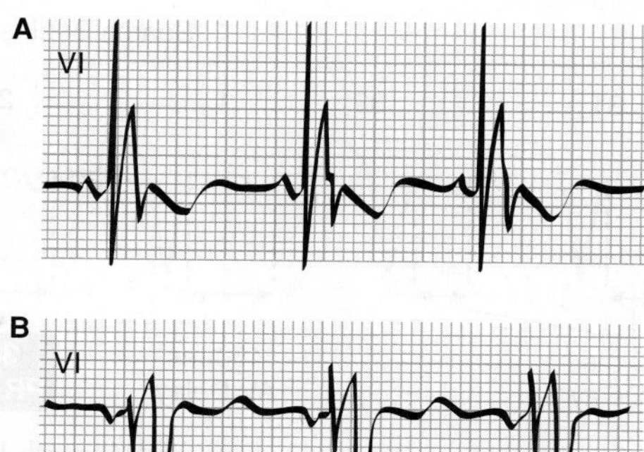

■ **Figure 28-30** Biventricular capture. **(A)** Lead V_1 showing a mostly upright paced complex with biventricular capture, common with RV lead in the RV apex. **(B)** Lead V_1 showing a predominantly negative paced complex, although somewhat narrower than a typical RV paced complex.

4. When capture is lost in both ventricles, the QRS resumes its prepaced shape and width, usually LBBB morphology with a QRS more than 120 milliseconds in width.

Further research is needed in this area to verify the accuracy of lead V_1 in biventricular pacemaker evaluation and to determine if other leads are helpful. Figure 28-31 is an example of loss of capture in a biventricular pacemaker.

Reducing Unnecessary RV Pacing. Pacing from the RV apex creates the same conduction abnormalities as LBBB and causes the same interventricular and intraventricular dysynchrony that occurs in LBBB. In addition, standard pacing from the RV apex increases the risk of HF and atrial fibrillation even in patients who do not have baseline LV dysfunction.[38–43] Atrial pacing and dual-chamber pacing both reduce the incidence of atrial fibrillation when compared to ventricular pacing alone; dual-chamber pacing has min-

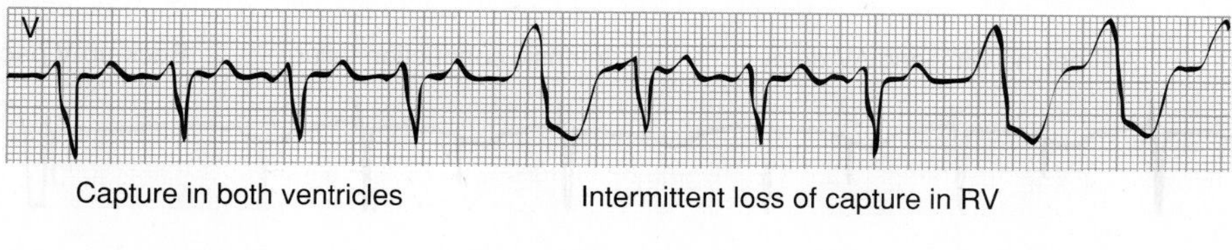

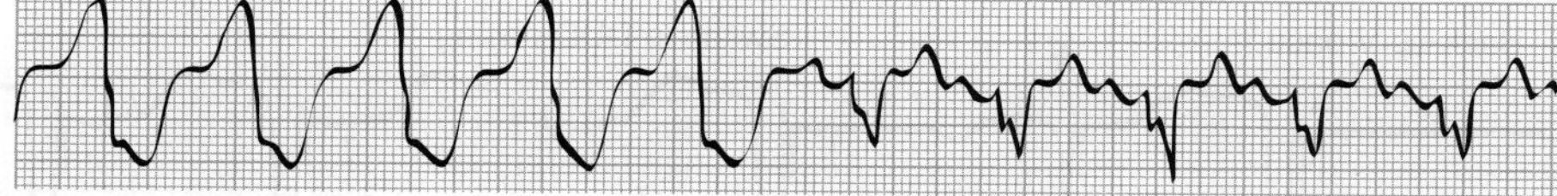

■ **Figure 28-31** Continuous strips showing loss of capture in one and then both ventricles in a biventricular pacemaker. The first half of the top strip illustrates biventricular capture. The second half of the top strip shows intermittent loss of capture in the RV, with a very wide RBBB morphology. The first half of the bottom strip continues to show loss of RV capture. The last half of the bottom strip shows loss of capture in both ventricles, with return to the patient's native LBBB morphology. (Modified from Medtronic [2001]. *Cardiac resynchronization therapy for heart failure management.* PowerPoint/Slide Presentation available from Medtronic, Minneapolis, MN or at www.medtronic.com.)

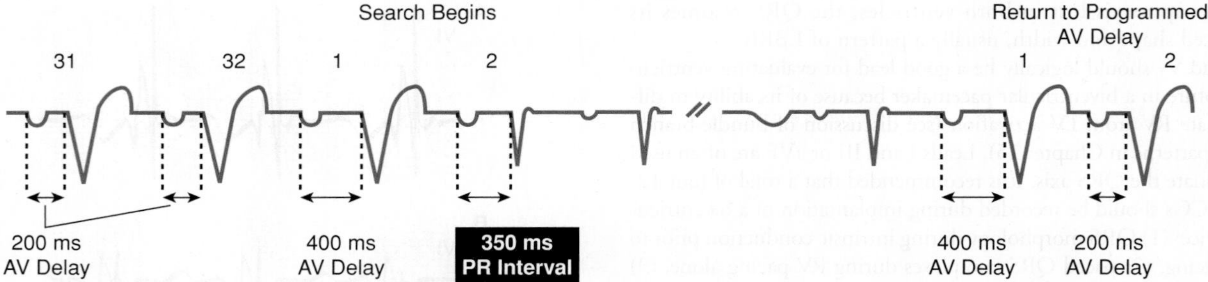

■ **Figure 28-32** Diagram of AV Search Hysteresis function. After 32 beats the AV delay extends to 400 milliseconds to encourage intrinsic conduction. On beat 2 intrinsic conduction occurs with a PR interval of 350 milliseconds; this will continue until intrinsic conduction fails. At the end of the strip, on beat 1 intrinsic conduction failed and a ventricular paced beat occurred at an AV delay of 400 milliseconds, returning the device to the programmed AV delay of 200 milliseconds. After another 32 beats the search will begin again. (From Boston Scientific brochure for Altrura Pacemaker, with permission.)

imal effect on HF and was associated with an increased risk of death and HF when compared to VVI pacing as a backup pacing mode in ICD patients.[40,44] A high percentage of ventricular pacing from the RV apex is thought to play a large role in the progression of HF by creating ventricular dysynchrony, and has been associated with increased risk of HF hospitalization and atrial fibrillation.[38,42,43] Although dual-chamber pacing maintains AV synchrony, which should improve ventricular function, it can also result in a high percentage of ventricular pacing because it paces the ventricle at the end of the AV delay in the absence of intrinsic AV conduction.

In the last few years, the recognition of the deleterious effects of RV pacing has led to efforts to reduce unnecessary RV pacing, including new pacing modes and functions to prevent RV pacing whenever possible. Some of these features to reduce ventricular pacing include AV search hysteresis (AVSH [Boston Scientific]), managed ventricular pacing (MVP [Medtronic]), and ventricular intrinsic preference (VIP [St. Jude]).

AV Search Hysteresis. AVSH is a feature of some dual-chamber pacemakers and ICDs that searches for the presence of intrinsic AV conduction by extending the AV delay by a programmable percentage in an effort to allow intrinsic conduction to occur rather than forcing RV pacing.[45,46] The device can be programmed to extend the AV delay every *x* cycles (*x* is a programmable number from 32 to 1024) to look for intrinsic AV conduction in the next eight cycles. If intrinsic conduction occurs during the search, the AV delay remains at the extended value and allows intrinsic conduction to continue until intrinsic conduction fails; then the device returns to its programmed AV delay until the next search begins. Figure 28-32 illustrates AVSH.

Managed Ventricular Pacing. MVP is a pacing mode in some dual-chamber pacemakers that paces the atrium only (AAI/R mode) while monitoring the ventricle for intrinsic conduction.[47] If intrinsic conduction fails (i.e. an atrial paced or sensed event that is not followed by an intrinsic QRS), a ventricular back-up pace occurs and AAI/R pacing continues. If loss of intrinsic conduction persists, the device switches from AAI/R to DDD/R for 1 minute. To test for return of intrinsic AV conduction, a ventricular pace is inhibited for one cycle; the conduction test is repeated at progressive time intervals (e.g. 1, 2, 4, 8, . . . minutes). If intrinsic conduction returns, the device switches back to AAI/R pacing with ventricular monitoring. Figure 28-33 is an example of MVP mode operation. VIP is a similar function in St. Jude devices.

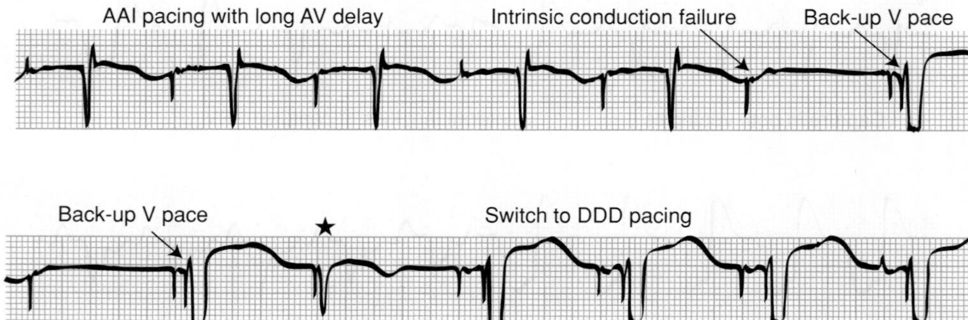

■ **Figure 28-33** MVP function. In the top strip the pacemaker is functioning in the AAI/R mode with a very long AV delay to allow intrinsic conduction with an A–R interval of 400 milliseconds. The sixth atrial pacing spike fails to conduct, triggering a backup ventricular pace at the end of the top strip. In the bottom strip, another backup ventricular pace occurs and the device switches to DDD pacing with a programmed AV delay of 160 milliseconds. DDD pacing will continue for a programmable number of minutes and then the AV delay will extend again to encourage intrinsic conduction. As long as intrinsic conduction is present the device will operate in AAI/R mode. The star beat appears to be a PVC that occurred right after the atrial pacing spike.

Potential Complications of Pacing

Pacemaker complications can be caused by implant-related problems or by malfunction of any part of the pacemaker system (e.g. lead problems or generator problems). The pacing lead must be in firm contact with the pulse generator for the system to work correctly. In a permanent pacing system, good contact between the lead connector pin and the pulse generator at the connector block of the pulse generator is dependent on a setscrew being tightened adequately during implantation; a loose setscrew can create problems with pacemaker output or sensing. In addition, normal pacemaker function can appear to be abnormal because of idiosyncrasies of specific devices or unusual programming, resulting in what appears to be abnormal pacing rates or changes in the AV interval.

Early complications of temporary or permanent pacemaker insertion are usually related to lead insertion and include pneumothorax or hemothorax, lead perforation (subclavian vein or myocardium), air embolus, and ventricular arrhythmias. Complications occurring later can include infection at the insertion site, endocarditis, hematoma formation, venous thrombosis, skin erosion over a permanent pulse generator, lead dislodgment or fracture, Twiddler syndrome, symptoms from pacemaker syndrome, and pacemaker failure.[23,48,49]

Pneumothorax can occur when the subclavian vein is used for lead insertion because the apex of the lung is located very near the subclavian vein, and lung injury is a possibility when accessing the vein. Pneumothorax may become manifest immediately or as long as 48 hours after implantation. Clinical signs of pneumothorax can include respiratory distress, absence of lung sounds on the affected side, chest pain, hypotension, elevated neck veins, and hypoxia.

Lead perforation may be asymptomatic or it can lead to cardiac tamponade if there is rapid accumulation of blood in the pericardium secondary to perforation of the RV wall. If the pacing lead perforates the septum and enters the LV, the ECG may show an RBBB pattern rather than the usual LBBB pattern that results from pacing the RV apex. Intercostal muscle or diaphragmatic stimulation by a perforated lead can cause hiccups or muscle twitching in the chest wall. The presence of a friction rub after implantation can indicate pericarditis or pericardial effusion caused by lead perforation.

Ventricular arrhythmias, either PVCs or runs of VT, can result from irritation of the ventricle by the pacing lead. PVCs that are caused by pacing lead irritation have the same morphology as paced beats because they originate from the same spot. Lead-induced arrhythmias most often occur within 24 to 48 hours of lead placement and usually resolve spontaneously.

Pacemaker system infection can involve just the pacemaker pocket or the entire generator and lead system and can occur early or late after implant. The use of prophylactic antibiotics and irrigation of the pacemaker pocket with antibiotics at the time of implant can reduce the incidence of infection. Infections involving the lead system can lead to endocarditis and usually require removal of the entire pacing system until the infection is resolved. Because patients are discharged so soon after implantation, they need to be taught to look for and report signs of infection: redness, swelling, or weeping of fluid from the pacemaker pocket; erosion of the pacemaker; and fever that is not related to the flu or other identifiable illness.

Twiddler syndrome is manipulation of a permanent pulse generator within its pocket by the patient. This can lead to rotation of the pacemaker and twisting of the leads, which can result in lead fracture or dislodgment. Patients should be cautioned to keep their hands away from the pacemaker pocket and to avoid manipulating the pulse generator.

Pacemaker syndrome refers to a constellation of symptoms resulting from inadequate timing of atrial–ventricular contraction. Symptoms include fatigue, jugular venous distention and pulsations in the neck, weakness, dizziness or near-syncope, hypotension, HF, and pounding in the chest. Symptoms may occur during periods of VVI pacing because of loss of AV synchrony or when retrograde conduction to the atria occurs, causing the atria to contract against closed AV valves. Contraction of the atria at a time when the AV valves are closed can activate stretch receptors in the atrial wall and pulmonary veins, resulting in a reflex vasodilation that causes hypotension and dizziness. The loss of AV synchrony causes loss of atrial contribution to ventricular filling and may be another cause of symptoms.

IMPLANTABLE CARDIOVERTER DEFIBRILLATORS

An implantable cardioverter defibrillator (ICD) is a battery powered electrical impulse generator that continuously monitors the heart rhythm and delivers either a life-saving shock or burst of rapid pacing to terminate a ventricular arrhythmia and restore normal rhythm. ICDs have been proven to prolong survival in patients who are receiving the device for treatment of ventricular arrhythmias, or receiving the ICD for primary prevention of sudden cardiac death. Two landmark studies the Multicenter Automatic Defibrillator Implantation Trial (MADIT II)[50] and the Sudden Cardiac Death in HF Trial (SCD-HeFT)[51] both demonstrated that patients with heart disease and decreased LV function could benefit from an ICD. The ICD provides safe and effective therapy for ventricular arrhythmias. The number of ICD implants have increased exponentially since first implanted in 1980. Technological advances have improved the function of the implantable defibrillator. Given the increasing numbers of patients with ICDs the goal of the chapter is to provide an understanding of the function of an ICD, appropriate ICD therapy, potential complications, and appropriate follow-up management.

Development

The implantable defibrillator was the brainstorm of Dr. Michel Mirowski. In the late 1960s, Mirowski conceived the idea of an automatic implantable defibrillator after a close friend died from repeated episodes of ventricular arrhythmias. The first experimental model was tested successfully in 1969, and after many years and much refining, the ICD was first implanted in humans in 1980.[52] The device was experimental until 1985 when it gained full U.S. Food and Drug Administration approval. The first generation devices were large (weighing 250 g and occupying a volume of 145 mL), requiring implantation in a subcutaneous abdominal pocket.

The earliest ICD systems required a thoracotomy approach. Patch electrodes were sutured to the pericardium over the apex of the heart, and either epicardial screw-in leads or an endocardial lead was placed for rate sensing and pacing. The leads were then tunneled to the pulse generator in the abdominal pocket.[53]

The first ICD was a nonprogrammable, shock-only device intended to treat VF. Once the device detected the arrhythmia and was completely charged the ICD was committed to deliver a shock. This first ICD was quickly modified to a second-generation device that had cardioversion capabilities.[54,55] The current

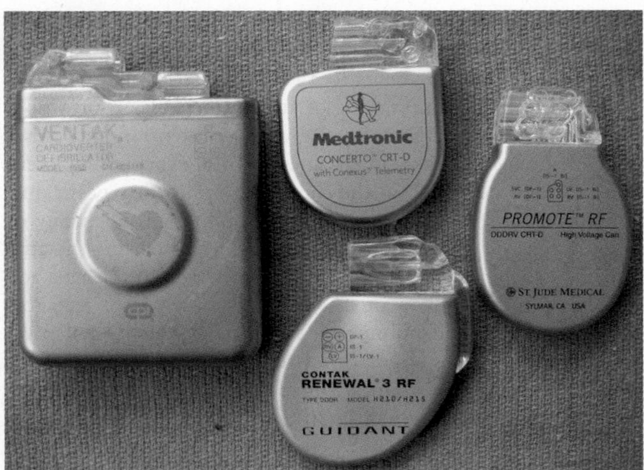

■ **Figure 28-34** ICDs showing the evolution in size. The largest one was the first-generation ICD that was implanted in the abdomen; the other three are current biventricular ICDs.

generations of defibrillators have evolved into a smaller, sophisticated device, much like a pacemaker (Fig. 28-34). Lead technology and the use of biphasic waveforms have made transvenous, nonthoracotomy systems the standard, eliminating the need for open-heart surgery. ICDs can deliver either high-energy or low-energy shocks, demand and rate-responsive pacing, antitachycardic pacing (ATP), and noninvasive electrical stimulation for electrophysiology studies (EPS). Extensive programmability and diagnostic data are characteristic of modern ICDs. Diagnostic data available include arrhythmia history, fluid level index, and heart rate variability all of which helps manage the cardiac patient.[55]

Indications for Use

Guidelines for ICD implantation are based on recommendations from a panel of experts who thoroughly review current scientific evidence with the intention to improve patient care. The American College of Cardiology Foundation (ACCF) and the American Heart Association (AHA) have jointly established guidelines since 1980. At the time of this writing, the most recent guidelines for management of patients with ventricular arrhythmias and prevention of SCD was published in 2006 by the ACC/AHA task force in conjunction with the European Society of Cardiology.[56] The current recommendations for ICD therapy to be considered include: (1) primary prevention for those patients who are at risk, but have not yet experienced a life-threatening arrhythmias or sudden cardiac "death" episode, or for secondary prevention when a patient has already experienced VT or VF; (2) for specific etiology of arrhythmia substrate; (3) the functional status of the patient; and (4) reduced LV ejection fraction. Classifications of recommendations are between classes I and III. Class I indication means that evidence supports an ICD to be beneficial, useful, and effective. Class II indicates there is conflicting evidence about usefulness/efficacy for an ICD. Class II is broken-down further: class IIa indicates weight of evidence in favor of ICD and class IIb indicates evidence is less established for ICD implantation. Class III indication means there is evidence to suggest the ICD would *not be* useful and in some cases may be harmful. The indications are then given level A, B, and C rankings. Level A indicates that data were derived from multiple, randomized clinical trials. Level B indicates data were derived from a single randomized trial or from well-designed, nonrandomized studies. Level C indicates that the consensus opinion of experts, or from case studies was the primary source of the recommendation.[56]

The rapid evolution of ICD technology, with the results of studies documenting efficacy of the ICD over antiarrhythmic drugs in both secondary and primary prevention of SCD, has led to the expansion of indications for the ICD.[55–57] Patients who receive an ICD usually fall into one of four categories: cardiac arrest survivors, those with spontaneous sustained VT, those with syncope of unknown origin with inducible VT/VF per electrophysiologic testing, and patients at high risk for future life-threatening arrhythmic events (see Display 28-4).

Sudden Cardiac Death Survivors

Ventricular arrhythmias are the cause of most sudden cardiac arrests.[58,59] Survivors of cardiac arrest, in the absence of acute MI, are at risk for a future event. Cobb et al.[60] report a 36% 1-year mortality rate in untreated patients who were successfully resuscitated, hospitalized, and discharged home. Follow-up data on ICD patients have shown that 42% to 60% of them have received ICD discharges for VT or VF in a follow-up period of 2 to 3 years.[61] Three landmark trials have shown the benefit of ICD therapy for the prevention of SCD in those patients who have experienced a cardiac arrest or have had documented hemodynamically significant VT. The Antiarrhythmics Versus Implantable Defibrillator (AVID) trial,[62] the Cardiac Arrest Study Hamburg (CASH),[63] and the Canadian Implantable Defibrillator Study (CIDS)[64] all established the benefit of ICD therapy as the first-line treatment option for patients with life-threatening arrhythmias. Before these studies, the ICD was used as a therapy option only for patients who continued to have life-threatening arrhythmias in combination with antiarrhythmic drug therapy. ICD therapy when compared with traditional antiarrhythmic drug therapy has been associated with mortality reductions between 23% and 54%; the improvement was due to reduction in sudden cardiac death.[55,56]

Sustained Ventricular Tachycardia

The ICD is also the first-line therapy in patients with spontaneous sustained monomorphic VT and structural heart disease. In patients without structural heart disease, the ICD is also a therapy option when alternative options have failed.[56] Patients with VT and an ICD may have other treatment options combined with ICD therapy, which include: (1) antiarrhythmic drug therapy to decrease ICD discharges, (2) surgical aneurysmectomy when a ventricular aneurysm is the substrate for VT, (3) radiofrequency catheter ablation of the VT foci, and (4) combination of antiarrhythmic drugs and radiofrequency catheter ablation.[56,65]

Therapy options with current ICDs are very beneficial in the VT patient. The ATP mode delivers an effective therapy in terminating monomorphic VT. ATP is not only effective but is painless; usually ATP is imperceptible to the patient. With ATP, the patient

(*text continues on page 686*)

DISPLAY 28-4 2006 Indications for Implantable Cardioverter-Defibrillator Therapy—ACC/AHA/ESC Practice Guidelines

Recommendations include chronic optimal medical therapy, and reasonable expectation of survival with good functional status for more than 1 year in all patients receiving ICDs.

	Class I	Class IIa	Class IIb	Class III
Level A **Data received from multiple clinical trials or meta-analyses**	Benefit > risk ICD implant should be performed for the following patients: 1. VF survivors if coronary revascularization cannot be carried out. 2. Primary prevention patients at least 40 days post-MI—with EF 30% to 40% and NYHA class II or III. 3. Patients with LV dysfunction due to prior MI who presents with VT. 4. Patients with nonischemic DCM and sustained VT/VF. 6. Patients who have survived SCD for secondary prevention of VF/VT. 7. Patients with long QT intervals and previous cardiac arrest. (ICD plus β-blocker)	Benefit > risk It is reasonable to perform ICD implant for the following patients: 1. Primary prevention for patients with HCM with one or more risk factors for sudden cardiac death. (Chapter 30, HCM).	Benefit ≥ risk ICD implant may be considered.	Risk ≥ benefit ICD implant should not be performed.
Level B **Data received from a single randomized trial or non-randomized studies**	1. Primary prevention for patients with nonischemic DCM who have EF <30% to 35%, who are NYHA class II or III. 2. Patients with congenital heart disease who have survived a cardiac arrest. 3. Patients with HCM who have sustained VT/VF. 4. Patients with arrhythmogenic RV cardiomyopathy with documented VT/VF. 5. Syncope of unknown cause with induced VT/VF at EP study.	1. Primary prevention patients at least 40 days post-MI—with EF 30% to 35% and NYHA class I. 2. Patients with congenital heart disease, unexplained syncope, and impaired LV function. 3. Patients that have QRS complex of at least 120 ms, and are NYHA functional class III or IV when combined with biventricular pacing. 4. Patients with long QT intervals experiencing syncope and/or VT while receiving β-blocker.	1. Primary prevention for patients identified with a genetic subtype such as LQT2, and LQT3 (ICD in combination with β-blockers).	
Level C **Only consensus opinion of experts, case studies, or standard of care**	1. Patients with congenital heart disease and VT not treated with catheter ablation or surgical resection. 2. Patients with infiltrative cardiomyopathy. 3. Patients with endocrine disorders who have persistent life-threatening VT/VF. 4. Patients with end-stage renal failure that has life-threatening VT/VF. 5. Patients with Brugada syndrome with previous cardiac arrest.	1. Patients post-MI with normal or near normal EF having recurrent sustained VT. 2. Patients with recurrent VT, normal or near normal LVEF and optimally treated heart failure. 3. Patients with unexplained syncope, decreased LV function, and nonischemic cardiomyopathy—with optimal medial treatment. 4. Patients with VT/VF who are not in acute phase of myocarditis. 5. Patients with HCM with one or more major risk factor.	1. Primary prevention in patients with nonischemic DCM, who have LVEF of less than or equal to 30% to 35% , who are NYHA functional class I.	1. Elderly Patients with projected life expectancy less than 1 year due to major comorbidities should not receive ICD. 2. Terminal illness with life expectancy less than one year.

(display continued on page 686)

DISPLAY 28-4 2006 Indications for Implantable Cardioverter-Defibrillator Therapy—ACC/AHA/ESC Practice Guidelines (continued)

Class I	Class IIa	Class IIb	Class III
6. Patients with catecholaminergic polymorphic VT with previous cardiac arrest.	6. Patients with arrhythmogenic RV cardiomyopathy. 7. Patients with Brugada syndrome and documented VT or Syncope—no prior cardiac arrest. 8. Patients with catecholaminergic polymorphic VT with syncope. 9. Patients with sustained VT(stable) with normal or near normal LV function and no structural heart disease.		3. Incessant VT/VF.

has fewer shocks, which is important as ICD shocks are painful and have been associated with significant anxiety, reduced QOL, and depression.[66,67] If ATP should fail, subsequent therapies do include shocks.

Syncope of Unknown Origin

Syncope in the setting of structural heart disease and inducible VT per electrophysiologic testing carries a high risk of SCD. Bass et al.[68] reported a sudden death rate of 48% at 3 years in patients with syncope of unknown origin and inducible sustained VT, compared with only 9% in patients with a negative EP study. Syncope with induced VT/VF is considered a class I indication for an ICD. Syncope in patients with structural heart disease in which all invasive and noninvasive examinations have failed to define a cause is likely to have an arrhythmic event. These events include syncope of unexplained cause, family history of sudden death, long QT interval and syncope in association with Brugada syndrome (RBBB and ST segment elevation).[56]

High-Risk Patients

Prophylactic ICD implantation is now justified in patients who are considered at high risk but have never had a spontaneous episode of sustained VT or VF. The goal is to prevent sudden death in the patient with LV ejection fraction of less than or equal to 30% and with history of MI (1 month after acute MI and 3 months after coronary artery revascularization surgery). The first randomized study to report primary prevention of SCD with direct comparison between the ICD and antiarrhythmic drugs was the MADIT. MADIT was designed as a prophylactic trial to determine if patients with coronary heart disease, LV dysfunction, and inducible VT, per electrophysiological testing, would have a better survival rate than those patients who were treated with conventional medical therapy. MADIT established that the incidence of cardiac arrest and total mortality were markedly reduced in the group of patients who received an ICD. The study was actually stopped early on advice of the Data and Safety Monitoring Board because the patients randomized to the ICD arm were found to have a 54% reduction in all-cause mortality compared with the patients receiving conventional therapy.[69]

Given the results of MADIT, Moss et al. reasoned that patients with previous history of MI and advanced LV dysfunction had substrate for life-threatening cardiac arrhythmias and would benefit from a prophylactic ICD without electrophysiological testing to confirm inducible VT. MADIT II, a randomized, controlled, clinical trial was designed to evaluate the benefit of the ICD in patients with a previous MI and an LV ejection fraction of 30% or less. The study began in 1997 and was stopped in November of 2001. Analysis revealed a 31% reduction in the risk of all-cause mortality in heart attack survivors due to ICDs.[50]

The SCD-HeFT was a randomized control trial that enrolled patients with either ischemic or nonischemic cardiomyopathy with LVEF less than or equal to 35%. The patients were evenly placed in three groups: conventional medial therapy plus placebo, conventional medical therapy plus amiodarone, and conventional medical therapy plus ICD. ICD therapy as compared with placebo was associated with 23% reduction in the risk of all-cause mortality.[51]

The Defibrillators in Nonischemic Cardiomyopathy Treatment Evaluation Trial (DEFINITE) enrolled patients with nonischemic dilated cardiomyopathy, EF <35%, with NYHA classes I and III HF. The patients were randomized to receive best medical therapy, with or without an ICD. The findings showed a trend toward reduced mortality in the ICD group (Display 28-5).[70]

These studies have expanded ICD indications for the patient with previous MI and advanced LV dysfunction, as well as those patients with nonischemic cardiomyopathy who definitely benefit from ICD therapy before sustaining a sudden cardiac arrest. Other groups of patients may also benefit from prophylactic ICD therapy. Those patients with idiopathic dilated cardiomyopathy, hypertrophic cardiomyopathy, long QT syndrome, Brugada

DISPLAY 28-5 Secondary and Primary Prevention Trials of Sudden Cardiac Death

Study	Randomization	Population	Main Finding
Secondary Prevention			
AVID[62] (n = 1016) 1997	Antiarrhythmic medications 97% amiodarone, 3% sotalol vs. ICD	Survived VT/VF SCA VT with syncope; VT with LVEF ≤40%	Reduction in total mortality with ICD, HR, 0.66; 95% CI
CIDS[64] (n = 659) 2000	Amiodarone vs. ICD	Survived VT/VF SCA; VT with syncope LVEF ≤35% and CL ≤400 ms (HR, 150)	Reduction in death from any cause with ICD therapy, HR, 0.85; 95% CI
CASH[63] (n = 288) 200	Antiarrhythmic medications propafenone (withdrawn)	Survived VT/VF SCA	Reduction in total mortality with ICD. HR, 0.82; 95% CI
Primary Prevention			
MADIT I[69] (n = 196) 1996	Antiarrhythmic therapy (74% amiodarone) vs. ICD	Prior MI; LVEF ≤35% asymptomatic NSVT; NYHA I-III; inducible VT refractory to procainamide on EPS	Reduction in total mortality with ICD 54% HR, 0.46; 95% CI
MADIT II[50] (n = 1232) 2002	Conventional therapy vs. ICD	Prior MI; LVEF ≤30%	Reduction in total mortality with ICD therapy 31%; HR, 0.69; 95% CI
DEFINITE[70] (n = 458) 2004	Conventional therapy vs. ICD	Nonischemic CM heart failure patients; NYHA classes I to III; EF <36% PVCs or NSVT	Trend in reduction in all cause mortality by 35%; HR, 0.65
DINAMIT[71] (n = 674) 2004	Acute MI patients, optimal therapy; with or without ICD	Acute MI 6 to 40 days; LVEF 35%; impaired Autonomic function	No difference seen in mortality at 2.5 years follow-up, HR, 1.08
SCD-HeFT[51] (n = 1676)	Conventional therapy vs. amiodarone vs. ICD	NYHA class II/III CHF ischemic and nonischemic LVEF ≤35%	Overall reduction in mortality with ICD 23%; HR, 0.77; 97.5 % CI

AVID, Antiarrhythmics Versus Implantable Defibrillators; CASH, Cardiac Arrest Study Hamburg; CI, confidence interval; CIDS, Canadian Implantable Defibrillator Study; DEFINITE, Defibrillators in Nonischemic Cardiomyopathy Treatment Evaluation; DINAMIT, Defibrillator in Acute Myocardial Infarction; HR, hazard ratio; MADIT I and II, Multicenter Automatic Defibrillator Trial; SCD-HeFT, Sudden Cardiac Death in Heart Failure Trial.

syndrome, and arrhythmogenic RV dysplasia have been shown to have better survival rates when treated with an ICD.[55–57]

Functional Characteristics

The ICD system consists of a pulse generator and defibrillation lead electrodes for arrhythmia detection and therapy delivery. ICD systems are implanted transvenously, like pacemakers, and no longer require cardiac surgery. However, devices that use defibrillation patches on the ventricle are still in use, and if these leads are still functional at the time of generator change for depleted battery, the original leads may be retained and used. In most ICD systems, the implanted pulse generator serves as part of the electrical pathway. The electrical current travels from the shocking coil on the RV lead to the ICD generator (Fig. 28-35).[55,72] In addition to internal defibrillation, today's ICD can provide all of the following: synchronized cardioversion, ATP, VVI, DDDR, and CRT pacing, telemetry, episode history logs, electrograms, activity levels, and transthoracic impedance reports. An example of cardiac heart failure diagnostics is shown in Figure 28-36. Defibrillators that provide CRT (CRT-D) (Fig. 28-37) are the newest type of defibrillators (Display 28-6).

The pulse generator is essentially a self-powered computer in a hermetically sealed titanium can. The operational circuitry consists of a battery, sense amplifier, control circuits (microprocessors, logic, and memory), high-voltage charging circuits, defibrillation

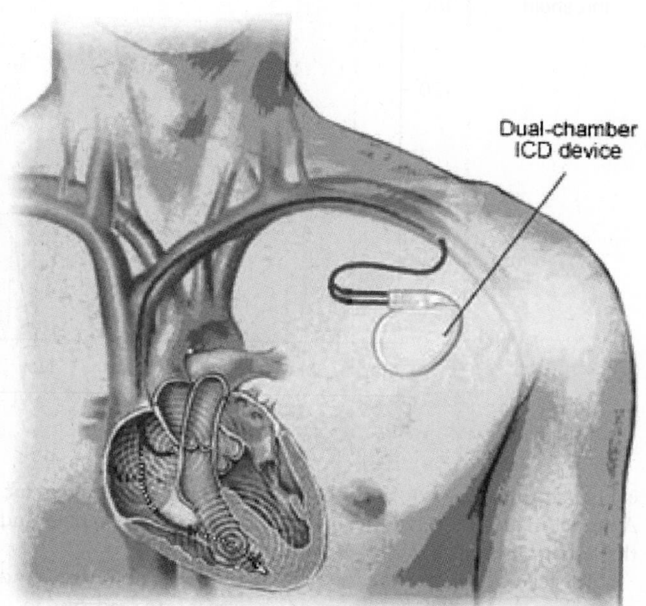

■ **Figure 28-35** Diagram from Guidant-Boston Scientific; showing current vectors from the shocking coils on the RV lead to the ICD. Reprinted with permission from Boston Scientific Corporation.

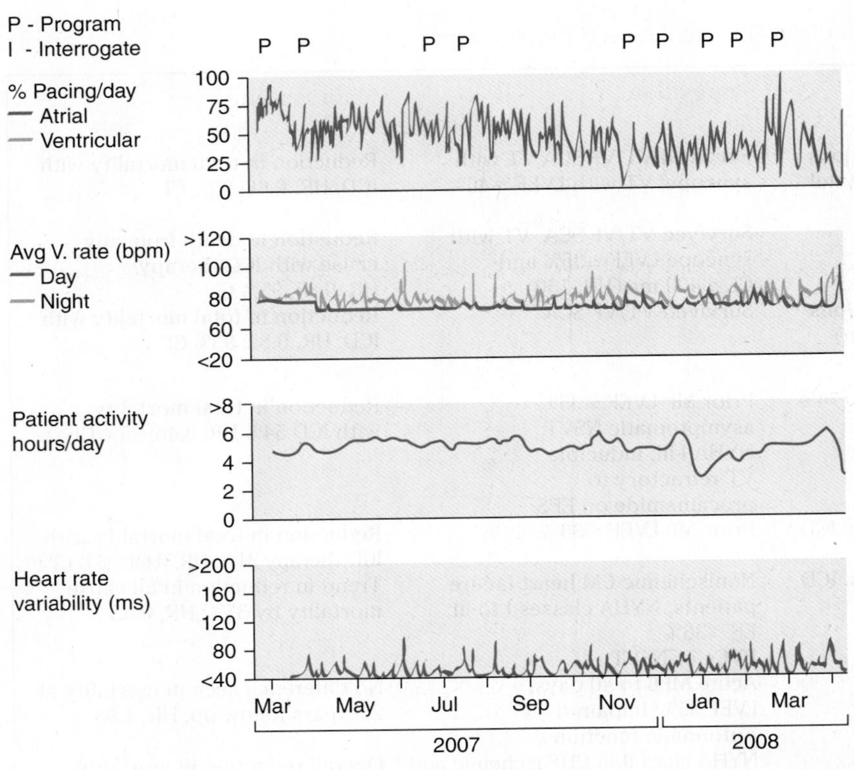

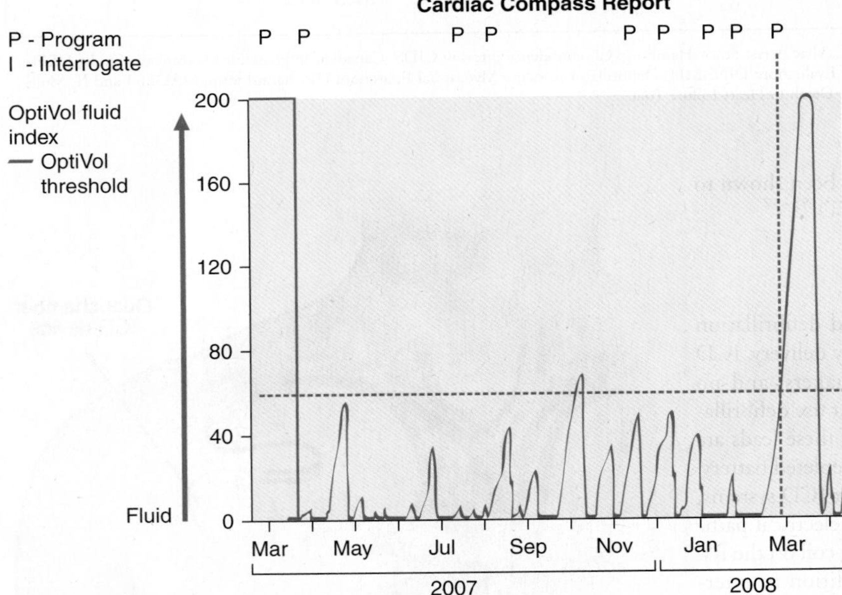

■ **Figure 28-36** Printout of Medtronic's Cardiac Compass report from an InSync Sentry 7299. The CRT-D monitors heart rate, activity level, heart rate variability, and fluid volumes. This data assists in managing the heart failure patient.

energy-storing capacitor, and a high-voltage output switch circuit. A header made of epoxy is the interface between the generator and the leads (Display 28-7).[72]

The lead system connects the generator to the heart. Lead technology has markedly improved; however, the lead system is the most vulnerable aspect of the ICD system and the most frequent cause of system failure. Long-term lead failure rate has been noted to be as high as 20% in 10-year-old leads. ICD lead failure may result in the ICD not properly sensing and delivering therapy resulting in syncope or sudden death. Lead failure may also cause the ICD to sense lead noise, causing inappropriate shocks, and subsequent psychological distress.[75]

ICD leads are now smaller, are steroid eluting to help achieve lower pacing thresholds, and provide better sensing, which is a critical function of the ICD.[76,77] When a single-chamber ICD is placed, only one lead is required and it is placed into the right ventricle in the same manner as a pacemaker lead. The ventricular lead has sensing and pacing

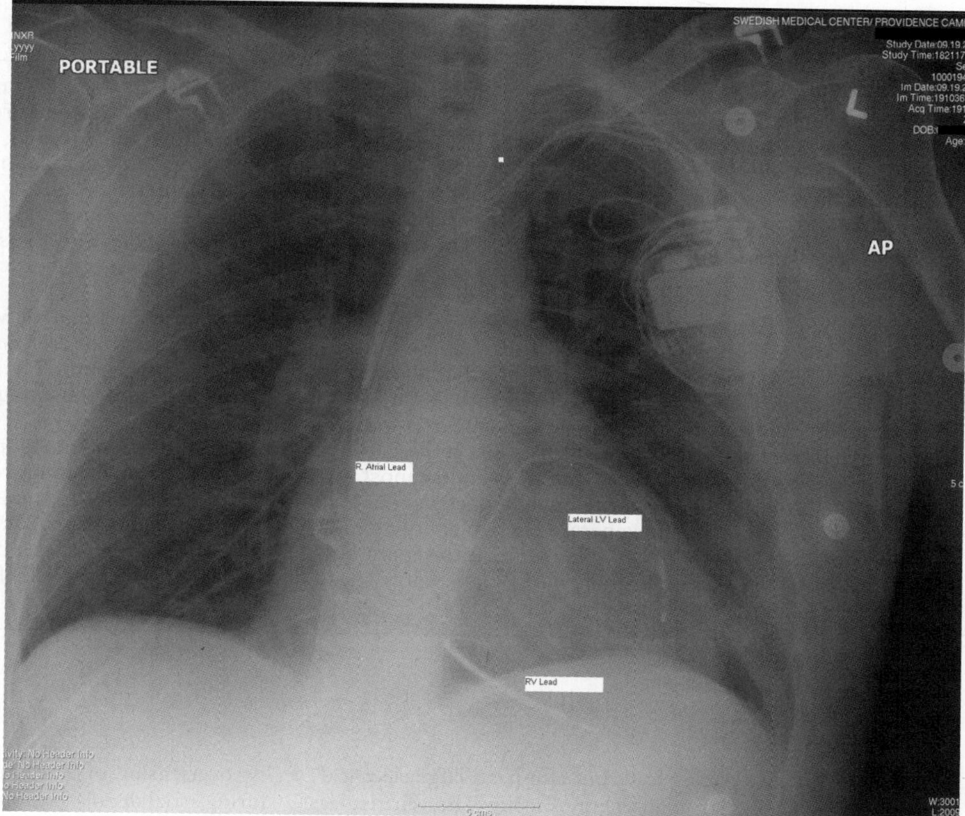

■ **Figure 28-37** X-ray film showing lead placement for cardiac resynchronization device. Three leads are placed into the heart; right atrial lead, right ventricular lead, and left ventricular lead.

DISPLAY 28-6 The Newest ICD—Cardiac Resynchronization Therapy-Defibrillators (CRT-D)

CRT is a term used to describe biventricular pacing. Biventricular pacing is used to improve mechanical efficiency of the heart. When both the left and right side of the heart are paced simultaneously contraction of the ventricles become coordinated overcoming the inefficiency associated with large conduction delays, particularly left bundle-branch block (LBBB). When LBBB is present there is a delay in the electrical conduction. This effects the mechanical action of the left ventricle and impairs systolic and diastolic function. At this time CRT devices are indicated in class III and IV heart failure patients, with a QRS interval >120 ms. Since left ventricular (LV) function and heart failure are predictors of sudden cardiac death the combination of CRT with implantable defibrillators provide additional benefit.

The most common lead placement for CRT-D devices is a right atrial lead, a coronary sinus pacing lead inserted into a distal coronary sinus tributary, which supplies the LV free wall, and a standard right ventricular ICD lead (Fig. 28-37) CRT involves sensing or pacing the right atrium followed by simultaneous pacing of the right and left ventricle. CRT-D devices combine all the pacing therapies of standard biventricular pacemakers with all the standard defibrillator therapies into one device.

The first controlled randomized study that clearly demonstrated improvement with heart failure patients was the Multicenter InSync Randomized Clinical Evaluation Trial (MIRACLE).[6] When patients received biventricular pacing there were significant improvements in all three primary endpoints: the 6-minute walk, New York Heart Association class (NYHA), and quality of life. Beneficial remodeling of the heart was also seen. LV size decreased and there was an increase in LV ejection fraction.

The Comparison of Medical Therapy, Pacing, and Defibrillation in Chronic Heart Failure (Companion Trial) enrolled patients with advanced heart failure, NYHA classes III and IV, LVEF less than or equal to 35%, QRS interval >120 ms, and PR interval >150 ms. The patients were enrolled in one of three groups: optimal medial therapy (OPT), OPT with cardiac resynchronization with pacing only (CRT-P) and OPT with cardiac resynchronization with defibrillation therapy (CDT-D). Risk of hospitalization or death from heart failure was reduced by 40% in the CRT-D group, and by 34% in the CRT-P group. All cause mortality was reduced by 36% in the CRT-D group when compared to optimal medical therapy.[34]

DISPLAY 28-7 The Makings of an ICD

Leads: Leads are insulated wires made from either silicone rubber or polyurethane, they connect the ICD to the patient's heart. There are five major components to a lead: (1) the electrode(s), (2) the conductor(s), (3) insulation, (4) connector pins, and (5) the fixation mechanism. The ICD system can have up to three leads placed, dependent on the system.
Casing: The casing, or outer shell of the ICD is made from titanium. Titanium is biocompatible, and highly resistant to penetration by body fluids. Titanium is stronger than steel, but up to 45% lighter.
Header: The top portion of the ICD is called the header; it is made of a see-through epoxy. The header has ports, which the connector pins of the lead(s) are inserted. The lead is secured into the header with the setscrew.
Setscrews: The leads are connected securely to the ICD with a small screw to ensure electrical contact between the lead and the ICD. At implant, a small sterile screwdriver is packaged with the ICD.
Circuitry: The ICD contains complex microelectronics (very small computer chips) that allows the ICD to process incoming signals, store information, and produce a response dependent on the signals that are processed. The microprocessors can respond to programming instructions that allow for changes after implantation. The circuits contain both read only memory (ROM) and random access memory (RAM). Just as in new computers, the amount of RAM in new ICDs is increasing rapidly, allowing for increased diagnostic information to be stored.
Battery: The internal power source for the ICD is the battery. Most ICD batteries are made from lithium silver vanadium oxide. The battery longevity is close to 5 years for most ICDs. Battery depletion is monitored regularly at follow-up visits. Once the battery reaches the elective replacement indicator (ERI), the entire ICD is replaced, not just the battery.
Capacitors: The ICD is able to generate enough energy to deliver a shock because the capacitors store an electrical charge. The capacitor is made of multiple conductors separated by insulators. Capacitors with high-voltage capabilities can charge up to 830 V in order to deliver a high-energy shock. It can take up to 15 seconds for the device to fully charge to the highest energy level, usually around 35 J.[73,74]

capabilities similar to pacing leads but also has a large electrical surface area for delivering high-energy shocks. The ventricular lead is usually a dual coil lead. When the lead is placed in the heart, the proximal coil is positioned at the level of the superior vena cava and the distal coil is positioned in the right ventricle. The defibrillation pathway that is used with most ICD implants today involves the titanium case of the pulse generator as the current flows from the distal defibrillation coil simultaneously to the ICD and the proximal coil. The generator is often referred to as an "active can" or "hot can." Using the generator to complete the defibrillation circuit has helped lower defibrillation thresholds known as defibrillation threshold testings (DFTs).[57,72] Early ICDs delivered shocks with a monophasic waveform, which was a single pulse at a given polarity and duration. Today's ICDs deliver shocks with a biphasic waveform. A biphasic shock has a negative and positive pulse, which lowered DFTs significantly. Lower thresholds result in higher rates of successful defibrillation, a higher margin of safety, and prolonged battery life.[78]

If a dual-chamber ICD is placed, a second lead is placed in the atrium. A dual-chamber system may be preferable in patients with a history of atrial fibrillation, for discrimination of arrhythmias. If the patient requires CRT therapy, a third lead is placed into the coronary sinus, which would then allow biventricular pacing (Fig. 28-38).

Sensing and Detection Enhancements

Recognizing ventricular arrhythmias is essential for the ICD; it is the *sensing* that measures the intracardiac electrograms signal from the lead electrodes. The sensing electrodes transmit each ventricular depolarization (R-wave) signal to the sense amplifier of the ICD. The main challenge for the sensing system is two fold. It must detect the very low amplitudes of VF while avoiding oversensing of T waves during repolarization and P waves during atrial depolarization. Other incoming signals that can be sensed include low-frequency noise, skeletal myopotentials, and EMI. ICD systems have either an automatic gain control or an auto-adjusting threshold feature that helps with proper sensing.[54,72]

The ICD primarily *detects* arrhythmias by looking at the cycle length, which is the time between R waves produced by ventricular depolarization. The cycle length represents the heart rate. The ICD can also be programmed to look at signal morphology, which helps in arrhythmia detection.[72] For the VF zone; ICD devices use rate criteria as the sole detection method. The use of rate criteria results in maximal sensitivity. The ICD charges the capacitor once the programmed amount of intervals is met (e.g. 8 to 12 intervals of a rate of 180 bpm). The ICD then delivers the shock after reconfirming the rate. If rate criteria are not met, the shock is aborted. The reconfirmation prevents unnecessary shocks for nonsustained events.

A VT zone can also be programmed into the ICD. Once again, rate is the primary detection method, but other detection enhancements can be programmed to increase specificity of VT detection, thus decreasing inappropriate shocks for supraventricular tachycardia and atrial fibrillation. One of the pitfalls of ICD detection is inappropriate shocks delivered for supraventricular arrhythmias. These optional detection features include sudden-onset criterion, an R-R interval stability criterion, an electrogram width criterion, and sustained rate duration. Dual-chambered pacemaker defibrillators also use atrial rate data (Fig. 28-39) and compare the atrial versus ventricular rate to help deliver appropriate therapy.[54] When VT episodes were reviewed in a dual-chamber ICD, the ventricular rate was noted to be faster than the atrial rate 80% of the time in most studies. ICDs either directly or indirectly compare atrial and ventricular rate as a first step in distinguishing SVT from VT.[79]

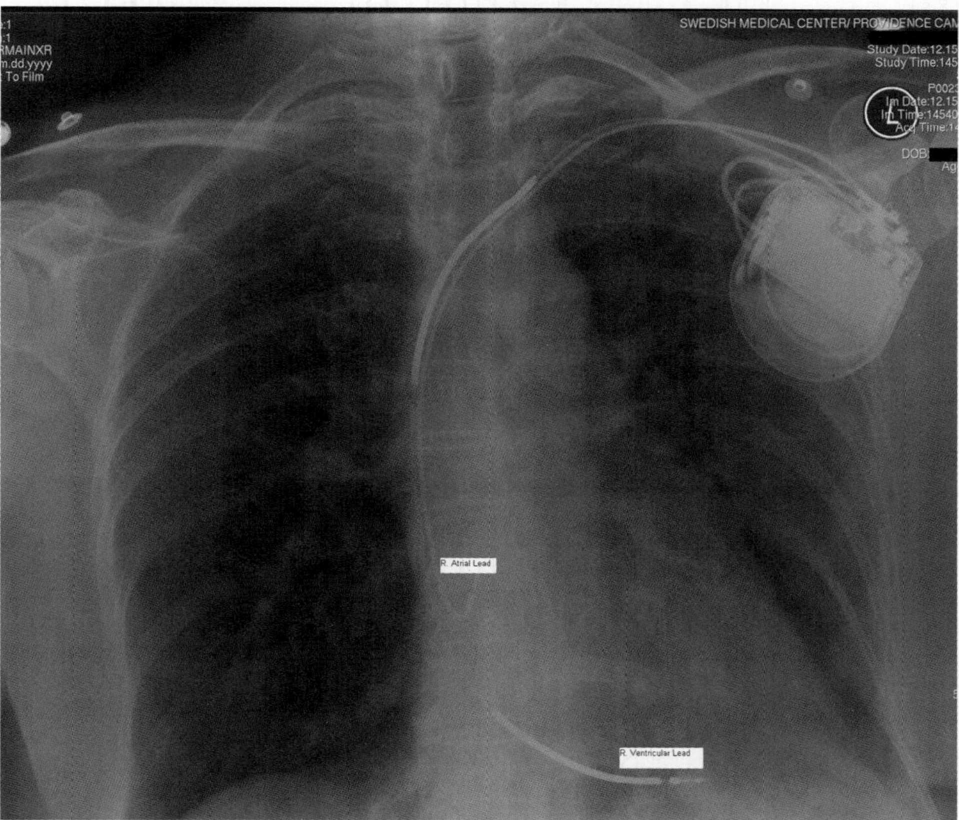

Figure 28-38 X-ray image showing dual-chamber ICD implant. Two leads are placed in the heart. Right atrial lead and a right ventricular lead. If a single chamber ICD were placed, only the right ventricular lead would be implanted.

Onset criterion is a feature used to distinguish sinus tachycardia from VT. When the patient is exercising and the ventricular rate increases gradually and subsequently goes into the VT zone, the ICD does not classify the tachycardia as VT. The ICD compares each cycle length interval and determines if the rate has increased faster than would be expected for a sinus increase.[79,80]

The rate stability criterion is used to help differentiate atrial fibrillation from VT. Atrial fibrillation has large cycle length variability, whereas VT cycle length varies minimally. When a fast ventricular response from atrial fibrillation meets the VT criteria and rate stability is programmed on, the ICD does not classify the fast rate as VT because it varies more than a monomorphic VT. Programming for stability varies among manufactures; it is usually programmed between 22 and 30 milliseconds.[54,80]

The electrogram width criterion (EGM width) measures the intracardiac electrogram and inhibits the ICD from detecting sinus tachycardia as VT. The ICD compares the width of the R wave with a programmed value. This algorithm uses digital signal processing to measure each beat and defines the rhythm as wide or narrow on the basis of its intracardiac morphology. If the R wave is narrow, the ICD classifies the tachycardia as sinus. If the R wave is wide, the ICD treats the tachycardia as VT. Electrogram width should be used cautiously or avoided in patients with a bundle-branch block or surface QRS width that exceeds 100 milliseconds. Patients who have had inappropriate shocks for SVT should have detection enhancements programmed on. Patient history and clinical arrhythmias should be reviewed, to allow for specific programming of detection enhancements.[80]

The Wavelet Dynamic Discrimination Criterion, known as "Wavelet," is an SVT discrimination algorithm in Medtronic ICDs. Wavelet is an electrogram template algorithm that automatically compares the morphology of tachycardia to the morphology of normal sinus beats. If the morphology is similar to the normal beat, the tachycardia would be classified as SVT. However, if the morphology of the tachycardia differs from the normal beat, then the tachycardia is classified as VT/VF. The Wavelet has replaced EGM width on all Medtronic single-chamber ICDs.[81]

With the addition of an atrial lead the potential to increase specificity of VT detection is increased. Dual-chamber ICDs have additional detection enhancements. Guidant-Boston Scientific devices have two additional programmable detection enhancements: (1) V rate greater than A rate and (2) atrial fibrillation rate threshold. Both of these detections work with stability and onset and are only applied in the VT zone. The V rate greater than A rate is based on the premise of AV dissociation and can only be VT. When V rate greater than A rate is programmed "on" and a VT occurs, other therapy inhibitors are bypassed and the ICD delivers therapy immediately. The AF rate threshold increases specificity by confirming AF from the atrial electrograms and withholding therapy for irregular ventricular rhythms.

Medtronic devices have PR logic pattern and rate analysis for SVT detection. The algorithm uses rate cut-off and stability and then applies PR logic to further categorize the arrhythmia. PR logic has three programmable parameters: (1) atrial fibrillation/atrial flutter, (2) sinus tachycardia, and (3) other 1:1 SVTs; each parameter

(*text continues on page 693*)

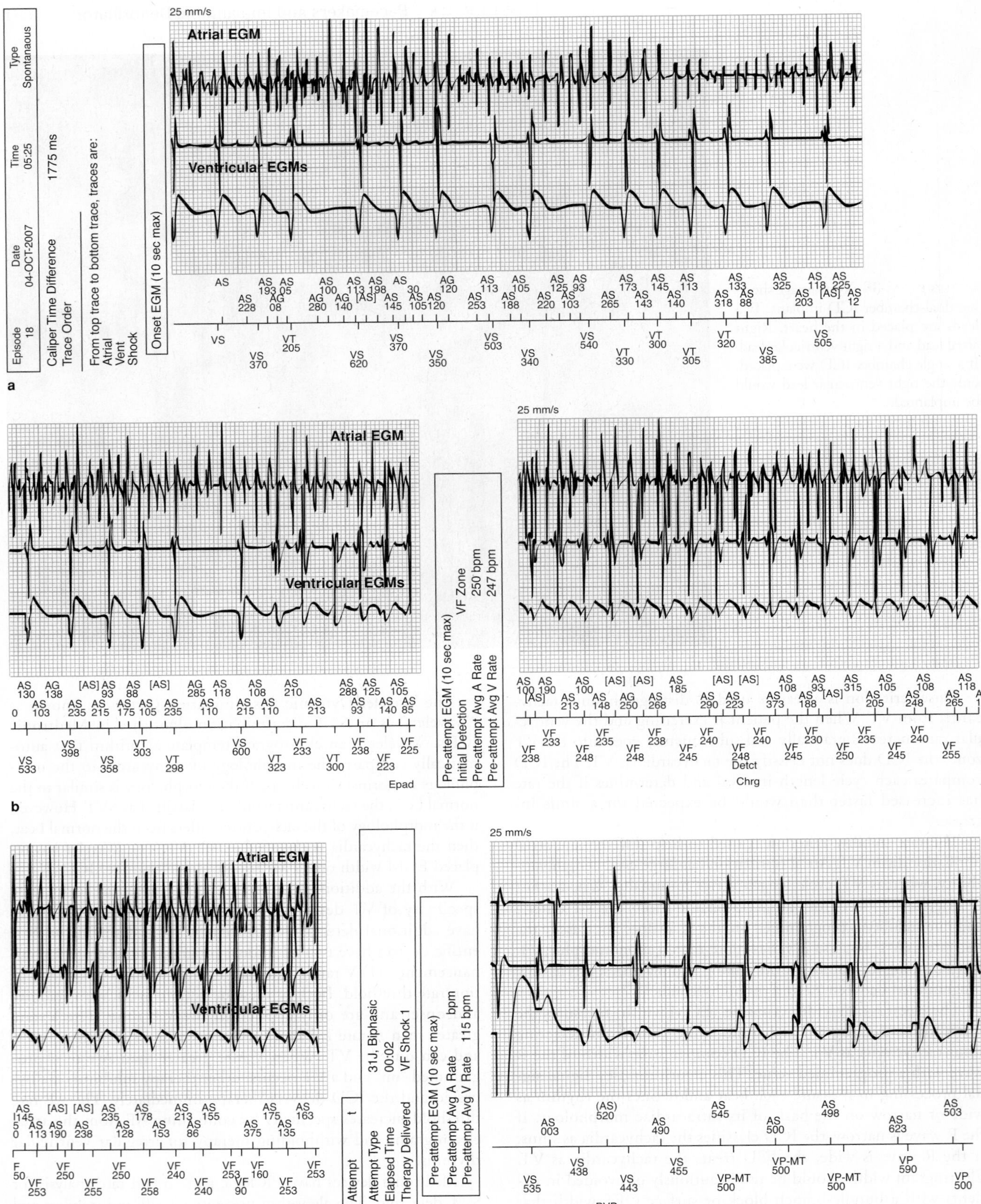

■ **Figure 28-39** Panel (A) shows tracing of rapid atrial fibrillation (AF); the atrial electrogram (EGM) shows the rapid atrial response of AF, and the slower but fast ventricular rhythm. Panel (B) shows the patient going into ventricular fibrillation. Note the morphology change on the ventricular EGM. Panel (C) shows a 31 J shock converting AF and VF to normal sinus rhythm. (Marker annotation for Guidant Vitality 2 DR ICD; AS, atrial sense; VS, ventricular sense; VT, ventricular tachycardia; VF, ventricular fibrillation; AS, atrial sense in total atrial refractory period; VP, ventricular pace; VP-MT, ventricular paced with atrial tracked at max tracking rate.)

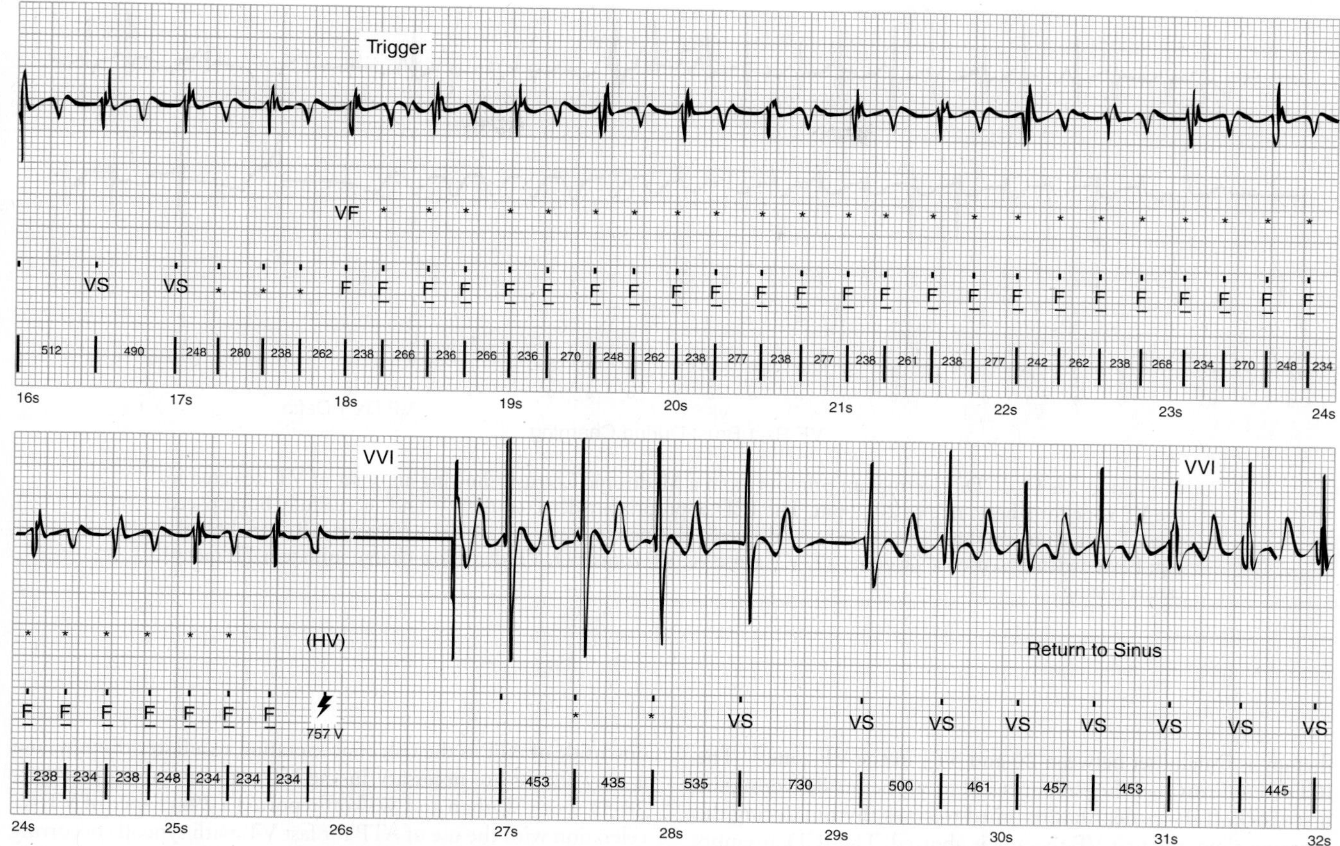

■ **Figure 28-40** ICD. Electrogram tracing shows an episode of sinus tachycardia that is detected as ventricular fibrillation. The ICD is counting the T wave of each beat. Special sensing changes were programmed to the ICD to eliminate the inappropriate shock. (Marker annotation for St. Jude Atlas; VS, ventricular sense; F, VF zone; HV and lightening bolt, high-voltage shock delivered.)

must be programmed "on" or "off." Once tachycardia is detected, the PR logic algorithm uses six elements in identification of VT versus SVT. The algorithm relies on rate (atrial and ventricular), pattern, regularity, AV dissociation, far-field R wave, and AF evidence.

St. Jude ICDs uses a feature called A–V rate branch to aid in diagnosis of SVT. It is a multitiered discrimination algorithm that assesses the atrial and ventricular rates. The arrhythmia is classified in one of three branches: V > A, V = A, and V < A. The rhythms that are classified as V > A are immediately treated for VT. If the arrhythmia is classified as V = A or V < A, other discriminators such as sudden onset, stability, and morphology discrimination can be utilized before therapy is delivered.[54,82]

Modes of Operation

ICDs can be programmed to detect one to three zones, one zone for VF and two different zones for VT. Therapies are programmed according to the detection zone. ICDs offer different types of tachyarrhythmia therapy depending on the manufacturer, including burst pacing, adaptive burst pacing or ramp pacing, incremental/decremental bursts, low-energy cardioversion, and defibrillation. Different zones allow the ICD to be programmed in a tiered or staged-therapy approach, allowing for maximum safety in the VF zone and less aggressive and less painful therapies in the VT zones. In addition to VT/VF therapy, the ICD has pacing abilities. Depending on the ICD system implanted, VVI pacing or DDDR pacing with mode switching is available.[54,72,80]

All newer devices have memory and electrogram storage capability. The ICD continuously stores parameter setting, device status, and significant information about the patient's arrhythmia. When the ICD programmer retrieves the data, it summarizes the data for display and printout. For each episode, up to maximum storage capacity, the ICD stores the ventricular electrogram for the single-chamber devices and stores atrial and ventricular electrograms for the dual-chamber devices. The ability to review stored electrograms from an episode has been especially helpful in differentiating between appropriate and inappropriate shocks. Once a cause has been determined, optimal programming can be performed to help eliminate inappropriate shocks (Fig. 28-40).[54]

Ventricular Fibrillation Therapy

When arrhythmias are detected in the VF zone, defibrillation is the only therapy option. Programming of the shock energy is based on DFT. The DFT is the minimum effective energy required to defibrillate the heart. To ensure that the ICD is effective, ICD shocks must be programmed above the DFT. Historically, a safety margin of 10 Joules (J) has been used; therefore, the first

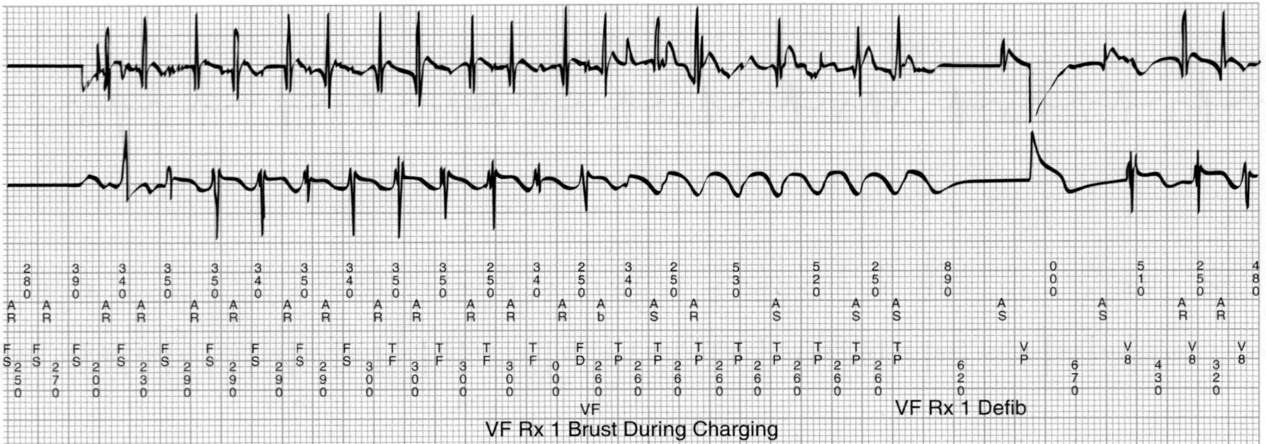

■ **Figure 28-41** ICD. Electrogram printout from a Medtronic Entrust, showing an onset of VT detected in the VF zone for a heart rate of 200 bpm. The ICD appropriately detected the VT and successfully burst paced the VT to a sinus rhythm. The pacing was delivered during charging. AR, Atrial refractory; AB, Atrial blanking; FS,ventricular sense in VF zone; TF, VT sense via VF zone; FD, VF detection-charge initiated; TP, tachycardia pacing)

therapy is usually set between 20 and 34 J in the VF zone.[80] The ICD reconfirms that the patient is still in VF before delivering the first shock. If the patient has returned to sinus rhythm during the charging time, the first VF therapy is aborted. The ICD attempts to deliver a synchronized shock to the R wave if at all possible.

There is a new feature in Medtronic ICDs that allows for ATP therapy in the VF zone while the ICD is charging. When VF is detected and the ICD starts to charge ATP, will be delivered. If the patient is still in the rapid ventricular arrhythmia, the ICD will deliver the programmed shock. If the ATP is successful, the ICD automatically aborts the shock, and the patient does not receive a painful shock. A charge saver feature is also available; if ATP during charging is successful, the ICD will automatically switch to ATP before charging with proven ATP efficacy. In patients with frequent VTs detected in the VF zone, this would eliminate frequent capacitor charges, which decreases battery longevity.[67] The ICD can take 8 seconds, sometimes longer to charge to energy levels above 30 J. Typically as the battery level decreases the charge time increases. The longer the ICD has been implanted, the longer the charge times will be prior to a delivered shock (Fig. 28-41).[67,83]

Ventricular Tachycardia Therapy

In contrast to treating arrhythmias in the VF zone, there are many more options when the ICD is programmed in the VT zone. Each VT episode can be treated with multiple therapies and is often treated in a step-wise fashion. The first therapy is often ATP, followed by low-energy cardioversion and, finally, by defibrillation if necessary to terminate the episode.[54,57,72,80] Most sustained monomorphic VTs are caused by re-entry and can be terminated by a timed pacing sequence. Pacing at a faster rate than the VT increases the probability of VT termination. ATP offers the patient the ability to terminate a tachycardia without a shock. ATP has shown to be effective in terminating VT 78% to 94% of the time when the heart rate is less than 200 bpm, and 75% effective when the VT rate is between 200 and 250 bpm.[66,84–86] The downside of ATP is the risk of acceleration to a faster rhythm, and is why shocks are necessary in the VT zone, as shown in Figure 28-39. Both Wathen and Wilkoff reported a 2% chance of VT acceleration with the use of ATP for fast VT, with syncope occurring in 2% of the patients.[85,86] Reviewing stored electrograms confirm that the onset of arrhythmias is primarily VT. Wathen et al. reported 1342 ventricular arrhythmic episodes with 90% recorded as VT (rates <200) and fast VT (FVT rates 200 to 250) and only 10% recorded as VF. ATP is very effective in treating VT, and prevents anxiety of receiving shocks and should be considered the preferred therapy for fast VT when programming the ICD.[85]

Antitachycardic pacing mode therapies can be set in the electrophysiology laboratory after VT has been induced and a specific ATP therapy has been proven successful in terminating the tachycardia. Another approach is programming the ICD empirically, modifying therapies as needed after the patient has a spontaneous VT.[85,86] A variety of pacing modes can be used to terminate the tachycardia. Each manufacturer has a slightly different approach to programming ATP. A common form of ATP is burst pacing, in which a group of paced beats is delivered at equal or fixed-cycle intervals that exceed the rate of the tachycardia. The number of beats in each burst and the number of burst sequences are programmed and vary from device to device. An adaptive burst, also called ramp pacing, is another frequently used ATP method. A ramp sequence consists of a set of pulses delivered at decreasing intervals to treat a detected episode of VT. Incremental/decremental bursts are another form of burst pacing in which the bursts alternate between incremental and decremental cycle lengths.[80]

Low-energy cardioversion is available on all devices and can be set as low as 0.1 J. The very-low-energy therapies are often determined by electrophysiology testing. Shocks that are under 2 J are much more comfortable for the patient and usually are perceived as small shocks Low-energy shocks may be delivered after ATP therapy has failed but may also be programmed as the initial therapy to terminate the tachycardia, particularly if ATP has been known to accelerate VT to VF. If low-energy cardioversion is unsuccessful, a high-energy shock is delivered.[87]

Bradycardia Pacing

Bradycardia pacing (VVI) is a standard feature available on all ICDs. Dual-chamber pacing, and biventricular pacing now comprise the majority of pacing in ICD patients. Review of data from the first year (2006) of the National ICD Registry revealed that 108,341 ICDs were placed and there were 23.4% single chamber, 38.8% dual-chamber, and 37.5% biventricular ICDs placed.[88] Pacing rate, hysteresis, sensitivity, pulse width, pulse amplitude, and blanking after pacing are all programmable. In the dual-chamber device, atrial tachycardia rate and mode-switch capabilities can also be programmed. Pacing thresholds during VT when ATP applied, and after defibrillation are usually higher than needed for bradycardia pacing, and they can be independently programmed in some of the devices.

Magnet Mode

All ICDs have a magnet mode, a feature that is activated when a magnet is placed over the pulse generator. Magnet modes allow for therapy to be suppressed in emergency situations when the patient is receiving inappropriate shocks. Some generators emit audible tones when a magnet is placed over the unit. Magnet response with pacemakers and ICDs are often very confusing. Generally, magnets disable only the VT/VF function of an ICD. Pacing function of the ICD will not be affected with magnet application except for ELA Medical, which paces DDD at 96 bpm.[89] Guidant magnet response can be programmed on or off, and in fact programming the magnet response off is required to correct an advisory alert in a subset of devices.[90] If a magnet is placed over the ICD, the patient should be monitored, as they are unprotected from life-threatening arrhythmias. Many facilities have polices requiring ICD interrogation pre- and postmagnet application (Display 28-8).

Device Implantation

ICD implants are preferably implanted in the left pectoral region as a result of the shock vector formed by the lead system and active can. The ICD in the unipolar system is known as the *active can* or *hot can.* There is more surface area covered with a shock when the system is placed on the left side and the current travels from the right ventricle to the active can on the left side. The lead is inserted in either the subclavian vein or the cephalic vein and advanced to the RV apex, using techniques similar to those for permanent pacemaker implantation. Defibrillation testing is completed once the lead is in place and secured. Delivering a small shock, approximately 1 J, to the vulnerable part of the T wave induces VF. Induction of VF is necessary to test whether the ICD can detect the fine fibrillatory waves of VF and if the programmed energy level of the ICD can convert the VF to sinus rhythm. If the first shock fails, a second shock at maximum output is delivered. If the second shock fails, a 200 to 360 J external shock is delivered. There are different techniques for DFT, but the 10 J safety margin for defibrillation is the acceptable "standard of care."[91] With the current "active can" ICD and biphasic waveform, it is very rare for implant criteria not to be met. The ICD may be implanted in the electrophysiology laboratory, catheterization laboratory, or OR. Anesthesia can be local or general, and the device can be placed subcutaneously or submuscularly. Most patients with an ICD placed transvenously are discharged on the day after surgery. A postimplantation noninvasive study is often performed before discharge to verify proper functioning of the device and to "fine-tune" the device programming.[80]

Complications

Postoperative complications have been reduced with the advent of the transvenous pectoral technique for ICD implantation. Complications reported by the national registry for ICD implant and prior to

DISPLAY 28-8 Critical Concepts: ICDS and Magnets

Magnets affect all ICDs. Magnets open the reed switch within the ICD, suspending detections or inhibiting therapy without a programmer. In an emergency place the magnet directly over the ICD to deactivate the shocking ability. *All* ICDs that are manufactured can be disabled while the magnet is applied (some may have the magnet feature programmed OFF.*) Interrogating the ICD with the programmer once the magnet is removed will assure all settings have been returned to normal programmed parameters.

- Cautery and other sources of strong EMI can be interpreted as an arrhythmia leading to shocks.
- Placing a magnet over the ICD for surgical procedures is an excellent way to ensure patient safety. In the event of a dangerous arrhythmia during surgery removing the magnet will usually return the ICD to normal function, treating the arrhythmia. It may not be possible to place the magnet over the ICD for all surgeries (shoulder, neck, and chest) as the magnet would be in the sterile field, in that setting the ICD needs to be programmed off.
- Inappropriate shocks can occur with lead damage. The ICD detects the noise from the damaged lead as an arrhythmia and can deliver multiple inappropriate shocks.
- In the event of an inappropriate shock confirmed by ECG monitoring, a magnet should be placed over the ICD to prevent further shocks until the device can be turned off.
- A magnet can be used to prevent further inappropriate shocks from rapid atrial fibrillation or SVT. Once it is determined that the patient is receiving shocks for atrial fib place a magnet over the ICD until the fast rates are controlled, or the ICD is programmed to detect the atrial arrhythmia and withhold therapy.

*Magnet response is a programmable feature in *Guidant-Boston Scientific* and *St. Jude Devices.* Only on rare occasion would the ICD be programmed to ignore magnets, or permanently disable therapies. Biotronik, ELA and Medtronic ICDs *always* suspend therapy when a magnet is applied; once the magnet is removed normal function returns. *Magnet information obtained by personal communication of all ICD company technical service departments, listed above.*

DISPLAY 28-9 Potential Complications of Implantable Cardioverter-Defibrillator

Adverse Events Associated with Surgery

- Subclavian stick complications
  - Pneumothorax
  - Hemothorax
  - Air embolism
  - Subclavian artery puncture
- Bleeding
- Right ventricular perforation
- Thromboemboli
- Venous occlusion
- Pericardial effusion/tamponade
- Pocket hematoma
- Hypotension—hemodynamic compromise
- Cerebrovascular accident
- Proarrhythmia

Adverse Events After System in Place

- System related
  - Lead dislodgement
  - Loose setscrew
  - Lead fracture
  - Lead insulation defect
  - Exit block
  - Premature battery depletion
- Chronic nerve damage
- Diaphragmatic stimulation
- Erosion of pulse generator
- Fluid accumulation/seroma
- Infection of the pocket/system
- Keloid formation
- Venous thromboembolism
- Endocarditis

hospital discharge occurred 3.63% of the time. Procedure related deaths were reported to be 0.02%. The two most common complications reported were hematoma, which occurred 1.27%, and lead dislodgement 1.01%.[88] Potential complications of ICD implantation are listed in Display 28-9. One of the most serious complications is infection of the ICD system. Removal of the entire ICD system is mandatory, and a long course of antibiotics is necessary.

Infection rates are higher after a generator replacement when compared to rates with initial implants,[92] Surgical revision of the ICD system may be necessary after lead dislodgment in the early recovery period (24 to 72 hours) or lead fracture, which is seen in long-term follow-up. Lead-related problems have been reported to be as high as 20% in 10-year-old leads. Patients with lead defects are often the younger more active patients. Lead fractures or insulation issues can lead to false sensing and inappropriate shocks.[72,73]

EMI can result in inappropriate discharge or inhibition of the ICD. These problems can be temporary or permanent. The delivery of inappropriate therapy can actually produce tachyarrhythmia. Sources of interference include, but are not limited to electrocautery, diathermy, hydraulic shock-wave lithotripsy, current-carrying conductors, arc welders, electrical smelting furnaces, and radiofrequency transmitters such as radar, high-voltage systems, theft prevention equipment, and high-powered electromagnetic fields. Magnetic resonance imaging is contraindicated because it may cause permanent damage to the ICD. Inadvertent contact between the generator and magnets should be avoided because changes in the magnetic field may inactivate the pulse generator or cause erratic functioning.[25] Tachyarrhythmia detection must be programmed *OFF* before subjecting the patient to procedures that induce strong EMI. If detections are turned OFF, the patient must be monitored. Once the procedure is completed, the ICD should be reprogrammed to the active mode. Placing a magnet over the ICD will inactivate it temporarily in most cases. Some ICDs can be programmed to ignore a magnet, and some have been programmed off due to a magnet switch problem. Placing a magnet over the ICD to temporarily disable shocks is also an option for disabling therapy. If a patient has a VT or VF episode, removing the magnet will allow the ICD to treat the arrhythmia quickly. If the ICD were programmed off, it takes a programmer and extra time to reactivate the ICD, delaying treatment time of the arrhythmia. Close communication with the patient's implanting physician should be made before determining deactivation technique of the ICD using a magnet or programmer. The facility performing the medical procedure should have a policy regarding preprocedure interrogation and disabling ICD therapies. Patient safety during the procedure to eliminate inappropriate shocks, and postprocedure to insure that the ICD has been programmed to the initial settings is crucial.

Antiarrhythmic medications are often used in conjunction with ICD therapy to decrease arrhythmia occurrence. The antiarrhythmic drugs can result in complications by changing the appearance or rate of the arrhythmia or by altering the DFT. The arrhythmia rate may be slowed below the cut-off rate so that the ICD fails to identify VT. Drugs could change the DFT, resulting in ineffective shocks. Amiodarone, for example, increases the threshold. Repeat EPS testing with the ICD may be required to reprogram VT zones capable of sensing and treating different VT after the addition of an antiarrhythmic.[93]

Standard Precautions

External Defibrillation

Patients with an ICD should be treated like any other patient without an ICD when sustained arrhythmias are present. ACLS with rapid defibrillation should be initiated when the ICD is ineffective or not delivering therapy.[83] ICDs are designed to withstand external defibrillation. However, possible circuit damage or loss of output may occur if the external paddle is placed to close to the device. If at all possible, the anterior–posterior approach should be used for external paddle placement (Fig. 28-42). Direct defibrillation could cause permanent damage to the ICD or the implanted leads. After external defibrillation the ICD should be interrogated to assess device function. During cardiac resuscitation when CPR is in progress shocks from the ICD may be felt, but will not harm rescuers.[81,93,94]

Pacemaker Interaction

With the advent of dual-chamber ICDs, the problems with device interactions between separate systems have been eliminated. If a patient has an older-model ICD in place and requires a temporary or permanent pacemaker in conjunction with the ICD, special care is required. For those patients who may still have an older system in place, unipolar pacemakers are contraindicated because the larger pacing pulse associated with unipolar lead systems may be mistaken by the ICD for the patient's intrinsic rhythm. Three

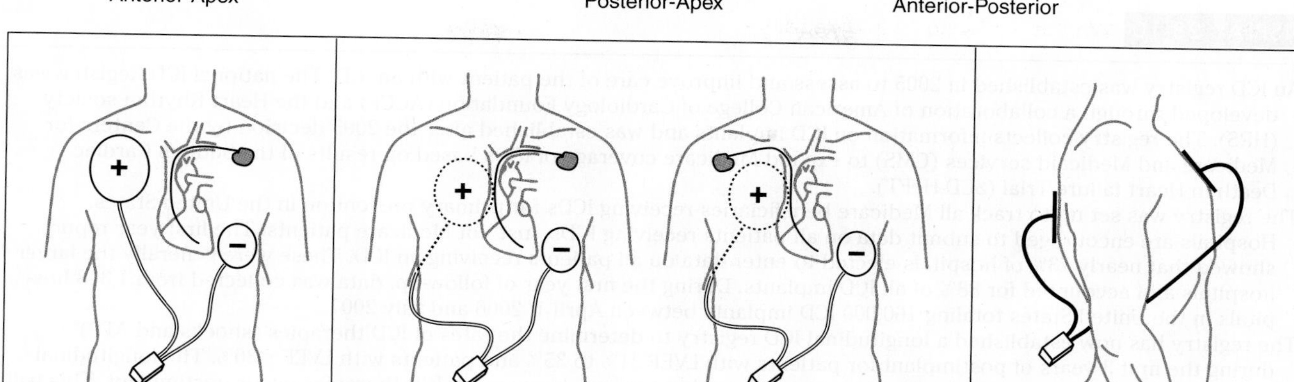

■ **Figure 28-42** ICD. For external cardioversion or defibrillation, the paddles should be positioned in the anterior–posterior position if at all possible. Ideally the external paddles should be kept 4 to 6 in away from the pulse generator. When the patient has a device in the left pectoral region, the anterior-apex position is acceptable.

unique complications have been observed in patients with *both* a permanent pacemaker and an ICD: (1) failure of the ICD to detect and treat VT/VF, as the ICD is counting pacer spikes only; (2) double counting of pacing spikes and QRS complexes, because the ICD thinks it is seeing VT and delivers a discharge; and (3) misinterpretation of ST segment elevation as a sinusoid pattern, resulting in discharge. To avoid potential complications with older-generation ICDs, single-chamber pacemakers with bipolar leads and lower voltages have been used.[83,95]

Preoperative and Postoperative Nursing Care

Consideration of the emotional response of the patient and family to the ICD is an important part of nursing care. Before surgery, an assessment of the patient's (and family's) knowledge level, support systems, and usual coping mechanisms should be made. Patients may have a high anxiety level because of categorization as a high-risk patient, EPS, impending surgery, and the ICD unit. With the introduction of a new therapy, the patient may have quality-of-life questions. "Will I be able to do more, and will I feel better?" Anxiety may be reduced through provision of ICD specific education, relaxation/stress management training, and group discussion and social support.[96–98]

Previous research has shown that ICD patients desire increased education about their device. Dougherty et al.[99] reported decreased anxiety levels in SCA patients who received combined education and telephone intervention by trained cardiovascular nurses. Nearly all patients (96%) randomized to the intervention group rated the intervention *very helpful*. Patients felt that the interventions were most helpful with resuming normal activities, exercise, managing symptoms and ICD shocks, and reducing anxiety.[99]

The patient should understand why the ICD is recommended and how it functions. ICD system models and patient education videotapes are available from the ICD manufacturers and are useful tools in providing visual and general information. Specific information regarding ICD efficacy, potential complications including ICD and lead failures, diagnostic information available and what happens when the patient receives a shock is an important component in patient intervention.[97] Specific postoperative instructions with precautions and limitation regarding the ICD implant should be reviewed with the patient prior to discharge. The patient and family members should also understand that the ICD does not prevent arrhythmias from occurring, but is there to correct the arrhythmia.

Postoperative care of the patient with an ICD is similar to the care of the patient after permanent pacemaker implantation. The patient should be informed that mild or moderate pain will be felt at the incision site. The patient's pain level and the incision site should be assessed and pain medications administered as needed. The patient should be instructed to minimize arm movements for the first 24 hours after implantation. Discharge instructions are an important aspect of postoperative nursing care. With transvenous ICD implants, hospital stays are much shorter, which limits the time available to teach patients. Written discharge instructions should be supplied to the patient and should include instructions about pain management, site assessment and care, what to do in the event of receiving a shock, when to notify the physician, the importance of carrying proper identification that allows medical personnel quickly to check the ICD with the correct programmer, avoiding magnetic fields, and cardiopulmonary resuscitation, as well as information regarding support groups.[99]

Instructions regarding ICD shocks should be thoroughly reviewed and understood. In follow-up of ICD patients whom had their device placed for secondary prevention, a chance of receiving a shock was 57% to 81% during a mean follow-up of 2.5 to 5 years.[83] Further data will be available in regards to ICD shocks in those patients who have had their ICD placed for primary prevention with the advent of the new United States National registry (Display 28-10). With ICD discharges, the patient will often have a sensation of their arrhythmia and wait for the ICD to deliver therapy. Patient perceptions of the discharge vary from minimal to very painful. The ICD shock is often described as a feeling of being punched or likened to a swift kick.[97] Patients with VF or a rapid VT may experience a syncopal event by the time the generator discharges.[85] Management of a single ICD shock, without syncope, dizziness, chest pain or shortness of breath does not

DISPLAY 28-10 What is the National ICD Registry?

An ICD registry was established in 2005 to assess and improve care of the patient with an ICD. The national ICD Registry was developed through a collaboration of American College of Cardiology Foundation (ACCF) and the Heart Rhythm society (HRS). The registry collects information on ICD implants and was established after the 2005 decision by the Centers for Medicare and Medicaid services (CMS) to expand Medicare coverage of ICDs based on results of the Sudden Cardiac Death in Heart failure Trial (SCD-HeFT).

The registry was set up to track all Medicare beneficiaries receiving ICDs for primary prevention in the United States. Hospitals are encouraged to submit data on all patients receiving ICDs, just not Medicare patients. The first year report showed that nearly 73% of hospitals elected to enter data on all patients receiving an ICD. These were generally the larger hospitals and accounted for 88% of all ICD implants. During the first year of follow-up, data was collected from 1,318 hospitals in the United States totaling 160,000 ICD implants between April 1, 2006 and July 2007.

The registry has now established a longitudinal ICD registry to determine the rates of ICD therapies (shocks and ATP) during the first 3 years of postimplant for patients with LVEF 31% to 35% and patients with LVEF ≤30%. The longitudinal registry will supply us with up to date information on what type, and how many ICD therapies occur postimplant. This will provide us with new information to share with ICD patients, particularly those receiving an ICD for primary prevention, which accounted for 79% of patients in the first year of the National ICD registry.[88]

necessarily require an emergent visit to the cardiologist's office or emergency room. The patient should notify their device following physician and may be instructed to call in a check with their remote monitoring equipment (see display remote monitoring). The ICD shock can be frightening to the patient. The patient should be reassured that occasional shocks are to be expected and reminded that they received the ICD because they are at risk for arrhythmias.

Once an appropriate shock has been determined the patient may need further work-up regarding their clinical condition. Often, no cause for the shock is determined and the patient just needs reassured that the ICD was effective in treating the arrhythmia. If a patient is having frequent shocks, the electrophysiologist may consider adjustments in medications, optimizing ICD programming, or proceeding with radiofrequency ablation.[57]

Psychosocial Issues

Anxiety and QOL

Evidence indicates the ICD patients experience some level of psychological distress and reduced QOL. After the ICD is implanted, specific fears and anxiety about the shock experience, device malfunction and/or death are the most common psychological symptoms reported by ICD patients.[96,98,100] ICD system (device and lead) alerts and recalls have become stressful events for the ICD patient and their families. There is no specific data on how the device recalls impact patients. Suggestions have been made to include risk for recalls in the informed consent process as a possible adverse event; informing patients that malfunctions are rare and that they have always occurred and will continue to occur. Patients should understand the importance of regular follow-up to recognize trends of a possible problem.[101]

Thomas et al. reviewed a total of 16 studies that related to QOL and the ICD patients.[98] QOL in ICD patients were reviewed in 14 studies, but only seven were reported to have a studied a comparison group. In the seven studies that did not include a comparison group, the data were inconclusive and limited. The ICD group led to desirable QOL for most patients in two studies, did not improve QOL in two studies, varied in two studies dependent on NYHA class or age, and worsened QOL in one study.

In the seven studies that did compare QOL with ICD patients to those patients with similar cardiac conditions, the QOL was reported to be similar in six studies. The comparison group of patients was receiving drug therapy, had pacemakers, or had coronary artery disease. In one study the ICD patients reported a higher QOL than did the patients receiving pharmacological therapy.

When ICD patients receive shocks they are more anxious, depressed, and have poorer QOL than patients who do not receive shocks as reported by the AVID investigators.[102] Shock experience is certainly a determinate of QOL as Wallace et al. report that the patients with the lowest anxiety and best QOL post-ICD implant are those who do not receive shocks and have a strong social support.[103] HF patients, who have CRT in conjunction with their ICD, have also been noted to have a significant improvement in QOL.[104]

Sears et al.[96] recently completed the first investigation of a stress and shock management intervention for ICD patients, consisting of either a 1-day 4-hour psychoeducational workshop, or a 6-weeks of 90-minute cognitive-behavioral sessions. The intervention was designed to address the cognitive and behavioral adaptation to a shock and the following distress that often occurs. All patients were followed for 4 months after they completed the randomized intervention. Physiologic markers (anxiety) and psychological markers (salivary cortisol) of distress were measured. Patients in both groups showed a reduction of anxiety and cortisol levels, and both groups showed a significant increase in patient acceptance of the ICD. These results suggest that patients can benefit from a cognitive-behavioral strategies and education to reduce anxiety after receiving shocks.

Taking care of the ICD patient can be difficult when they are receiving multiple shocks, but can also be rewarding as a special nurse/patient rapport develops. Interventions that have been shown to help reduce anxiety are ICD education, including having a set plans with specific instruction for when a shock occurs. Coping strategies for the ICD patient after they have received an ICD shock include positive thinking and follow-up debriefing with the device following health care team.[97] Support groups provide a forum for the patients to discuss their concerns and fears with one another and provide the nurse with an excellent opportunity for patient education.[98] Use of programs developed and implemented by nurses may decrease anxiety and depression in the ICD patient.[99] With a considerable increase in patients receiving ICDs, and very little data available on interventions there is a need for a large-scale clinical trial to determine the most optimal intervention to decrease anxiety, and increase QOL for the ICD patient.[96,100]

Automobile Driving

Patients with an ICD placed for secondary prevention of VT or VF, may be restricted from driving for up to 6 months. The main concern is the risk of an arrhythmic event or the delivery of a shock while driving. The length of the driving restriction depends on where the patient resides and state/country regulations. The patient who has an ICD placed for primary prevention should be restricted from driving for at least 1 week, until recovered from surgery. Thereafter, primary prevention patients would not have any driving restrictions unless they subsequently receive therapy for VT or VF. If they receive a shock, particularly in the setting of syncope they would be subject to the same driving restrictions as those patients who had an ICD placed for secondary prevention. Patients with ICDs, implanted for both primary and secondary prevention cannot be certified to drive commercially.[105] Driving restrictions can cause feelings of isolation, anger, and loss of autonomy, because driving is an important part of maintaining independence.[106] It is important for the patient to realize that the symptoms are associated with ventricular arrhythmias, not the ICD, which makes driving potentially dangerous. After 6 months, if the patient has not had an ICD discharge, he or she may resume noncommercial driving.

Patients may report discomfort with using a seatbelt, because the shoulder strap comes across the ICD implant site for a driver with a left pectoral implant and for a passenger with a right pectoral implant. Seatbelt shoulder protectors are recommended and can be found in stores selling auto parts, or can be ordered from medical supply companies. Simple padding can also be placed over the ICD. Patients should be encouraged to continue using seat belts.

Real Versus Phantom Shocks

Once a patient feels a shock they fall into one of three categories: (1) A shock was delivered appropriately for VT or VF. (2) A shock was delivered inappropriately due to sensing of a rapid supraventricular rhythm, electrical noise from EMI, or artifact from a fractured lead. (3) No shock was delivered and they perceived a phantom shock.[107] Patients are certain that they have received a shock, but when the ICD is interrogated, there is no record that a discharge has occurred. This phenomenon is known as a *phantom shock*. Phantom shocks, often occur as the patient is drifting off to sleep and more commonly in patients with previous ICD discharges.[108] It is important to spend time reassuring the patient and family. Patients may find it helpful to review interrogated printouts.

An ICD discharge can be frightening for both the patient and spouse, particularly if the shock occurs with sexual activity. The patient may need to have the tachycardia detection rate increased if sexual activity increases the heart rate enough to meet the detection criteria. Education and support regarding shocks should be provided to the patient. Professional counseling should be recommended for the patient and spouse with emotional concerns.

If the patient has had multiple ICD discharges during an occurrence of an "ICD storm," in which they experience three or more shocks in a 24-hour period, they will likely experience symptoms of anxiety. These patients should be reassured, but if symptoms persist, then referral to psychiatric specialists for treatment of depression and anxiety should be considered.[96]

Follow-up Care

Regular ICD follow-up is necessary to assess the patient's clinical status, ICD battery status, and device function. Review of stored electrograms provides diagnostic information for treated episodes of tachyarrhythmias. In general, there are two components of the follow-up: (1) assessment of the patient's status, reviewing the cardiovascular-medical condition of the patient as well as screening for medication changes and (2) the defibrillator and lead are assessed for normal device function.[93]

The ICD pulse generator is highly reliable but must be observed for battery status and charge times. When pulse generator defects do occur, they can be manifested by early battery depletion. Battery status is monitored at each follow-up visit (Fig. 28-43). If the device is close to its ERI, more frequent visits may be required. Episode data are reviewed and compared with the patient's clinical symptoms. Stored electrograms provide trending information on the frequency and severity, if any, of spontaneous ventricular arrhythmias (see Display 28-11) for information regarding remote follow-up.

The lead system is evaluated by testing lead impedance, completing pacing thresholds, and determining appropriate R-wave sensing. Evaluating the marker channel and real-time electrograms will identify appropriate R-wave sensing. Potential for lead problems can be identified if inappropriate sensing is noted. Chest radiographs should be used periodically for evaluation of system integrity.[93]

Episode data are reviewed and compared with the patient's clinical symptoms. Stored electrograms provide trending information on the frequency and severity, if any, of spontaneous ventricular arrhythmias.

Troubleshooting

Differentiating appropriate from inappropriate device function when a patient receives an ICD discharge or experiences symptoms such as syncope or palpitations can be challenging. Evaluation of a single ICD shock is usually performed in the outpatient clinic, or with remote monitoring. Multiple successive shocks constitute a medical emergency and require a hospital admission for evaluation.[57,72,93] The initial approach is two fold, *identifying* the problem, and *comforting* the patient. Are the shocks appropriate? What is the arrhythmia: SVT, VT, or sinus tachycardia? If the patient *does not* have a ventricular arrhythmia the ICD needs disabled, either with a magnet or with a programmer. If the patient is having incessant VT or VF antiarrhythmics, reprogramming of the ICD and ablation could be helpful.[57,93]

Approximately 20% to 30% of patients with ICDs that use heart rate only as the detection criterion receive an inappropriate shock, most commonly from atrial fibrillation or sinus tachycardia. Detection enhancement criteria using stability and sudden onset have been useful in decreasing shocks. The patient's medications are often adjusted. β-Blockers are used to decrease AV conduction; antiarrhythmics are used to decrease the frequency of atrial fibrillation. When stored electrograms are available, the appropriateness of ICD therapy can be evaluated immediately. The ICD also tracks nonsustained episodes, allowing the health care provider to know the frequency and severity of arrhythmias.[93]

If the patient is receiving multiple ICD discharges and not having clinical symptoms, then dislodged lead, fractured lead, or double counting of QRS and T waves should be suspected. The

Patient ICD and Lead Information

Physician:		Phone:		
ICD	Medtronic	Gem III DR 7275	PJM202	May 02, 2001
Atrial	Medtronic	5076 Capsur…	PJN050	May 02, 2001
RV/SVC	Medtronic	6947 Sprint…	TDA110	May 02, 2001

ICD Status

Battery Voltage (ERI=2.55 V, EOl=2.40 V)	2.56 V ERI	Oct 22, 2007
Last Full Energy Charge	11.20 sec	Sep 20, 2007
Last Capacitor Formation (Interval=2 month)		Sep 20, 2007

Lead Performance	**Atrial**	**Ventricular**	
Pacing Impedance	661 ohms	410 ohms	Oct 22, 2007
Defibrillation (HVB) Impedance		22 ohms	Oct 22, 2007

Parameter Summary

Type	Detection		Rx1	Rx2	Rx3	Rx4	Rx5	Rx6
VF	On	188–500 bpm	20 J	30 J	30 J	30 J	30 J	30 J
FVT	Off							
VT	Off							

SVT Criteria On; None

Modes		**Rates**		**A-V Intervals**	
Mode	DDI	Lower	40 ppm	Paced AV	180 ms

Lead Parameters	**Atrial**	**Ventricular**
Amplitude	3 V	3 V
Pulse Width	0.4 ms	0.4 ms
Sensitivity	0.3 mV	0.3 mV

Clinical Status: Since Sep 20, 2007

Episodes		**% Pacing**	
VF	0	AS-VS	100%
FVT	0	AS-VP	0%
VT	0	AP-VS	0%
SVT	0	AP-VP	0%
NST and others	1		
Mode Switch	0		

Observations (1)

- Battery Voltage is <= 2.55 V, ERI. Replacement of the ICD is recommended.

■ **Figure 28-43** ICD. Quick Look Report from a Medtronic Gem III DR. Report shows battery voltage at 2.55, which is the elective replacement indicator (ERI). The patient came in for follow-up because *Patient Alert Alarm* was triggered when battery dipped to 2.55. The alarm was programmed off, and the patient was scheduled for elective replacement of the ICD. Other information gleaned from Quick Look report: no episodes of VT, VF, one nonsustained event since last interrogated; 0% paced since last interrogated.

DISPLAY 28-11 What's New With Follow-up?

All major ICD companies now provide the ICD patients with equipment to call in their ICD interrogation over the phone. The patients following physician or nurse can then access follow-up data by logging onto a secure website. The data obtained is similar to the information that is obtained at the doctor's office. The system is ideal for patients who live in remote locations, need closer follow-up due to ICD or lead alerts, or have just received a shock. The stored electrograms can be reviewed promptly and without the patient having to go to the emergency room. Data retrieval can be made at any computer with Internet access.

The remote monitors are easy to use and the entire process only takes a few minutes. At this time all monitors are read-only system; no programming can be performed over the telephone. The monitors provide audible tones, indicator lights, or prompted commands to confirm that the transmission was successful.

Heart Rhythm Society encourages utilization of remote monitoring to provide earlier information regarding abnormal device behavior. Accurate information regarding specific device product performance would also be available for manufactures to review and report.[109]

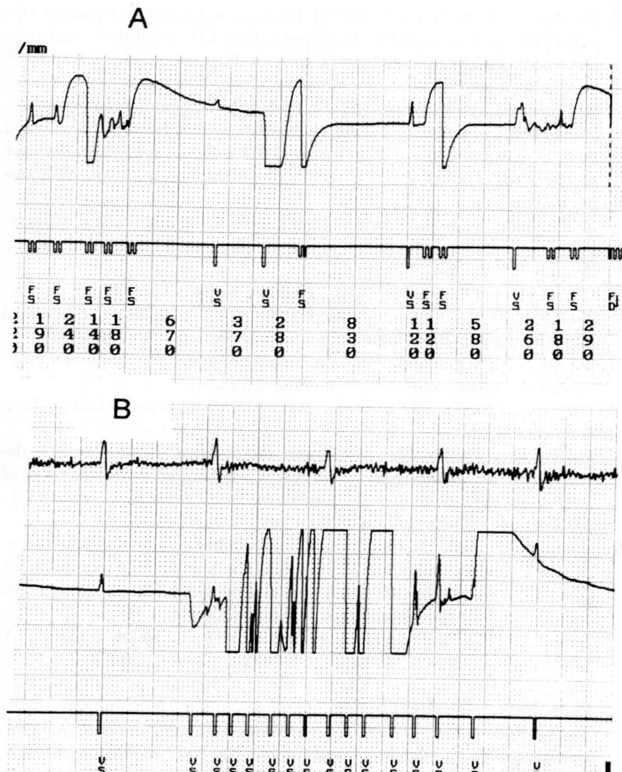

■ **Figure 28-44** ICD. Electrogram tracings showing artifact from fractured lead. Panel (A) shows intracardiac signal from stored electrograms, artifact signals and irregular cycle length confirm fracture. Panel (B) shows real-time recording while having patient move arm with detections suspended to reproduce artifact. This recording was from an older epicardial patch lead system and abdominal implant. The patient was admitted to hospital for placement of new ICD system. (Marker annotation for Medtronic Jewel 7202: VS, ventricular sense; FS, fibrillation sense; FD, fibrillation detection-charge initiated.)

patient should be instructed to call emergency medical services for transport to the hospital if having multiple shocks. When electrograms are available, interrogation of ICD can confirm fractured lead artifact (Fig. 28-44). In an emergency situation, placing a large ICD/pacemaker magnet over the ICD can deactivate the ICD, as mentioned. Magnets do not inhibit the bradycardia therapy that is programmed into the ICD. A chest radiograph may be able to provide information on lead fracture or insulation breaks and can diagnose a dislodged lead.[57,72,93]

Failure to deliver therapy is caused by failure to detect the arrhythmia. This failure could be caused by a sensitivity problem, a change in VT rate, deactivation of the device, or system failure. Inadvertent deactivation of the ICD is rare but potentially devastating. The device could be inadvertently deactivated with use of a magnet, or during a programming session. Therefore, a final interrogation with a printout should always be performed. Some ICDs (Guidant-Boston Scientific) can be programmed to turn *off* after a magnet has been placed over the ICD for approximately 30 seconds. Rarely, exposure to a strong magnetic field results in deactivation. Battery depletion and circuit failure could be other causes of the ICD failing to deliver therapy.

Frequent and thorough follow-up care can help detect potential problems early, preventing devastating results. ICDs have become sophisticated and complex, providing information on patient activity, heart rate, frequency of arrhythmia, as well as ICD status. ICDs have continued to improve, enhancing patient safety and comfort. Remote monitoring of ICDs can assist with regular follow-up, and many ICDs have warning beeps or tones to alert the patient of a change with their ICD system.

Special Considerations

Sex and Racial Differences

ICD therapy is recommended in all patients with HF and LV ejection fraction of 35% or less. Previous studies have shown a disparity in which patients receive costly cardiovascular technologies. Hernandez et al.[110] obtained data from the AHA, Get with the Guidelines Program between January 2005 and June 2007 using a 30% EF as implanting criteria. They compared baseline characteristics of patients that received ICD therapy with the characteristics of patients who did not receive ICD therapy. Review of the 13,034 patients eligible for ICD therapy resulted in the following findings: (1) the frequency of ICD therapy was low with only 35.4% of qualified patients receiving an ICD, (2) women were approximately 40% less likely than men to receive and ICD, and (3) black patients were approximately 30% less likely than white patients to receive an ICD.[110]

Awareness programs should address the recommendation for ICD therapy and the need for eliminating sex and racial disparities. Programs such a *Get with the Guidelines*[111] and the *National ICD registry*[88] provide nonbiased information on patients receiving ICD implants helping to reduce these disparities.

End of Life Issues

Decision about the deactivation of ICDs will become more common as the uses of ICDs are increasing. The primary concern for a terminally ill patient is the ICD could cause an unnecessary distressing death due to painful shocks. Deactivating an ICD by turning off the VT and VF therapies will not create discomfort; it would prevent treatment of a life-threatening ventricular arrhythmia. It is unknown how often patients are approached about end of life issues, and there are no set practice guidelines to address these issues. Discussions are needed to establish ethical criteria for end-of-life care in terminally ill or elderly patients with implanted devices.[112,113]

CONCLUSION

Tremendous technological advances have been made in the ICD since first implanted in 1980. The ICD is no longer a simple shock box. With the introduction of dual-chamber ICDs, many new programmable features are available. The ICD provides high-energy shocking capabilities for VF, ATP features for VT and fast VT, atrial therapies for atrial arrhythmias, and CRT for HF patients. Detection enhancements have improved dramatically. Inappropriate shocks have decreased. ICDs provide diagnostic data to assist the clinician in providing cardiac care to their patients. Diagnostic data such as activity levels, minimum and maximum heart rates, fluid level trends, and heart rate variability trends have become standard.

The future of device therapy will continue to evolve. Presently there are studies involving leadless ICDs.[114] A leadless system would minimize complication from multiple leads and could potentially increase the number of patients receiving ICDs, as it would be a less invasive option. ICDs are not just for cardiac arrest survivors. They are also placed as the first-line defense in prevention of sudden cardiac arrest from cardiac causes. For all eligible patients to receive an ICD, the benefits of the device need to be understood, and disparities need to be eliminated. Health care providers must become comfortable with the ICD and its capabilities and limitations.

REFERENCES

1. Epstein, A. E., DiMarco, J. P., Ellenbogen, K. A., et al. (2008). ACC/AHA/HRS 2008 guidelines for device-based therapy of cardiac rhythm abnormalities. A report of the American College of Cardiology/American Heart Association Task Force on Practice Guidelines (Writing Committee to Revise the ACC/AHA/NASPE 2002 Guideline Update for Implantation of Cardiac Pacemakers and Antiarrhythmia Devices). *Circulation, 117*, e350–e3408.
2. Vijayaraman, P., & Ellenbogen, K. A. (2008). Bradyarrhythmias and pacemakers. In V. Fuster, R. Walsh, R. O'Rourke et al. (Eds.), *Hurst's the heart* (8th ed.). New York: McGraw-Hill.
3. Hayes, D. L., & Zipes, D. P. (2008). Cardiac pacemakers and cardioverter-defibrillators. In P. Libby, R. O. Bonow, D. L. Mann, et al. (Eds.), *Braunwald's heart disease: A textbook of cardiovascular medicine* (8th ed., pp. 831–846). Philadelphia: Saunders Elsevier.
4. Trohman, R. G., Kim, M. H., & Pinski, S. L. (2004). Cardiac pacing: The state of the art. *The Lancet, 364*, 1701–1719.
5. Prinzen, F., Spinelli, J. C., & Auricchio, A. (2007). Basic physiology and hemodynamics of cardiac pacing. In K. A. Ellenbogen, N. G. Kay, C.-P. Lau, et al. (Eds.), *Clinical cardiac pacing, defibrillation, and resynchronization therapy* (3rd ed., pp. 291–335). Philadelphia: Saunders Elsevier.
6. Abraham, W. T., Fisher, W. G., Smith, A. L., et al., for the Miracle Investigatons. (2002). Cardiac resynchronization in chronic heart failure. *New England Journal of Medicine, 346*(24), 1845–1853.
7. Cazeau, S., Leclercq, C., Lavergne, T., et al. (2001). Effects of multisite biventricular pacing in patients with heart failure and intraventricular conduction delay. *New England Journal of Medicine, 344*(12), 873–880.
8. Saxon, L. A., De Marco, T., & Ellenbogen, K. A. (2007). Clinical trials of cardiac resynchronization therapy: Pacemakers and defibrillators. In K. A. Ellenbogen, N. G. Kay, C.-P. Lau et al. (Eds.), *Clinical cardiac pacing, defibrillation, and resynchronization therapy* (pp. 385–406). Philadelphia: Saunders Elsevier.
9. Albouaini, K., Rao, M., Alahmar, A., et al. (2008). Cardiac resynchronisation therapy: Evidence based benefits and patient selection. *European Journal of Internal Medicine, 19*, 165–172.
10. Goldenberg, I., & Moss, A. J. (2008). Implantable device therapy. *Progress in Cardiovascular Diseases, 50*(6), 449–474.
11. Saxon, L. A., Kumar, U. N., & De Marco, T. (2008). *Cardiac resynchronization therapy (biventricular pacing) in heart failure*. Retrieved August 12, 2008, from www.uptodateonline.com.
12. Cheng, J., & Arnsdorf, M. F. (2006). The role of pacemakers in the prevention of atrial fibrillation. *UpToDate*. Retrieved August 15, 2008, from www.uptodateonline.com.
13. Efremidis, M., Papps, L., Sideris, A., et al. (2008). Management of atrial fibrillation in patients with heart failure. *Journal of Cardiac Failure, 14*(3), 232–237.
14. Kalahasty, G., & Ellenbogen, K. A. (2008). The role of pacemakers in the management of patients with atrial fibrillation. *Medical Clinics of North America, 92*, 161–178.
15. Koebe, J., & Kirchof, P. (2008). Novel non-pharmacological approaches for antiarrhythmic therapy of atrial fibrillation. *Europace, 10*, 433–437.
16. Inoue, N., Ishikawa, T., Sumita, S., et al. (2006). Suppression of atrial fibrillation by atrial pacing. *Circulation, 70*, 1398–1401.
17. Bacik, B. M., Muller, D., & Corbisiero, R. (2006). Adaptive bi-atrial pacing improves the maintenance of sinus rhythm. *Pacing and Clinical Electrophysiology, 30*, 492–497.
18. Sulke, N., Silverbauer, J., Boodhoo, L., et al. (2007). The use of atrial overdrive and ventricular rate stabilization pacing algorithms for the prevention and treatment of paroxysmal atrial fibrillation: The Pacemaker Atrial Fibrillation Suppression (PAFS) Study. *Europace, 9*, 790–797.
19. Sheldon, R. S., & Hersi, A. (2007). Evolving indications for pacing: Hypertrophic cardiomyopathy, sleep apnea, long QT syndromes, and neurally mediated syncope syndromes. In K. A. Ellenbogen, G. N. Kay, C.-P. Lau, et al. (Eds.), *Clinical cardiac pacing, defibrillation, and resynchronization therapy* (3rd ed., pp. 473–498). Philadelphia: Saunders Elsevier.
20. Shanker, A., & Saksena, S. (2001). Cardiac pacemakers. In P. J. Podrid & P. R. Kowey (Eds.), *Cardiac arrhythmia: Mechanisms, diagnosis, and management* (2nd ed., pp. 323–356). Philadelphia: Lippincott Williams & Wilkins.
21. Reade, M. C. (2007). Temporary epicardial pacing after cardiac surgery: Part 1: General considerations in the management of epicardial pacing. *Anaesthesia, 62*, 264–271.
22. Bernstein, A. D., Daubert, J.-C., Fletcher, R. D., et al. (2002). The revised NASPE/BPEG generic code for antibradycardia, adaptive-rate, and multisite pacing. *Pacing and Clinical Electrophysiology, 25*, 260–264.
23. Barold, S. S., Stroobandt, R. X., & Sinnaeve, A. F. (2004). *Cardiac pacemakers step by step*. Malden, MA: Blackwell Futura.
24. Kenny, T. (2005). *The nuts and bolts of cardiac pacing*. Malden, MA: Blackwell Futura.
25. Pinski, S. L. (2007). Electromagnetic interference and implantable devices. In K. A. Ellenbogen, G. N. Kay, C.-P. Lau, et al. (Eds.), *Clinical cardiac pacing, defibrillation, and resynchronization therapy* (3rd ed., pp. 1149–1176). Philadelphia: Saunders Elsevier.
26. Wang, P. J., Chen, H., Okamura, H., et al. (2007). Timing cycles of implantable devices. In K. A. Ellenbogen, G. N. Kay, C.-P. Lau et al. (Eds.), *Clinical cardiac pacing, defibrillation, and resynchronization therapy* (3rd ed., pp. 969–1004). Philadelphia: Saunders Elsevier.
27. Love, C. J. (2007). Pacemaker troubleshooting and follow-up. In K. A. Ellenbogen, G. Kay, C.-P. Lau, et al. (Eds.), *Clinical cardiac pacing, defibrillation, and resynchronization therapy* (3rd ed., pp. 1005–1062). Philadelphia: Saunders Elsevier.
28. Tse, H.-F., & Lau, C.-P. (2007). Sensors for implantable devices: Ideal characteristics, sensor combinations, and automaticity. In K. A. Ellenbogen, G. N. Kay, C.-P. Lau, et al. (Eds.), *Clinical cardiac pacing, defibrillation, and resynchronization therapy* (3rd ed., pp. 201–233). Philadelphia: Saunders Elsevier.
29. Hasan, A., & Abraham, W. T. (2007). Cardiac resynchronization treatment of heart failure. *Annual Review of Medicine 58*, 63–74.
30. Flachskampf, F. A., & Voigt, J.-U. (2006). Echocardiographic methods to select candidates for cardiac resynchronisation therapy. *Heart, 92*, 424–429.
31. Sogaard, P., Egeblad, H., Pedersen, A. K., et al. (2002). Sequential versus simultaneous biventricular resynchronization for severe heart failure: Evaluation by tissue Doppler imaging. *Circulation, 106*, 2078–2084.
32. van Gelder, B. M., Bracke, F. A., Lakerveld, L. J. M., et al. (2004). Effect of optimizing the V-V interval on left ventricular contractility in cardiac resynchronization therapy. *American Journal of Cardiology, 93*(12), 1500–1503.
33. Young, J., Abraham, W. T., Smith, A. L., et al. (2003). Combined cardiac resynchronization and implantable cardioversion defibrillation in advanced chronic heart failure: The MIRACLE ICD Trial. *JAMA, 289*(20), 2685–2694.
34. Bristow, M., Saxon, L. A., Boehmer, J., et al., for the comparison of medical therapy. (2004). Cardiac-resynchronization therapy with or without an implantable defibrillator in advanced chronic heart failure. *New England Journal of Medicine, 350*(21), 2140–2150.
35. Cleland, J. G., Daubert, J.-C., Erdmann, E., et al. (2005). Cardiac Resynchronization in Heart Failure (CARE-HF) Study Investigators: The effect of cardiac resynchronization on morbidity and mortality in heart failure. *New England Journal of Medicine, 352*, 1539–1549.
36. Linde, C., Leclercq, C., Rex, S., et al. (2002). Long-term benefits of biventricular pacing in congestive heart failure: Results from the MUltisite STimulation in Cardiomyopathy (MUSTIC) study. *Journal of the American College of Cardiology, 40*(1), 111–118.
37. Barold, S. S., Herweg, B., & Giudici, M. (2005). Electrocardiographic follow-up of biventricular pacemakers. *Annals of Noninvasive Electrocardiology, 10*(2), 231–255.
38. Sweeney, M. O., Hellkamp, A., Ellenbogen, K. A., et al. (2003). Adverse effect of ventricular pacing on heart failure and atrial fibrillation among patients with normal baseline QRS duration in a clinical trial of pacemaker therapy for sinus node dysfunction. *Circulation, 107*, 2932–2937.
39. Sweeney, M. O., & Hellkamp, A. S. (2006). Heart failure during cardiac pacing. *Circulation, 113*, 2082–2088.
40. Wilkoff, B., Cook, J., Epstein, A., et al. (2002). Dual-chamber pacing or ventricular backup pacing in patients with an implantable defibrillator: The Dual chamber and VVI Implantable Defibrillator (DAVID) Trial. *JAMA, 288*(24), 3115–3123.

41. Lamas, G. A., Lee, K. L., Sweeney, M. O., et al. (2002). Ventricular pacing or dual-chamber pacing for sinus-node dysfunction. *New England Journal of Medicine, 346*(24), 1854–1862.
42. Ritter, O., Koller, M. L., Fey, B., et al. (2006). Progression of heart failure in right univentricular pacing compared to biventricular pacing. *International Journal of Cardiology, 110*, 359–365.
43. Manolis, A. S. (2006). The deleterious consequences of right ventricular apical pacing: Time to seek alternate site pacing. *Pacing and Clinical Electrophysiology, 29*(3), 298–315.
44. Healey, J. S., Morillo, C. A., & Connolly, S. J. (2007). Clinical trials of pacing modes. In K. A. Ellenbogen, G. N. Kay, C.-P. Lau, et al. (Eds.), *Clinical cardiac pacing, defibrillation, and resynchronization therapy* (3rd ed., pp. 337–356). Philadelphia: Saunders Elsevier.
45. Olshansky, B., Day, J., McGuire, M., et al. (2005). Inhibition of unnecessary RV pacing with AV search hysteresis in ICDs (INTRINSIC RV): Design and clinical protocol. *Pacing and Clinical Electrophysiology, 28*, 62–66.
46. Olshansky, B., Day, J. D., Moore, S., et al. (2007). Is dual-chamber programming inferior to single-chamber programming in an implantable cardioverter-defibrillator? Results of the INTRINSIC RV (Inhibition of Unnecessary RV Pacing With AVSH in ICDs) Study. *Circulation, 115*, 9–16.
47. Sweeney, M. O., Ellenbogen, K. A., Casavant, D., et al. (2005). Multicenter, prospective, randomized safety and efficacy study of a new atrial-based managed ventricular pacing mode (MVP) in dual chamber ICDs. *Journal of Cardiovascular Electrophysiology, 16*, 811–817.
48. Byrd, C. L. (2007). Managing device-related complications and transvenous lead extraction. In K. A. Ellenbogen, G. N. Kay, C.-P. Lau, et al. (Eds.), *Clinical cardiac pacing, defibrillation, and resynchronization therapy* (3rd ed., pp. 855–930). Philadelphia: Saunders Elsevier.
49. Bailey, S. M., & Wilkoff, B. L. (2006). Complications of pacemakers and defibrillators in the elderly. *American Journal of Geriatric Cardiology, 15*(2), 102–107.
50. Moss, A. J., Zareba, W., Hall, W. J., et al. (2002) for the Multicenter Automatic Defibrillator Implantation Trial II Investigators. Prophylactic implantation of a defibrillator in patients with myocardial infarction and reduced ejection fraction. *New England Journal of Medicine, 346*(12), 877–883.
51. Bardy, G. H., Lee K. L, Mark D. B., et al. (2005). Amiodarone or an implantable cardioverter defibrillator for congestive heart failure. *New England Journal of Medicine, 352*, 225–237.
52. Mirowski, M. (1985). The automatic implantable cardioverter-defibrillator: An overview. *American Journal of Cardiology, 6*, 461–466.
53. Gold, M. R. (2000). ICD therapy in the new millennium. *Cardiology Clinics, 18*(2), 375–389.
54. Swerdlow, C. D., Gillberg, J. M., & Olson, W. H. (2007). Sensing and detection. In K. A. Ellenbogen, G. N. Kay, C. P. Lau, et al. (Eds.), *Clinical cardiac pacing, defibrillation, and resynchronization therapy* (pp. 75–160). Philadelphia: Saunders Elsevier.
55. Goldberger, Z., & Lampert, R. (2006). Implantable cardioverter-defibrillators–expanding indications and technologies. *JAMA, 295*(7), 809–818.
56. Zipes, D. P., Camm, A. J., et al. (2006). ACC/AHA/ESC 2006 guidelines for management of patients with ventricular arrhythmias and the prevention of sudden cardiac death—executive summary. *Journal of the American College of Cardiology, 48*(5), 1064–1108.
57. Gehi, A. K., Mehta, D., & Gomes, J. A. (2006). Evaluation and management of patients after implantable cardioverter–defibrillator shock. *JAMA, 296*(23), 2839–2847.
58. Podrid, P. J., & Myerburg, R. J. (2005). Epidemiology and stratification of risk for sudden cardiac death. *Clinical Cardiology, 28*, 3–11.
59. Siddiqui, A., & Kowey, P. R. (2006). Sudden death secondary to cardiac arrhythmias: Mechanisms and treatment strategies. *Current Opinion in Cardiology, 21*, 517–525.
60. Cobb, L. A., Baum, R. S., Alvarez, H., et al. (1975). Resuscitation from out-of-hospital ventricular fibrillation: 4-year follow-up. *Circulation, 52*(Suppl. III), 23.
61. Cappato, R. (1999). Secondary prevention of sudden death: The Dutch Study, the Antiarrhythmic Versus Implantable Defibrillator Study. *American Journal of Cardiology, 83*(Suppl.), 68D–73D.
62. The Antiarrhythmics vs. Implantable Defibrillators (AVID) Investigators. (1997). A comparison of antiarrhythmic drug therapy with implantable defibrillators in patients resuscitated from near fatal ventricular arrhythmias. *New England Journal of Medicine, 337*, 1576–1583.
63. Kuck, K. H., Cappato, R., Siebels, J., et al. (2000). Randomized comparison of antiarrhythmic drug therapy with implantable defibrillators in patients resuscitated from cardiac arrest: The Cardiac Arrest Study Hamburg (CASH). *Circulation, 102*, 748–754.
64. Connolly, S. J., Gent, M., Roberts, R. S., et al. (2000). Canadian Implantable Defibrillator Study (CIDS): A randomized trial of the implantable cardioverter defibrillator against amiodarone. *Circulation, 101*, 1297–1302.
65. Engelstein, E. D. (2003). Prevention and management of chronic heart failure with electrical therapy. *American Journal of Cardiology, 91*(9A), 62–73.
66. Wathen, M. (2007). Implantable cardioverter defibrillator shock reduction using new antitachycardia pacing therapies. *American Heart Journal, 153*(4, Suppl. 1), 44–52.
67. Schoels, W., Steinhaus, D., Johnson, W. B., et al. (2007). Optimizing implantable cardioverter-defibrillator treatment of rapid ventricular tachycardia: Antitachycardia pacing therapy during charging. *Heart Rhythm, 4*(7), 879–885.
68. Bass, E. B., Elson, J. J., Fogoros, R. N., et al. (1988). Long-term prognosis of patients undergoing electrophysiologic studies for syncope of unknown origin. *American Journal of Cardiology, 62*, 1186–1191.
69. Moss, A., Hall, J., Cannom, D. et al., for the Multicenter Automatic Defibrillator Implantation Trial. (1996). Improved survival with an implanted defibrillator in patients with coronary disease at high risk for ventricular arrhythmia. *New England Journal of Medicine, 335*, 1933–1940.
70. Kadish, A., Dyer, A., Daubert, J. P., et al. (2004). Prophylactic defibrillator implantation in patients with non-ischemic dilated cardiomyopathy. *New England Journal of Medicine, 350*, 2151–2158.
71. Hohnloser, S. H., Kuck, K. H., Dorian, P., et al. (2004). Prophylactic use of an implantable cardioverter-defibrillator after acute myocardial infarction. *New England Journal of Medicine, 351*(24), 2481–2488.
72. Dimarco, J. P. (2003). Implantable cardioverter-defibrillators. *New England Journal of Medicine, 349*, 1836–1847.
73. Kroll, M.W., & Levine P. A. (2007). Pacemaker and implantable cardioverter-defibrillator circuitry. In K. Ellenbogen, G. N. Kay, C. P. Lau, et al. (Eds.), *Clinical cardiac pacing, defibrillation; and resynchronization therapy* (pp. 261–278). Philadelphia: Saunders Elsevier.
74. St. Jude Medical. (2005). What's Inside and ICD (Brochure). Sylmar, CA.
75. Kleemann, T., Becker, T., Doenges, S., et al. (2007). Annual rate of transvenous defibrillation lead defects in implantable cardioverter-defibrillators over a period of >10 years. *Circulation, 115*, 2474–2480.
76. Henry, P. D., & Pacifico, A. (2002). Defibrillator leads. In A. Pacifico (Ed.), *Implantable defibrillator therapy: A clinical guide* (pp. 43–62). Boston: Kluwer Academic Publishers.
77. Russo, A. M., & Marchlinski, F. E. (2007). Engineering and construction of pacemaker and implantable cardioverter-defibrillator leads. In K. Ellenbogen, G. N. Kay, C. P. Lau, et al. (Eds.), *Clinical cardiac pacing, defibrillation, and resynchronization therapy* (pp. 161–200). Philadelphia: Saunders Elsevier.
78. Bardy, G. H., Johnson, G., Poole, J. E., et al. (1993). A simplified, single-lead unipolar transvenous cardioversion-defibrillation system. *Circulation, 88*, 543–547.
79. Glikson, M., Swerdlow, C. D., Gurevitz, O. T., et al. (2005). Optimal combination of discriminators for differentiating ventricular from supraventricular tachycardia by dual chamber defibrillators. *Journal of Cardiovascular Electrophysiology, 16*, 732–739.
80. Zivin, A. Z., & Bardy, G. H. (2002). Device testing and programming at implant. In A. Pacifico (Ed.), *Implantable defibrillator therapy: A clinical guide.* (pp. 113–137). Boston: Kluwer Academic Publishers.
81. Klein, G. J., Gillberg, J. M., Tang, A., et al. (2006). Improving SVT discrimination in single-chamber ICDs: A new electrogram morphology based algorithm. *Journal of Cardiovascular Electrophysiology, 17*(12), 1310–1319.
82. Theuns, D. A., Rivero-Ayerza, M., Goedhart, D. M., et al. (2006). Evaluation of morphology discrimination for ventricular tachycardia diagnosis in implantable cardioverter-defibrillators. *Heart Rhythm Society, 3*(11), 1332–1338.
83. Russo, A. M., & Marchlinski, F. E. (2002). Long-term follow-up. In A. Pacifico (Ed.), *Implantable defibrillator therapy: A clinical guide* (pp. 161–243). Boston: Kluwer Academic Publishers.
84. Sweeney, M. O., Wathen, M. S., & Volosin, K. (2005). Appropriate and inappropriate ventricular therapies, quality of life, and mortality among primary and secondary prevention implantable cardioverter defibrillator patients: Results from the pacing fast VT Reduces Shock ThErapies (PainFREE Rx II) trial. *Circulation, 111*, 2898–2905.
85. Wathen, M. S., DeGroot, M. S., Sweeney, M. O., et al. (2004). Prospective randomized multicenter trial of empirical antitachycardia pacing versus shocks for spontaneous rapid ventricular tachycardia in patients with implantable cardioverter-defibrillators: Pacing fast ventricular tachycardia reduces shock therapies (PainFREE Rx II) trial results. *Circulation, 110*, 2591–2596.

86. Wilkoff, B. L., Ousdigian, K. T., Sterns. L. D., et al. (2006). A comparison of empiric to physician-tailored programming of implantable cardioverter-defibrillators. *Journal of the American College of Cardiology, 48*(2), 330–339.
87. Kenny, T. (2006). *The nuts and bolts of ICD therapy.* Waltham, MA: Blackwell Publishing.
88. Hammill, S. C., Stevenson, L. W., Kadish, A. H., et al. (2007). National ICD registry annual report 2006—Review of the registry's first year, data collected, and future plans. *Heart Rhythm Society, 4*(9), 1260–1263.
89. Rasmussen, M. J., Friedman, P. A., Hammill, S. C., et al. (2002). Unintentional deactivation of implantable cardioverter-defibrillators in health care settings. *Mayo Clinic Proceedings, 77,* 855–859.
90. Boston Scientific. (2006). Safety advisory: Original communication 23 June 2005. *CRM product performance report* (pp. 76–77). St. Paul, MN: Author.
91. Kroll, M. W., & Tchou, P. J. (2007). Testing and programming of implantable defibrillator functions at implantation. In K. A. Ellenbogen, G. N. Kay, C. P. Lau, et al. (Eds.), *Clinical cardiac pacing, defibrillation, and resynchronization therapy* (pp. 531–557). Philadelphia: Saunders Elsevier.
92. Allen, M. (2006). Review article: Pacemakers and implantable cardioverter defibrillators. *Anesthesia, 61,* 883–890.
93. Epstein, A. E. (2007). Troubleshooting of implantable cardioverter-defibrillator. In K. Ellenbogen, G. N. Kay, C. P. Lau, et al. (Eds.), *Clinical cardiac pacing, defibrillation, and resynchronization therapy* (pp. 1063–1086). Philadelphia: Saunders Elsevier.
94. McPherson, C. A., & Manthouos, C. (2004). Update in nonpulmonary critical care: Permanent pacemakers and implantable defibrillators—consideration for intensivists. *American Journal of Respiratory and Critical Care Medicine, 170,* 933–940.
95. Hayes, D. L. (2000). Electromagnetic interference and implantable defibrillators. In D. L. Hayes, M. A. Lloyd, & P. A. Friedman (Eds.), *Cardiac pacing and defibrillation: A clinical approach* (pp. 519–539). Elmsford, NY: Blackwell Publishing Inc.
96. Sears, S. F., Vasquez Sowell, L. D., Kuhl, E. A., et al. (2007). The ICD shock and stress management program: A randomized trial of psychosocial treatment to optimize quality of life in ICD patients. *Pacing and Clinical Electrophysiology, 30*(7), 858–864.
97. Sears, S. F., Shea, J. B., & Conti J. B. (2005). How to respond to an implantable cardioverter-defibrillator shock. *Circulation, 111,* e380–e382.
98. Thomas, S. A., Friedman, E., & Kao, C. W. (2006). Quality of life and psychological status of patients with implantable cardioverter defibrillators. *American Journal of Critical Care, 15*(4), 389–398.
99. Dougherty, C. M., Pyper, G. P., & Frasz, H. A. (2004). Description of a nursing intervention program after an implantable cardioverter defibrillator. *Heart and Lung, 33*(3), 183–190.
100. Pederson, S. S., Van Den Broek, K. C., & Sears, S. F. (2007). Psychological intervention following implantation of an implantable defibrillator: A review and future recommendations. *Pacing and Clinical Electrophysiology, 30*(12), 1546–1554.
101. Sears, S. F., & Conti, J. B. (2006). Psychological aspects of cardiac devices and recalls in patients with implantable cardioverter defibrillators. *American Journal of Cardiology, 98,* 565–567.
102. Schron, E. B., Exner, D. V., Yao, Q., et al. (2002). Quality of life in the antiarrhythmics versus implantable defibrillator trial: Impact of therapy and influences of adverse symptoms and defibrillator shocks. *Circulation, 105,* 589–594.
103. Wallace, R. L., Sears, S. F., Lewis, T. S., et al. (2002). Predictors of quality of life in long-term recipients of implantable cardioverter defibrillators. *Journal of Cardiopulmonary Rehabilitation, 22,* 278–281.
104. Abraham, W. T., Young, J. B., Leon, A. R., et al. (2004). Effects of cardiac resynchronization on disease progression in patient with left ventricular systolic dysfunction, an indication for an implantable cardioverter-defibrillator, and mildly symptomatic chronic heart failure. *Circulation, 110,* 2864–2868.
105. Epstein, A. E., Baessler, C. A., Curtis, A. B., et al. (2007). Addendum to "personal and public safety issues related to arrhythmias that may affect consciousness: Implication for regulation and physician recommendations: A medical/scientific statement from the American Heart Association and the North American Society of Pacing an Electrophysiology." A scientific statement from the AHA and Heart Rhythm Society. *Heart Rhythm, 4*(3), 386–393.
106. Cambre, S., & Silverman, M. E. (1993). Is it safe to drive with an automatic implantable cardioverter defibrillator or a history of recurrent symptomatic ventricular arrhythmias? *Heart Disease and Stroke, 2,* 179–181.
107. Stevenson, W. G., Chaitman, B. R., Ellenbogen, K. A. et al. (2004). AHA Science Advisory: Clinical assessment and management of patients with implanted cardioverter-defibrillators presenting to nonelectrophysiologists. *Circulation, 110,* 3866–3869.
108. Lloyd, M. A., Hayes, D. L, & Friedman, P. A. (2000). Troubleshooting. In D. L. Hayes, M. A. Lloyd, & P. A. Friedman (Eds.), *Cardiac pacing and defibrillation: A clinical approach* (pp. 345–451). Elmsford, NY: Blackwell Publishing, Inc.
109. Carlson, M. D. et al. (2006). Recommendations from the Heart Rhythm Society Task Force on Device Performance Polices and Guidelines. Endorsed by the American College of Cardiology Foundation (ACCF) and the American Heart Association (AHA) and the International Coalition of Pacing and Electrophysiology Organizations (COPE). *Heart Rhythm, 3*(10), 1250–1273.
110. Hernandez, A. F., Fonarow, G. H., Liang, L., et al. (2007). Sex and racial differences in the use of implantable cardioverter-defibrillators among patients hospitalized with heart failure. *JAMA, 298*(13), 1525–1532.
111. Smaha, L. A. (2004). The American Heart Association get with the guidelines program. *American Heart Journal, 148*(5), S46–S48.
112. Goldstein, N. E., Lampert, R., Bradley, E., et al. (2004). Management of implantable cardioverter defibrillators in end-of-life care. *Annals of Internal Medicine, 141,* 835–838.
113. Rich, M. W., Curtis, A. B. for the PRICE-IV Investigators. (2007). Fourth pivotal research in cardiology in the elderly (PRICE-IV) symposium—Electrophysiology and heart rhythm disorders in the elderly; mechanisms and management. *The American Journal of Geriatric Cardiology, 16*(5), 304–314.
114. Burke, M. C., Coman, J. A., Cates, A. W., et al. (2005). Defibrillation energy requirements using a left anterior chest cutaneous to subcutaneous shocking vector: Implication for a total subcutaneous implantable defibrillator. *Heart Rhythm, 2,* 1332–1338.

CHAPTER 29

Acquired Valvular Heart Disease

Denise Ledoux

DEFINITION, CLASSIFICATION, AND EPIDEMIOLOGY

Valvular heart disease continues to be a common source of cardiac dysfunction and mortality. Competent cardiac valves maintain a unidirectional flow of blood through the heart as well as to the pulmonary and systemic circulations. Diseased cardiac valves that restrict the forward flow of blood because they are unable to open fully are referred to as *stenotic.* Stenotic valves elevate afterload and cause hypertrophy of the atria or ventricles pumping against the increased pressure. Cardiac valves that close incompetently and permit the backward flow of blood are referred to as *regurgitant, incompetent,* or *insufficient.* Regurgitant valves cause an elevated volume load and dilation of the cardiac chambers receiving the blood reflux. Valvular dysfunction may be primarily stenotic or regurgitant, or may be "mixed," which refers to a valve that neither opens nor closes adequately. Valvular heart disease is usually described by the duration of the dysfunction (acute vs. chronic), the valves involved, and the nature of the valvular dysfunction (stenosis, insufficiency, or a combination of stenosis and insufficiency). The degree of cardiac dysfunction is defined by the New York Heart Association's (NYHA) Functional and Therapeutic Classification. Acquired valvular heart disease most commonly affects, and is most symptomatic with, the aortic and mitral valves. This chapter focuses on the mitral and aortic valves, with a brief discussion of tricuspid valve disease. Because the cause of pulmonic disease is primarily congenital, it is described in Chapter 31.

CAUSES OF ACQUIRED VALVULAR HEART DISEASE

Rheumatic Heart Disease

Rheumatic fever is an acute autoimmune disorder that results as a complication of streptococcal upper respiratory tract infections. Tissues involved in rheumatic fever include the lining and valves of the heart, skin, and connective tissue (Fig. 29-1). The group A β-hemolytic streptococcal organism is responsible for initial and recurrent attacks of rheumatic fever. Lymphatic channels from the tonsils are thought to transmit group A streptococci to the heart.

The incidence of rheumatic fever has declined to less than 1/100,000 in industrialized nations but remains higher than 100/100,000 in endemic, less developed countries.[1] Reasons for the decline in rheumatic fever include the use of antibiotics to treat and prevent streptococcal infections, as well as improved social conditions such as decreased crowding, better housing and sanitation, and access to health care. Rheumatic fever persists in underdeveloped countries in which socioeconomic conditions enable the spread of streptococcal bacteria and limit access to adequate health care. Acute rheumatic fever involves diffuse exudative and proliferative inflammatory reactions in the heart, joints, and skin.

Jones criteria, based on expert opinion rather than clinical trials, were introduced in 1944 for the diagnosis of rheumatic fever. Major diagnostic criteria include carditis, polyarthritis, chorea, erythema marginatum (pink skin rash), and subcutaneous nodules. Minor criteria include arthralgia, fever, and elevated C-reactive protein.[1]

Carditis is the most important clinical manifestation of acute rheumatic fever, causing inflammation of the endocardium, myocardium, and pericardium. Myocarditis is characterized by interstitial inflammation that may affect cardiac conduction. Endocarditis causes extensive inflammatory changes, resulting in scarring of the heart valves and acute heart failure. Warty lesions of eosinophilic material build-up at the bases and edges of the valves. As the lesions progress, granulation tissue and subsequent vascularization develop, and fibrosis occurs. The annulus, cusps, and chordae tendineae are scarred and, as a result, they thicken and shorten. Acute heart failure develops because of interstitial myocarditis. Fibrinoid degeneration develops, followed by the appearance of Aschoff nodules, the characteristic pathologic lesion of acute rheumatic fever. As Aschoff nodules heal, fibrous scars remain. In severe cases, death from acute heart failure may result. Carditis frequently does not cause any symptoms and is detected only when the patient seeks help because of arthritis or chorea.

Auscultatory signs of aortic and mitral insufficiency are frequently apparent. In more than 90% of patients with carditis, the mitral valve is affected. When the mitral valve is affected, there may be a high-pitched, blowing, pansystolic murmur. A Carey Coombs murmur, a low-pitched, mid-diastolic murmur of short duration, may be noted at the apex. The Carey Coombs murmur may be attributed to swelling and stiffening of mitral valve leaflets, increased flow across the valve, and alteration in left ventricular compliance.

Rheumatic fever can be prevented by aggressive treatment of the initial episode of streptococcal pharyngitis: penicillin G, 500 mg as the first dose and then 250 mg four times daily for a duration of 10 days. If the patient is allergic to penicillin, erythromycin or cephalosporins may be used. Effective antibiotic treatment started less than 10 days after the onset of infection almost completely eliminates the risk of rheumatic fever.[1]

Infective Endocarditis

Infective endocarditis is an endovascular infection that supports continuous bacteremia from the source of the infection, usually a vegetation on a heart valve.[2] While endocarditis is uncommon, affecting

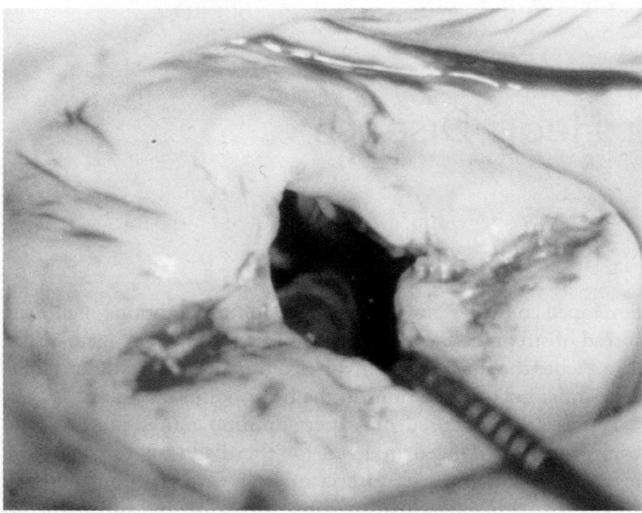

■ **Figure 29-1** Rheumatic mitral valve with leaflet thickening and commissural fusion. (From Alpert, J. S., Sabick, J., & Cosgrove, D. M. [1998]. Mitral valve disease. In E. J. Topol, R. M. Califf, J. M. Isner, et al. [Eds.], *Textbook of cardiovascular medicine* [p. 511]. Philadelphia: Lippincott-Raven.)

only 10,000 to 20,000 people in the United States each year, it may result in serious complications such as stroke, need for surgery, and death.[3] Although incidence of infective endocarditis is low, between 1.5 and 6 cases per 100 cases per year, morbidity and mortality are high.[4] In intravenous drug users, the risk for endocarditis is 2% to 5% per patient-year.[5] Rheumatic heart disease, calcific aortic stenosis, hypertrophic cardiomyopathy, congenital heart disease, and the presence of prosthetic heart valves predispose to endocarditis. Intravenous drug abusers are at risk for infective endocarditis caused by recurrent bacteremias related to injection from contaminated needles and localized infections at injection sites. Patients with long-term intravenous lines or dialysis catheters are also at increased risk. Acute endocarditis can also occur in normal heart valves from infection somewhere else in the body In patients with community-acquired, native valve endocarditis, *Staphylococcus aureus* exceeds streptococci as the causative pathogen.[5] Pathogens that are most commonly responsible for subacute endocarditis include streptococci, enterococci, coagulase-negative staphylococci, and the HACEK group of organisms (*Haemophilus* species, *Actinobacillus actinomycetemcomitans*, *Cardiobacterium hominis*, *Eikenella* species, and *Kingella kingae*). Clinical presentations of endocarditis range from fever and malaise to symptoms related to systemic emboli (Table 29-1).

The pathologic process of endocarditis requires that several conditions exist to permit infection to grow in the heart and to promote an environment that supports growth on the endocardial surface. For endocarditis to develop, there is first endocardial injury with thrombus formation at the site. Transient or persistent bacteremia allows bacteria to adhere to the injured surface. Infected vegetations result and may fragment and embolize.[5] The complications of infective endocarditis include congestive heart failure (CHF), paravalvular abscess formation, embolic events to the brain or other organs, sepsis, pericarditis, renal failure, and metastatic abscesses.[4] The reduction in mortality for infective endocarditis over the past 30 years from 25% to 30% down to 10% to 20% may be largely related to

Table 29-1 ■ CLINICAL MANIFESTATIONS OF INFECTIVE ENDOCARDITIS

Symptoms	Physical Examination Findings
Fever	Fever
Chills and sweats	Changing or new heart murmur
Malaise	Evidence of systemic emboli
Weight loss	Splenomegaly
Anorexia	Janeway lesions (small hemorrhages on palms or soles of feet)
Stroke symptoms	
Myalgias	Splinter hemorrhages (hemorrhagic streaks at finger nail tips)
Arthralgias	
Confusion	Osler's nodules (small, tender nodules on finger or toe pads)
CHF	

aggressive surgical intervention in cases complicated by CHF, invasive abscesses, and prosthetic valve infections.[6]

Blood cultures are an essential diagnostic tool in infective endocarditis. Three separate sets of blood cultures drawn from different venipuncture sites, obtained over 24 hours, usually identify the organism. Patients with infective endocarditis whose cultures remain negative may have fastidious organisms or may have received intravenous antibiotics before blood samples were drawn. In acute endocarditis, antibiotic therapy should be started after blood cultures have been obtained using strict aseptic technique and optimal skin preparation.[2] The clinical approach in acute endocarditis includes appropriate antibiotics and monitoring for complications (Display 29-1). The usual course is 6 full weeks of intravenous antibiotics. Patients who do not respond well to standard antibiotic therapy may be referred for surgical valve replacement (Display 29-2).

Echocardiography is frequently used to verify the presence of vegetations on the valves (Fig. 29-2). Transesophageal echocardiography (TEE) provides better resolution and can identify smaller vegetations than transthoracic echocardiography (TTE).[5] TEE is also useful to identify paravalvular leaks and annular abscesses seen in prosthetic valve endocarditis. Although TEE is more sensitive, some clinicians recommend to obtain TTE first and to perform TEE only if the TTE images are inadequate or suspicion of infective endocarditis remains high and the initial TTE was negative.[7]

DISPLAY 29-1 Clinical Approach to Endocarditis

- Establish diagnosis
  - Blood cultures
  - Physical examination findings
  - Echocardiography
  - Establish source that seeded endocarditis
- Start appropriate antibiotics based on blood cultures
- Monitor telemetry for conduction defects
- Treat valvular regurgitation with afterload reduction agents
- Repeat blood cultures 3 days after antibiotics started to ensure response
- Insert long-term intravenous access for antibiotics
- Monitor drug levels when appropriate
- Monitor for systemic emboli

DISPLAY 29-2 Indications for Cardiac Surgery in Infective Endocarditis

Heart failure with hemodynamic instability
Persistent bacteremia and fever despite optimal antibiotic therapy
Paravalvular abscess or fistula
Recurrence of endocarditis after full course of antibiotics
Systemic emboli
Heart failure due to prosthetic valvular dysfunction
Valve dehiscence (in prosthetic valvular endocarditis)
New conduction system defects
Fungal endocarditis

The American College of Cardiology/American Heart Association (ACC/AHA) guidelines now recommend antibiotic prophylaxis for patients with prosthetic cardiac valves or rings; previous endocarditis; unrepaired cyanotic congenital heart disease; repaired congenital heart disease with prosthetic material or residual defects adjacent to prosthetic device or patch; and cardiac transplant recipients.[8]

Miscellaneous Causes of Valvular Disease

Degenerative changes of the tissue, such as myxomatous degeneration, calcification, and changes associated with Marfan syndrome, can cause valvular dysfunction. Trauma or infection may affect the supportive or subvalvular apparatus. Dilation of the ventricles caused by chronically elevated preloading may dilate an atrioventricular valve opening to the point that the leaflets no longer approximate and the valve becomes incompetent. Coronary heart disease (CHD) and myocardial infarction can affect the papillary muscles of the right and left ventricles, causing either dysfunction caused by ischemia or frank flail of atrioventricular valve leaflets caused by papillary muscle rupture. Systemic diseases such as lupus erythematosus and scleroderma may also cause valvular dysfunction (see Display 29-3).

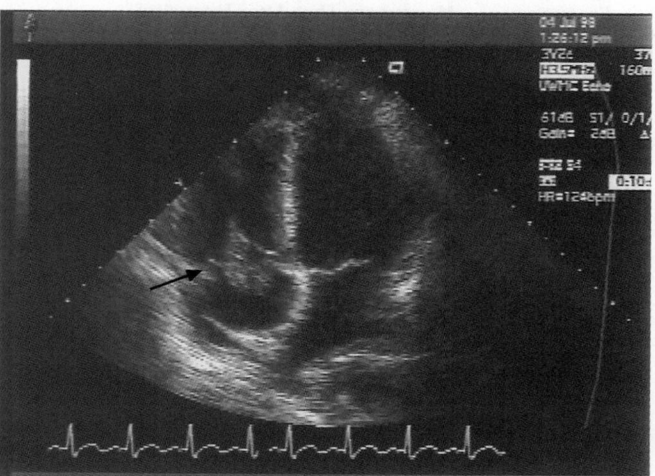

Figure 29-2 Two-dimensional echocardiogram view of vegetation on tricuspid valve in 27-year-old woman with endocarditis (*arrow*).

DISPLAY 29-3 Risk Factors for Infective Endocarditis

Recent dental procedure or periodontal disease
History of congenital heart disease
History of valvular heart disease
Long-term, in-dwelling intravenous line
Genitourinary infections or instrumentation
Prosthetic valve (mechanical or biologic)
History of intravenous drug abuse
Hemodialysis

DIAGNOSTIC TESTING FOR VALVULAR HEART DISEASE

The diagnosis of valvular heart disease is based on patient history, physical assessment, and diagnostic testing. Some tests, such as the electrocardiogram and the chest radiograph, may be relatively insensitive in diagnosing valvular heart disease, even though they are part of the standard screening tests in patients with heart dysfunction. Both TTE and TEE are used to identify and quantify valvular heart disease. Diagnostic findings for specific valvular lesions are noted in the sections discussing each abnormality.

MITRAL STENOSIS

Cause

The predominant cause of mitral stenosis is rheumatic fever. The mitral valve is the valve most often damaged by rheumatic carditis.[9] Rheumatic fever causes thickening and decreased mobility of the mitral valve leaflets associated with fusion of the commissures and destruction of normal leaflet structure. Other conditions that simulate the physiology of mitral stenosis include left atrial myxoma, ball-valve left atrial thrombus, large left atrial endocarditis vegetations, or cor triatriatum (three atria).[10]

Pathology

The rheumatic process causes the mitral valve to become fibrinous, resulting in leaflet thickening, commissural or chordal fusion, and calcification. As a result, the mitral valve apparatus becomes funnel shaped with a narrowed orifice. Fusion of the mitral valve commissures results in narrowing of the principal orifice, whereas interchordal fusion obliterates the secondary orifices.

Pathophysiology

Women have mitral stenosis more frequently than men. The normal mitral valve area is 4 to 6 cm^2. Once the cross-sectional area of the mitral valve is reduced to 2 cm^2 or less, a pressure gradient between the left atrium and left ventricle occurs. The reduced orifice impedes left atrial emptying. Increased left atrial pressure and dilation occurs along with left atrial hypertrophy in an attempt to maintain normal diastolic flow into the left ventricle. Increased left atrial pressure is transmitted to the pulmonary circuit, resulting in pulmonary hypertension and pulmonary congestion. Left atrial enlargement may lead to atrial fibrillation and worsening of symptoms related to the loss of atrial kick.[10] Patients have left-sided CHF without left ventricular dysfunction. Mitral stenosis has a sparing effect on the left ventricle. Symptoms of mitral stenosis are usually related to obstruction of the mitral valve rather than ventricular dysfunction. As pulmonary pressure increases, right-sided heart failure may occur.

Clinical Manifestations

Mild dyspnea on exertion occurs as the most common symptom of mild mitral stenosis (valve area of 1.6 to 2.0 cm^2). As mitral stenosis becomes more severe (valve area of 1 to 1.5 cm^2), dyspnea, fatigue, paroxysmal nocturnal dyspnea, and atrial fibrillation may occur. When mitral stenosis becomes severe (valve area of 1 cm^2 or less), symptoms include fatigue and dyspnea with mild exertion or rest. With advanced mitral stenosis, pulmonary hypertension and symptoms of right-sided heart failure occur (i.e., edema, hepatomegaly, ascites, elevated jugular venous pressure). Chest pain and hemoptysis may also occur. Increased left atrial pressure, atrial fibrillation, and stagnation of left atrial blood flow can result in the formation of mural thrombi, with resultant embolic events, including cerebral vascular accidents. Women who had previously been asymptomatic with mitral stenosis may become symptomatic and even experience severe hemodynamic decompensation during pregnancy due to increased cardiac output and increased heart rate. Tachycardia reduces diastolic filling time and worsens the mitral valve gradient while atrial fibrillation may precipitate pulmonary edema.[11]

Physical Assessment

In severe mitral stenosis, on auscultation, there are four typical findings including (1) an accentuated S_1; (2) an opening diastolic snap; (3) a middiastolic rumble noted best at the apex (in sinus rhythm), followed by presystolic accentuation; and (4) an increased pulmonic S_2 intensity associated with pulmonary hypertension (Table 29-2).

Patients with mitral stenosis may exhibit malar blush (pink discoloration of the cheeks). Patients with severe mitral stenosis may have weak pulses secondary to reduced cardiac output. The apical pulse is tapping in quality and is nondisplaced. A lower left parasternal lift or heave caused by right ventricular hypertrophy may be present. Cardiac rhythm is often irregularly irregular, indicating atrial fibrillation.

Diagnostic Tests

Echocardiography is used in the evaluation of mitral stenosis to (1) quantify the valve area and gradient; (2) quantify the degree of mitral insufficiency; (3) define the degree of left atrial enlargement; (4) assess mitral annular calcification; (5) assess pulmonary artery pressures and degree of pulmonary hypertension; and (6) evaluate right- and left-sided ventricular function. A TEE provides better detail of the mitral valve and better visualization of atrial thrombus than does TTE.[12]

Cardiac catheterization is used less in diagnosis of mitral stenosis as echocardiography techniques improve. Cardiac catheterization does allow for accurate assessment of valve area and can also identify associated mitral regurgitation. For patients with known or suspected CHD, coronary angiography can delineate coronary anatomy. Right heart catheterization can evaluate right heart and pulmonary artery pressures.

Electrocardiography is nonspecific and does not indicate the severity of mitral stenosis. If the patient remains in sinus rhythm and left atrial enlargement has occurred, characteristic P mitrale (broad, bifid P waves in leads II and V_1) may be identified. Right axis deviation and right ventricular hypertrophy may be noted in severe mitral stenosis. Atrial fibrillation is common in patients with long-standing mitral stenosis and is usually coarse in appearance.

Chest radiography correlates with the degree of mitral stenosis. As mitral stenosis becomes more severe, the chest radiograph demonstrates straightening of the left heart border caused by left

Table 29-2 ■ DIASTOLIC MURMURS IN ACQUIRED VALVULAR HEART DISEASE

Origin of Murmur	Auscultatory Location and Radiation	Configuration	Quality and Frequency	Maneuvers That Alter Intensity
Aortic insufficiency	Third and fourth left intercostal spaces	Decrescendo S_1 S_2 S_1	Blowing High pitched	Increases with isometric exercise and squatting Decreases with amyl nitrate and Valsalva maneuver
Mitral stenosis	Apex	Decrescendo Opening snap OS S_1 S_2 S_1	Rumbling Low pitched	Increases with expiration, squatting, amyl nitrate, and isometric exercise Decreases with Valsalva maneuver
Pulmonic insufficiency	Second left intercostal space	Crescendo-decrescendo S_1 S_2 S_1	Blowing High pitched	Increases with inspiration and amyl nitrate Decreases with Valsalva maneuver
Tricuspid stenosis	Parasternal at left fourth and fifth intercostal spaces	Decrescendo S_1 S_2 S_1	Rumbling Low pitched	Increases with inspiration, squatting, and amyl nitrate Decreases with Valsalva maneuver

atrial enlargement, elevation of the left mainstem bronchus caused by distention of the left atrium, and distribution of blood flow from the lower to upper lobes. Although heart size remains normal, central pulmonary arteries become prominent. Kerley B lines and interstitial edema are often present.

Medical Management

Medical therapy for mitral stenosis is aimed at preventing the complications of systemic embolization and bacterial endocarditis as well as atrial fibrillation if it occurs.[9] Patients who have asymptomatic mitral stenosis require only antibiotic prophylaxis. Patients with mild pulmonary congestion can be managed with diuretics alone. β-Blockers can be used to reduce heart rate and improve diastolic filling time. When patients have atrial fibrillation, digoxin, β-blockers, or calcium channel blockers can be used for ventricular response rate control. Patients with atrial fibrillation require anticoagulation to prevent thrombus formation in the atrium. Once the patient has symptoms of NYHA functional class III or IV despite adequate medical management, mechanical correction of mitral stenosis by balloon valvuloplasty or surgery should be performed.

Interventional and Surgical Management

Percutaneous Mitral Catheter Balloon Valvuloplasty

Percutaneous mitral catheter balloon valvuloplasty is an alternative, less invasive procedure than surgical treatment for mitral stenosis. Balloon valvuloplasty is performed in the cardiac catheterization laboratory by a cardiologist experienced with invasive techniques. A small balloon valvuloplasty catheter is introduced percutaneously at the femoral vein and passed into the right atrium. The catheter is then directed transseptally and positioned across the mitral valve. Mitral balloon valvuloplasty is recommended in patients with moderate-to-severe mitral stenosis that is symptomatic with favorable valve morphology.[10]

Inflation of either one large balloon (23 to 25 mm) or two smaller balloons (12 to 18 mm) stretches the valve leaflets (Fig. 29-3). Inflation of the balloon separates the fused commissures thus improving valve mobility. The best results from this technique to date have been in patients with rheumatic mitral stenosis with commissural fusion. An echocardiographic scoring system rates leaflet thickening, leaflet mobility, calcification, and

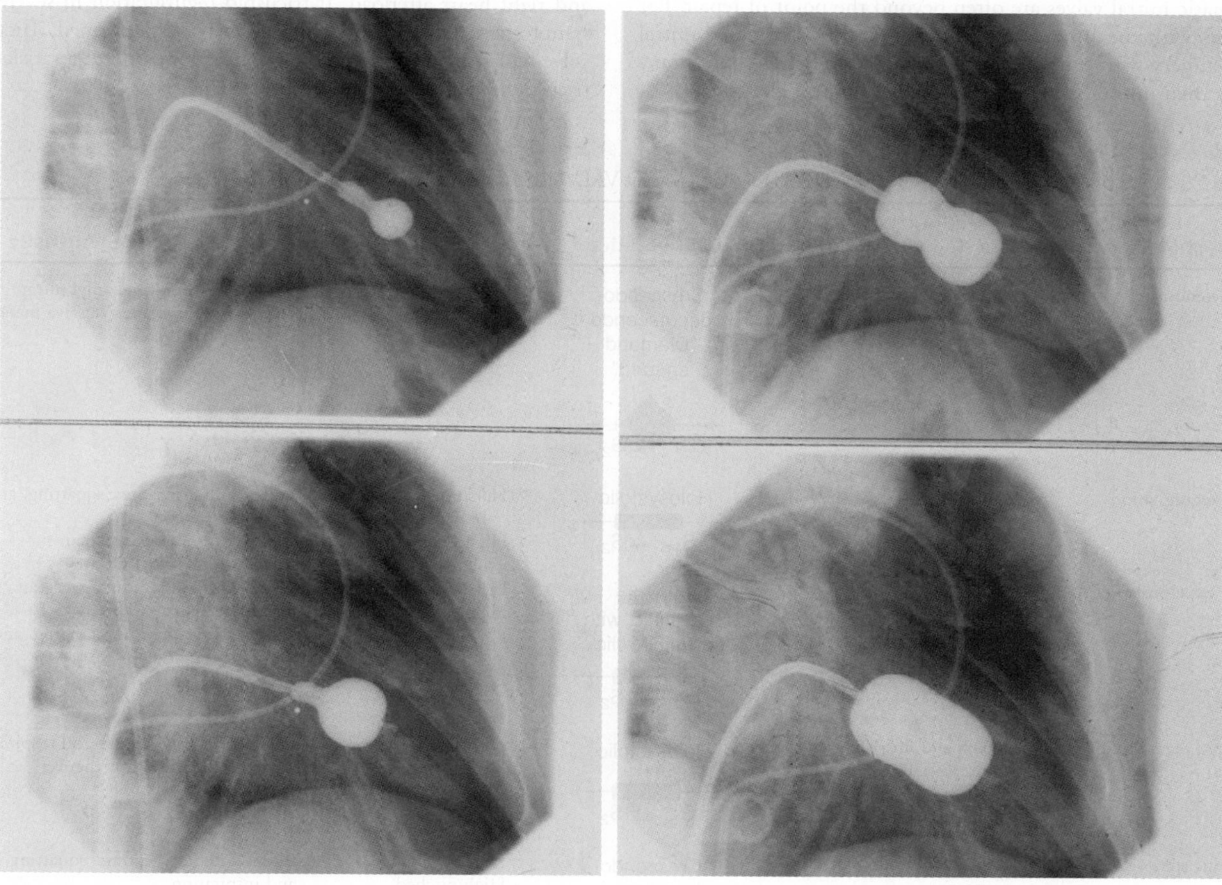

Figure 29-3 Mitral valvuloplasty: Inoue's technique. (A) Inflation of distal portion of balloon, which is then pulled back and anchored at the mitral valve. (B) Inflation of proximal and middle portions of balloon. At full inflation, the narrowed "waist" of the balloon has disappeared. (From Vahanian, A. S. [1998]. Valvuloplasty. In E. J. Topol, R. M. Califf, J. M. Isner, et al. [Eds.], *Textbook of cardiovascular medicine* [p. 2157]. Philadelphia: Lippincott-Raven.)

subvalvular deformity, with a maximum score of 4 in each division. Patients with a total echo score of ≤8 respond most favorably.[13] Balloon valvuloplasty has been associated with complications including systemic embolization (1% to 3%), severe mitral regurgitation (3% to 5%), and death (0% to 1%).[14] An atrial septal defect also may occur in as many as 10% of patients undergoing balloon valvuloplasty as a result of the transseptal approach, but the defect closes or decreases in most patients.[15] Results have been promising, with the average gradient reduction being approximately 18 to 6 mm Hg and, on the average, an increase in calculated valve area of 50% to 100%. Mitral balloon valvuloplasty is reserved for patients who continue to be symptomatic despite adequate medical therapy. Mitral balloon valvuloplasty may be used in women who experience hemodynamic decompensation during pregnancy due to mitral stenosis as it offers less risk to the fetus than mitral valve replacement and cardiopulmonary bypass.

Surgical Treatment

Surgical replacement of the mitral valve is required when there is severe mitral regurgitation coexisting with mitral stenosis or if the mitral stenosis is not amenable to percutaneous balloon valvuloplasty. Although some valves with mitral stenosis may be repaired by open commissurotomy and reconstruction, heavily calcified rheumatic mitral valves are often beyond the point of repair. For patients with coexistent tricuspid regurgitation, combined mitral valve surgery with tricuspid repair is related to better clinical outcomes than mitral balloon valvuloplasty alone.[16] The usual prosthetic valve of choice in mitral stenosis is a mechanical prosthesis, because patients already require life-long anticoagulation because of atrial fibrillation. For young women who wish to become pregnant, a bioprosthesis may be recommended.

TRICUSPID VALVE DISEASE

Tricuspid regurgitation is primarily "functional" rather than structural and occurs secondary to dilation of the right ventricle and the annulus of the tricuspid valve. Functional tricuspid regurgitation frequently accompanies mitral stenosis and pulmonary hypertension because of the increased pressure and volume load on the right ventricle. Symptoms include signs of right-sided heart failure, large V waves in their right atrial or central venous pressure trace, and pulsatile neck veins. Other causes of tricuspid regurgitation include trauma, infective endocarditis, right atrial tumor, and tricuspid valve prolapse. The murmur of tricuspid regurgitation is a holosystolic murmur heard along the left sternal border and may extend over the precordium, sounding like the murmurs of mitral regurgitation and ventricular septal defect (Table 29-3). Patients with mild tricuspid regurgitation normally do not require treatment. Medical treatment is aimed at reducing pulmonary artery pressures and right heart afterload. If tricuspid regurgitation in severe and symptomatic, tricuspid valve repair may be performed. Tricuspid valve replacement is uncommon and is done only if a satisfactory tricuspid repair cannot be accomplished.

Table 29-3 ■ SYSTOLIC MURMURS RELATED TO ACQUIRED VALVULAR HEART DISEASE

Origin of Murmur	Auscultatory Location and Radiation	Configuration	Quality and Frequency	Maneuvers That Alter Intensity
Aortic stenosis	Right second intercostal space Radiates to carotid arteries and apex	Crescendo-decrescendo "Diamond shaped" S_1 S_2	Harsh High pitched	Increases with squatting, amyl nitrate Decreases with standing, Valsalva maneuver, and isometric exercise
Mitral regurgitation	Apex Radiates to axilla and back	Holosystolic S_1 S_2	Harsh or blowing High pitched	Increases with expiration, squatting, and isometric exercise Decreases with Valsalva maneuver, standing, and amyl nitrate
Mitral valve prolapse	Apex Radiates to axilla and back	Mid- to late systolic, with systolic click S_1 Click S_2	Harsh High pitched	Increases with Valsalva maneuver, amyl nitrate, and inspiration Decreases with squatting, standing, and isometric exercise
Tricuspid regurgitation	Fourth and fifth left intercostal spaces Radiates to right parasternal border	Holosystolic S_1 S_2	Harsh High pitched	Increases with amyl nitrate and inspiration Decreases with Valsalva maneuver and standing
Pulmonic stenosis	Second left intercostal space Radiates to back	Crescendo-decrescendo "Diamond shaped" S_1 S_2	Harsh High pitched	Increases with amyl nitrate, squatting, and inspiration Decreases with Valsalva maneuver and standing

Acquired tricuspid stenosis is uncommon, recognized in approximately 5% of patients with rheumatic heart disease, and usually does not occur without involvement of the mitral valve.[17] Tricuspid stenosis has a pathologic process similar to that of mitral stenosis. The murmur of tricuspid stenosis is comparable to the murmur of mitral stenosis, including an opening snap followed by a diastolic rumble. The murmur of tricuspid stenosis is a diastolic decrescendo murmur along the left sternal border (see Table 29-2). Common symptoms of tricuspid stenosis include fatigue, minimal orthopnea, paroxysmal nocturnal dyspnea, hepatomegaly, and anasarca.

PROSTHETIC VALVES

Prosthetic cardiac valves have been used since the mid 1960s to treat acquired valvular heart disease. Because no "perfect" prosthetic valve exists, the patient with valvular heart disease is managed medically as long as it is safely feasible. Timing of valve replacement depends on the patient's functional status, ventricular dysfunction, and the natural course of the lesion.

Before a decision is made to use a particular valve, factors in valve design, specifically durability, thrombogenic potential, and hemodynamic properties, are weighed against annulus size and certain clinical conditions such as the desirability of long-term anticoagulation. Table 29-4 summarizes the characteristics considered in selection of prosthetic valves. Because of their proven durability, mechanical valves are most often chosen for patients younger than 65 to 70 years unless contraindicated (e.g., previous bleeding problems, desire to become pregnant, or poor compliance with medication and follow-up). Prosthetic heart valves differ in design, echocardiography image, and radiologic appearance (Fig. 29-4).

Mechanical Valves

Mechanical (nonbiologic) valves have excellent durability but are usually thrombogenic. Bileaflet and tilting-disk valves are the mechanical valves in common use today. Caged-ball valves are used less frequently in the United States but may be used in other areas of the world. In patients with aneurysm or dissection of the ascending aorta, composite grafts of conduit and mechanical valves may be used.

Bileaflet valves, such as St. Jude, ATS (advancing the standard), and the CarboMedic are low-profile valves that have centrally mounted leaflets attached to the seating ring with butterfly hinges. These hinges allow the leaflets to open to 85 degrees, making these valves the least obstructive of the mechanical valves. These valves are composed of pyrolytic carbon. With adequate anticoagulation, thromboembolic risk is low with bileaflet valves.

Table 29-4 ■ SELECTION OF TYPE OF PROSTHETIC VALVE BASED ON PATIENT CHARACTERISTICS

Biologic Valve	Mechanical Valve
History of bleeding	Age <65 years
Inability to take warfarin	Already on anticoagulation
Desire to become pregnant	History of embolic cerebral vascular accident
History of thrombosis with mechanical valve	History of atrial fibrillation
Age > 65 years	

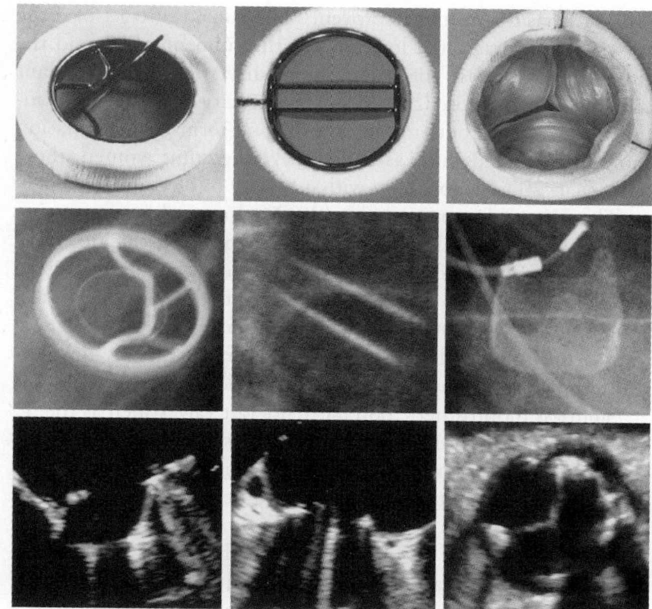

■ **Figure 29-4** Photographic (*top row*), radiographic (*middle row*), and echocardiographic (*bottom row*) appearance of prosthetic valves. From left to right: Bjork-Shiley single tilting disk, St. Jude's Medical bileaflet mechanical valve, and Carpentier–Edwards xenograft (radiographs courtesy of Dr. Carolyn van Dyke). (Adapted from Garcia, M. L. [1998]. Prosthetic valve disease. In E. J. Topol, R. M. Califf, J. M. Isner, et al. [Eds.], *Textbook of cardiovascular medicine* [p. 580]. Philadelphia: Lippincott-Raven.)

The *tilting-disk valve* is a low-profile valve consisting of a disk that sits in a seating ring; the flat or convexo-concave disk tilts in response to pressure changes. The Medtronic Hall valve is a tilting-disk valve commonly used today. Tilting-disk valves open to an angle of 60 to 75 degrees in relation to the seating ring. When open, tilting-disk valves produce a minor and major orifice for blood to pass through. Tilting disks have more central flow, but usually more turbulence, than caged-ball valves. Tilting disks close with an audible click. The technology for production of tilting-disk valves has evolved so that a single piece of metal is used to avoid welded struts.

Caged-ball valves have been used since the 1960s and have an excellent durability record. Changes in pressure cause the ball to move forward and back within its caged structure. Flow is directed laterally through the valve rather than centrally. Because of its high profile, the caged-ball valve prosthesis can become obstructive, especially when used in patients with small aortic roots or small left ventricles. The Starr–Edwards and the Sutter were two of the most commonly used caged-ball valves. Caged-ball prostheses have been largely abandoned in favor of lower-profile bileaflet valves.

Tissue Valves

Tissue (biologic) valves are characterized by having low rates of thrombotic episodes associated with their use. Porcine or bovine tissue is strengthened and made nonviable by treatment with glutaraldehyde. Homografts are tissue valves from cadavers. They are preserved cryogenically, but are difficult to procure, and their longevity has not been well proven. The main advantages of tissue valves are the associated low rates of thromboembolism and the subsequent decrease in patient morbidity when anticoagulant therapy is not required. Nonthrombogenicity is particularly important for those patients in whom long-term anticoagulation should be avoided, such as children, young adult women, those older than 70 years, or those with a history of bleeding.

The Hancock porcine valve, the Medtronic Mosaic porcine bioprosthesis (treated with α-oleic acid to retard calcification), and the Carpentier–Edwards porcine valve are xenografts using porcine aortic valves preserved with glutaraldehyde under pressure, mounted on a stent.[18] The Carpentier–Edwards pericardial bioprosthesis is made of leaflets fashioned from bovine pericardium fixed without pressure in glutaraldehyde.

Stentless bioprosthetic porcine xenograft valves such as the St. Jude Medical-Toronto, the Medtronic Freestyle Stentless, and the Edwards Prima Plus porcine bioprosthesis have been developed to improve the durability and enhance the hemodynamic performance of porcine aortic valves. Stentless aortic biological valves were developed secondary to the recognition that conventional bioprosthesis have limitations of long-term durability and residual obstruction that may impede left ventricular mass regression.[19] Use of the stentless aortic bioprosthesis has resulted in enhanced survival and hemodynamic superiority.[20] It is expected that reducing mechanical stress on valve leaflets, and the associated degeneration of the bioprosthesis, may be slowed.

Homografts or *allografts* from human cadavers are virtually free of any associated thrombosis. They are especially useful in patients with small aortic roots or in patients with active endocarditis. Earlier homografts were preserved with glutaraldehyde and demonstrated early failure. Homografts are now stored "fresh" after harvesting in an antibiotic solution and are then cryopreserved, increasing their longevity to at least 10 years. Valve failure is uncommon and usually the result of progressive valve incompetence.[21] Aortic allografts have demonstrated excellent freedom from thromboembolism, endocarditis, and progressive valve incompetence.[21] Because of lack of availability, use of homografts has been limited.

In the *Ross procedure* (also known as pulmonary autograft), the aortic valve is replaced with a pulmonary autograft, and the native pulmonary valve is replaced with a pulmonic allograft. Although this procedure introduced by Donald Ross in 1967 was originally developed for pediatric application, it has been expanded to adult surgery as well.[22] In patients undergoing the Ross procedure, the native pulmonary valve is excised and then implanted in the aortic position (autograft); a pulmonary homograft (allograft) is implanted into the pulmonic position (Fig. 29-5). The pulmonary autograft has been shown to be resistant to degeneration and calcification.[23] The actuarial freedom from pulmonary autograft valve replacement is 90% ± 3% at 13 years.[22] The Ross procedure cannot be performed in patients with bicuspid aortic valves or dilated aortic roots.[10] Although the Ross procedure has limited acceptance due to the complexity of the surgery and the replacement of both the aortic and pulmonic valves, in young adults who wish to avoid anticoagulation, it offers an alternative with favorable midterm results.[24]

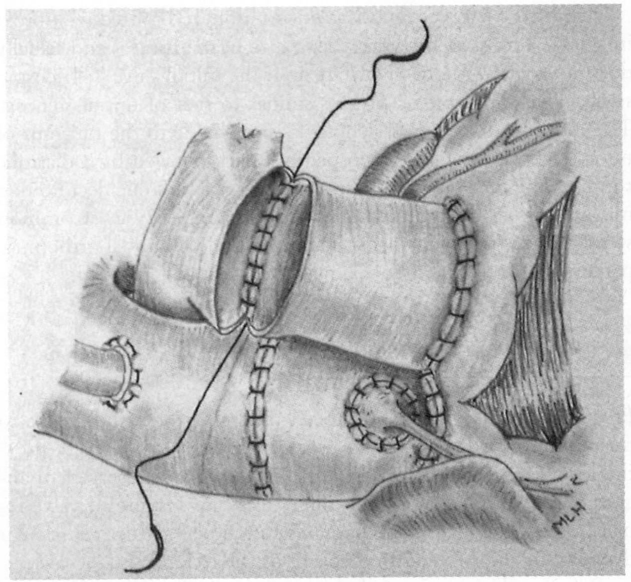

■ **Figure 29-5** Illustration of Ross procedure. Suture line of pulmonary homograft is shown. (From Elkins, R. C. [1998]. Valve repair and valve replacement in children, including the Ross procedure. In L. R. Kaiser, I. L. Kron, & T. L. Spray [Eds.], *Mastery of cardiothoracic surgery* [p. 947]. Philadelphia: Lippincott-Raven.)

Minimally Invasive Valve Surgery

Minimally invasive valve surgery is now used for both aortic valve replacement and mitral valve repair and replacement. Minimally invasive surgical approaches are possible because a wide assortment of technological advances, such as endoscopic and surgical equipment, have been developed to evolve towards more complex, video- and robot-assisted procedures.[25] Although patients undergoing minimally invasive valve surgery still require cardiopulmonary bypass, classic median sternotomy may be avoided, thus reducing pain, improving cosmetic results, and expediting recovery. Endoscopic mitral and tricuspid repair is feasible even after previous cardiac surgery.[26] As minimally invasive valve surgery continues to evolve, it will likely become a mainstay in the treatment of valvular heart surgery.

Aortic valve replacement can be performed through an upper "T" ministernotomy without intraoperative difficulties. Postoperative pain is reduced and recovery is expedited, with patients discharged to home as early as postoperative day 3.[27] Compared with patients with median sternotomy, patients undergoing mitral valve replacement through the right parasternal approach had a shortened length of stay and reduced direct hospital costs.[28] Most clinical series demonstrates that minimally invasive port-access approach to mitral valve surgery has low morbidity and mortality, with echocardiographic outcomes equivalent to conventional mitral valve surgery.[29] More recently, minimally invasive mitral valve surgery has evolved to include computer-assisted robotic techniques in current clinical trials. The da Vinci Surgical System allows the surgeon to operate from a console through an end-affecter using microwrist instruments, which are mounted on robotic arms, inserted through the chest wall.[30] For patients unsuitable for traditional aortic valve replacement due to comorbidities, percutaneous transarterial[31] or transapical aortic valve replacement are currently undergoing investigation. Catheter-based mitral valve repair for mitral regurgitation using clips that mimic the Alfieri stitch procedure or annuloplasty devices placed in the coronary sinus are also currently under investigation.[32,33]

Complications of Prosthetic Valves

Thromboembolism remains the most common complication of patients with prosthetic valves. Anticoagulant therapy with warfarin is begun in all patients 48 hours after surgery. All patients with mechanical valves require life-long anticoagulation because of the risk of thrombosis and embolization. The highest thromboembolic risk for mechanical and biologic valves occurs in the first few days to months after implantation, before the valve is fully endothelialized. The AHA and the ACC recommend international normalized ratio of 2.0 to 3.0 for mechanical aortic valves and international normalized ratio of 2.5 to 3.5 for mechanical mitral valves.[34] Tissue valves other than homografts also usually require anticoagulation for 6 to 12 weeks after surgery, after which patients have their therapy converted to aspirin. Homografts or the Ross procedure require no anticoagulation.

Prosthetic valvular thrombosis is a serious complication and can result in severe hemodynamic compromise. In patients with prosthetic valves who are not anticoagulated into a therapeutic range, thrombosis of the prosthetic valve can occur. Thrombus or pannus formation on the valve may occlude the orifice or entrap the pivoting mechanisms, causing acute stenosis or regurgitation. Symptoms of valve thrombosis include embolic events and CHF. If there are large thrombi or valve dysfunction, urgent or emergency valve replacement is usually indicated. Fibrinolytic therapy may be used for right-sided valve thrombosis or left-sided thrombosis with a small clot burden.[10]

Although symptoms of prosthetic valve endocarditis are similar to those of native valve endocarditis, the infection may be difficult to control with antibiotics alone because of the prosthetic material involved. *Early prosthetic valve endocarditis* (within the first 60 days) carries a high mortality rate. Early prosthetic valve endocarditis occurs in less than 1% of patients who have had valve replacements and frequently requires the patient to undergo additional operations.[35] The most common organism in early prosthetic valve endocarditis is *Staphylococcus epidermidis.* Fever, heart failure, new murmur, and embolic events are common manifestations. *Late prosthetic valve endocarditis* (more than 60 days after surgery) occurs most commonly in patients with bioprosthetic valves in the aortic position. The incidence is less than 1% per year and is generally caused by the same bacterial species that cause subacute bacterial endocarditis.[35]

Prosthesis malfunction is uncommon for the first 10 years after artificial valve implantation. The best-known problems with mechanical failures were those affecting the Bjork-Shiley convexo-concave tilting-disk valves first manufactured in 1978, with the peak incidence of valve failure in the 1981 to 1982 models. Subsequent modifications improved the valve area but also increased stress forces. Although these valves have been withdrawn from the market, approximately 40,000 had been implanted worldwide. Because acute valve strut fracture can be fatal, patients with these valves should be evaluated for partial strut fracture using high-resolution cineradiography. *Valve degeneration* is the primary complication of patients with tissue prostheses. Degeneration of biologic prostheses can occur as lipid or calcium deposits cause valve cusps to stiffen and become stenotic. Failure of tissue valves often occurs slowly over months to years and presents as progressive heart failure. Prosthetic valve degeneration and failure are most easily diagnosed with echocardiography.

Paravalvular leaks between the prosthetic ring and the annulus occur because of tearing of the suture line, spontaneously or after infection. Presence of a new murmur and signs of heart failure alert the clinician to paravalvular leaks. The patient's clinical course should be followed; when the leak becomes significant, surgical repair or replacement is indicated. Hemolysis may also accompany paravalvular leaks.

Hemolytic anemia is a consequence of shortened red cell survival time in all patients with prosthetic valves. Movement of the valve ball or disk causes varying degrees of destruction of the red blood cells. Hemolysis may also occur with paravalvular leak. Commonly, hemolysis is mild and the patient can compensate by increasing red blood cell production. Rarely, hemolytic anemia occurs. Chronic intravascular hemolysis results in loss of iron in the urine; iron deficiency anemia may result after several years.

MITRAL INSUFFICIENCY

Cause

Mitral insufficiency (also termed *regurgitation*) may be either chronic or acute (Table 29-5). Acute mitral regurgitation can be caused by endocarditis, myxomatous degeneration, rupture of chordae tendineae, papillary muscle disorders, prosthetic valve failure, or trauma.[10] Chronic mitral regurgitation may be the result of a number of abnormalities including, but not limited to, rheumatic heart disease, injury after radiation, cardiomyopathies, infiltrative disease, ischemic damage to the subvalvular apparatus, infective endocarditis, myxomatous degeneration, hypertrophic cardiomyopathy, diet-drug-induced lesions, or marked left ventricular dilation.[36]

Pathology

Primary mitral regurgitation occurs when the mitral valve annulus, leaflets, chordae, or papillary muscles are affected by ischemia, collagen disease, infection, calcification, trauma, or degenerative changes, causing incompetent coaptation of the mitral leaflets. Secondary mitral regurgitation occurs with ventricular dilation when ventricular geometry is changed, causing malalignment of the papillary muscles.

Table 29-5 ■ ETIOLOGIES OF ACQUIRED MITRAL REGURGITATION

Chronic Mitral Regurgitation	Acute Mitral Regurgitation
Rheumatic heart disease	Myocardial infarction causing:
Ischemia to subvalvular apparatus	Papillary muscle rupture or dysfunction
Infective endocarditis	Rupture of chordae
Myxomatous degeneration	Infective endocarditis
Hypertrophic cardiomyopathy	Trauma
Left ventricular dilation	Myxomatous degeneration with chordal rupture
Systemic lupus erythematosus	
Marfan syndrome	
Calcification of annulus	
Ankylosing spondylitis	
Scleroderma	
Ehlers–Danlos syndrome	
Prosthetic paravalvular leak	
Deterioration of prosthetic mitral valve	

Pathophysiology

Mitral regurgitation occurs as the result of inadequate closure of the mitral valve, allowing regurgitant flow back into the left atrium during each left ventricular systole. Its severity depends on the volume of regurgitant flow. Regurgitant flow also increases left atrial pressure, causing left atrial dilation and pulmonary congestion. During diastole, the regurgitant volume returns to the left ventricle and increases its volume load. In chronic mitral regurgitation, persistent volume overload results in progressive ventricular dilation and mild hypertrophy. Over time, chronic volume overload will result in systolic heart failure. In acute mitral regurgitation, neither the left atrium nor the ventricle has had sufficient time to adjust to the increased volume load. Left atrial pressure rises quickly, resulting in pulmonary congestion and edema.

Clinical Manifestations

Patients with acute versus chronic mitral regurgitation vary in clinical presentation and physical examination findings. In acute mitral regurgitation, symptoms progress rapidly. Symptoms are typically those of left ventricular failure. The patient is usually tachycardiac to compensate for the reduced forward stroke volume. Patients are dyspneic secondary to pulmonary congestion and edema; they are often orthopneic and have paroxysmal nocturnal dyspnea and poor exercise tolerance. Patients may also have signs of biventricular failure because right-sided failure may occur secondary to pulmonary hypertension. Patients with acute mitral regurgitation often present to the emergency department with reports of sudden inability to breathe. New-onset atrial fibrillation can occur. Patients with ischemic mitral insufficiency or papillary muscle rupture may also report chest pain.

During the compensatory phase of chronic mitral regurgitation, patients may be relatively asymptomatic for years. Initial signs of mitral regurgitation include exertional dyspnea, orthopnea, paroxysmal nocturnal dyspnea, cough, palpitations, new atrial fibrillation, and lower extremity edema. Symptoms may occur so gradually that patients may present subacutely to the clinic with symptoms as vague as fatigue and inability to sleep.

Physical Assessment

On examination, the most easily noted characteristic of either chronic or acute mitral regurgitation is the holosystolic murmur, which is heard best at the apex and radiates to the axilla (see Table 29-3). The murmur of mitral regurgitation may vary somewhat depending on the underlying cause. Patients may have an S_3 gallop in moderate-to-severe regurgitation caused by high diastolic flow into the ventricle. An S_4 gallop is uncommon in chronic mitral regurgitation. However, in acute mitral regurgitation, an S_4 gallop is common because the left atrium and ventricle are noncompliant. The patient with rheumatic heart disease may also have a diastolic murmur related to coexisting mitral stenosis.

Because of left ventricular dilation, patients with chronic mitral regurgitation have an easily palpated, left laterally displaced point of maximal impulse. Patients with a markedly enlarged left atrium may have a left parasternal lift because of anterior displacement of the apex. Patients with acute or decompensated chronic mitral regurgitation may be anxious and diaphoretic because of left ventricular failure. Blood pressure may be normal to low and pulse pressure may be narrowed secondary to decreased stroke volume. Jugular venous pressure can be normal or elevated in the patient with right-sided heart failure. Breath sounds can range from basilar crackles to dullness secondary to pleural effusion. In addition, hepatosplenomegaly, hepatojugular reflux, peripheral edema, and ascites may be present in the patient with right-sided heart failure.

Diagnostic Tests

TTE can identify the structural cause of the mitral regurgitation as well as gauge left atrial size, left ventricular dimensions and performance, pulmonary artery pressures, and right heart function. Color flow Doppler allows for the assessment of severity of regurgitation. TEE is better than TTE for defining mitral valve anatomy and discriminating prosthetic valves and paravalvular leaks.

Cardiac catheterization is used to identify coexisting coronary artery disease and to grade the severity of mitral regurgitation. Left ventriculography can assess left ventricular function and distinguish any wall motion abnormalities. Right heart catheterization quantifies pulmonary artery pressures and allows for evaluation of the large V waves in the pulmonary artery wedge tracing.

Electrocardiography in chronic mitral regurgitation may demonstrate left ventricular hypertrophy and left atrial enlargement or P mitrale (characterized by M-shaped P waves). Atrial fibrillation may occur with acute and chronic mitral regurgitation. Patients with ischemic papillary muscle dysfunction may demonstrate ischemic changes, and patients with papillary muscle rupture can show acute inferior, posterior, or anterior myocardial infarction.

Chest radiography in chronic mitral regurgitation shows left ventricular hypertrophy and left atrial enlargement. Calcification of the mitral valve annulus and apparatus may also be seen. In acute or decompensated chronic mitral regurgitation, pulmonary vascular redistribution and pulmonary edema can be observed. If the heart is of normal size, the degree of mitral regurgitation is so mild or so acute that eccentric left ventricular hypertrophy has not had time to develop.

Medical Management

Medical therapy for mitral regurgitation is geared toward afterload reduction to promote forward flow and minimize regurgitation into the left atrium and pulmonary vasculature. In patients with acute or decompensated chronic mitral regurgitation, intravenous vasodilators such as nitroprusside can reduce filling pressures and ventricular cavity size and promote forward flow with afterload reduction. Intravenous diuretics are used to reduce volume overload. In acutely ill patients refractory to medications, intra-aortic balloon counterpulsation can be used further to reduce afterload while maintaining coronary perfusion with diastolic augmentation.

In patients with chronic mitral regurgitation or those in acute heart failure who are being weaned from intravenous inotropes and vasodilators, other afterload-reducing agents, such as angiotensin-converting enzyme inhibitors, nitrates, or hydralazine, may be used. Diuretics can treat chronic and acute volume overload. Some practitioners continue to advocate the use of digoxin, especially for patients in atrial fibrillation. In the patient with chronic but compensated mitral valve regurgitation, mitral surgery can be safely deferred or avoided. The patient should be carefully monitored, however, and referred for mitral valve repair or replacement before significant left ventricular dysfunction or pulmonary hypertension occurs.

Surgical Management

Two surgical approaches are used to treat mitral regurgitation. Mitral valve repair uses reconstructive techniques as well as a rigid prosthetic ring to repair the mitral valve apparatus, thus sparing the valve and avoiding the consequences of valve replacement. Mitral valve replacement involves implantation of a prosthetic valve, either mechanical or bioprosthetic. The mitral valve apparatus is preserved whenever possible as it contributes to the preservation of left ventricular function (Fig. 29-6). In patients with chronic mitral regurgitation, mitral replacement should occur before the patient has had irreversible left ventricular dysfunction. Mitral valve replacement or repair can preserve left ventricular function and ejection fraction. Patients with NYHA class II symptoms should be considered for surgery.

In most patients, mitral valve repair may be undertaken for patients with mitral insufficiency as an alternative to replacement. Surgical techniques involve reconstructing the leaflets and annulus in such a way as to narrow the orifice. These procedures consist of direct suture of the valve cusps, repair of the elongated or ruptured chordae tendineae (chordoplasty), or repair of the valve annulus (annuloplasty). With an annuloplasty, the incompetent valve is remodeled using a ring prosthesis that is attached to the leaflets and the annulus. Mitral valve repair has demonstrated excellent short-term and long-term results with low perioperative mortality rate (not >2% in most reported series). In patients with acute mitral regurgitation secondary to myocardial infarction, coronary angiography should be performed to define coronary anatomy for concomitant coronary bypass surgery at the time of mitral valve repair or replacement.

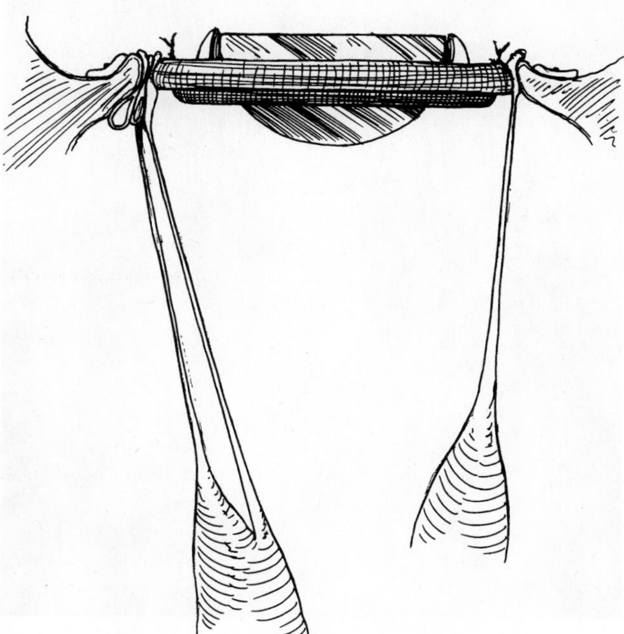

■ **Figure 29-6** Valve replacement with chordal preservation. (From Chitwood, W. R. [1998]. Mitral valve repair: Ischemic. In L. R. Kaiser, I. L. Kron, & T. L. Spray [Eds.], *Mastery of cardiothoracic surgery* [p. 321]. Philadelphia: Lippincott-Raven.)

MITRAL VALVE PROLAPSE

Cause

Mitral valve prolapse (MVP) refers to a variable clinical syndrome that is the result of a variety of pathologic mechanisms of one or more portions of the mitral valve leaflets and apparatus.[10] During ventricular systole, one or both of the mitral leaflets prolapse above the plane of the mitral valve annulus. MVP syndrome may also be known as Barlow syndrome, myxomatous valve syndrome, or click-murmur syndrome. The most common cause of MVP is myxomatous degeneration, but it is also caused by Marfan syndrome, Ehlers–Danlos syndrome, rheumatic heart disease, and ischemic papillary muscle dysfunction. MVP occurs twice as frequently in women as men but serious mitral regurgitation with MVP occurs more frequently in men older than 50 years.[10] MVP can be either nonfamilial or familial, transmitted as an autosomal trait.

Pathology

Patients with MVP have redundant myxomatous tissue with excess deposits of proteoglycans in the middle or spongiosa layer of the valve. Histologically, collagen fragmentation and disorganization as well as elastic fiber are present. Acid mucopolysaccharide material accumulates in the valve leaflets. The mitral valve leaflets, annulus, and chordae tendineae may also demonstrate disrupted collagen structure and extensive myxomatous change. While myxomatous changes occur most commonly in the mitral valve, they can also occur in the other cardiac valves.

Pathophysiology

Enlargement of the valve leaflets related to myxomatous degeneration causes systolic prolapse of one or both leaflets into the left atrium. Patients with MVP may have mitral regurgitation ranging in severity from none to severe. Persistent billowing of the valve causes stress to the underlying chordae and papillary muscles. Progressive mitral valvular degeneration can result in increasingly severe mitral regurgitation. If chordal rupture occurs, severe mitral regurgitation develops.

Supraventricular tachycardias (i.e., premature atrial contractions and paroxysmal supraventricular tachycardias) and ventricular arrhythmias may occur in patients with MVP. Although some patients with MVP have had sudden cardiac death, it is unclear what role MVP has in the cause. Patients with MVP may also have autonomic nervous system dysfunction; specifically, midbrain control of adrenergic and vagal responses may be abnormal.

Clinical Manifestations

Most patients with MVP are asymptomatic. Patients may have sharp, localized chest pain that is usually brief in duration. Patients may have equivocal symptoms of anxiety, fatigue, palpitations, chest pain, and orthostatic hypotension. The chest pain that occurs with MVP is often atypical and may be related to abnormal tension on papillary muscles.[10] As mitral regurgitation progresses, patients may note increasing dyspnea, fatigue, decreased exercise tolerance, orthopnea, and paroxysmal nocturnal dyspnea. Ruptured chordae with leaflet flail and acute mitral regurgitation result in symptoms of severe left ventricular failure.

Physical Assessment

The classic auscultatory finding of MVP is a midsystolic click with mid- to late systolic murmur (see Table 29-3). The murmur occurs secondary to regurgitant flow when the mitral valve leaflets fail to approximate. Patients with MVP may have the murmur or click or both. Findings may also vary over time. When the degree of mitral regurgitation is mild-to-moderate or less, heart rate and blood pressure may be normal. Additional physical findings may include thin body habitus, pectus excavatum, straight back syndrome, and scoliosis.

Diagnostic Tests

Echocardiography plays a key role in the diagnosis of MVP. Abnormal systolic motion of one or both of the mitral valve leaflets superior to the annular plane can be seen (Fig. 29-7). Doppler echocardiography gives additional evidence of valve regurgitation. TEE provides a more detailed look at the mitral valve and chordal structures.[12]

Cardiac catheterization can be used to rule out CHD as the origin of chest pain. Left ventriculography can demonstrate abnormal motion of the mitral valve and help determine the degree of regurgitation.

Electrocardiography is nondiagnostic. The electrocardiogram may be normal or have nonspecific ST-T-wave changes in the inferior leads (II, III, and aVF) and occasionally in the anterolateral leads (V_4 through V_6). The ST-T-wave changes may become more notable with exercise. Premature atrial and ventricular complexes may also be identified. *Exercise testing* may be used to help rule out the cause of the chest pain.

Chest radiography is often normal and is usually nondiagnostic for MVP. Patients with acute mitral regurgitation secondary to chordal rupture have pulmonary congestion but not cardiomegaly. Patients with chronic severe mitral regurgitation have an enlarged cardiac silhouette secondary to left atrial and left ventricular enlargement in addition to pulmonary congestion (Fig. 29-8).

Medical Management

Asymptomatic patients with MVP require no therapy. β-Blockers or calcium channel blockers may be used to help alleviate palpitations or chest pain syndrome.

Surgical Management

Patients with MVP and severe mitral regurgitation or flail leaflets should be evaluated for surgery. They often can undergo repair

A

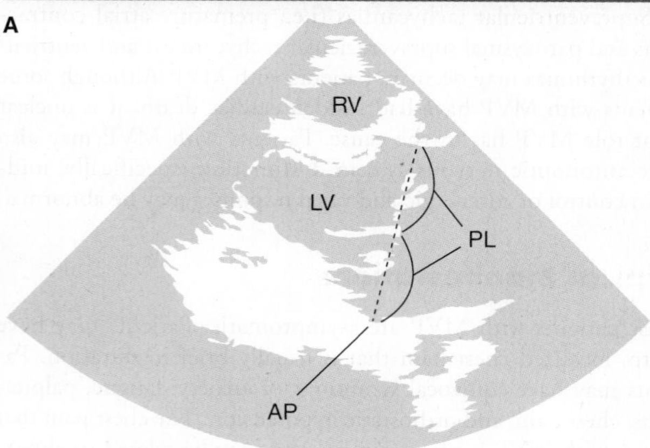

B

■ **Figure 29-7** (A) Long-axis echocardiographic view of mitral valve with bileaflet prolapse above the annular plane into the left atrium. (B) Illustration corresponding to echocardiogram. RV, right ventricle; LV, left ventricle; AP, annular plane; PL, prolapsing leaflet.

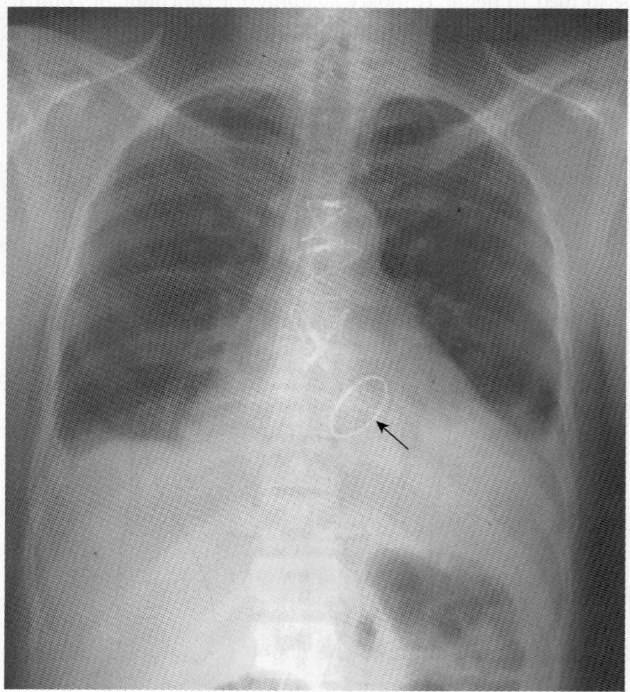

■ **Figure 29-8** Chest radiograph of 51-year-old male patient with history of MVP and repair (note annuloplasty ring marked with *arrow*). Patient's valve repair has failed and his mitral regurgitation is now severe. Patient is now in severe heart failure with notable bilateral pleural effusions and cardiomegaly.

rather than replacement. For discussion of surgical options, refer to the section on surgical intervention for mitral regurgitation.

Prognosis

MVP is usually a benign condition and most patients remain asymptomatic for their entire lives. Patients with progressive and symptomatic mitral regurgitation should be considered for mitral valve repair. In a small subset of patients, sudden cardiac death may occur secondary to arrhythmias. Patients with MVP and history of syncope, prolonged QT interval, palpitations, or dizziness should have further evaluation with arrhythmia monitoring.

AORTIC STENOSIS

Cause

Aortic stenosis is characterized by obstruction of the left ventricular outflow tract. Most commonly, left ventricular outflow obstruction is valvular, but it may be either supravalvular or subvalvular. Aortic stenosis is a gradually progressive disease that may have a long asymptomatic phase often lasting for decades that is then followed by a much shorter symptomatic phase with severe narrowing of the aortic valve orifice.[37] The age at which aortic stenosis becomes symptomatic is determined by the underlying cause. Aortic stenosis occurring from 1 to 30 years of age usually represents congenital aortic stenosis. Aortic stenosis presenting at the ages of 40 to 60 years is primarily rheumatic in origin or secondary to calcific aortic stenosis in a congenitally bicuspid aortic valve. In patients past the age of 60 to 70 years, calcific degenerative stenosis is the most prevalent cause. Of the causes of aortic stenosis, senile/degenerative calcific aortic stenosis is most common.

Pathology

In senile/degenerative calcific aortic stenosis, cumulative wear and tear leads to calcification on an otherwise normal aortic valve. Calcific deposits prevent the cusps from opening normally in systole, resulting in stenosis. Risk factors for the development of calcific aortic stenosis include male sex, elevated lipoprotein(a), height (inverse relation), hypertension, smoking, elevated low-density lipoprotein cholesterol, raised serum calcium, raised serum creatinine, and diabetes.[38] In patients with congenitally bicuspid aortic valves, abnormal flow through the valve leads to calcium deposition and restriction of cusp opening.

Pathophysiology

Aortic stenosis typically progresses over a period of years. As the valve cusps become less mobile, the valve orifice decreases in size, resulting in an increasingly higher left ventricular systolic pressure necessary to eject blood across the stenosed valve. Increased left ventricular afterload results first in compensatory concentric left ventricular hypertrophy. Although initially adaptive in aortic stenosis, left ventricular hypertrophy leads to decreased ventricular compliance and diastolic dysfunction. With the increased pressure gradient, blood from the left ventricle is ejected back into the left atrium worsening underlying mitral regurgitation. As aortic stenosis becomes severe, left ventricular systolic function may also decline, resulting in CHF.

Angina may result even in the absence of CHD because of an imbalance in myocardial oxygen supply and demand. Myocardial oxygen demand is increased secondary to increased left ventricular wall stress and muscle mass. Myocardial oxygen delivery is reduced as a result of decreased coronary perfusion pressure.

Syncope or near syncope can result secondary to reduced cerebral perfusion pressure, inappropriate left ventricular baroreceptor response, or arrhythmia. Orthostatic blood pressure changes may occur during exertion when arterial pressure drops because of systemic vasodilation in the setting of a fixed cardiac output. Increased left ventricular pressure may result in inappropriate baroreceptor response. Development of atrial fibrillation with rapid ventricular response may produce light-headedness or syncope due to loss of atrial kick and decline in cardiac output. Syncope at rest may be due to transient ventricular fibrillation that spontaneously converts.[10]

Clinical Manifestations

Patients with mild-to-moderate aortic stenosis are usually asymptomatic. As severe aortic stenosis develops, the most common initial symptom is dyspnea on exertion, followed by angina and near syncope or syncope. CHF also may occur as a result of ventricular dysfunction or increasing mitral regurgitation. Less commonly, sudden death, probably caused by ventricular fibrillation, may be the presenting clinical feature.

Physical Assessment

Aortic stenosis is most readily detected by auscultation of its classic mid-systolic (systolic ejection) murmur (see Table 29-3). As aortic stenosis progresses, the murmur peaks progressively later in systole and decreases in intensity as cardiac output falls. The murmur often radiates to one or both carotids. The murmur may be diminished at the base of the heart and radiate to the apex, which may be incorrectly thought to be mitral regurgitation (Gallavardin phenomenon). An S_4 gallop is usually present. The point of maximal intensity is sustained but may not be displaced. Blood pressure is normal-to-hypertensive until late in the disease progress. Jugular venous pressure is normal in most patients except in patients with severe aortic stenosis associated with heart failure. Reduction in stroke volume and cardiac output may cause diminished carotid upstrokes and late systolic peak (tardus) in severe or critical aortic stenosis.

Diagnostic Tests

Echocardiography is the principal modality used to diagnose and quantify aortic stenosis. Aortic valve pressure gradient can be measured, aortic valve area calculated, pulmonary artery pressures estimated, and left ventricular function and hypertrophy can be evaluated. Echocardiography is the most important diagnostic imaging technique used to diagnose and follow aortic stenosis.[12]

Cardiac catheterization is performed in patients with aortic stenosis primarily to rule out concomitant CHD. Left ventriculography can quantify the left ventricular ejection fraction. The transvalvular gradient can be established by direct pressure measurement. Right heart catheterization can better quantify pulmonary artery pressures and cardiac output.

Electrocardiography often shows a pattern of left ventricular hypertrophy, although its absence does not exclude the presence of critical aortic stenosis. Patients with aortic stenosis may demonstrate ST-T-wave changes typical of left ventricular strain. QRS voltage changes in the precordial leads correlates poorly with the severity of obstruction in aortic stenosis in adults.[10]

Exercise testing in patients with mild-to-moderate aortic stenosis with equivocal symptoms may be accomplished with caution in the hands of a cardiologist and can provide relevant information regarding exercise tolerance. In patients with known severe aortic stenosis and classic symptoms such as syncope, dyspnea, and chest pain, exercise testing carries increased risk of ventricular tachyarrhythmias and ventricular fibrillation and should not be performed.

Gated blood pool radionuclide scans provide information regarding ventricular function similar to echocardiography and left ventriculography. Gated pool scans may be useful in patients in whom left ventriculography cannot be performed (i.e., patients with elevated creatinine), or those in whom the left ventricle cannot be clearly imaged with echocardiography.

Chest radiography may be negative even in advanced disease. Heart size may be normal or only minimally enlarged. The left ventricular border and apex may be rounded, demonstrating a boot-shaped silhouette. Identifiable calcification of the aortic valve and aorta may be present. As disease progresses, left atrial enlargement, pulmonary hypertension, and CHF may become evident. Poststenotic dilation of the proximal ascending aorta may be noted along the right heart border in the posteroanterior chest radiograph (Fig. 29-9).

Medical Management

Because aortic stenosis is a mechanical problem, there is no effective medical management. The course of aortic stenosis varies in its progression; therefore, patients should be followed-up carefully by their health care providers with serial physical examinations and periodic echocardiography. Patients with mild aortic stenosis undergo echocardiography every 2 years. Patients with asymptomatic severe aortic stenosis are followed-up with serial echocardiograms every 6 to 12 months and should be taught to recognize the symptoms of worsening aortic stenosis, such as dyspnea, chest pain, and near syncope or syncope.

Interventional and Surgical Management

Percutaneous Aortic Catheter Balloon Valvuloplasty

Percutaneous aortic catheter balloon valvuloplasty is accomplished by passing a guide wire across the stenotic aortic valve into the apex of the left ventricle. A balloon-tipped catheter is advanced retrograde across the stenotic valve. The balloon is inflated, fracturing calcified nodules and separating the fused commissures. The aortic valve ring is also stretched to increase the size of the aortic valve orifice. Restenosis is a major problem in balloon aortic valvuloplasty in adults, occurring in approximately half of the patients within 6 months. Because of the high restenosis rate and high complication rates in early series, aortic balloon valvuloplasty

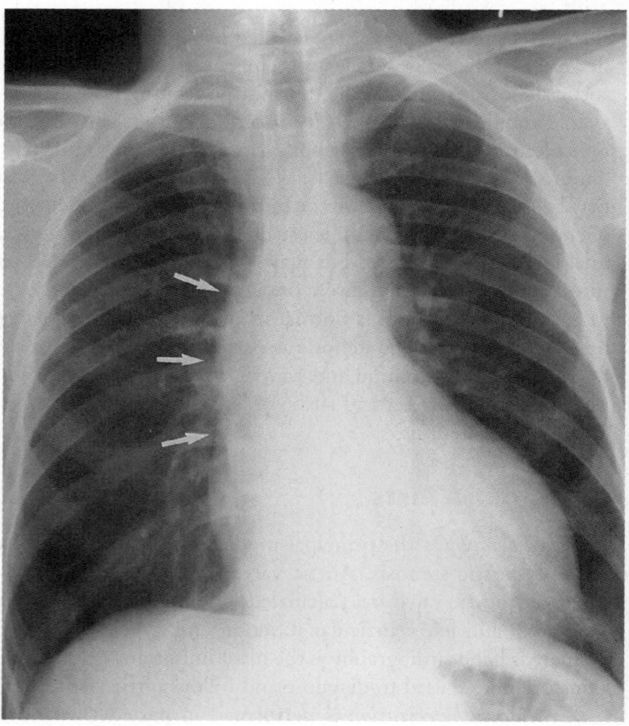

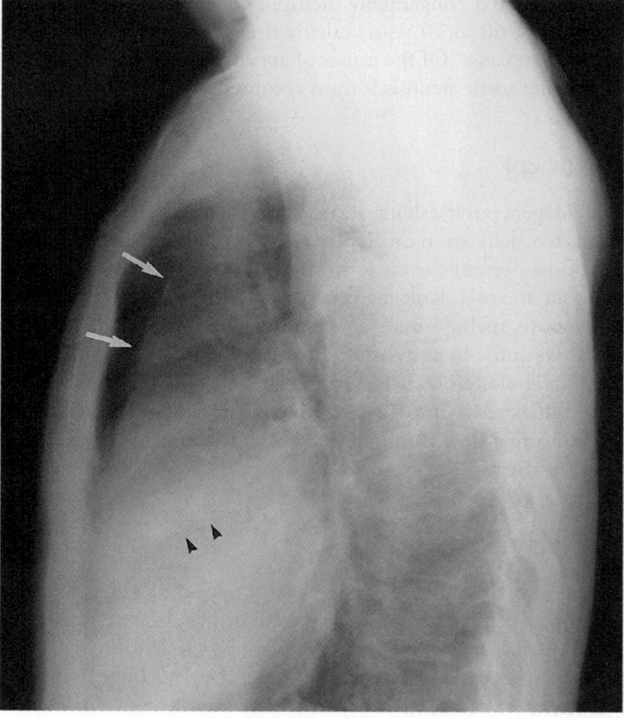

■ **Figure 29-9** (A) Posteroanterior chest radiograph showing rounded border of left ventricle (*arrows*). (B) Lateral chest radiograph showing calcified aortic valve (*arrowheads*) and filling of the retrosternal airspace with dilated ascending aorta (*arrows*). (From Boxt, L. M. [1998]. Plain film examination of the chest. In E. J. Topol, R. M. Califf, J. M. Isner, et al. [Eds.], *Textbook of cardiovascular medicine* [p. 511]. Philadelphia: Lippincott-Raven.)

in adults has been largely abandoned and is reserved for only those candidates unsuitable for surgery (i.e., older adults with heart failure or pregnant women).

Aortic Valve Replacement

Aortic valve replacement should be considered the treatment of choice for severe aortic stenosis in spite of age.[39] Aortic valve replacement for mechanical relief of obstruction to flow is the only effective treatment.[40] The natural history of aortic stenosis is used as a guide to determine the timing of aortic valve replacement surgery. Patients with asymptomatic aortic stenosis have nearly the same survival rate as the age-matched general population. Once the patient experiences symptoms of angina, syncope, or heart failure, there is an abrupt decline in survival rate. In patients presenting with CHF, only 50% survive 2 years. For patients who present with syncope, the 3-year survival rate is only 50% without aortic valve replacement. The average life expectancy of patients with apnea is only 5 years without aortic valve replacement.[41] Aortic valve replacement is recommended in all patients with severe, symptomatic aortic stenosis. Selection of aortic valve prostheses is discussed earlier in this chapter.

AORTIC INSUFFICIENCY

Cause

Aortic regurgitation may be caused by either intrinsic abnormalities of the aortic valve leaflets or disease of the aortic root. In rheumatic fever and endocarditis, the aortic leaflets are directly affected. In congenitally bicuspid valves, the larger cusp may become redundant, resulting in diastolic prolapse and progressive aortic regurgitation. The aortic valve may also become incompetent because of aortic root dilation. As the aortic root dilates, the aortic annulus becomes so large that the valve cusps no longer approximate, resulting in regurgitation.

Aortic root dilation is seen in patients with Marfan syndrome, rheumatic arthritis, ankylosing spondylitis, annuloaortic ectasia (associated with hypertension and aging), aortic dissection, syphilitic aortitis, and collagen vascular disease.

Pathology

Rheumatic fever leads to fibrinous infiltrates on the valve cusps, causing them to contract and become malaligned and incompetent. Patients with rheumatic disease may have a "mixed lesion" that includes both aortic regurgitation and aortic stenosis. In acute or subacute infective endocarditis of the aortic valve, tissue destruction of the leaflets causes cusp perforation or prolapse. Vegetations adherent to the aortic valve may also interfere with valve closure, causing incompetence. In patients with aortic root dilation or ascending aortic dissection, the aortic annulus becomes greatly enlarged, the aortic leaflets separate, and aortic incompetence follows.

Pathophysiology

Volume overload occurs secondary to regurgitant volume reentering the left ventricle from the aorta through the incompetent aortic valve. Retrograde flow occurs during diastole when left ventricular pressure is low and aortic pressure is high. The left ventricle is forced to pump the normal volume received from the left atrium as well as the regurgitant volume from the aorta.

Similar to mitral regurgitation, the hemodynamic presentation and the heart's ability to compensate differ depending on whether the aortic insufficiency is acute or chronic. In chronic aortic regurgitation, the left ventricle is subjected to pressure and volume overload. As a result, the left ventricle develops mild concentric hypertrophy to accommodate the pressure load and eccentric hypertrophy to compensate for the increased volume load. Patients with chronic aortic regurgitation may remain asymptomatic for years, until progressive left ventricular dilation and dysfunction result in CHF. In patients with acute aortic regurgitation, the left ventricle has not had time to compensate with either concentric or eccentric hypertrophy and cannot accommodate the large volume caused by acute aortic regurgitation. As a result, left ventricular and left atrial pressures rise sharply, causing acute CHF and pulmonary edema. Patients with acute aortic regurgitation usually require surgical intervention.

Clinical Manifestations

Patients with chronic aortic regurgitation are often asymptomatic for many years. Common symptoms of aortic regurgitation include fatigue and exertional dyspnea. Patients may report palpitations, dizziness, and the sensation of a forceful heartbeat, especially when lying on their left side. Angina may also be noted, but it occurs less frequently in aortic regurgitation than in aortic stenosis. As heart failure ensues, patients experience orthopnea, paroxysmal nocturnal dyspnea, and cough related to left-sided heart failure. With acute aortic regurgitation, symptoms of left-sided heart failure develop rapidly.

Physical Assessment

The typical murmur of aortic regurgitation is a high-pitched, early diastolic decrescendo murmur with a blowing quality (see Table 29-2). Patients also may have a physiologic murmur of mitral stenosis caused by the regurgitant aortic jet, which partially prevents mitral valve closure (Austin Flint murmur). As the severity of aortic regurgitation increases, the murmur becomes louder and longer. In chronic aortic regurgitation, the point of maximal impulse is displaced laterally. Systolic hypertension and decreased diastolic pressure create a widened pulse pressure. Patients with chronic aortic regurgitation may have a host of other physical findings that may not be present in acute aortic regurgitation (Table 29-6).

Table 29-6 ■ SPECIFIC PHYSICAL EXAMINATION FINDINGS IN AORTIC REGURGITATION

Sign	Physical Description
Quincke's sign	Pulsatile flushing/blanching of nail bed with application of gentle pressure
de Musset's sign	Bobbing of head with each pulse
Corrigan's pulse (waterhammer)	Sharp systolic upstroke and diastolic collapse of pulse
Müller's sign	Bobbing of uvula with each pulse
Traube's sign	"Pistol shot" sound auscultated over the femoral arteries
Duroziez's sign	Biphasic femoral bruit auscultated with mild pressure
Hill's sign	Blood pressure higher in arms than legs

Diagnostic Tests

Echocardiography is helpful in identifying the cause of aortic regurgitation. Echocardiography can indicate left ventricular volume overload by the increased internal diameter of the ventricular chamber during systole and diastole. Doppler echocardiography is the best noninvasive means to detect aortic regurgitation. TEE is especially useful in imaging the ascending and descending aorta in patients with suspected aortic dissection.

Cardiac catheterization should be performed to visualize and quantify the extent of regurgitation before surgery. However, physical findings and noninvasive tests are sufficient to establish the diagnosis of aortic insufficiency. In patients with known or suspected CHD, coronary angiography should be performed. In patients with aortic root dilation, aortic root angiography may be performed concurrently with coronary angiography.

Radionuclide imaging can be used to estimate ejection fraction and determine myocardial perfusion defects in patients with concomitant CHD.

Exercise testing may be used to establish exercise tolerance and to evaluate asymptomatic patients.

Electrocardiography may be normal in patients with acute aortic regurgitation or in patients with mild-to-moderate chronic regurgitation. Patients with moderate-to-severe chronic regurgitation may have left-axis deviation and a pattern of left ventricular strain (Q waves in leads I, aVL, and V_3 to V_6, with small R wave in V_1). Intraventricular conduction defects may occur with left ventricular dysfunction or annular abscess.

Chest radiography may show CHF only in the patient with acute aortic regurgitation because compensatory left ventricular dilation has not yet occurred. In chronic aortic regurgitation, the left ventricle enlarges in a leftward and inferior direction that causes little or no increase the transverse diameter.[10] Dilation of the ascending aorta and a widened mediastinum may be noted in patients with aortic dissection. In patients with a dilated aortic root or dissection, computed tomography or magnetic resonance imaging may be necessary to better delineate the ascending aorta, transverse arch, and proximal descending aorta.

Medical Management

Patients who have asymptomatic aortic regurgitation should have afterload reduction with vasodilators. Diltiazem and verapamil are contraindicated in aortic regurgitation because they have a more potent negative inotropic effect and may produce bradycardia, which may worsen heart failure. In addition to long-acting nifedipine and felodipine, angiotensin-converting enzyme inhibitors may be used to reduce afterload. Sodium nitroprusside reduces preload and afterload and can be used to stabilize patients with acute aortic regurgitation before surgery. Intra-aortic balloon counterpulsation cannot be used because inflation of the balloon during diastole would increase the regurgitant volume into the left ventricle, which acutely worsens left ventricular dilation and heart failure.

Surgical Management

Acute aortic regurgitation requires urgent aortic valve replacement. Without adequate time for compensatory mechanisms to develop, aortic regurgitation triggers rapid onset of CHF, tachycardia, and diminished cardiac output. It is desirable to treat patients with acute aortic regurgitation secondary to infective endocarditis with a minimum of 48 hours of appropriate intravenous antibiotics before implanting a prosthetic valve. In patients with active endocarditis who are hemodynamically unstable, use of cadaveric human aortic homografts may minimize the risk of prosthetic valve endocarditis. Patients who have aortic regurgitation caused by ascending aortic dissection or dilation require replacement of the ascending aorta as well.

In chronic aortic regurgitation, the aortic valve must be replaced before irreversible left ventricular dysfunction develops. In asymptomatic patients, it is usually recommended that the aortic valve be replaced when left ventricular function begins to deteriorate. Aortic valve replacement is recommended for the symptomatic patient when left ventricular ejection fraction drops to 0.50 or less, left ventricular systolic dimension is 55 mm or more, and left ventricular diastolic dimension is 75 mm or more.[10]

REFERENCES

1. Raju, B. S., & Turi, Z. G. (2008). Rheumatic fever. In P. Libby, R. O. Bonow, D. L. Mann, et al. (Eds.), *Braunwald's heart disease* (8th ed., pp. 2079–2086). Philadelphia: Saunders Elsevier.
2. Towns, M. L., & Reller, L. B. (2003). Diagnostic methods: Current best practices and guidelines for isolation of bacteria and fungi in infective endocarditis. *Cardiology Clinics, 21*, 197–205.
3. Cabell, C. H., Abrutyn, E., & Karchmer, A. W. (2003). Bacterial endocarditis: The disease, treatment, and prevention. *Circulation, 107*, e185–e187.
4. Sexton, D. J., & Spelman, D. (2003). Current best practices and guidelines: Assessment and management of complications in infective endocarditis. *Cardiology Clinics, 21*, 273–282.
5. Karchmer, A. W. (2008). Infective endocarditis. In P. Libby, R. O. Bonow, D. L. Mann, et al. (Eds.), *Braunwald's heart disease* (8th ed., pp. 1713–1737). Philadelphia: Saunders Elsevier.
6. Olaison, L., & Pettersson, G. (2003). Current best practices and guidelines: Indications for surgical intervention in infective endocarditis. *Cardiology Clinics, 21*, 235–251.
7. Sachdev, M., Peterson, G. E., & Jollis, J. G. (2003). Imaging techniques for diagnosis of infective endocarditis. *Cardiology Clinics, 21*, 185–195.
8. Nishimura, R. A., Carabello, B. A., Faxon, D. P., et al. (2008). ACC/AHA Guideline update on valvular heart disease: Focused update on infective endocarditis. *Circulation, 118*, 887–896.
9. Dalen, J. E., & Fenster, P. E. (2000). Mitral stenosis. In J. S. Alpert, J. E. Dalen, & S. H. Rahimtoola (Eds.), *Valvular heart disease* (3rd ed., pp. 75–112). Philadelphia: Lippincott Williams & Wilkins.
10. Otto, C. M., & Bonow, R. O. (2008). Valvular heart disease. In P. Libby, R. O. Bonow, D. L. Mann, et al. (Eds.), *Braunwald's heart disease* (8th ed., pp. 1625–1712). Philadelphia: Saunders Elsevier.
11. Warnes, C. A. (2008). Pregnancy and heart disease. In P. Libby, R. O. Bonow, D. L. Mann, et al. (Eds.), *Braunwald's heart disease* (8th ed., pp. 1967–1981). Philadelphia: Saunders Elsevier.
12. Brady, T. J., Grist, T. M., Westra, S. J., et al. (2003). Valvular. In T. J. Brady, T. M. Grist, S. J. Westra, et al. (Eds.), *Pocket radiologist: Cardiac top 100 diagnoses* (pp. 53–75). Salt Lake, UT: Amirsys.
13. Palacios, I. F., Sanchez, P. L., Harrell, L. C., et al. (2002). Which patients benefit from percutaneous mitral balloon valvuloplasty? *Circulation, 105*, 1465–1471.
14. Mayes, C. E., Cigarroa, J. E., Lange, R. A., et al. (1999). Percutaneous mitral balloon valvuloplasty. *Clinics in Cardiology, 22*, 501–503.
15. Mazur, W., Parilak, L. D., Kaluza, G., et al. (1999). Balloon valvuloplasty for mitral stenosis. *Current Opinion in Cardiology, 14*, 95–103.
16. Song, H., Kang, D. H., Kim, J. H., et al. (2007). Percutaneous mitral valvuloplasty versus surgical treatment of mitral stenosis with severe mitral regurgitation. *Circulation, 116*(Suppl. I), I-246–I-250.
17. Ewy, G. A. (2000). Tricuspid valve disease. In J. S. Alpert, J. E. Dalen, & S. H. Rahimtoola (Eds.), *Valvular heart disease* (3rd ed., pp. 377–392). Philadelphia: Lippincott Williams & Wilkins.
18. Jamieson, W. R. E. (2003). Update on new tissue valves. In K. L. Franco & E. D. Verrier (Eds.), *Advanced therapy in cardiac surgery* (pp. 177–195). Hamilton, Ontario, Canada: BC Decker.

19. Goldman, B. S., & Mallidi, H. (2003). Update on Stentless valves. In K. L. Franco & E. D. Verrier (Eds.), *Advanced therapy in cardiac surgery* (pp. 196–206). Hamilton, Ontario, Canada: BC Decker.
20. David, T. E., Puschmann, R., Ivanov, J., et al. (1998). Aortic valve replacement with the stentless and stented porcine valves: A case-match study. *Journal of Thoracic and Cardiovascular Surgery, 116*, 236–240.
21. Doty, J. R., Salazar, J. D., Liddicoat, J. R., et al. (1998). Aortic valve replacement with cryopreserved aortic allograft: Ten year experience. *Journal of Thoracic and Cardiovascular Surgery, 115*, 371–379.
22. Elkins, R. C. (2003). Pulmonary autograft. In K. L. Franco & E. D. Verrier (Eds.), *Advanced therapy in cardiac surgery* (pp. 156–167). Hamilton, Ontario, Canada: BC Decker.
23. Ross, D. N., Jackson, M., & Davies, J. (1987). Pulmonary autograft aortic valve replacement. *Circulation, 75*, 895–901.
24. Sievers, H. H., Hanke, T., Stierle, U., et al. (2006). A critical reappraisal of the Ross operation. *Circulation, 114*(Suppl. I), I-504–I-511.
25. Chitwood, W. R., & Rodriguez, E. (2008). Minimally invasive and robotic mitral valve surgery. In L. H. Cohn (Ed.), *Cardiac surgery in the adult* (pp. 1079–1100). New York: McGraw-Hill.
26. Cassleman, F. P., LaMeir, M., Jeanmart, H., et al. (2007). Endoscopic mitral and tricuspid valve surgery after previous cardiac surgery. *Circulation, 116*(Suppl. I),I-270–I-275.
27. Izzat, M. B., Yim, A. P., El-Zufari, M. H., et al. (1998). Upper T ministernotomy for aortic valve operations. *Chest, 114*, 291–294.
28. Cosgrove, D. M., Sabik, J. F., & Navia, J. L. (1998). Minimally invasive valve operations. *Annals of Thoracic Surgery, 65*, 1538–1539.
29. Sharony, R., Grossi, E. A., Ribakove, G. H., et al. (2003). Minimally invasive cardiac valve surgery. In K. L. Franco & E. D. Verrier (Eds.), *Advanced therapy in cardiac surgery* (pp. 147–155). Hamilton, Ontario, Canada: BC Decker.
30. Chitwood, W. R. (2003). Robot-assisted mitral valve surgery. In K. L. Franco & E. D. Verrier (Eds.), *Advanced therapy in cardiac surgery* (pp. 220–229). Hamilton, Ontario, Canada: BC Decker.
31. Webb, J. G., Pasupati, S., Humpheries, K., et al. (2007). Percutaneous transarterial aortic valve replacement in selected high-risk patients with aortic stenosis. *Circulation, 116*, 755–763.
32. Block, P. C. (2005). Percutaneous mitral valve repair. Are they changing the guard? *Circulation, 111*, 2154–2156.
33. Mack, M. J. (2006). Percutaneous mitral valve repair: A fertile field of innovative treatment strategies. *Circulation, 113*, 2269–2271.
34. Goldsmith, I., Turpie, A. C. G., & Lip, G. Y. (2002). ABC of Antithrombotic therapy: Valvular heart disease and prosthetic heart valves. *BMJ, 325*, 1228–1231.
35. Crawford, M. H., & Durack, D. T. (2003). Clinical presentation of infective endocarditis. *Cardiology Clinics, 21*, 159–166.
36. Enriquez-Sarano, M., Schaff, H. V., Tajik, A. J., et al. (2000). Chronic mitral regurgitation. In J. S. Alpert, J. E. Dalen, & S. H. Rahimtoola (Eds.), *Valvular heart disease* (3rd ed., pp. 113–141). Philadelphia: Lippincott Williams & Wilkins.
37. Cowell, S. J., Newby, D. E., & Prescott, R. J. (2005) A randomized trail of intensive lipid-lowering therapy in calcific aortic stenosis. *New England Journal of Medicine, 352*, 2389–2397.
38. Rajamannan, N. M., Gersh, B., & Bonow, R. O. (2003). Calcific aortic stenosis: From bench to bedside-emerging clinical and cellular concepts. *Heart, 89*, 801–805.
39. Hara, H., Pederson, W. R., Ladich, E., et al. (2007). Percutaneous balloon aortic valvuloplasty revisited: Time for a renaissance? *Circulation, 115*, e334–e338.
40. Carabello, B. A. (2007). Aortic stenosis, two steps forward, one step back. *Circulation, 115*, 2799–2800.
41. Ross, J., Jr., & Braunwald, E. (1968). Aortic stenosis. *Circulation, 38*(Suppl. V), 61–67.

CHAPTER 30 Pericardial, Myocardial, and Endocardial Disease

Margaret M. McNeill

Pericardial, myocardial, and endocardial diseases impact the health of populations across the globe, and can have a significant impact on cardiac function and therefore quality of life. These diseases translate into a tremendous economic burden; thus, it is therefore imperative for nurses to know the best practices for management of patients with pericardial, myocardial, and endocardial disorders in order to optimize patient outcomes.

PERICARDIAL DISEASE

The pericardium is a double-layered fibroserous sac that envelops the heart, covering almost the entire surface and part of the great vessels.[1] The pericardium is composed of two layers, the *serosa* and the *fibrosa*, which contain nerves, blood vessels, and lymphatics. The fibrous outer layer, also called the *parietal pericardium*, is attached to the sternum, great vessels, and diaphragm. The phrenic nerves innervate most of the parietal pericardium. A serosal layer of cuboidal cells one-cell-layer thick lines the pericardium. The monocellular serosa directly covers the heart surfaces and is also known as the *visceral pericardium* or the *epicardium*. The pericardial space between the layers normally contains 15 to 35 mL of serous pericardial fluid produced by the visceral pericardial cells.[2,3]

The pericardium is a relatively inelastic covering and it exerts a powerful restraining effect on the size of the heart in situations of acute volume overload.[2,4] The pericardium also exerts a mechanical effect that enhances normal ventricular interactions that contribute to the balance of right and left cardiac outputs.[5] The pericardium maintains the heart in a stable position and functionally optimum shape within the mediastinum. It acts as a barrier to inflammation from contiguous structures and contains defensive immunologic components.[5] The layer of pericardial fluid reduces friction on the epicardium and equalizes gravitational, hydrostatic, and inertial forces over the surface of the heart.[6] While the pericardium serves several functions, cardiac activity is normal if the pericardium is missing due to congenital absence or surgical removal.

Almost every known medical and surgical pathologic process can contribute to pericardial disease, either primarily involving the pericardium or with an indirect impact.[2] For unknown reasons, there is a predominance of men with pericardial disease.[7] The spectrum of pericardial diseases ranges from congenital defects, pericarditis, neoplasms, and cysts.[8] Pericarditis, pericardial effusion, and cardiac tamponade are the most important pericardial conditions to understand.

Pericarditis

Pericarditis is the inflammation of the pericardium surrounding the heart. The acute inflammatory process can produce either serous or purulent fluid, or a dense fibrinous material.[9] The possible sequelae of pericarditis include cardiac tamponade, recurrent pericarditis, and pericardial constriction.[10]

Acute clinically noneffusive or "*dry*" *pericarditis* refers to pericardial inflammation without a significant symptom-causing effusion, and is the most commonly recognized pericarditis. Acute inflammatory pericarditis usually lasts 1 to 3 weeks and does not lead to further problems. *Acute effusive pericarditis* is pericarditis in which an effusion is present in the pericardium.

Etiology

Pericarditis is caused by many different conditions. The etiological classification of pericardial diseases comprises infectious pericarditis, pericarditis in autoimmune diseases, postmyocardial infarction syndrome, and auto-reactive (chronic) pericarditis.[11] There has been a sharp decline in infectious pericarditis in the last few years, except in immunocompromised individuals, such as those with acquired immunodeficiency syndrome (AIDS).[12]

Viruses associated with pericarditis include influenza, coxsackie A or B, varicella, mumps, hepatitis B, mononucleosis, and human immunodeficiency virus (HIV).[7] Idiopathic pericarditis is thought often to be the result of viral pericarditis where the virus is never identified. Bacterial infections, such as tuberculosis, are rare in the United States, but have surged in incidence in regions of the world where HIV and AIDS are epidemic. Other bacteria that cause pericarditis include *Staphylococcus*, *Pneumococcus*, and *Streptococcus* species. *Aspergillosis* and *histoplasmosis* are among the fungal infections that can cause pericarditis.

Frequently, the patient's history indicates that a viral infection preceded the pericarditis. Sometimes the pericarditis itself is the first presenting symptom of a systemic disease, such as systemic lupus erythematosus or malignancy. In viral pericarditis, the pericardial fluid is most commonly serous, of low volume, and resolves spontaneously.[9] Exudative, hemorrhagic, and leukocyte-filled large effusions may be associated with neoplastic, tuberculous, and purulent pericarditis.[6]

Assessment Findings

The onset of symptoms can be acute, as is commonly seen in viral pericarditis, or insidious, as seen in uremic pericarditis. Acute viral pericarditis is nearly always preceded by a recent respiratory, gastrointestinal, or "flu-like" illness. A prodrome of fever, malaise, and myalgia is common in acute pericarditis, although older patients may not exhibit fever.[1]

A major symptom of pericarditis is chest pain that is retrosternal or left precordial, radiating to the trapezius ridge and varying with posture. The pain is transmitted through the phrenic nerves, and usually occurs on the left side. Shoulder pain should be distinguished from trapezius ridge pain by having the patient physically point to the specific site of pain. Frequently the chest pain caused by pericarditis induces shallow tachypnea as patients attempt to splint their chest movement.[2] The pain is generally worse when lying supine and is relieved by sitting.

A pericardial friction rub is pathognomonic for pericarditis, but is frequently not present, may come and go, and can vary in quality and intensity. Auscultation for a pericardial friction rub is accomplished with the diaphragm of the stethoscope at the left middle to lower sternal border during both inspiration and expiration, while the patient changes positions.[2] Often best heard at end expiration while the patient is leaning forward, the sound is classically a rasping or creaking with a triple cadence, but can also be bi- or monophasic.[1]

A diagnosis of acute pericarditis is made if the patient has a pericardial friction rub or chest pain, and widespread ST segment elevation on electrocardiography.[10] It is important to differentiate pericarditis from myocardial infarction (MI) and pulmonary embolism. Table 30-1 describes the different features from these three conditions.[10]

The pericardium itself does not produce electrical activity. The electrocardiogram (ECG) changes seen in pericarditis are a result of superficial inflammation of the myocardium underneath the pericardium. The ECG of a patient with pericarditis may be normal, atypically abnormal with nonspecific changes, or have a four-stage sequence that is diagnostic. Figure 30-1 shows the electrocardiographic manifestations of pericarditis.

In stage I, there are ST segment deviations, primarily due to inflammation on the ventricular surfaces. PR segment deviations are also usually present. Stage I is virtually pathognomonic of acute pericarditis when it involves all or almost all leads with early ST junction elevations that produce an appearance of T waves "jacked-up" on the QRS interval, but that is otherwise normal.[2] The ST segment is always depressed in aVR.[4]

In early stage II, the ST segments return to baseline, and PR segments may now be depressed. In late stage II, the T waves flatten and then invert. In stage III, the ECG is characteristic of diffuse myocardial injury. In stage IV, the ECG evolves back to the prepericarditis state.[2] Stage IV may last days or months.[4]

The changes seen in the ECG of a patient with pericarditis can occur over hours, particularly from stages I to II, or can take place over days or weeks, most often as stage III evolves to stage IV. Because of more prompt recognition and treatment of pericarditis, not all stages may be exhibited.[4] The ST elevation seen in pericarditis is usually distinguished from that of acute MI by the absence of Q waves, upward ST segments, and the absence of associated T wave inversion.[13] In research examining the cause of ST segment abnormalities in emergency department

Table 30-1 ■ FEATURES THAT DIFFERENTIATE PERICARDITIS FROM MYOCARDIAL ISCHEMIA OR INFARCTION AND PULMONARY EMBOLISM[10]

Symptom and Clinical Finding	Myocardial Ischemia or Infarction	Pericarditis	Pulmonary Embolism
Chest pain			
Location	Retrosternal	Retrosternal	Anterior, posterior, or lateral
Onset	Sudden, often waxing and waning	Sudden	Sudden
Character	Pressure-like, heavy, squeezing	Sharp, stabbing, occasionally dull	Sharp, stabbing
Change with respiration	No	Worsened with inspiration	In phase with respiration (absent when the patient is apneic)
Change with position	No	Worse when patient is supine; improved when sitting up or leaning forward	No
Radiation	Jaw, neck, shoulder, one or both arms	Jaw, neck, shoulder, one or both arms, trapezius ridge	Shoulder
Duration	Minutes (ischemia); hours (infarction)	Hours to day	Hours to day
Response to nitroglycerin	Improved	No change	No change
Physical examination			
Friction rub	Absent (unless pericarditis is present)	Present (in 85% of patients)	Rare; a pleural friction rub is present in 3% of patients
S_3 sound, pulmonary congestion	May be present	Absent	Absent
Electrocardiogram			
ST segment elevation	Convex and localized	Concave and widespread	Limited to lead III, aVF, and V_1
PR segment depression	Rare	Frequent	None
Q waves	May be present	Absent	May be present in lead III or aVF or both
T waves	Inverted when ST segments are still elevated	Inverted after ST segments have normalized	Inverted in lead II, aVF, or V_1 to V_4 while ST segments are elevated
Atrioventricular block, ventricular arrhythmias	Common	Absent	Absent
Atrial fibrillation	May be present	May be present	May be present

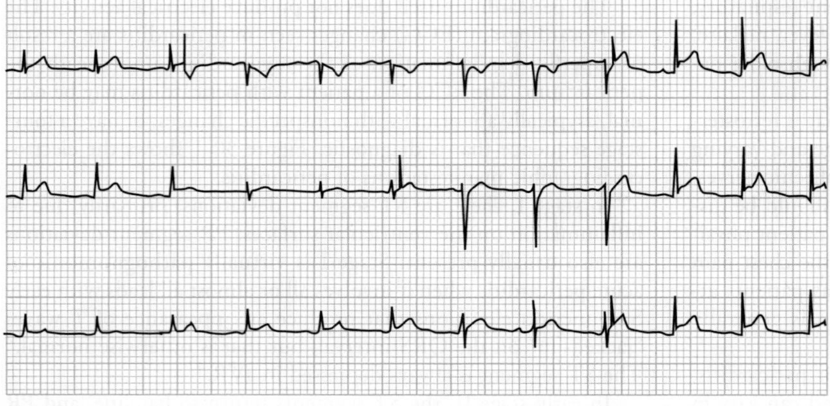

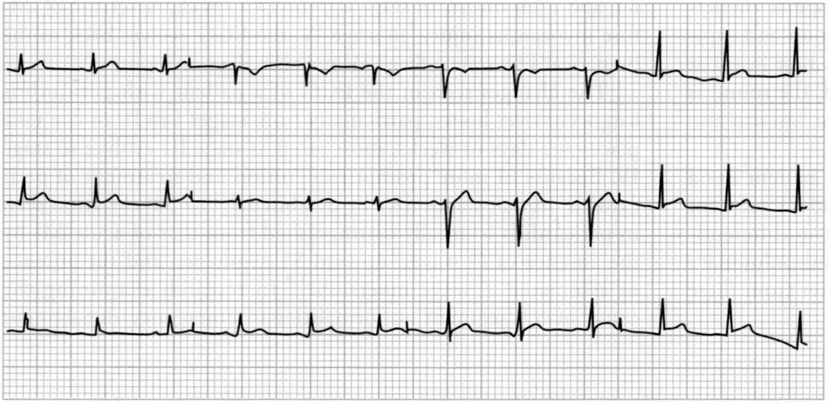

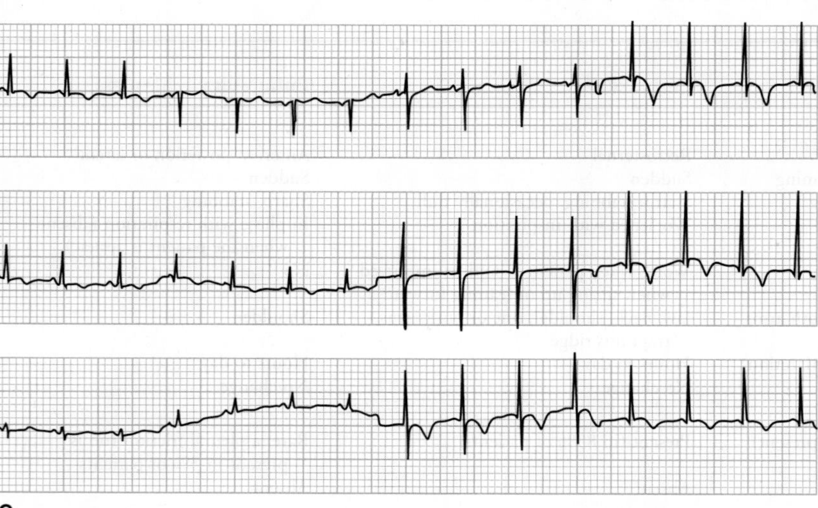

■ **Figure 30-1** ECG manifestations of pericarditis. **(A)** Typical, quasi-diagnostic stage I ECG: J (ST) elevated in all leads except AVL, depressed AVR and V1. PR segment deviated except in aVL where P is small. **(B)** Early stage II. J (ST) returning to baseline. **(C)** Stage III. T waves inverted in most leads and typically upright in aVRAVR and V1. (From Spodick, D. H. [1997g]. Electrocardiographic abnormalities in pericardial disease. In D. H. Spodick [Ed.], *The pericardium: A comprehensive textbook* [pp. 40–64]. New York: Marcel Dekker.)

chest pain patients, pericarditis was found in 1% of the study population.[14]

Evaluation of laboratory results almost always reveals an elevated erythrocyte sedimentation rate. Leukocytosis is present early but, depending on etiology, may give way to lymphocytosis. Serum cardiac enzymes are frequently normal unless the myocardium is involved, and then they give some indication as to the degree of involvement. In a study on viral or idiopathic pericarditis, troponin I elevation was frequently observed (32% of cases) and associated with young age, male gender, ST segment elevation, and pericardial effusion at presentation.[15] It is uncertain if elevated troponin I levels have any prognostic value.[15]

In some parts of the world, such as South Africa, tuberculosis is a major health problem, and can be complicated by tuberculosis pericarditis. The need for early diagnosis has led to emphasis on biochemical tests such as the pericardial adenosine deaminase test, and the use of interferon as an indicator of pericardial disease due to tuberculosis.[16]

Echocardiography is critical to assess the pericardium in pericardial disease. Computed tomography (CT) and magnetic resonance imaging (MRI) allow examination of the entire chest, so abnormalities that might be related to the pericardial findings can be assessed.

Medical Management

The goal of treatment in acute pericarditis is to relieve pain and prevent complications.[9] Treatment of the underlying cause is also a priority. Nonsteroidal anti-inflammatory drugs (NSAIDs) are the mainstay of treatment. Ibuprofen is preferred by many clinicians due to its rare side effects, favorable impact on coronary flow, and large dose range.[2] Depending on the severity and response, 300 to 800 mg every 6 to 8 hours may be initially required, and is best continued until the effusion is resolved, which may be days or weeks.[11] Aspirin (325 to 650 mg four times a day) is also commonly used to treat pericarditis.[3] Gastrointestinal protection during NSAID therapy is important.[3,11,17] Colchicine (0.5 or 6 mg b.i.d.) added to an NSAID or as monotherapy also appears to be effective in initial episodes, and to prevent recurrences.[11,12] Systemic corticosteroid therapy is recommended only in connective tissue diseases, autoreactive or uremic pericarditis.[3,11] Intrapericardial corticosteroids have been effective and do not cause systemic side effects.[11]

Pericarditis due to bacterial infections such as tuberculosis is treated by directing treatment to the cause. The mainstay of treatment of tuberculosis pericarditis in Africa is the 6-month course of antituberculosis drugs recommended by the World Health Organization.[18] Pericardiocentesis is recommended in all patients suspected of tuberculosis to facilitate diagnosis.[19]

Constrictive Pericarditis. Constrictive pericarditis results from a scarred, and often thickened and calcified pericardium that limits diastolic ventricular filling.[20] Tuberculosis is responsible for most cases of constrictive pericarditis in Africa and Asia.[21] Other causes of constrictive pericarditis are idiopathic, postradiation, and postsurgical.[22,23]

The often thickened, adherent pericardium restricts ventricular filling and limits chamber expansion and maximal diastolic volumes. End-diastolic pressures in all heart chambers are typically elevated and equalized. During classic constriction, Kussmaul's sign, inspiratory jugular venous distention, replaces the normal inspiratory venous "collapse" that reflects a normal inspiratory decrease of 3 to 7 mm Hg in right atrial pressure. This sign is a hallmark of constrictive pericarditis.[2] Patients present with signs of heart failure, although pulmonary edema is usually not a feature.[3,24]

A calcified pericardium is often visible on chest x-ray film.[25,26] CT, MRI, and echocardiography are tools also used to diagnose constrictive pericarditis.[3] CT allows detection of calcification that occurs in restrictive pericarditis.[5] Many abnormal findings can be seen on the echocardiogram that indicate constrictive pericarditis, such as premature opening of the pulmonic valve and rapid posterior motion of the left ventricular posterior wall in early diastole, with little or no posterior motion during the rest of diastole. However, these findings are not specific for constrictive pericarditis and can be caused by other conditions, such as restrictive cardiomyopathy (RCM).[27,28]

Pericardiectomy, surgical removal of the pericardium, is the treatment for symptomatic constrictive pericarditis.[24] The procedure may be either a total or a partial pericardiectomy. In a recent study, total pericardiectomy was associated with lower perioperative and late mortality, as well as a better hemodynamic condition for the patient.[22] Idiopathic etiology was associated with better outcomes in two studies.[22,24]

Recurrent Pericarditis. Recurrent pericarditis is a complication of acute pericarditis. Recurrence is diagnosed by recurrent pain and one or more of the following signs: fever, pericardial friction rub, ECG changes, effusion on echocardiography, and elevation of white blood count, C-reactive protein level, or the erythrocyte sedimentation rate.[17] The rate of recurrence is reported to vary from 15% to 50%. It is considered an autoimmune phenomenon.[17] Imazio et al.[17,29] found an increased risk of recurrence if corticosteroids were used during treatment of the first episode of pericarditis. Risk factors for recurrence in another study were identified as female gender, previous use of corticosteroids, and previous recurrent pericarditis.[30] Use of colchicine along with NSAIDs during a first episode of pericarditis has been found to decrease recurrence.[29]

Approximately 20% of pericarditis patients have a recurrence within months, or rarely, within years.[31] In a systematic review spanning 40 years of literature on patients with idiopathic recurrent pericarditis, the complication rate of pericardial tamponade was 3.5%, and no patients developed constrictive pericarditis.[32]

Pericarditis Associated With MI

Early Acute Post-MI Pericarditis. In the immediate period after MI, an early pericardial syndrome may develop and then resolve over a period of approximately 1 week. Pericardial involvement is correlated to infarct size.[33] The ECG shows a typical pattern of pericarditis and is helpful in differentiating between pericardial and ischemic pain. Pericardial friction rubs may be heard. As in all pericarditis, rubs are virtually 100% specific, but sensitivity depends on frequency of auscultation, because they tend to come and go over hours.[12] The course is usually benign, and treatment consists of aspirin or other NSAIDs. Treatment of MI with thrombolysis and mechanical revascularization appear to have reduced the incidence of this form of pericarditis by at least 50%.[33]

Dressler's Syndrome. Dressler's syndrome of chest pain, pleurisy, pericarditis with friction rub, severe malaise, moderate fever, and leukocytosis occurs 3 weeks to several months post-MI. The underlying pathologic process is unknown, but it is thought to reflect a late autoimmune reaction mediated by antibodies to circulating antigens.[34] In contrast to early post-MI pericarditis, inflammation is diffuse and not localized to the myocardial injury site.[33]

Pericardial Effusion

Pericardial effusion is an increased amount of fluid within the pericardial space. This fluid can be serous, serosanguineous, pus, lymph, or blood.[3]

Etiology

Many conditions cause acute pericarditis and pericardial effusions, including uremia, tuberculosis, neoplasms, and connective tissue diseases. The effusion may also be associated with acute idiopathic pericarditis. Pericardial effusions occur with heart failure and LVH, and are also common after cardiac surgery. Effusions associated with cardiac surgery usually resolve after a month.[6] In a population of patients in Italy, neoplastic etiology was found in 33 of 450 patients with acute pericardial disease (7.3%). Four percent of these patients presented with acute pericardial disease as the first manifestation of their malignancy.[35] Pericardial effusions are also seen secondary to uremia of renal failure and hypothyroidism. In a population of patients in Turkey, uremic pericarditis resulting from poorly controlled renal failure due to economic considerations was the most common cause of pericardial effusion.[20] Tuberculosis is responsible for approximately 70% of cases of large pericardial effusions in developing countries.[21]

Pathophysiology

The normal pericardium has a reserve capacity of 150 to 250 mL. An increase of volume of this amount in the pericardial space will not result in a major increase in intrapericardial pressure. Intrapericardial pressure will increase once this reserve volume is exceeded, and is also a function of how quickly the volume in the pericardial space accumulates. If fluid accumulates slowly, the normally stiff pericardium will stretch. However, if there is increased stiffness of the pericardium, as seen in constrictive pericarditis, small amounts of fluid will result in increased pericardial pressure. Once the intrapericardial pressure is elevated, the filling of the cardiac chambers becomes limited due to compression, resulting in hemodynamic effects.[5] Figure 30-2 shows the difference in effects of rapid versus slow effusion accumulation.[36]

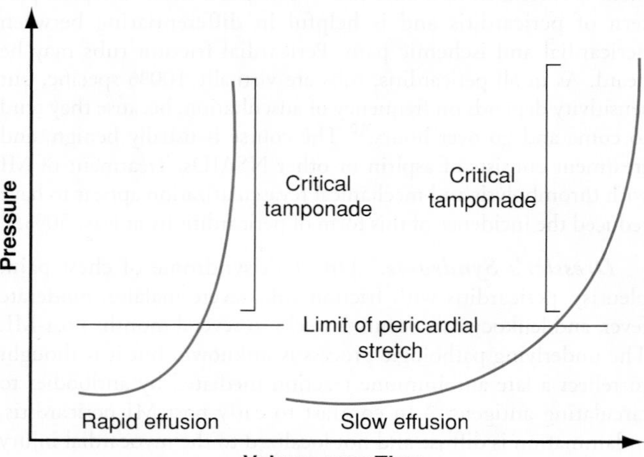

■ **Figure 30-2** Cardiac tamponade. Pericardial pressure–volume (or strain–stress) curves are shown in which the volume increases slowly or rapidly over time. In the left-hand panel, rapidly increasing pericardial fluid first reaches the limit of the pericardial reserve volume (the initial flat segment) and then quickly exceeds the limit of parietal pericardial stretch, causing a steep rise in pressure, which becomes even steeper as smaller increments in fluid cause a disproportionate increase in the pericardial pressure. In the right-hand panel, a slower rate of pericardial filling takes longer to exceed the limit of pericardial stretch, because there is more time for the pericardium to stretch and for compensatory mechanisms to become activated.

Assessment Findings

A 2003 task force of the American College of Cardiology, the American Heart Association, and the American Society of Echocardiography gave the use of echocardiography for evaluation of all patients with suspected pericardial disease an evidence class I recommendation.[37] Pericardial effusions are classified according to the distance between the left ventricular posterior wall and pericardium. Echocardiography can classify mild (<10 mm), moderate (10 to 20 mm), and severe (>20 mm) effusions.[3,20] "Noncompressing" effusions do not produce changes in CO or pulsus paradoxus. If the effusions are caused by a systemic disease, then the symptoms are related to that disease. A pericardial rub may or may not be appreciated. The ECG shows reduced voltage, and these changes are nonspecific and unreliable for diagnosis. Cardiomegaly on chest x-ray film may be observed if effusion is present. If the effusion is visible on radiography, then there is at least 250 mL of fluid accumulated.[2]

Medical Management

Pericardial effusion can be treated medically, with pericardiocentesis or with surgery.[20] Patients presenting for the first time with pericardial effusion are usually hospitalized to determine the cause of the effusion and to observe for the development of cardiac tamponade.[34] Medical management involves treatment of the pericarditis as discussed above with NSAIDs. Conservative treatment with clinical and echocardiographic monitoring is usually the approach for small or moderate effusions.[3] Uremic pericardial effusions are often treated with aggressive hemodialysis.[20]

Pericardiocentesis can be guided by fluoroscopy in the cardiac catheterization laboratory with ECG monitoring, or it can be conducted with echocardiography guidance.[20] This procedure is generally reserved for emergency situations where the patient is exhibiting symptoms of hemodynamic compromise as in cardiac tamponade, or for diagnostic purposes when tuberculosis is suspected.

Subxiphoid pericardiostomy and tube drainage can be performed under general or local anesthesia with sedation. During this procedure a small 2- to 4-cm piece of the pericardium is excised under direct vision. This sample can be analyzed. This subxiphoid incision is closed, and through a separate incision, a soft chest tube is placed in the pericardial cavity lateral to the right ventricle from the pericardiotomy, for postoperative drainage.[20]

Transcutaneous pericardioscopy and catheter drainage is another procedure to treat pericardial effusions. In this procedure general anesthesia is not needed. There is no need for an incision and therefore there is less pain, and several samples of the pericardium can be taken. However, small or posterior effusions are difficult to manage with this procedure, and it requires a clinician with a great deal of experience with the procedure.[20] Video-assisted transthoracic pericardial drainage, where a pericardial window is created, requires general anesthesia and single-lung ventilation. The window is not effective for longer-term drainage.[20]

Cardiac Tamponade

Cardiac tamponade is a life-threatening hemodynamic condition resulting from a pericardial effusion that has compressed the heart to restrict cardiac chamber filling. This restriction decreases cardiac output and causes heart failure. Cardiac tamponade can be caused by varying amounts of fluid. The speed of accumulation typically affects the severity of symptoms. Any scarring or thickening of the pericardium serves to amplify the effects of excess pericardial fluid on the heart.

Etiology

The most common causes of cardiac tamponade include effusions secondary to neoplasm, idiopathic pericarditis, acute MI resulting in pericarditis and/or cardiac rupture, catheter- or pacemaker-induced perforation of the right heart, coronary vessel perforation during percutaneous interventions, and cardiac surgery.[5] Trauma can also cause pericardial tamponade. Tamponade is reported in 15% of patients with idiopathic pericarditis but in as many as 60% of those with neoplastic, tuberculosis, or purulent pericarditis.[38]

Pathophysiology

Cardiac tamponade results from a pericardial effusion that increases intrapericardial pressure, compresses the heart, leading to diminished filling volumes and heart failure. If the effusion accumulates rapidly, as seen in trauma, then tamponade can occur with smaller volumes of 300 mL. Rapid accumulation does not allow time for the stiff pericardium to stretch. But an effusion that accumulates slowly, as seen in neoplasm, can be of as much as 1 L and still have little hemodynamic effect.[5] Slowly developing effusions allow time for the pericardium to be compliant and stretch.

The pressures measured by hemodynamic catheters are increased because the increased intrapericardial pressures are exerting an effect on the heart chambers. While increased pericardial pressure decreases cardiac volume, the measured pressure is still increased. In any cardiac condition, the measured filling pressure only reflects true preload when the chamber compliance, the pericardial space, and pericardial layers are normal.[5]

The decreased stroke volume results in neurohormonal compensatory responses to maintain organ perfusion. Increased sympathetic stimulation results in catecholamine release and increased contractility, tachycardia, and vasoconstriction. Sinus tachycardia reflects exhaustion of compensatory mechanisms and signals not only the presence of a hemodynamically important effusion, but may be indicative of impending hemodynamic collapse.[5]

Assessment Findings

A hemodynamically significant effusion may result in the symptoms of dyspnea, right heart failure, sinus tachycardia, and hypotension. Cardiac tamponade is a life-threatening condition that is diagnosed clinically by elevated jugular venous pressure, hypotension, and pulsus paradoxus in the setting of a pericardial effusion.[3] Although cardiac tamponade increases filling pressures, cardiac volumes are reduced. Right and left heart filling pressures are increased and equalized, but the amount of fluid in the pulmonary veins is modest. Therefore, in cardiac tamponade, lungs are typically clear despite profound shortness of breath.[5]

Pulsus paradoxus is defined as an inspiratory decrease in systolic blood pressure greater than 10 mm Hg.[5] Figure 30-3 depicts the mechanism of pulsus paradoxus as seen in pericardial tamponade.[5] It is easily observed on arterial line tracings and can be detected by using a sphygmomanometer. To measure the blood pressure change using a blood pressure cuff, inflate the cuff to 15 mm Hg above the highest systolic reading. The cuff is slowly deflated until the first Korotkoff sounds are heard. The sounds are heard only with some heartbeats; these are the ones occurring during expiration at that pressure. The other sounds are heard at a lower pressure during inspiration. Slowly deflate the cuff until all of the Korotkoff sounds can be heard. The difference between these two readings gives the size of the pulsus.[2]

Medical Management

The treatment of pericardial tamponade is pericardiocentesis, drainage of the fluid accumulated in the pericardium by needle paracentesis.[36] The use of echocardiographic imaging or fluoroscopy increases the safety and success of the procedure. Continuous hemodynamic monitoring of the effects of the procedure is critical. Surgery may be required if the cause of the tamponade is bleeding. A catheter can be placed for prolonged drainage.[36]

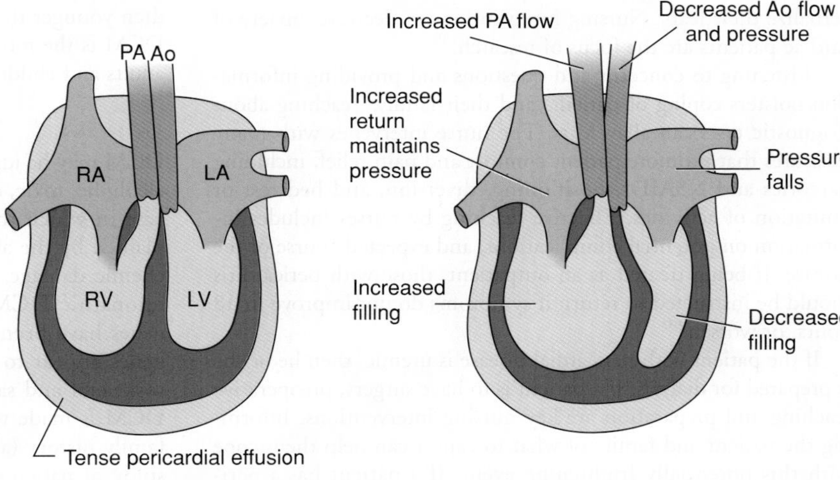

■ **Figure 30-3** Mechanism of pulsus paradoxus.

Nursing Management in Pericardial Disease

The nurse is perfectly positioned to recognize the symptoms of pericardial disease and the potential complications. The first priority of nursing management in pericardial disease is the recognition of the patient exhibiting hemodynamic compromise. It is critical that the patient maintain an adequate CO for organ perfusion. The nurse evaluates the patient's hemodynamic state, evaluating vital signs, symptoms, presence of pulsus paradoxus, and jugular venous distension. The nurse implements interventions that improve cardiac function, including oxygen, vasoactive medications, fluid management, and decreasing anxiety and stress. Nurses monitor for cardiac arrhythmias and evaluate their effects on the patient's condition. It is imperative that cardiac tamponade be diagnosed early, before hemodynamic collapse. Upon identification of a patient at risk, the nurse has the equipment readily available for an emergency pericardiocentesis. Close monitoring of the patient's condition during and after the procedure reveals any other complications.

The nurse who is knowledgeable of pericardial disease is able to identify the patients most at risk, such as those with renal failure or recent MI. Evaluation of history, physical exam, laboratory results, ECGs, and vital signs are key nursing interventions that have an enormous impact on the patient's outcome. A careful and skilled assessment is pivotal and points to the medical diagnosis of pericardial disease. To ensure appropriate treatment, the nurse needs to be aware of the subtle differences between symptoms of pericarditis and other conditions that cause chest pain, such as MI and pulmonary embolus. The characteristics of pericardial pain, including intermittent presence, location, quality, and the effect of position changes, are aspects of the patient's condition that nurses are best suited to assess. Because a pericardial friction rub is likely to come and go, and change in quality, the nurse is most likely to find the sound as the member of the health care team who is consistently and frequently evaluating the patient.

Anxiety is common among cardiac patients, has potentially serious consequences if untreated, and yet it is often not assessed or managed appropriately.[39] Emotional support and education can serve to decrease patient anxiety. Consistent care and a caring approach can encourage both the patient and family members to verbalize their fears. Nursing interventions to decrease anxiety of cardiac patients are the focus of research.[39]

Listening to concerns and questions and providing information bolsters coping of patients and their family. Teaching about diagnostic tests can allay fears. The nurse intervenes with many measures that promote patient comfort and pain relief, including narcotics and NSAIDs, positioning, diversion, and bed rest or limitation of activities. Effective teaching by nurses includes information on potential complications, and expected course of the disease. If being treated as an outpatient, those with pericarditis should be instructed to return if symptoms do not improve in 48 hours, or worsen.[40]

If the patient with pericardial disease is uremic, then he or she is prepared for dialysis. If a patient is to have surgery, preoperative teaching and preparation are key nursing interventions. Informing the patient and family of what to expect can help them cope with this potentially frightening event. If a patient has a pericardiectomy, pericardial window, or other cardiac surgery, close monitoring of hemodynamics after the surgical procedure is very important. Volume expanders and vasoactive medications may both be needed to maintain CO. The nurse is responsible for accurate hemodynamic measurements as this information is used to guide many treatment decisions. The nurse provides nursing care to prevent atelectasis and pneumonia, and monitors the surgical incision for infection. The nurse also monitors the effects of any other pharmacological therapy, such as NSAIDs, and is vigilant for side effects such as gastrointestinal upset or bleeding. The physician is notified if the desired effects of medical interventions are not seen or if side effects or complications arise.

CARDIOMYOPATHIES

The World Health Organization (WHO) defines cardiomyopathies as diseases of the myocardium associated with cardiac dysfunction. The WHO classification of cardiomyopathies includes dilated, hypertrophic, restrictive, and arrhythmogenic right ventricular cardiomyopathies.[41] The mortality rate in the United States due to cardiomyopathy is greater than 10,000 per year, with dilated cardiomyopathy (DCM) being the greatest contributor. The total cost of health care in the United States focused on cardiomyopathies is in the billions of dollars and limited success has been realized.[42] *Left ventricular noncompaction* is another type of cardiomyopathy that has recently gained attention. It may become a distinct classification in the future.[42] Noncompaction of the left ventricle is theorized to be due to myocardium embryogenesis of the endocardium and myocardium.[43]

Dilated Cardiomyopathy

DCM is characterized by dilation and impaired contraction of the left or both ventricles.[41] The diagnosis of DCM is made after exclusion of known, specific causes of heart failure.[44] DCM causes considerable morbidity and mortality, and it is one of the major causes of sudden cardiac death. DCM is the most common cardiomyopathy at 60% of the total cases.[45] Idiopathic DCM is the most common cause of congestive heart failure in the young with an estimated prevalence of at least 36.5 per 100,000 persons in the United States for adults.[46] The annual incidence of DCM in children younger than 18 years was 0.57 cases per 100,000 per year. DCM is the most common reason for cardiac transplantation in adults and children.[47]

Etiology

DCM may be idiopathic, familial/genetic, viral, and/or immune, alcoholic, toxic, or associated with recognized cardiovascular disease in which the degree of myocardial dysfunction is not explained by the abnormal loading conditions or the extent of ischemic damage.[41] It is estimated that 30% to 50% of cases of idiopathic DCM have a genetic origin.[45] Recently, multiple genes have been identified to be associated with DCM. These genes appear to encode two major subgroups of proteins; cytoskeletal and sarcomeric proteins.[42] The diagnosis of familial DCM is made when DCM is present in the setting of positive family history (at least two family members are affected).[48] In a study of patients with idiopathic DCM, a large number of patients were found to have had viral infections. These data suggest that myocardial persistence of various viruses, often presenting as multiple infections, may play a role in the pathogenesis of DCM far more frequently than suspected so far.[49] Another study found that adenovirus was the most common virus in the myocardium of children and adults with myocarditis and DCM.[50] Secondary causes of DCM include CAD, myocarditis, nutritional deficiency, systemic disease, cardiotoxins, puerperium, alcohol, and skeletal muscle wasting diseases.[46]

Pathophysiology

DCM is characterized by an increase in myocardial mass and a reduction in ventricular wall thickness. The heart assumes a globular shape and there is pronounced ventricular chamber dilatation, diffuse endocardial thickening, and atrial enlargement often with thrombi in the appendages.[46] The histological changes seen in DCM are nonspecific.[41] Familial DCM is caused by mutations in structural proteins comprising the myocyte cytoskeleton or sarcolemma.[46] Intraventricular conduction delay and LBBB commonly occur in patients with idiopathic DCM. When cardiomyopathy causes left ventricular failure, conduction abnormalities add further to LV dysfunction by compounding dyssynchrony in the contractile motion of the LV wall.[51]

Assessment Findings

Presentation of DCM is usually with heart failure, which is often progressive. The most typical symptoms include dyspnea, fatigue, and volume gain. A minority of patients report chest pain, which can signify epicardial coronary disease, subendocardial disease, or pulmonary embolism. Arrhythmias, thromboembolism, and sudden death are common, and may occur at any stage during the disease.[41] Complaints of abdominal discomfort or anorexia are frequent in late stages of the disease and suggest hepatomegaly or bowel edema, respectively. Other common late complications include thromboembolic events, which may be systemic, originating from the left atria and ventricle, or pulmonary thrombi from the lower extremities.[52] Mitral regurgitation is common in DCM, as are ventricular arrhythmias, particularly ventricular tachycardia, torsades de pointes, and ventricular fibrillation.[42] A recent study found strong evidence that glucose intolerance is a common characteristic of patients with idiopathic DCM.[53]

Echocardiography is a cornerstone in the evaluation and management of patients with DCM. Two-dimensional echocardiography is a valuable noninvasive technique to assess ventricular size and performance, and to evaluate associated valvular or pericardial abnormalities. Doppler echocardiography allows the evaluation of valvular regurgitation or stenosis, and the quantification of cardiac output.[52] This important information regarding the patient's condition helps guide therapy.

Cardiac catheterization usually reveals increased left ventricular end-diastolic pressures and pulmonary artery wedge pressures. Pulmonary hypertension may range from mild to severe. The right ventricle is frequently involved and enlarged, manifested with increased right ventricular end-diastolic pressures, right atrial pressures, and central venous pressures.[52]

Medical Management

The initial evaluation of patients presenting with DCM should focus on identifying reversible and secondary causes.[52] Medical management focuses on optimizing cardiac function. Treatment with neurohormonal antagonists to prevent disease progression and the use of diuretics to maintain the volume balance are the therapeutic cornerstones for the management of patients with DCM.[54] Medications identified through clinical trials as providing beneficial effects for patients with DCM include diuretics, angiotensin-converting enzyme (ACE) inhibitors or angiotensin receptor blockers if ACE intolerant, and β-blockers.[54] A recent study showed that β-blocker therapy (carvedilol) induced significant reductions in intraventricular dyssynchrony and improved contractility in DCM patients with heart failure and normal QRS.[55] Another study of the β-blocker carvedilol showed an improvement in coronary flow reserve and a reduction in stress-induced perfusion defects. These results suggest a favorable effect of the drug on coronary microvascular function in patients with idiopathic DCM.[56]

Successful treatment of the patient with alcoholic cardiomyopathy must include cessation of alcohol consumption, which can have significant benefits in improving symptoms of heart failure. Ongoing alcohol consumption significantly worsens the patient's prognosis. Additional therapy includes a regimen of neurohormonal blockers. Administration of thiamine is also indicated in the possibility that malnutrition may play a role in the presentation. Anticoagulation should only be considered in the presence of a clear-cut and pressing indication because of the increased risk of trauma, catastrophic bleeding, and increased anticoagulation caused by hepatic dysfunction related to alcohol abuse.[52]

In research on patients with severe, nonischemic DCM who were treated with ACE inhibitors and β-blockers, the implantation of a cardioverter defibrillator significantly reduced the risk of sudden death from arrhythmia.[57] This intervention has become an important mainstay of treatment. Cardiac resynchronization therapy (CRT) with biventricular pacing has emerged as a promising treatment for medically refractory heart failure.[55] CRT corrects dyssynchrony by synchronous pacing from transvenous pacing catheters implanted in the right atrium and right ventricle. The CRT device usually includes an implantable defibrillator.[51]

Patients with valvular heart disease, CHD, pericardial disease, or congenital heart defects should be considered for surgical correction. There are also other surgical approaches to DCM designed to restore chamber geometry or provide mechanical support. Procedures aimed at surgically remodeling of the heart include left ventricular reconstruction or implantation of external restraint devices. The CorCap Cardiac Support Device (Acorn Cardiovascular, Inc., St Paul, MN), one implanted device designed to provide support for the heart, was recently tested in a study funded by the developers to see if it improved heart failure in patients with DCM by preventing LV remodeling. This initial safety and efficacy trial of this device showed promising results.[58] Left ventricular assist devices provide aggressive mechanical support to patients with advanced decompensated heart failure.[54]

DCM is a leading reason for cardiac transplantation.[59] Although the incidence of ischemic cardiomyopathy is higher than DCM, these two diagnoses account for an equal number of performed cardiac transplantations. Cardiac transplantation becomes a possible treatment option when all medical therapies have been maximized, and no other surgical procedures will correct the underlying disease process.[60]

Recently new guidelines for management of heart failure were published in Europe and in the United States detailing medication management guidelines and clinical testing. The recommendations also include patient and family counseling, weight management and monitoring, dietary measures including sodium restriction, fluid management, exercise as tolerated, smoking cessation, and immunization for influenza.[54,61]

Hypertrophic Cardiomyopathy

Hypertrophic cardiomyopathy (HCM) is a familial cardiac disorder characterized by left and/or right ventricular hypertrophy, which is usually asymmetric and involves the interventricular septum.[41] The manifestations of HCM are complex and may include dynamic left ventricular outflow tract obstruction (LVOTO), mitral regurgitation, diastolic dysfunction, myocardial ischemia, and cardiac arrhythmias. Many individuals with HCM have a life expectancy similar to the general adult population, although there are subsets of patients that annual mortality rates up to 6%.[62] HCM is the single most common cause of athlete deaths in the United States, responsible for about one-third of the cases.[63]

Etiology

Familial disease with an autosomal dominant inheritance predominates. This disorder affects 1:500 of the population.[46] Mutations in sarcomeric contractile protein genes cause disease.[41,64] Mechanisms thought to lead to septal hypertrophy include reduced contractile dysfunction leading to compensatory hypertrophy of cardiac myocytes, insufficient levels of muscle ATP resulting in deranged sarcomere function, and the induction of growth factors that stimulate hypertrophy and fibrosis.[65]

Pathophysiology

In HCM, the left ventricular volume is typically normal or reduced, and systolic gradients are common. LVOTO is present in 30% to 50% of patients. LVOTO causes an increase in left ventricular systolic pressure, which leads to prolonged ventricular relaxation, increased left ventricular diastolic pressure, myocardial ischemia, and decreased cardiac output. The obstruction can be dependent on changes in preload, afterload, and contractility, so anything that influences these factors can affect the LVOTO.[64] Mitral valve regurgitation is due to systolic anterior motion of the mitral valve.[66] Typical morphological changes include myocyte hypertrophy and disarray surrounding areas of increased loose connective tissue.

Assessment Findings

HCM is diagnosed by echocardiography in the presence of left ventricular hypertrophy in the absence of other mechanical, metabolic, or genetic causes.[8,64] MRI can also aid in diagnosis.[8] Pressure gradients between the aorta and left ventricle greater than 30 mm Hg signify severe LVOTO. The preferred method of eliciting presence of latent gradients during and/or immediately following exercise is treadmill or bicycle exercise testing along with Doppler echocardiography. Knowledge of a latent gradient is very important to guide key management decisions.[8]

Classic findings in HCM include a systolic ejection murmur that becomes increasing loud during maneuvers that decrease preload, such as standing from a squatting position.[64] A mitral regurgitation murmur can be heard because the mitral leaflet is open as it is pulled into the left ventricular outflow tract during systole.[65]

The majority of patients are asymptomatic throughout life. However, some will present with severe symptoms of dyspnea, angina, and syncope.[64] The ECG will display signs of left ventricular hypertrophy. Ventricular arrhythmias and premature sudden death are common and appear to be genetically linked.[41,64] Atrial fibrillation is also commonly seen and thought to be due to atrial enlargement.[66]

Medical Management

Treatment strategies in HCM are directed toward prevention of sudden cardiac death and symptom relief.[67] An ICD and amiodarone are used to prevent sudden cardiac death in patients at high risk.[66] Risk factors for sudden cardiac death include sudden cardiac death in first-degree family members, unexplained syncope, abnormal blood pressure response to exercise, resting left ventricular outflow gradient greater than 30 mm Hg, ventricular ectopy, and massive LVH.[68,69] Pharmacological therapy is designed to increase diastolic filling and decrease LVOTO and gradient. Catecholamines exacerbate the LVOTO and increase the heart rate, reducing filling time, so they are the target of therapy. The medications used are β-blockers or calcium channel blockers, and the antiarrhythmic disopyramide.[66]

The goal of surgical intervention is to reduce permanently the LVOTO and gradient, thereby decreasing symptoms and improving quality of life. The size of the ventricular septum, and therefore the LVOTO, can be reduced through surgical myectomy or alcohol ablation.[66] Successful surgical myectomy results in marked improvement of symptoms. Percutaneous alcohol septal ablation was first reported in 1995, and involves the introduction of alcohol into a target septal perforator branch of the left anterior descending coronary artery to induce an MI within the proximal ventricular septum. This treatment results in a decrease in septal thickness. Improvement after septal ablation can occur immediately in the catheterization laboratory, or over hours or several months.[62] Patients are at risk for conduction problems so a temporary pacemaker is placed prior to the ablation. Some patients may require a permanent pacemaker.[70] There are no randomized clinical trials comparing surgery to ablation, therefore long-term outcomes for these strategies are unknown.[70,71]

Dual-chamber pacemaker therapy may be helpful to reduce symptoms in half of HCM patients. Patients with atrial fibrillation are aggressively treated to achieve a normal sinus rhythm. If atrial fibrillation is chronic, the ventricular rate is controlled with β-blockers, verapamil, or digoxin. Anticoagulation is also necessary.[62]

If the patient with HCM is hospitalized for deterioration, adequate volume and decreasing myocardial oxygen demands are important.[65] Positive inotropes and chronotropes should be avoided as they worsen LVOTO. Nitrates decrease preload so must be used with caution as that will also worsen LVOTO. β-Blockers are indicated. If hypotension is present, it should be managed with a purely α-adrenergic agonist medication such as phenylephrine.[64]

In the past, patients with HCM and LVOTO at rest were considered at risk for bacterial endocarditis and were prescribed appropriate antibiotic prophylaxis for dental and surgical procedures.[62,66,67,72] The new American Heart Association guidelines for infective endocarditis (IE) now recommend prophylaxis for a select group of patients.[97]

Because of the genetic nature of HCM, annually clinical screening of adolescent relatives aged 12 to 18 years, consisting of a history and physical examination, 12-lead ECG, and two-dimensional echocardiography is indicated. Because some individuals do not manifest HCM until adulthood, screening beyond adolescence is recommended every 5 years.[8] Patients are advised to avoid athletic competition and extremes of physical exertion.[67] Genetic testing may also be completed, but this testing is currently done in research laboratories, is very time-consuming and expensive, and not routinely available.[68,72]

Restrictive Cardiomyopathy

RCM is characterized by restrictive filling and reduced diastolic volume of either or both ventricles with normal or near-normal systolic function and wall thickness.[41] It is an uncommon type of cardiomyopathy in countries like the United States.[73]

Etiology

RCM may be idiopathic, or associated with other diseases, such as amyloidosis, and endomyocardial fibrosis.[41,73,74]

Pathophysiology

The pathophysiological feature that defines RCM is an increase in stiffness of the ventricular walls, which causes impaired diastolic filling of the ventricle and heart failure. In RCM, interstitial fibrosis may be present.[41] In early stages of RCM, systolic function may be normal, although deterioration in systolic function is usually observed as the disease progresses.[52]

Assessment Findings

Clinically, RCM mimics constrictive pericarditis. Symptoms include weakness, dyspnea, edema, and exertional chest pain. Patients with RCM frequently present with exercise intolerance because of an impaired ability to augment cardiac output during increasing heart rate because of the restriction of diastolic filling. With advanced disease, profound edema occurs that includes peripheral edema, hepatomegaly, ascites, and anasarca.[52] Physical examination reveals an elevated jugular venous pulse, often with the Kussmaul's sign, and an increasing jugular pressure during inspiration due to the restriction to filling. Both S_3 and S_4 heart sounds are common and the apical pulse is palpable (in contrast to constrictive pericarditis). Patients with RCM often develop atrial fibrillation. CT and MRI are valuable for differentiating constrictive and restrictive disease.

Medical Management

There is no known treatment for RCM, so therapy is supportive. It includes diuretics, corticosteroids, or anticoagulants, depending on the etiology and manifestations. Cardiac pacing may improve symptoms[75]

Arrhythmogenic Right Ventricular Cardiomyopathy

Arrhythmogenic right ventricular cardiomyopathy (ARVC) is also known as arrhythmic right ventricular dysplasia. ARVC is characterized by progressive fibrofatty replacement of right ventricular myocardium, initially with typical regional and later global right and some left ventricular involvement, with relative sparing of the septum.[41]

Etiology

Familial disease is common in ARVC, typically with autosomal dominant inheritance and incomplete penetrance. A recessive form has also been identified.[41,54] Several genes and gene loci are associated with ARVC.

Pathophysiology

The fibrofatty mechanism of this disease leads to the progressive loss of myocytes.[46] ARVC may also involve the left ventricle.[46] Structural and functional abnormalities of the right ventricle lead to arrhythmias and progressive right ventricular failure.[76]

Assessment Findings

Presentation of ARVC with arrhythmias and sudden death is common, particularly in the young, and may be precipitated by exertion.[41,46] ARVC accounts for up to 20% of cases of sudden cardiac death, and, importantly, among young athletes dying suddenly, the prevalence of this condition is high.[54]

The most common ECG abnormalities found in a U.S. cohort of ARVC patients were delayed S-wave upstroke and T-wave inversion. Thirty-one of 100 patients in this cohort experienced sudden cardiac death. Arrhythmic events are thought to be the most important events in ARVC, substantiated by the results in this cohort in which the prognosis was excellent once an ICD was instituted.[77] Another study showed that due to effective treatment of arrhythmias leading to sudden cardiac death, heart failure has emerged as an another major cause of death in patients with this disorder.[78]

Medical Management

The diagnostic criteria for ARVC involve features obtained from imaging, ECG, signal-averaged ECG and histological criteria, as well as a positive family history and a history of arrhythmias. Endomyocardial biopsy may offer valuable diagnostic information, but cardiac MRI is emerging as a more definitive diagnostic tool.[76] The main limitations of endomyocardial biopsy are a high false-negative rate because of sampling error, and absence from the right ventricular of the characteristic histological changes. Researchers have reported that characterization of the ventricular wall morphology with delayed enhancement gadolinium MRI correlated with histological findings and with inducibility of ventricular tachycardia during electrophysiological testing.[76]

Patients diagnosed with ARVC generally require an ICD. Antiarrhythmic therapy is appropriate prior to ICD insertion. Neurohormonal blockade with ACE inhibitors and β-adrenoreceptor antagonists is also recommended therapy. In individuals progressing to overt heart failure, management involves the same principles for the treatment of other forms of cardiomyopathy.[79] Consideration of heart transplantation is indicated for patients overt cardiac failure.[54]

Myocarditis

Myocarditis is an inflammatory disease of the myocardium. Myocarditis can be categorized as acute or chronic, and can lead to the development of DCM.[8] Myocarditis may be idiopathic, infectious, or autoimmune.[44] Primary or postviral myocarditis can be categorized by its clinical pathological manifestations. This includes fulminant, chronic active, eosinophilic, and giant cell myocarditis.[80] Fulminant myocarditis has a 2-week course, resulting either in full recovery, or death. Patients with chronic active myocarditis have ongoing inflammation and fibrosis, leading to RCM. Patients treated for the eosinophilic disorder respond to treatment. Giant cell myocarditis has a very poor prognosis despite aggressive treatment.[80]

Etiology

There are many etiologies of myocarditis. The cause may be viral, bacterial, fungal, protozoal, and parasitic. Toxins, hypersensitivity to medications, and immunological syndromes can also cause myocarditis.[81] Viruses are considered the predominant cause. Age-related and regional differences may be important when looking at the viral etiology of myocarditis.[81] HIV-related myocarditis is a significant problem for that patient population. Smallpox vaccination has also been associated with myocarditis.[82]

Pathophysiology

Myocarditis is the result of both myocardial infections and autoimmunity that results in active inflammatory destruction of myocytes. Inflammation of the myocardium affects its function, and heart failure can result.

Assessment Findings

The clinical appearance of myocarditis is varied; the features range from systemic symptoms of fever, myalgias, palpitations, and dyspnea, to arrhythmia, syncope, sudden death, acute right or left ventricular failure, cardiogenic shock, or DCM.[44,81] Myocarditis may resolve, or result in relapse, DCM requiring heart transplantation, or death.

Endomyocardial biopsy has been the gold standard for the diagnosis of myocarditis, but this technique is fraught with difficulties.[80] Other diagnostic criteria have been proposed that incorporate molecular techniques applied to the examination of the myocardium.[81] Contrast-enhanced MRI may become a valuable diagnostic tool.[81,83]

ECG, echocardiography, and measurement of serum troponin are additional required tests when myocarditis is suspected.[81] In myocarditis, the ECG can show low-voltage QRS complexes, ST segment elevation, or heart block. Nonsustained atrial or ventricular arrhythmias are common. An S_4 and systolic ejection murmurs may be heard on auscultation.

Medical Management

Supportive care is the first line of treatment in myocarditis. Management includes treatment of heart failure, with the goal of improving symptoms and hemodynamic status.[81] Many researchers have evaluated the use of immunosuppression in myocarditis, but the efficacy of routine use has not been established.[81,84,85] Intravenous (IV) immunoglobulin has also been given to treat viral myocarditis, but evidence does not support its use.[86]

Nursing Management in Cardiomyopathies and Myocarditis

The nurse can help in identifying the cause of cardiomyopathy or myocarditis through a careful and detailed nursing history. Advances in understanding of causes of cardiomyopathies make genetic counseling and screening strategies even more critical.[87] Advanced practice nurses are in a unique position to detect, educate, and treat familial diseases. As expert clinicians, they assess disorders from a holistic perspective using comprehensive physical examination and detailed history, including assessment of family history, psychosocial influences, and functional abilities.[66] The nurse must be attentive to family history so identification of a familial disease can be made and other family members might be screened. Young family members should be screened prior to participation in sports.[63] Genetic testing may identify those likely to develop the disease, although this testing is not a readily available option in most laboratories. Guidelines have been published recently for genetic testing in families where sudden cardiac death has occurred.[88] The nurse must probe to find out the concerns of the patient and the family, and try to address each of them.

It is crucial that the patient with a disease such as cardiomyopathy at high risk for sudden death wear a medical alert bracelet in case of emergency and that family members be trained in basic life support techniques.[89]

The nurse is also in the best position to monitor the patient for worsening of symptoms and for response to medical treatments. Evaluation of heart sounds, lung sounds, vital signs, and peripheral perfusion, as well as interpretation of laboratory results are key nursing responsibilities. Signs of congestion and decreased CO must be detected and reported early to ensure the most effective treatment. This assessment involves accurate hemodynamic measurements and assessments, which guide therapy. The nurse titrates medications and fluids to improve cardiac function, monitoring the effects and side effects. Patients with poor perfusion, as is seen in cardiac disease, are at increased risk for skin breakdown. The nurse is responsible for assessment and prevention of this complication. The nurse optimizes the patient's oxygenation through position changes, pulmonary toilet, monitoring and interpretation of arterial blood gases, and oxygen administration or ventilator management. Infection control is also critical. Because lethal arrhythmias can occur, emergency equipment should be readily available.

If a ventricular assist device is used in the course of treatment for cardiomyopathy or myocarditis, the nurse monitors the effects of this therapy. When the patient is to have surgery, preoperative education can allay many fears if the patient and family have an opportunity to ask questions and are prepared for the postoperative course. Teaching needs to be individualized, with determination of the best method for the patient and family. After surgery, the nurse is responsible for postoperative hemodynamic monitoring, pain control, and respiratory care. Recognition of symptoms of excess use of drugs or alcohol or withdrawal from these substances is necessary.[90] Complications need to be prevented or detected immediately. Patients with HCM who have undergone septal ablation must be monitored closely for conduction defects. The temporary pacemaker is employed as needed. Patients are also monitored for enzymes and ECG changes.

Emotional support and education are key components of nursing care of patients with cardiomyopathy and myocarditis. In a familial disease, a patient may be grieving for a family member while coping with his or her own new diagnosis. They may need assistance coping with this stressful crisis. Emotional needs are particularly important in cardiomyopathy because of its wide-ranging impact on the lives of both the patient and family. Individual counseling, support groups, or both can be effective.

The patient and his or her family must be educated about cardiomyopathy and myocarditis, its treatments and possible complications. To make the diagnosis, the patient undergoes many tests, such as echocardiography and cardiac catheterization. Each test that is done should be explained to the patient. The plan of care needs to be discussed and agreed on. If anticoagulants are used, side effects and their symptoms, as well as dietary interactions, need to be explained. Other dietary considerations must be addressed, such as fluid and salt restriction, and the nurse as a leader of the multidisciplinary team can ensure that the patient's multiple needs are met.

Research has shown the addition of a 1-hour, nurse educator-delivered teaching session at the time of hospital discharge resulted in improved clinical outcomes, increased self-care measure adherence, and reduced cost of care in patients with systolic heart failure.[91] As a leader of the health care team, the nurse can alert social workers, chaplains, mental health professionals, dieticians and others to the needs of the patient and coordinate the multidisciplinary care.

ENDOCARDIAL DISEASE

Infective Endocarditis

IE is a disease in which infective organisms invade the endothelial lining of the heart, usually involving one or more valves. The endocardium covers the valves and surrounds the chordae tendineae. Recently, the definition of IE has been expanded to include an infection of any structure within the heart including prosthetic valves, and implanted devices, as well as the valves and endothelium.[92] The infection that forms, an irregularly shaped echogenic mass adherent to the endothelial cardiac surface, often on the valve of the heart, is called *vegetation*.[92] Destruction, ulceration, or abscess formation can also occur. IE is the major endocardial disease. If left untreated, IE is fatal.[93]

Types

Native Valve Endocarditis. *Native valve endocarditis* (NVE), the most common type, is an infection seen in patients without prosthetic valves, but who usually have valvular or heart disease that predisposes them to IE.

The Intravenous Drug User. NVE is a severe complication of IV drug use. It is responsible for 5% to 20% of hospital admissions, and 5% to 10% of total deaths in those that use IV drugs.[92,94] IE in IV drug users is thought to be caused by infection introduced through contaminated needles or drugs. IE in these patients often involves the tricuspid valve.[92] In the IV drug user with IE, the valves were normal before infection in 75% to 93% of patients.[95]

Prosthetic Valve Endocarditis. The clinical index for suspicion is much higher for *prosthetic valve endocarditis* (PVE), which occurs more frequently than NVE. PVE is also much more likely to require surgery as part of the treatment. PVE represents 10% to 30% of all IE.

Infected Intracardiac Devices. During the 1990s there was a large increase in cardiac device implantations, such as pacemakers and ICDs. Accompanying this increase was a surge in IE related to these intracardiac devices, especially in elderly patients.[96]

Nosocomial Endocarditis. Nosocomial endocarditis is an infection of the cardiac endothelium related to health care.

Epidemiology

IE affects 15,000 patients every year and it has a mortality rate approaching 40%.[92] Rheumatic heart disease was the most common underlying condition predisposing an individual to endocarditis in developed countries, and this remains a common condition in developing countries.[97] Despite advances in health care, the incidence of IE has not decreased over the last few decades. This apparent paradox may be explained by an evolution in risk factors; while classic predisposing conditions such as rheumatic heart disease have been all but eradicated, new risk factors for IE have emerged. These include an increasing use of various intracardiac valvular prostheses and intravascular shunts, grafts, and other devices.[97] In a review of 26 publications, Moreillon and Que reported a median incidence of IE of 3.6 per 100,000.[98] In areas where there are many IV drug users, the incidence is higher.[92] The highest incidence of IE is reported in the elderly.[92]

Etiology

Streptococci and *staphylococci* account for 80% to 90% of IE cases in which identification of the organism is made.[92] *Staphylococcus aureus* is an important cause of IE, as the course is often fulminant, and this is frequently a nosocomial infection.[92] Enterococcus may cause up to 15% of IE cases.[92] Several other infectious organisms can also cause IE.

Pathophysiology

A complex series of events interplay to result in IE. Endothelial damage appears to be the first step, followed by platelet–fibrin deposition and formation of a lesion known as a nonbacterial thrombotic endocarditis. Bacteremia then allows bacterial colonization. Colonization allows formation of a vegetation as microorganisms adhere to the nonbacterial thrombotic endocarditis lesion.[92] Many of the clinical manifestations of IE result from the infected individual's immune response to the microorganism.[97]

Structural abnormality in a valve is commonly seen in IE. Mitral valve prolapse, aortic valve disease, and congenital heart disease exist in a large number of patients with IE.[92] Mechanical and prosthetic valves can also become infected.

Assessment Findings

The diagnosis of IE is based on clinical signs and symptoms, and demonstration of continued bacteremia.[92] In 1994, Durack et al.[99] proposed a set of diagnostic criteria for the diagnosis of IE that subsequently became known as the Duke criteria. According to the Duke criteria, persistent bacteremia with organisms typical for endocarditis and an oscillating mass on a valve (vegetation) make a clinically definitive diagnosis of IE. In the course of clinical practice, the diagnosis is suspected more often than it is confirmed. The Duke criteria include several minor criteria that also suggest IE, such as predisposition, fever, vascular phenomena such as septic pulmonary infarcts, and immunologic phenomena such as Osler's nodes. Transthoracic echocardiography with Doppler flow studies should be performed in everyone suspected of having endocarditis. In 2000, other researchers proposed several modifications to the Duke criteria, including the use of transesophageal echocardiogram.[100] If the clinical suspicion is high and the transthoracic echocardiogram is negative or inconclusive, a transesophageal echocardiogram should be obtained.[100]

Major criteria to diagnose IE includes at least two positive cultures of blood samples drawn greater than 12 hours apart, or all of three or a majority of four or more separate cultures of blood, with the first and last samples drawn at least 1 hour apart.[100] Blood cultures should be drawn from three different sites with 1 hour between each draw or, if time is limited, a total of 1 hour between the first and the last draw. Blood cultures isolate the organism, and positive cultures over time demonstrate true persistence. Meticulous site preparation is essential to avoid contamination.[101] Blood cultures can be negative in up to 15% of patients meeting criteria for IE diagnosis.[102] Other laboratory findings seen in IE can include normochromic normocytic anemia, elevated white blood cell count, and elevated erythrocyte sedimentation rate in almost all cases.[95]

Anemia, with red blood cell indices, a low serum iron level, and low serum iron-binding capacity, is found in 70% to 90% of patients. Anemia worsens with increased duration of illness and thus in acute IE may be absent. A leukocytosis with increased segmented granulocytes is common in acute IE. Thrombocytopenia occurs only rarely. While erythrocyte sedimentation rate is elevated in almost all patients with IE, the exceptions are those with CHF, renal failure, or disseminated intravascular coagulation.

Medical Management

The cornerstone of treatment of IE is early recognition and elimination of the infecting organism. Timely surgical intervention and anticipation and treatment of complications are also key concepts in the care of these patients. Antibiotics are usually bactericidal (versus ineffective bacteriostatic agents).[103] Antibiotic therapy is usually of a long duration. Published guidelines such as those from the American Heart Association and the European Society of Cardiology are valuable resources on the specifics of management of IE.[93,104]

All patients with IE should have an initial evaluation of cardiac function. Careful history and physical examination is paramount. Echocardiography is used to evaluate ejection fraction and valvular function. The most frequent complication of IE is congestive heart failure, usually the result of valvular insufficiency.[92] Valvular destruction is caused by the infection. Heart failure is the most common cause of death in IE, and is an indication for surgery.[103] Continuous close monitoring for symptoms of hemodynamic decompensation and heart failure is important as the aortic valve can sudden fail and pulmonary edema can abruptly develop. Left-sided IE involving the mitral valve frequently requires surgery as well.[103]

Valvular and perivalvular abscess, an extension of the infection, also requires surgical intervention.[92] Cardiac conduction problems may develop secondary to the abscess or infection, making cardiac rhythm monitoring essential.[103]

Vegetation emboli can cause stroke, especially from the mitral valve. Mycotic aneurysms result from septic embolization to an arterial intraluminal space or the vasa vasorum of the cerebral vessels. These aneurysms can have few symptoms, or may cause major neurological complications such as intracranial hemorrhage.[92] Angiography is valuable in assessing mycotic aneurysms. Placement of coils or neurosurgery to ligate or clip the aneurysm may be indicated.[103] Renal dysfunction is another commonly seen complication, and occurs due to localized infarctions and immune complex glomerlunephritis.[92]

Prevention

There has not been a placebo-controlled, multicenter, randomized, double-blinded study to evaluate the efficacy of IE prophylaxis in patients who undergo potentially risky dental, gastrointestinal, or genitourinary tract procedures.[97] There is no evidence about whether prophylaxis is effective or not against IE in patients undergoing dental procedures.[105] The American Heart Association has published new evidence-based guidelines for antimicrobial prophylaxis for IE.[97] The guidelines have radically changed regarding the recommendations for antibiotic prophylaxis in dental and other procedures. IE prophylaxis is now recommended only for those patients with underlying cardiac conditions associated with highest risk of adverse outcome from IE. These conditions include prosthetic cardiac valve, previous IE, specific forms of congenital heart disease, and cardiac transplantation with cardiac valvulopathy.[97] This prophylaxis for these select patients is recommended for all dental procedures that involve manipulation of gingival tissue or the periapical region of teeth or perforation of oral mucosa.[97] Prophylaxis is also "reasonable" for procedures on respiratory tract or infected skin, skin structures, or musculoskeletal tissue, for the same high-risk patients. Antibiotic prophylaxis is no longer recommended for gastrointestinal or genitourinal procedures. These new evidence-based guidelines are controversial, and are substantially different that from past recommendations.[106]

The association gave additional advice against body piercing for high-risk patients. Finally, the guidelines state that there should be greater emphasis placed on improving access to dental care and oral health in patients at risk for IE.[97]

Nursing Management in Infectious Endocarditis

Nurses need to be knowledgeable about IE and its symptoms and complications, the difficulty in making the diagnosis, and its far-reaching effects. A detailed history reveals risk factors, symptoms, prodromal illness, recent antibiotic therapy, and pre-existing renal disease. This information aids in the medical diagnosis. Determination of body piercing or tattooing is necessary. A careful physical examination may reveal the signs of IE, such as a murmur secondary to new-onset regurgitation. Patients that develop heart failure during IE may be managed with diuretics, and afterload reduction with nitroglycerin and ACE inhibitors.[107] The nurse manages the administration and monitoring of these medications.

Once the patient is diagnosed, the plan of care should be discussed with the patient and family. Management of the patient with IE is complex and requires a team of experts on infectious diseases, cardiology, cardiac surgery, respiratory therapy, nutritional medicine, social services, and nursing. Nurses can be effective leaders on this team, ensuring all the needs of the patient are met.

A lengthy hospitalization is likely, and patients need assistance with coping with hospitalization and the illness. IE is potentially life threatening, so information and emotional support are crucial. If it is indicated, a referral for drug addiction treatment should be completed. Drug addiction and alcohol abuse frequently engender strong negative feelings among nurses and physicians. The nurse must make care decisions in an ethical, professional manner, even when caring for patients who use IV drugs, do not follow recommendations, or do not take the prescribed medications.[108] In a recent study, it was found that consideration of drug abuse issues was frequently not incorporated into the plan of care in the intensive care unit.[109] Other issues in this population are an increased tolerance to analgesia, potential drug withdrawal, and behavior and adherence problems, and poly-substance abuse.[110,111]

The nurse manages oxygen therapy, ventilator care, and vasoactive medications and monitors fluid balance and ECGs. The nurse often obtains the blood for laboratory tests and blood cultures, and then interprets the results. The nurse is responsible for proper administration of antibiotics and monitoring for therapeutic levels and side effects. The nurse also manages the IV lines for the long course of antibiotics. If a pulmonary artery catheter is in place, accurate measurements and interpretations guide medical care. Meticulous handwashing, infection control, and early removal of invasive lines help to prevent nosocomial IE. The Center for Disease Control and the American Association of Critical-Care Nurses have both published guidelines to prevent catheter-related infections.[112,113]

Careful assessment facilitates early detection of complications. The nurse must know the symptoms of complications to facilitate rapid intervention. Preoperative teaching is necessary to prepare the patient undergoing surgery. During surgery, it is desirable to keep the family informed of the progress. After surgery, pulmonary hygiene and close hemodynamic monitoring are crucial. Idemoto and Kresevic[114] recently reviewed evidence-based practice, including pain management, infections, and patient education, and nurse-sensitive outcomes in postoperative cardiac patients. Monitoring for potential drug withdrawal if the patient is an IV drug user is also important. The signs of withdrawal include agitation, tachycardia, diaphoresis, and hypertension.[90]

Once the patient is ready for discharge, education is critical because the patient must be knowledgeable about recurrence of symptoms, such as fever and weight loss, antibiotic prophylaxis for certain high-risk procedures, and the need for keeping all health care providers informed that he or she is at increased risk for IE. The nurse should stress the importance of post-discharge follow-up and inform the patient about the need to obtain medical alert identification. The role of proper oral hygiene and dental health in IE should be emphasized during patient teaching.[97]

REFERENCES

1. Troughton, R. W., Asher, C. R., & Klein, A. L. (2004). Pericarditis. *Lancet, 363*(9410), 717–727.
2. Spodick, D. H. (1997). *The pericardium: A comprehensive textbook*. New York: Marcel Dekker, Inc.
3. Ivens, E. L., Munt, B. I., & Moss, R. R. (2007). Pericardial disease: What the general cardiologist needs to know. *Heart, 93*(8), 993–1000.
4. Ariyarajah, V., & Spodick, D. H. (2007). Acute pericarditis: Diagnostic cues and common electrocardiographic manifestations. *Cardiology in Review, 15*, 24–30.
5. Goldstein, J. A. (2004). Cardiac tamponade, constrictive pericarditis, and restrictive cardiomyopathy. *Current Problems in Cardiology, 29*(9), 503–567.
6. Hoit, B. D. (2007). Pericardial disease and pericardial tamponade. *Critical Care Medicine, 35*(8, Suppl.), S355–S364.
7. Carter, T., & Brooks, C. A. (2005). Pericarditis: Inflammation or infarction? *Journal of Cardiovascular Nursing, 20*(4), 239–244.
8. Maron, B. J., Ackerman, M. J., Nishimura, R. A., et al. (2005). Task Force 4: HCM and other cardiomyopathies, mitral valve prolapse, myocarditis, and Marfan syndrome. *Journal of the American College of Cardiology, 45*(8), 1340–1345.
9. Tingle, L. E., Molina, D., & Calvert, C. W. (2007). Acute pericarditis. *American Family Physician, 76*(10), 1509–1514.
10. Lange, R. A., & Hillis, L. D. (2004). Clinical practice. Acute pericarditis. *New England Journal of Medicine, 351*(21), 2195–2202.
11. Maisch, B., Seferovic, P. M., Ristic, A. D., et al. (2004). Guidelines on the diagnosis and management of pericardial diseases executive summary: The Task Force on the diagnosis and management of pericardial diseases of the European society of cardiology. *European Heart Journal, 25*(7), 587–610.
12. Spodick, D. H. (2003). Acute pericarditis: Current concepts and practice. *JAMA, 289*(9), 1150–1153.
13. Shabetai, R. (1998). Pericardial disease. In D. L. Brown (Ed.), *Cardiac intensive care* (pp. 469–475). Philadelphia: WB Saunders.
14. Brady, W. J., Perron, A. D., Martin, M. L., et al. (2001). Cause of ST segment abnormality in ED chest pain patients. *American Journal of Emergency Medicine, 19*(1), 25–28.
15. Imazio, M., Demichelis, B., Cecchi, E., et al. (2003). Cardiac troponin I in acute pericarditis. *Journal of the American College of Cardiology, 42*(12), 2144–2148.
16. Burgess, L. J., Reuter, H., Carstens, M. E., et al. (2002). The use of adenosine deaminase and interferon-γ as diagnostic tools for tuberculosis pericarditis. *Chest, 122*, 900–905.
17. Imazio, M., Demichelis, B., Parrini, I., et al. (2005). Management, risk factors, and outcomes in recurrent pericarditis. *American Journal of Cardiology, 96*(5), 736–739.
18. Ntsekhe, M., & Hakim, J. (2005). Impact of human immunodeficiency virus infection on cardiovascular disease in Africa. *Circulation, 112*(23), 3602–3607.
19. Mayosi, B. M., Burgess, L. J., & Doubell, A. F. (2005). Tuberculous pericarditis. *Circulation, 112*(23), 3608–3616.
20. Becit, N., Unlu, Y., Ceviz, M., et al. (2005). Subxiphoid pericardiostomy in the management of pericardial effusions: Case series analysis of 368 patients. *Heart, 91*(6), 785–790.
21. Syed, F. F., & Mayosi, B. M. (2007). A modern approach to tuberculous pericarditis. *Progress in Cardiovascular Diseases, 50*(3), 218–236.
22. Chowdhury, U. K., Subramaniam, G. K., Kumar, A. S., et al. (2006). Pericardiectomy for constrictive pericarditis: A clinical, echocardiographic, and hemodynamic evaluation of two surgical techniques. *Annals of Thoracic Surgery, 81*(2), 522–529.
23. Bellin, D., & Devine, P. (2007). Constrictive pericarditis: A cause of exertion-induced dyspnea in a soldier with a prior sternotomy. *Military Medicine, 172*(11), 1220–1223.
24. Bertog, S. C., Thambidorai, S. K., Parakh, K., et al. (2004). Constrictive pericarditis: Etiology and cause-specific survival after pericardiectomy. *Journal of the American College of Cardiology, 43*(8), 1445–1452.
25. Mobius-Winkler, S., & Walther, C. (2006). Images in clinical medicine. Cardiac constriction due to a calcified pericardium. *New England Journal of Medicine, 355*(17), e19.
26. Cavendish, J. J., & Linz, P. E. (2005). Images in cardiovascular medicine. Constrictive pericarditis from a severely calcified pericardium. *Circulation, 112*(11), e137–e139.
27. Goyle, K. K., & Walling, A. D. (2002). Diagnosing pericarditis. *American Family Physician, 66*(9), 1695–1702.
28. Nishimura, R. A. (2001). Constrictive pericarditis in the modern era: A diagnostic dilemma. *Heart, 86*, 619–623.
29. Imazio, M., Bobbio, M., Cecchi, E., et al. (2005). Colchicine in addition to conventional therapy for acute pericarditis: Results of the COlchicine for acute PEricarditis (COPE) trial. *Circulation, 112*(13), 2012–2016.
30. Imazio, M., Demichelis, B., Parrini, I., et al. (2004). Recurrent pain without objective evidence of disease in patients with previous idiopathic or viral acute pericarditis. *American Journal of Cardiology, 94*, 973–975.
31. American Heart Association. (2008). *Pericardium and pericarditis*. Retrieved January 28, 2008, from http://www.americanheart.org/presenter.jhtml?identifier = 4683.
32. Imazio, M., Brucato, A., Adler, Y., et al. (2007). Prognosis of idiopathic recurrent pericarditis as determined from previously published reports. *American Journal of Cardiology, 100*(6), 1026–1028.
33. LeWinter, M. M. (2007). Pericardial diseases. In P. Libby, R. O. Bonow, D. L. Mann, et al. (Eds.), *Braunwald's heart disease: A textbook of cardiovascular medicine*. Philadelphia: Saunders Elsevier.
34. Hoit, B. D. (2004). Diseases of the pericardium. In V. Fuster, R. W. Alexander, & R. A. O'Rourke (Eds.), *Hurst's the heart* (11th ed., pp. 2061–2085). New York: McGraw-Hill.
35. Imazio, M., Demichelis, B., Parrini, I., et al. (2005). Relation of acute pericardial disease to malignancy. *American Journal of Cardiology, 95*(11), 1393–1394.
36. Spodick, D. H. (2003). Acute cardiac tamponade. *New England Journal of Medicine, 349*(7), 684–690.
37. Cheitlin, M. D., Armstrong, W. F., Aurigemma, G. P., et al. (2003). ACC/AHA/ASE 2003 guideline update for the Clinical Application of Echocardiography: Summary article. A report of the American College of Cardiology/American Heart Association Task Force on Practice Guidelines (ACC/AHA/ASE Committee to Update the 1997 Guidelines for the Clinical Application of Echocardiography). *Journal of the American Society of Echocardiography, 16*(10), 1091–1110.
38. Permanyer-Miralda, G. (2004). Acute pericardial disease: Approach to the aetiologic diagnosis. *Heart, 90*(3), 252–254.
39. Moser, D. K. (2007). "The rust of life": Impact of anxiety on cardiac patients. *American Journal of Critical Care, 16*(4), 361–369.
40. Swart, S., & Tiffen, J. (2007). Acute pericarditis. *AAOHN J, 55*(2), 44–46.
41. Richardson, P., McKenna, W., Bristow, M., et al. (1996). Report of the 1995 World Health Organization/International Society and Federation of Cardiology Task Force on the Definition and Classification of cardiomyopathies. *Circulation, 93*(5), 841–842.
42. Towbin, J. A., & Bowles, N. E. (2006). Dilated cardiomyopathy: A tale of cytoskeletal proteins and beyond. *Journal of Cardiovascular Electrophysiology, 17*(8), 919–926.
43. Weiford, B. C., Subbarao, V. D., & Mulhern, K. M. (2004). Noncompaction of the ventricular myocardium. *Circulation, 109*(24), 2965–2971.
44. Caforio, A. L., Daliento, L., Angelini, A., et al. (2005). Autoimmune myocarditis and dilated cardiomyopathy: Focus on cardiac autoantibodies. *Lupus, 14*(9), 652–655.
45. Karkkainen, S., & Peuhkurinen, K. (2007). Genetics of dilated cardiomyopathy. *Annals of Medicine, 39*(2), 91–107.
46. Hughes, S. E., & McKenna, W. J. (2005). New insights into the pathology of inherited cardiomyopathy. *Heart,* 91(2), 257–264.
47. Towbin, J. A., Lowe, A. M., Colan, S. D., et al. (2006). Incidence, causes, and outcomes of dilated cardiomyopathy in children. *JAMA, 296*(15), 1867–1876.

48. Fatkin, D. (2007). Guidelines for the diagnosis and management of familial dilated cardiomyopathy. *Heart, Lung and Circulation, 16*(1), 19–21.
49. Kuhl, U., Pauschinger, M., Noutsias, M., et al. (2005). High prevalence of viral genomes and multiple viral infections in the myocardium of adults with "idiopathic" left ventricular dysfunction. *Circulation, 111*(7), 887–893.
50. Bowles, N. E., Ni, J., Kearney, D. L., et al. (2003). Detection of viruses in myocardial tissues by polymerase chain reaction. Evidence of adenovirus as a common cause of myocarditis in children and adults. *Journal of the American College of Cardiology, 42*(3), 466–472.
51. Friedewald, V. E., Jr., Boehmer, J. P., Kowal, R. C. (2007). The editor's roundtable: Cardiac resynchronization therapy. *American Journal Cardiology, 100*(7), 1145–1152.
52. Hare, J. M. (2007). The dilated, restrictive, and infiltrative cardiomyopathies. In P. Libby, R. O. Bonow, D. L. Mann, et al. (Eds.), *Braunwald's heart disease: A textbook of cardiovascular medicine* (8th ed.). Philadelphia: Saunders Elsevier.
53. Witteles, R. M., Tang, W. H., Jamali, A. H., et al. (2004). Insulin resistance in idiopathic dilated cardiomyopathy: A possible etiologic link. *Journal of the American College of Cardiology, 44*(1), 78–81.
54. Hunt, S., Abraham, W., & Chin, M. (2005). ACC/AHA 2005 guideline update for the diagnosis and management of chronic heart failure in the adult. *Circulation, 112*, e154–e235.
55. Takemoto, Y., Hozumi, T., Sugioka, K., et al. (2007). Beta-blocker therapy induces ventricular resynchronization in dilated cardiomyopathy with narrow QRS complex. *Journal of the American College of Cardiology, 49*(7), 778–783.
56. Neglia, D., De Maria, R., Masi, S., et al. (2007). Effects of long-term treatment with carvedilol on myocardial blood flow in idiopathic dilated cardiomyopathy. *Heart, 93*(7), 808–813.
57. Kadish, A., Dyer, A., Daubert, J. P., et al. (2004). Prophylactic defibrillator implantation in patients with nonischemic dilated cardiomyopathy. *New England Journal of Medicine, 350*(21), 2151–2158.
58. Mann, D. L., Acker, M. A., Jessup, M., et al. (2007). Clinical evaluation of the CorCap Cardiac Support Device in patients with dilated cardiomyopathy. *Annals of Thoracic Surgery,* 84(4), 1226–1235.
59. Bruce, J. (2005). Getting to the heart of cardiomyopathies. *Nursing, 35*(8), 44–47.
60. Robert Wood Johnson University Hospital. (2008). *Advanced heart failure and transplant cardiology program.* Retrieved January 30, 2008, from http://www.rwjuh.edu/medical_services/heart_failure_transplant.html.
61. Swedberg, K., Cleland, J., Dargie, H., et al. (2005). Guidelines for the diagnosis and treatment of chronic heart failure: Executive summary (update 2005): The Task Force for the Diagnosis and Treatment of Chronic Heart Failure of the European Society of Cardiology. *European Heart Journal, 26*(11), 1115–1140.
62. Maron, B. J., McKenna, W. J., Danielson, G. K., et al. (2003). American College of Cardiology/European Society of Cardiology clinical expert consensus document on hypertrophic cardiomyopathy. A report of the American College of Cardiology Foundation Task Force on Clinical Expert Consensus Documents and the European Society of Cardiology Committee for Practice Guidelines. *Journal of the American College of Cardiology, 42*(9), 1687–1713.
63. Maron, B. J., Thompson, P. D., Ackerman, M. J., et al. (2007). Recommendations and considerations related to preparticipation screening for cardiovascular abnormalities in competitive athletes: 2007 update: A scientific statement from the American Heart Association Council on Nutrition, Physical Activity, and Metabolism: Endorsed by the American College of Cardiology Foundation. *Circulation, 115*(12), 1643–1655.
64. Nishimura, R. A., & Holmes, D. R, Jr. (2004). Clinical practice. Hypertrophic obstructive cardiomyopathy. *New England Journal of Medicine, 350*(13), 1320–1327.
65. Elliott, P., & McKenna, W. J. (2004). Hypertrophic cardiomyopathy. *Lancet, 363*(9424), 1881–1891.
66. Jurynec, J. (2007). Hypertrophic cardiomyopathy: A review of etiology and treatment. *Journal of Cardiovascular Nursing, 22*(1), 65–73.
67. Sherrid, M. V. (2006). Pathophysiology and treatment of hypertrophic cardiomyopathy. *Progress in Cardiovascular Diseases, 49*(2), 123–151.
68. Ho, C. Y., & Seidman, C. E. (2006). A contemporary approach to hypertrophic cardiomyopathy. *Circulation, 113*, e858–e862.
69. Frenneaux, M. P. (2004). Assessing the risk of sudden cardiac death in a patient with hypertrophic cardiomyopathy. *Heart, 90*(5), 570–575.
70. Knight, C. J. (2006). Alcohol septal ablation for obstructive hypertrophic cardiomyopathy. *Heart, 92*(9), 1339–1344.
71. Olivotto, I., Ommen, S. R., Maron, M. S., et al. (2007). Surgical myectomy versus alcohol septal ablation for obstructive hypertrophic cardiomyopathy. Will there ever be a randomized trial? *Journal of the American College of Cardiology, 50*(9), 831–834.
72. Spirito, P., & Autore, C. (2006). Management of hypertrophic cardiomyopathy. *BMJ, 332*(7552), 1251–1255.
73. Seth, S., Thatai, D., Sharma, S., et al. (2004). Clinico-pathological evaluation of restrictive cardiomyopathy (endomyocardial fibrosis and idiopathic restrictive cardiomyopathy) in India. *European Journal of Heart Failure, 6*(6), 723–729.
74. Hassam, W., Fawzy, M., Helaly, S., et al. (2005). Pitfalls in diagnosis and clinical, echocardiographic, and hemodynamic findings in endomyocardial fibrosis. *Chest, 128*(6), 3985–3992.
75. Shah, K. B., Inoue, Y., & Mehra, M. R. (2006). Amyloidosis and the heart: A comprehensive review. *Archives of Internal Medicine, 166*(17), 1805–1813.
76. Tandri, H., Saranathan, M., Rodriguez, E. R., et al. (2005). Noninvasive detection of myocardial fibrosis in arrhythmogenic right ventricular cardiomyopathy using delayed-enhancement magnetic resonance imaging. *Journal of the American College of Cardiology, 45*(1), 98–103.
77. Dalal, D., Nasir, K., Bomma, C., et al. (2005). Arrhythmogenic right ventricular dysplasia: A United States experience. *Circulation, 112*(25), 3823–3832.
78. Hulot, J. S., Jouven, X., Empana, J. P., et al. (2004). Natural history and risk stratification of arrhythmogenic right ventricular dysplasia/cardiomyopathy. *Circulation, 110*(14), 1879–1884.
79. Buja, G., Estes, N. A., III, Wichter, T., et al. (2008). Arrhythmogenic right ventricular cardiomyopathy/dysplasia: Risk stratification and therapy. *Progress in Cardiovascular Diseases, 50*(4), 282–293.
80. Baughman, K. (2006). Diagnosis of myocarditis: Death of Dallas criteria. *Circulation, 113*, 593–595.
81. Magnani, J. W., & Dec, G. W. (2006). Myocarditis: Current trends in diagnosis and treatment. *Circulation, 113*(6), 876–890.
82. Eckart, R. E., Love, S. S., Atwood, J. E., et al. (2004). Incidence and follow-up of inflammatory cardiac complications after smallpox vaccination. *Journal of the American College of Cardiology, 44*(1), 201–205.
83. Skouri, H. N., Dec, G. W., Friedrich, M. G., et al. (2006). Noninvasive imaging in myocarditis. *Journal of the American College of Cardiology, 48*(10), 2085–2093.
84. Hia, C. P., Yip, W. C., Tai, B. C., et al. (2004). Immunosuppressive therapy in acute myocarditis: An 18 year systematic review. *Archives of Disease in Childhood, 89*(6), 580–584.
85. Chen, H., Liu, J., & Yang, M. (2006). Corticosteroids for viral myocarditis. *Cochrane Database of Systematic Reviews, 4*, CD004471. DOI: 004410.001002/14651858.CD14004471.pub14651852.
86. Robinson, J., Hartling, L., Vandermeer, B., et al. (2005). Intravenous immunoglobulin for presumed viral myocarditis in children and adults. *Cochrane Database of Systematic Reviews, 1,* CD004370. DOI: 004310.001002/14651858.CD14004370.pub.14651852.
87. Tang, W. H., & Francis, G. S. (2005). The year in heart failure. *Journal of the American College of Cardiology, 46*(11), 2125–2133.
88. Statement Development Group, Garratt, C. J., Elliott, P. M., et al. (2008). Clinical indications for genetic testing in familial sudden cardiac death syndromes: An HRUK Position Statement. *Heart, 94*(4), 502–507.
89. Vollman, M. W. (1995). Dynamic cardiomyoplasty: Perspectives on nursing care and collaborative management. *Progress in Cardiovascular Nursing, 10*(2), 15–22.
90. Baddigam, K., Pierantonio, R., Russo, J., et al. (2005). Dexmedetomidine in the treatment of withdrawal symptoms in cardiothoracic surgery patients. *Journal of Intensive Care Medicine, 20*(2), 118–123.
91. Koelling, T. M., Johnson, M. L., Cody, R. J., et al. (2005). Discharge education improves clinical outcomes in patients with chronic heart failure. *Circulation, 111*(2), 179–185.
92. Bashore, T., Cabell, C. H., & Fowler, V. (2006). Update on infective endocarditis. *Current Problems in Cardiology, 31*, 274–352.
93. Horstkotte, D., Follath, F., Gutschik, E., et al. (2004). Guidelines on prevention, diagnosis and treatment of infective endocarditis executive summary: The Task Force on Infective Endocarditis of the European Society of Cardiology. *European Heart Journal, 25*(3), 267–276.
94. Miro, J., del Rio, A., & Mestres, C. (2002). Infective endocarditis in intravenous drug abusers and HIV-infected patients. *Infectious Disease Clinics of North America, 16*, 273–295.
95. Karchmer, A., Bonow, R. O., Mann, D. L., et al. (2007). Infective endocarditis. In P. Libby (Ed.), *Braunwald's heart disease: A textbook of cardiovascular medicine* (8th ed.). Philadelphia: Saunders Elsevier.

96. Cabell, C. H., Heidenreich, P. A., Chu, V. H., et al. (2004). Increasing rates of cardiac device infections among Medicare beneficiaries: 1990–1999. *American Heart Journal, 147*(4), 582–586.
97. Wilson, W., Taubert, K. A., Gewitz, M., et al. (2007). Prevention of infective endocarditis: Guidelines from the American Heart Association: A guideline from the American Heart Association Rheumatic Fever, Endocarditis, and Kawasaki Disease Committee, Council on Cardiovascular Disease in the Young, and the Council on Clinical Cardiology, Council on Cardiovascular Surgery and Anesthesia, and the Quality of Care and Outcomes Research Interdisciplinary Working Group. *Circulation, 116*(15), 1736–1754.
98. Moreillon, P., & Que, Y. A. (2004). Infective endocarditis. *Lancet, 363*(9403), 139–149.
99. Durack, D. T., Bright, D. K., & Lukes, A. S. (1994). Duke Endocarditis Service new criteria for diagnosis of infective endocarditis: Utilization of specific echocardiographic findings. *American Journal of Medicine, 96,* 200–209.
100. Li, J. S., Sexton, D. J., Mick, N., et al. (2000). Proposed modifications to the Duke criteria for the diagnosis of infective endocarditis. *Clinical Infectious Diseases, 30*(4), 633–638.
101. Towns, M., & Reller, L. (2002). Diagnostic methods current best practices and guidelines for isolation of bacteria and fungi in infective endocarditis. *Infectious Disease Clinics of North America, 16,* 363–376.
102. Slater, M. S., Komanapalli, C. B., Tripathy, U, et al. (2007). Treatment of endocarditis: A decade of experience. *Annals of Thoracic Surgery, 83*(6), 2074–2079; discussion 2079–2080.
103. Sexton, D. J., & Spelman, D. (2003). Current best practices and guidelines. Assessment and management of complications in infective endocarditis. *Cardiology Clinics, 21*(2), 273–282, vii–viii.
104. Baddour, L. M., Wilson, W. R., Bayer, A. S., et al. (2005). Infective endocarditis: Diagnosis, antimicrobial therapy, and management of complications: A statement for healthcare professionals from the Committee on Rheumatic Fever, Endocarditis, and Kawasaki Disease, Council on Cardiovascular Disease in the Young, and the Councils on Clinical Cardiology, Stroke, and Cardiovascular Surgery and Anesthesia, American Heart Association: Endorsed by the Infectious Diseases Society of America. *Circulation, 111*(23), e394–e434.
105. Oliver, R., Roberts, G., & Hooper, L. (2004). Penicillins for the prophylaxis of bacterial endocarditis in dentistry. *Cochrane Database of Systematic Reviews, 2,* CD003813. DOI: 10.1002/14651858.CD003814. pub2.
106. Seto, T. B. (2007). The case for infectious endocarditis prophylaxis: Time to move forward. *Archives of Internal Medicine, 167*(4), 327–330.
107. Smith, M., Smith, T., & Davidson, B. (2007). Managing the infected heart. *Critical Care Nursing Clinics of North America, 19,* 99–106.
108. Maupin, C. R. (1995). The potential for noncaring when dealing with difficult patients: Strategies for moral decision making. *Journal of Cardiovascular Nursing, 9*(3), 11–22.
109. Broyles, L. M., Colbert, A. M., Tate, J. A., et al. (2008). Clinicians' evaluation and management of mental health, substance abuse, and chronic pain conditions in the intensive care unit. *Critical Care Medicine, 36*(1), 87–93.
110. Broyles, L., & Korniewicz, D. (2002). The opiate-dependent patient with endocarditis: addressing pain and substance abuse withdrawal. *AACN Clinical Issues, 13*(3), 431–451.
111. Jenkins, D. H. (2000). Substance abuse and withdrawal in the intensive care unit. *Surgical Clinics of North America, 80,* 1033–1053.
112. Centers for Disease Control and Prevention. (2002). *Guidelines for the prevention of intravascular catheter-related infections, 2002.* Retrieved January 31, 2008, from http://www.cdc.gov/ncidod/dhqp/gl_intravascular.html.
113. American Association of Critical-Care Nurses. (2005). *AACN practice alert: Preventing catheter related bloodstream infection.* Retrieved January 31, 2008, from http://www.aacn.org/AACN/practiceAlert.nsf/Files/CRBI/$file/Preventing%20Catheter%20Related%20Bloodstream%20Infections%209-2005.pdf.
114. Idemoto, B., & Kresevic, D. (2007). Emerging nurse-sensitive outcomes and evidence-based practice in postoperative cardiac patients. *Critical Care Nursing Clinics of North America, 19,* 371–384.

CHAPTER 31 Adult Congenital Heart Disease

Philip Moons / Mary M. Canobbio

Congenital heart disease is defined as gross structural abnormalities of the heart or intrathoracic great vessels that have actual or potential functional significance.[1] They include a wide spectrum of simple, moderate, and complex severity lesions.[2,3] Over the past five decades, advances in diagnosis and therapy, including palliative or corrective surgery, have resulted in increased survival of adults with congenital heart disease (ACHD). Surgical interventions have not only increased life expectancy of patients with defects that allow natural long-term survival but have also permitted survival of a large number of those with disorders previously fatal in childhood. Appropriate long-term management of this population requires an understanding of the anomalies and the residual effects of the surgical repair.

INCIDENCE AND PREVALENCE

The generally accepted incidence of congenital heart disease is 0.8%, although large variations in incidence data occur across studies.[4] Overall rates of congenital heart disease incidence in various studies have ranged from 4/1,000 to 75/1,000 live births,[4] depending on which heart defects are included in the assessment, the patient's age at diagnosis, and the study design (population studies or patient referral studies). Regardless, congenital heart defects do represent the most frequently occurring congenital disorder in newborns.[5–7] It is argued that the incidence of congenital heart disease remains stable over time.[4,8] However, some authors have found temporal trends in the occurrence of some heart defects[9] or in congenital heart disease overall.[5,10,11]

Since the first surgical procedure for the "blue baby" was performed over 50 years ago, the number of children surviving into adulthood has steadily increased. Today, because of the dramatic advances in diagnosis and medical therapies, including interventional procedures as well as cardiac surgical procedures, it is generally acknowledged that at least 85% of infants born with cardiovascular anomalies can expect to reach adulthood.[3] As a consequence of higher survival rates, the prevalence of ACHD has increased as well. The number of ACHD patients in the population has been estimated to be about 5,000 patients per million inhabitants.[2,12] For the first time in history, there are now more adults than children living with congenital heart defects, and this population is growing by approximately 5% per year.[13]

These data are important in that they are predictive of the increasing number of ACHD that will be presenting for care in adult health care settings. Unfortunately, the adult health care setting is neither well informed nor prepared to manage this growing subspecialty of cardiology. In future, nurses are required not only to provide care for the primary defect but also for the postoperative residua, sequelae, and complications, many of which become apparent in adulthood.

CATEGORIZATION OF CONGENITAL HEART DEFECTS

A variety of methods have been developed to classify congenital heart defects.[14–16] Some are based on the direction and magnitude of pulmonary blood flow or on a distinction between cyanotic and acyanotic heart defects. For the purpose of this discussion, we use a classification described by Jordan and Scott,[17] which is illustrated in Figure 31-1. A detailed review of all congenital heart defects is beyond the scope of this chapter; therefore, selected defects that commonly present in adult congenital heart disease practice are discussed here.

ACYANOTIC HEART DEFECTS WITH LEFT-TO-RIGHT SHUNT

This group of heart defects is characterized by a continuous flow of saturated blood from the left heart circulation to the right side of the heart. This left-to-right shunting is associated with an increased pulmonary blood flow.

Patent Ductus Arteriosus

Description

The ductus arteriosus is a vascular connection, which during fetal life directs blood flow from the pulmonary artery to the aorta, bypassing the lungs (Fig. 31-2). Functional closure of the ductus occurs within hours or days after birth, in some cases taking 6 months to several years to close. If the ductus remains patent, the direction of blood flow is reversed to left-to-right, because of high systemic pressure in the aorta. A patent ductus arteriosus (PDA), which can escape recognition until adulthood, accounts for about 10% of all cases of congenital heart disease and predominates in women. The incidence of PDA is higher at high altitude than at sea level. It is reported that the risk for PDA in individuals residing between 4,500 and 5,000 m is 30 times higher than in counterparts living at sea level.[18] This increased risk is due to a postnatal persistence of pulmonary hypertension. There is reversal of pulmonary hypertension after prolonged residence at sea level.[18]

The hemodynamic changes and clinical manifestations depend on the magnitude of the pulmonary blood flow. The amount of left-to-right shunt is related to the size of the ductal lumen and the resistance in the pulmonary vascular bed. When the ductus is small, the pulmonary artery pressure remains normal; when larger, aortic pressure is transmitted into the pulmonary trunk.

Pathophysiology

A PDA functions as an arteriovenous fistula, increasing the work of the left ventricle. The major complications are ventricular failure

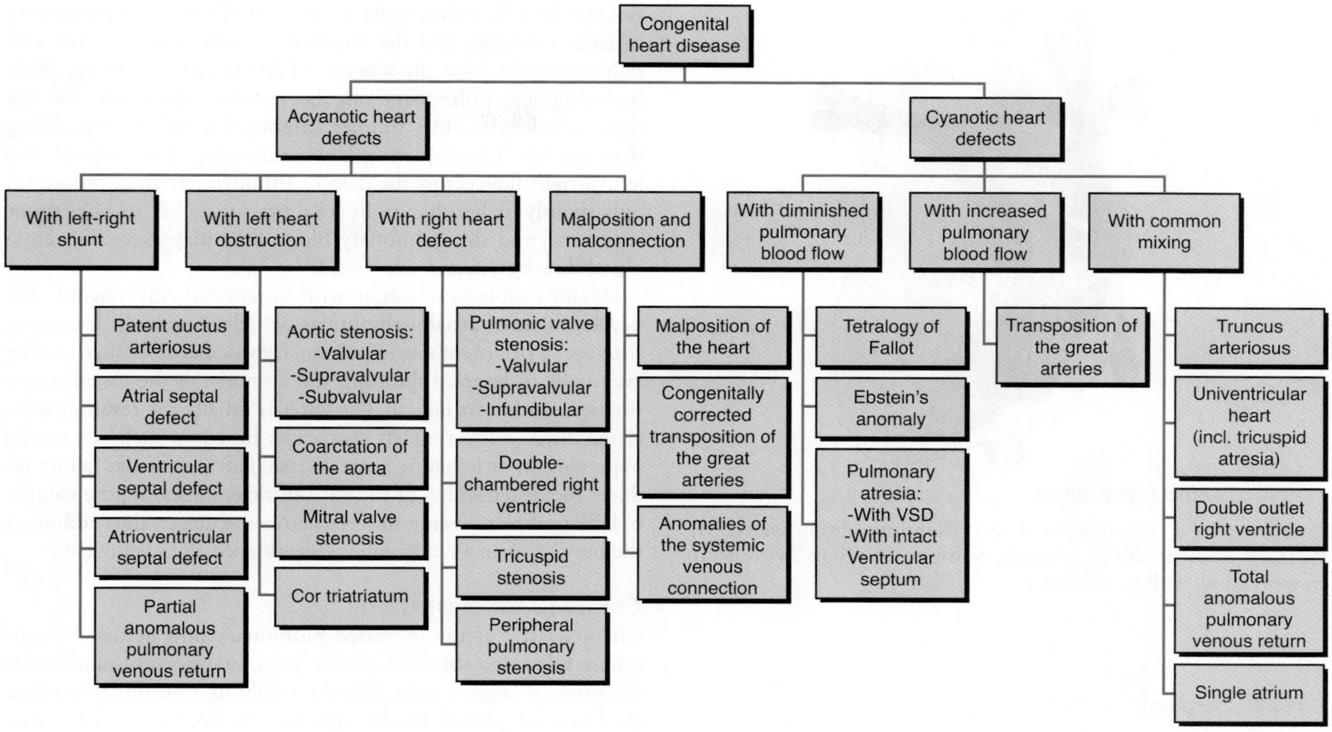

■ **Figure 31-1** Categorization of congenital heart defects.

and presence of increased pulmonary vascular disease. Adults with small left-to-right shunts from a persistent ductus have no symptoms and life expectancy is normal. Patients with large shunts and relatively low pulmonary vascular resistance are at risk for developing left ventricular failure, pulmonary vascular disease, and reversed shunting. In such cases, operation is advised. Once pulmonary resistance exceeds systemic pressure, patients are rendered inoperable.

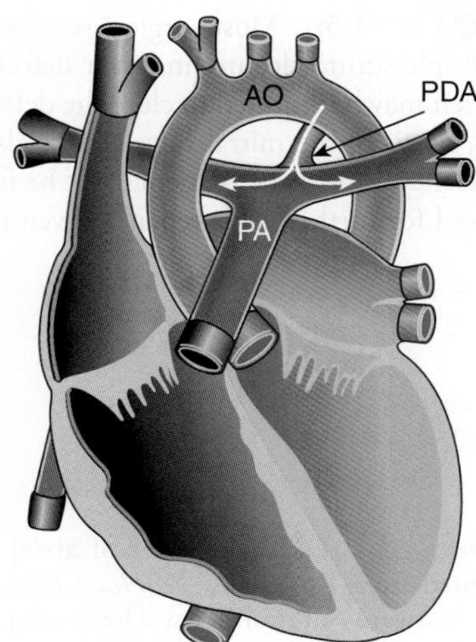

■ **Figure 31-2** Patent ductus arteriosus. AO= aorta; PDA=Patent Ductus Arteriosus; PA=Pulmonary artery (Reprinted from Everett, A. *PedHeart Resource*. 2009. Scientific Software Solutions. www.heartpassport.com., with permission.)

Clinical Manifestations

The clinical appearance characterizing a moderate or large PDA with normal pulmonary arterial pressure includes bounding peripheral pulses, a widened pulse pressure, with diastolic pressures as low as 30 to 50 mm Hg. The left ventricular impulse is hyperdynamic, and, if present, a systolic thrill may be palpated over the suprasternal notch area. A continuous loud "machinery" murmur accentuated in late systole is heard best in the first or second left intercostal space. In the setting of increased pulmonary vascular resistance, the diastolic component of the murmur disappears, leaving only the systolic component.

Patients with a moderate shunt may have no symptoms during infancy but may begin to develop fatigue, dyspnea, or palpitations during childhood or adulthood. Occasionally, the ductus arteriosus may become aneurismal, calcified, and rupture.[13]

Management

In the absence of pulmonary vascular disease, it is recommended that all PDAs be closed either by surgical ligation or by interventional catheterization using percutaneous closure devices. Patients with moderate to large size PDAs who go unrepaired are at risk for endarteritis, heart failure, and pulmonary hypertension. One third of these patients die by the age of 40 years; two thirds of them die by the age of 60 year.[13,19] Once closed, periodic long-term evaluation is recommended because residual problems such as pulmonary hypertension, atrial arrhythmias may develop particularly in those repaired later in life. Endocarditis prophylaxis in not required after surgical or device closure even if a residual shunt persists.[20]

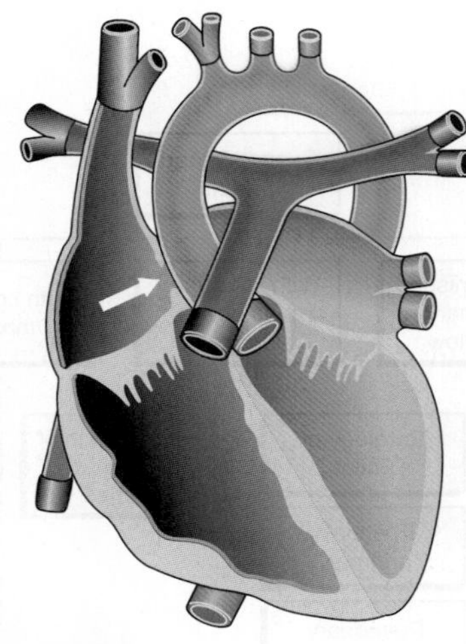

■ **Figure 31-3** Atrial septal defect. (Reprinted from Everett, A. *PedHeart Resource*. 2009. Scientific Software Solutions. www.heartpassport.com., with permission.)

Atrial Septal Defects

Description

Atrial septal defects (ASDs) are abnormal communications between the left and right atria (Fig. 31-3). They constitute 10% of all congenital heart anomalies. There is a female predominance.[14] They are differentiated by their occurrence within the septum. *Ostium secundum* ASD, the most common type, occurs in the central region of the fossa ovalis. *Ostium primum* ASD, which occurs low in the atrial septum, has an associated cleft anterior mitral valve with varying degree of mitral insufficiency. *Sinus venosus* ASD occurs in the upper part of the atrial septum near the entry of the superior vena cava and may be associated with the partial anomalous right pulmonary venous connection (Fig. 31-4). Owing to the trivial or absent physical signs, ASD may go undetected until the fourth or fifth decade.

Pathophysiology

The hemodynamic consequences of ASD are dependent on (1) the size and direction of the shunt; (2) the compliance of the left and right ventricles; and (3) the responsive behavior of the pulmonary vascular bed. In infancy, the persistence of increased pulmonary vascular resistance and the relatively equally compliant left and right ventricles limit the amount of left-to-right shunting. With increasing age, pulmonary vascular resistance decreases, and the right ventricle becomes thinner, offering less resistance to filling than the left. Consequently, the conditions are appropriate for left-to-right flow across the defect. Although left atrial pressure is only slightly higher than right atrial pressure, a left-to-right shunt is present, and the pulmonary blood flow may exceed systemic blood flow by three to four times.[21]

Major problems of adults with unrepaired ASD include the development of atrial arrhythmias, which increase in frequency with age; a persistent rise in pulmonary vascular resistance leading eventually to reversed shunting and cyanosis, or the Eisenmenger reaction; and heart failure. The latter is usually the result of associated diseases affecting left ventricular function, such as systemic hypertension or ischemic heart disease. Left ventricular failure reduces the distensibility of the left ventricle, increasing the volume of left atrial blood being shunted across the defect, thus adding to the burden of an already volume-overloaded right ventricle.

Clinical Manifestations

Characteristic of the increased pulmonary flow across the pulmonic valves is a soft mid-systolic pulmonic ejection murmur. If the shunt is large, a mild diastolic rumbling murmur is heard at the lower left sternal border, due to increased blood flow across the tricuspid valve. A second sound, which is widely split and does not vary with respiration, is consistent with a low pulmonary vascular resistance. Prominent right ventricle pulsations along the left sternal border and pulmonary artery are palpable. The presence of a systolic thrill reflects a large shunt or coexisting pulmonic stenosis. In ostium primum, there is the addition of the murmur of mitral regurgitation, a left ventricular impulse, and systolic thrill. In sinus venosus, the clinical findings are similar to the ostium secundum. Most patients with ASD remain asymptomatic but may complain of easy fatigability and exertional dyspnea.

Management

Closure of ASD is recommended if the pulmonary-to-systemic blood flow ratio (Q_p/Q_s) is $\geq$1.5:1. Most surgical repairs are performed in infancy by simple suture closure; in larger defects a pericardial or prosthetic patch may be required to close the defect. For *Ostium primum* defects, repair of the mitral valve cleft is also undertaken. If mitral insufficiency persists, the patient must be followed closely to determine need for further valve repair or even replacement.

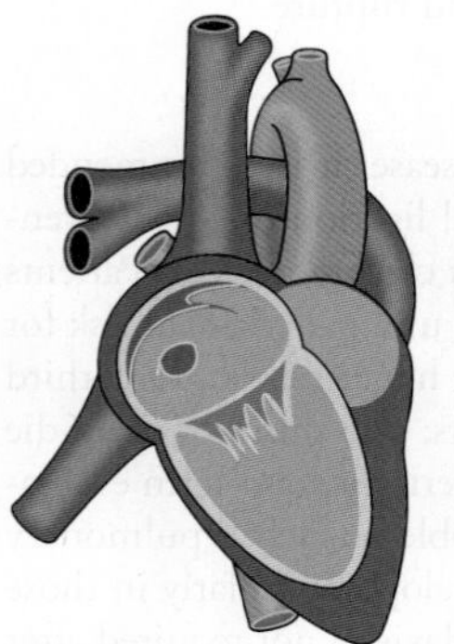

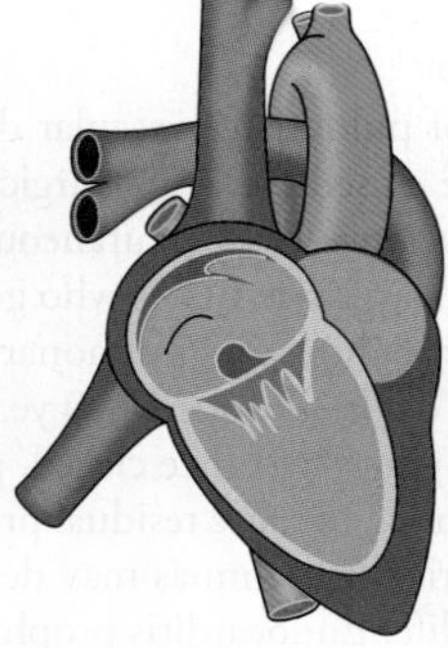

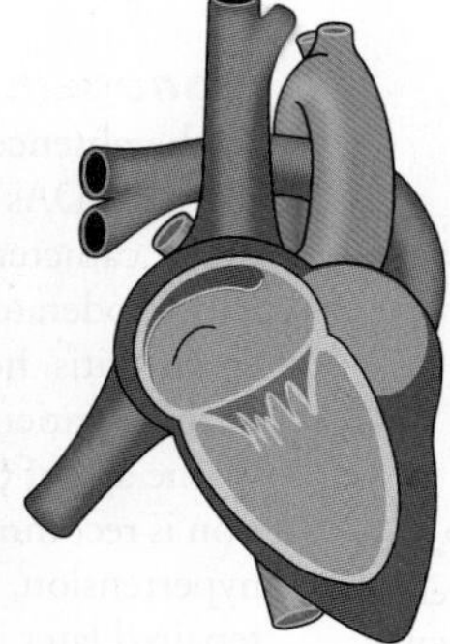

■ **Figure 31-4** Different types of atrial septal defects. (Reprinted from Everett, A. *PedHeart Resource*. 2009. Scientific Software Solutions. www.heartpassport.com., with permission.)

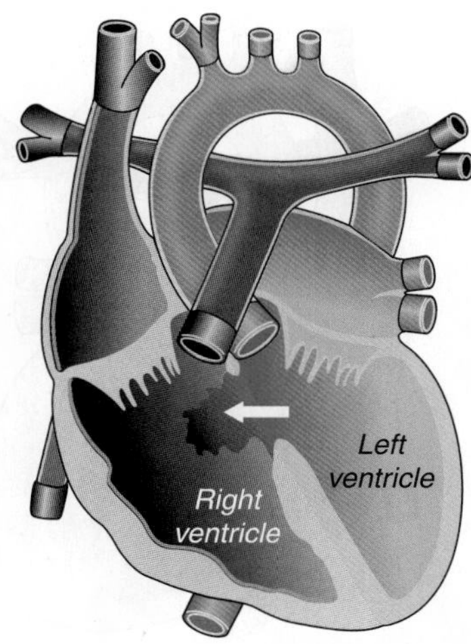

■ **Figure 31-5** Ventricular septal defect. (Reprinted from Everett, A. *PedHeart Resource*. 2009. Scientific Software Solutions. www.heartpassport.com., with permission.)

Today, transcatheter closure of ASD is the established method of closure for patients with secundum ASD with success rates of greater than 95% being reported.[22,23] While occurring infrequently, the long-term concerns for these devices include incomplete closure of the shunt, acute embolization of the devices, and the potential for thromboembolic complications.

Adults with simple ASD repaired in infancy and no residual effects may be followed at the community level. Patients with residual lesions or patients in whom the ASD is diagnosed in adulthood should be evaluated at a regional ACHD center. Indications for specialty care include pre- or postoperative arrhythmias, valvular and/or ventricular dysfunction, and elevated pulmonary pressures. Endocarditis prophylaxis is only indicated within the first 6 months after percutaneous closure with a device or surgical closure using prosthetic material.[20]

Ventricular Septal Defects

Description

Interventricular defects result in shunting of blood between right and left ventricles (Fig. 31-5). Ventricular septal defects (VSDs) are the most common heart defects, representing about 35% of all congenital cardiac anomalies.[4,14] There are three main categories of VSD, each classified according to its location: perimembranous VSD, muscular VSD, and subarterial VSD (Fig. 31-6). Perimembranous defects are the commonest type of defect accounting for 80% of all VSDs and occur in the membranous part of the ventricular septum and the surrounding muscular septum. A muscular VSD occurs in the muscular portion of the septum and accounts for approximately 15%. Subarterial VSDs occur in only 5% of cases and are located directly below the atrioventricular valves. VSDs are further categorized as either restrictive or unrestrictive. Restrictive VSDs are small defects resulting in a high-pressure gradient between right and left ventricle, while nonrestrictive VSDs are large defects in which the pressure between right and left ventricle is equalized. Unrestricted defects are typically repaired in childhood, but restrictive VSDs account for 7% of congenital heart defects found in adults. Isolated VSD occur with equal frequency in men and women. The 25 year follow-up indicates that the majority of patients managed medically or surgically, who do not develop Eisenmenger syndrom will fare well.[24,25]

Pathophysiology

Defects may be single or multiple, with the degree of shunting dependent on the size of the defect rather than the anatomic location. Defects vary in size from a millimeter or two in diameter to large openings with little or no septal wall, which behave physiologically like a single ventricle. Small isolated defects (<7 mm in diameter), and moderate-sized defects (7 mm to 1.25 cm) are considered to be restrictive. They have minimal hemodynamic changes and produce little or no symptomatology. But if moderate in size, it may be significant enough to produce some cardiac enlargement. If the defect is large (1.5 to 3 cm), systemic pressure in the right ventricle is equal or slightly lower than the left ventricle creating a left-to-right shunt and increased pulmonary blood flow (unrestricted VSD). This increase in blood flow is returned to the left heart, creating volume overload of both right and left ventricles. In addition, increased pulmonary blood flow may produce pulmonary hypertension. Because of the open communication between the two ventricles, systolic blood pressure in the pulmonary artery rises, equaling that in the aorta. If the pulmonary artery pressure continues to increase and pulmonary vascular resistance approaches or exceeds systemic pressure, shunt reversal (right to left) occurs, rendering the patient cyanotic and no longer a candidate for surgical correction. This syndrome is referred to as Eisenmenger reaction.

Clinical Manifestations

Clinical features depend on the volume of pulmonary blood flow, which in turn depends on the size of the defect and the pulmonary vascular resistance. A harsh holosystolic murmur and palpable thrill along the lower left sternal border may be the only findings

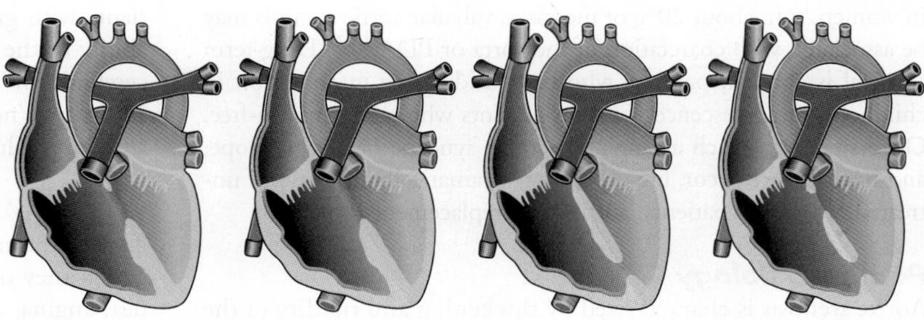

■ **Figure 31-6** Different types of ventricular septal defects. (Reprinted from Everett, A. *PedHeart Resource*. 2009. Scientific Software Solutions. www.heartpassport.com., with permission.)

of a small or moderate defect. A normal splitting second sound indicates the pulmonary arterial pressure is below systemic pressure. In large shunts, the murmur is lower in intensity, a mid-diastolic "flow murmur" and third heart sound are heard at the apex, and a right ventricular impulse is palpable.

Management

Patients with small VSD (<7 mm in diameter) have minimal hemodynamic changes and produce little or no symptoms. Therefore, they do not require surgical intervention. In the absence of high or fixed pulmonary vascular obstructive disease, surgical correction is indicated in patients with moderate to large left-to-right shunt. VSD closure will be considered if the Q_p/Q_s is higher than 2:1. According to the 2007 guidelines, endocarditis prophylaxis is no longer indicated, except for patients with prosthetic material (e.g. patch for VSD closure) with residua or within the first 6 months after an operation in which prosthetic material is placed.[20]

Patients with isolated, small VSDs or those with successful surgical repair require periodic follow-up visits every 3 to 5 years[26] may be cared for in general medical community. On the other hand, patients with residual defects or those who develop clinical sequelae such as right or left ventricular outflow tract obstruction, atrial or ventricular arrhythmias, or aortic regurgitation, annual cardiac evaluation is recommended. Patients who had late repairs of moderate-sized or large defects should have follow-up every 1 to 2 years to assess for left ventricular dysfunction and elevated pulmonary pressures.[26] Endocarditis prophylaxis in VSD is only indicated within the first 6 months after percutaneous closure with a device or surgical closure using prosthetic material.[20]

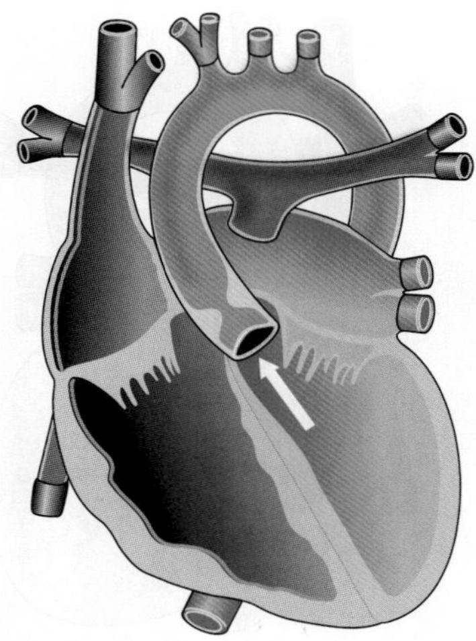

■ **Figure 31-7** Aortic stenosis. (Reprinted from Everett, A. *PedHeart Resource*. 2009. Scientific Software Solutions. www.heartpassport.com., with permission.)

ACYANOTIC HEART DEFECTS WITH LEFT HEART OBSTRUCTION

This category of heart defects is characterized by obstructed outflow of the left heart. These heart defects are associated with a normal pulmonary blood flow.

Congenital Aortic Stenosis

Description

The incidence of congenital aortic stenosis is 0.4 per 1,000 live births.[4] Congenital aortic stenosis is characterized by an obstruction to left ventricular outflow and can occur at three levels: valvular, supravalvular, or subvalvular (Fig. 31-7). The most common form is valvular aortic stenosis, which accounts for 3% to 6% of all cases of congenital heart disease. It is mostly the result of a bicuspid aortic valve. Congenital aortic stenosis occurs more frequently in men than in women.[13] In about 20% of the cases, valvular aortic stenosis may be associated with coarctation of the aorta or PDA.[13,27] Long-term survival is good in patients who have undergone intervention in childhood or adolescence[28] and in patients who are symptom-free. Once symptoms such as angina pectoris, syncope or near-syncope, and heart failure occur, life expectancy dramatically decreases if untreated.[13] In these patients, aortic valve replacement is required.

Pathophysiology

Aortic stenosis is characterized by thickening and rigidity of the valve tissue with a varying degree of commissure fusion in childhood and adolescence and calcification in adults. The adaptation response of chronic aortic stenosis is concentric hypertrophy, which can sustain large pressure gradients across the aortic valve without a drop in cardiac output, left ventricle dilatation, or development of symptoms. Peak systolic pressure gradients with a normal cardiac output reflect the severity of the obstruction. Mild obstruction produces a pressure gradient of <25 mm Hg (an aortic orifice of 0.8 cm^2/m^2 of body surface area); a moderate obstruction produces a gradient of 25 to 50 mm Hg (0.5 to 0.8 cm^2/m^2); stenosis that produces gradients >75 mm Hg (a body surface area of less 0.5 cm^2/m^2) reflects severe obstruction to left ventricular outflow. While resting cardiac output and stroke volume are generally within normal limits, the cardiac output increases with exercise. The gradient across the area of obstruction also increases with exercise, causing the obstruction to become more severe.

In severe aortic stenosis, the hemodynamic abnormalities produced by the obstruction to the left ventricle outflow increase myocardial oxygen demand, and the abnormally elevated pressure compressing the coronary perfusion pressure exceeds the coronary perfusion pressure, thereby interfering with coronary blood flow. As a result, significant stenosis may result in reduced subendocardial perfusion, particularly during exercise, leading to ischemia. Subendocardial ischemia plays a key role in the angina, syncope, ventricular arrhythmias, and sudden death reported in patients with aortic stenosis.[14] Exertional syncope, which can occur in patients with gradients exceeding 50 mm Hg, is related to the inability of the left ventricle to increase its output and to maintain cerebral flow during exercise. The onset of clinical symptoms in adults may not occur until the fourth or fifth decade and is usually the result of aortic valve calcification.

Clinical Manifestations

The symptoms of valvular aortic stenosis may be inconspicuous. When they occur, those most noted are fatigue, exertional dyspnea, angina, and syncope. With significant stenosis, a left ventricle lift may be palpable. A precordial systolic thrill is palpated over the base of the heart and is transmitted to the suprasternal notch and over both carotid arteries. The typical murmur of valvular aortic stenosis is a harsh, loud systolic murmur that begins after the first heart sound, rising to a peak (crescendo) and declining (decrescendo) before the second heart sound. The murmur radiates to the suprasternal notch and carotid arteries. A systolic ejection sound, which may be heard at the cardiac apex, implies a mobile valve and is found in mild to moderate stenosis. As calcification impairs valve mobility, the ejection sound decreases or vanishes completely.

Management

Asymptomatic patients with mild aortic stenosis and gradients <25 mm Hg may be treated medically. With higher gradients >50 mm Hg, balloon valvuloplasty may be successfully performed resulting in a 60% to 70% reduction in systolic gradient across the aortic valve. Balloon valvuloplasty is not recommended if aortic insufficiency is present, in patients with subvalvar stenosis or in adults with heavily calcified valves.[21] Symptomatic or asymptomatic patients with gradients >50 mm Hg are usually treated with surgical resection of subaortic fibrous ring leaving the aortic valve intact. For patients with a narrowed left ventricle outflow tract and small aortic valve annulus, the Ross–Konno surgical procedure maybe performed to relieve left ventricular obstruction to outflow.

Patients with discrete subvalvar aortic stenosis and mild gradients (<30 mm Hg) must be evaluated regularly to detect signs of progressive valve disease. This may be done by local practitioners. Patients with significant residual effects, however, should be followed in an adult congenital heart disease center every 1 to 2 years.[26] Prophylaxis against endocarditis is not required, unless prosthetic cardiac valves have been placed.[20]

Coarctation of the Aorta

Description

Coarctation of the aorta is a deformity of the aortic isthmus, characterized by narrowing either proximal or distal to the left subclavian artery where the ductus arteriosus joins the descending aorta (Fig. 31-8). Occasionally, the coarctation occurs above the origin of the right subclavian. Coarctation of the aorta represents 5% to 10% of all congenital cardiac anomalies[14] and occurs with greater frequency in men than in women.[13,27] It is strongly associated with bicuspid aortic valve, VSD, PDA, and initial valve abnormalities.[13] A noncardiac anomaly associated with coarctation of the aorta is an aneurysm of the circle of Willis.

Pathophysiology

The physiologic consequences of coarctation stem primarily from systemic hypertension. The increased resistance produced by aortic narrowing results in increased pressure in the aorta proximal to the coarcted area and a decreased pressure distal to the narrowing. Because renal artery blood flow is decreased, plasma renin release is stimulated, contributing further to the regulation of systemic arterial pressure. Complications in late adolescence and adulthood may include rupture of the aorta, seen more commonly in the second and third decades; endarteritis at the site of the coarctation; cardiac failure, which increases in incidence after the fourth decade; and cerebral hemorrhage due to rupture of an aneurysm of the circle of Willis.

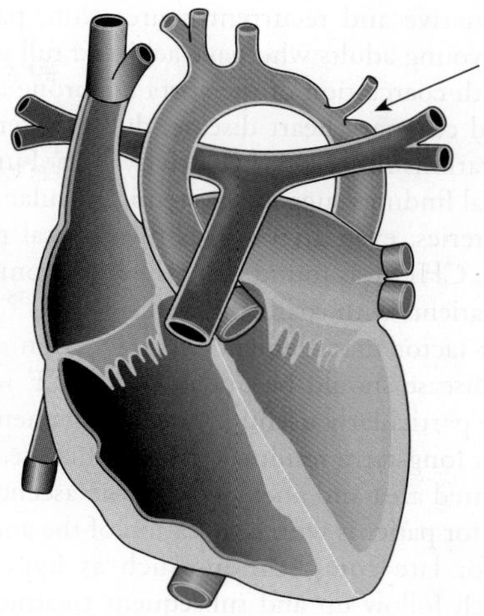

■ **Figure 31-8** Coarctation of the aorta. (Reprinted from Everett, A. *PedHeart Resource*. 2009. Scientific Software Solutions. www.heartpassport.com., with permission.)

Clinical Manifestations

Coarctation of the aorta is characterized by systemic hypertension with abnormal differences in the upper and lower extremities, pulses, and systolic blood pressure. As the patient grows older, systolic pressures rise more than diastolic, resulting in a widened pulse pressure. Arterial pressures may also vary between right and left arms depending on the zone of coarctation relative to the subclavian artery. In the presence of an anomalous right subclavian artery, the blood pressure in the right arm is lower than the left. When the coarctation involves the origin of the left subclavian artery, the blood pressure in the left arm is lower than the right. Differences between arm and leg blood pressure are accentuated further by exercise, with the brachial blood pressure rising, whereas the femoral pressure remains unchanged or may decrease. Often the patient exhibits forceful carotid and suprasternal pulsations resembling aortic regurgitation. Collateral arterial pulsations may be seen beneath the skin, particularly around the scapulae. Hypertensive retinopathy is rare. The femoral pulses may be delayed, diminished, or absent. A suprasternal thrill is common, but precordial thrills are uncommon. Palpation of the precordium reveals a left ventricle impulse that may vary from normal to the sustained heaving impulse of ventricular hypertrophy. Auscultatory signs consist of widespread, delayed systolic murmurs, caused by flow through collateral vessels, and the murmur at the site of coarctation. A mild late systolic murmur is heard best along the left sternal border toward the apex and in the suprasternal notch. An early diastolic murmur, suggestive of aortic regurgitation and an aortic ejection sound may be heard, particularly with a bicuspid aortic valve.

Management

Patients with mild coarctation pressure gradients (<30 mm Hg) may be treated medically, but should be followed carefully to monitor for an increase in the gradient. In patients with higher pressure gradients, surgical resection of the coarctation has been the treatment of choice during several decades. Since the 1990s, balloon angioplasty and stenting are more commonly used for treatment of native and recurrent coarctation, particularly in teenagers and young adults who have achieved full growth.[29]

Patients with coarctation of the aorta are prone to arterial hypertension and coronary heart disease, due to arterial wall stiffness and alterations in vascular reactivity.[30–33] Functional data and histological findings suggest a systemic vascular disease of the prestenotic arteries, even after successful surgical repair.[30,34] In several studies, CHD was found to be the most common cause of late death in patients with coarctation of the aorta.[35–38] Therefore, aggressive risk factor management for prevention of general acquired heart disease should be undertaken. ACE inhibitors and β-blockers are particularly useful in the management of these patients.[39] Other long-term residual effects include restenosis of the previously treated area and aneurysms of the ascending aorta.

Follow-up for patients with coarctation of the aorta is required to monitor for late complications such as hypertension and restenosis. Such follow-up and subsequent treatment should be scheduled every 1 to 2 years[26] in an adult congenital heart disease center. According to the 2007 guidelines on the prevention of infective endocarditis, antibiotic prophylaxis is only required within the first 6 months after placement of prosthetic material, or when residual defects occur at the site or adjacent to the site of prosthetic material.[20]

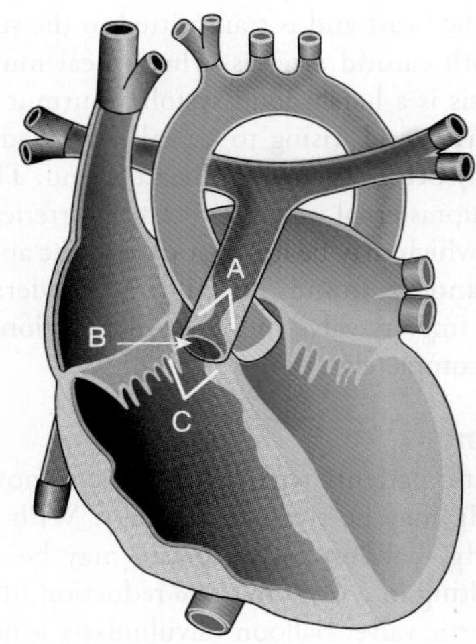

Figure 31-9 Pulmonic stenosis. A: supravalvular pulmonic stenosis; B: valvular pulmonic stenosis; C: infundibular stenosis (Reprinted from Everett, A. *PedHeart Resource*. 2009. Scientific Software Solutions. www.heartpassport.com., with permission.)

ACYANOTIC HEART DEFECTS WITH RIGHT HEART OBSTRUCTION

These defects are characterized by a right outflow tract obstruction. Although the outflow of the right heart is obstructed, pulmonary blood flow remains normal. The most commonly occurring heart defect in this category is a pulmonic valve stenosis.

Pulmonic Valve Stenosis

Description

Right ventricular outflow obstructive lesions constitute 25% to 30% of all congenital malformations of the heart. Pulmonic valve stenosis can occur at the valvular, subvalvular (infundibular or subinfundibular), or supravalvular level (stenosis of the pulmonary artery and its branches) (Fig. 31-9). It may occur as an isolated defect or in combination with other congenital cardiac defects, including VSD, ASD, or as part of the tetralogy of Fallot.[13] Life expectancy depends on the severity of the stenosis. Patients with mild pulmonary stenosis or patients who have undergone balloon valvuloplasty have an excellent survival.[40,41] They must, however, be periodically evaluated for mild residual pulmonary stenosis, or for pulmonary regurgitation which can occur as a result of the valvuloplasty. Long-term follow-up of these patients shows a survival rate similar to that of the general population; morbidity is rare, and risk of endocarditis is nonexistent.[42]

Pathophysiology

The clinical course of pure, isolated pulmonic valve stenosis is dependent on the degree of right ventricular obstruction. Most patients with mild pulmonic valve stenosis (peak right ventricle systolic outflow pressure gradients of 25 mm Hg) to moderate pulmonic valve stenosis (right ventricle systolic pressures of 75 mm Hg) are asymptomatic. Varying degrees of right ventricle hypertension may exist, but pulmonary blood flow remains normal. With moderate stenosis, easy fatigability may be the only complaint. The functional consequences of pulmonic valve stenosis are related to the degree of stenosis and the adaptive response of the right ventricle. The right ventricle hypertrophies in proportion to the degree of stenosis. Over time, changes in the right ventricle, such as myocardial fibrosis, infundibular stenosis, and subvalvular muscular hypertrophy, can lead to alterations in right ventricle function, which contributes further to the obstruction to the right ventricle outflow. Furthermore, with advancing age, a congenitally deformed pulmonic valve can become thickened, fibrotic, and even calcified, thus reducing valve mobility and increasing the degree of obstruction. In more severe cases, right atrial hypertrophy must be present and be of sufficient degree to open a previously patent foramen ovale leading to right to left shunting. Severe pulmonic valve stenosis eventually leads to tricuspid regurgitation and frank right ventricle failure.

Clinical Manifestations

Physical findings include a loud mid-systolic murmur heard along the left sternal border, at the second intercostal space, accompanied by a thrill during the ejection phase. A pulmonic ejection sound produced by the doming of the stenotic valve is present in mild to moderate cases but may be absent in severe pulmonic valve stenosis. Splitting of the pulmonic component of the second heart sound is present but diminished in intensity in mild stenosis. As the gradient increases, the pulmonic component becomes further delayed and softer or even inaudible.

Management

Patients with mild pulmonic stenosis (right ventricle pulmonary artery gradient 25 mm Hg) should be followed medically every 3 to 5 years,[26] but have no restrictions. Patients with moderate gradients (50 to 79 mm Hg) or severe gradient (80 mm Hg) are managed with balloon valvuloplasty. Restenosis is observed in 8% to 10% of the patients who underwent balloon dilatation.[43] Surgical valvotomy is indicated when the pulmonary valve is dysplastic rendering balloon valvuloplasty less effective. Valve replacement in the presence of significant obstruction with calcification of the pulmonic valve is seen in older adults. Prophylaxis against endocarditis is not required in patients with pulmonic valve stenosis, unless prosthetic cardiac valves have been placed.[20]

MALPOSITION AND MALCONNECTION

A number of defects are characterized by a malposition of the heart or a malconnection of the great vessels and are generally categorized as acyanotic defects (Fig. 31-1). A relevant heart defect in this category is a congenitally corrected transposition of the great arteries (CCTGA).

Congenitally Corrected Transposition of the Great Arteries

Description

CCTGA occurs only in 1% of all cardiac anomalies. CCTGA is also referred to as *L-transposition of the great arteries.* In CCTGA, the great arteries are reversed, whereby the aorta arises from the right ventricle and the pulmonary trunk from the left ventricle. However, the transposition is "congenitally corrected" by the fact that the ventricles are also inverted, with the right ventricle occupies the left side of the heart, and the left ventricle is on the right (Fig. 31-10). The circuit is physiologically correct, but the morphological right ventricle serves as the systemic ventricle. Since the atrioventricular valves follow the ventricles, the left-sided atrioventricular valve is the anatomical tricuspid valve, whereas the right-sided valve is the anatomical mitral valve. The coronary arteries also mirror the normal situation.

CCTGA is frequently associated with VSD (60%), a single-ventricle physiology (40%), pulmonic valve stenosis (30% to 50%), and tricuspid valve regurgitation due to an Ebstein-type configuration (25% to 30%). If a right-lo-left shunt is present, the patient should be classified as cyanotic. Surgical intervention is only indicated to repair associated anomalies such as VSD or pulmonary stenosis. While most cases are detected in childhood, many go unnoticed until clinical signs become apparent. Patients with corrected transposition without associated anomalies may reach adulthood, leading normal lives. Generally, 20-year survival rate of 75% in patients with CCTGA is reported.[44]

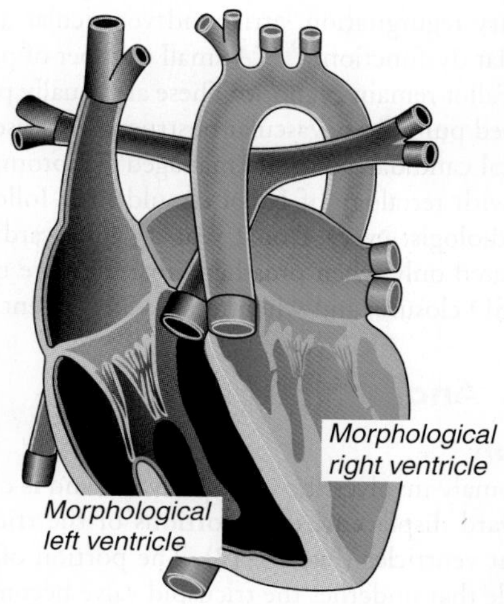

Figure 31-10 Congenitally corrected transposition of the great arteries. (Reprinted from Everett, A. *PedHeart Resource*. 2009. Scientific Software Solutions. www.heartpassport.com., with permission.)

Pathophysiology

The most common clinical sequelae and/or complications with CCTGA include right ventricular dysfunction, tricuspid regurgitation, residual left ventricle outflow obstruction, and complete heart block. Progressive right ventricle dysfunction resulting in heart failure is associated with increasing age, typically in the fifth decade, as the morphological right ventricle begins to fail as the systemic ventricle. Complete heart block, if not present at birth, is likely to develop at a rate of 2% per year, due to the unusual location and course of the atrioventricular node. In patients without associated lesions, it is expected that up to 27% are in need of a pacemaker. This percentage increased up to 45% in patients with associated heart defects.[45]

Clinical Manifestations

Adults with CCTGA present as one of two groups: (1) those diagnosed and repaired in infancy and now present with residual defects associated with a VSD or pulmonic stenosis, or (2) those with no associated lesions who have essentially remained asymptomatic but now have developed symptoms related to progressive right ventricle dysfunction or to atrioventricular valve regurgitation. This latter group of patients is often referred for evaluation of signs of pulmonary congestion or a systolic murmur at the apex of the heart or because of ECG abnormalities, including atrial tachycardias or an atrioventricular block. On examination, a right ventricular parasternal lift is common, along with a systolic murmur of tricuspid regurgitation heard best at the apex or left sternal border. In patients with residual pulmonary stenosis, a systolic ejection murmur may be heard at the upper left sternal border.

Management

The goal of treatment for the patients who underwent an operation and for those who did not undergo the operation is preservation of the systemic ventricle by avoiding dilatation and failure. Tricuspid valve replacement is recommended to avoid right ventricle volume overload and deterioration of right ventricle function. Tricuspid valvuloplasty is rarely successful because of recurrent regurgitation. Because of the high incidence of progressive heart block, pacemaker implantation is often indicated. Atrioventricular pacing is the preferred mode to preserve atrial transport function.[46]

Less commonly used is the double switch procedure whereby the morphological left ventricle becomes the systemic ventricle. This complex operation combines the atrial (Mustard or Senning) and the arterial switch procedures (Jatene) (see section "Complete Transposition of the Great Arteries"), or alternatively combines the atrial switch procedure and Rastelli operation. This long and extensive surgical operation has a high perioperative mortality, and carries a substantial risk for developing complications inherent to both atrial and arterial switch.

Patients with CCTGA should be followed regularly in a regional adult congenital heart disease center. The frequency is dependent upon the level of morbidity including ventricular dysfunction or tricuspid regurgitation. For those who remain asymptomatic, an annual evaluation that includes ECG and echocardiography is recommended.[26] Endocarditis prophylaxis is not required in the unrepaired patient, but is recommended in repaired patients with prosthetic material or artificial valves.[20]

CYANOTIC HEART DEFECTS WITH DIMINISHED PULMONARY BLOOD FLOW

Cyanotic heart defects are generally characterized by a right-to-left shunting, resulting in a flow of desaturated blood into the systemic circulation.

Tetralogy of Fallot

Description

Tetralogy of Fallot accounts for 10% of all congenital heart disease and has an equal sex distribution.[14] Whereas a wide anatomic and clinical spectrum exists, the classic cyanotic tetrad includes a nonrestrictive VSD, severe pulmonic stenosis causing obstruction to pulmonary blood flow, right ventricular hypertrophy, and various degrees of overriding or dextroposition of the aorta (Fig. 31-11). Today, surgical repair is undertaken in early childhood; however, natural survival of an unoperated adult is possible. Morbidity and mortality in adults with unrepaired tetralogy of Fallot result from cardiac failure; sudden death, presumably to arrhythmias; cerebral vascular accidents or brain abscess; and infective endocarditis.

Pathophysiology

The physiologic consequences of tetralogy of Fallot depend on the degree of pulmonary vascular resistance, which regulates pulmonary blood flow, the size of the VSD, and the systemic vascular resistance. The pulmonary stenosis is usually infundibular but may occur at the valvular level or in the pulmonary trunk and its branches. When the stenosis is mild, the shunt remains left-to-right with no cyanosis and is referred to as "acyanotic" tetralogy of Fallot. As pulmonic obstruction increases, the shunt reverses to right-to-left. Right ventricular hypertrophy develops due to resistance to the outflow. When total obstruction to pulmonary flow exists, and the pulmonary trunk and its branches are present, blood flow to the lung is mainly through enlarged bronchial arteries and, at times, also through a PDA. This severe form of tetralogy of Fallot is referred to as pulmonary atresia.

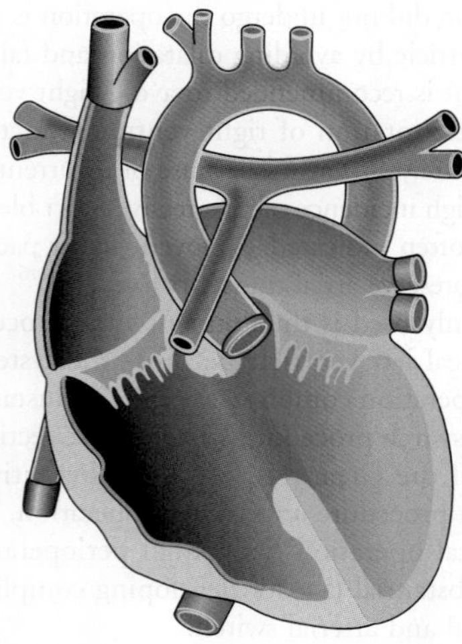

■ **Figure 31-11** Tetralogy of Fallot. (Reprinted from Everett, A. *PedHeart Resource*. 2009. Scientific Software Solutions. www.heartpassport.com., with permission.)

Clinical Manifestations

Typically the patient with tetralogy of Fallot has mild-to-moderate cyanosis and clubbing. The hyperpneic episodes ("hypoxic spells") associated with tetralogy of Fallot are virtually absent in the adult. The physical appearance is characterized by a small underdeveloped body size. If the patient has only mild cyanosis, development is normal. A loud systolic murmur over the third left sternal border with a thrill is characteristic; with severe tetralogy and marked decrease in pulmonary blood flow the murmur may be short and of low intensity. This is due to the absence of turbulent blood flow between the two high-pressure ventricles. When total obstruction (pulmonary atresia) is present, the murmur of the pulmonic stenosis vanishes and is replaced by a soft mid-systolic murmur. Continuous murmurs, an auscultatory sign of pulmonary atresia, indicate collateral circulation by way of bronchial arteries or presence of a PDA.

Management

The majority of patients born with tetralogy of Fallot have survived as a result of having undergone a series of surgical procedures. During infancy, a palliative systemic to pulmonary arterial shunt procedure would have been undertaken to permit pulmonary arterial blood flow and enhance oxygen saturation. Later in childhood, patients underwent complete surgical correction that included closure of the VSD and relief of the right ventricle outflow obstruction. Today, while palliative shunt procedures are still performed in selected cases, the majority of patients born with tetralogy of Fallot undergo reparative surgery in infancy.

Long-term survival following corrective repair ranges from 86% to 95% after 30 to 35 years.[47,48] However a number of residual complications must be monitored on a regular basis, including pulmonary regurgitation, atrial and ventricular arrhythmias, and ventricular dysfunction.[49,50] A small number of patients with tetralogy of Fallot remain cyanotic. These are usually patients who have developed pulmonary vascular obstructive disease and are no longer surgical candidates and are managed symptomatically.

Patients with tetralogy of Fallot should have follow-up visits with the cardiologist every 1 or 2 years.[26] Endocarditis prophylaxis is indicated only when prosthetic materials are used, for example for VSD closure, and when residua are present.[20]

Ebstein's Anomaly

Description

Ebstein's anomaly involves the tricuspid valve and is characterized by a downward displacement of portions of the tricuspid valve into the right ventricles (Fig. 31-12). The portion of the normal right ventricle that underlies the tricuspid valve becomes mechanically a part of the right atrium (atrialized right ventricle). As a result, the right atrium is exceptionally large, the right ventricle is small, and the tricuspid valve is incompetent. Ebstein's anomaly occurs in >1% of all congenital heart defects involving men and

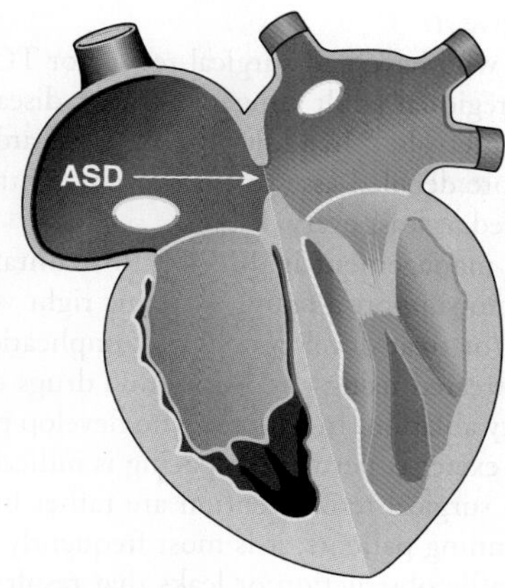

■ **Figure 31-12** Ebstein's anomaly. (Reprinted from Everett, A. *PedHeart Resource*. 2009. Scientific Software Solutions. www.heartpassport.com., with permission.)

women equally. In patients with Ebstein's anomaly, 80% have either an ASD or patent foramen ovale, often resulting in a right-to-left shunt.[50] In the presence of an atrial communication, central cyanosis may be present. Twenty percent of the patients with Ebstein's anomaly, however, are acyanotic. In addition, 25% of patients, one or more accessory atrioventricular pathways (Wolff–Parkinson–White) are found.[50]

The anomaly is compatible with a relatively long and active life. Patients with Ebstein's anomaly may live beyond age 50 years. The largest current long-term outcome study showed that the mean age of initial operation was 24 years (range 8 days to 79 years), and that the actuarial survival at 20 years postoperation was 71.2%.[51] The most common causes of death attributed to the malformation are heart failure, hypoxia, and arrhythmia. Sudden unexpected death tends to occur in adults rather than children and has been attributed to paroxysmal atrial arrhythmias to which this population is prone.

Pathophysiology

Hemodynamically abnormal function of the right heart is related to three problems: a malformed tricuspid valve, the atrialized portion of the right ventricle, and the reduced capacity of the pumping portion of the right ventricle. Ineffective emptying of the right atrium may result in an increase in right atrium volume and a right-to-left shunt through a patent foramen ovale or ASD. Tricuspid regurgitation caused by the malformed leaflets adds to the hemodynamic burden. Important complications associated with Ebstein's anomaly include supraventricular tachycardia resulting from Wolff–Parkinson–White bypass tracts.

Clinical Manifestations

Clinical features of Ebstein's anomaly may include effort intolerance due to dyspnea or fatigability. Progressive cyanosis and hypoxemia may occur as a result of a right-to-left atrial shunt. Because of the thin toneless atrialized right ventricle, the jugular pulse may be unimpressive despite tricuspid regurgitation. Auscultatory findings consist of a widely split first heart sound with a loud delayed second component. An S_3 is common due to abnormal filling characteristics of the functional right ventricle. In addition, an S_4 may be present, causing a quadruple rhythm. Murmurs vary from early systolic to holosystolic and are of medium frequency.

Management

Medical management of patients with Ebstein's anomaly is directed toward the prevention of complications and to the treatment of symptoms as they present themselves. Those patients with supraventricular tachycardia, or persistent atrial fibrillation or flutter may be treated with radiofrequency catheter ablation, although complete ablation of accessory pathways has a lower rate of success in patients with Ebstein's anomaly than in patients with a structurally normal heart.[52] Surgical repair of the tricuspid valve and closure of the ASD are recommended in symptomatic patients. Valve repair using annuloplasty ring is preferred to replacement, which is reserved for nonreparable valves. When required, a bioprosthetic valve is preferred to mechanical prosthesis.[50]

Patients with Ebstein's anomaly should have follow-up visits with the cardiologist every 1 or 2 years.[26] Endocarditis prophylaxis is needed both in repaired and unrepaired patients.[20]

CYANOTIC HEART DEFECTS WITH INCREASED PULMONARY BLOOD FLOW

There is only one heart defect that can be firmly classified under cyanotic heart defects with an increased pulmonary blood flow: a complete TGA.

Complete Transposition of the Great Arteries

Description

A complete transposition of the great arteries implies a reversal of the aorta and the pulmonary artery (Fig. 31-13). The aorta arises from the right ventricle and is located anterior to the pulmonary artery; with the pulmonary artery arising from the left ventricle.

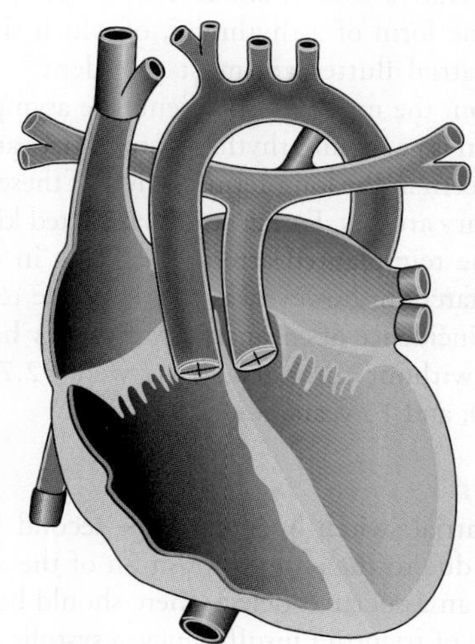

■ **Figure 31-13** Complete transposition of the great arteries (TGA). (Reprinted from Everett, A. *PedHeart Resource*. 2009. Scientific Software Solutions. www.heartpassport.com., with permission.)

Blood returning to the heart from the systemic circulation is ejected from the right ventricle into the aorta, sending unoxygenated blood back into the systemic circulation. Complete TGA, also referred to as *d-transposition of great arteries*, occurs in 5% to 8% of all congenital heart diseases. There is a male preponderance in patients with transposition of the great arteries, with a sex ratio of 1.5.[53] Natural survival is extremely rare, and survival into adulthood is dependent on the early use of palliative shunting procedures (atrioseptectomy, atrioseptostomy), pulmonary artery banding to regulate pulmonary flow, and, later, the atrial switch procedures known as the Mustard or Senning operation. Both of these procedures divert caval blood to the mitral valve and pulmonary venous blood to the tricuspid valve. In the Mustard procedure, venous blood is diverted to the mitral valve by means of an intra-atrial baffle. In the Senning procedure, a tunnel is created within the right atrium that carries caval blood to the mitral valve. While mid-term survival rates associated with the atrial switch procedures have been reasonably good, the commonly occurring complications of arrhythmias, baffle obstruction, and progressive failure of the systemic right ventricle have lead surgeons to replace the Mustard and Senning procedures with an arterial switch operation.[52–57] Carried out in an infant's first few weeks of life, the arterial switch procedure involves surgically detaching the coronary arteries from the aorta, then separating the aorta and pulmonary arteries above the semilunar valves. The aorta is then reimplanted to the stump of the pulmonary trunk, and the pulmonary artery is reimplanted to the stump of the aortic root. The coronary arteries are then anastomosed to the new aorta. While long-term survival data are limited, results appear to be very good.

Pathophysiology

For survivors of TGA who have undergone the Mustard or Senning operation, the preservation and integrity of the systemic right ventricle is the main concern. The long-term outlook for these patients is related to the demand placed on the right ventricle to support the systemic circulation. Additional long-term complications that may increase demand placed on the right ventricle include tricuspid regurgitation, sinus node dysfunction, atrial re-entrant tachycardia, and baffle obstruction or leaks. In a 20-year postoperative course, about 40% of the patients experience at least one form of arrhythmias, of which sinus node dysfunction and atrial flutter are most prevalent.[54] After arterial switch operation, the majority of patients are asymptomatic, ventricular function is good, and rhythm disturbances are uncommon. The major concern in the long-term survival of these patients is the status of coronary arteries. Earlier studies reported kinking and obstruction of the reimplanted arteries resulting in myocardial ischemia and infarction; however, as the operative techniques have improved, the incidence of coronary insufficiency has decreased.[21] Survival rates without coronary events were 92.7%, 91%, and 88.2% at 1, 10, and 15 years, respectively.[55]

Clinical Manifestations

Following an atrial switch operation, the second heart sound is usually single, due to the anterior position of the aortic valve. In the absence of an associated defect, there should be no murmurs. In the presence of tricuspid insufficiency, a systolic murmur is audible, and if due to the presence of a VSD, a pansystolic murmur is audible along the left sternal border. A harsh systolic ejection murmur along the left midsternal border will be heard in the setting of valvar or subvalvar pulmonary stenosis.

Management

All patients who have had surgical repair for TGA should be followed at a regional adult congenital heart disease center at 6 to 12 months intervals.[26] In addition to an echocardiogram, a cardiac MRI for more detailed assessment of right ventricular function is recommended at least every 3 years.

Medical management is directed to maintain right ventricle function or to support a failing systemic right ventricle as well as control and/or treat development of complications. Arrhythmias are mainly treated using antiarrhythmic drugs or by catheter radiofrequency ablation. In patients who develop poor chronotropic response to exercise, permanent pacing is indicated.

Data on surgical reintervention are rather limited.[56] In Mustard and Senning patients, it is most frequently performed in the setting of baffle obstruction or leaks that result in shunting. The latter is more often observed in patients after the Mustard operation than after the Senning operation.[54] Following the arterial switch operation, patients are monitored for right and left ventricle outflow tract obstruction in the supravalvular areas, due to suture line stenosis. If an outflow tract obstruction occurs, balloon angioplasty or surgical intervention with patch augmentation is the treatment of choice. Patients with transposition of the great arteries often have residual defects, therefore endocarditis prophylaxis is recommended.[20]

CYANOTIC HEART DEFECTS WITH COMMON MIXING

In certain heart defects there is common mixing of pulmonary and systemic venous blood within the heart or great vessels, resulting in desaturation of arterial blood.[17] Heart defects with common mixing are associated with or without obstruction of pulmonary blood flow. Patients with ventricular outflow obstruction have a diminished pulmonary blood flow, whereas those without ventricular outflow obstruction have an increased pulmonary blood flow.[17]

Truncus Arteriosus

Description

In this lesion, which occurs in >1% of all congenital heart diseases, the primitive trunk fails to divide into two great arteries (Fig. 31-14). Thus, a single great vessel emerges from the base of the heart through a single semilunar valve, straddling both ventricles over a large VSD. The truncus, which is the aorta, receives blood from both ventricles and gives rise to both pulmonary and systemic circulations, as well as coronary arteries. The second semilunar valve is absent but a short pulmonary trunk without a valve may emerge from the side of the truncus and give rise to the right and left pulmonary arteries (Type I), or both pulmonary arteries may arise directly from the posterior or lateral walls of the truncus (Type II). Pulmonary blood flow then arises entirely by way of collaterals from bronchial arteries or a PDA. In more than 80% of patients, a large VSD is also present.[58]

Survival rate of patients with truncus arteriosus is variable.[59] About 56% of the patients die in infancy or childhood before operation or during the immediate postoperative period.[60] Late mortality of hospital survivors, up to 20 years after the operation, is about 15%.[60,61] As a result, it is estimated that only 30% of the patients with truncus arteriosus will reach adulthood. Only patients

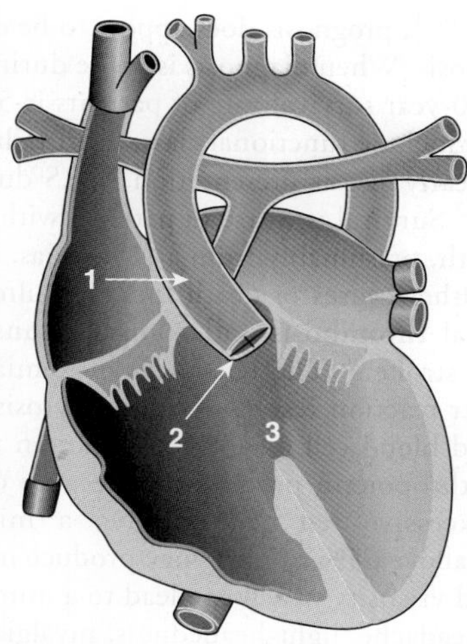

■ **Figure 31-14** Truncus arteriosus. 1: Common trunk; 2: Truncal valve; 3: VSD (Reprinted from Everett, A. *PedHeart Resource*. 2009. Scientific Software Solutions. www.heartpassport.com., with permission.)

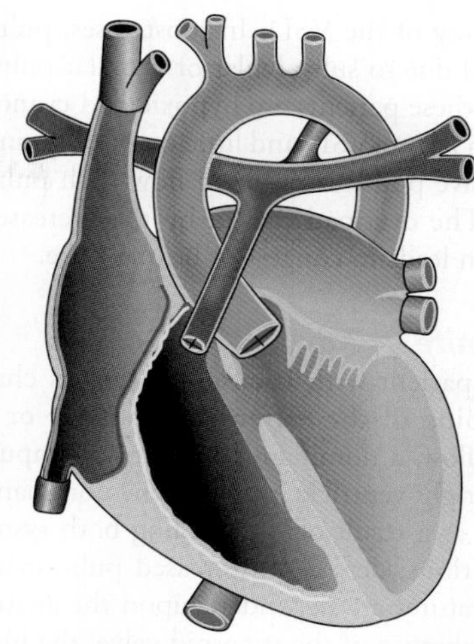

■ **Figure 31-15** Tricuspid atresia. (Reprinted from Everett, A. *PedHeart Resource*. 2009. Scientific Software Solutions. www.heartpassport.com., with permission.)

with regulated pulmonary circulation can survive into the third and fourth decades.[21]

Pathophysiology

The hemodynamic consequences of truncus arteriosus depend on the magnitude of pulmonary blood flow, which reflects the presence and the size of the pulmonary arteries and the resistance to flow through the lungs.[14] In the types with large unobstructed pulmonary arteries arising from the arterial trunk, pulmonary blood flow is greatly increased, clinically resembling patients with large VSD with left-to-right shunts.

Clinical Manifestations

Cyanosis, which may be mild or absent, occurs with increased pulmonary blood flow. Right ventricle pressure is equal to systemic pressure because both ventricles eject directly into the single trunk. The patient with mild cyanosis and a large pulmonary blood flow has a loud systolic murmur along the lower left sternal border. The second heart sound is single and loud. Diastolic flow murmurs may be present if truncus dilatation with resultant regurgitation is present. Variations may be caused by the resistance to flow into the pulmonary circuit (i.e., a higher resistance leads to shortening and softening of the murmur).

Management

Palliative procedures such as a bilateral pulmonary artery banding to restrict pulmonary blood flow have been performed with limited success in the past. Today, however, the majority of infants will undergo primary surgical repair which includes closure of the VSD, committing the truncus valve to the left ventricle, and thus serving as an aortic valve. In the right ventricle, a homograft or conduit is constructed connecting the right ventricle to the pulmonary artery. In some cases, replacement of the right ventricle–pulmonary artery homograft may be required as the conduits are subject to calcification or valve degeneration.

Patients require regular follow-up in a specialized adult congenital heart disease center,[26] with focus on any evidence of conduit stenosis or regurgitation, aortic root dilatation, branch pulmonary artery stenosis, residual VSD, ventricular dysfunction, truncal valve stenosis or regurgitation, arrhythmias, or pulmonary hypertension and right heart failure.[59] Both repaired and unrepaired patients are considered to have the highest risk of adverse outcome from endocarditis.[20] Therefore, antibiotic prophylaxis is recommended in all patients with truncus arteriosus.

Tricuspid Atresia

Description

Tricuspid atresia is the most common type of univentricular physiology. It is reported to occur in 1% to 2% of all congenital heart defects and occurs equally in men and women. However, there is a male preponderance in patients in whom the tricuspid atresia is associated with transposition of the great arteries.[62] Tricuspid atresia involves the absence of a tricuspid valve, resulting in a total right-to-left shunt at the atrial level by way of an obligatory ASD or foramen ovale (Fig. 31-15). In addition, there is a varying degree of hypoplasia of the right ventricle and an enlargement of the mitral valve and left ventricle. Whereas all types of tricuspid atresia have in common the absence of the tricuspid valve, various forms exist. One commonly used classification focuses on the relation of the great arteries, the degree of reduced pulmonary blood flow, and the size of the VSD.[63] The 20-year survival rate in patients with tricuspid atresia is about 60%.[64] Survival is determined by the adequacy of pulmonary blood flow and the pressure in the pulmonary vascular bed.[14]

Pathophysiology

In the most common form of tricuspid atresia, the VSD is small, the right ventricle is hypoplastic, and the great arteries are normally related. Because of the atretic tricuspid valve, systemic venous return crosses from the right atrium to the left atrium via an interatrial communication. Oxygenated and deoxygenated blood is mixed and redirected to the left ventricle, where blood is then ejected into the aorta, with some blood reaching the pulmonary circulation by way of the VSD. In most cases, pulmonary blood flow is restricted due to subvalvular or valvular pulmonary stenosis. As a result, these patients are hypoxic and cyanosed.

Patients with a large VSD and little or no pulmonary restriction will have excessive pulmonary blood flow with pulmonary artery hypertension. The overload caused by the increased pulmonary blood flow often leads to congestive heart failure.

Clinical Manifestations

Clinically, the patient with tricuspid atresia is characterized by cyanosis, clubbing of the extremities, normal or reduced pulmonary blood flow, a dominant left ventricle impulse, and a noticeably absent right ventricle impulse. The dominant left ventricle impulse occurs as a result of its handling both systemic and pulmonary circulations, despite a decreased pulmonary blood flow. The physical features are dependent upon the anatomic findings. Because of the absence of the tricuspid valve, the first heart sound is single. The presence or absence of a systolic murmur depends on the size of the VSD. If significant, a holosystolic murmur may be heard at the mid to lower left sternal border and can generate a precordial thrill. If the size of the VSD decreases, the murmur may change from holosystolic to early systolic.

Management

Survival beyond infancy without surgical intervention is rare. However, the palliative shunts such as Blalock and Taussig (subclavian artery to pulmonary artery) performed in infancy and the increasing success of the surgical procedures such as the Fontan, lateral tunnel and bidirectional Glenn have contributed to an increasing number of patients reaching adulthood. Introduced in 1971, the Fontan procedure has undergone a number of modifications. However, each provides an aorticopulmonary or atrioventricular connection. In patients who underwent a Fontan operation and who survived the perioperative period, 20-year survival rate was more than 80%.[65] However, the long-term concerns associated with these surgical procedures include the physiologic effects of persistent elevated right atrium pressure and elevated systemic venous pressure, and problems with stenosis or obstruction of the conduit used in the different connections.

Patients with tricuspid atresia require continuous long-term care in a regional ACHD.[26] In the setting of a Fontan physiology, endocarditis prophylaxis is imperative.[20]

EISENMENGER REACTION

Eisenmenger reaction occurs as a result of increased pulmonary vascular resistance and reversed or bidirectional shunts at the aorticopulmonary, ventricular, or atrial levels. It is associated with decreased oxygen saturation in the systemic circulation, cyanosis, and erythrocytosis. The term Eisenmenger reaction applies to a number of shunting defects that are hemodynamically similar because of the presence of pulmonary hypertension and an associated right-to-left shunt. It is usually a consequence of delayed operation and may go undetected until adolescence or adulthood when operation is no longer possible.

It is estimated that more than 50% of the patients with Eisenmenger reaction can reach the fifth decade of life,[66,67] and, although rare, patients living into the seventh decade have been reported.[68,69] While rates of survival are better than previously reported [24,70,71], prognosis does appear to be dependent on the age of diagnosis. When diagnosis is made during adulthood, the estimated 10-year survival rate of patients is 58%.[72] Predictors of mortality include functional class, heart failure, history of arrhythmias, early age at presentation, QRS duration, and QTc interval.[66,67] Survival is worse in patients with complex lesions. Sudden death, presumably from arrhythmias, is the usual cause of death. Other causes of death include pulmonary infarction from arterial thrombosis and complications of cerebral abscesses and stroke.[50] The chronic hypoxemia associated with Eisenmenger reaction results in erythrocytosis, an adaptive increase in red blood cell (>45%) production that is due to increased erythropoietin production. Because of the viscous effects of excessive red cell volume, a minor increase in hematocrit above 65% to 75% may produce marked increase in whole blood viscosity which can lead to a number of symptoms including headache, light-headedness, myalgias, and visual disturbances. Therapeutic phlebotomy is rarely required in stable "compensated" patients, but may be indicated in symptomatic patients with unstable hematocrits of 65% to 70%. When indicated, phlebotomy must be accompanied by crystalline or plasma exchange.[73]

While traditional medical management has had little to offer these patients, recent attention has been given to the use of selective pulmonary vasodilators in improving hemodynamics and exercise capacity in patients with pulmonary hypertension.[74] A number of approved and investigation therapies are now available, offering for the first time the potential for improved survival for these patients.

REFERENCES

1. Mitchell, S. C., Korones, S. B., & Berendes, H. W. (1971). Congenital heart disease in 56,109 births. Incidence and natural history. *Circulation, 43*, 323–332.
2. Hoffman, J. I., Kaplan, S., & Liberthson, R. R. (2004). Prevalence of congenital heart disease. *American Heart Journal, 147*, 425–439.
3. Warnes, C. A., Liberthson, R., Danielson, G. K., et al. (2001). Task Force 1: The changing profile of congenital heart disease in adult life. *Journal of the American College of Cardiology, 37*, 1170–1175.
4. Hoffman, J. I., & Kaplan, S. (2002). The incidence of congenital heart disease. *Journal of the American College of Cardiology, 39*, 1890–1900.
5. Dastgiri, S., Stone, D. H., Le Ha, C., et al. (2002). Prevalence and secular trend of congenital anomalies in Glasgow, UK. *Archives of Disease in Childhood, 86*, 257–263.
6. Tagliabue, G., Tessandori, R., Caramaschi, F., et al. (2007). Descriptive epidemiology of selected birth defects, Areas of Lombardy, Italy, 1999. *Population Health Metrices, 5*, 4.
7. Tan, K. H., Tan, T. Y., Tan, J., et al. (2005). Birth defects in Singapore: 1994–2000. *Singapore Medical Journal, 46*, 545–552.
8. Wren, C., Richmond, S., & Donaldson, L. (2000). Temporal variability in birth prevalence of cardiovascular malformations. *Heart, 83*, 414–419.
9. Pradat, P., Francannet, C., Harris, J. A., et al. (2003). The epidemiology of cardiovascular defects, Part I: A study based on data from three large registries of congenital malformations. *Pediatric Cardiology, 24*, 195–221.
10. Bosi, G., Garani, G., Scorrano, M., et al. (2003). Temporal variability in birth prevalence of congenital heart defects as recorded by a general birth defects registry. *Journal of Pediatrics, 142*, 690–698.
11. Calzolari, E., Garani, G., Cocchi, G., et al. (2003). Congenital heart defects: 15 years of experience of the Emilia-Romagna registry (Italy). *European Journal of Epidemiology, 18*, 773–780.
12. Marelli, A. J., Mackie, A. S., Ionescu-Ittu, R., et al. (2007). Congenital heart disease in the general population: Changing prevalence and age distribution. *Circulation, 115*, 163–172.
13. Brickner, M. E., Hillis, L. D., & Lange, R. A. (2000). Congenital heart disease in adults. First of two parts. *New England Journal of Medicine, 342*, 256–263.

14. Perloff, J. K. (2003). *The clinical recognition of congenital heart disease.* Philadelphia: WB Saunders.
15. Franklin, R. C., Anderson, R. H., Daniels, O., et al. (2002). Report of the Coding Committee of the Association for European Paediatric Cardiology. *Cardiology in the Young, 12,* 611–618.
16. Maruszewski, B., Lacour-Gayet, F., Elliott, M. J., et al. (2002). Congenital Heart Surgery Nomenclature and Database Project: Update and proposed data harvest. *European Journal of Cardiothoracic Surgery, 21,* 47–49.
17. Jordan, S. C., & Scott, O. (1994). *Heart disease in pediatrics.* Oxford: Butterworth-Heinemann.
18. Penaloza, D., & Arias-Stella, J. (2007). The heart and pulmonary circulation at high altitudes: Healthy Highlanders and chronic mountain sickness. *Circulation, 115,* 1132–1146.
19. Perloff, J. K. (1998). Survival patterns without cardiac surgery or interventional catheterization: A narrowing base. In J. K. Perloff & J. S. Childs (Eds.), *Congenital heart disease in adults* (pp. 15–53). Philadelphia: WB Saunders.
20. Wilson, W., Taubert, K. A., Gewitz, M., et al. (2007). Prevention of infective endocarditis: Guidelines from the American Heart Association: A guideline from the American Heart Association Rheumatic Fever, Endocarditis, and Kawasaki Disease Committee, Council on Cardiovascular Disease in the Young, and the Council on Clinical Cardiology, Council on Cardiovascular Surgery and Anesthesia, and the Quality of Care and Outcomes Research Interdisciplinary Working Group. *Circulation, 116,* 1736–1754.
21. Gersony, W. M., & Rosenbaum, M. S. (2002). *Congenital heart disease in the adult.* New York: McGraw-Hill.
22. Wilson, N. J., Smith, J., Prommete, et al. (2008). Transcatheter closure of secundum atrial septal defects with the Amplatzer septal occluder in adults and children—follow-up closure rates, degree of mitral regurgitation and evolution of arrhythmias. *Heart and Lung Circulation, 17*(4), 318–324.
23. Egred, M., Andron, M., Albouaini, K., et al. (2007). Percutaneous closure of patent foramen ovale and atrial septal defect: Procedure outcome and medium-term follow-up. *Journal of Interventional Cardiology, 20,* 395–401.
24. Kidd, L., Driscoll, D. J., Gersony, W. M., et al. (1993). Second natural history study of congenital heart defects. Results of treatment of patients with ventricular septal defects. *Circulation, 87,* I38–I51.
25. Roos-Hesselink, J. W., Meijboom, F. J., Spitaels, S. E., et al. (2004). Outcome of patients after surgical closure of ventricular septal defect at young age: Longitudinal follow-up of 22–34 years. *European Heart Journal, 25,* 1057–1062.
26. Landzberg, M. J., Murphy, D. J., Jr., Davidson, W. R., Jr., et al. (2001). Task Force 4: Organization of delivery systems for adults with congenital heart disease. *Journal of the American College of Cardiology, 37,* 1187–1193.
27. Aboulhosn, J., & Child, J. S. (2006). Left ventricular outflow obstruction: Subaortic stenosis, bicuspid aortic valve, supravalvar aortic stenosis, and coarctation of the aorta. *Circulation, 114,* 2412–2422.
28. Keane, J. F., Driscoll, D. J., Gersony, W. M., et al. (1993). Second natural history study of congenital heart defects. Results of treatment of patients with aortic valvar stenosis. *Circulation, 87,* I16–I27.
29. Rhodes, J. F., Hijazi, Z. M., & Sommer, R. J. (2008). Pathophysiology of congenital heart disease in the adult, Part II. Simple obstructive lesions. *Circulation, 117,* 1228–1237.
30. Vogt, M., Kuhn, A., Baumgartner, D., et al. (2005). Impaired elastic properties of the ascending aorta in newborns before and early after successful coarctation repair: Proof of a systemic vascular disease of the prestenotic arteries? *Circulation, 111,* 3269–3273.
31. Guerin, P., Jimenez, M., Vallot, M., et al. (2005). Arterial rigidity of patients operated successfully for coarctation of the aorta without residual hypertension. *Archives des Maladies du Coeur et des Vaisseaux, 98,* 557–560.
32. Vriend, J. W., de Groot, E., Bouma, B. J., et al. (2005). Carotid intima-media thickness in post-coarctectomy patients with exercise induced hypertension. *Heart, 91,* 962–963.
33. de Divitiis, M., Pilla, C., Kattenhorn, M., et al. (2001). Vascular dysfunction after repair of coarctation of the aorta: Impact of early surgery. *Circulation, 104,* I165–I170.
34. Sehested, J., Baandrup, U., & Mikkelsen, E. (1982). Different reactivity and structure of the prestenotic and poststenotic aorta in human coarctation. Implications for baroreceptor function. *Circulation, 65,* 1060–1065.
35. Cohen, M., Fuster, V., Steele, P. M., et al. (1989). Coarctation of the aorta. Long-term follow-up and prediction of outcome after surgical correction. *Circulation, 80,* 840–845.
36. Brouwer, R. M., Erasmus, M. E., Ebels, T., et al. (1994). Influence of age on survival, late hypertension, and recoarctation in elective aortic coarctation repair. Including long-term results after elective aortic coarctation repair with a follow-up from 25 to 44 years. *Journal of Thoracic and Cardiovascular Surgery, 108,* 525–531.
37. Toro-Salazar, O. H., Steinberger, J., Thomas, W., et al. (2002). Long-term follow-up of patients after coarctation of the aorta repair. *American Journal of Cardiology, 89,* 541–547.
38. Clarkson, P. M., Nicholson, M. R., Barratt-Boyes, B. G., et al. (1983). Results after repair of coarctation of the aorta beyond infancy: A 10 to 28 year follow-up with particular reference to late systemic hypertension. *American Journal of Cardiology, 51,* 1481–1488.
39. Gatzoulis, M. A., Swan, L., Therrien, J., et al. (2005). *Adult congenital heart disease: A practical guide.* Malden, MA: Blackwell Publishing Ltd.
40. Gersony, W. M., Hayes, C. J., Driscoll, D. J., et al. (1993). Second natural history study of congenital heart defects. Quality of life of patients with aortic stenosis, pulmonary stenosis, or ventricular septal defect. *Circulation, 87,* I52–I65.
41. Fawzy, M. E., Awad, M., Galal, O., et al. (2001). Long-term results of pulmonary balloon valvulotomy in adult patients. *Journal of Heart and Valve Diseases, 10,* 812–818.
42. Hayes, C. J., Gersony, W. M., Driscoll, D. J., et al. (1993). Second natural history study of congenital heart defects. Results of treatment of patients with pulmonary valvar stenosis. *Circulation, 87,* I28–I37.
43. Rao, P. S. (2007). Percutaneous balloon pulmonary valvuloplasty: State of the art. *Catheterization and Cardiovascular Interventions, 69,* 747–763.
44. Rutledge, J. M., Nihill, M. R., Fraser, C. D., et al. (2002). Outcome of 121 patients with congenitally corrected transposition of the great arteries. *Pediatric Cardiology, 23,* 137–145.
45. Graham, T. P., Jr., Bernard, Y. D., Mellen, B. G., et al. (2000). Long-term outcome in congenitally corrected transposition of the great arteries: A multi-institutional study. *Journal of the American College of Cardiology, 36,* 255–261.
46. Gatzoulis, M. A., Webb, G. D., & Daubeney, P. E. F. (2003). *Diagnosis and management of adult congenital heart disease.* Philadelphia: Churchill Livingstone.
47. Murphy, J. G., Gersh, B. J., Mair, D. D., et al. (1993). Long-term outcome in patients undergoing surgical repair of Tetralogy of Fallot. *New England Journal of Medicine, 329,* 593–599.
48. Jimenez, M., Espil, G., Thambo, J. B., et al. (2002). Outcome of operated Fallot's tetralogy. *Archives des Maladies du Coeur et des Vaisseaux, 95,* 1112–1118.
49. Cheung, M. M., Konstantinov, I. E., & Redington, A. N. (2005). Late complications of repair of tetralogy of Fallot and indications for pulmonary valve replacement. *Seminars in Thoracic and Cardiovascular Surgery, 17,* 155–159.
50. Brickner, M. E., Hillis, L. D., & Lange, R. A. (2000). Congenital heart disease in adults. Second of two parts. *New England Journal of Medicine, 342,* 334–342.
51. Brown, M. L., Dearani, J. A., Danielson, G. K., et al. (2008). The outcomes of operations for 539 patients with Ebstein anomaly. *Journal of Thoracic and Cardiovascular Surgery, 135,* 1120–1136.
52. Walsh, E. P. (2007). Interventional electrophysiology in patients with congenital heart disease. *Circulation, 115,* 3224–3234.
53. Francannet, C., Lancaster, P. A., Pradat, P., et al. (1993). The epidemiology of three serious cardiac defects. A joint study between five centres. *European Journal of Epidemiology, 9,* 607–616.
54. Moons, P., Gewillig, M., Sluysmans, T., et al. (2004). Long term outcome up to 30 years after the Mustard or Senning operation: A nationwide multicentre study in Belgium. *Heart, 90,* 307–313.
55. Legendre, A., Losay, J., Touchot-Kone, A., et al. (2003). Coronary events after arterial switch operation for transposition of the great arteries. *Circulation, 108*(Suppl. 1), II186–II190.
56. Dos, L., Teruel, L., Ferreira, I. J., et al. (2005). Late outcome of Senning and Mustard procedures for correction of transposition of the great arteries. *Heart, 91,* 652–656.
57. Losay, J., Touchot, A., Serraf, A., et al. (2001). Late outcome after arterial switch operation for transposition of the great arteries. *Circulation, 104,* I121–I126.
58. Jonas, R. A., & DiNardo, J. A. (2004). *Comprehensive surgical management of congenital heart disease.* London: Arnold.
59. Bashore, T. M. (2007). Adult congenital heart disease: Right ventricular outflow tract lesions. *Circulation, 115,* 1933–1947.
60. Williams, J. M., de Leeuw, M., Black, M. D., et al. (1999). Factors associated with outcomes of persistent truncus arteriosus. *Journal of the American College of Cardiology, 34,* 545–553.

61. Rajasinghe, H. A., McElhinney, D. B., Reddy, V. M., et al. (1997). Long-term follow-up of truncus arteriosus repaired in infancy: A twenty-year experience. *Journal of Thoracic and Cardiovascular Surgery, 113*, 869–878.
62. Rao, P. S. (1992). Demographic features of tricuspid atresia. In P. S. Rao (Ed.), *Tricuspid atresia*. Armonk, NY: Futura Publishing Co.
63. Edwards, J. E., & Burchell, H. B. (1949). Congenital tricuspid atresia: A classification. *Medical Clinics of North America, 33*, 1177–1196.
64. Sittiwangkul, R., Azakie, A., Van Arsdell, G. S., et al. (2004). Outcomes of tricuspid atresia in the Fontan era. *Annals of Thoracic Surgery, 77*, 889–894.
65. Khairy, P., Fernandes, S. M., Mayer, J. E., Jr., et al. (2008). Long-term survival, modes of death, and predictors of mortality in patients with Fontan surgery. *Circulation, 117*, 85–92.
66. Cantor, W. J., Harrison, D. A., Moussadji, J. S., et al. (1999). Determinants of survival and length of survival in adults with Eisenmenger syndrome. *American Journal of Cardiology, 84*, 677–681.
67. Diller, G. P., Dimopoulos, K., Broberg, C. S., et al. (2006). Presentation, survival prospects, and predictors of death in Eisenmenger syndrome: A combined retrospective and case-control study. *European Heart Journal, 27*, 1737–1742.
68. Rosenzweig, E. B., & Barst, R. J. (2002). Eisenmenger's syndrome: Current management. *Progress in Cardiovascular Disease, 45*, 129–138.
69. Su-Mei, A. K., & Ju-Le, T. (2007). Large unrepaired aortopulmonary window—survival into the seventh decade. *Echocardiography, 24*, 71–73.
70. Saha, A., Balakrishnan, K. G., Jaiswal, P. K., (1994). Prognosis for patients with Eisenmenger syndrome of various aetiology. *International Journal of Cardiology, 45*, 199–207.
71. Daliento, L., Somerville, J., Presbitero, P., et al. (1998). Eisenmenger syndrome. Factors relating to deterioration and death. *European Heart Journal, 19*, 1845–1855.
72. Oya, H., Nagaya, N., Uematsu, M., et al. (2002). Poor prognosis and related factors in adults with Eisenmenger syndrome. *American Heart Journal, 143*, 739–744.
73. Miner, P. D., & Canobbio, M. M. (1994). Care of the adult with cyanotic congenital heart disease. *Nursing Clinics of North America, 29*, 249–267.
74. Archer, S. L., & Michelakis, E. D. (2006). An evidence-based approach to the management of pulmonary arterial hypertension. *Current Opinion in Cardiology, 21*, 385–392.

PART V

Health Promotion and Disease Prevention

CHAPTER 32

Coronary Heart Disease Risk Factors

M. Kaye Kramer / Katherine M. Newton / Erika S. Sivarajan Froelicher

Coronary heart disease (CHD) is usually associated with one or more characteristics known as risk factors. A risk factor is "an aspect of personal behavior or lifestyle, an environmental exposure, or an inborn or inherited characteristic, which on the basis of epidemiologic evidence is known to be associated with" the occurrence of disease.[1]

Several aspects of the association between a potential risk factor and the disease are evaluated before an association is considered causal. These include the strength or magnitude of the association, the consistency or repeatability of the association, temporality (the cause precedes the disease), dose response (greater dose leads to greater likelihood of disease), the biologic and epidemiologic plausibility of the association, coherence of the potential cause with what is known about the disease, a decrease in the incidence of disease when the potential cause is eliminated, and experimental evidence.[2,3] Although few potential risk factors meet all of these criteria, the goal of epidemiologic investigations is to establish these characteristics. The results of epidemiologic studies of disease cause are frequently presented either as disease rates or as a relative risk. The relative risk is the rate of disease in a group exposed to a potential risk factor, divided by the rate of disease in an otherwise similar group that is unexposed to the risk factor.[3] For example, if the rate of fatal myocardial infarction (MI) in a group of smokers was 120 per 100,000 per year, and the rate in comparable nonsmokers was 60 per 100,000 per year, then the relative risk associated with smoking would be as follows:

$$\text{Relative risk} = \frac{\text{rate in exposed}}{\text{rate in unexposed}}$$

$$= \frac{120/[100{,}000 \text{ per year}]}{60/[100{,}000 \text{ per year}]}$$

$$= 2.0$$

The risk of MI is thus doubled in the smokers, or there is a 200% increase in risk compared with nonsmokers. A relative risk of 1.30 represents a 30% increase in risk; a relative risk of 3.0 represents a 300% increase, or a tripling of risk. United States death rates in 1998 from all cardiovascular diseases combined, acute MI, cancer, and other causes, for black and white women and men are presented in Figure 32-1. Cardiovascular disease continues to be the leading cause of death for black and white men and women throughout their life spans. Death rates from MI increase with age in men and women. CHD incidence in women lags approximately 10 years behind that in men, and there is approximately a 20-year lag for serious clinical events such as CHD mortality[4] (Fig. 32-2). Data from the Behavioral Risk Factor Surveillance System (BRFSS) in 2005 showed that the prevalence of a reported history of MI was highest for the American Indian/Alaskan Native population (7.4%) and lowest among Asians (2.9%) (Table 32-1).

CHD mortality rates have declined steadily since the late 1960s. From 1968 to 1984, CHD mortality declined at an average rate of 2% to 3% per year in all age groups, in both sexes, and in black and white subjects.[5] Overall, cardiovascular disease death rates declined 24.7% from 1994 to 2004.[4] There is ongoing speculation as to the cause of this decline in cardiovascular disease mortality, although multiple causes are likely. Decreases in case fatality rates have been documented. This indicates that changes in patient management, including more rapid access to emergency care and interventions that reduce infarct size and prevent death caused by arrhythmias, may account for some of the decline in CHD mortality.[6] One recent study which examined the decrease in CHD mortality between 1980 and 2000 determined that approximately 47% of the decrease was attributed to evidence-based medical treatments such as secondary preventive therapies after MI or revascularization, treatment for acute MI, angina and heart failure, and other therapies.[7] Approximately, 44% of the decrease was attributed to changes in risk factors in the population, such as decreases in total cholesterol, systolic blood pressure, physical inactivity, and smoking.

Cardiovascular disease risk factors have additive effects. The MI risk in a person with three major risk factors is higher than that of a person with two or one.[8] Furthermore, for any given combination of risk factors, at a given age, the risk is lower in women than in men; however, the risk for CHD increases dramatically in women after menopause.[9] In this chapter, the major known risk factors for cardiovascular disease are briefly reviewed.

DEMOGRAPHIC CHARACTERISTICS

CHD mortality rates increase exponentially with age for men and women (Fig. 32-2). Until the seventh decade of life, black men

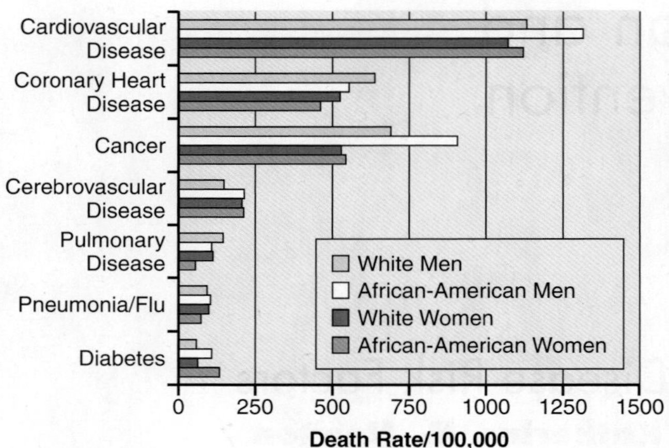

■ **Figure 32-1** U.S. death rates per 100,000 population for major causes of death by gender and race/ethnicity. (From Centers for Disease Control and Prevention: CDC Wonder. (October 1998). Available from http://wonder.cdc.gov/WONDER/mort.oo.ex./

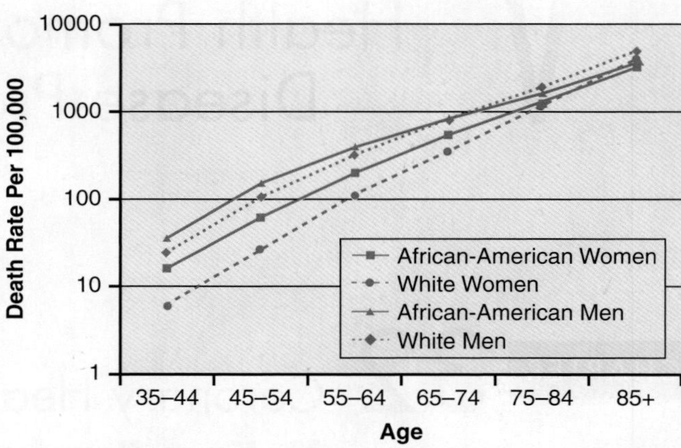

■ **Figure 32-2** U.S. coronary heart disease death rate per 100,000 population by age, gender, and race/ethnicity. (From Centers for Disease Control and Prevention: CDC Wonder. (October 1998). Available from http://wonder.cdc.gov/WONDER/mort.oo.ex./

have the highest rates of CHD mortality, followed by white men, black women, and white women. The rates in men converge at approximately the seventh decade, and those in women converge in the eighth decade. Further data about CHD rates by race/ethnicity come from analysis of death rates in California from 1990 to 2000.[10] The CHD death rates per 100,000 population were as follows: white women, 128; white men, 244; Hispanic women, 88; Hispanic men, 147; black women, 190; black men, 272; Chinese women, 56; Chinese men, 105; Japanese women, 55; Japanese men, 132; Asian-Indian women, 116; and Asian-Indian men, 201. Interestingly, when compared to the CHD death rates from 1985 to 1990 for the same populations, all groups showed a decrease with the exception of Asian-Indian women in which a 5% increase was noted.

Table 32-1 ■ PERCENTAGE OF RESPONDENTS AGED ≥18 YEARS WHO REPORTED A HISTORY OF MYOCARDIAL INFARCTION (MI) OR ANGINA/CORONARY HEART DISEASE (CHD), BY SELECTED CHARACTERISTICS—BEHAVIORAL RISK FACTOR SURVEILLANCE SYSTEM, UNITED STATES, 2005

Characteristic	No. of Respondents*	MI (%)†	95% CI§	Angina/CHD (%)¶	95% CI	MI or Angina/ CHD (%)**	95% CI
Age (yrs)							
18–44	128,328	0.8	0.7–0.9	1.1	0.9–1.2	1.6	1.5–1.8
45–64	137,738	4.8	4.5–5.0	5.4	5.2–5.6	7.7	7.4–8.0
≥65	87,351	12.9	12.5–13.3	13.1	12.6–13.5	19.6	19.1–20.1
Sex††							
Male	136,201	5.5	5.3–5.7	5.5	5.3–5.8	8.2	8.0–8.5
Female	219,911	2.9	2.8–3.0	3.4	3.3–3.6	5.0	4.9–5.2
Race/ethnicity††							
White, non-Hispanic	279,419	4.0	3.9–4.1	4.2	4.1–4.3	6.2	6.0–6.3
Black, non-Hispanic	27,925	4.1	3.8–4.5	3.7	3.4–4.1	6.2	5.7–6.7
Asian	5,974	2.9	1.7–4.7	3.3	2.2–4.8	4.7	3.3–6.5
Hispanic	25,539	3.6	3.1–4.2	5.0	4.5–5.7	6.9	6.3–7.7
American Indian/ Alaska Native	5,535	7.4	5.9–9.1	7.2	5.9–8.9	11.2	9.4–13.3
Multiracial	6,519	6.4	5.5–7.4	5.4	4.6–6.4	9.0	7.9–10.3
Education††							
Less than high school diploma	38,202	6.0	5.7–6.4	6.4	5.9–6.9	9.8	9.3–10.4
High school graduate	109,830	4.5	4.3–4.7	4.5	4.3–4.7	6.8	6.6–7.1
Some college	93,228	3.9	3.7–4.1	4.5	4.2–4.7	6.4	6.1–6.7
College graduate	113,944	2.9	2.8–3.2	3.6	3.4–3.8	5.0	4.7–5.2
Total††	**356,112**	**4.0**	**3.9–4.1**	**4.4**	**4.3–4.5**	**6.5**	**6.3–6.6**

*Sums of the sample sizes in each category might not add up to the total number of respondents because of unknown or missing information.
†Percentage of respondents who reported a history of MI.
§Confidence interval.
¶Percentage of respondents who reported a history of angina/CHD.
**Percentage of respondents who reported a history of MI, angina/CHD, or both.
††Weighted percentages are age adjusted to the 2000 U.S. standard population of adults.
Source: Morbidity and Mortality Weekly Report (MMWR) (2007). *Prevalence of Heart Disease—United States 2005, 56*(6), 115.

Surveillance data from the BRFSS suggest that marked disparities continue to exist in the overall prevalence, morbidity, and mortality associated with CVD and major CVD risk factors.[11] This report noted that the population subgroups most affected by disparity include those who are black, Hispanics/Mexican-Americans, persons with low socioeconomic status, and residents of the southeastern United States and the Appalachians. Furthermore, those with less than a high school education tend to have a higher burden of CVD and related risk factors regardless of race/ethnicity.

FAMILY HISTORY OF CARDIOVASCULAR DISEASE

A family history of CHD puts women and men at increased risk for CHD, probably from a combination of genetic and environmental factors.[12–15] This concept is reinforced in the findings from the INTERHEART study in which the odds ratio for an acute MI in people with a family history was about 1.5.[16] The population attributable risk rose from 90% with the other potentially modifiable risk factors under study (such as smoking, hypertension, etc.) to 91% with the addition of family history. Thus, a good portion of the effect of family history may be based on risk factors, which could be influenced by both environmental (lifestyle) and genetic factors. A history of MI in one first-degree relative doubles, and in two or more first-degree relatives triples MI risk.[15,17] MI risk is strongest when MI in relatives occurs before age 55 years but is still present when MI occurs after age 55 years.[15] The risk associated with a positive family history is independent of other known CHD risk factors.

Twin studies shed further light on the influence of family history on CHD risk. In a study of male and female Swedish monozygotic and dizygotic twins, among male twins the relative risk of CHD for monozygotic twins was 8.1, and the relative risk for dizygotic twins was 3.8 when one twin died of CHD before 55 years of age.[18] Among female twins, the relative risk of CHD for monozygotic twins was 15, and the relative risk for dizygotic twins was 2.6 when one twin died of CHD before 55 years of age. In monozygotic and dizygotic twins, as the age at which one twin died increased, the risk for CHD among the remaining twin decreased.

CIGARETTE SMOKING

In 2006, 45.3 million adults were current smokers, that is, 20.8% of the adult U.S. population (23.5% of men and 18.0% of women).[19] Smoking prevalence varies markedly by race/ethnicity and age (Fig. 32-3). In 2006, smoking rates for adults by race/ethnicity were as

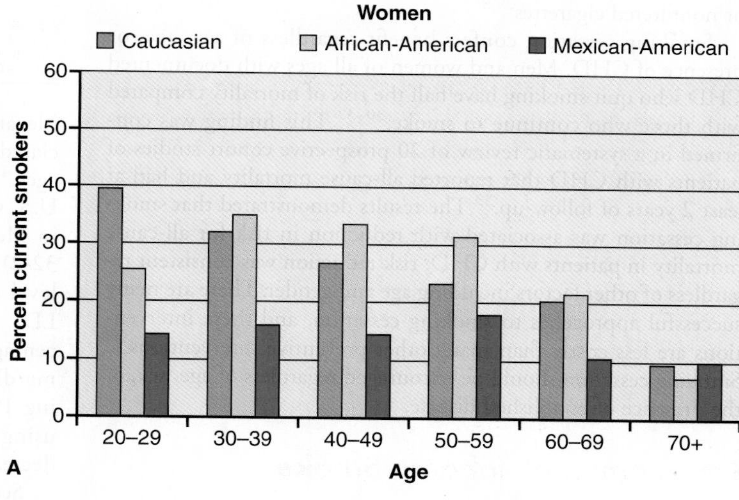

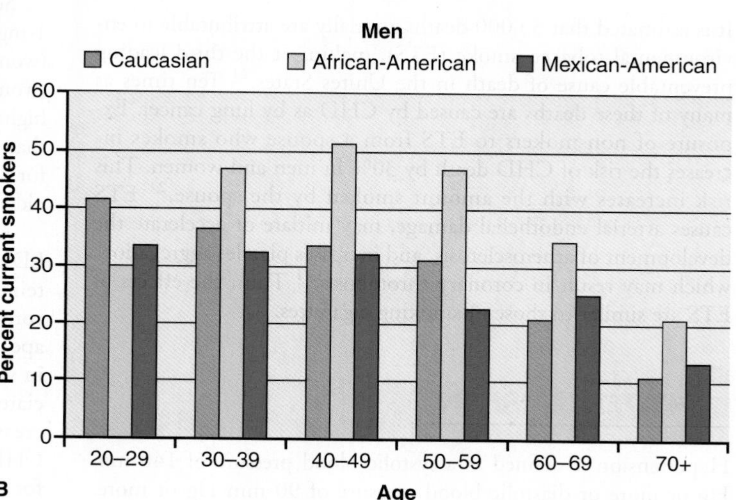

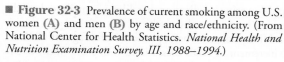

■ **Figure 32-3** Prevalence of current smoking among U.S. women (A) and men (B) by age and race/ethnicity. (From National Center for Health Statistics. *National Health and Nutrition Examination Survey, III, 1988–1994.*)

follows: American Indian/Alaskan Native, 32.4%; black or African American, 23.0%; non-Hispanic white, 21.9%; Hispanic, 15.2%; and Asian 10.4%.[19] Since 1965, rates of smoking in adults 18 years of age and older have declined by 50%.[4] Data from the Youth Risk Behavior Survey show that 23% of high school students were current smokers in 2005 (23% of female students and 22.9% of male students).[20] Cigarette use in this age group was stable or increased during the 1990s and then decreased significantly from the late 1990 to 2003, however, prevalence was unchanged during 2003 to 2005.

Smoking and CHD

Cigarette smoking is perhaps the most preventable known cause of CHD today, leading to more deaths from CHD than from either lung cancer or chronic obstructive pulmonary disease.[21] The CHD risk increases with number of cigarettes smoked, longer duration of smoking, and younger age at initiation of smoking.[22,23]

The CHD risk of male cigarette smokers is two (aged 60 years and older) to three (aged 30 to 59 years) times that of nonsmokers,[24] whereas women who are current smokers have up to four times the risk of first MI of those who have never smoked.[25–27] This elevation in the risk of MI and CHD death is sustained from youth into advanced age for men and women.[23,28] Smoking low-tar (<17.6 mg), low-nicotine (<1.2 mg), or filter cigarettes does not lower the risk of MI compared with high-tar, high-nicotine, or nonfiltered cigarettes[29,8]

Smoking cessation confers benefit regardless of sex, age, or presence of CHD. Men and women of all ages with documented CHD who quit smoking have half the risk of mortality compared with those who continue to smoke.[30–32] This finding was confirmed in a systematic review of 20 prospective cohort studies of patients with CHD that reported all-cause mortality and had at least 2 years of follow-up.[33] The results demonstrated that smoking cessation was associated with reduction in risk for all-cause mortality in patients with CHD; risk reduction was consistent regardless of other factors including age and gender. There are many successful approaches to smoking cessation, and these interventions are less costly than many other preventive interventions.[34] Smoking cessation should be encouraged regardless of age, sex, or the presence of established disease.

Environmental Tobacco Smoke

It is estimated that 53,000 deaths annually are attributable to environmental tobacco smoke (ETS), making it the third leading preventable cause of death in the Unites States.[21] Ten times as many of these deaths are caused by CHD as by lung cancer. Exposure of nonsmokers to ETS from a spouse who smokes increases the risk of CHD death by 30% in men and women. This risk increases with the amount smoked by the spouse.[21] ETS causes arterial endothelial damage, may initiate or accelerate the development of atherosclerosis, and increases platelet aggregation, which may result in coronary thrombosis.[21] Thus, the effects of ETS are similar to those of smoking cigarettes.

HYPERTENSION

Hypertension is defined as a systolic blood pressure of 140 mm Hg or more or diastolic blood pressure of 90 mm Hg or more. Hypertension carries particular importance as a cardiovascular risk factor for several reasons: it is highly prevalent, it is relatively simple to identify, it is a major risk for devastating cardiovascular outcomes, and control of hypertension is known to decrease its risk.[35] Prevalence of hypertension increases with age among white, black, and Mexican-American subjects (Fig. 32-4). The prevalence of hypertension is highest among black persons at all ages. Results from a cross-sectional analysis of data from the National Health and Nutrition Examination Survey (NHANES) 1999 to 2002 and NHANES III 1988 to 1994 showed that the prevalence of hypertension increased from 35.8% to 41.1% among black persons, with hypertension particularly high among black women (44%).[36] The prevalence of hypertension also increased among white persons from 24.3% to 28.1%. Hypertension is associated with three- to four-fold increases in the risk of CHD, stroke, and MI,[22,24,26] and it increases the risk of peripheral vascular disease, renal failure, and congestive heart failure in men and women across the life span.[24,37] The normalization of blood pressure dramatically decreases the risk of stroke, renal failure, cardiac failure, and coronary events.[38–40] Even in the elderly, control of hypertension confers major benefits against stroke, coronary events, and all cardiovascular events.[39,41] Hypertension and the nurse's role in its management are discussed in detail in Chapter 35.

SERUM LIPIDS AND LIPOPROTEINS

Elevated serum total cholesterol and LDL cholesterol are associated with an increased risk of CHD in men and women of all ages.[42–44] The prevalence of hypercholesterolemia is higher in U.S. women than in men, and higher in white and black than in Mexican-American subjects (National Center, 1997) (Table 32-2). CHD rates are lower for women than men at any given level of serum cholesterol.[42] Decreasing trends in total and LDL choletesterol levels have been noted over time; the percentage of adults with a total cholesterol level of at least 240 mg/dL during 1988 to 1994 decreased from 20% to 17% during 1999 to 2002.[45] The increase in the proportion of adults using lipid-lowering medication has likely contributed to the decreases that have been observed.

Serum HDL cholesterol has a protective effect against CHD. A 1-mg/dL increment in HDL is associated with a 2% (men) to 3% (women) decrement in total CHD risk, and a 3.7% (men) to 4.7% (women) decrement in CHD mortality.[46] At any given level of LDL, higher levels of HDL confer protection against CHD.[35] A level less than 40 mg/dL for adults is considered low HDL and increases risk for CHD. In 2005, for adults in the United States 20 years and older, the prevalence of HDL less than 40 mg/dL was 44.6 million.[4]

Attention has been focused on subfractions of HDL and LDL, the apolipoproteins (apoAI, apoAII, apoB), and lipoprotein(a) (Lp(a)). In a study of the predictors of premature CHD at coronary arteriography, Kwiterovich and associates[47] found that apoB was more strongly associated with an increase in CHD risk in women than in men, whereas ApoAI was more strongly associated with a decrease in CHD risk in men than in women. Increasing levels of Lp(a) are also associated with an increase in CHD risk.[48–51] In the Framingham Heart Study, the relative risk for CHD associated with elevated Lp(a) was 1.6 in women[49] and

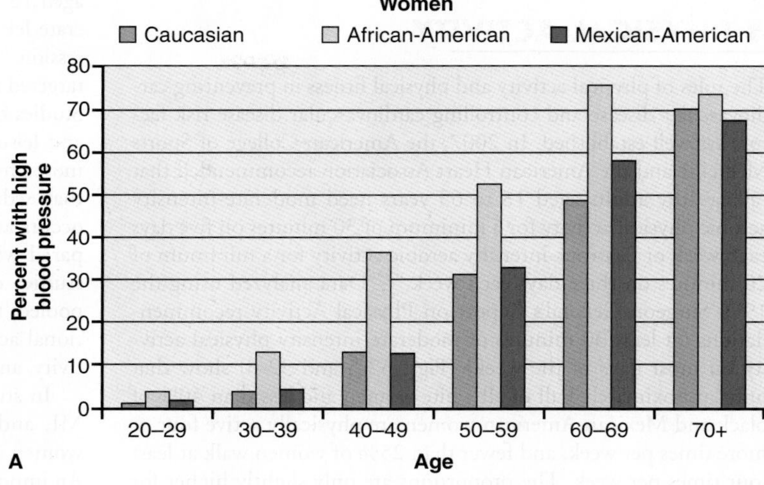

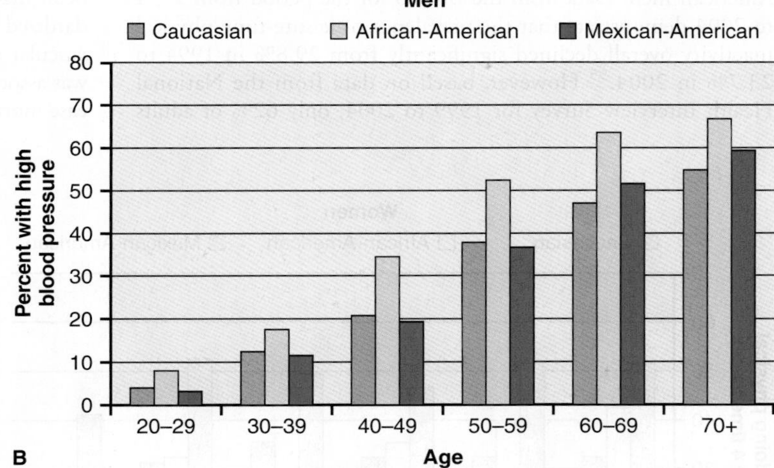

Figure 32-4 Prevalence of high blood pressure among U.S. women (A) and men (B) by age and race/ethnicity. (From National Center for Health Statistics. *National Health and Nutrition Examinations Survey, III, 1988–1994.*)

1.9 in men.[50] LDL subclass patterns also influence CHD risk. Compared with light, buoyant LDL, small, dense LDL is associated with a three-fold increase in the risk of MI.[48]

Serum cholesterol levels influence prognosis after MI. The risk for reinfarction is 3.7 times (men) to 9.2 times (women) as great when serum cholesterol levels are 275 mg/dL or greater, compared with levels of less than 200 mg/dL.[52] There is evidence that normalization of serum lipids and lipoproteins reduces the CHD mortality rate.[53] Hyperlipidemia and its management are discussed in more detail in Chapter 36.

Table 32-2 PREVALENCE OF HYPERCHOLESTEROLEMIA* AMONG U.S. WOMEN AND MEN BY AGE AND RACE/ETHNICITY

	White (%)		Black (%)		Mexican-American (%)	
Age Group	Women	Men	Women	Men	Women	Men
20–29	6.9	4.6	7.3	7.3	7.2	7.7
30–39	7.8	17.8	7.3	9.7	8.8	18.0
40–49	20.3	25.0	16.4	19.2	16.8	20.6
50–59	39.1	26.6	35.1	26.9	27.3	26.9
60–69	44.2	29.4	47.8	28.3	39.7	33.8
≥70	43.4	23.6	39.6	23.6	28.9	18.1

*On the basis of self-reported use of cholesterol-lowering medication or a total serum cholesterol value of ≥240 mg/dL.
From the National Center for Health Statistics, U.S. Department of Health and Human Services (DHHS). Third National Health and Nutrition Examination Survey, 1988–1994, NHANES III Data File (CD-ROM Series II, No. 1). Public Use Data File. Hyattsville, MD: Centers for Disease Control and Prevention, 1997.

PHYSICAL ACTIVITY

The roles of physical activity and physical fitness in preventing cardiovascular disease and controlling cardiovascular disease risk factors are well established. In 2007, the American College of Sports Medicine and the American Heart Association recommended that "all healthy adults aged 18 to 65 years need moderate-intensity aerobic physical activity for a minimum of 30 minutes on five days each week or vigorous-intensity aerobic activity for a minimum of 20 minutes on three days each week."[54] Data analyzed using the 1996 Surgeon General's Report on Physical Activity recommendations (at least 30 minutes of moderate-intensity physical activity on most days of the week) (Figs. 32-5 and 32-6) show that only approximately half of all white women and less than 40% of black and Mexican-American women are physically active four or more times per week, and fewer than 25% of women walk at least four times per week. The proportions are only slightly higher for American men. Data from the BRFSS for the period from 1994 to 2004 demonstrate that the prevalence of leisure-time physical inactivity overall declined significantly from 29.8% in 1994 to 23.7% in 2004.[55] However, based on data from the National Health Interview Survey for 1999 to 2004, only 62% of adults aged 18 years and older participated in at least some light to moderate leisure-time physical activity lasting 10 minutes or more per session.[4] Thus, a large proportion of the American public could be targeted for public health interventions to increase physical activity. Studies of the effects on cardiovascular disease of both on-the-job and leisure-time activity indicate that in general, people who are more physically active or physically fit tend to have CHD less often than sedentary or less fit people. CHD tends to be less severe and occurs at a later age among those who are physically active compared with those who are sedentary.[56] When data from cohort studies of occupational physical activity and CHD risk were pooled, the risk for CHD death for those with low-level occupational activity was almost twice that of those with high-level activity, and the MI risk was 40% higher in the sedentary group.[57]

In studies that included women, the risk for angina pectoris, MI, and sudden death was two to three times higher among women with the lowest compared with the highest activity level.[58] An important addition to understanding the benefits of fitness has been made by studies that measure physical fitness using standardized exercise tests and then compare fitness with later cardiovascular outcomes.[59–62] In these studies, a higher level of fitness was associated with a significantly lower rate of cardiovascular disease mortality in men and women,[59,62] all-cause mortality in men

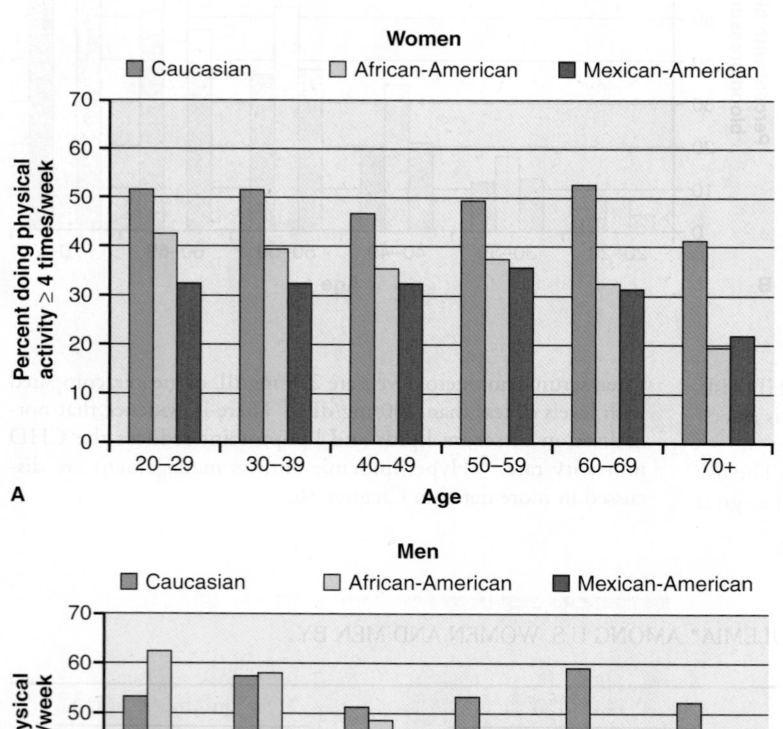

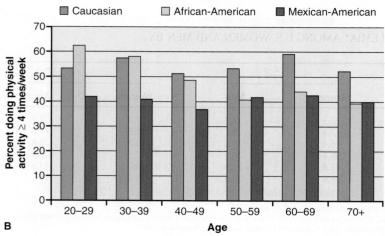

■ **Figure 32-5** Prevalence of physical activity at least four times per week among U.S. women (A) and men (B) by age and race/ethnicity. Physical activity: walking, jogging or running, bicycling, swimming, aerobics, dancing, calisthenics, garden/yard work, and/or lifting weights. (From National Center for Health Statistics. *National Health and Nutrition Examination Survey, III, 1988–1994.*)

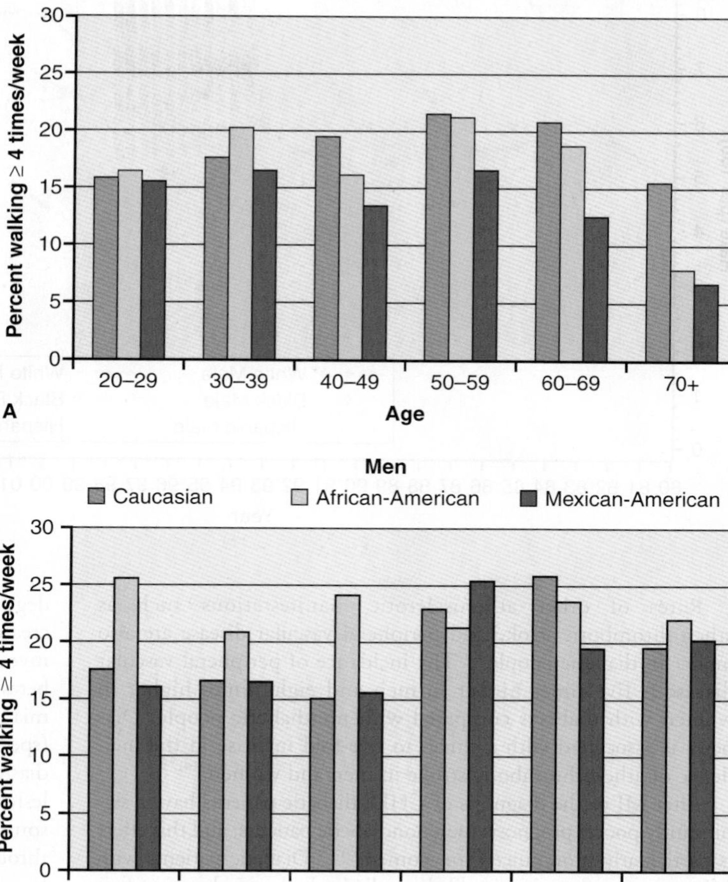

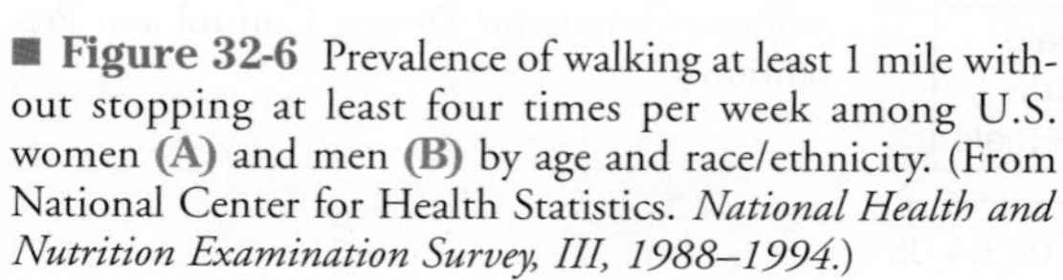
■ **Figure 32-6** Prevalence of walking at least 1 mile without stopping at least four times per week among U.S. women (A) and men (B) by age and race/ethnicity. (From National Center for Health Statistics. *National Health and Nutrition Examination Survey, III, 1988–1994.*)

and women,[59] and ischemic heart disease (fatal and nonfatal MI plus sudden death) in men.[62] Although pooled analyses from randomized trials of comprehensive cardiac rehabilitation suggest a 19% to 25% reduction in mortality rates associated with rehabilitation, it is difficult to dissociate the benefits of the exercise component of these programs from other lifestyle changes.[63,64] However, the potential benefits of a program of regular exercise after MI include an increase in exercise capacity, decrease in angina, improved control of other cardiovascular disease risk factors, decreased anxiety and depression, and increased self-esteem and sense of well-being.[64] A large systematic review and meta-analysis of randomized controlled trials of exercise-based rehabilitation for patients with CHD confirmed the benefits of exercise-based cardiac rehabilitation.[65] Exercise training is also recognized as an important adjunctive therapy, with similar benefits for those with a history of congestive heart failure.[66] Activity and exercise are discussed further in Chapter 37.

DIABETES MELLITUS

The American Diabetes Association diagnostic criteria for diabetes mellitus are random blood glucose of at least 200 mg/dL or fasting blood glucose of at least 126 mg/dL (Expert Committee, 1997). Currently over 23 million people or about 7.8% of the total U.S. population are estimated to have diabetes; about 17.9 million have been diagnosed and 5.7 million are unaware that they have the disease (Centers for Disease Control and Prevention, 2008). Approximately 90% to 95% of adults have type 2 diabetes; it is estimated that total diabetes prevalence will more than double between 2005 and 2050 (Narayan, 2006). Diabetes is more prevalent in minority populations. The prevalence of diabetes has been consistently higher in black and Hispanic than in white populations (Fig. 32-7). Prevalence tended to be higher in individuals aged 65 years and older, and lowest among those less than 45 years of age regardless of race.

Diabetes is associated with increased rates of virtually all forms of cardiovascular disease.[67] In men, diabetes is associated with a doubling in CHD incidence, and in women with diabetes, CHD incidence is five to seven times that of women without diabetes.[24,68] Diabetes doubles the rate of MI in men and increases the rate of MI in women four to six fold.[24,26,68] CHD and MI rates in diabetic women approach those of men of similar age, essentially eliminating the advantage found in nondiabetic women compared with men. This is true for white,[69] Mexican-American,[70] and Japanese[71] women. Ischemic heart disease mortality is doubled in men with diabetes and tripled in women with diabetes.[72]

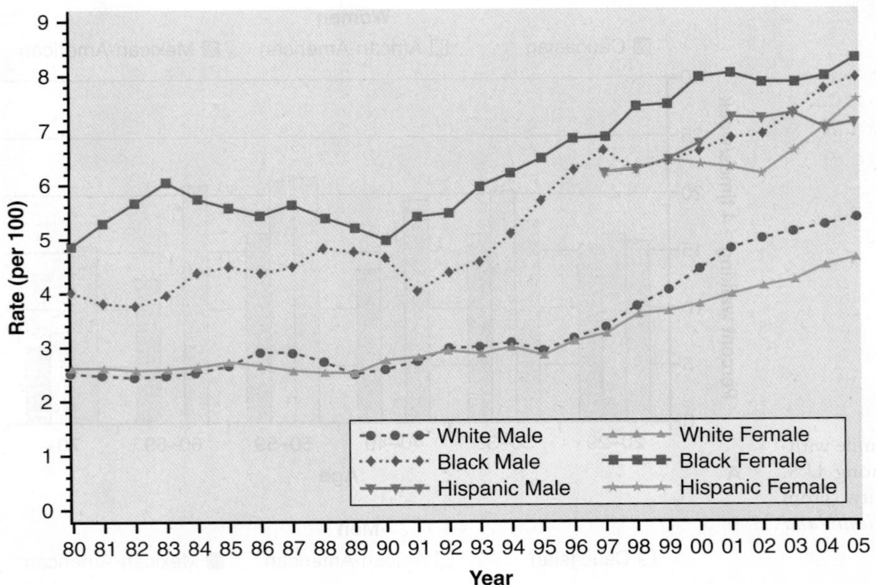

■ **Figure 32-7** Age-adjusted prevalence of diagnosed diabetes by race/ethnicity and sex, United States, 1980–2005. (From Centers for Disease Control and Prevention, National Center for Health Statistics, Division of Health Interview Statistics, data from the National Health Interview Survey. U.S. Bureau of the Census, census of the population and population estimates. Data computed by the Division of Diabetes Translation, National Center for Chronic Disease Prevention and Health Promotion, Centers for Disease Control and Prevention.)

Rates of other atherosclerotic manifestations such as atherothrombotic stroke and peripheral vascular disease are also higher in diabetic people.[24] The incidence of peripheral vascular disease is five times higher in men and eight times higher in women with diabetes compared with nondiabetic people. Diabetes is associated with a three- to five-fold increase in the incidence of atherothrombotic stroke in men and women.[24,73]

After MI or the diagnosis of CHD, diabetic patients have a significantly poorer prognosis than nondiabetic patients, and this effect is particularly pronounced for women.[74,75] Diabetic patients with MI are two to four times as likely to die in the hospital, more often have congestive heart failure and postinfarction angina pectoris, and more often extend their infarct than nondiabetic patients.[76]

Among survivors of an initial MI, the incidence of recurrent MI is increased by 30% in diabetic men and almost tripled in diabetic women, whereas fatal CHD is doubled in men and women.[77] During follow-up after MI, total mortality among diabetic patients is 1.5 to 3 times that of nondiabetic patients.[76] Results from the United Kingdom Prospective Diabetes Study showed that for those with diabetes, the risk of an MI being fatal increased with increasing hemoglobin (HbA_{1C})[78]; current practices are directed at reaching optimal levels of glucose control. Other studies have shown that intensive risk factor modification[79] and use of existing evidence-based therapies are important components in the outcome of acute coronary syndromes in those with diabetes.[80]

Insulin resistance, the primary pathologic process in type II diabetes, is also associated with CHD. Among nondiabetic adults in the Atherosclerosis Risk in Communities Study, women in the highest quintile of levels of fasting insulin had a three-fold increase in CHD risk compared with women in the lowest quintile of levels of fasting insulin; however, fasting insulin was not associated with the CHD risk in men.[81] In contrast, a study of Finnish men and women found that CHD prevalence increased with increasing fasting plasma insulin levels in diabetic and nondiabetic men and women.[82] A prospective study in England found a 60% increase in the risk of fatal and nonfatal MI among men in the tenth decile of serum insulin compared with the first to ninth deciles.[83] The differences in these findings in men appear to be related to the degree of insulin elevation; only severe elevations are related to increased risk. The mechanisms responsible for the acceleration of myocardial dysfunction and atherosclerosis associated with diabetes are the subject of great scrutiny.[84,85] Diabetes, hyperinsulinemia, and insulin resistance are associated with higher relative weight (specifically with a central body fat distribution); higher systolic and diastolic blood pressure; lower levels of HDL; and higher total cholesterol, HDL, and triglyceride levels.[8,84–86] These disturbances, sometimes called the "metabolic syndrome," appear to be linked through a complex set of genetic and environmental factors, and hypotheses about these associations are still being explored.

Although diabetes management has traditionally focused primarily on glycemic control, there is increasing recognition that interventions aimed at cardiovascular disease prevention, including behavioral interventions and pharmacotherapy aimed at treating overweight/obesity, hypertension, lipid disorders, and prothrombotic states, are critical in preventing cardiovascular complications among those with diabetes.[87–89] Recently the American Diabetes Association and the American Heart Association issued a joint statement to attempt to summarize the evidence supporting lifestyle and medical interventions that will prevent the development of CVD in people with diabetes.[90] The report highlighted similarities and differences in their prevention and treatment recommendations, but concluded in jointly supporting the aggressive use of lifestyle modifications to try to reduce or delay the need for medical intervention.

Recent trials have demonstrated that the onset of diabetes can be postponed or prevented through intensive lifestyle modification. In the Diabetes Prevention Program Study, an intensive lifestyle modification program aimed at modest weight loss (a goal of 7% loss in body weight) and physical activity (goal 150 minutes of brisk walking per week) in men and women at risk for diabetes decreased diabetes incidence by 58%. The average weight loss in the intervention group was 5.6 kg, versus 0.1 kg in the placebo group.[91] Similar results were reported from a Finnish study that used intensive lifestyle interventions to promote weight loss and increased physical activity in overweight persons with impaired glucose tolerance.[92] More recently, the Indian Diabetes

Prevention Programme demonstrated a 28.5% risk reduction for diabetes with lifestyle intervention in a high-risk Asian Indian population.[93] The DPP lifestyle intervention was also found to be effective in reducing risk factors for CVD[94] as well as components of the metabolic syndrome.[95] These results provide some of the most dramatic and powerful endorsements to date for primary prevention of diabetes through intensive behavioral intervention (see Chapter 39 for further discussion of diabetes).

BODY WEIGHT

The proportion of U.S. adults characterized as overweight and obese is reaching epidemic proportions. Widely, NIH Clinical Guidelines suggest that overweight and obesity be defined as a body mass index of 25.0 to 29.9 kg/m^2 and 30 or greater kg/m^2, respectively.[96] For example, an individual who is 5 ft 8 in tall would be overweight at 165 lb and obese at 200 lb. Using these definitions, the NHANES data surveys show that compared to data collected from 1976 to 1980, from 1999 to 2000 the age-adjusted prevalence of overweight and obesity in adults (BMI $\geq$25 kg/m^2) increased from 47% to 64.5%.[97] Further NHANES data from 2003 to 2004 indicate an increase to 66.3%. Prevalence of obesity (BMI $\geq$30 kg/m^2) and extreme obesity (BMI $\geq$40 kg/m^2) increased during these time periods as well. Data from the 2001 Behavioral Risk Factor Survey show that overweight and obesity increase with age, peaking at mid-life, and that the prevalence of obesity is highest in African-American and multiracial individuals, and lowest in Caucasians and those classified as "other" (Fig. 32-8). Of grave concern is the increased prevalence of overweight among children and adolescents in the United States. Using a definition of overweight based on gender- and age-specific BMI >95th percentile, compared to data collected from 1971 to 1974, from 2001 to 2004 the prevalence of overweight among children aged 6 to 11 years increased from 4% to 17.5%, and the prevalence among adolescents aged 12 to 19 years increased from 6.1% to 17%.[4] The potential long-term effects on diabetes and cardiovascular disease risks are staggering.

A positive association between obesity and CHD is expected. Hypertension, diabetes, and hypercholesterolemia are all more common in overweight people,[98] and weight reduction is an important therapy in the management of all CHD risk factors. Nevertheless, findings about the association between body weight and CHD risk are inconsistent. For example, despite the fact that body weight increased for black and white men and women from 1962 to 1980, cardiovascular mortality, stroke, and MI all decreased during this period.[99] In the Framingham Heart Study, men younger than age 50 years who were greater than 30% above ideal weight (determined by Metropolitan Life Insurance tables) had twice the incidence of CHD and acute MI compared with those less than 10% above ideal weight.[100] The findings were similar but of lower magnitude in those older than age 50 years.[100] In a Dutch study of BMI measured in men aged 18 years, the 32-year CHD mortality rate was more than doubled in those in the highest BMI category.[101] The relationship between obesity and mortality from CVD was further confirmed recently; however, no association between overweight and CVD was noted.[102]

Others have found no relationship between BMI and CHD mortality among white men, but a 70% increase in CHD mortality in black men in the 90th percentile of BMI compared with

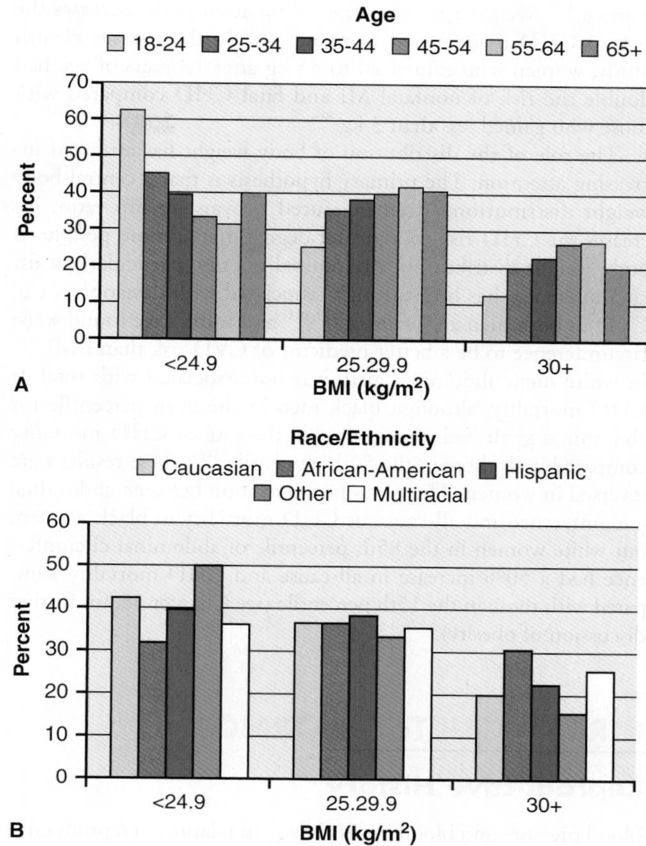

Figure 32-8 Prevalence of overweight and obesity among U.S. men and women (combined) by age (A) and race/ethnicity (B). (From National Center for Health Statistics.2001 Behavioral Risk Factor Survey. Available from http://apps.nccd.cdc.gov/brfss/display.asp? cat = RF&yr = 2001&qkey = 4409&state = US)

the 50th percentile. Still, other investigators have found no association between BMI and CHD death rates in black or white men.[103]

In women, relative weight predicts angina pectoris, CHD other than angina, CHD death, stroke, and congestive heart failure.[100] These relationships hold even among women of normal or near-normal weight; those with a BMI of 25 to 28.9 kg/m^2 and 23 to 24.9 kg/m^2 had a relative risk for CHD of 2.06 and 1.45, respectively, compared with women with a BMI less than 21 kg/m^2.[104] In the Framingham Heart Study, obese women (metropolitan relative weight >130%) aged 50 years or younger had a 2.4-fold increase in the CHD risk over 26 years of follow-up compared with lean women (metropolitan relative weight <110%).[100] The relationship between overweight and CHD is weaker among black women. In black women, BMI is unrelated to MI,[103,105,106] CHD death,[103,106] or all-cause mortality.[105,106]

Overweight also has a role in secondary prevention. Among women who have survived a first MI, a 1-unit increase in BMI is associated with a 3% increase in risk of reinfarction.[107]

Overweight continues to play a role in the elderly. Among men and women aged 65 years and older, the total mortality rate is as much as doubled in those above the 70th percentile of BMI compared with those in the 10th to 29th percentile, and the CHD mortality rate is increased by 50% in men and doubled in women.[108] Weight gain after the young adult years increases the risk of CHD in men and women.[86,100] In the Nurses Health Study, women who gained 20 to 35 kg after 18 years of age had double the risk of nonfatal MI and fatal CHD compared with those who gained less than 3 kg.[86]

The role of the distribution of body weight has attracted increasing attention. The primary hypothesis is that a central body weight distribution, often measured as waist-to-hip ratio, increases the CHD risk to a greater degree than a more peripheral body weight distribution. Abdominal obesity, particularly waist circumference, has been strongly associated with development of CVD in both men and women[109,110] and some have found waist circumference to be a better predictor of CVD risk than BMI.[111] In white men, abdominal girth was not associated with total or CHD mortality, although black men in the 90th percentile for abdominal girth had almost double the rate of CHD mortality compared with those in the 50th percentile.[106] These results were reversed in women. There was no association between abdominal circumference and all-cause or CHD mortality in black women, but white women in the 85th percentile of abdominal circumference had a 50% increase in all-cause and CHD mortality compared with those in the 15th percentile (see Chapter 38, for further discussion of obesity).

REPRODUCTIVE HORMONES

Reproductive History

Blood pressure and blood lipids change in relation to reproductive events. It is thus reasonable to investigate the potential impact of these events on the risk of CHD in women. Few studies have examined these factors, and their findings are contradictory. Nulliparous women appear to be at lower risk of CHD than parous women, and a woman's risk of CHD may increase with younger age at first birth.[26,112,113] Increasing parity may also increase CHD risk, perhaps because of the large changes in hormones associated with pregnancy.[113] Others, however, have found no differences in risk with parity and number of births.[114]

Earlier age at menopause increases CHD risk regardless of the mechanism of menopause. Among women who undergo bilateral oophorectomy, those younger than age 35 years have almost eight times the risk for nonfatal MI compared with natural menopause.[115] Premenopausal women of any age who undergo bilateral oophorectomy without estrogen replacement therapy have twice the risk of nonfatal MI and fatal CHD compared with premenopausal women of the same age.[116] At menopause, serum HDL levels decrease and LDL levels increase compared with premenopausal values.[117,118]

Oral Contraceptives

The increased risk for fatal and nonfatal MI in users of oral contraceptives (OCs) was first established in the 1960s and early 1970s. In these early studies, OC use was associated with an increased risk of nonfatal and fatal MI in young women.[119,120] Concurrent cigarette smoking acts synergistically with the risk from OCs, with the greatest risk occurring in women who smoke and are older than age 35 years.[25,121]

There are at least two mechanisms for the risk of cardiovascular events associated with OCs. First, OCs increase the risk of arterial and venous thromboembolism. The risk of arterial and venous thrombosis increases with the dosage of estrogen, whereas higher dosages of progestogens increase only the risk of arterial thrombosis.[122,123] The second possible mechanism for the association between OCs and CHD risk is the promotion of atherogenesis through unfavorable effects on blood pressure, serum lipids, and glucose tolerance.[124]

Dosages of estrogen and progestin in current OCs are considerably lower than those of the 1970s, and there appears to be little or no risk of MI or CHD death among users of newer OC formulations.[125–128] The exception is the finding in some[25,125] but not all[126] studies of continued high risk among women who are heavy cigarette smokers and OC users. A prospective cohort study in England and Scotland found a five-fold increase in the risk of MI among current smokers who used OCs.[125] It has been estimated that 9.7% of cases of nonfatal MI among women aged 35 to 44 years in the United States are caused by the combination of smoking and OC use.[129] However, a U.S. case-control study of low-dose OCs and MI risk in women aged 18 to 44 years found no increase in the risk among smokers.[126] Another more recent study examined mortality from all causes and CVD deaths in relation to OC use during a 14-year follow-up among Norwegian women who participated in a population-based health survey from 1985 to 1988.[130] The study found that women using OC of any type had no different adjusted total mortality (RR 0.87; 95% CI 0.46 to 1.65) or CVD mortality (RR 1.41; 95% CI 0.44 to 4.56) when compared with non-users. These findings support previous research, which has indicated that neither CHD mortality nor overall mortality is increased with OC use. Overall, OCs appear to offer a safe contraceptive alternative in terms of cardiovascular disease risk.

Postmenopausal Hormone Replacement Therapy

The public health implications of HRT have shifted dramatically with the publication of the findings from two landmark randomized, clinical trials: the Heart and Estrogen/Progestin Replacement Study (HERS) and the Women's Health Initiative. Despite the consistent findings of observational studies that HRT is associated with a 30% to 50% reduction in CHD events in women with[131] and without[116,132] preexisting CHD, the results of the first randomized trial of the effects of HRT on the CHD risk found no benefit.[133] The HERS study challenged our understanding of the effects of HRT in women with cardiovascular disease. There was a 50% increase in the relative risk of cardiovascular disease events in the first year of HRT use among women with established coronary disease. Overall, there was no difference in the likelihood of cardiovascular events between placebo and control. Because of the lack of overall benefit and the increased risk in the first year, the HERS investigators concluded that women with coronary disease should not initiate HRT.

The Women's Health Initiative consisted of two parallel randomized, double blind, placebo-controlled clinical trials of HRT which were designed to determine whether estrogen alone (for women with prior hysterectomy) or estrogen plus progesterone would reduce CVD events in "mostly healthy" women.[134] The estrogen plus progestin arm (planned duration 8.5 years) was stopped after an average of 5.2 years of follow-up because the overall risks outweighed the benefits of therapy.[135] Compared to women using placebo, women using estrogen plus progestin had a 29% increase in the risk of CHD, a 26% increase in the risk of breast cancer, a 41% increase in the risk of stroke, a doubling of risk of pulmonary embolus, a 37% decrease in the risk of colorectal cancer, and a 44% decrease in the risk of hip fracture. Although many of these findings were in the expected direction, the increase in the risk of CHD and stroke was unexpected. The study investigators concluded that HRT should not be used for the primary prevention of coronary disease. Like the estrogen plus progesterone arm of the study, the estrogen only arm was stopped prematurely after an average follow up of 6.8 years.[136] The results of this trial demonstrated that estrogen therapy significantly increased the risk for stroke, reduced the risk for hip and other fractures, and had no effect on CHD or overall mortality.

Further evidence against a cardiovascular benefit of HRT comes from the ERA trial.[137] In this randomized, controlled trial, neither unopposed estrogen nor estrogen plus progestin altered the progression of angiographically verified coronary disease compared to placebo after a mean of 3.2 ± 0.6 years. A similar trial showed no effect of HRT on progression of carotid atherosclerosis.[138] More recently, results from the Women's International Study of Long Oestrogen after Menopause trial, a multicenter, randomized, placebo controlled, double blind trial in the United Kingdom, Australia, and New Zealand, found that hormone replacement therapy increased CVD and thromboembolic risk when started many years after menopause.[139]

Thus, although trial data support a protective effect of HRT against fracture, and possibly colorectal cancer, concerns about breast cancer risk have been confirmed, and hopes that HRT would protect against cardiovascular disease and dementia have been reversed. The American College of Obstetricians and Gynecologists now recommends that HRT use should be limited to short-term therapy for vasomotor symptoms.[140]

FOLATE AND HOMOCYSTEINE

Homocysteine is an amino acid that is an intermediate byproduct of methionine metabolism. Homocysteine levels are higher in postmenopausal than in premenopausal women, lower in women than in men, positively correlated with age, and negatively correlated with serum/plasma levels of folic acid, vitamin B6, and vitamin B12.[141–144] Homocysteine levels of 5 to 15 μmol/L are considered normal, and elevations of 16 to 30, 31 to 100, and greater than 100 μmol/L are considered moderate, intermediate, or severe, respectively. Methylenetetrahydrofolate is an enzyme that contributes to the remethylation of homocysteine to methionine. This reaction requires folate as the substrate, and levels of dietary and blood folate are strong determinants of homocysteine levels.[145] Normally present in only small amounts (<10 μmol/L), homocysteine is highly toxic to the vascular endothelium. Homocysteine is associated with endothelial dysfunction, arterial intimal–medial thickening, wall stiffening, and a procoagulant activity.[146] People with homocysteinuria, a rare autosomal recessive condition in which homocysteine levels are severely elevated, are at extremely high risk for premature atherosclerosis.

Even mild elevations in homocysteine appear to be associated with increased CHD risk, and there is no specific threshold for the association between homocysteine and CHD risk. Numerous observation cohort and case-control studies have been conducted to evaluate the association between homocysteine and various manifestations of cardiovascular disease, including CHD, stroke, and peripheral vascular disease. The majority of studies show a positive association between homocysteine levels and these conditions.[143,146] Homocysteine levels are higher in women and men with angiographically confirmed obstruction of one or more major coronary arteries than in those with normal coronaries.[147,148] In the Framingham Heart Study, high plasma homocysteine concentrations and low concentrations of folate were associated with increased risk of extracranial carotid artery stenosis.[149] In Atherosclerosis Risk in Communities Study, the relative risk for carotid artery intimal–medial wall thickening among participants in the highest versus the lowest quintiles of plasma homocysteine was 3.2.[150]

In a 2-year prospective study, HRT was associated with an 11% decrease in homocysteine. The decrease was 17% in women with high homocysteine levels, whereas levels in women with low homocysteine did not change.[151] Increasing homocysteine after menopause may partially explain the increase in CHD risk associated with aging. Postmenopausal women have an excessive increase in homocysteine after a methionine load compared with premenopausal women, and folic acid supplementation decreases this increase in homocysteine after methionine loading.[152]

Despite evidence from observational studies that homocysteine is associated with an increased risk for cardiovascular disease, there is currently no evidence that lowering homocysteine levels decreases coronary morbidity and mortality. Several studies have failed to show a relationship between reduction in homocysteine levels and reduced CVD events or risks. The Vitamin Intervention for Stroke Prevention, a randomized controlled trial which included subjects with previous nondisabling cerebrovascular infarct, did not show any effect on vascular outcomes in the 2 years of study follow up despite moderate reduction in mean homocysteine levels.[153] Similarly, results from the Norwegian Vitamin trial, which evaluated the efficacy of lowering homocysteine levels with B vitamins in individuals with previous MI, did not find any effect upon lowering risk of recurrent cardiovascular disease despite a 27% reduction in homocysteine levels.[154] The Heart Outcomes Prevention Evaluation-2 trial, another randomized controlled trial that examined reduction in homocysteine levels using folic acid and B vitamins, failed to show a reduction in risk of major cardiovascular events in patients with vascular disease.[155] However, the debate regarding homocysteine continues; it has been suggested that longer trials are needed, as are trials focusing on those with higher homocysteine levels as well as achievement of greater reductions in homocysteine levels.[156,157] Therefore, because conclusive evidence for intervention does not yet exist, at this time, population-wide screening of homocysteine is considered inappropriate.[143,146,158,159]

ANTIOXIDANTS

Epidemiologic findings that antioxidants decrease CHD risk are supported by evidence that oxidized LDL is present in atherosclerotic lesions.[160,161] The accumulation of lipids in the arterial intima is the hallmark of early atherosclerotic lesions, and oxidation of LDL enhances its accumulation in the arterial wall lesions. Interest in the effects of antioxidants and CHD risk has centered on vitamins E and C and β-carotene.[160,162] Although observational studies suggested that consumption of foods high in β-carotene might reduce CHD risk,[46,163] the results of randomized trials in men[164] and men and women[165] show no benefit of β-carotene supplementation on CHD risk. Similarly, evidence that vitamin C reduces CHD risk is weak or lacking.[46,166,167] Recently the Women's Antioxidant Cardiovascular Study examined the effects of ascorbic acid (500 mg per day) and β-carotene (50 mg every other day) (as well as vitamin E) on the combined outcome of MI, stroke, coronary revascularization, or CVD death among 8,171 female health professionals aged 40 years and older.[168] All participants had a history of CVD or at least three risk factors for CVD; the participants were followed for a mean duration of 9.4 years. Results showed no overall effect of ascorbic acid, or β-carotene on the primary combined outcome, or on any of the individual secondary outcomes which included MI, stroke, coronary revascularization, or CVD death rate.

There is some evidence of cardiovascular benefit associated with vitamin E for women,[167,169,170] men[169] and in the elderly population.[171] Although a randomized trial of 50 mg of vitamin E in male smokers found only a 4% reduction in major coronary events,[172] a trial of patients with angiographically proven CHD, supplementation with 400 to 800 IU of vitamin E resulted in a 75% reduction in nonfatal MI compared with placebo.[173] These trials imply that supplementation at high doses may yield CHD protection. However, as mentioned above, in addition to investigating the effect of ascorbic acid and β-carotene in CVD prevention, the Women's Antioxidant Cardiovascular Study trial also examined the use of vitamin E (600 IU every other day) and found no effect on primary or secondary outcomes (RR, 0.94; 95% CI, 0.85 to 1.04 [$p = 0.23$]).[168]

Thus, while some evidence exists for the possible benefit of antioxidant supplementation in the prevention of CVD, the concept has not been proved and the results are somewhat inconsistent. In a recent review of the literature regarding antioxidant vitamin supplementation in cardiovascular diseases, the authors concluded that "although scientific rationale and observational studies are convincing, randomized primary and secondary intervention trials have failed to show any consistent benefit from the use of antioxidant supplements on CVD."[174] The United States Preventive Services Task Force states that the evidence is insufficient to recommend for or against the use of supplements of vitamins A, C, or E; multivitamins with folic acid; or antioxidant combinations for the prevention of cancer or cardiovascular disease. The The United States Preventive Services Task Force also recommends against the use of β-carotene supplements, either alone or in combination, for the prevention of cancer or cardiovascular disease.[175]

CONCLUSIONS

Outstanding progress has been made in our understanding of CHD risk factors and their management. The evidence against cigarette smoking, elevated serum cholesterol, and high blood pressure is strong, and sustained campaigns are underway to prevent and appropriately manage them. The importance of adequate physical activity and weight control is also acknowledged. Research continues on other emerging risk factors. The focus of future research will be on clarifying the role of these factors, particularly for women and ethnic minorities. In addition, as the rates of diabetes and obesity continue to rise in the United States and around the world, efforts directed toward translating prevention and risk-reducing strategies to the "real world" are absolutely essential.

REFERENCES

1. Last, J. M. (1988). *A dictionary of epidemiology* (2nd ed.). New York: Oxford University Press.
2. Kelsey, J. L., Thompson, W. D., & Evans, A. S. (1986). *Methods in observational epidemiology.* New York: Oxford University Press.
3. Rothman, K. J. (1986). *Modern epidemiology.* Boston: Little, Brown.
4. Rosamond, W., et al. (2008). Heart disease and stroke statistics—2008 update: A report from the American Heart Association Statistics Committee and Stroke Statistics Subcommittee. *Circulation, 117*(4), e25–e146.
5. Sempos, C., Cooper, R., Kovar, M. G., et al. (1988). Divergence of the recent trends in coronary mortality for the four major race–sex groups in the United States. *American Journal of Public Health, 78*, 1422–1427.
6. Pell, S., & Fayerweather, W. E. (1985). Trends in the incidence of myocardial infarction and associated mortality and morbidity in a large employed population, 1957–1983. *New England Journal of Medicine, 312*, 1005–1011.
7. Ford, E. S., Ajani, U. A., Croft, J. B., et al. (2007). Explaining the decrease in U.S. deaths from coronary disease, 1980–2000. *New England Journal of Medicine, 356*, 2388–2398.
8. Kannel, W. B., Doyle, J. T., Ostfeld, A. M., et al. (1984). Report of Inter-Society Commission for Heart Disease Resources: Optimal resources for primary prevention of atherosclerotic diseases. *Circulation, 70*, 181A.
9. Stangl, V., Bauman, G., & Stangl, K. (2002). Coronary atherogenic risk factors in women. *European Heart Journal, 23*(22), 1738–1752.
10. Palaniappan, L., Wang, Y., & Fortmann, S. P. (2004). Coronary heart disease mortality for six ethnic groups in California, 1990–2000. *Annals of Epidemiology, 14*(7), 499–506.
11. Mensah, G. A., Mokdad, A. H., Ford, E. S., et al. (2005). State of disparities in cardiovascular health in the United States. *Circulation, 111*(10), 1233–1241.
12. Burke, G. L., Savage, P. J., Sprafka, J. M., et al. (1991). Relation of risk factor levels in young adulthood to parental history of disease. The CARDIA study. *Circulation, 84*, 1176–1187.
13. Jousilahti, P., Puska, P., Vartiainen, E., et al. (1996). Parental history of premature coronary heart disease: An independent risk factor of myocardial infarction. *Journal of Clinical Epidemiology, 49*, 497–503.
14. Nyboe, J., Jensen, G., Appleyard, M., et al. (1989). Risk factors for acute myocardial infarction in Copenhagen: I. Hereditary, educational and socioeconomic factors. Copenhagen City Heart Study. *European Heart Journal, 10*, 910–916.
15. Roncaglioni, M. C., Santoro, L., D'Avanzo, B., et al. (1992). Role of family history in patient with myocardial infarction: An Italian case-control study. GISSI-EFRIM investigators. *Circulation, 85*, 2065–2072.
16. Yusuf, S., Hawken, S., Ounpuu, S., et al. Effect of potentially modifiable risk factors associated with myocardial infarction in 52 countries (the INTERHEART study): Case-control study. *The Lancet, 364*(9438), 937–952.
17. Friedlander, Y., Arbogast, P., Schwwartz, S. M., et al. (2001). Family history as a risk factor for early onset myocardial infarction in young women. *Atherosclerosis, 156*, 2101–2207.
18. Marenberg, M. E., Risch, N., Berkman, L. F., et al. (1994). Genetic susceptibility to death from coronary heart disease in a study of twins. *New England Journal of Medicine, 330*, 1041–1046.
19. Centers for Disease Control and Prevention. *Smoking and tobacco use.* Retrieved from http://www.cdc.gov/tobacco/data_statistics/tables/adult/table_2.htm
20. MMWR (2006, July 7). *Cigarette use among high school students—United States 1991–2005, 55*(26), 724–726. Retrieved from http://www.cdc.gov/mmwr/preview/mmwrhtml/mm5526a2.htm#tab1
21. Glantz, S. A., & Parmleyn, W. W. (1991). Passive smoking and heart disease: Epidemiology, physiology and biochemistry. *Circulation, 83*, 1–12.
22. Jensen, G., Nyboe, J., Appleyard, M., et al. (1991). Risk factors for acute myocardial infarction in Copenhagen: II. Smoking, alcohol intake, physical activity, obesity, oral contraception, diabetes, lipids, and blood pressure. *European Heart Journal, 12*, 298–308.
23. Slone, D., Shapiro, S., Rosenberg, L., et al. (1978). Relation of cigarette smoking to myocardial infarction in young women. *New England Journal of Medicine, 298*, 1273–1276.

24. Dawber, T. R. (1980). *The Framingham Study: The epidemiology of atherosclerotic disease.* Cambridge, MA: Harvard University Press.
25. Croft, P., & Hannaford, P. C. (1989). Risk factors for acute myocardial infarction in women: Evidence from the Royal College of General Practitioners' oral contraception study. *BMJ, 298*, 165–168.
26. LaVecchia, C., Franceshi, S., Decarli, A., et al. (1987). Risk factors for myocardial infarction in young women. *American Journal of Epidemiology, 125*, 832–843.
27. Rosenberg, L., Palmer, J. R., & Shapiro, S. (1990). Decline in the risk of myocardial infarction among women who stop smoking. *New England Journal of Medicine, 322*, 213–217.
28. LaCroix, A. Z., & Omenn, G. S. (1992). Older adults and smoking. *Clinics in Geriatric Medicine, 8*, 69–87.
29. Kaufman, D. W., Helmrich, S. P., Rosenberg, L., et al. (1983). Nicotine and carbon monoxide content of cigarette smoke and the risk of myocardial infarction in young men. *New England Journal of Medicine, 308*, 409–413.
30. Hermanson, B., Omenn, G. S., Kronmal, R. A., et al. (1988). Beneficial six-year outcome of smoking cessation in older men and women with coronary artery disease: Results from the CASS registry. *New England Journal of Medicine,* 319, 1365–1369.
31. LaVecchia, C., DeCarli, A., Franceshi, S., et al. (1987). Menstrual and reproductive factors and the risk of myocardial infarction in women under fifty-five years of age. *American Journal of Obstetrics and Gynecology,* 157, 1108–1112.
32. Salonen, J. T. (1980). Stopping smoking and long-term mortality after acute myocardial infarction. *British Heart Journal,* 43, 463–469.
33. Critchley, J., & Capewell, S. (2004). Smoking cessation for the secondary prevention of coronary heart disease. *Cochrane Database System Review, 1*, CD003041.
34. Cromwell, J., Bartosch, W. J., Fiore, M. C., et al. (1997). Cost-effectiveness of the clinical practice recommendations in the AHCPR guideline for smoking cessation. *JAMA, 278*, 1759–1766.
35. Kannel, W. B. (1987). Status of risk factors and their consideration in antihypertensive therapy. *American Journal of Cardiology, 59*, 80A–90A.
36. Ertz, R. P., Unger, A. N., Cornell, J. A., et al. (2005). Racial disparities in hypertension prevalence, awareness, and management. *Archives of Internal Medicine, 165*(18), 2098–2104.
37. Nastos, K., Charney, P., Charon, R. A., et al. (1991). Hypertension in women: What is really known? The Women's Caucus, Working Group on Women's Health of the Society of General Internal Medicine. *Annals of Internal Medicine, 115*, 287–293.
38. Hypertension Detection and Follow-up Program Cooperative Group. (1988). Persistence of reduction in blood pressure and mortality of participants in the hypertension detection and follow-up program. *JAMA, 259*, 2113–2122.
39. Medical Research Council Working Party. (1985). MRC trial of treatment of mild hypertension: Principal results. *BMJ, 291*, 97–104.
40. Ramsay, L. E., & Yeo, W. W. (1991). Hypertension and coronary artery disease: An unsolved problem. *Journal of Cardiovascular Pharmacology, 18*(Suppl.), S31–S34.
41. SHEP Cooperative Research Group. (1991). Prevention of stroke by antihypertensive drug treatment in older persons with isolated systolic hypertension: Final results of the systolic hypertension in the elderly program (SHEP). *JAMA, 265*, 3255–3264.
42. Bush, T. L., Fried, L. P., & Barrett-Connor, E. (1988). Cholesterol, lipoproteins and coronary heart disease in women. *Clinical Chemistry, 34*, 660–670.
43. Manolio, T. A., Pearson, T. A., Wenger, N. K., et al. (1992). Cholesterol and heart disease in older persons and women: Review of an NHLBI workshop. *Annals of Epidemiology, 2*, 161–176.
44. Wilson, P. W. F. (1990). High-density lipoprotein, low-density lipoprotein and coronary artery disease. *American Journal of Cardiology, 66*, 7A–10A.
45. Carroll, M. D., Lacher, D. A., Sorlie, P. D., et al. (2005). Trends in serum lipids and lipoproteins of adults, 1960–2002. *JAMA, 294*(14), 1773–1781.
46. Gaziano, J. M. (1994). Antioxidant vitamins and coronary artery disease risk. *American Journal of Medicine, 97*, 3A-18S–3A-28S.
47. Kwiterovich, P. O., Coresh, J., Smith, H. H., et al. (1992). Comparison of the plasma levels of apolipoproteins B and A-1, and other risk factors in men and women with premature coronary artery disease. *American Journal of Cardiology, 69*, 1015–1021.
48. Austin, M. A., Breslow, J. L., Hennekens, C. H., et al. (1988). Low-density lipoprotein subclass patterns and risk of myocardial infarction. *JAMA, 260*, 1917–1921.
49. Bostom, A. G., Cupples, L. A., Jenner, J. L., et al. (1996). Elevated plasma lipoprotein(a) and coronary heart disease in men aged 55 years and younger: A prospective study. *JAMA, 276*, 544–548.
50. Bostom, A. G., Gagnon, D. R., Cupples, L. A., et al. (1994). A prospective investigation of elevated lipoprotein(a) detected by electrophoresis and cardiovascular disease in women: The Framingham Heart Study. *Circulation, 90*, 1688–1695.
51. Stein, J. H., & Rosenson, R. S. (1997). Lipoprotein Lp(a) excess and coronary heart disease. *Archives of Internal Medicine, 157*, 1170–1176.
52. Wong, N. D., Wilson, P. W. F., & Kannel, W. B. (1991). Serum cholesterol as a prognostic factor after myocardial infarction: The Framingham Study. *Annals of Internal Medicine, 115*, 687–693.
53. Brown, G., Albers, J. J., Fisher, L. D., et al. (1990). Regression of coronary artery disease as a result of intensive lipid-lowering therapy in men with high levels of apolipoprotein B. *New England Journal of Medicine, 323*, 1289–1298.
54. Haskell, W. L., et al. (2007). Physical activity and public health: Updated recommendation for adults from the American College of Sports Medicine and the American Heart Association. *Circulation, 116*(9), 1081–1093.
55. MMWR (2005, October 7). *Trends in leisure-time physical inactivity by age, sex, and race/ethnicity—United States, 1994–2004, 54*(39), 991–994. Retrieved from http://www.cdc.gov/mmwr/preview/mmwrhtml/mm5439a5.htm
56. Haskell, W. L., Leon, A. S., Caspersen, C. J., et al. (1992). Cardiovascular benefits and assessment of physical activity and physical fitness in adults. *Medical Science Sports Exercise, 24*(Suppl.), S201–S220.
57. Berlin, J. A., & Colditz, G. A. (1990). A meta-analysis of physical activity in the prevention of coronary heart disease. *American Journal of Epidemiology, 132*, 612–628.
58. Douglas, P. S., Clarkson, T. B., Flowers, N. C., et al. (1992). Exercise and atherosclerotic heart disease in women. *Medical Science Sports Exercise,* 23(Suppl.), S266–S276.
59. Blair, S. N., Kohl, H. W., Paffenbarger, R. S., et al. (1989). Physical fitness and all-cause mortality: A prospective study of healthy men and women. *JAMA, 262*, 2395–2401.
60. Ekelund, L. G., Haskell, W. L., Johnson, J. L., et al. (1988). Physical fitness as a predictor of cardiovascular mortality in asymptomatic North American men: The Lipid Research Clinics mortality follow-up study. *New England Journal of Medicine, 319*, 1379–1384.
61. Slattery, M. L., & Jacobs, D. R. (1988). Physical fitness and cardiovascular disease mortality: The US Railroad Study. *American Journal of Epidemiology, 127*, 571–580.
62. Sobolski, J., Kornitzer, M., Backer, G. D., et al. (1987). Protection against ischemic heart disease in the Belgian physical fitness study: Physical fitness rather than physical activity? *American Journal of Epidemiology, 125*, 601–610.
63. Oldridge, N. B., Guyatt, G. H., Fischer, M. E., et al. (1988). Cardiac rehabilitation after myocardial infarction, combined experience of randomized clinical trials. *JAMA, 260*, 945–950.
64. Thompson, P. D. (1988). The benefits and risks of exercise training in patients with chronic coronary artery disease. *JAMA, 259*, 1537–1540.
65. Taylor, R. S., Brown, A., Ebrahim, S., et al. (2004). Exercise-based rehabilitation for patients with coronary heart disease: Systematic review and meta-analysis of randomized controlled trials. *The American Journal of Medicine, 116*(10), 682–692.
66. Pina, I. L., Apstein, C. S., Balady, G. J., et al. (2003). Exercise and heart failure, a statement from the American Heart Association Committee on Exercise, Rehabilitation, and Prevention. *Circulation, 107*, 1210–1225.
67. Howard, B. V., Rodriques, B. L., Bennett, P. H., et al. (2002). Prevention Conference VI: Diabetes and Cardiovascular Disease Writing Group I: Epidemiology. *Circulation, 105*, e132–e137.
68. Stampfer, M. J., Colditz, G. A., Willett, W. C., et al. (1987). Coronary heart disease risk factors in women: The Nurses' Health Study experience. In E. D. Eaker, B. Packard, N. K. Wenger, et al. (Eds.), *Coronary heart disease in women* (pp. 112–116). New York: Haymarket Doyma.
69. Orchard, T. J. (1996). The impact of gender and general risk factors on the occurrence of atherosclerotic vascular disease in non-insulin-dependent diabetes mellitus. *Annals of Medicine, 28*, 323–333.
70. Mitchell, B. D., Haffner, S. M., Huzuda, H. P., et al. (1992). Diabetes and coronary heart disease risk in Mexican-Americans. *Annals of Epidemiology, 2*, 101–106.
71. Kuczmarski, R. J., Flegal, K. M., Campbell, S. M. et al. (1994). Increasing prevalence of overweight among US adults: The National Health and Nutrition Examination Surveys, 1960 to 1991. *JAMA, 272*, 205–211.

72. Barrett-Connor, E., & Wingard, D. L. (1983). Sex differential in ischemic heart disease mortality in diabetics: A prospective population-based study. *American Journal of Epidemiology, 118*, 489–496.
73. Manson, J. E., Colditz, G. A., Stampfer, M. J., et al. (1991). A prospective study of maturity-onset diabetes mellitus and risk of coronary heart disease and stroke in women. *Archives of Internal Medicine, 151*, 1141–1147.
74. Khaw, K. T., & Barrett-Connor, E. (1986). Prognostic factors for mortality in a population-based study of men and women with a history of heart disease. *Journal of Cardiopulmonary Rehabilitation, 6*, 474–480.
75. Wong, N. D., Cupples, L. A., Ostfeld, A. M., et al. (1989). Risk factors for long-term coronary prognosis after initial myocardial infarction: The Framingham Study. *American Journal of Epidemiology, 130*, 469–480.
76. Stone, P. H., Muller, J. E., Hartwell, T., et al. (1989). The effect of diabetes mellitus on prognosis and serial left ventricular function after acute myocardial infarction: Contribution of both coronary disease and diastolic left ventricular dysfunction to the adverse prognosis. *Journal of the American College of Cardiology, 12*, 49–57.
77. Abbott, R. D., Donahue, R. P., Kannell, W. B., et al. (1988). The impact of diabetes on survival following myocardial infarction in men vs. women: The Framingham Study. *JAMA, 260*, 3456–3460.
78. Stevens, R. J., Coleman, R. L., Adler, A. I., et al. (2004). Risk factors for myocardial infarction case fatality and stroke case fatality in type 2 diabetes: UKPDS 66. *Diabetes Care, 27*(1), 201–207.
79. Murcia, A. M., Hennekens, C. H., Lamas, G. A., et al. (2004). Impact of diabetes on mortality in patients with myocardial infarction and left ventricular dysfunction. *Archives of Internal Medicine, 164*(20), 2273–2279.
80. Yan, R. T., Yan, A. T., Tan, M., et al. (2006). Underuse of evidence-based treatment partly explains the worse clinical outcome in diabetic patients with acute coronary syndromes. *American Heart Journal, 152*(4), 676–683.
81. Folsom, A. R., Szklo, M., Stevens, J., et al. (1997). A prospective study of coronary heart disease in relation to fasting insulin, glucose, and diabetes. *Diabetes Care, 20*, 935–942.
82. Rönnemaa, T., Kaakso, M., Pyörälä, K., et al. (1991). High fasting plasma insulin is an indicator of coronary heart disease in non–insulin-dependent diabetic patients and nondiabetic subjects. *Arteriosclerosis and Thrombosis, 11*, 80–90.
83. Perry, I. J., Wannamethee, S. G., Whincup, P. H., et al. (1996). Serum insulin and incident coronary heart disease in middle-aged British men. *American Journal of Epidemiology, 144*, 224–234.
84. Kaplan, N. M. (1989). The deadly quartet: Upper-body obesity, glucose intolerance, hypertriglyceridemia, and hypertension. *Archives of Internal Medicine, 149*, 1514–1520.
85. Simonson, D. C., & Dzau, V. J. (1991). Workshop IX: Lipids, insulin, diabetes. *American Journal of Medicine*, 90(Suppl. 2A), 85S–86S.
86. Manson, J. E., Colditz, G. A., Stampfer, M. J., et al. (1990). A prospective study of obesity and risk of coronary heart disease in women. *New England Journal of Medicine, 322*, 882–889.
87. Diabetes Control and Complications Trial Research Group. (1993). The effect of intensive treatment of diabetes on the development and progression of long-term complications in insulin-dependent diabetes mellitus: The Diabetes Control and Complications Trial Research Group. *New England Journal of Medicine, 329*, 977–986.
88. Gaede, P., Vedel, P., Larsen, N., et al. (2003). Multifactorial intervention and cardiovascular disease in patients with type 2 diabetes. *New England Journal of Medicine, 348*, 383–393.
89. Grundy, S. M., Garber, A., Goldberg, R., et al. (2002). Diabetes and cardiovascular disease writing group IV: Lifestyle and medical management of risk factors. *Circulation, 105*, e153–e158.
90. Buse, J. B., Ginsberg, H.N., Bakris G. L., et al. (2007). Primary prevention of cardiovascular diseases in people with diabetes mellitus: A scientific statement from the American Heart Association and the American Diabetes Association. *Diabetes Care, 30*(1), 162–172.
91. Diabetes Prevention Program Research Group. (2002). Reduction in the incidence of type 2 diabetes with lifestyle intervention or metformin. *New England Journal of Medicine*, 346, 393–403.
92. Tuomilehto, J., Lindstrom, J., Eriksson, J. G., et al. (2001). Finnish Diabetes Prevention Study Group. Prevention of type 2 diabetes mellitus by changes in lifestyle among subjects with impaired glucose tolerance. *New England Journal of Medicine, 344*(18), 1343–1350.
93. Ramachandran, A., Snehalatha, C., Mary, S., et al. (2006). The Indian Diabetes Prevention Programme shows that lifestyle modification and metformin prevent type 2 diabetes in Asian Indian subjects with impaired glucose tolerance (IDPP-1). *Diabetologia, 49*(2), 289–297.
94. The Diabetes Prevention Program Research, G. (2005). Impact of intensive lifestyle and metformin therapy on cardiovascular disease risk factors in the diabetes prevention program. *Diabetes Care, 28*(4), 888–894.
95. Orchard, T. J., Temprosa, M., Goldberg, R., et al. (2005). The Effect of metformin and intensive lifestyle intervention on the metabolic syndrome: The Diabetes Prevention Program Randomized Trial. *Annals of Internal Medicine, 142*(8), 611–619.
96. National Institutes of Health (NIH). (1998). *National Heart, Lung, and Blood Institute (NHLBI). Clinical guidelines on the identification, evaluation, and treatment of overweight and obesity in adults.* Bethesda, MD: HHS, Public Health Service (PHS).
97. Ogden, C. L., Carroll, M. D., Curtin, L. R., et al. (2006). Prevalence of overweight and obesity in the United States, 1999–2004. *JAMA, 295*(13), 1549–1555.
98. Van Itallie, T. B. (1985). Health implication of overweight and obesity in the United States. *Annals of Internal Medicine, 103*, 983–988.
99. Barrett-Connor, E. L. (1985). Obesity, atherosclerosis, and coronary artery disease. *Annals of Internal Medicine, 103*, 1010–1019.
100. Hubert, H. B., Feinleib, M., McNamara, P. M., et al. (1983). Obesity as an independent risk factor for cardiovascular disease: A 26-year follow-up of participants in the Framingham Heart Study. *Circulation, 67*, 968–977.
101. Hoffmans, M. D. A. F., Kromhout, D., & De Lezenne Coulander, C. (1989). Body mass index at the age of 18 and its effects on 32-yearmortality from coronary heart disease and cancer. *Journal of Clinical Epidemiology, 42*, 513–520.
102. Flegal, K. M., Graubard, B. I., Williamson, D. F., et al. (2007). Cause-specific excess deaths associated with underweight, overweight, and obesity. *JAMA, 298*(17), 2028–2037.
103. Keil, J. E., Sutherland, S. E., Knapp, R. G., et al. (1993). Mortality rates and risk factors for coronary disease in black as compared with white men and women. *New England Journal of Medicine, 329*, 73–78.
104. Willett, W. C., Manson, J. E., Stampfer, M. J., et al. (1995). Weight, weight changes, and coronary heart disease in women, risk within the "normal" weight range. *JAMA, 273*, 461–465.
105. Johnson, J. L., Heineman, E. F., Heiss, G., et al. (1986). Cardiovascular disease risk factors and mortality among black women and white women aged 40–64 years in Evans County, Georgia. *American Journal of Epidemiology, 123*, 209–220.
106. Stevens, J., Keil, J. E., Rust, P. F., et al. (1992). Body mass index and body girths as predictors of mortality in black and white women. *Archives of Internal Medicine, 152*, 1257–1262.
107. Newton, K. M., & LaCroix, A. Z. (1996). Association of body mass index with reinfarction and survival after first myocardial infarction in women. *Journal of Women's Health, 5*, 433–444.
108. Harris, T., Cook, E. F., Garrison, R. et al. (1988). Body mass index and mortality among nonsmoking older persons: The Framingham Heart Study. *JAMA, 259*, 1520–1524.
109. Li, T. Y., Rana, J. S., Manson, J. E., et al. (2006). Obesity as compared with physical activity in predicting risk of coronary heart disease in women. *Circulation, 113*(4), 499–506.
110. Rexrode, K. M., Buring, J. E., & Manson, J. E. (2001). Abdominal and total adiposity and risk of coronary heart disease in men. *International Journal of Obesity and Related Metabolic Disorders, 25*(7), 1047–1056.
111. Zhu, S., Wang, Z., Heshka, S., et al. (2002). Waist circumference and obesity-associated risk factors among whites in the third National Health and Nutrition Examination Survey: Clinical action thresholds. *American Journal of Clinical Nutrition, 76*(4), 743.
112. Beard, D. M., Fuster, V., & Annergers, J. F. (1984). Reproductive history in women with coronary heart disease: A case-control study. *American Journal of Epidemiology, 120*, 108–114.
113. Palmer, J. R., Rosenberg, L., & Shapiro, S. (1992). Reproductive factors and risk of myocardial infarction. *American Journal of Epidemiology, 136*, 408–416.
114. Colditz, G. A., Willett, W. C., Stampfer, M. J., et al. (1987). A prospective study of age at menarche, parity, age at first birth, and coronary heart disease in women. *American Journal of Epidemiology, 126*, 861–870.
115. Stampfer, M. J., Colditz, G. A., & Willett, W. C. (1990). Menopause and heart disease: A review. *Annals of the New York Academy of Science, 592*, 193–203.
116. Stampfer, M. J., & Colditz, G. A. (1991). Estrogen replacement therapy and coronary heart disease: A quantitative assessment of the epidemiologic evidence. *Preventive Medicine, 20*, 47–63.

117. Lindquist, O., Bengtsson, C., & Lapidus, L. (1985). Relationships between the menopause and risk factors for ischaemic heart disease. *Acta Obstetrica Gynecologica Scandia Supplement, 130*, 43–47.
118. Matthews, K. A., Meilhan, E., Kuller, L. H., et al. (1989). Menopause a risk factor for coronary heart disease. *New England Journal of Medicine, 321*, 641–646.
119. Mann, J. I., Vessey, M. P., Thorogood, M., et al. (1975). Myocardial infarction in young women with special reference to oral contraceptive practice. *BMJ, 2*, 241–245.
120. Mann, J. I., & Inman, W. H. W. (1975). Oral contraceptives and death from myocardial infarction. *BMJ, 2*, 245–248.
121. Jick, H., Dinan, B., & Rothman, K. J. (1978). Oral contraceptives and nonfatal myocardial infarction. *JAMA, 239*, 1403–1406.
122. Kelleher, C. C. (1990). Clinical aspects of the relationship between oral contraceptives and abnormalities of the hemostatic system: Relation to the development of cardiovascular disease. *American Journal of Obstetrics and Gynecology, 163*, 392–395.
123. Meade, T. W. (1988). Risks and mechanisms of cardiovascular events in users of oral contraceptives. *American Journal of Obstetrics and Gynecology, 158*, 1646–1652.
124. Rosenberg, L., Palmer, J. R., Lesko, S. M., et al. (1990). Oral contraceptive use and the risk of myocardial infarction. *American Journal of Epidemiology, 131*, 1009–1016.
125. Mant, J., Painter, R., & Vessey, M. (1998). Risk of myocardial infarction, angina and stroke in users of oral contraceptives: An updated analysis of a cohort study. *British Journal of Obstetrics and Gynaecology, 105*, 890–896.
126. Sidney, S., Siscovick, D. S., Petitti, D. B., et al. (1998). Myocardial infarction and use of low-dose oral contraceptives: A pooled analysis of 2 US studies. *Circulation, 98*, 1058–1063.
127. Stampfer, M. J., Willett, W. C., Colditz, G. C., et al. (1988). A prospective study of past use of oral contraceptive agents and risk of cardiovascular diseases. *New England Journal of Medicine, 319*, 1313–1317.
128. Stampfer, M. J., Willett, W. C., Colditz, G. C., et al. (1990). Past use of oral contraceptives and cardiovascular disease: A meta-analysis in the context of the Nurses' Health Study. *American Journal of Obstetrics and Gynecology, 163*, 285–291.
129. Goldbaum, G. M., Kendrick, J. S., Hogelin, G. C., et al. (1987). The relative impact of smoking and oral contraceptive use on women in the United States. *JAMA, 258*, 1339–1342.
130. Graff-Iversen, S., Hammar, N., Thelle, D. S., et al. (2006). Use of oral contraceptives and mortality during 14 years' follow-up of Norwegian women. *Scandinavian Journal of Public Health, 34*(1), 11–16.
131. Newton, K. M., LaCroix, A. Z., McKnight, B., et al. (1997). Estrogen replacement therapy and prognosis after first myocardial infarction. *American Journal of Epidemiology, 145*, 269–277.
132. Grodstein, F., & Stampfer, M. (1995). The epidemiology of coronary heart disease and estrogen replacement in postmenopausal women. *Progress in Cardiovascular Disease, 38*, 199–210.
133. Hulley, S., Grady, D., Bush, T., et al. (1998). Randomized trial of estrogen plus progestin for secondary prevention of coronary heart disease in postmenopausal women. Heart and Estrogen/progestin Replacement Study (HERS) Research Group. *JAMA, 280*, 605–613.
134. Design of the Women's Health Initiative clinical trial and observational study. The Women's Health Initiative Study Group. (1998). *Control Clinical Trials, 19*(1), 61–109.
135. Writing Group for the Women's Health Initiative Investigators. (2002). Risks and benefits of estrogen plus progestin in healthy postmenopausal women: Principal results from the Women's Health Initiative randomized controlled trial. *JAMA, 288*, 321–333.
136. Women's Health Initiative Steering, C. (2004). Effects of conjugated equine estrogen in postmenopausal women with hysterectomy: The Women's Health Initiative Randomized Controlled Trial. *JAMA, 291*(14), 1701–1712.
137. Herrington, D. M., Reboussin, D. M., Brosnihan, K. B., et al. (2000). Effects of estrogen replacement on the progression of coronary-artery atherosclerosis. *New England Journal of Medicine, 343*, 522–529.
138. Angerer, P., Strok, S., Kothny, W., et al. (2001). Effect of oral postmenopausal hormsone replacement on progression of atherosclerosis: A randomized, controlled trial. *Arteriosclerosis Thrombosis Vascular Biology, 21*, 262–268.
139. Vickers, M. R., MacLennan, A. H., Lawton, B., et al. (2007). Main morbidities recorded in the women's international study of long duration oestrogen after menopause (WISDOM): A randomised controlled trial of hormone replacement therapy in postmenopausal women. *BMJ, 335*(7613), 239.
140. ACOG. (2002). http: and www.acog.org/from_home/publications/press_releases/nr08-30-02.cfm. Alpha Tocopherol, Beta Carotene Cancer Prevention Study Group (1994). The effect of vitamin E and beta carotene on the incidence of lung cancer and other cancers in male smokers. *New England Journal of Medicine,* 330, 1029–1035.
141. Bates, C. J., Mansoor, M. A., van der Pols, J., et al. (1997). Plasma total homocysteine in a representative sample of 972 British men and women aged 65 and over. *European Journal of Clinical Nutrition, 51*, 691–697.
142. Dalery, K., Lussier-Cacan, S., Selhub, J., et al. (1995). Homocysteine and coronary artery disease in French Canadian subjects: Relation with vitamins B_{12}, B_6, pyridoxal phosphate, and folate. *American Journal of Cardiology, 75*, 1107–1111.
143. Malinow, M. R., Bostom, A. G., & Krauss, R. M. (1999). Homocyst(e)ine, diet, and cardiovascular diseases: A statement for healthcare professionals from the Nutrition Committee, American Heart Association. *Circulation, 99*, 178–182.
144. Selhub, J., Jacques, P. F., Wilson, P. W. F., et al. (1993). Vitamin status and intake as primary determinants of homocysteinemia in an elderly population. *JAMA, 270*, 2693–2698.
145. Schwartz, S. M., Siscovick, D. S., Malinow, M. R., et al. (1997). Myocardial infarction in young women in relation to plasma total homocysteine, folate, and a common variant in the methylenetetrahydrofolate reductase gene. *Circulation, 96*, 412–417.
146. Mangoni, A. A., & Jackson, S. H. (2002). Homocysteine and cardiovascular disease: Current evidence and future prospects. *American Journal of Medicine, 112*, 556–565.
147. Kang, S., Wong, P. W. K., Cook, H. Y., et al. (1986). Protein-bound homocysteine, a possible risk factor for coronary artery disease. *Journal of Clinical Investigation, 77*, 1482–1486.
148. Robinson, K., Mayer, E. L., Miller, D. P., et al. (1995). Hyperhomocysteinemia and low pyridoxal phosphate, common and independent reversible risk factors for coronary artery disease. *Circulation, 92*, 2825–2830.
149. Selhub, J., Jacques, P. F., Bostom, A. G., et al. (1995). Association between plasma homocysteine concentrations and extracranial carotid-artery stenosis. *New England Journal of Medicine, 332*, 286–291.
150. Malinow, M. R., Nieto, F. J., Szklo, M., et al. (1993). Carotid artery intimal-medial wall thickening and plasma homocysteine in asymptomatic adults. *Circulation, 87*, 1107–1113.
151. Van Der Mooren, M. J., Wouters, M. G., Blom, H. J., et al. (1994). Hormone replacement therapy may reduce high serum homocysteine in postmenopausal women. *European Journal of Clinical Investigation, 24*, 733–736.
152. Brattstrom, L. E., Hultberg, B. L., & Hardebo, J. E. (1985). Folic acid responsive postmenopausal homocysteinemia. *Metabolism, 34*, 1073–1077.
153. Toole, J. F., Malinow, M. R., Chambless, L. E., et al. (2004). Lowering homocysteine in patients with ischemic stroke to prevent recurrent stroke, myocardial infarction, and death: The Vitamin Intervention for Stroke Prevention (VISP) randomized controlled trial. *JAMA, 291*(5), 565–575.
154. Bonaa, K. H., Njolstad, I., Ueland, P. M., et al. (2006). Homocysteine lowering and cardiovascular events after acute myocardial infarction. *New England Journal of Medicine, 354*(15), 1578–1588.
155. The Heart Outcomes Prevention Evaluation. (2006). Homocysteine lowering with folic acid and B vitamins in vascular disease. *New England Journal of Medicine, 354*(15), 1567–1577.
156. Schwammenthal, Y., & Tanne, D. (2004). Homocysteine, B-vitamin supplementation, and stroke prevention: From observational to interventional trials. *The Lancet Neurology, 3*(8), 493–495.
157. Lonn, E. (2007). Homocysteine in the prevention of ischemic heart disease, stroke and venous thromboembolism: Therapeutic target or just another distraction? *Current Opinion in Hematology, 14*(5), 481–487.
158. Marcus, J., Sarnak, M. J., & Menon, V. (2007). Homocysteine lowering and cardiovascular disease risk: Lost in translation. *Canadian Journal of Cardiology, 23*(9), 707–710.
159. Wierzbicki, A. S. (2007). Homocysteine and cardiovascular disease: A review of the evidence. *Diabetes and Vascular Disease Research, 4*(2), 143–150.
160. Diaz, M. N., Frei, B., Vita J. A., et al. (1997). Mechanisms of disease, antioxidants and atherosclerotic heart disease. *New England Journal of Medicine, 337*, 408–416.
161. Steinbrecher, U. P. (1997). Dietary antioxidants and cardioprotection: Fact or fallacy? *Canadian Journal of Physiology and Pharmacology, 75*, 228–233.

162. Tribble, D. L. (1999). Antioxidant consumption and risk of coronary heart disease: Emphasis on vitamin C, vitamin E, and β-carotene. A statement from healthcare professionals from the American Heart Association. *Circulation, 99,* 591–595.
163. Tavani, A., Negri, E., Avanzo, B. D., et al. (1997). Beta-carotene intake and risk of nonfatal acute myocardial infarction in women. *European Journal of Epidemiology, 13,* 631–637.
164. Hennekens, C. H., Buring, J. E., Manson, J. E., et al. (1996). Lack of effect of long-term supplementation with beta carotene on the incidence of malignant neoplasms and cardiovascular disease. *New England Journal of Medicine, 334,* 1145–1149.
165. Omenn, G. S., Goodman, G. E., Thornquist, M. D., et al. (1996). Effects of a combination of beta carotene and vitamin A on lung cancer and cardiovascular disease. *New England Journal of Medicine, 334,* 1150–1155.
166. Kushi, L. H., Folsom, A. R., Prineas, R. J., et al. (1996). Dietary antioxidant vitamins and death from coronary heart disease in postmenopausal women. *New England Journal of Medicine, 334,* 1156–1162.
167. Rimm, E. B., & Stampfer, M. J. (1997). The role of antioxidants in preventive cardiology. *Current Opinion in Cardiology, 12,* 188–194.
168. Cook, N. R., Albert, C. M., Gaziano, J. M., et al. (2007). A randomized factorial trial of vitamins C and E and beta carotene in the secondary prevention of cardiovascular events in women: Results from the Women's Antioxidant Cardiovascular Study. *Archives of Internal Medicine, 167*(15), 1610–1618.
169. Rimm, E. B., Stampfer, M., Ascherio, A., et al. (1993). Vitamin E consumption and the risk of coronary heart disease in men. *New England Journal of Medicine, 328,* 1450–1456.
170. Stampfer, M. U., Hennekens, C. H., Manson, J. E., et al. (1993). Vitamin E consumption and the risk of coronary disease in women. *New England Journal of Medicine, 328,* 1444–1449.
171. Losonczy, K. G., Harris, T. B., & Havlik, R. J. (1996). Vitamin E and vitamin C supplement use and risk of all-cause and coronary heart disease mortality in older persons: The Established Populations for Epidemiologic Studies of the Elderly. *American Journal of Clinical Nutrition, 64,* 190–196.
172. Vitamo, J., Rapola, M. J., Ripatti, S., et al. (1998). Effect of vitamin E and beta carotene on the incidence of primary nonfatal myocardial infarction and fatal coronary heart disease. *Archives of Internal Medicine, 158,* 668–675.
173. Stephens, N. G., Parsons, A., Schofiled, P. M., et al. (1996). Randomized controlled trial of vitamin E in patient with coronary disease: Cambridge Heart Antioxidant Study. *Lancet, 347,* 781–786.
174. Riccioni, G., Bucciarelli, T., Mancini, B., et al. (2007). Antioxidant vitamin supplementation in cardiovascular diseases. *Annals of Clinical Laboratory Science, 37*(1), 89–95.
175. United States Preventive Services Task Force. (2003) Routine vitamin supplementation to prevent cancer and cardiovascular disease. *Nutrition in Clinical Care, 6*(3), 102–107.

CHAPTER 33

Psychosocial Risk Factors: Assessment and Management Interventions

Simone K. Madan / Erika S. Sivarajan Froelicher

Despite extensive research and advances in knowledge about coronary heart disease (CHD) over the past several decades, traditional risk factors and genetics fail to fully explain either the development or the course of the disease. Consistent with biopsychosocial models of health, studies have now shown that psychological and social factors are also related to the development of and recovery from CHD. In health schemas of the mind and body, emotions have often been linked to specific organs. The English language is replete with expressions that describe this assignation. For example, jubilation "makes the heart flutter" or anxiety causes "butterflies in one's stomach." Throughout the ages, the heart has been seen as the "seat of emotions." William Harvey (1578 to 1657), the English physician who first described the circulatory system, wrote, "Every affliction of the mind that is attended with either pain or pleasure, hope or fear, is the cause of an agitation whose influence extends to the heart."[1] In this chapter, we summarize the evidence that links psychological and social factors to CHD and describe how nurses can assess and manage selected psychosocial risk factors to promote cardiovascular and psychosocial health.

PSYCHOSOCIAL RISK FACTORS FOR CHD

Several psychosocial risk or prognostic factors have been identified for CHD: acute life events, anxiety, depression, hostility, job stress, low-perceived social support, social isolation, socioeconomic status, and Type A personality.[2–5] Of these, depression and low-perceived social support have been well established as independent risk factors for CHD, as shown in Table 33-1.[6]

Depression

The complex clinical diagnosis of depression, as defined in the Diagnostic and Statistical Manual of Mental Disorders, Fourth Edition,[7] classifies the disorders as either major or minor based, in part, on the number, frequency, and duration of symptoms and signs. In this chapter, the term *depression* will be all inclusive. Substantial empirical evidence from well-designed population studies[8,9] and review papers[2,4,10] have shown that depression is a risk factor for CHD. Furthermore, depression is also a prognostic factor for CHD patients,[2,4,10–16] and high prevalence rates of the disorder have been found in CHD populations. Studies have reported that 16% to 25% of the CHD population has depression, as compared with 6% of the general population.[11–14] Women in the general population are especially at higher risk because they are twice as likely to be depressed than men, thus one would expect the same gender distribution to be observed in the cardiac population,[17,18] and their depression leads to worse cardiovascular outcomes, especially in younger women.[19] Besides women, individuals with low income and less education experience significantly higher rates of depression.[17] Regardless of the severity of CHD, patients with depression are three to four times more likely to die in the first year after a myocardial infarction (MI) than those without depression.[20,21] Six months after an MI, patients with depression had a 17% event rate compared with 3% for nondepressed patients[20]; at 18 months, premature ventricular contractions and mortality were reported for 50% of patients with depression compared with 17% for those without.[22]

Combined depression and CHD is a significant challenge for patients recovering from a cardiac event. Depression can lead to social withdrawal and less participation in activities such as exercise.[23,24] Depressed patients have more difficulty adopting and maintaining healthy lifestyle behaviors,[25] and they consistently report higher smoking rates compared with nondepressed CHD patients.[11,26] For example, in older patients who suffered an MI, depression scores predicted the performance of risk-reducing, self-care behaviors.[27] In patients attending cardiac rehabilitation programs, anxiety, depression, and coping abilities predicted leisure-time activity and higher smoking cessation at 1-year follow up.[28] In relation to functional impairments, only 38% of patients with depression returned to work within 3 months of a cardiac event compared with 63% of nondepressed patients.[29] Depression is also associated with decreased compliance in taking medications[12,30] and a delay in seeking medical treatment, because affected patients often minimize the significance of cardiac symptoms.[31,32] Besides the individual health consequences of depression in CHD patients, tremendous economic costs affect society.[33] The cost of increased hospitalization admissions for recurrent cardiac events and longer hospital stays are also associated with higher emotional distress. The average hospital cost for a depressed cardiac patient is more than four times the cost of a nondepressed patient.[25]

Social Support

Social support is defined by the quality of the structure and function of social relationships. Structural support reflects the number and frequency of social interactions, social ties, and networks.[34,35] Functional support focuses on tangible aid, emotional comfort and care, and the value an individual places on the support.[34,35] Structural and functional support, however, fail to account for individual perceptions and beliefs about the support. Further, they do not account for (a) the social skills needed to elicit support from others; (b) how much support, if any, is needed or acceptable and who should provide it; (c) whether an individual is deserving of support; or (d) the concern of the cost of seeking

Table 33-1 ■ PSYCHOSOCIAL RISK FACTORS AND CHD: SUMMARY OF PROSPECTIVE STUDIES

	Number of Reports of Etiological Studies (n = 70)				Number of Reports of Prognostic Studies (n = 92)			
	−	0	+	++	−	0	+	++
Depression	0	8	5	9	0	16	7	11
Social support	0	3	4	2	0	7	4	10
Anxiety	0	4	1	3	1	9	4	4
Type A behavior/hostility	1	11	5	1	3	10	1	1
Work characteristics	0	3	5	5	0	2	2	0

−, Finding counter to hypothesis; 0, lack of clear association; +, moderate association (RR ≥1.50 and <2.00); ++, strong association (RR ≥ 2.00)
Borrowed with permission from Hemingway, H., Kuper, H., & Marmot, M. (2003). Psychosocial factors in the primary and secondary prevention of coronary heart disease: A systematic review. In S. Yusuf, J. A. Cairns, E. Fallen, B. J. Gersch, & A. J. Camm (Eds.), *Evidence based cardiology.* London: British Medical Journal Publishing.

support.[36] Individual differences must be considered because what one person may consider as valuable support, another person may consider a burden, engendering feelings of obligation or guilt. Gender or ethnic differences may influence attitudes and beliefs about support.[37] In the research substantiating the association between social support and CHD, the definition of social support is highly varied, ranging from marital status, or being single to measurement of social support that involves detailed complexity.

Social support from others decreased the incidence of cardiac events in men without CHD.[38] One important form of social support can be derived from a marital relationship. Marital relationships perceived as satisfactory are associated with decreased mortality.[39] Conversely, discordant marital relationships may precipitate poor health outcomes because social connections can also lead to stress if perceived needs or expectations are not met. A higher likelihood of mortality in cardiac patients has been associated with low-perceived support or lack of support for unmarried individuals.[40–42] In addition, lack of social support is also a risk factor if cardiac disease is already well established. Case et al.[43] examined social networks by comparing recurrent cardiac events in patients who had suffered an MI. Patients who lived alone had a 50% increased risk for subsequent events. In patients who had suffered an MI or were living with congestive heart failure or both, those with no sources of emotional support had a two-fold risk of a subsequent event.[44,45] An examination of gender differences discovered that high marital distress in women is associated with three times the risk of recurrent coronary events than in men.[46]

Low social support seems to blunt the desire for behavioral change in patients following an MI. Unmarried patients with high rates of smoking are less likely to stop smoking than married patients, and marital separation at the time of an MI decreases the likelihood that a patient will give up smoking.[47] Men receive more support for their participation in cardiac rehabilitation programs from their spouses than female cardiac patients do from their male partners.[48] During or after a hospital admission, distress can surface even in a satisfactory relationship if coping resources are challenged or if spouses become overprotective, which may be stressful for the patient.[49] Conversely, an MI can exacerbate distress in a tempestuous relationship if emotional or functional support are lacking, especially when nurturing is so important.[50] Researchers have suggested that being separated or divorced is an independent risk factor for MI.[9] Perhaps social support influences physiological and behavioral factors that promote "heart-healthy behaviors," reinforcing them and providing a sense of intimacy, belonging, while promoting competence and self-efficacy.[51] How social support protects a patient with CHD is not clearly understood, but it appears such protection exists.

Anxiety

High levels of anxiety are related to increased incidence of heart disease. Men who report two or more symptoms of anxiety are three times more likely to have a fatal CHD event than men without symptoms of anxiety.[52] Similar associations have been reported for phobic anxiety symptoms and for high levels of chronic worry among CHD patients.[52,53] Symptoms of anxiety during a hospital admission increase the risk of a recurrence of cardiac events independent of depression.[21] In patients who have experienced an acute MI, high levels of anxiety were associated with increased hospital complications, including acute ischemia, arrhythmias, functional impairments, reinfarction and sudden cardiac death.[52,54–56] Anxious cardiac patients without adequate support and education are more likely to smoke, to have higher cholesterol, hypertension and diabetes mellitus,[52] and can be fearful of physical activity.[57]

Hostility and Anger

After years of research on the relationship between Type A behavior and CHD, hostility and anger have emerged as risk factors for CHD.[58] Hostility has been redefined to include affective, behavioral, and cognitive components. *Expressive hostility* refers to overt anger, aggressive or rude behaviors, or assaultive behaviors.[59] *Potential for hostility* describes the tendency to experience anger and resentment in daily life.[59] Hostile cognitions include appraisals and perceptions of others as distrustful and attributions of frustration and mistreatment to others. Studies of hostility in adults have shown an association between hostility and CHD morbidity and mortality. Extremely hostile men, followed for 9 years, had a two-fold risk for an MI, even after controlling for behavioral risk factors such as alcohol use, body mass index, and smoking.[60–63] The link between anger and hostility and cardiac reactivity suggests an important physiologic pathway for triggering cardiovascular events. Expressing acute anger has been reported to lead to a coronary event within 2 hours.[64] Increased platelet aggregation and thrombogenesis,[65] plaque rupture, and occlusion have been hypothesized as the most likely mechanisms.[66] High levels of hostility have also been found predictive of restenosis after angioplasty.[67] If hostility is also a prognostic factor for CHD is not known.[4,58]

Acute Stress and Stressful Life Events

Convincing evidence exists that acute stress or stressful life events can trigger cardiac events. Observational studies on the incidence of cardiac events examined exposure to sudden stresses such as natural disasters. The incidence of fatal and nonfatal MIs in Los Angeles County significantly increased on the day of the Northridge earthquake compared with rates before and after the earthquake.[68] In contrast, mortality rates for other types of heart disease, such as cardiomyopathy or cerebrovascular disease, did not increase. Similar increases were observed after major Japanese earthquakes and the missile attacks on Israel during the 1991 Gulf War. These studies, however, could not exclude the effects of increased physical stress caused by exertion. Data from both the missile attacks against Israel and the Japanese earthquakes suggest that the incidence of MI and CHD mortality was greater in women than in men. Posttraumatic stress scores were also higher in Japanese women than in men, suggesting that mental stress could trigger these coronary events.[69,70] Some evidence suggests that in the hour after high levels of negative emotions, the risk for ischemic episodes doubles.[71] Some including Krieger[72] have suggested that lower socioeconomic groups appear to have increased incidence of CHD because of acute stress and exposure to stressful life events. It has been argued that they have less control over their environment, which leads to stress. Other factors, such as lack of access to medical care or engaging in unhealthy lifestyle behaviors, may be alternative explanations.

Acute stress can also lead to arrthymias and sudden cardiac death in patients with CHD.[73] The effects of mental stress have been evaluated during angiography by asking patients to solve arithmetic problems. Investigators found that stenosed coronary artery segments responded by dilating.[74] Studies using challenging video games that have a timing aspect have shown similar results. Comparisons of mental and physical activity stress tests found that mental stress produces higher diastolic blood pressure and lower heart rate responses than physical activity.[75] These studies suggest that ischemia caused by mental stress might occur because of inappropriate vasoconstrictor responses. Because exposure to severe stress cannot be ethically evaluated in experimental human studies, conclusive statements about its effects cannot be made.

Job Stress

Several observational studies have attempted to link chronic job stress with the precipitation of coronary events. Higher numbers of MIs occur in the early morning hours and are associated with increases in catecholamines. Weekly patterns suggest an approximately 20% increase in the incidence of MIs on Mondays, with the lowest rates occurring on Saturdays and Sundays.[76] Some relate this increased incidence with a person's return to his or her stressful workplace; others have suggested that lifestyle habits at work and at leisure account for this difference. Occupational stress has been posited as the explanation for the increase in CHD risk and mortality in blue-collar workers.[77–79] As more women enter the workforce, some have suggested that women will experience increased cardiovascular events.[80,81] When CHD risk factors were examined in middle-aged women in Rancho Bernardo, California, employed women had significantly lower lipids and glucose levels than unemployed women. In the same study, employed women tended to smoke fewer cigarettes and exercised more than unemployed women.[82] This suggests that factors other than employment explain observed associations. Low levels of support from coworkers and supervisors have also been associated with elevated blood pressure after accounting for other factors, such as cigarette smoking.[83] Such findings have led to the suggestion that workers who endure "job strain" (intense job demands with little control) would be more likely to develop CHD.[84] Studies using this assessment of job strain, however, have shown both positive and negative associations with CHD mortality.[85,86] Leading researchers suggest that other job factors, for example, little support from coworkers, job insecurity, and juggling family and job demands, likely influence a person's perception of employment as a stressor. Similarly, what one person experiences as stress, another may view as stimulating and exciting. All things considered, clearly substantiated evidence supporting the causal relationship between job stress and CHD is still absent.[2,87]

PATHOPHYSIOLOGICAL MECHANISMS FOR PSYCHOSOCIAL RISK FACTORS AND CHD

The neuroendocrine response theory, the behavioral mechanisms theory, or a combination of both offers the most likely explanation for the link between psychosocial risk factors and CHD. According to the neuroendocrine response theory, a state of physiological arousal occurs when a person is confronted by real or imagined threats or stressors.[88] "Fight-or-flight" describes these physiologic responses.[89] Neuroendocrine response systems are activated, triggering the release of cortisol and catecholamines (epinephrine [adrenaline] and norepinephrine) that initiate several physiologic responses (Fig. 33-1).

Circulating levels of plasma lipids are also increased and platelet and macrophage cells are activated to release chemotactic and cytotoxic substances. Cardiovascular responses include increased heart rate, blood pressure, muscle and myocardial oxygen demands, and accelerated blood flow. Increased blood flow triggers a cascade of endothelial vascular responses, including release of nitric oxide to promote vasodilation, stimulation of platelets to release chemoattractants and promote thrombosis, and activation of macrophages. Activated macrophages enhance phagocytic activity and have been implicated in the development of atherosclerotic foam cells and the destabilization and rupture of the fibrous cap surrounding atherosclerotic plaque.[90,91]

The neuroendocrine response theory has led to speculation about the connection between affective states and physiological responses. An association has been found between depression and increased nervous system activity,[92] which in turn can increase cardiovascular-disease-related death. Depressed cardiac patients have increased platelet reactivity,[93,94] and depressed patients following an MI have shown decreased heart rate variability.[95] The risk of sudden death after an MI is significantly higher in patients with a decrease in heart rate variability.[96] Lower heart rate variability and decreased parasympathetic nervous system activity in depressed patients has been associated with ventricular fibrillation.[22] Carney et al.[97] examined a subsample of ENRICHD patients and showed that low heart rate variability partially mediates

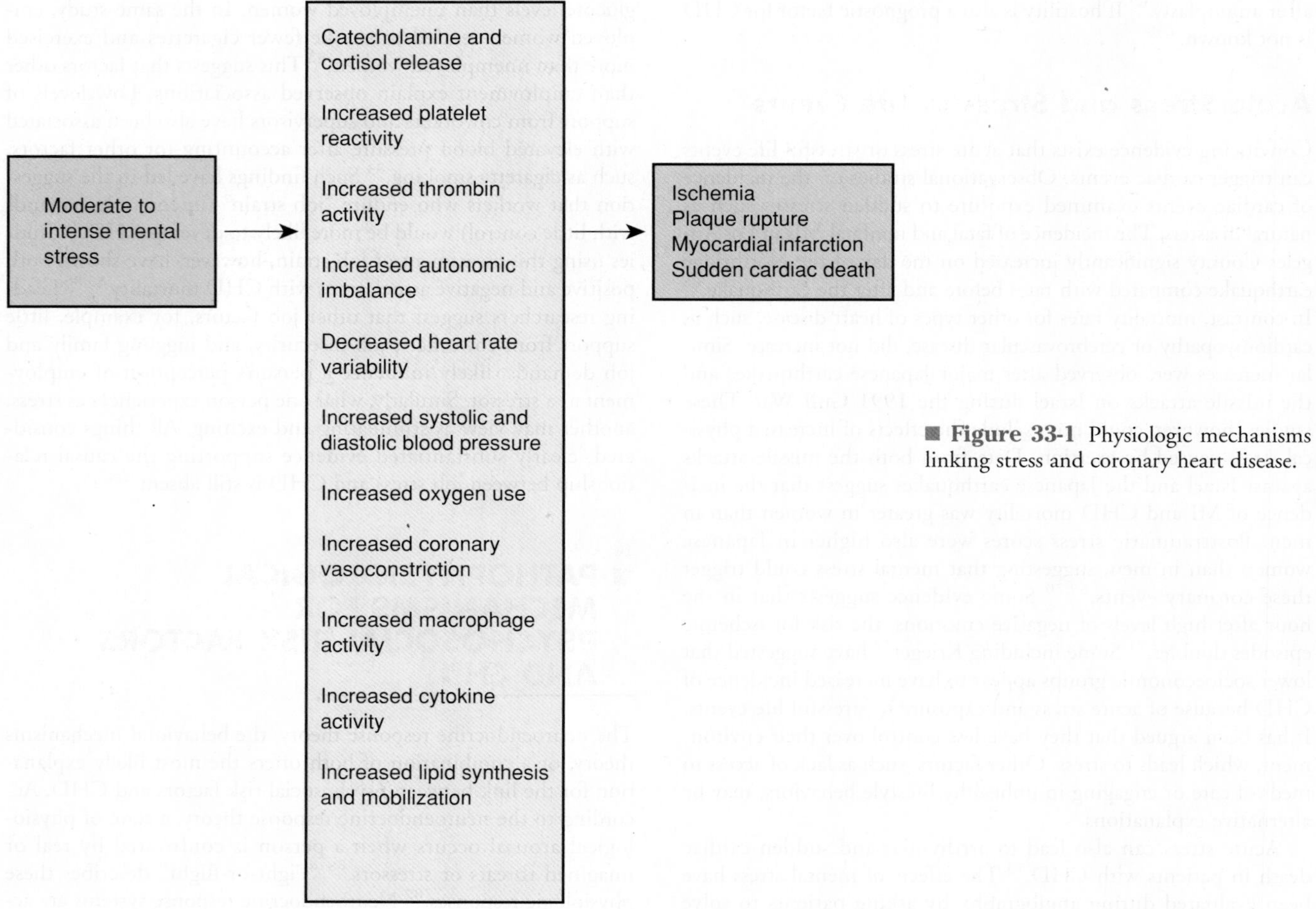

■ **Figure 33-1** Physiologic mechanisms linking stress and coronary heart disease.

the effect of depression on survival after an acute MI. Thus, treatment that improves depression and heart rate variability can also improve survival. Those with hostile traits usually have high blood pressure, heart rate, and neuroendocrine responses, such as cortisol release, in frustrating or harassing situations.[59] When the negative emotions of depression, anger, and anxiety were simultaneously evaluated in the same group of patients who suffered an MI, both depression and anxiety were significant independent predictors of subsequent cardiac events.[14] Dividing events into thrombogenic events (infarction or unstable angina) and arrhythmic events, the authors in this study found that anxiety and a history of depression were associated with thrombogenic events, while current depression and anger were associated with arrhythmic events. The authors speculate that mechanisms such as enhanced platelet adhesion leading to plaque instability and thrombosis might account for these results. These biologic pathways have yet to be tested.

Behavioral mechanism theories such as negative affective states also perpetuate behaviors such as social withdrawal, lack of pleasurable activities, chronic angry outbursts, and disconnection from support, which can adversely affect cardiac physiology. Also, patients who experience psychosocial risk factors may be less compliant with risk-reduction strategies, and their noncompliant behaviors may be the mechanism associated with the development of CHD and its prognosis. Longstanding negative behaviors, such as a high-calorie diet, inadequate self-care, inadequate sleep, lack of exercise, and smoking, are likely to contribute to the development of CHD and, unless modified following an MI, increase the susceptibility toward future events. Both of these theories may explain the link between psychosocial risk factors and CHD.

ASSESSMENT OF PSYCHOSOCIAL RISK FACTORS RELATED TO CHD

Nurses in any practice setting are encouraged to evaluate patients not only for the traditional risk factors but also for psychosocial risk factors. In the following discussion of subjective and objective assessment of depression, low-perceived social support, anxiety, and hostility and anger, note that several of these psychosocial risk factors may be present concurrently.

Screening for Depression

Depression has a complex variable definition, and measurement can often be difficult in patients with coexisting medical problems.[98] Jiang et al.[99] have questioned the sensitivity of the screening instruments for depression and have highlighted the difficulty of differentiating a normal grief response from a diagnosis of significant depression. Although the diagnosis of depression often requires the skill of a licensed mental health practitioner, nurses,

Table 33-2 ■ TWO-ITEM INSTRUMENT—DEPRESSION SCREEN

During the past *month*, have you often been bothered by . . .		
1. Little interest or pleasure in doing things?	Yes	No
2. Feeling down, depressed, or hopeless?	Yes	No

Adapted from McManus, D., Pipkin, S. S., & Whooley, M. A. (2005). Screening for depression in patients with coronary heart disease. (Data from the Heart and Soul Study.) *American Journal of Cardiology, 96*, 1076–1081.

given their extensive contact with cardiac patients, are in a pivotal role to recognize or screen for depression. Several brief and reliable screening tools for clinical purposes can be used by nurses to identify patients at high risk for depression:

1. The two-item instrument: This screening tool (Table 33-2) based on the Patient Health Questionnaire is a two-item instrument about depressed mood and anhedonia with yes/no responses and a higher sensitivity to identifying major depression.[100,101] The symptom duration is for a month. If no is the response to both questions, a patient is unlikely to have major depression. If yes is the answer to either question, a follow-up clinical interview is recommended.
2. The Patient Health Questionnaire-2: The Patient Health Questionnaire-2[102] is a two-item depressive symptom subscale of a longer version, Patient Health Questionnaire-9 described below (Table 33-3). The two items assess depressed mood and anhedonia. The symptom duration is for 2 weeks and the cutoff score is 3 or more with a score range of 0 to 6. This is a very suitable tool for quick and reliable screening.
3. The Patient Health Questionnaire-9: The Patient Health Questionnaire-9 is a self-report instrument[103] of nine items based on DSM-IV criteria with four possible responses ranging from 0 to 3 on each item (Table 33-3). The diagnosis of major depression is based on the presence of five or more of the nine symptoms present at least more than half the days in the past 2 weeks: in addition, one of the symptoms has to be depressed mood or anhedonia.
4. The Beck Depression Inventory: This frequently used, 21-question self-report scale[104] has been recommended for epidemiological studies of CHD patients.[33] Response scores for this first version, valid and reliable tool[105] can range from 0 to 63. A person who scores between 10 and 18 is considered *mildly depressed*, between 19 and 29 *moderately depressed*, and more than 30 *severely depressed*.

Although there are some good choices for brief screening tools available, a recent advisory statement by the American Heart Association has recommendations about the choice of screening instruments for depression in CHD patients. Lichtman et al.[106] recommend the use of the two-item instrument followed by the Patient Health Questionnaire-9, if one of the items on the two-item instrument meets criteria for depression.

Screening for Low-Perceived Social Support

The ENRICHD Social Support Instrument, a seven-item, five-point Likert scale (Table 33-4), is based on several other social support scales that are predictive of mortality.[107,108] This self-report instrument has items that assess for different types of support including structural, instrumental, and emotional support and takes about 5 minutes to complete. The criteria for low-perceived social support are based on five of the seven items (i.e., items 1, 2, 3, 5, and 6). The criteria are met if a score is less than or equal to 2 on at least two of the five items and a total score of less than 18. This tool can also be used for further clarification about a patient's social support system.

Timing the assessment of social support is crucial. Most individuals who are admitted to the hospital experience an atypical outpouring of support as family and friends respond to the crisis. Support can be more realistically assessed following discharge from the hospital.[109] Because people with few social ties and little

Table 33-3 ■ PATIENT HEALTH QUESTIONNAIRE-9: DEPRESSION MODULE

Over the Past *2 Weeks*, how Often have you been Bothered by any of the Following Problems?	Not at All 0	Several Days 1	More than Half the Days 2	Nearly Every Day 3
1. Little interest or pleasure in doing things				
2. Feeling down, depressed, or hopeless				
3. Trouble falling or staying asleep, or sleeping too much				
4. Feeling tired or having little energy				
5. Poor appetite or overeating				
6. Feeling bad about yourself—or that you are a failure or have let yourself or your family down				
7. Trouble concentrating on things, such as reading the newspaper or watching television				
8. Moving or speaking so slowly that other people could have noticed; or the opposite—being so fidgety or restless that you have been moving around a lot more than usual				
9. Thoughts that you would be better off dead or hurting yourself in some way				
If you checked off any problems on this questionnaire so far, how difficult have these problems made it for you to complete your work, take care of things at home, or get along with other people?	**Not difficult**	**Somewhat difficult**	**Very difficult**	**Extremely difficult**

Permission obtained from Pfizer. Kroenke, K., Spitzer, R. L., & Williams, J. B. W. (2001). The PHQ-9: Validity of a brief depression severity measure. *Journal of General Internal Medicine, 16*, 606–613.

Table 33-4 ■ ESSI: ENRICHD SOCIAL SUPPORT INSTRUMENT

	None of the Time	Little of the Time	Some of the Time	Most of the Time	All of the Time
1. Is there someone available to you whom you can count on to listen to you when you need to talk?	1	2	3	4	5
2. Is there someone available to you to give you advice about a problem?	1	2	3	4	5
3. Is there someone available to you who shows you love and affection?	1	2	3	4	5
4. Is there someone available to you to help you with daily chores?	1	2	3	4	5
5. Can you count on anyone to provide you with emotional support (talking over problems or helping you make a difficult decision)?	1	2	3	4	5
6. Do you have as much contact as you would like with someone you feel close to, in someone you can trust in, and confide?	1	2	3	4	5
7. Are you currently married, or living with a partner?	Yes			No	

Adapted from Mitchell, P. H., Powell, L., Blumenthal, J., et al. (2003). A short social support measure for patients recovering from myocardial infarction: The ENRICHD Social Support Inventory. *Journal of Cardiopulmonary Rehabilitation, 23*, 398–403.

structural support have a significantly poorer prognosis than those with complex social networks, the size and quality of the patient's network should also be evaluated. If the patient lives alone, he or she should be asked if they have someone who usually provides support (e.g., driving him or her to a doctor's appointment). Questions such as, "How many times a week do you visit with friends or relatives?" or "How many times a week do you attend a community or social event, such as church?" can elicit key information for evaluating social support.

Screening for Anxiety and Hostility

A few screening tools for anxiety and hostility are mentioned below but these can be more time-consuming and more useful in research rather than clinically. If time permits and there are concerns about anxiety, alcohol use, or other diagnoses, a nurse can also administer the Primary Care Evaluation of Mental Disorders (PRIME-MD), a diagnostic two-part instrument that combines 27 self-report screening questions and short clinical interview modules.[110] This is a practical and useful tool designed for primary care physicians (Table 33-5).

The three screening items for anxiety as mentioned in Table 33-5 are 20, 21, and 22. A yes response to one of these may lead to a more thorough interview or additional screening. Other anxiety screening tools for CHD patients include (a) the State Trait Anxiety Inventory, a 40-item standardized questionnaire for anxiety, that has been used in several nursing studies[111]; (b) the Crown-Crisp Experiential Index for excessive anxiety or phobias[112]; and (c) the Minnesota Multiphasic Personality Inventory-based Cook-Medley Hostility Inventory, a 50-item questionnaire. Williams & Williams[113] have adapted this questionnaire and scoring method for lay audiences. Patients can also use this resource for self-assessment and education.

As evident from the description above, depression and social support screening tools are more easily adapted for use by nurses; however, screening tools for anxiety and hostility could be further refined for use in acute settings. Nevertheless, the choice of a screening instrument depends on the patient population, patient readiness, clinician's skill and comfort, her or his clinical experience interpreting the instrument's results, available time, and resources.

Table 33-5 ■ PRIME-MD (PRIMARY CARE EVALUATION OF MENTAL DISORDERS), DIAGNOSTIC ASSESSMENT FOR DEPRESSION AND ANXIETY—PATIENT QUESTIONNAIRE

Instructions: This questionnaire will help your health provider better understand problems that you may have.

During the PAST MONTH, have you often been bothered by . . .

1. Stomach pain	Y	N
2. Back pain	Y	N
3. Pain in your arms, legs, or joints (knees, hips, etc.)	Y	N
4. Menstrual pain or problems	Y	N
5. Pain or problems during sexual intercourse	Y	N
6. Headaches	Y	N
7. Chest pain	Y	N
8. Dizziness	Y	N
9. Fainting spells	Y	N
10. Feeling your heart pound or race	Y	N
11. Shortness of breath	Y	N
12. Constipation, loose bowels or diarrhea	Y	N
13. Nausea, gas, or indigestion	Y	N
14. Feeling tired or having low energy	Y	N
15. Trouble sleeping	Y	N
16. The thought that you have a serious undiagnosed disease	Y	N
17. Your eating being out of control	Y	N
18. Little interest or pleasure in doing things	Y	N
19. Feeling down depressed or hopeless	Y	N
20. "Nerves" or feeling anxious or on edge	Y	N
21. Worrying about a lot of different things	Y	N
22. Have you had an anxiety attack (suddenly feeling fear or panic)	Y	N
23. Have you thought you should cut down your drinking of alcohol	Y	N
24. Has anyone complained about your drinking	Y	N
25. Have you felt guilty or upset about your drinking	Y	N
26. Was there ever a single day in which you had five or more drinks of beer, wine, or liquor	Y	N

Overall would you say your health is
- Excellent
- Very Good
- Good
- Fair
- Poor

Borrowed with permission from Spitzer, R., Williams, J. B., Linzer, M., et al. (1994). Utility of a new procedure for diagnosing mental disorders in primary care: The PRIME-MD 1000 study. *JAMA, 272*, 1749–1756.

Knowing that CHD patients can have one or more of the above-mentioned psychosocial manifestations, nurses should refer patients who meet the above diagnostic and assessment criteria to a licensed mental health professional for a complete "work up" and the initiation of appropriate treatment.

PSYCHOSOCIAL INTERVENTIONS IN CHD

Most research on psychosocial interventions has examined their effects on decreasing cardiac morbidity and mortality. The mixed results or small effect sizes from such inquiries in the last decade have been attributed to insufficient sample sizes; individual versus group-based interventions; heterogeneous targets of intervention—behavioral, physiological, or emotional distress reduction; variable length of treatment; and lack of biological or cardiac endpoints as outcome variables.[87,114] ENRICHD, a multicenter, randomized, controlled clinical trial, was the first large study to evaluate the effect of an intervention designed to reduce depression and improve social support on reducing CHD morbidity and mortality. Although the study's sample of 2,481 MI patients included a broad distribution of age, gender, ethnicity, and race, it was unable to demonstrate that treatment had a "mortality benefit."[3] The study, however, did show a statistically significant reduction in depression and improvement in social support, which improved the quality of life for those patients who received psychosocial intervention. Taylor[115] observed that the reduction in rates of death and reinfarction in the control and treatment groups as a result of early and aggressive treatment with cardiologic agents may have made it difficult to discern differences between the two groups. Another study, Sertraline Antidepressant Heart Attack Randomized Trial (SADHART), conducted concurrently to test if pharmacological management of depression alone could reduce CHD mortality, also failed to show improved survival.[116] Taylor,[115] however, noted that in the ENRICHD study the risk of death and recurrent MI was lower for those taking sertaline and receiving psychosocial interventions. Despite the mixed results, the role of depression and social support in the development and maintenance of cardiac disease is well established. Thus, developing and implementing psychosocial interventions to modify behavioral risk factors, decrease emotional distress (particularly depression), and improve quality of life are considered vital adjuncts to cardiac medical and surgical procedures.[3,87] Future trials, however, should track both physiological markers and changes in depressive symptoms, because correlating changes in depression and cardiovascular outcomes can be challenging.[98] Researchers should also investigate the effects of sustained intensity of treatment to address recurrent depression and to consider gender-specific treatments,[33] and the complex relationship between depression and mortality following an MI needs to be better understood to improve the timing of the depression intervention.[117]

As patients recover from coronary events, nurses have many opportunities to educate, motivate, facilitate, and provide psychosocial interventions. Such interventions should be initiated while patients are still in the hospital, because the first few months after a coronary event are critical for survival. An acute medical crisis often motivates patients to consider lifestyle changes. For example, one study showed that smoking cessation rates among MI patients were 70% compared with 9% for smokers in the general population.[118] Similarly, CHD patients may be more receptive to modifying their psychosocial risk factors. The ENRICHD study showed that patients' interest in treatment waned after awhile and that they often wanted to put the experience of their cardiac event behind them.[119] Thus, the critical time for intervention is within the first few months after an event when patients might still be motivated to make lifestyle changes. Most patients are receptive to education during the acute phase of a cardiac event. These interventions can provide a sense of control, decrease anxiety, and improve self-efficacy. The psychosocial management interventions described in the following section target physiological arousal, negative behaviors, and negative attitudinal cycles. Nurses are ideally suited to teach patients about these interventions.

Self-Monitoring Negative Reactions and Responses

With any intervention, nurses must determine how self-aware patients are of their behaviors and emotions. Acute coronary events are overwhelming and can lead to denial,[119] making it difficult for patients to understand their reactions to such an event. Even before an acute event, many patients are not attuned to or are uncomfortable with their emotional reactions, if they are considered harmful or unimportant.[120] Although it can be a useful coping response in the short term, denial, if it persists, can lead to avoidance or minimization of symptoms and lackadaisical effort in making lifestyle changes.[121,122] Also, it can lead to unchallenged negative assumptions and negative emotions that foster increased helplessness and hopelessness, impeding problem solving and possibly leading to social disconnectedness.

Cognitive-behavioral treatment enables patients to understand their reactions and to modify assumptions that lead to negative emotions and behaviors. This short-term structured treatment, which can be administered to individuals or groups, concentrates on current problems to develop mood management skills, new strategies to handle difficult situations, and self-therapy skills and can be applied to problems related to anxiety, anger, maladaptive behaviors besides depression, social isolation, and stress.[123] Cognitive behavior therapy[23] is an effective treatment for depression and evidence-based guidelines recommend its use for mild to moderate depression.[124,125]

Several studies of cardiac patients including ENRICHD [3,11,120,126–128] have used cognitive behavioral therapy (a) to raise patients' awareness of automatic assumptions about the MI, self, others, and the world; (b) to implement strategies and skill building that improve mood by evaluating assumptions, engaging in positive behaviors, practicing behavior drills, and improving interactions with others; and (c) to increase self-efficacy and self-esteem. Cognitive behavioral therapy emphasizes that stressful events, such as a coronary artery bypass graft or everyday stressors associated with recovery, can trigger negative reactions at multiple levels: attitudinal (thoughts), behavioral, emotional, and physiological. For example, a successful entrepreneur who experiences debilitating weakness following a coronary bypass surgery, may think "I am useless. I will never be able to work like before, I will have to quit." In such a state, the patient may become depressed, experience fatigue, sleep excessively, and when home, refuse to take his medication, exacerbating his physical symptoms. Negative thoughts may follow (Fig. 33-2).

Once aware of their assumptions, patients might re-evaluate their cognitions and improve their mood by seeking reliable information. Conversely, a lack of awareness may lead to prolonged

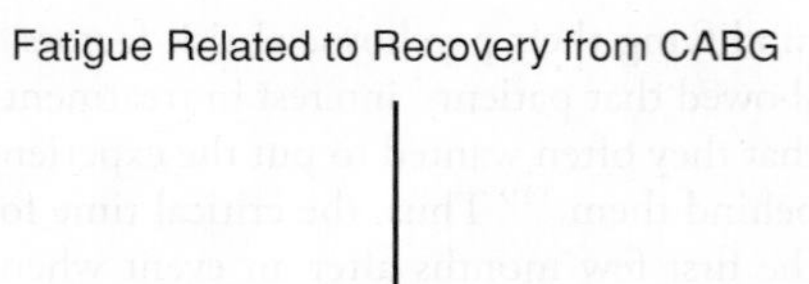
Fatigue Related to Recovery from CABG

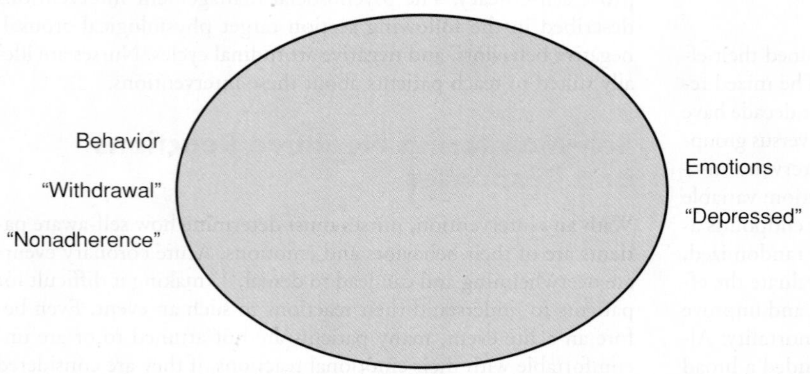
Thoughts: " I am useless or worthless, I will never be able to work like before, I will have tc quit"
Behavior
"Withdrawal"
"Nonadherence"
Emotions
"Depressed"
Physical Reactions - "Tired"

■ **Figure 33-2** An example of connections of thoughts and behaviors using cognitive behavioral model.

negative moods and a poor health outcome. Thoughts that perpetuate negative "heart health behaviours such as non-compliance with medication regimen can harm patients during their recovery from an acute coronary event. Consider these examples. First, a patient experiences chest tightness and aches associated with his surgery. Negative thoughts arise, "What if the doctor missed something?" or "Is this another heart attack?" leading to worry and anxiety. The patient's worry may manifest itself in behaviors such as frequently seeking reassurance. Once home, the patient's anxiety may surface in behaviors such as frequently calling the physician, avoiding being alone, avoiding engaging in activities, or excessively monitoring physical sensations, which only perpetuates the anxiety. Second, a patient who is the sole provider for his large family may feel discouraged by his fatigue. Fearful of losing his job, he returns to work prematurely and also resumes driving his three children to each of their schools before going to work. Assuming such commitments without social support while still recovering increases his fatigue, fear, and possibly leads to a slower recovery. Finally, a homemaker, committed to the care of her family and fearful of losing their affection, may dismiss fatigue and physical discomfort, overdoing her activities or postponing cardiac rehabilitation.

For receptive patients, nurses can increase their awareness of automatic and, often false, appraisals of stressful events. Patients can be encouraged to record their observations. If nurses have assessed patients' psychosocial risk factors and are attentive to their verbal and nonverbal communication, they can increase patient awareness of their automatic reactions by asking them nonconfrontational questions. Nurses can also teach their patients how automatic reactions affect their recovery, and patients must be taught that introspection is more effective when carried out in an inquisitive rather than a self-critical manner.[127,128]

Decreasing Physiological Arousal

Educating CHD patients about relaxation training and its direct effect on decreasing sympathetic nervous system arousal and increasing heart rate variability, which is associated with increased parasympathetic activity, can be useful to some patients in getting a relaxation effect. Relaxation training has been a standard part of many large research trials, such as the Recurrent Coronary Prevention Project, Project New Life, and ENRICHD[120,127–129] and can be used in clinical settings. This training can increase self-awareness of physical responses to daily stressors and decrease physiological arousal. Studies have shown the beneficial effects of practicing relaxation: decreased cortical arousal, decreased breathing rate, decreased sympathetic nervous system activity, increased heart rate variability, and improved sleep and emotional states.[130] Also, decreasing physiological arousal allows one to re-evaluate stress-related perceptions more neutrally.[131] Patient mastery of relaxation training depends on a clear understanding of its rationale, instruction by a nurse or other qualified health care provider, and supervised practice. Relaxation techniques are easy for patients to learn, can offer a sense of control, and can effectively manage pain in the acute care setting.[132] Nurses can provide patients with relaxation audiotapes, DVDs, CDs, MP3 files (whichever is feasible) in the hospital setting. Several relaxation methods are available[133] and vary based on their focus such as on breath, muscle groups, and pleasant imagery. Patients are commonly instructed to practice relaxation techniques every day for a 20-minute period, repeating the techniques for shorter periods throughout the day (Display 33-1). Many cardiac rehabilitation programs also include relaxation techniques that may be particularly useful for patients whose high arousal states are triggered by anxiety, anger, and depression.

Exercise is another method of managing physiological arousal. However, the first step—again—is to teach patients the rationale for exercise, which includes decreasing hypertension, decreasing weight, increasing heart rate variability, and decreasing heart rate and thereby oxygen demand, which raises the threshold for angina symptoms. Lowering the demand for oxygen and improving angina symptomse can motivate patients to make lifestyle changes.[134–136] Several studies have also reported that exercise can

DISPLAY 33-1 A Classic Example of a Relaxation Exercise

Transcendental Meditation

1. Sit quietly in a comfortable position.
2. Close your eyes.
3. Deeply relax all your muscles, beginning at your feet and progressing up to your face. Keep them relaxed.
4. Breathe through your nose. Become aware of your breathing. As you breathe out, say the word, "ONE," silently to yourself. For example, breathe IN . . . OUT, "ONE"; IN . . . OUT, "ONE"; etc. Breathe easily and naturally.
5. Continue for 10 to 20 minutes. You may open your eyes to check the time, but do not use an alarm. When you finish, sit quietly for several minutes, at first with your eyes closed and later with your eyes opened. Do not stand up for a few minutes.
6. Do not worry about whether you are successful in achieving a deep level of relaxation. Maintain a passive attitude and permit relaxation to occur at its own pace. When distracting thoughts occur, try to ignore them by not dwelling upon them and return to repeating "ONE." With practice, the response should come with little effort. Practice the technique once or twice daily, but not within two hours after any meal, since the digestive processes seem to interfere with the elicitation of the Relaxation Response.

Borrowed with permission from Benson, H. (1975). *The relaxation response* (pp. 114–115). New York: William Morrow.

decrease depressive symptoms in cardiac patients.[137] Exercise also seems to improve self-efficacy, decrease negative moods,[136] and provide social reinforcement.[138]

Interventions for Depression and Anxiety

Chronic stress increases vulnerability to develop depression and anxiety. These are often accompanied by negative lifestyle behaviors that further tax the cardiovascular system. These behaviors may include watching excessive television, web surfing, poor diet, and inadequate sleep, which increases vulnerability to more stress, creating a vicious cycle.[139] Treating depression and anxiety can improve compliance with medication and heart-healthy behaviors, such as exercise and better diet.[140]

Without question, depression and anxiety are associated with negative lifestyle behaviors: smoking, excessive drinking and eating, decreased exercise, hostile behaviors, and social withdrawal. Patients with moderate to severe depression are likely to have multiple negative behaviors and several failed attempts to changing their negative health behaviors. Such patients require psychiatric care. Patients with less severe depression often respond well to encouragement to engage in positive activities that increase their connection with others, increase their sense of accomplishment, or both. Examples include initiating contact with family and friends, sharing a meal with a friend, exercising with a friend, attending a lecture, or working on a home project. Scheduling such activities is a hallmark of cognitive behavioral treatment for depression.[23] The rationale for this intervention is that pleasant activities foster connections with others or give a sense of accomplishment, improving emotional states. However, what makes an activity satisfactory is based on personal preference.

Exercise is a valuable intervention for depression in CHD patients. In one study, those who adhered to exercise had greater reductions in anxiety and depression than nonadherers.[141,142] The relationship between adherence to exercise and improvement in psychological variables was also seen in a community study of older adults.[143] Participation in exercise was related to lower depression and anxiety.[136] Thus, exercise training as an intervention has the dual benefit of improved cardiovascular health and self-esteem[131] and helps patients who are anxious or depressed. Patients and their families must be taught about the benefits of exercise and encouraged to attend a cardiac rehabilitation program. For patients who are fearful of exercise, supervised trials of exercise can instill confidence in them and motivate them to try it.

Depression and anxiety are also perpetuated by negative perceptions, beliefs, and thoughts in response to stressful situations. The successful entrepreneur who becomes depressed after a coronary bypass surgery may perceive that his physical weakness is permanent and that he will never be able to work as he did before. For him, these perceptions are facts. During patient education, nurses can teach such patients how to correct these inaccurate and negative perceptions about recovery and their implications on future functioning. Patients can be encouraged to examine their reflex perceptions by questions and clarifications and to challenge the validity of their concerns. According to cognitive behavioral therapy for depression, this intervention is called "cognitive restructuring" or "realistic thinking." It evaluates and tests the evidence that supports or invalidates the depressive cognitions and assumptions.[23] Patients who are anxious about having another heart attack can be taught that obsessive worry about their physical symptoms is likely to increase anxiety and physiological arousal, which is not beneficial during recovery. Patients can be taught relaxation strategies and methods of worry control to decrease anxiety. In his book for the lay public on managing anxiety and fear, Bourne outlines several worry-control methods, such as postponing worry and checking physical symptoms and scheduling worry periods.[133]

Social Support Interventions

As educators, nurses can provide CHD patients functional support in terms of education and knowledge. Anticipatory guidance about CHD regarding the disease and the recovery process can alleviate stress for both patients and families. The benefits of support and its role as a buffer against stress can be discussed. However, patients' needs and desires for knowledge must be assessed. This is illustrated by research observations of patients with a repressive coping style. Those who received a great deal of information had a higher frequency of "heart alarms" and more medical complications.[144] Patients who actively deny that they have had a heart attack are not ready to receive a lot of information. Open-ended questions that allow patients to direct the flow of information should be used. A nurse can also provide emotional support by empathic listening and encouraging social interactions. Hospital admissions for cardiac problems make most patients apprehensive and fearful. Allowing patients and spouses to express these concerns can benefit both patients and their families and provide educational opportunities. Encouraging patients to eat with other patients, facilitating their access to social visits, and having family members prepare their favorite foods cook can promote connections with others and enhance perceived support.[145] For patients with few social ties or ties perceived to be unsupportive, Friedwald et al.[146] suggest referral to a cardiac rehabilitation program or to Mended Hearts, a national nonprofit organization that offers support services to patients with heart disease, may increase community contacts. Having a pet may also be beneficial. Patients referred to cardiac rehabilitation programs benefit by observing other patients recover and by maintaining contact with health care staff. Many CHD patients in rehabilitation programs develop lasting friendships with their counterparts. Such ties serve buffer the stresses of daily life.

Patients with existing support networks are likely to benefit by having family or significant others involved during their recovery in the hospital. Like CHD patients, spouses and significant others are likely to distort and make false assumptions about the recovery process during and after the medical emergency. Spouses can be significantly distressed by the hospital admission for several reasons: lack of control, fear of the unknown, fear of change in roles, self-blame for the event, and fear of loss.[147–149] Also, providing information before procedures occur and during rehabilitation can decrease the fear of uncertainty. Educating a spouse about his or her partner's MI, the course of treatment, and the recovery process can decrease over-protectiveness and over-involvement when the patient is discharged from the hospital.[150] Behavioral strategies that allow patients and families to rehearse or model experiences are useful. For example, treadmill exercise testing before discharge from the hospital, if observed by the spouse, has been shown to enhance the patient's self-esteem and to reduce spousal anxiety.[151] Rather than being overprotective in the recovery period, the spouse can provide positive support.

Intervention Strategies for Hostility and Anger

Hostility can often be an ingrained trait and resistant to change. In some cases, referral to a mental health specialist may be required. Hostile patients may be less compliant with risk factor modification and medical regimens. For example, when patients smoke to relieve episodes of anger or frustration, quit rates are lower than if they are able to control their expression of anger.[26] Evaluating adherence to health care recommendation and problem-solving strategies is important in all coronary patients, but they may be particularly important in people to excessive hostility and anger.

After establishing rapport with hostile or angry patients, nurses can teach them about the physiological effects of emotions. Socratic questioning works well: "Do you think that you often are angrier than others in similar situations or that you stay resentful for longer periods?" or "How do you think your anger and resentments affect your heart or your blood pressure?" This approach gives a nurse insight into a patient's understanding, to determine how best to share information without provoking anxiety, and to assess the patient's readiness to receive information. Eliciting feedback from patients also helps to assess how they are processing the information.

Hostile or angry patients should be informed about the effects of heightened cardiovascular and neuroendocrine responses that increase cortisol levels and plasma lipid levels. The effect of angry assumptions, thoughts, and behaviors in decreasing parasympathetic response should also be addressed. The benefits of exercise and relaxation training to decrease physiological arousal, decrease emotional arousal and increase parasympathetic response should be emphasized for patients with hostility and anger.[128] Patients should be encouraged to record their thoughts and feelings to become more aware of their hypercritical view of others as incompetent or untrustworthy. Such generalizations can be gently questioned so that patients' assumptions can be evaluated from a neutral perspective. Also, they can be questioned about the function of their anger and hostility,[152] and they can also learn when anger is justified and when it is not.[113]

The interventions used in most studies have involved group therapy programs with educational and behavioral strategies to assist patients in identifying and modifying their behaviors. One such strategy is the "Hook Intervention"[153] taught to patients with high autonomic reactivity to life's daily hassles, such as waiting in lines and being delayed in traffic. These patients frequently react to the unfairness of the external environment and unsuccessfully try to gain control over that environment through overt or covert impatient and hostile behaviors, which lead to further frustration and physiological arousal. Through practice, patients learn that daily hassles are hooks; they can choose to bite or they can ignore the bait, thus controlling their arousal levels. For example, a patient might identify routine behaviors such as speeding up when approaching a yellow light or passing cars or multitasking. Such patients can be instructed to modify their behavior or conduct experiments by driving in the slow lane, standing in a longer line, or doing one task at a time.

Patients who are hostile and angry tend to have unsatisfactory relationships and may have difficulty maintaining relationships.[154] Interventions can nurture social connectedness in these patients who either lack the skills to connect or fear the cost of these social connections, such as the risk of rejection and or diversion from goal-oriented activities.[128] These patients learn (a) to recognize their internal reactions in an interpersonal environment, (b) to practice expressing their feelings and listening in a reflective and empathetic way, (c) to practice assertiveness skills, such as saying no and delegating to others, and (d) to learn the difference between assertive and aggressive responses.[155] These programs, although costly and time consuming, have been shown to reduce hostility ratings.[156]

PHARMACOLOGICAL INTERVENTIONS FOR PSYCHOSOCIAL RISK FACTORS IN CHD

Besides interventions mentioned above, patients with psychosocial risk factors should also be evaluated for psychopharmacological interventions after a thorough assessment. The efficacy of antidepressants in treating clinical depression is well established. The Agency for Health Care and Policy Research's treatment guidelines recommend that moderate to severe depression and recurrent depression should be treated with antidepressants and psychotherapy.[125] Antidepressant treatment may also decrease anxiety and hostility, and is sometimes used to help patients stop smoking.[3,157–161] Given the availability of so many antidepressants and the potential side effects and drug interactions for CHD patients, consulting a psychiatrist is recommended. The empirically based medical consensus[162] is that selective serotonin reuptake inhibitors cause fewer side effects and have fewer contraindications for cardiac patients than tricyclic antidepressants, which increase orthostatic hypotension, increase heart rate,[163,164] and slow conduction (lethal for those with conduction problems). However, selective serotonin reuptake inhibitors can inhibit cytochrome P450 enzymes that help to metabolize drugs, such as antiarrhythmics, which are commonly given to CHD patients, and change plasma levels of these drugs.[165] Nurses should monitor patients who are taking these medications and consult pharmacology reference books to identify specific side effects and contradictions. Generally, sertraline and citalopram are considered safe and effective antidepressants for moderate, severe, and recurrent depression in CHD patients in the absence of other life-threatening medical conditions.[116,166] Furthermore, treatment by selective serotonin reuptake inhibitors may have cardioprotective effects such as reduce platelet/endothelial activation and improved autonomic functioning.[33,146,167]

SUMMARY

A multifaceted program that includes both psychosocial and traditional risk reduction strategies may provide the greatest benefit for men and women with CHD. Although behavioral strategies such as education, counseling, emotional support, and risk reduction may improve emotional states, psychosocial interventions should be implemented only after fully assessing a patient's beliefs and psychological and social needs. Education, counseling, modifying automatic assumptions, specific behavioral strategies, relaxation strategies, and emotional support can influence a patient's response to psychosocial factors. Treating the whole person is a fundamental tenety of the nursing profession. Managing CHD patients requires that nurses be attentive to all cardiovascular risk factors, including psychosocial factors.

Acknowledgment: *The authors thank the scholarly contribution of Joan M. Fair. She was one of the authors of this chapter for the previous edition.*

REFERENCES

1. Jenkins, C. D. (1978). Behavioral risk factors in coronary artery disease. *Annual Review of Medicine, 29*, 543–563.
2. Bunker, S. J., Colquhoun, D. M., Esler, M. D., et al. (2003). Stress and coronary heart disease: Psychosocial risk factors. *Medical Journal of Australia, 178*, 272–276.
3. ENRICHD Investigators. (2003). Enhancing recovery in coronary heart disease patients (ENRICHD) randomized trial: Effects of treating depression and low perceived social support on clinical events after myocardial infarction. *JAMA, 289*(23), 3106–3116.
4. Hemingway, H., & Marmot, M. (1999). Psychosocial factors in the etiology and prognosis of coronary heart disease. Systematic review of prospective cohort studies. *BMJ, 381*, 1460–1467.
5. Lynch, J., Kaplan, G., Salonen, R., et al. (1995). Socioeconomic status and carotid atherosclerosis. *Circulation, 92*, 1786–1792.
6. Hemingway, H., Kuper, H., & Marmot, M. (2003). Psychosocial factors in the primary and secondary prevention of coronary heart disease: A systematic review. In S. Yusuf, J. A. Cairns, E. Fallen, B. J. Gersch, & A. J. Camm (Eds.), *Evidence based cardiology.* London: British Medical Journal Publishing.
7. American Psychiatric Association. (1994). *Diagnostic and statistical manual of mental disorders* (4th ed.). Washington, DC: American Psychiatric Association.
8. Barefoot, J. C., & Schroll, M. (1996). Symptoms of depression, acute myocardial infarction, and total mortality in a community sample. *Circulation, 93*, 1976–1980.
9. Pratt, L. A., Ford, D. E., Crum, R. M., et al. (1996). Depression, psychotropic medication, and risk of myocardial infarction. Prospective data from Baltimore ECA follow-up. *Circulation, 94*, 3123–3129.
10. Frasure-Smith, N., & Lesperance, F. (2005). Reflections on depression as a cardiac risk factor. *Psychosomatic Medicine, 67*, S19–S25.
11. Carney, R. M., Rich, M. W., Tevelde, A., et al. (1987). Major depressive disorder in coronary artery disease. *American Journal of Cardiology, 60*, 1273–1275.
12. Carney, R. M., Rich, M. W., Freeland, K. E., et al. (1988). Major depressive disorder predicts cardiac events in patients with coronary artery disease. *Psychosomatic Medicine, 50*, 627–633.
13. Fielding, R. (1991). Depression and acute myocardial infarction: A review and reinterpretation. *Social Science Medicine, 32*, 1017–1027.
14. Frasure-Smith, N., Lesperance, F., & Talajic, M. (1996). Major depression before and after myocardial infarction: Its nature and consequences. *Psychosomatic Medicine, 58*, 99–110.
15. Frasure-Smith, N., & Lesperance, F. (2006). Recent evidence linking coronary heart disease and depression. *Canadian Journal of Psychiatry, 51*, 730–737.
16. Kuper, H., Marmot, M., & Hemingway, H. (2002). Systematic review of prospective cohort studies of psychosocial factors in the aetiology and prognosis of coronary heart disease. *Seminars in Vascular Medicine, 2*, 267–314.
17. Kessler, R. C., Berglund, P., Demler, O., et al. (2003). The epidemiology of major depressive disorder. *JAMA, 289*, 3095–3105.
18. Nolen-Hokesema, S. (1990). *Sex differences in depression*. Stanford: Stanford University Press.
19. Mallik, S., Spertus, J. A., Reid, K. J., et al. (2006). Depressive symptoms after acute myocardial infarction. Evidence for the highest rates in younger women. *Archives of Internal Medicine, 166*, 876–883.
20. Frasure-Smith, N., Lesperance, F., & Talajic, M. (1993). Depression following myocardial infarction: Impact on 6 month survival. *JAMA, 270*, 1819–1825.
21. Frasure-Smith, N., Lesperance, F., & Talajic, M. (1995). The impact of negative emotions on prognosis following myocardial infarction: Is it more than depression? *Health Psychology, 14*, 388–398.
22. Frasure-Smith, N., Lesperance, F., & Talajic, M. (1995). Depression and 18 month prognosis after a myocardial infarction. *Circulation, 91*, 999–1005.
23. Beck, A. T., Rush, A. J., Shaw, B. F., et al. (1979). *Cognitive therapy of depression.* New York: Guilford.
24. Cole, S. A., Christensen, J. F., Rajum, M. A., et al. (1997). Depression. In M. D. Feldman & J. F. Christensen (Eds.), *Behavioral medicine in primary care: A practical guide* (pp. 177–192). Norwalk, CT: Appleton & Lange.
25. Allison, T. G., Williams, D. E., Miller, T. D., et al. (1995). Medical and economic costs of psychological distress in patients with coronary artery disease. *Mayo Clinic Proceedings, 70*(8), 734–742.
26. Littman, A. B. (1993). Review of psychosomatic aspects of cardiovascular disease. *Psychotherapy and Psychosomatics, 60*, 148–167.
27. Conn, V. S., Taylor, S. G., & Wiman, O. (1991). Anxiety, depression, quality of life, and self-care among survivors of myocardial infarction. *Issues in Mental Health Nursing, 12*, 321–331.
28. Guiry, E., Conroy, R. M., Hickey, N., et al. (1987). Psychological response to an acute coronary event and its effect on subsequent rehabilitation and lifestyle change. *Clinical Cardiology, 10*, 256–260.
29. Wells, K. B., Stewart, A., Hays, R. D., et al. (1989). The functioning and well being of depressed patients. *JAMA, 262*, 914–919.
30. Carney, R. M., Freeland, K., Eisen, R., et al. (1995). Depression as a risk factor for cardiac events in established coronary heart disease: A review of possible mechanisms. *Annals of Behavioral Medicine, 17*, 142–149.
31. Blumenthal, J. A., & Williams, R. S. (1982). Physiological and psychological variables predict compliance to prescribed exercise therapy in patients recovering from myocardial infarction. *Psychosomatic Medicine, 44*, 519–527.
32. Finnegan, D. L., & Suler, J. R. (1985). Psychological factors associated with maintenance of improved health behavior in post coronary patients. *Journal of Psychology, 119*, 87–94.
33. Davidson, K. W., Kupfer, D. J., Bigger, J. T., et al. (2006). Assessment and treatment of depression in patients with cardiovascular disease: National Health, Lung and Blood Institute working group report. *Psychosomatic Medicine, 68*, 645–650.
34. Antonucci, T. C., & Johnson, E. H. (1994). Conceptualization and methods in social support theory and research as related to cardiovascular

disease. In S. A. Shumacker & S. M. Czajkowski (Eds.), *Social support and cardiovascular disease* (pp. 21–39). New York: Plenum.
35. Smith, C. E., Fernengel, K., Holcroft, C., et al. (1994). Meta-analysis of the associations between social support and health outcomes. *Annals of Behavioral Medicine, 16,* 352–362.
36. Vinokur, A., Schul, Y., & Caplan, R. D. (1987). Determinants of perceived social support: Interpersonal transactions, personal outlook and transient affective states. *Journal of Personal and Social Psychology, 53,* 1137–1145.
37. Pitula, C. R., Burg, M. M., & Froelicher, E. S. (1999). Psychosocial risk factors: Assessment and intervention for social isolation. In *Cardiac rehabilitation: A guide to practice in the 21st century* (pp. 279–286). New York: Marcel Dekker.
38. Ortho-Gomer, K., Rosengran, A., & Wilhelmsen, L. (1993). Lack of social support and incidence of coronary heart disease in middle-aged Swedish men. *Psychosomatic Medicine, 55,* 37–43.
39. Brecht, M. L., Dracup, K., Moser, D., et al. (1994). The relationship of marital quality and psychosocial adjustment to heart disease. *Journal of Cardiology Nursing, 9,* 74–85.
40. Ebrahims, S., Wannamethee, G., McCallum, A., et al. (1995). Marital status, change in marital status and mortality in middle-aged British men. *American Journal of Epidemiology, 142,* 834–842.
41. Gorkin, L., Schron, E. B., & Brooks, M. M. (1993). Psychosocial predictors of mortality in the Cardiac Arrthymia Supression Trial-1 (CAST-1). *American Journal of Cardiology, 71,* 263–267.
42. Williams, R. B., Barefoot, J. C., Califf, R. M., et al. (1992). Prognostic importance of social and economic resources among medically treated patients with angiographically documented coronary artery disease. *JAMA, 267,* 520–524.
43. Case, R. B., Moss, A. J., Care, N., et al. (1992). Living alone after myocardial infarction: Impact on prognosis. *JAMA, 267,* 515–519.
44. Berkman, L. F., Leo-Summers, L., & Horwitz, R. I. (1992). Emotional support and survival after myocardial infarction. *Annals of Internal Medicine, 117,* 1003–1009.
45. Krumholz, H. M., Butler, J., Miller, J., et al. (1998). Prognostic importance of emotional support for elderly patients hospitalized with heart failure. *Circulation, 97,* 958–964.
46. Ortho-Gomer, K., Wamala, S. P., Horsten, M., et al. (2000). Marital stress worsens prognosis in women with coronary heart disease. The Stockholm Female Coronary Risk Study. *JAMA, 284,* 3008–3014.
47. Rankin-Esquer, L. A., Miller, N. H., Myers, D., et al. (1997). Marital status and outcome in patients with coronary heart disease. *Journal of Clinical Psychology in Medical Settings, 4,* 417–435.
48. Nyamathi, A. M., Jacoby, A., Constancia, P., et al. (1992). Coping and adjustment of spouses of critically ill patients in cardiac disease. *Heart Lung, 21,* 160–166.
49. Coyne, J. C., & DeLongis, A. (1986). Going beyond social support—The role of social relationships in adaptation. *Journal of Consulting Clinical Psychology, 54,* 545–560.
50. Wishnie, H. A., Hackett, T. P., & Cassem, N. H. (1971). Psychological hazards of convalescence following myocardial infarction. *JAMA, 215,* 1292–1296.
51. Berkman, L. F. (1995). The role of social relations in health promotion. *Psychosomatic Medicine, 57,* 245–254.
52. Kawachi, I., Colditz, G. A., Ascherio, A., et al. (1994). Prospective study of phobic anxiety and risk of coronary heart disease in men. *Circulation, 89,* 1992–1997.
53. Kubzansky, L. D., Kawachi, I., Spiro III, A., et al. (1997). Is worrying bad for your heart? *Circulation, 95,* 818–824.
54. Ahern, D. K., Gorkin, L., Anderson, J. L., et al. (1990). Biobehavioral variables and mortality for cardiac arrest in the Cardiac Arrthymia Pilot Study (CAPS). *American Journal of Cardiology, 60,* 59–62.
55. Hayward, C. (1995). Psychiatric illness and cardiovascular disease risk. *Epidemiology Review, 17,* 129–138.
56. Moser, D. K., & Dracup, K. (1996). Is anxiety after myocardial infarction associated with subsequent ischemic and arrhythmic events? *Psychosomatic Medicine, 58,* 395–401.
57. Grace, S. L., Abbey, S. E., Shnek, Z. M., et al. (2002). Cardiac rehabilitation I: Review of psychosocial factors. *General Hospital Psychiatry, 24,* 121–126.
58. King, K. B. (1997). Psychologic and social aspects of cardiovascular disease. *Annals of Behavioral Medicine, 19*(3), 264–270.
59. Smith, T. W. (1992). Hostility and health: Current status of a psychosomatic hypothesis. *Health Psychology, 11,* 139–150.
60. Everson, S. A., Kauhanen, J., Kaplan, G. A., et al. (1997). Hostility and increased risk of mortality and acute myocardial infarction: The mediating role of behavioral risk factors. *American Journal of Epidemiology, 146,* 142–152.
61. Julkunen, J., Salonen, R., Kaplan, G. A., et al. (1994). Hostility and the progression of carotid atherosclerosis. *Psychosomatic Medicine, 56,* 519–525.
62. Kawachi, I., Sparrow, D., Spiro, A., et al. (1996). A prospective study of anger and coronary heart disease. *Circulation, 94,* 2090–2095.
63. Mittleman, M. A., Maclure, M., Sherwood, J. B., et al. (1995). Triggering of acute myocardial infarction onset by episodes of anger. *Circulation, 92,* 1720–1725.
64. Follick, M. J., Ahern, D. K., Gorkin, L., et al. (1990). Relation of psychosocial and stress reactivity variables to ventricular arrthymias in the cardiac arrthymia pilot study (CAPS). *American Journal of Cardiology, 66,* 63–67.
65. Malkoff, S. B., Muldoon, M. F., Zeigler, Z. R., et al. (1993). Blood platelet responsivity to acute mental stress. *Psychosomatic Medicine, 55,* 477–482.
66. Muller, J. E., Abela, G. S., Nesto, R. W., et al. (1994). Triggers, acute risk factors and vulnerable plaques: The lexicon of a new frontier. *Journal of the American College of Cardiology, 23,* 809–813.
67. Goodman, M., Quigley, J., Moran, G., et al. (1996). Hostility predicts restenosis after percutaneous transluminal coronary angioplasty. *Mayo Clinic Proceedings, 71,* 729–734.
68. Kloner, R. A., Leor, J., Poole, W. K., et al. (1997). Population-based analysis of the effect of the Northridge earthquake on cardiac death in Los Angeles County. *Journal of the American College of Cardiology, 30,* 1174–1180.
69. Kark, J. D., Goldman, S., & Epstein, L. (1995). Iraqi missile attacks on Israel. *JAMA, 273,* 1208–1210.
70. Suzuki, S., Sakamotot, S., Koide, M., et al. (1997). Hanshi-Awaji earthquake as a trigger for acute myocardial infarction. *American Heart Journal, 134,* 974–977.
71. Gullette, E., Blumenthal, J., Babyak, M., et al. (1997). Effects of mental stress on myocardial ischemia during daily life. *JAMA, 277,* 1521–1526.
72. Krieger, N. (1994). Influence of social call, race, and gender on the etiology of hypertension among women in the United States. In S. M. Czajkowski, D. R. Hill, & T. B. Clarkson (Eds.), Women, behavior, and cardiovascular disease (NIH Publication No. 94-3309, pp. 191–206). Rockville, MD: National Institute of Health.
73. Goldstein, M. G., & Niaura, R. (1992). Psychological factors affecting physical condition: Cardiovascular disease literature review. *Psychosomatics, 33,* 134–154.
74. Yeung, A. C., Vekshtein, V. I., Krantz, D. S., et al. (1991). The effect of atherosclerosis on the vasomotor responses of coronary arteries to mental stress. *New England Journal of Medicine, 325,* 1551–1556.
75. Rozanski, A., Bairy, C. N., Krantz, D. S., et al. (1988). Mental stress and the induction of myocardial ischemia in patients with coronary artery disease. *New England Journal of Medicine, 318,* 1005–1012.
76. Spielberg, C., Falkenhaln, D., Willich, S., et al. (1996). Circadian, day of week, and seasonal variability in myocardial infarction: Comparison between working and retired patients. *American Heart Journal, 132,* 579–585.
77. Hall, E. M. (1994). Multiple roles and caregiving stress in women. In S. M. Czajkowski, D. R. Hill, & T. B. Clarkson (Eds.), *Women, behaviour, and cardiovascular disease* (NIH Publication No. 94-3309, pp. 167–178). Rockville, MD: National Institute of Health.
78. Kivimaki, M., Leino-Arjas, P., Luukkonen, R., et al. (2002). Work stress and risk of cardiovascular mortality: Prospective cohort study of industrial employees. *BMJ, 325,* 857.
79. Kivimaki, M., Virtnanen, M., Elovainio, M., et al. (2006). Work stress in the etiology of coronary heart disease—A meta-analysis. *Scandinavian Journal of Work and Environmental Health, 32,* 431–432.
80. Dixon, J. P., Dixon, J. K., & Spinner, J. C. (1991). Tensions between career and interpersonal commitments as a risk factor for cardiovascular disease among women. *Women and Health, 17,* 33–57.
81. Thoerell, T. (1991). Psychosocial cardiovascular risks: On the double loads in women. *Psychotherapy and Psychosomatics, 55,* 81–89.
82. Kritz-Silverstein, D., Wingard, D., & Barrett-Connor, E. (1992). Employment status and heart disease risk factors in middle-aged women: The Rancho Bernardo Study. *American Journal of Public Health, 82,* 215–219.
83. Matthews, K., Cottington, E., Talbot, E., et al. (1987). Stressful work conditions and diastolic blood pressure among blue collar factory workers. *American Journal of Epidemiology, 126,* 280–291.

84. Schwartz, J., Pieper, C., & Krarasek, R. A. (1988). A procedure for linking psychosocial job characteristics data to health surveys. *American Journal of Public Health, 78*, 904–909.
85. Hlatky, M. A., Lam, L. C., Lee, K., et al. (1995). Job strain and the prevalence and outcome of coronary artery disease. *Circulation, 92*, 327–333.
86. Karasek, R., Baker, D., Marxer, F., et al. (1981). Job decision latitude, job demands and cardiovascular disease: A prospective study of Swedish men. *American Journal of Public Health, 71*, 694–705.
87. Smith, T. W., & Ruiz, J. M. (2002). Psychosocial influences on the development and course of coronary heart disease: Current status and implications for research and practice. *Journal of Consulting Clinical Psychology, 70*, 548–568.
88. Lazarus, R. S., & Folkman, S. (1984). *Stress, appraisal, and coping.* New York: Springer-Verlag.
89. Selye, H. (1956). *The stress of life.* New York: McGraw-Hill.
90. Adams, D. O. (1994). Molecular biology of macrophage activation: A pathway whereby psychosocial factors can potentially affect health. *Psychosomatic Medicine, 56*, 316–327.
91. McCarty, R., & Gold, P. E. (1996). Catecholamines, stress, and disease: A psychobiological perspective. *Psychosomatic Medicine, 58*, 590–597.
92. Veith, R. C., Lewis, N., Linares, O., et al. (1994). Sympathetic nervous system activity in major depression: Basal and desipramine-induced alterations in plasma norepinephrine kinetics. *Archives of General Psychiatry, 51*, 411–422.
93. Carney, R. M., Freedland, K. E., Miller, G. E. et al. (2002). Depression as a risk factor for cardiac mortality and morbidity: A review of potential mechanisms. *Journal of Psychosomatic Research, 53*, 897–902.
94. Musselman, D. L., Tomer, A., Manatunga, A. K., et al. (1996). Exaggerated platelet reactivity in major depression. *American Journal of Psychiatry, 153*, 1313–1317.
95. Carney, R. M., Blumenthal, J. A., Stein, P. K., et al. (2001). Depression, heart rate variability, and acute myocardial infarction. *Circulation, 104*, 2024–2028.
96. Kleiger, R. E., Miller, J. P., Bigger, J. T. et al. (1987). Multicenter post-infarction research group—Decreased heart rate variability and its association with mortality after myocardial infarction. *American Journal of Cardiology, 59*, 256–262.
97. Carney, R. M., Blumenthal, J. A., Freedland, K. E., et al. (2005). Low heart rate variability and the effect of depression on post-myocardial infarction mortality. *Archives of Internal Medicine, 165*, 1486–1491.
98. Joynt, K. E., & O'Connor, C. M. (2005). Lessons from SADHART, ENRICHD and other trials. *Psychosomatic Medicine, 67*, S63–S66.
99. Jiang, W., Alexander, J., Christopher, E., et al. (2001). Relationship of depression to increased risk of mortality and rehospitalization in patients with congestive heart failure. *Archives of Internal Medicine, 161*, 1849–1856.
100. McManus, D., Pipkin, S. S., Whooley, M. A., et al. (2005). Screening for depression with coronary heart disease. (Data from the Heart and Soul Study.) *American Journal of Cardiology, 96*, 1076–1081.
101. Whooley, M. A., Avins, A. I., Miranda, J., et al. (1997). Case finding instruments for depression: Two questions are as good as many. *Journal of General Internal Medicine, 12*, 439–445.
102. Kroenke, K., Spitzer, R. L., & Williams, J. B. W. (2003). The Patient Health Questionnaire-2—The validity of a two-item depression screener. *Medical Care, 41*, 1284–1292.
103. Kroenke, K., Spitzer, R. L., & Williams, J. B. W. (2001). The PHQ-9: Validity of a brief depression severity measure. *Journal of General Internal Medicine, 16*, 606–613.
104. Beck, A. T., Ward, C. H., Mendelson, M., et al. (1961). An inventory for measuring depression. *Archives of General Psychiatry, 4*, 53–63.
105. Beck, A. T., Steer, R. A., & Garbin, M. G. (1988). Psychometric properties of the Beck Depression Inventory: Twenty years of evaluation. *Clinical Psychiatry Review, 8*, 77–100.
106. Lichtman, J. H., Bigger, J. T., & Blumenthal, J. A. (2008). Depression and coronary heart disease: Recommendations for screening, referral and treatment. *Circulation, 118*(17), 1768–1775.
107. ENRICHD Investigators. (2001). Enhancing recovery in coronary heart disease (ENRICHD): Baseline characteristics. *American Journal of Cardiology, 88*, 316–322.
108. Mitchell, P. H., Powell, L., Blumenthal, J., et al. (2003). A short social support measure for patients recovering from myocardial infarction: The ENRICHD Social Support Inventory. *Journal of Cardiopulmonary Rehabilitation, 23*, 398–403.
109. Pitula, C. R., & Daugherty, S. R. (1995). Sources of social support and conflict in hospitalized depressed women. *Research in Nursing Health, 18*, 325–332.
110. Spitzer, R., Williams, J. B., Linzer, M., et al. (1994). Utility of a new procedure for diagnosing mental disorders in primary care: The PRIME-MD 1000 study. *JAMA, 272*, 1749–1756.
111. van Der Ploeg, H., Defares, P., & Spielberger, C. (1980). *Manual for the State Trait Anxiety Inventory.* Lisee, The Netherlands: Swets & Zeitlinger.
112. Kawachi, I., Sparrow, D., Vokona, S. P. S., et al. (1994). Symptoms of anxiety and risk of coronary heart disease: The Normative Aging Study. *Circulation, 90*, 2225–2229.
113. Williams, R. B., & Williams, V. P. (1993). *Anger kills: Seventeen strategies for controlling the hostility that can harm your health.* New York: Times Books.
114. Linden, W. (2000). Psychological treatments in cardiac rehabilitation: Review of rationales and outcomes. *Journal of Psychosomatic Research, 48*, 443–454.
115. Taylor, C. B., Youngblood, M. E., & Catellier, D. (2005). Effects of antidepressant medication on morbidity and mortality in depressed patients after myocardial infarction. *Archives of General Psychiatry, 62*, 792–798.
116. Glassman, A. H., O'Connor, C. M., Califf, R. M., et al. (2002). Sertraline treatment of major depression in patients with acute MI or unstable angina. *JAMA, 288*, 701–709.
117. Dickens, C., McGowan, L., Percival, C. et al. (2007). Depression is a risk factor for mortality after myocardial infarction. Fact or artefact. *Journal of the American College of Cardiology, 49*, 1834–1840.
118. Feinstein, R. E., Carey, L., Rabinowitz, P. M., et al. (1999). Cardiovascular and psychosocial risk factors reduction: Office-based interventions. In R. E. Feinstein & A. A. Brewer (Eds.), *Primary care psychiatry and behavioral medicine* (pp. 299–329). New York: Springer.
119. ENRICHD Investigators. (2001). Enhancing recovery in coronary heart disease (ENRICHD) study intervention: Rationale and design. *Psychosomatic Medicine, 63*, 747–755.
120. Billings, J. H., Scherwitz, L. W., Sullivan, R., et al. (1996). The Lifestyle Heart Trial: Comprehensive treatment and group support study. In R. Allan & S. Scheidt (Eds.), *Heart and mind: The practice of cardiac psychology* (pp. 233–253). Washington, DC: American Psychological Association.
121. Hackett, T. P., & Cassem, N. H. (1975). Psychological management of the myocardial patients. *Journal of Human Stress, 1*(30), 25–38.
122. Mayou, R. A., Foster, A., & Williamson, B. (1978). Psychosocial adjustment in patients after one year after myocardial infarction. *Journal of Psychosomatic Research, 22*(5), 447–453.
123. Beck, J. S. (1995). *Cognitive therapy: Basics and beyond.* New York: Guilford.
124. Elkin, I., Shea, M. T., Watkins, J. T., et al. (1989). National Institute of Mental Health Treatment of Depression Collaborative Research Program: General effectiveness of treatments. *Archives of General Psychiatry, 46*, 971–982.
125. Agency for Health Care Policy and Research. (1993). *Depression in primary care: Detection, diagnosis and treatment.* Rockville, MD: U.S. Department of Health and Human Services.
126. Allan, R., & Scheidt, S. (1998). Group psychotherapy for patients with coronary heart disease. *International Journal of Psychotherapy, 48*, 187–214.
127. Burell, G. (1996). Group psychotherapy in Project New Life: Treatment of coronary-prone behaviors for patients who have had coronary artery bypass graft surgery. In R. Allan & S. Scheidt (Eds.), *Heart and mind: The practice of cardiac psychology* (pp. 291–310). Washington, DC: American Psychological Association.
128. Bracke, P. E., & Thoresen, C. E. (1996). Reducing Type A behavior patterns: A structured-group approach. In R. Allan & S. Scheidt (Eds.), *Heart and mind: The practice of cardiac psychology* (pp. 255–290). Washington, DC: American Psychological Association.
129. ENRICHD Investigators. (2000). Enhancing recovery in coronary heart disease patients: ENRICHD study design and methods. *American Heart Journal, 139*, 1–9.
130. Freidman, R., Myers, P., Krass, S., et al. (1996). The relaxation response: Use with cardiac patients. In R. Allan & S. Scheidt (Eds.), *Heart and mind: The practice of cardiac psychology* (pp. 363–384). Washington, DC: American Psychological Association.
131. Benson, H. (1975). *The relaxation response.* New York: William Morrow.
132. Stuart-Shor, E. M. (1999). Stress management. In *Cardiac rehabilitation: A guide to practice in the 21st century* (pp. 287–294). New York: Marcel Dekker.

133. Bourne, E. J. (1995). *The anxiety and phobia workbook.* Oakland: New Harbinger.
134. Blumenthal, J. A., Sherwood, A., & Gullette, E. C. D. (2000). Exercise and weight loss reduce blood pressure in men and women with mild hypertension. Effects on cardiovascular, metabolic, and hemodynamic functioning. *Archives of Internal Medicine, 160,* 1947–1958.
135. Stahle, A., Nordlander, R., & Bergfeldt, L. (1999). Aerobic group training improves exercise capacity and heart rate variability in elderly patients with a recent coronary event. A randomized controlled study. *European Heart Journal, 20,* 1638–1646.
136. Stein, R. A. (1996). Exercise and patient with coronary heart disease. In R. Allan & S. Scheidt (Eds.), *Heart and mind: The practice of cardiac psychology* (pp. 385–396). Washington, DC: American Psychological Association.
137. Brosse, A. L., Sheets, E. S., Lett, H. S. et al. (2002). Exercise and the treatment of depression in adults: Recent findings and future directions. *Sports Medicine, 32*(12), 741–760.
138. Hughes, J. R. (1984). Psychological effects of habitual exercise: A critical review. *Preventive Medicine, 13,* 66–78.
139. Buselli, E. F., & Stuart, E. M. (1999). Influence of psychosocial factors and biopsychosocial interventions on outcomes after myocardial infarction. *Journal of Cardiovascular Nursing, 13,* 60–72.
140. Lane, D., Carroll, D., Lip, G. Y., et al. (1999). Psychology in coronary care. *Quarterly Journal of Medicine, 92,* 425–431.
141. Fontana, A. F., Kerns, R., Rosenberg, R., et al. (1986). Exercise training for cardiac patients: Adherence, fitness and benefits. *Journal of Cardiopulmonary Rehabilitation, 6,* 4–15.
142. Byrne, A., & Byrne, D. G. (1993). The effect of exercise on depression, anxiety, and other mood states. *Journal of Psychosomatic Research, 37,* 565–574.
143. King, A., Taylor, C. B., & Haskell, W. (1993). The effects of differing intensities and formats of twelve months of exercise training on psychological outcomes. *Health Psychology, 12,* 292–302.
144. Ell, K., & Dunkel-Schetter, C. (1994). Social support and adjustment to myocardial infarction, angioplasty and coronary artery bypass surgery. In S. A. Shumacker & S. M. Czajkowski (Eds.), *Social support and cardiovascular disease* (pp. 301–322). New York: Plenum.
145. Dossey, B. M. (1997). *Core curriculum for holistic nursing.* Gaithersburg, MD: Aspen Publishers.
146. Friedwald V. E., Arnold, L. W., Carney, R. M., et al. (2007). The Editor's Roundtable: Major depression in patients with coronary heart disease. *American Journal of Cardiology, 99,* 519–529.
147. Bedsworth, J. A., & Molen, M. T. (1982). Psychological stress in spouses of patients with myocardial infarction. *Heart Lung, 11,* 450–456.
148. Bramwell, L. (1986). Wives' experiences in the support role after husbands' first myocardial infarction. *Heart Lung, 15,* 578–584.
149. Gillis, C. L. (1984). Reducing family stress during and after coronary artery bypass surgery. *Nursing Clinics of North America, 19,* 103–111.
150. Doerr, B. C., & Jones, J. W. (1979). Effect of family preparation on the state of anxiety level in CCU patient. *Nursing Research, 28,* 315–316.
151. Taylor, C. B., Bandura, A., Ewart, C., et al. (1985). Exercise testing to enhance wives' confidence in their husbands' cardiac capacity soon after clinically uncomplicated myocardial infarction. *American Journal of Cardiology, 55,* 635–638.
152. Sotile, W. M. (1999). Psychosocial risk factors: Overview, assessment and intervention for anger and hostility. In *Cardiac rehabilitation: A guide to practice in the 21st century* (pp. 257–261). New York: Marcel Dekker.
153. Powell, L. H. (1996). The hook: A metaphor for gaining control of emotional reactivity. In R. Allan & S. Scheidt (Eds.), *Heart and mind: The practice of cardiac psychology* (pp. 313–327). Washington, DC: American Psychological Association.
154. Eriksen, W. (1994). The role of social support in the pathogenesis of coronary heart disease—A literature review. *Family Practice, 11,* 201–209.
155. Sotile, W. M. (1996). *Psychosocial interventions for cardiopulmonary patients. A guide for health professionals.* Champaign, IL: Human Kinetics.
156. Nunes, E. V., Frank, K. A., & Kornfeld, D. S. (1987). Psychologic treatment for the type A behavior pattern and for coronary heart disease: A meta-analysis of the literature. *Psychosomatic Medicine, 48,* 159–173.
157. Covey, L. S., Glassman, A. H., Stetner, F., et al. (2002). A randomized trial of sertraline as a cessation aid for smokers a history of major depression. *American Journal of Psychiatry, 159,* 1731–1737.
158. Lesprance, F., & Frasure-Smith, N. (2000). Depression in patients with cardiac disease. The role of psychosomatic medicine. *Journal of Psychosomatic Research, 48,* 379–392.
159. Sauer, W. H., Berlin, J. A., & Kimmel, S. E. (2001). Selective serotonin reuptake inhibitors and myocardial infarction. *Circulation, 104,* 1894–1898.
160. Shapiro, P. A., Lesperance, F., Frasure-Smith, N., et al. (1999). An open label preliminary trial of sertraline for treatment of major depression after acute myocardial infarction (the SADHART trial). *American Heart Journal, 137,* 1100–1106.
161. Strik, J. J. M. H., Hong, A., Lousberg, R., et al. (2000). Efficacy and safety of fluoxetine in the treatment of patients with major depression after first myocardial infarction. Findings from a double blind, placebo controlled trial. *Psychosomatic Medicine, 62,* 783–789.
162. Roose, S. P. (2001). Depression, anxiety and the cardiovascular system: The psychiatrist's perspective. *Journal of Clinical Psychiatry, 62*(8), 19–22.
163. Kannel, W. B., Kannel, C., Pattenbarger Jr., R. S., et al. (1987). Heart rate and cardiovascular mortality rate—The Framingham Study. *American Heart Journal, 113,* 1489–1494.
164. Roose, S. P., Laghrissi-Thode, F., Kennedy, J. S., et al. (1998). Comparison of paroxetine and nortriptyline in depression patients with ischemic heart disease. *JAMA, 279,* 287–291.
165. Taylor, C. B., & Cameron, R. P. (1999). Psychosocial risk factors: Assessment and intervention for depression. In *Cardiac rehabilitation: A guide to practice in the 21st century* (pp. 263–277). New York: Marcel Dekker.
166. Lesperance, F., Frasure-Smith, N., Koszycki, D., et al. (2007). Effects of citalopram and interpersonal psychotherapy on depression with coronary artery disease: The Canadian Cardiac Randomized Evaluation of Antidepressant and Psychotherapy Efficacy (CREATE) trial. *JAMA, 297,* 367–379.
167. Serebrauny, V. L., Glassman, A. H., Malinin, A. I. et al. (2003). Platelet endothelial biomarkers in depressed patients treated with the selective serotonin reuptake inhibitor sertraline after acute coronary events: the Sertraline Antidepressant Heart Attack Randomized Trial Study Group. *Circulation, 108,* 939–944.

CHAPTER 34

Smoking Cessation and Relapse Prevention

Min Sohn / Mark Hawk / Kirsten Martin / Erika S. Sivarajan Froelicher

Heart disease and stroke, both forms of cardiovascular disease (CVD), continue to be the first and third leading causes of death in the United States, respectively.[1] Smoking is the most preventable risk factor that contributes to premature death of coronary heart disease (CHD). More than 4,000 known toxins and carcinogens are found in tobacco smoke, which contributes to smoking being the single, most preventable cause of disease and premature death,[2] and also exposure to secondhand smoke also contributes to this risk.[3]

The U.S. adult smoking prevalence rate has decreased from 25% to 21% since the first publication of the guideline.[4] The number of current smokers being advised to quit smoking[5] in 2007 is twice the number it was in the 1990s[6] with a greater number of smokers receiving more concentrated cessation interventions.[7,8] While Chapter 32 describes smoking as a risk factor, we provide the assessment and management of smoking cessation in this chapter.

One of the major responsibilities of the nurse is health promotion; therefore, it is important that nurses be aware that they can play a major role in smoking cessation. There is a significant body of research that has documented the effectiveness of nurse-managed smoking cessation interventions, particularly in the hospitalized cardiovascular population.[9–19] "If the 2.2 million working nurses in the U.S. each helped one person per year quit smoking, nurses would triple the U.S. quit rate."[20]

Successful smoking cessation interventions usually have behavior modification as a core component. Behavioral modification skills include identifying areas of concern for patients, teaching patients strategies to cope with difficult situations, and role-playing strategies with patients to allow them to practice their new coping strategies. These behavioral modification skills usually are not part of most nursing school curricula.[21] Even when they are taught, there is rarely an opportunity for practice, feedback, and development of confidence in performing these skills. This chapter focuses on the important steps in smoking cessation interventions that should be provided to patients with CVD, with an emphasis on behavioral and pharmacologic approaches. After reading this chapter, the nurse, no matter what setting he or she practices in—intensive care unit, cardiac care unit, medical–surgical, labor and delivery, outpatient care—will posses the necessary knowledge to provide a smoking cessation intervention to every patient who smokes, every time the patient is encountered.

Permanent smoking cessation should be the goal for every intervention and every person who smokes. Achievement of this goal is difficult, however, because the nicotine in tobacco products is an addictive substance.[22] Smokers are physically and emotionally compelled to continue smoking even in the face of serious adverse health consequences. In addition, multiple quit attempts and failure to quit smoking despite high levels of motivation are common. The presence of withdrawal symptoms is another indicator of the addictive properties of nicotine. The criteria for diagnosis of nicotine withdrawal are met when any of the following symptoms commence within 24 hours of the abrupt cessation of nicotine use: dysphoric or depressed mood; insomnia; irritability, frustration, or anger; anxiety; difficulty concentrating; restlessness; decreased heart rate; or increased appetite or weight gain.[23] Rapid identification of these withdrawal symptoms and prompt intervention are important skills for all nurses, particularly hospital-based nurses, because these withdrawal symptoms may be so intense for a given patient that he or she is unable to make rational health care decisions and may leave the hospital against medical advice to relieve them with a cigarette.

HARMFUL EFFECTS OF SMOKING

Cigarette smoking, hypercholesterolemia, hypertension, and physical inactivity are considered the four major risk factors for CVD. What makes cigarette smoking unique among these risk factors is that it interacts synergistically with hypercholesterolemia and hypertension to increase greatly the risk for CHD. For example, in people who smoke and have hypercholesterolemia or hypertension, the risk for CHD is doubled. For people who have all three risk factors, the risk for CHD is quadrupled.[24]

In general, cigarette smoking accelerates atherosclerosis throughout the body, but this effect is most important in the coronary arteries, the aorta, and the carotid and cerebral arteries. Several mechanisms have been described to explain how cigarette smoking leads to atherosclerosis. These include (1) adverse effects on lipid profiles; (2) endothelial damage or dysfunction; (3) hemodynamic stress; (4) oxidative injury; (5) neutrophil activation; (6) enhanced thrombosis; and (7) increased blood viscosity.[25]

Although the acceleration of atherosclerosis is a major contributor to cardiovascular morbidity (e.g., aggravation of stable angina pectoris, vasospastic angina, intermittent claudication), a major focus in the population of smokers with CVD is how smoking mediates acute cardiovascular events (e.g., myocardial infarction [MI], sudden death, stroke) that lead to hospitalization. The smoking-related mechanisms thought to contribute to these events are (1) induction of a hypercoagulable state; (2) increased myocardial workload; (3) reduced oxygen-carrying capacity of the blood; (4) coronary vasoconstriction; and (5) catecholamine release.[25]

Nicotine and carbon monoxide, although only two of the more than 4,000 chemicals in cigarette smoke, are generally considered to be the major contributors to atherosclerotic disease.[26] Nicotine disrupts lipid metabolism, resulting in an increased level of low-density lipoprotein and a decreased level of high-density lipoprotein. Nicotine is also responsible for the increased platelet aggregation and hypercoagulability found in smokers. In addition, it leads to increased production of catecholamines, which in turn increases blood pressure, heart rate and contractility, and systemic vascular resistance, all of which result in increased myocardial oxygen demand.[25,27] Unfortunately, meeting this demand is difficult because cigarette smoking constricts large and small epicardial arteries and coronary resistance vessels, leading to a decrease in coronary blood flow.[28] In fact, in a study of patients with established CHD, Barry et al.[29] found that continued cigarette smoking was related to a 12-fold increase in the amount of total ischemia daily. Episodes of ischemic ST-segment depression occurred 3 times as often, and the duration was 12 times longer in smokers compared with nonsmokers (median duration of 24 min/24 h vs. 2 min/24 h). This increased ischemia may be related to the increased probability of recurrent coronary events in people who smoke. The increase in heart rate may also lead to endothelial injury, myocardial ischemia and MI, arrhythmias, and sudden death.[25]

Carbon monoxide interferes with oxygen transport, leading to a reduced supply of oxygen to the tissues, and, more important, to the myocardium at a time when the demand is high because of a higher heart rate.[26] Carbon monoxide interferes with the oxygen-carrying capacity of red blood cells by binding to hemoglobin, thereby reducing the amount of hemoglobin available for binding with oxygen and by impeding oxygen release from hemoglobin.[25] Carbon monoxide also increases the permeability of endothelial membranes, resulting in increased uptake of cholesterol that leads to atherogenesis.[27]

When the number of cigarettes smoked daily, the total number of years of smoking, the degree of inhalation, and the age of smoking initiation are considered, the risk for development of CHD is found to increase with increasing exposure to cigarette smoke. Overall, cigarette smokers have a two- to four-fold greater incidence of CHD than do nonsmokers, and cigarette smokers have a 70% greater death rate caused by CHD than do nonsmokers. Cigarette smokers also experience a two- to four-fold greater risk of sudden death than do nonsmokers.[27] The damage caused by cigarette smoking is not restricted to the heart alone. Cigarette smokers have a higher incidence of arteriosclerotic peripheral arterial disease and more severe atherosclerosis of the aorta than do nonsmokers,[26] as well as an increased rate of stroke and cerebrovascular disease.[27]

BENEFITS OF SMOKING CESSATION

The health benefits of smoking cessation on the cardiovascular system are well documented. The increased tendency to thrombus formation, coronary artery spasm, arrhythmias, and reduced oxygen supply are likely to reverse in a short time.[30] For example, evidence suggests that quitting smoking after an initial MI decreases a person's risk of death from CHD by at least 50% in the first year after quitting.[31]

This decline in risk appears to be independent of the severity of the MI.[32] In addition, reports from the Coronary Artery Surgery Study (CASS) indicate that smoking cessation significantly improves survival for people of all ages, including those older than 70 years.[33] In fact, after 1 year of abstinence from smoking, the excess risk of CHD related to smoking is cut in half and then gradually continues to decline over time. After 15 years of abstinence, the former smoker has achieved a risk level similar to that of a person who has never smoked. Smoking cessation also lowers the overall risk for stroke to that of a nonsmoker within 5 to 15 years of abstinence.[26]

Because the overall death rate and rate of reinfarction is higher in patients with established CHD, intensive smoking cessation intervention should be directed to this population. Nurses who provide care for patients with CVD in all practice settings must not miss the opportunity to encourage smokers to quit at every encounter. In addition to the smoking cessation efforts of public education, commercial programs, and worksite health promotion, efforts to assist patients who have manifestations of CHD in the primary care setting are worthwhile.

THEORETICAL FRAMEWORK FOR SMOKING CESSATION

The model we advocate for smoking cessation is the self-efficacy model based on social cognitive learning theory by Bandura.[34] Self-efficacy, in the case of smoking cessation, is defined as the smoker's level of confidence that he or she could refrain from smoking in various challenging or "risky" situations such as social situations (with friends in a cafe, when someone offers them a cigarette), emotional situations (when feeling tense or depressed), and habitual–addictive situations (when desiring a cigarette or when they are experiencing withdrawal symptoms).[35] The belief is that as risky situations are identified, strategies can be developed by the patient in conjunction with his or her health care provider that will help the patient to either avoid or cope with a given situation. Low self-efficacy is a strong predictor of relapse to smoking[16,36]; therefore, it behooves the health care provider to assess self-efficacy and provide coping skills and strategies to help the smoker successfully navigate those situations where they are most at risk to smoke.

Self-efficacy in various situations, however, is easily assessed in the clinical setting. It has recently been hypothesized, however, that self-efficacy is intertwined with the patient's smoking behaviors and fluctuates over the course of the quit attempt. In other words, when the patient is initially attempting to quit, self-efficacy may be low to moderate; as the patient successfully abstains from smoking, self-efficacy increases; self-efficacy may then decrease with a relapse and increase with renewed cessation. This cycle would continue to fluctuate until permanent smoking cessation has been achieved which would lead, theoretically, to continuously high self-efficacy. Unfortunately, self-efficacy has rarely been measured more than once or twice in a clinical trial, so this hypothesis requires further testing.[17] In the mean time, however, self-efficacy can be used clinically to help guide the intervention and is especially helpful in relapse prevention. The identification of risky situations, strategies to deal with risky situations, and relapse prevention are discussed in greater detail in the section titled "Relapse Prevention."

SMOKING CESSATION INTERVENTIONS IN THE CHD POPULATION

The recent trials have had larger study populations, used more clearly defined definitions for abstinence, and saliva or serum cotinine levels or expired carbon monoxide levels have been used to biochemically verify nonsmoking status. Only recently have randomized clinical trials been conducted in women with

CHD.[13–18,36–38] When the physician provides simple advice to the patient, the expected cessation rate in the general population is approximately 6% per year,[39] whereas group programs that use behavioral methods may achieve yearly cessation rates as high as 26% to 40%.[40] In the CHD population, in particular, the strong stimulus provided by a CHD event results in rates of smoking cessation that are higher than in most studies conducted in the general population.[41–43] In particular, studies on those patients having coronary artery bypass graft surgery show smoking cessation rates of approximately 50%,[44,45] whereas those undergoing coronary arteriography have smoking cessation rates of up to 62%.[46] Finally, studies of patients with an MI or angina pectoris reported smoking cessation rates of between 20% and 70%.[9,41,43,47,48]

A significant body of research has also focused on nurse-managed smoking cessation interventions that begin in the hospital and then continue with telephone follow-up after discharge from the hospital. The effectiveness of this type of intervention has been demonstrated in patients after MI[41] and cancer surgery[49] and in patients admitted to the hospital.[50]

In general, research indicates that those patients with high motivation or strong intention to quit,[45,46] more severe disease,[46] who were given strong advice to quit by their physician,[41,50] who have CVD[50] are male,[10] have made fewer attempts to quit in the past, and who had no difficulty refraining from smoking while in the hospital[45] achieved the highest smoking cessation rates. Patients with CHD who continue to smoke are in general younger,[51] female, unmarried/not living with a partner,[10,51] belong to a lower socioeconomic[10,52] and educational level, have a less negative attitude about smoking, smoke a greater number of cigarettes, and are more likely to be anxious or depressed.[52] Although effective interventions have been conducted to address some of these characteristics, interventions aimed at people of lower educational and socioeconomic status are still lacking.[53]

GENERAL TRENDS IN SMOKING CESSATION INTERVENTIONS

The public health approach to smoking cessation that has predominated in the smoking literature in the 1990s has primarily targeted populations or high-risk groups in their natural environments, such as worksites. Public health interventions are usually brief, low-cost, and are often provided by laypeople or through automated means (e.g., mail, contests).

Clinical approaches, however, are targeted to people who are self-referred or recruited, are most commonly applied in a medical or group setting, use trained professionals, and provide intensive multisession interventions. Because patients with CHD are at risk for recurrent cardiac events, such as another MI, a clinical approach is more cost-effective for this population—it is cheaper to help patients quit smoking than to hospitalize them for a repeat MI.[54]

Many intensive group smoking cessation programs are offered, but most smokers prefer to quit on their own or with individualized support.[55] For example, in a study of cardiovascular patients admitted to the hospital who were smoking at the time of admission, 86% expressed an interest in quitting. However, of the 86% who were interested in quitting, 79% stated they were interested in quitting on their own, with 50% expressing interest in the use of self-help materials. Fewer than 10% of patients endorsed a formal treatment program.[56] The international literature also supports these findings. One study of Korean men who were hospitalized with CVD found that 84% wanted to quit smoking, but 88% of them were interested in quitting on their own. However, surprisingly 51% were willing to participate in a formal, educational, smoking cessation program, if those programs were available during their hospitalization.[57,58]

The literature also supports the fact that 90% of all smokers eventually quit on their own, normally after three to four unsuccessful attempts.[59] It therefore behooves nurses to consider methods that may be individualized to patient needs, combining a clinical approach with multicomponent strategies without requiring patients to attend a formal treatment program.

TREATING TOBACCO USE AND DEPENDENCE: CLINICAL PRACTICE GUIDELINE

As the body of knowledge about the health consequences of smoking and the health benefits of smoking cessation grow, smoking cessation interventions play an even greater role in decreasing smoking-related cardiovascular morbidity and mortality. The Treating Tobacco Use and Dependence Guideline Panel of 1996, 2000, and 2008 developed clinical practice guidelines for tobacco cessation.[60–62] These guidelines provide an evidence-based recommendation for interventions for all smokers regardless of their intention to quit at the present time. The guidelines acknowledge that tobacco dependence is a chronic condition of dependence frequently requiring repeated interventions and that behavioral and pharmacologic interventions are cost-effective. The guidelines provide recommendations for primary care clinicians, smoking cessation specialists, and health care administrators, insurers, and purchasers. These recommendations are especially pertinent to the cardiovascular nurse because of the extensive contact nurses have with patients to initiate smoking cessation counseling.

So the guidelines[60–62] have established five major intervention steps also known as the "5As." These are (1) ask about tobacco use; (2) advise the patient to quit; (3) assess willingness to make a quit attempt; (4) assist in the quit attempt; and (5) arrange follow-up. Examples of how to implement a brief smoking cessation intervention outlined in the pocket guide, *Helping Smokers Quit: A Guide for Clinicians*[63] consistent with the guidelines[60–62] follow.

Step 1: Ask—Systematically Identify All Tobacco Users at Every Visit

To identify every smoker every time he or she is seen by a clinician, a system-wide structure must be put in place. It can be as simple as adding assessment of smoking status to the routine vital signs (heart rate, blood pressure, respiratory rate, temperature) at every visit. To ensure that the smoking status question is asked every time, preprinted progress notes can be used, vital sign stamps can be made, special stickers indicating smoking status can be placed on the outside of charts, and for those with computer charting, a query of smoking status can be inserted into the data collection tool. To obtain this information on patients who are hospitalized, smoking status must be asked as part of the routine admission questionnaire or, as in the outpatient setting, assessed with initial vital signs. It is especially important to identify hospitalized smokers because hospital policies prohibit smoking. If not identified, these patients may go through severe nicotine withdrawal unnecessarily, which may lead to noncompliance with treatments and, in the extreme case, a patient leaving against medical advice.

The roles of the nurse and the physician need to be clearly identified in each setting. It is thus important that physicians and nurses, as well as all other health care professionals, assess their level of comfort in offering advice and, if necessary, receive training on how to counsel people. Simply bringing up the subject may seem overwhelming to health care professionals. Simple ways to introduce the subject are shown in Display 34-1.

Step 2: Advise—Strongly Urge All Smokers to Quit

Smokers tend to deny anything but the most direct advice and clear-cut message about quitting. Therefore, the first step in the process of providing help to a smoker is to give him or her a clear, strong, and personalized message about quitting, such as "Your smoking is harming your health. As your nurse, I need to tell you that smoking is your major risk factor for cardiovascular disease. Continuing to smoke will lead to further cardiovascular disease and possibly death. Together, we must figure out how to help you become a nonsmoker." Clear and strong, however, is not enough. The message must be personalized. Make your message relevant to the smoker's current concerns about his or her health, disease status, family or social situation, age, sex, and past smoking behaviors. For example, if a patient is hospitalized for a coronary angioplasty, it is necessary for him or her to know that continued smoking is associated with an increased restenosis rate. Follow this with information about the health risks associated with continuing to smoke (see the section titled "Harmful Effects of Smoking") and the health and social benefits of smoking cessation (see the section titled "Benefits of Smoking Cessation"). Display 34-2 illustrates how a smoker may interpret an inadequate message.

DISPLAY 34-1 How to Ask About Smoking Status

Initial Assessment

"We're interested in knowing about your lifestyle and habits as they relate to your health. Have you ever smoked in your life? Are you still smoking?" or "Over the course of a lifetime, many people pick up the smoking habit. Have you ever smoked? Do you still smoke?"

Follow-Up

If the patient was not ready to quit at the last visit: "I'm sure it must be difficult, but have you seriously considered making an attempt to quit smoking since your last visit?"

If the patient was in the precontemplation stage at the last visit: "At your last visit, you were seriously thinking about quitting smoking. Were you able to cut down on the number of cigarettes you smoke, or were you successful at quitting since your last visit?"

If the patient was in the action stage at the last visit: "Have you had any problems in refraining from smoking since your last visit?"

DISPLAY 34-2 How a Smoker may Interpret an Inadequate Message

If You Say:	The Smoker May Think:
You probably should stop smoking.	I guess I don't have to stop smoking.
You are older, but stopping smoking may help anyway.	I don't have much time to live, so why stop smoking now?
The surgery has restored your circulation to normal.	Good. Now I don't have to quit smoking.

Step 3: Assess—Identify Smokers Willing to Make a Quit Attempt

After providing advice, it is important to determine if the patient is willing to quit smoking at this time. Willingness to quit can be measured through a simple yes/no question, such as "Are you willing to quit smoking now?" Another measure of a patient's willingness to quit smoking can be assessed using an intention question, "Do you intend to stay off cigarettes or other tobacco products in the next month?" The patient can respond on a 7-point scale ranging from 1 (*definitely no*) to 7 (*definitely yes*). Patients who score a three or less usually are not interested or ready to quit.[9] If the patient is willing to quit, provide a brief or more intensive intervention according to patient's preference.

If patients are unwilling to quit, it is important to determine why. In some cases, patients may not have enough information about associated risks. Whatever the barrier, providing help or solutions to anticipated problems may encourage the patient to think further about quitting, helping the patients to identify the barriers to quitting now.

If the patient clearly states that he or she is not willing to quit at the present time, do not give up; instead, provide a motivational intervention. The guidelines[60–62] recommends using the "5Rs": (1) relevance, (2) risks, (3) rewards, (4) roadblocks, and (5) repetition. To ensure that the 5Rs are as individualized and personally motivational as possible, it is important to have the patient self-identify in conjunction with the provider their own relevance, risks, rewards, and roadblocks. To make an intervention relevant and meaningful to a patient, discuss smoking cessation in light of the patient's disease status, family or social situation, age, sex, and other characteristics unique to the patient. Three types of risks should be addressed with the patient. Acute risks include shortness of breath and exacerbation of asthma. Long-term risks include heart attack, stroke, cancer, and chronic obstructive pulmonary disease. Environmental risks include risks that put the patient's children and other family members at risk for lung cancer, sudden infant death syndrome, and asthma. The rewards of smoking cessation should also be discussed with the patient. These include improved health, energy level, sense of smell and taste, self-esteem, economic savings, reduced wrinkling/aging of skin, modeling nonsmoking for children, as well as freedom from worry about the effect the patient's smoking has on his or her children and other family members. Roadblocks or barriers to quitting that need to be identified with the patient include withdrawal symptoms, fear of failure, weight gain, lack of social support, living with a smoker, depression, and loss of tobacco. Finally, repetition is included because the relevance, risks, and rewards need to be reviewed with the patient every time he or she is seen because on any given visit, the patient may finally be receptive to a smoking cessation intervention.

Step 4: Assist—Aid the Patient in Quitting

Setting a Quit Date and Planning for an Intervention

The first step in assisting the patient ready to quit smoking involves establishing a quit plan. Components of a quit plan include (1) setting a quit date; (2) telling family, friends, and coworkers about quitting and the desire for support; (3) anticipating challenges to remaining smoke free; and (4) removing tobacco products from home and work settings. In regard to setting a quit date, if a patient is motivated, setting a quit date within 2 weeks of meeting with the health care provider is most appropriate. Some patients, however, prefer to quit suddenly, or "cold turkey." If the smoker is identified in the hospital, setting a quit date is not necessary because the patient has become an ex-smoker because of the hospital smoking ban. Some programs have patients monitor the situations that cause them to smoke before they quit or reduce the number of cigarettes in the weeks before quitting. These techniques, however, although helpful to some, may simply prolong the process of quitting. Signing a contract at this point is a behavioral technique that has proved effective in helping patients to quit smoking. This process helps to formalize the smoker's commitment to quitting and can serve as a method by which the nurse extends support to the patient in this process. Contracts must be simple and explicitly written so that both parties agree with the stated terms, and they should specify the consequences of not adhering to the expected behavior (see the section titled "Harmful Effects of Smoking") and the rewards of successful adherence (see the section titled "Benefits of Smoking Cessation").

The guidelines[60–62] recommend that five major components be a part of a brief intervention. These include (1) provision of practical counseling such as problem solving, skills training, relapse prevention, and stress management; (2) provision of social support directly by the provider (intratreatment social support); (3) helping the patient obtain social support outside of the clinical setting (extratreatment social support); (4) recommending the use of approved pharmacotherapy, except in special circumstances; and (5) provision of supplementary materials. Practical counseling components include helping patients identify and anticipate "danger situations," such as events, activities, and internal states that increase the risk for smoking relapse, for example, negative affect, being with or living with another smoker, drinking alcohol, and stress. Coping strategies to review with patients include anticipatory planning, avoidance, and stress reduction. When providing practical counseling, it is also imperative to advise patients that smoking, even one puff of a cigarette, increases the likelihood of a complete relapse to smoking. Other information that is useful to patients attempting to quit smoking includes the addictive nature of smoking,[64] potential withdrawal symptoms, and that they can expect withdrawal symptoms to reach maximal intensity within 24 to 48 hours and then gradually subside over a 1- to 2-week period. The provision of intratreatment support is the simple act of providing the patient with encouragement, showing the patient that you care about them and their health, and giving the patient the opportunity to talk about their quit attempt (concerns, fears, successes). The provision of extratreatment social support includes encouraging family members and significant others to support the patient in the quit attempt and, if appropriate, providing a simultaneous smoking cessation intervention to household members who smoke. It is especially important to address this with women living with another smoker, because living with a smoker is a strong predictor of relapse in women.[16] It may also include role-playing with the patient how he or she will ask for the support that is needed, identifying and referring patient to community resources such as hotlines, Web sites, or group meetings, and helping patients find "cessation buddies" with whom they can work. Provision of effective pharmacotherapies is strongly recommended and is discussed in greater detail later. Finally, as the patient leaves the health care setting, it is strongly advised that they take with them supplemental information in the form of pamphlets that are culturally, racially, educationally, and age appropriate for the patient. Patients then need follow-up in the form of face-to-face or telephone contacts.[61,62]

When planning a smoking cessation intervention, the nurse should take into account the patient's desire for formal help. Literature on compliance suggests that when the patient participates in developing a personalized plan of action, greater follow-through is achieved (Chapter 40). Because most people choose individual methods for cessation, providing self-help materials is a low-cost method of intervention. When combined with strong advice by the nurse, these materials often double success rates. For the cardiac patient, the American Heart Association's *An Active Partnership for the Health of Your Heart* offers effective multimedia materials, including a videotape, audiotape, and workbook.[65] Other self-help materials, like those from the U.S. Department of Health and Human Services,[66] Tobacco Free Nurses,[63] the American Cancer Society, and the American Lung Association, along with information for the nurse, are listed at the end of this chapter.

Although most patients choose to quit on their own with minimal help, some patients prefer, and may benefit from, a group program that provides 8 to 10 weeks of behavior modification. Knowing available community resources and making them available to patients by providing them with a list of programs to choose from, including the intervention methods, costs, and a contact person, ensures that patients are adequately informed. The patient may also be encouraged to address the issue with his or her employer, because many larger employers offer smoking cessation programs as an employee benefit.

Occasionally, patients may decide that acupuncture or hypnosis is a viable alternative. The success rates of these types of smoking cessation interventions, however, have been shown to be no better than placebo.[61] Some patients, however, anecdotally report these methods to be helpful. If a patient chooses a group cessation program or an alternative intervention, referral should be made and follow-up scheduled to determine the success of the chosen intervention. It is important to note that although the majority of smokers will express the desire to quit on their own, this strategy has proven to be of limited success; therefore, it behooves the health care provider to encourage a combination of self-help and more intensive strategies including pharmacological therapy (Tables 34-1 and 34-2).

Table 34-1 ■ EFFECTIVENESS AND ABSTINENCE RATES FOR VARIOUS MEDICATIONS AND MEDICATION COMBINATIONS COMPARED TO PLACEBO AT 6-MONTH POSTQUIT (*N* = 86 STUDIES)

Medication	Number of Arms*	Estimated Abstinence Rate (95% CI)
Placebo	80	13.8
Monotherapies		
Varenicline (2 mg/day)	5	33.2 (28.9, 37.8)
Nicotine nasal spray	4	26.7 (21.5, 32.7)
High-dose nicotine patch (>25 mg) (these included both standard or long-term duration)	4	26.5 (21.3, 32.5)
Long-term nicotine gum (>14 weeks)	6	26.1 (19.7, 33.6)
Varenicline (1 mg/day)	3	25.4 (19.6, 32.2)
Nicotine inhaler	6	24.8 (19.1, 31.6)
Clonidine	3	25.0 (15.7, 37.3)

Reprinted from U.S. Department of Health and Human Services (2008) *Treating tobacco use and dependence: Clinical practice guideline, 2008 update.* Washington, DC: Government Printing Office.

Relapse Prevention

A major component of successful smoking cessation interventions for patients who have recently quit is relapse prevention training,[67] which involves (1) identifying the patient's high-risk situations; (2) providing skills training to help the patient cope with these situations; and (3) rehearsing the coping mechanisms. Relapse prevention is a key because the majority of relapses occur early after initiation of cessation, primarily within the first 3 months after treatment, but risk for relapse continues long after the initial quit date, leading many to conclude that there is no safe point beyond which relapse does not occur.[68] Although a variety of predictors for relapse have been identified, stress, high nicotine dependence, low self-efficacy, limited social support, etc., are the strongest clues to probable relapse within 60 days after cessation.[68]

The guidelines[61,62] divide relapse prevention into two categories, minimal practice interventions and prescriptive interventions. A minimal practice intervention should be provided to the patient who has recently quit every time their health care provider sees them. The provider must congratulate the patient on his or her successes, assist in problem solving and any difficulties that have occurred or are anticipated, and strongly encourage the patient to remain a nonsmoker. A prescriptive relapse prevention intervention is a more in-depth evaluation of potential high-risk situations, support systems, depression, withdrawal symptoms, and motivation to remain a nonsmoker and can be delivered in person or over the telephone.

Two useful ways to help patients identify their personal high-risk situations are self-monitoring and self-efficacy scales. Through self-monitoring, patients keep a record of each cigarette smoked, noting the time of day, situation during which they smoke, and a rating of mood. A thorough examination of this record can be used to identify patterns of smoking behavior. Self-efficacy scales, however, measure a patient's confidence to resist the urge to smoke in a variety of situations. Studies have shown that self-efficacy ratings in smoking are predictive of subsequent outcome and, when smoking is resumed, specific situations or contexts are frequently predictive of a relapse episode.[69] In fact, the specific context (negative affect, positive affect, restricted smoking, idle time, social/food situations, low arousal, and craving) with the lowest self-efficacy rating proves to be the best predictor of relapse or a sort of "Achilles heel."[70] A 14-item

Table 34-2 ■ SUGGESTIONS FOR THE CLINICAL USE OF PHARMACOTHERAPIES FOR SMOKING CESSATION*

Pharmacotherapy	Adverse Effects	Dosage	Duration
SR bupropion hydrochloride *Precaution* History of seizure, history of eating disorders	Insomnia, dry mouth, seizures	150 mg every morning for 3 days, then 150 mg twice daily (begin treatment 1–2 weeks prequit)	7–12 weeks Maintenance up to 6 months
Nicotine gum	Mouth soreness, dyspepsia	1–24 cigarettes/day: 2 mg gum (up to 24 pieces/day); ≥25 cigarettes/day: 4 mg gum (up to 24 pieces/day)	Up to 12 weeks
Nicotine inhaler	Local irritation of mouth and throat	6–16 cartridges/day	Up to 6 months
Nicotine lozenge	Nausea/heartburn	Time to first cigarette >30 min: 2 mg lozenge Time to first cigarette ≤30 min: 4 mg lozenge Between 4 and 20 lozenges/day	Up to 12 weeks
Nicotine nasal spray	Nasal irritation	8–40 doses/day	3–6 months
Nicotine patch	Local skin reaction, insomnia	Ex. 21 mg/24 h, 14 mg/24 h, 7 mg/24 h Ex. 15 mg/16 h	4 weeks then 2 weeks then 2 weeks 8 weeks
Varenicline *Precaution* Significant kidney disease Patients on dialysis	Nausea/trouble sleeping, abnormal or vivid/strange dreams, depressed mood and other psychiatric symptoms	0.5 mg/day for 3 days 0.5 mg twice/day for 4 days. Then, 1 mg twice/day (Begin treatment 1 week prequit)	3–6 months

*The information contained in this table is not comprehensive. See package inserts for additional information including safety information.

Reprinted from U.S. Department of Health and Human Services. (2008). *Treating tobacco use and dependence: Clinical practice guideline, 2008 update.* Washington, DC: Government Printing Office.

How confident are you that you can resist the urge to smoke in the 14 situations below?

Not at All Confident			Slightly Confident			Fairly Confident			Very Confident	
0%	10%	20%	30%	40%	50%	60%	70%	80%	90%	100%

1. When you feel bored or depressed ____________
2. When you see others smoking ____________
3. When you want to relax or rest ____________
4. When you just want to sit back and enjoy a cigarette ____________
5. When you are watching TV ____________
6. When you are driving or riding in a car ____________
7. When you have finished a meal or snack ____________
8. When you feel frustrated, worried, upset, tense, nervous, angry, anxious, or annoyed ____________
9. When you want to snack, but don't want to gain weight ____________
10. When you need more energy or can't concentrate ____________
11. When someone offers you a cigarette ____________
12. When you are drinking coffee or tea ____________
13. When you are in a situation where alcohol is involved ____________
14. When you feel smoking is part of your self-image ____________

■ **Figure 34-1** The Confidence Questionnaire (Modified Form). (Reprinted with permission from Condiotte, M. M., & Lichtenstein, E. [1981]. Self-efficacy and relapse in smoking cessation programs. *Journal of Consulting and Clinical Psychology, 49*, 648–658).

self-efficacy scale, which is a shorter version of the scale by Condiotte and Lichtenstein,[69] is illustrated in Figure 34-1.

Less than 70% confidence for a given efficacy item denotes a high-risk situation for which patients may require help.[9,14] Patients are taught to work on those situations in which they show the least confidence to resist smoking. After identification of high-risk situations, skills training helps people mobilize their resources by developing cognitive and behavioral strategies to cope with the situation. Tsoh et al.[71] recommend teaching patients to cope with urges to smoke by using the ACE (avoid, cope, escape) strategies. For example, if a patient does not feel ready to handle a risky situation, encourage the patient to avoid it until the patient's confidence in his or her ability to handle that particular risky situation improves. If a patient routinely watches football at a smoke-filled sports bar, tell him or her to invite some nonsmoking friends over to his or her home to watch the game. If a patient is going to a restaurant, he or she can ask to sit in the nonsmoking section, thereby avoiding the option to smoke. If a patient cannot avoid a risky situation, then coping with it is the next step. Possible coping strategies include distraction, incompatible behaviors, and positive self-talk. Distraction from the urge to smoke can be achieved by going for a walk, telephoning a friend, reading, or any other activity that gets the patient's mind off smoking until the urge subsides. Behaviors that are incompatible with smoking include chewing gum, snacking on low-calorie, low-fat foods, or engaging in tasks that occupy the hands, like knitting, sewing, woodworking, or crossword puzzles. Positive self-talk involves the patient telling himself or herself that he or she can continue to be a nonsmoker. For example, a patient may say, "I can do this. I am capable of remaining a nonsmoker. I have the power to improve my health by remaining a nonsmoker." Other things a patient can do include reminding himself or herself about the health risks of cigarette smoking, the health benefits of quitting, and the monetary savings.

If the patient cannot avoid or cope with a risky situation, escape is the next option. "Escape" means getting out of a risky situation without a puff. For example, if the patient is at a party with friends, the patient can socialize with nonsmokers in attendance instead of stepping outside with smokers. When dining out with others, escape can mean stepping outside while the others smoke after-dinner cigarettes. It is important to stress to the patient that a combination of strategies (ACE) is essential. By having many strategies, the patient decreases the risk of being caught in a situation he or she is not prepared to handle. The last step in relapse prevention training is practicing the coping response through rehearsal. Even though an urge may occur, if the patient is prepared to handle the situation, it decreases the likelihood that he or she will pick up a cigarette. One nursing responsibility includes practicing the different strategies to strengthen coping responses by role-playing with the patient a solution to handle the high-risk situation.

In addition to the strategies developed for specific situations, relapse prevention training focuses on general lifestyle modifications that help to enhance the patient's self-control.[67] Frequent assessment of dependence to smoking is useful and can guide the intensity of follow-up intervention. To measure the level of nicotine addiction, clinicians can ask to patients "time to first cigarette" in the morning. If patients smoke their first cigarette in the morning within 30 minutes of waking, it indicates a high level of nicotine dependence. Time to first cigarette is one of the six questions on the Fagerstrom Test for Nicotine Dependence,[72] and it is known that this single item reliably indicates the level of nicotine addiction (Fig. 34-2).[73] Exercise and relaxation techniques are two such strategies that have been used successfully to help patients develop a greater sense of self-control. In a study of patients after MI, smokers participating in an exercise training program combined with smoking cessation had greater cessation rates and smoked significantly fewer cigarettes than those who did not participate in such a program.[74] Exercise may also help reduce weight gain after quitting smoking and may minimize some withdrawal symptoms. For these reasons, patients should be encouraged to increase their activity levels through walking or other forms of exercise. Finally, patients who enjoy occasional social drinking should be encouraged to avoid using alcohol while attempting to become a

Question	Answers	Points
1. How soon after you wake up do you smoke your first cigarette?	Within 5 minutes	3
	6–30 minutes	2
	31–60 minutes	1
	After 60 minutes	0
2. Do you find it difficult to refrain from smoking in places where it is forbidden (e.g., in church, at the library, in the cinema, etc.)?	Yes	1
	No	0
3. Which cigarette would you hate most to give up?	The first on in the morning	1
	All others	0
4. How many cigarettes/day do you smoke?	10 or less	0
	11–20	1
	21–30	2
	31 or more	3
5. Do you smoke more frequently during the first hours after waking than during the rest of the day?	Yes	1
	No	0
6. Do you smoke if you are so ill that you are in bed most of the day?	Yes	1
	No	0

Total score ranges from 0 to 10.
Total score of greater than 7 indicates nicotine dependence.

■ **Figure 34-2** The Fagerstrom tolerance test. (Reprinted with permission from Heatherton, T., Kozlowski, L., Frecker, R., et al. [1991]. The Fagerstrom Test for Nicotine Dependence: A revision of the Fagerstrom Tolerance Questionnaire. *British Journal of Addiction, 86,* 1119–1127.)

nonsmoker, because alcohol consumption is an independent predictor of relapse to smoking.[75] Alcohol consumption and its relationship to smoking cessation are further discussed later.

Pharmacologic Therapy

The most important development since the last guideline has been the additional option of varenicline (Chantix), a nicotine receptor antagonist. The guidelines[61,62] recommend that *all* patients expressing the desire to quit smoking receive both counseling and pharmacotherapy, except when medication use is contraindicated or with specific populations in which medication use has not been shown to be effective such as pregnant or breast-feeding women, adolescents, smokeless tobacco users, light smokers (those smoking fewer than 10 cigarettes per day), and those with medical contraindications such as recent MI or worsening angina. Through meta-analysis, seven first-line pharmacotherapies were determined to be safe and efficacious, leading to cessation rates approximately double those of placebo. These are nicotine patch, nicotine gum, nicotine inhaler, nicotine nasal spray, nicotine lozenge, sustained-release (SR) bupropion and varenicline. Each of these first-line agents has received the U.S. Food and Drug Administration (FDA) *The 2008 Guideline* interestingly reported the different effectiveness among these agents. Comparing placebo as a reference group, combination therapy of nicotine patch and *ad libitum* nicotine replacement therapy (NRT) (gum or spray) presented highest abstinence rate followed by varenicline. However, other agents did not show statistically significant difference (Table 34-1). The nicotine patch, gum, and lozenge are available over the counter. The other forms of NRT are available by prescription only. The first-line agents are discussed below.

Varenicline. Varenicline (Chantix) is newly approved as a non-nicotine medication by the U.S. FDA for smoking cessation (Table 34-2).[62] Its mechanism of action is assumed to be a partial nicotine receptor agonist and antagonist effect. Varenicline is available by prescription only. The abstinence rates for varenicline are three times greater than for placebo, and varenicline is about one and a half times more effective than nicotine patch.

Like bupropion, smokers need to take varenicline 1 week before the quit date. Varenicline is well tolerated for periods up to 1 year.[76] Unlike bupropion, varenicline is not recommended for use in combination with NRT because of its nicotine antagonist properties. Varenicline is relatively well tolerated in most patients. However, recent studies reported incidents of exacerbations of preexisting psychiatric illness, schizophrenia, and bipolar illness, in patients who took varenicline.[77,78] Therefore, it is important that patients are carefully monitored while taking varenicline and this includes that patients be advised to tell their health care provider about any history of psychiatric illness prior to starting this medication. Clinicians need to monitor patients for any changes in mood and behavior when prescribing this medication. In February 2008, the FDA warned that depressed mood, agitation, changes in behavior, suicidal ideation, and suicide have been reported in patients attempting to quit smoking while using varenicline. In addition, varenicline should be used with caution in patients with severe renal dysfunction (creatinine clearance <30 mL/min), since varenicline is eliminated almost entirely unchanged in the urine.

Bupropion. Another alternative to NRT is SR bupropion (Zyban SR; GlaxoSmithKline, Research Triangle Park, North Carolina), an oral medication that comes in tablet form. This pharmacologic aid for smoking cessation has been used for many years to treat depression. The exact mechanism that promotes smoking cessation is unknown. Bupropion is, however, a weak inhibitor of neuronal uptake of dopamine, serotonin, and norepinephrine.[79] It is believed to affect the mesolimbic dopaminergic system and, therefore, mediates reward for nicotine use.[80] Like

NRT, bupropion produces cessation rates approximately double those of placebo (Table 34-1).

Unlike NRT, bupropion treatment should be initiated while the patient is still smoking, because it takes approximately 1 week of treatment to achieve steady-state blood levels of bupropion. A target quit date should be established in the second week of treatment to promote the highest likelihood of cessation. Treatment with bupropion SR should last a minimum of 7 to 12 weeks and can be maintained up to 6 months. Longer treatment has been shown to be effective and should be guided by an evaluation of the risks and benefits for the individual patient.

Bupropion is safe and effective for patients with CVD. Tonstad found in a randomized double-blind study of patients with CVD that there were adverse heart rate or blood pressure changes during treatment with bupropion and that cessation rates were twice that of placebo.[81,82]

Bupropion is contraindicated, however, in patients at high risk for seizure, previous head trauma, central nervous system tumor, anorexia nervosa, bulimia, previous seizure, or concomitant use with another medication that lowers the seizure threshold (antipsychotics, antidepressants, theophylline, systemic steroids).[79] Bupropion also interferes with the degradation of drugs such as tricyclic antidepressants, β-blockers, and antiarrhythmics such as flecainide.[83] Common side effects are insomnia and dry mouth; both symptoms are generally transient and usually resolve without intervention.[79,82,84,85] Thus, bupropion is generally well tolerated with discontinuation rates of 6% to 12% because of adverse events.[82]

Bupropion has been shown to decrease cravings associated with smoking cessation, which is an important piece of information to be aware of when considering pharmacologic interventions, because craving has been cited as a strong predictor of relapse to smoking cessation. Since craving was cited as the reason for relapse by 49.2% versus 22.4% of relapsers receiving placebo and bupropion SR, respectively,[86] bupropion has also been deemed effective at prolonging the median time to relapse, 156 days versus 65 days, when compared to placebo and it has been found to delay weight gain when used long-term.[87]

Nicotine Replacement Therapy. NRT is a pharmacologic therapy that provides either continuous or bolus dosing of nicotine through the skin (transdermal patch) or mucous membranes (gum, inhaler, nasal spray, lozenge). NRT has been used as a smoking cessation aid since the early 1990s and has consistently demonstrated an abstinence rate of approximately twice that of placebo.[62] Combination NRT is also appropriate for those patients unable to quit using a single first-line pharmacotherapeutic. The meta-analysis performed for the guideline[62] found that combination NRT therapy doubled the abstinence rate compared with NRT monotherapy.

NRT should be used with caution in those patients experiencing acute cardiovascular events such as recent MI (within the previous 2 weeks), serious arrhythmias, and unstable angina pectoris.[61,62] Establishment of a favorable risk-to-benefit ratio for NRT was based in part on the work of Benowitz,[88] who found that blood levels obtained during the use of 2-mg nicotine gum average 12 mg/mL, compared with peak levels without the gum of 35 to 54 mg/mL during smoking.[88] Moreover, in assessing the effects of transdermal nicotine in cardiac patients, multiple studies have found no association between the patch and acute cardiac events.[61] A review found that NRT constricts coronary arteries and alters hemodynamic profiles, leading to increased myocardial workload and oxygen demand. Cigarette smoking, however, precipitates acute cardiac events by three mechanisms: (1) it produces a hypercoagulable state and promotes thrombosis; (2) it delivers carbon monoxide, which limits oxygen delivery to the heart; and (3) it alters hemodynamic profiles. The reviewers also concluded that the alterations in hemodynamic profiles caused by NRT were less hazardous than those produced by cigarette smoking.[25] Therefore, it appears that the effects of NRT on the cardiovascular system are no greater and are probably less than the effects of cigarette smoking.[26]

The nicotine patch and gum are the most widely used forms. The choice of agent is based on patient preference; previous experience (good or bad) with a given form of NRT; whether the patient wears dentures, which precludes the use of nicotine gum; and whether the smoking habit is associated with oral gratification, which may favor the gum, lozenge, or inhaler. An alternative form of NRT that has not been widely used is the nicotine nasal spray. Widespread use may be prohibited by the common adverse effects of nicotine nasal spray, including headache, burning sensations in the nose or throat, watery eyes, nasal and throat irritation, sneezing, runny nose, cough, and sleep disturbances. These adverse effects usually begin on the first day of use but diminish over time.[89] Nicotine nasal spray, however, may be especially helpful for the highly addicted smoker due to its rapid onset of action.[90] The patch was the most preferred form of NRT followed by the spray, inhaler, and gum. It was noted, however, that women were more successful at quitting using the inhaler compared with quitting using the gum, and among those heavily addicted smokers the relapse rates to smoking were lower for those using the inhaler than for those using any other form of NRT.[91] The use of the nicotine patch and gum, the most commonly used forms of NRT are described in more detail in Display 34-3.

Although multiple studies have demonstrated the value of NRT in smoking cessation, the use of NRT remains relatively limited. Studies continue to document the underuse of NRT and several theories regarding potential barriers to prescription and use have been proposed. For example, the Women's Initiative for Nonsmoking (WINS) study revealed that of 142 women with CVD in the intervention group, 127 met the study criteria for NRT use, but the reported use of NRT by patients ranged from 9% (2-day follow-up) to 22% (90-day follow-up), even in light of the fact that NRT was available to the women free of charge. The researchers hypothesized that the intervention nurses may have been leery of recommending NRT because the Agency for Healthcare Policy and Research (AHCPR) had previously cautioned against use of NRT in patients with CVD or because of the lack of patient education regarding the myths of NRT such as trading one addiction for another.[18] Emmons et al.[92] also demonstrated a low level of use of NRT in hospitalized patients; only 7.1% of patients in a sample of 580 male and female smokers who were hospitalized used NRT. This finding is consistent with a study of African American smokers.[93] This study revealed that the major barriers of NRT use were concerns that using it would increase nicotine dependence and concerns about lack of control over drug delivery and absorption.

Another potential explanation for lack of use of NRT is reluctance on the part of health care providers to recognize cigarette

DISPLAY 34-3 Nicotine Replacement Therapy

Nicotine Gum

Nicotine chewing gum has been available in the United States since 1984, and has been available over the counter since 1997. It comes in 2- and 4-mg doses. It is a resin-based gum that releases nicotine into the bloodstream through the buccal mucosa inside the mouth. The success of nicotine gum is highly dependent on its proper use. It has been shown to be highly ineffective when dispensed without proper chewing instruction. Moreover, when nicotine gum is prescribed without any counseling or strong advice, it has been shown to produce very low cessation rates.[94]

Patients should start using the gum immediately as soon as they stop smoking. Although nicotine gum was originally prescribed to be taken on an as-needed basis, studies suggest that a regular schedule of taking the gum, normally one piece every 60 minutes during waking hours, ensures constant blood nicotine levels.[95] Side effects are also minimal and transient if the gum is administered properly. Most often, these side effects are limited to local mouth irritation, some gastrointestinal distress such as nausea and heartburn, palpitations, and jaw ache from excessive chewing.

An acidic environment in the mouth blocks nicotine absorption. Because the use of beverages such as colas, coffee, tea, and juices changes the oral pH to an acidic environment, these agents should not be used within 15 minutes of using the gum or during the first 15 minutes of chewing the gum.[96] Because nicotine gum is now available over the counter, it is imperative that teaching be done by the nurse or, alternatively, the patient should be encouraged to discuss proper use with a pharmacist. Nicotine chewing gum is normally used for a period of 3 to 6 months. A tapering schedule of at least 1 month is recommended. Weaning can be accomplished by decreasing the dosage, cutting gum pieces in half, and substituting sugarless gum for some of the doses. Nurses should also be aware that 8% to 25% of nicotine gum users who successfully quit smoking use the gum beyond the 6 months recommended for maximal use. Habitual use of the gum to deal with negative emotional states is often the cause of this prolonged use.[97] As noted previously, the prolonged use of the gum is preferred to smoking and has not been shown to be harmful.[61]

Nicotine Patch

The transdermal nicotine patch has been available in the United States by prescription since 1991 and over the counter since 1997. The nicotine patch produces a therapeutic effect by releasing a controlled amount of nicotine through the skin that is absorbed through the capillary bed.

The nicotine patch is designed to be worn for a period of 16 to 24 hours depending on the brand, with a recommended dose of 21 mg/24 h, or 15 mg/16 h. Lower doses (10–14 mg) are recommended for some cardiovascular patients, see above. Patches are designed to be changed daily and are normally recommended to be used for 8 weeks, with weaning beginning at 4 weeks. During the weaning period, the dose is reduced in a stepwise manner (i.e., 21, 14, and 7 mg) to 7 mg/24 h, or 5 mg/16 h, and finally discontinued.[98] The nicotine patch is often considered the preferred choice for patients because of ease of use. It requires little effort to apply the patch and coverage can be ensured for up to 24 hours.

The most frequent side effect of the nicotine patch is local skin redness, which occurs in approximately 35% to 54% of patients using the patch.[99–102] Severe skin reactions, which include rashes or eczema, have led to discontinuation of therapy in less than 7% of patients.[103,104] Other side effects reported, which occur much less frequently, include gastrointestinal problems of dyspepsia, abdominal pain, and diarrhea; muscle and limb weakness; paresthesia; nervousness; and vivid or disturbing dreams.[105]

smoking as an addiction. Cigarette smoking has clearly been found to be an addiction because it fulfills the requirements for addiction of (1) highly controlled or compulsive use; (2) psychoactive effects; and (3) drug-reinforced behavior.[22]

Step 5: Arrange—Schedule Follow-Up Contact

The guideline[62] concluded that reinforcement by numerous contacts and health care professionals leads to greater smoking cessation rates. Ideally, follow-up contact should occur soon after the established quit date, preferably within the first week and then again within the first month. Follow-up can be performed in person or by telephone. Important components of follow-up include congratulations on success, support, reinforcement, and problem solving. If the patient slipped or relapsed, follow-up provides the opportunity to review the circumstances that led to the slip or relapse, create a new plan to deal with a similar situation in the future, and establish a new quit date. Follow-up also allows the clinician to review and trouble-shoot any problems associated with the use of pharmacologic therapies.

Although a brief intervention is the minimum that all health care providers should offer their patients, the guidelines[61,62] clearly point out that implementation of a more intensive intervention is the goal because there is a strong dose–response relation between counseling intensity and success in smoking cessation. The meta-analyses conducted for the current guideline strongly indicate that there is a dose–response relationship between session length and abstinence rates, total amount of contact time and abstinence rates, and the number of sessions and treatment efficacy. In terms of session length, it was found that abstinence rates increase from 10.9 with *no* contact to 22.1 with longer counseling sessions (lasting >10 minutes). In terms of contact time, it was found that abstinence rates increase from 11.0 with *no* contact time to 28.4 with 91 to 300 minutes. In terms of number of sessions, abstinence rates double from 12.4 with no or one session to 24.7 with more than eight sessions. The guideline thus recommends four or more sessions lasting longer than 10 minutes for a total contact time of more than 30 minutes.

SPECIAL AREAS ON WHICH TO FOCUS

Stress

Patients may often relapse to smoking during stressful times, especially those involving emotional circumstances, such as arguments or a crisis situation with a spouse, family members, or coworkers.[75] The frequency and severity of distressing demands during everyday life have also been shown to be predictors of later relapse to smoking in both men and women.[106,107] Although some patients may need in-depth counseling to help them with such problems, simple relaxation training may produce a sense of increased control, which may in turn affect the patient's confidence to withstand the urge to smoke. Many patients can benefit from the use of inexpensive relaxation audiotapes that use simple instructions on how to use muscle tension and deep breathing exercises to achieve relaxation.

Depression

Current smokers have been found to have higher mean depression scores than never smokers in both men and women.[108] Smokers, in general, have had a significantly greater number of past episodes of major depression than average, and smokers with a history of major depression who quit smoking are seven times more likely to have a recurrence of major depression than do individuals who continue to smoke.[109] Depressive episodes occurring before smoking cessation have an inverse relationship with 6-month abstinence.[110] In other words, patients who have had a previous history of depression but are not depressed at the time smoking cessation is initiated have less success at quitting than do smokers who have never experienced depression. Higher depression scores are also related to lower self-efficacy for quitting, especially among men,[108] and decreases in self-efficacy, if they are going to occur, will most likely happen in the first 2 weeks after cessation.[110] Women experiencing depression were found to have more difficulty initiating a smoking cessation attempt, maintaining abstinence, and were likely to relapse to smoking significantly earlier than were nondepressed women.[111] Therefore, clinicians working with depressed smokers making a quit attempt may need to focus on enhancing self-efficacy and providing additional support in the first few weeks after cessation to prevent negative affect from significantly decreasing self-efficacy and increasing the likelihood of relapse. One thing that does bode well for smoking cessation is the finding that higher depression scores are related to a greater motivation to quit in women, a factor that clinicians must use in their favor.[108] Although there are multiple depression screening tools available in the literature, Whooley and Simon[112] have developed a very brief two-question case finding instrument that is quickly and easily used in the clinical setting to help guide plans for a smoking cessation intervention. The two questions are (1) during the past month, have you often been bothered by feeling down, depressed, or hopeless? and (2) during the past month, have you often been bothered by having little interest or pleasure in doing things? If the patient answers "no" to both questions, the patient is unlikely to have major depression. If the patient answers "yes" to either question, a follow-up clinical interview by a mental health professional is recommended; alternatively, a referral to either the primary care provider or a psychiatrist is indicated. Bupropion SR should be considered the first-line pharmacotherapeutic agent used in patients with current or past depression because it has been proven effective for both smoking cessation and depression therapy.[61]

Alcohol Use

Social situations that involve alcohol use are another predictor of relapse to smoking.[75] For this reason, nurses need to determine whether the smoker attempting to quit consumes excessive alcohol regularly. This information can be ascertained while taking a smoking history by using the simple four-item CAGE questionnaire (Fig. 34-3),[113] which is a screening tool for alcohol abuse. If a diagnosis of alcoholism is made, patients should be encouraged to seek treatment for alcoholism and smoking cessation simultaneously. Patients who are heavy social drinkers should also be encouraged to avoid alcohol or decrease their consumption substantially until they feel successful in their smoking cessation efforts.

Loss

For many patients, giving up smoking is like "losing a best friend." Nurses must help patients to recognize and understand the magnitude of this loss. Helping patients acknowledge how they feel about their loss and working with them to select new activities that provide immediate gratification is important. For example, patients should be encouraged to focus on old hobbies or select new hobbies. They can also develop reward systems for their daily success in remaining nonsmokers. Nurses should also encourage patients to build new activities into their daily schedules that also increase confidence as their focus shifts to new behaviors.

Weight Gain

The average weight gain after smoking cessation is approximately 6 to 10 lb, much of which is caused by metabolic changes that occur with cessation.[114] It appears weight gain is more often associated with those who smoke more cigarettes or have a history of weight problems.[115] In addition, those who quit smoking often crave sweet foods.[116]

Encouraging patients to be more active through daily exercise and helping them to identify low-calorie snacks and sweets can help

	YES	NO
1. Have you ever felt you ought to CUT DOWN on your drinking?	❑	❑
2. Have people ANNOYED you by criticizing your drinking?	❑	❑
3. Have you ever felt GUILTY about your drinking?	❑	❑
4. Have you ever had a drink first thing in the morning (EYE OPENER) to steady your nerves or get rid of a hangover?	❑	❑

Figure 34-3 The CAGE questionnaire. (Reprinted with permission from Ewing, J. A. [1984]. Detecting alcoholism: The CAGE questionnaire. *JAMA, 252,* 1905–1907.)

patients avoid excessive weight gain. Patients must also be aware that the risks of continued smoking far outweigh the risks of gaining a few pounds. Weight gain cannot be treated lightly because 67% of women in one study stated that they were very concerned or somewhat concerned about weight gain after cessation.[117] In another study, up to 75% of women and 35% of men reported an unwillingness to gain 5 or more pounds as a result of stopping smoking. In particular, more than half of women younger than 25 years and 39% of women older than 40 years stated that they were unwilling to gain any weight.[71] It is important to note that weight gain is not just a concern of women. Weight gain in the first 3 months after cessation was predictive of relapse to smoking for men. In fact, the risk of relapse increased by 17% for every kilogram of weight gained.[118] Providers must therefore openly discuss the possibility of weight gain but stress to the patient that the amount of weight gained is usually limited and that a program of exercise and a healthy diet can control weight gain.[61] In addition, current studies indicate that NRT, particularly the gum, and bupropion SR have been shown to at least delay postcessation weight gain.[61,62] In the case of bupropion SR, weight gain was actually significantly less compared with placebo, 3.8 kg versus 5.6 kg, respectively.[87]

Social Support

Support from a spouse or family members is directly related to quitting smoking and short-term maintenance of the nonsmoking behavior.[119] Women in particular give social support higher ratings of importance in smoking cessation than do men.[107] If family members or close friends smoke, it is important to initiate a plan to help the patient resist the temptation to smoke when around others who are smoking. It is imperative to prepare the patient for this situation if the family member or friend who smokes lives with the patient. Previous preparation is particularly important for women living with a smoker because the odds of relapsing are 2.5 times higher in this population.[16] The ideal situation, of course, is when the family member or friend attempts to quit at the same time the patient does; therefore, interventions that target other smokers in the household at the same time seem prudent. If this is not feasible, the nurse should counsel the family member or friend to (1) not smoke in the presence of the patient if possible; (2) remove all cigarettes and other tobacco products from the household; and (3) refrain from offering cigarettes to the patient who is trying to quit. Family members and friends should also be encouraged to provide daily positive reinforcement for patients successful at quitting. It may also be appropriate for the nurse to teach the patient some basic assertiveness skills, so that the patient is prepared to ask assertively that the family member or friend not smoke in his or her presence, not offer him or her cigarettes, and so forth. The Enhancing Recovery in Coronary Heart Disease Patients (ENRICHD) Social Support Instrument (ESSI) is a brief seven-item questionnaire that is useful in assessing social support in cardiac patients[120–122] and can help guide where emphasis should be placed when designing an individualized intervention when social support is low (Fig. 34-4).

Please read the following questions and circle the response that most closely describes your current situation.

1. Is there someone available to you whom you can count on to listen to you when you need to talk?

None of the time	A little of the time	Some of the time	Most of the time	All of the time
1	2	3	4	5

2. Is there someone available to give you good advice about a problem?

None of the time	A little of the time	Some of the time	Most of the time	All of the time
1	2	3	4	5

3. Is there someone available to you who shows you love and affection?

None of the time	A little of the time	Some of the time	Most of the time	All of the time
1	2	3	4	5

4. Is there someone available to help you with daily chores?

None of the time	A little of the time	Some of the time	Most of the time	All of the time
1	2	3	4	5

5. Can you count on anyone to provide you with emotional support (talking over problems or helping you make a difficult decision)?

None of the time	A little of the time	Some of the time	Most of the time	All of the time
1	2	3	4	5

6. Do you have as much contact as you would like with someone you feel close to, someone in whom you can trust and confide?

None of the time	A little of the time	Some of the time	Most of the time	All of the time
1	2	3	4	5

7. Are you currently married or living with a partner?

Yes No

■ **Figure 34-4** ESSI. (Reprinted with permission from Mitchell, P. H., Powell, L., Blumenthal, J., et al. [2003]. A short social support measure in patients recovering from myocardial infarction: The ENRICHD Social Support Inventory. *Journal of Cardiopulmonary Rehabilitation, 23*, 398–403.)

Vulnerable Populations

Vulnerable populations include, but are not limited to, the economically disadvantaged, underinsured or uninsured, migrant workers, immigrants, incarcerated, homeless, lesbian, gay, bisexual, or transgender populations, ethnic minorities, and infants and young children. These populations are vulnerable because of inadequate, inappropriate, or unavailable resources and/or inadequate knowledge of the numbers and needs of these populations as a result of inadequate census and research data.[53] In general, smoking cessation interventions have, for the most part, been successful in a variety of different types of populations from blue collar workers[123] to those enrolled in managed care medical programs[19]; therefore, it is in the best interest of the smoker no matter his or her age, ethnicity, lifestyle, or occupation to receive a smoking cessation intervention that is as individually tailored as possible. With time and further research, the hope is that current intervention strategies are found to be effective in these populations or that new strategies will be developed and found efficacious.

Women

The most recent Surgeon General's Report, *Women and Smoking,* reiterates the need for smoking cessation efforts targeted directly at women because approximately 3 million women in the United States have died since 1980 from a smoking-related disease.[124] Of even further concern is that the World Health Organization's Report, *Women and the Tobacco Epidemic: Challenges for the 21st Century,* confirms that the problem is not restricted to the United States.[125] Some researchers have found that women are less likely to quit smoking than men are,[46] whereas others have found similar cessation rates.[123,126] It is generally believed, however, that women respond differently to smoking cessation interventions. Some possible explanations are differences in physiology and behavioral and psychological factors. For example, the menstrual cycle may play a role in smoking cessation. The symptoms of menstrual distress include depression, irritability, anxiety, tension, decreased ability to concentrate, and weight changes, all of which are also symptoms of nicotine withdrawal. Withdrawal has been shown to be greater when the quit date is set during the luteal phase (ovulation to day before menses) of the menstrual cycle as opposed to the follicular phase (day 1 of menses to day 15). Therefore, it may be valuable to assess the menstrual cycle pattern before setting a quit date to reduce compounding withdrawal with normal menstrual distress.[127] Behavioral and psychological factors that play a major role in smoking cessation for women are fear of weight gain, low social support, reliance on cigarettes for control of negative affect or stress management, and self-efficacy in quitting.[107] These factors must be addressed when implementing a smoking cessation intervention with a woman. For example, the WINS study found that low self-efficacy and living with a smoker were predictive of smoking at 6 and 12 months of follow-up. In addition, women who perceived themselves to be in "fair" or "poor" health were more likely to be smokers at 12 months.[14] Furthermore, women who were 62 and older had higher abstinence rate than did those younger than 62 years. Their abstinence rates were 52% versus 38% and this difference was statistically significant.[37] Gritz et al. also found that a higher education level and a "white collar" job classification were also predictive of smoking cessation in a workplace-based study.[123] As always, it is best to tailor the intervention to the individual patient when possible. It is important to note, however, that women prefer to use a greater number and variety of quitting strategies, including individual strategies, like reading cessation materials, smoking substitutes, relaxation techniques, seeking support, hypnosis, and acupuncture than do men.[126] Specific benefits of smoking cessation we have found helpful to discuss with women include improved complexion, fewer wrinkles, no odor of cigarettes on their breath or in their hair or clothes, and better health for children and family members. Given the limited information on characteristics predictive of smoking cessation success in women and the limited number of women-only smoking cessation studies, the information on how specifically to support the female smoker in quitting is limited.

Nurses

Although nurses know that smoking has a negative impact on health, especially cardiovascular health, only 20% to 30% of nurses provide smoking cessation interventions to their patients.[6] One of the barriers to conducting smoking cessation interventions for nurses is the nurses themselves who continue to smoke.[128] The prevalence of smoking among nurses has been reported at approximately 15% for registered nurses and 28% for licensed vocational nurses.[129] Furthermore, nurses who smoked expressed guilt about their behavior and the public's perception, as well as feeling a lack of peer and management support regarding smoking cessation attempts.[130] A study also showed that nurses who smoke were perceived as taking more breaks and spending less time with patients than those who do not smoke.[131]

A program called Tobacco Free Nurses is an initiative funded by a grant from the Robert Wood Johnson Foundation. Tobacco Free Nurses is the first program to help nurses to quit smoking nationally and internationally and to support their patients' smoking cessation efforts. The program also provides a Web site (http://www.tobaccofreenurses.org) for all the resources that nurses need to support themselves and their patients in smoking cessation. The Tobacco Free Nurses initiative will provide a new and tremendous opportunity for nurses in various clinical settings to assist patients and their own nursing colleagues in smoking cessation.

International Considerations

In Chapter 43, Figure 43-2 shows the regions of the world with very high smoking prevalence, and given the long latency period between the exposure to tobacco and diseases most of these counties have not seen the devastating health consequences. Nurses and public health officials can play an important role acquiring the skills for counseling smokers to quit by using a guide for nurses to help smokers quit.[63] Setting up a systems approach to identify smokers for every health care encounter sends a powerful message to all smokers about the need for them to consider smoking cessation. Additionally the WHO convention framework legal policy statements can be used by Ministries of Health to combat aggressive cigarette advertisement for youths and adults.

SUMMARY

A systematic approach to smoking cessation leads to better outcomes. The measure of success should be based on the frequency with which the nurse asks about a patient's smoking status. Multicomponent strategies that include strong physician and nurse advice, self-help materials, behavioral counseling, pharmacologic therapy, and follow-up can be used to help the general population and those with CHD.

Acknowledgment: *We thank Nancy Houston Miller for contribution to the earlier editions of this chapter.*

REFERENCES

1. U. S. Department of Health and Human Services. (2004). *The health consequences of smoking: A report of the Surgeon General.* Atlanta, GA: Author.
2. World Health Organization. (2002). *Fact sheets, smoking statistics. Regional Office for the Western Pacific.* Retrieved from http://www.wpro.who.int/media_centre/fact_sheets/fs_20020528.htm
3. Centers for Disease Control and Prevention (CDC). (2005). Annual smoking-attributable mortality, years of potential life lost, and productivity losses–United States, 1997–2001. *Morbidity and Mortality Weekly Report, 54,* 625–628.
4. Centers for Disease Control and Prevention (CDC). (2007). State-specific prevalence of cigarette smoking among adults and quitting among persons aged 18–35 years–United States, 2006. *Morbidity and Mortality Weekly Report, 56,* 993–996.
5. Chase, E. C., McMenamin, S. B., & Halpin, H. A. (2007). Medicaid provider delivery of the 5A's for smoking cessation counseling. *Nicotine & Tobacco Research, 9,* 1095–1101.
6. Centers for Disease Control and Prevention (CDC). (1993). Physician and other health-care professional counseling of smokers to quit–United States, 1991. *Morbidity and Mortality Weekly Report, 42,* 854–857.
7. Quinn, V. P., Stevens, V. J., Hollis, J. F., et al. (2005). Tobacco-cessation services and patient satisfaction in nine nonprofit HMOs. *American Journal of Preventive Medicine, 29,* 77–84.
8. California Department of Health Services. *Smokers and quitting.* Retrieved from http://www.dhs.ca.gov/tobacco/documents/pubs/Cessation.pdf
9. Taylor, C. B., Houston-Miller, N., Killen, J. D., et al. (1990). Smoking cessation after acute myocardial infarction: Effects of a nurse-managed intervention. *Annals of Internal Medicine, 113,* 118–123.
10. Rice, V. H., Fox, D. H., Lepczyk, M., et al. (1994). A comparison of nursing interventions for smoking cessation in adults with cardiovascular health problems. *Heart & Lung, 23,* 473–486.
11. Wewers, M. E., Bowen, J. M., Stanislaw, A. E., et al. (1994). A nurse-delivered smoking cessation intervention among hospitalized postoperative patients–influence of a smoking-related diagnosis: A pilot study. *Heart & Lung, 23,* 151–156.
12. Taylor, C. B., Miller, N. H., Herman, S., et al. (1996). A nurse-managed smoking cessation program for hospitalized smokers. *American Journal of Public Health, 86,* 1557–1560.
13. Johnson, J. L., Budz, B., Mackay, M., et al. (1999). Evaluation of a nurse-delivered smoking cessation intervention for hospitalized patients with cardiac disease. *Heart & Lung, 28,* 55–64.
14. Froelicher, E. S., & Christopherson, D. J. (2000). Women's Initiative for Nonsmoking (WINS) I: Design and methods. *Heart & Lung, 29,* 429–437.
15. Martin, K., Froelicher, E. S., & Miller, N. H. (2000). Women's Initiative for Nonsmoking (WINS) II: The intervention. *Heart & Lung, 29,* 438–445.
16. Froelicher, E. S., Christopherson, D. J., Miller, N. H., et al. (2002). Women's Initiative for Nonsmoking (WINS) IV: Description of 277 women smokers hospitalized with cardiovascular disease. *Heart & Lung, 31,* 3–14.
17. Froelicher, E. S., & Kozuki, Y. (2002). Theoretical applications of smoking cessation interventions to individuals with medical conditions: Women's Initiative for Nonsmoking (WINS)—Part III. *International Journal of Nursing Studies, 39,* 1–15.
18. Mahrer-Imhof, R., Froelicher, E. S., Li, W. W., et al. (2002). Women's Initiative for Nonsmoking (WINS V): Under-use of nicotine replacement therapy. *Heart & Lung, 31,* 368–373.
19. Smith, P. M., Reilly, K. R., Houston Miller, N., et al. (2002). Application of a nurse-managed inpatient smoking cessation program. *Nicotine & Tobacco Research, 4,* 211–222.
20. *Tobacco Free Nurses.* (2008). Retrieved from http://www.tobaccofreenurses.org
21. Sarna, L., & Lillington, L. (2002). Tobacco: An emerging topic in nursing research. *Nursing Research, 51,* 245–253.
22. U.S. Department of Health and Human Services. (1988). *The health consequences of smoking: Nicotine addiction. A report of the Surgeon General* (DHHS Publication No. [CDC] 888406). Washington, DC: Government Printing Office.
23. American Psychiatric Association. (1994). *Diagnostic and statistical manual of mental disorders* (4th ed.). Washington, DC: Author.
24. U.S. Department of Health and Human Services. (1989). *Reducing the health consequences of smoking: 25 years of progress. A report of the Surgeon General* (DHHS Publication No. [CDC] 89-8411). Washington, DC: Government Printing Office.
25. Benowitz, N. L., & Gourlay, S. G. (1997). Cardiovascular toxicity of nicotine: Implications for nicotine replacement therapy. *Journal of the American College of Cardiology, 29,* 1422–1431.
26. Stillman, F. A. (1995). Smoking cessation for the hospitalized cardiac patient: Rationale for and report of a model program. *Journal of Cardiovascular Nursing, 9,* 25–36.
27. U.S. Department of Health and Human Services. (1983). *The health consequences of smoking: Cardiovascular disease. A report of the Surgeon General.* Washington, DC: Government Printing Office.
28. Quillen, J. E., Rossen, J. D., Oskarsson, H. J., et al. (1993). Acute effect of cigarette smoking on the coronary circulation: Constriction of epicardial and resistance vessels. *Journal of the American College of Cardiology, 22,* 642–647.
29. Barry, J., Mead, K., Nabel, E. G., et al. (1989). Effect of smoking on the activity of ischemic heart disease. *JAMA, 261,* 398–402.
30. Samet, J. M. (1991). Health benefits of smoking cessation. *Clinics in Chest Medicine, 12,* 669–679.
31. Sparrow, D., & Dawber, T. R. (1978). The influence of cigarette smoking on prognosis after a first myocardial infarction. A report from the Framingham study. *Journal of Chronic Diseases, 31,* 425–432.
32. Wilhelmsson, C., Vedin, J. A., Elmfeldt, D., et al. (1975). Smoking and myocardial infarction. *Lancet, 1,* 415–420.
33. Hermanson, B., Omenn, G. S., Kronmal, R. A., et al. (1988). Beneficial six-year outcome of smoking cessation in older men and women with coronary artery disease. Results from the CASS registry. *New England Journal of Medicine, 319,* 1365–1369.
34. Bandura, A. (1997). The anatomy of stages of change. *American Journal of Health Promotion, 12,* 8–10.
35. Dijkstra, A., de Vries, H., & Bakker, M. (1996). Pros and cons of quitting, self-efficacy, and the stages of change in smoking cessation. *Journal of Consulting and Clinical Psychology, 64,* 758–763.
36. Dornelas, E. A., Sampson, R. A., Gray, J. F., et al. (2000). A randomized controlled trial of smoking cessation counseling after myocardial infarction. *Preventive Medicine, 30,* 261–268.
37. Doolan, D. M., Stotts, N. A., Benowitz, N. L., et al. (2008). The Women's Initiative for Nonsmoking (WINS) XI: Age-related differences in smoking cessation responses among women with cardiovascular disease. *American Journal of Geriatric Cardiology, 17,* 37–47.
38. Rice, V. H., & Stead, L. (2006). Nursing intervention and smoking cessation: Meta-analysis update. *Heart & Lung, 35,* 147–163.
39. Kottke, T. E., Battista, R. N., DeFriese, G. H., et al. (1988). Attributes of successful smoking cessation interventions in medical practice. A meta-analysis of 39 controlled trials. *Journal of the American Medical Association, 259,* 2883–2889.
40. Schwartz, J. L. (1987). *Review and evaluation of smoking cessation methods: The United States and Canada, 1978–1985* (DHHS Publication No. [NIH] 87-2940). Washington, DC: Department of Health and Human Services, Public Health Service.
41. Burt, A., Thornley, P., Illingworth, D., et al. (1974). Stopping smoking after myocardial infarction. *Lancet, 1,* 304–306.
42. Mulcahy, R. (1983). Influence of cigarette smoking on morbidity and mortality after myocardial infarction. *British Heart Journal, 49,* 410–415.
43. Baile, W. F., Jr., Bigelow, G. E., Gottlieb, S. H., et al. (1982). Rapid resumption of cigarette smoking following myocardial infarction: Inverse relation to MI severity. *Addictive Behaviors, 7,* 373–380.
44. Crouse, J. R., III, & Hagaman, A. P. (1991). Smoking cessation in relation to cardiac procedures. *American Journal of Epidemiology, 134,* 699–703.
45. Rigotti, N. A., McKool, K. M., & Shiffman, S. (1994). Predictors of smoking cessation after coronary artery bypass graft surgery. Results of a randomized trial with 5-year follow-up. *Annals of Internal Medicine, 120,* 287–293.
46. Ockene, J., Kristeller, J. L., Goldberg, R., et al. (1992). Smoking cessation and severity of disease: The Coronary Artery Smoking Intervention Study. *Health Psychology, 11,* 119–126.
47. Havik, O. E., & Maeland, J. G. (1988). Changes in smoking behavior after a myocardial infarction. *Health Psychology, 7,* 403–420.
48. Scott, R. R., & Lamparski, D. (1985). Variables related to long-term smoking status following cardiac events. *Addictive Behaviors, 10,* 257–264.

49. Stanislaw, A. E., & Wewers, M. E. (1994). A smoking cessation intervention with hospitalized surgical cancer patients: A pilot study. *Cancer Nursing, 17*, 81–86.
50. Miller, N. H., Smith, P. M., DeBusk, R. F., et al. (1997). Smoking cessation in hospitalized patients. Results of a randomized trial. *Archives of Internal Medicine, 157*, 409–415.
51. Glasgow, R. E., Stevens, V. J., Vogt, T. M., et al. (1991). Changes in smoking associated with hospitalization: Quit rates, predictive variables, and intervention implications. *American Journal of Health Promotion, 6*, 24–29.
52. Ockene, J. K., Hosmer, D., Rippe, J., et al. (1985). Factors affecting cigarette smoking status in patients with ischemic heart disease. *Journal of Chronic Diseases, 38*, 985–994.
53. Hutchinson, K. M., & Froelicher, E. A. (2003). Populations at risk for tobacco-related diseases. *Seminars in Oncology Nursing, 19*, 276–283.
54. Krumholz, H. M., Cohen, B. J., Tsevat, J., et al. (1993). Cost-effectiveness of a smoking cessation program after myocardial infarction. *Journal of the American College of Cardiology, 22*, 1697–1702.
55. Fiore, M. C., Novotny, T. E., Pierce, J. P., et al. (1990). Methods used to quit smoking in the United States. Do cessation programs help? *Journal of the American Medical Association, 263*, 2760–2765.
56. Emmons, K. M., & Goldstein, M. G. (1992). Smokers who are hospitalized: A window of opportunity for cessation interventions. *Preventive Medicine, 21*, 262–269.
57. Sohn, M., Stotts, N. A., Benowitz, N., et al. (2007). Beliefs about health, smoking, and future smoking cessation among South Korean men hospitalized for cardiovascular disease. *Heart & Lung, 36*, 339–347.
58. Sohn, M., Benowitz, N., Stotts, N., et al. (2008). Smoking behavior in men hospitalized with cardiovascular disease in Korea: A cross-sectional descriptive study. *Heart & Lung, 37*, 366–379.
59. Pechacek, T. F. (1984). Modification of smoking behavior. In *Smoking and health: A report of the Surgeon General.* Washington, DC: Government Printing Office.
60. U.S. Department of Health and Human Services. (1996). *Treating tobacco use and dependence: Clinical practice guideline.* Washington, DC: Government Printing Office.
61. U.S. Department of Health and Human Services. (2000). *Treating tobacco use and dependence: Clinical practice guideline.* Washington, DC: Government Printing Office.
62. U.S. Department of Health and Human Services. (2008). *Treating tobacco use and dependence: Clinical practice guideline, 2008 update.* Washington, DC: Government Printing Office.
63. U.S. Department of Health and Human Services. (2008). *Helping smokers quit: A guide for clinicians.* Washington, DC: Government Printing Office.
64. Sohn, M., Hartley, C., Froelicher, E. S., et al. (2003). Tobacco use and dependence. *Seminars in Oncology Nursing, 19*, 250–260.
65. American Heart Association. (2002). *An active partnership for the health of your heart.* Dallas, TX: Author.
66. U.S. Department of Health and Human Services. (2003). *Pathways to freedom: Winning the fight against tobacco.* Atlanta, GA: Centers for Disease Control and Prevention.
67. Marlatt, A. G. (1982). Relapse prevention: A self-control program for the treatment of addictive behaviors. In R. B. Stuart (Ed.), *Adherence, compliance and generalization in behavioral medicine* (pp. 329–378). New York: Brunnel/Mazel.
68. Ockene, J. K., Emmons, K. M., Mermelstein, R. J., et al. (2000). Relapse and maintenance issues for smoking cessation. *Health Psychology, 19*, 17–31.
69. Condiotte, M. M., & Lichtenstein, E. (1981). Self-efficacy and relapse in smoking cessation programs. *Journal of Consulting and Clinical Psychology, 49*, 648–658.
70. Gwaltney, C. J., Shiffman, S., Norman, G. J., et al. (2001). Does smoking abstinence self-efficacy vary across situations? Identifying context-specificity within the Relapse Situation Efficacy Questionnaire. *Journal of Consulting and Clinical Psychology, 69*, 516–527.
71. Tsoh, J. Y., McClure, J. B., Skaar, K. L., et al. (1997). Smoking cessation. 2: Components of effective intervention. *Behavioral Medicine, 23*, 15–27.
72. Heatherton, T. F., Kozlowski, L. T., Frecker, R. C., et al. (1991). The Fagerstrom Test for Nicotine Dependence: A revision of the Fagerstrom Tolerance Questionnaire. *British Journal of Addiction, 86*, 1119–1127.
73. Fagerström, K. (2003). Time to first cigarette; the best single indicator of tobacco dependence? *Monaldi Archives for Chest Disease, 59*, 91–94.
74. Taylor, C. B., Houston-Miller, N., Haskell, W. L., et al. (1988). Smoking cessation after acute myocardial infarction: the effects of exercise training. *Addictive Behaviors, 13*, 331–335.
75. Shiffman, S. (1986). A cluster-analytic classification of smoking relapse episodes. *Addictive Behaviors, 11*, 295–307.
76. Oncken, C., Gonzales, D., Nides, M., et al. (2006). Efficacy and safety of the novel selective nicotinic acetylcholine receptor partial agonist, varenicline, for smoking cessation. *Archives of Internal Medicine, 166*, 1571–1577.
77. Freedman, R. (2007). Exacerbation of schizophrenia by varenicline. *American Journal of Psychiatry, 164*, 1269.
78. Kohen, I., & Kremen, N. (2007). Varenicline-induced manic episode in a patient with bipolar disorder. *American Journal of Psychiatry, 164*, 1269–1270.
79. GlaxoSmithKline. *Zyban prescribing information.* Retrieved from http://us.gsk.com/products/assets/us_zyban.pdf
80. Hays, J. T., & Ebbert, J. O. (2003). Bupropion for the treatment of tobacco dependence: Guidelines for balancing risks and benefits. *CNS Drugs, 17*, 71–83.
81. Smith, S. S., Jorenby, D. E., Leischow, S. J., et al. (2003). Targeting smokers at increased risk for relapse: Treating women and those with a history of depression. *Nicotine & Tobacco Research, 5*, 99–109.
82. Aubin, H. J. (2002). Tolerability and safety of sustained-release bupropion in the management of smoking cessation. *Drugs, 62*(Suppl. 2), 45–52.
83. Haustein, K. O. (2003). Bupropion: Pharmacological and clinical profile in smoking cessation. *International Journal of Clinical Pharmacology and Therapeutics, 41*, 56–66.
84. Holm, K. J., & Spencer, C. M. (2000). Bupropion: A review of its use in the management of smoking cessation. *Drugs, 59*, 1007–1024.
85. Bupropion (Zyban®) for smoking cessation. (1997). *Medical Letters on Drugs and Therapeutics, 39*, 77–78.
86. Durcan, M. J., Deener, G., White, J., et al. (2002). The effect of bupropion sustained-release on cigarette craving after smoking cessation. *Clinical Therapeutics, 24*, 540–551.
87. Hays, J. T., Hurt, R. D., Rigotti, N. A., et al. (2001). Sustained-release bupropion for pharmacologic relapse prevention after smoking cessation. A randomized, controlled trial. *Annals of Internal Medicine, 135*, 423–433.
88. Benowitz, N. L. (1988). Drug therapy. Pharmacologic aspects of cigarette smoking and nicotine addition. *New England Journal of Medicine, 319*, 1318–1330.
89. Hurt, R. D., Dale, L. C., Croghan, G. A., et al. (1998). Nicotine nasal spray for smoking cessation: Pattern of use, side effects, relief of withdrawal symptoms, and cotinine levels. *Mayo Clinic Proceedings, 73*, 118–125.
90. Schneider, N. G., Lunell, E., Olmstead, R. E., et al. (1996). Clinical pharmacokinetics of nasal nicotine delivery. A review and comparison to other nicotine systems. *Clinical Pharmacokinetics, 31*, 65–80.
91. West, R., Hajek, P., Nilsson, F., et al. (2001). Individual differences in preferences for and responses to four nicotine replacement products. *Psychopharmacology (Berl), 153*, 225–230.
92. Emmons, K. M., Goldstein, M. G., Roberts, M., et al. (2000). The use of nicotine replacement therapy during hospitalization. *Annals of Behavioral Medicine, 22*, 325–329.
93. Yerger, V. B., Wertz, M., McGruder, C., et al. (2008). Nicotine replacement therapy: perceptions of African-American smokers seeking to quit. *Journal of the National Medical Association, 100*, 230–236.
94. Cummings, S. R., Hansen, B., Richard, R. J., et al. (1988). Internists and nicotine gum. *JAMA, 260*, 1565–1569.
95. Killen, J. D., Fortmann, S. P., Newman, B., et al. (1990). Evaluation of a treatment approach combining nicotine gum with self-guided behavioral treatments for smoking relapse prevention. *Journal of Consulting and Clinical Psychology, 58*, 85–92.
96. Henningfield, J. E., Radzius, A., Cooper, T. M., et al. (1990). Drinking coffee and carbonated beverages blocks absorption of nicotine from nicotine polacrilex gum. *JAMA, 264*, 1560–1564.
97. Hajek, P., Jackson, P., & Belcher, M. (1988). Long-term use of nicotine chewing gum. Occurrence, determinants, and effect on weight gain. *JAMA, 260*, 1593–1596.
98. Agency for Healthcare Policy and Research: U.S. Department of Health and Human Services. (1996). *Clinical practice guideline: Smoking cessation* (Publication No. 96-0692). Washington, DC: Government Printing Office.
99. Marion Merrell Dow, Inc. (1991). *Nicoderm (nicotine transdermal system) prescribing information.* Kansas City, MO: Author.
100. Lederle Laboratories. (1992). *PROSTEP (nicotine transdermal system) prescribing information.* Wayne, NJ: Author.
101. Ciba-Geigy Corporation. (1992). *Habitrol (nicotine transdermal therapeutic system) prescribing information.* Edison, NJ: Author.
102. Parke-Davis. (1992). *Nicotrol (nicotine transdermal system) prescribing information.* Morris Plains, NJ: Author.
103. Rose, J. E., Levin, E. D., Behm, F. M., et al. (1990). Transdermal nicotine facilitates smoking cessation. *Clinical Pharmacology and Therapeutics, 47*, 323–330.

104. Daughton, D. M., Heatley, S. A., Prendergast, J. J., et al. (1991). Effect of transdermal nicotine delivery as an adjunct to low-intervention smoking cessation therapy. A randomized, placebo-controlled, double-blind study. *Archives of Internal Medicine, 151*, 749–752.
105. Transdermal nicotine for smoking cessation. Six-month results from two multicenter controlled clinical trials. Transdermal Nicotine Study Group. (1991). *JAMA, 266*, 3133–3138.
106. Romano, P. S., Bloom, J., & Syme, S. L. (1991). Smoking, social support, and hassles in an urban African-American community. *American Journal of Public Health, 81*, 1415–1422.
107. Gritz, E. R., Nielsen, I. R., & Brooks, L. A. (1996). Smoking cessation and gender: The influence of physiological, psychological, and behavioral factors. *Journal of the American Medical Women's Association, 51*, 35–42.
108. Haukkala, A., Uutela, A., Vartiainen, E., et al. (2006). Depression and smoking cessation: The role of motivation and self-efficacy. *Addictive Behaviors, 25*, 311–316.
109. Glassman, A. H., Covey, L. S., Stetner, F., et al. (2001). Smoking cessation and the course of major depression: A follow-up study. *Lancet, 357*, 1929–1932.
110. Cinciripini, P. M., Wetter, D. W., Fouladi, R. T., et al. (2003). The effects of depressed mood on smoking cessation: Mediation by postcessation self-efficacy. *Journal of Consulting and Clinical Psychology, 71*, 292–301.
111. Pomerleau, C. S., Brouwer, R. J., & Pomerleau, O. F. (2001). Emergence of depression during early abstinence in depressed and non-depressed women smokers. *Journal of Addiction Disorders, 20*, 73–80.
112. Whooley, M. A., & Simon, G. E. (2000). Managing depression in medical outpatients. *New England Journal of Medicine, 343*, 1942–1950.
113. Ewing, J. A. (1984). Detecting alcoholism. The CAGE questionnaire. *JAMA, 252*, 1905–1907.
114. Wack, J. T., & Rodin, J. (1982). Smoking and its effects on body weight and the systems of caloric regulation. *American Journal of Clinical Nutrition, 35*, 366–380.
115. Hall, S. M., Ginsberg, D., & Jones, R. T. (1986). Smoking cessation and weight gain. *Journal of Consulting and Clinical Psychology, 54*, 342–346.
116. Grunberg, N. E. (1982). The effects of nicotine and cigarette smoking on food consumption and taste preferences. *Addictive Behaviors, 7*, 317–331.
117. Pomerleau, C. S., Zucker, A. N., & Stewart, A. J. (2001). Characterizing concerns about post-cessation weight gain: Results from a national survey of women smokers. *Nicotine & Tobacco Research, 3*, 51–60.
118. Borrelli, B., Spring, B., Niaura, R., et al. (2001). Influences of gender and weight gain on short-term relapse to smoking in a cessation trial. *Journal of Consulting and Clinical Psychology, 69*, 511–515.
119. Cohen, S., Lichtenstein, E., Mermelstein, R., et al. (1988). Social support interventions for smoking cessation. In B. H. Gottlieb (Ed.), *Marshaling social support: Formats, processes, and effects*. Newbury Park, CA: Sage.
120. ENRICHD Investigators. (2001). Enhancing recovery in coronary heart disease (ENRICHD): Baseline characteristics. *American Journal of Cardiology, 88*, 316–322.
121. Mitchell, P. H., Powell, L., Blumenthal, J., et al. (2003). A short social support measure for patients recovering from myocardial infarction: The ENRICHD Social Support Inventory. *Journal of Cardiopulmonary Rehabilitation, 23*, 398–403.
122. Berkman, L. F., Blumenthal, J., Burg, M., et al. (2003). Effects of treating depression and low perceived social support on clinical events after myocardial infarction: The Enhancing Recovery in Coronary Heart Disease Patients (ENRICHD) Randomized Trial. *JAMA, 289*, 3106–3116.
123. Gritz, E. R., Thompson, B., Emmons, K., et al. (1998). Gender differences among smokers and quitters in the Working Well Trial. *Preventive Medicine, 27*, 553–561.
124. U. S. Department of Health and Human Services. (2001). *Women and smoking. A report of the Surgeon General.* Washington, DC: Government Printing Office.
125. World Health Organization. (2001). *Women and the tobacco epidemic. Challenges for the 21st century.* Geneva, Switzerland: Author.
126. Whitlock, E. P., Vogt, T. M., Hollis, J. F., et al. (1997). Does gender affect response to a brief clinic-based smoking intervention? *American Journal of Preventive Medicine, 13*, 159–166.
127. O'Hara, P., Portser, S. A., & Anderson, B. P. (1989). The influence of menstrual cycle changes on the tobacco withdrawal syndrome in women. *Addictive Behaviors, 14*, 595–600.
128. Wewers, M. E., Sarna, L., & Rice, V. H. (2006). Nursing research and treatment of tobacco dependence: State of the science. *Nursing Research, 55*, S11–S15.
129. U.S. Department of Commerce. (2001). *National Cancer Institute sponsored tobacco use supplement to the current population survey.* Washington, DC: Bureau of Labor Statistics.
130. Bialous, S. A., Sarna, L., Wewers, M. E., et al. (2004). Nurses' perspectives of smoking initiation, addiction, and cessation. *Nursing Research, 53*, 387–395.
131. Sarna, L., Bialous, S. A., Wewers, M. E., et al. (2005). Nurses, smoking, and the workplace. *Research in Nursing Health, 28*, 79–90.

PATIENT AND NURSING REFERENCES

Patient Materials

Complete guide to quitting
American Cancer Society
1599 Clifton Road NE
Atlanta, GA 30329
1(800) ACS-2345
www.Cancer.org

Help for smokers: Ideas to help you quit and *You can quit smoking*
Agency for Healthcare Research and Quality
Office of Health Care Information
540 Gaither Road
Rockville, MD 20850
http://www.ahcpr.gov/consumer/index.html#smoking

How can I quit and *An active partnership for the health of your heart*
American Heart Association
1-800-AHA-USA1 (242-8721)
www.AmericanHeart.org

Freedom from smoking
American Lung Association
1740 Broadway
New York, NY 10019
www.lungusa.org
(or call your local chapter of the American Lung Association)

Pathways to freedom: Winning the fight against tobacco
Centers for Disease Control and Prevention
1-800-CDC-INFO (800-232-4636)
www.cdc.gov

Materials and Web sites for Nurses

Treating tobacco use and dependence: Clinical practice guideline and *Treating tobacco use and dependence: Quick reference guide for clinicians*
Agency for Healthcare Research and Quality
Publications Clearinghouse
P.O. Box 8547
Silver Spring, MD 20907
(800) 358-9295

Nurses: Help your patients stop smoking
National Heart, Lung, and Blood Institute
P.O. Box 30105
Bethesda, MD 20824
NIH publication no. 92-2962
(301) 592-8573
www.nhlbi.nih.gov

The University of Wisconsin Center for Tobacco Research and Intervention
www.ctri.wisc.edu
Nursing Center for Tobacco Intervention
College of Nursing at Ohio State
www.con.ohio-state.edu/tobacco

Helping Smokers Quit: A Guide for Nurses
Tobacco Free Nurses
1-800-QUIT NOW
http://www.tobaccofreenurses.org

CHAPTER 35

Hypertension

Cheryl R. Dennison / Nancy Houston Miller / Susanna G. Cunningham

Hypertension (HTN), also known as high blood pressure (BP), is the most common risk factor for cardiovascular disease (CVD) in developed and developing countries. The prevalence of HTN in America is 73 million and many more individuals have prehypertension, which indicates they are at high risk for developing HTN.[1] Since the 1970s there has been a dramatic decrease in the mortality rate from hypertensive heart disease in Europe and the United States, primarily because of the development of effective antihypertensive drugs in conjunction with increased awareness, treatment, and control of HTN.[2,3] Despite this progress, worldwide, an estimated 7.1 million premature deaths are caused each year by HTN.[4]

EVIDENCE FOR MANAGEMENT

Definitions

BP has two components, which are continuous variables: systolic BP (SBP) and diastolic BP (DBP). Elevations in either SBP or DBP increase a person's risk for a clinical event. Death from both ischemic heart disease and stroke increases progressively and linearly from levels as low as 115 mm Hg SBP and 75 mm Hg DBP upward among individuals whose ages range from 40 to 89 years.[5] For every 20 mm Hg systolic and 10 mm Hg diastolic increase in BP, there is a doubling of mortality from ischemic heart disease and stroke.[5] Conversely, it is generally true that the lower the pressures, the lower the risk of morbidity and mortality, except in the relatively uncommon situations of sympathetic nervous system dysfunction or hypovolemia.

The word "hypertension" can be confusing to patients, who might believe that they are neither "tense" nor "hyper" and therefore unlikely to have HTN. For this reason, "high blood pressure" may be a better term to use when communicating with the public. HTN can be considered as a sign, a risk factor, and a disease.

Adults

As new research has become available, many countries have established guidelines on the detection, evaluation, and treatment of HTN.[6] Two widely promulgated guidelines defining normal and elevated BP levels were developed by The Joint National Committee of the National High Blood Pressure Education Program and the Guidelines subcommittee of the World Health Organization and the International Society of Hypertension.[4,7] These guidelines define HTN as SBP of ≥140 mm Hg and/or DBP of ≥90 mm Hg. Both reports recommend considering BP together with other risk factors for atherosclerotic CVD when making decisions about when to initiate treatment.

To reflect the curvilinear nature of the relationship between SBP and DBP and risk, "normal" BP, prehypertension, and two stages of HTN have been delineated as shown in Table 35-1.[7] Optimal or normal BP is <120/80 mm Hg. The term prehypertension (defined as BP 120–139/80–89 mm Hg) is intended to identify those individuals in whom early intervention by adoption of healthy lifestyles could reduce BP, decrease the rate of progression of BP to hypertensive levels with age, or prevent HTN entirely.[7] HTN (defined as BP ≥ 140/90 mm Hg) is classified as either Stage 1 (SBP 140 to 159 mm Hg and/or DBP 90 to 99 mm Hg) or Stage 2 (SBP ≥ 160 mm Hg and/or DBP ≥ 100 mm Hg). Isolated systolic HTN is defined as the occurrence of SBP at or greater than 140 mm Hg with DBP less than 90 mm Hg. The incidence of isolated systolic HTN increases dramatically with age and thus is of particular concern among older adults.[8] Types of HTN are classified as (1) systolic and diastolic HTN (either primary or secondary) and (2) isolated systolic HTN caused by increased cardiac output or increasing rigidity of the aorta.

Children

Criteria used for categorizing BP in adults are not applicable to children. The level of BP, which is considered normal, increases gradually from infancy to adulthood.[9] The definition of HTN in children and adolescents is based on the normative distribution of BP in healthy children.[10] Normal BP is defined as SBP and DBP less than 90th percentile for gender, age, and height. HTN is defined as average SBP or DBP at or greater than 95th percentile for gender, age, and height on at least three separate occasions. Children and adolescents with BP ≥ 120/80 mm Hg but less than 95th percentile should be considered prehypertensive. Tables listing BP levels by age and height percentile for boys and girls can be found in the Fourth Report on the Diagnosis, Evaluation, and Treatment of High Blood Pressure in Children and Adolescents.[10]

Epidemiology

Prevalence of HTN

Approximately 33.6%, or just over 73 million Americans have HTN.[1] Based on data from the National Health and Nutrition Examination Survey (NHANES), conducted between 2003 and 2004, 75% of hypertensive individuals were aware of their condition, and 65% were being treated for HBP. Of those treated, only 56.6% had achieved BP control (BP < 140/90 mm Hg). Only 37.5% of individuals being treated for both HTN and diabetes mellitus had achieved the lower goal BP of <130/80.[3] While the prevalence of HTN has increased, rates of HTN awareness, treatment, and control have also increased over the last decade.[2,3]

Age, Gender, and Weight

SBP and DBP levels correlate with age, height, and weight.[9] Evidence suggests that HTN begins in childhood, perhaps even *in*

Table 35-1 ■ CLASSIFICATION OF BLOOD PRESSURE FOR ADULTS

BP Classification	SBP (mm Hg)	DBP (mm Hg)
Normal	<120	and <80
Prehypertension	120–139	or 80–89
Stage 1 Hypertension	140–159	or 90–99
Stage 2 Hypertension	≥ 160	or ≥ 100

From Chobanian, A. V., Bakris, G. L., Black, H. R., et al. (2003). The Seventh Report of the Joint National Committee on Prevention, Detection, Evaluation, and Treatment of High Blood Pressure: The JNC 7 report. *JAMA, 289*(19), 2560–2572. (Erratum in *JAMA*, 2003, *290*[2], 197.)

utero, although a meta-analysis of 55 studies of birth weight and BP later in life did not support this so-called fetal origins hypothesis.[11–13] Because HTN in children is defined as a BP greater than the 95th percentile for a child of any given age and height, the initial incidence of HTN in children is automatically 5%. Normally, BP increases in children at a rate between 1 and 4 mm Hg per year for both SBP and DBP and then levels off after age 18 to 20 years. Children whose BP consistently falls above the 95th percentile for height, gender, and age are at risk for sustained HTN and should be evaluated and possibly treated.[10]

In adults, BP tends to increase with age.[2,3] The prevalence of HTN increases with advancing age to the point where more than half of the people aged 60 to 69 years and approximately three fourths of those aged 70 years and older are affected.[14] The age-related rise in SBP, often manifesting as isolated systolic HTN, is primarily responsible for an increase in both incidence and prevalence of HTN with increasing age.[8] Overall, women have a slightly higher prevalence of HTN (33.6%) than do men (33.2%).[1] However, the age-adjusted percent for women is 28%, and for men, it is 30%.[3] Although rates of HTN treatment are higher among women (58%) compared with men (52%), men achieved higher rates of HTN control (66%) than women (63%).[3]

Data from the Framingham and other epidemiologic studies have shown that as body weight increases, so do SBP and DBP in children and adults.[3,10,15–17] In the Bogalusa Study, children and adolescents who were overweight (body mass index [BMI] > 85th percentile) were 2.4 times more likely to have HTN than those with BMI less than the 85th percentile.[16] NHANES III data revealed that the prevalence of HTN in men and women with BMI < 25 kg/m^2 was 15%, whereas in men and women with a BMI ≥ 30 kg/m^2 prevalence was 42% and 38%, respectively.[15] This relationship between weight and BP is thought to be one of the reasons that BP increases with age.

Family History and Genetic Factors

Family history of HTN has been used as an indicator of genetic influence on HTN. With the progress on the human genome project, it is possible that we may be able to predict risk with more precision; however, expense and issues of privacy must also be considered. Depending on how a positive family history of HTN is defined, a person with a positive history has a relative risk for HTN of between 2.4 and 5.0.[18] The risks are greater when more family members have HTN and if these family members had HTN diagnosed before the age of 55 years. The risk associated with a positive family history is slightly greater for women than for men. The influence of family history is seen in children as well as adults.[19,20] Recent genetic studies suggest that rather than a single genetic variant, alleles at many different loci contribute to HTN, with the combinations of causative alleles varying between individuals. Among the most studied genetic markers for the pathogenesis of HTN are the renin–angiotensin system, salt intake, CVD, obesity and insulin resistance, the sympathetic nervous system, and endothelial dysfunction.[21]

Ethnic and Geographic Differences

Geographic differences in the prevalence of HTN have been described for different regions within the United States as well as across the world. When comparing across non-Hispanic White, non-Hispanic Black, and Mexican American ethnic groups in the United States, the prevalence of HTN was highest among non-Hispanic Black women (46.6%) and men (42.6%) and lowest among Mexican American women (31.4%) and men (28.7%).[1] Within the United States, HTN prevalence, associated stroke mortality, and all-cause mortality vary in geographic patterns and are higher in the Southeast than other regions of the United States. Ten of 11 states in the southeastern United States, the "Stroke Belt," have stroke mortality rates >10% above the national mean. Contributors to this pattern include geographic variations in obesity, physical inactivity, and salt and nutritional intake but not in HTN treatment or control.[2,3,22]

A review of the global burden of HTN revealed that regions with the highest estimated prevalence of HTN had roughly twice the rate compared with regions with the lowest estimated prevalence.[23] In men, the highest estimated prevalence was in the Latin America and Caribbean region, whereas for women the highest estimated prevalence was in the former socialist economies. The lowest estimated prevalence of HTN for both men and women was in the region "other Asian islands" (i.e., Korea, Thailand, and Taiwan).[23] Existing data suggest that the prevalence of HTN has increased in economically developing countries during the past decade.[23] Differences in HTN rates across regions may be caused by differences in BP measurement and treatment, genetics, lifestyle choices, or other confounding variables.

Income and Education

An inverse relationship between socioeconomic status, including educational level and income, and the prevalence of HTN has been documented.[24–27] The Atherosclerosis Risk in Communities Study of 10,091 Black and White Americans has even found a relationship between the stretch capacity (elasticity) of the carotid arteries and socioeconomic status, with persons in the lowest socioeconomic stratum having the greatest impairment of carotid elasticity.[28] The impact of socioeconomic status on BP and other cardiovascular risk factors is thought to be related to social, financial, and political barriers to health care and to adoption of low-risk lifestyles.[29,30]

Hemodynamics of HTN

BP is the product of the amount of blood pumped by the heart each minute (cardiac output) and the degree of dilation or constriction of the arterioles (systemic vascular resistance). Arterial BP is controlled over short time periods by the arterial baroreceptors that sense changes in pressure within major arteries and then through neurohumoral feedback mechanisms, which modulate heart rate, myocardial contractility, and vascular smooth muscle contraction to maintain BP within normal limits. Over longer time periods (hours to days), neurohumoral and direct renal regulation of vascular volume also play an important role in maintaining normal BP. Baroreceptors in low-pressure components of the cardiovascular system such as the veins, atria, and pulmonary circulation have a role in neurohumoral regulation of vascular volume.

HTN occurs because there is an increase in cardiac output and/or systemic vascular resistance.[31,32] It may be that either one or both are elevated. Because BP can be measured relatively easily and because it is not easy to measure cardiac output or systemic vascular resistance, we identify dysfunction of these variables as disorders of BP regulation. As discussion in several chapters of this book reveal, each of these variables, cardiac output and systemic vascular resistance, are themselves influenced by many factors. Given all the factors that can influence it, BP needs to be considered as an extremely complex variable.

The Causes of HTN

Despite decades of research, the main underlying cause of HTN is unknown. However, HTN has been linked to a family history and other factors, such as obesity, stress, excess sodium dysfunction, and sympathetic nervous dysfunction, which may all contribute to HTN. It is highly likely that in the future it will be the interaction of both genetic and environmental factors that play a role in the hypotheses of the causes of HTN.

Primary HTN is the term used to describe 90% to 95% of all cases of HTN for which the cause is unknown. Secondary HTN, which accounts for 5% to 10% of HTN cases, is linked to diseases of the kidney, endocrine system, vascular system, lungs, and central nervous system. These conditions are described below.

Primary HTN

The cause of primary HTN remains in question. BP is a complex variable involving mechanisms that influence cardiac output, systemic vascular resistance, and blood volume. HTN is caused by one or several abnormalities in the function of these mechanisms or the failure of other factors to compensate for these malfunctioning mechanisms. Currently, the genetic basis for rare types of HTN has been identified, and there is hope that soon these discoveries will lead to understanding of the cause or causes of most HTN.

Genetic factors and the environmental issues of obesity, stress, and excess sodium as well as sympathetic nervous system dysfunction may all contribute to HTN. Several hypotheses are linked to understanding the cause of HTN and include the following:

1. Dysfunction of the autonomic nervous system imbalance may be a cause due to the inheritance of genes predisposing an individual to increased sympathetic nervous activity.
2. Variations in renal sodium absorption also suggest that genes involved in rare inherited forms of HTN may be related to mutations in several genes that increase one's susceptibility to disorders of renal absorption of sodium, chloride, and water. To date, genes accounting for the vast majority of salt-sensitive HTN have not been identified.[21]
3. Dysfunction of the renin–angiotensin–aldosterone system results in an increase in renin–angiotensin–aldosterone activity resulting in extracellular fluid volume expansion and systemic vascular resistance. Angiotensin II has also been shown to act like a growth factor and a cytokine resulting in growth, differentiation, and apoptosis in vascular tissues. Studies have also identified gene coding for various components of the renin–angiotensin–aldosterone system and their roles in the development of HTN.[21]
4. Impaired vascular responsiveness, that is, impairments in vascular dilation and increased vascular contraction, due to the function of the endothelium, occurs in those individuals with HTN. Oxidative stress is also a critical factor in both HTN and atherogenesis.[33,34]
5. Insulin resistance may also play a role in the development of HTN. Insulin resistance may be the common factor that links HTN, diabetes, and other metabolic abnormalities. The metabolic syndrome of abdominal obesity, increased BP, dyslipidemia, and insulin resistance with or without impaired glucose tolerance plus prothrombotic and proinflammatory states may place individuals at high cardiovascular risk.

Secondary HTN

Secondary HTN affects between 5% and 10% of individuals with HTN, and a large number of children younger than 10 years have HTN due to a specific physiologic condition. In children younger than 10 years, the most common causes of persistent HTN are renal disease and vascular problems such as coarctation of the aorta. Common secondary causes of high BP in adults include chronic renal disease, renovascular disease, primary aldosteronism, and, increasingly, sleep apnea.[7] Display 35-1 summarizes the major secondary causes of HTN in both children and adults. Aspects of diagnosis and management of some of the more common conditions are highlighted here.

Renal Parenchymal Disease. Chronic renal disease causes HTN and, conversely, HTN contributes to the development of chronic renal disease. Three factors contribute to the development of HTN in those individuals with renal disease: loss of nephrons leading to retention of sodium, chloride, and water; decreased release of vasodilator substances such as nitric oxide; and activation of the renin–angiotensin system. NHANES III data indicates that 70% of all patients with chronic renal disease have HTN. Aggressive lowering of SBP may slow the progression of kidney disease, and clinicians must consider numerous options for treatment to reach goal BP.

Renovascular Disease. Renovascular HTN, found in 1% to 5% of all hypertensives, occurs when one or both of the renal arteries are diseased, leading to decreased perfusion of the kidneys. The most common cause of renal artery stenosis is atherosclerosis, which leads to renal ischemia, release of renin from juxtaglomerular cells of the kidney, and a secondary increase in BP.[35] Diagnosis of renal artery stenosis is made on the basis of difficult to control BP or deterioration in renal function or electrolyte imbalance and through identification of an abdominal bruit by physical examination. This is followed by the either magnetic resonance imaging or computed tomography and a renal angiogram with consideration of medical treatment, angioplasty, or surgery (which is the gold standard for severe renal artery stenosis).[36]

Primary Hyperaldosteronism. Primary aldosteronism is a disease characterized by excess secretion of aldosterone, caused by an adrenocortical adenoma, adrenal hyperplasia, adrenal carcinoma, or the cause may be unknown; in which case it is diagnosed as idiopathic hyperaldosteronism.[37] A common form of primary aldosteronism is a benign aldosterone producing adenoma. With high levels of aldosterone there is retention of

DISPLAY 35-1 Causes of Secondary Hypertension

Renal

Renal parenchymal disease
Renal vascular disease
Renin-producing tumors
Primary sodium retention (Liddle syndrome)
Increased intravascular volume

Endocrine

Acromegaly
Hypothyroidism
Hyperthyroidism
Hyperparathyroidism
Adrenal cortical
  Cushing syndrome
  Primary aldosteronism
  Apparent mineralocorticoid excess
Adrenal medulla
  Pheochromocytoma
  Carcinoid syndrome

Drugs and Exogenous Hormones

Neurological Causes

Increase intracranial pressure
Quadriplegia
Guillain-Barre syndrome
Idiopathic, primary, or familial dysautonomia

Obstructive Sleep Apnea

Acute Stress-Related Secondary Hypertension

Diseases of the Aorta
Rigidity of the aorta
Coarctation of the aorta

Pregnancy-Induced HTN

Isolated Systolic HTN Due to an Increased Cardiac Output

From Chiong, J. R., Aronow, W. S., Khan, I. A., et al. (2008). Secondary hypertension: Current diagnosis and treatment. *International Journal of Cardiology, 124*, 6–21.

sodium, chloride, and water resulting in an expanded extracellular fluid volume. This condition is now thought to be the cause of 5% to 13% of all cases of HTN.[37] Primary hyperaldosteronism may be difficult to diagnose due to low serum potassium, the most common sign being found in only one third of the cases.[37] The best screening test is now the plasma aldosterone to plasma renin activity ratio.[38] Clinicians should look for this condition in those patients younger than 50 years who appear to have resistant HTN or HTN with hypokalemia. Surgical removal of an adenoma reduces BP and if no tumor is present, medical treatment with aldosterone antagonists such as spironolactone is indicated.[38]

Pheochromocytoma. Pheochromocytomas are largely benign neuroendocrine tumors of the adrenal medulla and present in up to 6% of those individuals with HTN. Because excessive amounts of catecholamine occurs with these tumors, individuals may experience chest discomfort, tachycardia and palpitations, panic attack, and headaches.[35] A pheochromocytoma is normally diagnosed by undertaking measurement of urinary and plasma catecholamines, urinary metanephrine, and urinary vanillylmandelic acid. Nuclear imaging may also identify certain extra-adrenal tumors and once detected surgical intervention is needed.

Obstructive Sleep Apnea. An association between sleep apnea and systemic HTN has been reported since the 1970s. Increasingly this condition has gained more widespread attention due to the growing rate of obesity. Obstructive sleep apnea affects 2% to 4% of the general population, and more than 50% of those affected by it have HTN.[35] It is now a significant health problem causing disrupted sleep, memory loss, personality changes, decreased attention span, poor judgment, and frequent episodes of hypopnea (reduced chest movement with 4% or more decrease in oxyhemoglobin) and or apnea (cessation of airflow for 10 seconds or more).[39] A good medical history about sleep patterns is warranted and referral to a sleep disorder clinic needed to confirm the diagnosis. Treatment involves not only the use of continuous positive airway pressure, the most common approach to this condition, but also weight loss and treatment of concomitant HTN with medicines as needed.[39,40] Assessment of sleep patterns and snoring is also indicated for those individuals with resistant HTN.

Coarctation of the Aorta. Coarctation or narrowing of the lumen of the aorta is rare in adults but relatively common in children, accounting for 7% of all congenital CVD.[35,41] The most common narrowing occurs distal to the left subclavian artery.[42] Those individuals with coarctation of the aorta normally have high upper extremity BPs with low pressures in the lower extremities including weak femoral pulses.[43] If this condition is left untreated, it can cause left ventricular hypertrophy (LVH). Bruits may be present on physical findings, and screening tests, which include a transthoracic echocardiogram or contrast computed tomography/magnetic resonance imaging help to visualize this condition. Treatment includes surgical repair of the lesion or angioplasty. A comparison of the BP and left ventricular mass among patients who had surgical repair of a coarctation and controls found that these patients had significantly higher 24-hour ambulatory SBP and left ventricular mass compared with controls.[44] Thus, follow-up remains important in these patients.

Pregnancy-Induced HTN. HTN occurs in 5.9% of all pregnancies and is classified as preeclampsia–eclampsia, preeclampsia superimposed on chronic HTN, chronic HTN, or gestational HTN.[38] The cause of preeclampsia is not known but it includes proteinuria, renal insufficiency, impaired liver function, and abnormalities including thrombocytopenia, hemolysis, and fetal growth restriction.[45,46] Early diagnosis is critical and close monitoring of BP essential with treatment being directed at medicines with proven safety for each condition.

As shown in Display 35-1 numerous other causes of secondary HTN are noted. A careful history and physical examination, which is discussed in more detail under the section on management, will help reveal many of these secondary causes.

Clinical Manifestations of HTN

Signs and Symptoms

Unfortunately, there are few signs and no symptoms of HTN until it becomes very severe and target organ damage (TOD) has occurred. The major sign, obviously, is the presence of elevated BP based on the criteria for the definition HTN (see Table 35-1). Other signs and symptoms are described in the next section on complications of HTN.

DISPLAY 35-2 Cardiovascular Risk Factors

Major Risk Factors

Hypertension
Cigarette smoking
Obesity (body mass index ≥ 30 kg/m^2)
Physical inactivity
Dyslipidemia
Diabetes mellitus
Microalbuminuria or estimated GFR <60 mL/min
Age (older than 55 years for men and 65 years for women)
Family history of premature cardiovascular disease (men younger than 55 years or women younger than 65 years)

Target Organ Damage

Heart
- Left ventricular hypertrophy
- Angina or prior myocardial infarction
- Prior coronary revascularization
- Heart failure

Brain
- Stroke or transient ischemic attack
- Chronic kidney disease

Peripheral arterial disease
Retinopathy

GFR, glomerular filtration rate.
From Chobanian, A. V., Bakris, G. L., Black, H. R., et al. (2003). The Seventh Report of the Joint National Committee on Prevention, Detection, Evaluation, and Treatment of High Blood Pressure: The JNC 7 report. *JAMA, 289*(19), 2560–2572. (Erratum in *JAMA*, 2003, *290*[2], 197.)

Evaluation of hypertensive patients has three objectives: (1) to assess lifestyle and identify other cardiovascular risk factors or concomitant disorders that may affect prognosis and guide treatment (Display 35-2); (2) to reveal identifiable causes of high BP (Display 35-1); and (3) to assess the presence or absence of TOD and CVD (Display 35-2).[7] Morbidity and mortality associated with HTN are predominately the consequence of damage to a selected set of organs, known as "TOD," which include the blood vessels, heart, brain, kidneys, and eyes. Evidence of TOD is a serious prognostic indicator in a person with HTN. Mechanisms of TOD are described below.

Vascular Changes Associated With HTN

HTN can influence the endothelium, vascular smooth muscle, extracellular matrix, and connective tissue of the arteries. Alterations of vascular structure that occur during chronic HTN may be referred to as remodeling or hypertrophy.[47] Eutrophic inward remodeling, or "remodeling," refers to a decrease in lumen diameter without a change in the thickness of the arterial wall or the characteristic of the material within the vessel wall. In contrast, hypertrophic inward remodeling, or "hypertrophy," is defined as a decrease in lumen diameter associated with an increase in wall thickness and vessel wall material. In either case, narrowing of the vessel lumen is associated with increased vascular resistance.[48] Some of the factors that contribute to the hypertrophy and remodeling processes appear to be different. Mechanisms of hypertrophy may include increased arterial pulse pressure, sympathetic nerve activity, angiotensin II, genetic factors, endothelin-1, nitric oxide, and oxidative stress.[47,49] Mechanisms of remodeling may include intravascular pressure, angiotensin II, genetic factors, endothelin-1, $\alpha\beta\nu3$ integrins.[47]

Changes in the Vascular Endothelium. The vascular endothelium is the largest organ in the body.[50] Vascular endothelial cells are extremely active and play a critical role in regulation of blood vessel tone and cellular activity in the vascular wall. Endothelial cells modulate blood vessel tone by secreting a variety of dilator and constrictor substances. In addition to their effect on vascular tone, these substances and other factors produced by the endothelium, may also modify platelet aggregation, thrombogenicity of the blood, vascular inflammation, and oxidative stress and, over the long term, influence cell migration and proliferation with subsequent development and progression of atherosclerosis and its complications.[50]

Impaired endothelial vasodilation has been identified in persons with HTN and even in the normotensive children of hypertensive parents.[51,52] However, it is not yet clear whether endothelial dysfunction is a precursor of HTN or a sequel. Improved understanding of the molecular basis for endothelial dysfunction in HTN may provide a pathway to developing new therapies to reduce the impact of HTN. Other factors that cause endothelial dysfunction include aging, hyperlipidemia, insulin resistance/diabetes, tobacco use, physical inactivity, and hyperhomocysteinemia.[50]

Atherosclerosis. Atherosclerosis is a complex degenerative condition that is characterized by endothelial dysfunction and lipid accumulation in the endothelium and media, followed by wall thickening and outward remodeling, and later by luminal encroachment, thrombosis, and occlusion.[53] Atherosclerosis manifests as coronary heart disease, cerebrovascular, and peripheral arterial disease and is a major worldwide source of morbidity and mortality. Atherosclerotic plaque formation involves the interaction of genetic predisposition and environmental risk factors with diffuse vascular injury. Many of these factors are also involved in the pathogenesis of HTN. HTN promotes or accelerates all phases of the development of atherosclerotic lesions, from plaque formation to rupture.[53]

Heart. Parallel structural and functional changes in the large arteries (stiffness), cardiac mass (hypertrophy), and myocardial relaxation and filling (diastolic dysfunction) occur at an accelerated rate with chronic HTN. The pressure overload associated with HTN promotes left ventricular hypertrophy (LVH) that leads to left ventricular dysfunction and heart failure. HTN also promotes vascular endothelial and renal dysfunction that directly impacts the progression of heart failure, which in turn affects vascular endothelial and renal dysfunction.[54] Hypertensive individuals have a two- to four-fold increased risk of coronary heart disease and heart failure and those individuals with prehypertension have a 1.6- to 2.5-fold increased risk of CVD, both compared with those who are normotensive.[55,56] Aggressive HTN control can prevent the development of LVH and lead to regression of LVH. However, it remains controversial whether there are differential drug effects on reversing LVH related to HTN.

Kidney. HTN is both a cause and consequence of chronic kidney disease (CKD). The incidence and prevalence of CKD and end-stage renal disease, presumed to be secondary to primary HTN, have increased considerably over the past two decades and are particularly high among African Americans. HTN causes renal damage through multiple mechanisms.[57] One mechanism is ischemia with glomerular hypoperfusion causing glomerulosclerosis and subsequently tubulointerstitial fibrosis. Other mechanisms of injury, such as endothelial dysfunction, cholesterol oxidation, cigarette smoking, and proteinuria, act in concert with high systemic and glomerular capillary pressures to accelerate nephrosclerosis. While the presence of macroalbuminuria (proteinuria > 300 mg/day), indicates presence of kidney disease, even lower level microalbuminuria (30 to 300 mg/day) is associated with increased cardiovascular risk.

CKD mandates more aggressive treatment and lower target BP: <130/80 mm Hg in patients with diabetes or CKD and <120/75 mm Hg in patients with proteinuria >1 g/day.[7] Antihypertensive drugs classes differ in ability to lower proteinuria and slow the progression of CKD. Drugs that block the rennin–angiotensin system, that is, angiotensin-converting enzyme (ACE) inhibitors and angiotensin receptor blockers (ARBs), are the most potent antiproteinuric agents and also have been shown to be highly effective in slowing the progression of renal insufficiency.[58]

Eye. HTN has profound effects on the structure and function of the eye. Hypertensive retinopathy refers to a spectrum of microvascular signs in the retina related to HTN.[59] HTN initially causes retinal circulation vasospasm and increased vasomotor tone, which are reflected as the sign of generalized arteriolar narrowing. Persistent HTN leads to arteriosclerotic changes, including intimal thickening, media wall hyperplasia, and hyaline degeneration. This is seen as increasingly severe generalized arteriolar narrowing, arteriolar wall opacification, and focal narrowing. Thickening of the retinal arteriolar wall by these arteriosclerotic processes may compress the venules, resulting in the sign of AV nicking. In the presence of more acute elevations in BP, an exudative stage may occur, manifesting as microaneurysms, hemorrhages, hard exudates, and cotton wool spots. Optic disk swelling and macular edema may occur with severely elevated BP. These processes may not occur in the sequence described above. Numerous studies have confirmed the strong association between the presence of signs of hypertensive retinopathy and elevated BP.[59] The strongest evidence of the usefulness of the evaluation of hypertensive retinopathy for risk stratification is based on its association with stroke as the retinal circulation shares anatomical, physiological, and embryologic features with the cerebral circulation. A simplified classification of hypertensive retinopathy—none, mild, moderate, and malignant—according to the severity of the retinal signs is presented in Table 35-2.[59]

Table 35-2 ■ CLASSIFICATION OF HYPERTENSIVE RETINOPATHY

Retinopathy Grade	Description	Systemic Associations*
None	No detectable signs	None
Mild	One or more of the following signs: Generalized arteriolar narrowing, focal arteriolar narrowing, arteriovenous nicking, opacity ("copper wiring")	Modest association with risk of clinical stroke, subclinical stroke, coronary heart disease, and death
Moderate	Hemorrhage (blot, dot, or flame-shaped), microaneurysm, cotton–wool spot, hard exudate, or a combination of these signs	Strong association with risk of clinical stroke, subclinical stroke, cognitive decline, and death from cardiovascular causes
Malignant	Signs of moderate retinopathy plus swelling of the optic disk†	Strong association with death

*A modest association is defined as an odds ratio of greater than 1 but less than 2. A strong association is defined as an odds ratio of 2 or greater.
†Anterior ischemic optic neuropathy, characterized by unilateral swelling of the optic disk, visual loss, and sectorial visual field loss, should be ruled out.
From Wong, T. Y., & Mitchell, P. (2004). Hypertensive retinopathy. *New England Journal of Medicine, 351*, 2310–2317.

Brain. HTN has adverse consequences in the brain, including ischemia and hemorrhagic stoke, cognitive impairment/dementia, and encephalopathy. HTN contributes to the development of atherosclerotic plaques in the extracerebral and intracranial vessels as well as the process of microatheroma and hypertensive hyalinosis. Despite the brain's adaptive mechanisms to maintain cerebral blood flow, loss or reduction of blood flow results in stroke producing pathologic changes related to the duration and degree of ischemia. Research has documented the positive relationships between stroke and HTN as well as the reduction in stroke with HTN control.[5,60–63]

Cognitive impairment spans the spectrum from mild cognitive impairment to dementia. Cerebrovascular damage leading to cognitive impairment can occur not only from atherothrombosis but also through cerebral hemorrhage, hypoperfusion, and other arteriopathies. Longitudinal studies strongly suggest an adverse effect of elevated BP in middle age on cognitive functioning.[64] There is also an adverse effect of low BP in the older adults for development of dementia; however, studies suggest no deterioration in cognitive performance with antihypertensive therapy in older adults hypertensive individuals who are well. Hypertensive encephalopathy is a consequence of accelerated or malignant HTN. Encephalopathy occurs when the BP levels exceed the upper limit of autoregulation so that the cerebral arteries become dilated, disrupting the blood–brain barrier and leading to the formation of cerebral edema; local changes in ion and cytokine concentrations; and/or alteration in neural function.[65]

MANAGEMENT OF HTN

Assessment and Diagnosis

Diagnosis

HTN is relatively easy to diagnose. However, in part due to the lack of symptoms, an individual may not seek evaluation or treatment of HTN. In fact, more than 30% of the hypertensive population in the United States are unaware of their condition.[3] The awareness, treatment, and control rates for HTN in the United States between 1999 and 2004 are shown in Table 35-3. While the 37% HTN control rate in 2004 demonstrates continued improvement, it also clearly indicates a need for increased efforts on the part of health care professionals to better manage the treatment of HTN.[3]

BP Measurement. Accurate BP measurement is essential to classify individuals, to ascertain BP-related risk, and to guide HTN management.[66] Proper training of observers, positioning of the patient, and selection of cuff size are all essential. Because an individual's BP can vary markedly, diagnosis of HTN requires documentation of elevated BP (average of two or more BPs) on at least three separate occasions. Three measures of BP potentially could contribute to the adverse effects of HTN. The first is the average level, the second is the diurnal variation, and the third is the short-term variability. The measure of BP that is most clearly related

Table 35-3 ■ TRENDS IN AWARENESS, TREATMENT, AND CONTROL AMONG PARTICIPANTS WITH HYPERTENSION IN THE U.S. POPULATION, 1999 TO 2004

	National Health and Nutrition Examination Survey (%)		
	1999–2000	2001–2002	2003–2004
Awareness	69	71	76
Treatment	58	60	65
Control†	29	33	37

†Among all with hypertension
From Ong, K. L., Cheung, B., Man, Y. B., et al. (2007). Prevalence, awareness, treatment, and control of hypertension among United States adults 1999–2004. *Hypertension, 49*, 69–75.

to morbid events is the average level, although there is also accumulating evidence that suggests that hypertensive patients whose BP remains high at night (nondippers) are at greater risk for cardiovascular morbidity than dippers.[67] Less data are available to define the clinical significance of BP variability, although it has been suggested that it is a risk factor for cardiovascular morbidity.

The recognition of these limitations of the traditional clinic readings has led to two parallel developments: first, increasing use of measurements made out of the clinic, which avoids the unrepresentative nature of the clinic setting and also allows for increased numbers of readings to be taken; and second, the increased use of automated devices, which are being used both in and out of the office setting.[66,68] It is increasingly recognized that office measurements correlate poorly with BP measured in other settings and that they can be supplemented by self-measured readings taken with validated devices at home. There is increasing evidence that home readings predict cardiovascular events and are particularly useful for monitoring the effects of treatment.

Home BP Monitoring. Home BP monitoring overcomes many of the limitations of traditional office BP measurement and is both cheaper and easier to perform than ambulatory BP monitoring. Monitors using the oscillometric method are currently available and are accurate, reliable, easy to use, and relatively inexpensive. An increasing number of individuals are using them regularly to check their BP at home. Home BP monitoring has been endorsed by national and international guidelines and the American Heart Association recently provided detailed recommendations for their use.[68] Home BP monitoring has the potential to improve the quality of care while reducing costs.

White Coat HTN. Approximately 15% to 20% of people with stage 1 HTN have persistently elevated BP in the presence of a health care worker, particularly a physician. However, when BP is measured elsewhere, including at work, BP is not elevated. When this phenomenon is detected in patients not taking medications, it is referred to as white coat HTN. The commonly used definition is a persistently elevated average office BP of ≥140/90 mm Hg and an average awake ambulatory reading of <135/85 mm Hg.[66] Although it can occur at any age, it is more common in older men and women. The phenomenon responsible for white coat HTN is commonly referred to as the white coat effect and is defined as the difference between the office and daytime ambulatory BP; it is present in the majority of hypertensive patients. Its magnitude can be reduced (but not eliminated) by the use of stationary oscillometric devices that automatically determine and analyze a series of BPs over 15 to 20 minutes with the patient in a quiet environment in the office or clinic.

Masked HTN or Isolated Ambulatory HTN. The converse condition of normal BP in the office and elevated BPs elsewhere, such as at work or at home is somewhat less frequent than white coat HTN but more problematic to detect.[66] Lifestyle can contribute to this, for example, alcohol, tobacco, and caffeine consumption and physical activity away from the clinic or office.

Clinical Evaluation

The objectives of the medical assessment for HTN are to determine (1) diagnosis and stage of HTN, (2) secondary causes of HTN, (3) presence of TOD, (4) level of global CVD risk, and (5) the plan for individualized monitoring and therapy. The assessment should include a thorough history and physical examination, including orthostatic BP change. Display 35-3 lists many of the important variables to assess during the history and physical examination.[69] It is also important to ask the patient about any nontraditional remedies they may be using including herbs, vitamins, and other supplements. Display 35-4 lists the basic and optional laboratory tests recommended by the Joint National Committee on Prevention, Detection and Treatment of Hypertension (JNC 7) for the assessment of TOD.

Secondary HTN, a potentially curable condition, occurs in an estimated 5% to 10% of HTN cases; therefore, clinicians should evaluate for secondary causes (see Display 35-1).[35] Additional evaluation is recommended in patients whose age, severity of HTN, medical history, physical examination, or laboratory findings are suggestive of secondary HTN. Poor response to antihypertensive drug therapy or an accelerated phase of previously well-controlled HTN also indicates a need for further investigation.[7]

Prognosis

In the vast majority of cases, HTN cannot be cured. The relationship between BP and risk of CVD events is continuous, consistent, and independent of other risk factors.[7] For individuals aged 40 to 70 years, each increment of 20 mm Hg in SBP or 10 mm Hg in DBP doubles the risk of CVD across the entire BP range from 115/75 to 185/115 mm Hg.[5] The effectiveness of lifestyle and pharmacologic treatment in reducing BP has been demonstrated and substantial evidence indicates that controlling BP in hypertensive patients significantly lowers risk of CV morbidity and mortality.[5,70–72] A small reduction in BP could markedly reduce the risk of heart failure, stroke, and myocardial infarction.[7,73] The recent improvements in HTN control rates and decreased mean BPs, especially among the older adults, may help to decrease the incidence of strokes and heart attacks, which is highly encouraging.[3]

Prevention

The prevention of HTN is a major public health challenge. Many cases of HTN, cardiovascular and renal disease, and stroke might be prevented if the rise in BP with age could be prevented or diminished.[7] The six interventions that have been shown to delay or

DISPLAY 35-3 Important Aspects of the Patient's History

Duration of the Hypertension

Last known normal blood pressure
Course of the blood pressure

Prior Treatment of the Hypertension

Drugs: types, doses, side effects

Intake of Agents That May Interfere

Nonsteroidal antiinflammatory drugs
Oral contraceptives
Sympathomimetics
Adrenal steroids
Excessive sodium intake
Alcohol (>2 drinks/day)
Herbal remedies

Family History

Hypertension
Premature cardiovascular disease or death
Familial diseases: pheochromocytoma, renal disease, diabetes, gout

Symptoms of Secondary Causes

Muscle weakness
Spells of tachycardia, sweating, tremor
Thinning of the skin
Flank pain

Symptoms of Target Organ Damage

Headaches
Transient weakness or blindness
Loss of visual acuity
Chest pain
Dyspnea
Edema
Claudication

Presence of Other Risk Factors

Smoking
Diabetes
Dyslipidemia
Physical inactivity

Concomitant Diseases

Dietary History
Weight change
Fresh versus processed foods
Sodium
Saturated fats

Sexual Function

Features of Sleep Apnea
Early morning headaches
Daytime somnolence
Loud snoring
Erratic sleep

Ability to Modify Lifestyle and Maintain Therapy

Understanding the nature of hypertension and the need for regimen
Ability to perform physical activity
Source of food preparation
Financial constraints
Ability to read instructions
Need for care providers

From Kaplan, N. M. (2002). *Kaplan's clinical hypertension* (8th ed.). Philadelphia. Lippincott Williams & Wilkins.

prevent the onset of HTN are as follows: weight loss, sodium restriction, reduction in alcohol intake, increased exercise, potassium supplementation, and a diet high in fruits and vegetables.[74–80] Efforts to begin the lifestyle habits that prevent the development of HTN should begin during childhood.[76]

DISPLAY 35-4 Recommended and Optional Laboratory Tests and Diagnostic Procedures

Recommended

Urinalysis
Hematocrit
Blood chemistries
  Potassium, calcium, creatinine or estimated glomerular filtration rate, fasting glucose, fasting lipid profile
12-lead electrocardiogram

Optional

Urinary albumin excretion or
Albumin/creatinine ratio

From Chobanian, A. V., Bakris, G. L., Black, H. R., et al. (2003). The Seventh Report of the Joint National Committee on Prevention, Detection, Evaluation, and Treatment of High Blood Pressure: The JNC 7 report. *JAMA, 289*(19), 2560–2572. (Erratum in *JAMA,* 2003, *290*[2], 197.)

Treatment Options

The goal of therapy for patients with HTN is the prevention of morbidity and mortality related to the elevated BP, specifically the prevention of TOD and progression of atherosclerotic cardiovascular and renal disease.[7] Factors to consider in making treatment choices are any comorbid conditions, cost of treatment, patient preference, and potential impacts on the individual's quality of life. Figure 35-1 provides an algorithm for treatment of HTN in adults.[7] Treatment options, which will be described in greater detail below, include nonpharmacologic, or lifestyle modifications, and pharmacologic options. Treatment to achieve a goal BP, <140/90 or <130/80 mm Hg among those patients with diabetes mellitus or renal disease, is associated with reductions in CVD morbidity and mortality.

Nonpharmacologic Management of HTN

Adoption of a healthy lifestyle is recommended for all persons for the prevention of HTN and is an indispensable part of the management of those with HTN.[7] Well-established lifestyle modifications that lower BP include weight loss, increased physical activity, and dietary modifications including sodium restriction, a diet high in fruits and vegetables and potassium and reduction in alcohol intake.[79,80] A combined approach that aims to balance

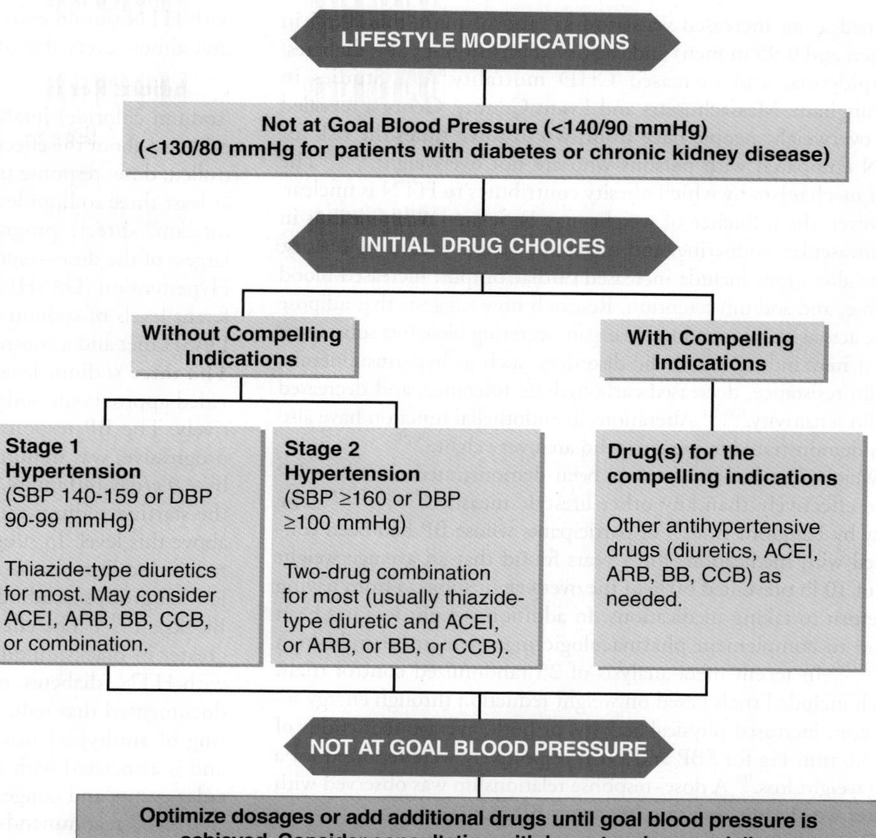

■ Figure 35-1 Algorithm for treatment of hypertension in adults. ACEI, angiotensin-converting enzyme inhibitor; BB, β-blocker; CCB, calcium channel blocker. (Chobanian, A. V., Bakris G. L., Black, H. R., et al. [2003]. The Seventh Report of the Joint National Committee on Prevention, Detection, Evaluation, and Treatment of High Blood Pressure: The JNC 7 report. *JAMA, 289*[19], 2560–2572. [Erratum in *JAMA, 290*(2), 197].)

energy intake with energy expenditure through a suitable dietary plan and physical activity is effective and an important component of weight loss and weight management. The JNC 7 recommendations for these lifestyle modifications are listed in Table 35-4.[7] In addition, persons with HTN are encouraged to modify their other risk factors for CVD such as dyslipidemia and smoking because of their additive impact on the rate of development and progression of atherosclerosis.

Weight Control. The results of many studies indicate a direct relationship between HTN and obesity.[17,81,82] There is also a correlation between the presence of excess abdominal adiposity

Table 35-4 ■ LIFESTYLE MODIFICATIONS TO MANAGE HYPERTENSION*,†

Modification	Recommendation	Approximate SBP Reduction (Range)
Weight reduction	Maintain normal body weight (body mass index 18.5–24.9 kg/m^2).	5–20 mm Hg/10 kg weight loss
Adopt DASH diet plan	Consume a diet rich in fruits, vegetables, and low fat dairy products with a reduced content of saturated and total fat.	8–14 mm Hg
Dietary sodium reduction	Reduce dietary sodium intake to no more than 100 mmol/day (2.4 g sodium or 6 g sodium chloride).	2–8 mm Hg
Physical activity	Engage in regular aerobic physical activity such as brisk walking (at least 30 min/day, most days of the week).	4–9 mm Hg
Moderation of alcohol consumption	Limit consumption to no more than two drinks (1 oz or 30 mL ethanol; e.g., 24 oz beer, 10 oz wine, or 3 oz 80-proof whiskey) per day in most men and to no more than one drink per day in women and lighter weight persons.	2–4 mm Hg

*For overall cardiovascular risk reduction, stop smoking.
†The effects of implementing these modifications are dose- and time dependent and could be greater for some individuals.
From Chobanian, A. V., Bakris, G. L., Black, H. R., et al. (2003). The Seventh Report of the Joint National Committee on Prevention, Detection, Evaluation, and Treatment of High Blood Pressure: The JNC 7 report. *JAMA, 289*(19), 2560–2572. (Erratum in *JAMA*, 2003, *290*[2], 197.)

(defined as an increased waist-to-hip ratio of more than 0.85 in women and 0.95 in men) and the development of HTN, diabetes, dyslipidemia, and increased CHD mortality.[83–87] Studies in Framingham, Massachusetts and Evans County, Georgia revealed that overweight people have from two to three times the risk for HTN compared with persons who are not overweight.[17,88] The exact mechanism by which obesity contributes to HTN is unclear. However, the influence of weight may be related to alterations in cardiovascular, endocrine, and metabolic factors caused by obesity. These alterations include increased cardiac output, increased blood volume, and sodium retention. Research now suggests that adipose tissue acts as a major endocrine organ, secreting bioactive substances which may induce metabolic disorders, such as hyperinsulinemia, insulin resistance, decreased carbohydrate tolerance, and decreased insulin sensitivity.[89–91] Alterations in endothelial function have also been demonstrated in persons who are overweight.[90,92]

Weight loss has consistently been demonstrated to reduce BP more effectively than any other lifestyle measure.[74–76,93–98] The study by Langford et al.[94] of participants whose BP had been controlled with medications for 5 years found that an average weight loss of 10 lb prevented 60% of the overweight subjects from having to return to taking medications. In addition, weight loss has been found to complement pharmacologic management of mild-high BP.[99,100] In recent meta-analysis of 25 randomized control trials, which included trials based on weight reduction through energy restriction, increased physical activity, or both, average reductions of 4.4/3.6 mm Hg for SBP and DBP, respectively were reported for a 5-kg weight loss.[98] A dose–response relationship was observed with greater weight loss resulting in greater BP reduction.

Counseling a hypertensive, overweight patient about weight reduction is important, both as a preventive measure as well as an independent or complementary treatment for high BP. The challenge for both clinicians and patients is supporting maintenance of weight loss, because longitudinal studies have shown that subjects who lose weight initially tend to gain back the weight over time.[76]

Physical Activity. A sedentary lifestyle is one of the risk factors for HTN.[80,101–105] There is increasing evidence showing inactivity in American adults. For example, in 2005 less than half of the U.S. adults met recommendations for physical activity.[80] The results of four meta-analyses on the effect of physical activity on HTN concluded that aerobic training does reduce BP.[106–109] The data indicate that physical fitness training had a graded influence on BP from a small influence on normotensive individuals to a larger impact on those with HTN. Other analyses indicate that persons who are physically active experience reduced cardiovascular and all-cause mortality rates.[110–122]

Physical activity is known to have a variety of metabolic and other effects that may partially explain its beneficial effects on BP. These include reduction in resting cardiac output and peripheral vascular resistance, a humoral mechanism contributing to reduction of the activity of the rennin–angiotensin–aldosterone system and sympathetic nervous system activity, and increase in prostaglandins with vasodilator effect.[80,109] Importantly, an effect of physical exercise on TOD has also been demonstrated. Two studies of 18 persons with HTN and LVH found that after 24 to 32 weeks of exercising at least three times per week, the participants had significant decreases in indices of LVH.[123] A confounding factor in many of these studies is that physical activity intervention is often combined with weight loss. It is recommended that persons with HTN should exercise moderately for a minimum of 30 minutes almost every day of the week.[7]

Sodium Restriction. In general, as the amount of dietary salt (sodium chloride) intake rises, so does BP.[79] The most persuasive evidence about the effects of salt on BP comes from rigorously controlled, dose–response trials.[124–126] Each of these three trials tested at least three sodium levels, and each documented statistically significant, direct, progressive dose–response relationships. The largest of the dose–response trials, the Dietary Approaches to Stop Hypertension (DASH)-Sodium trial, tested the effects of three different levels of sodium intake separately in two distinct diets: the DASH diet and a control diet more typical of what Americans eat. The three sodium levels (lower, intermediate, and higher) provided approximate sodium intakes of 1.5, 2.5, and 3.3 g, respectively. The BP response to sodium reduction, while direct and progressive, was nonlinear. Specifically, decreasing sodium intake by 0.9 g/day (40 mmol/day) caused a greater lowering of BP when the starting sodium intake was 100 mmol/day than when it was above this level. In subgroup analyses of the DASH-Sodium trial reduced sodium intake significantly lowered BP in each of the major subgroups studied (i.e., men, women, Blacks, and non-Blacks).[127,128] The effects of sodium reduction on BP tend to be greater in Blacks; middle-aged and older persons; and individuals with HTN, diabetes, or CKD.[79] In addition, clinical trials have documented that reduced sodium intake can lower BP in the setting of antihypertensive medication and facilitate HTN control and is associated with a reduced risk of atherosclerotic cardiovascular events and congestive heart failure.[79,129]

JNC 7 recommends a goal sodium intake of $\leq$100 mmol/day, which is equivalent to approximately 6 g of sodium chloride or 2.4 g of sodium per day.[7] In many of the clinical trials of sodium reduction, the goal levels of sodium intake were even lower than this recommended goal. To reduce salt intake, individuals should choose foods low in salt and limit the amount of salt added to food. However, because >75% of consumed salt comes from processed foods, any meaningful strategy to reduce salt intake must involve the efforts of food manufacturers and restaurants. It may help patients to know that it takes 8 to 12 weeks to adjust one's sense of taste to a lower intake of sodium.[130]

Diet High in Fruits and Vegetables. The DASH study examined the effects of an 8-week dietary intervention on BP in normotensive and hypertensive subjects.[77] The DASH diet emphasized fruits, vegetables, and low-fat dairy products; included whole grains, poultry, fish, and nuts; and was reduced in fats, red meat, sweets, and sugar-containing beverages. Accordingly, it was rich in potassium, magnesium, calcium, and fiber and was reduced in total fat, saturated fat, and cholesterol; it also was slightly increased in protein. In the 133 hypertensive subjects, the investigators found that adherence to a diet rich in fruits, vegetables, and low-fat dairy products and low in saturated and total fat resulted in a marked decline in both SBP and DBP. Compared with normotensive control subjects, those subjects with an SBP between 140 and 160 mm Hg and/or a DBP between 90 and 95 mm Hg had decreases in BP of $-11.4/-5.5$ mm Hg. There was no significant change in weight during the study in any of the study groups. The DASH diet included 8 to 10 servings per day of fruits and vegetables and 2.7 servings of low-fat dairy products. Subsequent clinical trials based on the DASH diets have shown that (1) adding salt reduction results in a significantly greater decrease in SBP and DBP and (2) the DASH diet can successfully be combined with other lifestyle modifications specifically limiting alcohol intake to 1 oz or less per day and increasing physical activity to a minimum of 180 minutes (3 hours) each week.[79,126,131] While the DASH diet is effective, adopting these dietary recommendations presents a great challenge for many individuals. Description of the DASH diet and sample menus is available on the National Heart, Lung, and Blood Institute Web site.

Reduction of Alcohol Intake. Observational studies and clinical trials have documented a direct, dose-dependent relationship between alcohol intake and BP, particularly as the intake of alcohol increases above two drinks per day.[79,132–135] Meta-analysis of 15 randomized controlled trials demonstrated that decreased consumption of alcohol (median reduction in self-reported alcohol consumption, 76%; range, 16% to 100%) reduced SBP and DBP by 3.3 and 2.0 mm Hg, respectively.[136] BP reductions were similar in nonhypertensive and hypertensive individuals. Importantly, the relationship between reduction in mean percentage of alcohol and decline in BP was dose dependent. However, there may be benefit to moderate levels of alcohol consumption. A case-control study of adults older than 40 years found a lower incidence of ischemic stroke in persons with an alcohol intake of one to two drinks per day compared with abstainers.[137]

JNC 7 recommends that alcohol consumption should be limited to ≤2 alcoholic drinks per day in most men and ≤1 alcoholic drink per day in women and lighter-weight persons.[7,79] A standard drink has been defined as approximately 14 g of alcohol, which is the amount contain in 12 oz of beer, 5 oz of wine, or 1.5 oz of distilled liquor such as vodka, gin, or scotch.

Control of Other Risk Factors. Any individual who has an elevated SBP or DBP has an increased risk for atherosclerotic CVD. In addition, longitudinal epidemiologic studies have shown that the major risk factors have an additive effect on the probability that an individual will have a morbid or mortal event.[138–141] Therefore, even though smoking cessation and improving dyslipidemia will not decrease BP, these interventions will reduce the risk of morbidity and mortality from atherosclerotic CVD.[142–148]

Pharmacologic Management

Since the 1960s, randomized, placebo-controlled, clinical trials have provided evidence that pharmacologic treatment of HTN reduces morbidity and mortality. The Veterans Administration Cooperative Group Studies on Antihypertensive Agents were the first studies in the United States demonstrating that drug treatment was extremely beneficial in people with moderate and severe HTN.[149,150] Subsequent clinical trials have explored the benefits of treatment in more representative populations as well as at lower BP levels. In addition, more recently, the value of lowering SBP to reduce risk has had a major impact on how we initiate pharmacotherapy and titrate and use additional therapies to control BP. The use of drugs in special populations also confers numerous treatment choices designed to treat HTN and reduce CVD risk and other TOD.

Two questions continue to remain paramount in the treatment of HTN. The first is how low should BP be lowered, and the second relates to the relative risks and benefits of the different classes of antihypertensive medications. The Hypertension Optimal Treatment (HOT) trial of 18,790 men and women, aged 50 to 80 years from 20 countries helped to respond to the issue of how low should BP be lowered.[151] Within this trial, subjects were randomly allocated to three target DBPs, 80, 85, and 90 mm Hg. Drug treatment included felodipine, a calcium channel antagonist, followed by the use of an ACE inhibitor or β-blocker and if needed a diuretic. In the last 6 months of the trial, the mean BPs in the three respective groups were 81, 83, and 85 mm Hg. When the relationship between BP and study outcomes was examined, the lowest risk for CVD events was a pressure of 138.5/82.6 mm Hg, for stroke 142.2/80 mm Hg, and for cardiovascular mortality 138.8/86.5 mm Hg. The greatest benefit from lowering of DBP was noted in diabetics where a pressure of ≤90 mm Hg was associated with 24.4 events, a pressure of ≤85 mm Hg with 18.6 events, and a pressure of ≤80 mm Hg associated with 11.9 events, all were statistically significant ($p = .005$). This trials provided strong evidence to support lower BP targets among hypertensive patients with diabetes. Follow-up studies have shown the very positive effects of lowering SBP and DBP in patients with renal disease, diabetes, and heart failure. The only cautionary note about lowering DBP lies with the population of older adults. The Rotterdam Study of 2,351 subjects showed that the risk of stroke increased significantly when DBP was reduced to <65 mm Hg.[152] A follow-up analysis of the Systolic Hypertension in the Elderly Program (SHEP) data also showed that people who suffered a CVD event had lower DBPs (65 mm Hg) than those who had no event (68 mm Hg).[153] However, the International Verapamil SR/Trandolapril (INVEST) study showed benefit when BP was lowered to 64 mm Hg in the older adults which included a reduction in CVD events.[154] Thus the question of the "J" curve (lowering BP too low to perfuse organs may increase CVD events) appears to remain but perhaps only in the older adults population and the research to date has been performed only in a small number of patients.[155]

The second question relates to the relative risks and benefits of different classes of antihypertensive medicines. Some experts believe that medicines like thiazide diuretics and β-blockers are as effective in lowering BP and reducing risk as newer agents such as ACEs, ARBs, and calcium channel blockers.[156] This led to the Antihypertensive and Lipid Lowering Treatment to Prevent Heart Attack Trial (ALLHAT), which followed 42,418 subjects, aged 55 years and older from 18 countries (623 sites in North America) who were randomly allocated to receive chlorthalidone, amlodipine, doxazosin, or lisinopril for an average of 4.9 years.[157] Additional agents including atenolol, clonidine, or reserpine and if necessary hydralazine could be added as necessary to maximum doses of the drugs originally assigned. The doxazosin arm was stopped early due to a significant increase in combined cardiovascular endpoints. At the end of the study period, there were no differences between the three treatment groups for the primary outcome, which was a combination of fatal coronary heart disease or nonfatal myocardial infarction or for all-cause mortality.[157] The study also showed the value of the thiazide diuretic on secondary endpoints. More strokes occurred in those patients assigned to lisinopril compared with those assigned to chlorthalidone (6.3% vs. 5.6%, $p = .02$). Heart failure was also more common in those patients receiving newer agents (chlorthalidone, 7.7%, amlodipine, 10.2%, lisinopril, 8.7%, $p < .0001$). Continued discussion, which relates to many follow-up studies today is around whether it is truly the specific agent or the reduction in BP that contributes to better outcomes. Just 2 months following the release of ALLHAT the results of the Second Australian National Blood Pressure Study (ANBP2) were published with contradictory results.[158] ANBP2 compared the efficacy of the diuretic hydrochlorothiazide with an ACE inhibitor, enalapril, in 6,083 subjects (50% women) aged 65 to 84 years who were followed over a median of 4.1 years. With identical reductions in BP (−26/12 mm Hg), the group treated with the ACE inhibitor had fewer cardiovascular events or deaths than the group treated with diuretics with a hazard ratio of 0.89 (95% confidence interval: 0.79 to 1.00). However, the primary endpoint for benefit was restricted to men, and the final publication states that this observation needs to be interpreted with caution and requires confirmation.[158] Although these studies were well designed, there were differences in designs, study populations, medications, and endpoints.

Following the release of these two major trials, another study in Europe, the Anglo-Scandanavian Cardiac Outcomes Trial—Blood Pressure Lowering Arm (ASCOT–BPLA), was published.[159] This trial was an open-label, controlled study of 19,257 hypertensive patients who were 40 to 79 years of age, with ≤3 other cardiovascular risk factors. Patients received either amlodipine or atenolol, titrated to maximum dose followed by perindopril with was added to amlodipine and bendroflumethiazide and potassium added to atenolol. If necessary, doxazosin was then added in both groups. The study was terminated at 5.5 years and no significant difference was found in the primary endpoint of nonfatal myocardial infarction and fatal coronary heart disease between those patients receiving amlodipine and those receiving atenolol (8.2 vs. 9.1 per 1,000 P = 0.105).[159] Secondary endpoints were better for the amlodipine group including total coronary endpoints, total cardiovascular procedures, cardiovascular mortality, stroke, peripheral arterial disease, and the development of diabetes. However, it has also been noted that in the amlodipine group both SBP and DBP demonstrated significant reductions, which may have been the contributing factor for better patient outcomes. What is notable from this study is that those patients treated in the amlodipine group had a reduction in cardiovascular events beginning as early as 1 month following treatment, again likely due to the greater decline in BP.

Since the ALLHAT, ANBP2, and ASCOT studies were done, there have been many other trials looking at the value of the five major classes of medications to treat HTN. Clearly, there may be beneficial effects from various agents in certain subpopulations and the need to consider using a medication with dual functions but the question of whether it is the agent that is critical or the lowering of SBP still remains. As noted by Frohlich, clinicians must consider coexisting conditions of their patients, health care resources, and the fact that most persons with HTN will need at least two classes of medications to control BP.[160] Clinicians must also consider that only 37% of all hypertensive patients are at goal BP and greater titration, use of multiple agents, and attention to national guidelines may all support better HTN control.[38]

Treatment Based on JNC 7 Guidelines

The current recommended guidelines from the JNC 7 provides an algorithm for the management of pharmacotherapy in hypertensive individuals.[7] As shown in Figure 35-1, on the basis of the results of ALLHAT and other trials, the JNC 7 expert panel recommends that unless there are other compelling reasons, thiazide diuretics should be the initial therapy in most persons with HTN.[7,157] Compelling indications for the use of other classes of antihypertensive medications in those patients with coexisting medical conditions broaden the choice of agents used in the treatment of patients with Stage 1 or 2 HTN. Table 35-5 includes the comorbid conditions that need to be considered when selecting medications for the person with HTN. In persons with Stage 2 HTN (≥160 mm Hg SBP or ≥100 mm Hg DBP) two medications are recommended for initial treatment with a thiazide diuretic recommended as the choice of one of these agents. Other factors that need to be considered when prescribing antihypertensive treatment include the cost, formulary, duration of action, frequency of adverse effects, patient preference, adherence, quality of life, and other medications the patient is using including over-the-counter agents that may be used for other conditions.

Seven classes of medications are available in the treatment of HTN including (1) diuretics; (2) adrenergic inhibitors including β-blocking agents, central-acting inhibitors, central α-agonists, α-adrenergic blockers, and combined α-adrenergic and β-adrenergic blockers; (3) vasodilators; (4) calcium channel blockers; (5) ACE inhibitors; (6) angiotensin II receptor blockers; and (7) ARBs. Table 35-6 lists the generic and trade names, usual doses,

Table 35-5 ■ CLINICAL TRIAL AND GUIDELINE BASIS FOR COMPELLING INDICATIONS FOR INDIVIDUAL DRUG CLASSES

	Recommended Drugs†						
Compelling Indication*	Diuretic	BB	ACEI	ARB	CCB	ALDO ANT	**Clinical Trial Basis‡,§**
Heart failure	•	•	•	•		•	ACC/AHA Heart Failure Guideline,[161] MERIT-HF,[162] COPERNICUS,[163] CIBIS,[164] SOLVD,[165] AIRE,[166] TRACE,[167] ValHEFT,[168] RALES[169]
Post-MI		•	•			•	ACC/AHA Post-MI Guideline,[170] BHAT,[171] SAVE,[172] Capricorn,[173] EPHESUS[174]
High coronary disease risk	•	•	•		•		ALLHAT,[157] HOPE,[175] ANBP$_2$,[158] LIFE,[176] CONVINCE[177]
Diabetes	•	•	•	•	•		NKF-ADA Guideline,[178] UKPDS,[179] ALLHAT[157]
Chronic kidney disease			•	•			NKF Guideline,[178] Captopril Trial,[180] RENAAL,[181] IDNT,[182] REIN,[183] AASK[184]
Recurrent stroke prevention	•		•				PROGRESS[185]

*Compelling indications for antihypertensive drugs are based on benefits from outcome studies or existing clinical guidelines; the compelling indication is managed in parallel with the BP.
†Drug abbreviations: ACEI, angiotensin-converting enzyme inhibitor; Aldo ANT, aldosterone antagonist; BB, β-blocker; CCB, calcium channel blocker.
‡Conditions for which clinical trials demonstrate benefit of specific classes of antihypertensive drugs.
§See list of references.
From Chobanian, A. V., Bakris, G. L., Black, H. R., et al. (2003). The Seventh Report of the Joint National committee on Prevention, Detection, Evaluation, and Treatment of High Blood Pressure: The JNC 7 report. *JAMA, 289*(19), 2560–2572. (Erratum in *JAMA*, 2003, *290*[2], 197.)

Table 35-6 ■ ORAL ANTIHYPERTENSIVE DRUGS*

Drug	Trade Name	Usual Dose Range, Total mg/day* (frequency per day)	Selected Side Effects and Comments*
Diuretics (partial list)			
Chlorthalidone (G)[†]	Thalitone	12.5–25 (1)	Short term: increases cholesterol and glucose levels; biochemical abnormalities: decreases potassium, sodium, and magnesium levels, increases uric acid and calcium levels; rare: blood dyscrasias, photosensitivity, pancreatitis, hyponatremia
Hydrochlorothiazide (G)	HydroDIURIL, Microzide	12.5–50 (1)	
Indapamide	Lozol	1.25–2.5 (1)	(Less or no hypercholesterolemia)
Metolazone	Mykrox	0.5–1.0 (1)	
	Zaroxolyn	2.5–5 (1)	
Polythiazide	Renes	2–4 (1)	
Loop Diuretics			
Bumetanide (G)	Bumex	0.5–2 (2)	(Short duration of action, no hypercalcemia)
Furosemide (G)	Lasix	40–80 (2)	(Short duration of action, no hypercalcemia)
Torsemide	Demadex	2.5–10 (1)	
Potassium-Sparing Agents			Hyperkalemia
Amiloride hydrochloride (G)	Midamor	5–10 (1–2)	
Triamterene (G)	Dyrenium	50–100 (1–2)	
Adrenergic Inhibitors			
Central Alpha Agonists			Sedation, dry mouth, bradycardia, withdrawal hypertension
Clonidine hydrochloride (G)	Catapres	0.1–0.8 (2)	(More withdrawal)
Guanfacine hydrochloride (G)	Generic	0.5–2 (1)	(Less withdrawal)
Methyldopa (G)	Aldomet	250–1,000 (2)	(Hepatic and "autoimmune" disorders)
Reserpine (G)	Generic	0.05–0.25 (1)	(Nasal congestion, sedation, depression, activation of peptic ulcer)
α-Blockers			Postural (orthostatic) hypotension
Doxazosin mesylate	Cardura	1–16 (1)	
Prazosin hydrochloride (G)	Minipress	2–20 (1–2)	
Terazosin hydrochloride	Hytrin	1–20 (1)	
β-Blockers			Bronchospasm, bradycardia, heart failure, may mask insulin-induced hypoglycemia; less serious: impaired peripheral circulation, insomnia, fatigue, decreased exercise tolerance, hypertriglyceridemia (except agents with intrinsic sympathomimetic activity)
Acebutolol[‡,§]	Sectral	200–800 (2)	
Atenolol (G)[§]	Tenormin	25–100 (1)	
Betaxolol[§] hyperchloride	Kerlone	5–20 (1)	
Bisoprolol fumarate[§]	Zebeta	2.5–10 (1)	
Metoprolol tartrate (G)[§]	Lopressor	50–100 (1–2)	
Metoprolol succinate[§]	Toprol XL	50–100 (1)	
Nadolol (G)	Corgard	40–120 (1)	
Penbutolol sulfate[‡]	Levatol	10–40 (2)	
Pindolol (G)[‡]	Visken	10–40 (2)	
Propranolol hydrochloride (G)	Inderal	40–160 (2)	
	Inderal LA	40–180 (1)	
Timolol maleate (G)	Blocadren	20–40 (2)	
Combined α- and β-Blockers			Postural hypotension, bronchospasm
Carvedilol	Coreg	12.5–50 (2)	
Labetalol hydrochloride (G)	Normodyne, Trandate	200–800 (2)	
Nebivolol	Bystolic	2.5–40 (1)	
Direct Vasodilators			Headaches, fluid retention, tachycardia
Hydralazine hydrochloride (G)	Apresoline	25–100 (2)	(Lupus syndrome)
Minoxidil (G)	Loniten	2.5–80 (1–2)	(Hirsutism)
Calcium antagonists			
Nondihydropyridines			Conduction defects, worsening of systolic dysfunction, gingival hyperplasia
Diltiazem hydrochloride	Cardizem LA	120–540 (1)	(Nausea, headache)
	Cardizem CD, Dilacor XR, Tiazac	180–240 (1)	
Verapamil hydrochloride	Isoptin SR, Calan SR Coer	120–360 (1–2)	(Constipation)
	(Verelan PM, Covera HS)	120–360 (1)	
Dihydropyridines			Edema of the ankle, flushing, headache, gingival hypertrophy
Amlodipine besylate	Norvasc	2.5–10 (1)	
Felodipine	Plendil	2.5–20 (1)	
Isradipine	DynaCirc CR	2.5–10, 5–20 (1)	
Nicardipine	Cardene SR	60–120 (2)	
Nifedipine	Procardia XL, Adalat CC	30–60 (1)	
Nisoldipine	Sular	10–40 (1)	
Angiotensin-Converting Enzyme Inhibitors			Common: cough; rare: angioedema, hyperkalemia, rash, loss of taste, leukopenia
Benazepril hydrochloride	Lotensin	10–40 (1–2)	
Captopril (G)	Capoten	25–100 (2)	
Enalapril maleate	Vasotec	2.5–40 (1–2)	
Fosinopril sodium	Monopril	10–40 (1)	
Lisinopril	Prinivil, Zestril	10–40 (1)	

(table continues on page 808)

Table 35-6 ■ ORAL ANTIHYPERTENSIVE DRUGS* (continued)

Drug	Trade Name	Usual Dose Range, Total mg/day* (frequency per day)	Selected Side Effects and Comments*
Moexipril	Univasc	7.5–30 (1)	
Perindopril	Aceon	4–8 (1–2)	
Quinapril hydrochloride	Accupril	10–40 (1)	
Ramipril	Altace	2.5–20 (1)	
Trandolapril	Mavik	1–4 (1)	
Angiotensin II Receptor Blockers			Angioedema (very rare), hyperkalemia
Candesartan	Atacand	8–32 (1)	
Eprosartan	Teveten	400–800 (1–2)	
Irbesartan	Avapro	150–300 (1)	
Losartan potassium	Cozaar	25–100 (1–2)	
Olmesartan	Benicar	20–40 (1)	
Telmisartan	Micardis	20–80 (1)	
Valsartan	Diovan	80–320 (1)	
Direct Renin Inhibitors			
Tekturna	Aliskiren	150–300 (1)	
Aldosterone Receptor Blockers			
Eplerenone	Inspra	50–100 (1–2)	Hyperkalemia
Spironolactone	Aldactone	25–50 (1–2)	Hyperkalemia, gynecomastia

*These dosages may vary from those listed in the *Physicians' Desk Reference* (51st edition), which may be consulted for additional information. The listing of side effects is not all-inclusive and side effects are for the class of drugs except where noted for individual drugs (in parentheses); clinicians are urged to refer to the package insert for a more detailed listing.
†(G) indicates generic available.
‡Has intrinsic sympathomimetic activity.
§Cardioselective.

and selected side effects of most of the common antihypertensive agents. Some of the most commonly used combinations are shown in Table 35-7. Combinations are often useful in simplifying therapy to increase adherence once the dose of medicines have been titrated appropriately and in Stage 2 HTN initially. Once an initial drug has been chosen, it is recommended that the patient begin with a low dose, which is titrated, or a new drug is added if BP goals are not achieved after a period of 1 to 2 months.[7] This becomes critically important as one of the failures of achieving better BP control is failure of health care professionals to titrate antihypertensive medications.[35]

A Few Issues Beyond JNC 7

Numerous studies have been undertaken since the release of the JNC 7 guidelines, which may add some relevance to changes that may occur with new guidelines. For example, there have been questions about whether to treat individuals with high-normal BP or prehypertensive individuals if they do not respond well to lifestyle changes. The Trial of Preventing Hypertension Study (TROPHY) was undertaken to determine if an ARB compared with a placebo in groups who had received lifestyle therapy would slow the progression of prehypertension to HTN defined as a BP of <140/90 mm Hg.[186] In this trial, the use of an angiotensin receptor blocker slowed the progression of prehypertension to HTN in the 2 years of the trial and the 2 years following the study when the drug was withheld. However, the authors stated very clearly that until this trial is confirmed with other studies, treatment should not be given to those individuals with pre-HTN unless there are other risk factors such as diabetes, CHD, or renal disease.

Should β-blockers be used as first-line agents is another issue that has surfaced since the JNC 7. Many of the European Guideline Committees have indicated that β-blockers should be used as second-line or even third-line agents due to their inability to reduce stroke as effectively as other medicines and reserved only for post-MI patients or those with angina.[187,188] The controversy continues as many of the studies were conducted in the older adults where it is known that β-blockers are not as effective in lowering BP as other agents. Moreover, in some studies, small doses of β-blockers were given once per day, which did not reduce BP to the same degree as newer agents.[189] Finally, newer vasodilating β-blockers have not been tested in outcome studies. In general, many experts now believe that nonvasodilating β-blockers should not be used as first-line agents unless one has a history of coronary heart disease.[189]

The relevant issues about medications and their use in special populations are discussed in more detail in the next section.

BP Management in Special Populations

Management of HTN is modified on the basis of individual characteristics as well as knowledge of HTN care for specific groups. The following section outlines additional information that guides the management of HTN in several special populations.

HTN in Older Adults. Individuals older than 60 years represent the most rapidly growing segment of the U.S. population. SBP increases almost linearly with age in industrialized societies as does the overall prevalence of HTN and the proportion of hypertensives with isolated systolic HTN.[7] Isolated systolic HTN is defined as SBP greater than 140 mm Hg with DBP less than 90 mm Hg. The incidence of isolated systolic HTN increases with age,

Table 35-7 ■ COMBINATION DRUGS FOR HYPERTENSION

Combination Type*	Fixed-Dose Combination, Mg†	Trade Name
ACEIs and CCBs	Amlodipine/benazepril hydrochloride (2.5/10, 5/10, 5/20, 10/20)	Lotrel
	Enalapril maleate/felodipine (5/5)	Lexxel
	Trandolapril/verapamil (2/180, 1/240, 2/240, 4/240)	Tarka
ACEIs and diuretics	Benazepril/hydrochlorothiazide (5/6.25, 10/12.5, 20/12.5, 20/25)	Lotensin HCT
	Captopril/hydrochlorothiazide (25/15, 25/25, 50/15, 50/25)	Capozide
	Enalapril maleate/hydrochlorothiazide (5/12.5, 10/25)	Vaseretic
	Fosinopril/hydrochlorothiazide 10/12.5, 20/12.5	Monopril HCT
	Lisinopril/hydrochlorothiazide (10/12.5, 15/12.5, 20/25)	Zestoretic
	Moexipril HCl/hydrochlorothiazide (7.5/12.5, 15/25)	Uniretic
	Quinapril HCl/hydrochlorothiazide (10/12.5, 20/12.5, 20/25)	Accuretic
ARBs and diuretics	Candesartan cilexetil/hydrochlorothiazide (16/12.5, 32/12.5)	Atacand HCT
	Eprosartan mesylate/hydrochlorothiazide (600/12.5, 600/25)	Teveten/HCT
	Irbesartan/hydrochlorothiazide (150/12.5, 300/12.5)	Avalide
	Losartan potassium/hydrochlorothiazide (50/12.5, 100/25)	Hyzaar
	Olmesartan medoxomil/hydrochlorothiazide 20/12.5, 40/12.5, 40/25	Benicar HCT
	Telmisartan/hydrochlorothiazide (40/12.5, 80/12.5)	Micardis/HCT
	Valsartan/hydrochlorothiazide (80/12.5, 160/12.5)	Diovan/HCT
ARBs and CCBs	Amlodipine/ valsartan (5/160, 10/160, 5/320, 10/320)	Exforge
	Amlodipine/olmesartan medoxomil (5/20, 10/20, 5/40, and 10/40)	Azor
BBs and diuretics	Atenolol/chlorthalidone (50/25, 100/25)	Tenoretic
	Bisoprolol fumarate/hydrochlorothiazide (2.5/6.25, 5/6.25, 10/6.25)	Ziac
	Propranolol LA/hydrochlorothiazide (40/25, 80/25)	Inderide
	Metoprolol tartrate/hydrochlorothiazide (50/25, 100/25)	Lopressor HCT
	Nadolol/bendrofluthiazide (40/5, 80/5)	Corzide
	Timolol maleate/hydrochlorothiazide (10/25)	Timolide
Centrally acting drug and diuretic	Methyldopa/hydrochlorothiazide (250/15, 250/25, 500/30, 500/50)	Aldoril
	Reserpine/chlorthalidone (0.125/25, 0.25/50)	Demi-Regroton or Regroton
	Reserpine/chlorothiazide (0.125/250, 0.25/500)	Diupres
	Reserpine/hydrochlorothiazide (0.125/25, 0.125/50)	Hydropres
Diuretic and diuretic	Amiloride HCl/hydrochlorothiazide (5/50)	Moduretic
	Spironolactone/hydrochlorothiazide (25/25, 50/50)	Aldactone
	Triamterene/hydrochlorothiazide (37.5/25, 50/25, 75/50)	Dyazide, Maxzide

*Drug abbreviations: ACEI, angiotensin-converting enzyme inhibitor; BB, β-blocker; CCB, calcium channel blocker.
†Some drug combinations are available in multiple fixed doses. Each drug dose is reported in milligrams.
From Chobanian, A. V., Bakris, G. L., Black, H. R., et al. (2003). The Seventh Report of the Joint National Committee on Prevention, Detection, Evaluation, and Treatment of High Blood Pressure: The JNC 7 report. *JAMA, 289*(19), 2560–2572. (Erratum in *JAMA,* 2003, *290*(2), 197.)

with the incidence in persons older than 70 years being 7%, and in persons older than 80 years the incidence was more than 25%.[190] Analysis of data from the Framingham Study and a 20-year follow-up of NHANES I participants revealed that even borderline systolic HTN was associated with significant morbidity and mortality.[191,192] In the Framingham Study, persons with borderline isolated SBP had increased risks for all CVD, coronary heart disease, stroke, transient ischemic attack, heart failure, and mortality from CVD. The hazard ratios for each of these were significantly greater than 1.0 (range 1.42 to 1.60) after the data had been adjusted for sex, decade of age, cholesterol level, BMI, cigarette smoking, and glucose intolerance.

Several large randomized trials have demonstrated the benefits of HTN control in the older adults.[193–197] Two meta-analyses of clinical trials on individuals older than 60 years found that treatment reduced the incidence of coronary heart disease by between 18% and 19%, stroke by 30% to 34%, and total mortality by 13%.[72,198] The largest study, the SHEP, had a population of 4,736 men and women older than 60 years with a mean baseline BP of 170/70 mm Hg.[196] The goal of this clinical trial was to determine drug efficacy, side effects, and eventual long-term outcomes related to morbidity and mortality from CVD. When the 17-mm Hg reduction in mean SBP in the treatment group was compared with the control group, there was a significant decrease in stroke. No serious short-term side effects occurred as a result of treatment. The Swedish Trial in Old Patients with Hypertension (STOP Hypertension) studied a group of 1,627 with systolic and diastolic HTN (mean entry BP 195/102 mm Hg).[199] In the group treated with diuretics or β-blockers, there was a mean decrease in BP of 27/9 mm Hg, with statistically significant decreases in fatal and nonfatal strokes and congestive heart failure. This study showed the benefit of treating older adults patients with systolic and diastolic HTN.

Treatment of the older adults is similar to that of younger patients. Emphasis can be put on the lifestyle management, including weight loss, sodium restriction, and exercise, because of the multiple benefits to older adults.[200] Physical activity, for example, offers not only reduction of BP but also weight management, reduced disability, and decreased mortality.[201,202] The same medications are used in the older adults, but lower initial doses are recommended, and there may be more comorbid conditions that will make one medication a better choice than another.[7] Cost will also be a factor because many older adults persons have a limited income. Because the older adults have an increased sensitivity to orthostatic hypotension, caution is required with drugs that may cause dizziness on standing, such as diuretics in large doses, peripheral adrenergic blockers, and α-blockers.[7]

HTN in Racial and Ethnic Minorities. Although the prevalence of HTN differs among ethnic groups, there is little evidence that the relationship of BP to TOD differs substantially by race or ethnicity.[203] Some risk factors, such as obesity, physical inactivity, and dietary excesses/deficiencies, confer quantitatively different risks for HTN in various ethnic groups, due to variability in prevalence across ethnic groups.[203] In addition to behavioral and socioeconomic factors, such as limited health care access, lack of health insurance, and transportation issues, failure of clinicians to treat HTN early and to continue treating it persistently to reach and maintain an appropriate target BP has also been demonstrated to contribute to racial and ethnic disparities in HTN care and control.[154,204,205] Recent NHANES data show HTN treatment rates as follows: non-Hispanic Whites, 54%; non-Hispanic Blacks, 55%; and Mexican Americans, 48%.[3] HTN control rates were significantly lower among treated ethnic minorities: non-Hispanic Whites, 68%; non-Hispanic Blacks, 52%; and Mexican Americans, 57%.[3] Limited data are available on the efficacy in different drugs in non-Black minorities but greater rates of ACE inhibitor side effects occur in some minorities: angioedema and cough in Blacks, cough and flushing in Asians.[203]

HTN in Pregnancy. HTN occurs in pregnancy either because of preexisting chronic HTN or because of the development of pregnancy-induced HTN including gestational HTN, preeclampsia, and eclampsia. HTN (>140/90 mm Hg) existing prior to pregnancy, develops before the 20th week of pregnancy, or that persists more than 6 weeks after delivery is considered chronic HTN.[206] Gestational HTN is defined as an elevated BP that usually occurs in the third trimester and is not accompanied by other signs and symptoms.[207] In preeclampsia and eclampsia, the elevated BP is considered as one of several signs and symptoms of an underlying disorder of organ perfusion. Edema and proteinuria usually occur with pregnancy-induced HTN.

JNC 7 and the recent Working Group Report on High Blood Pressure in Pregnancy recommend the use of β-blockers, methyldopa, or vasodilators for pregnant women.[7,206] ACE inhibitors are contraindicated because of their documented adverse effects on fetal growth and development. Because of the adverse effects of ACE inhibitors, ARBs have not been studied in pregnant women and their use is also contraindicated.[206] Methyldopa is considered the drug of choice because of the long experience with using it and the relative lack of adverse effects on mother and infant.[206]

HTN in Patients With Diabetes. Coexistent HTN contributes significantly to the development of CVD and associated premature morbidity among diabetics. Furthermore, among treated hypertensives, those with diabetes are significantly less likely to have controlled HTN compared to those without diabetes.[3] Numerous clinical trials including the United Kingdom Prospective Diabetes Study Group Study 39 (UKPDS39), the Losartan Intervention for Endpoint reduction in HTN Study (LIFE), the Heart Outcomes Prevention Evaluation (HOPE) Study, ALLHAT, and the Appropriate Blood Pressure Control in Diabetes (ABCD) Study have documented the benefits of treating HTN among individuals with diabetes.[157,175,179,206–209] Because of this documented reduction in mortality and progression to end-stage renal disease from treating HTN, the American Diabetes Association and JNC 7 have set goal BP for persons with diabetes at <130/80 mm Hg.[7,178] Lifestyle interventions are also recommended and include weight control and exercise, which are keys to BP control in persons with diabetes.[210–212] JNC 7 recommended the use of five drug classes, including diuretics, β-blockers, ACE inhibitors, ARBs, and calcium channel blockers for the treatment of HTN in the presence of diabetes.[7] Importantly, ACE inhibitors and ARBs have beneficial effects in diabetes beyond HTN control, including reducing renal dysfunction, CVD, and stroke.[7]

HTN with Renal Disease. Control of HTN has been shown to be extremely effective in preventing the progression of renal failure in persons with renal disease regardless of etiology.[211,213,214] JNC 7 has set the goal BP for persons with renal disease at <130/80 mm Hg.[7] Three or more optimally dosed antihypertensive medications are often needed to achieve the goal BP of <103/80 mm Hg. Dietary recommendations for potassium restriction must be considered for patients with more advanced renal disease. JNC 7 recommends use of ACE inhibitors and ARBs in treating persons with renal disease based on clinical trials demonstrating their effectiveness.[180–183,215,216]

Hypertensive Crisis. Hypertensive emergencies are characterized by severe elevations in BP (>180/120 mm Hg) complicated by evidence of impending or progressive target organ dysfunction.[7] Acute hypertensive crises are rare situations in which patients require immediate intervention to reduce BP. These crises may occur either in persons whose HTN previously was not diagnosed or in persons with known but poorly controlled HTN. Hypertensive crises have been classified into two types: hypertensive emergencies and urgencies. Hypertensive emergency occurs when end-organ damage is acute or imminent and immediate reduction in BP, usually via intravenous medication in an intensive care unit, is required. Hypertensive urgency occurs when the BP is critically high, with signs such as edema of the optic disk, but there is less evidence of TOD, so that BP reduction can occur over a longer period using oral antihypertensive medications.[7] There is a continuum from emergencies to urgencies and excellent assessment and judgment are required. Acute elevations of BP may occur after certain medications such as clonidine are discontinued or the individual either forgets to take or runs out of medication.[217]

JNC 7 recommends that persons with hypertensive urgency be treated immediately with oral combination therapy.[7] In the management of hypertensive emergencies, the goal is to reduce the pressure so that TOD from the HTN is prevented or minimized while preventing the cerebral or myocardial ischemia that could result from too rapid a reduction in pressure.[218] The parenteral drugs that may be used in hypertensive emergencies are listed in Table 35-8. One drug that is not recommended because of the high rate of adverse events that accompany its use is sublingual nifedipine.[219,220] Nitroprusside is also recognized as a medication with great potential toxicity that should used with great hesitancy.[220] After the BP has been brought under control, the patient who has experienced an HTN emergency or urgency will require extended expert outpatient HTN management.

Achieving BP Control

Despite the impressive array of effective lifestyle and pharmacologic treatments for HTN, the rates of HTN awareness, treatment,

Table 35-8 ■ PARENTERAL DRUGS FOR TREATMENT OF HYPERTENSIVE EMERGENCIES*

Dose	Action	Onset of Action	Duration of Drug	Adverse Effects†	Special Indications
Vasodilators					
Sodium nitroprusside	0.25–10 μg/kg/min as IV infusion† (maximal dose for 10 minutes only)	Immediate	1–2 minutes	Nausea, vomiting, muscle twitching, sweating, thiocyanate and cyanide intoxication	Most hypertensive emergencies; caution with high intracranial pressure or azotemia
Nicardipine hydrochloride	5–15 mg/h IV	5–10 minutes	1–4 hour	Tachycardia, headache, flushing, local phlebitis	Most hypertensive emergencies except acute heart failure; caution with coronary ischemia
Fenoldopam mesylate	0.1–0.3 μg/kg/min IV infusion	<5 minutes	30 minutes	Tachycardia, headache, nausea, flushing	Most hypertensive emergencies; caution with glaucoma
Nitroglycerin	5–100 μg/min as IV infusion‡	2–5 minutes	3–5 minutes	Headache, vomiting, methemoglobinemia, tolerance with prolonged use	Coronary ischemia
Enalaprilat	1.25–5 mg every 6 hours IV	15–30 minutes	6 hours	Precipitous fall in pressure in high renin states; response variable	Acute left ventricular failure; avoid in acute myocardial infarction
Hydralazine hydrochloride	10–20 mg IV 10–50 mg IM	10–20 minutes 20–30 minutes	3–8 hours	Tachycardia, flushing, headache, vomiting, aggravation of angina	Eclampsia
Diazoxide	50–100 mg IV bolus repeated, or 15–30 mg/min infusion	2–4 minutes	6–12 hours	Nausea, flushing, tachycardia, chest pain	Now obsolete; when no intensive monitoring available
Adrenergic Inhibitors					
Labetalol hydrochloride	20–80 mg IV bolus every 10 minutes 0.5–2.0 mg/min IV infusion	5–10 minutes	3–6 hours	Vomiting, scalp tingling, burning in throat, dizziness, nausea, heart block, orthostatic hypotension	Most hypertensive emergencies except acute heart failure
Esmolol hydrochloride	250–500 μg/kg/min for 1 minute, then 50–100 μg/kg/min for 4 minutes; may repeat sequence	1–2 minutes	10–20 minutes	Hypotension, nausea	Aortic dissection, perioperative
Phentolamine mesylate	5–15 mg IV	1–2 minutes	3–10 minutes	Tachycardia, flushing, headache	Catecholamine excess

*These doses may vary from those in the *Physicians' Desk Reference* (51st edition).
†Hypotension may occur with all agents.
‡Require special delivery system.
IV, intravenous; IM, intramuscular.
From Chobanian, A. V., Bakris, G. L., Black, H. R., et al. (2003). The Seventh Report of the Joint National Committee on Prevention, Detection, Evaluation, and Treatment of High Blood Pressure: The JNC 7 report. *JAMA, 289*(19), 2560–2572. (Erratum in *JAMA*, 2003, *290*(2), 197.)

and control remain low (see Table 35-3). This lack of success in managing HTN has many contributing factors.[205,221–224] Achieving HTN control requires concerted action by patients, providers, and health care organizations. Table 35-9 summarizes strategies to promote HTN control.

Role of Patients

The challenge for patients in achieving HTN control is to modify their lives in ways that support their treatment plan. Making the decision to control one's HTN is the critical factor that precedes lifestyle modification and HTN control.[225] Bakris et al.[226] recently identified key action steps required by each of these HTN care constituents to substantially improve BP control rates. Patients must take the following actions: (1) take an active and responsible role in personal health management, (2) be appropriately educated, (3) develop skills to monitor and control BP, (4) take a partnership role in treatment, and (5) resolve barriers to BP control. Chapters 44 and 46 include a review of strategies that have been demonstrated to be effective in helping patients control their risk factors for CVD.

Role of Health Care Providers

Health care providers in partnership with patients hold the keys to HTN control. The following is required of providers: (1) identify, prevent, and correctly treat HTN, (2) promote public and community awareness of HTN, (3) develop communication skills that empower patients, and (4) advocate improved access to health care.[226] The provider's responsibilities range from knowing and using the latest guidelines for HTN control to motivating the patient to follow the treatment plan. At a minimum, the challenges to a provider include correctly diagnosing the patient's condition; communicating the importance of HTN as a disease and as a risk

Table 35-9 ■ STRATEGIES TO PROMOTE HTN CONTROL

Actions	Specific Strategies
Actions by Patients	
Patients must engage in essential prevention and treatment behaviors.	
Decide to control risk factors.	Understand rationale, importance of commitment.
Negotiate goals with provider.	Develop communication skills.
Develop skills for adopting and maintaining recommended behaviors.	Use reminder systems.
Monitor progress toward goals.	Use self-monitoring skills.
Resolve problems that block achievement of goals.	Develop problem-solving skills, use social support networks.
Patients must communicate with providers about prevention and treatment services.	Define own needs on basis of experience. Validate rationale for continuing to follow recommendations.
Actions by Providers	
Providers must foster effective communication with patients.	
Provide clear, direct messages about importance of a behavior or therapy.	Provide oral and written instruction, including rationale for treatments. Develop skills in communication/counseling. Use tailoring and contracting strategies.
Include patients in decisions about prevention and treatment goals and related strategies.	Negotiate goals and a plan. Anticipate barriers to compliance and discuss solutions.
Incorporate behavioral strategies into counselling.	Use active listening. Develop multicomponent strategies (i.e., cognitive and behavioral).
Providers must document and respond to patient's progress toward goals.	
Create an evidence-based practice.	Determine methods of evaluating outcomes.
Assess patient's compliance at each visit.	Use self-report or electronic data.
Develop a reminder system to ensure identification and follow-up of patient status.	Use telephone follow-up.
Actions by Health Care Organizations	
Develop an environment that supports prevention and treatment interventions.	Develop training in behavioral science, office set-up for all personnel. Use preappointment reminders. Use telephone follow-up. Schedule evening/weekend office hours. Provide group/individual counselling for patients and families.
Provide tracking and reporting systems.	Develop computer-based systems (electronic medical records).
Provide education and training for providers.	Require continuing education courses in communication, behavioral counseling.
Provide adequate reimbursement for allocation of time for all health care professionals.	Develop incentives tied to desired patient and provider outcomes.
Adopt systems to incorporate innovations rapidly and efficiently into medical practice.	Incorporate nursing case management. Implement pharmacy patient profile and recall review systems. Use of electronic transmission storage of patient's self-monitored data. Obtain patient data on lifestyle behavior before visit. Provide continuous quality improvement training.

Adapted with permission from Miller, N. H., Hill, M. N., Kottke, T, et al. (1997). The multilevel compliance challenge: Recommendations for a call to action. *Circulation, 95*, 1085–1090.

factor for atherosclerosis; developing an effective treatment plan that fits the patient's lifestyle and economic situation; and evaluating the results of the therapy. To achieve these goals, the provider requires skills in assessment, diagnosis, communication, and behavioral counseling. Display 35-5 lists strategies for preventing, monitoring, and addressing problems of adherence to improve BP control.

The optimal management of HTN requires the collaboration of health care providers.[221,227] HTN care teams are diverse, with the patient as the central figure. Other members may include the nurse, health educator, community health worker, nutritionist, pharmacist, and physician. Nurses have a role in all aspects of HTN management, from measuring BPs to conducting research to setting national policy. The role of the individual nurse depends on his or her preparation and work experience. The successful use of nurses to manage patients with HTN has been reported in the literature since the 1970s.[228–232] The current era of cost containment and the preparation of advanced practice nurses create a receptive climate for further development of the nurses' role in HTN management. Successful HTN teams require expertise in communication, coordination, and an appreciation of the skills of each team member.

Clinician Inertia. A fundamental barrier to HTN control that must be addressed is clinician inertia. Clinician inertia occurs when clinicians who are treating HTN fail to increase the intensity of drug treatment even though they see the patient regularly and are aware that BP goals have not been achieved.[233,234] The causes of this problem are varied and include a lack of knowledge about the relative risks and benefits of rigorous HTN management and resistance to implement guidelines.[234–237] It is not sufficient merely to bring patients close to goal. Treatment guidelines explicitly indicate that most patients will require two or more antihypertensive agents to achieve HTN control.[7] The intensity of treatment (i.e., dose and/or selection of medication) must be increased until

DISPLAY 35-5 Preventing, Monitoring, and Addressing Problems of Adherence

Educate About Conditions and Treatment

Assess patient's understanding and acceptance of the diagnosis and expectations of being in care.
Discuss patient's concerns and clarify misunderstandings.
Inform patient of blood pressure level.
Agree with patient on a goal blood pressure.
Inform patient about recommended treatment and provide specific written information.
Elicit concerns and questions and provide opportunities for patient to state specific behaviors to carry out treatment recommendations.
Emphasize need to continue treatment, that patient cannot tell if blood pressure is elevated, and that control does not mean cure.

Individualize the Regimen

Include patient in decision making.
Simplify the regimen.
Incorporate treatment into patient's daily lifestyle.
Set, with the patient, realistic short-term objectives for specific components of the treatment plan.
Encourage discussion of side effects and concerns.
Encourage self-monitoring.
Minimize cost of therapy.
Indicate you will ask about adherence at next visit.
When weight loss is established as a treatment goal, discourage quick weight loss regimens, fasting, or unscientific methods, because these are associated with weight cycling, which may increase cardiovascular morbidity and mortality.

Provide Reinforcement

Provide feedback regarding blood pressure level.
Ask about behaviors to achieve blood pressure control.
Give positive feedback for behavioral and blood pressure improvement.
Hold exit interviews to clarify regimen.
Make appointment for next visit before patient leaves the office.
Use appointment reminders and contact patients to confirm appointments.
Schedule more frequent visits to counsel nonadherent patients.
Contact and follow up patients who missed appointments.
Consider clinician–patient contracts.

Promote Social Support

Educate family members to be part of the blood pressure control process and provide daily reinforcement.
Suggest small group activities to enhance mutual support and motivation.

Collaborate with Other Professionals

Draw on complementary skills and knowledge of nurses, pharmacists, dieticians, optometrists, dentists, and physician assistants.
Refer patients for more intensive counselling.

From National High Blood Pressure Education Program (1994). *The fifth report of the Joint National Committee on detection, evaluation, and treatment of high blood pressure* (NIH Publication No. 93-1088). Bethesda, MD: U.S. Department of Health and Human Services.

BP is at or below goal, with the requirement that treatment should also remain well tolerated.

Role of Health Care Organizations

Health care systems must be adequately resourced and structured to deliver effective HTN treatment and prevention and to promote public and professional education.[226] Specific strategies such as providing education for both providers and patients, setting standards of care, implementing computerized data systems, documenting the impact of care on patient outcomes, and determining which types of care are cost-effective while maintaining quality of life, that health care organizations can take to improve HTN control are included in Table 35-9.[221]

Role of the Community

Communities, including employers, can play an active role in HTN screening and education and promote and support health visits and follow-up care.[226] Community-based interventions in the United States and Europe have demonstrated that community action can reduce the risks of CVD.[238,239] The National High Blood Pressure Program provides resources to support the development of community programs with the goals of raising awareness of HTN risk factors, supporting entry into the health care system, and supporting individual's efforts to follow their HTN treatment plans.[7]

SUMMARY

In summary, HTN is a common risk factor for cardiovascular, renal, and cerebrovascular disease. HTN often occurs without symptoms and the cause is unclear in most cases. Effective treatment of HTN includes lifestyle modification and pharmacologic treatment. Although evidence-based guidelines for HTN prevention, detection, and treatment have been widely promulgated, HTN control rates remain suboptimal. Achieving further improvements in HTN control will require activated patients, providers, and healthcare organizations.

REFERENCES

1. American Heart Association. (2008). *Heart disease and stroke statistics—2008 update.* Dallas, TX: Author.
2. Hajjar, I., & Kotchen, T. A. (2003). Trends in prevalence, awareness, treatment, and control of hypertension in the United States, 1988–2000. *JAMA, 290*(2), 199–206.
3. Ong, K. L., Cheung, B., Man, Y. B., et al. (2007). Prevalence, awareness, treatment, and control of hypertension among United States adults 1999–2004. *Hypertension, 49*, 69–75.
4. World Health Organization, International Society of Hypertension Writing Group. (2003). World Health Organization (WHO)/International Society of Hypertension (ISH) statement on management of hypertension. *Journal of Hypertension, 21*, 1983–1992.

5. Lewington, S., Clarke, R., Qizilbash, N., et al. (2002). Age-specific relevance of usual blood pressure to vascular mortality: A meta-analysis of individual data for one million adults in 61 prospective studies. *Lancet, 360*(9349), 1903–1913.
6. Swales, J. D. (1993). Guidelines on guidelines. *Journal of Hypertension, 11*, 899–903.
7. Chobanian, A. V., Bakris, G. L., Black, H. R., et al. (2003). The Seventh Report of the Joint National Committee on Prevention, Detection, Evaluation, and Treatment of High Blood Pressure: The JNC 7 report. *JAMA, 289*(19), 2560–2572. (Erratum in *JAMA*, 2003, *290*[2], 197.)
8. Franklin, S. S., Jacobs, M. J., Wong, N. D., et al. (2001). Predominance of isolated systolic hypertension among middle-aged and elderly US hypertensives: Analysis based on National Health and Nutrition Examination Survey (NHANES) III. *Hypertension, 37*, 869–874.
9. Voors, A. W., Webber, L. S., & Berenson, G. S. (1978). Relationship of blood pressure levels to height and weight in children. *Journal of Cardiovascular Medicine, 3*, 911–918.
10. National High Blood Pressure Education Program Working Group on High Blood Pressure in Children and Adolescents. (2004). The fourth report on the diagnosis, evaluation, and treatment of high blood pressure in children and adolescents. *Pediatrics, 114*, 555–576.
11. Falkner, B. (2002). Birth weight as a predictor of future hypertension. *American Journal of Hypertension, 15*(2, Pt. 2), 43S–45S.
12. Huxley, R., Neil, A., & Collins, R. (2002). Unravelling the fetal origins hypothesis: Is there really an inverse association between birthweight and subsequent blood pressure? *Lancet, 360*(9334), 659–665.
13. Law, C. M., de Swiet, M., Osmond, C., et al. (1993). Initiation of hypertension in utero and its amplification throughout life. *BMJ, 306*, 24–27.
14. Burt, V. L., Whelton, P., Roccella, E. J., et al. (1995). Prevalence of hypertension in the US adult population. Results from the Third National Health and Nutrition Examination Survey, 1988–1991. *Hypertension, 25*, 305–313.
15. Brown, C. D., Higgins, M., Donato, K. A., et al. (2000). Body mass index and the prevalence of hypertension and dyslipidemia. *Obesity Research, 8*(9), 605–619.
16. Freedman, D. S., Dietz, W. H., Srinivasan, S. R., et al. (1999). The relation of overweight to cardiovascular risk factors among children and adolescents: The Bogalusa Heart Study. *Pediatrics, 103*(6, Pt. 1), 1175–1182.
17. Kannel, W. B., Brand, N., Skinner, J. J., Jr., et al. (1967). The relation of adiposity to blood pressure and development of hypertension: The Framingham study. *Annals of Internal Medicine, 67*, 48–59.
18. Hunt, S. C., & Williams, R. R. (1999). Genetics and family history of hypertension. In J. L. Izzo Jr. & H. R. Black (Eds.), *Hypertension primer* (2nd ed., pp. 218–221). Baltimore: Lippincott Williams & Wilkins.
19. Burke, V., Beilin, L. J., & Dunbar, D. (2001). Tracking of blood pressure in Australian children. *Journal of Hypertension, 19*(7), 1185–1192.
20. Fuentes, R. M., Notkola, I. L., Shemeikka, S., et al. (2000). Familial aggregation of blood pressure: A population-based family study in eastern Finland. *Journal of Human Hypertension, 14*(7), 441–445.
21. Marteau, J. B., Zaiou, M., Siest, G., et al. (2005). Genetic determinants of blood pressure regulation. *Journal of Hypertension, 23*, 2127–2143.
22. Howard, G., Prineas, R., Moy, C., et al. (2006). Racial and geographic differences in awareness, treatment and control of HTN: The reasons for geographic and racial differences in stroke study. *Stroke, 37*(5), 1171–1178.
23. Kearney, P. M., Whelton, M., Reynolds, K., et al. (2005). Global burden of hypertension: Analysis of worldwide data. *Lancet, 365*(9455), 217–223.
24. Daugherty, S. A. (1983). Hypertension detection and follow-up: Description of the enumerated and screened population. *Hypertension, 5*(Suppl. IV), IV1–IV43.
25. Holme, I., Helgeland, A., Hjermann, I., et al. (1976). Coronary risk factors and socioeconomic status: The Oslo study. *Lancet, 2*, 1396–1398.
26. Hypertension Detection and Follow-up Program Cooperative Group. (1987). Educational level and 5-year all-cause mortality in the hypertension detection and follow-up program. *Hypertension, 9*, 641–646.
27. Stamler, R., Shipley, M., Elliott, P., et al. (1992). Higher blood pressure in adults with less education: Some explanations from INTERSALT. *Hypertension, 19*, 237–241.
28. Din-Dzietham, R., Liao, D., Diez-Roux, A., et al. (2000). Association of educational achievement with pulsatile arterial diameter change of the common carotid artery: The Atherosclerosis Risk in Communities (ARIC) Study, 1987–1992. *American Journal of Epidemiology, 152*(7), 617–627.
29. Bolen, J. C., Rhodes, L., Powell-Griner, E. E., et al. (2000). State-specific prevalence of selected health behaviors, by race and ethnicity—Behavioral Risk Factor Surveillance System, 1997. *MMWR CDC Surveillance Summary, 49*(2), 1–60.
30. Jones, D. W. (1999). Socioeconomic status and blood pressure. In J. L. Izzo Jr. & H. R. Black (Eds.), *Hypertension primer* (2nd ed., pp. 242–243). Baltimore: Lippincott Williams & Wilkins.
31. Julius, S. (1988). Transition from high cardiac output to elevated vascular resistance in hypertension. *American Heart Journal, 116*, 600–606.
32. Lund-Johansen, P. (1991). Twenty-year follow-up of hemodynamics in essential hypertension during rest and exercise. *Hypertension, 18*(5, Suppl.), III54–III61.
33. Oparil, S., Zaman, M. A., & Calhoun, D. A. (2003). Pathogenesis of hypertension. *Annals of Internal Medicine, 139*, 761–776.
34. Dzau, V. (2005). The cardiovascular continuum and renin-angiotensin-aldosterone system blockade. *Journal of Hypertension. Supplement, 23*, S9–S17.
35. Chiong, J. R., Aronow, W. E., Khan, I. A., et al. (2008). Secondary hypertension: Current diagnosis and treatment. *International Journal of Cardiology, 124*, 6–21.
36. Harden, P. N., MacLeod, M. J., Rodger, R. S. C., et al. (1997). Effect of renal artery stenting on progression of renovascular renal failure. *Lancet, 349*, 1133–1136.
37. Young, W. F., Jr. (2003). Minireview: Primary aldosteronism–changing concepts in diagnosis and treatment. *Endocrinology, 144*(6), 2208–2213.
38. Chiong, J. R. (2008). Controlling hypertension from a public health perspective. *International Journal of Cardiology, 127*, 151–156.
39. Dart, R. A., Gregoire, J. R., Gutterman, D. D., et al. (2003). The association of hypertension and secondary cardiovascular disease with sleep-disordered breathing. *Chest, 123*(1), 244–260.
40. Unterberg, C., Luthje, L., Szych, J., et al. (2005). Atrial overdrive pacing compared to CPAP in patients with obstructive sleep apnoea syndrome. *European Heart Journal, 26*, 2568–2575.
41. Sinaiko, A. R. (1996). Current concepts: Hypertension in children. *New England Journal of Medicine, 335*, 1968–1973.
42. de Leeuw, P. W., & Birkenhäger, W. H. (1994). Coarctation of the aorta. In J. D. Swales (Ed.), *Textbook of hypertension* (pp. 969–979). Oxford, England: Blackwell Scientific.
43. Brickner, M. R., Hillis, L. D., & Lange, R. A. (2000). Congenital heart disease in adults. First of two parts. *New England Journal of Medicine, 342*, 256–263.
44. de Divitiis, M., Pilla, C., Kattenhorn, M., et al. (2003). Ambulatory blood pressure, left ventricular mass, and conduit artery function late after successful repair of coarctation of the aorta. *Journal of the American College of Cardiology, 41*(12), 2259–2265.
45. Zhang, J., Meikle, S., & Trumble, A. (2003). Severe maternal morbidity associated with hypertensive disorders in pregnancy: Diagnosis and treatment. *Hypertension in Pregnancy, 22*, 203–212.
46. Garovic, V. D. (2000). Hypertension in pregnancy: Diagnosis and treatment. *Mayo Clinic Proceedings, 75*, 1071–1076.
47. Baumbach, G. L. (2008). Mechanisms of vascular remodeling. In J. L. Izzo, D. Sica, & H. R. Black (Eds.), *Hypertension primer: The essentials of high blood pressure* (4th ed.). Philadelphia: Lippincott Williams & Wilkins.
48. Lindop, G. B. M. (1994). The effects of hypertension on the structure of human resistance vessels. In J. D. Swales (Ed.), *Textbook of hypertension* (pp. 663–669). Oxford, England: Blackwell Scientific.
49. Touyz, R. M., & Berry, C. (2002). Recent advances in angiotensin II signaling. *Brazilian Journal of Medical and Biological Research, 35*(9), 1001–1015.
50. Halcox, J. P. J., & Quyyumi, A. A. (2008). Endothelial function and cardiovascular disease. In J. L. Izzo, D. Sica, & H. R. Black (Eds.), *Hypertension primer: The essentials of high blood pressure* (4th ed.). Philadelphia: Lippincott Williams & Wilkins.
51. Panza, J. A. (1997). Endothelial dysfunction in essential hypertension. *Clinical Cardiology, 20*(11, Suppl. 2), II-26–II-33.
52. Taddei, S., Virdis, A., Mattei, P., et al. (1996). Defective L-arginine-nitric oxide pathway in offspring of essential hypertensive patients. *Circulation, 94*(6), 1298–1303.
53. Giles, T. D. (2008). Atherogenesis and coronary artery disease. In J. L. Izzo, D. Sica, & H. R. Black (Eds.), *Hypertension primer: The essentials of high blood pressure* (4th ed.). Philadelphia: Lippincott Williams & Wilkins.
54. Le Jemtel, T. H., & Ennezat, P. V. (2008). Pathogenesis of chronic heart failure. In J. L. Izzo, D. Sica, & H. R. Black (Eds.), *Hypertension primer: The essentials of high blood pressure* (4th ed.). Philadelphia: Lippincott Williams & Wilkins.
55. Kannel, W. B. (1996). Blood pressure as a cardiovascular risk factor: Prevention and treatment. *JAMA, 275*(20), 1571–1576.
56. Vasan, R. S., Larson, M. G., Leip, E. P., et al. (2001). Assessment of frequency of progression to hypertension in non-hypertensive participants in the Framingham Heart Study: A cohort study. *Lancet, 358*(9294), 1682–1686.

57. Anderson, S. (2008). Pathogenesis of nephrosclerosis and chronic kidney disease. In J. L. Izzo, D. Sica, & H. R. Black (Eds.), *Hypertension primer: The essentials of high blood pressure* (4th ed.). Philadelphia: Lippincott Williams & Wilkins.
58. National Kidney Foundation. (2004). K/DOQI clinical practice guidelines on hypertension and antihypertensive agents in chronic kidney disease. *American Journal of Kidney Disease, 43*(Suppl. 1), 1–290.
59. Wong, T. Y., & Mitchell, P. (2004). Hypertensive retinopathy. *New England Journal of Medicine, 351*, 2310–2317.
60. Collins, R., Peto, R., MacMahon, S., et al. (1990). Blood pressure, stroke, and coronary heart disease. Part 2, short-term reductions in blood pressure: Overview of randomised drug trials in their epidemiological context. *Lancet, 335*, 827–838.
61. Garraway, W. M., & Whisnant, J. P. (1987). The changing pattern of hypertension and the declining incidence of stroke. *JAMA, 258*, 214–217.
62. Gueyffier, F., Boutitie, F., Boissel, J. P., et al. (1997). Effect of antihypertensive drug treatment on cardiovascular outcomes in women and men. A meta-analysis of individual patient data from randomized, controlled trials. The INDANA Investigators. *Annals of Internal Medicine, 126*(10), 761–767.
63. MacMahon, S., Peto, R., Cutler, J., et al. (1990). Blood pressure, stroke, and coronary heart disease. Part 1, prolonged differences in blood pressure: Prospective observational studies corrected for dilution bias. *Lancet, 335*, 765–774.
64. Fotherby, M. D., Eveson, D. J., & Robinson, T. G. (2007). The brain in hypertension. In G. Lip & J. E. Hall (Eds.), *Comprehensive hypertension*. Philadelphia: Mosby, Elsevier.
65. Baumbach, G. L., & Heistad, D. D. (1999). Cerebrovascular disease in experimental models of hypertension. In J. D. Swales (Ed.), *Textbook of hypertension* (pp. 682–690). Oxford, England: Blackwell Scientific.
66. Pickering, T. G., Hall, J. E., Appel, L. J., et al. (2005). Recommendations for blood pressure measurement in humans and experimental animals. *Hypertension, 45*, 142–161.
67. Verdecchia, P., Schillaci, G., Borgioni, C., et al. (1996). Nocturnal pressure is the true pressure. *Blood Pressure Monitoring, 1*(Suppl. 2), S81–S85.
68. Pickering, T. G., Houston Miller, N., Ogedegbe, G., et al. (2008). Call to action on use and reimbursement for home blood pressure monitoring: Executive summary. A joint scientific statement from the American Heart Association, American Society of Hypertension, and Preventive Cardiovascular Nurses Association. *Hypertension, 52*, 1–9.
69. Kaplan, N. M. (2002). *Kaplan's clinical hypertension* (8th ed.). Philadelphia: Lippincott Williams & Wilkins.
70. UK Prospective Diabetes Study Group. (1998). Tight blood pressure control and risk of macrovascular and microvascular complications in type 2 diabetes: UKPDS 38. *BMJ, 317*, 703–713.
71. Curb, J. D., Pressel, S. L., Cutler, J. A., et al. (1996). Effect of diuretic-based antihypertensive treatment on cardiovascular disease risk in older diabetic patients with isolated systolic hypertension. Systolic Hypertension in the Elderly Program Cooperative Research Group. *JAMA, 276*, 1886–1892.
72. Staessen, J. A., Gasowski, J., Wang, J. G., et al. (2000). Risks of untreated and treated isolated systolic hypertension in the elderly: Meta-analysis of outcome trials. *Lancet, 355*, 865–872.
73. Staessen, J. A., Wang, J. G., & Thijs, L. (2003). Cardiovascular prevention and blood pressure reduction: A quantitative overview updated until 1st March 2003. *Journal of Hypertension, 21*, 1055–1076.
74. He, J., Whelton, P. K., Appel, L. J., et al. (2000). Long-term effects of weight loss and dietary sodium reduction on incidence of hypertension. *Hypertension, 35*(2), 544–549.
75. Stevens, V. J., Obarzanek, E., Cook, N. R., et al. (2001). Long-term weight loss and changes in blood pressure: Results of the Trials of Hypertension Prevention, phase II. *Annals of Internal Medicine, 134*(1), 1–11.
76. Whelton, P. K., He, J., Appel, L. J., et al. (2002). Primary prevention of hypertension: Clinical and public health advisory from The National High Blood Pressure Education Program. *JAMA, 288*(15), 1882–1888.
77. Appel, L. J., Moore, T. J., Obarzanek, E., et al. (1997). A clinical trial of the effects of dietary patterns on blood pressure. *New England Journal of Medicine, 336*, 1117–1124.
78. John, J. H., Ziebland, S., Yudkin, P., et al. (2002). Effects of fruit and vegetable consumption on plasma antioxidant concentrations and blood pressure: A randomised controlled trial. *Lancet, 359*(9322), 1969–1974.
79. Appel, L. J., Brands, M. W., Daniels, S. R., et al. (2006). Dietary approaches to prevent and treat hypertension: A scientific statement from the American Heart Association. *Hypertension, 47*, 296–308.
80. Haskell, W. L., Lee, I. M., Pate, R. R., et al. (2007). Physical activity and public health: Updated recommendation for adults from the American College of Sports Medicine and the American Heart Association. *Circulation, 116*, 1081–1093.
81. Garrison, R. J., Kannel, W. B., Stokes J., III, et al. (1987). Incidence and precursors of hypertension in young adults: The Framingham Offspring Study. *Preventive Medicine, 16*, 235–251.
82. Huang, Z., Willett, W. C., Manson, J. E., et al. (1998). Body weight, weight change, and risk for hypertension in women. *Annals of Internal Medicine, 128*, 81–88.
83. Blair, D., Habicht, J.-P., Sims, E. A., et al. (1984). Evidence for an increased risk for hypertension with centrally located body fat and the effect of race and sex on this risk. *American Journal of Epidemiology, 119*, 526–540.
84. Despres, J. P., Moorjani, S., Lupien, P. J., et al. (1990). Regional distribution of body fat, plasma lipoproteins, and cardiovascular disease. *Arteriosclerosis, 10*(4), 497–511.
85. Folsom, A. R., Prineas, R. J., Kaye, S. A., et al. (1990). Incidence of hypertension and stroke in relation to body fat distribution and other risk factors in older women. *Stroke, 21*, 701–706.
86. Haarbo, J., Hassager, C., Riis, B. J., et al. (1989). Relation of body fat distribution to serum lipids and lipoproteins in elderly women. *Atherosclerosis, 80*, 57–62.
87. Ostlund, R. E., Staten, M., Kohrt, W. M., et al. (1990). The ratio of waist-to-hip circumference, plasma insulin level, and glucose intolerance as independent predictors of the HDL_2 cholesterol level in elderly. *New England Journal of Medicine, 322*, 229–234.
88. Stamler, R., Stamler, J., Riedlinger, W. F., et al. (1978). Weight and blood pressure. Findings in hypertension screening of 1 million Americans. *JAMA, 240*(15), 1607–1610.
89. Manolio, T. A., Savage, P. J., Burke, G. L., et al. (1991). Correlates of fasting insulin levels in young adults: The CARDIA study. *Journal of Clinical Epidemiology, 44*(6), 571–578.
90. Muller-Wieland, D., Kotzka, J., Knebel, B., et al. (1998). Metabolic syndrome and hypertension: Pathophysiology and molecular basis of insulin resistance. *Basic Research in Cardiology, 93*(Suppl. 2), 131–134.
91. Katagiri, H., Yamada, T., & Oka, Y. (2007). Adiposity and cardiovascular disorders disturbance of the regulatory system consisting of humoral and neuronal signals. *Circulation Research, 101*, 27–39.
92. Yanai, H., Tomono, Y., Ito, K., et al. (2008). The underlying mechanisms for development of hypertension in the metabolic syndrome. *Nutrition Journal, 7*, 10.
93. Hypertension Prevention Trial Research Group. (1990). The Hypertension Prevention Trial: Three-year effects of dietary changes on blood pressure. *Archives of Internal Medicine, 150*, 153–162.
94. Langford, H. G., Blaufox, M. D., Oberman, A., et al. (1985). Dietary therapy slows the return of hypertension after stopping prolonged medication. *JAMA, 253*, 657–664.
95. Trials of Hypertension Prevention Collaborative Research Group. (1992). The effects of nonpharmacologic interventions on blood pressure of persons with high normal levels. Results of the Trials of Hypertension Prevention, Phase I. *JAMA, 267*, 1213–1220.
96. Trials of Hypertension Prevention Collaborative Research Group. (1997). Effects of weight loss and sodium reduction intervention on blood pressure and hypertension incidence in overweight people with high-normal blood pressure: The Trials of Hypertension Prevention, phase II. *Archives of Internal Medicine, 157*, 657–667.
97. Wassertheil-Smoller, S., Oberman, A., Blaufox, M. D., et al. (1992). The Trial of Antihypertensive Interventions and Management (TAIM) Study. Final results with regard to blood pressure, cardiovascular risk, and quality of life. *American Journal of Hypertension, 5*, 37–44.
98. Neter, J. E., Stam, B. E., Kok, F. J., et al. (2003). Influence of weight reduction on blood pressure: A meta-analysis of randomized controlled trials. *Hypertension, 42*, 878–884.
99. Neaton, J. D., Grimm, R. H., Prineas, R. J., et al. (1993). Treatment of Mild Hypertension Study: Final results. *JAMA, 270*, 713–724.
100. Oberman, A., Wassertheil-Smoller, S., Langford, H. G., et al. (1990). Pharmacologic and nutritional treatment of mild hypertension: Changes in cardiovascular risk status. *Annals of Internal Medicine, 112*, 89–95.
101. Arakawa, K. (1993). Hypertension and exercise. *Clinical Experience in Hypertension, 15*(6), 1171–1179.
102. Blair, S. N., Goodyear, N. N., Gibbons, L. W., et al. (1984). Physical fitness and incidence of hypertension in healthy normotensive men and women. *JAMA, 252*, 487–490.
103. Horan, M. J., & Lenfant, C. (1990). Epidemiology of blood pressure and predictors of hypertension. *Hypertension, 15*(2, Suppl.), I20–I24.
104. Ledoux, M., Lambert, J., Reeder, B. A., et al. (1997). Correlation between cardiovascular disease risk factors and simple anthropometric

measures. Canadian Heart Health Surveys Research Group. *Canadian Medical Association Journal, 157*(Suppl. 1), S46–S53.
105. Westheim, A., & Os, I. (1992). Physical activity and the metabolic cardiovascular syndrome. *Journal of Cardiovascular Pharmacology, 20*(Suppl. 8), S49–S53.
106. Fagard, R. H. (1993). Physical fitness and blood pressure. *Journal of Hypertension, 11*(Suppl. 5), S47–S52.
107. Kelley, G. A., & Kelley, K. S. (2000). Progressive resistance exercise and resting blood pressure: A meta-analysis of randomized controlled trials. *Hypertension, 35*(3), 838–843.
108. Whelton, S. P., Chin, A., Xin, X., et al. (2002). Effect of aerobic exercise on blood pressure: A meta-analysis of randomized, controlled trials. *Annals of Internal Medicine, 136*(7), 493–503.
109. Fagard, R. H., & Cornelissen, V. A. (2007). Effect of exercise on blood pressure control in hypertensive patients. *European Journal of Cardiovascular Prevention and Rehabilitation, 14*, 12–17.
110. Blair, S. N., Kohl, H. W., Paffenbarger, R. S., et al. (1989). Physical fitness and all-cause mortality: A prospective study of healthy men and women. *JAMA, 262*, 2395–2401.
111. Ekelund, L., Haskell, W. L., Johnson, J. L., et al. (1988). Physical fitness as a predictor of cardiovascular mortality in asymptomatic North American men. *New England Journal of Medicine, 319*, 1379–1384.
112. Erikssen, G., Liestol, K., Bjornholt, J., et al. (1998). Changes in physical fitness and changes in mortality. *Lancet, 352*, 759–762.
113. Ford, E. S., & DeStefano, F. (1991). Risk factors for mortality from all causes and from coronary heart disease among persons with diabetes. *American Journal of Epidemiology, 133*, 1220–1230.
114. Fried, L. P., Kronmal, R. A., Newman, A. B., et al. (1998). Risk factors for 5-year mortality in elderly: The Cardiovascular Health Study. *JAMA, 279*, 585–592.
115. Hakim, A. A., Petrovitch, H., Burchfiel, C. M., et al. (1998). Effects of walking on mortality among nonsmoking retired men. *New England Journal of Medicine, 338*, 94–99.
116. Kujala, U. M., Kaprio, J., Sarna, S., et al. (1998). Relationship of leisure-time physical activity and mortality: The Finnish Twin Cohort. *JAMA, 279*, 440–444.
117. Kushi, L. H., Fee, R. M., Folsom, A. R., et al. (1997). Physical activity and mortality in postmenopausal women. *JAMA, 277*, 1287–1292.
118. Paffenbarger, R. S., Jr., Hyde, R. T., Wing, A. L., et al. (1986). Physical activity, all-cause mortality, and longevity of college alumni. *New England Journal of Medicine, 314*, 605–613.
119. Salonen, J. T., Slater, J. S., Tuomilehto, H., et al. (1988). Leisure time and occupational physical activity: Risk of death from ischemic heart disease. *American Journal of Epidemiology, 127*, 87–94.
120. Sandvik, L., Erikssen, J., Thaulow, E., et al. (1993). Physical fitness as a predictor of mortality among healthy, middle-aged Norwegian men. *New England Journal of Medicine, 328*, 533–537.
121. Sherman, S. E., D'Agostino, R. B., Cobb, J. L., et al. (1994). Does exercise reduce mortality rates in the elderly? Experience from the Framingham Heart Study. *American Heart Journal, 128*, 965–972.
122. Sherman, S. E., D'Agostino, R. B., Cobb, J. L., et al. (1994). Physical activity and mortality in women in the Framingham Heart Study. *American Heart Journal, 128*, 879–884.
123. Kokkinos, P. F., Narayan, P., Colleran, J. A., et al. (1995). Effects of regular exercise on blood pressure and left ventricular hypertrophy in African-American men with severe hypertension. *New England Journal of Medicine, 333*, 1462–1467.
124. Johnson, A. G., Nguyen, T. V., & Davis, D. (2001). Blood pressure is linked to salt intake and modulated by the angiotensinogen gene in normotensive and hypertensive elderly subjects. *Journal of Hypertension, 19*, 1053–1060.
125. MacGregor, G. A., Markandu, N. D., Sagnella, G. A., et al. (1989). Double-blind study of three sodium intakes and long-term effects of sodium restriction in essential hypertension. *Lancet, 2*, 1244–1247.
126. Sacks, F. M., Svetkey, L. P., Vollmer, W. M., et al. Effects on blood pressure of reduced dietary sodium and the Dietary Approaches to Stop Hypertension (DASH) diet: DASH-Sodium Collaborative Research Group. *New England Journal of Medicine, 344*, 3–10.
127. Vollmer, W. M., Sacks, F. M., Ard, J., et al. (2001). Effects of diet and sodium intake on blood pressure: Subgroup analysis of the DASH-sodium trial. *Annals of Internal Medicine, 135*, 1019–1028.
128. Bray, G. A., Vollmer, W. M., Sacks, F. M., et al. (2004). A further subgroup analysis of the effects of the DASH diet and three dietary sodium levels on blood pressure: Results of the DASH-Sodium Trial. *American Journal of Cardiology, 94*, 222–227.
129. Cook, N. R., Cutler, J. A., Obarzanek, E., et al. (2007). Long term effects of dietary sodium reduction on cardiovascular disease outcomes: Observational follow-up of the trials of hypertension prevention (TOHP). *BMJ, 334*, 885.
130. Mattes, R. D. (1997). The taste for salt in humans. *American Journal of Clinical Nutrition, 65*(2, Suppl.), 692S–697S.
131. Appel, L. J., Champagne, C. M., Harsha, D. W., et al. (2003). Effects of comprehensive lifestyle modification on blood pressure control: Main results of the PREMIER clinical trial. *JAMA, 289*(16), 2083–2093.
132. Beilin, L. J., & Puddey, I. B. (1992). Alcohol and hypertension. *Clinical Experience in Hypertension [A], 14*(1–2), 119–138.
133. Cushman, W. C. (1999). Alcohol use and blood pressure. In J. L. Izzo Jr. & H. R. Black (Eds.), *Hypertension primer* (2nd ed., pp. 263–265). Baltimore: Lippincott Williams & Wilkins.
134. Klatsky, A. L., Friedman, G. D., Siegelaub, A. B., et al. (1977). Alcohol consumption and blood pressure Kaiser-Permanente Multiphasic Health Examination data. *New England Journal of Medicine, 296*(21), 1194–1200.
135. Thun, M. J., Peto, R., Lopez, A. D., et al. (1997). Alcohol consumption and mortality among middle-aged and elderly U.S. adults. *New England Journal of Medicine, 337*(24), 1705–1714.
136. Xin, X., He, J., Frontini, M. G., et al. (2001). Effects of alcohol reduction on blood pressure: A meta-analysis of randomized controlled trials. *Hypertension, 38*(5), 1112–1117.
137. Sacco, R. L., Elkind, M., Boden-Albala, B., et al. (1999). The protective effect of moderate alcohol consumption on ischemic stroke. *JAMA, 281*(1), 53–60.
138. Kannel, W. B., McGee, D., & Gordon, T. (1976). A general cardiovascular risk profile: The Framingham Study. *American Journal of Cardiology, 38*, 46–51.
139. Lerner, D. J., & Kannel, W. B. (1986). Patterns of coronary heart disease morbidity and mortality in the sexes: A 26-year follow-up of the Framingham population. *American Heart Journal, 111*, 383–390.
140. Luria, M. H., Erel, J., Sapoznikov, D., et al. (1991). Cardiovascular risk factor clustering and ratio of total cholesterol to high-density lipoprotein cholesterol in angiographically documented coronary artery disease. *American Journal of Cardiology, 67*, 31–36.
141. Otten, M. W., Teutsch, S. M., Williamson, D. F., et al. (1990). The effect of known risk factors on the excess mortality of black adults in the United States. *JAMA, 263*, 845–850.
142. Doll, R., & Peto, R. (1976). Mortality in relation to smoking: 20 years' observations on male British doctors. *BMJ, 2*, 1525–1536.
143. Grover, S. A., Paquet, S., Levinton, C., et al. (1998). Estimating the benefits of modifying risk factors of cardiovascular disease: A comparison of primary vs secondary prevention *Archives of Internal Medicine, 158*(6), 655–662. (Erratum in *Archives of Internal Medicine*, 1998, *158*[11], 1228.)
144. Hallstrom, A. P., Cobb, L. A., & Ray, R. (1986). Smoking as a risk factor for recurrence of sudden cardiac arrest. *New England Journal of Medicine, 314*, 271–275.
145. Hermanson, B., Omenn, G. S., Kronmal, R. A., et al. (1988). Beneficial six-year outcome of smoking cessation in older men and women with coronary artery disease. *New England Journal of Medicine, 319*, 1365.
146. Kawachi, I., Colditz, G. A., Stampfer, M. J., et al. (1993). Smoking cessation in relation to total mortality rates in women: A prospective study. *Annals of Internal Medicine, 119*, 992–1000.
147. LaCroix, A. Z., Lang, J., Scherr, P., et al. (1991). Smoking and mortality among older men and women in three communities. *New England Journal of Medicine, 324*, 1619–1625.
148. Shepherd, J., Cobbe, S. M., Ford, I., et al. (1995). Prevention of coronary heart disease with pravastatin in men with hypercholesterolemia. *New England Journal of Medicine, 333*, 1301–1307.
149. Veterans Administration Cooperative Study Group on Antihypertensive Agents. (1967). Effects of treatment on morbidity in hypertension: Results in patients with diastolic blood pressures averaging 115 through 129 mm Hg. *JAMA, 202*, 116–122.
150. Veterans Administration Cooperative Study Group on Antihypertensive Agents. (1970). Effects of treatment on morbidity in hypertension. II. Results in patients with diastolic blood pressure averaging 90 through 114 mm Hg. *JAMA, 213*, 1143–1152.
151. Hansson, L., Zanchetti, A., Carruthers, S. G., et al. (1998). Effects of intensive blood-pressure lowering and low-dose aspirin in patients with hypertension: Principal results of the Hypertension Optimal Treatment (HOT) randomised trial. *Lancet, 351*, 1755–1762.
152. Voko, Z., Bots, M. L., Hofman, A., et al. (1999). J-shaped relation between blood pressure and stroke in treated hypertensives. *Hypertension, 34*, 1181–1185.

153. Somes, G. W., Pahor, M., Shorr, R. I., et al. (1999). The role of diastolic blood pressure when treating isolated systolic hypertension. *Archives of Internal Medicine, 159*, 2004–2009.
154. Bakris, G. L., Gaxiola, E., Messerli, F. H., et al., for the INVEST Investigators. (2004). Clinical outcomes in the diabetes cohort of the International Verapamil SR-Trandolapril study. *Hypertension, 44*, 637–642.
155. Copley, J. B., & Rosario, R. (2005). Hypertension: A review and rationale for treatment. *Disease Management, 51*, 548–614.
156. Sawicki, P. T., & McGauran, N. (2006). Have ALLHAT, ANBP2, ASCOT-BPLA and so forth improved our knowledge about better hypertension control? *Hypertension, 48*, 1–7.
157. The ALLHAT Officers and Coordinators for the ALLHAT Collaborative Research Group. (2002). Major outcomes in high-risk hypertensive patients randomized to angiotensin-converting enzyme inhibitor or calcium-channel blocker vs diuretic: The Antihypertensive and Lipid-Lowering Treatment to Prevent Heart Attack Trial (ALLHAT). *JAMA, 288*(23), 2981–2997.
158. Wing, L. M., Reid, C. M., Ryan, P., et al. (2003). A comparison of outcomes with angiotensin-converting–enzyme inhibitors and diuretics for hypertension in the elderly. *New England Journal of Medicine, 348*(7), 583–592.
159. Dahlof, B., Sever, P. S., Poulter, N. R., et al. (2005). The Anglo-Scandanavian Cardiac Outcomes Trial—Blood Pressure Lowering Arm (ASCOT-BPLA): A multicentre randomized controlled trial. *Lancet, 366*, 895–906.
160. Frohlich, E. D. (2003). Treating hypertension-what are we to believe? *New England Journal of Medicine, 348*(7), 639–641.
161. Hunt, S. A., Baker, D. W., Chin, M. H., et al. (2001). ACC/AHA guidelines for the evaluation and management of chronic heart failure in the adult: Executive summary. A report of the American College of Cardiology/American Heart Association Task Force on Practice Guidelines (Committee to revise the 1995 Guidelines for the Evaluation and Management of Heart Failure). *Journal of the American College of Cardiology, 38*(7), 2101–2113.
162. Tepper, D. (1999). Frontiers in congestive heart failure: Effect of Metoprolol CR/XL in chronic heart failure: Metoprolol CR/XL Randomised Intervention Trial in Congestive Heart Failure (MERIT-HF). *Congestive Heart Failure, 5*(4), 184–185.
163. Packer, M., Coats, A. J., Fowler, M. B., et al. (2001). Effect of carvedilol on survival in severe chronic heart failure. *New England Journal of Medicine, 344*(22), 1651–1658.
164. A randomized trial of beta-blockade in heart failure. The Cardiac Insufficiency Bisoprolol Study (CIBIS). CIBIS Investigators and Committees. (1994). *Circulation, 90*(4), 1765–1773.
165. Effect of enalapril on survival in patients with reduced left ventricular ejection fractions and congestive heart failure. The SOLVD Investigators. (1991). *New England Journal of Medicine, 325*(5), 293–302.
166. Effect of ramipril on mortality and morbidity of survivors of acute myocardial infarction with clinical evidence of heart failure. The Acute Infarction Ramipril Efficacy (AIRE) Study Investigators. (1993). *Lancet, 342*(8875), 821–828.
167. Kober, L., Torp-Pedersen, C., Carlsen, J. E., et al. (1995). A clinical trial of the angiotensin-converting-enzyme inhibitor trandolapril in patients with left ventricular dysfunction after myocardial infarction. Trandolapril Cardiac Evaluation (TRACE) Study Group. *New England Journal of Medicine, 333*(25), 1670–1676.
168. Cohn, J. N., & Tognoni, G. (2001). A randomized trial of the angiotensin-receptor blocker valsartan in chronic heart failure. *New England Journal of Medicine, 345*(23), 1667–1675.
169. Pitt, B., Zannad, F., Remme, W. J., et al. (1999). The effect of spironolactone on morbidity and mortality in patients with severe heart failure. Randomized Aldactone Evaluation Study Investigators. *New England Journal of Medicine, 341*(10), 709–717.
170. Braunwald, E., Antman, E. M., Beasley, J. W., et al. (2002). ACC/AHA 2002 guideline update for the management of patients with unstable angina and non-ST-segment elevation myocardial infarction—Summary article: A report of the American College of Cardiology/American Heart Association task force on practice guidelines (Committee on the Management of Patients With Unstable Angina). *Journal of the American College of Cardiology, 40*(7), 1366–1374.
171. A randomized trial of propranolol in patients with acute myocardial infarction. I. Mortality results. (1982). *JAMA, 247*(12), 1707–1714.
172. Hager, W. D., Davis, B. R., Riba, A., et al. (1998). Absence of a deleterious effect of calcium-channel blockers in patients with left ventricular dysfunction after myocardial infarction: The SAVE Study Experience. SAVE Investigators. Survival and Ventricular Enlargement. *American Heart Journal, 135*(3), 406–413.
173. Dargie, H. J. (2001). Effect of carvedilol on outcome after myocardial infarction in patients with left-ventricular dysfunction: The CAPRICORN randomised trial. *Lancet, 357*(9266), 1385–1390.
174. Pitt, B., Remme, W., Zannad, F., et al. (2003). Eplerenone, a selective aldosterone blocker, in patients with left ventricular dysfunction after myocardial infarction. *New England Journal of Medicine, 348*(14), 1309–1321.
175. Yusuf, S., Sleight, P., Pogue, J., et al. (2000). Effects of an angiotensin-converting-enzyme inhibitor, ramipril, on cardiovascular events in high-risk patients. The Heart Outcomes Prevention Evaluation Study Investigators. *New England Journal of Medicine, 342*(3), 145–153.
176. Dahlof, B., Devereux, R. B., Kjeldsen, S. E., et al. (2002). Cardiovascular morbidity and mortality in the Losartan Intervention For Endpoint reduction in hypertension study (LIFE): A randomised trial against atenolol. *Lancet, 359*(9311), 995–1003.
177. Black, H. R., Elliott, W. J., Grandits, G., et al. (2003). Principal results of the Controlled Onset Verapamil Investigation of Cardiovascular End Points (CONVINCE) trial. *JAMA, 289*(16), 2073–2082.
178. Arauz-Pacheco, C., Parrott, M. A., & Raskin, P. (2003). Treatment of hypertension in adults with diabetes. *Diabetes Care, 26*(Suppl. 1), S80–S82.
179. Efficacy of atenolol and captopril in reducing risk of macrovascular and microvascular complications in type 2 diabetes: UKPDS 39. UK Prospective Diabetes Study Group. (1998). *BMJ, 317*(7160), 713–720.
180. Lewis, E. J., Hunsicker, L. G., Bain, R. P., et al. (1993). The effect of angiotensin-converting-enzyme inhibition on diabetic nephropathy. The Collaborative Study Group. *New England Journal of Medicine, 329*(20), 1456–1462.
181. Brenner, B. M., Cooper, M. E., de Zeeuw, D., et al. (2001). Effects of losartan on renal and cardiovascular outcomes in patients with type 2 diabetes and nephropathy. *New England Journal of Medicine, 345*(12), 861–869.
182. Lewis, E. J., Hunsicker, L. G., Clarke, W. R., et al. (2001). Renoprotective effect of the angiotensin-receptor antagonist irbesartan in patients with nephropathy due to type 2 diabetes. *New England Journal of Medicine, 345*(12), 851–860.
183. Randomised placebo-controlled trial of effect of ramipril on decline in glomerular filtration rate and risk of terminal renal failure in proteinuric, non-diabetic nephropathy. The GISEN Group (Gruppo Italiano di Studi Epidemiologici in Nefrologia). (1997). *Lancet, 349*(9069), 1857–1863.
184. Wright, J. T., Jr., Agodoa, L., Contreras, G., et al. (2002). Successful blood pressure control in the African American Study of Kidney Disease and Hypertension. *Archives of Internal Medicine, 162*(14), 1636–1643.
185. PROGRESS Collaborative Group. (2001). Randomised trial of a perindopril-based blood-pressure-lowering regimen among 6,105 individuals with previous stroke or transient ischaemic attack. *Lancet, 358*(9287), 1033–1041.
186. Julius, S., Nesbitt, S. D., Egan, B. M., et al. (2006). Trial of Preventing Hypertension (TROPHY) investigators. Feasibility of treating prehypertension with an angiotensin-receptor blocker. *New England Journal of Medicine, 354*, 1685–1697.
187. Mancia, G., De Backer, G., Dominiczak, A., et al. (2007). Guidelines for the management of arterial hypertension: The task force for the management of arterial hypertension of the European Society of Hypertension (ESH) and of the European Society of Cardiology (ESC). *Journal of Hypertension, 25*, 1105–1187.
188. Lindholm, L. H., Carlberg, B., & Samuelsson, O. (2005). Should beta-blockers remain first choice in the treatment of primary hypertension? A meta-analysis. *Lancet, 366*, 1545–1553.
189. Moser, M. (2008). Ten years and counting: The Journal of Clinical Hypertension. *Journal of Clinical Hypertension, 10*, 333–340.
190. Staessen, J., Amery, A., & Fagard, R. (1990). Isolated systolic hypertension in the elderly. *Journal of Hypertension, 8*, 393–405.
191. Qureshi, A. I., Suri, M. F., Mohammad, Y., et al. (2002). Isolated and borderline isolated systolic hypertension relative to long-term risk and type of stroke: A 20-year follow-up of the national health and nutrition survey. *Stroke, 33*(12), 2781–2788.
192. Sagie, A., Larson, M. G., & Levy, D. (1993). The natural history of borderline isolated systolic hypertension. *New England Journal of Medicine, 329*, 1912–1917.
193. Amery, A., Birkenyhäger, W., Brixko, P., et al. (1985). Mortality and morbidity results from the European working party on high blood pressure in the elderly trial. *Lancet, 1*, 1349–1354.
194. Dahlof, B., Lindholm, L. H., Hansson, L., et al. (1991). Morbidity and mortality in the Swedish Trial in Old Patients with Hypertension (STOP-Hypertension). *Lancet, 338*(8778), 1281–1285.

195. MRC Working Party. (1992). Medical Research Council trial of treatment of hypertension in elderly: Principal results. *BMJ, 304*(6824), 405–412.
196. SHEP Cooperative Research Group. (1991). Prevention of stroke by antihypertensive drug treatment in older persons with isolated systolic hypertension: Final results of the Systolic Hypertension in the Elderly Program (SHEP). *JAMA, 265*, 3255–3264.
197. Staessen, J. A., Fagard, R., Thijs, L., et al. (1997). Randomised double-blind comparison of placebo and active treatment for older patients with isolated systolic hypertension. *Lancet, 350*, 757–764.
198. MacMahon, S., & Rodgers, A. (1993). The effects of blood pressure reduction in older patients: An overview of five randomized controlled trials in elderly hypertensives. *Clinical Experience in Hypertension, 15*(6), 967–978.
199. Hansson, L., Lindholm, L. H., Ekbom, T., et al. (1999). Randomised trial of old and new antihypertensive drugs in elderly patients: Cardiovascular mortality and morbidity the Swedish Trial in Old Patients with Hypertension-2 study. *Lancet, 354*(9192), 1751–1756.
200. Black, H. R. (1999). Management of hypertension in older persons. In J. L. Izzo Jr. & H. R. Black (Eds.), *Hypertension primer* (2nd ed., pp. 430–432). Baltimore: Lippincott, Williams & Wilkins.
201. Lakka, T. A., Venalainen, J. M., Rauramaa, R., et al. (1994). Relation of leisure-time physical activity and cardiorespiratory fitness to the risk of acute myocardial infarction in men. *New England Journal of Medicine, 330*, 1549–1554.
202. Vita, A. J., Terry, R. B., Hubert, H. B., et al. (1998). Aging, health risks, and cumulative disability. *New England Journal of Medicine, 338*, 1035–1041.
203. Flack, J. M., Nassar, S. A., Britton, M., et al. (2007). Hypertension in racial and ethnic minorities. In G. Lip & J. E. Hall (Eds.), *Comprehensive hypertension.* Philadelphia: Mosby, Elsevier.
204. Douglas, J. G., Bakris, G. L., Epstein, M., et al. (2003). Management of high blood pressure in African Americans: Consensus statement of the Hypertension in African Americans Working Group of the International Society on Hypertension in Blacks. *Archives of Internal Medicine, 163*, 525–541.
205. Borzecki, A. M., Oliveria, S. A., & Berlowitz, D. R. (2005). Barriers to hypertension control. *American Heart Journal, 149*(5), 785–794.
206. Report of the National High Blood Pressure Education Program Working Group on High Blood Pressure in Pregnancy. (2000). *American Journal of Obstetrics and Gynecology, 183*(1), S1–S22.
207. Sibai, B. M. (1996). Treatment of hypertension in pregnant women. *New England Journal of Medicine, 335*(4), 257–265.
208. Lindholm, L. H., Ibsen, H., Dahlof, B., et al. (2002). Cardiovascular morbidity and mortality in patients with diabetes in the Losartan Intervention For Endpoint reduction in hypertension study (LIFE): A randomised trial against atenolol. *Lancet, 359*(9311), 1004–1010.
209. Mehler, P. S., Coll, J. R., Estacio, R., et al. (2003). Intensive blood pressure control reduces the risk of cardiovascular events in patients with peripheral arterial disease and type 2 diabetes. *Circulation, 107*(5), 753–756.
210. Ikeda, T., Gomi, T., Hirawa, N., et al. (1996). Improvement of insulin sensitivity contributes to blood pressure reduction after weight loss in hypertensive subjects with obesity. *Hypertension, 27*(5), 1180–1186.
211. Lazarus, J. M., Bourgoignie, J. J., Buckalew, V. M., et al. (1997). Achievement and safety of a low blood pressure goal in chronic renal disease. The Modification of Diet in Renal Disease Study Group. *Hypertension, 29*(2), 641–650.
212. Perseghin, G., Price, T. B., Petersen, K. F., et al. (1996). Increased glucose transport-phosphorylation and muscle glycogen synthesis after exercise training in insulin-resistant subjects. *New England Journal of Medicine, 335*, 1357–1362.
213. Klag, M. J., Whelton, P. K., Randall, B. L., et al. (1996). Blood pressure and end-stage renal disease in men. *New England Journal of Medicine, 334*, 13–18.
214. Klag, M. J., Whelton, P. K., Randall, B. L., et al. (1997). End-stage renal disease in African-American and white men. 16-year MRFIT findings. *JAMA, 277*(16), 1293–1298.
215. Giatras, I., Lau, J., & Levey, A. S. (1997). Effect of angiotensin-converting enzyme inhibitors on the progression of nondiabetic renal disease: A meta-analysis of randomized trials. Angiotensin-Converting-Enzyme Inhibition and Progressive Renal Disease Study Group. *Annals of Internal Medicine, 127*(5), 337–345.
216. Maschio, G., Alberti, D., Janin, G., et al. (1996). Effect of the angiotensin-converting-enzyme inhibitor benazepril on the progression of chronic renal insufficiency. The Angiotensin-Converting-Enzyme Inhibition in Progressive Renal Insufficiency Study Group. *New England Journal of Medicine, 334*(15), 939–945.
217. Neusy, A. J., & Lowenstein, J. (1989). Blood pressure and blood pressure variability following withdrawal of propranolol and clonidine. *Journal of Clinical Pharmacology, 29*(1), 18–24.
218. Vidt, D. G. (1999). Management of hypertensive emergencies and urgencies. In J. L. Izzo Jr. & H. R. Black (Eds.), *Hypertension primer* (2nd ed., pp. 437–440). Baltimore: Lippincott Williams & Wilkins.
219. Grossman, E., Messerli, F. H., Grodzicki, T., et al. (1996). Should a moratorium be placed on sublingual nifedipine capsules given for hypertensive emergencies and pseudoemergencies? *JAMA, 276*(16), 1328–1331.
220. Varon, J., & Marik, P. E. (2000). The diagnosis and management of hypertensive crises. *Chest, 118*(1), 214–227.
221. Miller, N. H., Hill, M., Kottke, T., et al. (1997). The multilevel compliance challenge: Recommendations for a call to action. A statement for healthcare professionals. *Circulation, 95*(4), 1085–1090.
222. Ebrahim, S. (1998). Detection, adherence and control of hypertension for the prevention of stroke: A systematic review. *Health Technology Assessment, 2*(11), 1–78.
223. Roter, D. L., Hall, J. A., Merisca, R., et al. (1998). Effectiveness of interventions to improve patient compliance: A meta-analysis. *Medical Care, 36*(8), 1138–1161.
224. Calhoun, D. A., Jones, D., Textor, S., et al. (2008). Resistant hypertension: Diagnosis, evaluation, and treatment. A scientific statement from the American Heart Association Professional Education Committee of the Council for High Blood Pressure Research. *Hypertension, 51*, 1403–1419.
225. Working Group to Define Critical Patient Behaviors in High Blood Pressure Control. (1979). Critical patient behaviors in high blood pressure control: Guidelines for professionals. *JAMA, 241*, 2534–2537.
226. Bakris, G., Bohm, M., Dagenais, G., et al. (2008). Cardiovascular protection for all individuals at high risk: Evidence-based best practice. *Clinical Research in Cardiology, 97*(10), 713–725.
227. Coordinating Committee of the National High Blood Pressure Education Program. (1984). Collaboration in high blood pressure control: Among professionals and with the patient. *Annals of Internal Medicine, 101*(3), 393–395.
228. Curzio, J. L., Rubin, P. C., Kennedy, S. S., et al. (1990). A comparison of the management of hypertensive patients by nurse practitioners compared with conventional hospital care. *Journal of Human Hypertension, 4*(6), 665–670.
229. Logan, A. G., Milne, B. J., Achber, C., et al. (1979). Work-site treatment of hypertension by specially trained nurses. A controlled trial. *Lancet, 2*(8153), 1175–1178.
230. Pheley, A. M., Terry, P., Pietz, L., et al. (1995). Evaluation of a nurse-based hypertension management program: Screening, management, and outcomes. *Journal of Cardiovascular Nursing, 9*(2), 54–61.
231. Schultz, J. F., & Sheps, S. G. (1994). Management of patients with hypertension: A hypertension clinic model. *Mayo Clinic Proceedings, 69*(10), 997–999.
232. Smith, E. D., Merritt, S. L., & Patel, M. K. (1997). Church-based education: An outreach program for African Americans with hypertension. *Ethnic Health, 2*(3), 243–253.
233. Rose, A. J., Berlowitz, D. R., Orner, M. B., et al. (2007). Understanding uncontrolled hypertension: Is it the patient or the provider? *The Journal of Clinical Hypertension, 9*(12), 937–943.
234. Rose, A. J., Shimada, S. L., Rothendler, J. A., et al. (2008). The accuracy of clinician perceptions of "usual" blood pressure control. *Journal of General Internal Medicine, 23*(2), 180–183.
235. Alderman, M. H., Furberg, C. D., Kostis, J. B., et al. (2002). Hypertension guidelines: Criteria that might make them more clinically useful. *American Journal of Hypertension, 15*(10, Pt. 1), 917–923.
236. Hyman, D. J., & Pavlik, V. N. (2001). Characteristics of patients with uncontrolled hypertension in the United States. *New England Journal of Medicine, 345*(7), 479–486.
237. Tu, K., Mamdani, M. M., & Tu, J. V. (2002). Hypertension guidelines in elderly patients: Is anybody listening? *American Journal of Medicine, 113*(1), 52–58.
238. Farquhar, J. W., Fortmann, S. P., Flora, J. A., et al. (1990). Effects of communitywide education on cardiovascular disease risk factors. The Stanford Five-City Project. *JAMA, 265*, 359–365.
239. Puska, P., Tuomilehto, J., Nissinen, A., et al. (1989). The North Karelia project: 15 years of community-based prevention of coronary heart disease. *Annals of Medicine, 21*(3), 169–173.

CHAPTER 36

Lipid Management and Cardiovascular Disease

Kathleen A. Berra / Joan M. Fair

Cardiovascular disease (CVD) is the leading cause of death for American women and men and is responsible for 35.2% of all deaths. Approximately one in every five Americans died from CVD in 2005. The death rates vary by gender, age, ethnicity, and socioeconomic status.[1] Importantly, the overall death rates from CVD declined by 24.7% from 1994 to 2004 likely as a result of improved risk factor surveillance and management.[1] Elevated serum cholesterol and, particularly, elevated low-density lipoprotein (LDL) cholesterol levels are significant modifiable risk factors associated with the development and progression of CVD. More than 106 million Americans have a blood cholesterol higher than the desirable level of 200 mg/dL.[1] Furthermore, more than 37 million Americans have a blood cholesterol more than 240 mg/dL, a level at which current treatment guidelines recommend the initiation of dietary or pharmacologic interventions.[1–3] The good news is that, in the United States, age-adjusted prevalence of high LDL cholesterol level in adults dropped from 26.6% in 1984 to 25.3% in 2004. This was associated with an increased awareness of the relationship between high LDL cholesterol and CVD (39.2% vs. 63%) and an increased use of pharmacological therapies to reduce high blood cholesterol (11.7% to 40.8%). The end result has been a decrease in overall death and disability from CVD.[1] This information demonstrates that both the incidence of high blood cholesterol and the benefits of treatment are substantial.

There is a large body of evidence, including animal studies,[4] observational studies,[5] and numerous clinical trials, that consistently point to a relationship between high blood lipids and CVD. A very recent example of this compelling relationship is the INTERHEART Study.[6] The INTERHEART study using data from 52 countries, showed that 90% of population-attributable risk is strongly associated with nine easily measured risk factors.[6] Two thirds (or 66%) of the population-attributable risks are accounted for by abnormal lipids (using the apo B/apo A-I ratio as a marker for abnormal lipids—a surrogate for LDL measure) and by current smoking. This association holds true for both men and women, across different geographic regions, and ethnic groups.[6] Table 36-1 summarizes the results of large randomized lipid-lowering primary and secondary prevention trials.[2,7–15] Meta-analyses of the cholesterol-lowering clinical trials estimated that a 10-mg/dL reduction in total cholesterol results in a 22% reduction in CVD incidence after 2 years of intervention, and a 25% reduction after 5 years.[3,16] There is some evidence that cholesterol lowering begun at an early age (e.g., age 40 years) may provide greater risk reduction than if started at a later age (e.g., age 70 years).[17] However, recent clinical trials including persons older than 65 years show benefit for CVD risk reduction in older populations.[14,18]

The Adult Treatment Panel III (ATP III) Guidelines were updated in 2004 in response to these important clinical trials.[3] This update highlighted the importance of lipid-lowering therapy in *high-risk* and *moderately high-risk* patients to achieve a 30% to 40% reduction in LDL cholesterol level, even if baseline levels were low or "normal" by current guidelines. An LDL goal of <100 mg/dL is now considered a reasonable option for patients designated at *high risk*. For those considered to be at very high risk an LDL goal of <70 mg/dL is proposed. The LDL goal of <70 mg/dL is suggested on the basis of the known elevated risk for heart attack and stroke in this group. This important ATP III update significantly expands both the numbers of persons needing treatment and redefines LDL treatment goals. Therapeutic Lifestyle Change (TLC) remains the cornerstone of treatment for all adults with elevated risk. TLC includes heart healthy nutrition, weight control, and regular physical activity. Initiation of pharmacologic therapies is based on risk classification.[3] See Table 36-2 for LDL goals and cut points for initiation of TLC and pharmacological therapies. Cardiovascular nurses need to understand the pathophysiology of dyslipidemia and should actively participate in the identification and management of lipid disorders.[19]

BLOOD LIPIDS: STRUCTURE AND FUNCTIONS

The complex relationships between genetic and metabolic mechanisms and the molecular interactions within the cell wall help explain the association between lipid abnormalities and CVD. The major lipid particles, cholesterol and triglycerides, both have important functions in the body. Cholesterol is an essential component of cell membranes, functioning to provide stability while permitting membrane transport; it is a precursor to adrenal steroids, sex hormones, and bile and bile acids. Triglycerides are the major source of energy for the body. Both cholesterol and triglycerides are insoluble molecules and must be transported in the circulation as lipoproteins.

Lipoproteins are complexes of nonpolar lipid cores (triglycerides and cholesterol esters) surrounded by a surface coat of polar lipids (phospholipids and free cholesterol) and specific proteins called apoproteins. Total cholesterol, for example, is composed of 18 different lipid and lipoprotein particles.[20] Lipoproteins can be classified according to their density, their migration on an electrophoretic field, or their lipid and apoprotein composition.[21]

During the 1980s, significant advances were made in determining the function of the apoproteins, the lipid processing enzymes, and lipoprotein receptors. Apoproteins function as more than transport vehicles; they have variant properties that activate enzyme systems or receptor sites to promote the catabolism or removal of lipoproteins from the circulation.[22] The functions of nine apoproteins in the lipid metabolic cascade have

Table 36-1 ■ SELECTED, RANDOMIZED, CLINICAL TRIALS USING STATIN THERAPY TO LOWER CHOLESTEROL

Trial	Number of Patients	Age (years)	Lipids (mean, mg/dL)	Average Length of Follow-up	Mean Lipid Reduction	Outcomes
Primary Prevention						
West of Scotland (WOSCOPS)*	6,595 men	45–64	TC: 272 LDL: 192	4.9 years	TC: ↓ 20% LDL: ↓ 26%	Nonfatal MI and CVD death: ↓ 31%
AFCAPS/TEXCAPS†	5,608 men 997 women		TC: 221 LDL: 150	5.2 years	TC: ↓ 18% LDL: ↓ 25%	Major coronary events (MI, unstable angina, or sudden cardiac death: ↓ 37%)
Primary and Secondary Prevention						
Heart Protection Study‡	15,454 men 5,082 women	40–80 (52% > 65)	TC: 228 LDL: 131‡‡	5.0 years	LDL ↓ 37 mg/dL	All cause mortality ↓ 13%, major vascular events ↓24% Coronary death rats ↓ 27%, nonfatal/fatal stroke ↓ 25% Nonfatal MI and coronary death ↓ 27%.
Prospective Study of Pravastatin in the Elderly at Risk§	2,804 men 3,000 women	70–82	TC: 150–350	3.2 years	LDL: ↓ 34%	Composite of: coronary death, nonfatal MI, fatal or nonfatal stroke ↓ 24%
Anglo-Scandinavian Cardiac Outcomes Trial-Lipid Lowering Arm‖	10,350 81% male	40–79	LDL: 132	3.3 (stopped early due to benefit)	LDL ↓ 29%	Total cardiovascular events ↓ 21% Total coronary events ↓ 29% Total fatal and nonfatal stroke ↓ 7%
Secondary Prevention						
Scandinavian Simvastatin Survival Study (4S)¶	3,617 men 427 women	35–70	TC LDL: 188	5.4 years	TC ↓ 28% LDL: ↓ 38%	CHD deaths: ↓ 42% Nonfatal MI and CVD death ↓ 37%
CARE#	4,159	Average 59	LDL: 139	3 years	LDL: ↓ 27%	Major coronary events ↓ 25% Coronary mortality ↓ 24% Total mortality ↓ 9%
LIPID**	9,014	31–75	LDL: 150	61 years	LDL: ↓ 25%	Major coronary events ↓ 29% Coronary mortality ↓ 24% Total mortality ↓ 23%
Pravastatin or Atorvastatin Evaluation and Infection—Thrombolysis in MI††	4,162	≥18	TC: ≤240 mg/dL Mean LDL: 106	24 months	LDL: ↓ 22% Pravastatin ↓ 51% Atorvastatin	Composite death from any cause, MI, hospitalization from unstable angina, revascularization, or stroke ↓ 16%

TC, total cholesterol; LDL, low density lipoprotein

*WOSCOPS: Shepherd, J., Cobbe, S. M., Ford, I., et al., for the West of Scotland Coronary Prevention Study Group. (1995). Prevention of coronary heart disease with pravastatin in men with hypercholesterolemia. *New England Journal of Medicine, 333*, 1301–1307.

†AFCAPS/TEXCAPS: Downs, J. R., Clearfield, M., Weis, S., et al., for the AFCAPS/TexCAPS Research Group. (1998). Primary prevention of acute coronary events with lovastatin in men and women with average cholesterol levels: Results of AFCAPS/TexCAPS. *JAMA, 279*, 1615–1622.

‡HPS: Heart Protection Study Collaborative Group. (2002). Heart Protection Study of cholesterol lowering with simvastatin in 20536 high-risk individuals: A randomised placebo-controlled trial. *Lancet, 360*, 7Y22.

§Shepherd, J., Blauw, G. J., Murphy, M. B., et al., PROSPER study group. (2002). Pravastatin in elderly individuals at risk of vascular disease (PROSPER): A randomised controlled trial. PROspective Study of Pravastatin in the Elderly at Risk. *Lancet, 360*, 1623–1630.

‖Sever, P. S., Dahlof, B., Poulter, N. R., et al., ASCOT investigators. (2003). Prevention of coronary and stroke events with atorvastatin in hypertensive patients who have average or lower-than-average cholesterol concentrations, in the Anglo-Scandinavian Cardiac Outcomes Trial–Lipid Lowering Arm (ASCOT-LLA): A multicentre randomised controlled trial. *Lancet, 361*, 1149–1158.

¶4S: Scandinavian Simvastatin Survival Study Group. (1994). Randomised trial of cholesterol lowering in 4444 patients with coronary heart disease: The Scandinavian Simvastatin Survival Study (4S). *Lancet, 344*, 1383–1389.

#CARE: Sacks, F. M., Pfeffer, M. A., Moye, L. A., et al., for the Cholesterol and Recurrent Events Trial Investigators. (1996). The effect of pravastatin on coronary events after myocardial infarction in patients with average cholesterol levels. *New England Journal of Medicine, 335*, 1001–1009.

**LIPID: Long-Term Intervention with Pravastatin in Ischaemic Disease (LIPID) Study Group. (1998). Prevention of cardiovascular events and death with pravastatin in patients with coronary heart disease and a broad range of initial cholesterol levels. *New England Journal of Medicine, 339*, 1349–1357.

††Cannon, C. P., Braunwald, E., McCabe, C. H., et al., for the Pravastatin or Atorvastatin Evaluation and Infection Therapy-Thrombolysis in Myocardial Infarction 22 Investigators. (2004). Intensive versus moderate lipid lowering with statins after acute coronary syndromes. *New England Journal of Medicine, 350*, 1495–1504.

‡‡Serum lipids were determined by direct LDL measurement method as baseline samples were nonfasting. If calculated by Friedewald (as in other trials) LDL would be ~15% higher.

been identified: apo A-I, apo A-II, apo B-100, apo B-48, apo C-I, apo C-II, apo C-III, apo E2, apo E3, apo E4, and lipoprotein(a), or Lp(a). In addition, the actions of several lipoprotein-processing enzymes (lipoprotein lipase [LPL], hepatic lipase [HL], lecithin cholesterol acyltransferase, and cholesteryl ester transfer protein [CETP]) and the function of cell receptors, including the LDL and chylomicron remnant receptor, are now established. These advances permit an understanding of lipid metabolism, as well as the abnormalities leading to elevated blood cholesterol.

Table 36-2 ■ GUIDELINES FOR INITIATION OF TLC AND/OR PHARMACOTHERAPIES—MODIFICATIONS BASED ON THE UPDATE TO ATP III[3]

Risk Category	LDL-C Goal	Initiate TLC	Consider Drug Therapy
1. *High Risk** CHD† or CHD Risk Equivalents‡ (10-year risk <20%)	<100 mg/dL optional goal <70 mg/dL	≥100 mg/dL	≥100 mg/dL <100 mg/dL: consider drug options
2. *Moderately High Risk* 10-year risk 10%–20%	<130 mg/dL	≥130 mg/dL	≥130 mg/dL 100–129 mg/dL: consider drug options
3. *Moderate Risk* 10-year risk <10%	<130 mg/dL	≥130 mg/dL	≥160 mg/dL
4. *Lower Risk* 0–1 risk factor	<160 mg/dL	≥160 mg/dL	≥190 mg/dL 160–189 mg/dL: LDL lowering drug optional

*Risk factors include cigarette smoking, hypertension (BP > 140/90 mm Hg or on antihypertensive medication), low HDL-C (<40 mg/dL), family history of premature heart disease (CHD in first-degree male relative < 55 years of age, or in a female relative > 65 years of age), and age (men ≥ 45 years of age and women ≥ 55 years of age).
†CHD includes history of MI, unstable angina, stable angina, coronary artery procedures (stenting, angioplasty, bypass surgery, or evidence of clinically significant myocardial ischemia.
‡CHD Risk Equivalents include manifestations of noncoronary forms of atherosclerotic disease (peripheral arterial disease, abdominal aortic aneurysm, and carotid artery disease (transient ischemic attach or stroke or carotid origin or > 50% obstruction in carotid artery), diabetes, and 2+ risk factors with 10-year risk for hard CHD > 20%.

LIPID METABOLISM AND TRANSPORT

The gut and liver are responsible for the production of the six principal lipoproteins. Exogenous lipoproteins are formed in the mucosa of the small intestine after digestion of dietary fats. During the digestive process, hydrolyzed products of ingested fats enter epithelial cells of the small intestine, where they are converted into triglycerides and cholesterol esters. These products are then aggregated into the lipoprotein complexes known as chylomicrons. Chylomicrons pass into small lymph vessels and reach the circulatory system through the thoracic duct. In the peripheral capillaries, chylomicrons are hydrolyzed by the enzyme LPL, located on the capillary endothelium. Free fatty acids and glycerol then enter adipose tissue cells. A cholesterol-rich chylomicron remnant (a second lipoprotein complex) is released into the circulation when lipolysis is nearly complete. Chylomicron remnants are cleared rapidly by the liver (Fig. 36-1).[23,24]

In the liver, the endogenous lipoprotein cascade begins with the production of very-low-density lipoproteins (VLDLs). Triglycerides are resynthesized from chylomicrons and packaged with specific apoproteins, apo B-100, apo C-I, apo C-II, and apo E, to form VLDL. Once VLDL is released into the circulation, intermediate-density lipoproteins (IDLs) and VLDL remnants are formed from VLDL lipolysis. This process takes place in the capillary endothelium and is mediated by LPL, the same enzyme responsible for the hydrolysis of chylomicrons. Apo C-II also acts as a cofactor in these processes.[25]

LDL receptors in the liver recognize and bind with apo E on the IDL particle and remove approximately half of the IDL from the circulation. The remainder is converted by HL into smaller cholesterol-rich lipoproteins known as LDL. Apo B-100 is the remaining protein left on the surface coat of LDL particles. The LDL receptors on cells of the liver and other organs that require cholesterol for structural and metabolic functions bind with apo B-100 and facilitate the removal of LDL from the blood. Figure 36-2 illustrates the endogenous pathway. The LDL particle is the major cholesterol-carrying lipoprotein in the blood and, consequently, the most atherogenic lipoprotein.[21] Under normal conditions, more than 93% of the cholesterol in the body is located in the cells, and only 7% circulates in the blood. Two thirds of the blood cholesterol is carried by LDL. Increased cellular uptake of cholesterol through the LDL receptor pathway suppresses the cell's own synthesis of cholesterol by inhibiting the hydroxymethylglutaryl coenzyme-A (HMG-CoA) reductase enzyme. This enzyme determines the rate of cholesterol synthesis. As cellular cholesterol levels increase, the activity of the LDL receptor is downregulated, and synthesis of new LDL receptors is inhibited.[26] These feedback control mechanisms serve as the rationale for determining the treatment of elevated blood cholesterol.

Several metabolic and genetic disorders can be related to elevated LDL cholesterol levels. Habitually high dietary intakes of saturated fats and cholesterol beyond that needed for cell functions result in blood levels of LDL beyond normal and result in

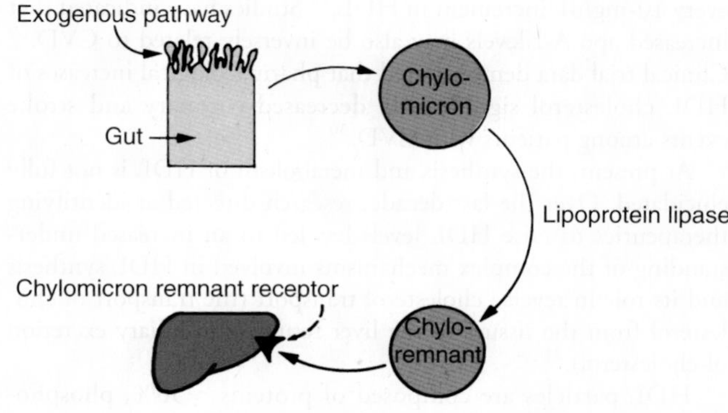

■ **Figure 36-1** The exogenous metabolism of lipoproteins and the transport of chylomicrons to the tissues and chylomicron remnants to the liver.

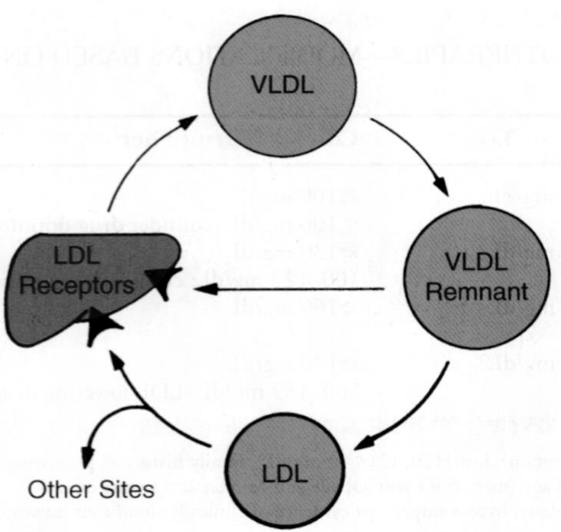

Figure 36-2 The endogenous lipid transport system originates in the liver. LDLs provide essential cholesterol to the tissue cells.

inhibited LDL receptor activity. High LDL levels also can result from a decrease in clearance of LDL because of a deficiency in LDL receptors. This deficiency may be caused by genetic abnormalities in the structure of the receptor binding sites (where apolipoproteins bind) or by a decrease in LDL receptors on the surface of cells. In addition, genetic mutation in apoproteins, particularly apo E and apo B-100, can result in decreased cholesterol clearance. The metabolic consequence is an increased blood level of this atherogenic lipoprotein and the synthesis of cholesterol within cells, a process normally suppressed by LDL uptake.

REVERSE CHOLESTEROL TRANSPORT

Studies have consistently observed a protective effect of high-density lipoprotein (HDL). For example, high levels of HDL have been associated with a reduced risk of CVD.[8,27] It has been suggested that the protective effect of HDL is greater than the atherogenic effect of LDL cholesterol. For men in the Framingham Heart Study, a 50% reduction in coronary risk was found with every 10-mg/dL increment in HDL.[28] Studies have indicated that increased apo A-I levels may also be inversely related to CVD.[29] Clinical trial data demonstrated that pharmacological increases of HDL cholesterol significantly decreased coronary and stroke events among patients with CVD.[30]

At present, the synthesis and metabolism of HDL is not fully elucidated. Over the last decade, research directed at identifying therapeutics to raise HDL levels has led to an increased understanding of the complex mechanisms involved in HDL synthesis and its role in reverse cholesterol transport (the transport of cholesterol from the tissues to the liver resulting in biliary excretion of cholesterol).[31]

HDL particles are composed of proteins ~50%, phospholipids ~30% and cholesterol ~25%, triglycerides ~5%, and assorted lipoprotein-processing enzymes.[31] The intestine and liver are responsible for synthesizing the precursors of HDL and its major lipoprotein, apo A-I to form incomplete (or nascent) lipid-poor HDL precursors. These precursors acquire excess cholesterol through a variety of mechanisms outlined below. One early step is the cholesterol efflux from macrophages mediated by the membrane protein, adenosine triphosphate binding cassette transporter A-1 (ABCA1), one of a family of proteins that transport molecules across cell membranes.[32] It is proposed that ABCA1 allows binding with apo A-I in nascent HDL to form more mature HDL particles.[33] Other steps include the action of the enzyme, lecithin cholesterol acyltransferase, which converts free cholesterol in the tissues into an HDL cholesteryl ester core.[34,35] Apo A-I has been shown to activate lecithin cholesterol acyltransferase and may influence the activity of the CETP. CETP facilitates the exchange of cholesterol esters for the triglycerides in apo B lipoproteins including LDL and VLDL.[36] Apo C-II is a cofactor for LPL. In the presence of circulating triglycerides, apo C-II moves from HDL to the triglyceride particle, activating LPL and promoting the catabolism of VLDL.[37] This mechanism, in part, explains the clinical observation of an inverse association between high triglycerides and low HDL levels. A third apoprotein, apo E, is thought to facilitate direct transfer of cholesterol esters to hepatocyte receptors.[37] Cholesterol esters are then excreted in bile or bile acids.[38]

Although the protective effect of HDL has been linked to its role in the reverse transport of cholesterol, it is clear that other factors, particularly genetic factors, determine coenzyme, apoprotein, and receptor activity. In fact, it is estimated that 50% to 70% of the variation in HDL is genetically determined influencing the receptor and enzyme activity involved in the catabolism of HDL.[39] Deletions or mutations of the apo A-I gene results in very reduced HDL levels (e.g., A-I Milano) and may be associated with increased atherosclerosis. One important recent discovery was that of the ABCA1 genetic defect manifested in Tangiers disease as a disorder with extremely low HDL levels and with accelerated cholesterol tissue deposition.[32,40]

Recent studies have found that plasma HDL levels are regulated by a class of enzymes including LPL, HL, and endothelial lipase (EL).[41] LPL is synthesized by adipose and skeletal muscle cells and acts primarily on the hydrolysis of triglycerides. HL is synthesized in the liver cells and acts on triglyceride and phospholipid catabolism. EL is synthesized in endothelial cells and appears to regulate HDL levels by preventing the transfer of triglycerides and remnant particles to HDL. Evidence includes genetically modified animal models that over express EL show a marked decrease in HDL levels[42] and human studies observing genetic variants in the EL gene in persons with high HDL levels.[39]

While we have gained a greater understanding of the role of HDL in reverse cholesterol transport, studies also suggest that HDL may have both pro- and anti-inflammatory properties and in the face of inflammatory states, HDL may be altered to become proinflammatory.[43,44] This may explain the finding that atherosclerosis (as an inflammatory disease) is observed even in persons with normal to high HDL levels. Studies have also suggested that HDL may act as an antioxidant, by preventing the oxidation of LDL, thus rendering it less atherogenic,[45,46] or by attenuating the expression of other enzymes and molecules that alter endothelial dilation and chemotactic properties.[47]

At present, there are two major subclasses of HDL based on density and apoprotein composition. HDL_3 is richer in apo A-II than HDL_2, which has a higher concentration of apo A-I.[29]

Production of apo A-I is higher in women than in men and is increased by exercise training, alcohol consumption, and estrogen administration.[21] Premenopausal women have more than three times the concentration of HDL_2 than do men. Studies have also suggested that HDL may act as an antioxidant, preventing the oxidation of LDL.[45,46]

LDL VARIANTS

LDL Particle Size

Mounting evidence suggests that the size of the LDL particle plays an important role in its atherogenicity. Particle size is determined by flotation rates after ultracentrifugation procedures. LDL can be separated into a small dense LDL particle (phenotype B) and a larger less dense LDL particle (phenotype A).[48] Clinical trial evidence suggests that people with a predominance of small dense LDL particles have a higher incidence of CVD and more accelerated progression of coronary lesions.[49] The exact mechanism of the negative influence of the small dense LDL particle is not completely understood. One possible explanation is that the smaller denser particles have a greater ability to penetrate the endothelial space and participate fully in the subendothelial atherosclerotic process. Small LDL particles also appear to be more susceptible to oxidation than larger LDL particles.[50] In addition, the small dense LDL particle is most commonly found in conjunction with a constellation of other factors, including hypertriglyceridemia, low HDL cholesterol, and insulin resistance.[51]

Research also suggests that it is possible to increase (alter) the size of the LDL particle to the larger (phenotype A) size by reducing triglycerides and normalizing insulin sensitivity. In addition, lipid-lowering drugs such as bile acid-binding resins, niacin, and the fibrates are reported to alter particle size favorably.[48]

Oxidized LDL

Ongoing research in lipid metabolism is investigating the issue of oxidation. Molecular biologists have established that modified or oxidized LDL is taken up more rapidly *in vitro* by monocytes and macrophages than is native LDL.[52] It has also been shown that Lp(a) is a primary carrier of oxidized LDL and account for the relationship between elevated Lp(a) and atherosclerosis.[53]

Oxidized LDL has been found to be cytotoxic, and it is postulated that this facilitates endothelial injury, leading to the development of fatty streaks and atherosclerotic lesions. Oxidative inhibitors can block the modification of LDL to an oxidized form. Studies are ongoing in this area but a clear understanding of oxidized lipids and CVD remains elusive.[54]

The Role of Lp(a)

Genetic researchers investigating variant LDL particles uncovered a lipoprotein, Lp(a), that is similar to LDL with each particle linked to a molecule of the atherogenic apo B-100 in a 1:1 ratio.[55] The attached protein, apolipoprotein(a) (apo[a]) is unique and is similar in DNA sequence to plasminogen, a substance that breaks up blood clots Recent prospective studies and meta-analysis have found elevated levels of Lp(a) are independent predictors of CVD. Lp(a) has also been detected in atherosclerotic plaques.[56] Lp(a) levels vary inversely to the size of the apo(a) protein. Those who are Black and South Asian have higher Lp(a) levels compared with those who are Caucasian or from other Asian populations.[57] Epidemiology studies suggest that Lp(a) levels above 25 to 30 mg/dL constitute CVD risk, further, it is estimated that 37% of those at high risk of CVD have elevated levels of Lp(a).[55] Currently only one therapeutic agent, niacin, lowers Lp(a) levels. A more complete understanding of the mechanisms by which Lp(a) influences atherosclerosis and the effect of apo(a) size is needed. Like Lp(a), there are a number of emerging lipid risk factors that may further explain the relationship of dyslipidemia to coronary heart disease (CHD) (Table 36-3).

Lipoprotein-Associated Phospholipase A_2 (Lp-PLA_2)

The search for biomarkers that identify those at risk for CVD has led to interest in Lp-PLA_2, an enzyme that hydrolyzes lipids and preferentially oxidized LDL thereby triggering inflammatory processes.[58] It is known that Lp-PLA_2 is produced by macrophages (prominent in the inflammatory atherosclerotic process) and mainly carried in circulation bound to LDL cholesterol. Clinical trial studies have observed a positive but inconsistent association between elevated Lp-PLA_2 and risk of CVD and stroke.[58] A cut-point of 235 ng/mL or more (greater than the 50th percentile from population studies) has been suggested as a level indicative of risk for CVD.[59]

CHOLESTEROL AND ENDOTHELIAL FUNCTION

Serum cholesterol levels and diets high in saturated fat have been associated with impairments in endothelial functioning. The endothelium acts to regulate vascular tone, platelet adhesion, thrombosis, and growth factors.[60] Studies have demonstrated that elevated cholesterol results in a reduced vasodilation response. Furthermore, when cholesterol is lowered, vasodilation responses improve.[61]

Elevated cholesterol also increases platelet aggregation and monocyte adhesion, factors that lead to thrombus formation and plaque rupture.[62] Continuing research suggests that the lipids influence a variety of endothelial responses that appear to contribute to the atherosclerotic process.

DYSLIPIDEMIC DISORDERS

Although the metabolic processes related to blood lipids are complex and influenced by both genetic and environmental factors, the management of dyslipidemia has been well characterized. National recommendations have been developed on the basis of the scientific evidence and taking into account the need for both primary and secondary prevention of CVD.[2,3] In general, lipid disorders can be characterized by the specific lipid abnormalities observed (see Table 36-3).

HYPERCHOLESTEROLEMIA

Hypercholesterolemia is the most common dyslipidemia and, in most people, decreased LDL clearance is responsible for the

Table 36-3 ■ LIPID ABNORMALITIES AND ASSOCIATED MECHANISMS

Lipid Abnormality	Mechanisms
Elevated total cholesterol	High dietary intake of saturated fat and cholesterol LDL receptor deficiency and other enzyme/receptor abnormalities.
Elevated LDL-cholesterol	LDL receptor deficiency Apoprotein B-100 genetic defect, other enzyme/receptor abnormalities. High dietary intake of saturated fat and cholesterol
Elevated triglycerides	Deficiency in LPL Obesity, physical inactivity, insulin resistance, glucose intolerance Excessive alcohol intake
Low HDL	Apoprotein A-I deficiency, other enzyme/receptor abnormalities Reduced VLDL clearance Cigarette smoking, physical inactivity Insulin resistance Elevated triglycerides Overweight and obesity Very high carbohydrate (CHO) intake (>60% total calories) Certain drugs (β-blockers, anabolic steroids, progestational agents)
Increased lipoprotein remnants (VLDL is a surrogate marker for Lipoprotein remnants when triglyceride (Tg) is >200 mg/dL)	Defective apolipoprotein E Seen in familial combined hyperlipidemia Level is genetically determined
Lp(a)	
Lipoprotein phospholipase A^2 (LpPLA^2)	An enzyme that hydrolyzes cholesterol and initiates inflammatory processes
Small LDL particles	Particle Size is determined by level of Triglycerides; LDL particle is denser and more atherogenic at higher levels of TG
HDL Subspecies	Low levels of HDL 2 and 3 increases CVD risk? Genetically determined versus lifestyle and other lipid levels
Apolipoprotein B	A potential marker for all atherogenic lipoprotein
Apolipoprotein A-I	Increased CVD risk when apo A-I is low
Combined dyslipidemias small, dense LDL, high triglycerides, low HDL elevated LDL and triglycerides	Defects in VLDL and LDL receptor activities coexisting with environmental influences such as obesity, physical inactivity, diet high in saturated fat, and cigarette smoking

National Cholesterol Education Program (2001).

observed abnormality. A high intake of dietary cholesterol and saturated fatty acids downregulates LDL receptor activity and receptor synthesis, resulting in decreased LDL clearance.[63]

Familial (Severe) Hypercholesterolemia

Severe hypercholesterolemia is caused most commonly by a genetic disorder and is known as familial hypercholesterolemia (FH). There are two types of FH, heterozygous and homozygous. Plasma LDL cholesterol normally binds to cell membrane receptors and is taken into the cell for several biologic functions. In heterozygous FH, there is one normal gene and one abnormal gene for the LDL receptor.

Because only half the normal number of LDL receptors are synthesized, LDL is removed from the blood at two thirds the normal rate.[26] The result is a two- to three-fold increase in blood LDL levels. One person in 500 is thought to have this genetic disorder, which eventually results in an increased risk for myocardial infarction (MI).[2,64] The homozygous form of FH develops when two abnormal genes are inherited. The one in one million persons who have this disorder have LDL levels six times normal and may have an MI as early as age 5 to 15 years.[2,26,48,64] In addition, a genetic defect related to apo B-100 results in marked elevations in LDL cholesterol.

Hypertriglyceridemia

The relationship between triglycerides and CVD is not entirely clear. Elevated serum triglyceride levels have been associated with CVD. However, the strength of the association is diminished when other CVD risks are accounted for, leading some to suggest that elevated triglycerides are a marker for other atherogenic factors.[65] Chylomicrons and VLDL are lipoprotein carriers of triglyceride and, whereas chylomicrons are not considered to be atherogenic, the remnants of VLDL catabolism are smaller particles that are richer in cholesterol esters.[65] These remnant particles, or IDL, are considered more atherogenic.[66]

Elevated triglycerides are frequently observed in people who also have low HDL levels and small dense LDL particles. This combination of lipid abnormalities is considered an atherogenic phenotype.[65] In addition, elevated triglycerides (and its associated small dense LDL particle size and low HDL cholesterol level) commonly exists with insulin resistance (with or without glucose intolerance), hypertension, obesity (particularly abdominal obesity pattern), and prothrombotic and proinflammatory states. This combination of risk factors is commonly called the metabolic syndrome and is linked to increased CVD risk.[2,3] See Table 36-4 for a summary of the metabolic syndrome characteristics. These associations suggest that elevated triglyceride levels may be a marker for other CVD risk factors. Diabetes also results in increased plasma triglyceride levels because of increased

Table 36-4 ■ CHARACTERISTICS OF THE METABOLIC SYNDROME

Risk Factor	Comments
Abdominal obesity (waist circumference)	Men: >102 cm (>40 in.) Women: >88 cm (>35 in.)
Triglycerides	≥150 mg/dL
HDL cholesterol	Men: <40 mg/dL Women: <50 mg/dL
Blood pressure	≥130/≥85 mm Hg
Fasting glucose	≥110–125 mg/dL

Adapted from Expert Panel on Detection, Evaluation, and Treatment of High Blood Cholesterol in Adults. (2001). Executive summary of the third report of the National Cholesterol Education Program (NCEP) Expert Panel on Detection, Evaluation, and Treatment of High Blood Cholesterol in Adults (Adult Treatment Panel III). *JAMA, 285*(19), 2486–2497.

VLDL. LDL cholesterol is more glycated in patients with diabetes compared with nondiabetic subjects. Glycated LDL particles have increased oxidative susceptibility.[65] HDL is often low in patients with diabetes as a result of increased HL triglyceride activity. Additionally, hyperglycemia is associated with significantly increased mortality in patients with acute coronary syndrome. The Heart Protection Study (HPS) further confirmed the importance of lipid management in persons with type 2 diabetes. HPS included 5,963 persons with diabetes (ages 40 to 80 years). Those subjects receiving simvastatin 40 mg/day had significant reductions of 25% for major coronary events including stroke and revascularization.[12]

High triglyceride levels are also related to high carbohydrate and alcohol intake. As a marker for CVD risk, the reduction of plasma triglyceride levels to less than 150 mg/dL is a desirable goal.[2,3] Although not designated as an independent risk predictor by ATP III, the importance of elevated triglycerides is recognized in a number of ways. In ATP III, triglyceride level is seen as a marker of elevated atherogenic remnant particle level thought to increase risk of CAD and as an indication of lipid and nonlipid risk factors in the metabolic syndrome.[2]

In addition, normal triglyceride level has been lowered to 150 mg/dL or less compared with[67] ATP II (see Table 36-5).[2] A new target for persons with elevated triglycerides is called "non-HDL cholesterol." Non-HDL cholesterol is the total cholesterol minus the HDL cholesterol. This number represents the sum of the LDL and the VLDL cholesterol in determining a treatment goal for LDL cholesterol. The goal for LDL cholesterol is 30 mg/dL higher in persons with triglycerides of 200 mg/dL or more. This is based on a normal VLDL value being 30 mg/dL.

Table 36-5 ■ ATP III CLASSIFICATION OF TRIGLYCERIDES (NCEP, 2001)

Triglyceride (Tg) Level (mg/dL)	Category
<150	Normal
150–199	Borderline high
200–499	High
≥500	Very high

Hypoalphalipoproteinemia

A familial HDL deficiency state, hypoalphalipoproteinemia, has been linked to premature CVD. Although high HDL levels may mobilize cholesterol from arterial luminal surfaces and return it to the liver, low HDL usually reflects an enzymatic or apoprotein abnormality affecting the catabolism of LDL or VLDL. (See section titled "Reverse Cholesterol Transport.") Alterations of the human apo A-I gene have been found in those with familial HDL deficiency and premature CVD.[68] This suggests that low HDL may represent a genetic marker for identifying those at risk for CVD. The abnormalities related to VLDL catabolism explain the common coexistence of low HDL with elevated triglycerides. Furthermore, when triglycerides are lowered, increases in HDL are observed. In the absence of a genetic deficiency (i.e., A-I Milano, Tangiers disease), lower HDL levels are related to environmental factors such as cigarette smoking and physical inactivity (see Table 36-3 for causes of low HDL cholesterol).

Although raising HDL-C by delaying catabolism (e.g., CETP inhibition) may not enhance reverse cholesterol transport, elevating HDL-C may have other cardioprotective benefits such as antioxidant, anti-inflammatory, and anticoagulant effects that all may improve endothelial function. At present, niacin is the most effective HDL-raising therapy. Although the mechanism by which niacin raises HDL level is not well understood, the predominant hypothesis is that niacin inhibits the holoparticle uptake of HDL, resulting in delayed catabolism.[69]

Combined Dyslipidemias

Combined dyslipidemias usually represent a combination of genetic lipoprotein or apoprotein defects and environmental effects. The specific lipid abnormalities observed provide clues to the genetic disorders. Table 36-3 summarizes observed lipid abnormalities and associated mechanisms. An understanding of these mechanisms guides the management of lipid abnormalities.

THE MANAGEMENT OF HIGH BLOOD CHOLESTEROL

Since the late 1980s, a large and convincing body of evidence has associated elevated blood lipids with CVD. Furthermore, clinical trials have demonstrated that reducing blood cholesterol is effective for both primary and secondary prevention of CVD. This research has prompted groups such as the National Institutes of Health, American Heart Association, and the American College of Cardiology to establish health policy guidelines for the detection and treatment of lipid disorders.[2,3,70–72]

Recommendations for the Detection of High Blood Cholesterol

Health policy recommendations for detection of high cholesterol include the measurement of total cholesterol and HDL cholesterol in all adults aged 20 years and older, with repeat measurement within 5 years. Total cholesterol less than 200 mg/dL is considered desirable; levels between 200 and 239 mg/dL are classified as borderline-high, and those more than 240 mg/dL are considered high

Table 36-6 ■ ESTIMATE OF 10-YEAR CVD RISK IN MEN (FRAMINGHAM POINT SCORES)

Age (years)	Points	HDL (mg/dL)	Points	Systolic BP (mm Hg)	Points: Untreated	Points: Treated
20–34	−9	≥60	−1	<120	0	0
35–39	−4	50–59	0	120–129	0	1
40–44	0	40–49	1	130–139	1	2
45–49	3	<40	2	140–159	1	2
50–54	6			≥160	2	3
55–59	8					
60–64	10					
65–69	11					
70–74	12					
75–79	13					

Total Cholesterol (mg/dL)	Points: Age 20–39 Years	Age 40–49 Years	Age 50–59 Years	Age 60–69 Years	Age 70–79 Years
<160	0	0	0	0	0
160–199	4	3	2	1	0
200–239	7	5	3	1	0
240–279	9	6	4	2	1
≥280	11	8	5	3	1
Nonsmoker	0	0	0	0	0
Smoker	8	5	3	1	1

Point Total	10-Year Risk (%)	Point Total	10-Year Risk (%)
<0	<1	9	5
0	1	10	6
1	1	11	8
2	1	12	10
3	1	13	12
4	1	14	16
5	2	15	20
6	2	16	25
7	3	≥17	≥30
8	4		

Adapted from Expert Panel on Detection, Evaluation, and Treatment of High Blood Cholesterol in Adults. (2001). Executive summary of the third report of the National Cholesterol Education Program (NCEP) Expert Panel on Detection, Evaluation, and Treatment of High Blood Cholesterol in Adults (Adult Treatment Panel III). *JAMA, 285*(19), 2486–2497.

blood cholesterol.[2] Measures of HDL less than 40 mg/dL are considered low and constitute a risk factor for CVD. HDL more than 60 mg/dL remains a "negative" risk factor and removes one risk factor from the overall risk profile. If total cholesterol is greater than 200 mg/dL or HDL is less than 40 mg/dL, then a full lipoprotein analysis is required and treatment is based on LDL levels.

Other nonlipid factors that contribute to CVD risk status also should be assessed, including cigarette smoking, hypertension, diabetes mellitus, a family history of premature heart disease, age (men younger than 45 years and women younger than 55 years), and the presence of other CVD "risk equivalents" (abdominal aortic aneurysm, peripheral vascular disease, Framingham risk score of 20% or more in 10 years, presence of multiple risk factors). Tables 36-6 and 36-7 provide scoring for determination of Framingham risk classification. In the update to ATP III in 2004, revised LDL goals for institution of TLC and pharmacotherapies were recommended[3] (see Table 36-8). In addition, risk classifications were redefined and include a *very-high-risk* category. The *very-high-risk* category includes persons with acute coronary syndrome or with existing CHD or CHD risk equivalents plus significantly elevated risk factors.

Recommended Goals for the Treatment of High Blood Cholesterol

The goal for cholesterol management is the achievement of an ideal LDL-C level based on risk category in all adults[3] (see Table 36-8). If the screening cholesterol is greater than 200 mg/dL and the person's risk profile predicts a risk of greater than 20% in 10 years, then a full lipid profile and evaluation is recommended. If CVD, CVD equivalents, and/or multiple risk factors are present, a full lipid profile is also recommended. Health policy guidelines strongly encourage consideration of risk status for both the evaluation and the treatment of elevated cholesterol. Risk factor reduction through TLC, such as weight reduction, dietary therapy, and increased physical activity, is the major therapy for CVD prevention in all adults including those at high risk or those with established CVD. When TLC fails to achieve desired LDL goal based on risk classification, pharmacological therapies are indicated.[3]

Table 36-7 ■ ESTIMATE OF 10-YEAR CVD RISK FOR WOMEN (FRAMINGHAM POINT SCORES)

Age (years)	Points
20–34	−7
35–39	−3
40–44	0
45–49	3
50–54	6
55–59	8
60–64	10
65–69	12
70–74	14
75–79	16

HDL (mg/dL)	Points
≥60	−1
50–59	0
40–49	1
<40	2

	Points	
Systolic BP (mm Hg)	Untreated	Treated
<120	0	0
120–129	1	3
130–139	2	4
140–159	3	5
≥160	4	6

	Points				
Total Cholesterol (mg/dL)	Age 20–39 Years	Age 40–49 Years	Age 50–59 Years	Age 60–69 Years	Age 70–79 Years
<160	0	0	0	0	0
160–199	4	3	2	1	1
200–239	8	6	4	2	1
240–279	11	8	5	3	2
≥280	13	10	7	4	2
Nonsmoker	0	0	0	0	0
Smoker	9	7	4	2	1

Point Total	10-Year Risk (%)	Point Total	10-Year Risk (%)
<9	<1	17	5
9	1	18	6
10	1	19	8
11	1	20	11
12	1	21	14
13	2	22	17
14	2	23	22
15	3	24	27
16	4	≥25	≥30

Adapted from Expert Panel on Detection, Evaluation, and Treatment of High Blood Cholesterol in Adults. (2001). Executive summary of the third report of the National Cholesterol Education Program (NCEP) Expert Panel on Detection, Evaluation, and Treatment of High Blood Cholesterol in Adults (Adult Treatment Panel III). *JAMA, 285*(19), 2486–2497.

EVALUATION OF THE PATIENT WITH ELEVATED CHOLESTEROL

It is appropriate that the patient with high blood cholesterol receive a thorough clinical evaluation in addition to a lipoprotein analysis. Several medical diagnoses have been associated with high cholesterol. Abnormal lipid profiles may be the first clue to undiagnosed endocrine disorders such as hypothyroidism or diabetes. A careful family history is also important. Genetic forms of hypercholesterolemia are relatively common in the general population; for example, FH has an estimated frequency of 1 in 500.[21] It is therefore advisable that first-degree relatives be screened for lipid disorders. Hyperlipidemia, like hypertension, is a relatively asymptomatic disorder and is usually first recognized by abnormal laboratory findings. Subcutaneous or tendinous lipid deposits, called xanthoma, are the one physical finding that may be prominent in severe lipid disorders. Xanthelasma palpebrarum are seen in the inner corner of eyelids and are associated with FH in approximately half of patients with this finding. Tendinous xanthomas are often found in extensor tendons of the hands and Achilles tendon. Planar xanthomas are lipid deposits in the webs of the hand and occur in children with FH. Corneal arcus is caused by cholesterol deposition within the corneal rim and can be seen as a white band around the cornea. This finding may be indicative of FH in younger people but may not be meaningful in the older adult.[22]

Table 36-8 ■ ATP III CLASSIFICATION OF LDL CHOLESTEROL

LDL Cholesterol Level (mg/dL)	Category
<100	Optimal
100–129	Near or above optimal
130–159	Borderline high
160–189	High
≥190	Very high

Adapted from ATP III.
Adapted from Expert Panel on Detection, Evaluation, and Treatment of High Blood Cholesterol in Adults. (2001). Executive summary of the third report of the National Cholesterol Education Program (NCEP) Expert Panel on Detection, Evaluation, and Treatment of High Blood Cholesterol in Adults (Adult Treatment Panel III). *JAMA, 285*(19), 2486–2497.

Certain types of hyperlipoproteinemia are characterized by abdominal pain. Possible causes for the abdominal pain include pancreatitis and hepatosplenomegaly. Abdominal pain of unknown origin also has been documented as a physical finding. This pain may be associated with ischemic bowel and is related to increased blood viscosity, macrophage ingestion of fat particles, or the effect of the size of the lipid particles on abdominal tissue.[22] Patients with chylomicronemia, or markedly elevated triglycerides levels, have a high risk for pancreatitis.

LIPOPROTEIN MEASUREMENT

The measurement of plasma lipids and lipoproteins is essential for the diagnosis of lipid abnormalities and for the identification of those at risk for CVD. These measurements also provide important feedback to the patient modifying his or her risk profile. The most common lipid analysis includes measurement of total cholesterol, total triglycerides, and HDL cholesterol. This allows calculation of LDL using the following equation: LDL = total cholesterol − (triglycerides ÷ 5) − HDL.[73] This indirect assessment of LDL can be used if triglycerides are less than 400 mg/dL. If triglycerides are more than 400 mg/dL, then LDL must be directly measured using the more complex and costly ultracentrifugation procedure.

To interpret the results of lipid measurements, some knowledge of the accuracy and precision of the measure is useful. One of the common scenarios encountered in lipid management is a laboratory report with values extremely different from the previously measured values, and the patient protests, "I have not been doing anything differently." Intraindividual cholesterol measurements have been shown to vary by 4% to 11% over a 1-year period.[74] Although there are several sources for variability or error in cholesterol measures, the most obvious is analytic variability, or laboratory error, which has been estimated to contribute one third to one half of the intraindividual variability. Laboratories must make their standardization criteria available and should strive to achieve less than 3% measurement variability. Biologic and physiologic factors constitute the other major source for measurement variability. To minimize measurement variability, the National Cholesterol Education Laboratory Standardization Panel recommends the following standards of practice[74]:

1. A stable lifestyle, including health status, diet, medication, and activity level, should be followed for at least 2 weeks before measurement.
2. Cholesterol measures should be made no sooner than 8 weeks after MI, surgical procedure, trauma, or an acute bacterial or viral infection.
3. In acute coronary syndrome, it is recommended that a lipid profile be collected at the earliest possible time during hospitalization.[75]
4. Blood collection procedures should include a 12-hour fast (except for water and usual medications) before sampling if lipid measures other than total cholesterol are to be performed.
5. The patient should sit quietly for 5 minutes before the venipuncture.
6. The sample should be obtained within 1 minute of tourniquet application.
7. Standardized procedures for processing and transporting samples should be followed.

DIETARY MANAGEMENT OF HYPERLIPIDEMIA

Evidence of the relationship between dietary intake, plasma cholesterol, and CVD has been steadily accumulating. Seminal population studies have shown that countries with the highest incidence of CVD and elevated blood cholesterol levels also have high dietary intakes of saturated fats.[76–79] Developing countries with a mean cholesterol level less than 150 mg/dL have a very low incidence of CVD and also have diets low in total fat, saturated fatty acids, and cholesterol.[77]

Diet Patterns and Lipid Effects

Epidemiology studies and randomized clinical trials have examined the relationship of dietary patterns including very-low fat, reduced saturated fat, vegetarian diets, and the Mediterranean diet with cardiovascular outcomes such as CVD events, mortality, or angiographic disease progression. In general, a benefit was observed if the dietary pattern was followed.[80] The goal of these low-fat dietary patterns was to reduce LDL blood concentrations. However, more recent studies of low-fat dietary plans have noted detrimental effects on other lipid parameters including reductions in HDL and increases in triglyceride levels leading to a controversy about which diet is best for CVD. The effects of diet on lipid parameters relates to the amount of fat, the type of fat, and whether fat is replaced with protein or carbohydrate. Sacks and Katan[81] have estimated the lipid effects of four common dietary plans: the average Western diet (38% total fat, 17% saturated fat, 42% carbohydrates), a 30% total fat diet, a 20% total fat diet, and the Mediterranean diet (a reduced saturated fat diet with increased use of vegetable oils such as olive oil, and increased intake of vegetables, fruits, and fish). Compared with the western diet, LDL is reduced by 6%, 12%, and 13% in each of the above-mentioned diet patterns, respectively. Conversely, HDL is reduced by 9%, 20%, and 9% in each diet pattern, respectively. The net result is that the cholesterol to HDL ratio increases in both lower fat diets but is lower with the Mediterranean diet.[81] Saturated fatty acids, with the exception of stearic acid, raise total and LDL cholesterol probably through a mechanism decreasing LDL receptor synthesis.[82] Studies suggest that diets high in monounsaturated fat relative to saturated fat provide a desirable plasma lipid profile, with lowering of total and LDL cholesterol and no reduction in HDL.[83] The major criticism of these studies has been that the addition of only unsaturated fats to the diet is not practical among free-living individuals. For example, food items high in stearic acid usually contain other highly saturated fatty acids as well. Studies also have found that *trans*-fats (partially hydrogenated unsaturated fats) raise LDL levels but show no effect on HDL levels, resulting in an even higher cholesterol to HDL ratio.[82]

The effect of other dietary additives on plasma lipids has also been studied. Dietary studies on the effect of increased omega-3 fatty acids either by fish intake or supplementation with fish oils have shown an effect on plasma lipids, primarily triglyceride lowering with concomitant increases in HDL.[84,85] The response is dose related and is sufficiently high that it is unlikely to be achieved using food choices only. Omega-3 fatty acids also exert antithrombotic effects through the thromboxane–prostaglandin pathways, resulting in decreases in platelet aggregation and vasoconstriction. Although the safety of consumption of large amounts of fish oils is an issue, most researchers agree that the inclusion of fish several times each week is a safe and prudent alternative. Plants sterols and stanols at doses of 2 g/day or greater can lower LDL cholesterol by 9% to 14%. Studies on other additives, such as soy protein, soluble fiber, antioxidants, and garlic, have been inconsistent and at best have shown very modest LDL (3% or less) reductions.[80]

The marked increase in obesity of the U.S. population has been attributed to increased consumption of carbohydrates as replacement for dietary fat and has further added to the diet controversy. In an effort to reduce dietary fat, Americans frequently select low-fat manufactured products containing sugar rather than choosing plant-based carbohydrate foods. This is evident in that the consumption of refined sugar has increased from 120 lb per person in 1970 to 150 lb per person in 1995, and fiber intake remains low.[86] Even those researchers who advocated diets high in monounsaturated fats are recommending lower consumption of refined carbohydrates and increased consumption of fruits and vegetables similar to the Mediterranean dietary pattern and the Dietary Approaches to Stop Hypertension (DASH) diet advocated for persons with hypertension.[80,87,88] Taken together, the above studies confirmed the effects of diet on blood lipids and have influenced the current dietary guidelines.

Dietary Recommendations

The goal of diet therapy is to reduce LDL cholesterol to desirable levels predicated by the person's CVD risk status while maintaining a nutritionally sound eating pattern. The most recent dietary recommendations from the American Heart Association include both dietary and healthy lifestyle recommendations.[89] The overarching recommendations call for (1) balancing calorie intake and physical activity to achieve desirable weight, (2) consuming a diet rich in fruits and vegetables, (3) using whole grain and high-fiber foods, (4) consuming fish two or more times per week, (5) restricting saturated fat to less than 7% of total calories, *trans*-fats to less than 1% of calories, and cholesterol intake to less than 300 mg/day, (6) use little or no salt, (7) restrict intake of sweetened beverages and foods with added sugar, and (8) use alcohol only in moderation. The major change in these goals recognizes the importance of a balanced diet and contrary to the previous National Cholesterol Education Program (NCEP) (NCEP III) diet plan, total fat intake is not restricted rather the quality of the fat is emphasized.[2] These dietary recommendations are consistent with the DASH and Mediterranean diets (see Table 36-9).

Table 36-9 ■ HEART HEALTHY DIETARY PLANS*

	AHA Healthy Lifestyle†	Mediterranean Diet‡	DASH Diet§
Fats and oils	Two to three servings a day Use vegetable or liquid oils. Examples: 1 tsp of soft margarine or vegetable oil. 2 tbsp mayonnaise. Saturated fat: Less than 7% of daily calories	Olive oil with each meal Used as the principal source of fat ~25%–35% of total calories Saturated fat: Less than 7% of daily calories	Two to three servings a day Saturated fat: Less than 6% of daily calories
Trans-fat	Less than 1% of daily calories. Minimize use of partially hydrogenated fats.	Very low—likely due to the absence of hydrogenated foods	Not specified
Lean meat, poultry, or fish	Less than 6 oz a day. Examples: grill or broil meats, trim fat. Fish intake ~8 oz a week, particularly of oily fish. Do not fry or serve with cream sauces.	Meat: four to five servings a month Poultry: one to three servings a week Fish: four to five servings a week	≤2 Servings a day Includes eggs
Whole grains	Six to eight servings a day. Examples: 1 slice of bread, 1 oz dry cereal, ½ cup cooked rice or pasta. At least half of the grains should be whole grains.	Nonrefined whole grains—eight servings a day	Seven to eight servings a day Include at least three servings of whole grains a day
Nuts, seed, legumes	Four to five servings a week. Examples: 2 tbsp peanut butter, or ½ oz of seeds, ½ cup of dried peas or beans.	Greater than four servings a week	Four to five a week
Vegetables	Four to five servings a day. Examples: 1 cup of leafy greens, ½ cup of raw or cooked vegetables	Two to three servings a day. Potatoes four to five servings a week	Four to five servings a day
Fruits	Four to five servings a day. Examples: 1 medium fruit, ¼ cup dried fruit, ½ cup fruit juice	Four to six servings a day.	Four to five a day
Fat-free or low-fat dairy products	Two to three servings a day: Use only low or non-fat products. Examples: 1 cup of milk, 1 cup of yogurt, 1½ oz of hard cheese.	One to two servings a day White cheese and yogurt intake more common than milk.	Two to three servings a day: Use only low or non-fat products.
Sweets and sugars	Five or less servings a week. Limit beverages with added sugar. Examples: ½ cup of sorbets or ices, 1 tbsp of jam, 1 tbsp sugar.	One to three servings a week	Limited
Alcohol	If consumed, use in moderation: 1 drink for women, 2 for men. Examples: 4 oz wine, 12 oz beer , 1½ oz spirits	One to two wine servings a day—accompanying meals	≤1 oz a day men, ≤½ oz women
Dietary cholesterol	<300 mg a day.	Not specified	≤150 mg a day

*Serving size examples are based on a 2000 daily caloric intake and require adjustment for other calorie intakes.
†American Heart Association Nutrition Committee, Lichtenstein, A. H., Appel, L. J., Brands, M., et al. (2006). Diet and Lifestyle Recommendations revision 2006: A scientific statement from the American Heart Association Nutrition Committee. *Circulation, 114*, 82–96.
‡Willett, W. C., Sacks, F., Trichopoulou, A., et al. (1995). Mediterranean diet pyramid: A cultural model for healthy eating. *American Journal of Clinical Nutrition, 61*, 1402S–1406S.
§Dietary Approaches to Stop Hypertension Diet available at: http://www.nhlbi.nih.gov/health/bublic/heart/hbp/dash/new_dash.pdf

The response to dietary intervention is variable and appears related not only to the specific fatty acid composition of the diet but to the level of plasma lipids. Persons with the higher lipid levels usually experience the greatest response to dietary interventions.[90]

Before initiating dietary change, an assessment of the patient's current dietary pattern and usual eating habits is necessary. Dietary assessments are based on subjective reports and are predisposed to problems of recall accuracy and reliability. Review articles on dietary assessment issues suggest that food frequency inventories or careful diet history provide the most accurate information on usual eating patterns.[91,92] Assessment tools are reported in the literature or can be obtained from agencies such as the American Dietetic Association, American Heart Association, the NCEP, the Preventive Cardiovascular Nurses Association, or product manufacturers.[93]

Dietary Change Strategies

For most patients, recommendations for dietary change are not sufficient to effect long-term dietary change. Substantial knowledge must be acquired and specific behavior skills must be learned and practiced. Required knowledge should include an understanding of the relationship between dietary fat, dietary cholesterol, and blood cholesterol; defining reasonable expectations for dietary change; understanding the differences in the quality of fats; ability to read and interpret food labels; sufficient knowledge about food items to estimate fat content of unlabeled items; and knowledge of food preparation methods that affect fat content. Because eating is a part of our social environment, the behavioral skills must be adapted to a variety of social settings, such as travel, eating out, celebrations, and the work environment. Patients should practice label reading and menu selections and questioning food preparers or servers. Anticipatory responses for avoiding high-fat foods in social situations should be explicitly identified. Adapting recipes and developing grocery shopping lists that include brand-name selections are also useful skills to learn.

Computer modeling techniques have been used to examine the effect of dietary fat reduction strategies to determine the most effective strategy for meeting dietary goal.[94] The strategies included substitution of low-fat counterparts for high-fat items, reduction in quantity of high-fat foods, replacement of high-fat foods with other types of foods (e.g., beans for meat), and modifying preparation techniques (e.g., broiling instead of frying). For men, the strategy of replacement was the single strategy that met the dietary goals. No single strategy was effective for women. The results suggest that the most significant changes occur using combinations of dietary strategies. Education alone is unlikely to facilitate dietary change. Studies examining educational interventions have found only a small relationship between knowledge, attitudes, and dietary behavior.[95]

When behavioral interventions were combined with educational strategies, more positive dietary outcomes were observed.[96–98] Behavioral strategies are based on the principles of social learning theory.[99] Social learning theory principles include examining the antecedents of the behavior (expectations and values placed on the behavior outcome), the skills and knowledge needed to perform the behavior, and the reinforcement contingencies associated with the behavior (rewards, feedback, and evaluation). Many behavioral techniques, such as self-monitoring, goal setting, defining alternatives and choices, evaluation, rewards, and feedback can be used to assist patients in the change process.[100–102]

Daily logs of food patterns, eating habits, environmental setting, and self-efficacy measures provide an opportunity for the patient to evaluate his or her own behavior and to receive feedback on specific successes or assistance in identifying undesirable patterns or trends. The antecedents to the behavior can be examined for positive or negative influences on dietary behavior. Small portable computers are available that can record dietary intake and give an immediate nutrient analysis. This type of device incorporates the techniques of self-monitoring, evaluation, and feedback and, in some cases, can supply alternative choices. Less sophisticated written records that detail the food item, amount, and type of preparation have also been shown to be adequate for the purposes of monitoring and changing behavior. It is not unusual for record-keeping alone to lead to altered behavior. Record analysis can also be useful in determining appropriate goals.

Many behaviorists view goal setting as a key element. The goal should be defined by the patient and should be one that is small, specific, and measurable. Nurses can assist the patient through the process, ensuring that these key goal attributes exist.

A variety of aids have been developed to assist personal monitoring and evaluation of food choices.[103,104] Booklets listing the grams of fat for typical portions of commonly consumed foods have been successfully used for this purpose.[105] These booklets usually are pocket-sized and are easily carried while grocery shopping or to restaurants, and they usually include a diary for recording personal daily intake. Behavior can be reinforced using evaluation and feedback techniques.

Feedback can be provided through analysis of food records and by measurement of blood lipids. It is possible to achieve plasma cholesterol reductions of 15% to 20% with adherence to a low-fat and low-cholesterol diet. However, given the individual variability of response, caution should be exercised in providing feedback based totally on plasma cholesterol measures. Feedback and rewards based on dietary behaviors are likely to provide more positive and long-lasting reinforcement.

WEIGHT CONTROL AND LIPID MANAGEMENT

The prevalence of obesity in the United States has increased since the late 1970s. It is estimated that more than one third (65 million) of adults have a body mass index (weight in kilograms divided by height in meters squared) greater than 31 and would be considered severely obese.[106] Because both LDL and the incidence of CVD are reduced in people who maintain a normal body weight, these data are alarming. Studies examining weight loss have reported varying effects on lipid profiles. A meta-analysis of 70 studies examining the effect of weight reduction on lipoproteins found that a 1-kg reduction in weight was associated with a 0.05-mmol/L decrease in total cholesterol (1 mmol/L = 38.67 mg/dL).[107] Significant decreases in LDL and triglyceride levels were also found.

The effect of weight loss on HDL varies, generally decreasing during the active weight-loss period and increasing after a period of stable reduced weight. Krauss et al. studied the effect of four diet patterns (a 54% carbohydrate, low-saturated fat diet, a 39% carbohydrate, low-saturated fat diet, a 26% carbohydrate, low-saturated fat diet and a 26% carbohydrate, high-saturated fat diet) consumed during a stable weight period and during a 5-week weight-loss period.[108] They observed significant increases in HDL after the weight-loss period for all diets combined with the largest decreases in lipid parameters including small dense LDL occurring with the 54% carbohydrate diet as compared to the 26% carbohydrate diet with low saturated fat content. The diet with the high-saturated fat content showed the smallest decrease in LDL cholesterol level as well as the lowest amount of weight loss[108] highlighting the importance of dietary restrictions of saturated fat. Of note, the DASH diet reported a 21% increase in HDL among men and a 33% increase among women.[109] The mechanisms postulated to account for these alterations in lipoproteins include decreased HMG-CoA reductase activity and enhanced cholesterol excretion in bile acids. The release of cholesterol from adipose tissues is also thought to inhibit hepatic synthesis of cholesterol.

For all patients with dyslipidemia, the secondary goal of diet intervention is weight reduction. Patients with dyslipidemia should be counseled to expect an initial reduction in HDL during active weight loss. Increased levels of physical activity may minimize the HDL reduction and facilitate weight loss.[110]

ALCOHOL AND LIPOPROTEINS

Moderate alcohol intake has been reported to be protective for CVD. France, a country with a low rate of CVD, has a markedly higher per capita consumption of alcohol, particularly of wine.[111] One possible mechanism for this protective effect may be related to the increase in HDL observed with alcohol intake. Researchers have established that moderate alcohol intake increases HDL_3, apo A-I, and apo A-II.[112,113]

Alcohol may also alter platelet aggregation and lower fibrinogen levels. Alcohol also increases catabolism of VLDL, the triglyceride-carrying lipoprotein. Patients with elevated triglyceride levels may have dramatic improvements in triglyceride levels with cessation of alcohol. Most researchers agree that the inverse association between alcohol intake and CVD risk is a consistent but weak association.[114] Recommendations to consume alcohol must therefore be considered cautiously, given the potential side effects of impaired judgment, decreased motor coordination, and possible addiction associated with alcohol use. The American Heart Association's recent "scientific advisory" on *Wine and Your Heart* concluded that until randomized clinical trials are undertaken, there is "little justification to recommend alcohol (specifically wine) as a cardioprotective strategy."[115]

PHYSICAL ACTIVITY AND LIPOPROTEINS

The American Heart Association has added physical inactivity to dyslipidemia, smoking, and hypertension as the fourth major modifiable risk factor for coronary artery and other vascular diseases.[71] Physical activity works through a variety of mechanisms to lower coronary risk. Regular physical activity aids in weight loss by increasing caloric output. Weight loss decreases serum triglycerides, which can result in increased levels of HDL cholesterol. Exercise improves glycemic control in type II diabetes by lessening insulin resistance and improving insulin sensitivity. In some people, exercise also lowers LDL cholesterol, although LDL reductions usually are modest. Regular physical activity has a positive influence on endothelial function. Research has shown that regular exercise can improve vasodilation responses and reduce platelet adhesion.[60] Given these beneficial effects, regular physical activity should be a part of the TLC interventions used to manage dyslipidemia (see Chapter 37).[116]

HORMONES AND LIPOPROTEINS

CHD develops in women almost a decade later in life than in men for reasons not entirely well understood. Several mechanisms have been suggested to account for this beneficial effect. Estrogen decreases LDL and increases HDL and apo A-I levels.[117] Estrogen use has been associated with lower Lp(a), reduced LDL oxidative susceptibility, and improved endothelial vasodilation responses.[117,118] Large, randomized, placebo-controlled clinical trials have examined the effect of hormone replacement therapy (HRT) for primary and secondary coronary artery disease prevention.

The Heart and Estrogen/Progestin Replacement Study (HERS) evaluated the influence of Premarin plus medroxyprogesterone acetate (MPA) versus placebo in 2,763 women with CVD at baseline.[119] After an average follow-up of 4.1 years, no differences were detected in acute MI and coronary death between the two groups. In addition, there was a pattern of early increased risk of CVD and thrombotic events with a pattern of late benefit in the women randomized to HRT. This increased risk seemed to occur primarily in the first year of treatment and there was a suggestion of potential benefit with long-term treatment (i.e., more than 4 years).[119] Because of this interesting potential late benefit, a follow-up study was undertaken. The investigators found that after 6.8 years of follow-up, use of estrogen–progestin did not significantly decrease the risk of primary or secondary CVD events in postmenopausal women with CVD. The effect of other doses and types of estrogen or estrogen only on CVD was not investigated in this trial; therefore, these conclusions can only be applied to women using this specific estrogen–progestin combination.[120]

The Women's Health Initiative (WHI), the largest study of primary and secondary prevention of heart disease in women ever undertaken reported a negative influence of HRT on breast cancer and cardiovascular risk in women. The WHI was a double-blind, randomized, placebo-controlled primary and secondary prevention trial examining the effects of estrogen and estrogen–MPA combination therapy on various cardiovascular, vascular, breast cancer, and other health outcomes. The Data and Safety Monitoring Board stopped the combined estrogen- plus-MPA arm of the trial because the rates of breast cancer in this group were significantly higher compared with placebo. They also found that the overall health risks of the estrogen–MPA combination, including increased risks for acute MI, thromboembolism, and stroke, far exceeded the benefits of the combination therapy.[121] This combined HRT was terminated 3 years earlier than its planned completion date of 2006. The increasing risk of breast cancer was the key factor that led the National Heart, Lung, and Blood Institute (NHLBI) to terminate the combined HRT arm of the study.[122] The breast cancer findings along with the negative CVD outcomes discredit short-term or long-term estrogen-plus-progestin use for women with and without CVD.[121,122] Women in the WHI with prior hysterectomy were randomized to the group receiving conjugated equine estrogen only versus the placebo group. After 6.8 years of follow-up, the use of conjugated equine estrogen was found to increase the risk of stroke and did not affect CVD incidence. As a result, conjugated equine estrogen is not recommended for prevention of chronic disease in postmenopausal women.[123] The 2007 AHA guidelines for the primary and secondary prevention of heart disease in women support these conclusions.[124]

PHARMACOLOGIC MANAGEMENT OF HYPERLIPIDEMIA

The primary rationale for the treatment of hyperlipidemia is the reduction of CVD morbidity and mortality. Studies using hypolipidemic drug therapy to achieve LDL reductions have demonstrated lower CVD morbidity and mortality and lower overall mortality rates.[8,10] Angiographic studies using lipid-lowering drugs have demonstrated less progression of angiographically determined CVD with reduction of LDL.[125–128] The rate of progression of CVD appears to be a dose-related response, with slower rates of progression associated with greater LDL lowering.

Meta-analytic techniques have been used to analyze lipid-lowering studies and suggest that the decrease in CVD mortality is offset by increased death rates from other causes, particularly cancer deaths and non-illness-related deaths such as injury deaths and suicides.[129–131] These meta-analyses did not include data from the more recent very large clinical trials investigating lipid-lowering drugs.[7,8,10] These studies did not observe any increase in cancer or non-illness-related deaths. Although the explanations for these findings remain controversial, the consensus of experts is that hypolipidemic drug therapy should always be instituted with nonpharmacologic interventions (TLC), including a low-fat, low-cholesterol diet, regular exercise, weight control, smoking cessation, control of hypertension, and control of blood glucose (in patients with diabetes). Hypolipidemic drug therapy requires careful consideration of individual risks as well as the benefits of such drug therapy. There is sufficient evidence that lowering LDL cholesterol, particularly with the use of HMG-CoA reductase inhibitors, in persons with known CAD and with CAD equivalents provides substantial benefit to reduced morbidity and mortality.

Lipid Criteria and Goals for Drug Therapy

Consideration of hypolipidemic drug therapy for primary prevention (i.e., in people without existing CVD) is indicated in those without CVD risk factors but with LDL levels of 190 mg/dL or more, or in people with 0 to 1 CVD risk factors and LDL levels of 160 mg/dL or more. The target goals of treatment should be to achieve LDL levels of less than 160 or 130 mg/dL, respectively. In secondary prevention (i.e., in patients with established CVD, with CVD equivalents, and/or a CVD risk of >20% in 10 years), drug therapy can be considered if LDL levels are more than 100 mg/dL and should be initiated if LDL levels are more than 130 mg/dL. The optimal LDL goal for all adults, in particular for those with established CVD[3], less than 100 mg/dL (see Table 36-10).

Classes of Hypolipidemic Drugs

The major classes of hypolipidemic drugs include the bile acid-binding resins, nicotinic acid, HMG-CoA reductase inhibitors (statins), fibric acid derivatives, and the intestinal absorption blockers. Individual response to each of these agents is variable, and each of the agents has potential side effects. Nursing can play a major role in the management of patients by assisting the patient to minimize side effects while promoting adherence to the regimen that achieves the desired lipid profile. In this section, the action, indications for use, and specific adherence strategies for each of the classes of hypolipidemic drugs are reviewed (Table 36-10).

Bile Acid-Binding Resins

Actions and Indications for Use. Bile acid-binding resins are insoluble in water and are not absorbed from the intestine. These agents bind with bile acids in the intestine, forming an insoluble complex. The enterohepatic circulation of bile acids is interrupted and fecal excretion of bile acids is increased. This results in increased synthesis of bile acids from hepatic cholesterol stores. Reduced hepatic cholesterol stimulates LDL receptor formation and increases HMG-CoA reductase activity, resulting in increased extraction of LDL from the bloodstream and a lower plasma concentration of LDL. Hepatic production of VLDL is also enhanced, resulting in increased triglyceride levels. The expected response to resin therapy is seen in 2 to 4 weeks and may result in a 20% to 25% reduction in LDL.[20]

Strategies for Increased Efficacy and Adherence. The major side effect of the bile acid-binding resins is constipation; the resins can be unpalatable, which may affect compliance. Resins come in both powder and tablet formulations. In powder form, the resins must be mixed with water. Because they are insoluble, they form a gritty solution. It is helpful to demonstrate the mixing process and allow the patient to taste the drug as part of the prescription process. If constipation develops, instruct the patient in the use of fiber, stool softeners, and other hygienic measures, such as increased fluid intake. Bile acid-binding resins should be taken with meals, particularly with the largest meal of the day, because intestinal bile acids are greatest during that time. Because these drugs are binding agents, they have the potential to bind and interfere with the absorption of other medications. Consequently, the patient should be instructed to take other medications 1 hour before or 4 hours after taking the resin. Reviewing the mechanism of action with the patient promotes adherence and a better understanding of the rationale for these instructions.

Nicotinic Acid (Niacin)

Actions and Indications for Use. Nicotinic acid, or niacin, is a vitamin B_3 derivative that in large doses blocks the release of free fatty acids from adipose tissues, resulting in less hepatic conversion of free fatty acids into triglycerides.[132]

The hepatic production of VLDL is also decreased. Because VLDL is converted to IDL and LDL, decreased VLDL levels lead to favorable reductions in these lipoproteins as well. Contraindications to use include active liver disease and peptic ulcer disease, and caution should be exercised when it is used in patients with diabetes and atrial arrhythmias.

Strategies for Increased Efficacy and Adherence. The most common side effect of nicotinic acid use is cutaneous flushing caused by a prostaglandin-mediated vasodilation effect on vascular smooth muscle. This effect can be minimized with the use of aspirin taken 30 minutes before the nicotinic acid

Table 36-10 ■ LIPID-LOWERING AGENTS

Drug Class	Average Lipid/ Lipoprotein Effects		Side Effects	Contraindications	Clinical Trial Results
HMG-CoA reductase inhibitors (statins)*	LDL-C	↓ 18%–60%	Myopathy	Absolute:	Reduced major coronary events, CVD deaths, need for coronary procedures, stroke, and total mortality
	HDL-C	↑ 5%–15%	Increased liver enzymes	Active or chronic liver disease	
	TG	↓ 7%–37%		Relative: Concomitant use with certain drugs†	
Bile acid sequestrants‡	LDL-C	↓ 15%–30%	GI distress	Absolute:	Reduced major coronary events and CVD deaths
	HDL-C	↑ 3%–5%	Constipation	Dysbetalipoproteinemia	
	TG	No change or an increase	Decreased absorption of offger drugs	TG > 400 mg/dL Relative: TG > 200 mg/dL	
Nicotinic acid§	LDL-C	↓ 5%–25%	Flushing	Absolute:	Reduced major coronary events and possibly total mortality
	HDL-C	↑ 15%–35%	Hyperglycemia	Chronic liver disease	
	TG	↓ 20%–50%	Hyperuricemia (or gout) Upper GI distress Hepatotoxicity	Severe gout Relative: Diabetes Hyperuricemia Peptic ulcer disease	
Fibric acid derivatives‖	LDL-C	↓ 5%–20%	Dyspepsia	Absolute:	Reduced major coronary events
	(May be increased in patients with high TG)		Gallstones Myopathy	Severe renal disease Severe hepatic disease	
	HDL-C	↑ 10%–20%	Unexplained non-CVD deaths in WHO study with clofibrate		
	TG	↓ 20%–50%			
Cholesterol absorption inhibitors††	LDL	↓ 18%	Adverse event profile similar to placebo	Known hypersensitivity to Ezetimibe	Studies in progress
	HDL	↑ 1%			
	TG	↑ 8%			

*Atorvastatin (10 to 80 mg), fluvastatin (20 to 80 mg), lovastatin (20 to 80 mg), pravastatin (20 to 80 mg), simvastatin (20 to 80 mg).
†Cyclosporine, macrolide antibiotics, antifungal agents, and cytochrome P450 inhibitors (fibrates and niacin should be used with appropriate caution).
‡Cholestyramine (4 to 16 g), colestipol (5 to 20 g), colesevelam (2.6 to 3.8 g).
§Immediate-release (crystalline) nicotinic acid (1.5 to 3 g), extended-release nicotinic acid (1 to 2 g), and sustained-release nicotinic acid (1 to 2 g).
‖Gemfibrozil (600 mg b.i.d.), fenofibrate (200 mg), clofibrate (1,000 mg b.i.d.).
††Not included in ATP III table of medications; approved for use after the guidelines were released.
Adapted from Expert Panel on Detection, Evaluation, and Treatment of High Blood Cholesterol in Adults. (2001). Executive summary of the third report of the National Cholesterol Education Program (NCEP) Expert Panel on Detection, Evaluation, and Treatment of High Blood Cholesterol in Adults (Adult Treatment Panel III). *JAMA, 285*(19), 2486–2497, and prescribing information for statins.

dose. Other less common side effects include abdominal discomfort; nausea; elevations in glucose, uric acid, and liver enzymes; reversible hepatotoxicity; and potentiation of atrial arrhythmias. Abdominal side effects are reduced if niacin is taken with meals. Niacin use must be monitored by a health professional, with liver enzymes measured before and periodically during therapy. Side effects can be minimized by starting at low doses and increasing the dose gradually. Written instructions, including a suggested dosage schedule, should be provided to the patient. The patient should be informed of the various side effects and instructed to contact a health professional if hepatotoxic side effects, such as flu-like symptoms and malaise, occur.[133]

CETP Inhibitor

Torcetrapib is a CETP inhibitor that has demonstrated a dose-dependent increase of HDL and, to a lesser extent, apo A-I, resulting in a marked increase in HDL particle size.[134] Unfortunately, torcetrapib results in a 3 to 4 mm Hg increase in blood pressure. In a large outcome trial with torcetrapib in CVD patients, torcetrapib was associated with an increase in total mortality.[135] There are other CETP-inhibitors that do not increase blood pressure and that are being studied in human trials.

HMG-CoA Reductase Inhibitors (Statins)

The statins inhibit HMG-CoA reductase, the rate-limiting enzyme in cholesterol synthesis. Reduced cholesterol synthesis in the hepatocytes stimulates increased LDL receptor activity, thereby promoting clearance of VLDL and LDL from the bloodstream.[136]

Strategies for Increased Efficacy and Adherence. The statins are well tolerated. Single daily doses may be sufficient to achieve lipid goals. If single-day dosage is used, lipid response has been shown to be greatest with evening use. Mild gastrointestinal symptoms and headaches are the most common side effects. Liver enzyme elevations occur in 1% to 2% of users and resolve with discontinuation of the drug. Myopathies (muscle aching, soreness, or weakness) associated with elevations in creatine kinase greater than three times the normal occur in 0.5% of users, but the incidence is increased when statins are used in combination with immunosuppressants, gemfibrozil, and niacin.[137] Patients should be instructed to report muscle aching. If such symptoms are present, liver aminotransferases and creatine kinase should be measured and the drug stopped.

Intestinal Absorption Inhibitors

A new class of medication (intestinal absorption blockers) has recently been released by the Food and Drug Administration (FDA). This medication (ezetimibe) acts by preventing the absorption of cholesterol at the intestinal brush border. The action of ezetimibe is similar to that of the plant stanols and sterols. This medication appears to be relatively "nonsystemic" in that it works exclusively in the intestine to block the uptake of cholesterol. Through this action, serum cholesterol is lowered, uptake by the liver of LDL is enhanced, and LDL levels decrease. This medication has been shown to lower LDL cholesterol alone or in combination with other cholesterol-lowering medications.[138,139]

Fibric Acid Derivatives

Fibric acid derivatives have been used as hypolipidemic agents. They act primarily to increase LPL activity, which enhances catabolism of VLDL and thereby reduces triglyceride levels.[137] Because of their limited LDL effect, these drugs are not considered first-line therapy for LDL lowering. They are effective in treating hypertriglyceridemia and low HDL cholesterol states.

General Adherence Strategies

It is estimated that 50% of patients discontinue drug therapy after 1 year and only one third adhere to dietary interventions beyond 1 year.[140,141] Factors related to nonadherence include lack of knowledge, misconceptions, beliefs and attitudes about the therapy, complexity of the regime, side effects, and the strength of the relationship between the patient and the health care provider.[141] Patient education should include information about the specific drug regime, how the drug works, when and how to use the drug, and how to minimize potential side effects. Barriers to medication adherence include faulty health perceptions. Beliefs and attitudes may interfere with adherence. Social and environmental barriers may include such problems as difficulty taking medication in social settings or restaurants and lack of equipment for mixing medication. It is appropriate to explore common beliefs, attitudes, and difficulties with the patient and develop strategies together to address these issues. Anticipation of potential side effects should also be explored. Studies indicate that adverse side effects and therapeutic ineffectiveness were the major reasons cited for discontinuing lipid-lowering drugs.[141]

Cues to action are important determinants of adherence to medication regimes. Ideal cues are ones that are a part of the patient's habitual routine. Because such cues are habitual, the patient may need assistance in recognizing possible cues. Monitoring and recording medication as it is taken can be useful in identifying potential cues. Feedback is a powerful reinforcer of behavior. Procedures for rapid lipid analysis should be used when possible. Communicating changes in blood lipid response and responding to side effect issues are essential components of lipid management and can often be accomplished by telephone. Consideration should be given to routine telephone contacts to promote adherence and increase the effectiveness of lipid management. Nursing case-managed intervention studies have demonstrated that adherence to lifestyle changes and lipid-lowering drug therapies can be achieved, perhaps caused in part by the strength of the relationship between the nurse and the patient.[126,142]

The nurse is in an excellent position to promote adherence. The focus of the intervention should include the concept of dyslipidemia as a "silent disease," one that is present for life but one for which treatment has been proven effective.

REFERENCES

1. American Heart Association Statistics Committee. (2008). Heart disease and stroke statistics 2008 update. *Circulation, 117*, e25–e146.
2. National Cholesterol Education Program (NCEP). (2001). *Expert Panel on Detection, Evaluation, and Treatment of High Blood Cholesterol in Adults* (Adult Treatment Panel III) (NIH Publication No. 01-3670). Bethesda, MD: U.S. Department of Health and Human Services.
3. Grundy, S. M., Cleeman, J. I., Bairey Merz, C. N., et al., for the Coordinating Committee of the NCEP. (2004). Implications of recent clinical trials for the NCEP Adult Treatment Panel III Guidelines. *Circulation, 110*, 227–239.
4. Armstrong, M. L., Warner, E. D., & Connor, W. E. (1970). Regression of coronary atheromatosis in rhesus monkeys. *Circulation Research, 27*, 59–67.
5. Anderson, K. M., Castelli, W. P., & Levy, D. (1987). Cholesterol and mortality: 30 years of follow-up from the Framingham Study. *JAMA, 257*, 2176–2180.
6. Yusuf, S., Hawken, S., Ôunpuu, S., et al. (2004). Effect of potentially modifiable risk factors associated with myocardial infarction in 52 countries (the INTERHEART study): Case-control study. *Lancet, 364*, 937–952.
7. Downs, J. R., Clearfield, M., Weis, S., et al. (1998). Primary prevention of acute coronary events with lovastatin in men and women with average cholesterol levels. *JAMA, 279*, 1615–1622.
8. Scandinavian Simvastatin Survival Study Group. (1995). Randomised trial of cholesterol lowering in 4444 patients with coronary heart disease: The Scandinavian Simvastatin Survival Study (4S). *Lancet, 344*, 1383–1389.
9. Sacks, F. M., Pfeffer, M. A., Moye, L. A., et al. (1996). The effect of pravastatin on coronary events after myocardial infarction in patients with average cholesterol levels. *New England Journal of Medicine, 335*, 1001–1009.
10. Shepherd, J., Cobbe, S. M., Ford, I., et al. (1995). Prevention of coronary heart disease with pravastatin in men with hypercholesterolemia. *New England Journal of Medicine, 333*, 1301–1307.
11. Long-Term Intervention with Pravastatin in Ischaemic Disease (LIPID) Study Group. (1998). Prevention of cardiovascular events and death with pravastatin in patients with coronary heart disease and a broad range of initial cholesterol levels. *New England Journal of Medicine, 339*, 1349–1357.
12. Heart Protection Study Collaborative Group. (2002). Heart Protection Study of cholesterol lowering with simvastatin in 20,536 high-risk individuals: A randomised placebo-controlled trial. *Lancet, 360*, 7–22.
13. Cannon, C. P., Braunwald, E., McCabe, C. H., et al. (2004). Intensive versus moderate lipid lowering with statins after acute coronary syndromes. *New England Journal of Medicine, 350*, 1495–1504.
14. Shepherd, J., Blauw, G. J., Murphy, M. B., et al. (2002). Pravastatin in elderly individuals at risk of vascular disease (PROSPER): A randomised controlled trial. PROspective Study of Pravastatin in the Elderly at Risk. *Lancet, 360*, 1623–1630.
15. Sever, P. S., Dahlof, B., Poulter, N. R., et al. (2003). Prevention of coronary and stroke events with atorvastatin in hypertensive patients who have average or lower-than-average cholesterol concentrations, in the Anglo-Scandinavian Cardiac Outcomes Trial–Lipid Lowering Arm (ASCOT-LLA): A multicentre randomised controlled trial. *Lancet, 361*, 1149–1158.
16. Gould, A. L., Rossouw, J. E., Santanello, N. C., et al. (1995). Cholesterol reduction yields clinical benefit: A new look at old data. *Circulation, 91*, 2274–2282.
17. Law, M. R. (1999). Lowering heart disease risk with cholesterol reduction: Evidence from observational studies and clinical trials. *European Heart Journal Supplement, 1*(Suppl. S), S3–S8.
18. Deedwania, P., Stone, P. H., Bairey Merz, C. N., et al. (2007). Effects of intensive versus moderate lipid-lowering therapy on myocardial ischemia in older patients with coronary heart disease. Results of the Study Assessing Goals in the Elderly (SAGE). *Circulation, 115*, 700–707.

19. Fletcher, B., Berra, K., Ades, P., et al. (2005). Management of abnormal blood lipids: A collaborative approach. *Circulation, 112,* 3184–3209.
20. Castelli, W. P. (1996). Lipids, risk factors and ischaemic heart disease. *Atherosclerosis, 124*(Suppl.), S1–S9.
21. Schaefer, E. J., & Levy, R. I. (1985). Pathogenesis and management of lipoprotein disorders. *New England Journal of Medicine, 312,* 1300–1310.
22. Gotto, A. M. (1983). High-density lipoproteins: Biochemical and metabolic factors. *American Journal of Cardiology, 54*(4), 2B–8B.
23. Grundy, S. M. (1984). Hyperlipoproteinemia: Metabolic basis and rationale for therapy. *American Journal of Cardiology, 54,* 20C–26C.
24. Grundy, S. M. (1984). Pathogenesis of hyperlipoproteinemia. *Journal of Lipid Research, 25,* 1611–1618.
25. Breslow, J. L. (1992). The genetic basis of lipoprotein disorders: Introduction and review. *Journal of Internal Medicine, 231,* 627–631.
26. Goldstein, J. L., & Brown, M. S. (1987). Regulation of low-density lipoprotein receptors: Implication for pathogenesis and therapy of hypercholesterolemia and atherosclerosis. *Circulation, 76,* 505–507.
27. Gordon, D. J., Probstfield, J. L., & Garrison, R. J. (1989). High density lipoprotein cholesterol and cardiovascular disease: Four prospective studies. *Circulation, 79,* 8–15.
28. Kannel, W. B. (1983). High-density lipoproteins: Epidemiologic profile and risks of coronary artery disease. *American Journal of Cardiology, 52*(4), 9B–12B.
29. Eisenberg, S. (1984). High-density lipoprotein metabolism. *Journal of Lipid Research, 25,* 1017–1054.
30. Asztalos, B. F., & Schaefer, E. (2003). HDL in atherosclerosis: Actor or bystander? *Atherosclerosis Supplements, 4,* 21–29.
31. Joy, T., & Hegele, R. A. (2008). Is raising HDL a futile strategy for atheroprotection? *Nature Reviews, 7,* 143–155.
32. Soumain, S., Albrecht, C., Davies, A. H., et al. (2005). ABCA1 and atherosclerosis. *Vascular Medicine, 10,* 109–119.
33. Curtiss, L. K., Valenta, D. T., Hime, N. J., et al. (2006). What is so special about apolipoprotein AI in reverse cholesterol transport? *Arteriosclerosis, Thrombosis and Vascular Biology, 26,* 12–19.
34. Gotto, A. M. (1983). Clinical diagnosis of hyperlipoproteinemia. *American Journal of Medicine, 74*(5A), 5–9.
35. Tall, A. R., & Small, D. M. (1978). Current concepts: Plasma high-density lipoproteins. *New England Journal of Medicine, 299,* 1232–1236.
36. Singh, I. M., Shishehbor, M. H., & Ansell, B. J. (2007). High-density lipoprotein as a therapeutic target. *JAMA, 298,* 786–798.
37. Miller, N. E. (1990). HDL metabolism and its role in lipid transport. *European Heart Journal, 11,* H1–H3.
38. Rifkind, B. M. (1991). *Drug treatment of hyperlipidemia.* New York: Marcel Dekker.
39. deLemos, A. S., Wolfe, M. L., Long, C. J., et al. (2002). Identification of genetic variants in endothelial lipase in persons with elevated high-density lipoprotein cholesterol. *Circulation, 106,* 1321–1326.
40. Rader, D. J. (2003). Regulation of reverse cholesterol transport and clinical implications. *American Journal of Cardiology, 92*(Suppl.), 43J–49J.
41. Cohen, J. C. (2003). Endothelial lipase: Direct evidence for a role in HDL metabolism. *Journal of Clinical Investigation, 111,* 318–321.
42. Ishida, T., Choi, S., Kundu, R. K., et al. (2003). Endothelial lipase is a major determinant of HDL level. *Journal of Clinical Investigation, 111,* 347–355.
43. Navab, M., Ananthramaiah, G. M., Reddy, S. T., et al. (2005). The double jeopardy of HDL. *Annals of Medicine, 37,* 173–178.
44. Ansell, B. J. (2007). Targeting the anti-inflammatory effects of high-density lipoprotein. *American Journal of Cardiology, 100*(Suppl.), 3N–9N.
45. Brown, B. G., Zhao, X. Q., Chait, A., et al. (1998). Lipid altering or antioxidant vitamins for patients with coronary disease and very low HDL cholesterol? The HDL-Atherosclerosis Treatment Study design. *Canadian Journal of Cardiology, 14,* 6A–13A.
46. Tall, A. R. (1998). Overview of reverse cholesterol transport. *European Heart Journal, 19,* A31–A35.
47. Assman, G., & Gotto, A. M. (2004). HDL cholesterol and protective factors in atherosclerosis. *Circulation, 109*(Suppl. III), 8–14.
48. Austin, M. D., Hokanson, J. E., & Brunzell, J. D. (1994). Characterization of low-density lipoprotein subclasses: Methodologic approaches and clinical relevance. *Current Opinion in Lipidology, 5,* 395–403.
49. Gardner, C. D., Fortmann, S. P., & Krauss, R. M. (1996). Small low-density lipoprotein particles are associated with the incidence of coronary artery disease in men and women. *JAMA, 276,* 875–881.
50. de Graaf, J., Hak-Lemmers, H., Hector, P., et al. (1991). Enhanced susceptibility to in vitro oxidation of the low-density lipoprotein subfractions in healthy subjects. *Arteriosclerosis and Thrombosis, 11,* 298–306.
51. Reaven, G. M., Chen, Y, D., Jeppesen, J., et al. (1993). Insulin resistance and hyperinsulinemia in individuals with small, dense, low-density lipoprotein particles. *Journal of Clinical Investigation, 92,* 141–146.
52. Steinberg, D., Parthasarathy, S., Carew, T. E., et al. (1989). Beyond cholesterol: Modification of low-density lipoprotein that increase its atherogenicity. *New England Journal of Medicine, 320,* 915–924.
53. Fraley A., & Tsimikas, S. (2006) Clinical applications of circulating oxidized low-density lipoprotein biomarkers in cardiovascular disease. *Current Opinion in Lipidology, 17,* 502–509.
54. Itabe, T. (2003). Oxidized low-density lipoproteins: What is understood and what remains to be clarified. *Biological & Pharmaceutical Bulletin, 26,* 1–9.
55. Koschinsky, M. L. (2006). Novel insights into Lp(a) physiology and pathogenicity: More questions than answers? *Cardiovascular & Hematological Disorders Drug Targets, 6,* 276–278.
56. Lawn, R. M. (1992). Lipoprotein (a) in heart disease. *Scientific American, 92*(6), 54–60.
57. Berglund, L., & Raakrishnan, R. (2004). Lipoprotein (a) An elusive cardiovascular risk factor. *Arteriosclerosis, Thrombosis, and Vascular Biology, 24,* 2219–2226.
58. McConnell, J. P., & Hoefner, D. M. (2006). Lipoprotein-associated phospholipase A2. *Clinical Laboratory Medicine, 26,* 679–697.
59. Lanman, R. B., Wolfert, R. L., Fleming, J. K., et al. (2006). Lipoprotein-associated phospholipase A2: Review and recommendation of a clinical cut point for adults. *Preventive Cardiology, 9,* 138–143.
60. Fair, J. M., & Berra, K. A. (1996). Endothelial function and coronary risk reduction: Mechanisms and influences of nitric oxide. *Cardiovascular Nursing, 32,* 17–22.
61. Treasure, C. B., Klein, J. L., Weintraub, W. S., et al. (1995). Beneficial effects of cholesterol-lowering therapy on the coronary endothelium in patients with coronary artery disease. *New England Journal of Medicine, 332,* 481–487.
62. Levine, G. N., Keaney, J. F., & Vita, J. A. (1995). Cholesterol reduction in cardiovascular disease. *New England Journal of Medicine, 332,* 512–521.
63. Brown, M. S., & Goldstein, J. L. (1986). A receptor-mediated pathway for cholesterol homeostasis. *Science, 232,* 34–47.
64. Austin, M. A., Brunzell, J. D., Fitch, W. L., et al. (1990). Inheritance of low density lipoprotein subclass patterns in familial combined hyperlipidemia. *Arteriosclerosis, 10,* 520–530.
65. Grundy, S. M. (1998). Hypertriglyceridemia, atherogenic dyslipidemia, and the metabolic syndrome. *American Journal of Cardiology, 81*(4A), 18B–25B.
66. Krauss, R. M. (1998). Atherogenicity of triglyceride-rich lipoproteins. *American Journal of Cardiology, 81*(4A), 13B–17B.
67. National Cholesterol Education Program (NCEP): The Expert Panel. (1993). Summary of the second report of the National Cholesterol Education Program Expert Panel on Detection, Evaluation, and Treatment of High Blood Cholesterol in Adults (Adult Treatment Panel II). *JAMA, 269,* 3015–3023.
68. Ordovas, J. M., Schaefer, E. J., Salem, D., et al. (1986). Apoprotein A-I gene polymorphism associated with premature coronary artery disease and familial hypoalphalipoproteinemia. *New England Journal of Medicine, 314,* 671–677.
69. Zhang, L. H., Kamanna, V. S., Zhang, M. C., et al. (2008). Niacin inhibits surface expression of ATP synthase[BETA] chain in HepG2 cells: Implications for raising HDL. *Journal of Lipid Research, 49,* 1195–1201.
70. Grundy, S. M., Balady, G. J., Criqui, M. H., et al. (1997). Guide to the primary prevention of cardiovascular diseases. *Circulation, 95,* 2329–2331.
71. Smith, S. C., Jr., Blair, S. N., Criqui, M. H., et al. (1995). Preventing heart attack and death in patients with coronary disease. *Circulation, 92,* 2–4.
72. Smith, S., Allen, J., Blair, S., et al. (2006). AHA/ACC guidelines for secondary prevention for patients with coronary and other atherosclerotic vascular disease: 2006 update. *Circulation, 113,* 2363–2372.
73. Friedewald, W. T., Levy, R. I., & Fredrickson, D. S. (1972). Estimation of the concentration of low-density lipoprotein cholesterol in plasma, with the use of preparative ultracentrifuge. *Clinical Chemistry, 18,* 499–502.
74. U.S. Department of Health and Human Services. (1990). *Recommendations for improving cholesterol measurement: A report from the Laboratory*

Standardization Panel of the National Cholesterol Education Program. Bethesda, MD: Author.

75. Antman, E. M., Hand, M., & Armstrong, P. W. (2008). 2007 focused update of the ACC/AHA 2004 guidelines for the management of patients with ST-elevation myocardial infarction: A report of the American College of Cardiology/American Heart Association Task Force on Practice Guidelines: Developed in collaboration with the Canadian Cardiovascular Society endorsed by the American Academy of Family Physicians: 2007 Writing Group to Review New Evidence and Update the ACC/AHA 2004 Guidelines on Behalf of the 2004 Writing Committee. *Circulation, 117,* 296–329.
76. Arntzenius, A. C., Kromhout, D., Barth, J. D., et al. (1985). Diets, lipoproteins, and the progression coronary atherosclerosis: The Lieden Intervention Trial. *New England Journal of Medicine, 312,* 805–811.
77. Keys, A. (1970). Coronary heart disease in seven countries. *Circulation, 41*(Suppl. I), 1–211.
78. Kushi, L. H., Lew, R. A., Stare, F. J., et al. (1985). Diet and 20 year mortality from coronary heart disease. *New England Journal of Medicine, 312,* 811–818.
79. McGee, D. L., Reed, D. M., & Yano, K., et al. (1984). Ten-year incidence of coronary heart disease in the Honolulu Heart Program: Relationship to nutrient intake. *American Journal of Epidemiology, 119,* 667–676.
80. Zarraga, G. E., & Schwarz, E. R. (2006). Impact of dietary patterns and interventions on cardiovascular health. *Circulation, 114,* 961–973.
81. Sacks, F. M., & Katan, M. (2002). Randomized clinical trials on the effects of dietary fat and carbohydrate on plasma lipoproteins and cardiovascular disease. *American Journal of Medicine, 113*(9B), 13S–24S.
82. Bonanome, A., & Grundy, S. M. (1988). Effect of stearic acid on plasma cholesterol and lipoprotein levels. *New England Journal of Medicine, 318,* 1244–1248.
83. Grundy, S. M., & Vega, G. L. (1983). Plasma cholesterol responsiveness to saturated fatty acids. *American Journal of Clinical Nutrition, 47,* 822–824.
84. Connor, W. E., Connor, S. L., & Connor, S. L. (1990). Diet, atherosclerosis, and fish oil. *Advances in Internal Medicine, 35,* 135–172.
85. Leaf, A., & Weber, P. C. (1988). Cardiovascular effects of n-3 fatty acids. *New England Journal of Medicine, 318,* 549–557.
86. Food Surveys Research Group and Agricultural Research Services. (1995). *Data tables: Results from USDA's 1995 Continuing Survey of Food Intakes by Individuals and 1995 Diet and Health Knowledge Survey, CSFI/DHKS, 1995.* Riverdale, MD: Department of Agriculture.
87. Connor, W. E., Connor, S. L., Katan, M. B., et al. (1997). Should a low-fat, high-carbohydrate diet be recommended for everyone? A clinical debate. *New England Journal of Medicine, 337,* 562–567.
88. Obarzanek, E., Sacks, F. M., Vollmer, W. M., et al. (2001). Effects on blood lipids of a blood pressure-lowering diet: The Dietary Approaches to Stop Hypertension (DASH) Trial. *American Journal of Clinical Nutrition, 74,* 80–89.
89. Lichtenstein, A. H., Appel, L. J., Brands, M., et al. (2006). Diet and lifestyle recommendations revision 2006. *Circulation, 114,* 82–96.
90. Kris-Etherton, P., Krummel, D., Russell, M. E., et al. (1988). The effect of diet on plasma lipids, lipoproteins, and coronary heart disease. *Journal of the American Dietetic Association, 88,* 1373–1400.
91. Freudenheim, J. L. (1993). A review of study designs and methods of dietary assessment in nutritional epidemiology of chronic disease. *Journal of Nutrition, 123,* 401–405.
92. Friedenreich, C. M., Slimani, N., & Riboli, E. (1992). Measurement of past diet: Review of previous and proposed methods. *Epidemiology Review, 14,* 177–196.
93. Connor, S. L., Gustafson, J. R., Sexton, R., et al. (1992). The diet habit survey: A new method of dietary assessment that relates to plasma cholesterol. *Journal of the American Dietetic Association, 92,* 41–47.
94. Smith-Schneider, L. M., Sigman-Grant, M. J., & Kris-Etherton, P. M. (1992). Dietary fat reduction strategies. *Journal of the American Dietetic Association, 92,* 34–38.
95. Axelson, M. L., Federline, T. L., & Brinberg, D. (1985). A meta-analysis of food- and nutrition-related research. *Journal of Nutrition Education, 17,* 51–54.
96. Crouch, S. J. F., Farquhar, J. W., Haskell, W. L., et al. (1986). Personal and mediated health counseling for sustained dietary reduction of hypercholesterolemia. *Preventive Medicine, 15,* 282–291.
97. Fraser, G. E., Schneider, L. E., Mattison, S., et al. (1988). Behavioral interventions from an office setting in patients with cardiac disease. *Journal of Cardiopulmonary Rehabilitation, 8,* 50–57.
98. Gorder, D., Dolecek, T. A., Coleman, G. G., et al. (1986). Dietary intake in the Multiple Risk Factor Intervention Trial (MRFIT): Nutrient and food group changes over 6 years. *Journal of the American Dietetic Association, 86,* 744–751.
99. Bandura, A. (1977). *Social learning theory.* Englewood Cliffs, NJ: Prentice-Hall.
100. Ewart, C. K. (1989). Changing dietary behavior: A social action theory approach. *Clinical Nutrition, 8,* 9–16.
101. McCann, B. S., Retzlaff, B. M., Dowdy, A. A., et al. (1990). Promoting adherence to low-fat, low-cholesterol diets: Review and recommendations. *Journal of the American Dietetic Association, 90,* 1414–1417.
102. Burke, L., & Fair, J. M. (2003). Promoting prevention: Skill sets and attributes of the health care providers who deliver behavioural intervention. *Journal of Cardiovascular Nursing, 18,* 256–266.
103. Buzzard, I. M., Asp, E. H., Chlebowski, R. T., et al. (1990). Diet intervention methods to reduce fat intake: Nutrient and food group composition of self-selected low-fat diets. *Journal of the American Dietetic Association, 90,* 42–50, 53.
104. Connor, S. L., Gustafson, J. R., Arthud-Wild, S. M., et al. (1986). The cholesterol/saturated-fat index: An indication of the hypercholesterolemic and atherogenic potential of food. *Lancet, 1*(8492), 1229–1232.
105. Pope-Cordle, J., & Katahn, M. E. (1991). *The T-factor fat gram counter.* New York: Norton.
106. Heini, A. F., & Weinsier, R. L. (1997). Divergent trends in obesity and fat intake patterns: The American paradox. *American Journal of Medicine, 102,* 259–264.
107. Dattilo, A. M., & Kris-Etherton, P. M. (1992). Effects of weight reduction on blood lipids and lipoproteins: A meta-analysis. *American Journal of Clinical Nutrition, 56,* 320–328.
108. Krauss, R. M., Blanche, P. J., Raulings, R. S., et al. (2006). Separate effects of reduced carbohydrate intake and weight loss on atherogenic dyslipidemia. *American Journal of Clinical Nutrition, 83,* 1025–1031.
109. Crawford, P., & Paden, S. L. (2006). What is the dietary treatment for low HDL cholesterol? *Journal of Family Practice, 55,* 1076–1078.
110. Wood, P. D., Stefanick, M. L., & Haskell, W. L. (1991). The effects on plasma lipoproteins of a prudent weight reducing diet with and without exercise in overweight men and women. *New England Journal of Medicine, 325,* 461–466.
111. Marmot, M. G. (1984). Alcohol and coronary disease. *International Journal of Epidemiology, 13,* 160–167.
112. Camargo, C. A., Jr., Williams, P. T., Vranizan, K. M., et al. (1985). The effect of moderate alcohol intake on serum apolipoproteins A-I and A-II. *JAMA, 253,* 2854–2857.
113. Haskell, W. L., Camargo, C., Williams, P.T., et al. (1984). The effect of cessation and resumption of moderate alcohol intake on serum high-density-lipoprotein subfractions. *New England Journal of Medicine, 310,* 805–810.
114. Stampfer, M. J., Colditz, G. A., Willett, W. C., et al. (1988). A prospective study of moderate alcohol consumption and the risk of coronary disease and stroke in women. *New England Journal of Medicine, 319,* 267–273.
115. Goldberg, I. J., Mosca, L., Piano, M. R., et al. (2001). Wine and your heart: A science advisory for healthcare professionals from the Nutrition Committee, Council on Epidemiology and Prevention, and Council on Cardiovascular Nursing of the American Heart Association. *Circulation, 103,* 472–475.
116. Thompson, P. D., Buchner, D., Pina, I. L., et al. (2003). Exercise and physical activity in the prevention and treatment of atherosclerotic cardiovascular disease. A statement from the council on clinical cardiology (Subcommittee on exercise, rehabilitation, and prevention) and the council on nutrition, physical activity, and metabolism (Subcommittee on physical activity). *Circulation, 107,* 3109–3116.
117. Campos, H., Wilson, P. W., Jiménez, D., et al. (1990). Differences in apolipoproteins and low-density lipoprotein subfractions in postmenopausal women on and off estrogen therapy: Results from the Framingham Offspring Study. *Metabolism, 39,* 1033–1038.
118. Sullivan, M. J. (1996). Estrogen replacement. *Circulation, 94,* 2699–2702.
119. Hulley, S. B., Grady, D., Bush, T., et al. (1998). Randomized trial of estrogen plus progestin for secondary prevention of coronary heart disease in post menopausal women. *JAMA, 280,* 605–613.

120. Grady, D., Herrington, D., Bittner, V., et al. (2002). Cardiovascular disease outcomes during 6.8 years of hormone therapy. Heart and Estrogen/replacement Study follow-up. *JAMA, 288*, 49–57.
121. The Writing Group for the Women's Health Initiative Investigators. (2002). Risks and benefits of estrogen plus progestin in healthy postmenopausal women. Principal results for the Women's Health Initiative Randomized Trial. *JAMA, 288*, 321–333.
122. Fletcher, S. W., & Colditz, G. A. (2002). Failure of estrogen and progestin therapy for prevention. *JAMA, 288*, 366–368.
123. The Women's Health Initiative Steering Committee. (2004). Effects of conjugated equine estrogen in postmenopausal women with hysterectomy. The Women's Health Initiative Randomized Controlled Trial. *JAMA, 291*, 1701–1712.
124. Mosca, L., Banka, C., Benjamin, E., et al. (2007). Evidence-based guidelines for cardiovascular disease prevention in women: 2007 Update. *Circulation, 115*, 1481–1501.
125. Brown, G., Albers, J. J., Fisher, L. D., et al. (1990). Regression of coronary artery disease as a result of intensive lipid-lowering therapy in men with high levels of apolipoprotein B. *New England Journal of Medicine, 323*, 1289–1298.
126. Haskell, W. L., Alderman, E. L., Fair, J. M., et al. (1994). Effects of intensive multiple risk reduction on coronary atherosclerosis and clinical cardiac events in men and women with coronary artery disease. *Circulation, 89*, 975–990.
127. Kane, J. P., Malloy, M. J., Ports, T. A., et al. (1990). Regression of coronary atherosclerosis during treatment of familial hypercholesterolemia with combined drug regimes. *JAMA, 264*, 3007–3012.
128. Watts, G. F., Lewis, B., Brunt, J. N., et al. (1992). Effects on coronary artery disease of lipid lowering diet, or diet plus cholestyramine, in the St. Thomas' Arteriosclerosis Regression Study (STARS). *Lancet, 339*, 563–569.
129. Hulley, S. B., Herman, T. B., Grady, D., et al. (1993). Should we be measuring blood cholesterol levels in young adults? *JAMA, 269*, 1416–1419.
130. Jacobs, D., Blackburn, H., Higgins, M., et al. (1992). The Conference on Low Cholesterol: Mortality associations. *Circulation, 86*, 1046–1060.
131. Muldoon, M. F., Manuck, S. B., & Matthews, K. A. (1990). Lowering cholesterol concentrations and mortality: A quantitative review of primary prevention trials. *BMJ, 301*, 309–314.
132. Schectman, G., McKinney, W. P., Pleuss, J., et al. (1990). Dietary intake of Americans reporting adherence to low cholesterol diet (NHANES II). *American Journal of Public Health, 80*, 698–703.
133. Kashyap, M. L., McGovern, M. E., Berra, K., et al. (1999). Long-term safety and efficacy of a once-daily niacin/lovastatin formulation for patients with dyslipidemia. *American Journal of Cardiology, 89*, 672–678.
134. Clark, R. W., Sutfin, T. A., Ruggeri, R. B., et al. (2004). Raising high-density lipoprotein in humans through inhibition of cholesteryl ester transfer protein: An initial multidose study of torcetrapib. *Arteriosclerosis, Thrombosis, and Vascular Biology, 24*, 490–497.
135. de Haan, W., de Vries-van der Weij, J., van der Hoorn, J. W., et al. (2008). Torcetrapib does not reduce atherosclerosis beyond atorvastatin and induces more proinflammatory lesions than atorvastatin. *Circulation, 117*, 2515–2522.
136. Tobert, J. A. (1987). New developments in lipid-lowering therapy: The role of inhibitors of hydroxymethylglutaryl-coenzyme A reductase. *Circulation, 76*, 534–538.
137. Gotto, A. M., & Pownall, H. J. (1992). *Manual of lipid disorders*. Baltimore: Williams & Wilkins.
138. Dujovne, C. A., Ettinger, M. P., McNeer, J. F., et al. (2002). Ezetimibe Study Group. Efficacy and safety of a potent new selective cholesterol absorption inhibitor, ezetimibe, in patients with primary hypercholesterolemia. *American Journal of Cardiology, 90*(10), 1092–1097.
139. Sudhop, T., & von Bergmann, K. (2002). Cholesterol absorption inhibitors for the treatment of hypercholesterolemia. *Drugs, 62*(16), 2333–2347.
140. Miller, N. H. (1997). Compliance with treatment regimens in chronic asymptomatic diseases. *American Journal of Medicine, 102*, 43–49.
141. Insull, W. (1997). The problem of compliance to cholesterol altering therapy. *Journal of Internal Medicine, 241*, 317–325.
142. Berra, K., Miller, N. H., & Fair, J. M. (2006). Cardiovascular disease prevention and disease management: A critical role for nursing. *Journal of Cardiopulmonary Rehabilitation, 26*(4), 197–206.

CHAPTER 37

Exercise and Activity

Jonathan Myers

Since the late 1950s, numerous scientific reports have examined the relationships between physical activity, physical fitness, and cardiovascular health. Expert panels convened by organizations such as the Centers for Disease Control and Prevention (CDC),[1] the American College of Sports Medicine (ACSM),[2] the Institute of Medicine (IOM),[3] and the American Heart Association (AHA),[4] along with the 1996 U.S. Surgeon General's Report on Physical Activity and Health,[5] have reinforced scientific evidence linking regular physical activity to various measures of cardiovascular health. The prevailing view in these reports is that more active or fit individuals tend to experience less coronary heart disease (CHD) than their sedentary counterparts, and when they do acquire CHD, it occurs at a later age and tends to be less severe.[1,2,5–7] Cardiac rehabilitation, as an industry, has evolved in large part because of the abundance of scientific evidence indicating that regular exercise improves physical function and reduces the risk of reinfarction and sudden death in patients with known CHD.[8–12] Despite this evidence, however, most adults in the United States remain effectively sedentary,[2,3,7] and the vast majority of patients who sustain a myocardial infarction (MI) are not referred to a cardiac rehabilitation program.[13] This is caused in part by the fact that physical activity is not currently integrated into the U.S. health care paradigm, and the majority of physicians fail to prescribe exercise to their patients.[14–17]

It is therefore incumbent on the nurse or other health care provider to encourage patients to become more physically active, to appreciate the role of rehabilitation in cardiac care, and to develop strategies that promote the adoption of physically active lifestyles in all their patients. This chapter describes the scientific evidence linking physical activity and health, summarizes the physiologic changes that occur with a program of regular exercise, and provides an outline for cardiac rehabilitation in the modern treatment era.

ROLE OF EXERCISE IN CARDIOVASCULAR HEALTH

Epidemiologic Evidence Supporting Physical Activity

It has been estimated that as many as 250,000 deaths per year in the United States are attributable to lack of regular physical activity.[18] Ongoing longitudinal studies have provided consistent evidence of varying strength documenting the protective effects of activity for a number of chronic diseases, including CHD,[4,5,8–10,12,19,20] type 2 diabetes,[20–24] hypertension,[25] osteoporosis,[26] and site-specific cancers.[27] In contrast, low levels of physical fitness or activity are consistently associated with higher cardiovascular and all-cause mortality rates.[2,4,5,19,20,28] Midlife increases in physical activity, through change in occupation or recreational activities, are associated with a decrease in mortality rates.[29]

The landmark epidemiologic work of the late Ralph Paffenbarger and associates among Harvard alumni[6,29–33] has been particularly persuasive in support of physical activity and therefore the development of the CDC, AHA, IOM, and ACSM guidelines. Table 37-1 illustrates the rates and relative risks of death over a 9-year period among 11,864 Harvard alumni by patterns of physical activity. Several findings in Table 37-1 are particularly noteworthy. The largest benefits in terms of mortality appear to occur by engaging in moderate activity levels; *moderate* is generally defined as activity performed at an intensity of 3 to 6 metabolic equivalents (METs) (a multiple of the resting metabolic rate), approximately equivalent to brisk walking for most adults.[34] Note also that regular moderate walking or sports participation is associated with 30% to 40% reductions in mortality compared with more sedentary individuals (relative risk of death 0.60 to 0.70). Likewise, the physical activity index, expressed as kilocalories per week (the sum of walking, stair climbing, and sports participation) suggests that a 40% reduction in mortality occurs by engaging in modest levels of activity (1,000 to 2,000 kcal/week, equivalent to three to five 1-hour sessions of activity), whereas only minimal additional benefits are achieved by engaging in greater-intensity activity. These findings agree closely with earlier results among 16,936 Harvard alumni assessed in the early 1960s and followed for all-cause mortality for nearly 20 years.[30] Similar results have been reported from large studies that have followed subjects for CHD morbidity and mortality in the range of 10 to 20 years among British civil servants,[35,36] U.S. railroad workers,[37] San Francisco longshoremen,[33] nurses,[38–40] physicians,[41] U.S. Veterans,[42] and other cohorts (for review, see Kohl[19] or Pedersen and Saltin[43]). Clearly, the evidence linking a physically active lifestyle and cardiovascular health is substantial.

Physiologic Fitness and Health

A growing number of studies have been published in which physical fitness, determined by standardized exercise testing, was determined among large samples of men and women who have been followed for the incidence of CHD morbidity and mortality for up to 10 years.[42,44–49] Each of these studies demonstrated that higher levels of fitness were associated with lower rates of CHD or all-cause mortality. It is important to note that these associations appear to be independent of other CHD risk factors. Also important is that the low levels of fitness in these studies did not appear to be associated with subclinical disease.

In a classic analysis, Blair et al.[44] assessed fitness by treadmill performance in 10,244 men and 3,120 women and followed them for 110,482 person-years (averaging >8 years) for all-cause mortality. These results are presented in Table 37-2. Mortality rates were lowest (18.6 per 10,000 man-years) among the most fit

Table 37-1 ■ RATES AND RELATIVE RISKS OF DEATH* AMONG HARVARD ALUMNI, BY PATTERNS OF PHYSICAL ACTIVITY

Physical Activity (weekly)		Person-Years (%)		No. of Deaths	Deaths per 10,000 Person-Years		Relative Risk of Death		p-Value of Trend
Walking (km)	<5	26		228	86.2		1.00		
	5–14	42		275	67.4		0.78		<.001
	15+	32		194	57.7		0.67		
Stair-climbing (floors)	<20	37		341	80.0		1.00		
	20–54	48		293	62.9		0.79		.001
	55+	15		80	59.6		0.75		
All sports play	None	12		156	88.9		1.00		
	Light only†	10		152	97.4		1.10		
	Light and moderate	36		208	59.7		0.67		<.001
	Moderate only‡	42		178	56.4		0.63		
Moderate sportsplay (h)	<1	30		308	92.9		1.00		
	1–2	41		126	58.2		0.63		<.001
	3+	29		64	43.6		0.47		
Index (kcal)§	<500	12		197	110.3		1.00		
	500–999	18		135	69.1		0.63		
	1,000–1,499	15	58	111	68.9	78.9	0.62	1.00	
	1,500–1,999	13		73	61.4		0.56		
	2,000–2,499	10		51	52.4		0.48		<.001
	2,500–2,999	8		44	64.6		0.59		
	3,000–3,400	6	42	36	74.7	55.4	0.68	0.70	
	3,500+	18		82	48.1		0.44		

*Age-adjusted.
†<4.5 METs intensity.
‡4.5 + METs intensity.
§Sum of walking, stair climbing, and all sports play.
From Paffenbarger, R. S., Hyde, R. T., Wing, A. L., et al. (1994). Some interrelations of physical activity, physical fitness, health, and longevity. In C. Bouchard, R. J. Shephard, T. Stephens (Eds.), *Physical activity, fitness, and health* (pp. 119–133), Champaign, IL: Human Kinetics.

and highest (64.0) among the least fit men, with the corresponding rates among the women 8.5 and 39.5 per 10,000 person-years, respectively. These findings closely parallel an earlier report among asymptomatic men from the Lipid Research Clinics (LRC) Mortality Follow-up Study,[50] in which each 2-SD decrement in exercise capacity was associated with a two- to five-fold higher CHD or all-cause death rate. More recent studies, including one from the LRC,[51] have reinforced the fact that these findings also apply to women who are healthy at the time of evaluation. Gulati et al.[52] suggested that the strength of exercise capacity in predicting risk of mortality was even greater among women than men, reporting a 17% reduction in risk for every 1-MET increase in fitness. In the LRC, nearly 3,000 asymptomatic women underwent exercise testing and were followed for up to 20 years.[51] A 20% decrease in survival was observed for every 1–MET decrement in exercise capacity. This study also pointed out the relative weakness of ischemic electrocardiogram (ECG) responses in predicting cardiovascular and all-cause mortality among women.

Table 37-2 ■ RATES AND RELATIVE RISKS OF DEATH* AMONG 10,244 MEN AND 3,120 WOMEN, BY GRADIENTS OF PHYSICAL FITNESS

	Men			Women		
Quintiles of Fitness†	No. of Deaths	Deaths Per 10,000 Man-Years	Relative Risk of Death‡	No. of Deaths	Deaths per 10,000 Woman-Years	Relative Risk of Death‡
1 (low)	75	64.0	1.00	18	39.5	1.00
2	40	25.5	0.40	11	20.5	.52
3	47	27.1	0.42	6	12.2	.31
4	43	21.7	0.34	4	6.5	.15
5 (high)	35	18.6	0.29	4	8.5	.22

*Age-adjusted.
†Quintiles of fitness determined by maximal exercise testing.
‡*p* Value for trend .05.
From Blair, S. N., Kohl, H. W., III, Paffenbarger, R. S., Jr., et al.(1989). Physical fitness and all-cause mortality: A prospective study of healthy men and women. *JAMA, 262,* 2395–2401.

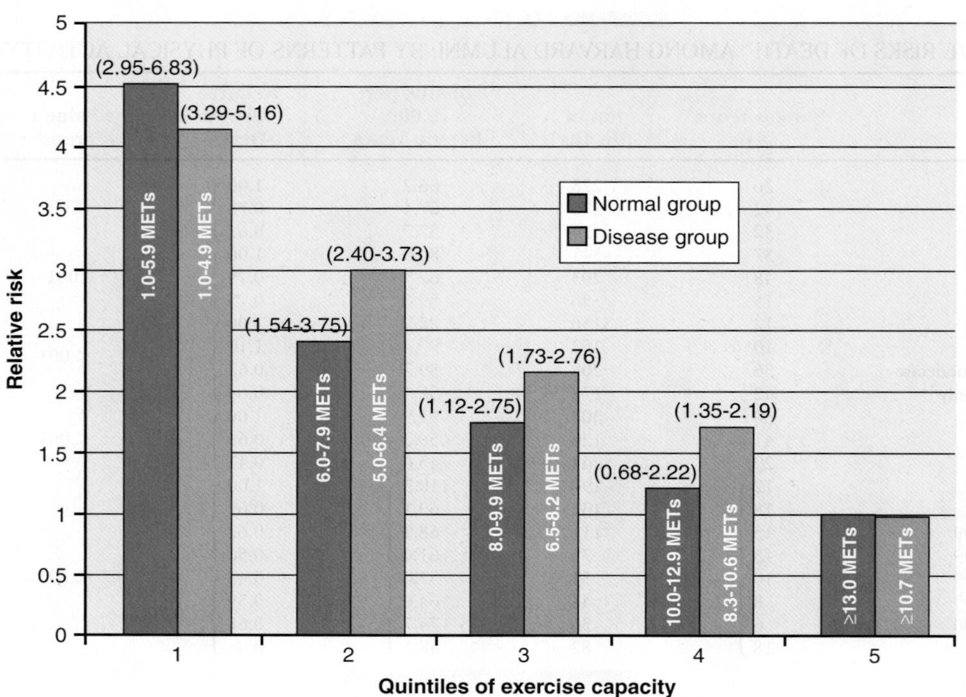

■ **Figure 37-1** Age-adjusted relative risks of mortality by quintiles of exercise capacity among normal subjects and patients with cardiovascular disease. The subgroup with the highest exercise capacity (group 5) is the reference category. For each quintile, the range of values for exercise capacity represented appears within each bar; 95% confidence intervals for the relative risks appear above each bar. (From Myers, J. N., Prakash, M., Froelicher, V. F., et al. [2002]. Exercise capacity and mortality among men referred for exercise testing. *New England Journal of Medicine, 346*, 793–853.)

This issue has also recently been addressed in clinical populations, for example, patients referred for exercise testing for clinical reasons.[42,45–47,52,53] In a study performed among the U.S. Veterans, 6,213 men underwent maximal exercise testing for clinical reasons and were followed for a mean of 6.2 years.[45] The subjects were classified into five categories by gradients of fitness. After adjustment for age, the researchers observed that the largest gains in terms of mortality were achieved between the lowest fitness group and the next lowest fitness group. Figure 37-1 illustrates the age-adjusted relative risks associated with the different categories of fitness. Among both normal subjects and those with cardiovascular disease, the least fit individuals had more than four times the risk of all-cause mortality compared with the most fit individuals. Importantly, an individual's fitness level was a stronger predictor of mortality than established risk factors such as smoking, high blood pressure, high cholesterol, and diabetes. Over the past few years, other cohorts, such as those from the Cleveland Clinic[53] and the Mayo Clinic,[46,47] have documented the importance of exercise capacity as a predictor of mortality among clinically referred populations. These clinically based studies confirm earlier observations from the Aerobics Center Longitudinal Study,[44] Framingham,[54] and the LRC Trial[50] among asymptomatic populations, underscoring the fact that fitness level has a strong influence on the incidence of cardiovascular and all-cause morbidity and mortality.

Public Health Policy Guidelines on Physical Activity and Health

Over the last 15 years, numerous consensus guidelines have been published from organizations concerning physical activity and health, including the World Health Organization, ACSM, AHA, CDC, and European Working Group on Exercise Physiology and Rehabilitation.[1–5,7,55,56] Among the most prominent of these was the U.S. Surgeon General's Report on Physical Activity and Health published in 1996. This document represented the strongest policy statement ever made by the U.S. Government concerning physical activity.[5] It represented a historic turning point redefining exercise as a key component to health promotion and disease prevention. The federal government mounted a multiyear educational campaign based on this report. In this report, the epidemiologic evidence supporting physical activity in the prevention of CHD morbidity and mortality is reviewed in detail. The document also outlines the quantity of exercise necessary to achieve these benefits. It is suggested that each person perform a moderate amount of activity daily, with the amount of activity emphasized rather than the intensity. The concept is that this offers people more opportunities for activities that fit into their daily lives. It is suggested that this moderate amount of activity be performed for 30 minutes or more on most, and preferably all, days of the week. These activities can take the form of brisk walking, yard work or other household chores, jogging, or a wide variety of recreational activities. Repeated intermittent or shorter bouts of activity (e.g., 10 minutes), including occupational, nonoccupational, or tasks of daily living, have similar cardiovascular and health benefits if performed at a level of moderate intensity with an accumulated duration of at least 30 minutes per day. Individuals who already meet these standards receive additional benefits from increasing this amount to more vigorous activity.

The concept that all individuals should incorporate 30 minutes of physical activity into their daily lives is a consistent theme in all of the recent consensus documents on physical activity and health throughout the world.[1–5,7,55,56] Despite this evidence, however, most adults in Western societies remain effectively sedentary,[7,17,18] and only a minority of patients who are eligible are referred to a cardiac rehabilitation program.[13] Given the dramatic increases over the last two decades in the prevalence of overweight, obesity, diabetes, and other conditions related in part to lack of physical activity,[28] the nurse or other health care provider's role is more critical than ever in terms of encouraging patients to become more physically active, and to develop strategies that promote the adoption of physically active lifestyles in all their patients.

"Health" Versus "Fitness" Benefits of Exercise

A noteworthy theme that is consistent in each of the aforementioned documents is that considerable health benefits are derived from moderate levels of activity; it is generally not necessary to engage in vigorous, sustained activity to derive many of these benefits. Before the release of these reports in the mid 1990s, consensus documents generally promoted the concept that exercise was thought to be effective only if an improvement in some measure of cardiopulmonary function was observed. In recent years, the philosophy on exercise as a means to this end ("fitness" measured by exercise capacity) has changed significantly. It is now appreciated that substantial health benefits can be achieved through relatively modest amounts of regular exercise, regardless of whether exercise results in a measurable improvement in exercise capacity. Epidemiologic studies have shown that death rates from cardiovascular and all causes are considerably lower even among people who engage in modest amounts of exercise, less than the threshold that was generally thought necessary to increase exercise capacity.[1–5,7,55,56] It is important for health professionals to be aware of the distinction between "health" and "fitness" when making activity recommendations to patients with cardiovascular disease, those at high risk for its development, and healthy adults. In addition to cardiopulmonary fitness, measures of fat and lean weight, bone density, glucose and insulin metabolism, blood lipid and lipoprotein metabolism, and quality of life should be included under the category of "health." A favorable profile for these variables represents a clear advantage in terms of health outcomes as assessed by morbidity and mortality statistics.

Role of Exercise in Secondary Prevention

During the 1970s and 1980s, numerous controlled trials addressed whether participation in a rehabilitation program influenced morbidity or mortality in patients with CHD. Although the results of these trials were inconclusive independently, most demonstrated a favorable trend for a lower mortality rate among patients who exercised compared with control subjects. For example, the National Exercise and Heart Disease Project was a controlled randomized trial in the United States on the effects of prescribed supervised exercise involving 651 men with acute MI.[57] The cumulative 3-year total mortality rates in this study were 7.3% and 4.6% for the control and exercise groups, respectively, whereas the rates for recurrent MI were 7.0% and 5.4%, respectively. Although this represented 37% and 24% reductions in mortality and reinfarction rates, respectively, for the exercise groups, more than twice as many patients would have been necessary in the study for these differences to be statistically significant. The lack of adequate sample size in this study is typical of the secondary prevention trials that have assessed mortality; although the trends are generally favorable, few have independently demonstrated that patients randomized to an exercise program have a significantly lower mortality compared with control subjects. However, two cardiac rehabilitation trials in Europe were noteworthy for their favorable morbidity and mortality outcomes. Vermuelen et al.,[58] in a study involving fewer than 100 patients, found that a 6-week rehabilitation program including comprehensive risk factor reduction and exercise resulted in a 50% lower rate of combined CHD morbidity and mortality in the rehabilitation compared with the control patients over a 5-year follow-up period. In the second of these multiple risk factor intervention trials, Kallio et al.[59] studied 375 consecutive male and female post-MI patients younger than 65 years in two clinical centers in Finland. After 3 years of follow-up, the cumulative CHD mortality rate was significantly lower in the intervention group compared with the control group (18.6% vs. 29.4%). This difference primarily reflected a reduction in sudden death in the intervention group during the first 6 months after MI. A favorable trend toward reduction in nonfatal reinfarctions also was observed in the intervention group.

An alternative but less rigorous scientific approach, in the absence of a definitive clinical trial, is to pool data from existing long-term, randomized, secondary prevention trials in which exercise training was a component. Several noteworthy meta-analyses have been published in which data from randomized clinical trials were pooled using the intention-to-treat principle.[9,10,60] In the trials included in these meta-analyses, intervention consisted of either a formal exercise program or exercise advice, generally in combination with multiple risk factor management, making it impossible to determine the independent contribution of exercise to subsequent morbidity and mortality. Nevertheless, patients randomized to active cardiac rehabilitation programs after an MI had statistically significant reductions of approximately 25% in 1- to 3-year rates of fatal cardiovascular events and total mortality compared with control patients (Table 37-3). However, significant

Table 37-3 ■ META-ANALYSIS OF CONTROLLED EXERCISE TRIALS IN PATIENTS WITH CHD

	No. of Events (%)	No. of Patients (%)		
	Treatment	Control	Pooled Odds Ratio (95% CI)	*p* Value
All-cause death	236/1823 (12.9)	289.1791 (16.1)	0.76 (0.63–0.92)	.004
Cardiovascular death	204/2051 (9.9)	252/1993 (12.6)	0.75 (0.62–0.93)	.006

From Oldridge, N. B., Guyatt, G. H., Fischer, M. E., et al. (1988). Cardiac rehabilitation with exercise after myocardial infarction. *JAMA*, 260, 945–950.

differences in general were not found in the rate of nonfatal recurrent reinfarctions in patients undergoing intervention compared with control patients.

Recently, Taylor et al.[12] performed an updated meta-analysis of rehabilitation trials among patients with CHD. While the aforementioned studies focused on research performed during the 1970s and 1980s, the latter study included trials performed through 2003. A total of 48 trials met the inclusion criteria, including 8,940 patients. Compared with usual care, cardiac rehabilitation was associated with reduced all-cause mortality (odds ratio = 0.80) and cardiac mortality (odds ratio = 0.74). In addition, participation in cardiac rehabilitation was associated with greater reductions in cholesterol, triglycerides, and systolic blood pressure. However, there were no differences between rehabilitation and usual care groups in nonfatal reinfarctions or revascularization rates. Importantly, the effect of rehabilitation on mortality was independent of chronic heart failure (CHF) diagnosis, type of rehabilitation, dose of exercise intervention, length of follow-up, trial quality, or trial publication data.

Physiologic Benefits of Exercise Training

Regular exercise increases work capacity. Hundreds of studies have been performed cross sectionally that document higher maximum oxygen consumption ($\dot{V}O_2max$) values among active versus sedentary individuals or between groups after a period of training. The magnitude of improvement in $\dot{V}O_2max$ with training varies widely, usually ranging from 5% to 25%, but increases as large as 50% have been reported. The degree of change in exercise capacity depends primarily on initial state of fitness and intensity of training. Training increases exercise capacity by increasing maximal cardiac output and the ability to extract oxygen from the blood. The physiologic benefits of a training program can be classified as morphologic, hemodynamic, and metabolic (Display 37-1). Many animal studies have demonstrated significant morphologic changes with training, including myocardial hypertrophy with improved myocardial function, increases in coronary artery size, and increases in the myocardial capillary-to-fiber ratio. However, such changes have been difficult to demonstrate in humans.[61] The major *morphologic* outcome of a training program in humans is probably an increase in cardiac size; however, this adaptation also appears to occur mainly in younger healthy people and is an unlikely outcome among individuals older than 40 years or in patients with heart disease. However, significant *hemodynamic* changes have been well documented among patients with heart disease after training. These include reductions in heart rate (HR) at rest and any matched submaximal workload, which is beneficial in that it results in a reduction in myocardial oxygen demand during activities of daily living (ADLs). Other hemodynamic changes that have been demonstrated after training include reductions in blood pressure, increases in blood volume, and increases in maximal oxygen uptake. The most important physiologic benefits of training among patients with heart disease occur in the skeletal muscle. The metabolic capacity of the skeletal muscle is enhanced through increases in mitochondrial volume and number, capillary density, and oxidative enzyme content. These adaptations enhance perfusion and the efficiency of oxygen extraction.[43,61,62] Finally, an important influence of training is a favorable effect on the risk profile in patients recovering from MI (Display 37-2). Although this may include such things as reductions in blood pressure, reductions in markers of inflammation (such as C-reactive protein), reductions in body weight, reductions in total cholesterol and low-density lipoprotein, and an increase in high-density lipoprotein, recent studies suggest that the most powerful influence of regular exercise may be an improvement in insulin sensitivity. It is also important to note that although the effect of exercise on any single risk factor may generally be small, the effect of continued regular exercise on overall cardiovascular risk, when combined with other lifestyle modifications such as proper nutrition, smoking cessation, and medication use, can be dramatic.

DISPLAY 37-1 Physiologic Adaptations to Physical Training in Humans

Morphologic Adaptations

Myocardial hypertrophy

Hemodynamic Adaptations

Increased blood volume
Increased end-diastolic volume
Increased stroke volume
Increased cardiac output
Reduced HR for any submaximal workload

Metabolic Adaptations

Increased mitochondrial volume and number
Greater muscle glycogen stores
Enhanced fat utilization
Enhanced lactate removal
Increased enzymes for aerobic metabolism
Increased maximal oxygen uptake

Cardiovascular Effects of Immobility

The deleterious physiologic effects of prolonged bed rest have been studied extensively. Since the late 1960s, these studies have been an important stimulus for cardiac rehabilitation. Although these effects are commonly attributed to the absence of regular physical activity, an additional important factor underlying the deconditioning of bed rest is the absence of normal hydrostatic pressure caused by orthostatic stress (i.e., caused by gravity). Thus, even short periods of bed rest (2 to 5 days) are accompanied not

DISPLAY 37-2 Changes in Risk Factors Influenced by Exercise Training

Decrease in blood pressure
Increase in high-density lipoprotein cholesterol level
Reduction in body weight
Psychological effects
 Less depression
 Reduced anxiety
Improved glucose tolerance
Reduction in inflammatory markers
Improved fitness level

DISPLAY 37-3 Physiologic Consequences of Prolonged Bed Rest

1. Loss of muscle mass, strength, and endurance
2. Decreased plasma and blood volume
3. Decreased ventricular volume
4. Increased hematocrit and hemoglobin
5. Diuresis and natriuresis
6. Venous stasis
7. Bone demineralization
8. Increased HR at rest and submaximal levels of activity
9. Decreased resting and maximum stroke volume
10. Decreased maximum cardiac output
11. Decreased maximal oxygen uptake
12. Increased venous compliance
13. Increased risk of venous thrombosis and thromboembolism
14. Decreased orthostatic tolerance
15. Increased risk of atelectasis, pulmonary emboli

only by reduced exercise capacity but also by reductions in muscle mass and strength, alterations in body fluid distribution, and orthostatic intolerance (Display 37-3). The importance of the absence of orthostatic stress on the deconditioning response has been documented by studies demonstrating that exercise training during bed rest is only partially effective or fails to maintain $\dot{V}O_2$max.[63,64]

Through much of the past century, patients were almost completely immobilized in bed for 6 to 8 weeks after MI. As recently as the 1960s, extended periods of bed rest were thought to facilitate myocardial healing for patients recovering from MI. Today, the converse is true. Carefully prescribed and supervised physical activity is recommended as soon as 1 day after the event to counteract the many negative physiologic effects of bed rest. In addition to their cardiovascular event, patients may be subjected to long periods of immobilization because of severe pain; musculoskeletal or nervous system impairment, including paralysis; generalized weakness; psychosocial problems, such as severe depression; and infectious disease. The extensive literature available on the deleterious effects of immobility has been reviewed elsewhere.[63,64]

CARDIAC REHABILITATION

Cardiac rehabilitation programs are designed to limit the physiologic and psychological effects of cardiac illness, reduce the risk for sudden death or reinfarction, control cardiac symptoms, stabilize the atherosclerotic process, and enhance the psychosocial and vocational status of selected patients. Cardiac rehabilitation services are typically prescribed for patients who (1) have had MI; (2) have had coronary revascularization (bypass surgery, percutaneous transluminal coronary angioplasty [PTCA], or stent placement); or (3) have chronic stable angina pectoris. In recent years, cardiac rehabilitation has been expanded to include patients who have CHF and those who have undergone valvular replacement, cardiac transplantation, or pacemaker implantation. Although the spectrum of patients who benefit from rehabilitation has widened, changes in health care economics have drastically altered the way in which cardiac rehabilitation is implemented. Hospital stays are shorter, progression through the program is more rapid, and much of "cardiac rehabilitation" as it was traditionally known has changed. Reimbursement patterns differ considerably from one state to another, and insurance coverage for rehabilitation services differs widely. With shorter periods of time for physicians and nurses to interact with and monitor patients and cover educational materials adequately, there is a greater need for structured outpatient programs in the home or community.

Historically, typical phases that were included in rehabilitation were phase I, which includes the coronary care unit and inpatient care during the first few days after the event; phase II, which involves convalescence, an outpatient program, or a home program; and phase III, which was usually a longer-term community-based or home program. The precise course of each program naturally depends on the individual's needs and clinical status.

In-Hospital Rehabilitation After a Myocardial Event

The purpose of beginning cardiac rehabilitation immediately after a myocardial event is to counteract the negative effects of deconditioning rather than to promote training adaptations. It also provides an ideal time to begin education and psychological support. These first 3 to 5 days after an MI or bypass surgery are critical for beginning these processes. The literature is replete with studies documenting the efficacy and safety of beginning activities and education soon after a coronary event in stable patients. Initially, it is worthwhile for the nurse, in concert with the primary physician, to medically evaluate the patient, including assessing the patient's clinical stability and the severity of the MI. Details concerning the diagnosis and management of MI are presented in Chapter 22. An overview of patient assessment is provided in the context of the patient being considered for cardiac rehabilitation.

History and Physical Examination

The tools for assessment begin with the history and physical examination. The first step in evaluating patients for cardiac rehabilitation is to determine whether the cardiovascular disease is stable. Each patient should be stratified into an appropriate risk category using information usually available from the history and physical examination, as well as diagnostic tests performed as part of the hospital course (Display 37-4).[65] Stability is determined primarily by the presence or absence of myocardial ischemia, CHF, and dysrhythmias.

The hallmark symptom of ischemia is chest pain. Most patients have chest pain of some type, and it is frequently ignored. Once patients are told about heart disease, their routine pains can become frightening. Clinically, it is important to separate nonischemic from ischemic chest pains. Chest pain that is unrelated to exercise or that is sharp is usually not attributable to ischemia, and not all chest pains should be called angina pectoris. Angina is considered unstable when it changes in pattern (i.e., occurs more frequently, at rest, or at lower workloads). It is important to note that as many as 25% of patients with acute MI have an atypical chest pain pattern, and some will have no chest pain at all. Ischemia can cause transient CHF, and increasing symptoms of CHF should be noted; these include sudden weight gain, edema in the lower

DISPLAY 37-4 General Guidelines for Risk Stratification

Low Risk (all must be present to be classified at lowest risk)

- Absence of significant LV dysfunction (i.e., EF > 50%).
- Uncomplicated MI or revascularization procedure.
- No resting or exercise-induced myocardial ischemia manifested as angina and/or ST-segment displacement.
- Absence of other symptoms during exercise (unusual shortness of breath, dizziness, light-headedness)
- No resting or exercise-induced complex arrhythmias.
- Functional capacity ≥7 METs on graded exercise test 3 or more weeks after clinical event.

Intermediate Risk (any one or combination of the following places a patient at moderate risk)

- Mild to moderately depressed LV function (e.g., EF 31%–49%).
- Functional capacity <5 to 6 METs on graded exercise test 3 or more weeks after clinical event.
- Failure to comply with exercise intensity prescription.
- Exercise-induced myocardial ischemia (1 to 2 mm ST-segment depression) or reversible ischemic defects (echocardiographic or nuclear radiography).
- Presence of angina or other symptoms occurring only at high levels of exercise (≥7 METs)

High Risk (any one or combination of the following places a patient at high risk)

- Severely depressed LV function (i.e., EF < 30%).
- Presence of angina or other significant symptoms occurring at low levels of exercise (≤5 METs)
- Complex ventricular arrhythmias at rest or increasing with exercise.
- Abnormal hemodynamic response to exercise (chronotropic incompetence or inability to appropriately increase systolic blood pressure during activity).
- History of sudden cardiac death.
- MI complicated by congestive heart failure, cardiogenic shock, and/or complex ventricular arrhythmias.
- Severe coronary artery disease and marked exercise-induced myocardial ischemia (>2.0 mm ST-segment depression).

extremities, dyspnea on exertion, and paroxysmal nocturnal dyspnea. Combinations of ischemia and CHF are more difficult to manage.

In general, patients can be categorized as those with myocardial damage, those with myocardial ischemia, or those with both. Initially, the ischemic threshold should be determined by the onset of angina pectoris or ST-segment depression at a particular HR, double product, or workload. When this threshold is clarified, the amount of mechanical damage should be determined.

Clinical clues, which suggest that the patient has myocardial damage, include a history of CHF, cardiogenic shock, a previous MI, a large anterior MI, cardiac enlargement, a large creatine kinase (CK) elevation, multiple Q waves, or underlying problems such as cardiomyopathy or valvular heart disease. These patients must be monitored for signs and symptoms of CHF, whereas patients with ischemia usually do not require such detailed observation. Patients with myocardial damage are limited by reduced maximal cardiac output, which leads to early fatigue and pulmonary symptoms, rather than by chest pain. An effort should be made to explain the symptoms related to CHF in such patients. In the patient with an MI, the symptoms could be caused by mitral valve insufficiency secondary to papillary muscle dysfunction, a dilated mitral annulus, or a dysfunctional myocardial segment supporting the mitral apparatus. Secondary processes include cardiomyopathy or a valvular defect. A rare explanation is ventricular septal defect resulting from septal infarction.

In addition to myocardial ischemia and dysfunction, the other key features of heart disease to consider are arrhythmias, valvular function, and exercise capacity. These five features are important because they not only help to determine the patients' prognosis but also help to determine the manifestation of symptoms. Patients should be evaluated for each of these for optimal management, including individualization of the rehabilitation program. The ECG, chest x-ray, and exercise test are next in importance. The exercise test is the key to prescribing exercise (discussed later). Specialized tests, including echocardiography, nuclear scans, and cardiac catheterization, can be used to confirm impressions, clarify incongruous clinical situations, or identify coronary anatomic patterns that necessitate revascularization.

Severity of the MI

Increases in risk for complications are generally associated with postinfarction ischemia and/or a history of previous MI. In addition to ischemia, postinfarction chest pain can be caused by anxiety and pericarditis. These factors can usually be distinguished by a careful history and an ECG. The ECG pattern predicts the clinical course and outcome surprisingly well. The greater the number of areas with Q waves and the greater the R wave loss, the larger the myocardial infarct. Non-Q wave MIs are usually less frequently associated with CHF or shock, but they can also be complicated, particularly when a previous MI has occurred.

The concept that an initial subendocardial infarction is incomplete and poses an increased risk has not been substantiated. Inferior infarcts are usually smaller, result in a smaller decline in ejection fraction, and are less likely to be associated with shock or CHF. Anterior infarcts are typically larger, are more often associated with significant wall motion abnormalities, and usually result in a greater decrease in ejection fraction. The perception that exercise may cause further ventricular damage among patients with anterior infarctions and associated left ventricular dysfunction has been refuted by a variety of imaging studies performed over the past 10 years.[61,66]

The size of an MI can be judged by the CK level, particularly by the MB fraction released (see Chapter 22) along with the troponin level. In general, the larger the amount of CK-MB released and the longer the CK level stays elevated, the larger the MI. The occurrence of CHF, shock, or pericarditis is also an indicator of a relatively large MI.

Complicated Versus Uncomplicated MIs

Whether an MI is *complicated* is important to consider because it can influence the clinical course and affect when a patient is stable enough to begin rehabilitation. Criteria for classifying an MI as complicated or uncomplicated are presented in Display 37-5. The rates of morbidity and mortality among postinfarction patients who have complicated clinical courses are much higher than

DISPLAY 37-5 Characteristics that Classify an MI as Being Complicated

- Congestive heart failure
- Cardiogenic shock
- Large MI—as determined by creatine phosphokinase, troponin, and/or ECG
- Pericarditis
- Dangerous arrhythmias, including conduction problems.
- Concurrent illnesses
- Pulmonary embolus
- Continued ischemia
- Stroke or transient ischemic attack

among those with uncomplicated MIs. The most important clinical predictors of complicated infarctions have been previous MI and the presence of CHF and/or cardiogenic shock. It is possible to assess risk at different temporal points, from presentation in the emergency department through the coronary care unit, as well as before discharge and during later follow-up. This is important because the clinical picture can change over time; a low-risk patient can become a high-risk patient and vice versa. These changes in risk are partially caused by the vicissitudes of the atherosclerosis process, reformation of thrombus, interventions, and disease–host interactions. For instance, a patient may present with premature ventricular contractions that can then disappear or worsen, chest pain may come and go, the ECG may change, or the enzymes may have a late peak. This makes it difficult to classify a patient strictly as high- or low-risk; risk stratification often requires good judgment by the patient's physician, along with that of the nursing staff. In addition, indicators signifying progress or regression of the patient's condition can change quickly during hospitalization. Importantly, any change in clinical status must be considered before initiating physical activity. The pace of rehabilitative steps must often be adjusted for a particular patient.

Psychosocial Considerations

Hospital admission for an acute MI is a stressful experience with a powerful impact. However, hospital discharge can be equally stressful after the patient has relied on the highly protective hospital support systems. Discharge into an uncertain future and into a home and work setting in which the patient may be considered a helpless invalid can be as damaging to the patient's self-esteem as the acute event itself. The nurse is faced with the difficult tasks of not only supervising the physical recovery of the patient but also maintaining morale, providing education, helping the family cope, providing support, and facilitating the return to a gratifying lifestyle. Studies have shown that psychosocial interventions, including such things as counseling, group therapy, behavior modification, stress management, and relaxation techniques, are effective in improving psychological well-being, reducing stress, and reducing type A behavior scores.[11,65]

It is also important to consider that a small percentage of patients will have no difficulty exercising on their own and might not need a formal exercise program. However, all patients can benefit from education and secondary risk reduction. Some patients benefit from exercising with a group, whereas others fare better by themselves. The approach to each patient must be individualized because patients' reactions to problems and their needs differ. In addition, nearly all patients will have one or more comorbidities, and any of these may require different clinical considerations and may also have a different psychosocial impact. For example, an increasing percentage of patients today will have obesity, diabetes, or both, and many will have musculoskeletal problems or other metabolic disorders. Triaging or management of these comorbidities often is within the purview of the cardiac rehabilitation team.

Education of the Patient

Education should be initiated before physical activities are begun; the patient may lack self-confidence and need affirmation that the activities are safe. Patient education during the acute phase usually consists of an explanation of the coronary care unit, the cardiac rehabilitation program, and the delivery of routine diagnostic and therapeutic modalities. The patient should be educated about the limitations imposed by the disease, the potential for improvement, and precautions to be observed. The program should be individualized for the patient depending on his or her clinical and psychosocial status. The medical status is determined largely by the severity of the MI, but the medical history must also be considered.

The activity and exercise component of inpatient education should involve teaching patients about activities they can do, as well as those they should be more cautious in doing, during the first few weeks of their rehabilitation. This differs somewhat between patients having cardiac surgery versus those with MI. The activity limitations after cardiac surgery involve sternal precautions and psychological adjustment to a major surgery. Those activities that put stress on the sternal incision are listed in Display 37-6. It is advisable for cardiac surgery patients to wait at least 4 to 6 weeks before driving a vehicle, partly because the sternal incision would be at risk in an impact. There is also some cognitive adjustment that needs to take place after a major surgery before the patient's reflexes are fully intact. Patients with MI have slightly different reasons for activity limitations. It may be necessary to return to activities gradually because of the added work placed on the healing myocardium. As mentioned, early mobilization of the patient with acute MI is now well accepted; however, there are important reasons to avoid sudden increases in myocardial oxygen demand during the first few weeks of rehabilitation. In addition, those patients who have undergone PTCA and stent placement are often cautioned to refrain from strenuous activity for a somewhat longer period, for example, approximately 6 weeks. A maximal exercise test is usually postponed until that time as well.

Patients should understand that the conditioning program for patients after MI and surgery should be gradual. Those in a walking program are usually instructed to continue the walking they have been doing in the hospital. In addition, the energy cost of

DISPLAY 37-6 Sternal Precautions and Activity Guidelines (for at least 6 weeks after Cardiac Surgery)

Do not lift more than 10 lb.
Do not push *up* as if getting out of bed or *out* as if pushing a cart.
No pulling.
No arm activities above the level of the heart.

DISPLAY 37-7 Energy Cost in Mets (Metabolic Equivalents) of Activities

Very Light Activity

1 MET
Resting
Eating
Writing
Hand sewing or knitting

2 METs
Light calisthenics (e.g., stretching)
Driving (can be higher under stressful conditions)
Light household activities (cooking, ironing)
Walking, 2.2 mph

3 METs
Self-care (washing, dressing)
Walking, 3.0 mph
Moderate household activities (e.g., sweeping, mopping, cleaning)

Light Activity

4 METs
Gardening (seeding)
Ballroom dancing
Canoeing, golf (without cart)

5 METs
Mowing lawn, power mower
Washing car
Heavy carpentry (scraping, painting—outdoors)

Moderate to Heavy Activity

6 METs
Shoveling snow
Digging
Sawing wood
Tennis
Skiing
Walking briskly on level, 5 mph

7 METs
Jogging, moderate pace
Carrying boxes
Skiing, general
Ice skating

8 METs
Cycling, 13 mph
Swimming, 40 yd/min
Level ski touring, 4 mph
Walking upstairs, briskly

Very Heavy Activity

10 METs
Swimming (crawl, 55 yd/min)
Cycle uphill

activities in METs should be explained to the patient (Display 37-7) and appropriate household or recreational activities should be recommended accordingly. Patients should also be taught how to take their HR and how to use the rating of perceived exertion (RPE) scale. This scale is useful because it is highly correlated with HR and, when given a range of RPE, the patient can then objectively judge his or her level of exercise exertion (Table 37-4).

Table 37-4 ■ 6 TO 20 AND 0 TO 10 BORG'S PERCEIVED EXERTION SCALES

Original Scale		Revised Scale	
6		0	Nothing
7	Very, very light	0.5	Very, very weak
8		1	Very weak
9	Very light	2	Weak
10		3	Moderate
11	Fairly light	4	Somewhat strong
12		5	Strong
13	Somewhat hard	6	
14		7	Very Strong
15	Hard	8	
16		9	
17	Very Hard	10	Very, very strong
18			Maximal
19	Very, very hard		
20			

From Borg, G. A. V. (1999). *Borg's perceived exertion and pain scales.* Champaign, IL: Human Kinetics.

Medications that may have an effect on HR or blood pressure should be discussed with the patient (i.e., β-blockers, calcium channel blockers). Patients also should be reminded when and how to take nitroglycerin and when to call for medical assistance. Inpatients' retention of information is low; therefore, it is important to repeat certain guidelines several times and also to provide written information. Patients should have a written walking or cycling program that includes mode, frequency, and duration of exercise. A copy of warm-up and cool-down exercises, preferably the same ones they were taught as an inpatient, can be helpful. A target HR should be provided (usually 20 beats/min above the standing resting HR for the initial phase after discharge); and an RPE scale should be provided, noting the appropriate intensity when exercising (10 to 12 is appropriate at the beginning). A chart to record HR, RPE, and symptoms can also be useful to track patients' adherence to the exercise prescription and to help determine appropriate progression. It is important that patients are familiar with precautions about exercise (Display 37-8). At the time of discharge, some method of contacting the patient for outpatient cardiac rehabilitation follow-up should be established, and appointments should be made for outpatient cardiac rehabilitation within 1 to 3 weeks after discharge.

Initiation of Inpatient Activity

Once the medical evaluation has been performed and the patient's clinical condition has been stabilized, inpatient activity can be initiated. The objectives for inpatient activity include the following:

- To educate the patient and family about the particular cardiac event and diagnostic tests and to prepare them for the stages of cardiac rehabilitation and returning to life at home

DISPLAY 37-8 General Guidelines and Precautions for Cardiovascular Exercise

1. Exercise only when feeling well. Wait 2 days until after a cold or flu. Never exercise when you have a fever.
2. Do not exercise vigorously soon after eating. Wait at least 2 hours.
3. Adjust exercise to the weather. Exercise in the cooler time of day on hot days. Exercise at a slower pace and drink more water than usual in hot weather.
4. Slow down for hills. Stay at the same level of exertion for hills.
5. Wear proper clothing and shoes.
6. Understand personal limitations. Find out from your physician what limitations to exercise you have.
7. Select appropriate exercise. Aerobic exercise should be a major component of activities. However, flexibility and strengthening exercises should also be considered for a well-rounded program.
8. Be alert for symptoms. If the following occur while exercising or immediately after, contact a physician before continuing exercise:
   a. Chest discomfort
   b. Faintness
   c. Shortness of breath during exercise to the point of uncomfortableness
   d. Discomfort in bones and joints either during or after exercise
9. Watch for the following signs of overexercising:
   a. Inability to finish
   b. Inability to converse during the activity
   c. Faintness or nausea after exercise
   d. Chronic fatigue
   e. Sleeplessness
   f. Aches and pains in the joints
10. Start slowly and progress gradually. Allow time to adapt.

From American Heart Association: Exercise Guidelines.

- To offset the deleterious physiologic and psychological effects of bed rest
- To return the patient to ADLs
- To provide additional medical surveillance for the patient
- To introduce the patient to behavior modification with the goal of reducing risk factors

To stratify the patient's risk for future cardiac rehabilitation (see Display 37-4). Patients experiencing MI, undergoing coronary artery bypass surgery, or undergoing PTCA are usually transferred from the cardiac or intensive care unit to a telemetry unit and sometimes to a general medicine or surgical unit. However, with decreased length of stays, many are discharged directly from the telemetry or step-down unit. The nurses on each of these units are usually the ones who orient and explain to the patient the processes involved in diagnosis and treatment of the specific cardiovascular event. Education about risk factor reduction and the important aspects of medical observation of the patient are discussed further in Chapter 32. As mentioned, before 1970, patients were generally relegated to strict bed rest after an acute MI. It was thought that any physical activity could lead to complications such as ventricular aneurysm formation, cardiac rupture, CHF, dysrhythmias, reinfarction, or sudden death.[67] It has become well established that complications are not increased with early ambulation. One of the important roles of inpatient cardiac rehabilitation is to counteract the detrimental physiologic effects of strict bed rest. There are also data demonstrating that activity during the in-hospital period may help to decrease anxiety and depression, improve self-esteem, and reduce type A behavior characteristics such as hostility and anger.[11,65]

Traditionally, progressive stepped programs have been used to increase activity levels while the patient was in the hospital, including early mobilization, range-of-motion exercises, and progressive activity. A sample step program is shown in Table 37-5. It should be noted that in the current health care climate, the time available for inpatient rehabilitation is far more limited. Thus, the

Table 37-5 EXAMPLE OF A PROTOCOL FOR PATIENT AMBULATION EARLYAFTER AN MI

Step	Nursing	Physical Therapy	Occupational Therapy	Dietary
Step 1 (bed rest)* 1 MET	Orient patient to cardiac care unit, use of commode (1.5); arms supported for upper extremity (UE) activities, decrease anxiety, advise patient of activity limitations	Lower extremity (LE), active range of motion and evaluation	UE, active range of motion and evaluation, introduction to sternal precautions and cardiac rehabilitation (CR) progress	
Step 2 survey (in room) 2 METs	Sit in chair for meals, and 20 minutes at a time, three to four times per day, personal ADLs at bedside or sink, answer patient questions as they arise	Walking in room, or 50 ft (2.0), warm-ups (WU) and cool-downs (CD) (2.5 to 3.0)	UE activity with shoulder flexion 45 degrees, 10 repetitions, education: activity guidelines and risk factor introduction	
Step 3 (short walking) 3 METs	Sitting shower (3.5), continue risk factor education	Walking 100 to 250 ft with WU and CD, instruction in independent walking	Increasing abduction to 90 degrees and 15 repetitions, continue energy conservation and showering guidelines	Introduction to heart healthy eating
Step 4 (long walking) 4 METs	Independent in ADLs and walking on ward, standing shower (3.7); discharge instruction: medicines, appointments, emergencies, review plans for risk factor reduction efforts	Walking 250 to 1000 ft three to four times per day, one flight of stairs (12 steps) (3.5 to 4.0) Given and taught home exercise program	Review of ADLs at home, work, and leisure (postsurgery and post-MI) activity precautions (sex, driving)	Review of dietary follow-up as needed

*MET estimates are in parentheses.

typical patient must be progressed more rapidly, and a greater emphasis must be placed on education, because exercise progression will often need to be accomplished independently by the patient.

While performing a program of education and increasing activity for the inpatient, measurable objectives should be established that are general and specific to each patient. Some examples of these objectives might include having the patient:

- Ambulate 1,000 ft around the unit two to three times per day before discharge
- Measure HR and relate RPE to activities performed
- Climb a flight of stairs without undue symptoms
- Relate upper extremity activity guidelines (sternal guidelines) after cardiac surgery
- Perform self-care ADLs
- Relate plans for resuming other ADLs (i.e., driving, sexual relations, and other strenuous life activities)
- Relate plan to perform walking or other exercise program at home

Although the progressive stepped concept has been widely used, approaches to increasing activity can differ considerably between programs and between patients. Inpatient activities should be individualized and can be specific to common activities the patient performs, in addition to walking. Because hospital stays have become shorter (3 to 5 days), it can be important to modify the inpatient program rapidly based on an individual patient's clinical status and needs.

Exercise Testing Before Hospital Discharge

The exercise test after an acute MI has been shown to be safe. When performed before discharge, it should be submaximal (e.g., limited to 5 or 6 METs) and should not exceed a Borg Scale level of 16. In many hospitals, a submaximal target HR is used (e.g., 110 beats per minute for patients using β-blockers). The protocol should be modified, given the reduced exercise tolerance of most patients recovering from an MI; individualized ramp or Naughton protocols are preferable. An example of a typical submaximal protocol is shown in Table 37-6. Later, when return to full activities is intended, the test can be symptom- and sign-limited.

The predischarge test has many benefits, including clarification of the response to exercise, development of an exercise prescription, and recognition of the need for medications or interventions.[68] It can also have a beneficial psychological impact on recovery and begins the rehabilitation process. The test is considered the first step in the outpatient cardiac rehabilitation exercise program. The prognostic value of the predischarge test has been debated. Meta-analysis has shown that a low exercise capacity or abnormal systolic blood pressure responses are better predictors of increased risk than is ST-segment depression.[69] However, ST-segment depression probably indicates increased risk in men who do not use digoxin and whose resting ECGs do not show extensive damage. The criterion of 2.0 mm or more ST-segment depression along with symptoms or abnormal hemodynamic responses appears to be useful for identifying higher risk patients who should be considered for cardiac catheterization and revascularization.

Table 37-6 ■ EXAMPLE PROTOCOL FOR LOW-LEVEL EXERCISE TESTING

Level	Speed (mph)	Gradient (%)	Time (min)	METs*
I	1.2	0	3	2.1 ± 0.4
II	1.2	3	3	2.4 ± 0.3
III	1.2	6	3	2.7 ± 0.3
IV	1.7	6	3	3.9 ± 0.5

*One MET is defined as the energy equivalent for an individual at rest in sitting position; represents the consumption of 3.5 to 4.0 mL of oxygen per kilogram of body weight per minute.

From Sivarajan-Froelicher, E. S., & Bruce, R. A. (1981). Early exercise test ing after MI. *Cardiovascular Nursing, 17*, 1–5.

Return to Work and Recreational Activities

The economic burden of cardiovascular disability has been enormous, and a great deal of effort has been directed toward vocational rehabilitation. Postdischarge activity recommendations, including determination of disability, are among the biggest challenges facing the health care provider. Historically, the patient's ability to return to work, to drive, and to be sexually active have been based on clinical judgments rather than on physiologic assessments. These decisions should be based on the consequence of the coronary event (e.g., ischemia, symptoms of CHF, or dysrhythmias), the nature of the patient's occupational or recreational activities, and the response to the predischarge exercise test.

In general, if patients do not exhibit any untoward responses to submaximal exercise testing and achieve 5 or more METs, it is unlikely that they will encounter difficulties during ADLs. More strenuous jobs or recreational pursuits should not be initiated until a symptom-limited exercise test can be performed and exercise capacity can be determined and related to the desired physical activities of the patient.

Factors that influence a patient's return to work include age, work history, severity of cardiac damage, financial compensation for illness, employer's ignorance of the patient's capabilities, termination of employment, and, most important, the patient's perception of his or her clinical status. Efforts of the rehabilitation team to help the patient develop a positive attitude, and a sense of well-being may facilitate appropriate vocational adjustments. The physician's attitude also greatly affects the patient's return to work; encouragement can be very beneficial.

Contraindications to Exercise Training

Absolute contraindications are the known or suspected conditions that prevent the patient from safely participating in an exercise program. These include unstable angina pectoris, dissecting aortic aneurysm, complete heart block, uncontrolled hypertension, decompensated CHF, uncontrolled dysrhythmias, thrombophlebitis, and other complicating illnesses[65,70] (Display 37-9). Relative contraindications, or those that can be superseded by clinical judgment, include frequent premature ventricular contractions, controlled dysrhythmias, intermittent claudication, metabolic disorders, and moderate anemia or

DISPLAY 37-9 Clinical Indications and Contraindications for Inpatient and Outpatient Cardiac Rehabilitation

Indications

- Medically stable post-MI
- Stable angina
- Coronary artery bypass graft surgery
- PTCA
- Compensated congestive heart failure
- Cardiomyopathy
- Heart or other organ transplantation
- Other cardiac surgery including valvular and pacemaker insertion (including implantable cardioverter defibrillator)
- Peripheral vascular disease
- High-risk cardiovascular disease ineligible for surgical intervention
- Sudden cardiac death syndrome
- End-stage renal disease
- At risk for coronary artery disease, with diagnoses of diabetes mellitus, hyperlipidemia, hypertension, etc.
- Other patients who may benefit from structured exercise and/or patient education (based on physician referral and consensus of the rehabilitation team)

Contraindications

- Unstable angina
- Resting systolic blood pressure >200 mm Hg or diastolic >110 mm Hg
- Blood pressure drop of >20 mm Hg with symptoms
- Moderate to severe aortic stenosis
- Acute systemic illness or fever
- Uncontrolled atrial or ventricular arrhythmias
- Uncontrolled tachycardia (>100 bpm)
- Uncompensated congestive heart failure
- Third-degree heart block (without pacemaker)
- Active pericarditis or myocarditis
- Recent embolism
- Thrombophlebitis
- Resting ST displacement (>2 mm)
- Uncontrolled diabetes
- Orthopedic problems prohibiting exercise
- Other metabolic problems

From American College of Sports Medicine. (2006). *Guidelines for exercise testing and prescription* (7th ed.). Philadelphia: Lippincott Williams & Wilkins.

pulmonary disease. Studies show that if these contraindications are considered, the incidence of exertion-related cardiac arrest in cardiac rehabilitation programs is extremely low, and because of the availability of rapid defibrillation, serious events rarely occur.

Outpatient Cardiac Rehabilitation

There have been multiple approaches to outpatient rehabilitation, and it has become necessary for programs to be more creative to provide outpatient rehabilitation in the current climate of reduced reimbursement. Traditionally, this phase begins 1 to 2 weeks after discharge from the hospital and may last from 1 to 4 months. Most commonly, patients attend group exercise sessions three times per week; however, frequency of exercise is often modified by the individual patient's overall goals, functional capabilities, reimbursement, proximity to the hospital or clinic, and personal commitment.

The first few exercise sessions after hospital discharge usually emphasize warm-up and cool-down activities, with only a modest aerobic component; some programs use direct electrocardiographic telemetry for the initial sessions to ensure safety. There is less emphasis today than in the past on the need for direct ECG monitoring (see later). A symptom-limited maximal exercise test is usually recommended approximately 6 weeks after the hospitalization to determine an appropriate exercise prescription and activity limitations.

At the beginning of the outpatient program, it is advisable to conduct a patient assessment, discuss the objectives of the program, and develop reasonable goals for the patient based on their needs, capabilities, and clinical condition. Usually the patient is scheduled for an initial interview, where baseline data are gathered and information about the program is given to the patient. At this initial interview the nurse should have reviewed the inpatient records so that the patient has been stratified into the appropriate risk category. In general, the objectives of the outpatient program include the following:

- Increase activity level and functional capacity
- Increase regular exercise participation
- Improve the patient's psychosocial status, depression, or anxiety through participation in exercise, education, or counseling when appropriate

Educate and support patients in other risk reduction efforts (i.e., stop smoking, control hypertension, normalize lipid values, and maintain healthy weight). The exercise prescription for outpatient rehabilitation is based on the exercise test and is described in detail below. A number of fundamental considerations are important when initiating outpatient rehabilitation. Although the typical outpatient session may last approximately 45 minutes, patients should work up to this duration gradually. It is preferable to focus on warm-up, stretching, range of motion, and cool-down exercises for the first three to six sessions and gradually increase the aerobic portion such that 30 to 45 minutes can be completed. Regardless of the duration of the aerobic portion, all exercise sessions should include warm-up and cool-down periods of 5 to 10 minutes. A variety of exercise modalities should be used, including those that use the upper and lower muscle groups. For example, patients may spend alternating periods using the treadmill, arm ergometer, cycle ergometer, or stair climber. Resistance exercise is also widely recommended today to assist the patient in restoring muscular strength, and complementing aerobic exercise with resistance training has been demonstrated to have favorable effects on cardiovascular endurance, hypertension, hyperlipidemia, and psychosocial well-being.[71]

Changes in reimbursement patterns have changed outpatient programs more than other components of cardiac rehabilitation. In some circumstances, only a few exercise or educational sessions are reimbursed. The transition from an outpatient to a home-based maintenance program now occurs more rapidly. Randomized trials have demonstrated that patients can return to work quickly and safely during rehabilitation and that participation in rehabilitation facilitates this process. It is also currently appreciated that only a small percentage of patients require continuous ECG monitoring during exercise. Efforts to reduce the cost of rehabilitation in addition to the recognition that most patients can exercise quite safely without continuous telemetry have brought about this change. Although the AHA guidelines suggest ECG monitoring for the first 6 to 12 sessions,[4] recommendations on this issue have varied widely. Patients who should be considered for longer ECG monitoring include those with a history of serious rhythm disorders, implantable cardioverter defibrillator implantation, CHF, and abnormal hemodynamic responses to exercise testing (e.g., exercise-induced hypotension).

Exercise Prescription for Outpatient Rehabilitation

Exercise prescription essentially describes the process whereby a person's recommended regimen of physical activity is designed in a systematic and individualized manner. An "individualized manner" implies specific strategies to optimize return to work or ADLs, reduction of risk factors for future cardiac events, and maximization of the patient's capacity to maintain an active lifestyle. The development of an appropriate exercise prescription to meet the individual patient's needs has a sound scientific foundation, but there is also an art to effective exercise programming.

The art of exercise prescription has become increasingly important in this era of cost containment (shorter rehabilitation), surgical and technologic advances (larger numbers of transplantations, pacemaker, or CHF participants than ever before), and the multitude of new medicines available. There is no single program that is best for all patients or even one patient over time; capabilities, vocational needs, and expectations differ among patients and can change with the passing of time. Thus, the art of exercise prescription relies on the nurse's abilities to synthesize the patient's pathophysiologic, psychosocial, and vocational factors and tailor them to the patient's needs and realistic goals. A final but important consideration is the selection of activities that the individual enjoys, which will provide the best chance that he or she will continue to perform safely after the formal rehabilitation program ends.

Principles of Exercise Prescription

Training implies adaptations of the body to the demands placed on it. A *training* effect is best measured as an increase in maximal ventilatory oxygen uptake, but not all institutions have gas exchange equipment and there are many ways to quantify functional outcomes of rehabilitation. For example, some patients after rehabilitation may be better suited to perform submaximal levels of activity for longer periods, remain independent, continue working, or rejoin their friends on the golf course. All of these can be important goals for a given patient and may occur even with a minimal change in maximal oxygen uptake.

The major ingredients of the exercise prescription are frequency, intensity, duration, mode, and rate of progression. In general, these principles apply for both the patient with heart disease and the healthy adult; however, the ways in which they are applied differ. On the basis of numerous studies performed since the 1950s, it is generally accepted that increases in maximal oxygen uptake are achieved if a person exercises dynamically for a period ranging from 15 to 60 minutes, three to five times per week, at an intensity equivalent to 50% to 80% of the maximum capacity. Dynamic exercises are those that use large muscle groups in a rhythmic manner, such as treadmill walking, cycle ergometry, rowing, stepping, and arm ergometry. As mentioned, short warm-up and cool-down periods are strongly encouraged for participants in cardiac rehabilitation programs. Again, however, an effective exercise prescription must consider the patient's goals, health status, and availability of time in addition to practical considerations such as cost, availability of equipment, and facilities.

Much of the art of exercise prescription clearly involves individualizing the exercise intensity. Typically, exercise intensity is expressed as a percentage of maximal capacity, either in absolute terms (i.e., workload or watts) or in relation to the maximal HR, maximal oxygen uptake, or perceived effort. Training benefits have been shown to occur with exercise intensities ranging from 40% to 85% of maximal oxygen uptake, which are generally equivalent to 50% to 90% of the maximal HR. However, the intensity that a given individual can maintain for a specified period of time varies widely. In general, the most appropriate intensity for most patients in rehabilitation programs is 50% to 70% of maximal capacity. The actual prescribed exercise intensity for the patient should naturally depend on goals, health status, length of time since infarction or surgery, symptoms, and initial state of fitness.

Training is a general phenomenon; there is no true threshold beyond which patients achieve benefits. Thus, as long as patients exercise safely, setting the exercise intensity is a less rigid practice than it was years ago. In addition, the patient's ability to tolerate activities can change daily. Other factors, such as time of day, environment, and time since medications were taken, can influence the patient's response to exercise, and the exercise prescription must be adjusted accordingly. It is also useful to use a window of intensity that ranges approximately 10% above and 10% below the desired level.

The graded exercise test is the foundation on which a safe and effective exercise prescription is based. To achieve a desired training intensity, oxygen uptake or some estimate of it must be quantified during a maximal or symptom-limited exercise test. Because HR is easily measured and is linearly related to oxygen uptake, it has become a standard by which training intensity is estimated during exercise sessions. The most useful method uses a measure known as the HR reserve. This method uses a percentage of the difference between maximum HR and resting HR and adds this value to the resting HR. For example, for a patient who achieves a maximum HR of 150 beats per minute, has a resting HR of 70 beats per minute, and wishes to exercise at intensity equivalent to 60% of maximum:

$$
\begin{aligned}
\text{Maximum HR} &= 150 \text{ bpm} \\
-\ \text{Resting HR} &= 70 \\
\text{HR range} &= 80 \\
\times\ \text{Desired intensity (60\%)} & \\
&= 48 \\
+\ \text{Resting HR} &= 70 \\
= \text{Training HR} &= 118
\end{aligned}
$$

A reasonable training HR range for this individual would be 115 to 125 beats per minute. This is also referred to as the Karvonen formula and is reliable for patients in normal sinus rhythm whose measurements of resting and maximum HRs are accurate. An estimated target HR for exercise should be supplemented by considering the patient's MET level relative to his or her maximum, the perceived exertion, and symptoms.

Patient Education in Outpatient Cardiac Rehabilitation

The education component in an outpatient rehabilitation program usually focuses on modifying risk factors for heart disease. Chapter 32 address risk factor modification in detail. Exercise, as mentioned previously, is usually the main focus of cardiac rehabilitation. However, exercise affects other alterable risk factors such as hypertension, abnormal lipids, obesity, smoking, and diabetes. During exercise, opportunities arise to teach informally about risk factor modification in all these areas. Teaching the patient about exercise is often performed formally through group presentations and informally as each patient progresses with their exercise sessions and as the home program evolves. Other issues can be addressed in formal classroom sessions, in short sessions after the exercise training periods, or by distributing educational materials. The home exercise prescription should be given to the patient soon after starting outpatient cardiac rehabilitation. Patients should be asked to exercise at home on the days they do not come to cardiac rehabilitation. The aim is to gradually have them exercising most days of the week for 30 or more minutes each time, as recommended by the AHA, Surgeon General Report, and ACSM guidelines. If they attempt to exercise every day, they will be most likely to achieve the recommended three to five times per week. When patients walk for exercise, they can be encouraged to gradually increase the duration to 60 minutes. Walking is the most common home exercise, but if the patient has access to other forms of exercise, then prescriptions should be given for these modes. Excellent references for home exercise include the *ACSM Fitness Book*,[72] *Take a Load off the Heart*,[73] and numerous other patient education materials that are available on the AHA and ACSM Web sites.

Safety of Exercise Training in Outpatient Cardiac Rehabilitation

The safety of outpatient cardiac rehabilitation has been well documented in both the United States and Europe. In 1986, Van Camp and Peterson sent questionnaires to 167 randomly selected cardiac rehabilitation centers.[74] Data were gathered on more than 51,000 patients who exercised more than 2 million hours from January 1980 to December 1984. During this time, there were only 21 cardiac resuscitations (three of which failed) and eight MIs. This amounts to 8.9 cardiac arrests, 3.4 infarctions, and 1.3 fatalities per one million hours of patient exercise. Surprisingly, ECG monitoring had little influence on complications, which suggests that the additional expense of telemetry may not be necessary.

In a 16-year follow-up from William Beaumont Hospital in Michigan, 292,254 patient-exercise-hours were recorded in phase II and III programs.[75] During this period, a total of five major cardiovascular complications occurred; the complication rate was one per 58,451 patient-exercise-hours. Over the last three decades, numerous other studies have confirmed the fact that exercise training is extremely safe in patients with cardiovascular disease. Despite the scarcity of serious events during exercise, appropriate medical personnel must be available to respond should an event occur.

Maintenance Program

Progression to an out-of-hospital maintenance program is desirable after patients have participated in a supervised program for a suitable period. The period of time required before patients move to a maintenance program can vary considerably, depending on reimbursement, the patient's stability, exercise capacity, and the individual patient's needs, but it rarely exceeds 12 weeks. The purpose of this phase is to maintain training adaptations, to prevent recurrence of events or symptoms, and to maintain progress. An important concept to instill in patients at this point in time is that continued maintenance of their exercise capacity and a physically active lifestyle is one of the most important determinants of future health outcomes.[2,5,32,43–45,55,56,62] It is important that patients understand how to monitor their exercise intensity, understand how to recognize symptoms, and have a basic knowledge of their particular disease and medications.

When making occupational activity recommendations for patients, it can be helpful to know the estimated energy requirements of various activities (see Display 37-7). With this knowledge, appropriate recommendations can be made, balancing patients' functional limitations with their need to return to work, desire to continue recreational activities, or both.

It is useful to perform an exercise test before the maintenance program to provide an outgoing exercise prescription, confirm the safety of exercise for a given patient, and assess risk for future cardiac events. Funding for this phase must often be borne by the patient because most types of health insurance do not cover it; however, mechanisms for follow-up should be in place. In recent years, programs have been developed in the Young Men's Christian Association (YMCA), gyms, and other community facilities that make it less expensive and more accessible for patients in need of maintenance programs.

Rehabilitation in Patients with CHF

Until the late 1980s, CHF was considered by many authorities to be a contraindication to participation in an exercise program. Today it is known that most patients with CHF derive considerable benefits from cardiac rehabilitation.[66] With improvements in therapy (i.e., thrombolysis, angiotensin-converting enzyme inhibitors, β-blockers, implantable cardioverter defibrillators), survival of patients with CHF has improved considerably, and more of these patients are candidates for rehabilitation. The incidence of CHF is increasing; it is currently approximately 500,000 per year in the United States. The numerous randomized trials performed during the 1990s in the United States and Europe indicated that the major physiologic benefit from training in CHF occurs in the skeletal muscle rather than in the heart itself.

The clinical approach to the patient with CHF who is considered for a rehabilitation program is similar to that for the post-MI patient described earlier, although several important differences are worth noting. While sudden cardiac events during exercise are extremely rare in all patients, the risk is higher in patients with CHF than in patients with normal left ventricular function. This is the population in whom serious arrhythmias occur most often. There are more medications to be considered that can influence exercise responses, including vasoactive, antiarrhythmic, inotropic, and β-blocking agents. Exercise capacity tends to be significantly lower than that in the typical patient with coronary disease.

Numerous hemodynamic abnormalities underlie the reduced exercise capacity commonly observed in CHF, including impaired HR responses, inability to distribute cardiac output normally, abnormal arterial vasodilatory capacity, abnormal cellular metabolism in skeletal muscle, higher-than-normal systemic vascular resistance, higher-than-normal pulmonary pressures, and ventilatory abnormalities that increase the work of breathing and cause exertional dyspnea.[66,76,77] Studies performed over the past decade have demonstrated that many of these abnormalities can be improved by exercise training.[62,66]

Most patients with reduced left ventricular function who are clinically stable and have reduced exercise tolerance are candidates for exercise programs. It is often necessary to exclude patients with signs and symptoms of right-sided failure or to treat them judiciously before entry into a program. An exercise test is particularly important before initiating the program to ensure safety of participation. Rhythm abnormalities, exertional hypotension, or other signs of instability should be ruled out. Expired gas exchange measurements are particularly informative in this group because they provide an improvement in accuracy and permit an assessment of ventilatory abnormalities that are common in this condition[76,78] (see Chapter 21). ECG monitoring during exercise is more often indicated in this group. Attention should be paid to daily changes in body weight, rhythm status, and symptoms.

Increasing numbers of patients have undergone cardiac transplantation for end-stage heart failure, and approximately 75% of these patients remain alive after 5 years. These patients are presently considered good candidates for rehabilitation programs. Because the transplantation patient's heart is denervated, some intriguing hemodynamic responses to exercise are observed. The heart is not responsive to the normal actions of the parasympathetic and sympathetic nervous systems. The absence of vagal tone explains the high resting HRs in these patients (100 to 110 beats per minute) and the relatively slow adaptation of the heart to a given amount of submaximal work. As a result, the delivery of oxygen to the working tissue is slower, contributing to earlier-than-normal metabolic acidosis and hyperventilation during exercise. Maximal HR is lower in transplantation patients than in normal subjects, which contributes to a reduction in cardiac output and exercise capacity.

A growing number of reports have addressed the effects of training after cardiac transplantation. These studies have demonstrated increases in peak oxygen uptake, reductions in resting and submaximal HRs, and improved ventilatory responses to exercise after periods of training. Whether the major physiologic adaptation to exercise is improved cardiac function, changes in skeletal muscle metabolism, or simply an improvement in strength remains to be determined. Psychosocial studies of rehabilitation in transplantation patients are lacking, as are studies of the effects of regular exercise on survival.

New Models of Cardiac Rehabilitation

Changes in reimbursement patterns over the past 15 years, along with the demonstration that clinical outcomes can be improved by multidisciplinary risk factor intervention,[79–81] have led to the development of new models of cardiac rehabilitation. The need for new approaches has also been fueled by the recent observations that a wider spectrum of patients can benefit from cardiac rehabilitation (e.g., valvular surgery, CHF, posttransplantation, peripheral vascular disease, postcardiac resynchronization therapy, and the elderly). Moreover, innovative strategies have been proposed to increase the proportion of eligible patients who receive cardiac rehabilitation services despite reductions in reimbursement. In addition, physicians have not been particularly effective in assisting patients in achieving defined risk factor goals,[14,16,82–85] and strategies have been suggested to facilitate a greater proportion of patients meeting evidence-based treatment guidelines.

Models that have been developed to meet these needs include the transformation of rehabilitation centers into "secondary prevention centers,"[79] the "inclusive chronic disease model,"[86] the implementation of affordable, evidence-based, comprehensive risk reduction in primary and secondary prevention settings,[79,87] home exercise programs,[88–90] and case-management systems.[91–94] The concept that cardiac rehabilitation should be the primary medium to implement comprehensive cardiovascular risk reduction has been embraced by the AHA,[80] the Agency for Health Care Policy and Research (AHCPR) Clinical Practice Guidelines,[11] and the American Association of Cardiovascular and Pulmonary Rehabilitation (AACVPR).[13,65] The recent AHA consensus statement on "Core Components of Rehabilitation/Secondary Prevention Programs"[80] defines specific evidence-based risk factor goals for management of lipids, blood pressure, weight, smoking cessation, diabetes management, and physical activity (Display 37-10). This model provides an integrated system that includes appropriate triage, education, counseling on lifestyle interventions, and long-term follow-up.

Several studies have demonstrated the efficacy of comprehensive risk factor management using a *case management* approach. In each of these studies, a nurse, as case manager, functions as the coordinator and point of contact who identifies, triages, provides surveillance on safety and efficacy, performs follow-up, and, in many instances, quantifies patient outcomes. Case management has been the cornerstone of recent multidisciplinary efforts to reduce cardiovascular risk. In addition, it has provided a framework for comprehensive management of existing disease, particularly for patients with CHF.[90–95] This approach involves the coordination of risk reduction strategies for targeted groups of patients by a single individual, most commonly a nurse or exercise physiologist, with appropriate medical supervision. The case management concept is based on the idea that risk factors are strongly interrelated, and an individualized, integrated approach to management will optimize care such that clinical outcomes will be improved and costs will be saved. The case management approach has been applied in various settings over the past decade and has been successful in reducing risk markers for coronary artery disease and improving outcomes in patients with existing disease. Some of the more prominent studies performed in recent years using case management approaches are described.

The Butterworth Heath System in Michigan reorganized their cardiac rehabilitation program to focus on improvement in long-term outcomes using a case-management model.[93] The model included the use of referral pathways, education sessions, and intervention by social workers as necessary. In addition, they added regular telephone follow-up to assess the effectiveness of the risk reduction interventions. One year after initiating the program, 77% of patients were on appropriate lipid-lowering therapy, 78% reported exercising at least 3 days per week, and 66% of previous smokers reported smoking cessation.

The MULTIFIT program of DeBusk et al.[91] has been a model for other case management programs, and its success led to it being adopted by the Kaiser Permanente Health Care System. MULTIFIT is a case-managed program for patients hospitalized

DISPLAY 37-10 Core Components for Cardiac Rehabilitation/Secondary Prevention Programs

Lipid Management

- Short-term: Assessment and modification of interventions until LDL < 100 mg/dL.
- Long-term: LDL < 100 mg/dL. Secondary goals include HDL > 40 mg/dL and triglycerides < 200 mg/dL.

Hypertension Management

- Short-term: Assessment and modification of interventions until BP is <140 mm Hg systolic and <90 mm Hg diastolic; in patients with heart failure, diabetes, and renal failure, BP < 130 mm Hg systolic and <85 mm Hg diastolic.
- Long-term: BP < 140 mm Hg systolic and <90 mm Hg diastolic; in patients with heart failure, diabetes, and renal failure, BP < 130 mm Hg systolic and <85 mm Hg diastolic.

Smoking Cessation

- Short-term: patient will demonstrate readiness to change by initially expressing decision to quit (contemplation) and selecting a quit date (preparation). Subsequently the patient will quit smoking and use of all tobacco products (action); adhere to pharmacotherapy, if prescribed; practice strategies as recommended; and resume cessation plan as quickly as possible when relapse occurs.
- Long-term: complete abstinence from smoking and use of all tobacco products at 12 months from quit date.

Weight Management

- In patients with BMI > 25 kg/m^2 and/or waist >40 in. in men (102 cm) and >35 in. (88 cm) in women.
- Establish reasonable short-term and long-term weight goals individualized to patient and associated risk factors (e.g., reduce body weight by at least 10% at a rate of 1–2 lb/week over a period of time up to 6 months).
- Short-term: Continued assessment and modification of interventions until progressive weight loss is achieved. Have patient participate in on-site weight loss program or provide referral to specialized nutrition weight loss programs such that weight goals are achieved.
- Long-term: adherence to diet and exercise program aimed toward attainment of established weight goal.

Diabetes Management

- In patients with diabetes:
  - Short-term: Develop a regimen of dietary adherence and weight control which includes: exercise, oral hypoglycemic agents, insulin therapy, and optimal control of other risk factors. Drug therapy should be provided and/or monitored in concert with primary healthcare provider.
  - Long-term: Normalization of fasting plasma glucose (80–110 mg/dL or HbA1C < 7.0), minimization of diabetic complications, control of associated obesity, hypertension (<130/85 mm Hg) and hyperlipidemia.
- Refer patients without known diabetes whose fasting glucose is ≥110 mg/dL to their primary healthcare provider for further evaluation and treatment.

Physical Activity Counseling

- Increased physical activity, which includes 20 to 30 minutes per day of moderate physical activity on 5 or more days per week, and increased activity in usual routines; for example, parking farther away from entrances, walking two or more flights of stairs, walking 15 minutes during lunch break.
- Increased participation in domestic, occupational, and recreational activities.
- Improved psychosocial well-being, reduction in stress, facilitation of functional independence, prevention of disability, and enhancement of opportunities for independent self-care to achieve recommended goals.

LDL, low-density lipoprotein; HDL, high-density lipoprotein, BP, blood pressure; BMI, body mass index; HBA1C, glycosylated hemoglobin.
From the AHA and AACVPR. (2007). Scientific statement on core components of cardiac rehabilitation secondary prevention programs: 2007 update. *Journal of Cardiopulmonary Rehabilitation, 27*, 121–129.

with acute MI in Northern California. Patients were randomized either to special risk reduction intervention by a nurse case manager or to usual care. The intervention patients received education and counseling regarding smoking cessation, regular physical activity, and nutrition. Medical management, such as lipid-lowering therapy, was instituted as indicated for risk factors not controlled by lifestyle change. Much of the intervention was mediated by phone and mail contact. The intervention group showed greater improvement at 6 months and 1 year in functional capacity, rate of smoking cessation, and changes in low-density lipoprotein-C compared with the usual care group, and subsequent analyses have shown MULTIFIT to be cost-effective.[95]

The Cardiac Hospital Atherosclerosis Management Program (CHAMP)[94] compared outcomes among 302 patients enrolled in a case-managed risk reduction intervention and compared them to 256 control patients. All were discharged from UCLA Medical Center with a diagnosis of coronary artery disease or other vascular disease. The case-managed approach emphasized close adherence to appropriate use of aspirin, β-blockers, angiotensin-converting enzyme inhibitors, and lipid-lowering agents, combined with outpatient exercise, nutrition, and smoking cessation counseling. After the study period, there was greater use of appropriate medications, an increase in the percentage of patients achieving a low-density lipoprotein-C level less than 100 mg/dL, a reduction in recurrent MI, and a lower 1-year mortality.

At Stanford, a randomized controlled trial funded by the National Institutes of Health (NIH) was performed to evaluate the efficacy of case-managed, physician-directed multi-risk factor intervention (the Stanford Coronary Risk Intervention Project [SCRIP]).[92] Case managers coordinated care along with a team of nutritionists, psychologists, and physicians to provide clinical and lifestyle interventions, attempting to achieve nationally recognized goals for risk factor reduction. Three hundred subjects were randomized to intervention or usual care groups. After the 4-year study period, the intervention group demonstrated an increase in exercise participation, reductions in dietary fat and cholesterol intake, reductions in systolic blood pressure, body mass index and blood lipids, an improvement in glucose tolerance, and a 27% reduction in Framingham Risk Score. These changes were associated with reductions in hospitalizations and coronary events. Angiographic results included less progression of coronary artery disease and greater stabilization of plaque in the intervention group. The home-based model of rehabilitation, validated at Stanford University in the 1980s,[88] has been used in many centers over the past 20 years. This approach uses home exercise that is either unmonitored or monitored via telephone or microprocessor. Some programs feature regular feedback via telephone or home visits, and recent approaches have used exercise monitoring devices such as pedometers, accelerometers, and HR recording devices to encourage and document compliance with prescribed exercise. Safety and efficacy of these home programs have been shown to be similar to those of more conventional programs.[88,89]

CLOSING COMMENT

Early and progressive ambulation of patients after an MI is now considered routine care. Despite the advent of new therapies in cardiovascular medicine, cardiac rehabilitation maintains an important place in reducing morbidity and mortality. The controlled exercise trials, when combined, demonstrate that the efficacy of rehabilitation in reducing mortality is similar to that of the best medical interventions. Moreover, cardiac rehabilitation has redirected interest to humanistic concerns, providing a balance for the emphasis on complex technology. It also provides an ideal environment for supervision of patients and for ensuring stability after an interventional procedure. Available data suggest that cardiac rehabilitation is economically sound.

Medicine is experiencing an evolution toward technologic efficacy and outcomes assessment. Health economists and legislators are reexamining the value placed on all forms of medical care. Although this movement has changed the way in which cardiac rehabilitation is implemented, studies have confirmed its value. Some of the ways in which the current economic environment has changed cardiac rehabilitation include lessening of direct ECG monitoring, shorter hospital stays, and more rapid progression to home programs. The frequency of interventions has lessened the morbidity associated with MI. Modifications in the way cardiac rehabilitation is implemented have encouraged greater referral to and participation in cardiac rehabilitation, and newer models of cardiac rehabilitation have brought a greater focus on secondary risk reduction, case management, and cost efficacy.

Data on efficacy, safety, and technologic advances in the treatment of cardiovascular disease have changed cardiac rehabilitation in such a way that a wider range of patients can benefit from these services than in the past. For example, patients with stable CHF, once excluded from cardiac rehabilitation programs, are now thought to be among those who benefit the most.[96] Patients who have had pacemakers, transplantation, bypass or valvular surgery, and claudication now comprise a significant fraction of those in many programs. Despite this fact, most eligible patients (approximately 80%) do not receive these services. It is clear that not all patients need all components of cardiac rehabilitation, but directing these services to patients who need them most remains one of the important challenges for the field.

Lastly, there has been a change in the public health care message toward physical activity as inherently beneficial regardless of objective measurements of fitness. This has led to a shift in focus from morbidity, mortality, and exercise capacity to issues related to maintaining an active lifestyle and optimizing the patient's capacity to perform the physical challenges offered by occupational or recreational activities. Further studies on costs, benefits, and other outcomes should solidify the role of cardiac rehabilitation in the clinical management of patients with cardiovascular disease.

REFERENCES

1. Centers for Disease Control and Prevention, U.S. Department of Health and Human Services. (1999). *Promoting physical activity: A guide for community action.* Champaign, IL: Human Kinetics.
2. Pate, R. R., Pratt, M. P., Blair, S. N., et al. (1995). Physical activity and public health: A recommendation from the Centers for Disease Control and Prevention and the American College of Sports Medicine. *JAMA, 273,* 402–407.
3. Institute of Medicine. (2002). *Dietary reference intakes for energy, carbohydrate, fiber, fat, fatty acids, cholesterol, protein, and amino acids.* Washington, DC: National Academy Press.
4. Fletcher, G. F., Balady, G., Blair, S. N., et al. (1996). Statement on exercise: Benefits and recommendations for physical activity programs for all Americans. A statement for health professionals by the Committee on Exercise and Cardiac Rehabilitation of the Council on Clinical Cardiology, American Heart Association. *Circulation, 94*(4), 857–862.
5. U.S. Public Health Service, Office of the Surgeon General. (1996). *Physical activity and health: A report of the Surgeon General.* Atlanta, GA: U.S. Department of Health and Human Services, Centers for Disease Control and Prevention, National Center for Chronic Disease Prevention and Health Promotion.
6. Paffenbarger, R. S., Hyde, R. T., Wing, A.L., et al. (1986). Physical activity, all-cause mortality, and longevity of college alumni. *New England Journal of Medicine, 314,* 605–613.
7. Haskell, W. L., Lee. I., Pate, R.., et al. (2007). Physical activity and public health: Updated recommendation for adults from the American College of Sports Medicine and the American Heart Association. *Medicine & Science in Sports & Exercise, 39,* 1423–1434.
8. Squires, R. W., & Hamm, L. F. (2006). Exercise and the coronary heart disease connection. In L. F. Hamm, K. Berra, & T. Kavanagh (Eds.), *AACVPR cardiac rehabilitation resource manual* (pp. 53–62). Champaign, IL: Human Kinetics.
9. O'Conner, G. T., Buring, J. E., Yusaf, S., et al. (1989). An overview of randomized trials of rehabilitation with exercise after myocardial infarction. *Circulation, 80,* 234–244.
10. Oldridge, N. B., Guyatt, G. H., Fischer, M. E., et al. (1988). Cardiac rehabilitation with exercise after myocardial infarction. *JAMA, 260,* 945–950.
11. Wenger, N. K., Sivarajan-Froelicher, E. S., Smith, L. K., et al. (1995). *Cardiac rehabilitation: Clinical practice guideline No. 17* (AHCOR Publication No. 96-0672). Rockville, MD: U.S. Department of Health and Human Services, Public Health Service, Agency for Health Care Policy and Research and the National Heart, Lung, and Blood Institute.
12. Taylor, R. S., Brown, A., Ebrahim, S., et al. (2004). Exercise-based rehabilitation for patients with coronary heart disease: Systematic review and meta-analysis of randomized controlled trials. *American Journal of Medicine, 116,* 682–692.
13. Thomas, R. J., King, M., Liu, L., et al. (2007). AACVPR/ACC/AHA 2007 performance measures on cardiac rehabilitation for referral to and delivery of cardiac rehabilitation/secondary prevention services. *Journal of Cardiopulmonary Rehabilitation and Prevention, 27,* 260–290.
14. Wee, C. C., McCarthy, E. P., Davis, R. B., et al. (1999). Physician counseling about exercise. *JAMA, 282,* 1583–1588.
15. Sherman, S. E., & Hershman, W. Y. (1993). Exercise counseling: How do general internists do? *Journal of General Internal Medicine, 8,* 243–248.
16. Damush, T. M., Stewart, A. L., Mills, K. M., et al. (1999). Prevalence and correlates of physician recommendations to exercise among older adults. *Journal of Gerontology A Biology Science Medicine Science, 54,* M423–M427.
17. Ribisl, P. M. (2001). Exercise: The unfilled prescription. *American Journal of Medicine and Sports, 3,* 13–21.

18. Mokdad, A. H., Marks, J. S., Stroup, D. F., et al. (2004). Actual causes of death in the United States, 2000. *JAMA, 291*, 1238–1245.
19. Kohl, H. W. (2001). Physical activity and cardiovascular disease: Evidence for a dose response. *Medicine & Science in Sports & Exercise, 33*(6, Suppl.), S472–S483.
20. Bassuk, S. S., & Manson, J. E. (2005). Epidemiological evidence for the role of physical activity in reducing risk of type 2 diabetes and cardiovascular disease. *Journal of Applied Physiology, 99*, 1193–1204.
21. Tanasescu, M., Leitzman, M. F., Rimm, E. B., et al. (2003). Physical activity in relation to cardiovascular disease and total mortality among men with type 2 diabetes. *Circulation, 107*, 2435–2439.
22. Myers, J. N., Atwood, J. E., & Froelicher, V. F. (2003). Active lifestyle and diabetes. *Circulation, 107*, 2392–2394.
23. Wareham, N. J. (2007). Epidemiological studies of physical activity and diabetes risk, and implications for diabetes prevention. *Applied Physiology, Nutrition, and Metabolism, 32*, 778–782.
24. LaMonte, M. J., Blair, S. N., & Church, T. S. (2005). Physical activity and diabetes prevention. *Journal of Applied Physiology, 99*, 1205–1213.
25. Fagard, R. H. (2001). Exercise characteristics and the blood pressure response to dynamic physical training. *Medicine & Science in Sports & Exercise, 33*(6, Suppl.) S484–S492.
26. Borer, K. T. (2005) Physical activity in the prevention and amelioration of osteoporosis in women: Interaction of mechanical, hormonal and dietary factors. *Sports Medicine, 35*, 779–830.
27. Thune, I., & Furberg, A. S. (2001). Physical activity and cancer risk: Dose response, all sites, and site-specific. *Medicine & Science in Sports & Exercise, 33*(6, Suppl.), S530–S550.
28. Lees, S. J., & Booth, F. W. (2004). Sedentary death syndrome. *Canadian Journal of Applied Physiology, 29*, 447–460.
29. Paffenbarger, R. S., Hyde, R. T., Wing, A. L., et al. (1993). The association of changes in physical-activity level and other lifestyle characteristics with mortality among men. *New England Journal of Medicine, 328*, 538–545.
30. Paffenbarger, R. S., Hyde, R. T., Wing, A. L., et al. (1984). Chronic disease in former college students: XXV. A natural history of athleticism and cardiovascular health. *JAMA, 252*, 491–495.
31. Paffenbarger, R. S., Blair, S. N., Lee, I., et al. (1993). Measurement of physical activity to assess health effects in free-living populations. *Medicine & Science in Sports & Exercise, 25*, 60–70.
32. Paffenbarger, R. S., Hyde, R. T., & Wing, A. L., et al. (1994). Some interrelations of physical activity, physiological fitness, health, and longevity. In C. Bouchard, R. J. Shephard, & T. Stephens (Eds.), *Physical activity, fitness, and health* (pp. 119–133). Champaign, IL: Human Kinetics.
33. Paffenbarger, R. S., Laughlin, M. E., Gima, A. S., et al. (1970). Work activity of longshoreman as related to death from coronary heart disease and stroke. *New England Journal of Medicine, 282*, 1109–1114.
34. Ainsworth, B. E., Haskell, W. L., Whitt, M. C., et al. (2000). Compendium of physical activities: An update of activity codes and ET intensities. *Medicine & Science in Sports & Exercise, 32*, S498–S504.
35. Morris, J. N., Kagan, A., Pattison, D. C., et al. (1966). Incidence and prediction of ischemic heart disease in London busmen. *Lancet, 2*, 552–559.
36. Morris, J. N., Everitt, M. G., Pollard, R., et al. (1980). Vigorous exercise in leisure-time: Protection against coronary heart disease. *Lancet, 2*, 1207–1210.
37. Slattery, M. L., Jacobs, D. R., & Nichaman, M. Z. (1989). Leisure time physical activity and coronary heart disease death: The U.S. Railroad Study. *Circulation, 79*, 304–311.
38. Rockhill, B., Willett, W. C., Manson, J. E., et al. (2001). Physical activity and mortality: A prospective study among women. *American Journal of Public Health, 91*, 578–583.
39. Hu, F. B., Stampfer, M. J., Solomon, C., et al. (2001). Physical activity and risk for cardiovascular events in diabetic women. *Annals of Internal Medicine, 134*, 96–105.
40. Li, T. Y., Rana, J. S., Willett, W. C., et al. (2006). Obesity as compared with physical activity in predicting risk of coronary heart disease in women. *Circulation, 113*, 499–506.
41. Lee, I. M., Hennekens, C. H., Berger, K., et al. (1999). Exercise and risk of stroke in male physicians. *Stroke, 30*, 1–6.
42. Myers, J., Kaykha, A., George, S., et al. (2004). Fitness versus physical activity patterns in predicting mortality in men. *American Journal of Medicine, 117*, 912–918.
43. Pedersen, B. K., & Saltin, B. (2006). Evidence for prescribing exercise as therapy in chronic disease. *Scandinavian Journal of Medicine & Science in Sports, 16*(Suppl. 1), 3–63.
44. Blair, S. N., Kohl, H. W., III, Paffenbarger, R. S., et al. (1989). Physical fitness and all-cause mortality: A prospective study of healthy men and women. *JAMA, 262*, 2395–2401.
45. Myers, J. N., Prakash, M., Froelicher, V. F., et al. (2002). Exercise capacity and mortality among men referred for exercise testing. *New England Journal of Medicine, 346*(11), 793–853.
46. Roger, V. L., Jacobsen, S. J., Pellikka, P. A., et al. (1998). Prognostic value of treadmill exercise testing: A population-based study in Olmsted County, Minnesota. *Circulation, 98*, 2836–2841.
47. Goraya, T. Y., Jacobsen, S. J., Pellikka, P. A., et al. (2000). Prognostic value of treadmill exercise testing in elderly persons. *Annals of Internal Medicine, 132*, 862–870.
48. Sui, X., LaMonte, M. J., Laditka, J. N., et al. (2007). Cardiorespiratory fitness and adiposity as mortality predictors in older adults. *JAMA, 298*, 2507–2516.
49. Aktas, M. K., Ozduran, V., Pothier, C. E., et al. (2004). Global risk scores and exercise testing for predicting all-cause mortality in a preventive medicine program. *JAMA, 292*, 1462–1468.
50. Ekelund, L. G., Haskell, W. L., Johnson, J. L., et al. (1988). Physical fitness as a predictor of cardiovascular mortality in asymptomatic North American men: The Lipid Research Clinics Mortality Follow-up Study. *New England Journal of Medicine, 319*, 1379–1384.
51. Mora, S., Redberg, R. F., Cui, Y., et al. (2003). Ability of exercise testing to predict cardiovascular and all-cause death in asymptomatic women. A 20-year follow-up of the Lipid Research Clinics Prevalence Study. *JAMA, 290*, 1600–1607.
52. Gulati, M., Pandey, D. K., Arnsdorf, M. F., et al. (2003). Exercise capacity and the risk of death in women. The St James Women Take Heart Project. *Circulation, 108*, 1554–1559.
53. Lauer, M. S., Pothier, C. E., Magid, D. J., et al. (2007). An externally validated model for predicting long-term survival after exercise treadmill testing in patients with suspected coronary artery disease and a normal electrocardiogram. *Annals of Internal Medicine, 147*, 821–828.
54. Kannel, W. B., Wilson, P., & Blair, S. N. (1985). Epidemiological assessment of the role of physical activity and fitness in development of cardiovascular disease. *American Heart Journal, 109*, 876–885.
55. Thompson, P. D., Buchner, D. M., Pina, I. L., et al. (2003). Exercise and physical activity in the prevention and treatment of atherosclerotic cardiovascular disease. A statement from the American Heart association Council on Clinical Cardiology (Subcommittee on Exercise, Rehabilitation, and Prevention) and the Council on Nutrition, Physical Activity, and Metabolism (Subcommittee on Physical Activity). *Circulation, 107*, 3109–3116.
56. World Health Organization. (2003). *Health and development through physical activity and sport.* Retrieved December 23, 2008, from www.whqlibdoc.who.int/hq/2003/who_nmh_pah_03.2.pdf.
57. Shaw, L. (1981). Effects of a prescribed supervised exercise program on mortality and cardiovascular morbidity in patients after myocardial infarction. *American Journal of Cardiology, 48*, 39–44.
58. Vermuelen, A., Lie, K., & Durber, D. (1983). Effects of cardiac rehabilitation after myocardial infarction: Changes in coronary risk factors and long term prognosis. *American Heart Journal, 105*, 798–801.
59. Kallio, V., Lamalainen, H., Hakkila, J., et al. (1979). Reduction of sudden deaths by a multifactorial intervention program after acute myocardial infarction. *Lancet, 2*, 1091–1094.
60. May, G. S., Eberlein, K. A., Furberg, C. D., et al. (1982). Secondary prevention after myocardial infarction: A review of long-term trials. *Progress in Cardiovascular Disease, 24*, 331–362.
61. Froelicher, V. F., & Myers, J. N. (2006). *Exercise and the heart* (5th ed.). Philadelphia: W.B. Saunders.
62. Duscha, B. D., Schulze, C., Robbins, J. L., et al. (2008). Implications of chronic heart failure on peripheral vasculature and skeletal muscle before and after exercise training. *Heart Failure Reviews, 13*, 21–37.
63. Myers, J. N. (1995). Physiologic adaptations to exercise and immobility. In S. L. Woods, E. S. Sivarajan-Froelicher, C. J. Halpenny, et al. (Eds.), *Cardiac nursing* (3rd ed., pp. 147–162). Philadelphia: JB Lippincott.
64. Pavy-Le Traon, E., Heer, M., Narici, M. V., et al. (2007). From space to earth: Advances in human physiology from 20 years of bed red studies (1986–2006). *European Journal of Applied Physiology, 101*, 143–194.
65. American Association of Cardiovascular and Pulmonary Rehabilitation. (2004). *Guidelines for cardiac rehabilitation and secondary prevention programs* (4th ed.). Champaign, IL: Human Kinetics.

66. Pina, I. L., Apstein, C. S., Balady, G. J., et al. (2003). Exercise and heart failure: A statement from the American Heart Association Committee on Exercise, Rehabilitation, and Prevention. *Circulation, 107*(8), 1210–1225.
67. Wood, P. (1968). *Diseases of the heart and circulation* (3rd ed.). London: Eyre and Spottiswood.
68. Sivarajan-Froelicher, E. S., Snydsman, A., Smith, B., et al. (1977). Low-level treadmill testing of 41 patients with acute myocardial infarction prior to discharge from hospital. *Heart & Lung, 6*, 975–980.
69. Froelicher, V. F., Perdue, S., Pewen, W., et al. (1987). Application of meta-analysis using an electronic spread sheet to exercise testing in patients after myocardial infarction. *American Journal of Medicine, 83*, 1045–1054.
70. American College of Sports Medicine. (2006). *Guidelines for exercise testing and prescription* (7th ed.). Baltimore: Lippincott Williams & Wilkins.
71. Graves, J. E., & Franklin, B. A. (2001). *Resistance training for health and rehabilitation.* Champaign, IL: Human Kinetics.
72. American College of Sports Medicine. (2003). *ACSM fitness book.* Champaign, IL: Human Kinetics.
73. Piscatella, J., & Franklin, B. A. (2003). *Take a load off your heart.* New York: Workman Publishing.
74. Van Camp, S. P., & Peterson, R. A. (1986). Cardiovascular complications of outpatient cardiac rehabilitation programs. *JAMA, 256*, 1160–1163.
75. Franklin, B. A., Bonzheim, K., Gordon, S., et al. (1998). Safety of medically supervised outpatient cardiac rehabilitation exercise therapy: A 16 year follow-up. *Chest, 114*, 902–906.
76. Myers, J. (2000). Effects of exercise training on abnormal ventilatory responses to exercise in patients with chronic heart failure. *Congestive Heart Failure, 6*, 243–249.
77. Clark, A. L., Poole-Wilson, P. A., & Coats, A. J. (1996). Exercise limitation in chronic heart failure: Central role of the periphery. *Journal of the American College of Cardiology, 28*, 1092–1102.
78. Arena, R., Myers, J., & Guazzi, M. (2008). The clinical and research applications of aerobic capacity and ventilatory efficiency in heart failure: An evidence-based review. *Heart Failure Reviews, 13*, 245–269. (Nov 7—e-pub).
79. Ades, P. A., Balady, G. J., & Berra, K. (2001). Transforming exercise-based cardiac rehabilitation programs into secondary prevention centers: A national imperative. *Journal of Cardiopulmonary Rehabilitation, 21*, 263–272.
80. Balady, G., Williams, M. A., Ades, P. A., et al. (2007). Core components of cardiac rehabilitation/secondary prevention programs 2007 update: A scientific statement from the American Heart Association Exercise, Cardiac Rehabilitation and Prevention Committee, the Council on Clinical Cardiology; the Council on Cardiovascular Nursing, Epidemiology and Prevention, and Nutrition, Physical Activity, and Metabolism; American Association of Cardiovascular and Pulmonary Rehabilitation. *Journal of Cardiopulmonary Rehabilitation and Prevention, 27*, 121–129.
81. Ades, P. (2001). Cardiac rehabilitation and secondary prevention of coronary heart disease. *New England Journal of Medicine, 345*, 892–902.
82. Cushman, W. C., & Basile, J. (2006). Achieving blood pressure goals: Why aren't we? *Journal of Clinical Hypertension, 12*, 865–872.
83. Sueta, C., Chowdhury, M., & Boccussi, S. (1999). Analysis of the degree of undertreatment of hyperlipidemia and congestive heart failure secondary to coronary artery disease. *American Journal of Cardiology, 83*, 1303–1307.
84. Myers, J. (2005). Physical activity The missing prescription. *European Journal of Cardiovascular Prevention and Rehabilitation, 12*, 85–86.
85. Schrott, H., Bittner, V., Vittinghoff, E., et al. (1997). Adherence to national cholesterol education program treatment goals in postmenopausal women with heart disease: The heart and estrogen/progestin replacement study (HERS). *JAMA, 277*, 1281–1286.
86. Ribisl, P. M. (2002). The inclusive chronic disease model: Reaching beyond cardiopulmonary patients. In J. Jobin, F. Maltais, P. Poirier, P. Leblanc, & C. Simard (Eds.), *Advancing the frontiers of cardiopulmonary rehabilitation* (pp. 29–36). Champaign, IL: Human Kinetics.
87. Gordon, N. F., Salmon, R. D., Mitchell, B. S., et al. (2001). Innovative approaches to comprehensive cardiovascular disease risk reduction in clinical and community-based settings. *Current Atherosclerosis Reports, 3*, 498–506.
88. DeBusk, R. F., Haskell, W. L., Miller, N. H., et al. (1985). Medically directed at-home rehabilitation soon after clinically uncomplicated acute myocardial infarction: A new model for patient care. *American Journal of Cardiology, 55*, 25–89.
89. Ades, P., Pashkow, F., Fletcher, G., et al. (2000). A controlled trial of cardiac rehabilitation in the home setting using electrocardiographic and voice transtelephonic monitoring. *American Heart Journal, 139*, 543–548.
90. Inglis, S. C., Pearson, S., Treen, S., et al. (2006). Extending the horizon in chronic heart failure: Effects of multidisciplinary, home-based intervention relative to usual care. *Circulation, 114*, 2466–2473.
91. DeBusk, R. F., Houston-Miller, N., Superko, H. R., et al. (1994). A case-management system for coronary risk factor modification after acute myocardial infarction. *Annals of Internal Medicine, 120*, 721–729.
92. Haskell, W. L., Alderman, E. L., Fair, J. M., et al. (1994). Effects of intensive multiple risk factor reduction on coronary atherosclerosis and clinical cardiac events in men and women with coronary artery disease. The Stanford Coronary Risk Intervention Project (SCRIP). *Circulation, 89*, 975–990.
93. Levnecht, L., Schriefer, J., Schriefer, J., et al. (1997). Combining case management, pathways, and report cards for secondary cardiac prevention. *Journal of Quality Improvement, 23*, 162–174.
94. Fonarow, G., Gawlinski, A., Moughrabi, S., et al. (2001). Improved treatment of coronary heart disease by implementation of a Cardiac Hospitalization Atherosclerosis Management Program (CHAMP). *American Journal of Cardiology, 87*, 819–822.
95. West, J. A., Miller, N. H., Parker, K., et al. (1997). A comprehensive management system for heart failure improves clinical outcomes and reduces medical resource utilization. *American Journal of Cardiology, 79*(1), 58–63.
96. Goebbels, U., Myers, J. N., Dziekan, G., et al. (1998). A randomized comparison of exercise training in patients with normal vs. reduced ventricular function. *Chest, 113*, 1387–1393.

CHAPTER 38

Obesity: An Overview of Assessment and Treatment

Lora E. Burke / Patricia K. Tuite / Melanie Warziski Turk

Obesity is a multifactorial disease involving complex interactions among genetic, metabolic, environmental, cultural, and psychosocial factors. Estimates from the 2003–2004 National Health and Nutrition Examination Survey (NHANES) indicate that 66.3% of the U.S. population is either overweight (body mass index [BMI] 25 to 29.9 kg/m^2) or obese (BMI ≥ 30 kg/m^2),[1] with significant increases in the overweight prevalence among children and adolescents, and obesity prevalence in men between 1999 and 2004.[2] In the United States today, obesity has become a pandemic, the most common nutritional problem, the second most preventable cause of death, a significant contributor to increased health care costs, and a condition that lessens life expectancy and reduces quality of life across the lifespan.[3] This medical condition is not limited to the United States, and the World Health Organization (WHO) has now deemed overnutrition to be a health concern.[4] Nearly 2.3 billion adults will be overweight and more than 700 million will be obese by 2015 according to estimates by the WHO. Despite overweight and obesity once being regarded as a problem of affluent countries, the prevalence of these conditions is on the increase in low- and middle-income countries, especially in metropolitan areas.[5] See Figure 38-1 for the estimated prevalence of obesity in several countries.

Obesity has been linked to a host of chronic disorders associated with heart disease, including type 2 diabetes, dyslipidemia, and hypertension.[6] It is associated with deleterious effects on the heart and circulatory system, contributing to an increased risk of arrhythmia, sudden death, congestive heart failure, and ischemic heart disease.[7,8] Moreover, several physiologic parameters that affect cardiovascular risk factors are associated with obesity, such as lipoprotein oxidizability, arterial blood pressure, hemostatic or fibrinolytic abnormalities, and C-reactive protein, a vascular inflammatory marker.[9,10] Obesity was established as a major risk factor for coronary heart disease (CHD) in 1998.

In the midst of the mounting evidence demonstrating the deleterious effects of obesity on health in general, and on the cardiovascular system in particular, research has demonstrated numerous benefits to health by as little as 5% to 10% reduction in initial weight.[6] However, survey data show that 33% of men and 46% of women are attempting to lose and maintain weight but approximately only 20% are using a combination of reduced caloric intake and at least 150 minutes of weekly physical activity during leisure time to achieve weight loss.[11] These facts highlight the importance of identifying the patient at risk and implementing an early treatment course that may prevent the development of obesity.

This major health problem began to receive increasing attention from the scientific community in the mid-1990s. Indeed, in 1997, a paper was published recognizing obesity as a chronic disease.[12] The work of several organizations and policymaking groups helped draw attention to obesity as a health concern; for example, the Institute of Medicine published criteria for evaluating weight-management programs and other organizations published guidelines for treatment.[13,14] In 1998, the National Heart, Lung, and Blood Institute (NHLBI) issued the *Evidence report*,[15] which provided empirically based guidelines for the identification, evaluation, and treatment of overweight and obesity in adults. The guidelines are being updated by the NHLBI in 2008. Today, other organizations are becoming involved in this increasing public health concern. America on the Move is a national nonprofit online organization whose goal is to improve the health of Americans by advocating small changes in eating and physical activity routines to promote weight loss or cessation of weight gain. This organization offers free web-based programs and tools to individuals, groups, and communities to encourage changes like decreasing daily caloric intake by 100 cal and increasing daily physical activity by 2,000 steps.[16] On the international level, the WHO began addressing the issue through the International Obesity Task Force.[17] However, despite all the attention given to this serious public health problem, this problem is not being addressed by clinicians or policymakers to the extent that previous health threats, such as the use of tobacco, have been addressed. When patients' visits to their family physicians were observed, only one in four received any nutritional counseling.[18] Health care professionals can help slow the trend of excess weight by educating and counseling their patients about maintaining a healthy weight and how to use healthy lifestyle measures to reduce excess weight.

This chapter draws on the growing volume of empirical literature pertaining to obesity and the evidence-based guidelines to provide an overview of treatment of overweight and obesity. It begins with a review of the process of identification and evaluation of a patient's risk status and the selection of appropriate treatment. The major components of treatment are covered: lifestyle modification, which includes dietary, exercise, and behavioral therapy; drug therapy; and surgical therapy. Finally, maintenance strategies to enhance long-term adherence to the lifestyle changes that facilitated the weight loss are reviewed.

IDENTIFICATION AND ASSESSMENT OF THE OVERWEIGHT OR OBESE PATIENT

Weight Status

In 1998, the United States adopted the cutoff points for the classification of overweight and obesity based on BMI developed by the WHO.[17] These criteria define normal weight as a BMI range of 18.50 to 24.99 kg/m^2, overweight as a BMI of

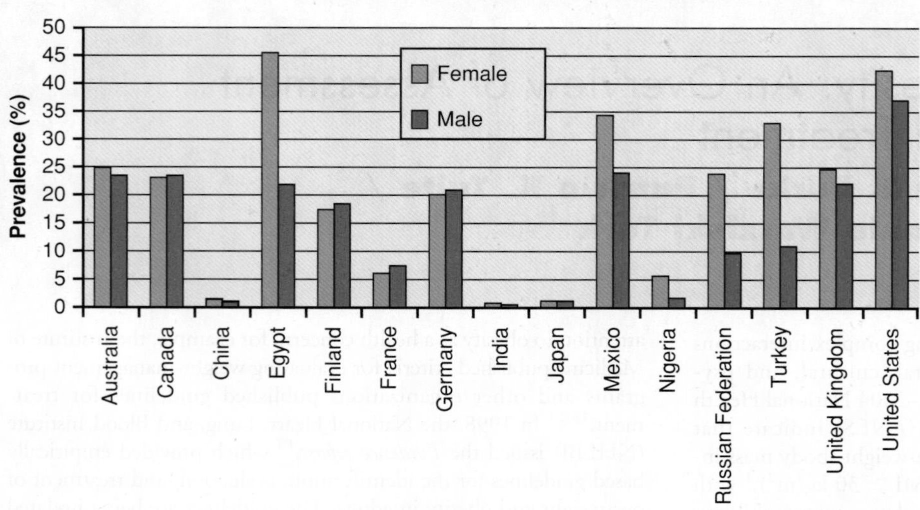

■ **Figure 38-1** Age-standardized estimates for obesity by country for persons aged ≥15 years in 2005. (Prevalence statistics taken from http://www.who.int/ncd_surveillance/infobase/web/InfoBasePolicyMaker/reports/Reporter.aspx?id=1.)

25.00 to 29.99 kg/m^2, and obese as a BMI of 30 kg/m^2 or more.[15,17] Further information specified that Asian populations have a higher amount of body fat than Caucasian populations at the same BMI. This information led the WHO to suggest that persons of Asian descent may have increasing but tolerable health risks at a BMI range of 18.50 to 23 kg/m^2, an elevated risk with a BMI between 23 and 27.5 kg/m^2, and a high risk at a BMI > 27.5 kg/m^2.[19] An evidence-based review concluded that BMI should be considered as another vital sign to screen for obesity and overweight and to decide upon treatment options[6] (see Display 38-1).

Waist (Abdominal) Circumference

Central or visceral obesity is an excess accumulation of fat in the abdomen that is out of proportion to total body fat.[15] Intra-abdominal obesity is considered more sensitive and specific than BMI as a predictor of obesity-related morbidity and mortality[20,21]; a large waist circumference increases the risk of myocardial infarction, heart failure, and death from all causes in patients with cardiovascular disease.[22] Visceral obesity can be measured more accurately by computed tomography or magnetic resonance imaging, but these are expensive and impractical for clinical assessment in a practitioner's office. NHLBI's evidence-based report recommended that waist circumference be included with the BMI in the clinical assessment.[15] Whether to use these criteria to determine treatment may be a clinical decision made on an individual patient basis. In addition, waist circumference can be a valuable marker to monitor progress in weight loss and provide feedback to the patient.

Waist circumference is a clinically acceptable method to assess the patient's visceral or abdominal fat content from baseline through weight loss treatment. Gender-specific cutoffs have been established to identify relative risk for development of obesity-associated risks factors. Men with a waistline circumference greater than 40 in. (102 cm) and women with a waistline circumference greater than 35 in. (88 cm) are at high risk for development of obesity-related morbidity (e.g., type 2 diabetes, dyslipidemia, and cardiovascular disease).[23] Because of an increased health risk associated with a smaller waist circumference in Asian populations, these cutoff points have been lowered for persons of Asian descent. South Asian and Chinese individuals have an increased risk at a waist circumference of ≥90 cm (35.5 in.) for men and ≥80 cm (31.5 in.) for women. Japanese men and women are at higher risk with a waist circumference of ≥85 cm (33.5 in.) and ≥90 cm (35.5 in.), respectively.[24,25] For Korean adults the suitable cutoff for waist circumference is 85 cm (33.5 in.) for women and 90 cm (35.5 in.) for men.[26] Patients of normal weight with increased waist circumference measurements may be at increased risk of cardiovascular disease. Because patients with a BMI of more than 35 kg/m^2 exceed the waist circumference cutoffs, these indicators of relative risk lose their predictive power, making it unnecessary to measure waist circumference in this group[15] (Table 38-1) for the classification of overweight and obesity with waist circumference incorporated in the relative risk assessment. See also Display 38-2.

DISPLAY 38-1 BMI Measurement Procedure

Weight and height measurements, required for the BMI determination, should be taken with the patient wearing undergarments and no shoes. Using the height and weight values, the BMI can be calculated or determined by available normograms.[15] The BMI is calculated as follows:

$$\text{BMI} = \text{weight (kg)}/\text{height (m)}^2$$

The BMI can be estimated in pounds and inches as follows:

$$[\text{weight (pounds)}/\text{height (inches)}^2]\ 704.5$$

Assessment of Cardiovascular Disease Risk Factors

Having established the patient's relative risk based on the overweight/obesity and abdominal obesity criteria, the third part of the assessment is determination of the patient's absolute risk status in terms of comorbid conditions or risk factors for cardiovascular disease.

Very High Absolute Risk

Patients who are overweight or obese or have abdominal obesity are considered at very high risk if they have the following disease

Table 38-1 ■ CLASSIFICATION OF OVERWEIGHT AND OBESITY BY BMI, WAIST CIRCUMFERENCE, AND ASSOCIATED RISK*

			Disease Risk* Relative to Normal Weight and Waist Circumference	
	BMI (kg/m2)	Obesity Class	Men ≤102 cm (≤40 in.) Women ≤88 cm (≤35 in.)	>102 cm (>40 in.) >88 cm (>35 in.)
Underweight	<18.5		—	—
Normal†	18.5–24.9		—	—
Overweight	25.0–29.9		Increased	High
Obesity	30.0–34.9	I	High	Very high
	35.0–39.9	II	Very high	Very high
Extreme Obesity	≥40	III	Extremely high	Extremely high

*Disease risk for type 2 diabetes, hypertension, and CVD.
†Increased waist circumference can also be a marker for increased risk even in persons of normal weight.
Original Source: WHO. (1997). *Preventing and managing the global epidemic of obesity. Report of the World Health Organization Consultation of Obesity.* Geneva, Switzerland: Author. Adapted from original source for National Heart, Lung, and Blood Institute. (1998). *Evidence report on detection, evaluation, and treatment of overweight and obesity.* Bethesda, MD: National Institutes of Health.

conditions: established CHD, presence of other atherosclerotic diseases (peripheral arterial disease, abdominal aortic aneurysm, or symptomatic carotid disease), type 2 diabetes, sleep apnea, or target organ damage in the hypertensive patient. People meeting these profiles require aggressive treatment to reduce their cardiovascular disease risk profiles (e.g., cholesterol-lowering therapy and blood pressure control).[15]

High Absolute Risk

Patients with obesity who have three or more of the following risk factors can be considered at high absolute risk for obesity-related comorbid conditions: cigarette smoking; hypertension; low-density lipoprotein (LDL)-cholesterol of 160 mg/dL or more, or 130 to 159 mg/dL in the presence of two or more other risk factors; high-density lipoprotein (HDL)-cholesterol less than 35 mg/dL; impaired fasting glucose; family history of premature CHD; and men aged 45 years or older or women aged 55 years or older or of postmenopausal status. The provider should follow the established guidelines in estimating absolute risk status and in treating the identified risk factors,[23] which are discussed in detail in other chapters.

Additional Factors That Increase Absolute Risk

The presence of additional risk factors (e.g., physical inactivity and elevated triglycerides) can increase a patient's absolute risk to a level higher than that estimated from the preceding categories.[15,27]

DISPLAY 38-2 Waist (Abdominal) Circumference Measurement Procedure

The patient should be dressed in undergarments or in an examining gown. Standing to the right of the patient, palpate the upper hipbone to locate the right iliac crest and draw a horizontal mark just above the upper border of the iliac crest. Cross that line with a vertical mark on the midaxillary line. Place the measuring tape in a horizontal plane (parallel to the floor) around the abdomen at the level of the marked point and hold the tape snug to, but not compressing the skin. Take the measurement at a normal minimal respiration.[15]

Elevated triglycerides in the patient with obesity may represent a common manifestation of a lipoprotein phenotype that includes elevated triglycerides, low HDL levels, and small LDL particles, a pattern considered atherogenic.[7,8, 27,28] There are several additional factors being investigated for their contribution to the risk profile associated with obesity, for example, excess visceral adiposity, hyperinsulinemia that accompanies insulin resistance, and adipose tissue-released proinflammatory cytokines such as interleukin-1, interleukin-6, tumor necrosis factor-α, resistin, or reduced adiponectin (anti-inflammatory).[3,29,30]

Cardiovascular-Related Conditions Influenced by Obesity

Several conditions related to cardiovascular disease are associated with increased body weight (Table 38-2), for example, CHD, hypertension, and congestive heart failure, and these may require additional medical management. The provider needs to address these conditions and make the patient aware that one's cardiovascular health is influenced by his or her weight. More importantly, discussing the significant impact of as little as a 5% reduction in weight may provide motivation for the patient to initiate behavior change for weight loss.

Undertreated Groups

Two groups that providers may be reluctant to treat are patients who are older than 65 years and smokers. However, elderly persons who are obese still suffer from an increased burden of disease such as hypertension, diabetes, osteoarthritis (OA) and decreased mobility.[31,32] Improved pulmonary function, a reduction in antihypertensive medications, and less pain from OA are benefits derived from intentional weight loss in the elderly people who are obese.[33] In particular, therapeutic goals for treatment of elderly patients with obesity should include decreasing abdominal fat and preserving muscle mass and strength.[34] Weight reduction improves functional status and reduces concomitant risk factors in the older population in a way similar to that in the younger adult[35]; therefore, this subgroup should at least receive interventions to prevent weight gain, if not achieve weight reduction. The overweight or obese smoker carries excess risk from obesity-associated risk factors. This patient should be advised to quit, and prevention of

Table 38-2 ■ CARDIOVASCULAR-RELATED CONDITIONS ASSOCIATED WITH OVERWEIGHT AND OBESITY

Condition	Details About Disease or Condition
CHD	Nurses' Health Study data reveal a 3.3-fold increase in risk for developing CHD with a BMI of >29 compared to women with a BMI of <21; a BMI between 27 and 29 has a relative risk of 1.8. Generally, risk increases as BMI increases.
Hypertension	BP is often increased in overweight persons. In the SOS, 44% to 51% were hypertensive at baseline. High BP in normal weight persons produces concentric hypertrophy of the heart with ventricular wall thickening; eccentric dilatation occurs in overweight individuals. The combination of hypertension and overweight leads to ventricular wall thickening and increased heart volume, and consequently to increased likelihood of heart failure.
Dyslipidemia (low HDL, high LDL, elevated triglycerides)	Weight gain is associated with increased LDL-cholesterol and reduced HDL; there is a positive correlation between triglyceride level and BMI.
Elevated plasma glucose, insulin resistance, and metabolic syndrome	The risk of type 2 diabetes increases with the duration of overweight and the degree of overweight, for example, in the Nurses' Health Study, women with a BMI of >35 had a 40-fold increase in relative risk. Risk for diabetes also increases with the amount of central adiposity.
	Weight gain increases diabetes risk; more than 60% of diabetes cases can be attributed to overweight.
	Obesity leads to increased insulin secretion and insulin resistance, which is considered the trademark of the metabolic syndrome. A central trait of the metabolic syndrome is increased central adiposity or visceral fat, which releases free fatty acids that impair insulin clearance by the liver and modified peripheral metabolism.
Increased waist circumference	Given similar levels of LDL cholesterol, CHD risk is significantly higher in persons with small dense LDL, which is associated with central body fat. A positive association has been shown between central adiposity and elevated triglycerides and decreased HDL.
Inflammation	Obesity is associated with an increase in circulating inflammatory markers, for example, cytokines (interleukin-6, interleukin-18, and P-selectin), as well as C-reactive protein (CRP). Excess cytokines, which are secreted by the adipose cells and called adipokines, are associated with insulin resistance and considered a predictor of atherosclerotic events. Levels of adiponectin and interleukin-10, anti-inflammatory cytokines, are reduced in the presence of weight gain and obesity. A reduction in CRP has been shown to be directly related to the amount of weight lost, fat mass, and change in waist circumference.
Congestive heart failure	Obese patients experience an increase in stroke volume and cardiac output resulting in hypertrophy of the left ventricle. This can occur with or without hypertension. These changes in the ventricle predispose an individual to left-sided heart failure and often dilated cardiomyopathy. An increase in BMI is also related to changes in the right side of the heart, most frequently due to an increase in pulmonary hypertension from sleep apnea.
Stroke	To adequately perfuse the higher volume of adipose tissue, obese persons have an increased total blood volume. Stroke and atrial fibrillation are more common in the obese patient due to dilatation of the atria from a higher fluid volume.
Thromboembolic events	A waist circumference >39 in. (100 cm) in men is related to an increase risk of venous thromboembolism. Women appear to have an increased risk of pulmonary embolism associated with an increased BMI, but this relationship is unclear in men.
Cardiac arrhythmias/ECG changes	The dilated cardiomyopathy that can be seen in obesity increases one's risk for sudden cardiac death. Obesity could also cause changes in the electrocardiogram. The heart can be somewhat displaced because of an elevated diaphragm while lying down. There is also a greater distance between the electrodes and the heart due to an increase in adipose tissue. One may see some ST-segment or T-wave abnormalities and left atrial abnormalities due to cardiac dilatation. A prolonged QT interval may also be seen, which predisposes one to cardiac arrhythmias.

weight gain should be addressed through lifestyle approaches, with the emphasis on smoking abstinence.[15] When attempting to address multiple behavior changes, rather than concurrent treatment, an improved outcome may result from a sequential approach that focuses on assisting the patient to stop smoking before initiating behavioral weight-management strategies.[36]

CLINICAL EVALUATION

Baseline assessment of the cardiac patient includes the BMI, waist circumference, and cardiovascular risk profile, as well as noncardiovascular conditions, for example, sleep apnea, OA, gallstones, and gynecologic abnormalities. These factors need to be evaluated so that obesity is treated in the context of the patient's risk profile and existence of comorbid conditions.[7] Weight loss frequently ameliorates risks by reducing blood pressure and triglycerides, as well as lessens the impact of other comorbid conditions. Therefore, risk factors should be addressed through weight loss treatment. The NHLBI *Evidence report*[15] includes an algorithm that addresses the treatment decisions based on that assessment (Fig. 38-2). This algorithm is focused on weight-related assessment and treatment and does not include evaluation for other disorders for which the patient may be seeing a health care provider. As noted in Figure 38-2, if the patient's BMI and waist circumference are in the normal range, these parameters should be measured again in 2 years. For the patient who is of normal weight, brief counseling about prevention of future weight gain should be provided. Knowing that weight gain can be expected from most patients, maintenance of weight is a positive outcome and patients should receive reinforcement for maintaining a healthy weight.

Clinical History

For the patient whose parameters are not normal, assessment needs to include the patient's history, including prior excess weight or weight fluctuations. If not done previously, a physical examination and laboratory measurements to assess lipid profile, glucose level, and related parameters need to be performed. The provider needs to identify existing cardiovascular disease and the presence of possible end-organ damage.

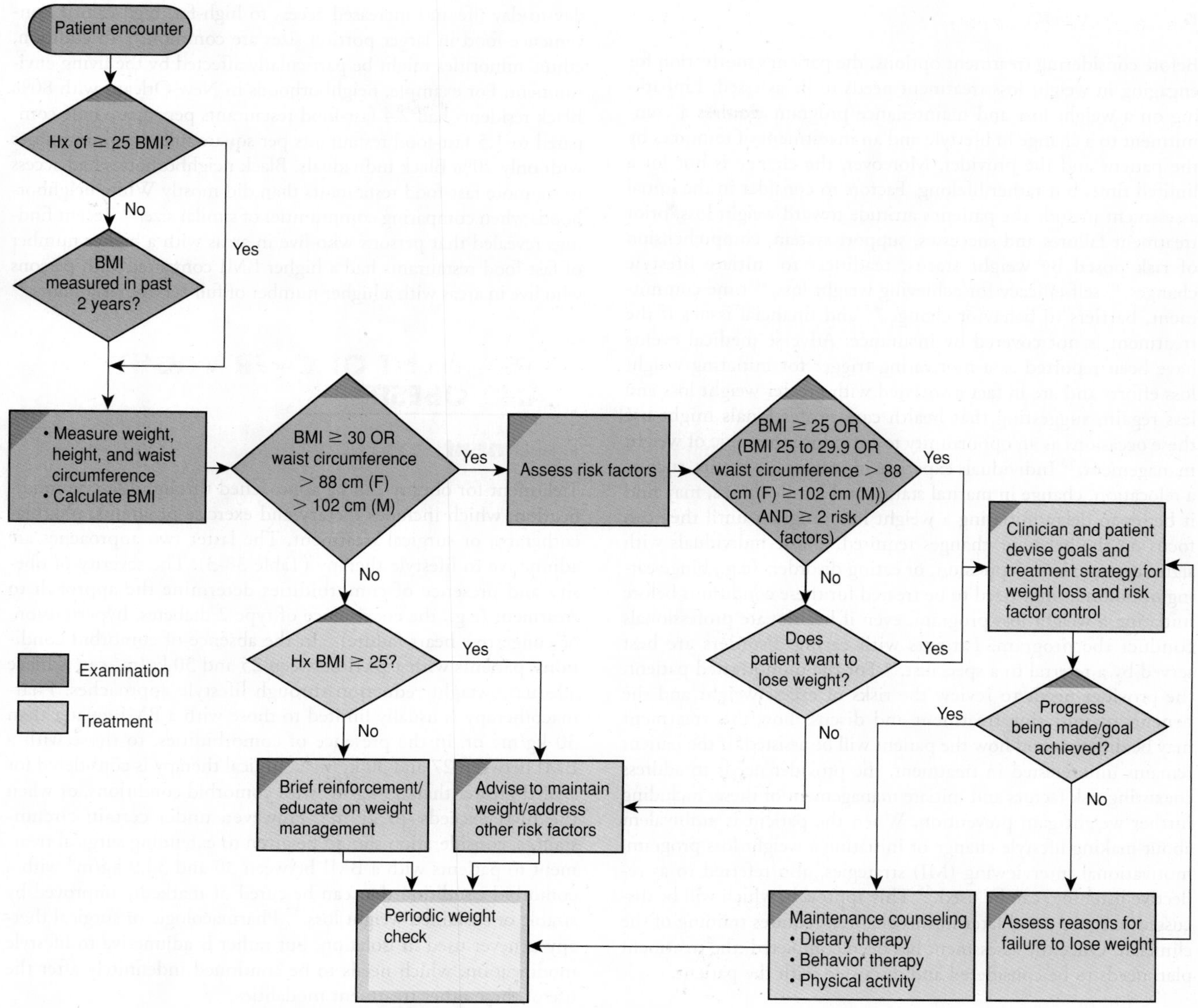

Figure 38-2 Treatment algorithm. This algorithm applies only to the assessment for overweight and obesity and subsequent decisions based on that assessment. It does not include any initial overall assessment for cardiovascular risk factors or diseases that are indicated. (Adapted from National Heart, Lung, and Blood Institute, Obesity Education Initiative Expert Panel on the Identification Evaluation and Treatment of Overweight and Obesity. [1998]. *Clinical guidelines on the identification, evaluation, and treatment of overweight and obesity in adults: The evidence report.* Bethesda, MD: National Institutes of Health.)

Eating and Physical Activity Patterns

A nutritional and physical activity assessment provides additional information that can be used in the treatment plan. This can be done by having the patient complete a 3-day food and activity diary, which should include two work and one nonwork or leisure-type days. When using a 3-day food and activity diary, the patient needs to be instructed on completion of the diary and the details to be included (e.g., exact amount of food eaten and inclusion of recipes or package labels if the food is unusual). Food frequency, 24-hour dietary recalls and activity questionnaires are another means of assessing past year food consumption or current level of physical activity.[37–39] During the 24-hour dietary recall, the trained interviewer asks the patient to recall every food and drink that was consumed in the previous 24 hours. The interview may be conducted either in-person or via the telephone, is usually unannounced, and typically takes 20 to 30 minutes to complete; this assessment tool may be more commonly used in a research setting.[37]

Patient Motivation

Before considering treatment options, the patient's motivation for engaging in weight loss treatment needs to be assessed. Embarking on a weight loss and maintenance program requires a commitment to a change in lifestyle and an investment of resources by the patient and the provider. Moreover, the change is not for a limited time, but rather lifelong. Factors to consider in the initial assessment include the patient's attitude toward weight loss, prior treatment failures and successes, support system, comprehension of risk posed by weight status, readiness to initiate lifestyle changes,[40] self-efficacy for achieving weight loss,[41] time commitment, barriers to behavior change,[42] and financial issues if the treatment is not covered by insurance. Adverse medical events have been reported as a motivating trigger for initiating weight loss efforts and are in fact associated with greater weight loss and less regain, suggesting that health care professionals might use these occasions as an opportunity to introduce the topic of weight management.[43] Individuals experiencing major life events, such as a relocation, change in marital status, and family illness, may find it better to delay initiating a weight loss program until they can focus on the behavior changes required. Those individuals with significant anxiety, depression, or eating disorders (e.g., binge eating or bulimia) may need to be treated for these conditions before initiating a weight loss program, even if health care professionals conduct the program. Patients with eating disorders are best served by a referral to a specialist.[44] For the unmotivated patient, the provider needs to review the risks of excess weight and the benefits of initiating treatment and discuss how this treatment may be different and how the patient will be assisted. If the patient remains uninterested in treatment, the provider needs to address coexisting risk factors and initiate management of these, including further weight gain prevention. When the patient is ambivalent about making lifestyle change or initiating a weight loss program, motivational interviewing (MI) strategies, also referred to as reflective listening, can be used.[45] This approach, which will be discussed in more detail later in this chapter, requires training of the clinician. Once the assessment has been completed, the treatment plan needs to be considered and discussed with the patient.

Provider Assessment of Patient's Objectives

The manner and attitude of the health care professional when addressing the patient's obesity and weight management may be an important determinant of the patient's receptivity. There is some evidence that health care professionals doubt a patient's motivation or ability to make lifestyle changes and thus might be nonsupportive of the patient's goals.[46] The patient needs to define the problem and the clinician needs to be nonjudgmental in discussing the behavior and the weight problem. When discussing treatment options with the patient, conveying an empathetic understanding of the challenges that come with the long-term lifestyle changes is important. Finally, eliciting the patient's objective for the treatment and mutually agreeing on a plan of action for the short- and long term will enhance the probability of a positive outcome.[47,48]

Environmental Barriers to Weight Loss

Environmental obstacles exist partially as a result of our technologically advanced society where reduced energy expenditure in day-to-day life and increased access to high-fat, high-calorie convenience food in larger portion sizes are common.[49] In addition, ethnic minorities might be particularly affected by the living environment. For example, neighborhoods in New Orleans with 80% Black residents had 2.4 fast-food restaurants per square mile compared to 1.5 fast-food restaurants per square mile in communities with only 20% Black individuals. Black neighborhoods had access to six more fast-food restaurants than did mostly White neighborhoods when comparing communities of similar size.[50] Recent findings revealed that persons who live in areas with a higher number of fast-food restaurants had a higher BMI compared with persons who live in areas with a higher number of full-service restaurants.[51]

TREATMENT OF OVERWEIGHT AND OBESITY

Treatment Approach

Treatment for obesity can be approached through lifestyle modification, which includes dietary and exercise programs, pharmacotherapy, or surgical treatment. The latter two approaches are adjunctive to lifestyle therapy (Table 38-3). The severity of obesity and presence of comorbidities determine the approach to treatment (e.g., the coexistence of type 2 diabetes, hypertension, or congestive heart failure).[7] In the absence of comorbid conditions, patients with a BMI between 25 and 30 kg/m^2 can achieve adequate weight reduction through lifestyle approaches. Pharmacotherapy is usually limited to those with a BMI greater than 30 kg/m^2 or, in the presence of comorbidities, to those with a BMI between 27 and 30 kg/m^2. Surgical therapy is considered for a BMI greater than 35 kg/m^2 with comorbid conditions, or when the BMI exceeds 40 kg/m^2. However, under certain circumstances, consideration should be given to extending surgical treatment to patients with a BMI between 30 and 34.9 kg/m^2 with a comorbid condition that can be cured or markedly improved by sizable or sustained weight loss.[52] Pharmacologic or surgical therapy is never used in isolation, but rather is adjunctive to lifestyle modification, which needs to be continued indefinitely after the use of these other treatment modalities.

Table 38-3 ■ APPROACHES TO TREATMENT OF OBESITY BY SEVERITY AND DISEASE RISK

BMI	Comorbid Conditions and/or CVD Risk Factors	Treatment Approaches[74]
25–30	Absent	Lifestyle modification*/Prevention of weight gain
27–30	≥2 Present†	Lifestyle modification + pharmacotherapy‡
>30	Absent	Lifestyle modification + pharmacotherapy‡
>35	≥2 Present	Consider surgical therapy‡
>40	Absent	Surgical therapy‡

*Lifestyle modification includes caloric restriction (400 kcal/day deficit), <30% fat diet, exercise at least 5 days/week, and behavioral therapy.

†Comorbid conditions warranting drug therapy: High BP, CHD, type 2 diabetes, congestive heart failure, and sleep apnea.

‡Pharmacotherapy and surgical therapy are adjunctive to lifestyle modification.

Goal of Treatment

The goal of weight loss is not to achieve some cosmetic standard of attractiveness, but rather to reduce morbidity and increase mobility and quality of life. The recommended initial weight loss goal is 10%;[6] however, improvement in obesity-related risk factors for CHD can be observed with as little as a 5% loss of initial weight. If a weight loss of ≥10% is not maintained, reductions in total and LDL-cholesterol revert toward baseline.[7,53] The rate of loss should be approximately 0.5 to 1 lb/week for the moderately obese and 1 to 2 lb/week in the severely obese.[54]

It is important to discuss treatment strategies and goals with the patient because these have to be arrived at through mutual decision making, and there could be a discrepancy between the provider's and the patient's goals.[55] An example would be a 55-year-old woman who has lower body obesity and no additional risk factors but may wish to lose a certain amount of weight that may be unrealistic. This patient may achieve the loss and feel better about her appearance, but if she is unable to sustain this loss, she will regain and feel like a failure. This person may benefit from guidance for a lower weight loss goal and exercise or a plan for stability of current weight. However, if this same woman had central adiposity or presence of risk factors, she should be counseled for achieving a 10% weight reduction. Another scenario might involve an individual without additional risk factors, but a desire to achieve a body weight that is significantly below her current weight and one she has not had since she was in her 20s. The achievement and maintenance of this goal weight is unlikely, as most individuals regain approximately one third of their lost weight in the year after treatment. A patient may benefit from an initial goal of 5% to 10% reduction, and if this is achieved, an additional goal can be established.

It is important for the provider to discuss with the patient what his or her goals are for weight loss. A patient may think that improved personal relationships or professional opportunities will result from achieving the weight loss goal, but this is rarely the case because more than just weight loss is usually necessary for such goals to be realized. The provider needs to emphasize to the patient the health benefits resulting from a 5% to 10% loss, and assist the patient in being realistic about weight loss outcomes.[55–57]

Once the patient and provider have agreed on the treatment approach and the initial goals, it is time to prepare the patient for the course of treatment. Orienting the patient to the active participation required for successful weight loss facilitates cooperation and adherence. Patients need to be instructed how to self-monitor food and caloric intake and expenditure, which requires reading food labels and at least initially, measuring food portions. Conveying understanding and support to the patient during the challenging course of weight loss and providing reinforcement for behavioral change can go a long way in sustaining the person's motivation.

Components of the Treatment

Lifestyle Modification

Lifestyle therapy encompasses three principal components: nutritional or dietary therapy, physical activity and daily activity, and behavioral therapy. The changes in the patient's dietary and activity habits are facilitated and reinforced through the behavioral strategies used in weight loss treatment. The following sections describe the three components of standard lifestyle modification for weight control.

Dietary Therapy

During weight loss treatment, the strongest determinant of the rate and amount of weight loss that will occur is the extent of the negative energy balance.[58] A key component of dietary therapy is a reduction in total caloric intake by 500 to 1,000 kcal/day, resulting in the patient consuming 800 to 1,500 kcal/day. This is referred to as a low-calorie diet and has been shown to reduce weight by 8% over 6 months. A deficit of 500 kcal/day results in a weight loss of 1 lb/week (1 lb is the equivalent of 3,500 kcal). Depending on the patient's baseline weight and the amount of weight loss desired, the patient may follow a diet ranging from 1,000 to 1,200 kcal for women and 1,200 to 1,800 kcal for men.[55] Programs using the lifestyle approach include nutritional education.[59] The focus of the instruction includes the energy value of food (e.g., fat contains 9 cal/g compared to protein and carbohydrates, which contain 4 cal/g), how to read labels, the three types of fat and the recommended distribution of these in the diet, methods to reduce fat and increase fiber and complex carbohydrate intake, and how to prepare food to reduce the addition of calories. Patients also are instructed on recipe modification and ordering from a restaurant menu; some programs include field trips to supermarkets to teach the participants how grocery shopping should be done.

An important component of dietary therapy is addressing both fat and caloric restriction. In general, a 20% to 30% fat diet is recommended and the patient is provided a daily fat gram goal along with the calorie goal.[59] The recommended diet composition is consistent with the Adult Treatment Panel Step I Diet[60] (Table 38-4).

Very-low-calorie diets, which are restricted to less than 800 kcal/day, are no longer recommended for several reasons. They provide inadequate nutrition unless supplemented, require medical supervision to monitor the patient's nutritional and electrolyte status, and increase the risk for development of gallstones. Furthermore, studies have shown that the rapid weight loss is followed by a rapid regain. A recent meta-analysis reported that long-term weight losses (average follow up was 1.9 years) were not different from the low-calorie diet with a mean weight loss of 6.3% ± 3.2% in the very-low-calorie diet groups compared with 5.0% ± 4.0% in the low-calorie diet groups.[61] The benefits of these weight loss plans do not outweigh the risks particularly when long-term outcomes are considered.

Table 38-4 ■ LOW-CALORIE STEP I DIET

Nutrient	Recommended Intake
Calories	Approximately 500 to 1,000 kcal/day reduction from usual intake
Total fat	≤30% of total calories
Saturated fatty acids	8% to 10% of total calories
Monounsaturated fatty acids	Up to 15% of total calories
Polyunsaturated fatty acids	Up to 10% of total calories
Cholesterol	<300 mg/day
Protein	Approximately 15% of total calories
Carbohydrate	≥55% of total calories
Sodium chloride	≤100 mmol/day (approximately 2.4 g of sodium or 6 g of sodium chloride)
Calcium	1,000 to 1,500 mg/day
Fiber	20 to 30 g/day

From National Heart, Lung, and Blood Institute Expert Panel. (1998). *Clinical guidelines on the identification, evaluation, and treatment of overweight and obesity in adults: The evidence report.* Bethesda, MD: National Institutes of Health.

Low-carbohydrate diets have received considerable attention in recent years by the lay public and the scientific community.[62,63] One of the biggest concerns about the low-carbohydrate diet, which is accompanied by a high fat and high protein intake, is its effects on coronary risk factors. However, the studies that have been conducted to evaluate this dietary approach to weight loss have found both benefits and disadvantages to the low-carbohydrate diet in terms of the effect on the lipid profile compared to a low-fat diet. Greater decreases in triglycerides and increases in HDL-cholesterol were noted in those individuals following the low-carbohydrate diet, but LDL-cholesterol decreased more in the low-fat diet groups.[62,63] Although greater short-term weight losses have been noted as a result of following a low-carbohydrate diet, long-term data are still lacking regarding the advantages of this diet for weight loss maintenance, with adherence to the dietary plan playing a more important role in weight loss than does the type of diet.[64] A recent report of a 12-month trial found a low-carbohydrate diet to be superior for weight loss at 12 months, although the mean weight loss was a moderate 4.7 kg.[65]

Another dietary plan for weight loss takes into consideration the glycemic index (GI) of food. The GI rates carbohydrate-rich food based upon whether the carbohydrate breaks down and is absorbed slowly (low GI) or quickly (high GI) during digestion, and the effect on blood glucose levels.[66] How rapidly glucose enters the blood and the resultant insulin response may cause considerable fluctuations in blood glucose, resulting in an individual's hunger returning more quickly.[67] Findings regarding weight loss and a low-GI diet have been equivocal. Some suggest that following a low-GI dietary plan has no significant weight loss benefit in either the short[68,69] or long term.[70] A review of six randomized controlled trials found greater reductions in body mass and total fat mass in those who received the low-GI diet compared with other diets, but the longest study was 6 months in length with a 6-month follow up assessment.[71] A low-glycemic load diet has been noted to have a favorable effect on HDL and triglycerides but not on LDL.[72] Additional information from longer studies is needed before conclusions can be drawn about this dietary plan.

Exercise and Physical Activity

Jakicic and Otto[58] describe the key to managing body weight in terms of energy balance; thus, theoretically, as long as energy intake equals energy expenditure, weight should be maintained. This is the premise for avoiding initial weight gain or preventing regain once weight loss occurs. They further state that in order to lose weight, one must create an energy imbalance that elicits an energy deficit.[58] Exercise can provide that increase in energy expenditure resulting in a deficit.

The amount of physical activity necessary for weight reduction is different from the amount of physical activity required for maintenance of one's health. Current recommendations from the American College of Sports Medicine (ACSM) and the American Heart Association (AHA) to improve health advise individuals between the ages of 18 and 65 years to participate in moderate intensity aerobic physical activity (walking at ~3.5 to 4.0 mph) for a minimum of 30 minutes 5 days/week or vigorous intensity aerobic activity (jogging or biking at 10 mph) for at least 20 minutes 3 days/week in order to maintain one's health.[73] A combination of both moderate and vigorous intensity activity is encouraged, although not necessary. The updated recommendations also suggest that individuals will benefit from activities that increase muscle strength two times per week (8 to 10 exercises using a resistance weight allowing for 8 to 12 repetitions per exercise). For adults older than 65 years it is important for the health care provider to instruct them to use ratings of perceived exertion to monitor their activity level. Older adults should not engage in exercise that is too vigorous for their age or the presence of potential comorbid conditions.[74]

The amount of activity to reduce one's body weight is greater than the above minimum requirements. Evidence suggests that ~450 min/week or at least 45 to 60 min/day is required for a weight loss at the rate of 0.5 kg/week.[75,76] The amount of physical activity needed to maintain weight loss is greater than 60 min/day or >2,500 kcal activity/week.[73,77] New recommendations from the ACSM and AHA state that one should participate in at least 60 to 90 minutes of moderate activity in order to prevent weight gain.[73] Long-term weight loss requires that individuals expend >2,500 kcal/week, but this level of activity is very difficult for both men and women to maintain once the treatment period ends.[77]

Various approaches are available for individuals beginning or expanding their exercise program. Adherence to exercise can be influenced by several factors, including the environment (e.g., supervised or group exercise classes vs. exercising at home) and the economic resources or neighborhood. A recent report from the NHANES data revealed that lower socioeconomic status has the strongest effect on reported physical activity.[78] A study from the Netherlands found that the neighborhoods of lower socioeconomic status individuals were often not conducive to exercise because of high traffic, poor lighting, and high crime rates.[79] However, under the right conditions, having a patient follow an independent exercise program at home may result in improved adherence and weight loss.[58] Another strategy that may improve exercise adherence as well as weight loss maintenance, includes having the patient use several short bouts (10 minutes) of exercise instead of the conventional long bout (20 to 40 minutes).[73]

Bish et al.[11] studied the behaviors of Americans trying to lose weight. They found that about 66% of both men and women use physical activity to assist with their weight loss. The proportion of those utilizing physical activity for weight loss increased among individuals with more education and decreased with increased age. Among women trying to lose weight, non-Hispanic Whites reported using physical activity more often than Hispanic and non-Hispanic Blacks.[11] Individuals who sought out regular care with their primary care providers were also more likely to use physical activity to assist with their weight loss.

Daily activity is another way of improving weight loss efforts. Incorporating activities that result in increased energy expenditure (e.g., using the stairs and walking) can help to increase overall caloric expenditure. Another approach is to encourage patients to decrease the amount of sedentary activities (i.e., watching TV or computer use) and replace them with activities such as gardening or recreational sports. Lifestyle activity can result in positive benefits on physical fitness and cardiovascular risk reduction.[58]

Depending on the patient's age, risk factor profile, and concomitant conditions and symptoms, exercise testing to assess cardiopulmonary function and presence of disease may be indicated. This needs to be determined before initiating an exercise program. Patients also require instruction on injury prevention, how to initiate and maintain an exercise program, proper attire, and weather conditions. The kind of activity or exercise and the amount of time spent engaged in it are recorded in the patient's diaries. Lists of activities and their caloric expenditure are provided to patients so that they can monitor progress toward their exercise goals.[73,74]

Behavioral Therapy

The treatment goal of obesity is to modify eating, physical activity, and cognition or thinking habits that contribute to one's weight problems.[53] Behavioral therapy helps overweight and obese individuals to develop a set of skills that can help regulate their weight.[55] The core of treatment is based on the principle of classical conditioning, which purports that stimuli are presented before or concurrent to a given behavior and then become associated with that behavior. As the events are paired more often, for example, eating high-fat snacks while watching TV, the association between the two becomes stronger and eventually one triggers the other. In behavioral treatment, the goal is to identify and extinguish the cues from the antecedent or stimulus. In the analysis of behavior that occurs in treatment, an individual examines the consequences or reinforcement value of eating and exercise and how to correct negative thoughts that prohibit one from reaching his or her goals.[53,59]

There are three distinguishing characteristics of behavioral treatment for weight loss: goal orientation, process orientation, and making small rather than large behavior changes.[53] Goals are specific, for example, the number of calories or fat grams per day that one should eat and the minutes spent in physical activity. Individuals record food eaten and exercise or physical activity performed in a daily diary and track behavior as to how it compares to the goals, which provides feedback on goal achievement. The process-oriented approach builds on the skill-building philosophy of weight management—that a set of skills can be learned that will enable individuals to identify what they wish to accomplish and what strategies can be learned to permit them to do this. Finally, this treatment approach advocates making small changes, which is based on the learning principle of successive approximation or shaping behavior.[53] Similar to the concept of enhancing self-efficacy, achieving small, incremental successes leads to gradually shaping new behaviors that are reinforced by success and improved self-confidence.[80]

The National Institutes of Health (NIH) treatment guidelines recommend a multidisciplinary approach; the team may include a psychologist, nutritionist, exercise physiologist, nurse, or physician.[15] Although no studies have evaluated the different health care professionals delivering the intervention, the guidelines suggest that providers avail themselves of the expertise offered by professionals who have counseled patients in this area.[15] Since 1974, standard behavioral treatment for weight loss has increased in duration from 8 weeks to an average of 31 weeks, with current research studies lasting 18 to 24 months.[63,81] The typical treatment program begins with weekly group sessions for 4 to 6 months, followed by a gradual decrease in frequency of group sessions, for example, biweekly for an additional 3 to 6 months followed by monthly sessions.[81,82] Behavioral therapy is usually delivered in a closed-group context, that is, the group is formed at the initiation of treatment and no new members are added thereafter. This approach facilitates the development of group cohesiveness, provides empathy and social support and also an acceptable level of competition among the group members.[55]

The Diabetes Prevention Program (DPP) was a 4-year, multicenter trial that targeted 7% weight reduction among individuals with impaired glucose tolerance and used personal coaches to deliver individual sessions.[83] An ongoing randomized, multicenter study, the Look AHEAD trial, tests an intensive lifestyle intervention that is similar to the DPP; however, this study combines individual and group meetings to achieve and maintain weight loss among those with type 2 diabetes.[84] One-year results reveal an average weight loss of 8.6% and improved CVD risk factors among the lifestyle intervention participants. Although the DPP trial, as well as a similar study that was conducted in Finland,[85] was highly successful in using lifestyle modification to achieve 7% weight loss and prevention of diabetes with individual treatment approaches, the group approach is more cost effective for clinical settings.[55] In one study, the use of groups demonstrated better results among those who were randomized to the group sessions than among those who were assigned to receive individual treatment even when that was the approach they preferred.[86] The treatment session usually follows a structured curriculum and also provides adequate time for discussion and problem solving among the group members. The structured content is similar to what is provided in the LEARN program[87] or the DPP protocol, which is available on the DPP Web site.[88] There is a set of behavioral strategies that are implemented in standard behavioral treatment programs to facilitate behavior change, which are described in detail below.

- ***Self-monitoring***—often considered the *sine qua non* of behavioral treatment.[59] It entails having individuals record their food intake, calories, fat grams, and time spent in physical activity in minutes and sometimes identifying the specific activity and its intensity. This requires patients to look up these values in books provided, which makes them aware of the caloric and fat content of food eaten. Self-monitoring may also include recording feelings or mood and circumstances of behavior. The self-monitoring exercise contributes to the functional analysis of behavior and helps individuals identify the barriers to changing behaviors and the high-risk situations they may encounter. Technology and the Internet have provided alternate methods to the paper-and-pencil diary. Dietary and physical activity software for personal digital assistants is available today, which eliminates the need to search for nutrient composition of food in a book since the software contains an extensive database of nutrients and physical activities.[89] Moreover, some software programs date-and-time stamp each entry so the interventionist or provider can determine if the person is recording in a timely manner.[89,90] In addition, programs are available on the Internet that provide the structure for self-monitoring, for example, www.FitDay.com, www.sparkpeople.com, and www.caloriecount.about.com. There is a growing body of evidence that supports the pivotal role self-monitoring plays in successful weight loss outcomes.[91,92]
- ***Goal setting***—patients are given goals for total calories, fat grams and percent of total calories, and energy expenditure through exercise. The goals need to be proximal, specific, and attainable. Goal setting theory predicts that under most circumstances setting specific goals leads to higher performance compared with none or vague goals.[80] Goals need to be specific in outcome, proximal in terms of attainment, and realistic in terms of the person's capability.[93] Success with short-term goals enhances self-efficacy.[94] Goals need to focus on behavior change, for example, substituting a piece of fruit for a high fat snack, rather than on physiological outcomes, for example, serum cholesterol, since behaviors are more directly under a patient's direct control and several factors can influence physiological changes. Goals that are difficult will not be attempted

while those viewed as too easy will not be taken seriously. Providing the patient with regular feedback on goal attainment instills a sense of learning and mastery.[95]

- ***Stimulus control***—considered the hallmark of behavioral therapy.[53] It is based on the assumption that environmental antecedents control behaviors, and that changing the environment to include positive cues for appropriate eating and exercise behaviors leads to desired behavior, for example, remove high-fat food and replace them with attractive fruits that are ready to eat, store other tempting food out of sight, restrict places of eating.[59]
- ***Problem solving***—using the approach described by D'Zurilla and Goldfried,[96] patients are taught four specific steps: identify the problem situation leading to inappropriate eating or exercise behavior, generate solutions, select one solution to test, and evaluate the use of the solution in resolving the problem. It is important that the provider or interventionist permit the participant or patient to generate the potential solutions and when possible, have the person role play or practice how he or she will implement one or two of the potential solutions, for example, interact with another person in a social setting when the person is insisting that the patient eat some food that are high in fat.
- ***Relapse prevention***—patients are taught that lapses are a natural occurrence and should be anticipated and planned for with strategies that can be used in coping with the situation, and thereby prevent relapses.[97] Relapse may become an issue during high-risk situations such as the holidays or vacations and it is helpful if the provider can discuss this in advance.
- ***Cognitive restructuring***—entails teaching patients about negative thoughts, rationalizations, comparisons with others, and all-or-none thinking, and how these thoughts serve the patient, for example, the person who sees that overeating once results in his or her "blowing the diet" and then proceeds to overeat for the remainder of the day because of feelings of disgust or despair. This strategy teaches patients how to counter these negative thoughts with more positive thinking and self-statements.[53,59]

Other strategies that can be used include contingency management, reinforcement, dealing with high-risk situations, stress management, and enlisting social support. Patient-centered counseling, an approach that focuses on encouraging patients to set goals, with input from the provider if needed, has been successful in helping patients make dietary behavioral changes and has potential in the treatment of these patients in primary care settings.[98] MI, a therapeutic strategy implemented to diminish ambivalence about behavior change and increase a person's motivation to take action,[45] is another strategy found to be beneficial in promoting weight loss. In this technique, the interventionist uses reflective listening to help patients identify and resolve uncertainty and increase internal motivation to change.[99] MI has been associated with increased adherence to a behavioral weight loss intervention in women with type 2 diabetes,[100] to dietary behavior changes,[101] and to more than an hour of additional weekly exercise in sedentary adults compared with those who did not receive MI.[102] In summary, the best results for treatment success are attained through a combination of dietary therapy, exercise and physical activity, and use of behavioral therapy.[53,59,83] In addition, recognition that obesity is a chronic disorder and requires ongoing treatment is the most important step to achieving long-term weight control.[6]

Acknowledging the chronicity of obesity and the limitations of conventional clinical settings to assist patients to manage their weight, alternative approaches have been evaluated that might reach a larger number of people and could provide ongoing support.[53,103,104] Use of the Internet to deliver a behavioral weight loss program permits weekly contacts and individualized feedback to participants and has been successful in achieving weight loss; however, interventions delivered by e-mail or the Internet generally are not as effective as on-site or face-to-face weight loss treatment programs.[55,105] Moreover, most of these programs enrolled White, well-educated women, limiting the generalizability of their findings.

Although the use of technology reduces participant burden by not requiring frequent visits to a study or clinical center, it does not reduce the expense of professional counselors. The widely available structured, commercial weight loss programs that advocate the use of sound, balanced eating plans as well as exercise and behavioral change serve a valuable role in supporting the large number of people who need guidance in weight loss. Although large numbers of individuals enroll in commercial programs such as Weight Watchers, which increasingly applies the behavioral strategies tested in the clinical trials conducted at academic centers, only one study has examined these programs.[103] While these programs require a fee payment and thus might not be an option for some segments of the population, they do provide ongoing support for weight loss and achieve good results. Thus, they fill a gap for needed long-term treatment that is not yet readily available in the primary care setting.

There are emerging findings from Great Britain of nurse-led programs for weight management in primary care settings.[106,107] Preliminary reports from the Counterweight Programme reveal that 34% of the patients who completed 12 months of treatment achieved a 5% weight loss.[107] In the United States, researchers and clinicians are collaborating to translate the findings of the highly successful DPP trial to practice settings,[108] and one small trial was successful in reducing weight and improving aerobic fitness and triglycerides in a workplace setting.[109] Yet, little translation of the DPP into practice has been reported.

Pharmacotherapy

Drug therapy for the treatment of obesity has a tainted history. Adverse events associated with the use of phentermine/fenfluramine, phenylpropanolamine, and ma huang include cardiac valvular abnormalities, stroke, and myocardial infarction, respectively. Only sibutramine and orlistat remain available for use.[110] Subsequently, the approval process of other antiobesity agents has been slowed. At the same time, these events brought attention to obesity as a chronic disorder, requiring ongoing treatment. Individuals who have markedly increased medical risks and who have been unsuccessful with nonpharmacologic therapy could benefit from adjunctive drug therapy. However, pharmacologic therapy for treatment of obesity has limited indications, which are treatment for patients with a BMI of $\geq$30 kg/m^2 in the absence of comorbid conditions, or for patients with a BMI of $\geq$27 kg/m^2 with concomitant morbidities such as diabetes, hypertension, or sleep apnea.

There are two categories of medications approved by the Food and Drug Administration (FDA) for the treatment of obesity: those that suppress appetite and those that reduce nutrient absorption. A third type of medication works through the endocannabinoid system (ECS), which influences food intake and the metabolism of lipids and glucose, but is not yet approved by FDA.[111] Numerous drugs that work through different mechanisms, originally developed for other indications, are undergoing clinical trial evaluation. These include bupropion, a reuptake inhibitor of norepinephrine, serotonin, and dopamine; topiramate and zonisamide, antiepileptic agents; and metformin, exenatide, and pramlintide, antidiabetic agents. Each of these drugs has been associated with small weight losses when used in the treatment of disorders for which they are indicated.[111] However, the pharmacological agents currently approved for the treatment of obesity are limited.

Two medications have long-term approval. Sibutramine acts centrally to block the reuptake of serotonin and noradrenaline, thereby reducing food intake and increasing thermogenesis.[110] A 10-mg daily dose of this drug has been shown to produce modest weight loss in several clinical trials, but its use is associated with increases in heart rate of approximately 4 to 6 beats per minute and increases of about 2 to 4 mm Hg in systolic and diastolic blood pressure.[112] Therefore, sibutramine must be used cautiously in persons with hypertension, stroke, and cardiovascular disease.[111] A second drug, orlistat, acts peripherally in the gastrointestinal tract to inhibit gastric and pancreatic lipases essential for digestion of fats, thereby decreasing fat absorption by approximately 30%.[113] It is also associated with decreased absorption of fat-soluble vitamins A, D, E, and K.[111] Orlistat requires a thrice daily 120-mg dosing with meals and adherence to a low-fat diet to prevent significant gastrointestinal side effects, including oily or loose stools and fecal incontinence. Therefore, patient adherence to the diet and medication must be monitored. A half strength formulation of orlistat is now available as the over-the-counter medication, Alli from GlaxoSmithKline. A meta-analysis reported that average 1-year weight losses relative to placebo were 4.5 and 2.9 kg for sibutramine and orlistat, respectively.[114]

Rimonabant, a drug under investigation for weight loss treatment, blocks the CB_1 cannabinoid receptors in the ECS. The ECS contributes to the control of energy homeostasis, and ECS overstimulation is linked to obesity.[115] CB_1 receptors were found to mediate the actions of marijuana and its appetite-stimulating effect.[116] A cannabinoid antagonist, rimonabant blocks the CB_1 receptors in the central nervous system, gastrointestinal tract, and adipose tissue that promote increased food intake.[110]

Large randomized clinical trials comparing rimonabant to placebo found that rimonabant produced significantly greater dose-dependent weight losses after 1 year.[117] The 20-mg dose also yielded significantly greater decreases in waist circumference and triglycerides and insulin resistance with increases in HDL-cholesterol compared with placebo.[118] However, rimonabant has been associated with depressive symptoms, and persons taking the 20-mg dose were 2.5 times more likely to stop taking the drug due to depressive mood disorders compared with those taking the placebo.[119] As a result of increased attention to the psychiatric side effects of new medications such as rimonabant, the FDA has required that drug companies now include a comprehensive assessment of suicide risk during the course of clinical trials.[120]

When medications are prescribed for weight loss, it is most likely that long-term use will be needed because obese individuals who lose weight using pharmacotherapy usually experience weight regain after the treatment is stopped.[112] For the total benefits of drug therapy to be realized, medication use needs to be accompanied by a program of behavior modification, a structured eating plan, and increased physical activity.[112] For example, Wadden et al. found that individuals who took sibutramine and participated in a 30-session lifestyle modification program lost 12.1 kg after 1 year compared with a 5.0-kg weight loss for those who only took sibutramine.[92] People who lose weight during the initial 6 months of drug therapy and maintain that loss without side effects may be considered successful and maintained on the drug with periodic follow-up to provide reinforcement and to monitor progress, side effects, weight, blood pressure, and laboratory values. Currently, FDA approval is for a 2-year course of treatment.

Bariatric Surgery

Morbid obesity is considered a major health problem with related economic consequences. Health care costs associated with obesity are in excess of $117 billion annually in the United States.[121] Bariatric surgery is now recognized as a viable treatment option for those with morbid obesity or those at high risk for obesity-related mortality or comorbidities.[121,122] In 2004, there was an 800% increase in the number of bariatric surgeries in the United States, increasing from 13,386 in 1998 to 121,055 in 2004.[123] These numbers have also increased world wide from 40,000 procedures in 1998 to 146,301 procedures in 2003.[124] Criteria established during the 1991 NIH consensus conference for bariatric surgery, which includes a BMI $\geq$40 kg/m^2 or a BMI of 35.0 to 39.9 kg/m^2 and a concomitant morbidity such as sleep apnea, uncontrolled diabetes, cardiovascular disease, or weight-related problems interfering with daily functioning are still reasonable today.[52]

There are numerous bariatric surgical procedures that include gastric bypass, gastric banding, and gastroplasty. Buchwald and Williams[124] reported the relative percentages of the most common procedures worldwide are: gastric bypass (65.11%), gastric banding (24.41%), vertical banded gastroplasty (5.43%), and the less frequently performed biliopancreatic diversion/duodenal switch (4.85%). The Roux-en-Y technique is the preferred approach to gastric bypass. It involves the construction of a gastric pouch of approximately 20 to 30 mL capacity that is attached to a Y-shaped limb of small bowel of different lengths. The proximal stomach is separated from the remaining part of the stomach with staples. Today, more than 90% of the gastric bypass surgeries are performed laparoscopically.[122,125] The gastric banding procedure is also done laparoscopically and involves placing a band around the upper part of the stomach approximately 1 to 2 cm below the gastroesophageal junction, forming a 30 mL gastric pouch.[125] The vertical banded gastroplasty involves partitioning the stomach with four parallel rows of sutures and applying a band at the opening between the upper gastric pouch and the body of the stomach. The biliopancreatic diversion involves removing three quarters of the stomach, preserving the pylorus, and constructing an ileoduodenostomy distal to the pylorus. The alimentary and biliopancreatic limbs have approximately the same length. In all of the procedures, vomiting is a common problem. Patients undergoing gastric restrictive procedures have an increased risk of experiencing dumping syndrome and nutritional deficiencies (particularly vitamin B_{12}, calcium, and iron).[122,125] The key complications associated with bariatric surgery include pulmonary embolus, respiratory failure, stomal obstruction or stenosis, bleeding, and gastrointestinal leaks from the breakdown of a staple/suture line. The level of risk depends upon the patient's age, BMI, surgical procedure used, and the presence of other comorbidities.[122]

Substantial weight loss can result from these surgical procedures. Indeed, these patients also had either reversal or significant improvement in type 2 diabetes, hyperlipidemia, hypertension, obstructive sleep apnea, weight-bearing OA, and depression.[121,126] The literature supports a mean percent excess weight loss between 47% and 70% for all procedures.[126,127] The most recent data from the Swedish Obesity Study (SOS), a large prospective controlled trial that began in 1987, found a significant difference between the control group and the surgical groups.[128] The average change in weight among the control group remained ±2% during the observation period, whereas in the three surgical groups the mean weight loss ± standard deviation reached the maximum after 1 to 2 years with gastric bypass 32% ± 8%, vertical banded gastroplasty, 25% ± 9% and gastric banding at 20% ± 10%. After 10 years, when compared to the baseline weight, losses were 25% ± 11% with bypass, 16% ± 11% with gastroplasty, and 14% ± 14% with banding; after 15 years, the weight losses consisted of 27% ± 12%, 18% ± 11%, and 13% ± 14%, respectively. Reports after 16 years of follow up revealed that patients in the surgery group had an overall lower mortality rate compared with the control group.[128]

Maintenance of Weight Loss

Successful long-term weight loss maintenance has been defined as intentionally losing at least 10% of one's initial body weight and maintaining that loss for at least 1 year.[129] Using this definition, successful weight loss maintenance occurs in approximately 20% of overweight or obese individuals who lose weight. Yet, 30% to 35% of the weight a person loses is often regained during the first year after treatment.[55] Because weight loss tends to level off after 6 months of treatment, the focus of weight-management programs are shifting from emphasizing only weight loss to introducing weight maintenance.[130] The greatest challenge remaining for health care professionals is not only assisting people to lose weight but also helping them to sustain the weight loss they have achieved.[131]

Some strategies associated with improved weight loss maintenance include extended contact with the provider, exercise/physical activity, and pharmacotherapy.[132] Ongoing follow-up to promote adherence to behavioral changes is consistent with the continuous care model for obesity as a chronic disease.[6] Continued contact with the treatment provider presents opportunities for discussion of problem-solving strategies for overcoming obstacles to long-term maintenance. Updated physical activity recommendations from the ACSM and the AHA specify that individuals should engage in 60 to 90 minutes of moderate-intensity physical activity each day in order to maintain weight loss.[73] Recently, individuals who reported expending more than 2,500 kcal/week in physical activity (approximately 75 minutes of daily walking) maintained an average weight loss of about 7 kg after 2.5 years compared with a <1 kg loss in those who expended less energy.[77] Other researchers have corroborated the finding that increased physical activity during weight maintenance supports sustained weight loss.[133–135] The use of obesity medications, orlistat and sibutramine, has also been shown to be beneficial for weight loss maintenance. In a recent meta-analysis, 80% to 100% of initially lost weight was maintained in 10% to 30% more sibutramine patients compared with those taking placebo.[136] A long-term study found that persons who received orlistat regained 2.4 kg less weight after 3 years in comparison to the placebo group.[137] After 2 years, the use of weight loss pharmacotherapy resulted in persons maintaining an average of 2% to 5% more of their lost weight than those who only received dietary and exercise interventions.[138]

Valuable information regarding weight loss maintenance has been obtained from the National Weight Control Registry, an ongoing registry of individuals who have been successful at losing and maintaining a minimum of 13.6 kg for at least 1 year.[139] Behavioral strategies used by these successful individuals include increasing physical activity, consuming a low-fat diet, regularly self-monitoring food eaten and body weight,[140] restricting the variety of food eaten,[141] consuming a consistent weekly diet,[142] eating breakfast,[143] and limiting the amount of time spent watching television.[144] The importance of self-weighing for weight maintenance has been confirmed by others who reported that a higher frequency of weighing was related to less weight regain.[130,145,146] Men belonging to the National Weight Control Registry report expending 3,293 kcal/week through physical activity while women report expending 2,545 kcal/week; these amounts are similar to walking 28 miles/week or about 1 hour of moderately intense activity daily.[140] This finding underscores the importance of exercise as a maintenance strategy; yet, adherence to exercise remains a problem.[77] Maintenance of weight loss requires long-term adherence to the numerous changes in lifestyle that created the initial weight loss.[132] Therefore, the provider needs to implement strategies to enhance adherence throughout the treatment and maintenance phases; these strategies for promoting adherence are detailed in Chapter 40 of this book.

SUMMARY

Obesity is a chronic medical condition with numerous adverse effects on the cardiovascular system and health-related quality of life. The significant increase in its prevalence and the epidemic of type 2 diabetes that is following it demand attention at all levels. The goal of treatment is reduced morbidity and improved health. Current treatment consists of lifestyle modification interventions and when indicated, pharmacotherapy or bariatric surgery. Since 1998, we have had evidence-based guidelines for use in the identification, evaluation, and treatment of overweight and obese patients in the clinical setting.[15] Although these guidelines are 10 years old and in the process of being updated, they still represent the standards of treatment and emphasize multidisciplinary approaches to the treatment of this chronic disorder. Practitioners can teach patients strategies for self-management, following the precedent established in treating similar conditions (e.g., hypertension, dyslipidemia, and diabetes). Similar to the role nurses play in the treatment of these chronic conditions, nurses need to take the lead in addressing the needs of this ever-growing subgroup of the population. To reduce the high prevalence of this chronic disorder, increased focus needs to be given to prevention of weight gain and sustaining the weight loss achieved.

Acknowledgment: *The authors were supported by grants R01 DK58387, R01 DK071817, and F31 NR 009750, National Institute of Health, National Institute of Diabetes, Digestive, and Kidney Disorders, and National Institute of Nursing Research.*

REFERENCES

1. Centers for Disease Control and Prevention. (2007). *Prevalence of overweight and obesity among adults: United States, 2003–2004.* Retrieved February 5, 2008, from http://www.cdc.gov/nchs/products/pubs/pubd/hestats/overweight/overwght_adult_03.htm
2. Ogden, C., Carroll, M., Curtin, L., et al. (2006). Prevalence of overweight and obesity in the United States, 1999–2004. *JAMA, 295*(13), 1549–1555.

3. Roth, J., Qiang, X., Marban, S. L., et al. (2004). The obesity pandemic: Where have we been and where are we going? *Obesity Research, 12*(Suppl. 2), S88–S101.
4. James, P. T. (2004). Obesity: The worldwide epidemic. *Clinics in Dermatology, 22*, 276–280.
5. World Health Organization. (2008). *Obesity and overweight.* Retrieved February 5, 2008, from http://www.who.int/mediacentre/factsheets/fs311/en/index.html
6. Orzano, A. J., & Scott, J. G. (2004). Diagnosis and treatment of obesity in adults: An applied evidence-based review. *Journal of the American Board of Family Practice, 17*(5), 359–569.
7. Klein, S., Burke, L. E., Bray, G. A., et al. (2004). Clinical implications of obesity with specific focus on cardiovascular disease. A statement for professionals from the American Heart Association Council on Nutrition, Physical Activity, and Metabolism. *Circulation, 110*, 2952–2967.
8. Poirier, P., Giles, T. D., Bray, G. A., et al. (2006). Obesity and cardiovascular disease: Pathophysiology, evaluation, and effect of weight loss: An update of the 1997 American Heart Association Scientific Statement on Obesity and Heart Disease from the Obesity Committee of the Council on Nutrition, Physical Activity, and Metabolism. *Circulation, 113*(6), 898–918.
9. Joshi, A. V., Day, D., Lubowski, T. J., et al. (2005). Relationship between obesity and cardiovascular risk factors: Findings from a multi-state screening project in the United States. *Current Medical Research and Opinion, 21*, 1755–1761.
10. Van Gaal, L. F., Wauters, M. A., & De Leeuw, I. H. (1997). The beneficial effects of modest weight loss on cardiovascular risk factors. *International Journal of Obesity and Related Metabolic Disorders, 21*(Suppl. 1), S5–S9.
11. Bish, C. L., Blanck, H. M., Serdula, M. K., et al. (2005). Diet and physical activity behaviors among Americans trying to lose weight: 2000 Behavioral Risk Factor Surveillance System. *Obesity Research, 13*(3), 596–607.
12. Rosenbaum, M., Leibel, R. L., & Hirsch, J. (1997). Obesity. *New England Journal of Medicine, 337*, 396–407.
13. Institute of Medicine. (1995). *Weighing the options criteria for evaluating weight-management programs.* Washington, DC: National Academy Press.
14. Shape Up American & American Obesity Association. (1996). *Guidance for treatment for adult obesity.* Bethesda, MD: Shape Up America.
15. National Heart, Lung, and Blood Institute, Obesity Education Initiative Expert Panel on the Identification Evaluation and Treatment of Overweight and Obesity. (1998). *Clinical guidelines on the identification, evaluation, and treatment of overweight and obesity in adults: The evidence report.* Bethesda, MD: National Institutes of Health.
16. America on the Move Foundation. (2008). *America on the Move: Steps to a healthier way of life.* Retrieved February 5, 2008, from http://aom.americaonthemove.org/site/c.krLXJ3PJKuG/b.1524891/k.C834/About_Us.htm
17. World Health Organization. (2000). *Preventing and managing the global epidemic of obesity: Report of a WHO consultation.* Retrieved February 20, 2008, from http://whqlibdoc.who.int/trs/WHO_TRS_894.pdf
18. Eaton, C. B., Goodwin, M. A., & Stange, K. C. (2002). Direct observation of nutrition counseling in community family practice. *American Journal of Preventive Medicine, 23*(3), 174–179.
19. WHO. Expert Consultation. (2004). Appropriate body-mass index for Asian populations and its implications for policy and intervention strategies. *Lancet, 363*(9403), 157–163.
20. Kuk, J. L., Katzmarzyk, P. T., Nichaman, M. Z., et al. (2006). Visceral fat is an independent predictor of all-cause mortality in men. *Obesity, 14*(2), 336–341.
21. Okura, T., Nakata, Y., Yamabuki, K., et al. (2004). Regional body composition changes exhibit opposing effects on coronary heart disease risk factors. *Arteriosclerosis, Thrombosis, and Vascular Biology, 24*(5), 923–929.
22. Dagenais, G. R., Yi, Q., Mann, J. F. E., et al. (2005). Prognostic impact of body weight and abdominal obesity in women and men with cardiovascular disease. *American Heart Journal, 149*(1), 54–60.
23. Grundy, S. M., Cleeman, J. I., Merz, C. N., et al. (2004). Implications of recent clinical trials for the National Cholesterol Education Program Adult Treatment Panel III guidelines. *Circulation, 110*(2), 227–239.
24. Alberti, K. G., Zimmet, P., Shaw, J., et al. (2005). The metabolic syndrome—A new worldwide definition. *Lancet, 366*(9491), 1059–1062.
25. Zimmet, P., Magliano, D., Matsuzawa, Y., et al. (2005). The metabolic syndrome: A global public health problem and a new definition. *Journal of Atherosclerosis and Thrombosis, 12*(6), 295–300.
26. Lee, S. Y., Park, H. S., Kim, D. J., et al. (2007). Appropriate waist circumference cutoff points for central obesity in Korean adults. *Diabetes Research and Clinical Practice, 75*(1), 72–80.
27. Pearson, T. A., Mensah, G. A., Alexander, R. W., et al. (2003). Markers of inflammation and cardiovascular disease: Application to clinical and public health practice: A statement for healthcare professionals from the Centers for Disease Control and Prevention and the American Heart Association. *Circulation, 107*(3), 499–511.
28. NIH Consensus Conference. (1993). Triglyceride, high-density lipoprotein, and coronary heart disease. NIH Consensus Development Panel on Triglyceride, High-Density Lipoprotein, and Coronary Heart Disease. *JAMA, 269*(4), 505–510.
29. Bergman, R. N., Kim, S. P., Hsu, I. R., et al. (2007). Abdominal obesity: Role in the pathophysiology of metabolic disease and cardiovascular risk. *The American Journal of Medicine, 120*(2, Suppl. 1), S3–S8.
30. Cottam, D. R., Mattar, S. G., Barinas-Mitchell, E., et al. (2004). The chronic inflammatory hypothesis for the morbidity associated with morbid obesity: Implications and effects of weight loss. *Obesity Surgery, 14*(5), 589–600.
31. Wannamethee, S. G., Shaper, A. G., Whincup, P. H., et al. (2004). Overweight and obesity and the burden of disease and disability in elderly men. *International Journal of Obesity, 28*(11), 1374–1382.
32. Kennedy, R. L., Webb, D., & Chokkalingam, K. (2004). Increasing prevalence of obesity: Implications for the health and functioning of older people. *Reviews in Clinical Gerontology, 14*(3), 235–246.
33. Zamboni, M., Mazzali, G., Zoico, E., et al. (2005). Health consequences of obesity in the elderly: A review of four unresolved questions. *International Journal of Obesity, 29*(9), 1011–1029.
34. Kennedy, R. L., Chokkalingham, K., & Srinivasan, R. (2004). Obesity in the elderly: Who should we be treating, and why, and how? *Current Opinion in Clinical Nutrition and Metabolic Care, 7*(1), 3–9.
35. Nelson, K. M., McFarland, L., & Relber, G. (2007). Factors influencing disease self-management among veterans with diabetes and poor glycemic control. *Journal of General Internal Medicine, 22*(4), 442–447.
36. Spring, B., Pagoto, S., Pingitore, R., et al. (2004). Randomized controlled trial for behavioral smoking and weight control treatment: Effect of concurrent versus sequential intervention. *Journal of Consulting and Clinical Psychology, 72*(5), 785–796.
37. Conway, J. M., Ingwersen, L. A., & Moshfegh, A. J. (2004). Accuracy of dietary recall using the USDA five-step multiple-pass method in men: An observational validation study. *Journal of the American Dietetic Association, 104*(4), 595–603.
38. Pereira, M. A., FitzerGerald, S. J., Gregg, E. W., et al. (1997). A collection of Physical Activity Questionnaires for health-related research. *Medicine & Science in Sports & Exercise, 29*(6, Suppl.), S1–S205.
39. Willett, W. (1998). *Nutritional epidemiology* (2nd ed.). New York: Oxford University Press.
40. Wee, C. C., Davis, R. B., & Phillips, R. S. (2005). Stage of readiness to control weight and adopt weight control behaviors in primary care. *Journal of General Internal Medicine, 20*(5), 410–415.
41. Warziski, M., Sereika, S., Styn, M. A., et al. (2008). Changes in self-efficacy and dietary adherence: The impact on weight loss in the PREFER study. *Journal of Behavioral Medicine, 31*(1), 81–92.
42. Burke, L. E., Styn, M. A., Elci, O. U., et al. (2007). How do barriers to healthy eating impact weight loss? *Circulation, 115*(8, Suppl.), 55.
43. Gorin, A. A., Phelan, S., Hill, J. O., et al. (2004). Medical triggers are associated with better short- and long-term weight loss outcomes. *Preventive Medicine, 39*(3), 612–616.
44. Hill, A. J. (2007). Obesity and eating disorders. *Obesity Reviews, 8*(Suppl. 1), 151–155.
45. Miller, W. R., & Rollnick, S. (2002). *Motivational interviewing: Preparing people for change.* New York: Guilford Press.
46. Brown, I. (2006). Nurses' attitudes towards adult patients who are obese: Literature review. *Journal of Advanced Nursing, 53*(2), 221–232.
47. Burke, L. E., & Fair, J. (2003). Promoting prevention: Skill sets and attributes of health care providers who deliver behavioral interventions. *Journal of Cardiovascular Nursing, 18*(4), 256–266.
48. Serdula, M. K., Khan, L. K., & Dietz, W. H. (2003). Weight loss counseling revisited. *JAMA, 289*(14), 1747–1750.
49. Booth, K. M., Pinkston, M. M., & Poston, W. S. (2005). Obesity and the built environment. *Journal of the American Dietetic Association, 105*(5, Suppl. 1), S110–S117.
50. Block, J. P., Scribner, R. A., & DeSalvo, K. B. (2004). Fast food, race/ethnicity, and income: A geographic analysis. *American Journal of Preventive Medicine, 27*(3), 211–217.
51. Mehta, N. K., & Chang, V. W. (2008). Weight status and restaurant availability. *American Journal of Preventive Medicine, 34*(2), 127–133.

52. Buchwald, H.; Consensus Conference Panel. (2005). Consensus conference statement bariatric surgery for morbid obesity: Health implications for patients, health professionals, and third-party payers. *Surgery for Obesity and Related Diseases, 1*(3), 371–381.
53. Wadden, T. A., Crerand, C. E., & Brock, J. (2005). Behavioral treatment of obesity. *Psychiatric Clinics of North America, 28*(1), 151–170.
54. Berkel, L. A., Poston, W. S., Reeves, W. S., et al. (2005). Behavioral interventions for obesity. *Journal of the American Dietetic Association, 105*(Suppl. 1), S35–S43.
55. Wadden, T. A., Butryn, M. L., & Byrne, K. J. (2004). Efficacy of lifestyle modification for long-term weight control. *Obesity Research, 12*(Suppl.), 151S–162S.
56. Foster, G. D., Makris, A. P., & Bailer, B. A. (2005). Behavioral treatment of obesity. *American Journal of Clinical Nutrition, 82*(1, Suppl.), 230S–235S.
57. Foster, G. D., Phelan, S., Wadden, T. A., et al. (2004). Promoting more modest weight losses: A pilot study. *Obesity Research, 12*(8), 1271–1277.
58. Jakicic, J. M., & Otto, A. D. (2005). Physical activity recommendations in the treatment of obesity. *Psychiatric Clinics of North America, 28*(1), 141–150.
59. Wing, R. R. (2004). Behavioral approaches to the treatment of obesity. In G. A. Bray, C. Bourchard, & W. P. T. James (Eds.), *Handbook of obesity: Clinical applications* (2nd ed., pp. 147–167). New York: Marcel Dekker.
60. National Cholesterol Education Program. (2001). *Third report of the National Cholesterol Education Program (NCEP) Expert Panel on Detection, Evaluation, and Treatment of High Blood Cholesterol in Adults (Adult Treatment Panel III).* Bethesda, MA: National Institutes of Health, National Heart, Lung, and Blood Institute.
61. Gilden Tsai, A., & Wadden, T. A. (2006). The evolution of very-low-calorie diets: An update and meta-analysis. *Obesity, 14*(8), 1283–1293.
62. Nordmann, A. J., Nordmann, A., Briel, M., et al. (2006). Effects of low-carbohydrate vs low-fat diets on weight loss and cardiovascular risk factors: A meta-analysis of randomized controlled trials. *Archives of Internal Medicine, 166*(3), 285–293.
63. Tay, J., Brinkworth, G. D., Noakes, M., et al. (2008). Metabolic effects of weight loss on a very-low-carbohydrate diet compared with an isocaloric high-carbohydrate diet in abdominally obese subjects. *Journal of the American College of Cardiology, 51*(1), 59–67.
64. Dansinger, M. L., Gleason, J. A., Griffith, J. L., et al. (2005). Comparison of the Atkins, Ornish, Weight Watchers, and Zone diets for weight loss and heart disease risk reduction: A randomized trial. *JAMA, 293*(1), 43–53.
65. Gardner, C. D., Kiazand, A., Alhassan, S., et al. (2007). Comparison of the Atkins, Zone, Ornish, and LEARN diets for change in weight and related risk factors among overweight premenopausal women: The A TO Z Weight Loss Study: A randomized trial. *JAMA, 297*(9), 969–977.
66. Brouns, F., Bjorck, I., Frayn, K. N., et al. (2005). Glycaemic index methodology. *Nutrition Research Reviews, 18*(1), 145–171.
67. Hare-Bruun, H., Flint, A., & Heitmann, B. L. (2006). Glycemic index and glycemic load in relation to changes in body weight, body fat distribution, and body composition in adult Danes. *American Journal of Clinical Nutrition, 84*(4), 871–879.
68. Aston, L. M., Stokes, C. S., & Jebb, S. A. (2008). No effect of a diet with a reduced glycaemic index on satiety, energy intake and body weight in overweight and obese women. *International Journal of Obesity, 32*, 160–165.
69. Sloth, B., Krog-Mikkelsen, I., Flint, A., et al. (2004). No difference in body weight decrease between a low-glycemic-index and a high-glycemic-index diet but reduced LDL cholesterol after 10-wk ad libitum intake of the low-glycemic-index diet. *American Journal of Clinical Nutrition, 80*(2), 337–347.
70. Das, S. K., Gilhooly, C. H., Golden, J. K., et al. (2007). Long-term effects of 2 energy-restricted diets differing in glycemic load on dietary adherence, body composition, and metabolism in CALERIE: A 1-y randomized controlled trial. *American Journal of Clinical Nutrition, 85*(4), 1023–1030.
71. Thomas, D. E., Elliott, E. J., & Baur, L. (2007). Low glycaemic index or low glycaemic load diets for overweight and obesity. *Cochrane Database of Systematic Reviews,* (3), Art. No. CD005105.
72. Ebbeling, C. B., Leidig, M. M., Feldman, H. A., et al. (2007). Effects of a low-glycemic load vs low-fat diet in obese young adults: A randomized trial. *JAMA, 297*(19), 2092–2102.
73. Haskell, W. L., Lee, I. M., Pate, R. R., et al. (2007). Physical activity and public health: Updated recommendation for adults from the American College of Sports Medicine and the American Heart Association. *Medicine & Science in Sports & Exercise, 39*(8), 1423–1434.
74. Nelson, M. E., Rejeski, W. J., Blair, S. N., et al. (2007). Physical activity and public health in older adults: Recommendation from the American College of Sports Medicine and the American Heart Association. *Medicine & Science in Sports & Exercise, 39*(8), 1435–1445.
75. Janiszewski, P. M., & Ross, R. (2007). Physical activity in the treatment of obesity: Beyond body weight reduction. *Applied Physiology, Nutrition, and Metabolism, 32*(2), 512–522.
76. U. S. Department of Health and Human Services. (2005). *Dietary guidelines for Americans 2005.* Retrieved February 21, 2008, from http://www.health.gov/dietaryguidelines/dga2005/document/pdf/DGA2005.pdf
77. Tate, D. F., Jeffery, R. W., Sherwood, N. E., et al. (2007). Long-term weight losses associated with prescription of higher physical activity goals. Are higher levels of physical activity protective against weight regain? *American Journal of Clinical Nutrition, 85*(4), 954–959.
78. Marshall, S. J., Jones, D. A., Ainsworth, B. E., et al. (2007). Race/ethnicity, social class, and leisure-time physical inactivity. *Medicine & Science in Sports & Exercise, 39*(1), 44–51.
79. van Lenthe, F. J., Brug, J., & Mackenbach, J. P. (2005). Neighbourhood inequalities in physical inactivity: The role of neighbourhood attractiveness, proximity to local facilities and safety in the Netherlands. *Social Science & Medicine, 60*(4), 763–775.
80. Rothman, A. J., Baldwin, A. S., & Hertel, A. W. (2004). Self-regulation and behavior change: Disentangling behavioral initiation and behavioral maintenance. In K. D. Vohs & R. F. Baumeister (Eds.), *The handbook of self-regulation: Research, theory, and applications* (pp. 130–148). New York: Guilford Press.
81. Burke, L. E., Choo, J., Music, E., et al. (2006). PREFER study: A randomized clinical trial testing treatment preference and two dietary options in behavioral weight management—rationale, design and baseline characteristics. *Contemporary Clinical Trials, 27*(1), 34–48.
82. Burke, L. E., Warziski, M., Styn, M. A., et al. (2008). A randomized clinical trial of a standard versus vegetarian diet for weight loss: The impact of treatment preference. *International Journal of Obesity, 32*, 166–176.
83. Wing, R. R., Hamman, R. F., Bray, G. A., et al. (2004). Achieving weight and activity goals among diabetes prevention program lifestyle participants. *Obesity Research, 12*(9), 1426–1434.
84. The Look Ahead Research Group. (2007). Reduction in weight and cardiovascular disease risk factors in individuals with type 2 diabetes: One-year results of the look AHEAD trial. *Diabetes Care, 30*(6), 1374–1383.
85. Laaksonen, D. E., Lindstrom, J., Lakka, T. A., et al. (2005). Physical activity in the prevention of type 2 diabetes: The Finnish Diabetes Prevention Study. *Diabetes, 54*(1), 158–165.
86. Renjilian, D. A., Perri, M. G., Nezu, A. M., et al. (2001). Individual versus group therapy for obesity: Effects of matching participants to their treatment preferences. *Journal of Consulting and Clinical Psychology, 69*(4), 717–721.
87. Brownell, K. D. (2004). *The LEARN Program for Weight Management* (9th ed.). Dallas, TX: American Health Publishing Company.
88. Diabetes Prevention Program Study Documents Website. (2001). *DPP protocol.* Retrieved February 23, 2008, from http://www.bsc.gwu.edu/dpp/protocol.htmlvdoc
89. Burke, L. E., Warziski, M., Starrett, T., et al. (2005). Self-monitoring dietary intake: Current and future practices. *Journal of Renal Nutrition, 15*(3), 281–290.
90. Burke, L. E., Music, E., Styn, M. A., et al. (2006). Using technology to improve self-monitoring in weight loss. *International Journal of Behavioral Medicine, 13*(Suppl.), 192.
91. Burke, L. E., Sereika, S. M., Music, E., et al. (2008). Using instrumented paper diaries to document self-monitoring patterns in weight loss. *Contemporary Clinical Trials, 29*(2), 182–193.
92. Wadden, T. A., Berkowitz, R. I., Womble, L. G., et al. (2005). Randomized trial of lifestyle modification and pharmacotherapy for obesity. *New England Journal of Medicine, 353*(20), 2111–2120.
93. Bandura, A. (1997). *Self-efficacy: The exercise of control.* New York: W.H. Freeman and Company.
94. Bandura, A., & Schunk, D. H. (1981). Cultivating competence, self-efficacy, and intrinsic interest through proximal self-motivation. *Journal of Personality and Social Psychology, 41*(3), 586–598.
95. Strecher, V. J., Seijits, G. H., Kok, G. J., et al. (1995). Goal setting as a strategy for health behavior change. *Health Education Quarterly, 22*(2), 190–200.
96. D'Zurilla, T. J., & Goldfried, M. R. (1971). Problem solving and behavior modification. *Journal of Abnormal Psychology, 78*(1), 107–126.
97. Marlatt, G. A., & Gordon, J. R. (1980). Determinants of relapse: Implications for the maintenance of behavior change. In P. Davidson &

S. Davidson (Eds.), *Behavioral medicine: Changing health lifestyles* (pp. 410–452). New York: Brunner/Mazel.

98. Glasgow, R. E., Goldstein, M. G., Ockene, J. K., et al. (2004). Translating what we have learned into practice: Principles and hypotheses for interventions addressing multiple behaviors in primary care. *American Journal of Preventive Medicine, 27*(2, Suppl. 1), 88–101.
99. Rubak, S., Sandbaek, A., Lauritzen, T., et al. (2005). Motivational interviewing: A systematic review and meta-analysis. *British Journal of General Practice, 55*(513), 305–312.
100. Smith West, D., DiLillo, V., Burzac, Z., et al. (2007). Motivational interviewing improves weight loss in women with type 2 diabetes. *Diabetes Care, 30*(5), 1081–1087.
101. Hoy, M., Lubin, M., Grosvenor, M., et al. (2005). Development and use of a motivational action plan for dietary behavior change using a patient-centered counseling approach. *Topics in Clinical Nutrition, 20*(2), 118–126.
102. Carels, R. A., Darby, L., Cacciapaglia, H. M., et al. (2007). Using motivational interviewing as a supplement to obesity treatment: A stepped-care approach. *Health Psychology, 26*(3), 369–374.
103. Heshka, S., Anderson, J. W., Atkinson, R. L., et al. (2003). Weight loss with self-help compared with a structured commercial program: A randomized trial. *JAMA, 289*(14), 1792–1798.
104. Tate, D. F., Jackvony, E. H., & Wing, R. R. (2006). A randomized trial comparing human e-mail counseling, computer-automated tailored counseling, and no counseling in an Internet weight loss program. *Archives of Internal Medicine, 166*, 1620–1625.
105. Weinstein, P. K. (2006). A review of weight loss programs delivered via the Internet. *Journal of Cardiovascular Nursing, 21*(4), 251–258.
106. Counterweight Project Team. (2005). Obesity impacts on general practice appointments. *Obesity Research, 13*(8), 1442–1449.
107. Counterweight Project Team. (2006). Nurse-led weight management: The Counterweight Programme. *Endocrine Abstracts, 11*, S101.
108. Kramer, M. K., Miller, R. G., Venditti, E. M., et al. (2008). DPP and the real world: Translating the Diabetes Prevention Program lifestyle intervention into primary care practice. *Under review*.
109. Aldana, S. G., Barlow, M., Smith, R., et al. (2005). The Diabetes Prevention Program: A worksite experience. *American Association of Occupational Health Nurses Journal, 53*(11), 499–505.
110. Bray, G. A., & Greenway, F. L. (2007). Pharmacological treatment of the overweight patient. *Pharmacological Reviews, 59*(2), 151–184.
111. Palamara, K. L., Mogul, H. R., Peterson, S. J., et al. (2006). Obesity: New perspectives and pharmacotherapies. *Cardiology in Review, 14*(5), 238–258.
112. Klein, S. (2004). Long-term pharmacotherapy for obesity. *Obesity Research, 12*(Suppl.), S163–S166.
113. Padwal, R. S., & Majumdar, S. R. (2007). Drug treatments for obesity: Orlistat, sibutramine, and rimonabant. *Lancet, 369*(9555), 71–77.
114. Li, Z., Maglione, M., Tu, W., et al. (2005). Meta-analysis: Pharmacologic treatment of obesity. *Annals of Internal Medicine, 142*(7), 532–546.
115. Osei-Hyiaman, D., DePetrillo, M., Pacher, P., et al. (2005). Endocannabinoid activation at hepatic CB1 receptors stimulates fatty acid synthesis and contributes to diet-induced obesity. *Journal of Clinical Investigation, 115*(5), 1298–1305.
116. Devane, W. A., Hanus, L., Breuer, A., et al. (1992). Isolation and structure of a brain constituent that binds to the cannabinoid receptor. *Science, 258*, 1946–1949.
117. Despres, J.-P., Golay, A., Sjostrom, L., et al. (2005). Effects of rimonabant on metabolic risk factors in overweight patients with dyslipidemia. *New England Journal of Medicine, 353*(20), 2121–2134.
118. Van Gaal, L. F., Rissanen, A. M., Scheen, A. J., et al. (2005). Effects of the cannabinoid-1 receptor blocker rimonabant on weight reduction and cardiovascular risk factors in overweight patients: 1-year experience from the RIO-Europe study. *Lancet, 365*(9468), 1389–1397.
119. Christensen, R., Kristensen, P. K., Bartels, E. M., et al. (2007). Efficacy and safety of the weight-loss drug rimonabant: A meta-analysis of randomised trials. *Lancet, 370*(9600), 1706–1713.
120. Harris, G. (2008). FDA requiring suicide studies in drug trials. *New York Times*, Retrieved February 1, 2008, from http://www.nytimes.com/2008/01/24/washington/24fda.html?pagewanted=2&_r=2&ei=5070&en=1cec78d043161c41&ex=1201842000&emc=eta1
121. Buchwald, H. (2005). The future of bariatric surgery. *Obesity Surgery, 15*(5), 598–605.
122. Steinbrook, R. (2004). Surgery for severe obesity. *New England Journal of Medicine, 350*(11), 1075–1079.
123. Zhao, Y., & Encinosa, W. (2007). *Bariatric surgery Utilization and outcomes in 1998 and 2004* (Statistical Brief No. 23). Rockville, MD: Agency for Healthcare Research and Quality.
124. Buchwald, H., & Williams, S. E. (2004). Bariatric surgery worldwide 2003. *Obesity Surgery, 14*(9), 1157–1164.
125. Elder, K. A., & Wolfe, B. M. (2007). Bariatric surgery: A review of procedures and outcomes. *Gastroenterology, 132*(6), 2253–2271.
126. Christou, N. V., Sampalis, J. S., Liberman, M., et al. (2004). Surgery decreases long-term mortality, morbidity, and health care use in morbidly obese patients. *Annals of Surgery, 240*(3), 416–423.
127. Buchwald, H., Avidor, Y., Braunwald, E., et al. (2004). Bariatric surgery: A systematic review and meta-analysis. *JAMA, 292*(14), 1724–1737.
128. Sjostrom, L., Narbro, K., Sjostrom, C. D., et al. (2007). Effects of bariatric surgery on mortality in Swedish obese subjects. *New England Journal of Medicine, 357*(8), 741–752.
129. Wing, R. R., & Hill, J. O. (2001). Successful weight loss maintenance. *Annual Review of Nutrition, 21*, 323–341.
130. Wing, R. R., Tate, D. F., Gorin, A. A., et al. (2006). A self-regulation program for maintenance of weight loss. *New England Journal of Medicine, 355*(15), 1563–1571.
131. Hill, J. O., Thompson, H., & Wyatt, H. (2005). Weight maintenance: What's missing? *Journal of the American Dietetic Association, 105*(5, Suppl. 1), S63–S66.
132. Perri, M. G., & Foreyt, J. P. (2004). Preventing weight regain after weight loss. In G. A. Bray & C. Bouchard (Eds.), *Handbook of obesity: Clinical applications* (2nd ed., pp. 185–199). New York: Marcel Dekker.
133. Befort, C. A., Stewart, E. E., Smith, B. K., et al. (2008). Weight maintenance, behaviors and barriers among previous participants of a university-based weight control program. *International Journal of Obesity, 32*(3), 519–526. (Advance online publication December 4, 2007, DOI: 10.1038/sj.ijo.0803769.)
134. Donnelly, J. E., Smith, B., Jacobsen, D. J., et al. (2004). The role of exercise for weight loss and maintenance. *Best Practice & Research. Clinical Gastroenterology, 18*(6), 1009–1029.
135. Villanova, N., Pasqui, F., Burzacchini, S., et al. (2006). A physical activity program to reinforce weight maintenance following a behavior program in overweight/obese subjects. *International Journal of Obesity, 30*(4), 697–703.
136. Rucker, D., Padwal, R., Li, S. K., et al. (2007). Long term pharmacotherapy for obesity and overweight: Updated meta-analysis. *BMJ, 335*(7631), 1194–1199.
137. Richelsen, B., Tonstad, S., Rossner, S., et al. (2007). Effect of orlistat on weight regain and cardiovascular risk factors following a very-low-energy diet in abdominally obese patients: A 3-year randomized, placebo-controlled study. *Diabetes Care, 30*(1), 27–32.
138. Franz, M. J., Vanwormer, J. J., Crain, A. L., et al. (2007). Weight-loss outcomes: A systematic review and meta-analysis of weight-loss clinical trials with a minimum 1-year follow-up. *Journal of the American Dietetic Association, 107*(10), 1755–1767.
139. Klem, M. L., Wing, R. R., McGuire, M. T., et al. (1997). A descriptive study of individuals successful at long-term maintenance of substantial weight loss. *American Journal of Clinical Nutrition, 66*(2), 239–246.
140. Wyatt, H. R., Phelan, S., Wing, R. R., et al. (2005). Lessons from patients who have successfully maintained weight loss. *Obesity Management, 1*(2), 56–61.
141. Raynor, H. A., Jeffery, R. W., Phelan, S., et al. (2005). Amount of food group variety consumed in the diet and long-term weight loss maintenance. *Obesity Research, 13*(5), 883–890.
142. Gorin, A. A., Phelan, S., Wing, R. R., et al. (2004). Promoting long-term weight control: Does dieting consistency matter? *International Journal of Obesity, 28*(2), 278–281.
143. Wyatt, H. R., Grunwald, G. K., Mosca, C. L., et al. (2002). Long-term weight loss and breakfast in subjects in the National Weight Control Registry. *Obesity Research, 10*(2), 78–82.
144. Raynor, D. A., Phelan, S., Hill, J. O., et al. (2006). Television viewing and long-term weight maintenance: Results from the National Weight Control Registry. *Obesity, 14*(10), 1816–1824.
145. Butryn, M. L., Phelan, S., Hill, J. O., et al. (2007). Consistent self-monitoring of weight: A key component of successful weight loss maintenance. *Obesity, 15*(12), 3091–3096.
146. Linde, J. A., Jeffery, R. W., French, S. A., et al. (2005). Self-weighing in weight gain prevention and weight loss trials. *Annals of Behavioral Medicine, 30*(3), 210–216.

CHAPTER 39

Diabetes Mellitus and Metabolic Syndrome

Beverly Dyck Thomassian

OVERVIEW OF DIABETES

The global epidemic of diabetes will challenge our generation to develop novel strategies to prevent and treat this life long condition. Every 10 seconds, two people develop diabetes and one person dies from diabetes-related causes. In 2007, 246 million people worldwide had diabetes. That number is expected to climb to 380 million by 2030.[1] In most developed countries, diabetes is the fourth or fifth leading cause of death and there is concern that it will become an epidemic in many developing and newly industrialized nations. City dwellers are at especially high risk since they tend to be less physically active and are more likely to be obese as compared to their rural counterparts.[2] Heart disease is the leading cause of death for all people with diabetes.[1] Heart disease, coupled with the other long-term complications including kidney, eye, and nerve disease, results in disability, reduced life expectancy, and enormous hearth burdens for virtually every society.[2] In 2007, the United Nations General Assembly recognized that diabetes "poses a severe risk for the families, Member States and the entire world" and passed a resolution declaring November 14 World Diabetes Day.[3]

In spite of this emerging epidemic, there is abundant evidence that diabetes can be prevented and its complications avoided. The challenge faced by health care providers is to increase awareness regarding diabetes risk factors, promote early identification, and provide treatment aimed at preventing complications and improving quality of life. The purpose of this chapter is to discuss (1) the natural history and pathophysiology of types 1 and 2 diabetes, (2) the relationship between insulin resistance and cardiovascular disease (CVD), (3) prevention of type 2 diabetes, (4) metabolic syndrome and cardiovascular complications, and (5) the goals of care and interventions aimed at complication prevention and mitigation.

Definition and Diagnosis

Diabetes can be caused by a variety of hormonal and cellular defects, which result in elevated blood glucose levels. A normal fasting glucose level is less than 110 mg/dL (6.1 mmol) according to the World Health Organization (WHO)[4] and the European Association for the Study of Diabetes (EASD).[5] According to the American Diabetes Association (ADA), normal fasting blood glucose is less than 100 mg/dL (5.7 mmol).[6] This level of fasting glucose is maintained in the body by an intricate balance of hormones, which work to maintain glucose levels at a steady state. Normally, insulin and other hormones are released in response to rising blood glucose levels. These powerful hormones activate cellular storage of glucose, amino acids, and triglycerides in target cells, including the liver, muscle, and fat, with the end result of normoglycemia. To keep glucose levels from falling too low, other hormones, such as glucagon, corticosteroids, growth hormone, and epinephrine, increase insulin resistance to maintain adequate circulating glucose. In the presence of diabetes, there is a diminished or absent insulin response and cellular resistance to insulin. These defects, coupled with a deficiency of other glucose lowering hormones, result in higher fasting and postmeal glucose levels.

To diagnose diabetes, either fasting plasma glucose, random glucose, or a post 75 g glucose challenge glucose level can be used. Currently, there is international consensus that a fasting blood glucose level of ≥126 mg/dL (7 mmol), or a random or post meal glucose tolerance level of ≥200 mg/dL (11.1 mmol) in the presence of symptoms of hyperglycemia confers a diagnosis of diabetes (Table 39-1).[5] Blood glucose levels that are higher than normal but do not reach the criteria for diabetes indicate future risk of diabetes and heart disease. This category of blood glucose is referred to as prediabetes and includes impaired fasting glucose and impaired glucose tolerance. Impaired fasting glucose is defined as fasting blood glucose of 100 to 125 mg/dL (5.6 to 6.9 mmol/L) by the ADA[6] and 110 to 125 mg/dL (6.0 to 6.9 mmol/L) by the EASD.[5] There is international consensus that impaired glucose tolerance is defined as blood glucose of 140 to 199 mg/dL (7.8 to 11.1 mmol/L) 2 hours after a 75 g glucose challenge. Uncontrolled, chronically elevated glucose, often termed "glucose toxicity," can lead to a multiplicity of vascular complications that start long before the diagnosis of diabetes is made. Identifying and treating hyperglycemia in its earliest stages is critical to prevent complications. Unfortunately, as many as 50% of people with diabetes worldwide remain undiagnosed and untreated.[1]

Prevalence and Consequence of Diabetes

The global prevalence of diabetes will double in the next 30 years due to population growth, urbanization, increasing prevalence of obesity, aging, and physical inactivity.[7] Table 39-2 illustrates the 10 countries with the highest prevalence estimates for diabetes in 2000 and 2030. The countries with the highest rates of diabetes include India, China, and the United States. In India, the crude prevalence rate is 9% in urban areas[8] and in the United States, 7% of the population is affected by diabetes.[9] In developing countries, the highest prevalence of diabetes is the middle productive years of 45 to 64 years of age range. In contrast, the majority of people with diabetes in developed countries are greater than 64 years of age.[7]

In the United States and globally, 90% to 95% of people with diabetes have type 2 and the majority of those are overweight.[9] Over 50% of the U.S. population is overweight and more than one billion people in the world are overweight, of which at least 300 million are obese.[2] The United States and other developing countries are experiencing an epidemic of type 2 diabetes in youth. This increase in type 2 diabetes in youth strongly correlates with increasing prevalence of childhood obesity.[10]

Table 39-1 ■ DIAGNOSTIC CRITERIA FOR DIABETES

1. FPG ≥126 mg/dL (7.0 mmol/L). Fasting is defined as no caloric intake for at least 8 h.*
   or
2. Symptoms of hyperglycemia and casual plasma glucose ≥200 mg/dL (11.1 mmol/L). Casual is defined as any time of day without regard to time since last meal. The classic symptoms of hyperglycemia include polyuria, polydipsia, and unexplained weight loss.
   or
3. 2-h plasma glucose ≥200 mg/dL (11.1 mmol/L) during an OGTT. The test should be performed as described by the World Health Organization, using a glucose load containing the equivalent of 75 g anhydrous glucose dissolved in water.*

*In the absence of unequivocal hyperglycemia, these criteria should be confirmed by repeat testing on a different day (5).
OGTT, oral glucose tolerance test.
From American Diabetes Association. (2008). Clinical practice recommendations: Diagnosis and classification of diabetes mellitus. *Diabetes Care, 31*(Suppl. 1), S12–S54.

From an ethnic perspective, type 2 diabetes is more common in the United States among Native American, Hispanic/Latino, non-Hispanic Black, African-American, and Pacific Islander populations.[11] Internationally, however, diabetes affects many diverse ethnic groups.[7] From a global and a local perspective, the human and economic costs of this epidemic are enormous. In the United States, one out of every 10 health care dollars is spent on treating diabetes and its complications. The total annual economic cost of diabetes in 2007 was estimated to be $174 billion. This includes direct costs of treating diabetes-related complications and indirect costs of lost workdays and disability.[12] The global burgeoning increase of diabetes will inevitably increase the rate of premature deaths from CVD as well as increase the prevalence of other diabetes complications.[7] Worldwide, one in 20 deaths is due to diabetes, which equals 3.2 million deaths annually. Globally, heart disease and stroke account for about 50% to 80% percent of deaths in people with diabetes and this chronic condition is the leading cause of blindness, amputation, and kidney failure.[2] The pace of growth and the complications of diabetes demand a concerted, global effort to focus on prevention and appropriate treatment of this epidemic. Multiple large-scale trials have proven that changes in diet, physical activity, or pharmacologic treatment can reduce the incidence of diabetes. Other trials document that complications of diabetes can be delayed or prevented through glucose control and risk factor management. The impressive results of these trials (which will be discussed later in this chapter) provide the impetus to focus on global prevention and aggressive treatment of this serious condition.

Table 39-2 ■ LIST OF COUNTRIES WITH THE HIGHEST NUMBERS OF ESTIMATED CASES OF DIABETES FOR 2000 AND 2030

	2000		2030	
Ranking	Country	People with Diabetes (millions)	Country	People with Diabetes (millions)
1	India	31.7	India	79.4
2	China	20.8	China	42.3
3	United States	17.7	United States	30.3
4	Indonesia	8.4	Indonesia	21.3
5	Japan	6.8	Pakistan	13.9
6	Pakistan	5.2	Brazil	11.3
7	Russian Federation	4.6	Bangladesh	11.1
			Japan	8.9
8	Brazil	4.6	Philippines	7.8
9	Italy	4.3	Egypt	6.7
10	Bangladesh	3.2		

From Wild, S., Roglic, G., Green, A., et al. (2004). Global prevalence of diabetes estimates for the year 2000 and projections for 2030. *Diabetes Care, 27*, 1047–1053.

PATHOPHYSIOLOGY OF DIABETES MELLITUS

Hormonal Regulation of Glucose Levels

The hallmark of diabetes is elevated blood glucose levels. This abnormal elevation is due to the decrease or absence of hormones that lower blood glucose and a cellular resistance to insulin. A review of normal fuel metabolism and the hormones responsible for glucose regulation follows.

Plasma glucose levels reflect the rate at which glucose is absorbed from the intestines and then removed from circulation to be stored as fuel. The first phase of fuel metabolism is called the fed state and encompasses the first 4 hours after ingestion of food. During this phase, the pancreas responds to increasing levels of circulating glucose by activating stored insulin called "proinsulin." Proinsulin is a protein composed of two chains "A" and "B" of amino acids, which are held together by a bridge called a connecting peptide (c-peptide). On pancreatic detection of elevating glucose, the connecting peptide of proinsulin cleaves off. The resulting activated insulin and c-peptide enter the bloodstream. This initial burst of insulin is referred to as first phase insulin response. First phase insulin is responsible for maintaining postmeal glucose within normal limits. Insulin then passes through the portal vein into the bloodstream. Once insulin enters the bloodstream, it has a half-life of a few minutes. However, since c-peptide has a longer half-life, it is can be measured by a blood test to determine how much endogenous insulin a person releases.

During these first 4 hours of the fed state, insulin promotes the storage of glucose as glycogen in the insulin-sensitive peripheral tissues, including hepatic and muscle cells. Insulin also promotes storage of amino acids as protein and excess glucose is stored as fat. The end result is a lowering of circulating blood glucose, lipids, and other energy substrates. Besides promoting the disposal of nutrients into cells, insulin has the critical role of suppressing glucagon. Glucagon, a hormone released by the α-cells of the pancreas, stimulates the release of stored glucose (glycogen) from the liver.

During this fed state, the β-cells of the pancreas also release the recently discovered hormone amylin, a 37-amino acid polypeptide.[13] Amylin compliments the action of insulin by preventing postmeal blood glucose excursions in several ways. Unlike insulin, it slows down gastric emptying, promotes a sense of satiety, and decreases the release of glucagon. People with type 1 diabetes make no amylin and those with type 2 make less than normal amounts.

Another group of newly discovered intestinal hormones, the incretins, are also released in response to nutrient ingestion. The incretins include glucose-dependent insulin-releasing peptide (GIP) and glucagon-like peptide-1 (GLP-1). GIP is secreted by the K cells of the upper intestine and GLP-1 is released from the L cells of the intestine.[13] Both are secreted in response to postmeal glucose elevations and stimulate β-cell insulin secretion. In addition to increasing glucose-dependent insulin secretion, incretin hormones inhibit glucagon secretion, slow gastric emptying, and increase feelings of satiety. Incretins help to keep postmeal blood glucose levels within normal ranges. Both GIP and GLP-1 are rapidly degraded by the enzyme dipeptidyl-peptidase-inhibitor-IV. (New therapies that imitate the incretins and inhibit their breakdown will be discussed in the section "Medication for Type 2 Diabetes.") People with type 1 diabetes make normal amounts of the incretins, while those with type 2 secrete less of this powerful glucose-lowering hormone.[13]

Four to 16 hours after eating, the body enters the phase II or the postabsorptive state. This phase most often occurs during sleep and marks the end of anabolism or energy storage and begins the phase of catabolism or energy production. During this phase, since the body is not exposed to food, it must revert to stored energy for fuel. Glucagon levels rise and insulin levels decrease to a steady state, often termed basal insulin release. The main function of insulin during this phase is not to promote energy storage, but to prevent hyperglycemia. The high levels of circulating glucagon increase the breakdown of glycogen stores in the liver (glycogenolysis) to ensure an adequate supply of glucose to the brain and other glucose-dependent tissues. In addition, fat cells (adipocytes) break down triglycerides and release free fatty acids (FFAs) to be used as energy by the liver and skeletal muscles. The brain will only use glucose for fuel due to its inability to use FFAs as fuel. Many individuals with type 2 diabetes experience morning fasting hyperglycemia due to the dominance of glycogen and the relative lack of insulin during this phase.[13]

In addition to glucagon, there are other catabolic hormones that increase the breakdown of stored fuel supplies and increase circulating glucose. They increase insulin resistance and glycogen breakdown, causing a net increase in blood glucose levels. The hormones released from the kidney, corticosteroids and epinephrine, are activated during flight-or-fight response or hypoglycemia. Other hormones including growth hormone and cortisol increase insulin resistance in early morning, causing many people with type 1 diabetes to experience the "dawn" phenomena, or an elevation in morning glucose.[14]

Glucose homeostasis is reliant on a complex interrelationship of hormones that activate anabolic and catabolic processes. When this precise balance is disrupted through the loss or dysfunction of insulin and other hormones, the end result is hyperglycemia.

Type 1 Diabetes Mellitus

Previously labeled "juvenile diabetes" or "insulin-dependent diabetes," type 1 diabetes affects approximately 10% of all people with diabetes.[6] The unique feature of type 1 is its' progressive autoimmunity resulting in complete destruction of the pancreatic β-cells. Although it can occur at any age, most new cases are expressed during childhood and puberty, when insulin-resistant pubertal hormones are at their peak. To express type 1 diabetes, a genetic propensity and an environmental trigger are necessary.[13] Research has not identified any one causative agent that triggers the autoimmune attack against the pancreas, but several agents are suspected.[15] Viral triggers such as enteroviruses, coxsackie virus B, congenital rubella, cytomegalovirus, and mumps are suspected culprits. However, these agents are only theorized to initiate the autoimmunity of type 1 diabetes, and research on causation is ongoing. From a prevention perspective, it appears that children who are breastfed are less likely to develop type 1 diabetes.[13]

When 90% of the pancreas is destroyed, there is no longer enough insulin available to maintain euglycemia and the symptoms of hyperglycemia are expressed. The rate of destruction of the β-cell mass with type 1 diabetes is rapid in youth and more gradual in the older age group.[13] Although the destruction of the β-cells is progressive, the onset of type 1 diabetes is usually abrupt. With only 10% of the pancreas working, there is no longer adequate insulin to maintain euglycemia. Without sufficient insulin to utilize glucose for energy, the body starts breaking down fat stores for fuel. The pace of this fat breakdown and resulting ketone bodies overwhelms the liver and, in a short time, it can no longer clear ketones at a fast enough pace. High levels of circulating ketones result in ketosis and acidosis—also called diabetes ketoacidosis. At this point, the body cells are starved for glucose and the person usually feels ill enough to seek medical help. Depending on the duration and severity of ketosis, the person with a new case of type 1 diabetes appears malnourished due to inability to store fuel, dehydrated due to osmotic diuresis, and may have abdominal pain and nausea from the ketone bodies. In an effort to blow off excess acids, the person may have rapid respirations and a their breath may smell fruity. Treatment includes fluids, insulin, electrolyte replacement, and patient and family education. Clinical presentation is usually enough to make a diagnosis of type 1 diabetes. If unsure, a diagnosis can be confirmed by antibody blood tests. Some tests used to confirm autoimmune β-cell destruction include antibodies to glutamic acid decarboxylase, islet cell autoantibodies, and insulin autoantibodies.[15] Patients with type 1 diabetes will require insulin replacement for the rest of their lives. There is ongoing investigation to evaluate if type 1 diabetes can be prevented or delayed in individuals at high risk of developing type 1 diabetes. To date however, large, randomized clinical trials have failed to demonstrate treatment effect.[16,17] These studies have improved the understanding of the immunopathogenesis and will hopefully lead to future strategies and treatments to prevent type 1 diabetes.

Type 2 Diabetes Mellitus

Unlike type 1 diabetes, type 2 diabetes (formerly referred to as adult onset or non-insulin-dependent diabetes) is not an autoimmune condition. Of all people with diabetes, 90% to 95% have type 2. Most people with type 2 diabetes are overweight and develop hyperglycemia as a result of insulin resistance and insulin deficiency. Besides being overweight, some of the risk factors for developing type 2 diabetes include physical inactivity, first-degree relative with diabetes, women who delivered a baby bigger than 9 lb (4.2 kg), or who had gestational diabetes. Other risk factors include hypertension, impaired glucose tolerance, elevated triglycerides, and other conditions associated with insulin resistance.[11] In addition to these risk factors, the social milieu into which a person is born can also increase or decrease the likelihood of the expression of type 2 diabetes. Social research reveals that people of lower socioeconomic status are more likely to express diabetes.[18] This may be due to a variety of factors including lack of access to safe places to exercise, limited knowledge of healthy eating, and increased prevalence of obesity. Being overweight and obese, especially central abdominal obesity, across all populations increases in the risk of diabetes. New research has discovered that abdominal adipose tissue acts as an endocrine organ, secreting chemical mediators that increase insulin resistance and inflammation.[19]

β-Cell Defects Associated With Type 2 Diabetes

Type 2 diabetes is a heterogeneous group of disorders that in combination result in hyperglycemia. These disorders include β-cell death, insulin resistance, excessive hepatic glucose release, and other hormonal deficiencies.[15]

The cause of β-cell mass death is not known. Studies suggest that about 40% of β-cell mass is lost in individuals with impaired glucose tolerance and 60% on clinical diagnosis of diabetes.[20] β-Cell loss starts 9 to 12 years before the diabetes is diagnosed.[15] The rate of β-cell death is much higher in people with diabetes, although the rate of new islet cell formation is unaffected.[13] Because of large clinical trials, such as the United Kingdom Prospective Diabetes Study, the natural history of type 2 diabetes is better understood. This study demonstrated that β-cell death in type 2 diabetes is progressive and continues over time.[21] Upon diagnosis of type 2 diabetes, regardless if the patient is lean or overweight, beta cell mass is decreased by half. This in part explains why 30% of people with type 2 diabetes eventually require insulin therapy.[22] In addition to β-cell death, there is diminished pancreatic sensitivity and insulin secretory response. This reduced response is caused by pancreatic overexposure to chronically abnormal high levels of blood glucose (sometimes termed glucose toxicity).[13] As insulin secretion decreases, blood glucose levels rise above normal and thus marks the beginnings of type 2 diabetes. However, more than β-cell death and insulin deficiency is to blame.

Insulin Resistance and Cardiometabolic Syndrome

Insulin Resistance. Insulin resistance refers to the inadequate response of the muscle, liver, and fat cells to insulin. As a result, glucose stays in circulation instead of being converted into energy through cellular metabolism.[5] People who are overweight and obese are more likely to be insulin resistant. Contrary to popular belief, insulin resistance is not due to deficient or malfunctioning insulin cell receptors. Studies show that people with diabetes have normal amount and function of insulin receptors.[13] The exact mechanism of insulin resistance is not understood but may be due to defective postinsulin receptor signal transduction mechanisms.[19]

Early in the process of diabetes, the pancreas oversecretes insulin in an effort to overcome insulin resistance and maintain euglycemia. Many people with insulin resistance have high levels of blood glucose and high levels of insulin circulating in their blood at the same time. As insulin resistance continues and β-cell loss worsens, blood glucose levels exceed normal levels. Morning glucose levels are elevated since there is not enough insulin to prevent nocturnal overproduction of glucose by the liver. Postmeal blood glucose levels are elevated due to several mechanisms. First, due to the defects of diabetes, the uptake of glucose by the muscle after meals is decreased by over 50%. Second, unchecked glucagon stimulates the liver to release glucose, even in a fed state. Finally, muscle and adipocytes (fat cells) are resistant to insulin, which results in high levels of FFAs. Elevated FFA worsens insulin resistance in the liver and muscle cells, increases the formation of glucose and impairs β-cell secretion. Dysfunctional adipocytes also produce chemical mediators that contribute to atherosclerosis and insulin resistance.[13] This unrestrained hyperglycemia further reduces insulin sensitivity and pancreatic insulin secretion.[15]

In addition to decreasing β-cell function and insulin resistance, other hormone dysfunction contributes to hyperglycemia. With type 2 diabetes, the β-cells are also under producing the glucose-lowering hormone, amylin. This hormone discovered in the 1980s is secreted in a 1:1 ratio with insulin and increases satiety and lowers postmeal glucagon release. People with type 2 diabetes make less than half the normal amount of amylin. The gut hormones GLP-1 and GIP that promote satiety and decrease postmeal glucagon release are also under produced. The enzyme that breaks down these hormones called dipeptidyl-peptidase-inhibitor-IV is overactive and decreases the bioavailability of these critical hormones adding to postmeal hyperglycemia.[23]

Metabolic Syndrome Overview. The term metabolic syndrome (sometimes termed insulin-resistant syndrome or cardiometabolic syndrome) refers to a clustering of risk factors that include abdominal obesity, dyslipidemia, hyperglycemia, and hypertension.[24] This syndrome is a major public health challenge worldwide since it is associated with a five-fold elevated risk of type 2 diabetes and a two- to three-fold risk of CVD.[25]

In 1998, Reaven described a syndrome based on insulin resistance, high circulating insulin levels, hyperglycemia, elevated very-low-density lipoprotein (VLDL), decreased high-density lipoprotein (HDL) cholesterol and high blood pressure.[26] Since then, there has been ongoing interest, research, and debate on definition and utility of the metabolic syndrome. The ADA and EASD have called into question the imprecision of the definition, the lack of certainty of the pathogenesis and its value in predicting CVD. These diabetes organizations stress the importance of evaluating and treating each cardiovascular risk factor; whether the person meets the diagnostic criteria for the metabolic syndrome or not.[27] Ongoing research is needed to determine the predictive benefit of diagnosing someone with metabolic syndrome. In addition, there is no one universal definition for the metabolic syndrome. The most commonly referred to definitions are the World Health Organization (WHO) definition developed in 1999,[28] the National Cholesterol Education Program Adult Treatment Expert Panel III (NCEP III) in 2001[29] and most recently the International Diabetes Federation (IDF)[30] consensus panel in 2005 which has developed a worldwide consensus of the definition of the metabolic syndrome. In 2003, the American College of Endocrinology (ACE) published a position statement in collaboration with American Association of Clinical Endocrinologists (AACE) on "insulin resistance syndrome"[31] (their preferred term) which avoids using a set of criteria to define metabolic syndrome, but instead focuses on the cluster of abnormalities that are more likely to occur in individuals who are insulin resistant/hyperinsulinemic and stress that diagnosis should be based on clinical judgment informed by the evaluation of risk factors. In their position paper, they specifically strive to distinguish insulin-resistant syndrome from type 2 diabetes and CVD, since their stated clinical focus is to identify individuals at risk BEFORE such consequences occurred. In addition to these philosophical differences, they also use body mass index (BMI) rather than waist circumference to measure central obesity and introduce ethnicity as a risk factor.

Metabolic Syndrome Definitions. The WHO definition of metabolic syndrome requires the presence of insulin resistance as identified by either type 2 diabetes, impaired fasting glucose, or impaired glucose tolerance plus at least two of the following:

- BMI >30 kg/m^2 and/or waist to hip ratio >0.90 in men or >0.85 in women.
- Serum triglycerides ≥50 mg/dL (1.7 mmol/L) or HDL cholesterol <35 mg/dL (0.9 mmol/L) in men and <39 mg/dL (1.0 mmol/L) in women.
- Raised arterial blood pressure ≥140/90 mm Hg.
- Urinary albumin excretion rate >20 μg/min or albumin to creatine ratio ≥30 mg/g.

According to the NCEP III, hyperglycemia is not the critical factor to enter the risk stratification for metabolic syndrome; instead, adults who are diagnosed with metabolic syndrome must have *three* or more of the following:

- Waist circumference >40 in (102 cm) in men and >35 in (88 cm) in women.
- Serum triglycerides ≥150 mg/dL (1.7 mmol/L).
- Blood pressure ≥130/≥85 mm Hg.
- HDL cholesterol <40 mg/dL (103 mmol/L) in men and <50 mg/dL (1.29 mmol/L) in women.
- Fasting glucose ≥110 mg/dL (6.1 mmol/L).

Here, there is a shift from waist to hip ratio to waist circumference and elevated glucose levels may be included but are not critical for diagnosis of diabetes. In this stratification, the risk factors carry a similar weight.

The IDF organized a consensus panel to create a worldwide definition of metabolic syndrome. The results of the consensus group were presented in 2005 in Berlin at the First International Conference on prediabetes and the metabolic syndrome. This new definition of metabolic syndrome is more user friendly for those in clinical practice. While the underlying cause of the metabolic syndrome is still the subject of intense debate, the IDF consensus statement identifies both abnormal abdominal fat distribution and insulin resistance as critical, interrelated causes. To be defined as having metabolic syndrome, the IDF definition requires the following: central obesity (defined as waist circumference >37 in (94 cm) in European men and >31.5 in (88 cm) for European women with ethnicity specific values for other groups, *plus two of the following four additional factors*:

- Raised triglycerides: >150 mg/dL (1.7 mmol/L) or specific treatment for this lipid abnormality.
- Reduced HDL cholesterol: <40 mg/dL (1.03 mmol/L) in men and <50 mg/dL (1.29 mmol/L) in women or specific treatment for this lipid abnormality.
- Raised blood pressure: systolic BP ≥130 mm Hg or diastolic BP ≥85 or treatment of previously diagnosed hypertension.
- Raised fasting plasma glucose level FPG ≥100 mg/dL (5.6 mmol/L) or previously diagnosed diabetes. If above 100 mg/dL or 5.6 mmol/L, oral glucose tolerance test is strongly recommended but not necessary to define the presence of the syndrome.

With the creation of an international definition, it is now possible to estimate the prevalence of metabolic syndrome and make comparisons between nations. According to the IDF, up to 25% of the world's adults have metabolic syndrome.[1]

Although debate exists about which definition of the metabolic syndrome is the best, in clinical practice it is important to assess for insulin resistance, risk factors for heart disease, and diabetes in all patients. The position of ACE highlights a main feature of insulin resistance; it is not only associated with heart disease and diabetes, but with a multitude of other conditions that interlink with increased risk of hyperglycemia and vascular disease. According to ACE, risk factors that increase the likelihood of the insulin resistance syndrome include the following:

- Diagnosis of CVD, hypertension, polycystic ovary syndrome, nonalcoholic fatty liver disease, or acanthosis nigricans
- Family history of type 2 diabetes or glucose intolerance
- Non-Caucasian ethnicity
- Sedentary lifestyle
- BMI >25.0 kg/m^2 (or waist circumference >40 in (102 cm) in men and >35 in (88 cm) in women)

Some authors have argued that since there is no unifying cause of the syndrome and that the CVD or diabetes risk prediction is no greater than the sum of its parts and treatment of the syndrome is no different from treatment of its components, that we put aside the metabolic syndrome as a unique disease. Instead, until the relationship and etiology of the clustering of these risk factors is better understood, the focus should be on assessing for the well-known diabetes and heart disease risk factors and treating according to guidelines with a special emphasis on regular exercise and weight management.[27] This alternative perspective being promoted by the ADA is called the cardiometabolic risk initiative. The risk factor map (Fig. 39-1) describes a pathway from obesity to insulin resistance to type 2 diabetes and/or CVD. It is designed to highlight the individual risk factors and their interrelationships. The ADA is also promoting the use of a well-validated global risk assessment tool called Diabetes Personal Health Decisions (Diabetes PHD)[32] that is a user friendly online algorithm that can provide a personalized risk assessment based on user health data (including height, weight, lipid level, family history, blood pressure, etc.). In addition to providing a risk assessment, it also provides strategies to decrease risk through lifestyle and pharmacologic interventions. Improvements and patient outcomes should certainly improve as the understanding of the complex interrelationships between insulin resistance, obesity, heart disease, and hyperglycemia expand.

Prevention of Type 2 Diabetes

Since even mildly elevated blood glucose levels indicate greater risk for heart disease and the development of diabetes, it is critical to identify people at risk for developing type 2 diabetes and provide risk reduction interventions. People at risk for type 2 diabetes are easily identified through standardized risk assessments, blood glucose measurements, or by ascertainment of family history, lifestyle, and BMI or waistline measurements.[5] The risk of developing diabetes is a complex interaction of genetics and lifestyle. A person at risk of diabetes who is not overweight and exercises regularly has less chance of developing diabetes during their lifetime than their counterpart who leads a sedentary lifestyle and is overweight. Certainly, if a particular family has several members with type 2 diabetes, this may be due to not only genetic susceptibility but also shared environment and similar lifestyles, demonstrating that a combination of genetics and behavioral influences work to increase or decrease risk of disease expression.[13]

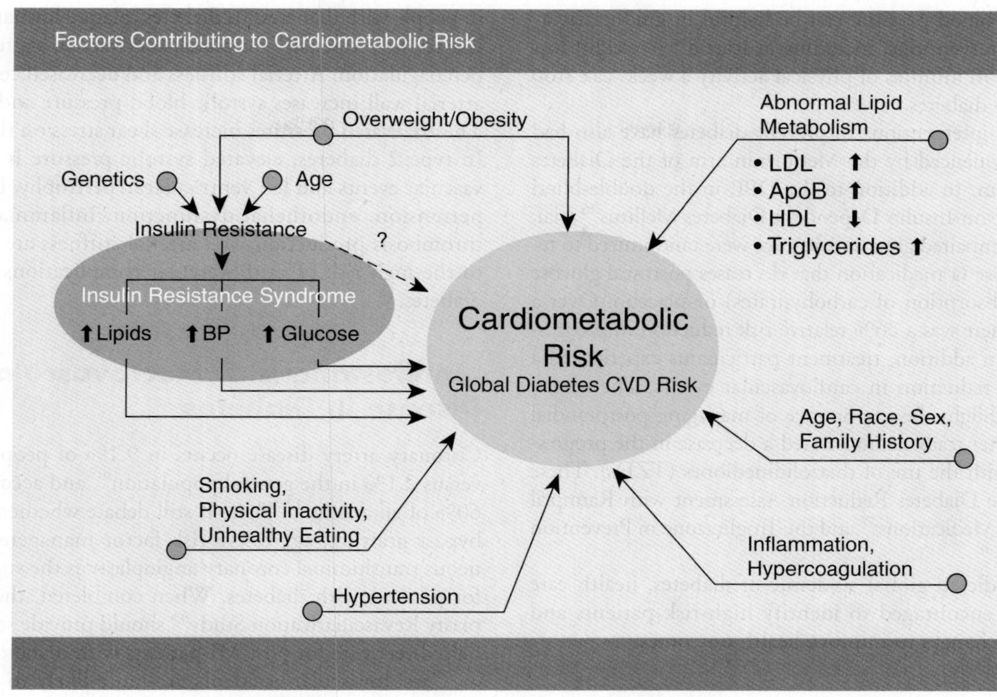

■ **Figure 39-1** The cardiometabolic risk initiative.

The expression of type 2 diabetes is a reflection of many years of metabolic dysregulation, including impaired glucose tolerance, lipid abnormalities, and insulin resistance. For people with impaired glucose tolerance on the metabolic pathway to diabetes, carefully conducted clinical studies have demonstrated that these individuals can prevent the expression of type 2 diabetes by more than 50% through lifestyle changes alone. Other studies have demonstrated risk reduction through pharmacologic interventions. An understanding of the interventions and outcomes of these trials can provide health care professionals with strategies and tools to help instruct and motivate their clients with impaired glucose tolerance to take action to prevent the onset of diabetes.

Four major studies have examined the effects of lifestyle changes for people at risk with diabetes. These studies demonstrated a 31% to 63% risk reduction and include the Malmo Study in Finland,[33] the Da Qing Study from China,[34] the Finnish Diabetes Prevention Study,[35] and the U.S. based Diabetes Prevention Program.[16] Although the design for each study is slightly different, each program identified people with impaired glucose tolerance and assigned participants to either a control or a intervention group. In the Finnish study which included 522 participants, the intervention groups received detailed counseling by a nutritionist with the goal of reducing weight by at least 5%. This was achieved by reducing total fat intake to <30% of calories and saturated fat to <10% of calories, increasing fiber intake to at least 15 g per 1000 calories and participating in at least 30 minutes a day of physical activity. Participants received seven individual sessions with the nutritionist during the first year and one session every 3 months thereafter. They also received individually tailored guidance on increasing physical activity. In this 3-year study, the incidence of progressing to diabetes was 11% in the lifestyle intervention group and 23% in the control group. This equaled a 58% reduction in risk of developing diabetes in the intervention group. The reduction in the incidence of diabetes was directly associated with the degree of change in lifestyle.

The goal of the U.S. Diabetes Prevention Program was to determine the safest and most effective approach to preventing progression to type 2 diabetes among an ethnically diverse group of individuals with impaired glucose tolerance. In addition to lifestyle intervention, this 3-year trial with over 3,000 participants also included a pharmacologic intervention (metformin) compared to placebo. The lifestyle goals were similar to the Finnish study, to lose at least 7% of body weight by decreasing daily caloric intake by 500 to 1000 calories with less than 25% of calories from fat and participating in 150 minutes of physical activity a week. Participants met with a lifestyle coach 16 times in the first 24 weeks to review a 16-lesson curriculum which included detailed instruction on diet, physical activity, and behavioral modification strategies. Every month participants also met in person or by phone with the lifestyle coach to address specific barriers to adherence and if desired they could attend group classes. The results confirmed the Finnish findings. Among the lifestyle intervention group, there was a 58% reduction in developing diabetes over a 3-year period.

The metformin arm of the Diabetes Prevention Program compared the results of 850 mg of metformin twice daily versus a placebo. Metformin was nearly ineffective in individuals over 60 years old or those with BMI less than 30. However, a 31% overall risk reductions in developing diabetes was observed in the Metformin group.

In addition to decreasing the risk of developing diabetes, most of the studies also documented improvements in other clinical outcomes such as blood pressure, lipids, and participants required dose reductions in blood pressure and lipid medications.

For overweight patients with a family history of type 2 diabetes or CVD, assessment of risk and measurement of fasting glucose levels, lipids, and blood pressure can be helpful in guiding treatment. Lifestyle interventions, including at least a 5% weight loss and engaging in 150 minutes of physical activity a week, can stop the progression to diabetes.

Pharmacologic interventions to prevent diabetes have also had some success as evidenced by the Metformin arm of the Diabetes Prevention Program. In addition to the DPP, in the double-blind Study to Prevent Non-Insulin Dependent Diabetes Mellitus[36] trial, participants with impaired glucose tolerance were randomized to receive either acarbose (a medication that decreases postmeal glucose by delaying the absorption of carbohydrates) or placebo. Over a 3.3-year period, there was a 36% relative risk reduction in progression to diabetes. In addition, treatment participants experienced a 53% relative risk reduction in cardiovascular events. The results from this trial highlight the importance of managing postprandial glucose levels. Other trials demonstrated a decrease in the progression to diabetes with the use of thiazolidinediones (TZDs). These studies include the Diabetes Reduction Assessment with Ramipril and Rosiglitazone Medications[37] and the Troglitazone in Prevention of Diabetes Study.[38]

Given the predicted global epidemic of diabetes, health care professionals are encouraged to identify high-risk patients and promote lifestyle changes to improve health outcomes.

MACROVASCULAR COMPLICATIONS OF DIABETES

The NCEP III has termed diabetes a coronary heart disease risk equivalent.[40] CVD is the major cause of mortality and morbidity for individuals with diabetes and is the largest contributor to the direct and indirect costs of diabetes.[11] Given the prevalence and severity, an understanding of the pathophysiology and manifestations of CVD will be presented. Risk reduction and treatment will be addressed in "Goals of the Diabetes Care" section.

Pathophysiology of Macrovascular Disease in Diabetes

Hyperglycemia is associated with defects in the vascular endothelium, the lining of the blood vessels, and chemical mediators that increase vascular dysfunction. Current research has shown that the vascular endothelium is an active endocrine organ that secretes a number of factors, which provide an environment that inhibits the adhesion of leukocytes, platelets, prevents clot formation, and inhibits vasopasm.[13] A bioactive substance of particular importance is nitric oxide (NO). NO causes vasodilatation and platelet inhibition, reduces vascular wall inflammation, prevents vasoconstriction and thrombus formation.[5] However, in the presence of cardiovascular risk factors and hyperglycemia, levels of NO are diminished and there is decreased vasodilatation in response to NO. This defect contributes to the high prevalence of hypertension associated with hyperglycemia.

Diabetes also increases the inflammatory response often seen in damaged vessels due to oxidative stress, diminished NO production, and high postmeal circulating levels of FFAs. Inflammatory mediators enhance the creation of foam cells, decrease plaque stability, and increase risk of plaque rupture triggering acute thrombotic events. Cardiovascular risk is closely linked to the platelet dysfunction and coagulation disorders commonly seen in people with diabetes. In diabetes, plaque formation is amplified due to the propensity for platelet activation, aggregation, and hypercoagulation. Arterial stiffness and decreased compliance of the arterial wall increases systolic blood pressure and pulse pressure. These elevated pressures increase shear stress on the endothelium. In type 2 diabetes, elevated systolic pressure is associated with vascular events and left ventricular hypertrophy. In summary, hypertension, endothelial dysfunction, inflammation, increased thrombosis production, and arterial stiffness are all contributors to the high risk of cardiovascular complications associated with diabetes.[13]

Manifestations of Macrovascular Disease in Diabetes

Coronary artery disease occurs in 9.1% of people with diabetes versus 2.1% in the general population[40] and accounts for 56% to 60% of all deaths.[13] There is still debate whether coronary artery bypass grafting, aggressive risk factor management or percutaneous transluminal coronary angioplasty is the superior treatment for patients with diabetes. When completed, the Bypass Angioplasty Revascularization Study[41] should provide some answers and help direct care for post-MI patients with diabetes.

Cerebrovascular accidents are more likely to occur in people with diabetes at a younger age and when there is a history of myocardial infarction. Stroke occurs in 6.6% of the diabetes population and 1.8% in persons without diabetes.[40] Management includes vascular surgery or management of risk factors, with a special focus on managing hypertension, smoking cessation, and initiation of antiplatelet therapy.[13]

Diabetes increases the risk of the development of congestive heart failure (CHF), especially in women;[13] 7.9% of people with diabetes have CHF, versus 1.1% in the general population. [40] Possible mechanisms for this increased risk include decreased ventricular elasticity due to cross-linking of collagen, inflammatory cytokines, and oxidative stress. Other risk factors include hypertension, hyperglycemia, and endothelial inflammation. The end result is diminished relaxation of the ventricle and impaired diastolic filling, both of which increase the risk of developing CHF.[13]

Peripheral arterial disease (PAD) affects approximately 20% to 30% of people with diabetes and is frequently under diagnosed and under treated.[42] Assessment of PAD includes determining if the patient suffers from intermittent claudication and measuring ankle brachial index. Main risk factors for development of PAD include tobacco use and diabetes. Since people with diabetes and PAD are at increased risk for lower extremity complications including amputations and cardiovascular events, it is important to help patients identify and reduce vascular risk factors.

NURSING MANAGEMENT OF DIABETES

Nurses are positioned to play a pivotal role in curbing the diabetes epidemic. Nurses can initiate diabetes detection initiatives, such as evaluation of all glucose levels in the hospital or outpatient settings to find those who are undiagnosed. In the clinical setting, they can review patient's history, symptoms, and lab values to determine if they are at risk for prediabetes, undiagnosed diabetes, or heart disease. Important nursing roles include explaining the importance of treating hyperglycemia and encouraging at risk patients to seek follow-up care from their provider. Providing patients with a written record of abnormal glucose levels and encouraging follow-up testing is critical.

Since diabetes occurs throughout the lifespan, it is important to tailor education to meet the needs of patients and families. Nursing care includes providing the patient and family with skills to cope with both the medical and psychosocial issues that often coexist with a new diagnosis of diabetes. Younger clients with newly diagnosed type 1 diabetes benefit from management by a diabetes specialist or endocrinologist.[15] The patient and family members also benefit from the expertise of a mental health professional to deal with the emotional impact of a new diagnosis of diabetes.[43]

Since the majority of people with diabetes are over 65 years of age, age is an important factor in patient assessment.[42] Given the high rate of comorbidities for older people with diabetes, they often require a long list of medications to manage not only diabetes, but hypertension, hyperlipidemia, and other conditions. Many older clients on fixed incomes cannot afford all of their prescribed medications. Nurses can encourage patients to collaborate with their pharmacist and provider to determine the safest and most economical strategy to manage their medications. Older clients are also at risk for depression, feelings of isolation, physical limitations, and lack of transportation and other barriers to self care.[13] Identification of these barriers and provision of resources and support can improve adherence and quality of life for these patients.

For patients with new or longstanding diabetes, nurses play an important role in informing the patient of the goals of care for diabetes specifically focusing on A_{1c}, blood pressure and cholesterol, the "ABCs of diabetes care."[44] (This will be discussed in the next section.) Nurses can reinforce with patients that meeting these goals of care will improve every day quality of life and reduce the risk of long-term complications, especially heart disease. Focusing on the positive outcomes helps motivate patients to action. In addition, nurses can assist patients to identify one or two achievable and measurable goals. This helps patients focus on concrete activities that will directly improve their health and ultimately increase their feelings of self-efficacy and independence. Diabetes is largely a self-managed condition that requires an informed and motivated patient supported by the expertise and encouragement of nurses and an interdisciplinary team.

Goals of Diabetes Care

Glycemic Control

Getting glucose levels as close to normal as possible reduces the risk of diabetes complications. In diabetes, two measurements reflect glucose control, the A_{1c} and daily blood glucose testing. A landmark study in 1993, the Diabetes Control and Complications Trial demonstrated that intensive insulin management and maintaining an A_{1c} of less than 7% reduced the development of microvascular (retinopathy, nephropathy, and neuropathy) complications in people with type 1 diabetes by up to 75%.[45] The A_{1c} test provides a 3-month overview of overall glucose control and is a reliable predictor of diabetes-related complications (Table 39-3). In type 2 diabetes, the Kumamoto study[46] and the United Kingdom Prospective Diabetes Study[47] also demonstrated significant reductions in complications with intensive diabetes management. Each of these large clinical trials demonstrated that treatment regimens that lower A_{1c} to 7% (about 1% above the upper limits of normal) reduce microvascular complications. Further analysis suggests that lowering the A_{1c} from 7% to 6% is associated with further risk reduction.[11] Since intense glucose control also increases the risk of hypoglycemia, the benefit of a lower A_{1c} level must be weighed against the risk. As such, glucose and A_{1c} goals are individualized based on the patient's self-care ability and risk profile. To evaluate achievement of glucose levels, A_{1c} is measured every 3 to 6 months (more often if above goal and less often if within goal range).[11] The ADA A_{1c} goal is less than 7% for everyone, but a more stringent glycemic goal (normal A_{1c}) may be appropriate for certain individuals.[11] The IDF and the AACE set the A_{1c} goal at 6.5%.[15,48] As with the ADA, the A_{1c} goal is individualized based on hypoglycemic risk and the patient's self-care ability.

Table 39-3 ■ ESTIMATED AVERAGE GLUCOSE

A1c(%)	mg/dl*	mmol/l†
5	97 (76–120)	5.4 (4.2–6.7)
6	126 (100–152)	7.0 (5.5–8.5)
7	154 (123–185)	8.6 (6.8–10.3)
8	183 (147–217)	10.2 (8.1–12.1)
9	212 (170–249)	11.8 (9.4–13.9)
10	240 (193–282)	13.4 (10.7–15.7)
11	269 (217–314)	14.9 (12.0–17.5)
12	298 (240–347)	16.5 (13.3–19.3)

Data in parentheses are 95% CIs.
*Linear regression eAG (mg/dl) = 28.7 × A1C–46.7.
†Linear regression eAG (mmol/l) = 1.59 × A1c − 2.59.
From D.M. Nathan, J Kuenen, R Borg, H Zheng, D Schoenfeld, R J. Heine for the A1c-Derived Average Glucose (ADAG) Study Group (2008). Translating the A1C Assay Into Estimated Average Glucose Values. *Diabetes Care August 2008 vol. 31 no. 8 1473–1478.*

In addition to this long-range view of glycemia, people with diabetes are also encouraged to check blood glucose levels in the home setting. Home testing provides a snapshot of glucose level at any given moment. This information provides immediate feedback on the effectiveness of the treatment plan, including the interaction of medications, food choices and quantity, and exercise. The frequency of checking is based on the type of diabetes, individual ability, and the negotiated goals. For patients with type 1 diabetes, ADA and AACE recommend testing at least three times a day. For patients with type 2 diabetes, the frequency of testing is based on the stability of glucose levels, patient ability and willingness, and therapeutic goals. To get a complete picture, it is important to evaluate premeal blood glucose levels and 1 to 2 hour postmeal levels. The goals for premeal blood glucose levels are 70 to 130 mg/dL (ADA) and less than 110 mg/dL (AACE and IDF). One to 2 hours after a meal, blood glucose goals are less than 180 mg/dL (ADA), less than 145 mg/dL (IDF), and less than 140 mg/dL (AACE). Patients and providers work together to determine safe and realistic targets and then negotiate strategies to achieve goals.

Blood Pressure Goals and Treatment

People with type 2 diabetes are up to three times as likely to have hypertension and hypertension is often found in those with type 1.[5] Hypertension amplifies the effects of hyperglycemia and increases the risk of diabetes complications. Many randomized trials[49,50] have demonstrated that blood pressure control reduces morbidity and mortality and is cost-effective. The internationally agreed upon goals are systolic blood pressure ≤130 mm Hg and diastolic blood pressure ≤80 mm Hg.[5,11,15,51] If tolerated, an even lower blood pressure may be attempted.[5] Blood pressure should be measured each office visit and home blood pressure monitoring devices may also be beneficial.[52] Promoting lifestyle changes including weight reduction, reducing sodium and alcohol intake, and regular exercise can help lower blood pressure. However, they are generally insufficient by themselves to achieve blood pressure goals.[51] According to the ADA, if blood pressure goals are not met within 3 months through lifestyle intervention then pharmacologic intervention is warranted. Studies have shown that the use of antihypertensives not only provide renal protection, but can help reduce endothelial inflammation and reduce the risk of CAD.[15,51] Most people with diabetes require combination therapy to lower blood pressure and improve outcomes.[15,51] Effective first line agents include angiotensin-converting enzyme (ACE) inhibitor and/or angiotensin receptor blocker. The IDF also includes β-adrenergic blockers as a first line agent, although the AACE strongly argues against their use due to accumulating literature that questions their benefit. If one class is not tolerated, than the other should be substituted. According to ADA, if blood pressure control is not achieved with one or a combination of these, a diuretic may be added. In addition, the ADA and EASD note that for patients with a prior myocardial infarction, the addition of β-blockers reduces mortality.

Cardiovascular Risk Protection

Since CVD is the major cause of mortality and morbidity in people with diabetes, assessment and aggressive management of CVD risk factors is a core part of care.[5] Risk assessment of CVD should be performed at diagnosis and at least annually thereafter. Areas to assess include history of heart disease, BMI and abdominal adiposity, presence of hypertension, smoking, dyslipidemia, family history of premature heart disease, and presence of microalbuminuria (a marker of heart disease).[53]

People with diabetes typically present with abnormal, atherogenic lipid profiles, including small dense LDLs, elevated triglycerides, and low HDL levels. This profile increases the risk of heart disease and requires aggressive treatment. The goals for lipids are as follows: For LDL, ADA states the level should be less than 100 mg/dL. The EASD and IDF goal is slightly lower at <95 mg/dL (2.5 mmol/L). Both the ADA and EASD agree, that for those with overt CVD an LDL cholesterol goal of <70 mg/dL (1.8 mmol/L) is desirable. This more aggressive goal is in line with the National Cholesterol Education Adult Treatment Program III. The goal for HDL cholesterol is greater than 40 mg/dL (1.0 mmol/L). The ADA and EASD guidelines recommend a slightly higher target for women of 50 g/dL (1.3 mmol/L) and 46 mg/dL (1.2 mmol/L), respectively. Triglyceride targets are less than 200 mg/dL (2.3 mmol) according to the IDF. The EASD and ADA triglyceride goals are more stringent at less than 150 mg/dL (1.7 mmol/L).

Lifestyle treatment to lower the risk of heart disease includes reduction of saturated fat, trans fat, and cholesterol intake, weight loss if indicated, and increased physical activity. Patients who smoke should receive education, support, and pharmacologic intervention if appropriate to quit smoking.[54] In addition to these lipid-lowering measures, pharmacologic therapy to achieve lipid goals is a priority. In the Heart Protection Study,[55] patients over 40 years of age who were treated with a statin reduced their risk of coronary artery events by 25%, independent of baseline LDL levels. Based on the results of this study and others which had similar findings, the IDF guidelines state that statin therapy should be initiated in people over 40 years of age with diabetes or all those with diabetes and heart disease. The EASD state that statin therapy should be considered in adults with type 2 diabetes and heart disease regardless of baseline LDL cholesterol with a treatment target of <70 mg/dL (1.8 mmol). For patients with diabetes without CVD, if total cholesterol is >135 mg/dL (3.5 mmol/L) statin therapy should be considered aiming to reduce LDL by 30% to 40%. The ADA guidelines state that statin therapy should be added to lifestyle therapy regardless of baseline lipid levels for patients with diabetes if they have overt CVD or if they are over 40 years of age and have one or more CVD risk factors. For patients without CVD and under 40 years of age, statin therapy should be added to lifestyle in LDL is >100 mg/dL (2.6 mmol/L). Even though these goals to initiate treatment are slightly different, research has demonstrated that statin therapy is a powerful primary and secondary intervention that effectively lowers LDL and prevents cardiovascular events. Triglycerides and HDL usually improve in response to lower LDL and glucose levels. According to the EASD and IDF if goals are not met, a specific inhibitor of cholesterol absorption, ezetimibe, can be added in addition to lifestyle and statin therapy. All agree that if goals are still not met, a combination of fenofibrates and nicotinic acid (niacin) may be considered.

In addition to lipid lowering, there is international agreement regarding provision of aspirin therapy to as an antiplatelet agent. The EASD also recommends the use of ADP receptor-dependent platelet activation (clopidogrel) in addition to aspirin for patients with acute coronary syndrome and the ADA recommends its addition for those with severe and progressive CVD. The ADA cautions against aspirin therapy for patients under 30 years of age due to lack of evidence of benefit and for patients under 21 years of age due to associated risk of Reye's syndrome.

Aggressive management of glucose and cardiovascular risk factors can improve daily quality of life and long-term complications for people with diabetes. Informing patients of the goals and steps to achieve these goals can dramatically improve outcomes.

Strategies to Achieve Glucose Control

Lifestyle Management

Since many of the risk factors associated with diabetes can be improved by changes in lifestyle, it is important to encourage healthy eating and exercise when working with patients with diabetes. All patients with diabetes should meet with a health care professional trained in the principles of nutrition at the time of diagnosis and on an ongoing basis to assess their current nutritional status and develop an individualized meal plan that works within the context of their life and addresses their particular risk factors.[56] Some basic initial recommendations include limiting foods with high amounts of sugars and fats—especially saturated and trans fats and teaching patient to monitor intake of carbohydrate-containing foods.[57] Eating fresh fruits, vegetables, and whole grains and limiting alcohol should also be encouraged. Weight loss of 5% to 7% of current body weight reduces insulin resistance and other risk factors and can be accomplished gradually through calorie reduction and regular physical activity. In addition to healthy eating, exercise is also a cornerstone of diabetes self care. Besides helping with weight maintenance, exercise also reduces cardiac risk factors and improves an individual's sense of well-being. Introduce physical activity gradually, based on the person's willingness, ability, and cardiac risk factors. Current recommendations include accumulation of 150 minutes of exercise a week, however goals should be individualized and structured so that they are achievable and realistic.[11,46] Particular attention should be paid to proper footwear and injury prevention for anyone with diabetes nerve disease or a history of feet problems.[58]

People with diabetes who succeed in weight loss and exercise regularly may need to decrease their dose of glucose lowering medications and insulin. Ongoing monitoring of glucose levels and symptoms will provide the feedback needed to make adjustments. While lifestyle changes can lower glucose levels, due to the progressive nature of diabetes, most people will need pharmacologic intervention to keep their diabetes and risk factors at target.[46] The next section provides a review of pharmacologic interventions to help achieve glycemic goals.

Medication for Type 2 Diabetes

Secretagogues. There are two categories of secretagogues or medications that increase insulin release. Sulfonylureas are the oldest class of oral medications used to treat type 2 diabetes. The most commonly used agents in this class include glyburide, glipizide, and glimiperide. The main action of these agents is to stimulate pancreatic insulin secretion. They effectively lower A_{1c} by approximately 1.0% to 2.0%.[15] The main concerns with this class include weight gain and hypoglycemia. In addition, since these drugs are excreted renally, the duration of action may be prolonged in those with kidney failure. All patients taking these medications are at risk for hypoglycemia, so instruction on symptoms and treatment of low blood glucose is imperative, especially for elderly patients or those with renal dysfunction.

Meglitinides. A newer addition to the secretagogue category is the meglitinides, which include repaglinide, and nateglinide. Like sulfonylureas, these agents reduce glucose by stimulating a burst of insulin from the pancreas. Unlike the sulfonylureas, the meglitinides target postmeal blood glucose since they start working in 15 to 30 minutes and last for 1 to 2 hours.[15] They lower A_{1c} by approximately 1.5%.[59] These medications are given three times a day with meals. As with the sulfonuylureas, teaching points include identification and treatment of hypoglycemia and the possibility of weight gain. Patients should also be instructed to skip a dose of their medication if they plan to skip a meal.

Incretin Mimetics. People with type 2 diabetes have lower than normal circulating amounts of the gut hormone or incretin GLP-1 that is normally released by the L cells of the intestine.[23] The medications in this class mimic the action of GLP-1 and lower glucose levels by increasing insulin release in response to food, decreasing postmeal glucagon release, slowing the rate of digestion, and promoting satiety. In addition to lowering A_{1c} by 0.8% to 9%, many patients taking this medication experience a weight loss of 2 to 3 kg over 6 months.[15] The incretin mimetic exenatide is injected twice a day before meals. There is a longer acting version of exenatide LAR in the pipeline that would require only once weekly injections.[60] Only people with type 2 diabetes can benefit from exenatide, since it promotes insulin release from the pancreas. Teaching points include giving injections about 60 minutes before meals and nausea as a potential side effect. There is no risk of hypoglycemia with exenatide, unless it is used in combination with a secretagogue or insulin.

DPP-4 Inhibitors. These oral agents promote the effectiveness of the incretin hormone GLP-1, since it blocks the dipeptidyl peptidase-4 inhibitor (DPP-4) enzyme which deactivates GLP-1. Like the incretin mimetics, the end result is an increase in glucose-dependent insulin production, prevention of postmeal rise in glucagon, and a slowing of gastric emptying.[23] Currently sitagliptin is the only approved DPP-4 inhibitor in the United States; however, a newer DPP-4 inhibitor, vildagliptin, has been approved for use in the European Union. Although this class only lowers A_{1c} by 0.6% to 0.8%, it has the advantage of no associated weight gain or hypoglycemia.[15] The dose of these agents may need to be reduced in the presence of kidney or liver failure.

Biguanides. The biguanide metformin is recommended as a first line agent upon diagnosis of type 2 diabetes.[59] The primary action of metformin is to decrease hepatic glucose production. It is very effective and lowers A_{1c} by approximately 1.0% to 2.0%. It is usually taken twice daily, however there is a long-acting formulation which is taken once daily. In addition to lowering glucose, metformin also lowers LDL and triglycerides and increases HDL levels. Metformin will not cause weight gain and often contributes to weight loss.[15] To avoid decrease gastrointestinal upset (nausea, anorexia, and diarrhea), instruct patients to take metformin with meals. To prevent the risk of lactic acidosis, metformin should be avoided in patients who are at risk for renal impairment, those with liver failure, excessive alcohol use, and congestive heart failure requiring medication. Metformin should be held during intravenous contrast dye studies and during any acute illness that might cause renal dysfunction or tissue hypoperfusion[61] (AADE).

Thiazolidinediones. This class of agents increases insulin sensitivity in target tissues and decreases insulin resistance. The two TZDs available include rosiglitazone and pioglitazone. In addition to lowering A_{1c} up to 1.5%, (AACE) this class also modestly reduces blood pressure, enhances fibrinolysis, and improves endothelial function. These agents are usually used in combination with another class of glucose lowering medications and can take up to 8 weeks to reach their maximal effect (AADE). Teaching points include advising patients to inform their provider if they experience unusual weight gain or edema when starting these medications. TZDs should not be used in patients with congestive heart failure (New York Heart Association class III or IV cardiac disease and functional capacity). Rosiglitazone and pioglitazone both have black box warnings, highlighting the increased risk of CHF secondary to fluid retention.[62] In addition, due to the findings of a 2007 meta-analysis of rosiglitazone, the Food and Drug Administration issued a warning that rosiglitazone is associated with an increased risk of heart attack and heart failure-related deaths.[63] TZDs should be avoided in patients with hepatic failure. As such, evaluate baseline liver enzymes on initiation of therapy and if patients exhibit any signs of hepatic dysfunction. Women taking TZDs are also at greater risk of peripheral fractures.

Glucosidase Inhibitors. These medications delay carbohydrate absorption and are helpful in decreasing postprandial hyperglycemia. The glucosidase inhibitors include acarbose and miglitol. Patients take this medication with the first bite of food at each meal and experience reductions in A_{1c} levels of about 0.5% to 1.0%.[59] These medications are better tolerated when dosing is

Table 39-4 ■ PHARMACOKINETICS OF AVAILABLE INSULIN PREPARATIONS

Insulin, Generic Name (Brand Name)	Onset	Peak	Effective Duration
Rapid-acting, Bolus			
Insulin aspart injection (NovoLog) Insulin lispro injection (Humalog) Insulin glulisine injection (Apidra)	5 to 15 min	30 to 90 min	<5 h
Short-acting, Bolus			
Regular	30 to 60 min	2 to 3 h	5 to 8 h
Intermediate, basal			
NPH	2 to 4 h	4 to 10 h	10 to 16 h
Insulin detemir injection (Levemir)*,† (3)	3 to 8 h	No peak	5.7 to 23.2 h
Long-acting, basal			
Insulin glargine injection (Lantus)*,†	2 to 4 h‡	No peak	20 to 24 h

*May require two daily injections in patients with type 1 diabetes mellitus.
†Assumes 0.1 to 0.2 U/kg per injection. Onset and duration may vary significantly greatly by injection site.
‡Time to steady state.
NPH, neutral protamine Hagedorn.
Adapted from American Association of Clinical Endocrinologists. (2007). Medical guidelines for clinical practice for the management of diabetes mellitus. *Endocrine Practice, 13.*

started at a low range with gradual increase since they can cause severe flatulence and abdominal discomfort.

Given its action, people with chronic intestinal diseases, inflammatory bowel disease, or bowel obstruction should not take this class of medication. If a patient is taking a secretagogue and/or insulin and a glucosidase inhibitor, they need to treat hypoglycemia with oral glucose (dextrose) such as glucose tablets to reverse hypoglycemia. Products containing sucrose (table sugar, candy, and sodas) are not effective because this class of agents will delay absorption.

Amylin Analogs. Pramlintide is the synthetic version of the human amylin, a hormone that lowers blood glucose by suppressing glucagon production, slowing gastric emptying, and increasing satiety. It is only available in injectable form and is given before meals to lower postmeal glucose levels. Patients with type 1 or 2 on insulin therapy can utilize this therapy that lowers A_{1c} by about 0.5% to 7% and often result in weight loss.[59] Teaching points include reduction of rapid-acting insulin dose by about 50% while starting amylin therapy to reduce the potential of hypoglycemia, which is most common after 3 hours of injection. This medication frequently causes nausea and should not be used in patients with gastroparesis or hypoglycemia unawareness.[15]

Insulin Replacement Therapy

Many patients regard the need to start insulin therapy as a personal failure to successfully manage their diabetes. Avoiding the threat of insulin therapy if patients do not comply with self-care changes is critical, since this puts a negative light on a very powerful and effective hormone that will always lower blood glucose levels. Since only 50% of U.S. adults with diabetes have A_{1c} levels less than the target of 7% [41] in spite of a wealth of oral medications, there is a movement to initiate insulin therapy earlier in patients with type 2 diabetes.[59]

Understanding the normal cycle of insulin release is helpful to determine strategies to replace insulin in a therapeutic and effective manner.[64] An average person releases about 0.5 to 0.1 units of insulin per kg per day.[13] This insulin release happens in two different and overlapping phases. The first phase bolus insulin is released in response to glucose elevations associated with meals. This bolus of insulin serves to regulate the blood glucose from the ingested meals to prevent postprandial (after meal) hyperglycemia. People with type 1 secrete no insulin in response to meals and people with type 2 secrete less than normal. Replacement of this insulin is accomplished by the use of the short-acting insulin (regular) or the rapid-acting insulins including aspart, lispro, and glulisine (Table 39-4). The dose of this insulin is adjusted depending on the patient's glucose level prior to a meal and the amount of carbohydrate they plan to eat.

Small amounts of basal insulin are released throughout the day to maintain between meal and nighttime blood glucose levels at target range. People with type 1 diabetes secrete no basal insulin and those with type 2 diabetes secrete diminished amounts. In type 2 diabetes, this lack of basal insulin is most often reflected in elevated fasting glucose levels. Insulins that imitate the basal insulin release include the intermediate-acting insulin, NPH, and (or) long-acting insulins such as glargine or detemir.[65] The dose of insulin is based on the patient's weight, morning glucose levels, and usually compromises about half the total dose.[13]

People with diabetes who are more on insulin therapy are more likely to reach glucose goals with thoughtful insulin management strategies that include a combination of bolus and basal insulins.

SUMMARY

Diabetes is a global epidemic that will continue to affect the lives of millions of people, their families, and health care systems. The evidence is overwhelming that diabetes can be prevented through lifestyle changes and medications. In addition, aggressive risk factor management, with particular focus on blood glucose, lipid, and blood pressure control can mitigate the complications associated with diabetes. By promoting prevention, early treatment and risk reduction of diabetes, nurses and health care professionals can improve diabetes outcomes in their own backyard and globally. Educating individuals and their families, promoting changes in delivery of care, tracking outcomes and working within communities to promote access to safe places to exercise and healthy foods are all activities that health care professionals can participate in to raise awareness and motivate change. Nurses and health care providers, through advocacy, education, and one-to-one personal care and connection to people with diabetes and their families, will help to slow the pace of this global epidemic, one person at a time.

REFERENCES

1. International Diabetes Federation (IDF). (2007). *Diabetes alas.* Belgium: International Diabetes Federation.
2. World Health Organization. (2004). *Diabetes Action Now: An initiative of the World Health Organization and International Diabetes Foundation.* Geneva: Switzerland.
3. United Nations General Assembly Resolution 61/225. World Diabetes Day 18 January 2007.
4. World Health Organization. (2006). *Definition and diagnosis of diabetes mellitus and intermediate hyperglycemia: Report of a World Health Organization and International Diabetes Federation.* Geneva, Switzerland.
5. Lars Ryde'n, L., Standl, E., Bartnik, M., et al. (2007). Guidelines on diabetes, pre-diabetes, and cardiovascular disease: The Task Force on Diabetes and Cardiovascular Disease of the European Society of Cardiology (ESC) and the European Association for the Study of Diabetes (EASD). *European Heart Journal, 28,* 88–136.
6. American Diabetes Association. (2008). Clinical practice recommendations: Diagnosis and classification of diabetes mellitus. *Diabetes Care, 31*(Suppl. 1), S12–S54.
7. Wild, S., Roglic, G., Green, A., et al. (2004). Global prevalence of diabetes estimates for the year 2000 and projections for 2030. *Diabetes Care,* 27, 1047–1053.
8. The Indian Task Force on Diabetes Care in India. Accessed January 31, 2008 from http://diabetesindia.com/diabetes/itfdci.htm
9. National Institute of Diabetes and Digestive and Kidney Diseases. (2005). *National Diabetes Statistics fact sheet: General information and national estimates on diabetes in the United States.* Bethesda, MD: U.S. Department of Health and Human Services, National Institute of Health.
10. Eppens, M., Craig, M., Cusumano, J., et al. (2006). Prevalence of diabetes complications in adolescents with type 2 compared with type 1 diabetes. *Diabetes Care, 29,* 1300–1306.
11. American Diabetes Association. (2008). Clinical practice recommendations: Standards of medical care. *Diabetes Care, 31.* (Suppl.1), S14.
12. American Diabetes Association. (2008). Economic costs of diabetes in the United States in 2007. *Diabetes Care, 31,* 1–20.
13. American Association of Diabetes Educators. (2006). *Art and science of diabetes self-management education: A desk reference for health care professionals.* Chicago, Illinois.
14. Carroll, M. F., & Schade, D. S. (2005). The dawn phenomenon revisited: Implications for diabetes therapy. *Endocrine Practice, 11*(1), 55–64.
15. American Association of Clinical Endocrinologists. (2007). Medical guidelines for clinical practice for the management of diabetes mellitus. *Endocrine Practice, 13.*
16. Knowler, W. C., Barret-Connor E., Fowler, S. E., et al. (2002). Reduction in the incidence of type 2 diabetes with lifestyle intervention or metformin. *New England Journal of Medicine, 346,* 393–403.
17. Gale, E. A., Bingley, P. J., & Emmett, C. L. (2004). European Nicotinamide Diabetes Intervention Trial (ENDIT): A randomised controlled trial of intervention before the onset of type 1 diabetes. *Lancet, 363* (9413), 925–931.
18. Rabi, D., Edwards, A., Southern, D., et al. (2006). Association of socioeconomic status with diabetes prevalence and utilization of diabetes care services. *BMC Health Service Research, 6,* 124. Retrieved January 22, 2008, from http://www.pubmedcentral.nih.gov/articlerender.fcgi?artid=1618393
19. Fowler, M. (2007). Classification of diabetes: Not all hyperglycemia is the same. *Clinical Diabetes, 25,* 74–76.
20. Fowler, M. (2007). Diabetes magnitude and mechanisms. *Clincal Diabetes, 25,* 25–28.
21. UK Prospective Diabetes Study Group (UKPDS). (1998). Effect of intensive blood-glucose control with metformin on complications in overweight patients with type 2 diabetes. *The Lancet, 352,* 854–865.
22. Inzucchi, S. E., Reed, J. W., Fagan, T. F., et al. (2006). Achievement of ADA Guidelines among U.S. adults with diabetes: NHANES. *Clinical Insights in Diabetes, 9*(3), 1–4.
23. Hinnen, D., Nielsen, L., Waninger, A., et al. (2006). Incretin mimetics and DPP-IV inhibitors: New paradigms for the treatment or type 2 diabetes. *The Journal of the American Board of Family Medicine, 19*(6), 612–620.
24. Lorenzo, C., Williams, K., Hunt, J., et al. (2007). The National Cholesterol Education Program-Adult Treatment Panel III, International Diabetes Federation, and World Health Organization Definitions of the Metabolic Syndrome as Predictors of Incident Cardiovascular Disease and Diabetes. *Diabetes Care, 30,* 8–13.
25. Zimmet, P. Z., George, K., Alberti, M., et al. (2005). Mainstreaming the metabolic syndrome: A definitive definition. *The Medical Journal of Australia, 184*(4), 175–176. Retrieved December 16, 2007, from http://www.mja.com.au/public/issues/183_04_150805?zim10442_fm.html
26. Reaven, G. M. (1988). Banting lecture. Role of insulin resistance in human disease. *Diabetes 37,* 1595–1607.
27. Kahn, R., Buse, J., Ferrannino, E., et al. (2005). The Metabolic syndrome: Time for a critical appraisal. *Diabetes Care, 28*(9), 2289–2304.
28. WHO Consultation. (1999). *Definition, diagnosis and classification of diabetes mellitus and its complications.* Geneva, World Health Organization. Report 99.2.
29. National Cholesterol Education Program (NCEP). (2001). Executive summary of the third report of the National Cholesterol Education Program Expert Panel on detection, evaluation, and treatment of high blood cholesterol in adults. *JAMA,* 285, 2486–2497.
30. Alberti, K. G., Zimmet P., & Shaw, J. (2005). The metabolic syndrome—A new world definition. *The Lancet, 366,* 1059–1062.
31. American Association of Clinical Endocrinologists. (2003). ACE position statement on the insulin resistance syndrome. *Endocrine Practice, 9*(3), 240–252.
32. American Diabetes Association Website. http://www.diabetes.org/diabetesphd
33. Eriksson, K. F., & Lindgarde, F. (1991). Prevention of type 2 diabetes mellitus by diet and physical exercise. The 6 year Malmo feasibility study. *Diabetologia, 20,* 891–898.
34. Pan, X. R., Li, G. W., Hu, Y. H., et al. (1997). Effects of diet and exercise in preventing NIDDM in people with impaired glucose tolerance. *Diabetes Care, 20,* 537–544.
35. Tuomilehto, J., Lindstrom, J., Eriksson J. G., et al. (2001). Prevention of type 2 diabetes mellitus by changes in lifestyle among subjects with impaired glucose tolerance. *New England Journal of Medicine, 344,* 1343–1350.
36. Chiasson, J. L., Josse, R. G., Gomis, R., et al. (2002). Acarbose for prevention of type 2 diabetes mellitus: The STOP-NIDDM randomised trial. *The Lancet, 359,* 2072–2077.
37. Gerstein, H. C., Yusuf, S., Bosch, J., on behalf of the DREAM trial investigators (2006). Effect of rosiglitazone on the frequency of diabetes in patients with impaired glucose tolerance or impaired fasting glucose: A randomised controlled trial. *The Lancet, 368,* 1096–1105.
38. Buchanan, T. A., Xiang, A. H., & Peters, R. K. (2002). Preservation of pancreatic B-cell function and prevention of type 2 diabetes by pharmacological treatment of insulin resistance in high-risk Hispanic women. *Diabetes, 51,* 2769–2803.
39. National Cholesterol Education Program (NCEP). (2002). Third Report of the National Cholesterol Education Program (NCEP) Expert Panel on Detection, Evaluation, and Treatment of High Blood Cholesterol in Adults (Adult Treatment Panel III). *Circulation, 106,* 3143–3421.
40. American Association of Clinical Endocrinologists. (2007). *State of diabetes Complications in America.* A Comprehensive Report Issued by the American Association of Clinical Endocrinology.
41. Bypass Angioplasty Revascularization Investigation (BARI) 2 Diabetes: A clinical study. On the internet at www.bari2D.org. University of Pittsburgh, Epidemiology data center 2006. Accessed January 21, 2008.
42. Childs, B. P., Cypress, M., & Spollett, G. (2005). *Complete nurse's guide to diabetes care.* Virginia: American Diabetes Association (Nurses guide).
43. Young-Hyman, D. (2004). Psychosocial factors affecting adherence, quality of life, and well-being: Helping patients cope. In *Medical management of type 1 diabetes (162–182).* Alexandria, VA: American Diabetes Association.
44. *Know your ABCs of diabetes—NCBDE.* http://ndep.nih.gov/diabetes/control/control.htm
45. The Diabetes Control and Complications Trial (DCCT) Research Group. (1993). The effect of intensive treatment of diabetes on the development and progression of long-term complications in insulin-dependent diabetes mellitus. *New England Journal of Medicine, 329,* 977–986.
46. Ohkubo, Y., Kishikawa, H., Araki, E., et al. (1995). Intensive insulin therapy prevents the progression of diabetic microvascular complications in Japanese patients with non-insulin-dependent diabetes mellitus: A ran-

domized prospective 6-year study. *Diabetes Research and Clinical Practice, 28*, 103–117.

47. UK Prospective Diabetes Study Group (UKPDS). (1998). Intensive blood-glucose control with sulphonylureas or insulin compared with conventional treatment and risk of complications in patients with type 2 diabetes. *The Lancet, 352*, 837–853.
48. International Diabetes Federation (IDF). (2005). *Global Guidelines for Type 2 Diabetes Chapter 6: Glucose control levels*. Brussels: International Diabetes Federation.
49. International Diabetes Federation (IDF). (2005). *Global Guidelines for Type 2 Diabetes Chapter 11: Blood pressure control*. Brussels: International Diabetes Federation.
50. UK Prospective Diabetes Study Group (UKPDS). (1998). Tight blood pressure control and risk of macrovascular and microvascular complications in type 2 diabetes. *BMJ, 317*, 703–713.
51. Hansson, L., Zanchetti, A., Carruthers, S. G., et al. (1998). Effects of intensive blood-pressure lowering and low-dose aspirin in patients with hypertension: Principal results of the Hypertension Optimal Treatment (HOT) randomised trial. *The Lancet, 351*, 1755–1762.
52. Heart Outcomes Prevention Evaluation Study Investigators (HOPE). (2000). Effects of ramipril on cardiovascular and microvascular outcomes in people with diabetes mellitus: Results of the HOPE study and MICRO-HOPE substudy. *Lancet, 355*, 253–259.
53. International Diabetes Federation (IDF). (2005). *Global guidelines for type 2 diabetes. Chapter 12: Cardiovascular risk protection*. Brussels: International Diabetes Federation.
54. American Diabetes Association (ADA). (2004). Smoking and diabetes. *Diabetes Care, 27*, S74–S75.
55. Collins, R., Armitage, J., Parish, S., & Heart Protection Study Collaborative Group. (2004). Effects of cholesterol-lowering with simvastatin on stroke and other major vascular events in 20536 people with cerebrovascular disease or other high-risk conditions. *The Lancet, 363*, 757–767.
56. International Diabetes Federation (IDF). (2005). *Global guidelines for type 2 diabetes. Chapter 5: Lifestyle management*. Brussels: International Diabetes Federation.
57. American Diabetes Association (ADA). (2008). Nutrition recommendations and interventions for diabetes—2008. *Diabetes Care, 31*, S61–S78.
58. American Diabetes Association (ADA). (2004). Preventative foot care in diabetes. *Diabetes Care, 27*, S63–S64.
59. Nathan, D. M., Buse, J. B., Davidson, M. B., et al. (2006). Management of hyperglycemia in type 2 diabetes: A consensus algorithm for the initiation and adjustment of therapy: A consensus statement from the American Diabetes Association and the European Association for the Study of Diabetes. *Diabetes Care, 29*, 1963–1972.
60. American Diabetes Association (ADA). (2007). Once-weekly exenatide safe and effective. *DOC News, 4(7)*. Retrieved January 16th, 2008, from http://docnews.diabetesjournals.org/cgi/content/full/4/7/18-a?ck=nck
61. Misbin, R. I. (2004). The phantom of lactic acidosis due to metformin in patients with diabetes. *Diabetes Care, 27*, 1791–1793.
62. Singh, S., Loke, Y. K., & Furberg, C. D. (2007). Long-term risk of cardiovascular events with rosiglitazone: A meta-analysis. *JAMA, 298*, 1189–1195.
63. Nissen, S. E., & Wolski, K. (2007). Effect of rosiglitazone on the risk of myocardial infarction and death from cardiovascular causes. *New England Journal of Medicine, 356*, 2457–2471.
64. Mooradian, A. D., Bernbaum, M., Albert, S. G., et al. (2006). Narrative review: A rational approach to starting insulin therapy. *Annals of Internal Medicine, 145*, 125–134.
65. Rosenstock, J., Dailey, G., Massi-Benedetti, M., et al. (2005). Reduced hypoglycemia risk with insulin glargine: A meta-analysis comparing insulin glargine with human NPH insulin in type 2 diabetes. *Diabetes Care, 28*, 950–955.

CHAPTER 40

Adherence to Cardiovascular Treatment Regimens

Lora E. Burke / Kyeongra Yang / Sushama D. Acharya

Adherence or compliance has been studied extensively in recent decades.[1–4] The terms *adherence* and *compliance* have been used interchangeably in the literature; however, more recently the use of *adherence* has superseded compliance.[5] Compliance is viewed by many as having a negative connotation that implies an authoritarian relationship between the provider and the patient with the provider issuing instructions that the patient is expected to follow. *Adherence* is similar but is seen as recognizing the rights of the patient to chose and thus removes the concept of blame.[6] *Concordance*, a term used mainly in the United Kingdom, has been more broadly defined and today ranges from prescribing and communicating to supporting the patient in medication taking, and includes consideration for the preferences and beliefs of the patient.[6] Today, it seems to be more widely recognized that the patient is only one part of the equation when adherence is considered. Numerous factors may play a part in adherence, which involves the health care professional, the system or organization in which care is delivered, and the patient, for example, the provider's suboptimal use of evidence-based treatment guidelines or the health organization's practices that present barriers to the patient's attempts to being adherent.[7]

Other terms that sometimes are considered synonymous or related include self-management and disease management.[5,7] Heart failure disease management focuses on educating patients about adherence, monitoring symptoms that may warn of decompensation, factors that may precipitate an exacerbation, and being seen in close follow-up by nurses specialized in heart failure care. Broader than adherence or compliance, self-management includes general strategies and behaviors that contribute to disease management, improved health, and prevention or reduction of complications rather than mainly focusing on following specific regimen components.[8,9]

This chapter reviews adherence and the significance of nonadherence in the management of the cardiac patient. Methods used to assess adherence across the behaviors of medication taking, dietary self-management, following an exercise program, and smoking cessation are reviewed. Factors that influence adherence and strategies to enhance adherence are discussed and guidelines for implementing educational and behavioral strategies are provided.

SIGNIFICANCE OF NONADHERENCE

A number of pharmacologic therapies are used in the prevention, as well as the acute and chronic management of cardiovascular disease (CVD). However, the extent to which these therapies can be demonstrated to be efficacious in clinical trials and later effective when prescribed by practitioners can be influenced by the patient's adherence to the treatment regimen,[10] which is less than ideal in both clinical trial and clinical practice settings. The survival benefits of several drugs have been demonstrated in large-scale clinical trials. However, it has been shown repeatedly that 50% of individuals prescribed statins will discontinue the therapy within 6 months[10] or stop taking the drug for an extended period.[11] A quantitative review of 50 years of research in patient adherence revealed that the average nonadherence rate is 24.8%; the highest adherence rates are among patients with HIV disease, arthritis, gastrointestinal disorders, and cancer, the lowest are among patients with pulmonary disease, diabetes, and sleep disorders.[12] Approximately 31% of hypertensive participants in a Veterans Affairs study reported unintentional nonadherence mainly due to carelessness or forgetfulness and 9% reported intentional nonadherence.[13] The rates of nonadherence to treatment recommendations are found to be 20% to 40% for acute illness, 30% to 60% for chronic illness, and 80% for prevention.[14] The most common preventable cause of rehospitalization in the heart failure population is nonadherence to the regimen.[15] In the United States, 33% to 69% of medication-related hospital admissions are the result of poor medication adherence, resulting in an annual cost of $100 billion.[10] These statistics illustrate how medication nonadherence is a major health problem; however, it is not limited to the United States.

Nonadherence is a ubiquitous problem that spans across continents and treatment regimens. Indeed, the magnitude of this problem was underscored by the World Health Organization (WHO) convening a panel of experts to examine its prevalence and develop an evidence-based report on treatment strategies. The panel reported that adherence to long-term therapies in developed countries is approximately 50% and is much lower in developing countries. Poluzzi et al.[16] reported 69% adherence during the second year and 60% during the third year of antihypertensive therapy among Italian adults. A study among Asian Pacific Americans (Japanese, Filipino, Chinese, Korean, and part-Hawaiian; $N =$ 28,395) showed that Japanese living in Hawaii were 21% more likely to adhere to antihypertensive medications than white population while individuals of Korean, Hawaiian, and Filipino descent were less likely to adhere than white population, after controlling for patient's education and physician characteristics such as specialty, gender, and race.[17] Among all ethnic groups in this sample, overall adherence rates were less than 60%.

Several risk factors associated with CVD are related to lifestyle; however, adherence to public health recommendations for dietary and physical activity habits is also lacking. Generally, Americans exceed the dietary fat limit by 2% to 5%, depending on ethnic group and exceed the 2,400 mg of sodium per day guideline by

1,000 mg. In contrast, the reported intake of dietary fiber is at approximately 50% to 75% of the recommended intake.[18] Results from the behavioral risk factor surveillance system revealed that 50.01% of adults engaged in regular activities and that 13.5% were physically inactive.[19] In general, white population reported being more physically active than black population and Hispanics. The dietary excess and physical activity deficiency rates are reflected in the prevalence of overweight and obesity in the United States and other westernized countries; the most recent reports indicate a combined prevalence of 66% for the United States.[20]

The poor rates of smoking has been relatively static with an estimated 23.9% men and 18.1% women current smokers in the United States as indicated by National Health Interview Survey. The highest proportion of smokers were American Indian or Alaska Native adults (25%) followed by black (21%), white (21%), and Asian populations (13%).[21] Worldwide more than one third of the population is estimated to be smokers.[22] Studies suggest that smoking cessation rates remain low with the majority of self-quitters relapsing within the first 8 days of initial cessation, and that only about 3% to 5% of self-quitters are able to successfully achieve abstinence for 6 to 12 months after initial cessation.[23] Among those who participate in a formal treatment program, relapse during or after treatment is usual and might require treatment several times.[24]

The duration of treatment is usually a factor influencing compliance, with an initial decline in adherence observed in the first year followed by a gradual decline over time. This pattern is observed repeatedly among those participating in long-term programs, for example, weight loss programs.[25] The prevention and treatment of CVD requires ongoing management of lifestyle habits and, increasingly, inclusion of pharmacologic therapy, such as aspirin, hyperlipidemic agents, β-blockers, or calcium channel blockers. In the absence of sustained adherence, the benefits of prevention or treatment cannot be realized. This may be critical among patients who have had solid organ transplantation. A meta-analysis of 147 studies revealed that average nonadherence rates to immunosuppressants, diet, exercise, and other health care requirements ranged from 19 to 25 cases per 100 patients per year; failure to exercise was highest among heart recipients.[26]

In the clinical arena, nonadherence at any point in the treatment continuum poses a threat to satisfactory outcomes. Medication nonadherence has been associated with increased risk of coronary heart disease, precipitated episodes of heart failure, late organ rejection among heart transplant recipients, and mortality. The literature emphasizes the mediating effects of adherence on clinical outcomes, and the impact nonadherence can have on morbidity and mortality associated with CVD regardless of when it occurs in the treatment continuum.[7,12,26]

In the research arena, nonadherence affects therapy evaluation before its introduction into the clinical setting. Incomplete adherence to the treatment under study underestimates its efficacy, and the diminished effect reduces the study's power to detect a difference between treatment groups, thus preventing the study from meeting the assumptions of the projected sample size. In this situation, when nonadherence to the study protocol results in diminished effect, additional subjects are required. Furthermore, nonadherence to the treatment protocol may mask side effects or result in an overestimation of optimal dosage.[1,27–29] Finally, intermittent or varying adherence to the study protocol may reflect varying adherence to concomitantly prescribed therapeutic modalities, which may affect study outcomes.[30]

METHODS OF MEASUREMENT

Assessment of adherence needs to be incorporated into each clinical encounter. It is important that the clinician separate adherence from therapeutic or clinical outcome, which can be affected by a myriad of variables besides adherence. For example, inadequate control of serum cholesterol may be due to inadequate drug dosage, individual variation in pharmacokinetic factors of different drugs, daytime or seasonal variations in measurement values, or personal factors. Conversely, the absence of symptoms or achievement of goal does not confirm adherence. Clinical outcomes are indirect measures of adherence, whereas patient behaviors (e.g., weight loss, exercise, taking the medication) are direct measures of adherence. Both direct and indirect measures have inherent advantages and disadvantages.[31,32] Unfortunately, it is difficult to measure behavior directly, and thus there is a great reliance on self-reported behavior. Table 40-1 summarizes the numerous measurement methods and the advantages and disadvantages of their use.

Adherence assessment can be conducted through numerous methods. However, a weakness common to all forms of measurement is a bias toward overestimation of adherence.[31] One of the reasons for this measurement error is that the period being measured is usually not representative of the patient's usual behavior. Research has shown that patients' adherence varies in relation to the clinical appointment, with adherence increasing immediately prior to and after the visit.[33] An example of this would be the patient taking medicines very closely to how they were prescribed, or closely following a low-cholesterol eating plan for the 7 days prior to the clinic appointment. Thus, when the patient is asked to report on his or her behavior, the report may be influenced by the individual's recollection of the most recent behavior and thus overestimates adherence for the longer period.[31] Cramer's research also showed that the patient was more adherent in the 7 days following the appointment, and then adherence again tapered off until a week prior to the next appointment.[34] A variety of methods are available to measure adherence in the clinical setting. These include self-report, biologic and electronic measures, pill counts, and records such as pharmacy refills.

Self-Report Measures

Self-report measures consist of interviews, structured questionnaires, and diaries, which can be in either paper-and-pencil or electronic formats. This form of adherence assessment is used most frequently, which is probably explained by its ease of administration and low cost.

Interviews

Interviews, often used in the research setting to assess adherence behavior at each contact, can easily be conducted in the clinical setting. A brief interview scale was developed to assess global medication compliance among hypertensive patients. The four-item scale developed by Morisky and colleagues pertains to areas of omission, such as forgetting, being careless, and stopping the medication when feeling better or when feeling worse. The literature would suggest that the scale is used more often as a questionnaire.

Adherence can also be ascertained through a 7-day recall interview by asking the patient to report the number of pills and the times at which these were taken for each day of the week before

Table 40-1 ■ METHODS OF ADHERENCE MEASUREMENT AND FEATURES OF THEIR USE

Measurement Method	Behaviors*	Advantages	Disadvantages
Self-report			
Interview	All behaviors	Inexpensive, provides details	Tends to over-report adherence
24-hour recall	All behaviors	Increased accuracy due to short recall period	Under representation of time may increase bias if recall day is atypical
Questionnaire	All behaviors	Numerous scales available, inexpensive, does not influence behavior	Requires literacy; may be lengthy, needs to be sensitive and appropriate to age, gender, reading level, and ethnicity, can be easily distorted
Diaries	All behaviors	Provides detail of circumstances of behavior	May influence the behavior, may under- or over-report adherence, subject to recall bias if not recording not done timely, requires cooperation of patient, requires patient literacy
Biologic outcomes (serum, urine, or saliva level of drug or its metabolite)	Medication-adherence, diet, smoking cessation	May provide a validation of behavior	Are indirect measures of adherence, only measures adherence close to time of measurement, expensive
Electronic monitors (electronic event monitors, heart rate monitors, accelerometers, SenseWear Arm Bands, electronic diaries: PDAs, glucometers)	Medication taking, exercise, smoking cessation, pain control, symptoms, food intake	Provides detailed pattern of adherence, provides data on unsupervised exercise; diaries provide data on adherence to recording protocol, record closer to occurrence of behavior, e.g. eating, smoking. Results in decreased recall bias, records in naturalistic setting	Cost prohibits widespread use, use of the monitoring device may influence behavior, requires cooperation of patient
Pill counts	Medication taking	Inexpensive, easy to conduct	Over estimates, does not provide pattern of adherence
Pharmacy records	Medication taking	Provides another source of adherence data, easy to obtain data	Not available universally, requires use of 1 pharmacy, does not provide data on adherence pattern

*Medication taking, eating, exercise, smoking cessation.

the visit. However, these tend to provide an overestimation of adherence.[35] When comparing self-reported interview adherence to electronic measured adherence, Dunbar-Jacob et al.[35] found 97% adherence reported in the interview compared with 84% adherence measured by an unobtrusive electronic event monitor.

Assessing dietary adherence requires a determination of what the person eats and the degree to which the food intake approximates the recommended diet.[36] The most widely used and rigorous measure of dietary adherence in population studies is the 24-hour dietary recall, where individuals are asked to recall their food and beverage intake in the previous day.[37] The recall is conducted unannounced so that individuals cannot change eating habits in anticipation of the recall. This method allows more exact description of foods (e.g., brands, degree of fat modification) but also requires interviewer skill at prompting recall and eliciting detail. Benefits of the 24-hour recall are increased accuracy because of the shortened recall period and reduced patient burden compared to recording in a food diary, but a disadvantage is that there may be increased bias if the recall is conducted for days on which the eating pattern is atypical.[37] To compensate for this weakness, some studies have multiple 24-hour dietary recalls (from 3 to 7) performed on nonconsecutive days to account for daily variations in food intake; however, three is most typical.

In order to improve accuracy in reporting dietary intake, various techniques have been employed to help individuals estimate their intake accurately. One such example includes the United States Department of Agriculture automated multiple-pass method (AMPM), a five-step multiple-pass 24-hour dietary recall method.[38] It is a computer assisted 24-hour dietary recall designed to provide better cues for respondents' cognitive processes. The AMPM has been shown to provide valid measures of total energy and nutrient intake among healthy normal weight women[38] and obese women.[39] Based on the AMPM approach, the Nutrition Data System for Research is a comprehensive software program available for research purposes for dietary data collection and analysis through 24-hour dietary recalls, food records, menus, and recipes. It also features optional dietary supplement data that may be included with 24-hour dietary recalls or food records. This software was developed by the Nutrition Coordinating Center at the University of Minnesota and is updated annually to reflect marketplace changes and new analytic data. It contains values for 155 nutrients, nutrient ratios, and food components and includes over 18,000 foods, including ethnic foods and over 8,000 brand products (NDSR, 2006 to 2007, University of Minnesota, Minneapolis). Additional software programs are available to collect dietary data, for example, the United States Department of Agriculture Nutrient Database for Standard Reference (Washington, DC), ProNESSy (Princeton, NJ), and Food Processor (Salem, OR). All these programs provide summarization of dietary data and detailed reports of macronutrients (carbohydrate, fat) and micronutrients (vitamins, minerals).

Adherence to exercise regimens may also be assessed through 7-day physical activity recall interviews. One study reported a very weak association between the 7-day physical activity recall and the energy expenditure as assessed by doubly labeled water.[40] However, on balance, self-report measures provide the most practical and cost-effective method for assessing adherence. Interviews may be guided by established questionnaires, for example, the Paffenbarger, the Physical Activity Recall, and the Modified Activity Questionnaire.

Nicotine dependence was assessed through the nicotine dependence module of the Composite International Diagnostic Interview.[41] The Composite International Diagnostic Interview is a comprehensive and standardized instrument to assess the presence of nicotine dependence in the past year and a lifetime history of nicotine dependence. It is reported to provide reliable and valid psychiatric diagnosis of nicotine dependence based on the *International Classification of Diseases* (*ICD-10*) and the *Diagnostic and Statistical Manual of Mental Disorder* (*DSM-IV*).[42]

Questionnaires

Questionnaires are available to assess adherence across multiple behaviors. Although there are numerous scales available for assessment of eating and exercise behaviors, few exist for medication-taking behavior. The Morisky scale, first published in 1986, has been adapted by several investigators and used as a paper-and-pencil questionnaire in several populations, including those being treated for hypercholesterolemia, rheumatoid arthritis, and HIV. This scale, for which adequate psychometric properties have been reported, was used recently in a study of medication adherence among older Chinese immigrants[43] and patients taking cardiovascular medications.[44,45] Shalansky et al.[45] recommended rewording the questions, increasing the number of items, and the use of graded response options to improve the scale's consistency. Rottlaender et al.[46] used the scale and found that 83% of the patients reported they were absolutely compliant to their medication regimen but the Morisky score indicated high adherence in only 52% of the sample. Similarly, the Morisky questionnaire revealed lower adherence rates than that measured by pill count.[47]

Dietary adherence can be measured by several established questionnaires including the Connor Diet Habit Survey, the Eating Pattern Questionnaire, and food frequency questionnaires (FFQ). The first two questionnaires focus on fat intake and have reported psychometric properties when used in cardiac and general populations.[48,49] However, the FFQ is now the most commonly used dietary measure to provide estimates of usual dietary intake over time (typically 6 months to a year) in large epidemiological studies.[50] FFQs include a list of foods with a frequency response section to report how often and how much each food item was consumed. Examples of FFQ are the Harvard/Willett FFQ, National Cancer Institute's Diet History Questionnaire (DHQ), and the Fred Hutchinson FFQ. The Fred Hutchinson FFQ was updated in 2001 and has a separate questionnaire for men and women. The DHQ was recently updated in 2007 to reflect changes in food availability. Both Fred Hutchinson FFQ and the DHQ are available in English and Spanish. Although FFQs provide a relatively inexpensive and standardized way of collecting dietary information, their major limitation is the number and types of items listed thereby reducing its utility among ethnic groups.[37] It becomes very important for the FFQ to be culture-specific to capture dietary intake of specific racial/ethnic groups. FFQs have been adapted and validated to assess the diet of diverse populations,[51] US Chinese women,[52] South Asians in the UK,[53] and elderly populations of low socioeconomic status.[54] A regionally specific FFQ has been developed for white and black adults residing in the southern region of the United States.[55]

Measurement of physical activity, which continues to receive high priority in the public health field, has relied primarily on the questionnaire.[56,57] Exercise assessment questionnaires, which are subjective measures, have been validated by objective measures of physical activity, such as measures of total energy expenditure (doubly labeled water), estimates of physical fitness (heart rate), or measures of physical motion by accelerometers.[57] A beneficial trait of the questionnaire is that it does not influence the behavior being measured, and although less precise than the objective measures, it estimates activity relative to others in the population. The questionnaire may range from one item to an array of questions covering a wide range of occupational and leisure activities, and may cover varying time intervals. A compilation of physical activity questionnaires and a review of their psychometric properties was published, providing an excellent resource for anyone wishing to measure exercise adherence.[58] In selecting a questionnaire, the investigator must consider characteristics of the population, such as gender, age, culture, and the outcome of interest. Most of the activity questionnaires were developed with men's activities in mind making them less sensitive to differences in physical activity levels in women.[57] The Kaiser Physical Activity Survey, which includes questions on household/care giving activities, is available to measure physical activity in women.[59] The 7-day Physical Activity Recall and the Paffenbarger Physical Activity Questionnaire are widely used for various groups including patients in cardiac rehabilitation programs,[60] male veterans,[61,62] individuals in the National Weight Control Registry,[63] and adults with a body mass index greater than 27.[64] The Community Healthy Activities Model Program is a valid and reliable questionnaire to estimate physical activity among middle- and older-aged adults.[65]

The most common measure of nicotine dependence among cigarette smokers is the Fagerstorm Tolerance Questionnaire (FTQ),[66] which was designed to estimate the degree of nicotine dependence in smoking. The Fagerstrom Test for Nicotine Dependence (FTND) is a shortened version of FTQ that emphasizes cigarette consumption and time to first cigarette after awakening.[67] Recently, the Cigarette Dependence Scale (CDS-12) has been proposed as a good alternative to FTND for measuring nicotine dependence with better validity and internal consistency than FTND.[68]

In summary, questionnaires with a shorter time interval are less vulnerable to recall bias and easier to validate with objective measures. However, using a shorter time frame reduces the likelihood of obtaining a picture of usual behavior, because eating and exercise patterns may vary by season. Reliability and validity are affected by the person's ability to store and retrieve information, and by potential influence of the interviewer or respondent bias.[69,70]

Diaries

Daily diaries for food intake or exercise circumvent the bias of recall, but require training and cooperation of the patient or study participant, which limits its use to highly motivated, literate individuals. While diaries may be used as part of an intervention to achieve awareness of one's behavior, the focus here is on assessment of adherence. Food and exercise diaries are often used periodically and cover a 3- or 7-day period, including one nonwork or leisure day. Recording for extended periods (i.e., over 3 days) may reduce accuracy, and the recording may begin to influence the recorder's behavior. Several investigators[71–73] have used diaries to measure exercise and dietary adherence. Wickel[74] reported high convergent validity for the Bouchard activity diary with an accelerometry-based monitor. However, when comparing self-report (questionnaire) to doubly labeled water data, Walsh et al.[75] demonstrated that sedentary overweight women overreported their exercise in comparison to normal weight control counterparts.

Issues of concern with self-report measures include response biases due to social desirability, deliberate and nondeliberate errors in recall or reporting; for example, underreporting food consumption[76,77] and overreporting energy expenditure[75,78] are common phenomenon among obese subjects. Moreover, there are concerns specific to self-report of eating and exercise behaviors. It is difficult for individuals to accurately estimate the portion size and components of mixed foods. Because there are so many dimensions of exercise, it is a challenge for individuals to accurately characterize the type of exercise, its frequency, duration, and intensity.[78] Staff need to be trained on how to teach participants to record the information, and potential problems with memory and social desirability need to be reduced. For example, recording the behavior immediately reduces forgetting and conveying an expectation of a full range of behaviors may help reduce less than truthful reports. Despite their limitations, self-report measures are common, easy to use, inexpensive, and provide information on the circumstances surrounding the good or poor adherence.

Biologic Measures

Adherence is often reported in terms of biologic end points, such as serum cholesterol or glycosylated hemoglobin level. Other biologic assays frequently used include serum, urine, or saliva level of a drug or its metabolites. Examples include antihypertensive medication adherence measured by serum bromide level,[79] dietary adherence measured by urine sodium,[80] smoking cessation by serum or saliva thiocyanate or cotinine,[81] and exercise by direct or indirect calorimetry and maximal oxygen uptake.[82] Doubly labeled water ($^2H_2{}^{18}O$), a procedure that requires the subject to ingest water enriched with ^{18}O and ^2H isotopes, is the most accurate measurement of total energy expenditure available,[83] but is too costly to be used on a widespread basis.[84] A limitation of biologic assays is that daily variability in compliance cannot be detected. Instead, they indicate if the person has been adherent close to the time of assessment and may serve as a validation of the behavior. Moreover, biological measures are not available for many drugs and dietary factors; moreover, biologic assays may be influenced by many other factors such as ethnic differences in urinary sodium excretion.[85]

Electronic Monitoring

Technology has provided tools for ongoing and detailed assessment of adherence behavior. Electronic methods include unobtrusive electronic medication monitors, heart rate monitors, electronic motion detectors for exercise (pedometers, accelerometers, SenseWear Armband), and electronic diaries for self-report data.[86] The Medication Event Monitor System (MEMS; APREX, a division of AARDEX Ltd., Union City, CA), consists of an electronic chip housed inside the medication bottle cap, provides date and time data on medication bottle openings and closures. This assessment is based on the assumption that bottle opening leads to pill removal and ingestion.[87,88] An additional applications of an electronic monitor for medication use includes the IDAS II (Intelligent Drug Administration System, Bang and Olufsen Medicom, Denmark) that accommodates blister pill packs.[88] This new device uses visual and audible reminders to the patients to enhance adherence. Similar to the MEMS, the IDAS II has been demonstrated to be acceptable to people with hypertension.[88] Santschi et al.[88] reported that there was a tendency for patients using the IDAS II to take their drug more regularly.

Several devices measure exercise adherence. The Polar® monitor can be worn during ambulatory exercises (walking, bicycling). It includes a microprocessor that measures and sequentially stores average heart rate values, which provide data on adherence to the exercise prescription (Polar Electro, Inc., Lake Success, NY).[89,90] Pedometers are used to measure steps and miles during ambulatory activity and are the most inexpensive objective monitoring device for physical activity. However, pedometer accuracy is influenced by walking speed; there was significant improvement in pedometer accuracy in fast pace walking, compared to that in slow pace walking.[91–93] Electronic accelerometers are motion sensors that register body accelerations and decelerations, and thus provide a direct and objective measure of movement intensity and frequency during physical activity. The Actigraph accelerometer (Manufacturing Technologies Inc., Fort Walton Beach, FL) and the Caltrac accelerometer (Muscle Dynamics Corp., Torrance, CA) were used to assess physical activity levels among adults with congenital heart disease,[94] and among individuals of all ages from the 2003 to 2004 National Health and Nutritional Examination Survey.[95] The SenseWear®Armband (BodyMedia, Inc., Pittsburgh, PA) is a relatively new product that monitors physical activity and energy expenditure. It is worn on the upper right arm. It includes a two-axis accelerometer, heat flux sensor, galvanic skin response sensor, skin temperature sensor, and a near-body ambient temperature sensor, which enables it to measure heat produced by the body as a result of basic metabolism and from all forms of physical activity. Data are stored up to 12 days and can be uploaded to a personal computer for analysis using the SenseWear® Software. This device has been shown to reliably determine energy expenditure in both the active and resting state, and thus measures activity adherence in an unsupervised setting.[96–99]

Electronic hand-held diaries are available to answer a set of programmed questions, report symptoms or cravings, when prompted by a sound,[100] or to record eating and physical activity behaviors.[65,70,77,101,102] Because recalling events or symptoms is plagued by biases and inaccuracies, the electronic diaries attempt to avoid this barrier by having individuals record experiences close to the time of their occurrence.[103] Moreover, these monitoring devices permit objective measurement of adherence to a recording schedule under naturalistic conditions. An added benefit is that the data are directly entered by the person and later uploaded to a computer for analysis. Acceptability of the hand-held computers has been reported as excellent.[65,104,105] Stone et al.[86] compared the use of a paper diary equipped with a light sensor to record the day and time of diary openings with an electronic diary (similar to a personal digital assistant). They found that 95% of participants using the personal digital assistant (PDA) recorded in the diary while 90% using the sensor embedded paper diary reported that they recorded in the diary but in reality, only 11% recorded.[86] Burke et al.[106] used the same sensor embedded diaries as the ones used by Stone and Shiffman and found that study participants often falsified the date and times of their recordings so that it appeared that they were recording on a daily basis when in reality they were recording several days of behavior at one time.[69,106] Other innovative approaches to self-monitoring include the use of web sites for patients to log onto and record behaviors.[107,108] In addition, programs are available on the Internet that provide the structure for self-monitoring, for example, www.FitDay.com, www.sparkpeople.com, and www.caloriecount.com. In summary, electronic monitors provide a detailed picture of the temporal pattern of adherence, from medication taking to self-reporting symptoms or eating or physical activity behaviors.

With the advancement of technology, more products and software programs are available for assessing adherence in the person's naturalistic environment.

Pill Counts and Pharmacy Refills

Unique to the assessment of medication-taking adherence, these measures provide opportunities for alternative or concurrent measurement methods. The pill count is done by tabulating pills remaining from a previous dispensing for a specific interval, and comparing that number with what should have been remaining. An adherence rate is calculated by dividing the number that should have been taken by the number prescribed and multiplying by 100. This method tends to overestimate adherence. An early study reported that the pill count rate of adherence was 94%, compared with 84% for the medication event monitor.[35] A recent study compared the pill count to the four-item Morisky questionnaire and reported that the pill count data suggested that 90% of participants took 80% or more of their study drug while the Morisky scale showed that 56% reported high adherence and 44% reported medium adherence.[47] A study conducted in Brazil showed that neither the pill count nor the Morisky scale had good positive predictive value for adherence.[109] In the age of managed care and large organizations filling prescriptions, pharmacy refill records are commonplace. However, the disadvantage with the pill count and pharmacy record is that they do not provide information on the pattern of adherence, that is, how the individual is taking the medication on a daily basis and if the interdose intervals vary so much that a therapeutic drug level cannot be maintained. Several factors may influence the pattern of medication taking, for example, forgetfulness, variations in the patient's schedule.

Summary

Despite the limitations of self-report measures of adherence, there remains value in this assessment approach, particularly to complement objective measures; however, how the provider poses the question is of utmost importance. First, one needs to give the patient permission to be nonadherent, and second, one needs to ask the patient and respond to the patient's answer in a nonjudgmental way. Introducing the question with *I know it must be difficult to take all these medicines and to also remember when to take each one. Often, people forget to take their medications, how often do you forget to take them? How often do you not take your medicine because of side effects that you think are related to the medicines?* Similar questions can be posed related to diet, physical activity, and smoking cessation.

Because adherence varies over time, ongoing assessment of adherence is essential. Moreover, adherence cannot be assumed, nor can the clinician make a clinical judgment that adherence is present. Use of one or more of these methods provides the clinician or researcher some indication of adherence and possibly information regarding the circumstances surrounding nonadherence. In general, it is recommended that more than one method be used concurrently.

DETERMINANTS OF ADHERENCE

There are factors that are consistently identified as related to adherence, and, most importantly, they can be addressed through interventions. They can be divided into four categories: patient-related, regimen-related, provider-related, and process-oriented or system-related, however, there may be overlap across categories (Table 40-2). Although some of these factors are not remedial, one needs to keep these in mind when developing interventions to improve adherence.

Patient Related

Self-efficacy for disease management and medication adherence can be significantly affected by several factors, including the patient's perceived disease severity,[110] self-concept, and the perceived role of medications, for example, taking medication may make a person feel weak or ill.[111] Other factors include prior adherence behavior, for example, early appointment canceling, history of not following the prescribed regimen, hospitalization for nonadherence; also absence of supportive others and satisfaction with the provider.[112] Motivation has been identified as an influencing factor; however, the source of motivation (intrinsic vs. extrinsic) for the initiation and maintenance of behavior may vary.[113,114] Two additional factors include skills for implementing the regimen and health literacy. Skills acquisition, for example, learning how to follow a complex medication regimen or make prescribed dietary changes requires that the patient receive training and opportunity for practice and feedback before adherence is expected. Health literacy is necessary for understanding the regimen and for informed decision making.[115] Finally, a factor that has a positive impact on adherence is conscientiousness.[116,117]

Regimen Related

A simpler regimen (e.g., fewer medications per day) is associated with higher levels of adherence in multiple cultures.[46,118] However, in some circumstances, twice daily dosing may be superior to single daily dosing, for example, if an individual misses one or two sequential days of a single daily dose medication, the therapeutic concentration in the plasma may be insufficient and the interadministration interval may exceed the drug's duration of action. One study reported that the probability of missing a single daily dose was twice as high as the probability of sequential omission of a two or three times per day dose.[119] A factor that has been reported as one of the best predictors of low adherence is medication side effects.[109]

Provider Related

A working alliance, defined as the cognitive and emotional aspect of the physician–patient relationship showed a strong, positive relationship with the patient's adherence.[112] Continuity of provider care and follow-up leads to improved adherence.[11,120] In addition, medication adherence can be improved when the provider clearly communicates the details of the regimen and the expected side effects.[121]

System Related

The frequency at which the prescription needs to be refilled can influence adherence, for example, one study found that patients with a 60-day prescription of statin reported more adherence than those with 30-day prescription.[122] In contrast, some patients may find the cost of a longer term prescription prohibitive and thus

Table 40-2 ■ STRATEGIES TO ENHANCE ADHERENCE ACROSS THE FOUR CATEGORIES OF FACTORS AFFECTING ADHERENCE

Determinants	Strategies
Patient related	
Prior adherence behavior	If history of nonadherence, monitor appointment keeping, reinforce importance of adherence to prescribed treatment/intervention from initiation to maintenance phase, provide reminder of appointment (phone call, postcard, electronic mail), immediately follow-up on every missed appointment to prevent patient dropping out of system.
Self-efficacy, self-concept	Instill in patients confidence they can achieve treatment goals; implement self-efficacy enhancing strategies: set specific, short-term, attainable goals, provide opportunities for practice, provide credible models performing similar behaviors via use of videotapes or classes, verbally persuade patients they are capable of achieving treatment or adherence goals, provide feedback on accomplished behavior changes.
Presence of social support	If applicable, include other support in education and counseling, assist patient to enlist support of others (e.g., have an exercise "buddy").
Knowledge and comprehension of treatment regimen	Provide instructions in small amounts over time, follow up with printed materials, reinforce over time, and regularly assess patient recall and understanding.
Skills to implement treatment regimen	Assess patient's skill, use self-monitoring to reveal baseline habits; refer for training as needed, e.g., dietitian to learn how to make dietary changes. Ask patient to describe how to do something, e.g., how to take several medications that may require specific time intervals between doses.
Low literacy level	Provide explicit instructions in basic terms, keep instructions brief and use simple terms, ask patient to restate instructions, assess patient's recall and comprehension of new concepts. Use color coding to help identify concepts, e.g., green for permissible foods, red for foods to avoid and yellow for ones to limit. Apply a similar rule for reporting symptoms. Demonstrate as much of regimen as feasible.
Cognitive impairment	Provide simple instructions with a copy in writing, teach patient how to use cues, set up reminder systems, use pill organizers; include significant other in counseling sessions if possible. Keep instructions brief and simple.
Impaired vision or hearing	Let patient know you are approaching and identify self, speak slowly and in a normal voice, face patient when speaking; use visual aids with large print and pictures, provide video aids to reinforce materials. Enlist assistance of person to assist patient with limitations, e.g., remove pills from bottle and place in pill organizer, use labels with large print on medicine bottle.
Conscientiousness	Commend for attention to details of following regimen and for adherent behavior.
Motivation	Assess if ambivalence is present; if so, apply strategies guided by motivational interviewing. Provide frequent reinforcement for positive behaviors as a means to maintain motivation.
Older age and living alone	Involve available support system in educational and counseling sessions, arrange for home visit follow-up. When possible, set up telephone follow-up plan.
Satisfaction with provider and care received	Convey a nonjudgmental attitude when assessing adherence, maintain an open dialogue, develop treatment plan with the patient's input and assess satisfaction with treatment plan over time.
Health literacy	Prepare the reading materials that match with patient's literacy level, ask patient to restate instructions, assess patient's recall and comprehension of new concepts.
Ethnicity	Ask the person about cultural or religious customs that have implications for treatment adherence. Develop a regimen plan acknowledging cultural preferences; be sensitive to religious implications for dietary restrictions. Determine the extent that the person understands English and obtain assistance when indicated.
Regimen-related factors	
Prescription size/duration, stability of regimen over time	Ask the patient about ability to have prescriptions refilled monthly vs. every 2 to 3 months, and the rules for copay; write prescription according to what best fits patient's needs. Acknowledge the challenge of taking medication; periodically reinforce importance of maintenance of adherence, provide rewards, reduce visit frequency, consider phone follow-up with longer intervals between visits.
Cost	Prescribe less expensive or generic brand and seek sources for additional help.
Presence of side effects	Assess for presence of side effects, discuss how they can be managed, if necessary modify treatment plan.
Presence of comorbidities leading to polypharmacy	Be aware of the complexity that polypharmacy and multiple lifestyle changes add to a regimen, set priorities for what needs to be addressed in treatment, introduce additional components as time and condition permit. Emphasize the importance of not missing pills that are once daily.
Provider-related factors	
Communication style and attitude of provider	Actively listen and demonstrate sensitivity to patient's feelings and situation, respect patient's right to exercise choice, use patient-centered counseling strategies and seek the patient's input.
Continuity with health care providers	Develop system to provide continuity in service where patient's treatment goals, regimen components and progress (lab values, weight) are recorded for easy review.
Provider's teaching/counseling skills	Use nontechnical language the patient can understand, ask patient questions to assess comprehension. Augment the printed material with discussion of its content; determine if patient has read it. Follow-up and ask patient about recall over time. Seek education/training in improving counseling skills.
System-related/process-oriented factors	
Ease of arranging/receiving care	Reduce the length of time patients need to wait to get an appointment, reduce waiting time in clinics. Facilitate low turnover of staff, involve staff in patient related activities, have staff assist/reinforce adherence message.
Availability of reimbursement or amount of required copay for services, drugs	Develop treatment regimen that fits within patient's insurance plan and reinforce the importance of adherence.
Ability to follow and track patient's progress toward goal	Develop system for practice/clinic where patient's treatment goal, regimen components and progress (lab values, weight) are recorded for easy review. If possible, provide patient a copy. Create reminder system. Use telemedicine strategies to follow patient between visits.
Supportive environment for adherence-enhancing strategies	Have prompts and reminders on patient record to remind provider and staff to follow up on adherence, e.g., have patient complete brief questionnaire to track patient's progress or changes in lifestyle habits while waiting for appointment. Have educational materials available to give patients, video films for patients to watch in the waiting room, e.g., how to prepare low fat meals, how to shop for healthy eating, how to exercise properly. Incorporate nursing case management system into clinic.

may be more adherent with a short-term prescription.[123] Moreover, medication nonadherence has been associated with the limited availability of reimbursement after exceeding the cap amount among Medicare beneficiaries; this system-related restraint can lead to poorer adherence.[124]

MODELS OF BEHAVIOR CHANGE

Improving adherence to treatment regimens remains one of the greatest challenges facing health care professionals. Various models of behavior change have guided studies examining the factors that influence adherence and also trials that have tested interventions. Earlier models included operant learning, which focused on the environment and used stimulus control strategies to restructure the environment. More recently, cognitive-motivational models have focused on beliefs, intentions, self-efficacy, self-regulation, and readiness to change. Intervention strategies used in the cardiac population have frequently been guided by social cognitive theory, which is based on an underlying assumption that behavior, the environment, and cognition function as interacting determinants with a bidirectional influence on each other.[125] Using the cognitive-motivational models, studies have examined the influence of health beliefs, intentions, illness perception, and barriers to adherence. Since these constructs explained little variance of behavior change related to adherence, additional constructs such as self-efficacy were added to the models, which have increased the explained variance in behaviors.

Self-efficacy is described as the perception of one's abilities to mobilize the motivation, cognitive resources, and courses of action required to meet given situational demands.[126] Thus, it is concerned not with a person's skills, but with the person's judgments of what he or she can do with those skills. Self-efficacy is behavior specific, that is, a person may feel highly efficacious in one behavior domain (eating healthy) but have low self-efficacy in another domain (exercising). There are four sources of efficacy: (1) mastery performance—the most powerful source comes from achievement of a series of subgoals, (2) modeling or vicarious learning—observing another person perform a task, (3) physiologic cues—making inferences from autonomic arousal or other symptoms, and (4) verbal or social persuasion—convincing others they possess the capability to achieve their goals.[125] These sources have implications for the application of self-efficacy based interventions. Outcome expectancy, one's perception of whether actually performing the behavior will lead to the desired outcome, represents the second component of the self-efficacy construct.[126]

Sustained adherence to medication taking and lifestyle changes can lead to reduced morbidity and mortality; however, the rates of improved adherence that result from interventions are often not translated into maintenance.[127,128] Adoption and maintenance of new behaviors pose challenges for most individuals. Because the beneficial effects of adherence to risk reduction strategies are not realized immediately, long-term adherence is essential.

The psychological factors that enable individuals to adopt new behaviors are not necessarily the same as those that enable one to persist for the long term.[129] An individual's assessment of the benefits of initiating behavior change that would improve adherence needs to compare favorably to their current situation; moreover, the person needs to have favorable expectancies regarding future outcomes.[129] However, a person's decision to maintain that behavior is influenced by the outcomes associated with the new behaviors and if they are sufficiently advantageous to sustain the behavior. If the person shares this perception, the decision to persist with the new behavior depends on the person's perceived satisfaction with the new behaviors' outcomes, for example, fewer symptoms due to improved medication adherence, being less fatigued after weight loss. Thus, if the individual's experiences do not meet those expectations, they will be dissatisfied and less motivated to sustain the behavior. From a practical perspective, if the person has high expectations of the outcomes of an intervention, the person will be motivated to initiate change; however, if those expected outcomes are not fulfilled, the dissatisfaction will undermine maintenance of the new adherence behavior. Thus, maintenance requires an environment that is supportive of healthy choices. Implementation of several strategies can reinforce behavior change and maintenance.

Based on research guided by the models of behavior change, a list of strategies for use in assisting patients to improve and maintain adherence to behavior change follows.

ADHERENCE-ENHANCING STRATEGIES

Goal Setting

Mastery performance, the strongest source of self-efficacy, centers on goal achievement. According to Kanfer's model of self-regulation, learning and maintaining the behavior are enhanced by self-control. Self-control is also the mechanism by which the control of behavior is shifted from external sources to that maintained by the individual.[130,131] Self-control operates through self-observation, specifying an unambiguous goal, criteria for performance, and a procedure for evaluating the performance or behavior against the criteria, and self-reward. Goal setting appears to be the most important consideration in achieving self-control. Goal setting entails working with the patient in developing realistic and attainable goals that are specific in terms of the expected outcome and proximal in terms of achievement. Goals that are unrealistic or too difficult for the patient will not be tried while those that are vague or too easy will be ignored. The goal, which should be developed in collaboration with the provider, needs to include what will be done, when, and how: for example, "will walk for 15 minutes three times a week for the next 2 weeks." As each subgoal is reached, the duration, frequency, or intensity of the next goal is increased, and reinforcement is provided for the achievement, which leads to mastery and enhanced self-efficacy.[125] It is recommended that goals focus on behaviors, which are under the control of the individual, rather than on physiological outcomes that can be influenced by several factors, for example, setting a goal for reducing fat in the diet by 5% rather than targeting an LDL cholesterol level. In order to change behaviors, individuals need to pay adequate attention to their own actions, as well as the conditions under which they occur and their immediate and long-term effects.[130] Therefore, successful self-regulation depends in part on the fidelity, consistency, and temporal proximity of self-monitoring one's behavior.

Self-Monitoring

A key technique in approaches to behavioral change, self-monitoring requires the patient to record behavior (e.g., eating, exercise, smoking behaviors, or medication taking) and use this information for behavioral analysis (i.e., the patient and provider can identify problem behaviors that could be altered or high-risk situations that can be anticipated and modified). The provider reviews the self-monitoring record and provides reinforcement for progress and/or maintenance. An alternative to the paper-and-pencil diary exists today in the form of a PDA; dietary and physical activity software programs are available for use on PDAs, which facilitate easier access to information on nutrient composition of foods and permits identifying the type and duration of exercise performed.[70] This format has also been pilot tested for use in medication adherence[132] and in recording eating and exercise behaviors.[104] There is increasing evidence that self-monitoring is related to better outcomes in behavioral intervention studies.[133,134] An immediate benefit of self-monitoring is that the patient develops an acute awareness of his/her current behavior and how this may be inconsistent with one's health-related goals. Kanfer has described self-regulation as a process having three distinct stages: self-monitoring, self-evaluation, and self-reinforcement, and suggests that changing habits requires developed self-regulatory skills.[130,131] The behavioral strategy of self-monitoring is central to this process, and includes deliberate attention to some aspect of an individual's behavior and recording details of that behavior.

Reinforcement

Giving positive feedback to the patient on progress made, supporting self-motivation by highlighting accomplishments, encouraging continued progress, and instilling confidence in the person's capability of meeting a goal all constitute reinforcement. When providing positive feedback, focus on the behavior that the person has achieved rather than on the clinical outcome. Having a diary to review provides a mechanism to relay support. The self-reinforcement component comes from the provider in assisting the patient to attribute the progress to his/her own efforts rather than to the provider.

Self-Efficacy Enhancement

Self-efficacy enhancement strategies are based on the sources of self-efficacy and include providing opportunities for successful performance or mastery, which can be achieved through realistic goal setting. Provide feedback and praise for progress (achieving specific goals) can be done though review of self-monitoring materials; convince the person that he or she is capable of performing the activity through verbal persuasion, and interpret symptoms of physiologic response, such as breathlessness due to inactivity and diminished symptoms after a program of regular exercise. Several of the above-described strategies are very effective in increasing self-efficacy.

Motivational Interviewing

This is a directive, client-centered counseling style for helping patients examine and resolve ambivalence about behavior change. In settings where time and possibly clinician expertise is limited, an abbreviated version of the technique can be applied. Motivational interviewing has four core principles: express empathy, develop a discrepancy, roll with resistance and support self-efficacy. It is through the technique of reflecting listening that the interviewer helps individuals identify and resolve uncertainty, thereby increasing intrinsic motivation to change.[135] Motivational interviewing has been shown to be effective across a wide range of health-related behaviors and population groups, including weight loss,[136,137] adherence to treatment and follow-up,[137] increasing physical activity,[138] improving medication adherence among hypertensive blacks,[139] and smoking cessation.[140] A meta-analysis of 72 trials showed a significant effect of motivational interviewing on outcomes such as blood cholesterol, blood pressure, and weight loss in 74% of the studies.[135] One needs to obtain training in the application of this strategy, which is available at professional meetings and academic centers.

Stimulus Control

Using information recorded in the diary on the circumstances of the behavior allows identification of the antecedent or trigger for problem behaviors. The patient is counseled to remove the stimuli and to restructure the environment to minimize the will power needed to overcome strong stimuli, for example, remove unhealthy foods from view and have healthy foods visible and readily available, have exercise equipment in a place that is easy to access, have morning medications near the coffee maker.

Modeling Behavior

The patient can observe a credible model perform a task or have an activity demonstrated, which may be done by watching a video or live action. It is important that the patient find the model credible and the activity feasible, such as observing fellow patients exercising in cardiac rehabilitation programs, or a cooking or exercise demonstration.

Social Support

Social support includes enlisting others to assist the patient through the behavior change process, and inclusion of supportive others from various aspects of the patient's life (e.g., family, friends, coworker, community). The purpose of this strategy is to have supportive allies in place during successes and failures. This may take the form of enlisting a "buddy" for exercise or eating behavior change, or having someone there for reinforcement. Social support has been shown to be important in behavior change, but particularly in programs of dietary and physical activity change; also the presence of a supportive other can be instrumental in improving medication adherence.

Ongoing Contact

Continued contact through mail, telephone, or the Internet has consistently demonstrated improved adherence in maintaining behavior change. The mail can be used as a method of ongoing contact by having patient's return weekly diaries of eating, exercise, or medication-taking behaviors, which could be followed by a brief phone call to provide feedback. This technique adds the accountability factor and encourages ongoing communication with the provider. Similarly, the telephone provides ongoing support and assistance with problem solving. A brief phone call to the patient can provide encouragement that may help the patient sustain the behavior during a challenging period. Regular telephone contacts need to have a structure in terms of purpose, what is to be accomplished, approximate time allowed, and a schedule of when the calls should occur. Scripting or outlining the main steps to follow in the contact can help maintain a focus and ensure that each point is addressed. Because of the increasingly busy lives of patients, it may be more difficult to have regular phone contacts; however, more people are using the Internet (e.g., discussion board or e-mails) as a means of ongoing contact.[108] When considering initiating a telephone or telemedicine follow-up system, the provider needs to consider the purpose or goal of the system, if these can be met given the frequency and duration of the planned contacts, and the costs in terms of staff time. One study reported a large effect size following the use of telephone calls and provider feedback for improving adherence to lipid-lowering medication therapy.[141]

Cueing

Cueing consists of setting up a system of reminders or cues to perform certain activities (e.g., a sticker to remind the person to take a medication, or setting out exercise shoes as a prompt to exercise on a busy day). This strategy is used frequently to improve medication adherence.

Habit Building

Habit building is derived from the stimulus control model and is based on the premise that a large amount of behavior is automatic and responsive to stimuli. It further suggests that behavior can be modified by establishing a relationship between the behavior stimulus and the target behavior, such as pairing a new behavior (medication taking) with an established behavior (brushing teeth). Using cues, as described previously, is a related strategy. These techniques may be particularly helpful when in an unusual environment (e.g., traveling). Pairing the medication bottle with the toothpaste or adding a note to the travel alarm clock may prevent an episode of nonadherence.

Contracting

A form of public commitment, contracting involves the patient in the development of the plan and clearly specifies in writing what is expected, the time frame, and any conditions for a reward if the goal is achieved. The contract needs to specify a behavior rather than the health outcome, and should specify the incremental steps necessary to achieve a goal that is attainable and valued by the patient. A contingency reward may be included for achievement of the goal. This needs to be a reward valued by the person and reinforcing to the healthier behavior, such as a new outfit or fun activity for someone in a weight reduction program, but not food or a dinner at their favorite restaurant.

Problem Solving

Problem solving involves several steps, beginning with identification or acknowledgment of a problem, defining the problem, generating potential solutions, selecting one solution or set of actions to resolve the problem, and then evaluating the success of the attempt to resolve the problem.[142] This technique is integral to maintenance of behavior change and is facilitated by reviewing self-monitoring records and identifying high-risk situations. Anticipatory problem solving can help a patient prepare for an upcoming situation, such as a major social event or vacation. It is ideal if the provider can have the patient role play the interactions that might occur in a social situation and how the person would use the new strategy.

Relapse Prevention

Based on the work of Marlatt and Gordon,[143] the relapse prevention technique emphasizes that slips or lapses are natural occurrences in the process of behavior change. Patients are taught to anticipate high-risk situations and to identify ways to cope with the situation. When possible, patients should practice problem solving to develop these skills better and rehearse the strategies they would use to resolve the threat to adherence or maintenance. Patients need to be reminded lapses will occur and not to be discouraged or give up the entire behavior change program because of one slip.

Tailoring the Regimen

Tailoring the regimen addresses the patient's capability to carry out the plan, that is, what is realistic for the patient to achieve in behavior change. It includes accommodating the patient's schedule for appointments, being sensitive to cultural issues in recommending dietary change or other behaviors, and being sensitive to literacy as well as to financial constraints in general. It is an important consideration in medication-taking compliance (e.g., considering the costs, memory requirements, and schedule when prescribing a drug that may be available in numerous dosing forms).

Use of Frequent, Short Bouts, Home-based, or Moderate-Intensity Exercise Sessions

There is ample evidence of using frequent, short bouts to induce exercise benefits. Accumulated exercise using short bouts (2×15 min, 3×10 min) has similar benefits in aerobic fitness and weight loss with that of one 30-min bout of exercise. The effectiveness of this approach to improving VO_{2max} was demonstrated among healthy sedentary adults in Hong Kong[144] and Canada.[145] In a recent paper published by the American College of Sports Medicine and American Heart Association,[146] the duration of short bouts was more clearly defined. Exercise short bouts, lasting 10 or more minutes, are recommended to meet the minimum 30 minutes of moderate intensity physical activity level on five days per week. Individuals can be reassured that they can be flexible in planning their exercise routine by using the short-bout approach. Patients often do better in terms of long-term adherence and fewer injuries if they are instructed to follow a moderate-intensity exercise program.

Use of External Cognitive Aids

External cognitive aids include appointment reminder letters, follow-up letters for missed appointments, reminder cards for medication refill, medication calendars or reminder charts, and unit-of-use packaging of pills. Any of these strategies can enhance adherence to appointment keeping and to medication taking. Appointment reminder calls and letters are used effectively in most long-term clinical trials.

Nurse Case-Managed Care

Serving as case managers, nurses provide clinic and telephone follow-up, initiate therapy for risk reduction, and provide counseling for behavior change (e.g., smoking cessation, dietary change). Use of this treatment model has demonstrated improved clinical outcome in studies of patients with coronary heart disease in which several of the previously described strategies were incorporated into the treatment plan.[147–149] More recently, nurses have been managing patients with heart failure through clinics and through follow-up care at home.[150–152]

Patient-Centered Counseling

Patient-centered counseling is an intervention developed by Ockene et al.[153] and is based on provider training in the technique. The counseling approach includes advising the patient about nutrition change, assessing strengths and barriers, reviewing the patient's FFQ that was completed in the waiting room, developing a plan for change, and arranging follow-up. The intervention took 8 to 10 minutes of the clinic visit time, has been successful in helping patients make dietary behavioral changes, and has potential in primary care settings. These investigators have applied this model of care to other health conditions such as alcohol addiction.

Model of Self-Management of Chronic Disease

An updated approach to management of chronic disease and improved adherence has been presented by Bodenheimer et al.[154,155] This has been referred to as a Chronic Care Model and more recently a Teamlet Model of Primary Care has been presented. The latter approach involves the clinician with health coach assistants; the latter spend time with the patient prior to and following the clinical visit and also provide intervisit follow-up. The health coach engages the patient in collaborative goal setting and developing an action plan for whatever regimen needs to be addressed. Enhancement of self-efficacy is also considered.

Non Face-to-Face Approaches

Keeping in mind the barriers to face-to-face intervention (work schedules, travel, childcare, etc.), recent studies have examined the effectiveness of interventions without face-to-face contact, such as telephone and the use of the Internet. Pierce et al.[156] reported long-term adherence to a high-vegetable dietary pattern with the one-on-one intervention delivered over the telephone. A review of weight-loss interventions delivered over the Internet found that those programs that emphasized dietary and physical activity changes, used cognitive-behavior strategies and provided personalized feedback and support were most effective.[157] Advantages of Internet-based interventions are that they are available at any time, may provide tailored information and messages, and provide privacy and anonymity. However, literacy, language, culture, and limited skills may preclude individuals from utilizing Internet-based interventions.

EDUCATIONAL STRATEGIES TO IMPROVE ADHERENCE

Didactic, cognitive interventions may be used to transmit information about the disease process or the treatment regimen. Often a behavior change requires educating the patient about the regimen, such as how to follow a low-fat diet or initiate an exercise program. The underlying aim may be to increase the person's knowledge in the expectation that behavior change will follow. However, the association between knowledge and behavior is small. A recent systematic review of intervention studies to improve medication adherence reported that adherence increased most consistently with behavioral interventions, particularly those that reduced the dosing demands.[158] Past reports have indicated that educational interventions alone do not yield positive results.[159] Supplementing educational interventions with improving tolerability of the regimen and motivational approaches were effective and improved adherence by 41%.[159] A multifactorial intervention approach focusing on drug adherence, lifestyle modification and conversations with the provider (patient education) was more successful in BP control than provider education and provider education and alert,[160] suggesting a more interdisciplinary approach with behavioral strategies increases the effectiveness of the intervention. Additionally, feedback and specific instructions using the MEMS resulted in a higher compliance adherence to bupropion-SR for smoking cessation when compared to the control group indicating that interventions using feedback may have a positive effect on medication-taking behavior.[161] A list of guidelines for delivering educational interventions is presented in Display 40-1. It is important to also incorporate into the intervention the behavioral strategies previously described.

DISPLAY 40-1 Guidelines to Follow in Delivering Educational Interventions

- Keep instructions specific to the activity
- Assess the reading level of material; make sure it is understandable, accurate, and appropriate
- Review material for cultural relevance and acceptability
- Be aware of religious restrictions related to diet
- Deliver informational material over time and provide in small amounts
- Provide verbal instructions in small amounts
- Avoid the use of jargon or technical terms
- Use printed materials to supplement and reinforce verbal instructions
- Permit family members or other sources of support to sit in or participate in session, arrange for extra space when this occurs
- Encourage questions of patient and ask patient questions to determine level of understanding; permit sufficient time for the person to answer
- Focus on the regimen, not the disease
- Utilize a variety of media formats (videotapes, interactive computer programs, visual illustrations, reliable websites sources, e.g., American Heart Association)
- Provide demonstrations to augment verbal instructions
- Provide for patient or relative giving return demonstrations and practice opportunities, e.g., mixing medications, taking nitroglycerin, completing diaries, counting pulse, reading prescription or food label
- Utilize community resources, e.g., American Heart Association, local health department or hospital for health classes, cardiac rehabilitation programs

QUESTIONNAIRES RELEVANT TO ADHERENCE-ENHANCING INTERVENTIONS

Most interventions to improve adherence focus on one or more of the constructs of social cognitive theory (i.e., self-regulation and self-efficacy). Research has produced several psychometrically sound instruments to measure the constructs that may influence adherence across several behavioral domains. Because of their behavioral specificity, self-efficacy scales have been developed for several behavioral domains, including following a general cardiac diet and exercise program[162–164] for adhering to a cholesterol-lowering diet,[48,49] for following a weight-loss diet,[165–167] for smoking cessation,[168] and for medication taking.[169] Instruments have been developed that apply the processes of change to risk reduction behavior, including an instrument that measures readiness for change to a low-fat diet[170] and one to measure future success in smoking cessation.[171] These represent just a few of the self-administered scales that can be used in the clinical or research setting. An extensive database of health behavior questionnaires is available at Health and Psychosocial Instruments; access may vary by academic institutions.

BUILDING A THERAPEUTIC RELATIONSHIP WITH THE PATIENT

Working with a patient to ensure adequate adherence at the initiation of treatment, and over the long term either to enhance compliance or remediate poor adherence, requires good rapport and clear communication lines between the patient and provider. Having a good therapeutic relationship allows ongoing assessment of the patient's adherence and also provides an environment conducive to the patient confiding in the provider when barriers to adherence arise. The patient needs to be queried regularly if he or she has any concerns about the condition or the treatment, and should be commended for seeking and following through on the treatment process.

Listening reflectively to the patient and being supportive can facilitate communication. The provider should listen more than talk, and listen with interest. Encourage the patient to express problems he or she anticipates having or has encountered in implementing the treatment. Acknowledge how difficult the new, possibly complex, treatment is and the demands it places on the patient, for example, "I am sure all of this is overwhelming to you. What concerns you the most about your treatment?" Assist the patient to identify barriers to implementing or following the treatment, such as no available time or place where he or she can exercise safely, or, for the patient who needs to quit smoking, a spouse who smokes and has no intentions of quitting. Determine what the patient's view of the treatment is, and clarify what the patient's responsibilities will be in carrying out the treatment. If possible, give priority to the patient's goal in the treatment plan. If ambivalence is present, try to help the patient resolve it, and use the strategies of motivational interviewing that have been described previously in this chapter.

When it is time to begin working on the treatment plan, the provider may begin by acknowledging the challenge, "I know how difficult it is to make changes in long-established eating habits. We are asking you to make changes gradually over time and will work with you in making those changes. What may we do to assist you with this?" and "What would you like to focus on first?" Express confidence in the patient's ability to implement the treatment, and in the treatment having a beneficial effect if it is followed. Assist the patient gradually to assume responsibility for the treatment. Involve the patient in development and implementation of the treatment plan. Before closing the session, review with the patient exactly what will be done: "Now let's go over this plan once more just to make sure I have given you all the information you need. What is the medication you're going to be taking?" Or, to avoid putting the patient in an awkward position: "The name of the drug is ... Now please tell me how many pills you plan to take and when. Are there any symptoms you should report to us?" In follow-up sessions, acknowledge each time how difficult it is to take medications or follow whatever treatment regimen has been recommended (e.g., smoking cessation, dietary change, or regular exercise) and assess how the patient is doing. The nurse may say, "I know it can be difficult to remember to take your pills each time. Do you find that you forget to take your pills sometime?" or "Sometimes when patients feel better, they skip their medications. Do you ever skip taking your pills when you feel good?" A general question may also be asked, such as "Tell me about your medicines and how you are taking them." Ask the patient to go through each medication and describe how many pills are being taken and when. The same general questions can be applied to other behaviors or activities. Regular follow-up on previously discussed regimen plans conveys to the patient that the behavior is important and so is adherence to it.

An important part of follow-up is providing encouragement and reinforcement. The nurse needs to acknowledge the difficulties the patient faces, but also must be firm regarding the importance of the treatment and continue to instill confidence in the patient. Reinforcement should be given for the behavior change made, not for the clinical outcome. Providing information on clinical outcomes (e.g., blood cholesterol levels) can be an additional reinforcement to the patient, showing the progress he or she has made in changing behavior and its positive effects on health. However, focusing only on the clinical outcomes does not acknowledge the behavioral efforts made by the patient, and moreover, clinical outcomes such as serum cholesterol can be influenced by several intervening variables such as concomitant medications or laboratory changes.

The greatest challenge in adherence is to assist the patient to maintain the behavioral changes for the long term. As noted previously, there is a decline in adherence during the first year of treatment, with continued erosion over time. This decline is usually accelerated in the absence of any contact with the health care professional. Thus, adherence needs to be addressed at each visit with the previously suggested questions. Slips, lapses, or relapse can be expected and should be prevented when possible. A slip is missing the treatment for a very brief period, for example, one or two doses of medication missed, a lapse is when the person does not adhere for three to four days, and a relapse is usually when a person stops following the treatment regimen for at least a week. If there is an indication the patient is lapsing, additional attention needs to be provided. It may take the form of periodic telephone contacts and/or mail contact. This may include the patient reporting on progress made toward a goal, or the nurse assisting with problem solving in difficult situations, correcting any further problems, providing reinforcement for attempts and progress, and helping the patient set new goals, if appropriate. It may help to have the patient self-monitor behavior for a period and have these records returned before each phone call, or have the patient bring them in at each visit. It is important that these diaries or records be reviewed and used in pointing out positive behaviors and making suggestions for healthier behaviors.

SUMMARY

Inadequate adherence to the recommended treatment plan remains a significant, ubiquitous problem facing health care professionals in all settings and populations worldwide. Research has demonstrated the efficacy of pharmacological and behavioral treatment for an array of conditions. However, a wide separation exists between evidence-based recommendations and the actual treatment being prescribed.[141] This gap reflects providers not recognizing patients' need for treatment, not prescribing the best drug or dose, and not involving the patient in the choice of treatment. Moreover, the effectiveness of the treatments that have been prescribed has been undermined by less than ideal adherence. Progress has been made in the measurement of adherence and in identifying strategies that may enhance adherence. However, measurement methods remain limited and some are unaffordable or impractical for widespread clinical use. The simple measures that exist may be as revealing (e.g., asking the patient directly how often he or she does not perform a behavior or monitoring appointment nonattendance) but often are not used or heeded. Although research is ongoing on strategies to improve adherence, there remains a huge gap between what is known and beneficial and what is applied in clinical practice. Thus, the poor rates of adherence have remained relatively static.[76,117,118]

Not only are the intervention strategies applied in the clinical setting not enough to significantly affect adherence, but some interventions are labor intensive and thus not easily implemented in a practice setting. Furthermore, the nurse faces additional challenges because of the changing health care environment, including shortened length of hospital stay, increased level of acuity of patients during their hospitalization and at discharge, reduced number of visits after acute events, and increasingly complex treatment regimens that patients need to learn how to implement. However, the nurse is often in the best position to address adherence. As nursing assumes an expanded role in an array of settings, the nurse often assumes responsibility for patient education, ensuring that the patient understands the regimen, and for arranging needed follow-up. Additionally, the voluminous body of literature on *adherence, compliance, persistence* and *concordance* verify the increasingly greater attention being given to this important issue related to care delivery and clinical outcomes. The identification of the different levels of factors that affect adherence, for example, patient, regimen, provider, and system, also provide evidence that this is no longer viewed as a 'patient problem' but rather one that each member of the health care teams needs to assume responsibility for and address.

The nursing profession has shown leadership in promoting patient education in past decades, and more recently in advancing the case-management role. It is time again for nursing to take the lead and intervene to improve adherence. This requires looking at how health care is provided and determining where interventions need to be directed (i.e., at the level of the system, the provider, the treatment regimen, or the patient). Most likely, all four components of the system need to be addressed when making changes to facilitate improved adherence. Moreover, the changes need to be addressed over the continuum of care provision, particularly during the maintenance phase, when nonadherence is most likely to become an issue.

Acknowledgment: *The authors were supported by grant 5RO1 DK071817, National Institute of Health, National Institute of Diabetes, Digestive, and Kidney Disorders.*

REFERENCES

1. Burke, L. E., Dunbar-Jacob, J. M., & Hill, M. N. (1997). Compliance with cardiovascular disease prevention strategies: A review of the research. *Annals of Behavioral Medicine, 19*(3), 239–263.
2. Burke, L. E., & Ockene, I. S. (2001). *Compliance in healthcare and research.* Armonk, NY: Futura.
3. Sackett, D. L., & Haynes, R. B. (1976). *Compliance with therapeutic regimens.* Baltimore: The Johns Hopkins University Press.
4. Sackett, D. L., & Snow, J. C. (1979). The magnitude of adherence and nonadherence. In R. B. Haynes, D. W. Taylor, & D. L. Sackett (Eds.), *Compliance in health care* (pp. 11–22). Baltimore: Johns Hopkins University Press.
5. Horne, R. (2006). Compliance, adherence, and concordance: Implications for asthma treatment. *Chest, 130*(1, Suppl.), 65S–72S.
6. Tilson, H. H. (2004). Adherence or compliance? Changes in terminology. *Annals of Pharmacother, 38*(1), 161–162.
7. Whellan, D. J., & Hamad, E. (2007). Natural history, adherence, or iatrogenic insult: Repeat hospitalizations as a predictor of survival. *American Heart Journal, 154*(2), 203–205.
8. Clark, R. A., Inglis, S. C., McAlister, F. A., et al. (2007). Telemonitoring or structured telephone support programmes for patients with chronic heart failure: Systematic review and meta-analysis. *BMJ, 334*(7600), 942.
9. McAlister, F. A., Stewart, S., Ferrua, S., et al. (2004). Multidisciplinary strategies for the management of heart failure patients at high risk for admission: A systematic review of randomized trials. *Journal of the American College of Cardiology, 44*(4), 810–819.
10. Osterberg, L., & Blaschke, T. F. (2005). Adherence to medication. *New England Journal of Medicine, 353*(5), 487–497.
11. Brookhart, M. A. P. A., Schneeweiss, S., Avorn, J., et al. (2007). Physician follow-up and provider continuity are associated with long-term medication adherence: A study of the dynamics of statin use. *Archives of Internal Medicine, 167*(8), 847–852.
12. DiMatteo, M. R. (2004). Variations in patients' adherence to medical recommendations: A quantitative review of 50 years of research [see comment]. *Medical Care, 42*(3), 200–209.
13. Lowry, K. P., Dudley, T. K., Oddone, E. Z., et al. (2005). Intentional and unintentional nonadherence to antihypertensive medication. *The Annals of Pharmacotherapy, 39*(7), 1198–1203.
14. Christensen, A. J. (2004). Patient adherence to medical treatment regimens: Bridging the gap between behavioral science and bio-medicine. *Current Perspectives in Psychology.* New Haven: Yale University Press.
15. Granger, B. B., Moser, D., Harrell, J., et al. (2007). A practical use of theory to study adherence. *Progress in Cardiovascular Nursing, 22*(3), 152–158.
16. Poluzzi, E., Strahinja, P., Vargiu, A., et al. (2005). Initial treatment of hypertension and adherence to therapy in general practice in Italy. *European Journal of Clinical Pharmacology, 61*(8), 603–609.
17. Taira, D. A., Gelber, R. P., Davis, J., et al. (2007). Antihypertensive adherence and drug class among Asian Pacific Americans. *Ethnicity & Health, 12*(3), 265–281.
18. USDA. (2008). Nutrient intake from food: Mean amount consumed per individual by race/ethnicity and age, one day, 2003–2004. Retrieved March 2, 2008, from http://www.ars.usda.gov/ba/bhnrc/fsrg.
19. CDC. (2007). Prevalence of fruit and vegetable consumption and physical activity by race/ethnicity—United States 2005. *Morbidity and Mortality Weekly Report, 56*(13), 301–304.
20. Ogden, C., Carroll, M., Curtin, L., et al. (2006). Prevalence of overweight and obesity in the United States, 1999–2004. *JAMA, 295*(13), 1549–1555.
21. CDC. (2006). Summary health statistics for U.S. adults: National Health Interview Survey 2005. *Vital Health Statistics.*
22. WHO. (2008). *The facts about smoking and health.* Retrieved March 2, 2008, from http://www.wpro.who.int/media_centre/fact_sheets/fs_20060530.htm.
23. Hughes, J. R., Keely, J., & Naud, S. (2004). Shape of the relapse curve and long-term abstinence among untreated smokers. *Addiction, 99*(1), 29–38.
24. Aveyard, P., & West, R. (2007). Managing smoking cessation. *BMJ, 335*(7609), 37–41.

25. Acharya, S. D., Elci, O. U., Sereika, S. M., et al. (2009). Examination of adherence to a multi-component behavioral weight loss treatment program. *Journal of Patient Preference and Adherence, 3*, 1–10.
26. Dew, M. A., DiMartini, A. F., De Vito Dabbs, A., et al. (2007). Rates and risk factors for nonadherence to the medical regimen after adult solid organ transplantation. *Transplantation, 83*(7), 858–873.
27. Burke, L. E. (2001). Electronic monitoring. In L. E. Burke & I. S. Ockene (Ed.), *Compliance in healthcare and research.* Armonk, NY: Futura Publishing Company, Inc.
28. Schron, E., & Czajkowski, S. M. (2001). Clinical trials. In L. E. Burke & I. S. Ockene (Eds.), *Compliance in healthcare and research* (pp. 237–246). Armonk, NY: Futura Publishing Company, Inc.
29. Sereika, S. M., & Dunbar-Jacob, J. (2001). *Analysis of electronic event monitored adherence.* Armonk, NY: Future Publishing Company Inc.
30. Urquhart, J. (1991). *Patient compliance as an explanatory variable in four selected cardiovascular studies.* New York: Raven Press.
31. Dunbar-Jacob, J., & Sereika, S. (2001). Conceptual and methodological problems. In L. A. Burke & I. S. Ockene (Ed.), *Compliance in healthcare and research.* Ormonk, NY: Futura Publishing Company, Inc.
32. Urquhart, J. (2001). Biological measures. In L. E. Burke & I. S. Ockene (Ed.), *Compliance in healthcare and research.* Armonk, NY: Futura Publishing Company, Inc.
33. Cramer, J. A., Scheyer, R. D., & Mattson, R. H. (1990). Compliance declines between clinic visits. *Archives of Internal Medicine, 150*, 1509–1510.
34. Cramer, J. A., Mattson, R. H., Prevey, M. L., et al. (1989). How often is medication taken as prescribed? A novel assessment technique. *JAMA, 261*(22), 3273–3277.
35. Dunbar-Jacob, J., Burke, L. E., Rohay, J. M., et al. (1997). How comparable are self-report, pill count, and electronically monitored adherence data? *Circulation, 96*(8, Suppl.), I738.
36. Dixon, L. B., Subar, A. F., Peters, U., et al. (2007). Adherence to the USDA Food Guide, DASH Eating Plan, and Mediterranean dietary pattern reduces risk of colorectal adenoma. *Journal of Nutrition, 137*(11), 2443–2450.
37. Tucker, K. L. (2007). Assessment of usual dietary intake in population studies of gene-diet interaction. *Nutrition, Metabolism and Cardiovascular Diseases, 17*(2), 74–81.
38. Blanton, C. A., Moshfegh, A. J., Baer, D. J., et al. (2006). The USDA automated multiple-pass method accurately estimates group total energy and nutrient intake. *Journal of Nutrition, 136*(10), 2594–2599.
39. Conway, J. M., Ingwersen, L. A., Vinyard, B. T., et al. (2003). Effectiveness of the US Department of Agriculture 5-step multiple-pass method in assessing food intake in obese and nonobese women. *American Journal of Clinical Nutrition, 77*(5), 1171–1178.
40. Fuller, Z., Horgan, G., O'reilly, L. M., et al. (2007). Comparing different measures of energy expenditure in human subjects resident in a metabolic facility. *European Journal of Clinical Nutrition, 62*, 560–569.
41. Shaffer, H. J., Nelson, S. E., LaPlante, D. A., et al. (2007). The epidemiology of psychiatric disorders among repeat DUI offenders accepting a treatment-sentencing option. *Journal of Consulting and Clinical Psychology, 75*(5):795–804.
42. American Psychiatric Association. (2000). *Diagnostic and statistical manual of mental disorders* (text revision, 4th ed.). Washinton, DC: Author.
43. Li, W. W., Wallhagen, M. I., & Froelicher, E. S. (2008). Hypertension control, predictors for medication adherence and gender differences in older Chinese immigrants. *Journal of Advanced Nursing, 61*(3), 326–335.
44. Natarajan, N., Putnam, R. W., Yip, A. M., et al. (2007). Family practice patients' adherence to statin medications. *Canadian Family Physician, 53*(12), 2144–2145.
45. Shalansky, S. J., Levy, A. R., & Ignaszewski, A. P. (2004). Self-reported Morisky score for identifying nonadherence with cardiovascular medications. *Annals of Pharmacother, 38*(9), 1363–1368.
46. Rottlaender, D., Scherner, M., Schneider, T., et al. (2007). Polypharmacy, compliance and non-prescription medication in patients with cardiovascular disease in Germany. *Deutsche Medizinische Wochenschrift, 132*(4), 139–144.
47. Elm, J. J., Kamp, C., Tilley, B. C., et al. (2007). Self-reported adherence versus pill count in Parkinson's disease: The NET-PD experience. *Movement Disorders, 22*(6), 822–827.
48. Burke, L. E., Dunbar-Jacob, J., Sereika, S., et al. (2003). Development and testing of the Cholesterol-Lowering Diet Self-Efficacy Scale. *European Journal of Cardiovascular Nursing, 2*(4), 265–273.
49. Burke, L. E., Kim, Y., Senuzun, F., et al. (2006). Evaluation of the shortened cholesterol-lowering diet self-efficacy scale. *European Journal of Cardiovascular Nursing, 5*, 264–274.
50. Rutishauser, I. H. (2005). Dietary intake measurements. *Public Health Nutrition, 8*(7A), 1100–1107.
51. Matt, G. E., Rock, C. L., & Johnson-Kozlow, M. (2006). Using recall cues to improve measurement of dietary intakes with a food frequency questionnaire in an ethnically diverse population: An exploratory study. *Journal of the American Dietetic Association, 106*(8), 1209–1217.
52. Tseng, M., & Hernandez, T. (2005). Comparison of intakes of US Chinese women based on food frequency and 24-hour recall data. *Journal of the American Dietetic Association, 105*(7), 1145–1148.
53. Sevak, L., Mangtani, P., McCormack, V., et al. (2004). Validation of a food frequency questionnaire to assess macro- and micro-nutrient intake among South Asians in the United Kingdom. *European Journal of Nutrition, 43*(3), 160–168.
54. Quandt, S. A., Vitolins, M. Z., Smith, S. L., et al. (2007). Comparative validation of standard, picture-sort and meal-based food-frequency questionnaires adapted for an elderly population of low socio-economic status. *Public Health Nutrition, 10*(5), 524–532.
55. Tucker, K. L., Maras, J., Champagne, C., et al. (2005). A regional food-frequency questionnaire for the US Mississippi Delta. *Public Health Nutrition, 8*(1), 87–96.
56. Jakicic, J. M., Wing, R. R., & Winters-Hart, C. (2002). Relationship of physical activity to eating behaviors and weight loss in women. *Medicine & Science in Sports & Exercise, 34*(10), 1653–1659.
57. Kriska, A. M., & Caspersen, C. J. (1997). Introduction to a collection of physical activity questionnaires. *Medicine and Science in Sports and Exercise, 29*, S5–S9.
58. Pereira, M. A., FitzerGerald, S. J., Gregg, E. W., et al. (1997). A collection of Physical Activity Questionnaires for health-related research. *Medicine & Science in Sports & Exercise\, 29*(6, Suppl.), S1–S205.
59. Sternfeld, B., Wang, H., Quesenberry, C. P., Jr., et al. (2004). Physical activity and changes in weight and waist circumference in midlife women: Findings from the Study of Women's Health Across the Nation. *American Journal of Epidemiology, 160*(9), 912–922.
60. Hughes, A. R., Mutrie, N., & Macintyre, P. D. (2007). Effect of an exercise consultation on maintenance of physical activity after completion of phase III exercise-based cardiac rehabilitation. *European Journal of Cardiovascular Prevention and Rehabilitation, 14*(1), 114–121.
61. Cooper, T. V., Resor, M. R., Stoever, C. J., et al. (2007). Physical activity and physical activity adherence in the elderly based on smoking status. *Addictive Behaviors, 32*(10), 2268–2273.
62. Dubbert, P. M., Vander Weg, M. W., Kirchner, K. A., et al. (2004). Evaluation of the 7-day physical activity recall in urban and rural men. *Medicine & Science in Sports & Exercise, 36*(9), 1646–1654.
63. Catenacci, V. A., Ogden, L. G., Stuht, J., et al. (2008). Physical activity patterns in the National Weight Control Registry. *Obesity, 16*(1), 153–161.
64. Dunn, C. L., Hannan, P. J., Jeffery, R. W., et al. (2006). The comparative and cumulative effects of a dietary restriction and exercise on weight loss. *International Journal of Obesity, 30*(1), 112–121.
65. King, A. C., Ahn, D. K., Oliveira, B. M., et al. (2008). Promoting physical activity through hand-held computer technology. *American Journal of Preventive Medicine, 34*(2), 138–142.
66. Fagerstrom, K. O., & Schneider, N. G. (1989). Measuring nicotine dependence: A review of the Fagerstrom Tolerance Questionnaire. *Journal of Behavioral Medicine, 12*(2), 159–182.
67. John, U., Riedel, J., Rumpf, H. J., et al. (2006). Associations of perceived work strain with nicotine dependence in a community sample. *Occupational and Environmental Medicine, 63*(3), 207–211.
68. Etter, J. F. (2005). A comparison of the content-, construct- and predictive validity of the cigarette dependence scale and the Fagerstrom test for nicotine dependence. *Drug and Alcohol Dependence, 77*(3), 259–268.
69. Burke, L. E., Sereika, S. M., Music, E., et al. (2008). Using instrumented paper diaries to document self-monitoring patterns in weight loss. *Contemporary Clinical Trials, 29*(2), 182–193.
70. Burke, L. E., Warziski, M., Starrett, T., et al. (2005). Self-monitoring dietary intake: Current and future practices. *Journal of Renal Nutrition, 15*(3), 281–290.
71. Wadden, T. A., Berkowitz, R. I., Womble, L. G., et al. (2005). Randomized trial of lifestyle modification and pharmacotherapy for obesity. *New England Journal of Medicine, 353*(20), 2111–2120.
72. Carels, R. A., Darby, L. A., Rydin, S., et al. (2005). The relationship between self-monitoring, outcome expectancies, difficulties with eating and

exercise, and physical activity and weight loss treatment outcomes. *Annals of Behavioral Medicine, 30*(3), 182–190.

73. Burke, L. E., Warziski, M., Styn, M. A., et al. (2008). A randomized clinical trial of a standard versus vegetarian diet for weight loss: The impact of treatment preference. *International Journal of Obesity, 32*, 166–176.
74. Wickel, E. E., Welk, G. J., & Eisenmann, J. C. (2006). Concurrent validation of the Bouchard Diary with an accelerometry-based monitor. *Medicine & Science in Sports & Exercise, 38*(2), 373–379.
75. Walsh, M. C., Hunter, G. R., Sirikul, B., et al. (2004). Comparison of self-reported with objectively assessed energy expenditure in black and white women before and after weight loss. *American Journal of Clinical Nutrition, 79*(6), 1013–1019.
76. Johnson, R. K., Friedman, A. B., Harvey-Berino, J., et al. (2005). Participation in a behavioral weight-loss program worsens the prevalence and severity of underreporting among obese and overweight women. *Journal of the American Dietetic Association, 105*(12), 1948–1951.
77. Yon, B. A., Johnson, R. K., Harvey-Berino, J., et al. (2006). The use of a personal digital assistant for dietary self-monitoring does not improve the validity of self-reports of energy intake. *Journal of the American Dietetic Association, 106*(8), 1256–1259.
78. Colley, R. C., Hills, A. P., O'Moore-Sullivan, T. M., et al. (2008). Variability in adherence to an unsupervised exercise prescription in obese women. *International Journal of Obesity (London), 32*(5), 837–844.
79. Braam, R. L., van Uum, S. H., Lenders, J. W., et al. (2008). Bromide as marker for drug adherence in hypertensive patients. *British Journal of Clinical Pharmacology, 65*(5), 733–737.
80. Leiba, A., Vald, A., Peleg, E., et al. (2005). Does dietary recall adequately assess sodium, potassium, and calcium intake in hypertensive patients? *Nutrition, 21*(4), 462–466.
81. Pärna, K., Rahu, M., Youngman, L. D., et al. (2005). Self-reported and serum cotinine-validated smoking in pregnant women in Estonia. *Maternal and Child Health Journal, 9*(4), 385–392.
82. St-Onge, M., Mignault, D., Allison, D. B., et al. (2007). Evaluation of a portable device to measure daily energy expenditure in free-living adults. *American Journal of Clinical Nutrition, 85*(3), 742–749.
83. Schoeller, D. A. (1988). Measurement of energy expenditure in free-living humans by using doubly labeled water. *Journal of Nutrition, 118*(11), 1278–1289.
84. Allison, D. B. (1995). *Handbook of assessment methods for eating behaviors and weight related problems: Measures, theory, and research.* Thousand Oaks, CA: Sage.
85. Charlton, K. E., Steyn, K., Levitt, N. S., et al. (2005). Ethnic differences in intake and excretion of sodium, potassium, calcium and magnesium in South Africans. *European Journal of Cardiovascular Prevention and Rehabilitation, 12*(4), 355–362.
86. Stone, A. A., Shiffman, S., Schwartz, J. E., et al. (2002). Patient non-compliance with paper diaries. *BMJ, 324*(7347), 1193–1194.
87. Girvin, B. G., & Johnston, G. D. (2004). Comparison of the effects of a 7-day period of non-compliance on blood pressure control using three different antihypertensive agents. *Journal of Hypertension, 22*(7), 1409–1414.
88. Santschi, V., Wuerzner, G., Schneider, M. P., et al. (2007). Clinical evaluation of IDAS II, a new electronic device enabling drug adherence monitoring. *European Journal of Clinical Pharmacology, 63*(12), 1179–1184.
89. Gamelin, F. X., Baquet, G., Berthoin, S., et al. (2008). Validity of the polar s810 to measure R-R intervals in children. *International Journal of Sports Medicine, 29*(2), 134–138.
90. Gamelin, F. X., Berthoin, S., & Bosquet, L. (2006). Validity of the polar S810 heart rate monitor to measure R-R intervals at rest. *Medicine & Science in Sports & Exercise, 38*(5), 887–893.
91. Cyarto, E. V., Myers, A. M., & Tudor-Locke, C. (2004). Pedometer accuracy in nursing home and community-dwelling older adults. *Medicine & Science in Sports & Exercise, 36*(2), 205–209.
92. Melanson, E. L., Knoll, J. R., Bell, M. L., et al. (2004). Commercially available pedometers: Considerations for accurate step counting. *Preventive Medicine, 39*(2), 361–368.
93. Storti, K. L., Pettee, K. K., Brach, J. S., et al. (2008). Gait speed and step-count monitor accuracy in community-dwelling older adults. *Medicine & Science in Sports & Exercise, 40*(1), 59–64.
94. Dua, J. S., Cooper, A. R., Fox, K. R., et al. (2007). Physical activity levels in adults with congenital heart disease. *European Journal of Cardiovascular Prevention and Rehabilitation, 14*(2), 287–293.
95. Troiano, R. P., Berrigan, D., Dodd, K. W., et al. (2008). Physical activity in the United States measured by accelerometer. *Medicine & Science in Sports & Exercise, 40*(1), 181–188.
96. Jakicic, J. M., Marcus, M., Gallagher, K. I., et al. (2004). Evaluation of the SenseWear Pro Armband[TM] to assess energy expenditure during exercise. *Medicine & Science in Sports & Exercise, 36*(5), 897–904.
97. Malavolti, M., Pietrobelli, A., Dugoni, M., et al. (2007). A new device for measuring resting energy expenditure (REE) in healthy subjects. *Nutrition, Metabolism and Cardiovascular Diseases, 17*(5), 338–343.
98. Papazoglou, D., Augello, G., Tagliaferri, M., et al. (2006). Evaluation of a multisensor armband in estimating energy expenditure in obese individuals. *Obesity, 14*(12), 2217–2223.
99. Welk, G. J., McClain, J. J., Eisenmann, J. C., et al. (2007). Field validation of the MTI actigraph and BodyMedia Armband monitor using the IDEEA monitor. *Obesity, 15*(4), 918–928.
100. le Grange, D., Gorin, A., Dymek, M., et al. (2002). Does ecological momentary assessment improve cognitive behavioural therapy for binge eating disorder? A pilot study. *European Eating Disorders Review, 10*, 316–328.
101. Glanz, K., Murphy, S., Moylan, J., et al. (2006). Improving dietary self-monitoring and adherence with hand-held computers: a pilot study. *American Journal of Health Promotion, 20*(3), 165–170.
102. Sevick, M. A., Zickmund, S., Korytkowski, M., et al. (2007). Design, feasibility, and acceptability of an intervention using personal digital assistant-based self-monitoring in managing type 2 diabetes. *Contemporary Clinical Trials, 29*(3), 396–409. Epub 2007 Sep 26.
103. Stone, A. A., & Shiffman, S. (2002). Capturing momentary, self–report data: A proposal for reporting guidelines. *Annals of Behavioral Medicine, 24*, 236–243.
104. Burke, L. E., Music, E., Styn, M. A., et al. (2006). Using technology to improve self-monitoring in weight loss. *International Journal of Behavioral Medicine, 13*(Suppl.), 192.
105. Music, E., Choo, J., Styn, M. A., et al. (2006). Feasibility study: Using PDA-based DietMate Pro® for dietary self-monitoring. *Annals of Behavioral Medicine, 31*(Suppl.), S058.
106. Burke, L. E., Sereika, S., Choo, J., et al. (2006). Ancillary study to the PREFER trial: A descriptive study of participants' patterns of self-monitoring: Rationale, design and preliminary experiences. *Contemporary Clinical Trials, 27*(1), 23–33.
107. Baer, A., Saroiu, S., & Koutsky, L. A. (2002). Obtaining sensitive data through the Web: An example of design and methods. *Epidemiology, 13*(6), 640–645.
108. Tate, D. F., Jackvony, E. H., & Wing, R. R. (2006). A randomized trial comparing human e-mail counseling, computer-automated tailored counseling, and no counseling in an Internet weight loss program. *Archives of Internal Medicine, 166*, 1620–1625.
109. Prado, J. C., Jr., Kupek, E., & Mion, D., Jr. (2007). Validity of four indirect methods to measure adherence in primary care hypertensives. *Journal of Human Hypertension, 21*(7), 579–584.
110. DiMatteo, M. R., Haskard, K. B., & Williams, S. L. (2007). Health beliefs, disease severity, and patient adherence: A meta-analysis. *Medical Care, 45*(6), 521–528.
111. Vlachopoulos, S. P., & Neikou, E. (2007). A prospective study of the relationships of autonomy, competence, and relatedness with exercise attendance, adherence, and dropout. *The Journal of Sports Medicine and Physical Fitness, 47*(4), 475–482.
112. Fuertes, J. N., Mislowack, A., Bennett, J., et al. (2007). The physician-patient working alliance. *Patient Education* and *Counseling, 66*(1), 29–36.
113. Capdevila Ortís, L., Niñerola Maymí, J., Cruz Feliu, J., et al. (2007). Exercise motivation in university community members: A behavioural intervention. *Psicothema, 19*(2), 250–255.
114. Jones, M., Jolly, K., Raftery, J., et al. (2007). 'DNA' may not mean 'did not participate': A qualitative study of reasons for non-adherence at home- and centre-based cardiac rehabilitation. *Family Practice, 24*(4), 343–357.
115. Gazmararian, J. A., Kripalani, S., Miller, M. J., et al. (2006). Factors associated with medication refill adherence in cardiovascular-related diseases: A focus on health literacy. *Journal of General Internal Medicine, 21*(12), 1215–1221.
116. Stilley, C. S., Sereika, S., Muldoon, M. F., et al. (2004). Psychological and cognitive function: Predictors of adherence with cholesterol lowering treatment. *Annals of Behavioral Medicine, 27*(2), 117–124.
117. Tinker, L. F., Rosal, M. C., Young, A. F., et al. (2007). Predictors of dietary change and maintenance in the Women's Health Initiative Dietary Modification Trial. *Journal of the American Dietetic Association, 107*(7), 1155–1166.

118. Grégoire, J., Moisan, J., Guibert, R., et al. (2006). Predictors of self-reported noncompliance with antihypertensive drug treatment: A prospective cohort study. *The Canadian Journal of Cardiology, 22*(4), 323–329.
119. Comte, L., Vrijens, B., Tousset, E., et al. (2007). Estimation of the comparative therapeutic superiority of QD and BID dosing regimens, based on integrated analysis of dosing history data and pharmacokinetics. *Journal of Pharmacokinetics & Pharmacodynamics, 34*(4), 549–558.
120. Yiannakopoulou, E. C., Papadopulos, J. S., Cokkinos, D. V., et al. (2005). Adherence to antihypertensive treatment: A critical factor for blood pressure control. *European Journal of Cardiovascular Prevention and Rehabilitation, 12*(3), 243–249.
121. Tarn, D. M., Heritage, J., Paterniti, D. A., et al. (2006). Physician communication when prescribing new medications. *Archives of Internal Medicine, 166*(17), 1855–1862.
122. Batal, H. A., Krantz, M. J., Dale, R. A., et al. (2007). Impact of prescription size on statin adherence and cholesterol levels. *BMC Health Services Research, 7,* 175.
123. Gellad, W. F., Haas, J. S., & Safran, D. G. (2007). Race/ethnicity and nonadherence to prescription medications among seniors: Results of a national study. *Journal of General Internal Medicine, 22*(11), 1572–1578.
124. Hsu, J., Price, M., Huang, J., et al. (2006). Unintended consequences of caps on Medicare drug benefits. *New England Journal of Medicine, 354*(22), 2349–2359.
125. Bandura, A. (1986). *Social foundations of thought and action: A social cognitive theory.* Englewood Cliffs: Prentice Hall.
126. Bandura, A. (1997). *Self-efficacy: The exercise of control.* New York: W.H. Freeman and Company.
127. Murray, M. D., Young, J., Hoke, S., et al. (2007). Pharmacist intervention to improve medication adherence in heart failure: A randomized trial. *Annals of Internal Medicine, 146*(10), 714–725.
128. Vrijens, B., Belmans, A., Matthys, K., et al. (2006). Effect of intervention through a pharmaceutical care program on patient adherence with prescribed once-daily atorvastatin. *Pharmacoepidemiology and Drug Safety, 15*(2), 115–121.
129. Rothman, A. J., Baldwin, A. S., & Hertel, A. W. (2004). Self-regulation and behavior change: Disentangling behavioral initiation and behavioral maintenance. In K. D. Vohs & R. F. Baumeister (Eds.), *The handbook of self-regulation: Research, theory, and applications* (pp. 130–148). New York: Guilford Press.
130. Kanfer, F. H. (1991). *Self-management methods* (4th ed.). New York: Pergamon Press.
131. Kanfer, F. H. (1996). Motivation and emotion in behavior therapy. In K. S. E. Dobson & K. D. E. Craig (Eds.), *Advances in cognitive-behavioral therapy.* Thousand Oaks, CA: SAGE Publications.
132. Sereika, S. M., Colbert, A. M., Erlen, J. A., et al. (2006). Monitoring medication taking behavior in HIV patients using an electronic diary. *International Journal of Behavioral Medicine, 13*(Suppl.), 192.
133. Burke, L. E., Choo, J., Warziski, M., et al. (2004). Self-monitoring among subjects in a weight loss study. *European Journal of Cardiovascular Nursing, 4*(1), 64–65.
134. Wadden, T. A., Crerand, C. E., & Brock, J. (2005). Behavioral treatment of obesity. *Psychiatric Clinics of North America, 28*(1), 151–170.
135. Rubak, S., Sandbaek, A., Lauritzen, T., et al. (2005). Motivational interviewing: A systematic review and meta-analysis. *British Journal of General Practice, 55*(513), 305–312.
136. Carels, R. A., Darby, L., Cacciapaglia, H. M., et al. (2007). Using motivational interviewing as a supplement to obesity treatment: A stepped-care approach. *Health Psychology, 26*(3), 369–374.
137. Smith West, D., DiLillo, V., Burzac, Z., et al. (2007). Motivational interviewing improves weight loss in women with type 2 diabetes. *Diabetes Care, 30*(5), 1081–1087.
138. Hardcastle, S., Taylor, A., Bailey, M., et al. (2008). A randomised controlled trial on the effectiveness of a primary health care based counselling intervention on physical activity, diet and CHD risk factors. *Patient Education and Counseling, 70*(1), 31–39.
139. Ogedegbe, G., Schoenthaler, A., Richardson, T., et al. (2007). An RCT of the effect of motivational interviewing on medication adherence in hypertensive African Americans: Rationale and design. *Contemporary Clinical Trials, 28*(2), 169–181.
140. Soria, R., Legido, A., Escolano, C., et al. (2006). A randomised controlled trial of motivational interviewing for smoking cessation. *British Journal of General Practice, 56*(531), 768–774.
141. Marquez Contreras, E., Casado Martinez, J. J., Corchado Albalat, Y., et al. (2004). Efficacy of an intervention to improve treatment compliance in hyperlipidemias. *Atención Primaria, 33*(8), 443–450.
142. D'Zurilla, T. J., & Goldfried, M. R. (1971). Problem solving and behavior modification. *Journal of Abnormal Psychology, 78*(1), 107–126.
143. Marlatt, G. A., & Gordon, J. R. (1980). Determinants of relapse: Implications for the maintenance of behavior change. In P. Davidson & S. Davidson (Eds.), *Behavioral medicine: Changing health lifestyles* (pp. 410–452). New York: Brunner/Mazel.
144. Macfarlane, D. J., Taylor, L. H., & Cuddihy, T. F. (2006). Very short intermittent vs continuous bouts of activity in sedentary adults. *Preventive Medicine, 43*(4), 332–336.
145. Osei-Tutu, K. B., & Campagna, P. D. (2005). The effects of short- vs. long-bout exercise on mood, VO2max, and percent body fat. *Preventive Medicine, 40*(1), 92–98.
146. Haskell, W. L., Lee, I. M., Pate, R. R., et al. (2007). Physical activity and public health: Updated recommendation for adults from the American College of Sports Medicine and the American Heart Association. *Circulation, 116*(9), 1081–1093.
147. Allen, J. (1996). Coronary risk factor modification in women after coronary artery bypass surgery. *Nursing Research, 45*(5), 260–265.
148. DeBusk, R., Miller, N. H., Superko, R., et al. (1994). A case-management system for coronary risk factor modification after acute myocardial infarction. *Annals of Internal Medicine, 120*(9), 721–729.
149. Haskell, W. L., Alderman, E. L., Fair, J., et al. (1994). Effects of intensive multiple risk factor reduction on coronary atherosclerosis and clinical cardiac events in men and women with coronary artery disease the Stanford Coronary Risk Intervention Project (SCRIP). *Circulation, 89,* 975–990.
150. Bowles, K. H., Ratcliffe, S. J., Holmes, J. H., et al. (2008). Post-acute referral decisions made by multidisciplinary experts compared to hospital clinicians and the patients' 12-week outcomes. *Medical Care, 46*(2), 158–166.
151. McCauley, K. M., Bixby, M. B., & Naylor, M. D. (2006). Advanced practice nurse strategies to improve outcomes and reduce cost in elders with heart failure. *Disease Management, 9*(5), 302–310.
152. Sisk, J. E., Hebert, P. L., Horowitz, C. R., et al. (2006). Effects of nurse management on the quality of heart failure care in minority communities: a randomized trial. *Annals of Internal Medicine, 145*(4), 273–283.
153. Ockene, I., Hayman, L., Pasternak, R., et al. (2002). Task Force 4. Adherence issues and behavioral changes: Achieving a long-term solution. *Journal of the American College of Cardiology, 40*(4), 630–640.
154. Bodenheimer, T., & Laing, B. Y. (2007). The Teamlet Model of Primary Care. *Annals of Family Medicine, 5*(5), 457–461.
155. Bodenheimer, T., Lorig, K., Holman, H., et al. (2002). Patient self-management of chronic disease in primary care. *JAMA, 288*(19), 2469–2475.
156. Pierce, J. P., Newman, V. A., Natarajan, L., et al. (2007). Telephone counseling helps maintain long-term adherence to a high-vegetable dietary pattern. *Journal of Nutrition, 137*(10), 2291–2296.
157. Saperstein, S. L., Atkinson, N. L., & Gold, R. S. (2007). The impact of Internet use for weight loss. *Obesity Reviews, 8*(5), 459–465.
158. Kripalani, S., Yao, X., & Haynes, R. B. (2007). Interventions to enhance medication adherence in chronic medical conditions: A systematic review. *Archives of Internal Medicine, 167*(6), 540–550.
159. Haynes, R. B., Yao, X., Degani, A., et al. (2005). Interventions to enhance medication adherence. *Cochrane Database System Review,* (4), CD000011.
160. Roumie, C. L., Elasy, T. A., Greevy, R., et al. (2006). Improving blood pressure control through provider education, provider alerts, and patient education: A cluster randomized trial. *Annals of Internal Medicine, 145*(3), 165–175.
161. Schmitz, J. M., Sayre, S. L., Stotts AL, et al. (2005). Medication compliance during a smoking cessation clinical trial: A brief intervention using MEMS feedback. *Journal of Behavioral Medicine, 28*(2), 139–147.
162. Hickey, M. L., Owen, S. V., & Froman, R. D. (1992). Instrument development: Cardiac diet and exercise self-efficacy. *Nursing Research, 41*(6), 347–351.
163. Resnick, B., & Jenkins, L. S. (2000). Testing the reliability and validity of the Self-Efficacy for Exercise scale. *Nursing Research, 49*(3), 154–159.
164. Sallis, J. F., Pinski, R. B., Grossman, R. M., et al. (1988). The development of self-efficacy scales for health-related diet and exercise behaviors. *Health Education Research, 3*(3), 283–292.
165. Clark, M. M., Abrams, D. B., Niaura, R. S., et al. (1991). Self-efficacy in weight management. *Journal of Consulting and Clinical Psychology, 59,* 739–744.

166. Glynn, S. M., & Ruderman, A. J. (1986). The development and validation of an eating self-efficacy scale. *Cognitive Therapeutic Research, 10,* 403.
167. Warziski, M., Sereika, S., Styn, M. A., et al. (2008). Changes in self-efficacy and dietary adherence: The impact on weight loss in the PREFER study. *Journal of Behavioral Medicine* (Epub ahead of print), DOI: 10.1007/s10865–10007-19135-10862.
168. Baer, J. S., Holt, C. S., & Licktenstein, E. (1986). Self-efficacy and smoking reexamined: Construct validity and clinical utility. *Journal of Clinical Consulting Psychology, 54,* 846–852.
169. De Geest, S., Abraham, I., Gemoets, H., et al. (1994). Development of the long-term medication behaviour self-efficacy scale: Qualitative study for item development. *Journal of Advanced Nursing, 19,* 233–238.
170. Bowen, D. J., Meischke, H., & Tomoyasu, N. (1994). Preliminary evaluation of the processes of changing to a low-fat diet. *Health Education Research Theory and Practice, 9,* 85–94.
171. Kristeller, J. K., Rossi, J. S., Ockene, J. K., et al. (1992). Processes of change in smoking cessation: A cross-validation study in cardiac patients. *Journal of Substance Abuse, 4,* 263–276.
172. Simpson, R. J., Jr. (2006). Challenges for improving medication adherence. *JAMA, 296*(21), 2614–2616.
173. Piette, J. D., Heisler, M., Krein, S., et al. (2005). The role of patient-physician trust in moderating medication nonadherence due to cost pressures. *Archives of Internal Medicine, 165*(15), 1749–1755.
174. Piette, J. D., Heisler, M., & Wagner, T. H. (2004). Cost-related medication underuse: Do patients with chronic illnesses tell their doctors? *Archives of Internal Medicine, 164*(16), 1749–1755.

CHAPTER 41

Complementary and Alternative Approaches in Cardiovascular Disease

Eleanor F. Bond / Shannon M. Latta

Complementary and alternative medicine (CAM) health care approaches are commonly used by patients with cardiovascular problems to promote health or to treat cardiovascular or other diseases or symptoms. Despite CAM's substantial influence, much remains unknown about the therapeutic efficacy of CAM methods and interactions with mainstream clinical care. There is a need for systematic investigation of the safety, efficacy, and interactions of CAM with conventional therapies. It is important that scientists consider CAM issues when they design trials of conventional therapies. In the past, U.S. conventional health care profession schools such as nursing schools have given insufficient attention to CAM. This pattern is changing as educators, researchers, care providers, and patients become aware of CAM approaches. It is important that health care providers understand the power and limitations of CAM approaches and integrate this information into their care delivery.

This chapter describes some CAM therapies commonly used to promote cardiovascular health and treat cardiovascular disease. It summarizes the evidence regarding efficacy, untoward effects, and interactions with conventional treatments. Included are suggestions regarding assessing a patient's underlying health beliefs and CAM use, and also suggestions relating to integration of CAM into clinical nursing management.

CAM DEFINITIONS AND CHARACTERISTICS

The National Institutes of Health's National Center for Complementary and Alternative Medicine (NCCAM)[1] defines *CAM* as "a group of diverse medicine and health systems, practices, and products that are not presently considered part of conventional medicine." *Conventional health care,* in turn, is defined by NCCAM as those practices currently used by medical doctors and other Western health care providers.[1] As evidence emerges regarding CAM, these practices and therapies are integrated into conventional Western health care approaches; they are then no longer considered to be part of CAM. Thus, the categorization of practices and therapies as CAM continually evolves. For example, exercise prescriptions, once considered an alternative approach, are now a core element of conventional clinical management of diabetes mellitus, heart disease, arthritis, cancer-related fatigue, and bone health. In a similar way, cognitive-behavioral therapies, once part of CAM, are now a component of allopathic care, for example, for irritable bowel syndrome.

Terms used in discussing CAM include the following:

Allopathic medicine denotes conventional health care approaches as taught in a country's medical and nursing schools.

Alternative medicine approaches are those used in place of conventional health practices.

Complementary medicine approaches are those used in conjunction with conventional health practices.

Holistic health care approaches emerge from viewing the patient's physical condition and emotional responses in the context of his environment and support system (family, home, communities). Nursing models are typically holistic.

Integrative health care combines elements of CAM and allopathic health care.

Traditional medicine denotes health behaviors and traditions of people indigenous to a particular region. Traditional health practices are typically based on experience and knowledge accumulated over thousands of years. Traditional medical systems are typically based on cultural perceptions of the universe, religious beliefs, and bodily function. In the United States, "traditional" sometimes is used to refer to allopathic or conventional medicine (although that use will not be applied in this chapter). More commonly in North America the term "traditional medicine" denotes the spiritual and health care practices of American Indians, Alaska Natives, and Canada's First Nations people.

Whole (*or alternative*) *medical systems* are defined by NCCAM as being built on complete systems of theory and practice. Generally, these systems have evolved separately from conventional Western medicine. Some whole medical systems have evolved in other cultures (Traditional Chinese Medicine [TCM], Ayurveda); others have been developed within Western cultures (naturopathy, homeopathy).

CAM DOMAINS

According to NCAAM, CAM practices can be categorized into four major domains: *mind–body interventions, biologically based practices, manipulative and body-based methods,* and *energy medicine.* These domains are described in Table 41-1. *Whole medical systems* typically include treatment approaches from several of the CAM domains.

PREVALENCE OF CAM

In all areas of the world, traditional healing systems compete with the allopathic biomedical model. According to the World Health Organization,[2] at least 80% of the developing world uses traditional healing systems as their primary source of health care. While developing countries are striving toward improving health

Table 41-1 ■ CAM DOMAINS

Domain	Definition	Examples
Mind–body interventions	Techniques to facilitate the mind's capacity to affect bodily function and symptoms	Meditation, hypnosis, prayer and mental healing, biofeedback, yoga, some types of dance, music, or art therapy
Biologically based practices	Natural products	Botanicals, special dietary remedies, aromatherapy, minerals, hormones
Manipulative and body-based methods	Movement or manipulation of the body	Chiropractic or osteopathic manipulation, massage therapy, reflexology.
Energy medicine	Manipulation of energy fields originating within the body (biofields) or application of external energy fields to the body.	Tai chi, qi gong, reiki, use of external electric or magnetic fields

outcomes by adopting allopathic medicine, the growing trend in industrialized countries is to reclaim traditional healing systems and adopt CAM modalities.

In the 2002 National Health Interview Survey (NHIS) of more than 31,000 Americans, more than one third of adults used some form of CAM during the past 12 months (this number excludes the use of prayer for health reasons).[3] Similar findings were reported in earlier estimates.[4,5] The number of visits to CAM providers increased by nearly 50% from 425 million in 1990 to 629 million visits in 1997. American health care consumers spent between $36 billion and $47 billion for CAM therapies in 1997.[4,6] Problems most commonly treated with CAM approaches are back or neck problems, head or chest colds, joint pain and stiffness, anxiety, and depression.[3] The most common CAM modalities used are natural products (18.9%), deep breathing exercises (11.6%), meditation (7.6%), chiropractic care (7.5%), yoga (5.1%), massage (5.0%), and diet-based therapies (3.5%).[3]

Use of CAM modalities is common in other countries as well as the United States. Although many countries have adopted Western health practices, often traditional health approaches persist. In some countries, such as Korea, there has been a resurgence of interest in traditional healing practices. Integration of CAM and Western health approaches vary widely within and between countries. Sometimes the two systems are integrated; sometimes they are separate and parallel. Immigration from countries where CAM therapies are common has increased the demand for equivalent treatments in the United States and Canada.

Several factors contribute to CAM use in North America. Many chronic health problems are only partially managed by allopathic approaches, leading patients to seek alternative care to fill the perceived gap. Most CAM users (59.4%) believe that CAM combined with conventional medical treatment is beneficial to health.[3] CAM approaches are appealing to some consumers because they are viewed as less invasive and "drug-like."[7] Patients sometimes express the belief that dietary supplements and herbal products are "natural," and thus "safe." Patients sometimes express dissatisfaction with what is perceived to be technologically and disease-focused medicine. Astin et al.[5] found that patients report their most powerful motivator in seeking CAM treatment is a desire for a provider approach that more closely matches their personal values, beliefs, and philosophy of health and wellness. The CAM caregiver approach often involves less emphasis on a disease model and more emphasis on healing, overall health, and the patient–caregiver relationship. In CAM venues, that relationship is likely to be more of a partnership than a hierarchical association. CAM approaches may provide the patient with an increased sense of individual responsibility and control over health problems. The trend for the U.S. third-party payers to cover CAM therapies has also contributed to increased CAM use.

CAM Use in Specific Populations

Use of CAM varies by gender, racial and ethnic status, age, geographic region, socioeconomic status, health status, and profession. Surveys have demonstrated that those using CAM are more likely to be female, of Asian or Native American racial background, and older. Also linked with more CAM use are the following factors: Western United States residence, more years of education, higher socioeconomic status, and increased number of chronic health conditions.[3,4,8]

To characterize the ethnic/racial variation in the utilization of CAM versus conventional Western medicine, Xu and Farrell[9] accessed data in the 1996 and 1998 Medical Expenditure Panel Survey of 46,673 respondents, stratified by ethnic group. They found that Native Americans are the most likely to substitute CAM practices for conventional health care; Asian populations also very commonly use CAM methods,[8] particularly massage, herbal medicine, traditional Asian medicine, and spiritual healing instead of or in conjunction with conventional health care.[9] Hispanic populations use CAM; they are likely to substitute herbal therapies, massage, and spiritual healing for conventional health care. African Americans tend to use spiritual healing, nutritional approaches, and massage to complement conventional medicine.[9] Non-Hispanic White populations use chiropractic, acupuncture, and nutritional advice in conjunction with conventional approaches and use spiritual healing, prayer, and other CAM modalities as substitutes. It is not clear that surveys of minority cultures accurately reveal CAM use. Consumption of certain foods, botanical products, and spices for medicinal purposes is a routine dietary practice in many cultures and not identified as CAM; similarly, meditative or structured exercises are not so identified. There is need for culturally sensitive methods to evaluate CAM usage in clinical and research populations.

Many health care providers use CAM therapies to manage their own health. Burg et al.[10] surveyed faculty at a major U.S. health science university regarding their personal use of CAM therapies. About half of the respondents indicated that they had themselves used one or more CAM therapies. Highest overall use was by allied health faculty, followed by nursing, dental, pharmacy, and medical faculty. Fontaine[11] suggests that nurses' CAM use is related to the profession's emphasis on self-care.

CAM Use for Cardiovascular Health

Patients with cardiovascular disease commonly use CAM approaches to treat their conditions, treat a coexisting noncardiovascular problem, or for health promotion. Saydah and Eberhardt[12] evaluated 2002 NHIS data to identify CAM use patterns among chronically ill adults. They found that having a chronic illness diagnosis increased the likelihood that adults would use CAM. Nearly half of adults with cardiovascular disease (46.4%) and more than half of adults with two or more chronic diseases (55%) reported using CAM. Xu and Farrell[9] evaluated survey data from 46,673 persons; hypercholesterolemia and hypertension were among the top 10 conditions or diseases of persons using CAM. Using 2002 NHIS data, Bell et al.[13] noted that of those with hypertension, less than 10% were using CAM to treat that condition; rather, they sought other health improvements.

In a telephone questionnaire, patients in a Canadian cardiovascular disease registry reported much higher CAM use than has been reported in the United States: 64% of those surveyed used CAM; most commonly used were herbal remedies and nutritional supplements. Acupuncture was used by 12% and chiropractic care by 11% of the patients. Most cardiac patients were using CAM treatments for cardiac or vascular disease, but some were using the treatments for noncardiac conditions such as arthritis or psychological symptoms. Patients generally reported believing that the treatments were safe, proven effective, and that their health was improving because of the treatments.[14]

Xu and Farrell[9] noted that patients with elevated cholesterol commonly used nutritional (33%), herbal (32%), and massage (28%) remedies. Those with hypertension reported using spiritual (31%), herbal (31%), and nutritional (26%) modalities. Another survey revealed that those individuals with hypertension commonly used nutritional supplements (coenzyme Q10, vitamin E), herbal products (hawthorn), and relaxation techniques.[4]

Ai and Bolling[15] conducted a telephone survey of mixed gender middle-aged and older patients on the day before scheduled cardiac surgery to elicit information about CAM use. Of 225 patients, more than 80% used CAM. Most commonly used approaches were relaxation techniques, lifestyle/diet modification, megavitamins, spiritual healing, massage, herbal remedies, and imagery. CAM usage was higher in those with more education and in those with better functional status; men and women used CAM equally. Former cigarette smokers, patients with more comorbidities, and those with heart failure were more likely to use CAM than those with cardiac arrhythmias or coexisting cerebrovascular disease.

Patient Disclosure of CAM Use

Many Americans use CAM, but they often do not inform their primary care providers about their CAM use.[3,12] A small study of older people, many with cardiac abnormalities, revealed that 35% had not told their providers about their CAM use.[16] Another 40% of the participants reported that their primary care provider was aware of the CAM use, but was not supportive. Montbriand[17] reported that most health care providers believe that they are aware of their patients' CAM use, but in actuality only 50% of their elderly patients had informed their providers. Another study queried nonemergent patients visiting the emergency department of a major metropolitan medical center in the Western United States.[18] Most patients were using some type of CAM, but less than half of those patients had mentioned this usage to their primary care provider; this is notable in that the sampling method produced only subjects in the process of seeking conventional health care services. Another study, a survey of adults aged 50 years and older, revealed that only one in five CAM users had discussed their CAM usage with their providers.[19]

Rationales for nondisclosure of CAM practices include the following: the provider does not need to know; the patient had not seen their provider since starting the CAM treatment; the patient did not think of telling the provider; the provider never asked; the patient perceived that the provider would not take the CAM approach seriously or would disapprove; there was insufficient time during the visit; and the provider lacked knowledge about CAM.[18] In the Brown[19] study of patients aged 50 years and older, the few who had discussed CAM usage with their providers initiated the topic themselves.

Patients who reported speaking to their physicians about CAM asked specific questions. In Brown's study,[19] it was found that only the minority of patients discussed CAM with their providers, but those who did sought specific advice. They sought CAM recommendations and had questions about CAM therapy effectiveness, medication interactions, and safety of a CAM therapy.[19] The majority of Brown's subjects reported that they turned to family or friends for information and advice about CAM use rather than talking to a health care professional.[19]

The common use of CAM as a complement to conventional health practices, the increased use of multiple prescription drugs, and the reluctance of patients to discuss their CAM practices with their health care providers leaves patients vulnerable to poor health outcomes related to drug interactions, side effects, or other problems.

WHOLE MEDICAL SYSTEMS

Whole medical systems include multiple approaches and use various modalities to maintain or restore health. Some whole medical systems (e.g., Ayurveda, TCM, Traditional Native American Healing, Traditional Korean Medicine) are based on ancient cultural beliefs and practices of a population group; other whole medical systems (e.g., homeopathy, naturopathy, chiropractic) developed concurrently with conventional Western medicine, but are based on different principles and beliefs. Many whole medicine systems incorporate beliefs about the mind–body–spirit connection and are inherently holistic in approach. The following briefly summarizes some features of several common whole medical systems.

Ayurvedic Medicine (AM)

Literally, *Ayurveda* means "science of life." This traditional medicine system originated in India thousands of years ago; it is commonly practiced in South Asia and is growing in popularity in the West. Historically, AM was one of the first medical systems to acknowledge the importance of the mind–body connection. The human body is considered a replica of the universe and composed of the same basic matter (earth, water, air, fire, space). Nonmaterial aspects of the person include *Sattva* (consciousness, intelligence),

Rajas (motion, action), and *Tamas* (inertia resisting motion, action). Diagnoses are based on history, observation, palpation, and inspection, particularly of the pulse, tongue, eyes, and nails. Therapeutic goals in AM are to maintain or restore harmony between the individual and cosmic forces (mind, body, spirit). This involves increasing *Sattva* while reducing *Rajas* and *Tamas*. The AM approach is holistic; treatments are customized to match the individual's characteristics (i.e., constitutional type or *Prakruti*). Appropriate food, sleep, and sexual activity are pillars of good health in AM. Many treatments utilize vegetable-based botanicals such as cardamom, cinnamon, and turmeric. Treatments emphasize mental and physical hygiene and discipline, adherence to moral and spiritual values, massage, exercise, meditation, herbs, sunlight exposure, and controlled breathing. Strict adherence to diet (*Yama*) and behavior (*Niyama*) is part of AM. Treatments include accessing pressure regions (*Marma*), similar to acupuncture. Meditation and yoga exercises are essential components of AM, with stress on the ability to bend, flex, extend, and stretch. Physical fitness from the AM viewpoint involves a capacity to withstand heat, cold, hunger, thirst, and fatigue.

Traditional Chinese Medicine

TCM has been practiced for thousands of years; it relates health to concepts about a person's energy. The practitioner's role is to guide the patient toward restored energy balance and, thus, health. Several types of energy are involved. *Qi* (pronounced *chee*) is the energy of life. In disease, qi is imbalanced. Related to qi are *yin* (associated with cold, moist, internal aspects) and *yang* (associated with heat, dry, external aspects). Yin and yang are constantly interrelated; when imbalanced, illness results (Fig. 41-1). Qi flows along channels called *meridians* (Fig. 41-2). Disease blocks qi flow and upsets the balance between yin and yang. In TCM, *five elements* (water, fire, earth, wood, metal) describe a person's physical and emotional characteristics. TCM assessment involves history taking and physical examination, particularly of the tongue, pulse, and abdomen. Treatments prescribed include *acupuncture*, the inserting of needles at specific points along the meridians to improve qi flow (Fig. 41-3). *Moxibustion* treatments involve holding a burning herb to provide heat along a meridian. *Cupping* treatments involve placing a warmed glass over the skin; as the cup cools, the resulting vacuum pulls blood toward the area. Other TCM treatments include consuming proper foods (*nutrition*), preparing and ingesting Chinese herbs (*herbal medicine*), massaging, and exercising the body through prescribed movements such as *qi gong* and *tai chi*. Herbs have energies and are characterized as *yin* or *yang*. Herbs with cold energy treat hot syndromes; herbs with hot energy treat cold syndromes. For example, anemia or weak pulse might be considered a cold syndrome; treatments would warm the blood and strengthen the energy.

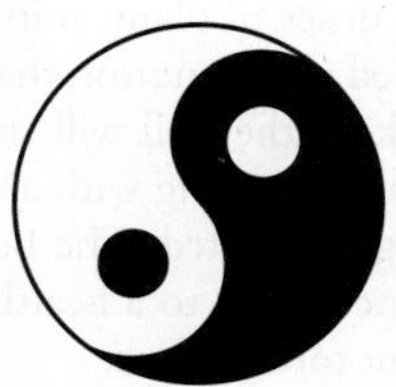

■ **Figure 41-1** Yin-yang symbol. In TCM, yin and yang are constantly interrelated forces; disease results when these forces are imbalanced. Yin is associated with cold, moist, and internal aspects and yang is associated with heat, dry, and external aspects. (From Lewis, S. M., Heitkemper, M. M., & Dirksen, S. R. [2004]. *Medical surgical nursing: Assessment and management of clinical problems* [6th ed.]. St. Louis: Mosby; used with permission.)

Traditional Native American Healing

Native American healing methods are based on the accumulated knowledge and skills from hundreds of generations of traditional healers. The medicine person (traditional healer) holds a place of honor within the tribe; he or she is chosen by their tribe, by an older healer, by a tribal medical society, or as a result of a personal vision quest. Practices are typically not written down. They are handed down verbally from one practitioner to another and not shared with those outside of the group. Mastery of the Native American healing requires many years of training and disciplined spiritual practice. Native American healing practices were illegal in the United States between 1887 and 1978, but traditions were handed down and practiced covertly. Today, Native Americans are more likely to use traditional healing than other ethnic and racial groups.[9] The majority of the two million Native American and Alaska Native people consult with traditional healers regardless of whether they live on or off the reservation.[9]

Tribal groups vary in terms of rituals and ceremonies but, in general, disease is believed to relate to problems of the person's spirit. The underlying Native American belief system conceptualizes each person as consisting of mind, body, and spirit. Wellness involves harmony between the three components of the inner self and with the outer universe. Illness is attributed to negative mental, physical, or spiritual activity, or to imbalances of the environment; violation of a sacred or tribal taboo could be involved. Interventions are designed to heal the spirit; they include energy field manipulation, sweats, religious ceremony (song, dance), herb lore, and sand painting. In Native American culture, medicine and religion are not separate, but one concept. Most traditional religious ceremonies are also healing ceremonies because spirituality is the cornerstone of healing practices. Typically, each person is believed responsible for his own health care. Healing ceremonies implicitly include family, patient, the traditional healer, and tribal members. The traditional healer may include rituals, prayers, singing, sweat lodge, body manipulation, or herbal remedies as part of the healing process.

Chiropractic Medicine

Chiropracty is the fourth largest health care profession in the United States with 53,000 active practitioners in 2006.[20] Chiropractors have 4 to 5 years of postbaccalaureate education including at least 4,500 supervised classroom, laboratory, and clinical hours; they are licensed and regulated in all 50 of the United States and in more than 30 other countries.

Chiropracty focuses on manipulation of the structure of the body to influence the body's innate ability to restore and optimize health. Special emphasis is placed on spinal alignment. Care is provided by realignment of subluxations through manipulations of joints and vertebrae. Subluxation or a subluxation complex is defined as an abnormal function of a joint and the associated muscles, nerves, tendons, ligaments, and discs. Treatment goals for chiropractic joint realignment include restoration of proper

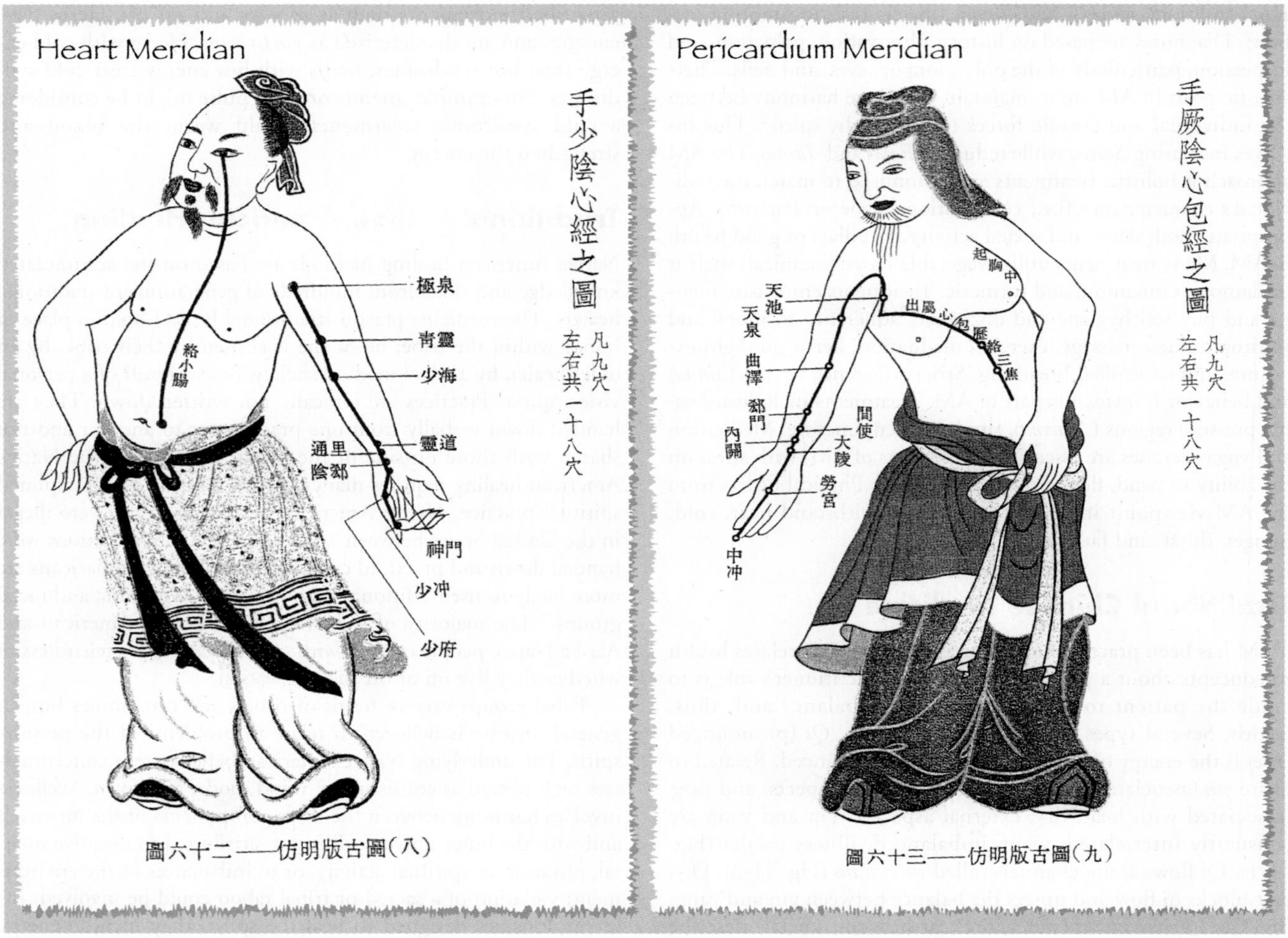

■ **Figure 41-2** Meridian flow chart for the heart and the pericardium. In TCM, the Oi, or life energy, flows along meridians. Illustrated are meridians associated with *(A)* the heart and *(B)* pericardium. (Adapted from Choi, Y. W. [1973]. *The topography of the fourteen meridians.* Pasadena, CA: Cunningham Press; with permission.)

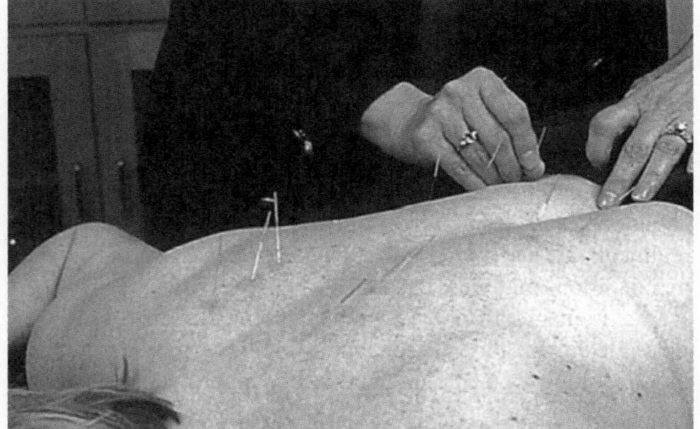

■ **Figure 41-3** Person receiving acupuncture treatment. (From Lewis, S. M., Heitkemper, M. M., & Dirksen, S. R. [2004]. *Medical surgical nursing: Assessment and management of clinical problems* [6th ed.]. St. Louis: Mosby; used with permission.)

alignment, control of pain, and, ultimately, restoration of proper body functions.[21]

Homeopathic Medicine

Homeopathic medicine was founded by Samuel Hahnemann, a 19th-century German physician and chemist. Treatments involve prescription of minute doses of plant, mineral, or animal materials. Homeopathy is based on the notion that "like cures like," that is, a substance that sickens the well will stimulate innate healing powers to cure a patient presenting with a similar disease pattern. Substances used are highly diluted. The belief is that dilute concentrations of a substance given to a healthy person may have an opposite effect in a symptomatic one.

Naturopathic Medicine

Naturopathic medicine is a primary health care system designed around the principle of supporting the patient's inherent healing capacity. It emphasizes the body's natural healing powers and personal responsibility for prevention and treatment of diseases.

Treatments are designed to amplify the natural tendency of the body to heal and eliminate toxins from the body.

Naturopathic remedies include diet and clinical nutrition counsel, particularly, use of naturally processed foods and herbs. Other therapies involve application of heat, water, air, or electricity; physiotherapy, acupuncture, or manipulations; homeopathy; and psychotherapy and counseling.

Naturopathic physicians normally provide primary care and do not perform major surgery, dispense pharmaceutical prescriptions (other than botanicals or body-based substances), or use radioactive substances for diagnosis or treatment.

Osteopathic Medicine

Osteopathy was developed by Andrew Taylor Still, a physician who became disillusioned with allopathic medicine after three of his children died in the meningitis epidemic of 1864. His goal was to establish practices to treat disease and promote health, rather than treat symptoms. He developed osteopathic manipulative treatment and established his own medical schools. There are currently about 20 schools of osteopathic medicine in the United States today; their graduates become fully licensed physicians, Doctors of Osteopathy. Three principles guide osteopathy, as follows: (1) the body is a unit designed to move, (2) structure and function are reciprocally interrelated by motion, and (3) the body possesses self-regulatory and self-healing mechanisms which are enhanced by the unrestricted motion of blood and body chemicals.[21]

MIND–BODY INTERVENTIONS FOR CARDIOVASCULAR HEALTH

There are several types of mind–body interventions used to improve health. Some mind–body interventions are based on a belief that the content of thoughts, beliefs, and emotions affects physical functioning; therapies are thought to improve health by evoking a more positive attitude. Other mind–body approaches promote health by freeing the mind of troubling thoughts or by focusing thought so as to exclude usual mental patterns (e.g., meditation or yoga; prayer, music, dance, or art therapy). Some mind–body therapies involve teaching the patient to control and regulate physical functioning and reduce stress responses (e.g., biofeedback).

Meditation

Meditation involves mental discipline, replacing typical thought patterns with a deeper state of relaxation or awareness. It has been a healing and/or spiritual practice in many cultures and religions for more than 5,000 years.[22] Meditation goals sometimes include improved self-awareness, higher levels of consciousness, strengthened mental focus, or more relaxed frame of mind.[23] It often involves focusing, centering, and relaxing the mind and body by using techniques such as listening to the breath, repeating a phrase (called a *mantra*), avoiding thought, or focusing thought. Meditation usually involves focusing on the breath or using a specific breathing pattern. Generally, meditation practices require training to tame, quiet, or focus the mind and achieve a state of detached awareness.[23]

Meditation has been employed in cardiovascular disease as a method of regulating the stress response and physiological variables, such as blood pressure, heart rate, and peripheral vascular resistance, often linked with cardiovascular problems. Meditative techniques have been recommended to reduce heart rate, lower blood pressure, reduce body weight, or improve the lipid profile. However, it is not clear whether meditation has long-term effects on cardiovascular health. The Agency for Health Care Research and Quality (AHRQ) published a comprehensive review of 817 studies of health applications of meditation published between 1956 and 2005.[23]

Evidence reviewed in the AHRQ summary suggests that meditation can evoke acute lowering of blood pressure in both healthy adults and in those with hypertension. Zen Buddhist meditation (compared with a blood pressure monitoring group) was associated with lowering diastolic blood pressure by approximately 6 mm Hg. Similarly, Transcendental Meditation was associated with small decreases in systolic (weighted mean difference 4.3 mm Hg) and diastolic (weighted mean difference 3.1 mm Hg) blood pressure when compared to progressive muscle relaxation. Some mind-body interventions also involve energy medicine. Qi gong involves breathing and movements which focus the mind and move qi through channels or meridians in the body. In two trials, hypertensive patients taught qi gong were compared with subjects on a waiting list. The qi gong groups displayed a substantial reduction in blood pressure (average systolic drop 17.8 mm Hg; diastolic 12 mm Hg) compared to those waitlisted. Tai chi is another form of focusing the mind and completing structured movements. Tai chi, yoga plus biofeedback, and yoga alone were each superior to no treatment or health education in decreasing systolic blood pressure; yoga alone and yoga plus biofeedback reduced diastolic blood pressure when compared with groups receiving no treatment.[23]

Two trials reviewed in the AHRQ analysis (total of 99 participants) demonstrated that tai chi was more effective than another exercise in reducing resting heart rate. In two other studies, yoga was compared with lipid-lowering medications in reducing cholesterol. One study followed patients for 4 months; the drugs were more effective than yoga in reducing total and low-density lipoprotein (LDL) cholesterol. Another study followed patients for a year; the yoga and drug groups had similar reductions in cholesterol.[23]

Meditation studies are difficult to compare. Studies vary in type and duration. Often the descriptions of the physical aspects of the meditation techniques or training paradigms are incomplete, making it difficult to judge the integrity of the interventions. Another concern is the lack of standards of dosage, including frequency or number of sessions to achieve desired results. It is difficult to judge if the intervention (meditation) is delivered as designed since it is an internal process. However, there are no documented adverse effects for meditation, thus the possibility of positive outcomes outweigh the risk of harm.

Biofeedback

Biofeedback methods are effective in acutely altering physiological parameters such as heart rate, blood pressure, body temperature, and heart rate variability (a measure of the variation in the beat to beat interval). Long-term effects are less well established. In one randomized study of 38 hypertensive subjects, heart rate variability-based biofeedback in combination with emotional-response retraining to manage the stress response was associated with reduced blood pressure 3 months following training.[24]

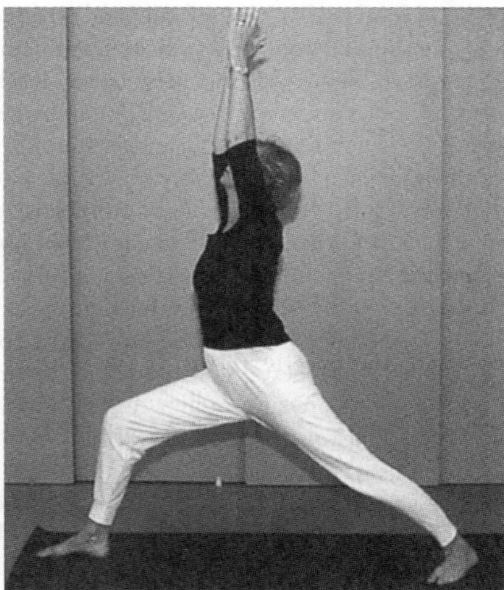

■ **Figure 41-4** Yoga posture. (From Lewis, S. M., Heitkemper, M. M., & Dirksen, S. R. [2004]. *Medical surgical nursing: Assessment and management of clinical problems* [6th ed.]. St. Louis: Mosby; used with permission.)

Yoga

The term *yoga* derives from a Sanskrit word meaning to join or unite. Yoga methods include physical and mental disciplines designed to produce unity (e.g., unity of the body with the mind, of the mind with the soul, of the individual with a higher power). Unity is thought to result in a happy, balanced, useful life, and possibly improved health. Yoga methods include *Asanas* (yoga postures) (Fig. 41-4), *Pranayamas* (regulated breathing), *Mudras* (hand gestures), and *Mantras* (chanted words). Several small studies suggest that yoga techniques can improve cardiac health. Vempati and Telles[25] studied healthy young adult males; yoga was associated with acute reductions in heart rate and sympathetic tone (indicated by heart rate variability). Yoga lifestyle changes have been associated with improved cardiovascular risk factors such as lower-body weight and improved lipid profile and blood pressure regulation.[26–28] Good experimental yoga studies are needed but difficult to design.

BIOLOGICALLY BASED TREATMENTS

Herbal and dietary remedies are commonly used to treat cardiac and vascular disease. Aromatherapy is also considered a biologically based therapy, although there is scant literature on the use of aromatherapy for cardiac conditions.

Herbal Remedies

Herbal products are derived from plants. For thousands of years, plant extracts have been to improve health. Some ancient herbs (e.g., aspirin, reserpine, digitalis, caffeine) are now mainstays of conventional pharmacotherapy. Care providers can refer to the *Natural Medicines Comprehensive Database* Web site, http://www.naturaldatabase.com, for up-to-date information about herbal products used by their patients.

Several factors are important to keep in mind when considering use of herbal remedies. Plant preparations do not have uniform active ingredient composition; labeling can be confusing. The concentrations of active compounds in a plant vary according to climate, soil conditions, and growing season. Plant components (e.g., flowers, leaves, stems) vary in concentration and proportion of active compounds. Extraction methods vary, producing highly variable concentrations of active ingredients. For example, hawthorn products (see section titled "Hawthorn") are usually described as containing a certain amount (mg) of extract from the plant. The extract can be from flowers or leaves or both. Extractions can be performed using water, ethanol, or methanol; each of these methods results in different quantities and ratios of active ingredients. When Vierling et al.[29] tested the activity of the various hawthorn extractions on contractility of a strip of aortic tissue, the pharmacologic effects were remarkably diverse. Thus, it is difficult to standardize a dose of hawthorn; the same is true with many other herbal products.

Often, herbal products contain multiple ingredients. For example, the *Natural Medicines Comprehensive Database* lists more than 100 patented compounds containing hawthorn, each with variable coingredients. In many cases, the specific active ingredient from a plant has not been identified, making it impossible to achieve uniformity between products.

Another consideration involves contaminants. For example, products sometimes contain heavy metals (e.g., lead, chromium) or toxins or microbial elements (e.g., *Fusarium*, *Aspergillus*). Because testing, labeling, and manufacturing regulatory standards are significantly less rigorous with herbal than with pharmaceutical products, the consumer is not well protected.

The 1994 *Dietary Supplement and Health Act* permits the sale of herbal products that are not toxic as long as no claims are made related to therapeutic efficacy. Regulations mandating quality control are lacking. In 2003, in an attempt to try to improve product purity, potency, and consistency, the United States Food and Drug Administration proposed rules called *good manufacturing practices* to guide herbal product manufacturing practices. These rules have not been mandated. However, some herbal product manufacturers have adopted voluntary good manufacturing practices. U.S. Pharmacopoeia is an independent group that serves as the official standard-setting body for all U.S. medicines; some herbal manufacturers have sought U.S. Pharmacopoeia certification. Patients can be directed to seek products with the USP logo indicating the product has passed stringent quality-control standards (Fig. 41-5).

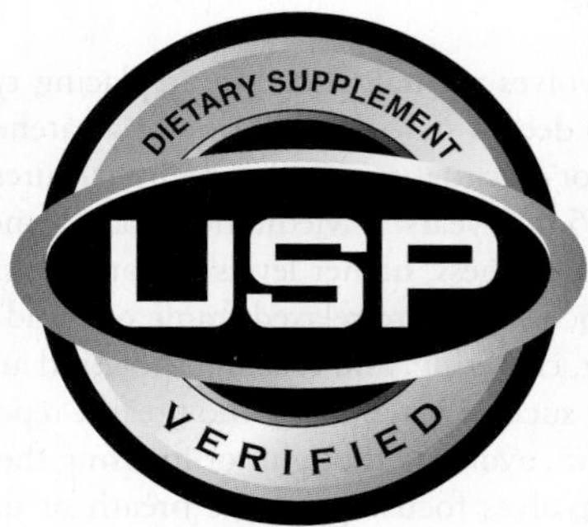

■ **Figure 41-5** USP logo. This label on a dietary supplement indicates the product in the container has passed the stringent purity, potency, and consistency standards set forth by U.S. Pharmacopeia. (From the U.S. Pharmacopeia website. [http://www.usp-dsvp.org/, retrieved November 12, 2003]; used with permission.)

There are special concerns related to cardiac patients and herbal remedies. Cardiac conditions generally require clinical surveillance by a licensed care provider. It is unwise for patients with heart failure to self-medicate, whether for cardiac or noncardiac conditions. Herbal products can alter drug absorption. For example, guar gum and psyllium reduce absorption of some pharmaceutical or herbal remedies. Some herbal remedies are associated with drug interactions. For example, several herbs increase the bleeding risk for patients taking anticoagulants. Bleeding has been reported with the use of gingko biloba, garlic, and the Chinese herbs danshen and dong quai.

One compound merits special comment related to potential adverse cardiac effects. Aconite (sometimes called "chuanwu" or "caowu") is used in TCM to treat neuromuscular and arthritic-related pain conditions. Aconite contains diterpenoid alkaloids, which are toxic to neurons and to the heart. Fatal cardiac arrhythmias (bradycardia, hypotension, ventricular tachycardia, supraventricular tachycardia, bidirectional tachycardia, heart block, *torsade de pointes*) have been reported with the herb. There is no known antidote. Atropine may be helpful if there are bradyarrhythmias. Electrical cardioversion tends not to work in aconite poisoning.

Two herbal remedies commonly prescribed today in heart failure include *Crataegus oxyacantha* (hawthorn) and *Terminalia arjuna.* Although both of these products appear relatively safe and somewhat effective, self-medication poses risk for interactions with conventional clinical management paradigms.

Hawthorn

Hawthorn (also known as maybush, maythorn, or may; the formal name is *C. oxyacantha*) is traditionally used as a cardiac tonic. The German Commission E approves use of hawthorn leaf and flower extracts for patients with New York Heart Association (NYHA) class II heart failure. Hawthorn has been recommended to treat angina, hypertension, hypotension, arrhythmias, heart failure, hyperlipidemia, atherosclerosis, and gastrointestinal symptoms. A poultice of the hawthorn fruit is sometimes used to treat skin lesions.

A *Cochrane Systematic Review*[30] summarizes a meta-analysis of the evidence relating to the therapeutic efficacy of hawthorn extracts in heart failure. In 14 trials hawthorn was used, generally as an adjunct to conventional clinical management of patients with NYHA classes I to III. Hawthorn extracts compared favorably with placebo in that treated patients demonstrated increased exercise tolerance. Pressure-rate product (an index of myocardial oxygen consumption) decreased, indicating improvement. Shortness of breath and fatigue improved with hawthorn treatment compared with placebo.

Hawthorn preparations have positive inotropic effect on the myocardium. This is likely due to phosphodiesterase inhibition activity (similar to amrinone, milrinone). However, because the myocardial cell refractory period is lengthened with hawthorn, preparations are antiarrhythmic (unlike other phosphodiesterase inhibitors which are typically proarrhythmic). Hawthorn preparations reduce peripheral vascular resistance (i.e., afterload), possibly the reason that myocardial oxygen consumption is reduced. Other clinical actions attributed to hawthorn include increased coronary blood flow and reduced lipid levels; it has been suggested to have antibacterial, spasmolytic, and analgesic effects. Several studies have demonstrated that standardized leaf and flower extracts (known as LI 132 or WS 1442) improve ejection fraction, exercise tolerance, and reduce subjective symptoms in patients with NYHA class II heart failure.[31,32] Tauchert[33] reported that WS 1442, when combined with diuretics, improved exercise tolerance and reduced symptoms in patients with NYHA class III heart failure. When patients treated with hawthorn extract (900 mg/day; LI 132) were compared with those treated with captopril (37.5 mg/day), both groups increased their maximal exercise significantly and similarly.[33]

There could be risks if hawthorn is taken in conjunction with drugs and herbs containing cardiac glycosides (i.e., digoxin preparations, black hellebore, Canadian hemp root, digitalis leaf, hedge mustard, figwort, lily of the valley roots, motherwort, oleander leaf, pheasant's eye plant, pleurisy root, squill bulb leaf scales, strophanthus seeds), since the effects could be additive. There have been reports of interactions with anticoagulants and antihypertensives. Other botanical products with potential cardioactive properties include calamus, cereus, cola, coltsfoot, devil's claw, European mistletoe, fenugreek, fumitory, ginger, Panax ginseng, white horehound, mate, parsley, quassia, scotch broom flower, shepherd's purse, and wild carrot. Hawthorn taken in combination with these or with cardioactive drugs could amplify or counteract the activity of those herbs or drugs. However, Daniele et al.[34] completed a systematic review of the adverse events associated with hawthorn and concluded that the products are relatively safe. Side effects reported include gastrointestinal symptoms, dizziness, sleep problems, fatigue, rash (particularly on the hands), and palpitations. According to the *Cochrane Review*, no data are available related to mortality or cardiac-related morbidity: no rigorous trials have monitored long-term outcomes such as cardiac death, nonfatal myocardial infarction, and hospitalization.

T. arjuna Tree Bark

The bark of the *T. arjuna* tree (sometimes called Indian almond) has been used in India as a cardiac tonic for more than 3,000 years. Its stem bark possesses glycosides, flavonoids, tannins, and minerals (calcium, magnesium, zinc). Glycosides have a positive inotropic effect. Flavonoids have antioxidant, anti-inflammatory, and lipid-lowering effects. *T. arjuna* has been used to treat coronary artery disease, angina, heart failure, and hypercholesterolemia. It has sometimes been used as an antibacterial, antimutagen, or aphrodisiac. Related products made from the fruit of *Terminalia chebula* and *Terminalia belerica* are used in AM as a "health harmonizer" or to balance the vital humors. No large-scale, long-term, well-controlled studies of the efficacy of *T. arjuna* in cardiac disease have been published, but there are many small studies. Dwivedi and Agarwal[35] conducted small clinical trials in patients with angina, comparing usual care (in this case, nitrates, aspirin, and/or a calcium channel blockers) with and without powdered *T. arjuna* bark for 3 months. Patients receiving *T. arjuna* bark experienced less angina compared with patients receiving the usual care.[35,36] In another small study, patients with severe refractory congestive heart failure (treated with digitalis, diuretics, vasodilators) had reduced symptoms and improved left ventricular function when *T. arjuna* was added to the treatment regimen.[37] Studies are needed analyzing the efficacy of *T. arjuna* in combination with more recently recommended conventional regimens with demonstrated efficacy in heart failure (i.e., β-blockers, angiotensin-converting enzyme inhibitors). The mechanism of action for *T. arjuna* is not known. The herb is thought to be relatively safe, but it may increase blood pressure.

Nutraceuticals and Other CAM Dietary Approaches to Cardiovascular Health

Nutraceuticals derive their name from "nutrition" plus "pharmaceutical." The term refers to food extracts claimed to have therapeutic effect. Among the nutraceuticals used in cardiac conditions are omega-3 fatty acids, red yeast rice, coenzyme Q10, garlic, niacin, and plant sterols. Dietary approaches are important adjuncts to the treatment of cardiovascular diseases, including hypertension, although some of these approaches are associated with risk.

Omega-3 Fatty Acids

Omega-3 and omega-6 fatty acids are essential nutrients, not synthesized by the human body; thus, they must be obtained through diet or supplements. Omega-3 Fatty acids have anti-inflammatory, antiarrhythmic, and antithrombotic properties, different from omega-6 fatty acids, which are proinflammatory. There are three types of omega-3 fatty acids: eicosapentaenoic acid (EPA), docosahexaenoic acid, and α-linolenic acid (ALA). Fat-rich fish (e.g., salmon, trout, herring, sardines) are the primary source of EPA and docosahexaenoic acid, while ALA generally derives from plant sources such as ground flax seed, flax seed oil, walnuts, tofu, and soy or from omega-3 enriched eggs. Generally, evidence suggests that 0.5 to 1.8 g/day of docosahexaenoic acid and EPA either as fatty fish or as supplements significantly reduces cardiac mortality and morbidity. For ALA, intakes of 1.5 to 3.0 g/day are possibly helpful. The American Heart Association recommends at least two weekly servings of fish (particularly fatty fish) as well as inclusion of ALA food sources; fish recommendations should take into account federal and state advisories related to environmental pollutants such as methylmercury and polychlorinated biphenyls.

It has long been known that Eskimos and some other populations with high dietary intake of omega-3 fatty acids have lower heart disease rates.[38] Bucher et al.[39] conducted a meta-analysis of 11 studies comparing dietary or supplemental omega-3 fatty acids to placebo. Subjects in the omega-3 groups had significantly reduced risk of fatal myocardial infarction (risk ratio 0.7), sudden death (risk ratio 0.7), and all-cause mortality (risk ratio 0.8). A large study, the Gruppo Italiano per lo Studio della Sopravvivenza nell'Infarto Miocardico (GISSI) trial, was included in the meta-analysis. The GISSI trial studied more than 11,000 subjects who had experienced a myocardial infarction within the past 3 months. Subjects were randomly assigned to one of four groups: fish oil (1 g daily), vitamin E (300 mg daily), both fish oil and vitamin E, or neither. Subjects receiving fish oil had significantly reduced risk of sudden death at 4 months (relative risk 0.47) and at 42 months.[40,41] The fish oil group also had reduced risk of vascular and coronary death beginning at 8 months. Other prospective trials report a similar inverse relationship between fish oil intake and coronary events.[42,43] In the U.S. Physicians' Health Study of more than 20,000 men, those who consumed more than one fish serving weekly had 52% less risk of sudden death compared with those consuming fish less than once monthly.[44,45]

A systematic literature review of various lifestyle interventions to reduce blood pressure supports the use of fatty fish to reduce blood pressure in hypertensive individuals.[46] A meta-regression analysis of 36 randomized trials endorsed the efficacy of fish oil in reducing blood pressure.[47] Median fish oil intake was 3.7 g daily, significantly greater than the average fish oil (EPA, docosahexaenoic acid) intake in Western countries (<250 mg/day, less than one serving of fatty fish per week). Fish oil was found to reduce systolic blood pressure by 2.1 mm Hg and diastolic blood pressure by 1.6 mm Hg. Blood pressure reduction tended to be greater in persons older than 45 years and in those with hypertension (BP ≥ 140/90 mm Hg). The antihypertensive effect did not appear to be dose dependent. The effect was noted in one trial at a relatively low dose of 180 mg/day. It has been suggested that fish oil may influence the arteries, reducing blood pressure by evoking vasodilation. Older meta-analyses from the 1990s show a dose–response reduction of blood pressure of 3.4/2.0 mmHg with 5.6 grams of fish oil per day, reduction of 5.5/3.5 mm Hg in trials of 3 g/day, and 2.1/1.6 mm Hg with 3.7 g/day in hypertensive patients.[48] Blood pressure reductions associated with the Dietary Approaches to Stop Hypertension (DASH) diet may in part be attributed to increased fish intake.[47] It is reasonable to recommend several servings of fatty fish per week for the treatment of hypertension. A fish oil supplement may be an adequate alternative.

The mechanism underlying the effect of omega-3 fatty acids on blood pressure could be due to the lowering of serum triglyceride levels; this in turn causes an increase in LDL particle size.[49–51] Triglyceride concentration is a determinant of LDL concentration; thus, fish oil is expected to lower LDL as well.

Side effects of high levels of fish oil consumption include gastrointestinal effects (nausea, bloating, flatulence, eructation). It has been suggested that fish oil worsens glycemic control in patients with type 2 diabetes mellitus[52]; however, a meta-analysis found that hemoglobin A1C was not adversely affected with fish oil consumption.[53] Vitamin E levels decrease with high doses of omega-3 fatty acids.[54,55] Some fish oil preparations (e.g., cod liver oil) contain large amounts of fat-soluble vitamins and could cause vitamin A or D toxicity. Fish products may be contaminated with toxins such as mercury or pesticides if the fish were caught in contaminated waters. Mercury is more likely to contaminate fish tissue than to contaminate fish oil products. Fish oils (as all oils) have a high-caloric content and can contribute to weight gain. Because fish oils could possibly lower blood pressure, there is potential for additive effects in patients treated with antihypertensive drugs. There is also a potential for additive antithrombotic effects. Caution is needed for patients with pathological conditions inhibiting clotting and in patients taking aspirin, warfarin, clopidogrel (Plavix), or herbs such as garlic or ginseng. Fish oil levels were associated with reduced stroke risk in one study,[56] but another study suggested that very high dietary fish oil consumption increased the risk of hemorrhagic stroke.[57]

Flaxseed

Whole flaxseed has been linked with lowered serum cholesterol in subjects without[58,59] and with hypercholesterolemia.[60,61] Flaxseed products are also used for noncardiac uses, for example, to treat constipation, arthritis, cancer, anxiety, benign prostatic hyperplasia, vaginitis, obesity, and dry eyes. Flaxseed oil contains the omega-3 fatty acid ALA, linoleic acid, and oleic acid. Linoleic acid and ALA are required to maintain cell membrane structure. ALA is associated with lower incidence of cardiac disease and improved outcomes in cardiac patients.[62] Flaxseed oil might decrease platelet aggregation.[62,63] Linoleic acid is an omega-6 fatty acid; it possibly reduces the risk of ischemic stroke.[64] Flaxseed oil may have anti-inflammatory effects; this in turn could slow the progression of coronary vascular disease. ALA suppresses production of interleukin-1, tumor necrosis factor, leukotriene B4, and oxygen-free radicals by polymorphonuclear leukocytes and monocytes.[62] ALA from flaxseed oil might have antitumor effects.

Chinese Red Yeast Rice

Chinese red yeast rice, called *Xuezhikang,* is the fermentation product resulting when red yeast (*Monascus purpureus*) is grown on rice. Ancient documents from the Tang Dynasty (800 AD) describe the product; the Ming Dynasty (1368–1644) pharmacopoeia *Ben Cao Gang Mu* notes that the product evokes mild useful circulatory improvements.[65] Red yeast rice remains common in the Chinese and Japanese diets (e.g., in Peking duck). Animal[65,66] and human studies[67] note reductions in serum cholesterol and triacylglycerol concentrations. Heber et al.[67] conducted a randomized, double-blind, repeated-measures, controlled trial of 46 men and 37 women (ages 34–78 years) with moderate hypercholesterolemia. Half of the subjects took 600 mg of red yeast rice in a capsule; the control group took a similar-appearing placebo capsule; all subjects were counseled to consume American Heart Association Step 1 diet. Triacylglycerol and LDL cholesterol were significantly reduced in the test group (by approximately 16% and 7%, respectively) compared with the placebo control group; high-density lipoprotein cholesterol did not change. Improvements were noted at 8 and 12 weeks. Several subjects in the placebo group noted adverse effects (headaches, pneumonia, rash); one test subject noted chest pain. None of the subjects had abnormal liver or renal function studies during the trial (these complications are reported for red yeast rice). The menopausal status of the women was not discussed, nor was results separated for men versus women. Because ovarian hormone state is known to affect lipid metabolism, studies are needed explicating the interaction of this dietary component with ovarian hormone status.

Red yeast rice contains various monacolins (including monacolin K, also known as lovastatin, an HMG-CoA reductase inhibitor that is an allopathic drug prescribed to lower serum cholesterol). Also present in red yeast rice are sterols, isoflavone glycosides, and monounsaturated fatty acids. It is likely that the cholesterol-lowering effects are caused by multiple active ingredients, not just the monacolin K. In the study by Heber et al.,[67] the monacolin K concentration consumed by the test group was lower than that in clinical trials of lovastatin alone,[68] yet the lipid reductions were almost as large. This could suggest that other red yeast rice ingredients contribute to its therapeutic effect. More studies are needed to determine the efficacy, mechanism, and safety of red yeast rice.

Many precautions are needed if the patient is taking red yeast rice. Side effects associated with red yeast rice include gastrointestinal symptoms and liver problems[69,70]; anaphylaxis has been reported after inhalation.[71] Because they have a similar chemical composition, red yeast rice has a potential to cause the same side effects and drug interactions that are associated with HMG-CoA reductase drugs such as lovastatin. Similar to lovastatin, rhabdomyolysis has been reported with red yeast rice.[72] The effects of red yeast rice and HMG-CoA reductase-inhibiting drugs could be additive. It is well known that grapefruit products can increase the serum levels of lovastatin by inhibiting the cytochrome P450-based drug metabolism[73]; the same is likely to be true of red yeast rice. Incorrect fermentation can result in the presence of citrinin (nephrotoxin) in red yeast rice products.[74] American College of Cardiology recommends not using red yeast rice.[75]

Garlic

Garlic is used to treat various cardiac and vascular conditions, but there is controversy about its effectiveness. Some studies have shown that garlic reduces hyperlipidemia, but other studies have shown no benefit.[76,77] In a meta-analysis of 45 randomized clinical trials, Stevinson et al.[78] concluded that when used for 4 to 25 weeks, garlic usually lowers total cholesterol levels by 4% to 12%. However, the six studies judged to be the most rigorous failed to show a significant difference between the garlic and placebo groups. By comparison, "statin" drugs typically decrease cholesterol levels by 17% to 32%. Garlic's antihyperlipidemic effects are possibly caused by a component of garlic (*S*-allyl cysteine), likely an HMG-CoA reductase inhibitor.[79,80] HMG-CoA reductase inhibitors inhibit hepatic cholesterol synthesis; statin-type drugs and red yeast rice act via a similar mechanism.

Garlic is sometimes used to improve hypertension. There is some evidence that garlic can modestly reduce blood pressure by 2% to 7% after 4 weeks of treatment.[81] This effect is thought to be caused by nitric oxide release, which relaxes smooth muscle, causing vasodilatation. Garlic is sometimes used as an anticoagulant.[82,83] Other medicinal applications of garlic include antifungal, antibacterial, anthelmintic, antiviral, antispasmodic, diaphoretic, expectorant, and immunostimulant. These effects are not proven.[84]

It is difficult to compare studies of garlic and to achieve consistent dosing. There are several active ingredients present; it is not always clear which component might induce a therapeutic effect. Because some components are more labile than others, this issue complicates clinical trials and treatment recommendations. Garlic's pharmacologic properties are attributed to organosulfur compounds, particularly allicin and ajoene. Alliin is an odorless compound in the garlic bulb. When the bulb is crushed, the cells release an enzyme called allinase. Allinase converts alliin to the unstable, odiferous compound, allicin, and then to ajoene. The compounds present in a garlic preparation depend on how the products are prepared. Processes that macerate the garlic clove increase allinase activity. Freeze-dried garlic may contain little or no allicin. Gastric acids may degrade products without enteric coating before the active ingredients are absorbed. When heat and steam distillation are used to produce garlic oil from crushed garlic, allicin is converted to less biologically active allyl sulfides. Garlic is sometimes aged to reduce the content of sulfur compounds and the odor commonly associated with garlic. However, the process of producing odorless aged garlic extract reduces the alliin content to only 3% of what is typically contained in fresh garlic. Aged garlic extract is usually standardized to *S*-allyl cysteine, another major organosulfur constituent in garlic, but this is not the compound thought to be the most biologically active. All these factors make it difficult to know what dose of garlic the patient is receiving.

Garlic is associated with noxious breath and body odor; it can burn the skin and irritate the gastrointestinal track. Garlic's effects could be additive with warfarin. Patients taking cyclosporine are advised to avoid garlic because it may activate the liver enzyme (cytochrome P450 3A4), which metabolizes cyclosporine.[85] Other drugs that are potentially affected by this mechanism include some calcium channel blockers (diltiazem, nicardipine, verapamil), chemotherapeutic agents (etoposide, paclitaxel, vinblastine, vincristine, vindesine), antifungals (ketoconazole, itraconazole), glucocorticoids, alfentanil (Alfenta), cisapride (Propulsid), fentanyl (Sublimaze), lidocaine (Xylocaine), losartan (Cozaar), fexofenadine (Allegra), midazolam (Versed), the protease inhibitor saquinavir, and others.

Coenzyme Q10

Coenzyme Q10 is a fat-soluble vitamin-like compound occurring naturally in the heart, liver, pancreas, and kidney. Some foods such as soybean oil contain the compound. Commercial preparations are made from fermented beets, sugar cane, and yeast. Coenzyme Q10 has antioxidant properties and serves as a cofactor in some metabolic cycles; it contributes to adenosine triphosphate (ATP) production. It is used extensively in Japan, Europe, and Russia to treat cardiovascular diseases including heart failure, angina, hypertension, and doxorubicin (Adriamycin)-induced cardiotoxicity. Several studies suggest that coenzyme Q10 in combination with conventional therapy improves quality of life, improves symptoms such as dyspnea, edema, and insomnia, and decreases the number of hospitalizations in patients with New York Heart Association class II–IV heart failure.[86,87] Other studies found no effect on exercise tolerance or on ejection fraction.[88] Coenzyme Q10 may enhance the efficacy of antihypertensives in lowering blood pressure.[89] A meta-analysis of 12 trials (three random control trials) supported the conclusion that coenzyme Q10 has good potential to lower blood pressure in hypertensive patients.[90] Coenzyme Q10 may be most effective when endogenous levels are low, as they are in some types of heart failure. Coenzyme Q10 has also been recommended for some noncardiac diseases including Huntington disease, Parkinson disease, chronic fatigue syndrome, alopecia, and topically for periodontal infection. Coenzyme Q10 is generally considered safe; side effects include gastrointestinal symptoms and are typically minimal. It should be used cautiously in combination with pharmaceutical antihypertensives because the effects can be additive.

Protein

Several epidemiologic studies have reported lowering of the blood pressure with increased dietary protein. A meta-analysis of nine population-based cross-sectional studies supports an inverse association between protein intake and elevated blood pressure in men and women; a stronger effect is noted in men. Both human and animal studies show decreased blood pressure with increased dietary protein, regardless of the protein type, although a greater effect is noted with animal-based protein.[91] In a randomized, double-blind, multicenter, controlled trial, soybean protein supplementation was associated with reduced diastolic (2.7 mm Hg) and systolic (4.3 mm Hg) pressure after 12 weeks in persons with prehypertension or hypertension; the effect was greater in those with hypertension.[92]

Increasing fiber (in the form of psyllium) and protein (in the form of soy) was shown to have a cumulative effect lowering blood pressure in a small randomized trial. Subjects on the combined diet showed a decrease in systolic pressure by about 8 mm Hg and a decrease in diastolic pressure by 2 mm Hg.[93] Increasing daily protein intake, regardless of source, has been associated with at least modest reductions in blood pressure.

Calcium

Calcium in the form of dairy products or as supplements may decrease blood pressure in hypertensive adults. A cross-sectional, population-based study conducted in France found that both dairy and calcium supplements significantly and independently reduce blood pressure.[94] Clinical trials have also supported the use of calcium as a supplement to lower blood pressure, but the effects have been small. A 6-week randomized crossover study of 60 hypertensive patients showed an average reduction of only 1 to 2 mm Hg in blood pressure with calcium supplementation.[95] More research is needed to establish if milk has properties that decrease blood pressure separate from calcium to strengthen the support of dairy in dietary recommendations for hypertensive patients.

Other Dietary Recommendations

Diets rich in magnesium may be linked with lower blood pressure and cardiovascular risk.[75] The DASH diet was developed by the National Institutes of Health to improve cardiac health. It emphasizes a high-fiber diet rich in fruits, vegetables, low-fat dairy; it is low in saturated fat, total fat, and cholesterol. It includes six to eight servings of whole grains, four to five servings of fruit, four to five servings of vegetables, two to three servings of low or non-fat dairy, three to six servings of lean meat, poultry or fish, two to three teaspoons of oil, and less than two sweets per day; four to five servings of nuts, seeds, or beans weekly are recommended; it does not include recommendations related to omega-3 fatty acids.[96] The DASH diet was associated with 8 to 14 mm Hg drop in systolic blood pressure. Reduced sodium intake (<2.4 g sodium/day) and limiting alcohol consumption (less than two drinks per day for men, less than one drink per day for women) were also associated with minor reductions in blood pressure.[97]

MANIPULATIVE, BODY-BASED METHODS AND ENERGY THERAPIES

Many cultures and religions believe that there is a life force, or energy moving within the body or emanating from the body, and that this energy can be manipulated by conscious and unconscious efforts. In Hindu philosophy this energy is *prana*, in Chinese philosophy *qi*, in Japanese philosophy *ki*. These approaches are difficult to test and there are no large-scale trials of these approaches. Manipulative and body-based methods (e.g., chiropractic manipulation, massage therapy, reflexology) and energy therapies (e.g., reiki, therapeutic touch) could improve cardiac disease, possibly by promoting relaxation and blunting stress responses. A study probed the feasibility of such a study of chiropractic adjustments and massage.[98] A randomized controlled trial of frequent massage (three times per week) given to hypertensive patients lowered their blood pressure with increased effect noted with continued intervention.[99] Tai chi and qi gong, type of energy therapy, have been prescribed as a low-impact exercise in cardiac rehabilitation; it is equivalent to approximately 3 metabolic equivalent tasks.[100]

Acupuncture is another form of energy therapy; it may be helpful in reducing blood pressure in patients with hypertension.[101] Acupuncture is associated with risk of transmission of infectious diseases, including hepatitis, HIV infection, and AIDS.

Healing touch is a nonverbal communication technique, a mechanism used by care providers to be present in the moment

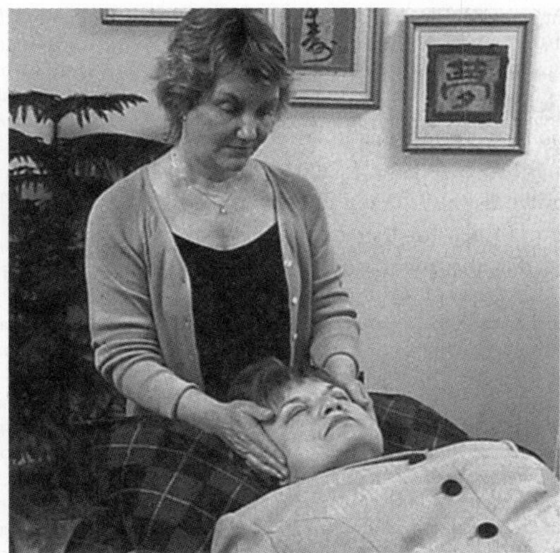

■ **Figure 41-6** Therapeutic touch. (From Lewis, S. M., Heitkemper, M. M., & Dirksen. S. R. [2004]. *Medical surgical nursing: Assessment and management of clinical problems* [6th ed.]. St. Louis: Mosby; used with permission.)

with a patient who is experiencing physical or psychological pain. Nurses with specialized training sometimes practice this form of energy therapy (Fig. 41-6). Healing touch could potentially improve the provider–patient relationship, promote relaxation, reduce the stress response, or alter cardiac variables. More studies are needed of the efficacy in cardiac diseases.

LEGAL ASPECTS OF CAM

Most forms of CAM require specialized training and licensure. Naturopathy, TCM, acupuncture, homeopathy, and chiropractic medicine all require years of training. Other therapies such as massage therapy, reiki, therapeutic touch, and yoga require some, but less, extensive training. License regulations vary from state to state. Nurses who are making referrals or assisting patients to evaluate various treatment approaches should become familiar with the state regulatory statutes.

INTEGRATION OF CAM INTO NURSING ASSESSMENT AND CLINICAL MANAGEMENT

It is important to specifically query patients regarding their CAM usage. Metz et al.[102] evaluated the intake interviews of 196 cancer patients. Each patient received a standard medical history and physical examination including queries about over-the-counter treatments. After completion of the usual interview, patients were asked explicit questions about use of CAM treatments. Although only 13 patients (6.6%) initially disclosed CAM treatments; after directed questioning, an additional 66 patients (36%) disclosed CAM treatments. Thus, CAM usage should be integrated into the health interview rather than relying on the patient to initiate it. The nurse or health care provider should approach the interview with an attitude of being willing to learn from the patient as well as being able to teach. The nurse should proceed in an open, nonjudgmental fashion, avoiding terms that suggest disapproval, such as "unproven." The nurse should ask the patient how well the remedy has worked or not worked before stating an opinion. It may be appropriate to ask the patient's permission to coordinate with the other therapists. Some suggested questions are as follows:

1. What are your values and beliefs related to health and illness?
2. Are there health practices that are part of your cultural, spiritual, or religious beliefs?
3. What therapies have you used to maintain or improve your health?
4. Have you consulted with or been treated by a naturopathic, acupuncturist, or homeopathic provider? (Elicit specific details.)
5. Have you consulted with any specialized healers, such as practitioners of oriental medicine or Native American healing practices?
6. Do you meditate or practice yoga or tai chi?
7. Have you used any herbal treatments?
8. Have you tried any dietary modifications such as increasing your consumption of vitamins or fish oils?
9. Have you consulted with a chiropractor or massage therapist?
10. Do you use magnets or crystals to alter your health status?
11. Why did you select this approach?
12. What is your attitude toward conventional medical care?

Nursing Management Related to CAM

Some CAM approaches are within the scope of nursing practice and can be integrated into the plan of care. Massage, relaxation therapy, or music therapy may be useful adjuncts to the care plan. Some nurses conduct reiki and therapeutic touch treatments. As with any procedure, the nurse should acquire training in the correct applications of the procedure, review the evidence that the therapy is useful, devise a means to evaluate the efficacy of the treatment, and act in conjunction with institutional protocols and procedures. There is considerable need for patient education in regard to CAM approaches. Patients often use products or approaches that they learn about from laypeople, the Internet, or television advertisements. The nurse can assist the patient with weighing the risks and benefits of CAM treatment approaches and help them identify licensed and certified providers of CAM therapies.

SUMMARY

The widespread and increasing use of CAM by the consuming public amplifies the imperative for health care professionals to become familiar with the range of CAM care options, the role CAM plays in health promotion, the interaction between CAM and conventional medicine and nursing, and the potential for adverse outcomes. Unfortunately, nursing curricula traditionally have not included CAM education. This breach in the education of direct care providers has obvious consequences in the care delivered to patients. At the same time, there is a clear need for research into the efficacy of CAM practices either as sole therapies or as adjuvant treatments in health promotion and disease management.

REFERENCES

1. National Center for Complementary and Alternative Medicine. (2007). What is complementary and alternative medicine (CAM)? *NCCAM Publication No. D347.* Retrieved February 10, 2008, from http://nccam.nih.gov/health/whatiscam/
2. World Health Organization. (2007). *Fact sheet No. 326.* Retrieved April 1, 2008, from http://www.who.int/mediacentre/factsheets/fs326/en/
3. Barnes, P. M., Powell-Griner, E., McFann, K., et al. (2004). Complementary and alternative medicine use among adults: United States, 2002. *Advanced Data, 27*(343), 1–19.
4. Eisenberg, D. M., Davis, R. B., Ettner, S. L., et al. (1998). Trends in alternative medicine use in the United States, 1990–1997. *JAMA, 280,* 1569–1575.
5. Astin, J. A., Pelletier, K. R., Marie, A., et al. (2000). Complementary and alternative medicine use among elderly persons: One-year analysis of a Blue Shield Medicare supplement. *Journal of Gerontology Series A: Biological Science and Medical Science, 55*(1), M4–M9.
6. Centers for Medicare & Medicaid Services. (1997). *National health expenditures survey.* Retrieved April 20, 2008, from www.cms.hhs.gov/statistics/nhe
7. Swartzman, L.C., Harshman, R. A., Burkell, J., et al. (2002). What accounts for the appeal of complementary/alternative medicine, and what makes complementary/alternative medicine alternative? *Medical Decision Making, 22,* 431–450.
8. Nahin, R. L., Dahlamer, J. M., Taylor, B. L., et al. (2007). Health behaviors and risk factors in those who use complementary and alternative medicine. *BioMed Central Public Health, 7*(217), 1–9.
9. Xu, K. T., & Farrell, T. W. (2007). The complementary and substitution between conventional and mainstream medicine among racial and ethnic groups in the United States. *Health Services Research, 42*(2), 811–824.
10. Burg, M. A., Kosch, S. G., Neims, A. H., et al. (1998). Personal use of alternative medicine therapies by health science center faculty. *JAMA, 280*(18), 1563.
11. Fontaine, K. L. (2000). *Healing practices, alternative practices for nursing.* Upper Saddle River, NJ: Prentice-Hall.
12. Saydah, S. H., & Eberhardt, M. S. (2006). Use of complementary and alternative medicine among adults with chronic diseases: United States 2002. *The Journal of Alternative and Complementary Medicine, 12*(8), 805–812.
13. Bell, R. A., Suerken, M. S., Grzywacz, J. G., et al. (2006). CAM use among older adults age 65 and older with hypertension in the United States: General use and disease treatment. *The Journal of Alternative and Complementary Medicine, 12*(9), 903–909.
14. Wood, M. J., Stewart, R. L., Merry, H., et al. (2003). Use of complementary and alternative medical therapies in patients with cardiovascular disease. *American Heart Journal, 145*(5), 806–812.
15. Ai, A. L., & Bolling, S. F. (2002). The use of complementary and alternative therapies among middle-aged and older cardiac patients. *American Journal of Medical Quality, 17*(1), 21–27.
16. Williamson, A. T., Fletcher, P. C., & Dawson, K. A. (2003). Complementary and alternative medicine: Use in an older population. *Journal of Gerontological Nursing, 29*(5), 20–28.
17. Montbriand, M. J. (2000). Senior and health professionals' perceptions and communication about prescriptions and alternative therapies. *Canadian Journal on Aging, 19*(1), 35–36.
18. Li, J. Z., Quinn, J. V., McCullock, C. E., et al. (2004). Patterns of complementary and alternative medicine use in ED patients and its association with healthcare utilization. *American Journal of Emergency Medicine, 22*(3), 187–191.
19. Brown, H. W. (2007). *Complementary and alternative medicine: What people 50 and older are using and discussing with their physicians.* Washington, DC: AARP.
20. U.S. Department of Labor: Bureau of Labor Statistics. (2007). *Chiropractors.* Retrieved May 28, 2008, from http://www.bls.gov/oco/pdf/ocos071.pdf.
21. Kligler, B., & Lee, R. A. (2004). *Integrative medicine: Principles for practice.* New York: McGraw-Hill, Medical Publishers Division.
22. Walters, J. D. (2002). *The art and science of Raja Yoga: Fourteen steps to higher awareness.* Delhi: Motilal Banarsidass Publishers.
23. Ospina, M. B., Bond, K., Karkhaneh, M., et al. (2007). *Meditation practices for health: State of the research. Evidence report/technology assessment No. 155.* (Prepared by the University of Alberta Evidence-based Practice Center under Contract No. 290-02-0023, AHRQ Publication No. 07-E010). Rockville, MD: Agency for Healthcare Research and Quality.
24. McCraty, R., Atkinson, M., & Tomasino, D. (2003). Impact of workplace stress reduction program on blood pressure and emotional health in hypertensive employees. *Journal of Alternative and Complementary Medicine, 9*(3), 355–369.
25. Vempati, R. P., & Telles, S. (2002). Yoga-based guided relaxation reduces sympathetic activity judged from baseline levels. *Psychology Report, 90*(2), 487–494.
26. Mahajan, A. S., Reddy, K. S., & Sachdeva, U. (1999). Lipid profile of coronary risk subjects following yogic lifestyle intervention. *Indian Heart Journal, 51*(1), 37–40.
27. Manchanda, S. C., Narang, R., Reddy, K. S., et al. (2000). Retardation of coronary atherosclerosis with yoga lifestyle intervention. *Journal of the Association of Physicians of India, 48*(7), 687–694.
28. Schmidt, T., Wijga, A., Von Zur Muhlen, A., et al. (1997). Changes in cardiovascular risk factors and hormones during a comprehensive residential three month kriya yoga training and vegetarian nutrition. *Acta Physiologica Scandinavia Supplement, 640,* 158–162.
29. Vierling, W., Brand, N., Gaedcke, F., et al. (2003). Investigation of the pharmaceutical and pharmacological equivalence of different Hawthorn extracts. *Phytomedicine, 10*(1), 8–16.
30. Pittler, M. H., Guo, R., & Ernst, E. (2008). Hawthorn extract for treating chronic heart failure. *Cochrane Database of Systematic Reviews, 23*(1), CD005312.
31. Schmidt, U., Kuhn, U., Ploch, M., et al. (1994). Efficacy of the Hawthorne (Crataegus) Preparation LI 132 in 78 patients with chronic congestive heart failure defined as NYHA functional class II. *Phytomedicine, 1,* 17–24.
32. Zapfe, G. (2001). Clinical efficacy of crataegus extract WS 1442 in congestive heart failure NYHA class II. *Phytomedicine, 8,* 262–266.
33. Tauchert, M. (2002). Efficacy and safety of crataegus extract WS 1442 in comparison with placebo in patients with chronic stable New York Heart Association class-III heart failure. *American Heart Journal, 143,* 910–915.
34. Daniele, C., Mazzanti, G., Pittler, M. H., et al. (2006). Adverse event profile of *Crataegus* spp.: A systematic review. *Drug Safety, 29*(6), 523–535.
35. Dwivedi, S., & Agarwal, M. P. (1994). Antianginal and cardioprotective effects of Terminalia arjuna, an indigenous drug, in coronary artery disease. *Journal of the Association of Physicians of India, 42*(4), 287–289.
36. Dwivedi, S., & Jauhari, R. (1997). Beneficial effects of Terminalia arjuna in coronary artery disease. *Indian Heart Journal, 49*(5), 507–510.
37. Bharani, A., Ganguly, A., & Bhargava, K. D. (1995). Salutary effect of Terminalia Arjuna in patients with severe refractory heart failure. *International Journal of Cardiology, 49*(3), 191–199.
38. Rissanen, T., Voutilainen, S., Nyyssonen, K., et al. (2000). Fish oil-derived fatty acids, docosahexaenoic acid and docosapentaenoic acid, and the risk of acute coronary events: The Kuopio ischaemic heart disease risk factor study. *Circulation, 102,* 2677–2679.
39. Bucher, H. C., Hengstler, P., Schindler, C., et al. (2002). N-3 polyunsaturated fatty acids in coronary heart disease: A meta-analysis of randomized controlled trials. *American Journal of Medicine, 112,* 298–304.
40. Marchioli, R., Barzi, F., Bomba, E., et al. (2002). Early protection against sudden death by n-3 polyunsaturated fatty acids after myocardial infarction: Time-course analysis of the results of the Gruppo Italiano per lo Studio della Sopravvivenza nell'Infarto Miocardico (GISSI)-Prevenzione. *Circulation, 105,* 1897–1903.
41. GISSI Group (Gruppo Italiano per lo Studio della Sopravvivenza nell'Infarto miocardico). (1999). Dietary supplementation with n-3 polyunsaturated fatty acids and vitamin E after myocardial infarction: Results of the GISSI-Prevenzione trial. *Lancet, 354,* 447–455.
42. Kromhout, D., Bosschieter, E. B., & de Lezenne Coulander, C. (1985). The inverse relation between fish consumption and 20-year mortality from coronary heart disease. *New England Journal of Medicine, 312*(19), 1205–1209.
43. Daviglus, M. L., Stamler, J., Orencia, A. J., et al. (1997). Fish consumption and the 30-year risk of fatal myocardial infarction. *New England Journal of Medicine, 336*(15), 1046–1053.
44. Albert, C. M., Campos, H., Stampfer, M. J., et al. (2002). Blood levels of long-chain n-3 fatty acids and the risk of sudden death. *New England Journal of Medicine, 346,* 1113–1118.
45. Albert, C. M., Hennekens, C. H., O'Donnell, C. J., et al. (1998). Fish consumption and risk of sudden cardiac death. *JAMA, 279*(1), 23–28.

46. Dickinson, H. O., Mason, J. M., Nicolson, D. J., et al. (2006), Lifestyle interventions to reduce raised blood pressure: A systematic review of randomized controlled trials. *Journal of Hypertension, 24*(2), 215–233.
47. Geleijnse, J. M., Giltay, E. J., Grobbee, D. E., et al. (2002). Blood pressure response to fish oil supplementation: Metaregression analysis of randomized trials. *Journal of Hypertension, 20*(8), 1493–1499.
48. Covington, M. B. (2004). Omega-3 fatty acids. *American Family Physician, 70*(1), 133–140.
49. Mori, T. A., Burke, V., Puddey, I. B., et al. (2000). Purified eicosapentaenoic and docosahexaenoic acids have differential effects on serum lipids and lipoproteins, LDL particle size, glucose, and insulin in mildly hyperlipidemic men. *American Journal of Clinical Nutrition, 71*, 1085–1094.
50. Contacos, C., Barter, P. J., & Sullivan, D. R. (1993). Effect of pravastatin and omega-3 fatty acids on plasma lipids and lipoproteins in patients with combined hyperlipidemia. *Arteriosclerosis Thrombosis, 13*, 1755–1762.
51. Suzukawa, M., Abbey, M., Howe, P. R., et al. (1995). Effects of fish oil fatty acids on low density lipoprotein size, oxidizability, and uptake by macrophages. *Journal of Lipid Research, 36*, 473–484.
52. Vessby, B., & Boberg, M. (1990). Dietary supplementation with n-3 fatty acids may impair glucose homeostasis in patients with non-insulin-dependent diabetes mellitus. *Journal of Internal Medicine, 228*, 165–171.
53. Farmer, A., Montori, V., Dinneen, S., et al. (2001). Fish oil in people with type 2 diabetes mellitus. *Cochrane Database Systematic Review,* 3, CD003205.
54. Schectman, G., Kaul, S., Cherayil, G. D., et al. (1989). Can the hypotriglyceridemic effect of fish oil concentrate be sustained? *Annals of Internal Medicine, 110*, 346–352.
55. Brown, J. E., & Wahle, K. W. (1990). Effect of fish oil and vitamin E supplementation on lipid peroxidation and whole blood aggregation in man. *Clinica Chimica Acta, 193*, 147–156.
56. Yamori, Y., Nara, Y., Mizushima, S., et al. (1994). Nutritional factors for stroke and major cardiovascular diseases: International epidemiological comparison of dietary prevention. *Health Report, 6*, 22–67.
57. Pedersen, H. S., Mulvad, G., Seidelin, K. N., et al. (1999). N-3 fatty acids as a risk factor for haemorrhagic stroke. *Lancet, 353*, 812–813.
58. Cunnane, S. C., Ganguli, S., Menard, C., et al. (1993). High alpha-linolenic acid flaxseed (Linum usitatissimum): Some nutritional properties in humans. *British Journal of Nutrition, 69*, 443–453.
59. Cunnane, S. C., Hamadeh, M. J., Liede, A. C., et al. (1995). Nutritional attributes of traditional flaxseed in healthy young adults. *American Journal of Clinical Nutrition, 61*, 62–68.
60. Bierenbaum, M. L., Reichstein, R., & Watkins, T. R. (1993). Reducing atherogenic risk in hyperlipemic humans with flaxseed supplementation: A preliminary report. *Journal of the American College of Nutrition, 12*(5), 501–504.
61. Jenkins, D. J., Kendall, C. W. C, Vidgen, E., et al. (1999). Health aspects of partially defatted flaxseed, including effects on serum lipids, oxidative measures, and ex vivo androgen and progestin activity: A controlled, crossover trial. *American Journal of Clinical Nutrition, 69*, 395–402.
62. Prasad, K. (1997). Dietary flax seed in prevention of hypercholesterolemic atherosclerosis. *Atherosclerosis, 132*, 69–76.
63. Allman, M. A., Pena, M. M., & Pang, D. (1995). Supplementation with flaxseed oil versus sunflower seed oil in healthy young men consuming a low fat diet: Effects on platelet composition and function. *European Journal of Clinical Nutrition, 49*(3), 169–178.
64. Iso, H., Sato, S., Umemura, U., et al. (2002). Linoleic acid, other fatty acids, and the risk of stroke. *Stroke, 33*(8), 2086–2093.
65. Li, C., Zhu, Y., Wang, Y., et al. (1995). *Monascus purpureus*-fermented rice (red yeast rice): a natural food product that lowers blood cholesterol in animal models of hypercholesterolemia. *Nutrition Research, 18*, 71–81.
66. Wei, W., Li, C., Wang, Y., et al. (2003). Hypolipidemic and anti-atherogenic effects of long-term Cholestin (*Monascus purpureus*-fermented rice, red yeast rice) in cholesterol fed rabbits. *Journal of Nutrition and Biochemistry, 14*(6), 314–318.
67. Heber, D., Yip, I., Ashley, J. M., et al. (1999). Cholesterol-lowering effects of a proprietary Chinese red-yeast-rice dietary supplement. *American Journal of Clinical Nutrition, 69*, 231–236.
68. Downs, J. R., Clearfield, M., Weis, S., et al. (1998). Primary prevention of acute coronary events with lovastatin in men and women with average cholesterol levels: Results of AFCAPS/TexCAPS. Air Force/Texas Coronary Atherosclerosis Prevention Study. *JAMA, 279*(20), 1615–1622.
69. Roselle, H., Ekatan, A., Tzeng, J., et al. (2008). Symptomatic hepatitis associated with the use of herbal red yeast rice. *Annals of Internal Medicine, 149*(7), 516–517.
70. Robbers, J. E., & Tyler, V. E. (1999). *Tyler's herbs of choice: The therapeutic use of phytomedicinals.* New York: The Haworth Herbal Press.
71. Wigger-Alberti, W., Bauer, A., Hipler, U. C., et al. (1999). Anaphylaxis due to *Monascus purpureus*-fermented rice (red yeast rice). *Allergy, 54*, 1330–1331.
72. Prasad, G. V., Wong, T., Meliton, G., et al. (2002). Rhabdomyolysis due to red yeast rice (*Monascus purpureus*) in a renal transplant recipient. *Transplantation, 74*, 1200–1201.
73. Kantola, T., Kivisto, K. T., & Neuvonen, P. J. (1998). Grapefruit juice greatly increases serum concentrations of lovastatin and lovastatin acid. *Clinical Pharmacological Therapy, 63*, 397–402.
74. Heber, D., Lembertas, A., Lu, Q. Y., et al. (2001). An analysis of nine proprietary Chinese red yeast rice dietary supplements: Implications of variability in chemical profile and contents. *Journal of Alternative and Complement Medicine, 7*, 133–139.
75. Vogel, J. H. K., Bolling, S. F., Olshansky, B., et al. (2005). Integrating complementary medicine into cardiovascular medicine. *Journal of the American College of Cardiology, 46*(1), 184–221.
76. Isaacsohn, J. L., Moser, M., Stein, E. A., et al. (1998). Garlic powder and plasma lipids and lipoproteins, a multicenter, randomized, placebo-controlled trial. *Archives of Internal Medicine, 158*, 1189–1194.
77. Berthold, H. K., Sudhop, T., & von Bergmann, K. (1998). Effect of a garlic oil preparation on serum lipoproteins and cholesterol metabolism. *JAMA, 279*(23), 1900–1902.
78. Stevinson, C., Pittler, M. H., & Ernst, E. (2000). Garlic for treating hypercholesterolemia: a meta-analysis of randomized clinical trials. *Annals of Internal Medicine, 133*, 420–429.
79. Yeh, Y. Y., & Liu, L. (2001). Cholesterol-lowering effect of garlic extracts and organosulfur compounds: Human and animal studies. *Journal of Nutrition, 131*(3s), 989S–93S.
80. Gebhardt, R., & Beck, H. (1996). Differential inhibitory effects of garlic-derived organosulfur compounds on cholesterol biosynthesis in primary rat hepatocyte cultures. *Lipids, 31*, 1269–1276.
81. Silagy, C., & Neil, A. (1994). Garlic as a lipid lowering agent—A meta-analysis. *Journal of the Royal College of Physicians (London), 28*, 39–45.
82. Rahman, K., & Billington, D. (2000). Dietary supplementation with aged garlic extract inhibits ADP-induced platelet aggregation in humans. *Journal of Nutrition, 130*(11), 2662–2265.
83. Chutani, S. K., & Bordia, A. (1981). The effect of fried versus raw garlic on fibrinolytic activity in man. *Atherosclerosis, 38*, 417–421.
84. Natural Medicines Comprehensive Database. (2008) Retrieved October 10, 2008, from http://www.naturaldatabase.com
85. Piscitelli, S. C., Burstein, A. H., Welden, N., et al. (2002). The effect of garlic supplements on the pharmacokinetics of saquinavir. *Clinics in Infectious Disease, 34*, 234–238.
86. Morisco, C., Trimarco, B., & Condorelli, M. (1993). Effect of coenzyme Q10 therapy in patients with congestive heart failure: A long-term, multicenter, randomized study. *Clinical Investigation, 71*(Suppl. 8), S134–S136.
87. Hofman-Bang, C., Rehnqvist, N., Swedberg, K., et al. (1995). Coenzyme Q10 as an adjunctive treatment of congestive heart failure. *Journal of Cardiac Failure, 1*, 101–107.
88. Mortensen, S. A. (2000). Coenzyme Q10 as an adjunctive therapy in patients with congestive heart failure. *Journal of the American College of Cardiology, 36*, 304–305.
89. Singh, R. B., Niaz, M. A., Rastogi, S. S., et al. (1999). Effect of hydrosoluble coenzyme Q10 on blood pressures and insulin resistance in hypertensive patients with coronary artery disease. *Journal of Human Hypertension, 13*, 203–208.
90. Rosenfeldt, F. L., Haas, S. J., Krum, H., et al. (2007). Coenzyme Q10 in the treatment of hypertension: A meta-analysis of the clinical trials. *Journal of Human Hypertension, 21*(4), 297–306.
91. Liu, L., Ikeda, K., Sullivan, D. H., et al. (2002). Epidemiological evidence of the association between dietary protein intake and blood pressure: A meta-analysis of published data. *Hypertension Research, 25*, 689–695.
92. He, J., Gu, D., Wu, X., et al. (2005). Effect of soybean protein on blood pressure: A randomized, controlled trial. *Annals of Internal Medicine, 43*, 1–9.
93. Burke, V., Hodgson, J. M., Beilin, L. J., et al. (2001). Dietary protein and soluble fiber reduce ambulatory blood pressure in treated hypertensives. *Hypertension, 38*(4), 821–826.

94. Ruidavets, J., Bongard, V., Simon, C., et al. (2006). Independent contribution of dairy products and calcium intake to blood pressure variations at a population level. *Journal of Hypertension, 24*(4), 671–681.
95. Kwano, Y., Yoshimi, H., Matsuoka, H., et al. (1998). Calcium supplementation in patients with essential hypertension: Assessment by office, home, and ambulatory blood pressure. *Journal of Hypertension, 16*(11), 1693–1699.
96. National Heart Lung and Blood Institute. (2008). *Your guide to lowering high blood pressure.* Retrieved on May 11, 2008 from http://www.nhlbi.nih.gov/hbp/prevent/h_eating/h_eating.htm
97. Chobanian, A. V., Bakris, G. L., Black, H. R., et al. (2004). *The Seventh Report of the Joint National Committee on Prevention, Detection, Evaluation, and Treatment of High Blood Pressure (complete version)* (NIH Publication No. 04-5230). Rockville, MD: U.S. Department of Health and Human Services.
98. Plaugher, G., Long, C. R., Alcantara, J., et al. (2002). Practice-based randomized controlled-comparison clinical trial of chiropractic adjustments and brief massage treatment at sites of subluxation in subjects with essential hypertension: Pilot study. *Journal of Manipulative Physiological Therapy, 25*(4), 221–239.
99. Olney, C. M. (2005). The effect of therapeutic massage in hypertensive persons: A preliminary study. *Biological Research Nursing, 7*(2), 98–105.
100. Chao, Y. F., Chen, S. Y., Lan, C., et al. (2002). The cardiorespiratory response and energy expenditure of Tai-Chi–Qui-Gong. *American Journal of Chinese Medicine, 30*(4), 451–461.
101. Guo, W., & Ni, G. (2003). The effects of acupuncture on blood pressure in different patients. *Journal of Traditional Chinese Medicine, 23*(1), 49–50.
102. Metz, J. M., Jones, H., Devine, P., et al. (2001). Cancer patients use unconventional medical therapies far more frequently than standard history and physical examination suggest. *Cancer Journal, 7*(2), 149–154.

CHAPTER 42

Disease Management Models for Cardiovascular Care

Nancy Houston Miller / Erika S. Sivarajan Froelicher

Since the mid-1990s disease management programs have served as an important method of caring for patients with chronic illness to improve patient outcomes, increase quality of life, and decrease health care utilization and cost. Disease management has been adopted on the basis of results of numerous randomized controlled trials showing that patients with cardiovascular conditions such as heart failure, coronary heart disease, diabetes, and hypertension are better supported through methods involving a team approach, coordinated delivery of care, systematic education, and documentation of outcomes directed at improving program delivery. The trend toward caring for patients through disease management programs has spread rapidly and now involves not only researchers, but also numerous health care organizations, the government, and for-profit organizations that are attempting to improve chronic disease care and reduce costly emergency department visits and hospitalizations. Data from managed care organizations indicate that at least 88% of such organizations have implemented at least one disease management program.[1]

In a health care system faced with an overburden of chronic illnesses, disease management is a concept likely to enable Americans to live differently in the future. It is necessary in any society whose population is growing older and a health care system that is focused on managing the acute aspects of illness. By 2030 it is expected that one in five Americans will enter the age group older than 65 years.[2] Moreover, life expectancy has increased 44% between 1900 and 1950, 13% between 1950 and 2000, and is projected to increase by 9% between 2000 and 2050. In 1997, the average life expectancy was 79 years for women and 74 years for men. As of 2005, only 8 years later, life expectancy was 80 years for women and 75 years for men.[3] Life expectancy at ages 65 and 85 years has also increased substantially over the past 50 years; women who survive to age 65 years can expect to live to age 84 years, and those who survive to age 85 years can expect to live to age 92 years.[4] Although the average American then can expect to live much longer, will their quality of life enable them to enjoy both independence and function?

In 2005 more than 133 million Americans had one or more chronic conditions.[5] This figure is expected to increase by 1% per year through the year 2030, where the number will increase by 46 million Americans.[5] Moreover, women will experience the major burden of chronic diseases. Many of these conditions are related to the vascular system including hypertension, which is the leading chronic condition in those younger and older than 65 years and heart disease, which is the leading cause of death in both men and women.[5] Other chronic conditions most prevalent in those older than 65 years include pulmonary disease, diabetes, arthritis, and chronic mental disorders. Treatment is complicated by the coexistence of multiple medical conditions and the social and psychological sequelae that accompany them.[5]

It is estimated that three quarters of all health care expenditures go to caring for individuals with chronic conditions. With health care expenditures exceeding $1.7 trillion and 15% of the gross domestic product,[6] numerous health care plans, including Medicaid and Medicare have implemented disease management programs to improve high-cost care. Whether disease management programs will succeed in significantly lowering the costs associated with managing chronic disease remains to be seen as the evidence of cost-effectiveness remains limited.[7] Advanced Practice Nurses are well positioned to take on the challenge of disease management, as they constitute the largest group of health care professionals, with more than 2.4 million employed in the United States.[8]

The resources to manage those with an acute illness are quite different from those with a chronic condition. Acute care services are provided primarily by physicians and nurses, often in intensive, hospital-based care requiring the use of expensive technology. In contrast, effective chronic care requires a comprehensive approach that combines social, educational, vocational, and medical services provided in a variety of settings that increasingly focus on the home as the setting of care. The scope of chronic care is broad, encompassing social, community, and personal services as well as medical and rehabilitative care. The management of chronic conditions also requires a network of health care professionals including nurses, social workers, family, and caregivers. Finally, much of chronic care requires education and support of patients and family members to maximize self-management.

In the late 1990s, in a review of the literature, Wagner et al.[9] identified five important elements associated with improved outcomes for those with chronic conditions such as hypertension and diabetes. Successful programs tended to be those that (1) incorporated guidelines and protocols in practice; (2) used a multidisciplinary team with careful allocation of tasks and ongoing patient contact; (3) provided counseling, education, information feedback, and other support to patients; (4) offered access to necessary clinical expertise such as referral to specialists, collaborative care models, and computer-decision support; and (5) used supportive information systems that offer reminders for preventive care and follow-up as well as feedback to providers on patient compliance and service use. Various disease management models have been developed to meet the needs of those with chronic conditions, incorporating many of these elements associated with chronic care delivery. Moreover, a systems approach to care delivery is needed to enhance long-term adherence (see Chapter 40).[10] This chapter focuses on various models of disease management, including clinic and nurse case management approaches developed for cardiovascular care. Elements important to care delivery are discussed.

DISEASE MANAGEMENT: DEFINITION AND MODELS

Disease management is a term that has been used for more than a decade to encompass the way in which care is delivered to individuals, but more specifically to groups of patients. Many associate the term with managed care and a way to control health care services.[11] Although numerous definitions for this term exist, Ellrodt et al.[12] define disease management as an approach to patient care that emphasizes coordinated comprehensive care along a continuum of disease and across health care delivery systems.

The most comprehensive definition for disease management has been developed by the Disease Management Association of America (DMAA), a nonprofit trade association.[13] However, not all programs meet the standards held by this organization. The DMAA states that disease management is a system of coordinated health care interventions and communications for populations with conditions in which patient self-care efforts are significant. Disease management components include the following: (1) population identification processes; (2) evidence-based practice guidelines; (3) collaborative practice models, which include nurses, physician, and other support service providers; (4) patient self-management education; (5) process and outcomes measurement, evaluation, and management; and (6) routine reporting and feedback. This organization suggests that full-service disease management involves all six components. More recently recognizing the significant variation in the heterogeneous variation of disease management programs, the American Heart Association developed taxonomy for disease management that may serve as a guide to help individuals involved in developing programs and attempting to identify factors associated with effectiveness.[14] This taxonomy provides a framework for reporting on disease management which offers specific details to help the reader note all aspects of the delivery of care. It is highlighted in Figure 42-1.

In addition to numerous definitions used for disease management and the many models that exist fall under the rubric of disease management. Case management was a term used early in the course of managing patients with chronic illness with a primary focus of managing patients at high risk for expensive outcomes. Case managers often undertake a broad assessment of the medical, functional, social, and emotional needs of individuals developing written plans of care and incorporating community resources to support individuals. Education about symptom management, compliance with medications, diet and medical follow-up, and ways of accessing the emergency department are often part of the care provided by case managers. Case managers may also be involved in care coordination, which is another term that is often used to specify how these individuals integrate the efforts of medical and social service providers.[15]

Another model of disease management offers programs that are specific to patient-focused diagnoses such as heart failure or diabetes. Often undertaken by nurses, these disease management programs follow guidelines for a particular disease, utilize standardized education related to the disease, and often use technology to monitor a patient's condition. Follow-up is often long-term as well noting that conditions like heart failure and diabetes are

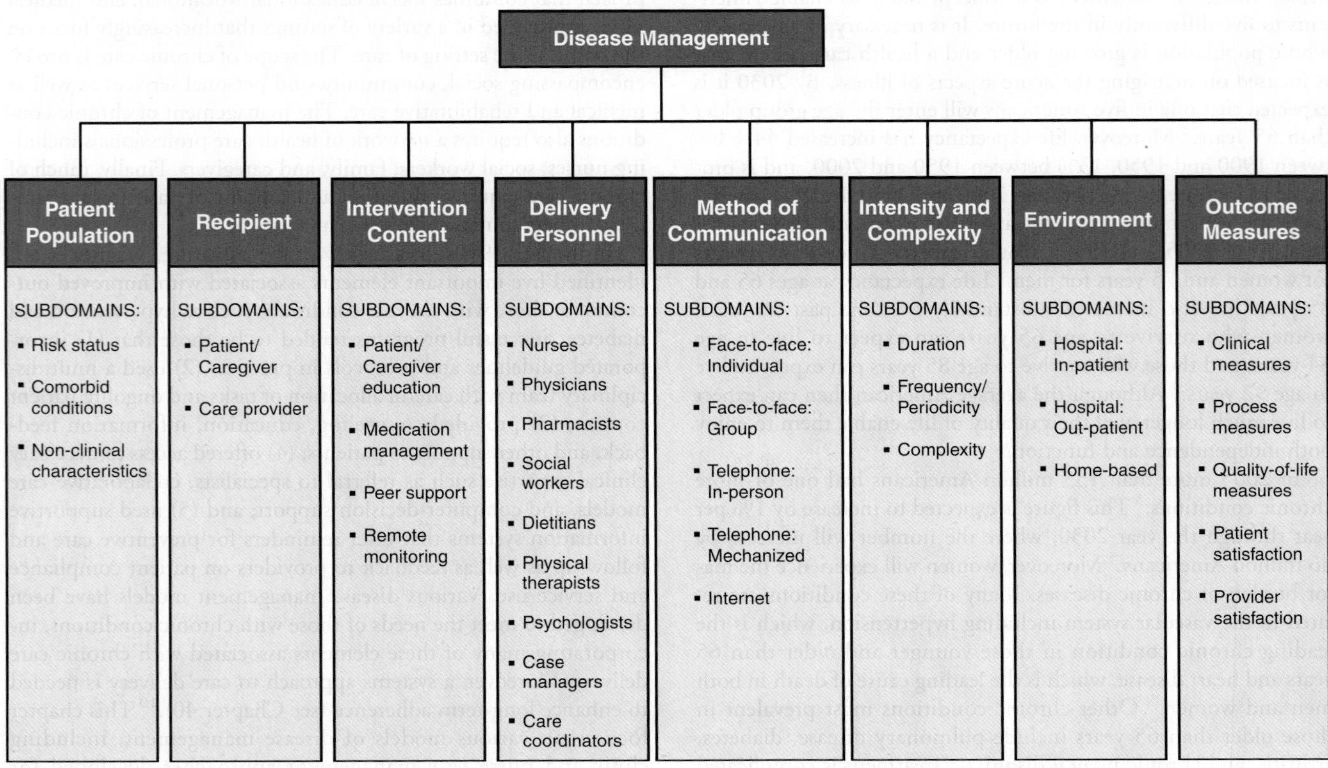

Figure 42-1 The American Heart Association's taxonomy for disease management.

not amenable to care and that patients are likely to lapse into old behaviors.

Disease management is also often provided by a group of individuals focused on providing multidisciplinary care. Utilizing numerous health care providers such as nurses, pharmacists, social workers, dieticians, and others, multidisciplinary care teams may facilitate the transition from hospital to long-term care at home.[14] Each individual of the multidisciplinary team offers unique services to provide lifestyle interventions and health care. These teams may employ "coaching" a term coined in disease management to support behavior modification.

Finally, Ed Wagner and colleagues at Group Health Cooperative of Puget Sound have developed the chronic care model embraced by large organizations such as Kaiser Permanente of Northern California and Health Partners Medical Group in Minneapolis, Minnesota, which is the most comprehensive form of disease management focused on changing an entire system of care delivery. Operationalized, the chronic care model addresses the community, health care system, and provider organization and ensures that six elements are in place to ensure optimal care. These elements include (1) community resources and policies, (2) health care organization, (3) self-management support, (4) delivery system design, (5) decision support, and (6) clinical information systems. A large focus for this type of disease management is geared toward coordinating activities within primary care.[16]

Models of Disease Management in Cardiovascular Care by Nurses

Since the early 1970s, unique models for delivering care to individuals with chronic conditions by nurses have evolved. Much of this early work in disease management occurred in hypertension control in the United States and Europe.[17,18] Most often, attempts were made to deliver high-quality care in various settings that were convenient to the population being studied. In one of the first disease management programs,[18] patients with hypertension, diabetes, or cardiac disease chose to be followed by specially trained nurses in decentralized clinics close to their homes or in a hospital-based outpatient clinic for chronic disease that was staffed by internists. Patients had similar sociodemographic and clinical characteristics. After 2 years, hypertension control rates were superior in those patients cared for by specially trained nurses, and they had 50% fewer hospital admission days. The authors of this study attributed the success of the nurse-run clinics to greater follow-up and time devoted to helping patients manage their chronic conditions.

In another early trial,[17] nurses played a key role in the screening and follow-up of individuals within a work site setting in New York City. Nurses screened and enrolled patients over an 11-day period and followed up hypertensive individuals over 1 year. Working closely with a medical director, they performed an initial medical history, obtained preliminary laboratory data, and followed treatment algorithms, initiating and titrating medications for hypertension treatment. Diuretics were chosen as first-line therapy for hypertension treatment, and after controlling blood pressure to goal, patients were seen for review of therapy and were monitored for compliance every 3 months by the nurses. At the end of the year, 84% of the work site had been screened, 97% of those followed up by the nurses remained in therapy, and 81% succeeded with optimal blood pressure lowering. The cost per patient of $100 offset the costs associated with hypertension, including the time lost from work.

These early studies suggested that the convenience of helping individuals manage their health in settings conducive to work and home offered an optimal opportunity for disease management to be brought to the patient. Since the 1970s, disease management by nurses has been applied not only to hypertension,[17–26] but also to other aspects of cardiovascular management, including dyslipidemia,[27–30] tobacco dependence,[31–35] diabetes,[36–40] coronary artery disease,[41–54] and heart failure.[55–71] Much of the early work before the term disease management was coined occurred in managing patients after myocardial infarction using a multidisciplinary approach to managing risk factors, adherence to diet, exercise, medications, and medical regimens to improve functioning and quality of life through the provision of individual and group education, counseling, and behavioral interventions, which included the patient and family as part of rehabilitation.[72]

The largest number of studies related to disease management are in heart failure, in which considerable interest has arisen about how to care for a large and growing population of high-risk patients with the most costly cardiovascular condition (see Chapter 24). The aforementioned body of work and the reviews conducted by investigators in the area of heart failure,[73–77] diabetes,[78–80] and hypertension[81] offer insights and guidance to nurses on the application of disease management systems for care delivery. Disease management systems have now also been used in randomized controlled trials[21,27,28,39] and clinical practice settings,[11] which include younger,[28] older,[49,66,82] and minority populations,[83,84] clinics,[41,59] hospitals,[32–34] work sites,[17] home-based[39,43] and cardiac rehabilitation settings,[46,85] and the use of multidisciplinary[44,47,65] or physician–nurse teams[41,71] to direct care delivery. Moreover, these disease management programs have been shown to effectively reduce multiple risk factors,[36,43,46,47] improve quality of life,[41,62] and functional status,[59] increase short-term compliance,[10] reduce total admissions, and cardiovascular readmissions,[49,63,65,67] improve survival,[68] reduce days of hospitalizations,[55,68] and reduce rehospitalization costs.[49,86]

Disease Management in Low-Income Populations

Recent work has shown the benefit of disease management in low-income and minority populations who may be at greatest risk of cardiovascular disease. For example, Sisk et al.[83] randomly allocated 406 Hispanic and Black patients with systolic dysfunction from four Harlem hospitals to receive usual care or nurse case management over a period of 12 months. Bilingual nurse case managers counseled patients in the intervention group about sodium intake, fluid buildup, medication adherence, and self-management symptoms, and in addition served as a bridge between patients and physicians. At the end of 12 months, patients who were managed by nurses had fewer hospitalizations (143 vs. 180, adjusted difference, −0.13 hospitalization/person year, 95% CI −0.24 to −0.001 hospitalization/person year) than patients receiving usual care. In addition, they had better functioning and quality of life based on the Minnesota Living with Heart Failure Questionnaire[87] and the Medical Outcomes Study (MOS) short-form.[88] Other investigators report challenges when working with minority populations, such as Mexican Americans who travel to and from the United States to Mexico making interventions sporadic and unsystematic in this population.[89] Stafford and Berra highlight the barriers and facilitators of effective case management in multiethnic, low-income populations, and offer important suggestions for future work based on experiences with such populations.[84]

Is Disease Management Cost-Effective?

The majority of work in the area of the cost-effectiveness of disease management is still in its infancy. Due to the burden of heart failure and the high costs associated with 2.5 million readmissions annually, much of the evaluation of costs has been conducted in this population. Chan et al.[90] applied a Markov model to assess the incremental life expectancy and cost of disease management to both low- and high-risk patients. They looked at the cost of providing disease management to all patients for a period of 15 years and found that the average coverage at 15 years was $12,882 per life-year saved with 95% CI of $6,486 to $29,293 per life-year saved. The incremental cost-effectiveness ratio of extending care to all patients was $9,700 per life-year gained and having universal coverage quadrupled life-years saved as compared with only those at high risk. Disease management is likely to be cost-effective in the long-term, with $50,000 per life-year gained as the benchmark for cost-effectiveness.[90] While one of the pitfalls of some disease management programs is the focus on a single disease condition, it has also been shown that few studies have looked at the clustering of chronic conditions and the cost-effectiveness of managing multiple conditions. The work of Naylor et al. suggest that advance practice nurses may not only be able to reduce costs associated with caring for patients with heart failure, but may significantly reduce the costs of caring for those patients who often have five to six comorbid conditions.[91]

Future Research by Nurses

Research is still needed to determine the most cost-effective models, how to support long-term adherence including the frequency of interactions to ensure maintenance of health behavior changes, and if improved outcomes in reduction in rehospitalizations are achieved through disease management programs. Nurses who have conducted numerous successful trials are also well positioned to disseminate and study the translation of these models into clinical practice settings.

Approaches to disease management have shown promise and documented the leadership and contribution nurses can make in the care of patients with cardiovascular health problems. Although the names of such models may differ, the specific components, format, and distribution of health care professionals contributing to the multidisciplinary approaches vary by setting and scope of practice according to various health care professional practice acts, geographic region, payors, and by nationality. Examples of beneficial models have been cited from Europe, Australia, the United States, and Canada.

COMPONENTS OF DISEASE MANAGEMENT SYSTEMS

Identifying a Patient Population

Effective disease management involves a process of identifying at-risk populations, coordinating systems of care delivery, obtaining outcomes, and managing outcomes most appropriately to improve care. The process is shown in Figure 42-2. Most often, disease management programs are developed for chronic conditions that are costly, such as coronary artery disease, diabetes, heart failure, renal failure, and chronic obstructive pulmonary disease. Populations are moderate-risk to high-risk individuals. They may be identified through hospital discharge records as high users of care,[49] through health plan databases when the aim is to reduce costs associated with a certain conditions,[36] or through a team of individuals such as nurses and physicians aiming to improve the quality of care through a quality-improvement process to meet national guidelines.[44]

Disease management is most effective when there are incentives tied to outcomes. For example, the goal of managed care organizations may be to reduce rehospitalizations for heart failure as reimbursement for patients readmitted within 30 days of hospitalization may be low. Thus, a program for patients with heart failure must consider a clear understanding of why patients are being admitted so frequently. For a health plan, the goal may be to ensure that all individuals' cardiovascular risk factors are screened and to focus on intensive disease management programs for those

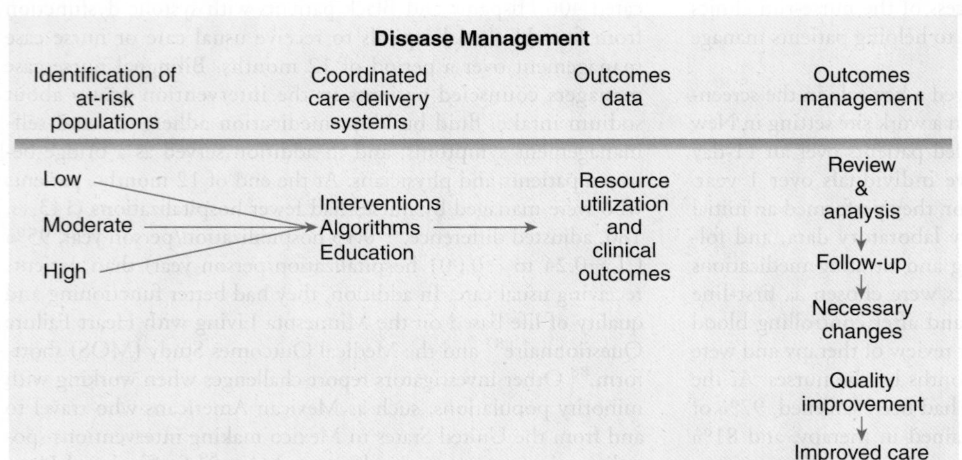

Figure 42-2 The process of disease management.

individuals with multiple risk factors who are at greatest risk for future cardiovascular events. Noting that it may be costly to include all patients in disease management programs, organizations, such as Kaiser Permanente of Northern California, have focused their chronic disease efforts by subgrouping populations, offering lower-risk individuals educational and supportive services individually or in groups, and offering moderate-to-high risk individuals what they term "care management." Their experience is invaluable to those considering the development of disease management efforts.

Once a population in need has been identified, it is critical to learn as much as possible about the population. Knowing the demographic (age, gender, race, socioeconomic, and cultural) characteristics of the population being addressed enables one to structure appropriate and effective interventions. Moreover, being sensitive to the educational, social, and cultural needs of the individual and populations is critical to success.

Coordinating Delivery Systems for Disease Management

Although disease management models have operated in a variety of settings including clinics, hospitals, and work sites, investigators have also used telephones and the Internet to deliver care and structure interactions with the patient to optimize care within the home setting.[43,92,93] Although there is much diversity related to structured interventions among these programs, most have incorporated patient education, multidisciplinary or physician–nurse teams, and specialized follow-up. Furthermore, the development of algorithms and protocols for delivering structured care has been crucial to the success of disease management systems.

Disease management involves a process of care delivery. Because the process of care delivery is different from the typical structure within an office visit or hospital that is well known to most health care professionals; many different models for care delivery in disease management exist today. Although populations differ, interventions have varied, such as a single face-to-face visit with telephone follow-up to comprehensive management teams comprising multiple team members.[75,86] Moreover, few have been able to specify which components are most important to overall outcome.[74] Although this is because of the system's approach to care uses multiple interventions, specifying primary and secondary goals is key to developing intervention activities. Goals for a disease management program are often to improve patient and caregiver knowledge of the disease, enhance self-management through skill building, increase medication and treatment adherence, and improve health-related outcomes.[52,54,94,95]

Education as a Part of Disease Management

Education is a key intervention component of disease management. Most often, education entails lifestyle changes including diet, exercise, and smoking cessation, as well as ways to self-monitor a disease condition, including taking medication, recognizing important signs and symptoms, and daily monitoring of indicators such as weight, glucose, or blood pressure. The format for education differs from one program to another. Some have used face-to-face individualized education,[36,43] whereas others have used a group approach followed by individualized education.[39,53,54] A review of programs offering structured educational interventions for cardiovascular disease[96] found that more than two thirds of successful programs, many directed by nurses, were focused on behavioral approaches directed at skill building. Rather than providing information, these programs succeeded by offering a range of health behavior skills, such as contracting, goal setting, self-monitoring, feedback, and problem solving.[97] Many used theories of stages of change,[98] social learning (most specifically, self-efficacy),[99,100] and relapse prevention training[95,96,101] to plan successful educational interventions. In addition, offering educational materials in multiple formats (e.g., print, audio, and video) has also been shown to increase adherence to long-term behavioral changes. Adult learners differ in their preferred ways of gaining knowledge and skills and these multimedia approaches giving them an opportunity for reinforcement of information.[97]

Developing educational interventions based on the critical behaviors to be changed is key to successful disease management efforts. For example, Stewart et al.[67] formulated a disease management program educating patients in a single face-to-face visit about medication use behaviors to improve heart failure outcomes. The goal of the intervention was to focus on the problems associated with medication adherence for each patient after hospital discharge. With support of a pharmacist and a nurse in a single face-to-face visit in the home, Stewart planned an approach to manage each individual's problems associated with medication use and sought methods for improving adherence. Patients with multiple problems were offered additional support through telephone calls by the pharmacist. At the end of 18 months and 4 years, this disease management intervention resulted in decreased hospitalizations, improved survival, and lower cost associated with heart failure.[68,102] The authors attribute the success of the intervention to the focused problem solving and tailoring for each individual patient and the additional efforts applied to more difficult patients through individualization of care.[67]

The success of educational interventions for disease management appears to be related to individualized approaches to education, offering multiple formats, use of behavioral approaches, and a focus on more intensive education in those with the greatest need.

Medical Management of Care Delivery: Protocols and Algorithms

In addition to education, one of the main objectives of disease management programs is to ensure that patients are using prescribed medication regimens that optimize outcomes. Irrespective of disease state, this may be actualized through careful dose titration of medications. Strong emphasis has also been placed on the achievement of high adherence rates to prevent exacerbation of symptoms or deterioration of outcomes known to impact future risk.[57] Although national guidelines, such as those developed by the National Institutes of Health,[103,104] the American Heart Association,[105] and the American Diabetes Association,[106] are a starting point for decisions about initiating pharmacotherapy, they are often insufficient in supplying the important aspects of dose titration necessary for disease management, especially in severely ill populations such as those with heart failure. Thus, protocols or algorithms that delineate appropriate dosing and that are developed from formulary decisions of institutions are key to managing medications effectively in disease management programs. Nurses have played important roles in the management of the pharmacological aspects of disease management. Many State Nurse Practice Acts require that nurses follow strict protocols for managing medications in an outpatient setting that must be updated annually.[107] Moreover, the development of protocols for medication management is often a shared responsibility of nurses, physicians, and pharmacists within the local institution offering the disease management program. Advanced Practice Nurses are in an excellent position to help manage the pharmacologic aspects of disease management and have often taken on this role as case managers.

Structuring Interventions: The Process of Coordinating Care

Interventions that focus on education and medication management as part of any disease management program must be structured in a way to optimize outcomes. As previously mentioned, there is large variation in the frequency of interactions with patients, the use of face-to-face visits versus telephone follow-up, how much follow-up is needed, whether in-home monitoring can support health care professionals and the number of health care professionals including the expertise of nurses required for disease management. However, several investigators suggest that the most important factors to be addressed in making decisions about how to structure the frequency of interactions to the following: (1) understanding the needs of the patient population based on problems (e.g., lack of adherence, material support, frequent hospitalizations, inadequate risk factor control); (2) deciding whether face-to-face, group, or individual interventions will enhance overall success, or whether telephone or electronic encounters are sufficient to enhance motivation; (3) determining if home visits are needed; (4) noting what the time-frame is for problematic behaviors and lack of adherence; and (5) considering how much tailoring is needed to support individual patients. Irrespective of whether face-to-face interventions or telephone or electronic encounters are used, most often interactions occur more frequently in the early phases of disease management programs and are designed to taper-off as patients and family members learn how to better self-manage behaviors and pharmacotherapies. Many groups have successfully operationalized disease management in research settings through several studies[33,49,52–54,67–69,91,97,108] and offer their experience, whereas others who have had success in clinical practice settings for more than 10 years[11,72,109,110] offer important perspectives on the structuring of interventions and the coordination of care delivery.

Communication With Physicians and Other Personnel

The frequency of interactions with other personnel in the disease management team is important to overall care. One of the failures of the current system in the United States in managing those with chronic conditions has been the frequency of visits to multiple physician providers and the lack of communication among them. In disease management models, nurses most often assume the role of coordinating care between two or more providers. Electronic medical records within large systems have often facilitated that communication. However, full integration of these systems in most health care settings has yet to be realized. In some instances, the disease management program is situated outside the usual health care delivery system that the patient is enrolled in, or a database for disease management is separate from the existing paper-based or electronic medical record. Thus, to facilitate clear communication about ongoing management, letters updating physicians and documentation of care within the medical record become crucial. These can be facilitated through computer-generated reports highlighting clinical progress to physicians and the development of standard tools for receiving responses from physicians. The frequency of phone-based interactions and the format for receiving information about the care being delivered to patients as part of disease management should be addressed as part of the development of algorithms and protocols. Interactions with physicians most often relate changes in symptoms and medications and need to be addressed by the team. Physician champions who can facilitate problem solving and offer expertise to nurses in the absence of primary care or specialty physicians facilitates success with program implementation.

Anticipating the needs of patients and family members, nurses also plays a role in coordinating the care delivered by other health care professionals such as social workers, pharmacists, dietitians, and psychologists. These disciplines offer specialized expertise in defined fields often required for managing long-term chronic conditions. Overseeing the presence of social isolation and depression is very important. The need for economic and material support, and continued education related to diet and medications, is necessary for improvement of patient outcomes such as reduction in utilization.

Measuring Clinical and Resource Utilization Outcomes

Irrespective of a research or clinical initiative in disease management, collecting data on outcomes is crucial to evaluating a program. Many disease management programs collect process and outcome data including resource utilization, quality of life, patient satisfaction,[111] physician satisfaction, and program costs, which is important to substantiate the need for these programs. Health insurance companies and payers of care are most interested in outcomes associated with a reduction in emergency department visits, in hospitalizations or rehospitalizations, length of hospital stay, and costs of care. This type of information is obtained from financial records or review of medical records and insurance information. Keeping accurate process data in an individual database that is part of the disease management program assists in determining whether adequate pharmacologic treatment was delivered, thus ultimately influencing outcomes.

Quality of life is most often measured within the research setting. However, patients and family members place high value on the improvement of quality of life as an outcome of disease management programs. Thus, measurement of this outcome is important in clinically based programs. Although researchers have difficulty agreeing on what constitutes overall quality of life, comprehensive tools exist to measure many of the important components including biologic or physiologic indicators, symptoms, functioning, health perceptions, and overall well being. Some of the most commonly used tools include the MOS Short Form-36 Item Questionnaire (SF-36)[112,113] and the Sickness Impact Profile.[94,114] Shorter tools such as the Short-Form 12,[88] a modification of the SF-36, are much easier to administer in clinical practice settings but do not provide measurements of changes that are offered through longer instruments.

Although general quality-of-life questionnaires can be useful, disease-specific tools are more valuable in defining patient outcomes. For example, the Minnesota Living with Heart Failure tool, which measures multiple domains of quality of life in heart failure patients and contains 21 items, correlates well with assessments of dyspnea and fatigue, is important in this population.[115] Finally, others suggest that using both a general and a disease-specific measure of quality of life may enhance results. Smith et al.[6] reported on the quality of life in 1,069 community-dwelling patients in south Texas who were randomly assigned to disease management versus a control group. Health-related quality of life was based on the MOS 36-item Short Form Health Survey (SF-36)[112,113] measured at 6-month intervals. Although there was a positive effect of the intervention on self-reported improvement in quality of health at 6 and 12 months, this was not sustained. This is the largest study conducted to date that evaluated quality of life in heart failure patients; the authors concluded that lack of a disease-specific measure to serve as a comparison was regrettable not available.[6]

Measuring functional status of patients, which may be significantly impacted as a result of disease management programs, should also be considered in developing outcome measures for disease management. The Duke Activity Status Instrument (DASI)[116] is an example of a simple self-administered questionnaire that correlates well with functional activities in heart failure subjects. Other tools that measure symptoms and function include the Canadian Cardiovascular Society (CCS) Functional Classification used for functional disability and angina[117] and the Seattle Angina Questionnaire.[118]

Measures of patient satisfaction can be an important marketing tool for disease management program. Most large organizations are committed to measuring patient satisfaction as part of quality assurance.[119] However, there are no prevalent, systematic, or validated approaches for measuring patient satisfaction within the disease management industry. One exception is a tool measuring satisfaction in individuals participating in diabetes disease management programs. Thus, a clear need to develop a standardized approach to the assessment of patient satisfaction is needed.

Measuring overall program satisfaction and satisfaction with individual key components of the program may be helpful not only to administrators but also to enhancing program delivery. As noted earlier, assessment of patient satisfaction has also been initiated as part of quality-assurance assessments.[111] Likewise, brief physician satisfaction surveys may help program administrators in monitoring and can lead to restructuring of aspects of a disease management program. Because these programs are designed to support the physician's care, physician satisfaction surveys should measure items such as help in improving self-management, a reduction in physician's time for various aspects of care, and support in achieving national guidelines for quality care such as those established by the Joint Committee on the Accreditation of Health Care Organizations (www.jcaho.org) or the National Committee for Quality Assurance (NCQA).[120,121]

Finally, many process measures enable disease management personnel to better understand the important aspects of program delivery. Observing the frequency of face-to-face or telephone contacts, length of contacts, and the type of daily tasks performed, completed through time-analysis records, enable one to determine the need for program restructuring. This type of process evaluation is helpful in determining whether nonclinical tasks could be allocated to other personnel so nurses are performing the most important clinical tasks. Process measures also enable one to determine the actual implementation of intervention activities, important to outcomes.

Outcomes Management

Outcomes management includes using evaluation data to make necessary changes in program implementation for continued quality improvement. Although the goal of a disease management model may not be to lower the cost of care, specific outcomes such as reducing the frequency of physician visits for those in a disease management program may be an important outcome of a busy health maintenance organization. Moreover, increased patient satisfaction as a result of the program may enable payers to retain patients in their delivery system, thus increasing competition among health industry providers. Finally, looking for more efficient ways to deliver the program to a larger number of patients is often a goal for those actively involved in disease management efforts. Because groups like Kaiser Permanente of Northern California have succeeded in offering disease management to large numbers of patients for more than a decade, they offer insights about achievable outcomes that are useful to those planning new programs and large system changes.[122]

Program Marketing

Whereas the clinical aspects of disease management are critical to success, continual marketing of the program to hospital administrators, payers, physicians, and other health care professionals is important to sustaining a program. Important marketing activities include (1) a plan for recruiting program participants using brochures, flyers, letters, and other announcements, which are continually maintained; (2) updating administrators and decision makers about program implementation through quarterly, biannual, or annual reports and presentations; and (3) ensuring that physicians and other health care professionals outside the disease management program are continually informed of program delivery changes, successes, and program volume. Satisfied patients and family members are often willing to write letters to key decision makers about the value of the program to their overall care.

TRAINING AND JOB QUALIFICATIONS FOR DISEASE MANAGEMENT

Managing a caseload of patients as part of disease management requires sound clinical expertise and a number of other important qualifications. Qualifications for those involved in these programs include strong physical assessment skills, interpersonal skills (warmth, empathy, good listening and problem solving, and an ability to work with families and a multidisciplinary team), the ability to work independently, leadership capability (advocate for patients and families, the disease manager's role, and the program), and good organizational skills (ability to use information systems and time-management skills). Knowledge of and skills in conducting groups is essential when the program is offered in a group format.[72] Most often, nurses have bachelor degrees or master degrees and have been specially trained for the position. Many are Advanced Practice Nurses specializing in case management or disease management. A strong background in cardiovascular nursing (minimum 3 years) and cardiac rehabilitation are desirable qualifications for disease management.

Core competencies in chronic disease management may be mastered through a curriculum that includes knowledge of the disease process, medical management of risk factors, treatment protocols, lifestyle and psychosocial interventions, information systems, and institutional operations. Patient education and behavioral counseling skills include motivational interviewing and adherence counseling. An ability to operationalize treatment protocols surrounding the initiation and titration of medications, symptom management, documentation in medical records, and coordination of care are core competencies that must be mastered. Like those involved in public health and community nursing, disease management nurses must be committed to following patients and families on a long-term basis.

Much of the training for disease management occurs on the job, although more schools of nursing are offering classes that support skills for disease management. Best practice programs[109] offer in-depth training to nurses managing multiple risk factors occurring over 2 weeks. Didactic lecture, role playing, and case study presentation are followed by 1 week of preceptorship training with other experienced disease management nurses in the field. Nursing organizations, such as the Preventive Cardiovascular Nurses Association (PCNA),[123] are committed to educating nurses to take on expanded roles in preventive cardiovascular nursing. They offer regional and national training, web-based continuing education online (CEU) courses and important publications including cardiovascular guidelines and tools that support those undertaking disease management roles.

THE UNRESOLVED ISSUES FOR DISEASE MANAGEMENT

Although disease management has not yet reached widespread application in clinical practice, it holds promise as a new way of delivering care to those at high risk for and those with established cardiovascular disease. The success of using nurses to coordinate disease management programs has most often resulted in more frequent medication changes, an increase in the use of combination drug regimens, less expensive medications, and an increase in short-term adherence. These results are in large part because of the use of defined protocols and increased patient contact time for education and behavioral counseling. In addition, a greater achievement of goals such as a reduction in blood pressure, cholesterol, and glucose control has been realized. A by-product of comprehensive care in patients has produced a reduction in utilization for all causes (emergency department visits and hospitalizations), something not expected by many in the field.[124] As noted in Display 42-1, organizations implementing disease management programs for more than 10 years suggest several important lessons for those developing new programs. In addition, Stewart and Horowitz[69] have highlighted a number of factors that appear to be important in the overall development of those disease management programs that successfully reduced rehospitalization rates and costs for heart failure. These are highlighted in Display 42-2.

DISPLAY 42-1 Important Lessons for Program Implementation in Disease Management

- Physician leadership/support is key to program viability
- Ongoing marketing is essential
- Program modifications save time and resources
- Protocols require annual updates and alignment with national guidelines
- Defining caseload requirements and reevaluating is necessary for quality control

Many challenges continue to confront those involved in disease management, offering future opportunities for research and for those conducting clinical programs. Disease management programs have typically focused on what is often called a "single disease state" or "carve out." These specialty programs for high-cost patient populations treat only a single chronic condition such as diabetes or heart failure. However, many individuals have predisposing risk factors and comorbid conditions that determine their functional status and prognosis. For example, more than half of all rehospitalizations for heart failure are caused by coexisting conditions that impact the disease, such as hypertension and coronary artery disease, or unrelated conditions, such as chronic obstructive pulmonary disease.[92] Moreover, the overlap of cardiovascular risk factors (dyslipidemia, obesity, hypertension, and smoking) is significant. Thus, the need for managing multiple risk factors concurrently is noteworthy and requires continued research. As adherence to guidelines by physicians and systems becomes more common place, allowing achievement of better patient outcomes, a more central role for nurses in disease management is likely to reside with an elderly and aging population that is burdened by multiple diseases and associated conditions. Naylor et al. have started to addressed many of the factors associated with the older adults,[49,91,108] early findings suggest promise for the future.

A second challenge relates to intervention components and the duration of follow-up. Although disease management models focus on multiple interventions, there is large variation in the

DISPLAY 42-2 Key Features of Successful Programs of Care in CHF

- A commitment to individualized health care
- A multidisciplinary approach to managing the patient
- A major role for a specialist nurse to assess patient needs and provide for ongoing management within a supportive multidisciplinary environment
- At least one home visit for a comprehensive assessment of the patients circumstances
- The promotion of self-care behaviors
- Increased levels of monitoring in "high-risk" patients
- The application of optimal, evidence-based pharmacological treatment with flexible protocols for changes in patient status and titration to maximal tolerated doses.

Adapted with permission from Stewart, S., & Horowitz, J. (2003). Specialist nurse management programmes: Economic benefits in the management of heart failure. *Pharmacoeconomics, 21*(4), 225–240.

frequency of contact, the context for what is provided to patients, and whether patients are followed-up for 1 month, 1 year, or indefinitely. To date, few programs have analyzed the most important components of their programs, and few have compared the effectiveness of different programs or the individual components or combinations of components within programs.[125] It is likely that those who demonstrate high accountability through good patient outcomes at a reasonable cost and that also offset the high costs of acute exacerbations will likely prevail. Finally, web-based technology now affords the opportunity for health care professionals to follow-up patients over an extended period of time.

Does home telemonitoring for chronic disease improve patient outcomes? The use of electronic blood pressure monitors, blood glucose meters, and voice recognition technology offers data that can be concealed during infrequent office visits. A *Cochrane Review* evaluated the use of home telemonitoring on improvement of patient outcomes.[126] Their review suggests that irrespective of nationality, socioeconomic status, or age, patients are relatively adherent with telemonitoring programs and technologies. Studies in patients with cardiological problems showed significant benefit on clinical outcomes from the use of such devices. However, research is still needed on the cost-effectiveness of the use of these technologies, the impact on service utilization, and the acceptance by health care professionals such as case managers.

Although disease management models have been effectively implemented in research and clinical practice, it is likely that such programs will be delivered only to subgroups of patients in the future, because of cost. Peer support models for self-management of chronic conditions have also been tested.[127,128] These offer significant promise as an alternative modality supporting self-management of symptoms in individuals with chronic conditions. The Chronic Disease Management Program is a community-based, peer-led program designed to help those individuals with chronic conditions such as cardiovascular disease, arthritis, pulmonary disease, and stroke. This program, which is offered to 10 to 15 participants over 7 weeks in 2.5-hour group sessions and led by a trained peer leader, focuses on improving self-management skills based on self-efficacy theory, drawing on peers for support. Weekly sessions focus on action planning and feedback, modeling of behaviors and problem solving by participants for one another, group problem solving, and individual decision making. Supported by a program guide entitled "*Living a Healthy Life with Chronic Conditions*," weekly content includes the following: adopting exercise programs; use of cognitive symptom management techniques, such as guided relaxation and distraction; fatigue and sleep management; use of medications and community resources; managing the emotions of fear, anger, and depression; training in communication with health care professionals and others; health-related problem solving; and decision making.

In a study of 831 subjects, Lorig et al.[127] found that compared with baseline, for each of 2 years, emergency department and outpatient visits were reduced ($p = .05$) and self-efficacy improved in those attending the sessions ($p = .05$). This model, now widely used by health care organizations in the United States and abroad, offers another important alternative for disease management. The question remains whether the high cost of training the peer teachers who frequently are unavailable after their initial orientation versus investing in nursing professionals who can and will sustain such programs remains to be seen. Also, in persons with multiple chronic conditions, the extent to which a peer education program is safe has also not been addressed.

A final important challenge facing disease management relates to the transitional aspects of care and the health care delivery system. Acute care that has been linked to the hospital must truly be linked to the delivery of chronic care. A problem confronting some patients has been the perceived loss of control over the health care system.[129] Nelson found that impersonal service, health care system navigation, and, for many, feeling discounted by the medical care system are problems many older adults patient face today. Conversely, feeling cared for and receiving support were frequently cited by those patients participating in nurse case management. Structured appropriately, disease management models must help to support a successful transition from home to hospital and other settings. Ensuring a smooth transition with the disease manager operating in partnership with the patient at the center is likely to reduce the sense of loss of control for patients and families. More opportunities will arise to improve care as communication technologies improve and our capability to monitor patients in the home environment is extended.

In summary, disease management models offer the promise of better care for millions of individuals with multiple risk factors and known cardiovascular diseases. Although much has been studied, the challenge of implementation of those models showing improved outcomes must continue, and further research is needed about best methods for dissemination. Much of this challenge rests in the hands of nurses who participate in research in disease management and those who are in newly defined disease management roles.

REFERENCES

1. Lazarus, A. (2001). The promise of disease management. *Psychiatric Services, 52*, 161–171.
2. National Center for Health Statistics. (1999). *Health, United States 1999.* Hyattsville, MD: U.S. Government Printing Office.
3. Centers for Disease Control. National Center for Health Statistics. (2006). *Deaths. Preliminary data for 2005.* Retrieved June 5, 2008, from www.nlm.nih.gov/medlineplus/healthstatistics.html.
4. The Robert Wood Johnson Foundation. (2000). *Health and healthcare 2010: The forecast, the challenge.* Princeton, NJ: The Robert Wood Johnson Foundation.
5. The Robert Wood Johnson and Johns Hopkins University Partnerships for Solutions. (2002*). Chronic conditions: Making the case for ongoing care.* Princeton, NJ: The Robert Wood Johnson Foundation.
6. Smith, B., Forner, E., Zaslow, B., et al. (2005). Disease management produces limited quality of life improvements in patients with congestive heart failure: Evidence from a randomized controlled trial in community-dwelling patients. *American Journal of Managed Care, 11*, 701–713.
7. Goetzel, R., Ozimkowski, R., Villagra, V., et al. (2005). Return on investment in disease management: A review. *Health Care Financing Review, 26*, 1–19.
8. Berra, K. B., Houston Miller, N., Fair, J. (2006). Cardiovascular disease prevention and disease management. *Journal of Cardiopulmonary Rehabilitation, 26*, 197–206.
9. Wagner, E. H., Austin, B., & Von Korff, M. (1996). Organizing care for patients with chronic illness. *Milbank Quarterly, 74*(4), 511–542.
10. Miller, N. H., Hill, M. N., Kottke, T., et al. (1997). The multilevel compliance challenge: Recommendations for a call to action. A statement for healthcare professionals. *Circulation, 95*, 1085–1990.
11. Unger, B. T., & Warren, D. A. (1999). Case management in cardiac rehabilitation. In N. K. Wenger, L. K. Smith, E. S. Froelicher, et al. (Eds.), *Cardiac rehabilitation: A guide to practice in the 21st century* (pp. 327–341). New York: Marcel Dekker.
12. Ellrodt, G., Cook, D. J., Lee, J., et al. (1997). Evidence-based disease management. *JAMA, 278*, 1687–1692.
13. Disease Management Association of America. (2008). *The definition of disease management.* Retrieved June 13, 2008, from http://www.dmaa.org/definition.html.
14. Krumholz, H. M., Riegel, B., Phillips, C. O., et al. (2006). A taxonomy for disease management: A scientific statement from the American Heart

Association Disease Management Taxonomy Writing Group. *Circulation, 114,* 1432–1445.
15. Flarey, D. L., & Blancett, S. S. (1996). Case management: Delivering care in the age of managed care. In D. L. Flarey & S. S. Blancett (Eds.), *Handbook of nurse case management.* Gaithersburg, MD: Aspen Publishing.
16. Bodenheimer, T., Wagner, E., & Grumbach, K. (2002). Improving primary care for patients with chronic illness. *JAMA, 288,* 1775–1779.
17. Alderman, M. H., & Shoenbaum, E. F. (1975). Detection and treatment of hypertension at the work site. *New England Journal of Medicine, 293,* 65–68.
18. Runyan, K. W., Jr. (1975). The Memphis Chronic Disease Program. Comparison in outcome and the nurse's extended role. *JAMA, 231,* 264–267.
19. Denver, E. A., Barnard, M., Woolfson, R. G., et al. (2003). Management of uncontrolled hypertension in a nurse-led clinic compared with conventional care for patients with Type 2 diabetes. *Diabetes Care, 26,* 2256–2260.
20. Gabbay, R. A., Lendel, I., Saleem, T. M., et al. (2006). Nurse case management improves blood pressure, emotional stress and diabetes complication screening. *Diabetes Research and Clinical Practice, 71,* 28–35.
21. Hill, M. N., Bone, L. J., Hilton, S. C., et al. (1999). A clinical trial to improve high blood pressure care in young urban black men. *American Journal of Hypertension, 12,* 548–554.
22. Logan, A. G., Milne, B. J., Achber, C., et al. (1979). Work-site treatment of hypertension by specially trained nurses. A controlled trial. *Lancet, 2,* 1175–1178.
23. Perry, H. M., Schnapner, J. W., Meyer, G., et al. (1982). Clinical program for screening and treatment of hypertension in veterans. *Journal of the National Medical Association, 74,* 433–444.
24. Pheley, A. M., Terry, P., Peitz, L., et al. (1995). Evaluation of a nurse-based hypertension management program: Screening, management, and outcomes. *Journal of Cardiovascular Nursing, 9,* 54–61.
25. Reichgott, M. J., Pearson, S., & Hill, M. N. (1983). The nurse practitioner's role in complex patient management: Hypertension. *Journal of the National Medical Association, 75,* 1197–1204.
26. Tobe, S. W., Pylypchuk, G., Wentworth, J., et al. (2006). Effect of nurse-directed hypertension treatment among First Nations people with existing hypertension and diabetes mellitus: The Diabetes Risk Evaluation and Microalbuminuria (DREAM) randomized controlled trial. *Canadian Medical Association Journal, 174,* 1–6.
27. Allen, J., Blumenthal, R. S., Margolis, S., et al. (2002). Nurse case management of hypercholesterolemia in patients with coronary heart disease: Results of a randomized clinical trial. *American Heart Journal, 144,* 678–686.
28. Becker, D. M., Rqueno, J. V., Yook, R. M., et al. (1998). Nurse mediated cholesterol management compared with enhanced primary care in siblings of individuals with premature coronary disease. *Archives of Internal Medicine, 158,* 1533–1539.
29. Blair, T. P., Bryant, J., & Bocuzzi, S. (1988). Treatment of hypercholesterolemia by a clinical nurse using a stepped-care protocol in a nonvolunteer population. *Archives of Internal Medicine, 148,* 1046–1048.
30. Shaffer, J., & Wexler, L. F. (1995). Reducing low-density lipoprotein cholesterol levels in an ambulatory care system. *Archives of Internal Medicine, 155,* 2330–2335.
31. Hollis, J. F., Lichtenstein, E., Vogt, T. M., et al. (1993). Nurse-assisted counseling for smokers in primary care. *Annals of Internal Medicine, 118,* 521–525.
32. Martin, K., Froelicher, E., & Houston Miller, N. (2000). Women's Initiative for Nonsmoking (WINS) II: The intervention. *Heart & Lung, 29,* 438–445.
33. Miller, N. H., Smith, P. M., DeBusk, R. F., et al. (1997). Smoking cessation in hospitalized patients. Results of a randomized trial. *Archives of Internal Medicine, 157,* 409–415.
34. Rigotti, N. A., McKool, K. M., & Shiffman, S. (1994). Predictors of smoking cessation after coronary artery bypass graft surgery: Results of a randomized trial with 5-year follow-up. *Annals of Internal Medicine, 120,* 287–293.
35. Taylor, C. B., Miller, N. H., Killen, J. D., et al. (1990). Smoking cessation after acute myocardial infarction: Effects of a nurse-managed intervention. *Annals of Internal Medicine, 13,* 118–123.
36. Aubert, R. E., Herman, W. H., Waters, J., et al. (1998). Nurse case management to improve glycemic control in diabetic patients in a health maintenance organization. *Annals of Internal Medicine, 129,* 605–612.
37. Peters, A. L., Davidson, M. B., & Ossorio, R. C. (1995). Management of patients with diabetes by nurses with support of specialists. *HMO Practice, 9,* 8–13.
38. Piette, J. D., Weinberger, M., Kraemer, F. B., et al. (2001). Impact of automated calls with nurse follow-up on diabetes treatment outcomes in a Department of Veterans Affairs Health Care System. *Diabetes Care, 24,* 202–208.
39. Taylor, C. B., Houston Miller, N., Reilly, K. R., et al. (2003). Evaluation of a nurse-care management system to improve outcomes in patients with complicated diabetes. *Diabetes Care, 26,* 1058–1053.
40. Weinberger, M., Kirkman, M. S., Samsa, G. P., et al. (1995). A nurse-coordinated intervention for primary care patients with non-insulin-dependant diabetes mellitus: Impact on glycemic control and health-related quality of life. *Journal of General Internal Medicine, 10,* 59–66.
41. Campbell, N. C., Ritchie, L. D., Thain, J., et al. (1998). Secondary prevention in coronary heart disease: A randomized trial of nurse led clinics in primary care. *Heart, 80*(5), 447–452.
42. Cupples, M. E., & McKnight, A. (1994). Randomized controlled trial of health promotion in general practice for patients at high cardiovascular risk. *BMJ, 309*(6960), 993–996.
43. DeBusk, R. F., Miller, N. H., Superko, H. R., et al. (1994). A case management system for coronary risk factor modification following acute myocardial infarction. *Annals of Internal Medicine, 120,* 721–729.
44. Fonarow, G. C., Gawlinksi, A., Moughrabi, S., et al. (2001). Improved treatment of coronary heart disease by implementation of a Cardiac Hospitalization Atherosclerosis Management Program (CHAMP). *American Journal of Cardiology, 87,* 819–822.
45. Fonorow, G., Gawlinski, A., & Watson, K. (2003). Inhospital initiation of cardiovascular protective therapies to improve treatment rates and clinical outcomes: The University of California–Los Angeles, Cardiovascular Hospitalization Atherosclerosis Management Program. *Critical Pathways in Cardiology, 2,* 61–70.
46. Gordon, N. F., English, C. D., Contractor, A. S., et al. (2002). Effectiveness of three models for comprehensive cardiovascular disease risk reduction. *American Journal of Cardiology, 89,* 1263–1268.
47. Haskell, W. L., Alderman, E. L., Fair, J. M., et al. (1994). Effects of intensive multiple risk factor reduction on coronary atherosclerosis and clinical cardiac events in men and women with coronary artery disease. The Stanford Coronary Risk Intervention Project (SCRIP). *Circulation, 89,* 975–990.
48. Murchie, P., Campbell, N., Ritchie, L. D., et al. (2003). Secondary prevention clinics for coronary heart disease: Four year follow up of a randomized controlled trial in primary care. *BMJ, 326,* 84.
49. Naylor, M., Brooten, D., Campbell, R., et al. (1999). Comprehensive discharge planning and home follow-up of hospitalized elders. *JAMA, 281*(7), 613–620.
50. O'Malley, P. G., Feurstein I. M., & Taylor, A. J. (2003). Impact of electron beam tomography, with or without case management, on motivation, behavioral change, and cardiovascular risk profile. *JAMA, 289*(17), 2215–2223.
51. Pozen, M. W., Stechmiller, J., Harris, W., et al. (1977). A nurse rehabilitator's impact on patients with myocardial infarction. *Medical Care, 15,* 830–837.
52. Sivarajan, E. S., Bruce, R. A., Almes, M. J., et al. (1981). In-hospital exercise after myocardial infarction does not improve treadmill performance. *New England Journal of Medicine, 305,* 357–362.
53. Sivarajan, E. S., Bruce, R. A., Lindskog, B. D., et al. (1982). Treadmill test responses to an early exercise program after myocardial infarction: A randomized study. *Circulation, 65,* 1420–1428.
54. Sivarajan, E. S., Newton, K. M., Almes, M. J., et al. (1983). Limited effects of out-patient teaching and counseling after myocardial infarction: A controlled study. *Heart & Lung, 12,* 65–73.
55. Benatar, D. B., Ghitelman, M., & Avitall, J. (2003). Outcomes of chronic heart failure. *Archives of Internal Medicine, 163,* 347–351.
56. Blue, L. L., McMurray, E., Davie, J. J., et al. (2001). Randomized controlled trial of specialist nurse intervention in heart failure. *BMJ, 323,* 715–718.
57. Cline, C. M. J., Israelsson, B., Willenheimer, R. B., et al. (1998). Cost effective management programme for heart failure reduces hospitalization. *Heart, 80,* 442–446.
58. Ekman, I., Andersson, B., Ehnforst, M., et al. (1998). Feasibility of a nurse-monitored, outpatient-care programme for elderly patients with moderate-to-severe, chronic heart failure. *European Heart Journal, 19,* 1254–1260.

59. Fonarow, G., Stevenson, L. W., Walden, J. A., et al. (1997). Impact of a comprehensive heart failure management program on hospital readmission and functional status of patients with advanced heart failure. *Journal of the American College of Cardiology, 30,* 725–732.
60. Jaarsma, T., Halfens, R., Huijer Abu-Saad, H., et al. (1999). Effects of education and support on self-care and resource utilization in patients with heart failure. *European Heart Journal, 20,* 673–682.
61. Jaarsma, T., van der Wal, M. H., Lesman-Leegle, I., et al. (2008). Effect of moderate or intensive disease management program on outcomes in patients with heart failure. *Archives of Internal Medicine, 168,* 316–324.
62. Kasper, E., Gerstenblith, G., Hefter, G., et al. (2002). A randomized trial of the efficacy of multidisciplinary care in heart failure outpatients at high risk of hospital readmission. *Journal of the American College of Cardiology, 39*(3), 471–480.
63. Kornowski, R., Zeeli, D., Averbuch, M., et al. (1995). Intensive homecare surveillance prevents hospitalization and improves morbidity rates among elderly patients with severe congestive heart failure. *American Heart Journal, 129,* 762–766.
64. Laramee, A. S., Levinsky, S. K., Sargent, J., et al. (2003). Case management in a heterogeneous congestive heart failure population. *Archives of Internal Medicine, 163,* 809–817.
65. Reigel, B. C., Kopp, Z., LePetri, B., et al. (2002). Effect of a standardized nurse case-management telephone intervention on resource use in patients with chronic heart failure. *Archives of Internal Medicine, 162,* 705–712.
66. Rich, M. W., Beckham, V., Wittenberg, C., et al. (1995). A multidisciplinary intervention to prevent the readmission of elderly patients with congestive heart failure. *New England Journal of Medicine, 333*(18), 1190–1195.
67. Stewart, S., Horowitz J., & Pearson, S. (1998). Effects of a home-based intervention among patients with congestive heart failure discharged from acute hospital care. *Archives of Internal Medicine, 158,* 1067–1072.
68. Stewart, S., Marley, J. E., & Horowitz, J. D. (1999). Effects of a multidisciplinary, home-based intervention on planned readmissions and survival among patients with chronic congestive heart failure: A randomized controlled study. *Lancet, 354,* 1077–1083.
69. Stewart, S., & Horowitz, J. (2003). Specialist nurse management programmes. *Pharmacoeconomics, 21*(4), 225–240.
70. Weinberger, M., Oddone, E., & Henderson, W. G. (1996). Does increased access to primary care reduce hospital readmissions? *New England Journal of Medicine, 334*(22), 1441–1447.
71. West, J., Miller, N. H., Parker, K. M., et al. (1997). A comprehensive management system for heart failure improves clinical outcomes and reduces medical resource utilization. *American Journal of Cardiology, 79*(1), 58–63.
72. Sivarajan, E. S., & Newton, K. M. (1984). Symposium on cardiac rehabilitation: Exercise, education and counseling for patients with coronary artery disease. *Clinics of Sports Medicine, 2,* 349–369.
73. McAlister, F. A., Lawson, F., Teo, K. K., et al. (2001). A systematic review of randomized trials of disease management programs in heart failure. *American Journal of Medicine, 110*(5), 378–384.
74. Philbin, E. (1999). Comprehensive multidisciplinary programs for the management of patients with congestive heart failure. *Journal of General Internal Medicine, 14,* 130–137.
75. Rich, M. W. (2001). Heart failure disease management programs: Efficacy and limitations. *American Journal of Medicine, 110*(5), 410–412.
76. Reigel, B., & LePetri, B. (2001). *Improving outcomes in heart failure. Heart failure disease management models* (pp. 267–281). Gaithersburg, MD: Aspen Publishing.
77. Whellan, D., Hassleblad, V., Peterson, E., et al. (2005). Metanalysis and review of heart failure disease management randomized controlled trials. *American Heart Journal, 149,* 722–729.
78. Ingersoll, S., Valente, S. M., & Roper, J. (2005). Nurse care coordination for diabetes. A literature review and synthesis. *Journal of Nursing Care Quality, 20,* 208–214.
79. Loveman, E., Royle, P., & Waugh, N. (2005). Specialist nurses in diabetes mellitus. *Cochrane Database System Review,* (2), CD003286.
80. Renders, C. M., Valk, G. D., Griffin, S., et al. (2003). *Interventions to improve the management of diabetes mellitus in primary care, outpatient and community settings.* Amsterdam: Institute for Research in Extramural Medicine. (Cochrane Review).
81. Curzio, J. L., & Beevers, M. (1997). The role of nurses in hypertension care and research. *Journal of Human Hypertension, 11,* 541–550.
82. Del Sindaco, D., Pulignano, G., Minardi, G., et al. (2007). Two-year outcome of a prospective, controlled study of a disease management programme for elderly patients with heart failure. *Journal of Cardiovascular Medicine, 8,* 324–329.
83. Sisk, J. E., Hebert, P. L., Horowitz, C. R., et al. (2006). Effects of nurse management on the quality of heart failure care in minority communities. *Annals of Internal Medicine, 145,* 273–283.
84. Stafford, R. S., & Berra, K. B. (2007). Critical factors in case management: Practical lessons from a cardiac case management program. *Disease Management, 10,* 197–207.
85. Vale, M. J., Jelinek, M. V., Best, J. D., et al. (2003). Coaching patients on achieving cardiovascular health (COACH): A multicenter randomized trial in patients with coronary heart disease. *Archives of Internal Medicine, 163,* 2775–2783.
86. Stewart, S., Vanderbrock, A. J., Pearson, S., et al. (1999). Prolonged beneficial effects of a home-based intervention on unplanned readmissions and morality among patients with congestive heart failure. *Archives of Internal Medicine, 159,* 257–261.
87. Rector, T. S., Kubo, S. H., & Cohn, J. N. (1993). Validity of the Minnesota living with heart failure questionnaire as a measure of therapeutic response to enalapril or placebo. *American Journal of Cardiology, 71,* 1106–1107.
88. Jenkinson, C., Layte, R., Jenkinson, D., et al. (1997). A shorter form health survey: Can the SF-12 replicate results from the SF-36 in longitudinal studies. *Journal of Public Health, 19,* 179–186.
89. Reigel, B., Carlson, B., Glaser, D., et al. (2006). Randomized controlled trial of telephone case management in Hispanics of Mexican origin with heart failure. *Journal of Cardiac Failure, 12,* 211–219.
90. Chan, D. C., Heidenreich, P. A., Weinstein, P. A., et al. (2008). Heart failure disease management programs: A cost-effectiveness analysis. *American Heart Journal, 155,* 332–338.
91. Naylor, M. D., Brooten, D. A., Campbell, R. L., et al. (2004). Transitional care of older adults hospitalized with heart failure: A randomized, controlled trial. *Journal of the American Geriatric Society, 52,* 675–684.
92. DeBusk, R. F., Houston Miller, N., Parker, K., et al. (2004). Care management for low-risk patients with heart failure. *Annals of Internal Medicine, 141,* 606–613.
93. Chaudhry, S. I., Phillips, C. O., Stewart, S. S., et al. (2007). Telemonitoring for patients with chronic heart failure: A systematic review. *Journal of Cardiovascular Failure, 13,* 56–62.
94. Ott, C. R., Sivarajan, E. S., Newton, K. M., et al. (1983). A randomized study of early cardiac rehabilitation: The sickness impact profile as an assessment tool. *Heart & Lung, 12*(2), 162–170.
95. Sivarajan Froelicher, E., & Kozuki, Y. (2002). Application of theory to smoking cessation intervention. Women's Initiative for Non-smoking IV. *International Journal of Nursing Studies, 39,* 1–15.
96. Mullen, P. D., Mains, D. A., & Velez, R. (1992). A meta-analysis of controlled trials of cardiac patient education. *Patient Education and Counseling, 19,* 143–162.
97. Miller, N. H., & Taylor, C. B. (1995). Education, communication and methods of intervention. In E. Giles & S. Moore (Eds.), *Lifestyle management for patients with coronary heart disease* (pp 21–30). Champaign, IL: Human Kinetics.
98. Prochaska, J. O., & DiClemente, C. C. (1983). Stages and process of self-change of smoking: Toward an integrative model of change. *Journal of Consulting and Clinical Psychology, 51,* 390–395.
99. Bandura, A. (1997). *Self-efficacy: The exercise of control.* New York: W. H. Freeman.
100. Bandura, A. (1977). *Social learning theory.* Englewood Cliffs, NJ: Prentice-Hall.
101. Marlatt, G. A., & Gordon, J. R. (1985). *Relapse prevention: Maintenance strategies in the treatment of addiction.* New York: Guilford Press.
102. Stewart, S., & Horowitz, J. (2002). Home-based intervention in congestive heart failure: Long term implications on readmission and survival. *Circulation, 105,* 286–296.
103. Expert Panel on Detection, Evaluation, and Treatment of High Blood Cholesterol in Adults. (2001). Executive Summary of the third report of the National Cholesterol Education Program (NCEP). *JAMA, 285,* 2486–2497.
104. Chobanian, A. V., Bakris, G. L., Black, H. R., et al. (2003). Seventh report of the Joint National Committee on Prevention, Detection, Evaluation and Treatment of High Blood Pressure. *Hypertension, 42,* 1206–1252.
105. Smith, S. C., Allen, J., Blair, S. N., et al. (2006). AHA/ACC Guidelines for secondary prevention for patients with coronary and other atherosclerotic vascular disease: 2006 update. *Circulation, 113,* 2363–2372.

106. American Diabetes Association. (2007). Clinical practice recommendations. *Diabetes Care, 30,* S4–S41.
107. Board of Registered Nurses State of California. Retrieved from www.rn.ca.gov.
108. Naylor, M., Brooten, D., Jones, R., et al. (1994). Comprehensive discharge planning for the hospitalized elderly: A randomized clinical trial. *Annals of Internal Medicine, 120,* 999–1006.
109. Miller, N. H., Warren, D., & Myers, D. (1996). Home-based cardiac rehabilitation and lifestyle modification: The MULTIFIT model. *Journal of Cardiovascular Nursing, 11*(1), 76–87.
110. Von Korff, M., Gruman, J., Schaefer, J., et al. (1997). Collaborative management of chronic illness. *Annals of Internal Medicine, 127*(12), 1097–1102.
111. Attkinsson, C. C., & Greenfield, T. K. (1996). The client satisfaction questionnaire (CSQ) scales and the services satisfaction scale-30 (SSS-30). In L. I. Sederer & B. Dickey (Eds.), *Outcomes assessment in clinical practice* (pp. 120–128). Baltimore: Williams and Wilkins.
112. Stewart, A. L., Hays, R. D., & Ware, J. E. (1988). The MOS short form general health survey: Reliability and validity in a patient population. *Medical Care,* 724–735.
113. Tarlov, A. R., Ware, J., Greenfield, S., et al. (1989). The medical outcomes study: An application of methods for monitoring the results of medical care. *JAMA, 262,* 925–930.
114. Bergner, M., Bobbitt, R. A., Carter, W. B., et al. (1981). The sickness impact profile: Development and final revision of a health status measure. *Medical Care, 19,* 787–805.
115. Wilson, J. R., Rayos, G., Yeoh, T. K., et al. (1995). Dissociation between exertional symptoms and circulatory function in patients with heart failure. *Circulation, 92,* 47–53.
116. Hlatky, M., Boineau, R. E., Higginbotham, M. B., et al. (1989). A brief self-administered questionnaire to determine functional capacity (the Duke Activity Status Index). *American Journal of Cardiology, 64,* 651–654.
117. Campeau, L. (1976). Grading of angina pectoris [letter]. *Circulation, 54,* 522–523.
118. Spertus, J. A., Winder, J. A., Dewhurst, T. A., et al. (1995). Development and evaluation of the Seattle Angina Questionnaire: A new functional status measure for coronary artery disease. *Journal of the American College of Cardiology, 25,* 333–341.
119. Sen, S., Fawson, P., Cherrington, G., et al. (2005). Patient satisfaction measurement in the disease management industry. *Disease Management, 8,* 288–300.
120. Joint Commission on Accreditation of Healthcare Organizations. *Disease-specific care certification.* Retrieved June 17, 2008, from www.jcaho.org/dscc/index.htm
121. National Committee for Quality Assurance. (2002). *The state of health care quality 2002, health plan employer information and data set (HEDIS).* Washington, DC: Author.
122. Fireman, B., Bartlett, J., & Selby, J. (2004). Can disease management reduce health care costs by improving quality? *Health Affairs, 23,* 63–75.
123. Preventative Cardiovascular Nurses Association. Madison, WI. Retrieved June 17, 2008, from www.pcna.net
124. Ades, P., Kottke T., Houston Miller, N., et al. (2002). 33rd Bethesda Conference: Preventive cardiology: How can we do better? Task force #3—getting results: Who where and how? *JACC, 40*(4), 615–630.
125. Grady, K. L., Dracup, K., Kennedy, G., et al. (2000). Team management of patients with heart failure: A statement for healthcare professionals from the cardiovascular nursing council of the American Heart Association. *Circulation, 102,* 2443–2456.
126. Pare, G., Jaana, M., & Sicotte, C. (2007). Systematic review of home telemonitoring for chronic diseases: The evidence base. *Journal of the American Medical Information Association, 14,* 269–277.
127. Lorig, K., Ritter, P., Stewart, A., et al. (2001). Chronic disease self-management program. 2-year health status and health care utilization outcomes. *Medical Care, 39*(11), 1217–1223.
128. Lorig, K., Sobel, D. S., Stewart, A. L., et al. (1999). Evidence suggesting that a chronic disease self-management program can improve health status while reducing hospitalization: A randomized trial. *Medical Care, 37*(1), 5–14.
129. Nelson, J., & Arnold-Powers, P. (2001). Community case management for frail, elderly clients: The nurse case managers role. *Journal of Nursing Administration, 31*(9), 444–450.

CHAPTER 43 Global Cardiovascular Health

Kawkab Shishani / Erika S. Sivarajan Froelicher

INTRODUCTION TO GLOBAL HEALTH

In recent years, medicine worldwide has witnessed an "epidemiologic transition." Morbidity and mortality from chronic diseases have gradually eclipsed infectious diseases.[1] The World Health Organization (WHO) has reported that chronic diseases have now reached epidemic proportions. Of the 58 million deaths from all causes worldwide in 2005, cardiovascular disease (CVD) caused approximately 17.5 million deaths (Fig. 43-1), which is three times more than those caused by infectious diseases, including HIV/AIDS, malaria, and tuberculosis combined.[2] Although CVD is declining in developed countries, it is rising in developing countries.[3] Furthermore, 80% of deaths caused by CVD occur in developing countries.[2] The experience of developed countries in preventing CVD could slow the rapid increase in lifestyle-related risks in developing countries.[4–8]

Besides the morbidity and premature mortality caused by CVD, the impaired quality of life caused by the functional and psychological consequences of this chronic disease poses economic and social threats to society.[3] Thus, the impact of CVD is greatest in developing countries, where financial resources are limited and professionals with expertise in CVD prevention, treatment of risk factors, and rehabilitation are few. But the significant burden of CVD morbidity and mortality can be prevented.[9] Health care professionals in developing countries should learn from the risk prediction and preventive intervention standards, protocols, and procedures that WHO has implemented in Europe[10] and in the Americas.[11] Furthermore, the countries that participated in the Catalonia Declaration[6] and the Victoria Declaration[7] have established networks of health care experts from developed countries to help them develop comprehensive health policies and to ensure efficient and cost-effective public health services. The Catalonia and Victoria Declarations also emphasized the influential role of women in reducing CVD risk factors.

The etiology of CVD is multifactorial. Knowledge of the risk factors is derived mainly from the developed countries. To validate these findings on a global basis, the INTERHEART study, a case-control study, compared risk factors for acute myocardial infarction in 52 countries. In 15,152 cases and 14,820 controls, modifiable behavioral risk factors such as smoking, regular physical activity, dietary patterns, obesity (waist/hip ratio), alcohol consumption, and blood apolipoprotein subfractions of cholesterol were examined. Odds ratios (OR) were estimated for the risk factors of myocardial infarction: smoking: OR = 2.87, population attributable risk (PAR) 35.7%; regular physical activity: OR = 0.86, PAR 12.2%; daily consumption of fruits and vegetables: OR = 0.70, PAR 13.7%; and abdominal obesity: OR = 1.12, for top versus lowest tertile and OR = 1.62 for middle versus lowest tertile, PAR 20.1% for top two tertiles versus lowest tertile. All risk factors were significant predictors of acute myocardial infarction ($p < .01$).[12]

CONTROLLING THE CVD EPIDEMIC

According to the WHO,[2] the key modifiable lifestyle or behavioral risk factors for CVD worldwide are smoking cessation, regular physical activity, and diet. A systematic review of the causes of mortality from CVD revealed that four factors improved prognosis and three of them were associated with lifestyle changes: smoking cessation, physical activity, and dietary modification.[13] In developing countries, prevention and control measures to decrease exposure to these risk factors are relatively less advanced.[14] Primary and secondary prevention involving medications are not addressed in this chapter because nurses in many parts of the world do not have prescriptive authority. The patient education and compliance component of medication monitoring (see Chapter 40) are contained in the chapters for hypertension (see Chapter 35) and lipids (see Chapter 36). Risk reduction decreases morbidity in patients with CVD. Thus, the guidelines of American Heart Association (AHA) for primary prevention recommend that risk factor assessment of diet, smoking, and physical activity in adults should begin at age 20 years.[4] The European Society of Cardiology (ESC) promulgated similar guidelines based on European Action to reduce morbidity and mortality in those individuals at high risk and to safeguard the health of those at low risk by advocating their adoption of healthy lifestyles.[5] Although more women than men die from CVD, women are less frequently assessed for risk. Thus, the AHA and ESC emphasize risk assessment in women with particular attention to smoking, obesity, and the use of oral contraceptives.[5,15]

Smoking Cessation Interventions

Developing countries have the largest proportion of smokers in the world and rates of smoking in these countries are rising (Fig. 43-2). In contrast, the rates of smoking in developed countries have been declining dramatically.[16] This decline can be attributed to aggressive public policies that have imposed higher taxes on cigarettes, increasing their cost, and laws restricting smoking in public places. The combination of higher costs, inconvenience, and restrictions on the advertising and sale of cigarettes to minors has drastically reduced smoking rates in many areas of the world. The first international convention treaty to address health dealt with tobacco use.[3] It is not surprising then that the burden of disease associated with smoking is higher in developing countries than in developed countries. One study of several countries in the Eastern Mediterranean Region that examined the prevalence of complications in patients with hypertension showed that complication

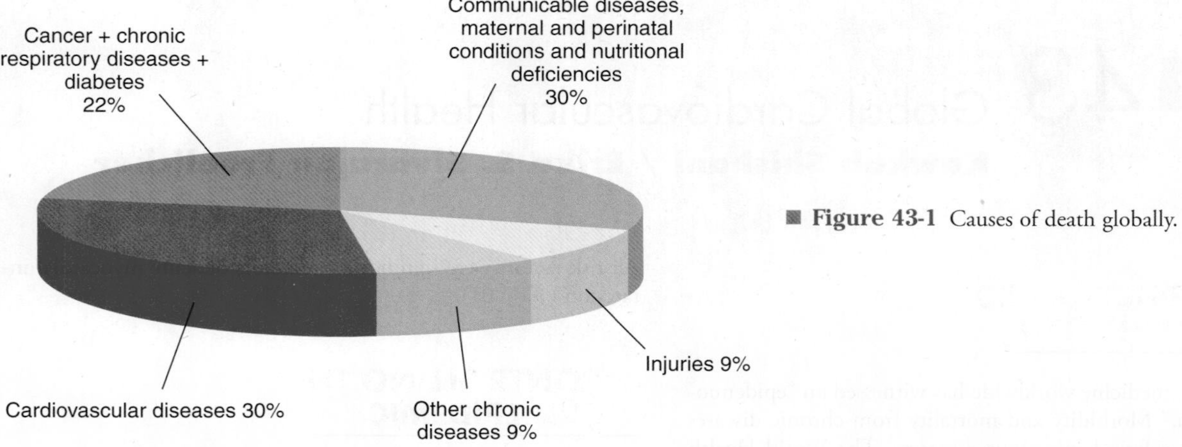

■ **Figure 43-1** Causes of death globally.

rates were significantly higher among smokers than among nonsmokers.[17] The water pipe, also known as *argeela, arghileh, narghile, nargile, nargileh, hubbly-bubbly, sheesha, shisha,* and *goza,* is a popular form of smoking that is practiced socially in many regions in the world. This activity usually involves two or more people who share the same water pipe.[18] Although a common misconception persists that smoking a water pipe is not as harmful as smoking cigarettes, one episode of smoking a water pipe produces as much tar as smoking 20 cigarettes. One study found that water pipe smoke contains an abundance of chemicals known to be risk factors for cancer and CVD; the ratio of carbon monoxide to nicotine was 50:1 as compared with 16:1 for cigarettes.[19] An analysis of studies done in Arab countries reveals that 31% to 57% of the population smokes a water pipe[20,21] and that more women than men use tobacco in this way.[22] Among the reasons for this practice is the perception that smoking a water pipe causes fewer adverse health effects and is safer than cigarettes, it is a social activity, and it is considered attractive.[22] Nonetheless, this practice may have serious consequences. Women who smoke a water pipe in their homes expose their children to its fumes, which may adversely impact the health of these "passive smokers."

Health care professionals must make smoking prevention and cessation high priorities in their practices. Details on smoking cessation interventions are provided in Chapter 34. Such counseling must consider individual differences and use culturally appropriate and sensitive methods. Not all forms of pharmacologic aids for smoking cessation are available globally and may be costly. Nurses also can work with nongovernmental organizations to ban smoking. The WHO's Code of Practice on Tobacco Control for Health Professional Organizations adopted in Geneva in 2004 encourages and supports nurses to promote tobacco-free cultures.[23]

Health care professionals must be proactive in helping their patients to quit smoking. Nurse educators can have a major influence on tobacco control by teaching their students about smoking prevention and smoking cessation for those who are already smokers. To successfully aid smokers who wish to quit, however, nurses often need more resources. An excellent and valuable resource that offers references and education around the clock to nurses is the www.tobaccofreenurses.org Web site. A discussion of effective smoking cessation interventions is provided in Chapter 34.

Although health care professionals can be effective role models, those who smoke—and continue to smoke—undermine their credibility and persuasiveness as smoking-cessation counselors. When many smokers are advised to quit, they often resist claiming, "My doctor smokes" or "Doctors smoke." For this reason, health care professionals who smoke must be targeted for smoking-cessation interventions. This approach has a desirable secondary benefit: Anecdotal evidence suggests that health care professionals who have successfully quit smoking are among the best smoking-cessation interventionists.

Physical Activity

Regular physical activity reduces the risk of CVD morbidity in general and of CVD mortality in particular.[24] The risk in physically inactive people is about double. Developed and developing countries, however, vary in their perceptions of physical activity. In developed countries, routine and recreational activities are considered physical activity (see Chapter 37)[25]; in developing countries, occupational and nonrecreational activities are considered physical activity.[26] Regardless of how physical activity is defined, the proportions of people who are physically inactive is increasing in many regions of the world.[27,28] According to the INTERHEART study, the regions with the least physically active populations are China (20.3%), Africa (10.1%), and the Middle East.[17] Being physically active, however, presumes that a person is engaged in regular moderate exercise, such as walking, cycling, or gardening, at least five times a week or more.[29]

Physical activity is exceptionally important because it has a direct salutary effect on body systems and risk factors, such as high blood pressure, low-density lipoproteins, and high-density lipoproteins, and contributes to the reduction of excess weight and general fitness. Specific recommendations for increasing physical activity and exercise can be found in Chapter 37. Culturally appropriate environments (e.g., climate) and the cultural suitability of exercising outdoors or in groups of mixed genders are also discussed. According to the WHO, physical activity in the workplace is recommended when other means for maintaining activity are not available.[30]

Diet

Besides recommending food for energy and nutrition, the United States Department of Agriculture Food Guide Pyramid also

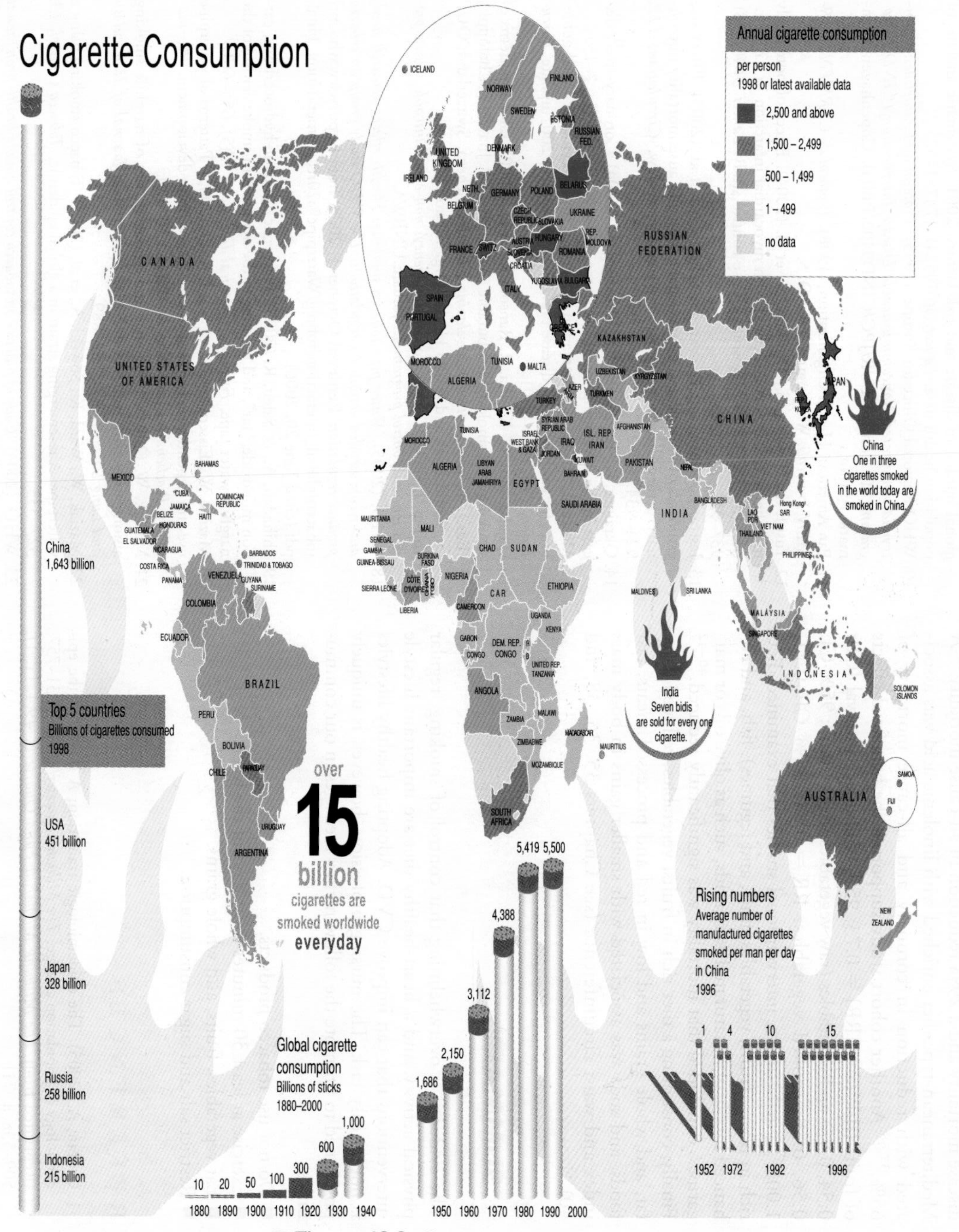

Cigarette Consumption
Annual cigarette consumption
per person
1998 or latest available data
2,500 and above
1,500 – 2,499
500 – 1,499
1 – 499
no data
Top 5 countries
Billions of cigarettes consumed
1998
China
1,643 billion
USA
451 billion
Japan
328 billion
Russia
258 billion
Indonesia
215 billion
over
15
billion
cigarettes are
smoked worldwide
everyday
Global cigarette
consumption
Billions of sticks
1880–2000
10 20 50 100 300 600 1,000
1,686 2,150 3,112 4,388 5,419 5,500
1880 1890 1900 1910 1920 1930 1940
1950 1960 1970 1980 1990 2000
China
One in three
cigarettes smoked
in the world today are
smoked in China.
India
Seven bidis
are sold for every one
cigarette.
Rising numbers
Average number of
manufactured cigarettes
smoked per man per day
in China
1996
1 4 10 15
1952 1972 1992 1996
CANADA
UNITED STATES
OF AMERICA
BRAZIL
RUSSIAN
FEDERATION
CHINA
INDIA
AUSTRALIA
KAZAKHSTAN
INDONESIA
SUDAN
EGYPT
ALGERIA

■ **Figure 43-2** Cigarette consumption.

recommends a high-quality diet that contains limited amounts of fat, saturated fat, cholesterol, sodium, and refined sugars and ample servings of fruits, vegetables, and whole grain products.[31,32] Although high intakes of fat, salt, and refined sugar have not been a concern for developing countries, recent global trends toward eating unhealthy fast food make these problems increasingly relevant for these countries as well.[33,34] In China, the gastronomic change to a "Western diet" has been linked to a dramatic increase in the CHD mortality rate.[35]

On the other hand, dietary modifications have been shown to slow the progression of CVD. Consumption of oily fish at least twice a week demonstrated a 32% reduction in coronary heart disease mortality and a 29% reduction in all-cause mortality.[36] A Mediterranean-type diet enriched with linolenic acid was associated with reduction in coronary and all-cause mortality of 65%.[37,38] Another cohort study supported the beneficial effects of fruits (risk ratio [RR] = 0.73; 95% confidence interval [CI]: 0.54, 0.98) and vegetables (raw vegetables: RR = 0.67; 95% CI: 0.56, 0.79; cooked vegetables: RR = 0.84; 95% CI: 0.71, 1.00).[39] Furthermore, interventional studies that examined diets rich in fibers (fruits, vegetables, nuts, and legumes), fish, and enhanced intake of unsaturated fatty acids, such as olive oils or margarines, concluded that mortality was significantly reduced.[40–42] Finally, consuming a diet rich in fruits, vegetables, reduced dairy fat, and whole grains and low in red and processed meats, fast foods, and soda was associated with smaller gains in body mass index and waist circumference (see Chapters 35, 36, 38, and 40).[43]

SUMMARY

The evidence is overwhelming that control of smoking, regular physical activity, and a heart-healthy diet are important lifestyle interventions that can improve CVD. Adopting healthy lifestyles is not an easy task. The nursing profession, however, is uniquely positioned to promote the following key messages in our communities:

- Do not use tobacco products.
- Exercise at least 30 minutes most days of the week.
- Eat vegetables, fruits, and whole grains.
- Restrict salt and sugar consumption.

REFERENCES

1. Omran, A. (2005). The epidemiologic transition: A theory of the epidemiology of population change. *The Milbank Quarterly, 83*(4), 731–757. (Reprinted from *The Milbank Memorial Fund Quarterly, 49*(4, Pt. 1), 509–538, 1971)
2. WHO. (2005). *Preventing chronic diseases: A vital investment.* Retrieved October 10, 2008, from http://www.who.int/chp/chronic_disease_report/contents/en/index.html
3. WHO. (2003). *The world health report 2003.* Retrieved October 10, 2008, from http://www.who.int/whr/2003/en/Chapter6-en.pdf
4. Pearson, T., Blair, S., Daniels, S., et al. (2002). AHA guidelines for primary prevention of cardiovascular disease and stroke: 2002 update: Census panel guide to comprehensive risk reduction for adult patient with coronary or other atherosclerotic vascular diseases. *Circulation, 106,* 388–391.
5. Graham, I., Atar, D., Borch-Johnson, K., et al. (2007). European guidelines on cardiovascular disease prevention in clinical practice: Executive summary. *European Journal of Cardiovascular Prevention & Rehabilitation, 14*(Suppl. 2), E1–E40.
6. Advisory Board Second International Heart Health Conference. (1995). *The Catalonia declaration investing in heart health. Declaration of the Advisory Board of the Second International Heart Health Conference, Barcelona, Catalonia (Spain). June 1, 1995.* Retrieved October 1, 2008, from http://www.internationalhearthealth.org/Publications/catalonia1995.pdf
7. International Heart Health Conference Advisory Board. (1992). *The Victoria Declaration on heart health.* Declaration of the Advisory Board of the International Heart Health Conference, Victoria, Canada, May 28, 1992. Retrieved October 1, 2008, from http://www.internationalhearthealth.org/Publications/victoria_eng_1992.pdf
8. New Zealand Guidelines Group (NZGG). (2002). *Cardiac rehabilitation.* Retrieved October 1, 2008, from http://www.nzgg.org.nz/guidelines/0001/cardiac_rehabilitation.pdf
9. Lopez, A. D., Mathers, C. D., Ezzati, M., et al. (2006). Global and regional burden of disease and risk factors, 2001: Systematic analysis of population health data. *Lancet, 367*(9524), 1747–1757.
10. WHO Regional Office for Europe. (1995). *Protocol and guidelines: Countrywide Integrated Noncommunicable Disease Intervention (CINDI) Programme* (Document EUR/JPC/CIND9402/PB04). Copenhagen, Denmark: Author.
11. Pan American Health Organization. (1998). *Protocol de CARMEN (CARMEN Protocol).* Washington, DC: OPS.
12. Yusuf, S., Hawken, S., Ounpuu, S., et al. (2004). Effect of potentially modifiable risk factors associated with myocardial infarction in 52 countries (the INTERHEART study): Case-control study. *Lancet, 364*(9438), 937–952.
13. Iestra, J., Kromhout, D., van der Schouw, Y., et al. (2005). Effect size estimates of lifestyle and dietary changes on all-cause mortality in coronary artery disease patients: A systematic review. *Circulation, 112,* 924–934.
14. Okrainec, K., Banerjee, D., & Eisenberg, M. (2004). Coronary artery disease in the developing world. *American Heart Journal, 148*(1), 7–15.
15. Mosca, L., Banka, C., Benjamin, E., et al. (2007). Evidence-based guidelines for cardiovascular disease prevention in women: 2007 update. *Circulation, 115,* 1481–1501.
16. Gajalakshmi, C. K., Jha, P., Ranson, K., et al. (2000). Global patterns of smoking and smoking-attributable mortality. In P. Jha & F. Chaloupka (Eds.), *Tobacco control in developing countries.* Geneva, Switzerland: OUP for World Bank and World Health Organization.
17. Yousef, J. (2003). *Evaluation of the Agency's non-communicable disease prevention and control programme.* Jordan: UNRWA.
18. WHO. (2005). *Water pipe tobacco smoking: Health effects, research needs and recommended actions by regulations. The WHO study group on tobacco product regulation.* Retrieved October 1, 2008, from http://www.who.int/tobacco/global_interaction/tobreg/Waterpipe%20recommendation_Final.pdf (cited June 20, 2006).
19. Shihadeh, A., & Saleh, R. (2005). Polycyclic aromatic hydrocarbons, carbon monoxide, "tar", and nicotine in the mainstream smoke aerosol of the narghile water pipe. *Food and Chemical Toxicology, 43*(5), 655–661.
20. Maziak, W., Eissenberg, T., & Ward, K. D. (2005). Patterns of waterpipe use and dependence: Implications for intervention development. *Pharmacology, Biochemistry, and Behavior, 80*(1), 173–179.
21. Maziak, W. (2004). Prevalence and characteristics of narghile smoking among university students in Syria. *International Journal of Tuberculosis and Lung Diseases, 8*(7), 882–889.
22. Maziak, W., Ward, K., Soweid, A., et al. (2004). Tobacco smoking using a waterpipe: A re-emerging strain in a global epidemic. *Tobacco Control, 13,* 327–333.
23. WHO. (2004). *Code of practice on tobacco control among health professional organizations.* Retrieved October 1, 2008, from http://www.who.int/tobacco/research/cessation/code_practice_en.pdf (cited June 20, 2006).
24. AHA. (2007). *Physical activity and cardiovascular health fact sheet.* Retrieved October 1, 2008, from http://www.americanheart.org/presenter.jhtml?identifier=820
25. Kriska, A. M., Knowler, W. C., La Porte, R. E., et al. (1990). Development of questionnaire to examine relationship of physical activity and diabetes in Pima Indians. *Diabetes Care, 13,* 401–411.
26. Forrest, K., Bunker, C., Kriska, A., et al. (2000). Physical activity and cardiovascular risk factors in a developing population. *Medicine & Science in Sports & Exercise, 33,* 1598–1604.
27. Bunker, C. H., Ukoli, M. U., Nwankwo, M. U., et al. (1992). Factors associated with hypertension in Nigerian civil servants. *Preventive Medicine, 21,* 710–722.

28. Kaufman, J. S., Owoaje, E. E., Rotimi, C. N., et al. (1999). Blood pressure change in Africa: Case study from Nigeria. *Human Biology, 71*, 641–657.
29. CDC. (2007). *How active do adults need to be to gain some benefit?* Retrieved October 1, 2008, from http://cdc.gov/nccdphp/dnpa/physical/recommendations/adults.htm
30. WHO. (2003). *The world health report 2003—Shaping the future.* Retrieved October 1, 2008, from http://www.who.int/whr/2003/en/index.html
31. Haines, P., Siega-Riz, A., & Popkin, B. (1999). The Diet Quality Index revised: A measurement instrument for populations. *Journal of the American Dietetic Association, 99*, 697–704.
32. Welsh, S., Davis, C., & Shaw, A. (1992). Development of the Food Guide Pyramid. *Nutrition Today, 27*, 12–23.
33. Popkin, B. M. (1994). The nutrition transition in low-income countries: An emerging crisis. *Nutrition in Review, 52*, 285–298.
34. WHO. (1996). *Preparation and use of food-based dietary guidelines. WHO technical report, series 880. Report of a joint FAO/WHO consultation.* Geneva, Switzerland: Author.
35. Critchley, J., Liu, J., Zhao, D., et al. (2004). Explaining the increase in coronary heart disease mortality in Beijing between 1984 and 1999. *Circulation, 110*, 1236–1244.
36. Burr, M. L., Fehily, A. M., Gilbert, J. F., et al. (1989). Effects of changes in fat, fish and fibre intakes on death and myocardial re-infarction: Diet and Re-infarction Trial (DART). *Lancet, 2*, 757–761.
37. Ebrahim, S., Davey Smith, G., McGabe, C., et al. (1999). What role for statins? A review and economic model. *Health Technology Assessment, 3*, i–iv, 1–91.
38. Kris-Etherton, P., Eckel, R. H., Howeard, B. V., et al. (2001). Lyon Diet Heart Study: Benefits of a Mediterranean-lifestyle, National Cholesterol Education Program/American Heart Association Step I dietary pattern on cardiovascular disease. *Circulation, 103*, 1823–1825.
39. Barzi, F., Woodward, M., Marfisi, R. M., et al. (2003). Mediterranean diet and all-causes mortality after myocardial infarction: Results from the GISSI-Prevenzione trial. *European Journal of Clinical Nutrition, 57*, 604–611.
40. De Lorgeril, M., Renaud, S., Mamelle, N., et al. (1994). Mediterranean alpha-linolenic acid-rich diet in secondary prevention of coronary heart disease. *Lancet, 343*, 1454–1459.
41. De Lorgeril, M., Salen, P., Martin, J. L., et al. (1999). Mediterranean diet, traditional risk factors, and the rate of cardiovascular complications after myocardial infarction: Final report of the Lyon Diet Heart Study. *Circulation, 99*, 779–785.
42. Singh, R. B., Rastogi, S. S., Verma, R., et al. (1992). Randomised controlled trial of cardioprotective diet in patients with recent acute myocardial infarction: Results of one year follow up. *BMJ, 304*, 1015–1019.
43. Newby, P. K., Muller, D., Hallfrisch, J., et al. (2003). Dietary patterns and changes in body mass index and waist circumference in adults. *American Journal of Clinical Nutrition, 77*, 1417–1425.

RELATION OF RIGHT ATRIAL AND PULMONARY ARTERY PRESSURES TO ECG FINDINGS

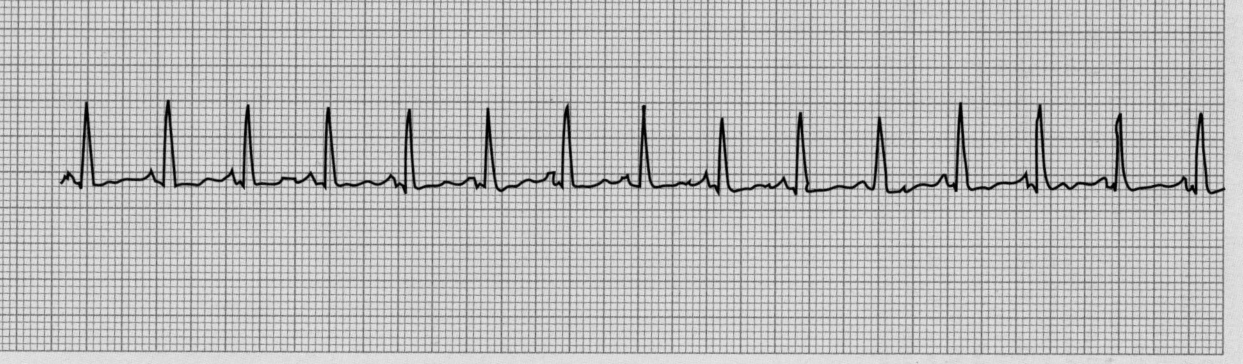

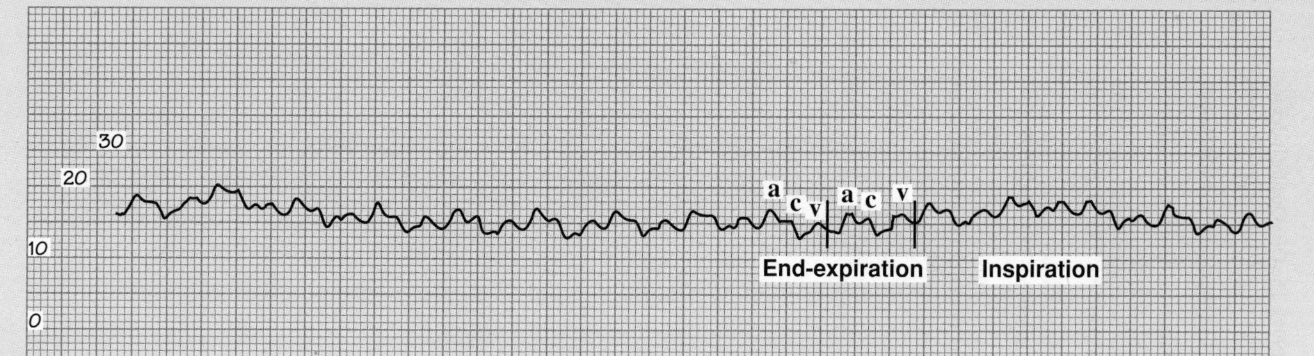

Pressures/waveforms	Mechanical Event	ECG Findings	Example
RA Pressure (2–6 mm Hg)			
a wave	RA systole	80–100 msec after P wave	
x descent	RA relaxation	(Downslope of the a wave)	
c wave	Tricuspid valve closure	After the QRS (follows the a wave by a time interval = PR)	**Interpretation:** RAP tracing from patient on mechanical ventilation. The RAP is a mean pressure (bisect an end-expiratory waveform so that the areas above and below are equal). RAP = 15 mm Hg
v wave	RA filling against closed tricuspid valve	Peak of the T wave	
y descent	RA emptying with opening of tricuspid valve (onset of RV diastole)	(Downslope of the v wave)	

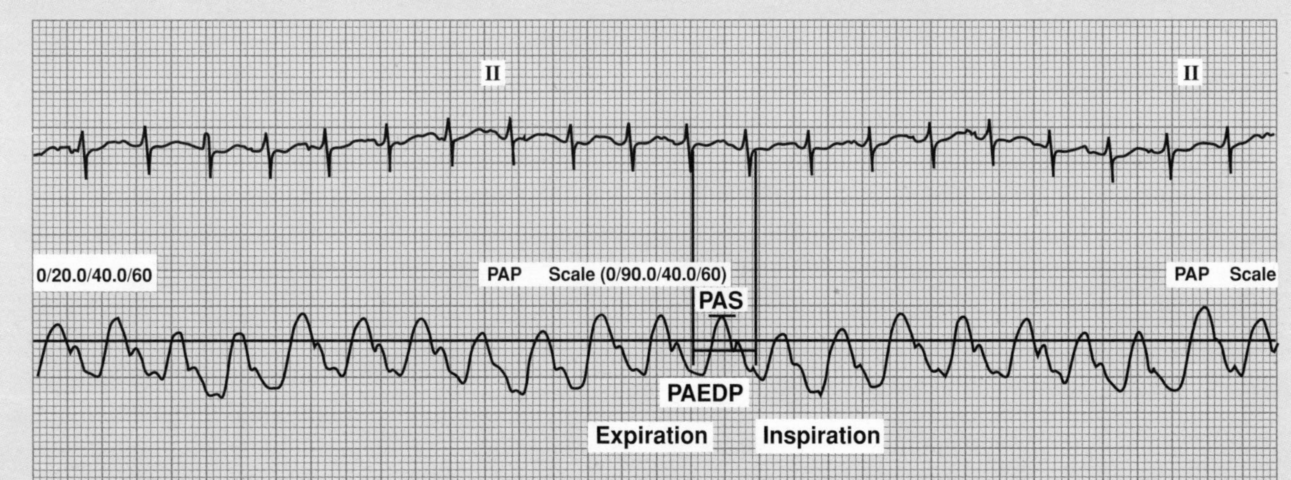

PA Pressures			
Systolic (15–25 mm Hg)	RV ejection of blood into pulmonary vasculature		
Diastolic (8–12 mm Hg)	Indirect indicator of LV end-diastolic pressure	T wave (read at peak of waveform 0.08 seconds after onset of QRS (Determine by bisecting the wave)	**Interpretation:** PA pressure waveform from spontaneously breathing patient
Mean (9–18 mm Hg)			

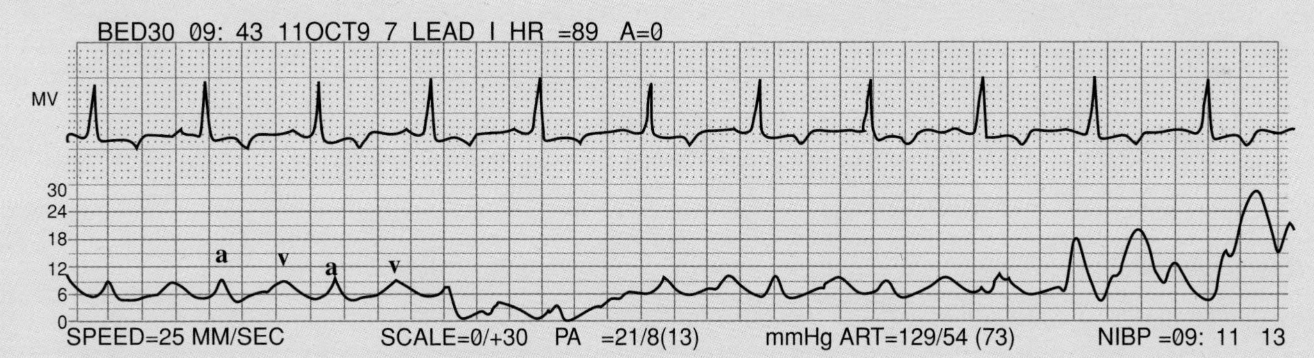

PAWP (6–12 mm Hg)			
a wave	Left atrial systole		**Interpretation:** PAWP tracing from spontaneously breathing patient. The PAWP is a mean pressure (bisect an end-expiratory waveform so that the areas above and below are equal). PAWP = 6 mm Hg
x descent	Left atrial relaxation	Approximately 200 ms after p wave (Downslope of the a wave)	
v wave	Left atrial filling against closed mitral valve	T-P interval	
y descent	Left atrial emptying associated with opening of mitral valve (onset of LV diastole)	(Downslope of the v wave)	

LA, left atrial; PA, pulmonary artery; RA, right atrial. Bridges, E. J. (2000). Monitoring pulmonary artery pressures: Just the facts. *Critical Care Nurse,* 20(6), 59–80.

Index

Note: Page numbers followed by *f* indicate figures, *t* tables, *d* display, and *ncp* nursing care plan.

B

D

I

N

O

P

W

X

Y

Z

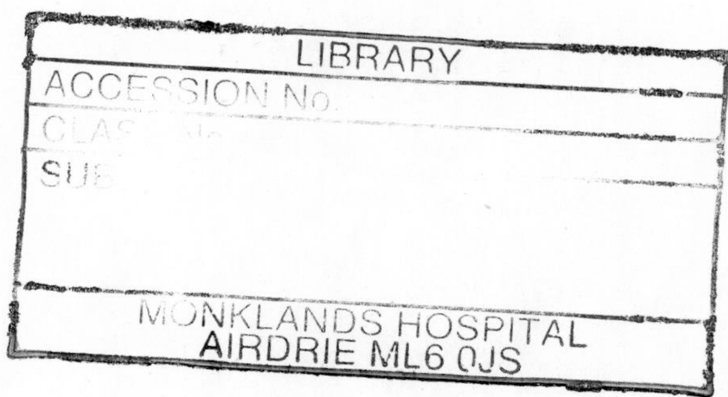

HEMODYNAMIC INDICES

Indices/Equations	Normal Values
Preload	
Right atrial pressure (RAP) or central venous pressure (CVP)	2–6 mm Hg
Pulmonary artery end-diastolic pressure (PAEDP)	8–12 mm Hg
Pulmonary artery wedge pressure (PAWP)	6–12 mm Hg
Afterload	
Systolic blood pressure (SBP)	120 mm Hg
Systemic vascular resistance (SVR)	800–1200 dynes/sec/cm^{-5}
$SVR = \frac{MAP - RAP}{CO} \times 80$	
Systemic vascular resistance index (SVRI)	1900–2400 dynes/sec/cm^{-5}/m^2
$SVRI = \frac{MAP - RAP}{CI} \times 80$	
Force of Contraction	
Stroke volume (SV)	60–180 mL/beat
$SV = \frac{CO \times 1000}{HR}$	
Stroke Volume Index	33–47 mL/beat/m^2
$SVI = \frac{CI \times 1000}{HR}$	
Right ventricular stroke work index (RVSWI)	5–10 gm-m/m^2/beat
$RVSWI = SVI(MAP - CVP) \times 0.0136$	
Left ventricular stroke work index (LVSWI)	45–65 gm-m/m^2/beat
$LVSWI = SVI(MAP - PAWP) \times 0.0136$	
Right Heart Function	
Right ventricular ejection fraction	40%–60%
Right ventricular end-systolic index	30–60 mL/m^2
Right ventricular end-diastolic volume index	60–100 mL/m^2
Functional Indices	**Predictive Value (Preload Dependence)**
RAP Variation (ΔRAP)	ΔRAP > 1
Systolic Pressure Variation (ΔPs)	>12–15 mm Hg associated with hypovolemia
$\Delta Ps\% = 100 \times (Ps_{max} - Ps_{min})/[(PS_{max} + Ps_{min})/2]$	Increase in ΔPs > 4 mm Hg indicative of blood loss > 10%
ΔDown	>2–5 mm Hg indicative of hypovolemia No absolute predictive value identified
Pulse Pressure Variation (ΔPp)	
$\Delta Pp\% = [(PP_{max} - PP_{min})/(PP_{max} + PP_{min})/2] \times 100$	>13%
Stroke Volume Variation (SVV)	>Neurosurgical patients 9.5% (Vt = 10 mL/kg)
$SVV = SVV_{max} - SVV_{min}/SVV_{mean}$	>13% (septic shock)
Aortic Blood Flow Velocity	>12% (septic shock)
$\Delta V_{peak}(\%) = 100 \times (Vpeak_{max} - Vpeak_{min})/[Vpeak_{max} + Vpeak_{min})/2]$	

CONVERSIONS TO SYSTÉME INTERNATIONAL (SI) UNITS

Component	System	Present Reference Intervals	Present Unit	Conversion Factor	SI Reference Intervals	SI Unit Symbol
Alanine aminotransferase (ALT)	Serum	5–40	U/L	1.00	5–40	U/L
Albumin	Serum	3.9–5.0	mg/dl	10	39–50	g/L
Alkaline phosphatase	Serum	35–110	U/L	1.00	35–110	U/L
Aspartate aminotransferase (AST)	Serum	5–40	U/L	1.00	5–40	U/L
Bilirubin	Serum					
Direct		0–0.2	mg/dl	17.10	0–4	μmol/L
Total		0.1–1.2	mg/dl	17.10	2–20	μmol/L
Calcium	Serum	8.6–10.3	mg/dl	0.2495	2.15–2.57	mmol/L
Carbon dioxide, total	Serum	22–30	mEq/L	1.00	22–30	mmol/L
Chloride	Serum	98–108	mEq/L	1.00	98–108	mmol/L
Cholesterol	Serum					
Age <29 yr		<200	mg/dl	0.02586	<5.15	mmol/L
30–39 yr		<225	mg/dl	0.02586	<5.80	mmol/L
40–49 yr		<245	mg/dl	0.02586	<6.35	mmol/L
>50 yr		<265	mg/dl	0.02586	<6.85	mmol/L
Complete blood count	Blood					
Hematocrit						
Men		42–52	%	0.01	0.42–0.52	1
Women		37–47	%	0.01	0.37–0.47	1
Red cell count						
Men		4.6–6.2 × 10^6	/mm^3	10^6	4.6–6.2 × 10^{12}/L	
Women		4.2–5.4 × 10^6	/mm^3	10^6	4.5–5.4 × 10^{12}/L	
White cell count		4.5–11.0 × 10^3	/mm^3	10^6	4.5–11.0 × 10^9/L	
Platelet count		150–300 × 10^3	/mm^3	10^6	150–300 × 10^9/L	
Cortisol	Serum					
8AM		5–25	μg/dl	27.59	140–690	nmol/L
8PM		3–13	μg/dl	27.59	80–360	nmol/L
Cortisol	Urine	20–90	μg/24 hr	2.759	55–250	nmol/24 hr
Creatine kinase	Serum					
High CK group (black men)		50–250	U/L	1.00	50–520	U/L
Intermediate CK group (nonblack men, black women)		35–345	U/L	1.00	35–345	U/L
Low CK group (nonblack women)		25–145	U/L	1.00	25–145	U/L
Creatinine kinase isoenzyme, MB fraction	Serum	>5	%	0.01	>0.05	1
Creatinine	Serum	0.4–1.3	mg/dl	88.40	35–115	μmol/L
Men		0.7–1.3	mg/dl	88.40		
Women		0.4–1.1	mg/dl	88.40		
Digoxin, therapeutic	Serum	0.5–2.0	ng/ml	1.281	0.6–2.6	nmol/L
Erythrocyte indices	Blood					
Mean corpuscular volume (MCV)		80–100	$microns^3$	1.00	80–100	fL
Mean corpuscular hemoglobin (MCH)		27–31	pg	1.00	27–31	pg
Mean corpuscular hemoglobin concentration (MCHC)		32–36	%	0.01	0.32–0.36	1